GYNAECOLOGY

For Elsevier

Commissioning Editor: *Michael Houston*
Development Editors: *Rachael Harrison with Louise Cook*
Project Manager: *Jagannathan Varadarajan*
Designer: *Kirsteen Wright*
Illustration Manager: *Gillian Richards*
Marketing Manager (UK): *Richard Jones*

FOURTH EDITION

GYNAECOLOGY

Robert W Shaw CBE, MBChB, MD, FRCOG, FRCS (Ed), FRANZCOG (Hon), FACOG (Hon), FRCPI (Hon)
Professor of Obstetrics and Gynaecology
Nottingham University, Nottingham, UK

David Luesley MA, MD, FRCOG
Lawson-Tait Professor of Gynaecological Oncology
Department of Obstetrics and Gynaecology
City Hospital NHS Trust, Birmingham, UK

Ash Monga MB BS, FRCOG
Consultant Gynaecologist and Urogynaecologist
Department of Obstetrics and Gynaecology
Southampton University Trust Hospital, Southampton, UK

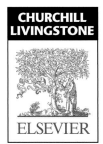

Edinburgh   London   New York   Oxford   Philadelphia   St Louis   Sydney   Toronto   2011

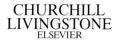

CHURCHILL LIVINGSTONE an imprint of Elsevier Limited
© 2011, Elsevier Limited. All rights reserved.

First edition 1992
Second edition 1997
Third edition 2003
Fourth edition 2011
  Reprinted 2011

No part of this publication may be reproduced or transmitted in any form or by any means, electronic or mechanical, including photocopying, recording, or any information storage and retrieval system, without permission in writing from the publisher. Details on how to seek permission, further information about the Publisher's permissions policies and our arrangements with organizations such as the Copyright Clearance Center and the Copyright Licensing Agency, can be found at our website: **www.elsevier.com/permissions**.

This book and the individual contributions contained in it are protected under copyright by the Publisher (other than as may be noted herein).

Notices
Knowledge and best practice in this field are constantly changing. As new research and experience broaden our understanding, changes in research methods, professional practices, or medical treatment may become necessary. Practitioners and researchers must always rely on their own experience and knowledge in evaluating and using any information, methods, compounds, or experiments described herein. In using such information or methods they should be mindful of their own safety and the safety of others, including parties for whom they have a professional responsibility.

With respect to any drug or pharmaceutical products identified, readers are advised to check the most current information provided (i) on procedures featured or (ii) by the manufacturer of each product to be administered, to verify the recommended dose or formula, the method and duration of administration, and contraindications. It is the responsibility of practitioners, relying on their own experience and knowledge of their patients, to make diagnoses, to determine dosages and the best treatment for each individual patient, and to take all appropriate safety precautions.

To the fullest extent of the law, neither the Publisher nor the authors, contributors, or editors, assume any liability for any injury and/or damage to persons or property as a matter of products liability, negligence or otherwise, or from any use or operation of any methods, products, instructions, or ideas contained in the material herein.

ISBN-13: *978-0-7020-3120-5*

British Library Cataloguing in Publication Data

Gynaecology. — 4th ed.
  1. Gynecology.
  I. Shaw, Robert W. (Robert Wayne) II. Luesley, David. III. Monga, Ash K.
618.1–dc22

Library of Congress Cataloging in Publication Data
A catalog record for this book is available from the Library of Congress

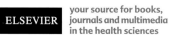 **ELSEVIER** your source for books, journals and multimedia in the health sciences
www.elsevierhealth.com

Working together to grow libraries in developing countries

www.elsevier.com | www.bookaid.org | www.sabre.org

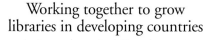 ELSEVIER BOOK AID International Sabre Foundation

The publisher's policy is to use **paper manufactured from sustainable forests**

Printed in China
Last digit is the print number: 9 8 7 6 5 4 3 2

Contents

Preface to the fourth edition   ix

List of Contributors   xi

SECTION A: Basic principles and investigations

1. Surgical anatomy   1
Adrian Lower

2. Hysteroscopy   17
Nazar N. Amso, Richard J. Penketh and Asmita Patwardhan

3. Laparoscopy   36
Alan Farthing and Alexandra Lawrence

4. Diathermy and lasers   48
Priya Agrawal and Fiona Reid

5. Imaging techniques in gynaecology   59
Nandita deSouza and David Cosgrove

6. One-stop gynaecology: the role of ultrasound in the acute gynaecological patient   80
Kevin Jones and Tom Bourne

7. Preoperative care   93
Kate P. Stewart and Saad A. Amer

8. Principles of surgery and management of intra-operative complications   105
Angus McIndoe

9. Postoperative care   116
Saad A. Amer

10. Hormones: their action and measurement in gynaecological practice   128
Scott McGill Nelson and Jurgis Gedis Grudzinskas

11. Biosynthesis of steroid hormones   145
Anthony E. Michael and Robert Abayasekara

12. Principles and new developments in molecular biology   156
Raheela Khan

SECTION B: Reproductive medicine

13. Sexual differentiation — normal and abnormal   166
D. Keith Edmonds

14. Disorders of puberty   182
Adam Balen

15. Control of hypothalamic-pituitary-ovarian function   197
Robert W. Shaw

16. Amenorrhoea, oligomenorrhea and hypothalamic-pituitary dysfunction   212
Hilary O.D. Critchley, Andrew Horne and Kirsty Munro

17. Ovulation induction 231
Maria Vogiatzi and Robert W. Shaw

18. Polycystic ovary syndrome 251
Adam Balen

19. Fertilization and implantation 265
Hayden Homer and Alison Murdoch

20. Disorders and investigation of female reproduction 278
Mark Hamilton

21. Disorders of male reproduction 292
Richard A. Anderson and D. Stewart Irvine

22. Assisted reproduction treatments 312
Kannamannadiar Jayaprakasan and James Hopkisson

23. Sporadic and recurrent miscarriage 335
William M. Buckett and Lesley Regan

24. Tubal disease 353
Ertan Saridogan, Essam El Mahdi and Ovrang Djahanbakhch

25. Ectopic pregnancy 363
Neelam Potdar and Justin C. Konje

26. Hirsutism and virilisation 382
Julian Barth

27. Premenstrual syndrome 391
Sungathi Chandru, Radha Indusekhar and P.M. Shaughn O'Brien

28. Menopause 405
Margaret Rees

29. Fertility control 422
Catherine A. Schünmann and Anna F. Glasier

30. Psychosexual medicine 440
Susan V. Carr

31. Menstruation and menstrual disorders 448
Sujan Sen and Mary Ann Lumsden

32. Uterine fibroids 473
Gareth Weston and David L. Healy

33. Endometriosis 488
Robert W. Shaw

SECTION C: Benign and malignant tumours

34. Epidemiology of gynaecological cancer 509
Peter Sasieni, Alejandra Casteñón and Jack Cuzick

35. The genetics and molecular biology of gynaecological cancer 522
Martin Widschwendter, Simon Gayther and Ian J. Jacobs

36. Principles of radiotherapy and chemotherapy 539
Nawaz Walji and Indrajit Fernando

37. Novel therapies in gynaecological cancer 554
Debra Josephs, Susannah Stanway and Martin Gore

38. Premalignant diseases of the genital tract 566
Esther Moss, Charles W. Redman and Raji Ganesan

39. Cancer of the uterine cervix 582
Kavita Singh and Janos Balega

40. Benign disease of the vulva and the vagina 599
Allan Maclean and Wendy Reid

41. Malignant disease of the vulva and the vagina 613
Shing Shun N. Siu and David Luesley

42. Malignant disease of the uterus 629
Sudha S. Sundar and Suhail Anwar

43. Gestational trophoblastic tumours 650
Thomas Newsom-Davis and Michael J. Seckl

44. Benign tumors of the ovary 668
Ulises Zanetto and Gabrielle Downey

45. Carcinoma of the ovary and fallopian tube 678
Sean Kehoe

46. Benign disease of the breast 689
Paul TR Thiruchelvam, William E. Svensson and John Lynn

47. Malignant disease of the breast 707
Paul TR Thiruchelvam, William E. Svensson and John Lynn

48. Supportive care for gynaecological cancer patients: psychological and
emotional aspects 750
Karen Summerville

SECTION D: Urogynaecology

49. Classification of urogynaecological disorders 767
Stuart L. Stanton and Ash Monga

50. The mechanism of continence 771
Ash Monga and Abdul Sultan

51. Urodynamic investigations 783
Philip Toozs-Hobson and Matthew Parsons

52. Urethral sphincter incompetence 798
Fiona Reid and Anthony RB Smith

53. The overactive bladder syndrome 813
Dudley Robinson and Linda Cardozo

54. Voiding difficulties 836
L. Bombieri and Robert Freeman

55. Pelvic organ prolapse 849
Colin A. Walsh and Mark Slack

56. Frequency, urgency and the painful bladder 864
Michelle M. Fynes and Stergios K. Doumouchtsis

57. Fistulae 874
Paul Hilton

58. Urinary tract infection 896
Charlotte Chaliha and Michael R. Millar

59. Lower intestinal tract disease 907
Karen Nugent

60. Sexual dysfunction in urogynaecology 919
Ranee Thakar

SECTION E: Women's reproductive health

61. Chronic pelvic pain 929
William Stones

62. Pelvic inflammatory disease 942
Nazar N. Amso and Anthony Griffiths

63. Non-HIV Sexually transmitted infections 955
Daniel P. Hay and Eimear P. Kieran

64. Human immunodeficiency syndrome 979
Saurabh V. Phadnis and Margaret A. Johnson

65. Forensic gynaecology 988
Helen Margaret Cameron

66. Violence against women 1002
Mary Hepburn and Kirstyn Brogan

67. Lesbian and bisexual women's health issues 1009
Julie Fish and Susan Bewley

68. Evidence-based care in gynaecology 1017
Arri Coomarasamy and Siladitya Bhattacharya

Index 1025

This fourth edition of *Gynaecology* looks to the challenges we face in our specialty in the 21st century. Healthcare provision has changed a great deal even in the first decade of this century, and so too has this textbook to address these issues. We look to update our readers of all the major advances since the previous edition.

We have two new editors — Professor David Luesley who is overseeing the Gynaecological Oncology, Section 3, and Mr Ash Monga who edits the Urogynaecology, Section 4. Both are recognised subspecialists in their respective fields and bring, not only their personal perspectives to their sections, but also have recruited many new chapter contributors to reflect the increasing number of subspecialists being appointed in gynaecology.

Recognising the multidisciplinary nature of much of the care we now offer our patients to ensure access to other medical staff with allied expertise to our own and to improve our patients' outcomes, is reflected in contributions from many other colleagues from other medical specialities.

We have reviewed carefully previous chapter headings, content, style and length. This has meant the amalgamation of some previous chapters to reflect changing emphasis in the practice of gynaecology, the recognition of increased day case operative laparoscopic and hysteroscopic procedures. There has also been an increased role and use of medical therapies in many areas of reproductive medicine. This has opened up the field of what some may call a separate special-ity of 'medical gynaecology'. This shift away from surgery as the prime treatment choice for many gynaecology problems has implications for future surgical training of our juniors and the realisation that many may not be undertaking major gynaecological procedures in their future careers.

The publication of the human genome in 2006 and the increased application of molecular biological techniques in research is beginning to unearth the cellular and molecular basis of many gynaecological benign and malignant conditions. However, it is early days of such work and we await the potential advances in new therapies which may come from this increased understanding of pathogenesis and for 'regenerative medicine' from stem cell work and gene therapy to become realities in terms of treatment potential.

Each chapter has been rewritten, we have many new authors and adopted a new presentation with greater use of colour illustrations. This book will serve equally well as a comprehensive text for the already established specialist in gynaecology as well as a useful source for trainees preparing for specialist examinations.

We hope that you will both find its contents useful and enjoy reading the book as much as we have enjoyed collating and editing its contents.

Robert Shaw
David Luesley
Ash Monga

List of Contributors

Robert Abayasekara BSc (Hons), MA (Cantab), PhD
Senior Lecturer in Physiology
Department of Veterinary Basic Sciences
Royal Veterinary College
London, UK

Priya Agrawal MD
Specialist Registrar in Obstetrics and Gynaecology
St Mary's Hospital
London, UK

Saad A Amer MRCOG, MSc, MD
Associate Professor and Consultant Gynaecologist
University of Nottingham
Royal Derby Hospital
Nottingham, UK

Nazar N Amso PhD, FRCOG
Clinical Senior Lecturer
Obstetrics & Gynaecology
Cardiff University School of Medicine
Cardiff, UK

Richard A Anderson MD, PhD, FRCOG
Professor of Clinical Reproductive Science
Centre for Reproductive Biology
University of Edinburgh
Edinburgh, UK

M Suhail Anwar MBBS, BSc, MRCP (UK), MRCP (Ireland), FRCR (UK)
Consultant Clinical Oncologist
The Cancer Centre
University Hospital
Birmingham NHS Foundation Trust
Birmingham, UK

Janos Balega MD, MRCOG
Consultant Gynaecological Oncologist
Pan-Birmingham Gynaecology Cancer Centre
Birmingham, UK

Adam Balen MD, FRCOG
Professor of Reproductive Medicine & Surgery
Leeds Teaching Hospitals
Leeds, UK

Julian Barth MD, FRCP, FRCPath
Consultant in Chemical Pathology & Metabolic Medicine
Clinical Biochemistry
Leeds General Infirmary
Leeds, UK

Susan Bewley MD, MA, FRCOG
Consultant Obstetrician/Maternal Fetal Medicine and Honorary Senior Lecturer
Kings Health Partners
London, UK

Siladitya Bhattacharya MD, FRCOG
Professor of Reproductive Medicine
Head, Section of Applied Clinical Sciences
Division of Applied Health Sciences
School of Medicine and Dentistry
University of Aberdeen
Aberdeen Maternity Hospital
Foresterhill, Aberdeen, UK

L Bombieri MD, MRCOG
Consultant Obstretician & Gynaecologist
Derriford Hospital
Plymouth, UK

Tom Bourne FRCOG PhD
Consultant Gynaecologist
Queen Charlotte's and Chelsea Hospital London, UK;
Visiting Professor, Department of Obstetrics and Gynecology
Katholieke Universiteit
Leuven, Belgium

Kirstyn Brogan MRCOG
Consultant Obstetrician
Ayrshire Maternity Unit
Kilmarnock, Scotland

William M Buckett
Consultant Gynaecologist
St Mary's Hospital
London;
Honorary Senior Lecturer
Imperial College
London, UK

Helen Margaret Cameron MB BS, FRCOG
Consultant Obstetrician and Gynaecologist
Sunderland Royal Hospital
Sunderland, UK

Linda Cardozo MD, FRCOG
Professor of Urogynaecology,
King's College Hospital,
London, UK

Susan V. Carr MBChB, MPhil, FFRHC
Head of Psychosexual Service,
Royal Womens Hospital,
Melbourne, Australia

Alejandra Casteñón MD, MSc
Epidemiologist
Cancer Research UK Centre for Epidemiology, Mathematics and Statistics
Wolfson Institute of Preventive Medicine
Bart's and The London School of Medicine
Queen Mary University of London
London, UK

Charlotte Chaliha MB BChir, MA, MD, MRCOG
Consultant Obstetrician and Gynaecologist,
Sub-specialist in Urogynaecology,
Royal London and St Bartholomew's Hospitals,
London, UK

Sungathi Chandru MD, MRCOG
Locum consultant
Birmingham Heartlands Hospital
Birmingham, UK

Arri Coomarasamy MB ChB, MD, MRCOG
Senior Lecturer and Subspecialist in Reproductive Medicine and Surgery.
Consultant Gynaecologist.
School of experimental and Clinical Medicine
University of Birmingham
Birmingham, UK

David Cosgrove MA, MSc, FRCR, FRCP
Senior Research Fellow and Emeritus Professor
Imaging Sciences Department
Imperial College,
Faculty of Medicine
Hammersmith Hospital
London, UK

Hilary O. D. Critchley BSc, MBChB, MD, FRCOG, FRANZCOG, FMedSci
Professor of Reproductive Medicine
University of Edinburgh;
Honorary Consultant Gynaecologist
Centre for Reproductive Biology
Edinburgh, UK

Jack Cuzick PhD
John Snow Professor of Epidemiology, Head of Department
Cancer Research UK Centre for Epidemiology, Mathematics and Statistics
Queen Mary University of London
Wolfson Institute of Preventive Medicine
London, UK

Nandita deSouza MD, FRCR
Professor of Translational Imaging
Co-director MRI Unit
Institute of Cancer Research and Royal Marsden Hospital
Sutton, UK

Ovrang Djahanbakhch Tip Doktoru FRCOG, MD
Consultant
Barts and the London NHS Trust
London, UK

Gabrielle Downey MD, FRCOG
Consultant Gynaecology
Department of Obstetrics & Gynaecology
City Hospital NHS Trust
Birmingham, UK

Stergios K. Doumouchtsis PhD, MRCOG
Subspecialty Training Fellow in Urogynaecology
Senior Specialist Registrar in Obstetrics and Gynaecology
Department of Obstetrics and Gynaecology
Pelvic Reconstructive Surgery and Urogynaecology Unit
St George's Hospital, St George's University of London
London, UK

D Keith Edmonds MB ChB, FRCOG, FRANZCOG
Clinical Programme Director
Women's and Children's Services
Queen Charlotte's and Chelsea Hospital
Imperial College Healthcare
London, UK

Essam El Mahdi MB BS
Department of Obstetrics and Gynaecology
Royal Free and University College Medical School
London, UK

Alan Farthing MB BS, MD, MRCOG, FRCOG
Honorary Senior Lecturer
Imperial College of Science & Medicine;
Consultant Gynaecologist
Imperial NHS Trust
London, UK

Indrajit Fernando FRCP, FRCR
Consultant Clinical Oncologist
Birmingham Oncology Centre
Queen Elizabeth Hospital
Birmingham, UK

Julie Fish PhD
Reader in Social Work and Health Inequalities,
School of Applied Social Sciences
De Montfort University
The Gateway
Leicester, UK

Robert Freeman MD, FRCOG
Consultant Gynaecologist
Derriford Hospital
Plymouth, UK

Michelle M Fynes MD, MRCOG, DU
Director of the Department of Urogynaecology and Pelvic Floor Reconstruction
St Georges Hospital
London, UK

Raji Ganesan MB BS, MD, FRCPath
Consultant Histopathologist
Birmingham Women's NHS Foundation Trust
Birmingham, UK

Simon Gayther PhD
Reader and Head Translational Research Laboratory
Research Department of Women's Cancer UCL
London, UK

Anna F Glasier BSc, MD, DSc, FRCOG, FFPRHC, OBE
Lead Clinician for Sexual Health in NHS Lothian
Honorary Professor at the Universities of Edinburgh and London
Edinburgh, UK

Martin Gore PhD, FRCP
Consultant Medical Oncologist
Department of Medicine
The Royal Marsden NHS Foundation Trust
London, UK

Anthony Griffiths MRCOG, Dip Med Ed
Consultant Obstetrician & Gynaecologist
University Hospital of Wales
Cardiff, UK

Jurgis Gedis Grudzinskas MD, FRCOG, FRACOG
Consultant Obstetrician & Gynaecologist
Department of Obstetrics & Gynaecology, Women and Childrens Directorate
The Royal London Hospital;
Department of Obstetrics and Gynaecology (Reproductive Physiology Laboratory)
St Bartholomew's Hospital
London, UK

Mark Hamilton MD, FRCOG
Consultant/Clinical Senior Lecturer, Subspecialist in Reproductive Medicine
University of Aberdeen
Aberdeen Maternity Hospital
Foresterhill
Aberdeen, UK

Daniel P Hay BSc, DM, MRCOG
Associate Professor in Obstetrics & Gynaecology
University of Nottingham,
Derby City General Hospital
Derby, UK

David L Healy PhD, FRANZCOG, CREI
President – Elect, International Federation of Fertility Societies
Chairman
Department of Obstetrics & Gynaecology
Monash University
Victoria
Australia

Mary Hepburn BSc, MD, MRCGP, FRCOG
Consultant Obstetrician and Gynaecologist,
Princess Royal Maternity
Glasgow, Scotland

Paul Hilton MB BS, MD, FRCOG
Consultant Gynaecologist and Urogynaecologist
Directorate of Women's Services
Royal Victoria Infirmary
Newcastle upon Tyne, UK

Hayden Homer MBBS, MRCOG, PhD
Wellcome Trust Clinician Scientist
Subspecialty Fellow in Reproductive Medicine
Institute for Women's Health
University College London
London UK

James Hopkisson MD, MRCOG
Consultant Gynaecologist and Subspecialist in Reproductive Medicine
Clinical Director,
NURTURE
University of Nottingham
Nottingham, UK

Andrew Horne MB ChB, PhD, MRCOG, DF, SRH
Clinician Scientist and Honorary Consultant in Obstetrics and Gynaecology
Centre for Reproductive Biology
Queen's Medical Research Institute
Edinburgh, UK

Radha Indusekhar MRCOG
Consultant in Obstetrics and Gynaecology
University Hospital of North Staffordshire
Stoke-on-Trent, UK

D Stewart Irvine MD, FRCOG
Deputy Director of Medicine
NHS Education for Scotland
Edinburgh, Scotland

Ian J Jacobs MD, FRCOG
Chair, Research Department of Women's Cancer UCL;
Dean, Faculty of Biomedical Sciences
University College London
London, UK

Kannamannadiar Jayaprakasan PhD, MRCOG
Subspecialty Trainee in Reproductive Medicine
NURTURE
University of Nottingham
Nottingham, UK

Margaret A Johnson MD, FRCP
Professor of HIV Medicine
Royal Free and UCL Medical School
London, UK

Kevin Jones BSc (Hons), MSc, MB ChB, MRCOG, MD
Consultant Gynaecologist
Swindon and Marlborough
NHS Trust's Great Western Hospital
Swindon, UK

Debra Josephs MB ChB, BSc, MRCP
Specialist Registrar in Medical Oncology Guy's and
St Thomas' Hospital
London, UK

Sean Kehoe MA, MD, DCH, FRCOG
Lead in Gynaecological Oncology, Fellow of St Peters College, Oxford
Oxford Gynaecological Cancer Centre,
Churchill Hospital
Oxford , UK

Raheela Khan BSc(Hons), PhD
Associate Professor
School of Graduate Entry Medicine & Health
University of Nottingham
Royal Derby Hospital
Nottingham, UK

Eimear P Kieran MRCOG
Consultant
Derby City General Hospital,
Derby, UK

Justin C Konje MD, FRCOG
Professor of Obstetrics and Gynaecology
Reproductive sciences Section, Department of Cancer Studies and Molecular Medicine
University of Leicester and University Hospitals of Leicester
Leicester
Leicester, UK

Alexandra Lawrence
MD, MRCOG
St Bartholomew's Hospital,
London
Queens Hospital, Romford
London, UK

Adrian Lower FRCOG
Consultant Gynaecologist
Princess Grace Hospital
London, UK

David Luesley MA, MD, FRCOG
Lawson-Tait Professor of
Gynaecological Oncology
Department of Obstetrics and
Gynaecology
City Hospital NHS Trust
Birmingham, UK

Mary Ann Lumsden BSc Hons,
MB BS, MRCOG, MD, FRCOG
Honorary Consultant
Obstetrician and
Gynaecologist,
NHS Greater Glasgow and
Clyde;
Professor of Medical Education
and Gynaecology
Head of the Section of
Reproductive & Maternal
Medicine
Acting Head of Division of
Developmental Medicine
University of Glasgow
Glasgow, UK

John Lynn MS, FRCS
Consultant Breast and
Endocrine Surgeon
Bupa Cromwell Hospital
London, UK

Allan MacLean MD, FRCOG,
FRCP(Edin)
Professor of Obstetrics and
Gynaecology
University College London
Royal Free Campus
London, UK

Angus McIndoe PhD,
FRCS, MRCOG
Consultant Gynaecologist &
Gynaecological Oncologist,
Hammersmith Hospital,
The Wellington Hospital,
Rapid Diagnostics Clinic
London, UK

Anthony E Michael BSc, PhD
Reader in Reproductive Science
(and Deputy Head of Graduate
School)
Academic Section of Obstetrics
and Gynaecology
St George's University of
London
London, UK

Michael R Millar MB ChB, MA,
MD, FRCPath
Head of the Department of
Infection
Barts and the London NHS
Trust
London

Ash Monga BM BS, FRCOG
Consultant Gynaecologist and
Urogynaecologist
Department of Obstetrics and
Gynaecology
Southampton University Trust
Hospital
Southampton, UK

Esther Moss MRCOG, MSc
Subspecialty trainee in
Gynaecological Oncology
Pan-Birmingham
Gynaecological Cancer Centre
Birmingham, UK

Kirsty Munro MB ChB
Clinical Research Fellow in
Obstetrics and Gynaecology
University of Edinburgh;
Centre for Reproductive
Biology
Edinburgh, UK

Alison Murdoch BSc, MD,
FRCOG
Professor of Reproductive
Medicine
Newcastle Fertility Centre at
Life
International Centre for Life
Newcastle-Upon-Tyne, UK

Scott McGill Nelson BSc, DFFP,
MRCOG, PhD
Muirhead Professor of
Obstetrics & Gynaecology
Western Infirmary
Glasgow, UK

Thomas Newsom-Davis BSc,
MRCP, PhD
Clinical Lecturer in Medical
Oncology
Department of Medical
Oncology
Imperial College Healthcare
NHS Trust
London, UK

Karen Nugent MA, MS, Med,
FRCS
Honorary Consultant
Coloproctologist and Senior
Lecturer
Professorial Surgical Unit
Southampton University
Southampton, UK

Matthew Parsons MB ChB,
MRCOG
Consultant, Departments of
Obstetrics, Gynaecology,
Urogynaecology
Birmingham Women's Hospital
Birmingham, UK

Asmita Patwardhan MD,
MRCOG
Consultant Gynaecologist and
obstetrician
University Hospital of Wales
Cardiff, UK

Richard J Penketh FRCOG
Consultant Obstetrician and
Gynaecologist
University Hospital of Wales
Cardiff, UK

Saurabh V Phadnis MB, BS
Clinical Research Fellow
Royal Free Centre for HIV
Medicine
London, UK

Neelam Potdar MD, MRCOG
Clinical Lecturer and
Subspecialty Trainee in
Reproductive Medicine
Reproductive Sciences Section,
Department of Cancer Studies
and Molecular Medicine
University of Leicester and
University Hospitals of
Leicester
Leicester, UK

P M Shaughn O'Brien DSc, MD,
FRCOG
Professor of Obstetrics and
Gynaecology
Academic Obstetrics and
Gynaecology
New Maternity Hospital
University Hospital of North
Staffordshire
Stoke on Trent, UK

Charles W Redman MD, FRCSE,
FRCOG, MMedEd
Consultant Gynaecological
Oncologist
University Hospital of North
Staffordshire
Stoke-on-Trent, UK

Margaret Rees MA, DPhil,
FRCOG
Visiting Professor,
University of Glasgow and
Adjunct Associate Professor,
Department of Obstetrics,
Gynecology and Reproductive
Sciences,
University of Medicine and
Dentistry of New Jersey,
Editor in Chief Maturitas,
Reader in Reproductive
Medicine
Honorary Consultant Medical
Gynaecologist
Nuffield Department of
Obstetrics and Gynaecology
John Radcliffe Hospital
Oxford, UK

Lesley Regan MD, FRCOG
Professor of Obstetrics and
Gynaecology,
Imperial College;
Head
Recurrent Miscarriage Clinic
St Mary's Hospital
London, UK

Fiona Reid MD, MRCOG
Consultant Urogynaecologist
The Warrell Unit
St Mary's Hosptial
Manchester, UK

Wendy Reid MB BS, FRCOG
Consultant gynaecologist
Royal Free Hospital
London, UK

Dudley Robinson MD, MRCOG
Consultant Urogynaecologist
Department of Urogynaecology
Kings College Hospital
London, UK

Ertan Saridogan PhD, MRCOG
Consultant in Reproductive
Medicine and Minimal Access
Surgery
University College London
Hospitals,
The Portland Hospital
London, UK

Peter Sasieni BA, MA, MS, PhD
Professor, Department of
Mathematics, Statistics and
Epidemiology
Imperial Cancer Research Fund
London, UK

Catherine A Schünmann MB
ChB, MD, MRCOG, DFFP
Subspeciality Trainee in Sexual
& Reproductive Health
Square 13 Sexual &
Reproductive Health Clinic
Aberdeen, UK

Michael J Seckl PhD, FRCP
Professor of Molecular Cancer
Medicine
Director of the Charing Cross
Gestational Trophoblastic
Disease Centre
Department of Medical
Oncology
Charing Cross Hospital
London

Sujan Sen
Gynaecologist & Obstetrician
Glasgow and Greater Clyde
Health NHS Trust
Glasgow, UK

**Robert W Shaw CBE, MBChB,
MD, FRCOG, FRCS (Ed),
FRANZCOG (Hon), FACOG
(Hon), FRCPI (Hon)**
Professor of Obstetrics and
Gynaecology
Nottingham University
Nottingham, UK

Kavita Singh MD, MRCOG
Consultant Gynaecological
Oncologist
Pan-Birmingham Gynaecology
Cancer Centre
Birmingham, UK

Shing Shun N. Siu MRCOG
Consultant Gynaecologist
Department of Obstetrics and
Gynaecology
Prince of Wales Hospital,
Shatin, Hong Kong

**Mark Slack MB BCh, MMed,
MRCOG, FCOG(SA)**
Consultant Gynaecologist
Department of Urogynaecology
and Reconstructive Pelvic
Surgery
Addenbrooke's Hospital,
Cambridge University Hospital
NHS Foundation Trust
Cambridge, UK

Anthony R B Smith
Consultant Urogynaecologist
Department of Urological
Gynaecology
Saint Mary's Hospital for
Women & Children
Manchester
United Kingdom

**Stuart L Stanton FRCS, FRCOG,
FRANZCOG(Hon)**
Consultant Urogynaecologist,
Pelvic Reconstruction and
Urogynaecology Unit
St George's Hospital Medical
School
London, UK

**Susannah Stanway MB ChB,
MRCP**
Specialist Registrar
The Royal Marsden Hospital
London, UK

Kate P Stewart MB BS
Specialist Registrar in
Obstetrics and Gynaecology
Royal Derby Hospital
Derby, UK

William Stones MD, FRCOG
The Puribai Kanji Jamal
Professor
Chair Department of Obstetrics
and Gynaecology
Aga Khan University Nairobi
Nairobi, Kenya

Abdul Sultan MD, FRCOG
Reader at St George's University
of London
Consultant Obstetrician and
Gynaecologist
Mayday University Hospital
Croydon, UK

Karen Summerville MSc, RGN
Registered Independant Nurse
Presenter
Senior Macmillan Clinical
Nurse Specialist Gynaecological
Cancers
Imperial College Health Care
NHS Trust
Queen Charlotte's and Chelsea
Hospitals
London
UK

**Sudha S Sundar M Phil,
MRCOG**
Senior Lecturer/Hon NHS
Consultant
Academic Department of
Gynaecological Oncology
Pan-Birmingham
Gynaecological Cancer centre,
City Hospital,
Birmingham School of Cancer
Sciences
University of Birmingham
Birmingham, UK

**William E Svensson LRCPSI,
FRCSI, FRCR**
Consultant Radiologist and
Reader in Breast Imaging
Imperial College Healthcare
NHS Trust (Charing Cross,
Hammersmith and St Mary's
Hospitals)
London, UK

Ranee Thakar MD, MRCOG
Consultant Obstetrician and
Gynaecologist (Urogynaecology
Subspecialist)
Mayday University Hospital
Croydon, UK

**Paul TR Thiruchelvam BSc
MBBS, PhD, MRCS**
CR:UK / RCS Clinical Research
Fellow & Surgical Registrar NW
Thames
Imperial College School of
Medicine
Hammersmith Hospital
London, UK

**Philip Toozs-Hobson MD,
FRCOG**
Consultant Urogynaecologist
Birmingham Women's Hospital
Birmingham, UK

Maria Vogiatzi MD
Specialist Registrar
Directorate of Women's and
Children's Services
Obstretrics and Gynaecology
Derby, UK

**Nawaz Walji MB ChB,
MRCP, FRCR**
Specialist Registrar Clinical
Oncology
The Cancer Centre
Queen Elizabeth Hospital
Vincent Drive
Birmingham, UK

Colin A Walsh MRCOG
Department of Obstetrics and
Gynaecology
St George's Hospital
Kogarah, New South Wales,
Australia

**Gareth Weston MB BS, MPH,
PhD, FRANZCOG, CREI**
Senior Lecturer Centre for
Women's Health Research,
Department of Obstetrics and
Gynaecology
Monash University
Melbourne, Australia

**Martin Widschwendter MD,
MRCOG**
UCL Professor in Women's
Cancer
Consultant Gynaecological
Oncologist
Department of Gynaecological
Oncology
UCL EGA Institute for
Women's Health
University College London
London, UK

Ulises Zanetto MD
Consultant Histopathlogist
Department of Pathology
City Hospital, Birmingham, UK

Surgical anatomy

Adrian Lower

Chapter Contents

INTRODUCTION	1	THE URETHRA	8
THE OVARY	1	THE SIGMOID COLON	8
THE FALLOPIAN TUBE	3	THE RECTUM	8
THE UTERUS	3	PELVIC MUSCULOFASCIAL SUPPORT	9
THE VAGINA	5	BLOOD SUPPLY TO THE PELVIS	11
THE VULVA	5	NERVE SUPPLY TO THE PELVIS	13
THE URETER	7	LYMPHATIC DRAINAGE OF THE PELVIS	14
THE BLADDER	7	KEY POINTS	16

Introduction

A clear understanding of the anatomy of the female pelvis is essential to successful gynaecological surgery and the avoidance of surgical morbidity. The close relationships between the reproductive, urinary and gastrointestinal tracts must be appreciated, together with the pelvic musculofascial support, vascular and lymphatic circulations, and neurological innervation. It is important to understand the effect of pneumoperitoneum on the anatomy and relationships of the pelvis, and the opportunities afforded by a retroperitoneal approach in minimal access techniques. Figure 1.1 shows a panoramic view of the pelvis from the umbilicus during a laparoscopy. The probe is lifting the right ovary, displaying the right pelvic side wall and ureter (arrows).

The Ovary

The size and appearance of the ovaries depend on both age and the stage of the menstrual cycle. In the young adult, they are almond shaped, solid and white in colour, 3 cm long, 1.5 cm wide and approximately 1 cm thick. The long axis is normally vertical before childbirth; after this, there is a wide range of variation, presumably due to considerable displacement in the first pregnancy.

The ovary is the only intra-abdominal structure not to be covered by peritoneum. Each ovary is attached to the cornu of the uterus by the ovarian ligament, and at the hilum to the broad ligament by the mesovarium, which contains its supply of vessels and nerves. Laterally, each is attached to the suspensory ligament of the ovary with folds of peritoneum which become continuous with that over the psoas major.

Structure

The ovary has a central vascular medulla, consisting of loose connective tissue containing many elastin fibres and non-striated muscle cells, and an outer thicker cortex, denser than the medulla and consisting of networks of reticular fibres and fusiform cells, although there is no clear-cut demarcation between the two. The surface of the ovary is covered by a single layer of cuboidal cells, the germinal epithelium. Beneath this is an ill-defined layer of condensed connective tissue, the tunica albuginea, which increases in density with age. At birth, numerous primordial follicles are found, mainly in the cortex but some in the medulla. With puberty, some form each month into Graafian follicles which, at later stages of their development, form corpora lutea and ultimately atretic follicles, the corpora albicantes (Figure 1.2).

Relations

Anteriorly lie the fallopian tubes, the superior portion of the bladder and the uterovesical pouch; posteriorly is the pouch of Douglas. The broad ligament and its content are related inferiorly, whilst superior to the ovaries are the bowel and the omentum. The lateral surface of the ovary is in contact with the parietal peritoneum and the pelvic side walls.

Vestigial structures

The vestigial remains of the mesonephric duct and tubules are always present in young children, but are variable structures in adults. The epoophoron, a series of parallel blind tubules, lies in the part of the broad ligament between the mesovarium and the fallopian tube, the mesosalpinx. The tubules run to the rudimentary duct of the epoophoron, which runs parallel to the lateral fallopian tube. A few rudimentary tubules, the paroophoron, are occasionally seen in the broad ligament, between the epoophoron and the uterus.

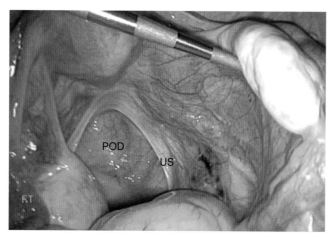

Figure 1.1 View of the pelvis with uterus anteverted from laproscopy. Right ovary turned over with probe to expose right pelvic sidewall. FT, fallopian tube; POD, pouch of Douglas; US, uterosacral ligament.

In a few individuals, the caudal part of the mesonephric duct is well developed, running alongside the uterus to the internal os. This is the duct of Gartner.

Age-related changes

During early fetal life, the ovaries are situated in the lumbar region near the kidneys. They gradually descend into the lesser pelvis and, during childhood, they are small and situated near the pelvic brim. They are packed with primordial follicles. The ovary grows in size until puberty by an increase in the stroma. Ova are first shed around the time of onset of menstruation, and ovulation is usually established within a couple of years.

After the menopause, the ovary atrophies and assumes a smaller, shrivelled appearance. The fully involuted ovary of old age contains practically no germinal elements.

Blood supply

The main vascular supply to the ovaries is the ovarian artery, which arises from the anterolateral aspect of the aorta just below the origin of the renal arteries. The right artery crosses the anterior surface of the vena cava, the lower part of the abdominal ureter and then, lateral to the ureter, enters the pelvis via the infundibulopelvic ligament. The left artery crosses the ureter almost immediately after its origin and then travels lateral to it, crossing the bifurcation of the common iliac artery at the pelvic brim to enter the infundibulopelvic ligament. Both arteries then divide to send branches to the ovaries through the mesovarium. Small branches pass to the ureter and the fallopian tube, and one branch passes to the cornu of the uterus where it freely anastomoses with branches of the uterine artery to produce a continuous arterial arch (see Figure 1.3).

The ovarian and uterine trunks drain into a pampiniform plexus of veins in the broad ligament near the mesovarium,

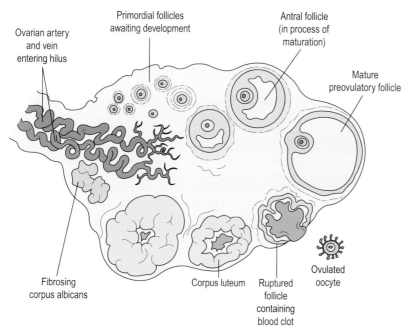

Ovarian artery and vein entering hilus

Primordial follicles awaiting development

Antral follicle (in process of maturation)

Mature preovulatory follicle

Ovulated oocyte

Fibrosing corpus albicans

Corpus luteum

Ruptured follicle containing blood clot

Figure 1.2 Diagrammatic section of an ovary and schematic representation of the cycle of follicular maturations.

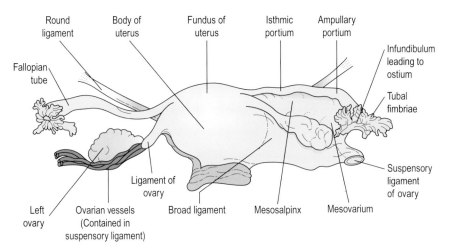

Round ligament
Body of uterus
Fundus of uterus
Isthmic portium
Ampullary portium
Fallopian tube
Infundibulum leading to ostium
Tubal fimbriae
Suspensory ligament of ovary
Left ovary
Ovarian vessels (Contained in suspensory ligament)
Ligament of ovary
Broad ligament
Mesosalpinx
Mesovarium

Figure 1.3 Posterosuperior aspect of the uterus and the broad ligament as seen from the umbilicus at laparoscopy.

which can occasionally become varicose. The right ovarian vein drains into the inferior vena cava, the left usually into the left renal vein.

The Fallopian Tube

The uterine or fallopian tubes are two oviducts originating at the cornu of the uterus which travel a rather tortuous course along the upper margins of the broad ligament. They are approximately 10 cm in length and end in the peritoneal cavity close to the ovary. This abdominal opening is situated at the end of a trumpet-shaped lateral portion of tube, the infundibulum. This opening is fringed by a number of petal-like processes, the fimbriae, which closely embrace the tubal end of the ovary. This fimbriated end has an important role in fertility.

Medial to the infundibulum is the ampulla which is thin walled and tortuous, and comprises at least half of the length of the tube. The medial third of the tube, the isthmus, is relatively straight. The tube has narrowed at this point, from approximately 3 mm at the abdominal opening to 1–2 mm. The final centimetre, the interstitial portion, is within the uterine wall.

Structure

The tubes are typical of many hollow viscera in that they contain three layers. The outer serosal layer consists of peritoneum and underlying areolar tissue. This covers the whole tube apart from the fimbriae at one end and the interstitial portion at the other. The middle muscular layer consists of outer longitudinal fibres and inner circular fibres. This is fairly thick at the isthmus and thins at the ampulla.

The mucous membrane is thrown into a series of plicae or folds, especially at the infundibular end. It is lined with columnar epithelium, much of which contains cilia which, together with the peristaltic action of the tube, help in sperm and ovum transport. Secretory cells are also present, as well as a third group of intercalary cells of uncertain function.

Relations

These are similar to those of the ovary (see above). Medially, the fallopian tube, after arching over the ovary, curves around its tubal extremity and passes down its free border.

Blood supply

The fallopian tube is supplied by branches from the vascular arcade formed by the ovarian artery laterally and a branch of the uterine artery medially.

The Uterus

The uterus is shaped like an inverted pear, tapering inferiorly to the cervix and, in the non-pregnant state, is situated entirely within the lesser pelvis. It is hollow and has thick muscular walls. Its maximal external dimensions are approximately 9 cm long, 6 cm wide and 4 cm thick. The upper expanded part of the uterus is termed the 'body' or 'corpus'. The area of insertion of each fallopian tube is termed the 'cornu' and that part of the body above the cornu, the 'fundus'. The uterus tapers to a small central constricted area, the isthmus, and below this is the cervix, which projects obliquely into the vagina and can be divided into vaginal and supravaginal portions (Figure 1.4).

The cavity of the uterus has the shape of an inverted triangle when sectioned coronally; the fallopian tubes open at the upper lateral angles (Figure 1.5). The lumen is apposed anteroposteriorly. The constriction at the isthmus where the corpus joins the cervix is the anatomical internal os.

Structure

The uterus consists of three layers: the outer serous layer (peritoneum), the middle muscular layer (myometrium) and the inner mucous layer (endometrium).

The peritoneum covers the body of the uterus and, posteriorly, the supravaginal portion of the cervix. This serous coat is initimately attached to a subserous fibrous layer, except laterally where it spreads out to form the leaves of the broad ligament.

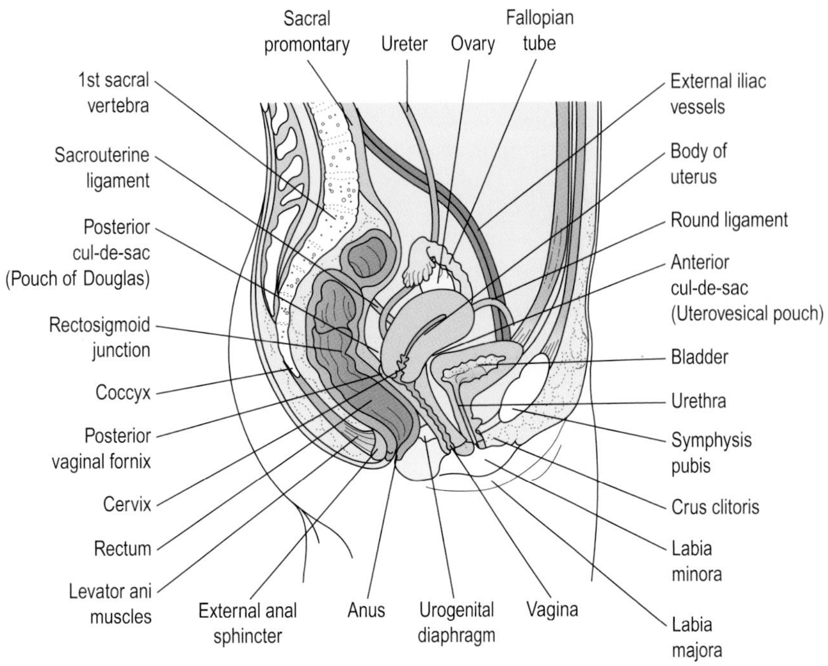

Figure 1.4 Median sagittal section through a female pelvis.

Sacral promontary
Ureter
Ovary
Fallopian tube
1st sacral vertebra
External iliac vessels
Sacrouterine ligament
Body of uterus
Posterior cul-de-sac (Pouch of Douglas)
Round ligament
Anterior cul-de-sac (Uterovesical pouch)
Rectosigmoid junction
Bladder
Coccyx
Urethra
Posterior vaginal fornix
Symphysis pubis
Cervix
Crus clitoris
Rectum
Labia minora
Levator ani muscles
External anal sphincter
Anus
Urogenital diaphragm
Vagina
Labia majora

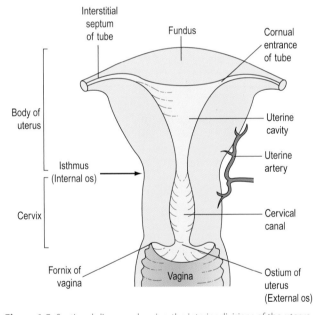

Interstitial septum of tube
Fundus
Cornual entrance of tube
Body of uterus
Uterine cavity
Uterine artery
Isthmus (Internal os)
Cervix
Cervical canal
Fornix of vagina
Vagina
Ostium of uterus (External os)

Figure 1.5 Sectional diagram showing the interior divisions of the uterus and its continuity with the vagina.

The muscular myometrium forms the main bulk of the uterus and comprises interlacing smooth muscle fibres intermingling with areolar tissue, blood vessels, nerves and lymphatics. Externally, these are mostly longitudinal but the larger intermediate layer has interlacing longitudinal, oblique and transverse fibres. Internally, they are mainly longitudinal and circular.

The endometrium forms the inner layer and is not sharply separated from the myometrium: the tubular glands dip into the innermost muscle fibres. A single layer of columnar epi-thelium covers the endometrium. Ciliated prior to puberty, this columnar epithelium is mainly lost due to the effects of pregnancy and menstruation. The endometrium undergoes cyclical histological changes during menstruation and varies in thickness between 1 and 5 mm.

The cervix

The cervix is cylindrical in shape, narrower than the body of the uterus and approximately 2.5 cm in length. It can be divided into the upper, supravaginal and lower vaginal portions. Due to anteflexion or retroflexion, the long axis of the cervix is rarely the same as the long axis of the body. Anterior and lateral to the supravaginal portion is cellular connective tissue, the parametrium. The posterior aspect is covered by the peritoneum of the pouch of Douglas. The ureter runs approximately 1 cm laterally to the supravaginal cervix. The vaginal portion projects into the vagina to form the fornices.

The upper part of the cervix mainly consists of involuntary muscle, whereas the lower part is mainly fibrous connective tissue.

The mucous membrane of the endocervix has anterior and posterior columns from which folds radiate out, the arbor vitae. It has numerous deep glandular follicles which secrete a clear alkaline mucus, the main component of physiological vaginal discharge. The epithelium of the endocervix is cylindrical and also ciliated in its upper two-thirds, and changes to stratified squamous epithelium around the region of the external os. This change may be abrupt or there may be a transitional zone up to 1 cm in width.

Position

The longitudinal axis of the uterus is approximately at right angles to the vagina and normally tilts forwards; this is termed 'anteversion'. The uterus is usually also flexed forwards on itself at the isthmus; this is termed 'anteflexion'. In approximately 20% of women, this tilt is not forwards but backwards, termed 'retroversion' or 'retroflexion'. In most cases, this does not have pathological significance and the uterus is mobile.

Relations

Anteriorly, the uterus is related to the bladder and is separated from it by the uterovesical pouch of peritoneum. Posteriorly is the pouch of Douglas plus coils of small intestine, sigmoid colon and upper rectum. Laterally, the relations are the broad ligament and that contained within it. Of special importance are the uterine artery and the ureter, running close to the supravaginal cervix.

Age-related changes

The disappearance of maternal oestrogenic stimulation after birth causes the uterus to decrease in length by approximately one-third and in weight by approximately one-half. The cervix is then around twice the length of the body of the uterus. At puberty, however, the corpus grows much faster and the size ratio reverses; the body becomes twice the length of the cervix. After the menopause, the uterus undergoes atrophy, the mucosa becomes very thin, the glands almost disappear and the walls become less muscular. These changes affect the cervix more than the corpus, so the cervical lips disappear and the external os becomes more or less flush with the vault.

The Vagina

The vagina is a fibromuscular tube which extends posterosuperiorly from the vestibule to the uterine cervix. It is longer in its posterior wall (approximately 9 cm) than anteriorly (approximately 7.5 cm). The vaginal walls are normally in contact, except superiorly, at the vault, where they are separated by the cervix. The vault of the vagina is divided into four fornices: posterior, anterior and two lateral. These increase in depth posteriorly. The mid-vagina is a transverse slit and the lower portion has an H-shape in transverse section.

Structure

The skin of the vagina is firmly attached to the underlying muscle and consists of stratified squamous epithelium. There are no epithelial glands present and the vagina is lubricated by mucus secretion from the cervix and Bartholin's glands. The epithelium is thick and rich in glycogen, which increases in the postovulatory phase of the cycle. Doderlein's bacillus is a normal commensal of the vagina, breaking down the glycogen to form lactic acid and producing a pH of approximately 4.5. This pH has a protective role for the vagina in decreasing the incidence of pyogenic infection.

The muscle layers consist of an outer longitudinal and inner circular layer, but these are not distinctly separate and are mostly spirally arranged and interspersed with elastic fibres.

The hymen

The hymen is a thin fold of mucous membrane across the entrance to the vagina. It has no known function. There are usually one or more openings in it to allow menses to escape. If these are not present, a haematocolpos will form with the commencement of menstruation. The hymen is usually, but not always, torn with first intercourse but can also be torn digitally or with tampons. It is certainly destroyed in childbirth and only small tags, carunculae myrtiformes, remain.

Relations

The upper posterior vaginal wall forms the anterior peritoneal reflection of the pouch of Douglas. The middle third is separated from the rectum by pelvic fascia and the lower third abuts the perineal body.

Anteriorly, the upper vagina is in direct contact with the base of the bladder, whilst the urethra runs down the lower half in the midline to open into the vestibule; its muscles fuse with the anterior vaginal wall.

Laterally, at the fornices, the vagina is related to the attachment of the cardinal ligaments. Below this are the levator ani muscles and the ischiorectal fossa. Near the vaginal orifice, the lateral relations include the vestibular bulb, bulbospongiosus muscle and Bartholin's gland.

Age-related changes

Immediately after birth, the vagina is under the influence of maternal oestrogen so the epithelium is well developed. Acidity is similar to that of an adult and Doderlein's bacilli are present. After a couple of weeks, the effects of maternal oestrogen disappear, the pH rises to 7 and the epithelium atrophies.

At puberty, the reverse occurs. The pH becomes acid again, the epithelium undergoes oestrogenization and the number of Doderlain's bacilli increases markedly. The vagina undergoes stretching during coitus, and especially childbirth, and the rugae tend to disappear.

At the menopause, the vagina tends to shrink and the epithelium atrophies.

The Vulva

The female external genitalia, commonly referred to as the 'vulva', include the mons pubis, the labia majora and minora, the vestibule, the clitoris and the greater vestibular glands (Figure 1.6).

Labia majora

The labia majora are two prominent folds of skin with underlying adipose tissue bounding either side of the vaginal opening. They contain numerous sweat and sebaceous glands, and correspond to the scrotum of the male. Anteriorly, they fuse together over the symphysis pubis to form a deposition of fat, the mons pubis. Posteriorly, they merge with the perineum. From puberty onwards, the lateral aspects of the labia majora and the mons pubis are covered with coarse hair. The inner aspects are smooth but have numerous sebaceous follicles.

Labia minora

The labia minora are two small vascular folds of skin, containing sebaceous glands but devoid of adipose tissue, which lie within the labia majora. Anteriorly, they divide into two to form the prepuce and frenulum of the clitoris. Posteriorly, they fuse to form a fold of skin termed the 'fourchette'. They are not well developed before puberty, and atrophy after the

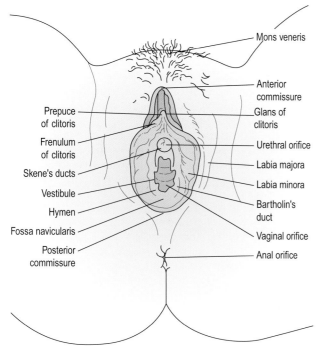

Figure 1.6 Female external genitalia with the labia majora and minora separated.

menopause. Their vascularity allows them to become turgid during sexual excitement.

Clitoris

This is a small erectile structure, approximately 2.5 cm long, homologous with the penis but not containing the urethra. The body of the clitoris contains two crura, the corpora cavernosa, which are attached to the inferior border of the pubic rami. The clitoris is covered by ischiocavernosus muscle, whilst bulbospongiosus muscle inserts into its root. The clitoris has a highly developed cutaneous nerve supply and is the most sensitive organ during sexual arousal.

Vestibule

The vestibule is the cleft between the labia minora. The vagina, urethra, paraurethral (Skene's) duct and ducts of the greater vestibular (Bartholin's) glands open into the vestibule (see Figure 1.7). The vestibular bulbs are two masses of erectile tissue on either side of the vaginal opening, and contain a rich plexus of veins within bulbospongiosus muscle. Bartholin's glands, each about the size of a small pea, lie at the base of each bulb and open via a 2 cm duct into the vestibule between the hymen and the labia minora. These glands secrete mucus, producing copious amounts during intercourse to act as a lubricant. They are compressed by contraction of the bulbospongiosus muscle.

Perineal body

This is a fibromuscular mass occupying the area between the vagina and the anal canal. It supports the lower part of the vagina and is of variable length. It is frequently torn during childbirth.

Age-related changes

In infancy, the vulva is devoid of hair and there is considerable adipose tissue in the labia majora and the mons pubis

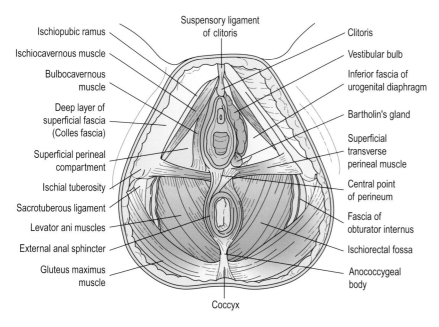

Figure 1.7 Dissection of the female perineum to show the bulb of the vestibule and the greater vestibular gland on the right; on the left side of the body, the muscles superficial to these structures have been left *in situ*.

which is lost during childhood but reappears during puberty, at which time hair grows. The vaginal opening tends to widen and sometimes shorten after childbirth. After the menopause, the skin atrophies and becomes thinner and drier. The labia minora shrink, subcutaneous fat is lost and the vaginal orifice becomes smaller.

The Ureter

The ureters are a pair of muscular tubes which convey urine to the bladder by peristaltic action. They are between 25 and 30 cm in length, and approximately half of their course lies within the abdomen and half within the pelvis. Each has a diameter of approximately 3 mm but there are slight constrictions as they cross the brim of the lesser pelvis and when they enter the bladder.

Structure

The ureter has three layers. The outer fibrous coat merges inferiorly with the bladder wall. The middle muscular layer has outer circular and inner longitudinal non-striated fibres, plus a further outer longitudinal layer along the lower third of the ureter. The inner mucous coat is lined with transitional epithelium and is continuous with the mucous membrane of the bladder below.

Relations and course

Throughout its abdominal course, the ureter travels retroperitoneally along the anteromedial aspect of the psoas major and is crossed by the ovarian vessels. The right ureter passes down just laterally to the inferior vena cava, and must be carefully retracted away if dissection of the nodes of the inferior vena cava is necessary.

The ureter enters the pelvis anterior to the sacroiliac joints and crosses the bifurcation of the common iliac artery. It then passes along the posterolateral aspect of the pelvis, running in front of and below the internal iliac artery and its anterior division, medial to the obturator vessels and nerves.

On reaching the true pelvis, the ureter turns forwards and medially, passing lateral to the uterosacral ligaments. It then travels through the base of the broad ligament and, lateral to the cervix, is crossed superiorly from the lateral to the medial side by the uterine artery. It continues, running approximately 1.5 cm lateral to the cervix, anterolateral to the upper part of the vagina and, passing slightly medially, enters the bladder at the trigone.

Surgical injury

The ureter can be damaged during gynaecological surgery at a number of points in its course. It can be injured near the pelvic brim where it is adjacent to the ovarian vessels or lower, near the cervix, where it crosses beneath the uterine vessels. The dangers are greater when the pelvis is distorted by fibroids or ovarian cysts, or the ureter's course is displaced by a broad ligament cyst. Damage can occur through the ureter being cut, crushed or ligated, and occasionally it may be devitalized by extensive dissection, especially at

Wertheim's hysterectomy. Occasionally, it is injured by high sutures near the cervix in a pelvic floor repair.

The Bladder

The bladder is a muscular reservoir capable of altering its size and shape depending on the amount of fluid it holds. It is a retroperitoneal viscus and lies behind the symphysis pubis. When empty, it is the shape of a tetrahedron, with a triangular base or fundus and a superior and two inferolateral surfaces. The two inferolateral surfaces meet to form the rounded border which joins the superior surface at the apex. The base and the inferolateral surface meet at the urethral orifice to form the bladder neck. As the bladder fills, it expands upwards and outwards and becomes more rounded. Normal bladder capacity is between 300 and 600 ml, but it can, in cases of urinary retention, contain several litres and extend as far as the umbilicus.

Vesical interior

The mucous membrane of the bladder is only loosely attached to the underlying muscular coat, so that it becomes irregularly folded when the bladder is empty. A triangular area, the trigone, is immediately above and behind the urethral opening; the posterolateral angles are formed by the ureteric orifices (Figure 1.8). The mucous membrane here is redder in colour, smooth and attached firmly to the underlying muscle. The superior boundary is slightly curved, the interureteric ridge.

The ureteric orifices are slit-like and approximately 2.5 cm apart in the contracted bladder. They enter the bladder at an oblique angle which helps to prevent reflux of urine during filling.

Structure

The wall of the bladder is in three layers. The outer serous coat, the peritoneal covering, is only present over the fundus. The muscular layer, the detrusor muscle, consists of three

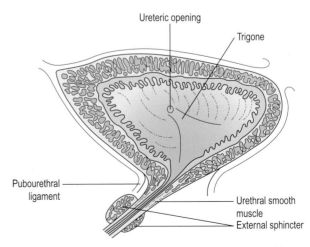

Figure 1.8 Except where it is fixed at its base, the bladder is a highly distensible structure. Urinary continence probably depends on the physical relations of the fixed/mobile junction.

layers of non-striated muscle, inner and outer longitudinal layers and a middle circular layer.

The mucous membrane is entirely covered by transitional epithelium which is responsive to ovarian hormonal stimulation. There are no true glands in this layer.

Relations

Superiorly, the bladder is covered by peritoneum. This extends forwards on to the anterior abdominal wall and sideways on to the pelvic side walls where there is a peritoneal depression, the paravesical fossa. As the bladder fills, the peritoneum is displaced upwards anteriorly, so that suprapubic catheterization of the full bladder can take place without the peritoneal cavity being entered. Anteriorly, below the peritoneal reflection is the loose cellular tissue of the cave of Retzius.

Posteriorly, the base of the bladder is separated from the upper vagina by the pubocervical fascia. Above this is the supravaginal portion of the cervix. The peritoneal reflection is at the isthmus of the uterus to form a slight recess, the uterovesical pouch, which often contains coils of intestine.

Surgical injury

The bladder may occasionally be opened during abdominal hysterectomy. The trigone, being in close relation with the upper vagina and the anterior fornix, is rarely damaged and perforation is usually 3–4 cm above it and can be easily repaired without damage to the ureter. If the injury is not noted, however, a vesicovaginal fistula may result. Damage may also occur during anterior colporrhaphy or vaginal hysterectomy, especially if a previous repair has been performed.

The Urethra

The urethra begins at the internal meatus of the bladder and runs anteroinferiorly behind the symphysis pubis, immediately related to the anterior vaginal wall. It is approximately 4 cm long and 6 mm in diameter. It crosses the perineal membrane and ends at the external urethral orifice in the vestibule, approximately 2.5 cm behind the clitoris. Skene's tubules, draining the paraurethral glands, open into the lower urethra. These glands are homologous to the male prostate.

There are no true anatomical sphincters to the urethra. The decussation of vesical muscle fibres at the urethrovesical junction acts as a form of internal sphincter, and continence is normally maintained at this level. Urethral resistence is mainly due to the tone and elasticity of the involuntary muscles of the urethral wall and this keeps it closed except during micturition. Approximately 1 cm from its lower end, before it crosses the perineal membrane, the urethra is encircled by voluntary muscle fibres, arising from the inferior pubic ramus, to form the so-called 'external sphincter'. This sphincter allows the voluntary arrest of urine flow.

Structure

The urethra has mucous and muscular coats. Near the bladder, the mucous membrane is lined by transitional epithelium which gradually converts into non-keratinizing stratified squamous epithelium as it approaches the external urethral meatus. The muscular layer, consisting of inner longitudinal and outer circular fibres, is continuous with that of the bladder.

Relations

Anteriorly, the urethra is separated from the symphysis pubis by loose cellular tissue. Posteriorly is the anterior vaginal wall plus Skene's tubules. Laterally is the urogenital diaphragm, bulbospongiosus muscle and the vestibular bulb.

The Sigmoid Colon

The pelvic or sigmoid colon is continuous with the descending colon and commences at the brim of the pelvis. It forms a loop approximately 40 cm in length and lies in the lesser pelvis behind the broad ligament. It is entirely covered by peritoneum, which forms a mesentery, the sigmoid mesocolon, which diminishes in length at either end and is largest at mid-segment. The lower end of the colon is continuous with the rectum at the level of the third sacral vertebra.

Structure

The mucous membrane of the colon is thrown into irregular folds and is covered by non-ciliated columnar epithelium. Separated from this layer by areolar tissue is the muscle layer. This is arranged as an inner circular layer and an outer longitudinal layer which has three narrow bands, the taeniae coli. These bands are shorter than the general surface of the colon and therefore give it its typical sacculated appearance. A series of small pieces of fat, the appendices epiploicae, are attached to the serous coat.

Relations

The position and shape of the pelvic colon vary considerably and hence so do its relations. Inferiorly, it rests on the uterus and the bladder. Above and on the right are the coils of ileum; below and on the left is the rectum. Posterior relations also include the ureter, internal iliac vessels, piriformis muscle and sacral plexus, all on the left side. Lateral relations include the ovary, external iliac vessels and obturator nerve.

The Rectum

The rectum, which begins at the level of the third sacral vertebra, moulds to the concavity of the sacrum and the coccyx; its anteroposterior curve forms the sacral flexure of the rectum. It is approximately 12 cm in length. The lower end dilates to form the ampulla which bulges into the posterior vaginal wall and then continues as the anal canal. When distended, the rectum has three lateral curves; the upper and lower are usually convex to the right, and the middle is convex to the left. Peritoneum covers the front and sides of the upper third of the rectum and the front of the middle third. The lower third is devoid of peritoneum.

Structure

Unlike the sigmoid colon, there are no sacculations, appendices epiploicae or mesentery. The taeniae coli blend approximately 5 cm above the junction of the rectum and colon, and form two bands, anterior and posterior, which descend the rectal wall. When the rectum is empty, the mucous membrane is thrown into longitudinal folds which disappear with distension. Permanent horizontal folds are also present and are more pronounced during distension. The lining is of mucus-secreting columnar epithelium.

Anal canal

The anal canal is approximately 3 cm long and passes downwards and backwards from the rectum. It is slit-like when empty but distends greatly during defaecation. This is aided by the presence of fat laterally in the ischiorectal fossa. Anteriorly, the anal canal is related to the perineal body and the lower vagina; posteriorly, it is related to the anococcygeal body.

For most of its length, it is surrounded by sphincteric muscles which are involved in the control of defaecation. The action of the levator ani muscles which surround it is also important in the control mechanism. The internal sphincter is involuntary and is a thickening of the circular muscle of the gut wall enclosing the anal canal just above the anorectal junction. The external sphincter is voluntary and composed of three layers of striated muscle.

Relations

The relations of the rectum are particularly important because they can be felt on digital examination. Posteriorly are the lower three sacral vertebrae, the coccyx, median sacral and superior rectal vessels. Posterolateral relations are the piriformis, coccygeus and levator ani muscles, plus the third, fourth and fifth sacral and coccygeal nerves. Below and lateral to the levator ani muscle is the ischiorectal fossa (Figure 1.9).

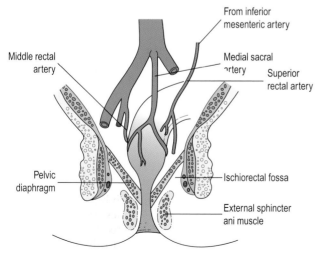

Figure 1.9 The rectum has a rich anastomotic blood supply from the median sacral, the internal iliac and the inferior mesenteric arteries; this arrangement is reflected in its venous drainage.

Anteriorly, above the peritoneal reflection lie the uterus and adnexa, upper vagina and pouch of Douglas with its contents. Below the reflection, it is related to the lower vagina.

Pelvic Musculofascial Support

Pelvic peritoneum

Posteriorly, the peritoneum is reflected from the rectum on to the posterior wall of the vagina, at which point it is in close contact with the outside world; a fact that can be used both diagnostically and therapeutically. It then passes upwards over the cervix and the uterus to form the rectouterine pouch, the pouch of Douglas.

The peritoneum then passes over the fundus of the uterus and down its anterior wall to reach the junction of the body and cervix, where it reflects over the anterior wall of the bladder, forming a shallow recess, the uterovesical pouch. The peritoneum in front of the bladder is loosely applied to the anterior abdominal wall so that it strips away as the bladder fills. Suprapubic catheterization of the distended bladder can therefore be performed without entering the peritoneal cavity.

On either side of the uterus, a double fold of peritoneum passes to the lateral pelvic side walls, the broad ligament. These two layers, anteroinferior and posterosuperior, enclose loose connective tissue, the parametrium. At the upper border, between the two layers, is the fallopian tube. The mesentery between the broad ligament and the fallopian tube is called the mesosalpinx, and that between the broad ligament and the ovary, the mesovarium (see Figure 1.3). Beyond the fallopian tube, the upper edge of the broad ligament, as it passes to the pelvic side wall, forms the infundibulopelvic ligament, or suspensory ligament of the ovary, and contains the ovarian blood vessels and nerves. Between the fallopian tube and the ovary, the mesosalpinx contains the vestigial epoophoron and paroophoron. After crossing the ureter, the uterine vessels pass between the layers of the broad ligament at its inferior border. They then ascend the ligament medially and anastomose with the ovarian vessels.

Pelvic ligaments

The round ligaments, a mixture of smooth muscle and fibrous tissue, are two narrow flat bands which arise from the lateral angles of the uterus and then pass laterally, deep to the anterior layer of the broad ligament, towards the lateral pelvic side wall. They then turn forwards towards the deep inguinal ring, crossing medial to the vesical vessels, obturator vessels and nerve, obliterated umbilical artery and external iliac vessels. They finally pass through the inguinal canal to end in the subcutaneous tissue of the labia majora. Together with the uterosacral ligaments, the round ligaments help to keep the uterus in a position of anteversion and anteflexion.

The ovarian ligaments, which are fibromuscular cords of similar structure to the round ligament, lie within the broad ligament and each runs from the cornu of the uterus to the medial border of the ovary. Together, the round and ovarian

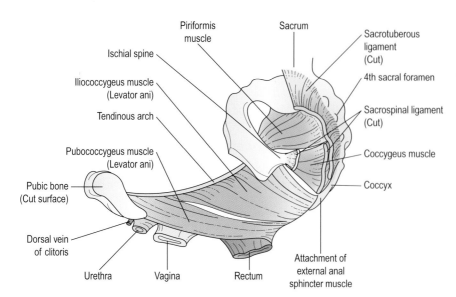

Piriformis muscle

Ischial spine

Iliococcygeus muscle (Levator ani)

Tendinous arch

Pubococcygeus muscle (Levator ani)

Pubic bone (Cut surface)

Dorsal vein of clitoris

Urethra

Vagina

Rectum

Sacrum

Sacrotuberous ligament (Cut)

4th sacral foramen

Sacrospinal ligament (Cut)

Coccygeus muscle

Coccyx

Attachment of external anal sphincter muscle

Figure 1.10 Pelvic musculature. Muscles leave the pelvis either above the superior ramus of the pubis or through the greater or lesser sciatic foramina. Nerves and vessels also leave via the obturator foramen.

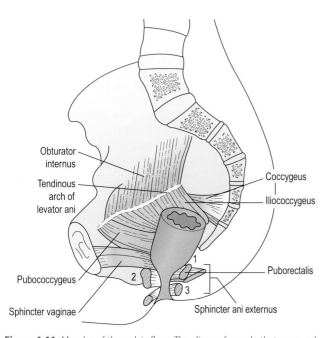

Obturator internus

Tendinous arch of levator ani

Pubococcygeus

Sphincter vaginae

Coccygeus

Iliococcygeus

Puborectalis

Sphincter ani externus

Figure 1.11 Muscles of the pelvic floor. The slings of muscle that surround and separate the major body effluents have an important role as sphincters. 1, rectum; 2, internal anal sphincter; 3, external anal sphincter.

ligaments form the homologue of the gubernaculum testis of the male.

In addition, there are also condensations of pelvic fascia on the upper surface of the levator ani muscles, the so-called 'fascial ligaments', composed of elastic tissue and smooth muscle. They are attached to the uterus at the level of the supravaginal cervix and, being extensive and strong, have an important supporting role. The transverse cervical or cardinal ligaments pass laterally to the pelvic side wall and their posterior reflection continues around the lateral margins of the rectum as the uterosacral ligaments. They insert into the periostium of the fourth sacral vertebra. These ligaments provide the major support to the uterus above the pelvic dia-

phragm, helping to prevent uterine descent. The uterosacrals also help to pull the supravaginal cervix backwards in the pelvis to assist in anteflexion. Anteriorly, the pubocervical fascia is more of a fascial plane than a distinct ligament. It extends beneath the base of the bladder, passing around the urethra and inserting into the body of the pubic symphysis. It supports the bladder base and the anterior vaginal wall.

Pelvic musculature (Figures 1.10 and 1.11)

The levator ani and coccygeus muscles on either side, together with their fascial coverings, form the pelvic diaphragm which separates the structures in the pelvis from the perineum and the ischiorectal fossa. This diaphragm, together with all the tissue between the pelvic cavity and the perineum, makes up the pelvic floor. In lower mammals, the diaphragm represents the abductor and flexor muscles of the tail; in humans, who have an erect attitude, these muscles help to provide support to the pelvic viscera.

The levator ani is a wide, thin, curved sheet of muscle which arises anteriorly from the pelvic surface of the body of the pubic bone, the ischial spine and the tendinous arch of the obturator fascia between the two. The muscle fibres converge across the midline. The levator ani can be divided into three parts: puborectalis, which is most medial, encircling the rectum and vagina, and acting as support and additional sphincter for both; pubococcygeus, the strongest part of the muscular component, which is slung from the pubis to the coccyx; and iliococcygeus, the most posterior, also attached to the coccyx.

The posterior part of the pelvic floor is made up of coccygeus muscle, a thin, flat, triangular muscle, lying on the same plane as the iliococcygeal portion of the levator ani. It arises from the ischial spine and inserts into the lower sacrum and the upper coccyx. Like the levator ani, it acts by supporting the pelvic viscera.

Most of the side wall of the lesser pelvis is covered by the fan-shaped obturator internus muscle which is attached to the obturator membrane and the neighbouring bone. The fibres run backwards and turn laterally at a right angle to

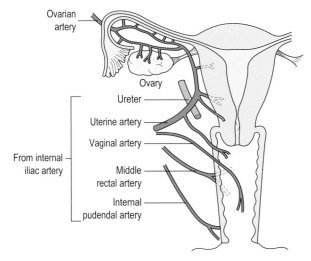

Figure 1.12 The urogenital diaphragm. The floor of the pelvis slopes steeply forwards and plays an important role in continence and childbirth.

emerge through the lesser sciatic foramen. The side wall is covered medially by the obturator fascia (Figure 1.12).

The ischiorectal fossa, the wedge-shaped space lateral to the anus, is bounded laterally by the obturator internus and superomedially by the external surface of the levator ani. The base is the perineal skin. The fossa extends forwards, almost to the pubis, and backwards almost to the sacrum, where it is widest and deepest. The posterior boundary is made up by the sacrotuberous ligament and the gluteus maximus muscle, and the anterior boundary by the upper surface of the deep fascia of the sphincter urethrae muscle. It crosses the midline in front of the anal canal.

The musculature of the urogenital region can be divided into two groups, the superficial and deep muscles. Superficially, there are three muscles: the bulbospongiosus, the sphincter vaginae, which surrounds the vaginal orifice, posteriorly being continuous with the perineal body and anteriorly attaching to the corpora cavernosa of the clitoris; the ischiocavernosus, covering the unattached surface of the crus of the clitoris; and the superficial transverse perineal muscle. The deep muscles are the deep transverse perineal muscle, starting from the inner surface of the ischial ramus and passing to the perineal body, and the sphincter urethrae, surrounding the membranous urethra. These layers, and their fascial component, constitute the urogenital diaphragm.

The perineal body or central perineal tendon is a fibromuscular mass lying between the anal canal and the vagina. Superficially, it contains insertions of transverse perineal muscles and fibres of the external anal sphincter and, on a deeper plane, the levator ani muscle. It supports the lower part of the vagina and is frequently torn during childbirth.

Blood Supply to the Pelvis

Abdominal aorta

The abdominal portion of the aorta commences as it passes between the crura of the diaphragm at the level of the body of the 12th thoracic vertebra. It runs downwards to the left of the midline along the front of the vertebral column, and bifurcates at the level of the body of the fourth lumbar vertebra to form the right and left common iliac arteries. The inferior vena cava runs immediately on its right. In the lower part of its course, ovarian and inferior mesenteric branches arise from the front of the aorta, and median sacral and lumbar branches arise from the back of the aorta.

Inferior mesenteric artery

The inferior mesenteric artery arises 3–4 cm above the bifurcation of the aorta. It descends at first in front of the aorta, then to the left of it, to cross the left common iliac artery medial to the left ureter, and continues in the mesentery of the sigmoid colon into the lesser pelvis. During its course, it gives off a left colic branch which supplies the left half of the transverse colon and descending colon, and a sigmoid branch supplying the sigmoid colon. In the lesser pelvis, it continues as the superior rectal artery, supplying the upper rectum and anastomosing with the middle and inferior rectal branches. The inferior mesenteric artery can occasionally be traumatized during para-aortic lymph node dissection and will bleed freely. Transection, however, is not of serious consequence to the blood supply to the lower bowel due to considerable anastomotic connections.

Common iliac artery

After the aortic bifurcation, the two common iliac arteries run a distance of 4–5 cm before again bifurcating to form internal and external iliac branches on either side. The left artery runs partly lateral and partly in front of the corresponding iliac vein. On the right side, the slightly longer artery runs in front of the lowermost portion of the inferior vena cava and the terminations of the two common iliac veins, and then anterior to the right common iliac vein. The bifurcation of the common iliac artery is in front of the sacroiliac joint. The ureter lies in front of the bifurcation at this point.

External iliac artery and its branches

The external iliac arteries are larger than the internal iliac vessels and run obliquely and laterally down the medial border of the psoas major. At a point midway between the anterior superior iliac spine and the symphysis pubis, the artery enters the thigh behind the inguinal ligament and becomes the femoral artery. At this point, it is lateral to the femoral vein but medial to the nerve. The ovarian vessels cross in front of the artery just below the bifurcation, as does the round ligament. The external iliac vein is partly behind the upper part of the artery, but medial in its lower part.

The external iliac artery gives off two main branches. The inferior epigastric artery ascends obliquely along the medial margin of the deep inguinal ring, pierces the transversalis fascia and runs up between the rectus abdominis muscle and its posterior sheath, supplying the muscle and sending branches to the skin. It anastomoses with the superior epigastric artery above the level of the umbilicus. The deep circumflex artery runs posteroinferior to the inguinal ligament to the anterior superior iliac spine, and then pierces and supplies the transversus abdominis and internal oblique muscles.

Once the external iliac artery has pierced the thigh and become the femoral artery, it almost immediately gives off an external pudendal branch which supplies much of the skin of the vulva, anastomosing with the labial branches of the internal pudendal artery.

Internal iliac artery and its branches

The internal iliac arteries are 4 cm long and descend to the upper margin of the greater sciatic foramen where they divide into anterior and posterior divisions (Figure 1.13). In the fetus, they are twice as large as the external iliac vessels and ascend the anterior wall to the umbilicus to form the umbilical artery. After birth, with the cessation of the placental circulation, only the pelvic portion remains patent; the remainder becomes a fibrous cord, the lateral umbilical ligament. The ureter runs anteriorly down the artery and the internal iliac vein runs behind.

The posterior division has three branches which mainly supply the musculature of the buttocks. The iliolumbar artery ascends deep to the psoas muscle and divides to supply the iliacus and the quadratus lumborum. The lateral sacral arteries descend in front of the sacral rami and supply the structures of the sacral canal. The superior gluteal artery is the direct continuation and leaves the lesser pelvis through the greater sciatic foramen to supply much of the gluteal musculature.

The anterior division has seven main branches. The superior vesical artery runs anteroinferiorly between the side of the bladder and the pelvic side wall to supply the upper part of the bladder. The obturator artery passes to the obturator canal and thence to the adductor compartment of the thigh. Inside the pelvis, it sends off iliac, vesical and pubic branches (Table 1.1).

The vaginal artery corresponds to the inferior vesical artery of the male. It descends inwards, low in the broad ligament to supply the upper vagina, base of the bladder and adjacent rectum. It anastomoses with branches of the uterine artery to form two median longitudinal vessels, the azygos arteries of the vagina, one descending in front and the other behind.

The uterine artery passes along the root of the broad ligament and crosses above and in front of the ureter approximately 2 cm from the cervix. It then runs tortuously along the lateral margin of the uterus between the layers of the broad ligament. It supplies the cervix and the body of the uterus and part of the bladder, and one branch anastomoses with the vaginal artery to produce the azygos arteries. It ends by anastomosing with the ovarian artery (Figure 1.14). The branches of the uterine artery pass circumferentially around the myometrium, giving off coiled radial branches which end as basal arteries supplying the endometrium.

The middle rectal artery is a small branch passing medially to the rectum to vascularize the muscular tissue of the lower rectum and anastomose with the superior and inferior rectal arteries.

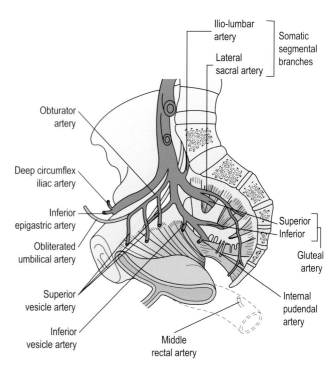

Figure 1.13 The blood supply to the pelvic viscera is derived in the main from the internal iliac artery.

Table 1.1 Arterial supply of the pelvic organs

Organ	Artery	Origin
Ovary	Ovarian	Aorta
	Uterine	Internal iliac
Fallopian tube	Ovarian	Aorta
	Uterine	Internal iliac
Uterus	Uterine	Internal iliac
	Ovarian	Aorta
Vagina	Vaginal	Internal iliac
	Uterine	Internal iliac
	Internal pudendal	Internal iliac
	Middle rectal	Internal iliac
Vulva	Internal pudendal	Internal iliac
	External pudendal	Internal iliac
Ureter	Renal	Aorta
	Ovarian	Aorta
	Uterine	Internal iliac
	Superior vesical	Internal iliac
	Inferior vesical	Internal iliac
Bladder	Superior vesical	Internal iliac
	Inferior vesical	Internal iliac
Urethra	Inferior vesical	Internal iliac
	Internal pudendal	Internal iliac
Sigmoid colon	Left colic	Inferior mesenteric
Rectum	Superior rectal	Inferior mesenteric
	Middle rectal	Internal iliac
	Inferior rectal	Internal pudendal (internal iliac)

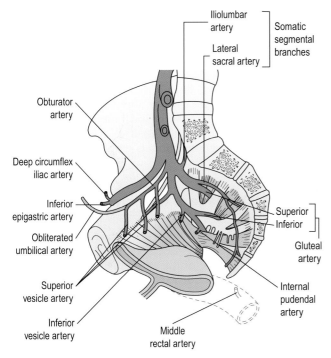

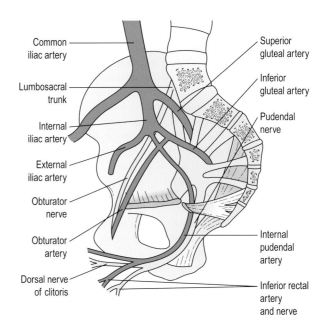

Figure 1.14 The uterus has an anastomotic supply from both the ovarian and uterine arteries, both vessels running in the broad ligament.

Figure 1.15 Pelvic nerves and blood supply of the pudenda. The major nerve is the pudendal, but it is supplemented by the posterior cutaneous nerve of the thigh, and the ilioinguinal and genitofemoral nerves.

The internal pudendal artery, the smaller of the two terminal trunks of the internal iliac artery, descends anterior to the piriformis and, piercing the pelvic fascia, leaves the pelvis through the inferior part of the greater sciatic foramen, crosses the gluteal aspect of the ischial spine and enters the perineum through the lesser sciatic foramen (Figure 1.15). It then traverses the pudendal canal with the pudendal nerve, approximately 4 cm above the ischial tuberosity. It then proceeds forwards above the inferior fascia of the urogenital diaphragm and divides into a number of branches. The inferior rectal branch supplies the skin and musculature of the anus, and anastomoses with the superior and middle rectal arteries; the perineal artery supplies much of the perineum, and small branches supply the labia, vestibular bulbs and vagina. The artery terminates as the dorsal artery of the clitoris.

The inferior gluteal artery, the larger terminal trunk, descends behind the internal pudendal artery, traverses the lower part of the greater sciatic foramen and, with the superior gluteal artery, supplies much of the buttock and the back of the thigh.

Nerve Supply to the Pelvis

Autonomic nerves (see Figure 1.15)

The internal pelvic organs are supplied by both the sympathetic and the parasympathetic autonomic nervous systems and this represents their sole innervation. As they descend into the pelvis, branches from the lower part of the lumbar sympathetic trunk join the aortic plexus of sympathetic nerves and ganglia as it continues downwards over the bifurcation of the aorta to form the superior hypogastric plexus. This then divides to form the right and left inferior hypogastric or pelvic plexuses, which lie lateral to the rectum and further subdivide into two, anteriorly innervating the base of the bladder and urethra and posteriorly innervating the uterus, cervix, vagina, sigmoid colon and rectum.

The parasympathetic nerves enter the pelvis through the second, third and fourth sacral nerves. The preganglionic fibres are distributed through the pelvic plexus, and the parasympathetic ganglia are situated close to, or in the walls of, the viscera concerned. With the exception of the ovaries and fallopian tube, which are supplied directly by nerves from the preaortic plexus travelling along the ovarian vessels, all internal pelvic organs are supplied via the pelvic plexuses.

Somatic nerves

The lumbar plexus is formed by the anterior primary rami of the first three lumbar nerves, part of the fourth nerve and a contribution from the 12th thoracic (subcostal) nerve. It lies on the surface of the psoas major and gives off a number of major branches.

The iliohypogastric and ilioinguinal nerves both arise from the first lumbar nerve. The former gives branches to the buttock, while the latter supplies the skin of the mons pubis and the surrounding vulva. The genitofemoral nerve arises from the first and second lumbar nerves, its femoral branch supplying the upper thigh, whilst its genital branch supplies the skin of the labium majus. The lateral femoral cutaneous nerve arises from the second and third lumbar nerves, and also supplies the thigh.

The femoral nerve is the largest branch, coming from the second, third and fourth lumbar nerves. It descends in the groove between the psoas and iliacus muscles and enters the thigh deep to the inguinal ligament, lateral to the femoral artery, to supply the flexors of the hip, the extensors of the knee and numerous cutaneous branches including the saphenous nerve. The obturator nerve also comes from the second, third and fourth lumbar nerves, and passes downwards, medial to the psoas into the pelvis, to supply the adductor muscles of the hip.

The lumbosacral trunk comes from the fourth and fifth lumbar nerves, and passes medial to the psoas into the pelvis to join the anterior primary rami of the first three sacral nerves to form the sacral plexus in front of the piriformis muscle. From this plexus, a number of branches emerge. The most important of these are the sciatic nerve — a large nerve formed from the fourth and fifth lumbar nerves and the first, second and third sacral nerves — which leaves the pelvis through the lower part of the greater sciatic foramen to supply the muscles of the back of the thigh and the lower limb, and the pudendal nerve, formed from the second, third and fourth sacral nerves.

The pudendal nerve leaves the pelvis between the piriformis and coccygeus muscles and curls around the ischial spine to re-enter the pelvis through the lesser sciatic foramen where, medial to the internal pudendal artery, it lies in the pudendal canal on the lateral wall of the ischiorectal fossa. The point where the nerve circles the ischial spine is the region in which a pudendal block of local anaesthetic is injected.

The pudendal nerve gives a number of terminal branches. The inferior rectal nerve gives motor and sensory fibres to the external anal sphincter, anal canal and skin around the anus. The perineal nerve passes forwards below the internal pudendal artery to give labial branches, supplying the skin of the labia majora, the deep perineal nerve supplying the perineal muscles and the bulb of the vestibule. The dorsal vein of the clitoris passes through the pudendal canal, giving a branch to the crus and piercing the perineal membrane 1–2 cm from the symphysis pubis. It supplies the clitoris and surrounding skin.

Lymphatic Drainage of the Pelvis

In the pelvis, as elsewhere in the body, the lymph nodes are arranged along the blood vessels. The lateral aortic lymph nodes lie on either side of the aorta; their efferents form a lumbar trunk on either side which terminates at the cisterna chylia. Those structures which receive their blood supply directly from branches of the aorta, i.e. the ovary, fallopian tube, upper ureter and, in view of arterial anastomoses, uterine fundus, drain directly into the lateral aortic group of nodes.

The lymph drainage of most other structures within the pelvis is via more outlying groups of lymph nodes associated with the iliac vessels. The common iliac lymph nodes are grouped around the common iliac artery and are usually arranged in medial, lateral and intermediate chains. They receive efferents from the external and internal iliac nodes, and send efferents to the lateral aortics (Figure 1.16).

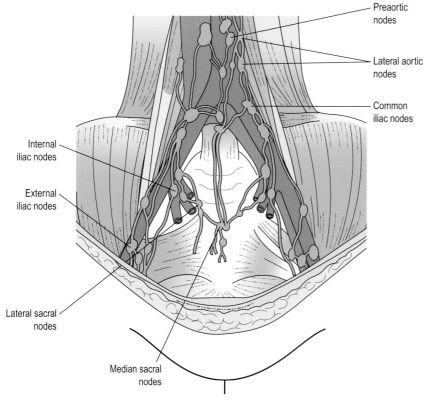

Figure 1.16 The lymph vessels and nodes of the pelvis.

Preaortic nodes

Lateral aortic nodes

Common iliac nodes

Internal iliac nodes

External iliac nodes

Lateral sacral nodes

Median sacral nodes

Table 1.2 Lymphatic drainage of the pelvis

Organ	Lymph nodes
Ovary	Lateral aortic nodes
Fallopian tube	Lateral aortic nodes Superficial inguinal nodes External and internal iliac nodes
Corpus uteri	External and internal iliac nodes Superficial inguinal nodes Lateral aortic nodes
Cervix	External and internal iliac nodes Obturator node Sacral node
Upper vagina	External and internal iliac nodes Obturator node Sacral nodes
Lower vagina	Superficial inguinal nodes
Vulva	Superficial inguinal nodes Internal iliac nodes (deep tissues)
Ureter	Lateral aortic nodes Internal iliac nodes
Bladder	External and internal iliad nodes
Urethra	Internal iliac nodes
Sigmoid colon	Preaortic nodes
Upper rectum	Preaortic nodes
Lower rectum and canal	Internal iliac nodes
Anal orifice	Superficial inguinal nodes

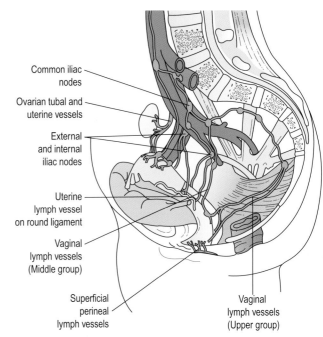

Figure 1.17 The lymphatic drainage of the female reproductive organs. *Semi-diagrammatic after Cunéo and Marcille 1901, Bull. Soc. Anat. Paris 3,653.*

The external iliac nodes lie on the external iliac vessels and are in three groups: lateral, medial and anterior. They collect from the cervix, upper vagina, bladder, deeper lower abdominal wall and inguinal lymph nodes. Inferior epigastric and circumflex iliac nodes are associated with these vessels and can be considered to be outlying members of the external iliac group (Table 1.2).

The internal iliac nodes, which surround the internal iliac artery, receive afferents from all the pelvic viscera, deeper perineum, and muscles of the thigh and buttock. The obturator lymph node, sometimes present in the obturator canal, and the sacral lymph nodes on the median and lateral sacral vessels can be considered to be outlying members of this group (Figure 1.17).

The upper group of superficial inguinal lymph nodes forms a chain immediately below the inguinal ligament. The lateral members receive afferents from the gluteal region and adjoining lower anterior abdominal wall. The medial members drain the vulva and perineum, lower vagina, lower anal canal, adjoining anterior abdominal wall and uterus owing to lymph vessels that accompany the round ligament to the anterior abdominal wall. The lymphatics on either side of the vulva communicate freely, emphasizing the importance of removing the whole vulva in cases of malignant disease. The superficial lymph nodes send their efferents to the external iliac lymph nodes, passing around the femoral vessels or traversing the femoral canal.

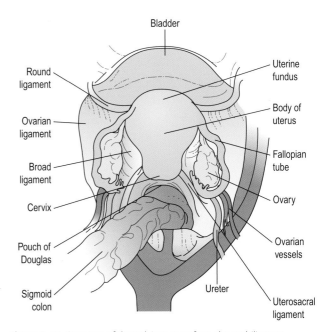

Figure 1.18 Overview of the pelvis as seen from the umbilicus at laparoscopy.

The deep inguinal (femoral) lymph nodes, varying from one to three, are on the medial side of the femoral vein. They receive efferents from the deep femoral vessels and some from the superficial inguinal nodes; one, the node of Cloquet, is thought to drain the clitoris. Efferents from the deep nodes pass through the femoral canal to the external iliac group (Figure 1.18).

KEY POINTS

1. Knowing the course of pelvic migration of the ovaries is important in understanding the consequences of maldescent.

2. The sizes of the uterus and the cervix, and their ratio, change with age and parity.

3. The uterine artery is a branch of the internal iliac artery that crosses above the ureter and passes medially in the base of the broad ligament to reach the supravaginal portion of the cervix. It divides to pass superiorly alongside the body of the uterus, and inferiorly to supply the vagina and cervix.

4. The ovarian artery arises from the aorta at the level of the second lumbar vertebra. The right ovarian vein drains into the inferior vena cava, while the left ovarian vein drains into the left renal vein.

5. The inferior epigastric artery is a branch of the external iliac artery and ascends between the rectus muscle and the posterior rectus sheath, where it should be avoided during insertion of laparoscopic ports.

6. The ureter crosses the pelvic brim at the bifurcation of the common iliac artery and descends on the lateral pelvic side wall, where it is at risk during oophorectomy.

7. The ureter runs beneath the uterine vessels in the base of the broad ligament and emerges close to the supravaginal portion of the cervix (1.0–1.5 cm), where it is at risk during the ligation of pedicles at hysterectomy.

8. The internal urethral sphincter comprises two loops of smooth muscle fibres that pass around the vesical neck.

9. The term 'external urethral sphincter' refers to paraurethral striated muscle that is under voluntary control and includes the external, circular layer of urethral muscle together with the compressor urethrae and the urethrovaginal sphincter.

10. The pudendal nerve leaves the pelvis between the piriformis and coccygeus muscles, passes around the ischial spine and re-enters the pelvis via the lesser sciatic foramen, where it lies medial to the internal pudendal artery in the lateral wall of the ischiorectal fossa.

CHAPTER 2

Hysteroscopy

Nazar N. Amso, Richard J. Penketh and Asmita Patwardhan

Chapter Contents

INTRODUCTION	17
HISTORICAL DEVELOPMENT	17
DIAGNOSTIC INDICATIONS	17
CONTRAINDICATIONS	18
INSTRUMENTATION	19
TECHNIQUE OF DIAGNOSTIC HYSTEROSCOPY	20
PATHOLOGY SEEN AT DIAGNOSTIC HYSTEROSCOPY	21
HYSTEROSCOPIC SKILLS	21
TREATMENT OF THE ENDOMETRIAL CAVITY WITHOUT INTRACAVITY LESIONS	29
HYSTEROSCOPIC STERILIZATION	31
COMPLICATIONS OF HYSTEROSCOPY AND PROCEDURES	31
LATE COMPLICATIONS	33
NEWER DEVELOPMENTS	33
KEY POINTS	34

Introduction

Over the last century, uterine surgery has evolved from being dominated by hysterectomy to a range of less invasive procedures that have the common principle of conserving the uterus and reducing procedural morbidity. Disorders of the uterine cavity leading to abnormal uterine bleeding, infertility and pain affect the majority of women during their lifetime. The ability to view the uterine cavity has enabled the accurate diagnosis and treatment of numerous conditions. The quest to improve diagnostic and therapeutic capabilities has led to the widespread acceptance of modern gynaecological endoscopy.

Historical Development

Bozzini was the first to look into the cavity of a hollow organ, the bladder, in 1805. This was achieved with long tubes assisted by external illumination. In 1853, Desormeaux made the first satisfactory endoscope, but it was Panteleoni who performed the first satisfactory hysteroscopy in 1869 (Panteleoni 1869). Inability to distend the uterus and lack of proper illumination caused poor visualization and lack of widespread acceptance until Lindemann renewed Rubin's attempts to use carbon dioxide in the 1970s (Lindemann 1972).

Over the last three decades, improved optics and video monitoring systems have encouraged gynaecologists to learn this skill. Increased use and better understanding of electrosurgery have enabled significant developments in operative hysteroscopy. Smaller-diameter hysteroscopes have enabled hysteroscopy without anaesthesia, and outpatient hysteros-copy is now firmly established. 'See and treat' in an outpatient hysteroscopy clinic is a reality in modern gynaecological practice.

Diagnostic Indications

Abnormal uterine bleeding

Menstrual abnormality is one of the most common reasons for referral to the gynaecological outpatient department. Menometrorrhagia, dysmenorrhoea and intermenstrual bleeding are the most common. After the menarche, such problems are usually dysfunctional, and hysteroscopy is rarely indicated. In postmenopausal patients, bleeding is a worrying symptom and warrants urgent attention as the patient is anxious to exclude endometrial cancer. Outpatient hysteroscopy offers rapid diagnosis and reassurance. In women of reproductive age, abnormal uterine bleeding can be associated with hormonal disturbances or pathology such as fibroids and polyps. Cervical polyps may be associated with endometrial polyps in 26.7% of patients (Stamatellos et al 2007), and exclusion of endometrial pathology is important.

Infertility

Hysteroscopy is a reliable method to detect and potentially treat submucous fibroids, endometrial polyps, intrauterine adhesions and endometritis. Congenital anomalies are infrequent but are associated with infertility. Abnormalities of the endometrium and organic intrauterine pathologies are important causes of failed in-vitro fertilization/embryo transfer cycles. A recent meta-analysis has shown potential benefits of performing pretreatment hysteroscopy in patients being referred for IVF (El-Toukhy et al 2008).

Intrauterine synechiae (Asherman's syndrome)

Intrauterine adhesions can lead to infertility, recurrent miscarriage, hypomenorrhoea or amenorrhoea. Adhesions are caused by trauma to the endometrial basal layer, during evacuation of retained products of conception or may be secondary to infections (e.g. tuberculosis).

Fibroids and polyps

Submucus fibroids and polyps, which occlude the cervix or the tubal ostia, may hamper sperm progression and interfere with implantation.

Müllerian anomalies

Patients with a uterine structural anomaly may have normal fertility or present with infertility. Hysteroscopy may reveal arcuate, subseptate, septate, bicornuate or uterus didelphis. Hysterosalpingography, ultrasonography and laparoscopy are additional valuable tools to investigate these patients once an anomaly has been found.

Recurrent miscarriage

The aetiology of recurrent miscarriage is poorly understood. Intrauterine pathology such as fibroids, polyps, Asherman's syndrome or congenital abnormalities may be detected in up to 33% of infertile couples (Romano et al 1994). Implantation of an embryo over the septum or fibroid can also fail due to the poor blood supply in these parts of the uterus.

Foreign body

Missing threads of an intrauterine contraceptive device (IUCD) or a deeply embedded coil may need to be removed under hysteroscopic guidance. Apart from anxiety, these patients may present with menstrual irregularities and pain.

Chronic pelvic pain

Patients with chronic pain can pose a difficult challenge to the gynaecologist. Obstructive uterine anomaly may be associated in 40% of these patients (Schifrin et al 1973). Concomitant hysteroscopy may reveal polyps, fibroids, adhesions and septate uterus which may contribute to the patient's symptoms.

Contraindications

Infection

Hysteroscopy in the presence of acute pelvic infection can lead to spread of infection with the distension medium flowing through the tubes, spreading the infection to the peritoneal cavity. The only exception is when infection is secondary to a lost IUCD, which should be removed hysteroscopically under antibiotic cover.

Pregnancy

Pregnancy is another contraindication, although embryoscopy prior to 10 weeks of gestation has been performed as an aid to prenatal diagnosis. Pregnancy leads to increased uterine softening and vascularity, increasing the risks of bleeding, uterine perforation and miscarriage. Hysteroscopy during pregnancy may occasionally be performed to remove a coil where the tails are not visible.

Malignancy

Hysteroscopy is contraindicated in the presence of cervical cancer. However, it is a gold standard procedure in patients with endometrial cancer as it aids directed biopsy.

Bleeding

Diagnostic hysteroscopy may be performed in the presence of bleeding, but the view is likely to be poor. Hysteroscopy is best performed in the mid-to-late proliferative phase when the endometrium is thinnest. If this is difficult to arrange, preoperative hormonal treatment with progesterone can help to postpone or control bleeding.

Cardiopulmonary disorders

Patients with these medical conditions are at higher risk of anaesthetic when recognized hysteroscopic complications, such as gas embolism and fluid overload, occur. Outpatient hysteroscopy under local anaesthetic is therefore the treatment of choice for such patients.

Cervical stenosis

Patients who have a history of cervical surgery or difficult uterine entry in the past are at increased risk of cervical trauma, perforation and false passage during the performance of a hysteroscopy. Prostaglandins inserted 2 h before hysteroscopy may help to soften the cervix, allowing easy dilatation and entry into the uterine cavity, although the evidence is limited for their value in postmenopausal patients (Crane and Healey 2006).

Instrumentation

Inadequate instrumentation resulting in poor visualization and reduced safety is not only dangerous, but will potentially give erroneous results. Good-quality hysteroscopes, cameras and driver units are basic requirements for good visualization of the uterine cavity. Appropriate fluid monitoring systems and energy sources, such as laser or diathermy, are essential for operative hysteroscopy (Figure 2.1).

Before commencing any hysteroscopic procedure, one must ensure that the stack system (Figure 2.2) is fully functional. This includes the telescope, surgical instruments, camera drive unit, camera head, light source, light lead, monitor, electrosurgical generator and image recording equipment. If a simultaneous laparoscopy is required, two stack systems should be made available. It is essential to assemble the equipment to ensure that it works prior to use. The distension medium, suction machine, fluid measurement apparatus and connecting tubing must be checked.

Fluid should be allowed to flow through the giving set to remove all air bubbles.

Optical systems

Rigid telescopes

Panoramic hysteroscopy is performed with the help of a distension medium, and is common practice. The majority of hysteroscopists use rigid telescopes. Improved technology has allowed significant reduction in the outer diameter (as low as 2.5 mm, including the inflow sheath). The outer diameter of operative hysteroscopes using monopolar electrosurgery may be up to 10 mm. This includes the telescope with the working element, inflow sheath (inner) and outflow sheath (outer). Smaller-diameter operative scopes (Figure 2.3) measure 5 mm and consist of a 5 French operative channel communicating with the outflow sheath. This allows instruments of 5F diameter (e.g. the bipolar electrode, laser fibre, mechanical scissors and grasper) down the operative channel. The telescopes may be forward view (0°) or oblique view (angled scopes 12, 30, 70 or 90°).

Flexible telescopes

Flexible hysteroscopes offer the advantage of negotiating the scope along the uterine cavity with a 'no touch technique'. The tip can bend up to 110°, allowing easy uterine entry with minimal discomfort. Improved optics helps the image quality to be comparable with small rigid scopes. The risk of uterine perforation is reduced as the scope is able to

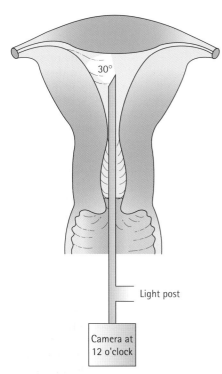

Figure 2.1 Clinical anatomy of the uterus, showing the relation between the angle of the telescope, the light lead and the camera orientation.

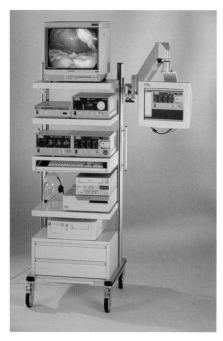

Figure 2.2 Stack system.

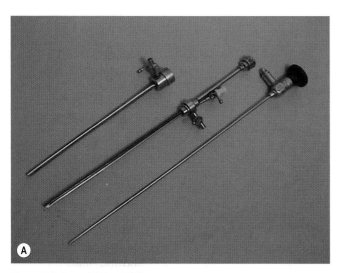

Figure 2.3 Bettochhi hysteroscope.

negotiate the angle between the cervix and the uterus. The disadvantage is that continuous flow irrigation is not currently available for flexible hysteroscopy.

Hysteroscopic sheaths

For diagnostic panoramic hysteroscopy, a single sheath for inflow is sufficient. This enables a smaller outer diameter and outpatient hysteroscopy without anaesthesia. Operative hysteroscopy needs separate sheaths for inflow and outflow. The inflow sheath carries the distension medium to the tip of the telescope, from where it is withdrawn via the outer sheath (Figure 2.4). Fluid circulates over the tip of the telescope to maintain a clear view.

Camera and stack system

The hysteroscopic image is visualized on a monitor with the help of a camera connected to a camera drive unit. The image clarity of a single chip camera is perfectly adequate. Special weighted cameras are available and facilitate orientation, but the same camera as is used for laparoscopy is equally appropriate. It is important to 'white balance' the camera system to ensure that the colours are displayed correctly (see Figure 2.2).

Light source

A minimum power of 150 W is essential to obtain a clear image. It is essential to have a spare bulb and to know how to change it, as it can fail in the middle of a procedure. After use and between cases, if the light source is not going to be used for a short while, the bulb intensity should be turned down. Switching the light source on and off frequently reduces the bulb life.

Light lead

The optic fibres running along the light lead need careful handling and should never be rolled or kinked as the fibres break. Damaged fibres do not transmit light from the source, and give rise to poor illumination. The light lead should be checked before starting any procedure.

Monitor

The wiring and controls of the camera drive unit are often complex. The hysteroscopist should be familiar with the setting up of the system and able to rectify simple faults. One should always check that the monitor is displaying the appropriate image before commencing the procedure.

Image recording equipment

Images taken before and after the procedure can help patients to understand their clinical condition, and allow comparison with images obtained at a later date. Recorded images can serve as evidence in defence if there is a claim of medical negligence against the surgeon. Recordings of various hysteroscopic procedures can become useful teaching aids for trainees.

Distension medium

The anterior and posterior uterine walls are in apposition. In order to obtain a view, the uterine cavity has to be dis-

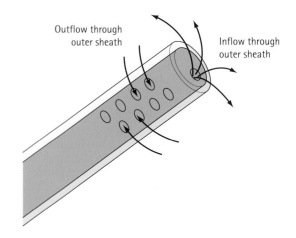

Figure 2.4 Continuous flow concept.

tended with gas or fluid. Carbon dioxide can be effective for diagnosis, and is delivered via a pressure reduction system or hysteroflator which is designed to give a maximum flow rate of 100 ml/min and a maximum pressure of 200 mmHg (note: a laproflator must not be used). An alternative is to use a liquid distension medium (e.g. normal saline or Hartmann's solution) which is appropriate for diagnosis and some operative procedures. Monopolar electrosurgery requires a non-conductive distension medium such as 1.5% glycine. However, it should be remembered that once the solution becomes contaminated with blood, its function as an insulator is reduced. Fluid can be pressurized via a roller pump (with maximum flow rate of 500 ml/min and maximum pressure of 200 mmHg), gravity or a pressure infusion bag cuff system. For diagnosis, gravity or a 50-ml syringe connected to a giving set via a three-way tap provides very good control of the distension pressure. Dextran 70 (Hyskon) is no longer used due to anaphylactic reactions.

Technique of Diagnostic Hysteroscopy

Clinical anatomy of the uterus

The uterine cavity is flat in its anterior/posterior dimension as, when not distended, the anterior and posterior endometrial surfaces are apposed to each other. The cervical canal is essentially round, but once the cavity is entered, the lateral dimension widens until it is at its broadest at the fundus. The cavity extends laterally towards the tubal ostia (see Figure 2.1). The fundal dome may be flat, concave or convex on its interior surface. Indeed, a proportion of uteri have a pronounced fundal convexity, a so-called 'arcuate deformity'.

Endometrial preparation

A diagnostic hysteroscopic examination is best performed without medical preparation of the endometrium. The endometrium will be at its thinnest in the immediate postmenstrual phase, and at its most vascular in the premenstrual phase. Abnormal bleeding is a common indication for diagnostic hysteroscopy, and whilst it is often possible to time the examination such that bleeding is not occurring, light bleeding need not preclude successful examination of the endometrial cavity. When prolonged heavy bleeding occurs, norethisterone 5 mg three times daily for 7–10 days may be given prior to the examination. It is rarely necessary to use a gonadotrophin-releasing hormone (GnRH) analogue prior to a diagnostic procedure, but one to three doses are employed prior to endometrial ablation, or to shrink a vascular fibroid prior to operative hysteroscopic resection.

Anaesthesia

In the majority of cases, the smallest modern diagnostic hysteroscopes require no anaesthetic whatsoever. A crucial factor is good communication between the gynaecologist and the patient, with thorough preoperative counselling and the support of a skilled nurse who is able to complement the operator in explaining things to the patient. The role of local anaesthetic gels is open to question. They are inexpensive and certainly lubricate and cause the external os to open. They probably have little anaesthetic effect other than as a psychological adjunct to the gynaecologist's reassurance.

Where facilities do not exist for outpatient hysteroscopy, the procedure is carried out in the operating theatre. Whilst a 5-mm rigid diagnostic hysteroscope can be passed through the cervix in the majority of women of reproductive age, this can prove extremely difficult in postmenopausal women and cervical dilatation is often needed. This requires a paracervical block, a regional anaesthetic or a general anaesthetic. The choice of anaesthetic method will, of course, be decided in conjunction with the anaesthetist and the patient. The choice will, in part, be determined by the patient's state of health and whether any additional procedures are planned. It must be remembered, however, that those patients who are at risk of endometrial cancer in the postmenopausal period are often more obese and suffer from cardiovascular and airways disease. These render them at high risk from the anaesthetic point of view. Such patients provided a major stimulus to the establishment of outpatient diagnostic and, in some cases, therapeutic hysteroscopy services.

Positioning

Hysteroscopy can be performed on a general operating table equipped with lithotomy poles or Lloyd Davies supports. Care must be taken to avoid excessive pressure from the leg supports on neurovascular structures, and if there is limitation of joint movement owing to hip or knee pathology, the final position of the patient will have to be modified.

In the outpatient setting, a colposcopy chair is desirable. This allows a comfortable modified lithotomy position with minimum loss of dignity. It is essential that the patient should be kept covered until the examination is due to start.

Procedure

Inpatient/general anaesthetic

A pelvic examination is performed in order to determine the size and direction of the uterus. The vulva and vagina are cleaned with antiseptic solution, and the anterior lip of the cervix is grasped with a vulsellum forceps. The majority of rigid hysteroscopes offer a fore/oblique view ranging from 12 to 90°. By convention, the direction of the view is away from the light post. The camera system is attached to the scope with the camera orientated correctly and the light post either up or down such that the angled view is in the vertical plane. It is easier to follow the cervical canal if the scope is orientated to view along the direction of the canal (i.e. forwards and downwards in a retroverted retroflexed uterus). Crucial to obtaining a thorough hysteroscopic examination is an understanding of how rotation of the hysteroscope allows the area of uterine wall under inspection to be changed. The authors suggest holding the camera in one hand and maintaining the position of the camera fixed in relation to the vertical plane. Rotation of the scope by manipulating the light post with the other hand allows the view to be manipulated appropriately.

Insertion of the hysteroscope through the cervical canal should be performed under direct vision and, in the first instance, without cervical dilatation or the passage of a sound. This allows examination of the cervical canal and inspection of undamaged endometrium. Once instruments have been passed into the uterine cavity, they cause damage to and stripping of the endometrium, which can then give appearances suggestive of polyp formation. The image of the cervical canal during passage of the scope is, of course, dependent on the viewing angle of the scope. A 0° scope requires the cervical canal to be kept in the middle of the field of view during insertion to maintain the direction of travel of the scope parallel to the direction of the cervical canal. When an angled viewing scope is used, the position of the cervical canal in the field of view has to be offset in order to maintain the direction of travel of the hysteroscope parallel with the direction of the cervical canal. This is why orientation of the light post relative to the orientation of the camera is a crucial step in the assembly of the equipment, but it is often overlooked.

Once the cervical canal is passed, a panoramic view of the uterine cavity is obtained. Uterine distension at a flow rate of 40–60 cc/min with pressure between 40 and 80 mmHg achieves good visualization. The scope is advanced towards the fundus and rotated to allow inspection of the tubal ostia. The scope can then be withdrawn and readvanced whilst rotating it to enable systematic inspection of each uterine wall in turn.

Potential problems include blood accumulating in the cavity and obscuring the view. This can occur during diagnosis when the seal between the hysteroscope and the cervix is very tight, preventing outflow of distension medium. The passage of a dilator 1 mm greater than the outer diameter of the hysteroscope allows flow and clearance of the contaminating blood. If a large polyp is present in the endometrial cavity, it is possible to inspect the cavity without realizing that the polyp is there because the polyp fills the cavity and the scope has been passed beyond the tip of the polyp before inspection begins (Figure 2.5). Suspicion should be aroused if the endometrial surfaces are different in colour, and careful inspection of the panoramic view of the cavity during insertion and removal of the scope will avoid missing a large polyp as the tip of it will be seen. A thorough examination of the uterine cavity should allow inspection of both tubal ostia. A record of this in the operation notes demonstrates that the operator has obtained a good view.

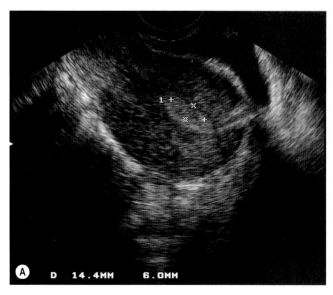
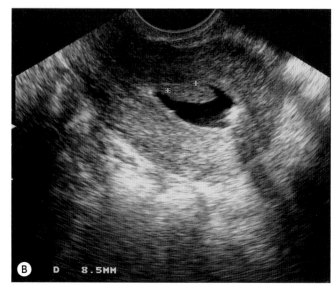

Figure 2.5 (A) Transvaginal sonography showing polyp. (B) Sonohysterography with polyp clearly outlined.

Postoperative care

The majority of the recovery process after a diagnostic hysteroscopy relates to recovery from the anaesthetic. A small amount of vaginal bleeding is not unusual following hysteroscopy, and the patient should be warned about this. Occasionally, cramping period-like pains are experienced; these should settle within 48 h and respond to paracetamol or a non-steroidal anti-inflammatory drug such as mefenamic acid. Persistent pain and bleeding may suggest a complication such as endometritis, and the patient should seek medical help. The provision of a postprocedure information leaflet is good practice.

Hysteroscopy in outpatients

Provision of hysteroscopy combined with transvaginal ultrasound in outpatients provides a very efficient method of assessing women with pre- and postmenopausal bleeding. As mentioned above, many patients who require a hysteroscopy pose significant risk for general anaesthesia, and are best managed under local or no anaesthetic (Valli et al 1998). In addition, there are many advantages to the patient, including shorter time at the hospital and more rapid return to normal activity. There are also cost advantages to the hospital, as an outpatient clinic is clearly a less expensive environment than an operating theatre (Marsh et al 2004).

Choice of equipment

Choice of equipment will vary with the prior experience of the operator and the facilities available for disinfection/sterilization of the instruments. Rod lens hysteroscopes may be autoclaved, necessitating the provision of an adequate number of scopes for a session of activity. Fibreoptic hysteroscopes, whether rigid or flexible, cannot be autoclaved and must be sterilized with ethylene oxide or closed liquid disinfection systems.

In reality, there are disadvantages and advantages of every system. Rigid autoclavable scopes tend to be of larger diameter, necessitating cervical dilatation in a proportion of cases. The advantage is clarity of view and a fore/oblique view allowing easier examination of the cornua. Flexible scopes are delicate and more expensive, but allow steering through the cervical canal and angulation to allow full inspection of the uterine cavity without any anaesthesia (Kremer et al 1998) (Figure 2.6A). Fibreoptic rigid scopes can be of very small diameter (1.2 mm in a 2.5-mm diagnostic sheath (Figure 2.6B). They are 0° so viewing of the cornua is more difficult, but they are relatively easy to pass through stenosed postmenopausal cervices, leading to a very low failure rate. The Versascope system provides a disposable sheath which can be distended by the passage of a 5 French instrument. This means that a change of sheath is not required to convert a diagnostic procedure into an operative procedure.

Hysteroscopy technique

In the outpatient setting, the authors favour a Cusco's speculum to bring the cervix into view prior to introduction of the hysteroscope. This allows manipulation of the position of the cervix with the speculum as the scope is inserted to straighten the cervical canal. Rarely, it is necessary to grasp the cervix with a single-toothed tenaculum. Others use no speculum at all when performing vaginoscopy, and locate the cervix before inserting the hysteroscope into it. With the patient awake and the gynaecologist concentrating on passing the scope through a difficult cervix, the role of the attending nurse is paramount (Prather and Wolfe 1995). The nurse should have a good knowledge of the procedure, excellent communication skills and be able to maintain a rapport with the patient during the procedure. Preprocedure explanatory leaflets and a brief discussion help to reassure the patient, who often finds that the procedure causes less discomfort than is anticipated. Patients vary in their wish to see the television screen during the procedure, but the majority find it reassuring and helpful to be able to view the image of the uterine cavity. This also allows easier explanation of any pathology found.

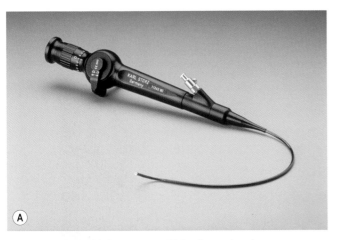
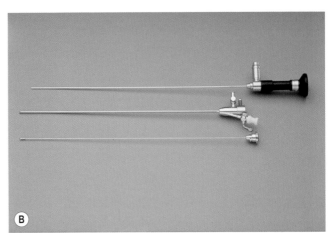

Figure 2.6 (A) Flexible hysteroscope. (B) Rigid outpatient hysteroscope.

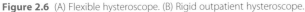

Endometrial sampling

Endometrial sampling that only yields a small percentage of the endometrium causes discomfort that is often greater than that of the hysteroscopy. It is not indicated in all cases, and in particular should be avoided in patients with post-menopausal bleeding in whom the endometrium is found to be atrophic on hysteroscopy. An 'inadequate for diagnosis — malignancy cannot be excluded' report on histology confounds the picture and leads to further unnecessary procedures. Hysteroscopically-directed biopsy often results in a sample which is so small that it is difficult for the pathologist to orientate.

Pathology Seen at Diagnostic Hysteroscopy

The diagnostic hysteroscopist should familiarize him-/herself with the normal appearances of the endometrium during the phases of the endometrial cycle and during the menopause (Figure 2.7). The endometrium should be assessed for colour, texture, vascularity and thickness. An impression of thickness can be gained by pressing the surface of the endometrium with the end of the hysteroscope. Post-menopausal atrophy is characterized by very thin pale endometrium, often accompanied by a ridged appearance.

Endometrial polyps (Figure 2.8A) can vary considerably in appearance, and the observer should define the position and size of the base of the polyp to aid subsequent operative hysteroscopy. Fibroids (Figure 2.8B) have a characteristic whitish appearance, and often have clearly visible surface vessels. Submucous fibroids which bulge significantly into the uterine cavity may remain covered with endometrium, but do not often have an appearance similar to that of a fibroid polyp. An assessment should be made of the relative proportion of the fibroid which is bulging into the endometrial cavity, as this determines whether it is likely to be resectable during a single operative procedure or may require multiple attempts.

A uterine septum (Figure 2.8C) may be seen dividing the cavity into two halves, while intrauterine adhesions (Figure 2.8D) can lead to complete disruption of the cavity. An IUCD (Figure 2.8E) is the most common foreign body seen at diagnostic hysteroscopy.

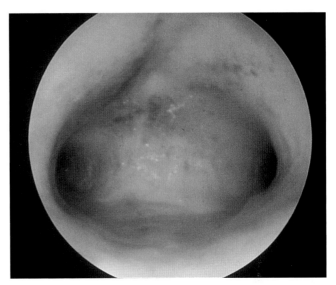

Figure 2.7 Premenstrual endometrium.

Hyperplastic endometrium is thickened, often polypoid and has increased vascularity (Figure 2.9). Endometrial cancer is often friable, sometimes has a lobed appearance and may appear necrotic. It should be suspected in post-menopausal patients where only a poor view is obtained due to excessive bleeding. Tamoxifen causes a specific pattern of hyperplasia associated with a vesicular appearance.

Hysteroscopic Skills

The Royal College of Obstetricians and Gynaecologists (RCOG) report on minimal access surgery categorized skill levels in training in both laparoscopy and hysteroscopy (Royal College of Obstetricians and Gynaecologists 1994). Hysteroscopic procedures were divided into three levels, with the first level covering diagnostic and simple procedures such as the removal of a foreign body (Box 2.1). The second level contains operative procedures, such as resection or ablation of the endometrium, and removal of polyps and fibroids. Advanced procedures (third level) include repeated

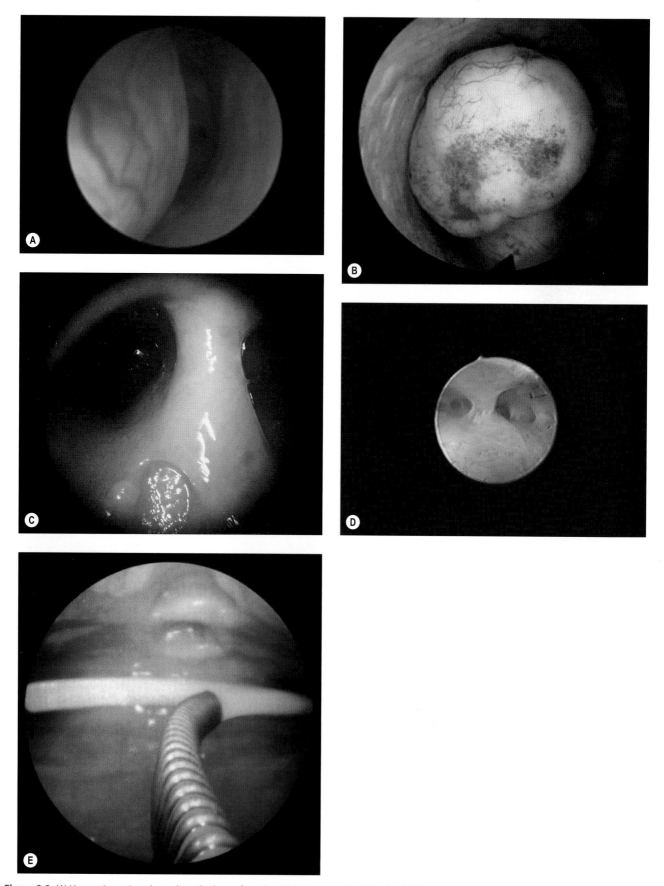

Figure 2.8 (A) Versapoint spring electrode at the base of a polyp. (B) Submucous fibroid polyp. (C) Intrauterine septum. (D) Intrauterine adhesion. (E) Intrauterine foreign body.

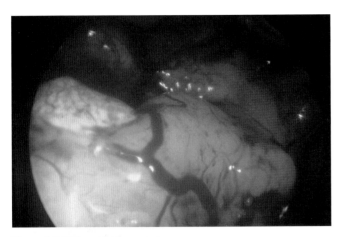

Figure 2.9 Endometrial hyperplasia.

Box 2.1 Stratification of hysteroscopic procedures by level of training

Level 1. Diagnostic procedures
- Diagnostic hysteroscopy plus target biopsy
- Removal of simple polyp
- Removal of IUCD

Level 2. Minor operative procedures
- Proximal fallopian tube cannulation
- Minor Asherman's syndrome
- Removal of pedunculated fibroid or large polyp

Level 3. More complex operative procedures requiring additional training
- Division/resection of uterine septum
- Endoscopic surgery for major Asherman's syndrome
- Endometrial resection or ablation
- Resection of submucous leiomyoma
- Repeat endometrial resection or ablation

Source: Royal College of Obstetricians and Gynaecologists (RCOG) 1994 Report of Working Party on training in gynaecological endoscopic surgery, RCOG Press, London.

resection or ablation, and treatment of extensive uterine synechiae. The RCOG established a subcommittee of the training committee to supervise training in minimal access surgery, and has since designed an advanced training module in benign gynaecological surgery which covers both diagnostic and operative hysteroscopy. It is mainly aimed at senior specialist registrars in obstetrics and gynaecology in their final 2 years of training. By completion of the module, ideally within 1 year, trainees are expected to have reached independent competence in performing both diagnostic and operative hysteroscopy. The trainee has to register with their preceptor and training programme director, who supervise and train the trainee in the practical aspects of outpatient diagnostic and operative hysteroscopy.

In addition, the trainee has to attend a practical training course in hysteroscopy. It is also recommended that trainees should attend the hands-on skills station in a training laboratory.

Training and learning curve

Hysteroscopy is a relatively simple surgical skill to learn, provided that the surgeon undergoes a structured training process. It is clear that familiarity with equipment and knowledge of the basic underlying principles should be imparted early in the training process. To this end, the basic skills course in obstetrics and gynaecology provides an introduction to these skills. Manipulating hysteroscopes and a camera system on models allows an early grasp of the basic principles of the orientation, and allows the trainee to progress rapidly to successful diagnostic hysteroscopy on anaesthetized patients. Outpatient diagnostic hysteroscopy requires considerable skill, confidence and familiarity with the equipment. It should be reserved for consultants and senior trainees with a specific interest.

It has been shown that achieving the operative hysteroscopy skills has a steep learning curve. A recent survey of trainees registered for the hysteroscopy module showed that the 1-year target for obtaining the special skills module was difficult to achieve, with the most evident cause being the inability to acquire the expected operative hysteroscopy standard within the intended time (Shoukrey et al 2008).

Therapeutic strategy for benign disease

Identification of ocal intracavity lesions

- Fibroids.
- Polyps.
- Uterine anomalies.
- Foreign bodies.

Dysfunctional uterine bleeding

While focal intracavity lesions need operative hysteroscopic treatment, treatment of abnormal uterine bleeding has changed over the last few years. These conservative non-hysteroscopic treatments will be reviewed later in this chapter.

Indications for operative hysteroscopy

- Polyp or fibroid more than 2 cm in diameter.
- Uterine adhesions.
- Uterine anomalies.

Instrumentation for operative hysteroscopy

Operative hysteroscopy generally requires a larger instrument and a continuous flow sheath. In addition, a source of energy is used to perform the required manipulations.

Mechanical

Scissors and grasping forceps are passed down the operating channel of the hysteroscope, and can be used to cut the stalk of simple polyps, which are then grasped with forceps for removal (Figure 2.10). Lost foreign bodies such as IUCDs can be removed in a similar fashion.

Monopolar electrical

Monopolar electrosurgery requires flow of radiofrequency electric current from the active tip of the instrument through

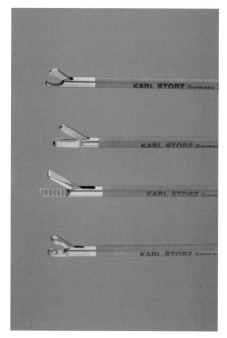

Figure 2.10 Mechanical instruments for operative hysteroscopy.

the patient to the large surface area return plate. The electrical effect depends on both current density and the waveform provided by the generator. Simple instruments for use with monopolar diathermy include a polyp snare and simple electrodes, which can be passed down a 5 French operating channel. A dedicated continuous flow hysteroscope is required for more sophisticated operative instruments, including a resection loop, knife, rollerball and cylinder (Figure 2.11).

Trancervical resection of the endometrium (TCRE) is a popular technique for endometrial destruction in which the loop is used to cut away the prepared endometrium down to the myometrium. Figure 2.12A demonstrates the loop in use, and the transverse myometrial fibres can be seen clearly. Movement of the loop within the hysteroscope sheath and withdrawal of the scope itself allow long strips of endometrium to be resected. Removal of the tissue strips maintains a clear view. Most operators start with the posterior wall in order that the resected tissue strips do not obscure the working area. Considerable training is needed to ensure safe use of this technique. Difficult areas to treat include the cornua where the myometrium is thin, and the fundus where the resection loop has to be bent forwards in order to achieve a cutting effect in front of the tip of the hysteroscope. Cornual

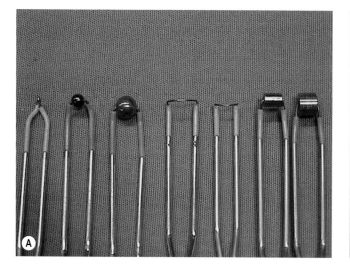

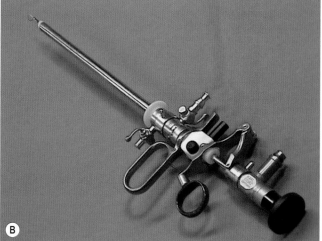

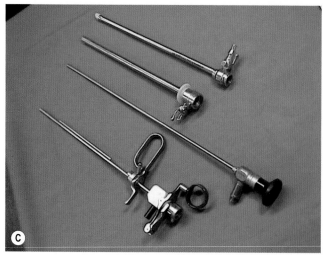

Figure 2.11 (A) Working elements for operative hysteroscopy. (B) Assembled resectoscope. (C) Components of resectoscope.

The same instrument is used for resection of submucous fibroids and fibroid polyps, whilst the knife is employed for the treatment of Asherman's syndrome and uterine septae. The resectoscope system is inexpensive as it uses reuseable electrodes, which are autoclavable. A careful watch must be kept on the fluid balance during the procedure, as overload of 1.5% glycine solution may lead to significant complications. More than 1 l of solution lost into the patient poses significant risk, and the procedure should be abandoned if such levels of fluid loss are significantly exceeded. Laser destruction is an alternative (Figure 2.12C).

Bipolar electrosurgery

Versapoint (Figure 2.13A) is a 5 French electrode. It requires a dedicated electrosurgery generator, which pulses the electrical energy through the saline irrigation medium from the active electrode tip to the larger return sleeve (Figure 2.13B). This creates a vapour pocket around the active electrode, and when tissue enters the vapour pocket, the high current density causes vaporization of the tissue. This device has been used for vaporizing fibroids and polyps. It is suitable for use under local anaesthetic, particularly in conjunction with the Versascope. The Versapoint resection system, a larger version using similar technology, is suitable for the removal of larger fibroids under general anaesthetic (Figure 2.13C). Bipolar electrodes appear to have a safer profile compared with monopolar electrodes because of the unchanged serum sodium. Irrigant consumption has been reported to be significantly higher in the two bipolar groups, without any side-effects during or after the procedure. Furthermore, the TCRE loop appears to be superior to the Versapoint loop in terms of operating time and amount of tissue removed (Berg et al 2009).

Endometrial destruction

The in-vivo studies of Duffy et al (1992) demonstrate that rollerball coagulation results in thermal necrosis to a depth of 3.3–3.7 mm. The depth of cut with a resection loop is 3–4 mm. Endometrial thickness, however, varies from 3 to 12 mm during the menstrual cycle. Therefore, satisfactory ablation can only be achieved if surgery is performed in the immediate postmenstrual phase. This leads to a shorter duration of surgery, greater ease of surgery and a high rate of postoperative amenorrhoea (Sowter et al 2001).

A national survey of the complications of endometrial destruction for menstrual disorders, the MISTLETOE study (Overton et al 1997), compared the different surgical techniques for endometrial destruction. Combined diathermy resection appeared safer than resection alone, but laser and rollerball ablation were the safest. Fibroids were associated with associated increased operative haemorrhage. Increasing operative experience was associated with fewer uterine perforations in the loop resection alone group, but had no effect on operative haemorrhage in any group. Cumulative failure rate at 1 year for combined resection and rollerball ablation was lowest at 15%, compared with 20% for resection or rollerball ablation alone, and 32% for laser ablation.

Comparison of endometrial destruction methods with hysterectomy revealed that they have less postoperative morbidity, shorter hospital stay, and quicker return to work, normal activity and sexual intercourse compared with

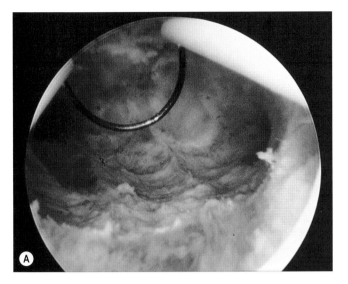

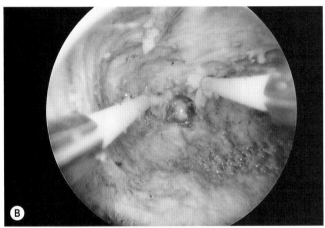

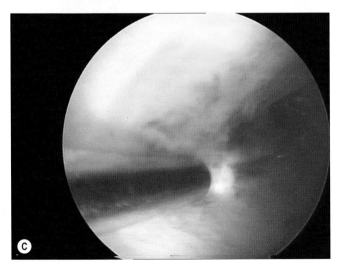

Figure 2.12 (A) Endometrial resection. (B) Rollerball ablation. (C) Laser ablation.

endometrium may be ablated with a rollerball and combined with resection of the remaining endometrium (Figure 2.12B). A Scandinavian study (Furst 2007) reported long-term follow-up of TCRE. This showed 80% patient satisfaction, and 20% of patients required hysterectomy at the end of 10 years.

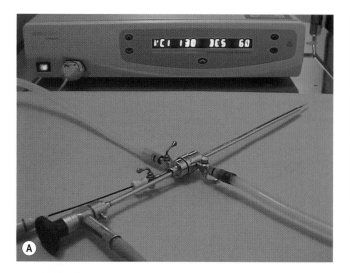

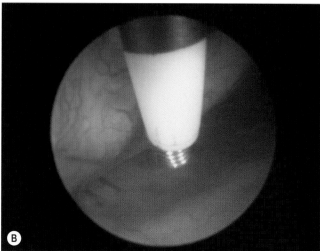

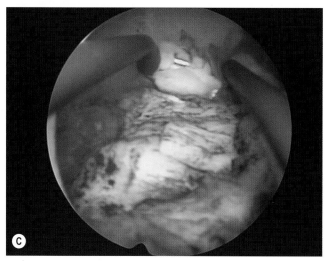

Figure 2.13 (A) Bettochhi with Versapoint. (B) Versapoint spring electrode at polyp base. (C) Versapoint resection system.

hysterectomy, but patient satisfaction may be slightly higher following hysterectomy (Pinion et al 1994).

As with all ablation techniques, success is dependent on the proximity of the menopause, with postoperative amenorrhoea rates being highest in the older age group. Adenomyosis is a major cause of failure.

Non-operative methods of endometrial ablation and the use of the levonorgestrel-releasing intrauterine device (LNG IUS) for the treatment of menorrhagia have decreased the use of endometrial resection to treat dysfunctional uterine bleeding. The LNG IUS results in a smaller mean reduction in menstrual blood loss than TCRE and women are not as likely to become amenorrhoeic, but there is no difference in the rate of satisfaction with treatment (Lethaby et al 2005). In fact, in the meta-analysis of six randomized clinical trials, the efficacy of the LNG IUS in the management of heavy menstrual bleeding appears to have similar therapeutic effects to endometrial ablation up to 2 years after treatment (Kaunitz et al 2009).

Polypectomy and myomectomy

Hysteroscopic polypectomy and myomectomy are dependent on the experience of the operator and the size and posi-

tion of the fibroid. Removal of the polyp can be as difficult as detaching it. If the polyp is small enough, grasping it with forceps, pulling it against the end of the scope and then withdrawing the whole scope can be effective. An alternative is to remove the detached polyp blindly using polyp forceps. This is often difficult and serves to illustrate the futility of blind techniques.

Fibroids under 2 cm in size can be resected in one sitting. For larger fibroids or those where more than half is intramural, a two-stage procedure may be necessary. In the first stage, the protruding portion of the fibroid is removed, followed by transhysteroscopic myolysis of the intramural portion (Donnez and Nisolle 1992). Subsequently, GnRH agonist therapy for 8 weeks shrinks the uterine cavity, extruding the intramural portion of the fibroid, which is then easily removed at the second stage to complete the myomectomy. Complete removal of the fibroid is associated with improved long-term results (Wamsteker et al 1993).

Uterine adhesions and septae

The division of dense uterine synechiae (Figure 2.14) and uterine septae requires considerable skill and is often

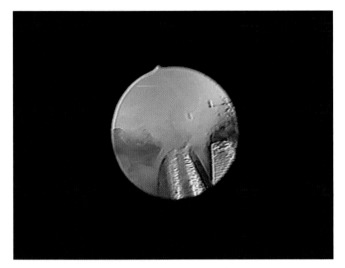

Figure 2.14 Division of intrauterine synechiae with scissors.

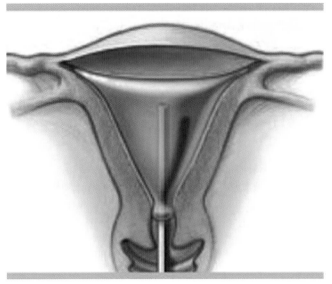

Figure 2.15 Thermal balloon ablation system.

performed under laparoscopic guidance, which ensures that thermal or electrical energy is not allowed to penetrate through the myometrium, damaging the adjacent bowel. Careful assessment prior to division of uterine septae is essential to prevent perforation at the fundus. The hysteroscopic appearances of a septate uterus and a uterus didelphys can be similar, and any attempt to resect the septum will clearly lead to disaster in the latter case. Careful ultrasound evaluation helps to differentiate between the two, but this has not yet replaced laparoscopic assessment. After adhesiolysis, an IUCD may be inserted for 3 months to prevent reformation of the adhesions. Similarly, postoperative hormone therapy may be initiated to help endometrial development and prevent further adhesion formation (Gordon et al 1995).

Operative hysteroscopy in the outpatient unit will be feasible in future. Authors have carried out transcervical resection procedures under local anaesthetic in daycare settings and have found a high level of patient satisfaction. A recent study has shown that this procedure is feasible with the availability of a mini-resectoscope (Papalampros et al 2009).

Treatment of the Endometrial Cavity without Intracavity Lesions

Menorrhagia has always been a major health problem in premenopausal women. Its treatment has evolved from hysterectomy at one end of spectrum to less invasive procedures at the other. All the treatment modalities aim to destroy the basal endometrium, preventing its regeneration. First-generation techniques use operative hysteroscopy procedures. Second-generation devices have been developed to achieve the results of first-generation techniques using simpler procedures. The use of these techniques obviates the need of hysteroscopic expertise, general anaesthesia and dilatation of the cervix, and therefore can be applied more widely.

Second-generation techniques have shown comparable quality-of-life improvements and patient satisfaction rates with first-generation techniques, along with comparable success rates and complication profiles (Lethaby et al 2005).

Thermal balloon ablation (Thermachoice, Gynaecare Ethicon Ltd, Somerville, NJ, USA)

Thermachoice is a silicone balloon catheter system which is inserted into the uterine cavity and inflated with 5% dextrose solution to achieve a pressure of 160–180 mmHg. The dextrose is heated to a temperature of 87° when the treatment cycle starts and continues for 8 min.

The procedure does not require any dilatation and is feasible to perform in an outpatient setting (Andersson and Mints 2007, Clark and Gupta 2004). The National Institute for Health and Clinical Excellence (NICE) has approved and validated the clinical safety and effectiveness of thermal ablation (see Figure 2.15).

A large multicentre observational study showed a significant reduction in the severity and duration of menstrual loss (Amso et al 1998). Thermachoice achieved a reduction in menstrual blood loss that was comparable with the first-generation techniques. In a long-term multicentre study, Thermachoice showed an 86% probability of avoiding a hysterectomy at 4–6-year follow-up (Amso et al 2003).

Other thermal balloons used in ablation are Cavaterm and Thermablate.

Cryoablation (Her Option, Uterine Cryoablation Therapy System, Cryo-gen Inc., San Diego, CA, USA)

The principle of cryotherapy is used for cryoablation. Liquid nitrogen is used to produce extreme cooling, producing an iceball at the tip of the cryoprobe. The probe is moved from one cornua to the other and through the entire cavity in a series of freeze–thaw cycles. Ultrasound guidance is needed to monitor the position and the depth of the probe. Tissue necrosis of 9–12 mm is achieved using this method in a 4-min cycle. The procedure is recommended as quick, easy and feasible for outpatient settings. However, severe abdominal cramping and vaginal pain, prolonged tiredness and perimenopausal symptoms were some of the major side-effects and late complications.

Free fluid ablation (Hydrothermablator, Boston Scientific, Natick, MA, USA)

In this technique, circulating hot saline solution is instilled into the uterus under direct hysteroscopic guidance. The saline is heated to 90°C and circulated for 10 min. A randomized controlled trial comparing Hydrothermablator with rollerball ablation (Townsend et al 2003) showed similar success rates as other second-generation devices (see Figure 2.16).

Impedance bipolar radiofrequency ablation (NovaSure, Novacept, Palo Alto, CA, USA)

Bipolar radiofrequency under impedence control is used for endometrial ablation. The bipolar current provides shallower ablation in the cornual region and deeper ablation in the main cavity. The device is a three-dimensional conformable bipolar gold-plated mesh mounted on an expandable frame. After insertion, bipolar radiofrequency energy travels between the electrodes and initial electrical pulses vaporize the low-impedance endometrium. As the energy travels deeper into the muscle and begins to desiccate the superficial myometrium, the resistance grows. The system automatically terminates the procedure when an impedance of 50 ohm is reached, signifying adequate ablation.

The device can be inserted into the uterus with a cavity length between 4 and 12 mm. The mean ablation time is 90 s. Ablation is based on physical tissue characteristics and not on temperature, pressure or time. This is claimed to achieve high ablation success rates regardless of endometrial thickness. Hence, pretreatment is not necessary. The short duration of the procedure makes it feasible for use in the outpatient setting under local anaesthetic.

Efficacy was reported in two randomized controlled trials and two case series (Abbott et al 2003). Amenorrhoea rates in these four studies ranged from 41% to 59% at 12 months, with higher amenorrhoea rates in the impedance controlled procedure. Continuing menorrhagia rates ranged from 3.9%

to 14% at 12 months. There was also evidence to suggest that the majority of patients were satisfied following the procedure, and that quality of life had improved. At 3-year follow-up (Gallinat 2004), hysterectomy was avoided in 97% of women, 65% of whom were amenorrhoeic. Five-year follow-up of a randomized controlled trial comparing NovaSure and Thermachoice endometrial ablation showed that bipolar radiofrequency ablation was superior to thermal ablation (Kleijn et al 2008).

Microwave endometrial ablation (MEA, Mircosulis Plc, Waterlooville, UK)

The MEA device utilizes low-power, high-frequency microwave energy to generate heat and destroy the endometrium. The probe is inserted into the uterine cavity and moved from side to side with the temperature maintained at 75–80°C to ablate the endometrium.

MEA was compared with TCRE in a well-designed randomized controlled trial (Cooper et al 1999), and was reported to have a significantly shorter mean operative time than TCRE (11.4 vs 15.0 min, $P = 0.001$), and comparable satisfaction and acceptability. Improved quality of life 1 year after treatment was reported for both groups. These results were sustained at 2-year follow-up. At 5-year follow-up, both techniques achieved significant and comparable improvements in menstrual symptoms and health-related quality of life (Cooper et al 2005). High rates of satisfaction with and acceptability of treatment were achieved following TCRE, but these rates were significantly lower than those following MEA. The long-term data after a further 5 years of follow-up, when combined with the trial's operative findings and the known costs of both procedures, led the authors to conclude that MEA is a more effective and efficient treatment for heavy menstrual loss than TCRE (Sambrook et al 2009).

Complications of second-generation ablation devices

Minor immediate postoperative complications are common with second-generation ablation techniques and include pelvic pain, endometritis, urinary tract infection, nausea, vomiting, haematometra and pelvic inflammation. Reported serious complications included sepsis, adnexal/uterine necrosis, lower genital tract thermal injury and one death. Many of these resulted from non-compliance with the manufacturers' instructions and other avoidable factors. A 2005 update of a Cochrane review (Lethaby et al 2005) concluded that equipment failure, nausea, vomiting and uterine cramping were more likely with second-generation ablation techniques but these were less likely to be associated with fluid overload, uterine perforation, cervical lacerations and haematometra than conventional ablation and resection techniques. Overall, they compared favourably with TCRE. Most of the second-generation devices (Cavaterm, Thermachoice, NovaSure, Cryoablation) require a relatively normal uterine cavity with a depth of less than 12 cm to complete the treatment satisfactorily. Free fluid ablation (Hydrothermablator) and MEA can be performed when the uterine cavity is irregular, although complete septate or bicornuate uteri are contraindications to undertaking the procedures. Pretreatment is not generally required.

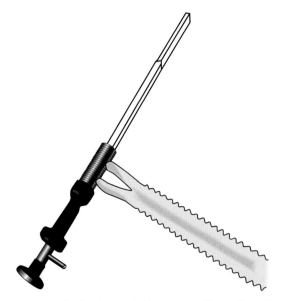

Figure 2.16 Free fluid endometrial ablation system (Boston Scientific, Natwick, MA, USA).

Each device has its relative strengths and weaknesses, and no single device can be preferred over another in all circumstances. Clinicians should consider the safety and effectiveness figures, applicability to the outpatient environment, and evidence of quality-of-life improvement, applied on an individualized basis after full discussion with the patient and taking her preferences into account, as well as equipment availability and skill. Ongoing audit of a department's success rates compared with the published figures ensures that patient selection and surgical strategy are appropriate. A survey of preferences and practices of endometrial ablation/resection for menorrhagia in UK showed that second-generation devices were preferred over first-generation devices. Thermal balloon ablation was the most favoured procedure (Deb et al 2008).

Hysteroscopic Sterilization

Essure system

A safe, simple and highly effective alternative to invasive procedures for interval tubal sterilization is now possible using a hysteroscopic approach. The Essure permanent birth control device (Conceptus Inc., San Carlos, CA, USA) is a combined metallic and fibre coil placed into the cornua hysteroscopically. Approval for its use has been granted by the US Food and Drug Administration (FDA) and NICE. The dynamic outer coil made of nickel titanium alloy includes an inner flexible coil (stainless steel). The device is delivered into the fallopian tube in a tightly wound or 'low profile' position, where the two coils are tightly opposed and held in place with a wire before being released in the tubal lumen. The rapidly expanding outer coil fills the tubal lumen (Figure 2.17), anchoring the device in place. The polyethylene terephthalate fibres induce a benign localized tissue response consisting of inflammation and fibrosis, which leads to obliteration and occlusion of the tubal lumen in approximately 3 months (Valle et al 2002, Abbott 2007). The procedure is preferably done in the proliferative stage of the menstrual cycle. The procedure can be performed under local anaesthetic (paracervical nerve block with lidocaine 1%) in the outpatient setting (Sinha et al 2007). Hysteroscopy is then performed and tubal access is established. During insertion, the microinsert is maintained in a 'wound down' configuration by a release catheter, which is enclosed in a transparent delivery catheter. A guide wire is attached to the inner coil to facilitate device placement. The device is then deployed in the proximal tubal ostium with a single-handed release mechanism, and the guide wire is detached and withdrawn. Follow-up pelvic X-ray or hysterosalpingogram is recommended 3 months after insertion to confirm correct placement of the device or tubal occlusion. An occlusion rate of 100% has been shown at the end of 1 year with no pregnancies reported (Kerin et al 2003).

A comparison of the Essure permanent birth control device and laparoscopic sterilization (Duffy et al 2005) reported reduced hospital stay, less pain, better patient acceptability, higher patient satisfaction levels and fewer adverse events with the Essure procedure. A separate study of the direct costs associated with the Essure procedure compared with laparoscopic sterilization indicated that there is a cost advantage to Essure, although indirect costs were not considered in this model (Levie and Chudnoff 2005).

Although outpatient sterilization offers many potential advantages, uptake is currently affected by cost, additional follow-up and the 3-month delay in providing permanent fertility control. Long-term results are still awaited.

Alternative techniques and future developments

The Adiana procedure (Adiana Inc., Redwood City, CA, USA and Hologic, Inc., Bedford, MA, USA) involves bipolar ablation of the proximal fallopian tube followed by the placement of a synthetic matrix, subsequently leading to tubal occlusion. The device is currently being investigated in an FDA study in the USA, Australia and Mexico (Johns 2005) (Figure 2.18).

Complications of Hysteroscopy and Procedures

Surgeon related

Inadequate training and lack of experience can lead to avoidable, but potentially major, complications, such as uterine perforation, haemorrhage and other visceral injuries.

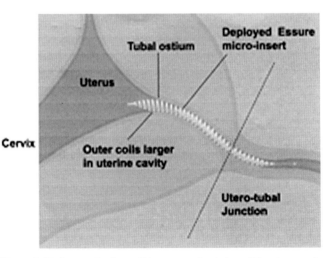

Figure 2.17 Essure microinsert. This cross-sectional view of the uterus and fallopian tube shows the device placed across the uterotubal junction (external).

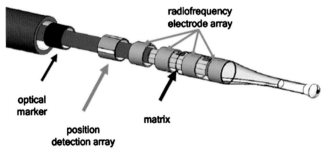

Figure 2.18 Adiana hysteroscopic delivery catheter.

Distension medium

There are different types of distension media used for hysteroscopy. Carbon dioxide may lead to gas embolism, which can lead to hypotension, tachycardia and arrhythmias, which can be fatal. Fortunately, this is a rare complication and should not occur provided the correct pressure insufflator is used.

Electrolyte imbalance from excessive absorption of non-electrolytic liquid distension medium such as 1.5% glycine can lead to hypervolaemia and hyponatraemia; a deficit of 1 l requires caution and surgery should be discontinued at 1.5 l. If the patient is asymptomatic with normal serum electrolytes and haematocrit, observation is sufficient. However, patients may develop bradycardia, hypertension, nausea, vomiting, headache, confusion, agitation and visual disturbances. This is due to water moving across the blood–brain barrier, leading to cerebral oedema. If hyponatraemia is present with haemodilution, a loop diuretic (e.g. frusemide) and restricted fluid intake may be helpful. This symptom complex has been described in the past as 'post-TURP syndrome' (TURP, transurethral resection of prostate). Careful assessment of fluid input and output is critical, particularly if glycine is used.

Haemorrhagic

Bleeding during hysteroscopy is caused by inadvertent trauma or by the operative steps disturbing the endometrium. Thick and vascular endometrium is likely to cause heavy bleeding. Preoperative endometrial thinning to decrease the vascularity is recommended practice. Bleeding can be controlled during surgery by coagulating the vessels under direct vision, or after surgery by inflating a Foley balloon in the uterine cavity with 5 ml of normal saline. The balloon is then deflated 6 h after surgery. If bleeding has settled, the catheter should be left in place for 1–2 h before discharging the patient. If not, the balloon can be left for a maximum of 24 h. If bleeding continues despite tamponade by the Foley balloon, hysterectomy may become necessary. In the MISTLETOE study, 1% of women undergoing endometrial resection required an emergency hysterectomy.

Bleeding is likely to occur during endometrial ablation, myomectomy, adhesiolysis and septum resection. Polyps are unlikely to bleed significantly. Arterial bleeding is pulsatile and should be stopped immediately using electrosurgery. The distension medium can suppress venous ooze. The cavity should be viewed after the pressure is reduced to check for haemostasis after operative hysteroscopy, and the hysteroscopist should always be prepared to control bleeding, which can happen unexpectedly.

Traumatic

At the beginning of any hysteroscopy, due care must be taken while grasping the cervical lip as good grip ensures that the tenaculum does not cut through. Dilatation of the cervix, if needed, is a blind procedure. If one is not careful, a false passage may be created and, occasionally, perforation of the cervical canal. This is more likely to occur when the cervix is scarred and stenosed following previous surgery, and some surgeons prefer to soften the cervix with vaginal prostaglandins 2 h before surgery. Rarely, the dilator can give way suddenly, resulting in perforation of the fundus.

Introducing the hysteroscope under direct vision, as described above, minimizes the chance of cervical trauma or uterine perforation during introduction of the scope.

Uterine perforation

Uterine perforation occurs in approximately 1% of women undergoing endometrial ablation (Lewis 1994). It can happen due to entry of the scope into a false passage, when the scope is against the fundus, or while using the energy sources without visualizing the electrode. It is suspected if excessive bleeding is noted before the procedure is commenced, if the scope goes freely into the uterine cavity, or if the fluid distension pressure stays low or decreases suddenly. Rarely, a loop of bowel or omentum may be seen.

The energy source should only be activated while withdrawing the active tip, keeping the working element constantly under vision, which decreases the risk of perforation.

The distension medium tends to stretch the uterine wall, which is normally 2–2.5 cm thick. This has to be understood while performing operative hysteroscopy to avoid myometrial damage and decrease the risk of perforation. Extra care should be taken while operating near the uterine cornu as this is the thinnest portion of the uterine wall. Cornual injuries are likely to be full thickness with an additional risk to bladder, bowel and pelvic vessels.

As soon as perforation is suspected, the procedure should be stopped. Diagnostic hysteroscopy may be attempted, but the visualization will be poor due to inadequate distension and bleeding. Laparoscopy will help in assessment of the perforation site. The majority of injuries can be managed conservatively. In the event of heavy bleeding, haemostasis should be achieved by coagulation or by suturing the perforation. Diagnostic hysteroscopy may be completed under laparoscopic control. If perforation occurs during an operative hysteroscopy, it is wise to defer the procedure.

Infections

Diagnostic hysteroscopy is less likely to cause infection. During operative hysteroscopy, blood and tissue debris becomes a focus of infection. Energy applied to tissue leads to necrotic tissue in the uterine cavity. Infection leads to blood-stained offensive discharge, which is accompanied by fever, generally feeling unwell and raised white cell count. A high degree of suspicion in postoperative patients with deteriorating symptoms is crucial for early diagnosis. Prophylactic antibiotics should be considered for many operative hysteroscopy procedures.

Anaesthetic and energy source related

These complications are rare but still need to be discussed with patients. Patients at high anaesthetic risk will need a thorough explanation of the risks involved, and should be offered the alternative of having the procedure under local anaesthetic.

Late Complications

Infertility

Neosynechiae formation after hysteroscopic surgery may lead to Asherman's syndrome, and adhesions can reform after adhesiolysis. Infertility may persist despite treatment of the suspected cause.

Abnormal menstrual bleeding

Hysteroscopic surgery performed in the younger age group (40–45 years) is more likely to fail than that performed in older age groups. Counselling to ensure realistic postoperative expectations is crucial to improve patient satisfaction.

Pregnancy

Patients undergoing endometrial ablation should be made aware of the need to use contraception as sterility cannot be guaranteed.

Cancer

Cervical cancer is a contraindication for hysteroscopy, but endometrial cancer is not. Failure of endometrial ablation and lack of endometrial thinning despite agents (e.g. GnRH analogues and danazol) should raise suspicion. Inability to shrink a fibroid by preoperative GnRH analogue treatment is another cause for concern. There is no evidence of retrograde spread with the fluid or gaseous distension media, or of any adverse effects on the activity of the malignant cells. Similarly, histology of all specimens obtained at hysteroscopic surgery must be reviewed. Sarcomatous change in a fibroid occurs in less than 1% of patients, but must be ruled out. Endometrial chips obtained at resection may occasionally reveal malignancy.

Haematometra and pyometra

Collection of blood in the uterine cavity followed by infection can occur after hysteroscopic surgery due to cervical stenosis. This can be prevented by avoiding ablation near the internal os. Occasionally, haematometra may occur after commencement of hormone replacement therapy (Dwyer et al 1991).

Postablation sterilization syndrome

Endometrial ablation in women with a history of sterilization can occasionally lead to postoperative pain. Active endometrium between the scarred uterine cavity and the tubal block leads to haemorrhagic tubal distension during menses. This leads to stretching of the intramural and isthmic portion of the tube with resultant pain. The presentation of this condition can be similar to an ectopic pregnancy.

Consent issues

Thorough preoperative explanation and counselling, including detailed explanation of the pathophysiology of the underlying gynaecological condition, treatment options available and their risks and benefits, is essential to ensure a successful operative experience for the patient as well as the surgeon. This is best started during the outpatient consultation when the decision for hysteroscopy is taken, and followed by giving an information leaflet with a helpline telephone number to clarify any further doubts.

Newer Developments

Diagnostic hysteroscopy is now well established in the outpatient setting in many UK hospitals. The current challenge is to extend the service to include operative work and to transfer other procedures, discussed above, from the theatre to the outpatient treatment suite. Hysteroscopy is thus becoming a skill which requires senior medical or nurse specialist input. As the number of hysteroscopies carried out under general anaesthetic declines, the importance of utilizing all training opportunities for junior medical staff cannot be overstated.

KEY POINTS

1. Hysteroscopy is a well-established tool in modern gynaecology due to its unique advantage of direct visualization of the uterine cavity.
2. Advantages include decreased morbidity and quicker recovery (for the patient), diagnosis and treatment in the outpatient department (for the surgeon), and resultant cost benefits (for the healthcare system).
3. Contraindications include cervical cancer, pelvic infection, heavy uterine bleeding, pregnancy, and inexperienced or untrained surgeon.
4. Uterine distension, essential for panoramic hysteroscopy, is achieved using media such as carbon dioxide, normal saline, Ringer's lactate, 5% dextrose, sorbitol or 1.5% glycine.
5. Pathology such as fibroids, polyps, adhesions or uterine septum can be seen and then treated using mechanical scissors, laser or electrosurgery (monopolar or bipolar).
6. Hysteroscopic myomectomy is successful in controlling menorrhagia in approximately 93% of women. Adhesiolysis leads to improved fertility in 60.5% of cases and menstruation in over 80% of cases.
7. Abnormal uterine bleeding is the most common indication for hysteroscopy. Partial or complete endometrial ablation can be performed using a resection loop, rollerball, bipolar technology or laser.
8. Endometrial ablation offers a conservative alternative to hysterectomy, although one would like to improve the current amenorrhoea rates of 15% to 40% and success rates of 70% to 75%.
9. Each second-generation endometrial ablation device has its relative strengths and weaknesses, and no single device can be preferred over another in all circumstances. Clinicians should consider the published safety and effectiveness figures, applicability to the outpatient environment, and evidence of

quality-of-life improvement before selecting which device to use in their department.

10. Preoperative endometrial thinning with danazol or GnRH analogues helps by shrinking the tissue and decreasing vascularity, thereby leading to reduced blood loss, reduced operating time and decreased fluid absorption.

11. Histological assessment of the tissue obtained at endometrial ablation, myomectomy or polypectomy is important to detect the occasional underlying malignancy or other abnormal histology.

12. Endometrial histology is also essential before any form of endometrial ablation, and is desirable for patients with postmenopausal bleeding.

13. Technological development has enabled hysteroscopy in the outpatient setting, which has led to the widespread introduction of 'one-stop hysteroscopy clinics' where patients with abnormal uterine bleeding are clerked, assessed, investigated and potentially treated in full at the same visit.

14. Other indications for hysteroscopy include infertility, foreign body and chronic pelvic pain.

15. Complications during hysteroscopy include cervical or uterine trauma, haemorrhage, infection, fluid overload, gas embolism and uterine perforation with injury to other pelvic viscera.

16. Important late complications include failure to relieve presenting symptoms, infertility, pregnancy with associated complications and cancer.

17. The above complications are rare and avoidable. However, they are potentially serious and hence the surgeon must understand the working principles of the hysteroscopic equipment, including the energy source used, and undergo a structured training programme.

18. Adequate explanation and consent improves patient satisfaction and decreases litigation when complications occur.

19. The training process includes acquiring knowledge, working on laboratory models, attending a well-recognized structured course and assisting experts. Initial procedures are undertaken under general anaesthesia, followed by daycase procedures under local anaesthesia, and finally performing diagnostic and then operative hysteroscopy in the outpatient setting.

20. Hysteroscopic sterilization using Essure is an effective method applicable to the outpatient setting, but its cost is inhibiting its widespread use.

References

Abbott J 2007 Transcervical sterilization. Current Opinion in Obstetrics and Gynecology 19: 325–330.

Abbott J, Hawe J, Hunter D, Garry R 2003 A double-blind randomized trial comparing the Cavaterm(™) and the NovaSure(™) endometrial ablation systems for the treatment of dysfunctional uterine bleeding. Fertility and Sterility 80: 203–208.

Andersson S, Mints M 2007 Thermal balloon ablation for the treatment of menorrhagia in an outpatient setting. Acta Obstetricia et Gynecologica Scandinavica 86: 480–483.

Amso NN, Stabinsky SA, McFaul P, Blanc B, Pendley L, Neuwirth R 1998 Uterine thermal balloon therapy for the treatment of menorrhagia: the first 300 patients from a multi-centre study. International Collaborative Uterine Thermal Balloon Working Group. British Journal of Obstetrics and Gynaecology 105: 517–523.

Amso NN, Fernandez H, Vilos G et al 2003 Uterine endometrial thermal balloon therapy for the treatment of menorrhagia: long-term multicentre follow up study. Human Reproduction 18: 1082–1087.

Berg A, Sandvik L, Langebrekke A, Istre O 2009 A randomized trial comparing monopolar electrodes using glycine 1.5% with two different types of bipolar electrodes (TCRis, Versapoint) using saline, in hysteroscopic surgery. Fertility and Sterility 91: 1273–1278.

Clark TJ, Gupta JK 2004 Outpatient thermal balloon ablation of the endometrium. Fertility and Sterility 82: 1395–1401.

Crane JM, Healey S 2006 Use of misoprostol before hysteroscopy: a systematic review. Journal of Obstetrics and Gynaecology Canada 28: 373–379.

Cooper KG, Bain C, Parkin DE 1999 Comparison of microwave endometrial ablation and transcervical resection of the endometrium for treatment of heavy menstrual loss: a randomised trial. The Lancet 354: 1859–1863.

Cooper KG, Bain C, Lawrie L, Parking DE 2005 A randomised comparison of microwave endometrial ablation with transcervical resection of the endometrium: follow-up at a minimum of five years. BJOG: an International Journal of Obstetrics and Gynaecology 112: 470–475.

Deb S, Flora K, Atiomo W 2008 A survey of preferences and practices of endometrial ablation/resection for menorrhagia in the United Kingdom. Fertility and Sterility 90: 1812–1817.

Donnez J, Nisolle M, Smets M et al 2001 Hysteroscopy in the diagnosis of specific disorder. In: Donnez J, Nisolle M (eds) An Atlas of Operative Laparoscopy and Hysteroscopy. Parthenon, London, pp 403–409.

Donnez J, Nisolle M 1992 Hysteroscopic surgery. Current Opinion in Obstetrics and Gynecology 4: 439–446.

Duffy S, Marsh F, Rogerson L et al 2005 Female sterilisation: a cohort controlled comparative study of ESSURE versus laparoscopic sterilisation. BJOG: an International Journal of Obstetrics and Gynaecology 112: 1522–1528.

Dwyer N, Fox R, Mills M, Hutton J 1991 Haematometra caused by hormone replacement therapy after endometrial resection. The Lancet 338: 1205.

El-Toukhy M, Sunkara K, Coomarasamy A, Grace J, Khalaf Y 2008 Outpatient hysteroscopy and subsequent IVF cycle outcome: a systematic review and meta-analysis. Reproductive Biomedicine Online 16: 712–719.

Erian J 1994 Endometrial ablation in the treatment of menorrhagia. British Journal of Obstetrics and Gynaecology 101 (Suppl 11): 19–22.

Finikiotos G 1994 Hysteroscopy: a review. Obstetrical and Gynecological Survey 49: 273–283.

Furst SN 2007 Ten year follow up of endometrial ablation for menorrhagia. Acta Obstetricia et Gynecologica Scandinavica 86: 334–338.

Gallinat A 2004 NovaSure impedance controlled system for endometrial ablation: three-year follow-up on 107 patients. American Journal of Obstetrics and Gynecology 191: 1585–1589.

Gordon AG, Lewis BV, De Cherney AH 1995 Gynecologic Endoscopy, 2nd edn. Mosby Wolfe, London.

Johns D 2005 Advances in hysteroscopic sterilization: report on 600 patients enrolled in the Adiana EASE pivotal trial. Journal of Minimally Invasive Gynecology 12 (Suppl): S39–S40.

Kaunitz AM, Meredith S, Inki P, Kubba A, Sanchez-Ramos L 2009 Levonorgestrel-releasing intrauterine system and endometrial ablation in heavy menstrual bleeding: a systematic review and meta-analysis. Obstetrics and Gynecology 113: 1104–1116.

Kleijn J, Engels R, Bourdrez P, Mol BWJ, Bongers MY 2008 Five-year follow-up of a randomised controlled trial comparing NovaSure and ThermaChoice endometrial ablation. BJOG: an International Journal of Obstetrics and Gynaecology 111: 193–198.

Kerin JF, Cooper JM, Price T et al 2003 Hysteroscopic sterilization using a micro-insert device: results of a multicentre phase II study. Human Reproduction 18: 1223–1230.

Kremer C, Barik S, Duffy S 1998 Flexible outpatient hysteroscopy without anaesthesia: a safe, successful and well tolerated procedure. British Journal of Obstetrics and Gynaecology 105: 672–676.

Lethaby A, Hickey M, Garry R 2005 Endometrial destruction techniques for heavy menstrual bleeding. An update of Cochrane Database of Systematic Reviews 2: CD001501. Cochrane Database of Systematic Reviews 4: CD001501.

Lewis BV 1994 Guidelines for endometrial ablation. British Journal of Obstetrics and Gynaecology 101: 470–473.

Levie MD, Chudnoff SG 2005 Office hysteroscopic sterilization compared with laparoscopic sterilization: a critical cost analysis. Journal of Minimally Invasive Gynecology 12: 318–322.

Lindemann HJ 1972 The use of CO2 in the uterine cavity for hysteroscopy. International Journal of Fertility 17: 221–225.

Marsh F, Kremer C, Duffy S 2004 Delivering an effective outpatient service in gynaecology. A randomised controlled trial analysing the cost of outpatient versus daycase hysteroscopy. BJOG: an International Journal of Obstetrics and Gynaecology 111: 243–248.

Overton C, Hargreaves J, Maresh M 1997 A national survey of the complications of endometrial destruction for menstrual disorders: the MISTLETOE study. Minimally invasive surgical techniques — laser, endothermal or endoresection. British Journal of Obstetrics and Gynaecology 104: 1351–1359.

Panteleoni D 1869 On endoscopic examination of the cavity of the womb. The Medical Press and Circular 8: 26–27.

Papalampros P, Gambadauro P, Papadopoulos N, Polyzos D, Chapman L, Magos A 2009 A mini-resectoscope: a new instrument for office hysteroscopic surgery. Acta Obstetricia et Gynecologica Scandinavica 88: 227–230.

Pinion SB, Parkin DE, Amramovich DR et al 1994 Randomised trial of hysterectomy, endometrial laser ablation and transcervical endometrial resection for dysfunctional uterine bleeding. BMJ (Clinical Research Ed.) 309: 979–983.

Prather C, Wolfe A 1995 The nurse's role in office hysteroscopy. Journal of Obstetrics, Gynecology, and Neonatal Nursing 24: 813–816.

Romano F, Cicinelli E, Anastasio PS, Epifani S, Fanelli F, Galantino P 1994 Sonohysteroscopy versus hysteroscopy for diagnosing endouterine abnormalities in fertile women. International Journal of Gynecology and Obstetrics 45: 253–260.

Royal College of Obstetricians and Gynaecologists (RCOG) 1994 Report of Working Party on training in gynaecological endoscopic surgery. RCOG Press, London.

Sambrook A, Bain C, Parkin D, Cooper K 2009 A randomised comparison of microwave endometrial ablation with transcervical resection of the endometrium: follow-up at a minimum of 10 years. BJOG: an International Journal of Obstetrics and Gynaecology 116: 1033–1037.

Schifrin BS, Erez S, Moore JG 1973 Teenage endometriosis. American Journal of Obstetrics and Gynaecology 116: 973–980.

Shoukrey M, Fathulla BI, Samarrai T 2008 Hysteroscopy training in the UK: the trainees' perspective. Gynecological Surgery 5: 213–219.

Sinha D, Kalathy V, Gupta JK, Clark TJ 2007 The feasibility, success and patient satisfaction associated with outpatient hysteroscopic sterilisation. BJOG: an International Journal of Obstetrics and Gynaecology 114: 676–683.

Sowter MC, Singla AA, Lethaby A 2001 Pre-operative endometrial thinning agents before hysteroscopic surgery for heavy menstrual bleeding. Cochrane Database of Systematic Reviews 1.

Stamatellos I, Stamatopoulos P, Bontis J 2007 The role of hysteroscopy in the current management of the cervical polyps. Archives of Gynecology and Obstetrics 276: 299–303.

Townsend DE, Duleba AJ, Wilkes MM 2003 Durability of treatment effects after endometrial cryoablation versus rollerball electroablation for abnormal uterine bleeding: two-year results of a multicenter randomised trial. American Journal of Obstetrics and Gynecology 188: 699–701.

Valle RF, Cooper J, Kerin J 2002 Hysteroscopic tubal sterilization with the Essure nonincisional permanent contraception. Obstetrics and Gynecology 99 (Suppl): 11.

Valli E, Zupi E, Marconi D, Solima E, Nagar G, Romanini C 1998 Outpatient diagnostic hysteroscopy. Journal of the American Association of Gynecologic Laparoscopists 5: 397–402.

Wamsteker K, Emanuel MH, de Kruif JH 1993 Transcervical hysteroscopic resection of submucous fibroids for normal uterine bleeding: results regarding the degree of intramural extension. Obstetrics and Gynaecology 82: 736–740.

CHAPTER 3

Laparoscopy

Alan Farthing and Alexandra Lawrence

Chapter Contents			
INTRODUCTION	36	PORT ENTRY	39
HISTORY	36	TEACHING AND LEARNING	41
THEATRE SET-UP	36	COMPLICATIONS OF LAPAROSCOPY	45
SURGICAL TEAM	37	USES OF LAPAROSCOPY	45
EQUIPMENT	37	KEY POINTS	46

Introduction

Laparoscopy (Greek *lapar* meaning flank) is a technique utilized by surgical gynaecologists around the world to great effect. Advances in the technique over the past two decades have revolutionized gynaecological surgery and provided a vastly improved service for patients. At the same time, some of these advances have been associated with considerable controversy, and many opinions are forcefully expressed without much factual basis. This chapter aims to discuss the basics of laparoscopy and its application, providing some of the evidence from the literature where possible.

History

Examination of the body cavities using instrumentation has been practised by clinicians over many centuries. Most of the early techniques involved inspection of the bladder and urethra (Bozzini 1805). Light sources were introduced initially with alcohol flames (Desmoreaux 1865), and subsequently the incandescent light bulb. The first inspection of the peritoneal cavity was through the posterior fornix in the early 20th Century (von Ott 1901). Examination of other cavities was described soon afterwards (Jacobaeus 1910), with carbon dioxide used for insufflation more than a decade later (Zollikoffer 1924). The first diagnosis of an ectopic pregnancy followed (Hope 1937), as did female sterilizations. Veress first reported the spring-loaded insufflation needle as a technique for introducing a pneumothorax in patients with tuberculosis (Veress 1938).

Further advances were relatively slow with few clinicians inspired by the new techniques. The first description of sterilization in English was not until 25 years later (Steptoe 1967). Few therapeutic procedures were performed laparoscopically, although the technique gained widespread support for diagnosis.

The revolution in therapeutic techniques probably started with the report of the first laparoscopic hysterectomy (Reich et al 1989) and, with advances in instrumentation, light sources and camera systems, continued apace throughout the 1990s. However, a few practitioners attempted procedures that were beyond either their surgical training or ability, and responsible bodies rapidly concluded that regulation was required. The Royal College of Obstetricians and Gynaecologists (RCOG) established its training guidelines in 1994 with certification for those trained to perform at different levels. This has been repeatedly modified to bring the UK training into line with practice in other European countries.

Theatre Set-Up

When setting up a theatre for laparoscopic surgery, a number of factors need to be considered. First, both the surgeon and the assistant need to have an excellent view of the operating area. Second, the surgeon needs to be in a comfortable position, and third, the instrumentation needs to be arranged systematically and consistently.

The authors believe that the television screen should be placed between the patient's legs if the camera is inserted at the umbilicus. Figure 3.1 demonstrates that the view displayed on the screen is in the same direction in which the patient is lying and the surgeon operating. Many experienced surgeons place the television screen directly in front of themselves and behind the assistant. Under these circumstances, the surgeon is operating in a different direction to which he or she is looking; not only is this uncomfortable and ergonomically disadvantageous, but all images have to be transposed through 90 degrees, adding to the difficulties of hand–eye coordination. The additional advantage of placing the monitor between the patient's legs is that only one screen is required.

DOI: 10.1016/B978-0-7020-3120-5.00003-5

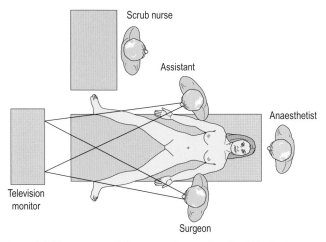

Figure 3.1 Theatre set-up is important. The monitor should be in the same plane as the surgical field, i.e. a straight line from the surgeon through the surgical field also passes through the monitor.

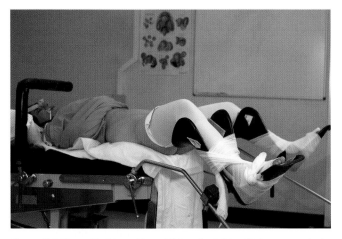

Figure 3.2 The patient is positioned flat on the table with legs supported. A bar is placed over the endotracheal tube to protect this from being dislodged and to support the assistant's arm.

The scrub nurse should stand in a consistent position, and instrumentation such as bipolar diathermy, scissors, graspers and suction irrigation should be placed reliably within easy reach of the surgeon. The scrub nurse should be within sight of the television screen, enabling anticipation of the next instrument required. A protective bar placed across the table prevents the assistant's arm from resting on the upper part of the patient and potentially dislodging the endotracheal tube (Figure 3.2).

Surgical Team

A coordinated surgical team is essential for safe laparoscopic procedures. An experienced anaesthetist can allow a state of permissive hypercapnia whilst the patient is in a steep Trendelenberg position. Careful positioning on a non-slip mattress decreases the tendency of the patient to slide up the bed. A well-stocked laparoscopic trolley will decrease overall operating time by minimizing the delay whilst staff find the required instruments.

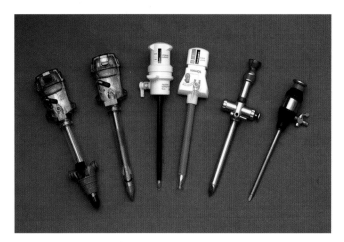

Figure 3.3 A selection of trocars used in laparoscopic surgery.

Equipment

Laparoscopic surgeons are totally dependent on their equipment. Any laparoscopic procedure can only be performed safely if clear images are presented to the surgeon. The quality of the image is dependent on the weakest link in a long series of technologically advanced items. It is essential that laparoscopic surgeons are familiar with the function and adjustments of the imaging systems that they use, and it is this complicated equipment that provides the majority of the cost of laparoscopic surgery.

It is primarily the vast improvement in technology that has led to the increase in the number of procedures performed using laparoscopic techniques; however, there is scope for further improvement in laparoscopic equipment and robotics. Three-dimensional viewing systems and automated assistants may enhance the current instrumentation.

The following items are essential.

Trocars

Many different types of trocar are available, which vary in size, length and design of the tip (Figure 3.3). The 12 mm, 10 mm and 5 mm trocars are used most commonly in gynaecological surgery. When performing complicated surgery, there can be many changes of instrument down any individual port. For this reason, the trocars have to be able to grip the abdominal wall, and there are various designs to facilitate this. Some of the more modern trocars have a type of 'fish scale', whilst others utilize a screw thread which can grip more effectively but increases the diameter of the incision. The trocar tip can be conical, pyramidal or a single flat blade in design. They create different sized and shaped incisions in the fascia, with the single flat blade and conical dilating tip producing the smallest defect. Optical trocars have a blunt clear dome-shaped tip housing a crescent-shaped blade. They allow a controlled sharp dissection of the abdominal wall layers under direct vision. These trocars can be inserted prior to insufflation and may be useful in obese patients with thick abdominal walls. Trocars may be disposable or reusable. Many laparoscopic surgeons have been persuaded to use disposable trocars because of their constantly sharp tips, the so-called safety devices to retract the tip when through the full thickness of the abdominal wall and to avoid contamination between patients. However, most surgical units find the cost of disposable trocars prohibitive for use with every case.

Laparoscopes

The laparoscopes most commonly used in gynaecological surgery are of 10 mm, 5 mm or, occasionally, 3 mm diameter. The 10 mm laparoscopes provide the largest images with the optimal illumination, although the new generation of 5 mm laparoscopes can provide an image equal to their 10 mm relatives from only a few years ago. The laparoscope is a high-precision engineered instrument which requires careful handling, both during operations and in the sterilization process between cases. It contains both a fibreoptic bundle for light transmission and a series of lenses to transfer the image back to the eyepiece. Modern laparoscopes consist of a hybrid rod lens system, although the 3 mm laparoscope utilizes a high-quality fibreoptic bundle. The hybrid rod lens system at 3 mm diameter would be too easily damaged. Most surgeons utilize a laparoscope which projects an image that appears at 0 degrees to the shaft of the scope; however, laparoscopes that project an image from 30 or 70 degrees are also available. Although these laparoscopes rarely cause problems for the surgeon, they can cause difficulty in coordination of the image by the assistant who is holding the laparoscope and camera device.

Light source and lead

The weakest link in the endoscopic equipment chain is often the light lead. This fibreoptic cable is often used for months or years after many of its cables are damaged. It also requires careful maintenance and will inevitably require replacement in time. A number of light sources exist and many surgeons still utilize the halogen system, despite the fact that this has been superseded by the more powerful xenon light source.

Camera system

Modern camera systems are an essential part of the laparoscopic surgeon's equipment. There are few surgeons around the world who continue to operate by looking directly down the eyepiece of the laparoscope, even for minor diagnostic procedures. There is a clear advantage in being able to project the image on to a television screen that is visible to all members of the surgical team. Together with the ergonomic advantages of not having to stoop over the patient, this means that camera systems are now commonplace. The image seen through the eyepiece of the laparoscope is converted into electrical signals by a charge-coupled device housed in the camera head. These electrical signals are then processed by the camera control facility which is, in turn, connected to the television monitor. Cameras may contain one or three charge-coupled devices, each of which is colour specific, recording only one of the three primary colours. Most modern camera systems enable collection of digital images which are projected on to a digital monitor, although hybrid set-ups can co-exist. Some camera heads incorporate remote buttons to allow the operator to control various features of the imaging system, such as taking prints, operat-

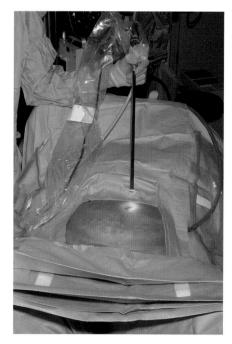

Figure 3.4 A sterile bag can be used for placement of the camera head and cable.

ing the video recorder or white balancing. Some cameras are autoclavable but the majority of surgeons will place the camera system inside a sterile plastic sheath before connecting to the laparoscope (Figure 3.4).

Recording equipment

The modern laparoscopic surgery theatre should contain a video recorder and still photo facility for the purpose of producing images of any procedure. Many educational and training videos have been produced and are extremely valuable. Patients may appreciate a copy of their operation and some surgeons believe it is important to create a medicolegal record of the procedure for possible future reference. There is no reason why laparoscopic surgery should be treated any differently to open surgery, and surgeons who do not record their procedures on a video can hardly be regarded as neglecting the medical records. Within gynaecology, the majority of medicolegal claims are connected with laparoscopic sterilization, and most surgeons would regard photographs of the clips occluding each fallopian tube to be a sensible precaution.

Television monitor

Many different television monitors are available, but the majority are 20 inches in size. High-definition monitors coupled with a digital camera have led to improvements in display. The monitor should be the last piece of equipment that is adjusted if the image is of poor quality, and is possibly the least important in determining a good view of the surgical field.

Insufflator

As laparoscopic surgical techniques have advanced, there has been a significant improvement in the technology of insufflators. They should provide a maximum flow rate of approximately 35 l/min with continuous monitoring of volume, flow rate and intra-abdominal pressure. Safety devices should ensure that the maximum pressure setting is not exceeded, and most modern insufflators have an alarm to notify the surgeon. Some insufflators additionally provide smoke evacuation, either controlled by the surgeon with a foot pedal or with a direct link through to the diathermy or laser device. The insufflator needs to have simple and easily interpreted display panels. The laparoscopic surgeon will refer to the insufflator when creating the pneumoperitoneum and, at this vital part of the procedure, needs to know where to look for the information he or she is seeking.

Operating instruments

There are innumerable types of operating instruments, and individual surgeons will have their own preferences. Essentially, the instruments can be divided into the jaws, the shaft and the handles. Jaws have been designed which mimic all the instrumentation available for open surgery, plus many others. Examples are shown in Figure 3.5. The shafts may be of 10, 5 or 3 mm diameter and may or may not contain a diathermy attachment. For non-disposable instrumentation, it is often the shaft that is the most difficult part of the instrument to keep clean and maintain. Handles come in a variety of ergonomic designs, according to surgeon preference. Handles may be ratcheted or non-ratcheted in a variety of ways. Most non-disposable instruments have a detachable handle in order to convert an instrument into one with or without a ratchet. Surgeons have their favourite graspers and, as with most situations, it is more important to be familiar with an instrument and to know its limitations than it is to have a wide variety of instrumentation that is less familiar.

Laparoscopic operating equipment is expensive and has a relatively short shelf-life in comparison with open instrumentation. It is essential that any theatre budget takes this into consideration and that laparoscopic surgeons are not asked to continue working with blunt and non-functioning instruments. The more complex problems of decontamination and sterilization of these precision instruments

mean that they require careful maintenance by a specialist team.

Port Entry

A variety of techniques have been described for insufflation in order to allow the surgeon to view the pelvic and abdominal contents through the laparoscope. A great deal of discussion has occurred, particularly in medicolegal circles, regarding which is the safest technique. Complication rates for laparoscopy are so low that individual surgeons are unlikely to be able to evaluate the various entry techniques in their own practice. However, the number of laparoscopies performed is so high that the overall effect of an inferior technique could be significant for a number of patients around the country each year. Traditionally, gynaecologists are familiar with the closed technique, having performed many diagnostic laparoscopies in their training. General surgeons perform fewer laparoscopies, and these are usually for major procedures. They are usually more familiar with the open technique. Each technique has its persuasive advocates basing their arguments on a combination of scientific evidence and personal bias. Methods of port entry were examined by a recent Cochrane review which concluded that there was no evidence that one method was superior (Ahmad et al 2008).

Site of entry

There are three main sites of entry into the peritoneal cavity. The most common site is at the umbilicus, with some clinicians using a suprapubic approach and others utilizing Palmer's point (in the mid-clavicular line in the ninth intercostal space).

At the umbilicus, the abdominal wall is at its thinnest. A subumbilical incision is preferred by some clinicians, but there appears to be no logic to this. If the umbilicus is to be used, there is little point in inserting either the Veress needle or primary trocar at a point where the abdominal wall has expanded. In addition, an intraumbilical incision is cosmetically superior (Figure 3.6). The left upper quadrant of the peritoneal cavity is where the fewest intraperitoneal

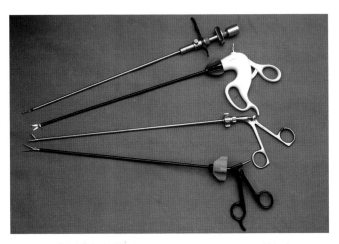

Figure 3.5 A selection of laparoscopic scissors, graspers and bipolar diathermy of 5 mm diameter.

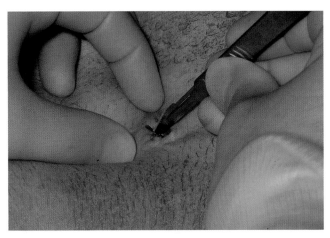

Figure 3.6 An incision is made intraumbilically.

adhesions occur. For this reason, Palmer suggested the ninth intercostal space as an insertion point for insufflation and brief inspection of the peritoneal cavity. A number of clinicians utilize this entry point when they suspect that periumbilical adhesions may be present.

Closed laparoscopy

A vertical incision is made intraumbilically, with the angle of the Veress needle insertion varying according to the body mass index (BMI) of the patient, from 45 degrees in non-obese women to 90 degrees in obese women (Figure 3.7). Most clinicians stabilize the anterior abdominal wall by grasping it with the left hand, while the right hand inserts the Veress needle. Experienced laparoscopists can feel the Veress needle pass through the layers of the anterior abdominal wall, and will usually be able to tell whether the Veress needle is correctly positioned. At this point, a number of techniques have been described to assist in demonstrating that the Veress needle is correctly positioned. A syringe can be used to aspirate from the Veress needle to identify visceral contents. Alternatively, a droplet of water or saline can be placed on the end of the Veress needle and the negative intra-abdominal pressure causes this to be sucked in. A syringe placed on the end of the Veress needle and containing water or saline, but without its plunger, will usually allow the solution to drip into the peritoneal cavity if correctly positioned. Once insufflation is commenced, the filling pressure can be observed and uniform distension of the abdominal cavity can be determined by percussion. In particular, the area over the liver becomes resonant to percussion when pneumoperitoneum is created. 'Waggling' of the Veress needle from side to side should be avoided as this can enlarge a 1.6 mm puncture injury to an injury of up to 1 cm in viscera or blood vessels.

It is important to create pneumoperitoneum of a set pressure rather than volume. The size of the intraperitoneal cavity varies greatly between individuals. The purpose of insufflation is to provide a cushion between the anterior abdominal wall and the important underlying structures when the primary trocar is inserted. Phillips et al (1999) demonstrated that an intraperitoneal pressure of 25 mmHg

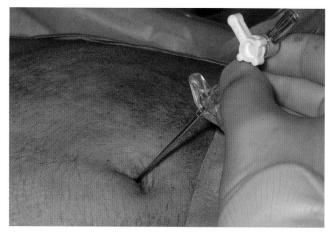

Figure 3.7 The Veress needle is placed intraumbilically and directed towards the pouch of Douglas during insertion.

was necessary in order to maintain the gas bubble during insertion of the primary trocar. It is extremely important that this pressure is then reduced to 15 mmHg or less for the rest of the operation. Ventilation difficulties are not encountered at this initial filling pressure, as the patient is flat and the pressure of this level is only maintained for a short period of time.

Direct entry

Direct trocar insertion without pneumoperitoneum using an optical trocar can be employed but there is insufficient evidence to suggest any benefit over the open or closed techniques (Ahmad et al 2008). A disadvantage of this technique is that any inadvertent visceral perforation is guaranteed to be of significant size, unlike damage caused by the Veress needle. Direct entry is increasingly employed in the morbidly obese undergoing gastric bypass surgery.

Open laparoscopy

The Hasson entry technique was first described in 1971 (Hasson 1971). A vertical incision is placed intraumbilically and the various layers of the abdominal wall are incised using two Langenbeck retractors on either side to assist with visualization. Once the rectus sheath is incised, a suture is inserted on either side of the incision into the sheath. The peritoneum is opened, a blunt Hasson cannula is inserted directly into the peritoneal cavity and insufflation is commenced. A seal is usually created utilizing the sutures in the rectus sheath and tightening around a cone attached to the Hasson cannula.

Comparison of complications

A vast number of laparoscopies using the closed technique have been performed over many years. A collection of over 350,000 procedures has calculated the risk of bowel damage to be 0.4/1000 and the risk of major vessel injury to be 0.2/1000. The most common bowel injury is to the transverse colon, while the most common vascular injury is to the right common iliac artery (Clements 1995).

There are no comparable data on such a large number of patients for open laparoscopy. One rationale of the Hasson technique is to identify intraperitoneal and bowel adhesions at entry into the peritoneal cavity, thus avoiding blind insertion of a trocar into a visceral structure, but this was not supported by a recent Cochrane review (Ahmad et al 2008). More logically, the Hasson technique avoids major vessel damage. Population-based studies are an inappropriate way of comparing the two techniques, as many clinicians only use the open laparoscopy approach if they think there is a danger of intraperitoneal adhesions. They are therefore selecting a high-risk group of patients on which to perform this technique. Studies that have been published with large numbers suggest that bowel damage in the open laparoscopy group is equivalent to that in the closed laparoscopy group (Chapron et al 1998).

Advocates of the open laparoscopy approach maintain that the time taken to achieve pneumoperitoneum is equivalent to that of the closed laparoscopy approach (Pickersgill et al 1999).

Ten percent of patients will have intra-abdominal adhesions, with 5% having severe adhesions containing bowel around the umbilicus. Ninety-two percent of these patients with severe adhesions will have had a previous laparotomy, with the vast majority following midline incisions (Garry 2000). Although not all visceral perforations caused by laparoscopy are the result of negligence, it would seem prudent for clinicians to take previous midline laparotomies into consideration when performing a laparoscopy. It is important that those advocates of closed laparoscopy are able to perform open laparoscopy when their own technique fails. There is currently no conclusive proof that one technique is safer than the other, and a huge randomized controlled trial would be necessary to detect small safety differences between the two techniques.

Teaching and Learning

The RCOG recognized at an early stage that teaching and learning laparoscopic surgery was important for safe practice. A system of recognized preceptors who are qualified to teach laparoscopic techniques has been established and is maintained by the RCOG. This is an area which is currently in a state of flux. The RCOG has recently developed a basic surgical skills course and an advanced training skills module in benign gynaecological laparoscopy. Achievement of the module requires proficiency in oophorectomy, ovarian cystectomy and treatment of peritoneal and ovarian endometriosis. Other units around the country have set up courses such as the University of Surrey's MSc which teaches skills for treating complex endometriosis.

Many trainers have recognized the value of simulating exercises in the training of laparoscopic surgeons, so laboratories have been established to teach and assess practical skills in a variety of centres around the country. Hand–eye coordination exercises are now widespread and many are quite imaginative. Computer simulations play an increasing part in the training of laparoscopic surgeons. Exercises based on surgical procedures are available through the i-sim® system (www.isurgicals.com). Simulators have been shown to improve surgical performance whilst learning a new technique (Aggarwal et al 2006). It is perfectly logical to assume that, in the future, surgeons will have to demonstrate their competence on these virtual reality systems before being allowed to operate on patients. Reproducible tests of dextrous ability can be used as part of the assessment process when determining which candidate should be appointed to a particular specialty post.

Laparoscopic suturing

Laparoscopic suturing can be avoided in many procedures, but is an important skill for the advanced laparoscopic surgeon. Many experienced open surgeons are reluctant to pass through the sometimes humiliating learning curve required in order to master suturing techniques. However, it is simply a matter of 'practice making perfect' and laparoscopic suturing is an ideal exercise for the simulator.

Sutures are usually introduced through the accessory ports, and care needs to be taken to ensure that the needle is observed for the entire time it is in the peritoneal cavity.

Laparoscopic suturing is less forgiving than suturing at open surgery, and this is classically demonstrated with the curved needle. The correct surgical technique is to insert the tip of the needle into the tissue and then rotate the needle through the tissue in an arc that follows the exact curve of the needle. The needle holder needs to be at right angles to the needle in order to fulfil this task. Poor surgical technique at open surgery often involves surgeons pushing a curved needle in a straight line through the tissues, rather than rotating it through.

Some surgeons prefer to use a straight needle when suturing laparoscopically as this passes through the ports more easily. The principle of suture insertion remains the same by passing the needle through the tissues in a direction that mimics the shape of the needle.

Once the suture is appropriately placed, a knot can be tied either intracorporeally or extracorporeally, according to the individual surgeon's preference and familiarity. Knots of adequate strength can be tied by either method.

Pre-tied sutures

The endo-loop is a simple technique for applying a suture to a pedicle, pushing down a pre-tied knot (Figure 3.8). These pre-tied sutures employ a Roeder knot and are extremely useful either as a time-saving device or for less-experienced laparoscopic surgeons.

Stapling

Mechanical stapling devices have helped to revolutionize laparoscopic surgery and encouraged a generation of surgeons to utilize these precision instruments (Figures 3.9 and 3.10). The device usually inserts three lines of carefully arranged titanium staples, either side of a knife tract, which allows the tissue to be divided when the staples are fired. It is an extremely efficient and rapid instrument, but its major disadvantage is its diameter which requires a 12 mm port. They do need to be applied with great care, and the surgeon needs to ensure that only the desired tissue is secured within the jaws of the device. In the use of this instrument, the surgeon has to be particularly aware that the view on the

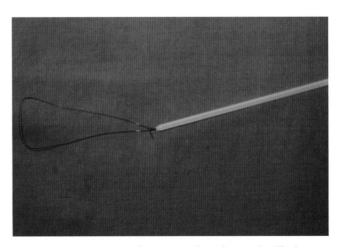

Figure 3.8 A pre-tied Roeder knot mounted on a knot pusher. The loop is placed over the pedicle and the knot pushed tight by advancing the plastic pusher.

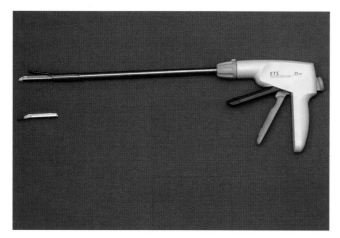

Figure 3.9 The stapling device. The white handle is fixed, the grey lever closes the instrument and the black lever fires the staples and knife.

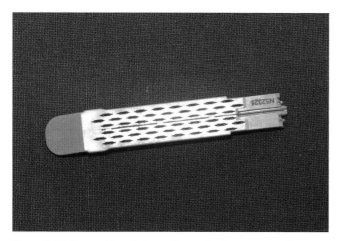

Figure 3.10 The cartridge of the stapling device shows six rows of titanium staples separated in the centre by the knife tract.

monitor is only provided in two dimensions. The tips of the stapling device must be visualized before firing.

Specimen removal

Many laparoscopic operations are initially straightforward, such as an oophorectomy for a large ovarian cyst. Very often, the most difficult part of the procedure is actually removing the specimen without increasing the size of the incisions in the abdominal wall. A number of devices have been employed in order to make this extraction easier. The most commonly used specimen retrieval system utilizes a bag such as the Endo-catch bag in Figure 3.11. The bag comes pre-folded and springs open once inserted into the abdominal cavity, allowing the specimen to be inserted. The edges of the bag are brought to the surface and the specimen removed without spilling its contents into the peritoneal cavity. A large cyst can be deflated extracorporeally for easy removal.

For larger cysts and more solid structures, such as fibroids, alternative methods of specimen removal may be necessary. A posterior colpotomy can be extended with ease to 4 or 5 cm diameter without increasing discomfort or recovery

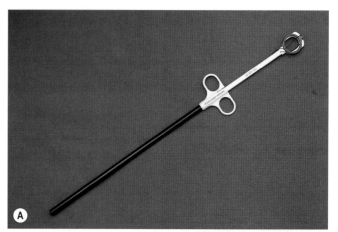

A

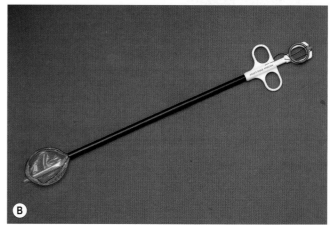

B

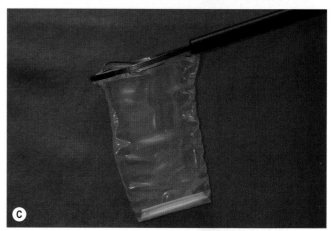

C

Figure 3.11 The bag specimen retrieval system. Advancing the white plunger pushes the bag out of the introducer. The wire around the neck of the bag springs open.

time for the patient. Large-volume specimen bags can be inserted through the posterior fornix and wrapped around large ovarian cysts or fibroids. The neck of the bag can be brought through the incision in the posterior fornix, and the specimen either morcellated or deflated through a much larger incision than is required for the abdominal ports. Figures 3.12–3.20 demonstrate the removal of a 7 cm pedunculated fibroid using a posterior colpotomy. Initially, the fibroid is fixed with a suture to avoid it being displaced into

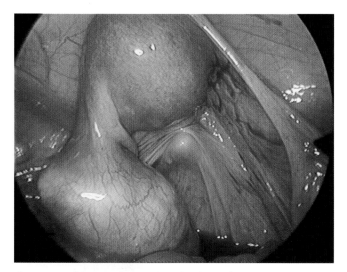

Figure 3.12 This uterus has a pedunculated 7 cm fibroid arising from the left side of the fundus. An instrument can be seen causing an indentation in the posterior fornix.

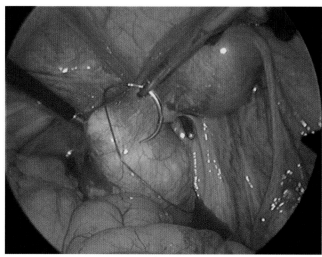

Figure 3.13 A suture has been introduced through the posterior fornix and is passed through the fibroid to fix the specimen.

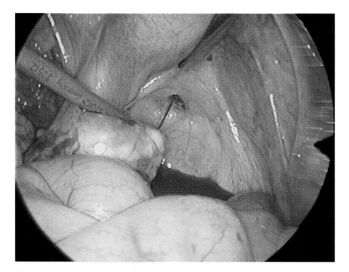

Figure 3.14 The suture is returned to the posterior fornix.

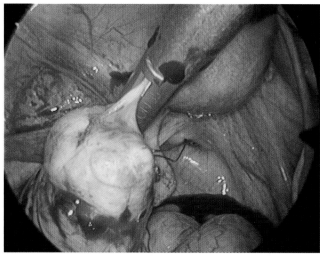

Figure 3.15 A staple is placed over the pedicle of the fibroid which is divided.

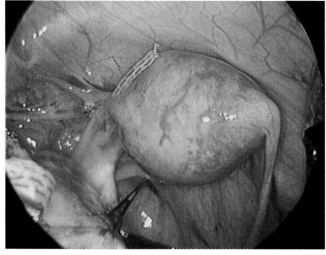

Figure 3.16 The staple provides an effective haemostatic and excisional device. Despite the patient being in a steep Trendelenburg position, the separated fibroid remains fixed by the suture through the posterior fornix.

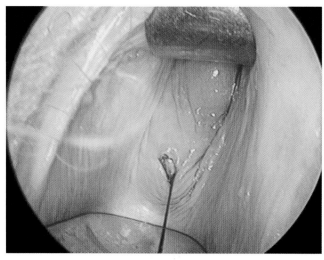

Figure 3.17 The view vaginally shows the suture passing through into the peritoneal cavity.

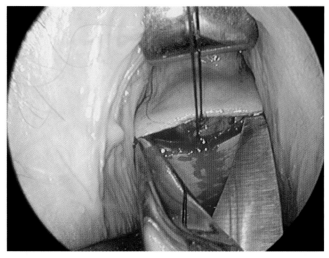

Figure 3.18 The incision in the posterior fornix is enlarged to 3–4 cm.

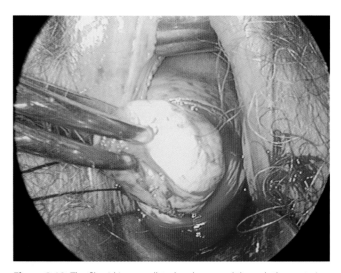

Figure 3.19 The fibroid is morcellated and removed through the posterior fornix incision.

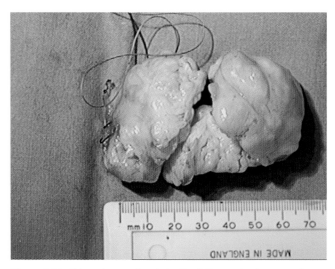

Figure 3.20 Although morcellated, the fibroid is completely removed without the need to extend the abdominal incisions.

the upper abdomen under the influence of gravity once it is disconnected from the uterus (Figures 3.13–3.14). A straightforward Endo-GIA staple disconnects the fibroid from the uterus and the fibroid is brought down to the posterior colpotomy by pulling on the suture (Figures 3.15–3.17). Transvaginally, the posterior colpotomy is extended and the fibroid morcellated to remove the specimen (Figures 3.18 and 3.19). The posterior colpotomy is repaired either vaginally or laparoscopically with precision.

Mechanical morcellators are an alternative way of removing the fibroids or the fundus and body of the uterus if a subtotal hysterectomy is performed. Extreme care needs to be taken with mechanical morcellators as they are dangerous if the wrong tissue is grasped inadvertently. They require considerable patience and are another piece of expensive theatre equipment.

Energy sources

Many energy sources are available for use with laparoscopic instruments. Bipolar and monopolar diathermy are widely available and reliable. The use of lasers is covered elsewhere in this text (see Chapter 4). Newer methods of tissue division and vessel sealing include the Harmonic Scalpel® and the Ligasure® system. Progress in this area of technology has allowed many diagnostic laparoscopies to be converted into effective therapeutic treatment.

Gasless laparoscopy

It is possible to operate within the peritoneal cavity without distending it using carbon dioxide (Chin et al 1993, Wood et al 1994). A rigid mechanical support is required in order to elevate the anterior abdominal wall so that the viscera can be identified. The advantages of gasless laparoscopy are the avoidance of insufflators causing possible gas emboli, and the use of simpler trocars. However, most gasless laparoscopy techniques require extra portals in order to insert the mechanical device for visualization. It is not a technique that has become widespread.

Robotic techniques

Robots were first used in humans to carry out a transurethral resection of the prostate in 1991 at Imperial College, London (Davies et al 1997). The controls of modern robots have an intuitive ease of use, and complex manoeuvres such as suturing can be easily mastered. Physiological movement can be digitally subtracted from the camera signal to give a still image on the screen; for example, cardiac pulsation can be dampened down. The surgeon can be remote from the patient, even in another continent. In an era of consumer-driven health care, there is increasing demand for the most up-to-date equipment. Disadvantages of the robot include limited haptic feedback so the operator is unable to gauge the force applied to the tissue. The robot is an expensive and complex piece of equipment requiring careful maintenance, and in the event of a malfunction, the surgeon must be prepared to complete the operation either laparoscopically or as an open procedure. Operations performed robotically include radical prostatectomy, beating heart bypass grafts and radical hysterectomy.

Complications of Laparoscopy

The complications associated with port entry have been mentioned earlier in this chapter, and this is generally the most dangerous time for the patient. However, laparoscopic surgery can have many of the same complications as open surgery, depending on the complexity of any procedure. A list of possible complications is seen in Box 3.1.

Once access has been obtained and the laparoscope inserted, accessory ports have to be placed. These need to avoid the inferior epigastric vessels which supply the anterior abdominal wall. They can invariably be visualized even in the most obese of patients by remembering that they originate from the external iliac vessels as they enter the femoral canal, and then run laterally to the obliterated umbilical vessels. The authors usually place a left accessory port lateral to the inferior epigastric vessels and a further port suprapubically. This allows the right-handed surgeon to operate in a straight line whilst opposing the instruments sufficiently for them to work together. Placing the right port lateral to the inferior epigastric vessels means that the surgeon will have to reach over the patient to an instrument that is then aimed back towards the pelvis. This position is uncomfortable for long procedures.

Once the accessory trocars are inserted, complications will depend on the procedure and will be similar to open surgery. During steep Trendelenburg tilt, the pressure required to ventilate the patient will increase and carbon dioxide absorption can be a problem in those with borderline pulmonary function. As with any type of surgery, trust and understanding between the anaesthetist and the surgeon are essential.

Damage to visceral structures can occur during any procedure, but they can be more difficult to recognize with laparoscopic surgery. Dense adhesions may involve the bowel and therefore the use of diathermy should be limited. Inadvertent diathermy damage by direct current transfer, or direct or capacitive coupling may occur.

Postoperatively, patients should be more mobile and make a quicker recovery as a result of smaller abdominal wounds. Serious complications such as unrecognized visceral injury may occur in the first few days and it is essential that these are rectified immediately. All surgeons get complications and any surgeon who does not believe it possible that their patient could sustain a complication from a laparoscopic procedure is a potentially dangerous surgeon. As a general rule, all patients should continue to improve from 24 h after any laparoscopic procedure. If this does not occur, consideration should be given to intraoperative visceral injury, and the patient should be investigated further with possible return to theatre before they collapse.

Medium- and long-term laparoscopic complications are rare. Incisional hernias have been reported, particularly in slim patients where larger (10–12 mm) ports are used lateral to the rectus muscle. These can usually be avoided by closure of the rectus sheath and ensuring that when removing the primary trocars at the same time as the pneumoperitoneum, no omentum has been drawn into the wound.

Uses of Laparoscopy

Diagnostic

All gynaecologists perform diagnostic laparoscopies for multiple indications. It is a common investigation for pelvic pain, infertility, assessment of pelvic masses and in trials to assess clinical efficacy of treatment. There is virtually no indication for a diagnostic laparotomy in current medical practice. All clinicians would agree that a diagnostic laparoscopy is a quick, easy and safe way of assessing the peritoneal cavity, while causing minimal discomfort and allowing rapid recovery for the patient.

Therapeutic

If a therapeutic laparoscopic procedure can be performed with ease and without putting the patient in increased danger, there is no question about its efficacy. Clinicians would agree that a diagnostic laparotomy is unnecessary, has a long recovery period and significant minor morbidity. It is therefore logical to extend this principle into the area of therapeutics. There are many procedures that are clearly better performed laparoscopically, and these should be made available to all patients. It is the responsibility of health authorities, hospital administration and local clinicians to ensure that this logical and sensible approach is available for their patients. Examples of procedures that should normally be performed laparoscopically are given in Box 3.2.

Obese and infirm patients recover significantly better after a laparoscopic procedure compared with an open procedure. A high BMI, previously regarded as a relative

---

Box 3.1 Complications of laparoscopy

Primary trocar insertion

Bowel injury: transverse colon, small bowel

Vessel injury: common iliac arteries or veins, aorta, inferior vena cava

Bladder perforation

Damage to omentum

Surgical emphysema from extraperitoneal gas

Vasovagal reflex during gas insertion

Gas embolism

Secondary trocar insertion

Inferior epigastric vessel injury

Bowel injury

During the procedure

Anaesthetic complications: ventilatory problems, CO_2 absorption

Visceral injury: recognized, unrecognized, direct, secondary to diathermy, etc., contamination of operative field

Haemorrhage: circulatory compromise, visual loss

Equipment failure: cameras, lighting, diathermy, staples, sutures, etc.

Postoperative

Fluid balance

Pain relief

Thromboembolic

Unrecognized visceral injury

Port site hernia

> **Box 3.2** Therapeutic procedures that should routinely be performed laparoscopically
>
> Laser ablation of endometriosis (Sutton et al 1994)
> Salpingectomy (Yao and Tulandi 1997)
> Removal of ovarian cysts (Audebert 1998)
> Minor adhesiolysis
> Sterilization

contraindication, should be viewed as an indication for a laparoscopic approach.

The debate about laparoscopic surgery becomes more involved when examining more complex gynaecological procedures. There is no doubt that the vast majority of procedures can be performed laparoscopically, but not all procedures should be. The dilemma is in determining which patient fits into which category, and that will sometimes depend on the surgeon. This is not the place to discuss at length the use of laparoscopy in various operations. Laparoscopy is merely the route by which a procedure is performed. It is the appropriate operation rather than the route that is perhaps more important.

The debate concerning the route most suitable for a hysterectomy is an excellent example of the difficulties in determining where laparoscopic surgery is best used. For many years, the surgeon has had a choice of the vaginal or the abdominal route for removing a patient's uterus. The rates of vaginal hysterectomy vary enormously depending on the country in which a patient is treated. However, the circumstances in which a vaginal or abdominal hysterectomy is most suitable are still unclear.

The frequently quoted paper from Dicker et al (1982), where one-third of hysterectomies were performed vaginally, demonstrates a faster recovery time and lower minor morbidity rate by this route. Major morbidity was infrequent in both groups, but considerably higher in the vaginal hysterectomy group. It seems logical that an easy vaginal hysterectomy would have minimal major complications and provide the patient with the shortest recovery period. However, as the procedure becomes more difficult, the possibility of major complications increases. Judging when to dismiss the advantages of shorter recovery and look for the lower major morbidity rate is an issue that has not been standardized.

It is most desirable to perform a vaginal hysterectomy under the easiest circumstances, but when the procedure is extremely difficult, an abdominal hysterectomy is preferable. At some point between these two extremes, the lines cross.

Laparoscopic hysterectomy was introduced in an attempt to make some of the more difficult vaginal hysterectomies easier. As a consequence, many patients who would have otherwise had an abdominal hysterectomy were offered a laparoscopic hysterectomy or a laparoscopic-assisted vaginal hysterectomy. The effects of the route of hysterectomy were examined in 1347 women in the eVALuate study (Garry et al 2004). The trial had two arms; one arm compared abdominal with laparoscopic hysterectomy, and the second underpowered arm compared vaginal and laparoscopic routes. The abdominal arm showed a higher risk of complications including ureteric injuries and conversion to laparotomy with the laparoscopic route, but also less pain and a shorter hospital stay. The vaginal arm showed a longer duration of operation with the laparoscopic route compared with the vaginal route. The trial has been criticized for the low number of laparoscopic hysterectomies performed by each surgeon. The complications may have been higher due to the learning curve of the surgeons. In addition, conversion to open surgery was recorded as a major complication, which may have encouraged surgeons to persist against their better judgement.

With a decrease in the number of hysterectomies being performed and significantly reduced surgical experience as a trainee, the opportunity to learn these techniques is limited. The vast majority of gynaecologists performing this surgery are inevitably self-taught. There are no scientifically reproducible data to show which factors should determine whether a patient has a vaginal, laparoscopic or abdominal hysterectomy. Indeed, the indications would be different for individual surgeons with varied surgical expertise; as such, the debate continues.

There will obviously be some instances where one procedure is clearly preferable. Where prolapse exists, a vaginal hysterectomy is preferable. Where multiple intraperitoneal adhesions are expected or ovarian malignancy is diagnosed, an abdominal approach is superior. For most stage I endometrial cancers where the peritoneal cavity needs to be inspected, washings taken, ovaries removed and possibly lymph node sampling performed, a laparoscopic hysterectomy is superior.

As with the majority of situations, the real truth lies somewhere between the two extremes. Clinicians who have avoided learning laparoscopic surgical techniques need to accept that they have significantly improved the care of many patients and should be readily available. Conversely, some of the proponents of laparoscopic surgery need to accept that there is nothing clever about a procedure that results in increased serious morbidity.

KEY POINTS

1. As a result of smaller incisions, uncomplicated operations performed laparoscopically result in faster recovery and less postoperative pain.
2. The equipment required for laparoscopic surgery should be of good quality and well maintained.
3. Systematic training of surgeons is required using courses, simulators and a log of the case load.
4. The single most dangerous time in any laparoscopic procedure is usually the insertion of the primary trocar. An understanding of anatomy and surgical principles is necessary in order to minimize the risk.
5. Various techniques are available to make laparoscopic surgery easier. These include staples, pre-tied knots, specimen retrieval bags and robots.
6. Virtually all operations can be performed laparoscopically, but not all should be.

References

Aggarwal R, Tully A, Grantcharov T et al 2006 Virtual reality simulation training can improve technical skills during laparoscopic salpingectomy for ectopic pregnancy. BJOG: an International Journal of Obstetrics and Gynaecology 113: 1382–1387.

Ahmad G, Duffy JM, Phillips K, Watson A 2008 Laparoscopic entry techniques. Cochrane Database of Systematic Reviews 2.

Audebert AJM 1998 Laparoscopic ovarian surgery and ovarian torsion. In: Sutton C, Diamond MP (eds) Endoscopic Surgery for Gynecologists. WB Saunders, Philadelphia.

Bozzini P 1805 Der lichtleiter odere beschreibung einer eingachen vorrichtung und ihrer anwendung zur erleuchung innerer hohlen und zwischeraume deslebenden animaleschen corpses. Landes-Industrie-Comptoi, Weimer.

Chapron C, Querleu D, Bruhat MA et al 1998 Surgical complications of diagnostic and operative gynaecological laparoscopy: a series of 29,966 cases. Human Reproduction 13: 867–872.

Chin AK, Moll FH, McColl MB, Reiv H 1993 Mechanical peritoneal retraction as a replacement for carbon dioxide pneumoperitoneum. Journal of the American Association of Gynecologic Laparoscopists 1: 62–66.

Clements RV 1995 Major vessel injury. Clinical Risk 1: 112–115.

Davies BL, Harris SJ, Arambula-Cosio F, Mei Q, Hibberd RD 1997 The Probot — an active robot for prostate resection. Proceedings of the Institute of Mechanical Engineers, Part H, Jl. Engineering in Medicine 211: 317–326.

Dicker RC, Scally MJ, Greenspan JR et al 1982 Hysterectomy among women of reproductive age — trends in USA 1970–78. JAMA: the Journal of the American Medical Association 248: 323–327.

Desmoreaux AJ 1865 De l'endoscopie et de sas applications au diagnostic et au traitement des affections de l'uretre et de la vessie. Baillière, Paris.

Dingfelder JR 1978 Direct laparoscopic trocar insertion without prior pneumoperitoneum. Journal of Reproductive Medicine 21: 45–47.

Garry R 2000 Towards evidence based laparoscopic entry techniques: clinical problems and dilemmas. Gynaecological Endoscopy 8: 315–326.

Garry R, Fountain J, Mason S et al 2004 The eVALuate study: two parallel randomised trials, one comparing laparoscopic with abdominal hysterectomy, the other comparing laparoscopic with vaginal hysterectomy. BMJ (Clinical Research ed.) 328: 129.

Hasson HM 1971 A modified instrument and method for laparoscopy. American Journal of Obstetrics and Gynecology 110: 886–887.

Hope R 1937 The differential diagnosis of ectopic pregnancy in peritoneoscopy. Surgery, Gynecology and Obstetrics 64: 229–234.

Jacobaeus HC 1910 Uber due Moglichkeil die Zystoskopie bei Untersuchlung seroser Hohlungen anzerwerden. Munchener Medizinische Wochenschrift 57: 2090–2092.

Phillips G, Garry R, Kumar C, Reich H 1999 How much gas is required for initial insufflation at laparoscopy? Gynaecological Endoscopy 8: 369–374.

Pickersgill A, Slade RJ, Falconer GF, Attwood S 1999 Open laparoscopy: the way forward. BJOG: an International Journal of Obstetrics and Gynaecology 106: 1116–1119.

Reich H, DeCaprio J, McGlynn F 1989 Laparoscopic hysterectomy. Journal of Gynecologic Surgery 5: 213–216.

Steptoe PC 1967 Laparoscopy in Gynaecology. E&S Livingstone, Edinburgh.

Sutton CJG, Ewen SP, Whitelaw N, Haines P 1994 Prospective, randomised, double-blind controlled trial of laser laparoscopy in the treatment of pelvic pain associated with minimal, mild, and moderate endometriosis. Fertility and Sterility 62: 696–700.

Veress J 1938 Neues instrument fur ausfuhrung von brust-oder brachpunktionen und pneumothoraxbehandlung. Deutsche Medizinische Wochenschrift 104: 1480–1481.

von Ott D 1901 Ventroscopic illumination of the abdominal cavity in pregnancy. Zhurnal Akrestierstova I Zhenskikh Boloznei 15: 7–8.

Wood G, Maher P, Hill D 1994 Current states of laparoscopic associated hysterectomy. Gynaecological Endoscopy 3: 75–84.

Yao M, Tulandi T 1997 Current status of surgical and nonsurgical management of ectopic pregnancy. Fertility and Sterility 67: 421–433.

Zollikoffer R 1924 Zur Laparoskopie. Schwizerische Medizinische Wochenschrift 15: 264–265.

CHAPTER 4

Diathermy and lasers

Priya Agrawal and Fiona Reid

Chapter Contents			
INTRODUCTION	48	CONCLUSIONS	58
DIATHERMY	48	KEY POINTS	58
LASERS	52		

Introduction

For many years, diathermy was the technique of choice for tissue resection and destruction in both gynaecology and general surgery. The advent of the laser in the 1960s threatened this supremacy, but, during the last decade, advances in diathermy have led to a more balanced position between the two modalities. The aim of this chapter is to briefly explain the operation of these instruments, tissue effects, common system types, some of the safety aspects involved and practical clinical use of both techniques in gynaecology.

Diathermy

Diathermy has been used in surgical procedures for over 100 years (d'Arsonval 1893) for cutting and coagulation of tissues. Harvey Cushing pioneered the use of electrosurgery in neurosurgery, using a generator designed by Bovie in the 1920s, and this name is still synonymous with diathermy to some surgeons.

Although diathermy is still a much-used tool in surgical practice, few surgeons have received formal training in its use. Operating theatres will often have a variety of diathermy units for which 'standard' settings are used without reference to the operating conditions. In conventional open surgery, this has only presented a few hazards. The development of laparoscopic and hysteroscopic surgery has greatly increased the number of applications for electrosurgery and has presented new dangers. Only by having an understanding of the principles of this energy source will surgeons avoid the risk of injury to the patient, theatre staff and themselves.

Electrosurgery refers to both types of diathermy, monopolar or bipolar, in which current passes through the patient's tissue. In monopolar diathermy, the active electrode and return electrode are some distance apart. In bipolar diathermy, the two electrodes are only millimetres apart. Electrocautery refers to the use of a heating element in which no current passes through the patient.

Monopolar diathermy

In monopolar diathermy, one electrode is applied to the patient who becomes part of the circuit. The surface area of the electrode plate is much greater than the contact area of the diathermy instrument to ensure that heating effects are confined to the end of the active electrode (Figure 4.1). The advantage of monopolar diathermy is that it can be used to cut as well as to coagulate tissues.

Tissue effects of diathermy

When household electrical current of 50 Hz frequency passes through the body, it causes an irreversible depolarization of cell membranes. If the current is sufficiently large, depolarization of cardiac muscles will occur and death may result. If household current is modified to a higher frequency, above 200 Hz, depolarization does not occur; instead, ions are excited to produce a thermal effect. This is the basis of diathermy. Figure 4.2 illustrates how the frequency of a current influences the effects on the body.

Factors which influence the effect of diathermy

- Diathermy current
  - Current density
  - Size of the current
- Current waveform
  - Cutting and coagulation current
- Type of tissue
  - Tissue moisture
- Duration of application
- Size and shape of diathermy electrode

Diathermy current

The amount of damage or thermal injury that diathermy produces is determined by the current density and the size of the current.

DOI: 10.1016/B978-0-7020-3120-5.00004-7

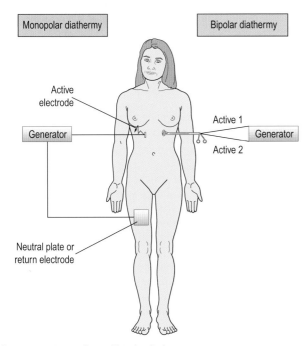

Figure 4.1 Monopolar and bipolar diathermy systems.

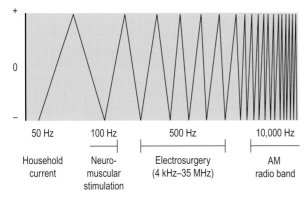

Figure 4.2 Current frequency spectrum.

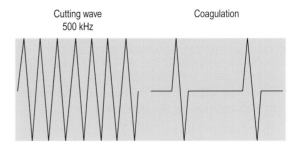

Figure 4.3 Cutting and coagulation waveforms.

approach allows for control of this voltage (voltage regulation).

The resistance of tissue varies particularly with its water content. Dry tissue has high resistance and moist tissue has lower resistance. Thus, during diathermy of an area of tissue, it is desiccated by the thermal effect and its resistance will increase. To prevent the current flow from falling, some modern electrosurgical units will increase the voltage output. The surgeon should be aware of this because there are additional hazards to working with higher voltages. Insulation failure, capacitance coupling and direct coupling are all more likely with a higher voltage.

Cutting and coagulation

Coagulation and cutting can be achieved by changing the area of contact or the waveform of the current. The cutting waveform is a low-voltage, higher frequency current but the area of contact is the main factor and a cutting effect is achieved when the cutting electrode is not quite in contact with the tissue so that an electrical arc is formed. This causes the water in the cells to vaporize and the cells to explode as they come into contact with the arc. The power and current levels will rise when cutting takes place inside a liquid-filled, relatively non-conductive cavity such as the bladder or uterus. The surgeon must be aware that if the resistance increases when using cutting current (e.g. when cutting through the cervix with a wire loop), some generators will produce a higher voltage to maintain current flow against the increased resistance.

When the electrode is brought into direct contact with tissue and the waveform is modulated, coagulation occurs rather than vaporization. An intermittent waveform is used and thus bursts of thermal energy are interspersed with periods of no energy (Figure 4.3). For the power delivered to the tissue to remain constant, the electrosurgical unit must deliver a higher voltage to compensate for the episodes when no energy is delivered (up to 90% of the time with pure coagulation current). Thus, whilst cutting current at 50 W power will produce a high-frequency current of approximately 200–1000 V, a coagulation current may produce over 3000 V to deliver the same wattage to the tissue. The coagulating effect is produced by slower desiccation and shrinkage of adjacent tissue, producing haemostasis. The higher voltage produced by coagulation current carries a higher risk of inadvertent discharge of energy.

If a mixture of the two types of waveform is employed, the advantages of both techniques are exploited. This is normally termed 'blended' output and many combinations are possible.

The current density at the tip of a needle electrode will be very high because the current is concentrated into a small point. The plate used for the return electrode in monopolar diathermy has a large surface area of contact, resulting in a much lower current density. Any thermal effect will therefore be widely dissipated. This highlights the need for the whole surface of the plate to be attached securely to the body. If the plate becomes partially detached, the current density will be greater in the remaining attached part and a burn may result.

The size of the current is influenced by the voltage potential and the resistance to current flow according to the following equation:

$$\text{Current (amps)} = \text{potential (volts)/impedance or tissue resistance (ohms)}$$

Turning up the power output of an electrosurgical unit will increase the size of the diathermy current if the resistance remains constant. Some electrosurgical units can automatically alter the voltage potential to keep the current constant if the resistance changes; however, an alternative design

Type of tissue

Tissue moisture is the major factor affecting tissue resistance; the higher the moisture content, the lower the resistance and the higher the current flow. The cervix in a postmenopausal woman will have lower water content than that of a young nulliparous woman. A lower wattage will be required to perform a loop biopsy in the latter case.

Duration of application

The longer the duration of application of electrosurgical current, the greater the extent of thermal injury. Research on uterine tissue shows that the duration of exposure of the tissue to current, rather than the wattage used, was the most important factor in producing tissue damage (Duffy et al 1991).

Size and shape of the diathermy electrode

The smaller the point of contact, the greater the current density. Thus, if the points of diathermy scissors are brought close to tissue, a cutting effect will result, whilst if the convex part of the scissor blades is used, a lower current density will result in a coagulating effect. Similarly, when using a wire loop to biopsy the cervix, the thickness of the wire or the diameter of the loop will influence the current. A thicker wire will need a higher current than a finer wire to produce a cutting effect because of the lower current density.

Heat and tissue injury

Diathermy current produces thermal injury to tissues. The temperature generated will dictate the degree of injury (Table 4.1). If carbon is seen on the tip of the diathermy electrode, the surgeon can assume that, at some stage, a temperature of 200 °C has been reached.

Bipolar diathermy

In bipolar diathermy, the current flows between two electrodes positioned a short distance apart because both contacts are on the surgical instrument. Lower power is employed since high power would damage the tips of the instrument. This is safer because the current flow is limited to a small area and lower power is used, but a cutting effect cannot be achieved. These features encourage some surgeons to employ bipolar diathermy exclusively in the laparoscopic environment. However, there is still a small risk of aberrant current flow because the patient, table and diathermy machine are all earthed. In addition, the tissue temperatures

are much higher (340 °C) and this factor alone can cause unexpected effects.

Bipolar current produces tissue desiccation and has been used commonly in tubal sterilization. More recently, in laparoscopic surgery, its value in coagulating major vascular pedicles has led to its use in laparoscopic hysterectomy and laparoscopic salpingectomy for ectopic pregnancy. The lower power employed also leads to less heat spread to adjacent tissues, which reduces the risk of injury to nearby delicate structures. Engineers are endeavouring to produce reliable bipolar dissectors and scissors to compete with the range of monopolar diathermy instruments available.

Instruments are now available which coagulate a pedicle with bipolar current and utilize a non-electrosurgical blade to cut the pedicle. These instruments are often referred to as tripolar instruments, although this is a misnomer.

Bipolar instrumentation has also been introduced into hysteroscopic surgery. A bipolar electrode may be employed in the outpatient setting for the removal of endometrial polyps. The distension medium used with these devices is saline rather than glycine. Saline is isotonic and therefore reduces the risk of fluid overload associated with a hypotonic solution such as glycine.

Short-wave diathermy

Electrode redesign has led to an interest in the use of short-wave diathermy for its tissue destructive effect (Phipps et al 1990). It has been used in endometrial ablation. In this, the two electrodes form a capacitor in the output circuit with the patient providing the dielectric medium between the two plates. Frequencies of approximately 27 MHz are employed with power levels of approximately 500 W. By altering the shape and size of the electrodes, heating effects may be localized or diffused as required. However, care must be exercised as the effects are not always predictable.

Diathermy safety

Three major safety issues with the use of monopolar diathermy have become apparent with the evolution of electrosurgery in laparoscopic surgery. Each of them involves inadvertent discharge of diathermy current. These issues are:

- insulation failure;
- direct coupling; and
- capacitive coupling.

Insulation failure

Defects in insulation are most likely to cause a discharge of current when higher power is employed. The use of coagulation current carries a greater risk than cutting current. Insulation failure can occur at any point from the electrosurgical unit to the active electrode. The most common site of failure is in the instrument that contains the active electrode. With conventional surgical instruments, the most common site is the joint on diathermy graspers where repeated use wears away the insulation material. Any insulation breakdown, seen as sparks from the joint area, is usually clearly visible because the whole instrument is within the surgeon's field of view. This contrasts with laparoscopic surgery where the field of view is much smaller and only a small part of the

Table 4.1 The degree of injury caused at different temperatures

Temperature (°C)	Tissue effect
44	Necrosis
70	Coagulation
90	Desiccation
200	Carbonization

instrument containing the active electrode may be visible. Repeated discharges from a break in the insulation may occur without the surgeon being aware. Damage to insulation most commonly occurs when moving an instrument through the laparoscopic port. Although the port valve may cause damage, the most likely cause is scraping against the sharp edge of the inner end of the port, particularly one constructed of metal.

Concern about insulation failure has fuelled the debate about disposable and reusable instruments. Disposable instruments clearly have an advantage in that the insulation sheath does not have to withstand both repeated use and repeated cleaning cycles. However, disposable instruments are built to much less robust specifications and the insulating material may not withstand harsh treatment in a long case. It is important that surgeons and theatre nurses are constantly vigilant for evidence of trauma to insulation, and reusable instruments must be checked on a regular basis both during and between cases.

Whilst a metal port may cause more trauma to the instruments passing through it, it will allow discharge of diathermy current in the event of insulation failure. The large area of port contact with the skin should enable the current to be dissipated without serious thermal injury. A plastic port would not facilitate such a discharge and the current might therefore flow to adjacent bowel, causing damage that may not be recognized at the time. Sigmoid colon is the most vulnerable piece of bowel because of its proximity to a left lateral port. If a metal port cannula is used, a plastic retaining sleeve must not be used because this prevents any discharged diathermy current passing through the skin back to the ground plate.

Direct coupling

Direct coupling involves the transmission of diathermy current from one instrument to another. Many surgeons use direct coupling to coagulate small vessels which have been grasped with a small forceps, when opening a wound for example. The diathermy instrument is then placed against the small forceps and the pedal pressed. Such a practice carries a real risk of a diathermy burn to the surgeon or assistant. If the surgeon's glove has a perforation, the diathermy current may flow through the surgeon to ground either through the feet or through contact with the operating table. The surgeon should also be aware that theatre gowns do not provide insulation against high-frequency diathermy current.

The risk of direct coupling will be reduced in laparoscopic surgery if insulated instruments alone are used when diathermy is employed. Since many instruments, such as needle holders, are not commonly produced with insulation, this may restrict instrument choice. The risk of direct coupling to a metal port is increased when the working part of the laparoscopic instrument is large. The surgeon must always try to keep the whole of the metal part visible when using diathermy so that any inadvertent discharge will be seen.

Capacitive coupling

The concept of capacitive coupling is new to most gynaecologists. A capacitor consists of two conductors separated by an insulator. A metal instrument surrounded by an insulated sheath passing through a metal port is a capacitor. When a current passes through the instrument, a capacitive current may develop in the metal port, particularly if it is insulated from the skin. The higher the current passing through the instrument, the greater the capacitive current. If the port is insulated from the skin (by a plastic sleeve), capacitive current may be discharged to adjacent bowel, causing thermal injury. In common with insulation failure, the sigmoid colon is most vulnerable to capacitive current injury due to its proximity to a left lateral port.

A capacitive current can also develop in a gloved hand holding a non-insulated instrument through which diathermy current is passed. This risk is greater if the hand is moist and there is contact between the surgeon and the operating table or the floor.

Other safety issues

Current flow to adjacent organs

The current will follow the path of least resistance, and, if a non-target tissue such as bowel lies in contact with target tissue, the current will flow through the tissue with least impedence. In addition, the impedence will rise as the target vessels desiccate, and the current may then flow to an alternative earth, usually but not necessarily in contact with the pedicle. If the current flows through bowel, damage will result which may not be recognized at the time.

Surgical clothing

Operating theatre gowns do not provide insulation against high-frequency electrosurgical currents. This means that there is always a risk of discharge of electrosurgical current through to the operating table.

Operating theatre footwear used to provide 'antistatic' protection. Antistatic theatre shoes were used to prevent build-up of static electricity, which could spark and ignite volatile anaesthetic gases. Since such agents are no longer employed in anaesthesia, there is no need for antistatic footwear. Non-antistatic footwear will generally provide higher resistance between the surgeon and ground, and will therefore reduce the risk of discharge through the surgeon to ground.

Electrosurgical unit

The surgeon should be familiar with the electrosurgical unit in the theatre. Many departments have different units available with different settings and features. The power delivered by a numerical setting may vary greatly in different machines. Many units divide the power output in settings from 1 to 10. Position 5 in one unit may represent a different power output to position 5 in another unit. In addition, there will not always be equal differences between the unit settings, so there may be a different change in output between positions 1 and 2 than between positions 8 and 9. Modern units have overcome this hazard by indicating the power setting on a digital display.

Changes in electrosurgical unit

Prior to 1970, all electrosurgical units had a 'grounded design' which provided numerous potential alternative pathways for the discharge of diathermy current to ground, e.g. electrocardiogram leads. In 1970, isolated electrosurgery units were introduced. This meant that the ground electrode discharge returned to the electrosurgical unit. Thus, the whole circuit of electrosurgical current passed through the unit. Whilst this arrangement reduced the risk of inappropriate grounding routes, it did not solve the risk of burns from poor contact of the ground electrode with the patient. Poor contact leads to the development of high current density areas and a subsequent heating effect.

After 1980, some electrosurgical units employed a return electrode monitoring system, which detects failure of contact of the return electrode. Return electrode burns will be significantly reduced with this system.

Since 1990, the growth of minimal access surgery has increased the risk of inadvertent discharge from the active electrode through insulation failure or capacitive coupling. The Active Electrode Monitoring system now marketed by Encision provides an additional protective shield on the active electrode instrument, which picks up discharge of current from any point other than the active part of the electrode and inactivates the unit if such current is detected.

Electrosurgical equipment set-up

It is critically important to be certain that the diathermy ground plate is securely attached in the correct position. Whilst modern machines will give a warning signal when the plate is incorrectly attached, many machines will function if there is partial attachment. Partial attachment may lead to severe burns.

The positioning of the diathermy leads to and from the operating table needs care and attention. Capacitance current can develop alongside the diathermy lead delivering current to the active electrode anywhere along its length. Diathermy leads should not be secured with metal clips to the theatre gowns covering the patients.

Theatre staff must be trained in the use of electrosurgical equipment. Protocols should be in place regarding who attaches the equipment and who switches the machine on. If a patient's position is changed during the course of an operation, the electrosurgical unit should be switched off prior to the move, and the attachment of the ground electrode should be checked after repositioning.

Risk of fire/explosion

Flammable materials should not be used for skin preparation in gynaecological surgery. Theatre gowns can soak up such solutions which may also pool in the vagina or under the buttocks. Fires have been reported caused by sparks from diathermy current igniting flammable cleansing material.

Pacemakers

Monopolar diathermy should be avoided in patients with internal or external catheter pacemakers. There is a risk of inducing a rhythm disturbance, damage to the device or even electrical burns around the device. If monopolar diathermy is used, short bursts in the cutting mode are advisable. The pacemaker should not lie in the pathway of the diathermy current, but this will not guarantee safety as it is known that radiofrequency current can radiate away from a straight pathway. The electrosurgical unit should be placed as far away from the pacemaker as possible because of the risk of 'noise' from the generator. When diathermy is required, a bipolar instrument should be used whenever possible.

Neuromodulators

Implanted neuromodulators are being increasingly employed for the treatment of lower urinary and lower gastrointestinal tract dysfunction. Monopolar or bipolar diathermy should not be employed when these devices have been implanted without consultation with the manufacturer. Similarly, deep brain stimulators may be implanted to treat patients with Parkinson's disease.

Keloid scarring

Keloid scarring has high tissue resistance so the diathermy ground electrode should not be placed over an area of keloid.

Joint prostheses

The joint prosthesis most commonly encountered by a gynaecologist is in the hip joint. If the prosthesis is unilateral, the diathermy ground plate should be sited on the opposite side. If bilateral prostheses are present, the ground plate should be placed on the flank. If a ground plate is sited over a prosthesis, current may be concentrated through the prosthesis in a preferential pathway and also in the tissue between the plate and the prosthesis, and a thermal injury may occur.

Lasers

A laser is a device capable of producing near-parallel beams of monochromatic light, either visible or invisible, at controlled intensities. This light can be focused, thus concentrating its energy, so that it can be utilized to treat various conditions. The term 'laser' is an acronym for 'Light Amplification by the Stimulated Emission of Radiation'. The process of stimulated emission was foreshadowed by Einstein at the turn of the century, but it was not until 1960 that the first optical device was constructed (Maiman 1960). Since that time, many lasers have been made but comparatively few have found their way into gynaecological practice.

Basic laser physics

A laser consists of three main elements: a power supply, an excitable medium and an optical resonator (Figure 4.4). Atoms or molecules within the medium are raised to high-energy states (Figure 4.5A) by the power supply, and, under normal circumstances, these would decay to the ground state by the emission of energy as photons (Figure 4.5B). By confining the process to an optical cavity and restricting the decay paths, stimulated emission (Figure 4.5C) can take place. This process produces a build-up of photons (light) at a particular wavelength inside the cavity. The laser output is a small fraction of this which is allowed to escape from one end of the cavity.

Many substances have been found to be suitable laser media — solids, liquids, gases or metallic vapours — but the basic principles remain the same. A more detailed explanation of laser physics is provided elsewhere (Carruth and McKenzie 1986).

The radiation emitted is monochromatic (if only one decay path is involved), coherent and collimated. Collimation, or the near-parallel nature of laser light, can be exploited in many ways and is the main feature which makes such devices useful in the medical world. A single convex lens placed in the beam will bring it to a sharp focus, the size of which is dependent upon the width of the collimated beam. The use of different lenses or varying the lens-to-tissue distance alters the diameter of the beam at the point of contact with the tissue (Figure 4.6). This is referred to as changing the spot size.

The most important determinant of the effects of a laser upon tissue is the power density. This can be calculated approximately as:

$$PD = 100 \times W/D^2 \ [W/cm^2]$$

where PD is power density, W is power output in watts and D is the effective diameter of the spot in millimetres. D can be measured by firing a short low-power pulse at a suitable target. The power density can be altered by changing either the power or the spot size, but the latter has the greater effect.

Light–tissue interaction

Light impinging on tissue is subject to the normal laws of physics. Some of the light is reflected and some is trans-

mitted through the air–tissue barrier and passes into the tissue where it is scattered or absorbed. Obviously the extent to which each process dominates is dependent upon the physical properties of the light and the tissue. The theory of light–tissue interaction is not as well developed as that of ionizing radiation (Wall et al 1988), but enough is known to explain the macroeffects upon which most laser treatments depend.

At very-low-energy density levels (power density × time), say below 4 J/cm², a stimulating effect on cells has been observed, but above this level, the effect is reversed and suppression occurs (Mester et al 1968). As the energy density rises to 40 J/cm², indirect cell damage can take place if any sensitizing agents present become activated (e.g. haematoporphyrin derivative). Direct tissue damage does not take place until approximately 400 J/cm², when the first thermal effects appear and photocoagulation occurs. Another 10-fold increase in energy density results in complete tissue destruction as it is sufficient to raise the cell temperature rapidly to 100°C, causing tissue vaporization. Obviously these are general observations and other properties of the incident beam will have an influence, but the general 10-fold relationship alluded to above holds although other parameters may be varied. Amongst the most important of these are

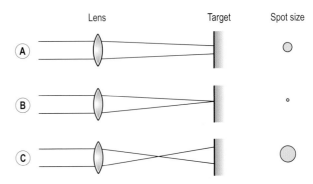

Figure 4.6 Changing the focal length of the focusing lens while keeping the lens-to-tissue distance constant alters the spot size, the diameter of the beam at the point of contact with the tissue. (A) The focal length of the lens is greater than the lens-to-tissue distance. (B) The focal length of the lens is the same as the lens-to-tissue distance, i.e. the laser is focused on the tissue. (C) The focal length of the lens is less than the lens-to-tissue distance.

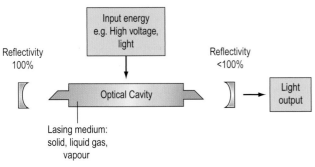

Figure 4.4 Typical laser systems.

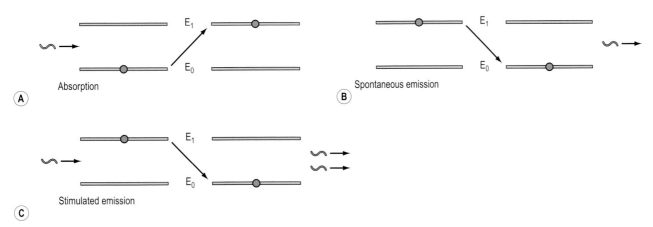

Figure 4.5 Basic atomic processes. (A) Absorption of a photon of energy. (B) Spontaneous emission of a photon. (C) Stimulated emission of an additional photon of energy. ～, photon; E_0, lower energy state; E_1, higher energy state; ●, particle.

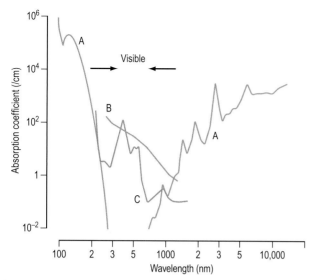

Figure 4.7 Absorption characteristics of (A) water, (B) melanin and (C) haemoglobin at different wavelengths.

Source: With kind permission from Springer Science+Business Media: Lasers in Medical Science, Photophysical processes in recent medical laser developments: a review, 1:47–66, 1986, Boulnois J.

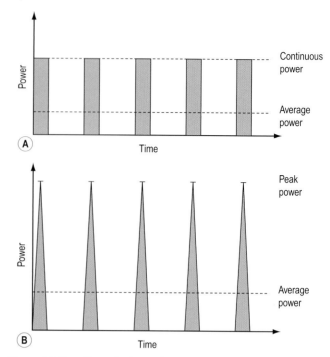

Figure 4.8 The effects of pulse irradiation.

the wavelength and the pulsatile nature of the radiation involved.

The wavelength absorption characteristics of various body tissues are reasonably well understood, qualitatively if not quantitatively. Figure 4.7 shows the absorption curves for water, melanin and haemoglobin which, to a large extent, will determine the curves for tissue as a whole. In the ultra-violet and the middle-to-far infrared spectrum, absorption by water predominates whereas melanin and haemoglobin effects take over in the visible range. From this graph, it is easy to see that a particular laser, operating at a fixed wavelength, will be preferentially absorbed by one tissue constituent and its effects will be different from those of another laser with a different wavelength.

So far, it is implied that the laser is operated continuously for long enough for thermal effects to appear [continuous wave (CW) mode]. However, it is relatively simple, by means of a shutter or a controllable power supply, to switch the energy on and off rapidly (pulse mode). In general, the medical definition of a pulse is a burst of energy lasting 0.25 s or less. This does not correspond to the physics definition of a pulse, and care must be taken to avoid confusion. Methods of generating these pulses differ between lasers and the tissue effects can also vary. The reason for this phenomenon is shown in Figure 4.8.

Figure 4.8A shows the output from a CW laser which is modulated by a perfect shutter. The average power delivered to the tissue can be calculated from a knowledge of the CW power, the pulse repetition rate and width. In the case of an electronically controlled high-pulse power system where the time–power curve is not so closely defined (Figure 4.8B), it is much more difficult to determine the average power delivered. It is necessary to measure the energy of the pulse and the pulse repetition rate. The peak power, although impressive, is almost irrelevant.

The effects on tissue of this pulsatile radiation are to reduce the pure thermal effects (lower average power input) whilst maintaining and sometimes enhancing the vaporization potential. Provided the pulse repetition rate is sufficiently low to allow heat dissipation to take place between pulses, the tissue temperature will stabilize at a lower value. These effects are analogous to those induced by modulation in diathermy output which leads to the differences between cutting and coagulation diathermy referred to earlier.

Very short pulses, such as those produced by Q-switched lasers, can cause electromechanical breakdown in tissues because of the extremely high energy densities obtainable. In the early days, these lasers were tested in gynaecology but untoward side-effects were noted (Minton et al 1965).

Common laser systems

Two laser systems established themselves in gynaecological practice during the 1980s:

- the carbon dioxide (CO_2) laser; and
- the neodymium:yttrium aluminium garnet (Nd:YAG) laser.

These will be described in detail, with a further section devoted to other types of laser which are now entering general usage after extensive research.

Carbon dioxide laser

This is the system which has been most used in gynaecology since it was used for the first time in 1973 for the treatment of cervical erosions. This has been because of its clinical stability, ease of use, reliability and easy serviceability. It is a precise laser, especially in ultrapulse mode, making it useful for division of adhesions and accurate and safe vaporization of deposits of endometriosis (Sutton 1993). Although a major drawback is that its output cannot be transmitted by fibres, it has so far not been totally displaced by other lasers but is rivalled by modern diathermy equipment.

As the name implies, the active lasing medium is CO_2 gas. Efficiencies of 15% energy conversion to light output have been achieved. In fact, an analyser has used this ability to detect CO_2 in the breath! The first generation of CO_2 lasers used a flowing gas system with high-voltage direct current excitation. A gas mixture of CO_2, nitrogen and helium has been used to help achieve and maintain lasing conditions. Sealed tube lasers are now available with radiofrequency low-voltage discharges being used for excitation. This has made the machines smaller and removed the need for gas bottles.

The output radiation of 10.6 μm wavelength is well into the infrared region of the spectrum. This radiation is absorbed rapidly by tissue water, and therefore cuts and vaporizes more easily than it coagulates. Most of the incident radiation is absorbed within approximately 0.03 mm of the surface and intense heating occurs. Coagulation will only take place in small blood vessels less than 0.5 mm in diameter, but haemostasis can be facilitated by reducing the power density so that the zone of thermal damage around the central crater is wider.

As the 10.6 μm laser is invisible, an aiming beam must be used so that the operator can see where the therapeutic beam is going to have its effect. A helium–neon (HeNe) laser emitting at 628 nm (red) is incorporated into the system and optically aligned so that it coincides with the therapeutic beam. This alignment can degenerate and should be checked regularly.

As yet, there is no commercially available fibre which can transmit 10.6 μm light efficiently, so most commercial systems use some form of articulated arm. At each joint, there is a mirror which is adjusted so that the beam stays central despite movement between the two adjacent limbs of the arm. The choice of the mirror material is limited because of the need to reflect both the infrared CO_2 beam and the red HeNe aiming beam. It is possible to use waveguide delivery systems to avoid the use of mirrors, but this limits the manoeuvrability of the complete system.

The final delivery to the operation site can be carried out in two ways, both incorporating a focusing lens. For hand-held surgery, the lens at the end of a straight delivery tube focuses the beam on the operative field approximately 1 cm from the end of the tube. The lens-to-tissue distance can thus be varied at will so that the spot size will be changed within a narrow range (Figure 4.9A). Colposcopic delivery involves a mirror after the focusing lens which brings the beam into line with the viewing axis of the colposcope. This mirror is at the end of a joystick so that the beam may be moved around within the field of view (Figure 4.9B). Originally the spot size was changed using lenses of different focal lengths and so was limited to three or four predetermined sizes. Nowadays, the use of zoom optics allows infinite adjustment over a limited range (0.5–4 mm).

Power outputs of these lasers can be from a few watts up to 100 W continuous. Most commercial systems in gynaecology produce up to 25–35 W as this, coupled with a variable spot size, provides power densities of up to 6000 W/cm², sufficient for tissue cutting and vaporization at a controllable rate. The extra power provided by instruments producing 40–60 W is useful for dealing with patients who bleed during the procedure. Higher peak powers are available with modulation being employed to keep tissue temperatures within acceptable limits but with 'cleaner' cuts.

Neodymium:yttrium aluminium garnet laser

This device is a solid-state laser with the active neodymium ions being incorporated in an artificial crystal YAG. Pumping is achieved by energy input from a parallel gas discharge lamp, usually a water-cooled krypton tube, with the output radiation being refocused into the laser crystal. Output power levels up to 100 W continuous can be achieved, but, with a conversion efficiency of 1% or so, nearly 10 kW of input power is needed.

The energy produced is at a wavelength of 1.06 μm and is thus in the near-infrared. As such, it can be transmitted easily down a flexible fibreoptic delivery system and delivered to

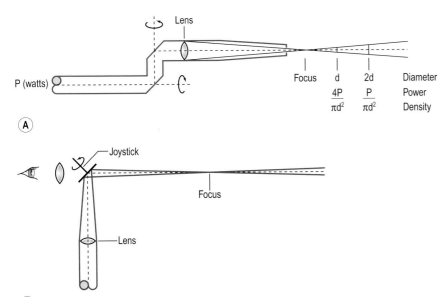

Figure 4.9 Laser delivery systems. (A) Hand-held. (B) Colposcopically controlled.

many more anatomical sites than the CO_2 laser. The emergent radiation has lost its collimation and will diverge quite rapidly. Most fibres have a coaxial flow of gas, usually CO_2, to keep debris away from the end of the fibre. This is particularly necessary where contamination with blood or blood products may make continuous operation difficult.

As with the CO_2 laser, 1.06 μm Nd:YAG radiation is invisible. An HeNe laser (or other light source) needs to be incorporated into the device as an aiming beam. This is also a very useful safety feature as near-infrared radiation can cause irreparable damage to the retina. The Nd:YAG laser is easy to operate as a Q-switched laser. An optoelectronic switch is incorporated inside the laser cavity and the lasing action is prevented for a large percentage of the time. The photon energy therefore builds up to an even higher level than normal, and when the switch is eventually opened, a massive pulse of energy is delivered. The switch can then be closed and the process repeated. This type of action has found a use in ophthalmology where, by focusing the pulse to a very small spot, electromechanical breakdown of tissue can be induced with minimal surrounding damage.

The Nd:YAG laser has a greater depth of penetration and is more suited to hysteroscopic surgery (Sutton 1993). Hysteroscopic procedures include removal of fibroids and polyps, transsection of uterine septae, lysis of adhesions and endometrial ablation.

Other laser systems

Many other laser systems are used in medicine and the time period from research to common usage seems to be getting shorter. It is neither possible nor desirable to give a complete list, but some of the following examples have potential benefits for gynaecological surgery.

Metal vapour lasers

As their name implies, metal vapour lasers consist of a container filled with a heated and vaporized metal in an inert gas atmosphere at low pressure. The electrical discharge used must be pulsed because the necessary conditions cannot be sustained long enough for true CW operation to take place. Two types of metal vapour laser have found a use in medicine — copper and gold. The copper vapour laser produces two beams at 510 and 578 nm at up to 25 W power output. These by themselves are not particularly useful, although the green can be used as a substitute for the argon laser in dermatology. The output is ideally suited to act as an optical pumping source for a dye laser, which can be tuned to provide radiation for photodynamic therapy.

Photodynamic therapy

Photodynamic therapy is a treatment for certain tumours (Spikes and Jori 1987). It relies upon selective retention in tumour tissues of a drug (photosensitizer), such as haematoporphyrin derivative, which only becomes active on exposure to light of a particular wavelength. This provides highly selective tissue necrosis. Each photosensitizer has a particular spectrum of action requiring light of the appropriate wavelength for maximum absorption and effect. Clinically used sensitizers work between 420 nm (blue) and 780 nm (deep red). Longer wavelengths penetrate deeper (blue 1–2 mm and red >5 mm). As there are many decay pathways

available, the output is multi-wavelength, but a narrow wavelength range can be selected with suitable optical devices. The copper vapour and dye laser combination can produce over 5 W of red light at 630 mm, which is an absorption peak of haematoporphyrin derivative.

The other metal vapour device is the gold laser. The output of this is at 627.8 nm, a close match to the dye laser, without the added complication of two devices in series.

Argon laser

The argon laser, producing light at 488 nm (blue) and 514.5 nm (blue/green), is particularly favoured by ophthalmologists. The green output of the KTP laser (potassium titanyl-phosphate, 532 nm) has been more useful in gynaecology. The output is derived by taking the Nd:YAG beam and frequency and doubling it in a KTP crystal, thus providing the surgeon with a choice of wavelengths (or even a mixture of the two). The advantages of the light lasers, argon and KTP lasers, over the CO_2 laser is their selective absorption by haemoglobin, less smoke plume production and an easy delivery system that uses lower power settings. They have been considered to be more suitable for treatment of ovarian endometriomas and ectopic pregnancies, as the CO_2 laser energy is strongly absorbed by the water molecule and is rendered ineffective in the presence of blood (Sutton 1993). The main disadvantage of the light lasers is the need to wear special protective glasses which can distort the view of the pelvis.

Ultraviolet lasers

Research into ultraviolet lasers has produced systems which seem to rely on non-thermal mechanisms for tissue destruction. These are the excimer lasers, a term derived from 'excited dimmer', where the active medium is made from a combination of two substances which do not normally combine, such as a rare gas and a halide. These lasers have found a place in ophthalmology, and their potential for precise tissue removal offers the microsurgeon a very powerful tool.

The early use of lasers in gynaecology was in the treatment of cervical intraepithelial neoplasia, but subsequently spread to most other areas of the lower reproductive tract. The use of the laser in treatment of intraepithelial neoplasia of the genital tract is described in Chapter 38. Similar diathermy techniques are described in the same chapter.

We are under pressure to decrease health costs, so alternative, less-expensive technology has reduced the use of laser technology in recent years. However, lasers are still used in various clinical settings in obstetric and gynaecological surgery. Some examples include intrauterine laser ablation of placental vessels for the treatment of twin–twin transfusion syndrome (Robyr et al 2005), and ovarian drilling for ovulation induction in patients with anovulatory polycystic ovary syndrome (Farquhar et al 2007). Other uses are being investigated, but the evidence on safety and efficacy outcomes thus far is insufficient to support use in a non-research environment. Examples of these include laparoscopic laser myomectomy and percutaneous laser therapy for fetal tumours. There are also controversial areas regarding the use of lasers which have entered commercial gynaecology without much regulation or scientific evaluation, such as laser vaginal rejuvenation.

Laser safety

All laser systems in current use have no way of distinguishing between patient and operator. The desired effect on a patient can be a serious accident to the surgeon. The subject of the safe construction and operation of lasers in medicine and surgery is thus very important and must be understood by all involved. This section is biased in favour of UK regulations, but the situation is similar in most European countries and the USA, although, of course, regulatory bodies and documents will have different guises.

All lasers sold in the UK must conform to three basic standards. Electrical safety requirements are detailed in BS EN 60601-1-1 (British Standards Institution 2001) and non-ionizing radiation hazards are covered by BS EN 60825-1 and BS EN 60601-2-22 (British Standards Institution 1996, 2007). A further publication by the Medicines and Healthcare Products Regulatory Agency (2008) outlines good laser practice together with some additional equipment safety features. All these publications should be considered by a laser protection adviser (a health authority or trust appointee) who will assist each user in specifying and installing lasers in clinical surroundings. Although the requirements will vary from laser to laser and from site to site, the following sections outline the major considerations involved.

Nature of hazard

The body is divided into two regions for hazard analysis: the eye and the skin. In the visible region, which extends into the near-infrared, the eye is the organ at greatest risk. Outside this range, the eye is no different from the skin, except that corneal damage can lead to visual loss although the retina itself may be undamaged.

Radiation entering the eye is focused on the retina, and the power density can increase by up to 5×10^5 times so that a $50 \ W/m^2$ corneal incident beam can become $25 \ mW/m^2$ on the retina, with disastrous and irreparable results. Maximum permitted exposure levels are laid down by the regulations and are set well below known damage thresholds. Manufacturing and administrative controls are written to prevent operators, assistants and patients from accidentally receiving radiation in excess of these limits. There are separate values for the skin and the eye, with the latter being the more stringent.

Control of hazards

Lasers are currently classified into four groups from Class 1 to 4, with Class 1 being the least hazardous and Class 4 being the most hazardous. Class 3 is also subdivided into two classes, 3A and 3B. It is the manufacturers' responsibility to classify a laser, but, once this is done, it will rarely be changed. Stringent safety precautions must be introduced when Class 3 and 4 lasers are in use. Most medical lasers are Class 3B or 4 and do need such safeguards. Aiming beams are usually Class 1 or 2 and present a minimal hazard.

In addition to classifying the laser, manufacturers must ensure that the equipment complies with the specification for its particular class. Generally all systems will have a key control and some way of monitoring the power being delivered to the patient. It should also indicate, either visually or audibly, when the laser shutter is opened and the maximum permitted exposure is exceeded.

Administrative controls are framed to ensure that the equipment is then used safely. A set of local rules must be drawn up which specify who is allowed to use a laser and where it can be used. A laser controlled area must be defined and the activities within that area must be controlled. There must be no possibility of radiation in excess of the maximum permitted exposure level passing out of the area, even if this means blocking windows and doors. Warning signs must be exhibited at the entrance to the laser controlled area, and door interlocks can be used but are not obligatory. Examples of such local rules can be found in other texts (Stamp 1983, Medicines and Healthcare Products Regulatory Agency 2008).

All personnel within the laser controlled area must either be protected from the radiation by the inherent optical properties of the operating equipment or must wear appropriate spectacles. For example, any common translucent glass is impervious to CO_2 laser radiation. Precautions for the Nd:YAG laser are more complicated, and special eyewear for observers and filters to protect the operator from back-reflection through a delivery system are required. Obviously such devices cannot be used when the aiming beam is derived from the therapeutic beam. In this case, an additional safety shutter is required to protect the surgeon during treatment. Precautions against eye damage must be rigorously implemented for all present, including the patient.

Fire is an ever-present hazard with the use of Class 4 lasers and simple precautions must be observed. Aqueous instead of spirit-based solutions should be used and paper drapes should be avoided. CO_2 radiation is readily absorbed by water, and by keeping swabs soaked in water or saline, tissues adjacent to the operation site can be protected. A suitable fire extinguisher should always be available. Greater care must be exercised in the presence of inflammable anaesthetic gases. Endotracheal tubes have been ignited by a laser with serious results (Bandle and Holyoak 1987). While this situation is not likely to be encountered in gynaecology, inflammable gases may be passed rectally by the patient during laser treatment of the lower genital tract, posing a theoretical risk of explosion.

A by-product of laser treatment (and diathermy to a certain extent) is a plume of smoke and debris, with a characteristic odour. This must be evacuated and collected from as near as possible to the impact zone for two important reasons. First, the emission of smoke is likely to obscure the operating site. This is particularly true in cervical or vaginal surgery. Second, doubts have been raised over the viability of particles contained within the plume (Garden et al 1988). Although the evidence is not overwhelming, it is essential that the smoke should be adequately extracted and filtered.

Unintentional reflections of the laser beam striking an instrument can be dangerous. Although it is very unlikely that radiation reflected in this way will be sufficiently focused to cause damage, it is sensible to ensure that the instruments are not highly polished and scatter any incident radiation. It should not be assumed that the reflecting qualities of a surface are the same at visible and far-infrared wavelengths, so care should be exercised in the choice of speculae and other operating instruments.

Conclusions

Diathermy techniques have improved markedly and have replaced laser techniques developed in the 1970s and 1980s on economic grounds. However, there is still a place for the use of lasers in gynaecology, particularly as new devices are made available and as yet unknown light–tissue interactions are discovered and exploited. Interactions between light, tissue and drugs hold much promise.

KEY POINTS

1. Monopolar diathermy uses electric currents to cut or coagulate. Bipolar diathermy can only be used for coagulation; however, bipolar cutting devices are in development.

2. Great care must be taken to prevent accidental burns during diathermy use. Current can flow to organs not in direct contact with the active electrode.

3. Insulation failure, direct coupling and capacitive coupling are the three major safety issues in the use of diathermy.

4. Lasers produce near-parallel beams of monochromatic light.

5. The beam can be focused by a lens to alter the diameter of the beam at the point of contact with the tissue (the spot size).

6. The power density is the most important determinant of the effects of the laser upon tissue.

7. The greater the power density, the less the thermal effect and the less the haemostatic property of the beam.

8. The beam of a CO_2 or an Nd:YAG laser is invisible so a guiding HeNe laser is required.

9. The eye must be protected from accidental exposure to laser energy. This is especially important with Nd:YAG endoscopic systems.

References

Bandle AM, Holyoak B 1987 Laser incidents. In: Mosely H, Haywood JK (eds) Medical Laser Safety. Institute of Physical Sciences in Medicine, London, pp 47–57.

Boulnois J 1986 Photophysical processes in recent medical laser developments: a review. Lasers in Medical Science 1: 47–66.

British Standards Institution 1996 Medical Electrical Equipment. Particular Requirements for Safety. Specification for Diagnostic and Therapeutic Laser Equipment. BS EN 60601-2-22. BSI, London.

British Standards Institution 2001 Medical Electrical Equipment. Collateral Standard. Safety Requirements for Medical Electrical Systems. BS EN 60601-1-1. BSI, London.

British Standards Institution 2007 Safety of Laser Products. Equipment Classification and Requirements. BS EN 60825-60821. BSI, London.

Carruth JAS, McKenzie AL 1986 Medical Lasers, Science and Clinical Practice. Adam Hilger, Bristol.

d'Arsonval MA 1893 Production de courants de haute frequence et de grande intensite: leurs effects physiologiques. Comptes Rendus Societe de Biologie 9: 122–124.

Duffy S, Reid PC, Smith JHF, Sharp F 1991 In vitro studies of uterine electrosurgery. Obstetrics and Gynaecology 78: 213–220.

Farquhar C, Lilford RJ, Marjoribanks J, Vandekerckhove P 2007 Laparoscopic 'drilling' by diathermy or laser for ovulation induction in anovulatory polycystic ovary syndrome. Cochrane Database of Systematic Reviews 18: CD001122.

Garden JM, O'Banion MK, Shelnitz LS et al 1988 Papillomavirus in the vapour of carbon dioxide laser treated verrucae. JAMA: the Journal of the American Medical Association 259: 1199–1202.

Maiman TH 1960 Stimulated optical radiation in the ruby. Nature 187: 493–494.

Medicines and Healthcare Products Regulatory Agency 2008 Guidance on the Safe Use of Lasers, IPL Systems and LEDs. MRHA, London.

Mester E, Ludany G, Vajda J et al 1968 Uber die Wirkung von Laser-Strahlen auf die Bakteriemphagozytose der Leukozyten. Acta Biologica et Medica Germanica 21: 317–321.

Minton JP, Carlton DM, Dearman JR et al 1965 An evaluation of the physical response of malignant tumour implants to pulsed laser radiation. Surgery, Gynaecology and Obstetrics 121: 538–544.

Phipps JH, Lewis BV, Roberts T et al 1990 Treatment of functional menorrhagia by radiofrequency-induced thermal endometrial ablation. The Lancet 335: 374–376.

Robyr R, Quarello E, Ville Y 2005 Management of fetofetal transfusion syndrome. Prenatal Diagnosis 25: 795.

Spikes JD, Jori G 1987 Photodynamic therapy of tumours and other diseases using porphyrins. Lasers in Medical Science 2: 3–15.

Stamp JM 1983 An introduction to medical lasers. Clinical Physics and Physiological Measurement 4: 267–290.

Sutton C 1993 Lasers in infertility. Human Reproduction 8: 133–146.

Wall BF, Harrison RM, Spiers FN 1988 Patient Dosimetry Techniques in Diagnostic Radiology. Institute of Physical Sciences in Medicine, York.

CHAPTER 5

Imaging techniques in gynaecology

Nandita deSouza and David Cosgrove

Chapter Contents

INTRODUCTION	59	SAFETY ISSUES	76
METHODOLOGY	59	CONCLUSIONS	77
CLINICAL APPLICATIONS	62	KEY POINTS	77

Introduction

Since the discovery of X-rays by Roentgen in 1895, there has been an explosion in technology for imaging the human body; in addition to ionizing radiation, high-frequency sound (Wade 1999), radiolabelled pharmaceuticals and non-ionizing radiation in strong magnetic fields are used. The parallel expansion in computer technology has enabled the development of cross-sectional imaging using computed tomographic (CT) techniques, and three-dimensional imaging using magnetic resonance imaging (MRI) data.

Methodology

X-ray techniques

Standard radiographs are obtained by placing the patient between an X-ray source and a photographic film. Images are produced by the attenuation of X-ray photons by the patient. As a result, structures of interest are often obscured by the attenuation of photons by other overlying structures. A basic limitation of the standard X-ray technique is the effect of scattered photons adding to the image noise and degrading the quality of the final image. Various manoeuvres have been adopted to reduce this effect, such as scatter grids. The linear tomograph is obtained by the synchronous movement of the X-ray tube and the film, causing a blurring of the overlying and underlying structures while leaving the plane of interest in focus. This procedure increases the detection of lesions such as chest metastases.

Contrast studies

To increase contrast in the soft tissues, an iodine-containing agent may be injected into the lumen of a cavity such as the uterus and fallopian tubes (hysterosalpingogram) or blood vessels (angiogram). Such contrast agents are widely available in ionic and (more expensive) non-ionic forms. The less toxic non-ionic preparations are preferred.

Ultrasound

In Glasgow in 1950, Ian Donald used an industrial flaw detector, designed for testing the integrity of steel boilers, to demonstrate that the massive abdominal swelling of one of his patients was fluid and not solid (Kurjak 2000). A large ovarian cyst that proved to be benign was subsequently removed. Since then, the rapid and continuing evolution of ultrasound technology has led to a proliferation of applications in almost all aspects of medicine and surgery.

Ultrasound waves are generated by a piezoelectric crystal mounted in a transducer housing, and the whole construction is referred to as a 'probe'. Piezo materials respond to an applied voltage by changing thickness, and produce electrical signals of a few millivolts when compressed. In the final image, the resolution along the beam is determined by the wavelength, while the resolution across it depends on the width of the beam, which is improved by focusing using combinations of lenses and electronic mechanisms.

The time from transmission of the ultrasound pulse to receipt of an echo is translated into depth using the speed of sound in tissue. Echoes arise wherever the pulse of ultrasound encounters an interface between tissues of different acoustic impedance, which may simplistically be regarded as changes in density. Thus, homogeneous materials such as clear fluids are echo-free, while low-level echoes are given by the interfaces between the various components of soft tissue structures. Stronger echoes result from the interface between fibrous tissues (high impedance) and fatty tissues (low impedance), and maximal echoes are given by interfaces between soft tissues and bone or gas, both of which are effectively opaque to ultrasound. To form a real-time image, the beam is electronically swept through a region of tissue and the images are pie-shaped (sector and curved arrays) or rectangular (linear probes).

The choice of frequency is a compromise between the spatial resolution and the depth of penetration required. The higher the frequency, the better the resolution, but the

DOI: 10.1016/B978-0-7020-3120-5.00005-9

greater the attenuation of the beam within the tissues. Hence, for abdominal scanning, frequencies of between 3.5 and 5 MHz are commonly employed. Probes designed for intra-cavitary and intraoperative use employ higher frequencies (8–15 MHz) because the organs of interest are closer to the transducer. This enables higher resolution images to be obtained, and also allows study of the movement of structures when pressure is applied to the probe, which gives important diagnostic clues on their relative mobility. The drawbacks of transvaginal scanning are practical (intolerance of the probe by the very young and old, and in the presence of scarring) and diagnostic (the depth of view is limited to approximately 70 mm) (Bennett and Richards 2000). By sweeping an array through the tissues, a three-dimensional scan can be created; while most useful in obstetrics to visualize complex structures such as the fetal face, it also displays uterine anatomy well (Alcazar and Galvan 2009).

The interactivity of ultrasound is an important feature; it is effectively an extension of clinical examination. Ultrasound also provides numerous views during the real-time examination and facilitates guided needle biopsies. However, it has many limitations, notably the variable image quality, that frustrate its application. An important problem is the complete barrier posed by bowel gas, which is why a full bladder is required for transabdominal scanning.

Doppler operates by detecting the change in frequency of ultrasound echoes caused by movement of the target. In the simplest system, this is done continuously with only minimal control of the beam direction. Continuous wave Doppler is well suited to fetal heart monitoring, especially because movements of the fetus do not interrupt the signal. In gynaecology, the vessels of interest are small so precise placement of the Doppler sample is a prerequisite. This can be achieved with pulsed Doppler. The Doppler gate is superimposed on a real-time image that allows the target to be pinpointed (Figure 5.1). The Doppler signal depicts a range of blood velocities occurring in the selected vessel over time. Output can be audio or as a strip chart on which intensity indicates the strength of the signal at each velocity in the spectrum. A variety of measurements can be made from these tracings, the most useful of which are systolic/diastolic velocity ratios. These are measures of the arteriolar resistance to flow, with a low value indicating low vasomotor tone, typical of the placenta and the corpus luteum. This pattern also occurs in inflammation and malignancy. High indices are typical of inactive tissue, such as the resting uterus. Doppler can be used to measure fetal and uteroplacental blood flow, thereby producing physiological information (Brinkman and Wladimiroff 2000).

In colour Doppler scanning, the same process is applied across an area of interest. The velocity signals are presented as a colour-coded overlay, superimposed on the real-time scan (Figure 5.2). Although the Doppler information is less rich than with spectral Doppler (only the mean velocity or the amount of flow is depicted), the angiogram-like map provides information on the morphological arrangement of the vascular tree, and its sensitivity allows vessels as small as approximately 1 mm in diameter to be detected. Colour Doppler is often used to locate a vessel to guide placement of the spectral Doppler gate for haemodynamic analysis.

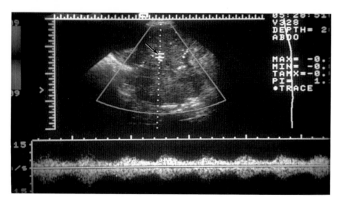

Figure 5.1 Spectral Doppler. In this scan of an ovarian cancer, the Doppler gate (arrow) has been positioned on the tumour. The spectral tracing is in the lower portion of the figure and shows the typical low-resistance pattern of malignant neovascularization with marked diastolic flow.

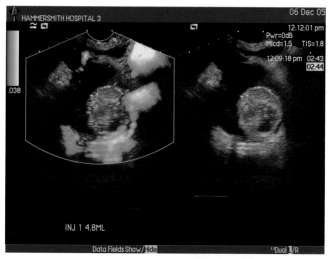

Figure 5.2 Colour Doppler of an ovarian carcinoma. On colour Doppler, flow signals are colour coded and presented as an overlay on the grey-scale image in the left-hand panel of this transvaginal scan, while the right-hand panel shows the grey-scale image on its own. The neovascularization in this ovarian carcinoma is shown as knots of colour. Apart from providing a graphic display of vascularity, a useful feature of colour Doppler is to guide placement of the gate for spectral Doppler tracings.

A recent advance has been the introduction of contrast agents for ultrasound in the form of microbubbles for injection. Not only does the signal improvement they produce allow smaller vessels to be detected, but they can be visualized in grey scale to reveal regions of flow in real time. In addition, they can be used as tracers by tracking a bolus as it crosses a tissue of interest, and this may yield valuable functional information.

Computed tomography

The sensitivity of conventional radiography may be improved by using a radiation detector such as a scintillation crystal and a photomultiplier tube. By measuring the attenuation of a finely collimated beam of radiation, passing through the patient at multiple angles, it has been possible to produce images of very high quality. A computer uses the attenuation of each beam passing through the patient to calculate the attenuation coefficient for each area of tissue in the cross-section of interest. The final images are reconstructed using a filtered back-projection technique and displayed in grey scale as a series of attenuation units (with values between +500 and −500) in a matrix of 512 × 512 or 1024 × 1024 elements. The reconstruction of data is limited to the transverse (transaxial) plane. This imaging technique revolutionized modern medicine in the 1970s, but its impact on gynaecology has been less marked.

Magnetic resonance imaging

MRI depends upon the magnetic properties of certain atomic nuclei which, when placed within a magnetic field and stimulated by radio waves of a specific frequency, will absorb and then re-emit some of this energy as a radio signal. This phenomenon of nuclear magnetic resonance (NMR) was first described by Felix Bloch and Edward Purcell in 1946. NMR as a basis for an imaging technique was proposed some 30 years later by Lauterbur.

Nuclei possessing magnetic properties have an odd number of protons or neutrons. The charged particles are spinning, which causes them to behave as tiny bar magnets. If placed within a magnetic field, a majority of protons will line up in the direction of the magnetic field. In addition, their axes are tilted and caused to rotate like small gyroscopes. The frequency of this precessional movement is directly proportional to the strength of the applied field and is called the 'Larmor frequency'. The hydrogen proton gives a relatively high signal due to its abundance in biological tissues. Other potential NMR isotopes include ^{13}C, ^{23}Na, ^{19}F and ^{31}P.

If a pulse of radio waves is imposed on the nuclei, a strong interaction or 'resonance' will occur when the frequency coincides with the precessional frequency of the nuclei. The energy absorbed by the nuclei is then re-emitted as a signal that can be detected in a receiver coil situated around the sample. The initial strength of this signal is proportional to the proton density of the sample. It will then decay in an exponential fashion as the disturbed protons relax back to their original state. The T_1 relaxation time is described as the time taken for the stimulated protons to return to their initial state. The T_2 relaxation time is that taken for the precessing nuclei to get out of step with one another. A variety of sequences of radio wave pulses have been devised so that the resulting signal is weighted to different degrees by the proton density and the T_1 and T_2 relaxation times.

The contrast between different tissues in MRI can be manipulated by altering the pattern of radio waves applied. This is done by changing the time constants associated with the different sequences of radio waves: the repetition time, echo time or inversion time. A further advantage of MRI is the ability to obtain images in multiple planes, such as sagittal, coronal or oblique planes, without moving the patient.

The female pelvis is suitable for MRI examination because of the minimal effect of respiratory motion on the pelvic organs. By placing the receiver coil adjacent to the tissue of interest (e.g. endovaginally to maximize signal from the cervix), very-high-resolution images of an area of interest may be obtained. However, as the data to produce a set of images are accumulated over 5–10 min, patients are required to remain still during this time. If multiple sequences and multiple planes are employed, the total imaging time may exceed 30 min which reduces patient tolerance. However, newer faster pulse sequences with breath-hold techniques and improved computer software are greatly reducing scan times. Recently, open design MR scanners and production of MR-compatible equipment has produced an explosion in the field of 'interventional MRI'. This has expanded the applications of MRI from being purely diagnostic to its use during treatment, such as for placing brachytherapy implants (Popowski et al 2000) or monitoring thermal ablative therapy.

Radionuclide imaging

Unlike the other imaging modalities, radionuclide imaging provides physiological rather than anatomical detail. Modern gamma cameras are capable of accurately imaging the distribution of administered radiopharmaceuticals, and the use of tomographic systems for single photon emission tomography has improved image resolution. In gynaecological oncology, radiolabelled monoclonal antibodies may be employed in the localization of malignancies (radioimmunoscintigraphy) and in their treatment (radioimmunotherapy).

The purity and specificity of monoclonal antibodies gives them an important role in tumour detection and possibly in the targeting of antitumour agents. Different anticytokeratin antibodies may help in distinguishing a primary ovarian adenocarcinoma from a metastatic adenocarcinoma, especially of colorectal origin (McCluggage 2000). These antibodies have also helped to clarify the origin of the peritoneal disease in most cases of pseudomyxoma peritonei. In recent years, several studies have also investigated the value of a variety of monoclonal antibodies in the diagnosis of ovarian sex cord stromal tumours, and in the distinction between these neoplasms and their histological mimics. Of these, anti-alpha-inhibin and CD99 appear to be of most diagnostic value (Choi et al 2000). Antibodies should always be used as part of a larger panel and not in isolation.

The antibodies or antibody fragments are radiolabelled with a gamma-emitting radionuclide such as ^{99m}Tc, ^{131}I, ^{123}I or ^{111}In. A subcutaneous test dose is no longer given because of the immune response it may generate in the patient. If ^{131}I or ^{123}I is employed, oral potassium iodide is given to block thyroid uptake of free radioactive iodide. In addition, blood pool subtraction techniques are required for ^{131}I studies to simulate the non-tumour distribution of labelled antibody. This is not necessary for ^{123}I- or ^{111}In-labelled preparations.

Following injection of the antibody, a gamma camera provides serial images of the distribution and uptake of radiolabelled antibody between 18 and 72 h after the antibody has been administered. The radionuclide ^{111}In is ideally suited for tomographic studies using images produced by a gamma camera mounted on a gantry which rotates through 360°. The images are reconstructed by computer in the same manner as X-ray CT. ^{111}In-labelled antibody is taken up into the liver, spleen, bone marrow and, occasionally, adrenal

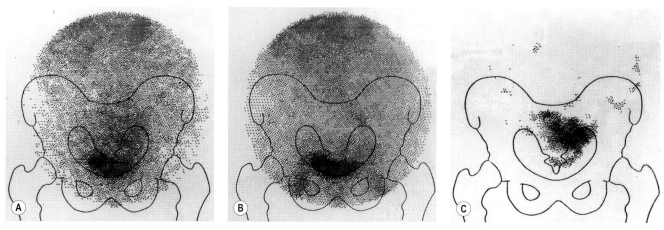

Figure 5.3 Radionuclide scan: primary ovarian carcinoma. Anterior view of the pelvis with 80 MBq ^{111}In-labelled OC-125.

glands but is a more suitable radiolabel than [131]I. Excretion of ^{111}In into the bladder has not been a problem, although non-specific bowel uptake may account for false-positive results. An example of an ^{111}In study is shown in Figure 5.3. A central area of increased uptake is apparent at the site of a primary ovarian cancer.

[18]FDG ([18]fluorodeoxyglucose) is a non-specific positron-emitting tracer. It is an analogue of glucose, thereby reflecting metabolism and detecting the increased glycolysis associated with several tumour types. It gains entry into cells by membrane transporter proteins, such as Glut-1, which are expressed in many tumours. It is phosphorylated intra-cellularly to FDG-6-phosphate and retained within malignant cells. Tumour hypoxia may also increase [18]FDG accumulation via activation of glycolysis. The quantitative parameter used is typically a standardized uptake value (SUV), which represents the tissue activity within a region of interest corrected for the injected activity and the patient's body weight. A new lesion (Figure 5.4) or a rise in SUV within a lesion indicates disease progression. Whether this can be used as a marker for early therapy remains to be proven.

Angiography

Diagnostic and therapeutic angiography have made great strides in recent years with the development of catheters whose tips can be manipulated. This allows considerable control over the guidance of these catheters into selected vessels. In parallel with this, ingenious devices have been devised which can be introduced via these catheters for purposes as diverse as angioplasty and embolization.

In gynaecological practice, the main use of angiography is the control of pelvic bleeding, but both the diagnosis of pelvic venous thrombosis and the prevention of subsequent pulmonary embolism are important roles for this exciting new technique. Pelvic arteriovenous malformations are most readily diagnosed and treated with angiography, and pelvic varices causing chronic pain may be managed in the same way. Selective sampling of gonadal venous blood and steroid hormone assay can be valuable in the preoperative assessment of phenotypic women with chromosomal abnormalities and intra-abdominal gonads of uncertain nature.

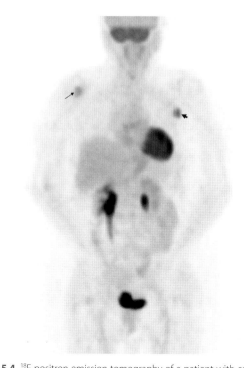

Figure 5.4 ^{18}F positron emission tomography of a patient with cervical cancer showing metastatic deposits with increased glucose uptake in left axilla (short arrow) and right scapula (long arrow).
de Souza NM, Brosens JJ, Schwieso JE, Paraschos T, Winston RM. The potential value of magnetic resonance imaging in infertility. Clin Radiol 1995; 50(2):75–79, with permission of Elsevier.

Clinical Applications

Normal anatomy and variations

Uterus

The normal uterine cavity is delineated as a triangular structure on hysterosalpingography, with the cornua and the internal cervical os as the corners. Intracavitary abnormalities, both congenital and acquired, such as internal septations and divisions may be defined using this technique (Figure 5.5). Similar information can be acquired with ultrasound following instillation of saline into the uterine cavity (hysterosonography) (van den Brule et al 1998).

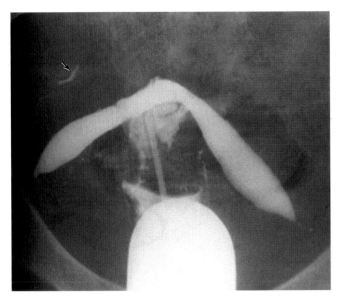

Figure 5.5 Hysterosalpingogram: contrast outlining the cavities of a bicornuate uterus. Free spill into the peritoneal cavity can be seen on the right (arrow).

On ultrasound, the uterine cavity is normally represented by a bright line of apposition of the endometrial layers, although occasionally a trace of fluid can be seen at menstruation. Persistent fluid or fluid in a non-menstruating woman is abnormal. In adolescence, it may be caused by vaginal atresia, where the upper vagina dilates more than the uterus so that haematocolpos dominates the picture, while in postmenopausal women, cervical stenosis, either fibrotic or malignant, must be considered. Ultrasound is also useful in detecting the position of an intrauterine device; provided the coil lies in the uterus, it is easy to locate, but a coil that has penetrated through the myometrium is obscured by echoes from bowel gas (Figure 5.6).

The entire uterus can be imaged using ultrasound (Figure 5.7) and its size measured accurately. This is useful in precocious or delayed puberty and in planning brachytherapy. The endometrium is seen as an echogenic layer of uniform texture, often with a fine echo-poor margin. Its thickness varies through the menstrual cycle from 12 mm premenstrually (double-layer thickness) to a thin line after menstruation. The endometrium gradually thins after menopause unless supported by hormones.

The morphology of the normal uterus, however, is best defined on MRI where its zonal architecture may be recognized (Hricak et al 1983). On T_2-weighted images, the endometrium is seen as a central high-signal stripe which increases in thickness in the secretory phase of the menstrual cycle. The inner myometrium (junctional zone) is of lower signal intensity than the outer myometrium on T_2 weighting, and correlates histologically with a layer of more densely packed smooth muscle.

Fallopian tubes

The patency of the fallopian tubes may be demonstrated on hysterosalpingography where filling and free spill into the peritoneal cavity may be seen (Figure 5.5). Ultrasound contrast salpingography is currently being evaluated to reduce

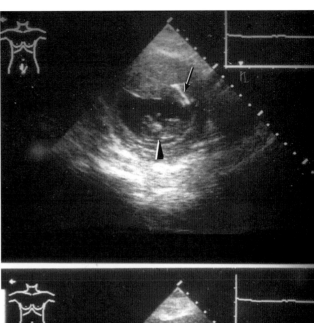

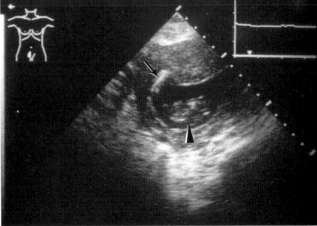

Figure 5.6 Two views of an intrauterine device in the uterine cavity (arrows) with a coexisting pregnancy (arrowheads).

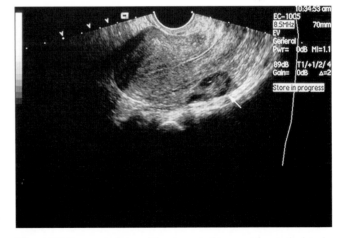

Figure 5.7 Transvaginal scan of the uterus. In this scan, taken in the luteal phase of the cycle, the secretory endometrium is seen as an echogenic band in comparison with the relatively echo-poor myometrium.

the radiation dose to the ovaries in patients trying to conceive. Normal uterine tubes cannot be demonstrated on ultrasound, but instillation of microbubble contrast agents into the uterus and tubes permits their visualization and can be used as an initial screening test for tubal patency. Although the anatomical detail is less than that offered by conventional X-ray salpingography and false-positive results occur, this technique of ultrasound salpingography seems likely to find an important role as an initial screen; if the tubes are demonstrated to be patent, no further investigation is necessary and this should result in a reduction of radiation exposure (Van Voorhis 2008).

The normal fallopian tubes are too small in calibre and of too variable a course to be reliably imaged using a cross-sectional technique such as CT or MRI.

Ovaries

The ovaries are best imaged with ultrasound (either transabdominal or, preferably, transvaginal). Changes in their appearance can be correlated with their functional status. Infantile ovaries are small (except in the neonate when hypertrophy and follicles stimulated by maternal hormones may be a surprising finding) and they enlarge before puberty. Follicular development begins before menstruation, but these cycles and those at the menopause are often imperfect

so that follicles may persist and continue enlarging for several months. Normally, ovulation occurs at a follicle size of 20–25 mm diameter and the echo-free follicle is replaced by a corpus luteum which can be cystic or solid. Corpora lutea produce a confusing variety of appearances, whose only consistent feature is their transience (Figure 5.8A–C). In doubtful cases, a rescan at 6 weeks to image them at a different phase of the cycle may be needed to resolve their identity. The postmenopausal ovary is usually too small to identify with ultrasound.

On CT and MRI, the normal ovaries are often difficult to define, but may be recognized on short inversion recovery MRI sequences as very-high-signal foci in the adnexae.

Ovarian varices

The pelvic congestion syndrome is one of many causes of chronic pelvic pain, and is associated with the presence of large varices within the broad ligaments (Liddle and Davies 2007). When pelvic symptoms are severe, there may be gross dilatation of the ovarian veins, with reflux down into the

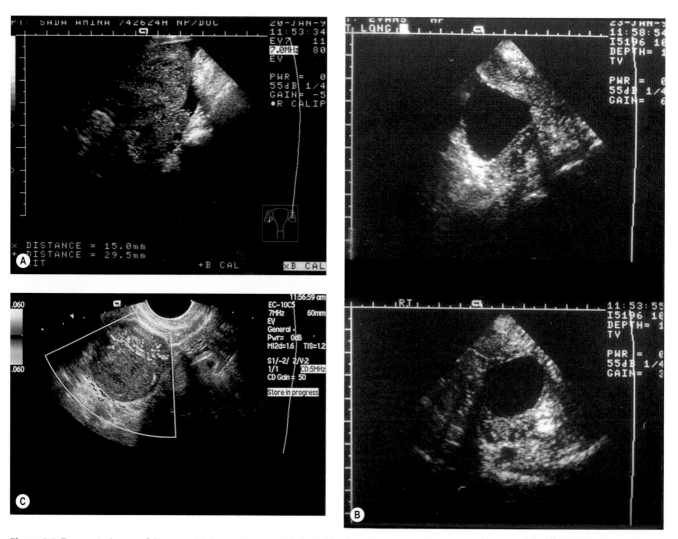

Figure 5.8 Transvaginal scans of the ovary. (A) An inactive ovary is indicated by the caliper marks. It is surrounded by a small amount of free fluid and contains minute developing follicles. (B) Two views of an ovary containing a 3-cm simple cystic structure which presumably represents an unruptured follicle. (C) An ovary in the luteal phase containing a solid corpus luteum.

pelvis and often into the legs. These vessels are best demonstrated by selective ovarian venography, although they may also be imaged with Doppler ultrasound (Haag and Manhes 1999). Venography is performed via a femoral or internal jugular venous approach, and the ovarian veins are selectively catheterized with an appropriately shaped angiographic catheter. Satisfactory retrograde opacification of pelvic varices is achieved by injecting contrast medium through the selectively placed catheter with the patient almost upright on a tilting table, while the Valsalva manoeuvre is performed.

Treatment of this condition is primarily surgical and consists of venous ligation. Symptomatic relief has been reported following transcatheter ovarian vein embolization (Ganeshan et al 2007).

Investigation of female infertility

The success of in-vitro fertilization (IVF) has been due, in part, to the correct timing of ovulation and subsequent oocyte recovery that ultrasound can provide. Using transabdominal scanning, ovarian follicles of 3–5 mm diameter can be visualized. They appear as echo-free structures amidst the more echogenic ovarian tissue. Their rate of growth is linear and the mean diameter prior to ovulation is 20 mm (range 18–24 mm). Structures within the follicle, such as the cumulus oophorus, can also be visualized. Following ovulation, internal echoes appear because of bleeding. Free fluid may also be observed in the pouch of Douglas.

Transvaginal sonography has largely replaced the transabdominal approach in infertility practice because of the superior anatomical display and because it allows precisely guided aspiration of follicles and fluid in the pouch of Douglas. More precise measurement of follicles is possible, and the corpus luteum is easily recognized. In the midluteal phase, it appears as an oval structure 30–35 mm long and 20–25 mm wide with a wide variety of sonographic appearances (Baerwald et al 2005). Endometrial reflectivity patterns have been proposed as another way to assess ovulation (Randall et al 1989). Ultrasound can only provide presumptive evidence of ovulation/pregnancy. The collection of secondary oocytes constitutes definitive evidence of ovulation. The appearance of internal echoes before the follicle reaches 18 mm or continuous enlargement to 30–40 mm indicates follicular failure.

Ultrasound is also useful for accurate timing of artificial insemination, while a postcoital test can help to differentiate between inadequate sperm penetration and poor mucus production in the presence of immature follicles. Ultrasound scanning is also employed to monitor patients on clomiphene therapy, and there is good correlation between follicular diameter and plasma oestradiol concentration. Ovarian hyperstimulation syndrome is uncommon if gonadotrophin therapy is monitored by ultrasound in conjunction with measurements of plasma oestradiol levels.

The waveforms of blood flow in vessels supplying the ovaries of women undergoing IVF have been studied using transvaginal power Doppler ultrasound (Palomba et al 2008). The observation of blood flow patterns did not improve any reproductive outcomes and is currently not advocated in IVF programmes.

MRI is valuable in the investigation of infertility where uterine pathology is suspected, and provides a particularly high diagnostic yield in patients with dysmenorrhoea and menorrhagia (deSouza et al 1995). It should be part of the investigation of patients with persistent unexplained infertility awaiting costly procedures such as gamete intrafallopian transfer and IVF. MRI should also be used before myomectomy in order to differentiate between leiomyoma and adenomyoma, as attempts to perform a myomectomy on a localized adenomyoma often result in extensive uterine damage.

Adenomyosis and endometriosis

The diagnosis of adenomyosis is often suggested by symptoms of hypermenorrhoea and dysmenorrhoea, but similar symptoms are also produced by leiomyomas. Hysterosalpingography may show multiple small tracks of contrast extending into the myometrium but is now obsolete. Ultrasound in skilled hands may be useful (Dueholm and Lundorf 2007).

Adenomyosis is best demonstrated on T_2-weighted MRI, with which two patterns (focal and diffuse) can be recognized (Hricak et al 1992, Byun et al 1999). In focal adenomyosis, there is a localized ill-defined mixed-signal-intensity mass (adenomyoma) within the myometrium (Figure 5.9). Diffuse adenomyosis presents with diffuse or irregular thickening of the junctional zone, often with underlying high-signal foci (Figure 5.10). Pathologically, this represents smooth muscle hypertrophy and hyperplasia surrounding a focus of basal endometrium. It is the smooth muscle changes that are easily recognized by MRI rather than the foci of heterotopic glandular epithelium. Values for junctional zone thickness from >5 to >12 mm have been suggested for the diagnosis of adenomyosis. In the authors'

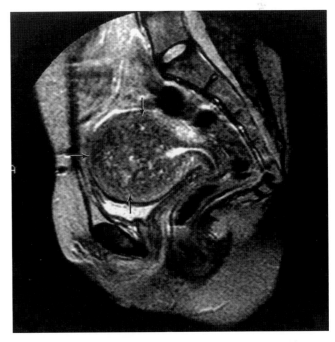

Figure 5.9 Focal adenomyoma. T_2-weighted spin-echo (SE 2500/80) midline sagittal section through the uterus, demonstrating a large ill-defined mixed-signal intensity mass characteristic of an adenomyoma (arrows).

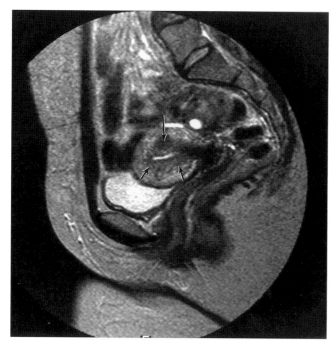

Figure 5.10 Diffuse adenomyosis. T$_2$-weighted spin-echo (SE 2500/80) midline sagittal section through the uterus, showing thickening and irregularity of the low-signal band of the junctional zone (short arrows). Diffuse infiltration of a mixed-signal lesion (long arrow) is seen in the posterior wall.

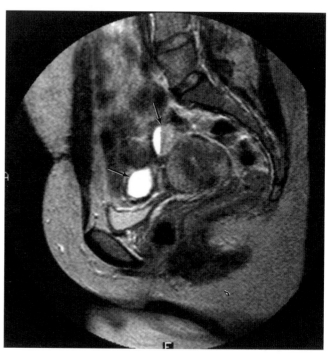

Figure 5.11 Endometriotic deposits. T$_2$-weighted spin-echo (SE 2500/80) midline sagittal image; fluid levels are seen in cystic lesions with mixed-signal intensity suggestive of haemorrhage (arrows).

experience, however, the thickening of the junctional zone that is described in adenomyosis (Reinhold et al 1999) is not diagnostic of adenomyosis on its own; it may be seen in hypermenorrhoea where no pathological evidence for adenomyosis has subsequently been shown. In these instances, absolute values for junctional zone widths are unhelpful (Hauth et al 2007), and ratios to the width of the outer myometrium or the cervical stroma may be more meaningful.

The lesions of endometriosis are difficult to detect with imaging techniques, mainly because of their small size. Only larger endometriomas can be detected on ultrasound and are seen as well-defined spaces, most commonly in the adnexal region (Figure 5.11). The role of MRI in the diagnosis of endometriosis also depends on the site of the endometriotic implants; deposits on the ovarian cortex are much more readily identified than small peritoneal deposits. The latter are recognized at laparoscopy but may be missed on MRI (Brosens et al 2004). Endoscopic ultrasound has been advocated to improve the diagnosis of endometriotic infiltration into the digestive tract (Dumontier et al 2000). MRI is particularly valuable in detecting deep enclosed endometriosis typically found in the uterosacral ligaments and rectovaginal septum (Figure 5.12) commonly associated with pelvic pain. Deep pelvic endometriosis consists mainly of fibromuscular rather than endometrial tissue (Del Frate et al 2006), and often goes undetected on visual inspection of the pelvic cavity because of its position. However, MRI lacks sensitivity in detecting rectal endometriosis if the rectum is not distended (Kinkel et al 1999). More recently, there have been isolated reports correlating an increased junctional zone thickness with endometriosis in patients with infertility (Kunz et al 2000).

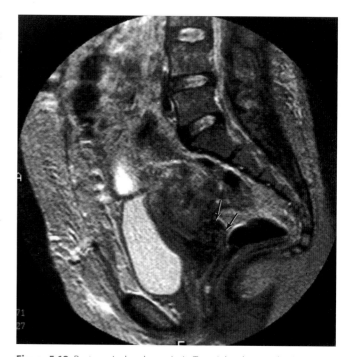

Figure 5.12 Rectovaginal endometriosis. T$_2$-weighted spin-echo (SE 2500/80) sagittal section demonstrating a rectovaginal mass (arrows) in a patient with laparoscopically proven endometriosis. This was not detected at laparoscopy because it is retroperitoneal.

Leiomyomas

The most common cause of disturbance of the normal uniform echo texture of the myometrium is fibroids. Generally, a focal thickening occurs and their position in the uterus can be determined. Submucosal fibroids, or the polyps they may produce, can be mistaken for endometrial thickening, although occasionally the way they move with normal uterine contractions is diagnostic. Instillation of saline into the uterine cavity, a form of ultrasound contrast, provides much more information about intracavitary lesions. Pedunculated or broad ligament fibroids frequently masquerade as extrauterine masses. The echo texture of fibroids is very variable, in accordance with their histological spectrum. A characteristic is calcification which is easily recognized on ultrasound as intensely reflective foci with accompanying acoustic shadowing.

MRI has been reported to be superior to ultrasound for the diagnosis of leiomyomas (Ascher et al 1994). Characteristic well-defined low-intensity masses are seen within the myometrium on T_2-weighted scans, often with high-signal foci within them. There are no completely reliable features that distinguish fibroids from leiomyosarcomas on ultrasound or MRI, and even Doppler has proved disappointing here. In those patients presenting with more advanced disease, alterations in the lesion margins may suggest malignant change.

Ectopic pregnancy

Traditionally, ultrasound has been used to exclude an ectopic pregnancy by demonstrating an intrauterine pregnancy, but this sign is unreliable in assisted pregnancy because the likelihood of coexistent intra- and extrauterine pregnancies is not negligible. The positive diagnosis of ectopic pregnancy requires the demonstration of an extrauterine fetal heart. Secondary features that may be recognized are an adnexal mass with peritrophoblastic Doppler signals, free fluid in the pelvis and increased endometrial thickness. With a combination of these features, the negative predictive value of an ultrasound examination may be 96%. However, significant problems can arise in distinguishing an ectopic pregnancy with a pseudogestational sac from an early normal or failed intrauterine pregnancy.

The role of ultrasound in the diagnosis of ectopic gestations has been strengthened by the use of transvaginal probes and the introduction of Doppler. A weakness of transabdominal scanning was the difficulty in demonstrating the sac itself, because of gas in overlying or adherent bowel. With transvaginal scanning, the adnexal sac can be demonstrated and women at high risk can be monitored through the first few weeks of pregnancy (Figure 5.13). Early ectopic sacs can be treated by injection of potassium chloride or methotrexate under ultrasound guidance. This approach is especially useful in IVF programmes where sparing the uterine tubes is important.

Infections

Ultrasound is useful in the diagnosis and management of ovarian abscesses, where shaggy walled cavities can be demonstrated in the adnexal region (Figure 5.14). They usually have a vascular pseudocapsule that can be demonstrated on colour Doppler. However, in pelvic inflammatory disease without abscess formation, the ultrasonic changes are too subtle to make this a useful technique. Monitoring the effects of antibiotic treatment on tubo-ovarian abscesses may be useful, although, in some cases, sterile cavities persist for

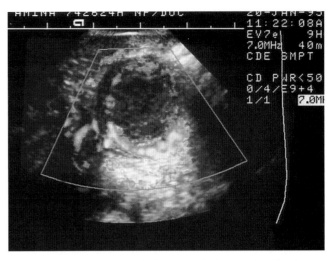

Figure 5.13 Ectopic gestation. In this transvaginal scan, colour signals are seen around the ectopic sac using power Doppler.

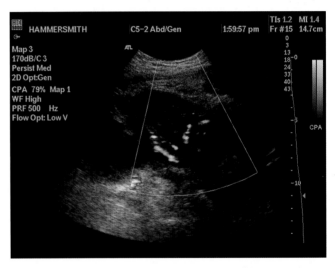

Figure 5.14 Tubo-ovarian abscess. The irregular walls of this cavity are vascularized as part of the inflammatory response.

many weeks after signs of infection have been controlled. The hydrosalpinx that complicates pelvic inflammatory disease is seen as a funnel-shaped cavity in the adnexal region with thin walls and no internal echoes.

Venous thrombosis

Diagnosis

A relatively common complication of pregnancy and gynaecological malignancies, deep venous thrombosis is most easily diagnosed using colour Doppler ultrasound and this should be the investigation of first choice. Visualization of the iliac veins may be difficult and some patients will have to proceed to contrast venography. If colour Doppler ultrasound has shown the femoral veins to be clear of thrombus, this is most easily performed by puncturing these vessels directly, which allows excellent opacification of the iliac veins and thus a confident diagnosis or exclusion of thrombosis, which can be difficult when contrast is injected into foot veins.

Inferior vena cava filter insertion

The indications for insertion of an inferior vena cava filter are listed in Box 5.1. The procedure is easily performed via femoral or jugular venous punctures, and some devices may even be inserted through a sheath introduced into an antecubital fossa vein. The majority of these filters are inserted permanently; short-term placement is possible, however, and is most commonly indicated in the late stages of pregnancy (when free-floating thrombus is demonstrated or when a recent pulmonary embolus has occurred), or prior to surgical removal of a large pelvic tumour which has caused compression and thrombosis of one or both iliac veins. Two types of short-term filter may be used: temporary and retrievable.

- Temporary filters are mounted on a long catheter and are placed via an internal jugular or antecubital fossa venous approach into the infrarenal inferior vena cava above the thrombus (Figure 5.15). The device is then sutured in place. They can only be left *in situ* for approximately 10 days and should then be removed because of the risk of infection.
- Retrievable filters are designed for permanent placement and are inserted via an internal jugular venous approach. One such device is the Günther Tulip filter (William Cook Europe, Bjaeverskov, Denmark) which has a hook on its superior aspect. This may be grasped with a loop snare and withdrawn into a sheath prior to its removal. These devices can be removed after 10 days, but this is associated with more potential complications as some endothelialization of the filter is likely to have occurred at this time and the filter limbs may be partially fixed to the caval wall.

Haemorrhage

Haemorrhage from the genital tract may complicate parturition or may be associated with benign (e.g. uterine arteriovenous malformation) or malignant (e.g. cervical carcinoma) disease. Traditional surgical therapy of severe pelvic haemorrhage consists most commonly of unilateral or bilateral internal iliac artery ligation, although in the case of primary postpartum haemorrhage, hysterectomy is more often performed.

There is a strong argument in favour of angiography and embolization prior to arterial ligation or hysterectomy in

---

Box 5.1 Indications for inferior vena cava filter placement

- Recurrent pulmonary emboli despite anticoagulation
- Pulmonary embolic disease in a patient in whom anticoagulation is contraindicated
- Free-floating pelvic or inferior vena caval thrombus
- Prophylaxis during surgery (see text)
- Previous life-threatening pulmonary embolism

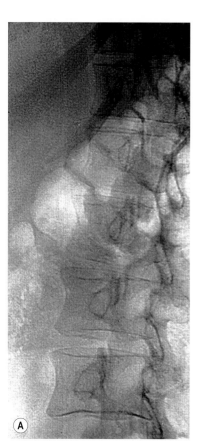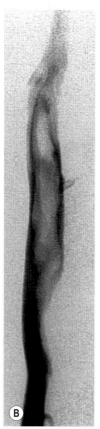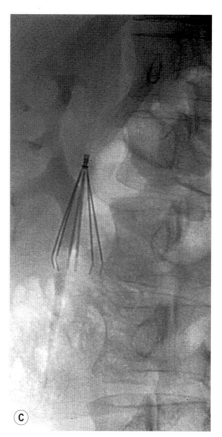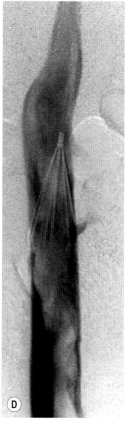

Figure 5.15 Temporary vena caval filter insertion above free-floating thrombus. (A) Control film. (B) Inferior vena cavogram using digital subtraction demonstrates a large free-floating thrombus. (C, D) A temporary filter has been placed on top of the thrombus using a right internal jugular approach. The plastic catheter on which the filter is mounted is barely visible.

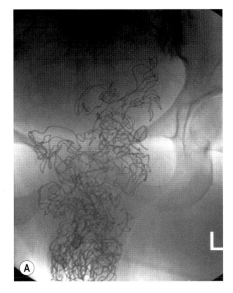

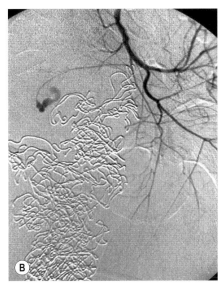

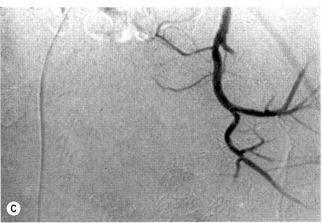

Figure 5.16 Severe postpartum haemorrhage in a patient who had been explored twice vaginally and who continued to bleed in spite of vaginal packing. (A) Control film showing a large pack in pelvis. (B) Selective internal iliac arteriogram demonstrates brisk extravasation of contrast from a branch of the anterior division. This was selectively catheterized and occluded with polyvinyl alcohol particles. (C) Postembolization arteriogram demonstrates occlusion of the bleeding vessel with no further extravasation of contrast.

hospitals having the necessary expertise. Bleeding sites are often impossible to localize at surgery (hence the necessity for non-specific ligation of the internal iliac artery), but are usually easily identified at angiography; selective occlusion of the haemorrhaging vessel can then be performed with a much higher likelihood of controlling bleeding (Figure 5.16). Previous internal iliac artery ligation does not necessarily prevent successful arterial embolization but may make the procedure technically more difficult (Collins and Jackson 1995).

Embolization is very successful in a variety of gynaecological disorders complicated by bleeding. For certain conditions (e.g. uterine arteriovenous malformations, bleeding from recurrent cervical carcinoma), this should be considered as the procedure of first choice (Figure 5.17). In others, it may be life-saving when more conventional treatment has failed.

Cervical carcinoma

The cervix

In cervical carcinoma, precise staging of the primary disease provides a prognosis, allows the institution of correct treatment and permits comparison of different treatment proto-

cols. Clinical staging, applied according to the system of the International Federation of Gynecology and Obstetrics, is subjective and is still widely used. Imaging with ultrasound does not improve the accuracy of clinical staging (Fotopoulou et al 2008), with poor image quality and difficulty in interpretation as the major problems. Although transrectal ultrasound produces clearer views of the cervix, definition of tumour from normal cervix is still poor. The same difficulty limits the value of CT because the normal cervix and cervical carcinomas have similar attenuation values, so the tumour can only be recognized if it alters the contour or size of the cervix (Subak et al 1995). MRI is now widely recognized as the staging modality of choice.

Several studies confirm the accuracy of MRI in the staging of early cervical cancer in comparison to surgical staging (Whitten and deSouza 2006). The primary tumour is best assessed using T_2-weighted MRI, which is superior to CT in detection (sensitivity 75% vs 51%, $P < 0.005$) and staging (accuracy 75–77% vs 32–69%, $P < 0.025$) (Kim et al 1993, Ozsarlak et al 2003).

The resolution of the primary tumour on MRI may be further improved by using intracavitary receiver coils. Endorectal coils give high-resolution images of the posterior cervix, but the anterior margin of the tumour and its relation to the bladder base is often difficult to define because

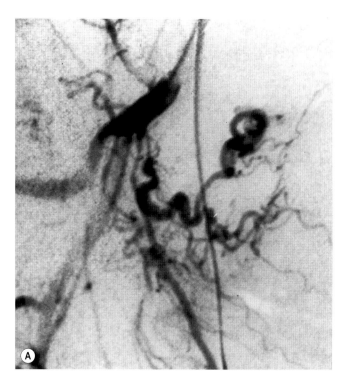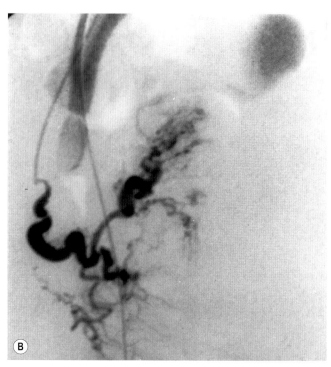

Figure 5.17 Embolization of an area of neovascularity in the right side of the pelvis due to recurrent carcinoma of the cervix in a patient with persistent bleeding. (A) Selective right internal iliac arteriogram using digital subtraction shows encasement of the origin of the right uterine artery which supplies an extensive area of neovascularity. (B) The right uterine artery has been selectively catheterized prior to embolization. Note the marked irregularity of this vessel due to involvement by tumour. Embolization performed with polyvinyl alcohol particles gave excellent control of bleeding.

of drop-off of signal. Endovaginal coils give very-high-resolution images of the cervix and adjacent parametrium (deSouza et al 1996). The distortion of the low-signal ring of inner stroma may be apparent, and any breaks in the ring representing tumour extension may be identified (Figure 5.18A,B).

With MRI, the invasion of cervical cancer may be assessed in three planes: the coronal and axial planes are used for determining parametrial invasion, the axial plane is used for determining extension into the bladder and rectum, and the sagittal plane is used for extension into the uterine body, bladder and rectum (Sala et al 2007). Fast spin-echo T_2-weighted sequences provide the best image contrast (Figure 5.19). MRI is also accurate in the prediction of myometrial tumour involvement and in showing the relationship of the tumour to the internal os, and hence the patient's suitability for trachelectomy (Peppercorn et al 1999). Volume (three-dimensional) imaging also provides the information necessary to calculate tumour volumes, which is of prognostic significance. Volumes obtained with MRI correlate well with those obtained by histomorphometric methods, but only weakly with clinical stage (Burghardt et al 1989). The volumetry of the tumour also gives a more accurate prediction of parametrial invasion and lymph node involvement (Burghardt et al 1992). Measuring tumour volume on MRI is of paramount importance; it has been shown that it is the size of tumour burden that determines the outcome rather than invasion beyond the anatomical margins of the uterus (Soutter et al 2004). Dynamic contrast-enhanced studies have been used for assessment of tumour angiogenesis (Hawighorst et al 1999), and the rate of contrast uptake has

been shown to correlate with microvessel density in the tumour. However, no correlation with tumour aggressiveness has been demonstrated (Postema et al 1999) and these images are not used routinely. Recently, diffusion-weighted MRI has shown higher accuracy than T_2-weighted imaging alone for tumour detection (Charles-Edwards et al 2008).

Parametrium

CT and MRI have both been used to assess parametrial spread. False-positive diagnoses may arise from misinterpreting inflammatory parametrial soft tissue strands associated with a tumour as actual tumour invasion on both CT and MRI. A comparison of the assessment by these modalities with histological findings after radical hysterectomy showed an accuracy rate for parametrial involvement of 87–90% for MRI, 55–80% for CT and 82.5% for examination under anaesthesia (Kim et al 1993). Extracervical extension on MRI is best defined using T_2-weighted fast spin-echo sequences transverse to the cervix (deSouza et al 1998). Fat-suppression techniques do not provide additional benefits (Lam et al 2000). Contrast enhancement has not proved beneficial; in a series of 73 patients, fast spin-echo T_2-weighted images had an accuracy of 83% for determining parametrial extension (compared with 65% for T_1-weighted gadolinium-enhanced images and 72% for T_1-weighted gadolinium-enhanced fat-suppressed images). The high negative predictive value (95%) for the exclusion of parametrial tumour invasion was the principal contributor to the staging accuracy obtained with fast spin-echo T_2-weighted imaging (Sironi et al 2002). MRI therefore yields valuable informa-

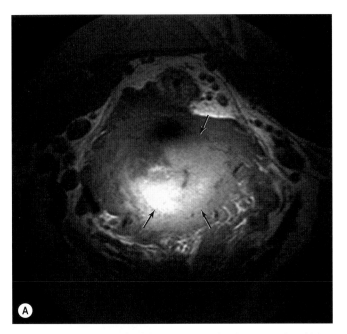

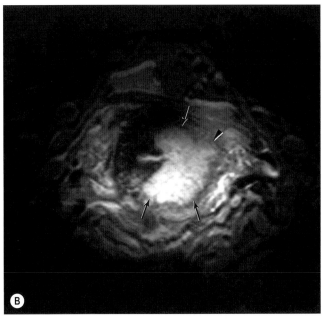

Figure 5.18 Carcinoma of the cervix. (A) T_1-weighted (SE 780/20) and (B) T_2-weighted (SE 2500/80) transverse spin echo through the cervix showing a large intermediate-signal-intensity mass mainly on the left. There is distortion and displacement of the normal low-signal band of inner stroma (arrows). A break in this stromal ring indicating parametrial extension is seen on the T_2-weighted images (arrowhead in B).

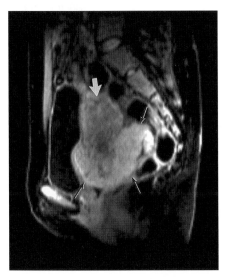

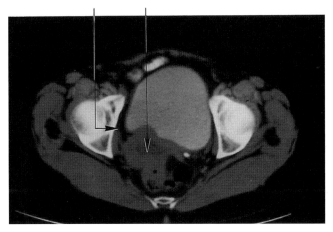

Figure 5.20 Computed tomography scan of stage IIIb cervical carcinoma.

Figure 5.19 Carcinoma of the cervix: a sagittal magnetic resonance image using a newly developed double inversion recovery sequence through the pelvis. A large carcinoma is seen (arrows) abutting but not invading the bladder base anteriorly and the rectal wall posteriorly. The uterus lies immediately cranial (large arrow).

tion for treatment planning and should be used routinely in conjunction with clinical staging to determine the appropriate therapy in patients with cervical carcinoma.

An intravenous urogram is now obsolete as part of the staging process as it is has been superseded by MRI.

Nodal involvement

The role of lymphangiography in the staging of cervical cancer is obsolete, with up to 71% false-positive results

and 16% false-negative results. Percutaneous fine-needle aspiration biopsy of nodes had been used to improve the results obtained with pelvic lymphangiography, but this has been replaced by CT. The major drawback for epithelial tumours is that nodes must be enlarged to be detectable. Thus, metastases less than 2 cm in diameter will not be identified.

Some studies have shown an improvement in pelvic lymph node evaluation with MRI compared with CT (accuracy 88% vs 83%, $P < 0.01$) (Kim et al 1993). However, like CT, this relies on changes in the size of the lymph nodes (Figure 5.20) since the tumour deposits themselves are not highlighted.

A lymph-node-specific MR contrast agent has been developed that allows the identification of malignant nodal infiltration independent of the lymph node size. This novel

MR contrast agent is classified as a nanoparticle (mean diameter 30 nm), and is composed of an iron oxide core, coated with low-molecular-weight dextran (ultrasmall particles of iron oxide, USPIO). The particles, administered intravenously, are taken up by macrophages in the reticuloendothelial system, predominantly within the lymph nodes. Uptake of USPIO results in marked loss of signal intensity (darkening) of the node on T_2- and T_2^*-weighted sequences because of a susceptibility artifact caused by the iron. Metastatic tissue within a node displaces the normal macrophages, thus preventing uptake of contrast agent, and the node continues to remain high in signal intensity. A significant increase in sensitivity with no loss of specificity has been demonstrated for the detection of malignant lymph nodes with USPIOs in patients with cervical and endometrial cancer (Rockall et al 2005). On a node-by-node basis, the sensitivity increased from 29% using standard size criteria to 93% using USPIO criteria. On a patient-by-patient basis, sensitivity increased from 27% using standard size criteria to 100% using USPIO criteria.

The role of positron emission tomography (PET) for detecting metastatic pelvic lymph nodes remains unproven. Small single-centre studies claim 91–96% sensitivity and 96–100% specificity for detecting nodes involved with tumour (Reinhardt et al 2001, Loft et al 2007), while results from other studies are much poorer (Williams et al 2001). Urinary residues of ^{18}FDG in the ureters remain a source of false-positive results. Quantitation suggests that a SUV_{max} ≥3.3 for lymph nodes is a significant adverse factor in those patients with nodal enlargement (Yen et al 2008).

Distant spread

Even with advanced pelvic spread, involvement of distant sites is the exception rather than the rule. Patients with stage I and II cervical cancer do not need to have bone scans.

A chest X-ray is a routine pretreatment investigation, but the yield of lung metastases at first presentation is likely to be no more than 2%.

Assessing response and recurrence

In conjunction with clinical examination, MRI can provide an objective assessment of the effects of surgery or radiotherapy. Serial MRI may be used before and after primary radiation therapy to assess tumour response (Akin et al 2007), and is increasingly important with the increased use of cytotoxic regimes. CT and ultrasound have limited ability to differentiate between fibrosis and tumour. While some say that infiltration of the parametrium may be easily recognizable, it is difficult to differentiate fibrosis after treatment from tumour recurrence. The use of contrast agents in detecting recurrent disease has proved disappointing; overall, diagnosis is best with unenhanced T_2-weighted images, but particularly in patients with treatment complications (e.g. fistula formation), contrast enhancement does help (Hricak et al 1993).

PET-CT is increasingly used in identifying pelvic recurrence with sensitivity, specificity and accuracy of 92.0%, 92.6% and 92.3%, respectively (Kitajima et al 2008). PET-CT is also able to detect lung metastasis, local recurrence, peritoneal dissemination, para-aortic lymph node metastasis and pelvic lymph node metastasis, and is a useful comple-mentary tool for obtaining good anatomical and functional localization of sites of recurrence during follow-up of patients with cervical cancer.

Endometrial carcinoma

Primary tumour

Thickening of the endometrium is characteristic of endometrial carcinoma and is well demonstrated on transvaginal ultrasound (Figure 5.21). However, specificity is low, although Doppler may help to distinguish hormonal causes of thickening (weak signals) and malignancy which gives marked colour and spectral Doppler signals (Weber et al 1998). Three-dimensional power Doppler has been reported to improve detection of endometrial carcinoma in patients with postmenopausal bleeding (Alcazar and Galvan 2009).

In patients already proven to have an endometrial cancer, myometrial extension has important prognostic and therapeutic implications. Myometrial invasion may be classified as absent, superficial or deep, and this can be assessed with high-resolution ultrasound probes. In a study of 75 patients, ultrasound had a diagnostic accuracy of 73% (Berretta et al 2008). Errors occurred when the tumour was exophytic and had significant extension into the uterine cavity. False-positive results also occur if the uterine cavity is distended with pus or blood when a subendometrial hypoechoic halo may be seen. Ultrasound assessment of the integrity of the echo-poor layer can be improved by the use of transvaginal or transrectal sonography. However, ultrasound has been superseded by MRI.

Changes in uterine blood flow have been used to detect endometrial cancer using endometrial thickness (including tumour), and the pulsatility index (PI) derived from flow velocity waveforms recorded from both uterine arteries and from within the tumour (Bourne et al 1991) found an overlap in endometrial thickness between women with endometrial cancer and those without, but the PI was invariably lower in women with postmenopausal bleeding caused

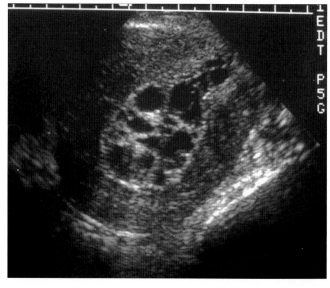

Figure 5.21 Transvaginal ultrasound image of cystic hyperplasia of the endometrium. The grossly thickened endometrium is clearly seen, together with the cystic spaces, in this patient on tamoxifen.

by endometrial cancer than in those with other reasons for bleeding. Blood flow impedance is inversely related to the stage of the cancer. However, although PI values in healthy women increase slightly with age, they decrease with oestrogen replacement therapy, so although Doppler studies may be helpful in the detection of endometrial cancer, allowance must be made for oestrogen replacement therapy.

CT has been used to stage endometrial cancer which is seen as a hypodense lesion in the uterine parenchyma (Hardesty et al 2001), or as a fluid-filled uterus due to tumour obstruction of the endocervical canal or vagina. These findings, however, are non-specific and are easily confused with leiomyomata, intrauterine fluid collections and extension of a cervical carcinoma into the uterine body. In addition, a central lucency may occur in normal postmenopausal women.

MRI represents the best method of assessing a patient with an endometrial cancer, with advantages over other radiological techniques. Figure 5.22 is a series of MRI scans of patients with endometrial cancer. On the T_2-weighted pulse sequence,

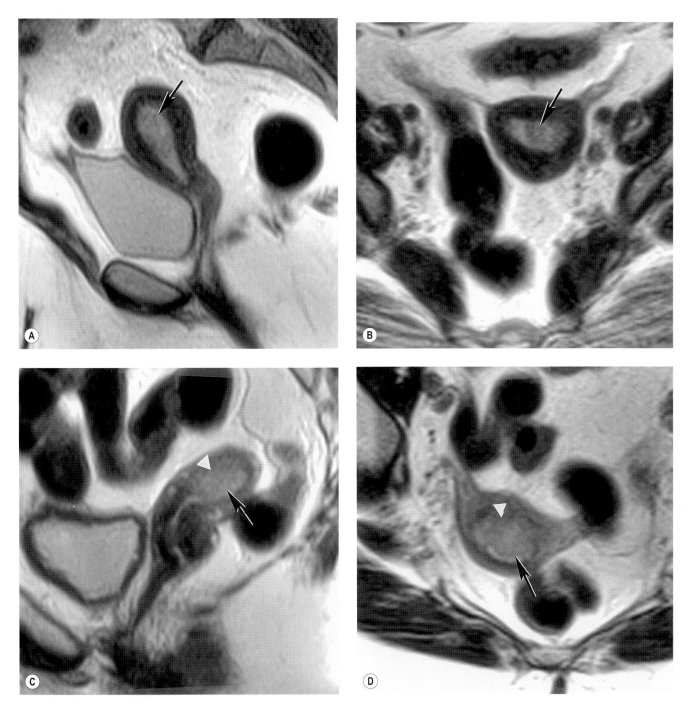

Figure 5.22 Magnetic resonance imaging scans (T_2) of two patients with endometrial cancer. The sagittal (A) and transverse (B) views in the first patient show tumour filling the endometrial cavity (arrows), but the surrounding low-signal-intensity junctional zone is intact. In the second patient, the sagittal (C) and transverse (D) views show tumour filling the endometrial cavity (arrows) with breach of the low-intensity junctional zone (arrowheads) and extension of tumour into the myometrium.

the tumour has a signal intensity similar to that of normal endometrium, but showing some degree of variability. The high signal makes the tumour quite distinct from the surrounding myometrium, which possesses an intermediate-signal intensity. In a premenopausal uterus, however, it may be difficult to differentiate tumour from adenomatous hyperplasia or indeed from the high signal of normal endometrium. Contrast-enhanced T_1-weighted MRI improves the ability to assess the depth of myometrial invasion by endometrial tumour (Koyama et al 2007, Sala et al 2009). MRI has been found to have a sensitivity of 57% and a specificity of 96% for tumour confined to the endometrium, a sensitivity and specificity of 74% for superficial invasion, and a sensitivity and specificity between 83–88% and 72–85%, respectively, for deep penetration (Sironi et al 1992, Cabrita et al 2008). However, the degree of invasiveness may be overestimated for exophytic polypoid tumours with significant extraluminal extension (Chung et al 2007, Sanjuan et al 2008). Powell et al (1986) first described the low-signal band of inner myometrium to be thinned or absent in those patients with deeply invasive tumours, and this correlated well with the pathological measurement of myometrial invasion.

The sagittal plane is the most appropriate for examination of a patient with primary endometrial cancer, as this provides a longitudinal view of the uterus which will include both corpus and cervix. Using the sagittal plane also provides the opportunity to assess anterior invasion of the tumour into the bladder and posteriorly to the rectum. Critical review and expert consensus of MRI protocols by the European Society of Urogenital Radiology, from 10 European institutions, and published literature between 1999 and 2008 indicated that high-field MRI should include at least two T_2-weighted sequences in sagittal, axial oblique or coronal oblique orientation. High-resolution post-contrast images acquired at 2 min ± 30 s after intravenous contrast injection are optimal for the diagnosis of myometrial invasion. If cervical invasion is suspected, additional slice orientation perpendicular to the axis of the endocervical channel

is recommended. Due to the limited sensitivity of MRI to detect lymph node metastasis without lymph-node-specific contrast agents, retroperitoneal lymph node screening with precontrast sequences up to the level of the kidneys is optional. The likelihood of lymph node invasion and the need for staging lymphadenectomy are indicated by high-grade histology at endometrial tissue sampling and by deep myometrial or cervical invasion detected by MRI (Kinkel et al 2009).

FDG-PET has been shown to display a higher sensitivity (96.7%) than CT/MRI (83.3%) for identifying primary and extrauterine (83.3% vs 66.7%) lesions, although no difference in specificity emerged between the two modalities (both 100%) (Suzuki et al 2007). For lymph node evaluation, MRI and FDG-PET are equivalent — sensitivity (91.5% vs 89.4%), specificity (33.3% vs 50.5%), accuracy (84.9% vs 84.9%), positive predictive value (91.5% vs 93.3%) or negative predictive value (33.3% vs 37.5%) (Park et al 2008) — which does not justify the use of PET-CT in disease staging.

Recurrent disease

Transrectal sonography has been investigated in cases where recurrent endometrial cancer is suspected (Savelli et al 2004). Physical examination may be difficult because of postsurgical fibrosis. Infiltration into the surrounding connective tissues and organs such as the rectum and bladder can be identified, and transrectal ultrasound can be used to guide transvaginal or transperineal fine-needle biopsy. As with recurrent cervical cancer, CT, MRI or PET-CT may be used to detect recurrent disease and metastatic carcinoma to omentum or lymph nodes.

Choriocarcinoma

Choriocarcinomas (gestational trophoblastic tumours) are characteristically hypervascular and this can be detected with colour Doppler (Figure 5.23) (Sebire and Seckl 2008). On spectral Doppler, they have a very low resistance index and this is useful for monitoring response to chemotherapy,

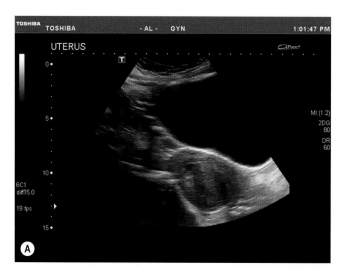
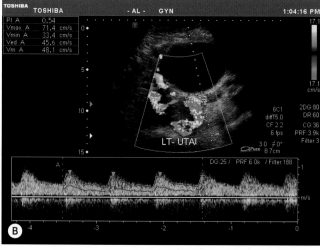

Figure 5.23 Choriocarcinoma. A bulky uterus of non-specific pattern was seen on grey-scale ultrasound of this choriocarcinoma (A). (B) The colour Doppler study shows the marked tumour vascularity. The spectral Doppler sample volume has been placed over the left uterine artery and reveals fast flow with minimal pulsatility, indicating lack of normal resistance to flow. This results in a low pulsatility index, changes in which can be used to monitor response to treatment.

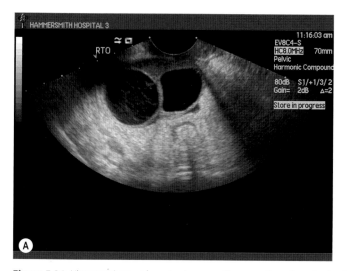
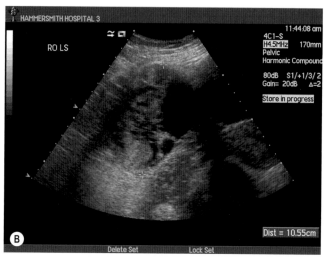

Figure 5.24 Ultrasound scan of ovarian tumours. The smooth walls and echo-free contents of the benign cystic mass in (A) (arrowhead) are very different from the complex appearance of the 10.5 cm carcinoma in (B). The second cyst in (A) contains uniform low-level echoes, probably representing debris.

although ultrasound is not very sensitive in their initial diagnosis since the characteristic snow-storm appearance of the multiple cystic spaces is only present in 40% of cases.

Ovarian carcinoma

In patients with ovarian cancer, the dramatic difference in cure between patients with local disease (80–90%) and distant disease (15–25%) means that imaging to detect ovarian cancer early is desirable.

The ovary

Ultrasound has been explored as a screening method for carcinoma of the ovary in an attempt to detect early disease (Menon and Jacobs 2000, Sato et al 2000). Early studies demonstrated a poor yield: out of 5479 women screened, five women with primary stage I cancer and four women with metastatic disease of the ovary were diagnosed (Campbell et al 1989). The overall rate of false-positive results was 2.3% and the likelihood of a positive scan being a primary ovarian cancer was one in 67. A scoring system has been evolved which reduces the number of false-positive results which otherwise occur due to confusion with unusual-appearing corpora lutea and benign tumours (Timmerman et al 1999). The improved resolution of transvaginal scanning permits a more detailed morphological examination (Figure 5.24A,B). This has been tested in a study of 25,000 asymptomatic postmenopausal women, of whom 740 had raised CA125 levels and were referred for ultrasonography; an ovarian volume of 8.8 ml was used as a cut-off for normality. All 20 cancers had abnormal morphology consisting of complex cysts, although there were numerous false-positive results. The positive predictive value was approximately 20% (Menon et al 2000).

Benign lesions are unilocular or multilocular with thin septae and no nodules, whereas malignant lesions are often multilocular with thick septae and nodules. The use of transvaginal colour flow imaging has been advocated, but these studies have been variously reported as disappointing or useful (Varras 2004). Initially, a low resistance index (less than 0.4) was advocated as the best discriminator, but this has proved unreliable and a high peak velocity may be a

better feature. At present, the role of ultrasound in screening, although attractive, remains unvalidated (Partridge et al 2009) and the results of larger trials are awaited. Additional specificity might be gained by adding contrast agents.

In ovarian cancer staging, MRI and CT are more sensitive than ultrasound (95%, 92% and 69%, respectively) for detecting peritoneal metastases, especially in the subdiaphragmatic spaces and hepatic surfaces (Tempany et al 2000). Either modality therefore can be used to stage advanced ovarian cancer. The potential of PET to identify metabolically active tumour that does not appear on morphological studies is promising. In one study, the PET-CT scan indicated a different disease distribution compared with CT alone in 55% of patients, and changed therapeutic management in 34% (Soussan et al 2008). Therefore, although current evidence for its utility is limited, PET-CT may be of major importance in staging ovarian cancer in the future.

As a tumour arising from a non-essential organ that is initially confined to the peritoneal cavity, ovarian cancer makes an attractive target for monoclonal antibodies. An antibody to CA125 has been assessed in monitoring the course of the disease (Sok et al 2009). However, antibodies are often limited by problems that include antibody specificity, stability and immunoreactivity, as well as patient reaction to the antibodies used. Antibodies coupled to drugs or biological toxins are also under investigation. Some antibodies may have direct antitumour effects through binding to biologically active receptors or through immune receptor functions. The use of antibody fragments, chimeric antibodies and genetically engineered antibodies is also under active investigation (Badgwell and Bast 2007).

Pelvic and abdominal spread

CT is the most useful imaging modality for demonstrating macroscopic recurrence, and can spare patients a second-look laparotomy. A variety of manifestations can be seen with CT, each of which can have a spectrum of appearances including ascites, peritoneal seeding, and visceral and nodal metastases (Forstner 2007). Ultrasound may also be used to detect ascites and liver metastases. MRI should be

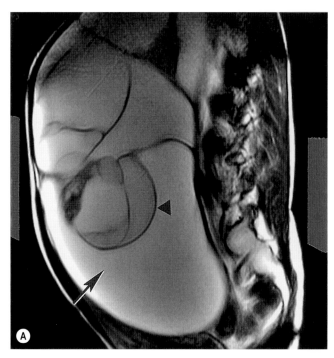
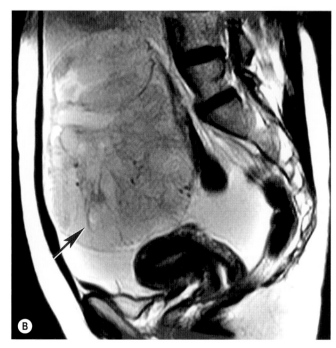

Figure 5.25 Magnetic resonance imaging scans (T$_2$) of two patients with ovarian cancer. Sagittal views show a predominantly cystic mass in (A) with a solid component around the rim of the tumour. In (B), the mass is largely solid with a small cystic component.

performed in women with questionable macroscopic recurrent tumour and negative CT examination (Figure 5.25), although neither modality can exclude microscopic disease. Newer whole-body diffusion-weighted MRI measurements are looking extremely promising in identifying peritoneal spread (Kyriazi et al 2009). PET-CT may also prove to be of benefit, although quoted accuracy reflects local expertise at image interpretation: lesion-based sensitivity and accuracy of FDG-PET/CT vs MRI has been recorded as 43% and 86%, and 75% and 94%, respectively ($P < 0.05$) (Kim et al 2007), indicating that FDG-PET/CT is not as useful as MRI for detecting local pelvic recurrence and peritoneal lesions in ovarian cancer recurrence. In contrast, in a recent meta-analysis of 34 studies comparing CA125, PET alone, PET-CT, CT and MRI, PET-CT had the highest pooled sensitivity (0.91, 95% confidence interval 0.88–0.94). The area under the curve (AUC) was 0.9219, 0.9297, 0.9555, 0.8845 and 0.7955, respectively. Results of pairwise comparison between each modality demonstrated that AUC of PET, whether interpreted with or without the use of CT, was higher than that of CT or MRI ($P < 0.05$) (Gu et al 2009).

Immunoscintigraphy of ovarian cancer lesions has been performed mainly with ^{99m}Tc, ^{111}In and ^{123}I labelled with HMFG1, HMFG2, OC-125, B72.3, H17E2, OVTL3, MoAb170, Mov18 and other monoclonal antibodies (MoAbs). Improved targeting has resulted in a highly sensitive and specific method. However, it is not yet known which type of MoAb most usefully supplements conventional diagnostic methods in staging or measurement of treatment response (Kalofonos et al 2001).

Safety Issues

Although the majority of imaging procedures described are largely non-invasive, some modalities involve exposing the patient to ionizing radiation. This is one of the reasons why techniques such as ultrasound and MRI have received so much attention in obstetrics and gynaecology. Nevertheless, ultrasound necessitates irradiation of the patient with sound waves (mechanical vibrations), and MRI involves the application of strong and rapidly changing magnetic fields combined with radio waves. Careful studies have failed to reveal harmful effects from the clinical use of ultrasound or MRI investigations, but each modality has an associated risk which must be appreciated.

With ultrasound and MRI, the main biological effect is of the conversion of the interrogating source of energy (sound, magnetic flux, radio waves) into heat. The American Institute for Ultrasound in Medicine has issued the following guidelines: 'In the low megahertz frequency range there have been no demonstrated significant biological effects of ultrasound in mammalian tissues exposed in vivo to intensities below 100 mW/cm^2'. Higher powers do damage tissue (mainly by heating, a feature used in physiotherapy), but at diagnostic levels the heating is minimal and removed continuously by the blood circulation. Spectral Doppler delivers the highest intensity, and this is compounded by the fact that the beam is trained on to a target for longer periods of time than in imaging. It seems prudent to restrict scanning, especially spectral Doppler, to genuine clinical indications and to use it for the shortest time and at the lowest intensity needed to make the diagnosis.

As early as 1896, reports were made of a visual sensation of light flashes induced by exposure to changing magnetic fields. However, the main hazards associated with rapidly changing magnetic fields are those from magnetic implants. Patients with cardiac pacemakers or aneurysm clips constitute an absolute exclusion to being scanned. Other metallic implants must be considered on an individual basis. Other hazards arise from electroconvulsion and atrial fibrillation, hence caution should be exercised with epileptic patients and those who have recently suffered from myocardial infarction. Guidelines for the use of MRI have been laid down by the National British Radiological Protection Board (1984).

Before deciding to carry out any imaging investigation, however, a clinical decision has to be made concerning whether the benefits accrued from the results of the investigation outweigh any possible risk to the patient from the procedure to be undertaken.

Conclusions

Advances in medical imaging are occurring at a rapid rate, mainly due to the development of sophisticated imaging techniques, computer software and display systems. Ultrasound, with its flexibility and relatively low cost, retains an integral diagnostic role in gynaecology, with transvaginal sonography a routine adjunct to a bimanual pelvic examination. MRI provides superior soft tissue contrast of the pelvic organs and leads to an increase in detection, improved staging and assessment of a range of disease processes including cancer. The technology needed to overcome the major disadvantages of long scanning times and claustrophobic scanners is well advanced. MR spectroscopy remains largely unexplored in gynaecology, but is an exciting prospect for the future. The various imaging modalities are complementary to each other, and the appropriate choice to produce the greatest diagnostic return while minimizing the risk to the patient should be sought.

KEY POINTS

1. Ultrasound examination is dependent upon both the technical expertise of the ultrasonographer and an understanding of the patient's history and clinical findings.

2. Ultrasound is the technique of choice for imaging the endometrial cavity and the ovaries, but it cannot distinguish reliably between benign and malignant disease.

3. Ultrasound is very valuable in monitoring ovulation induction and is used in directing egg collection for IVF.

4. Ultrasound can be valuable in identifying an ectopic gestation.

5. MRI gives the best images of endometrial carcinoma and adenomyosis. It may identify endometriosis that cannot be visualized in any other way.

6. MRI is the best method for imaging cervical carcinoma, especially when an endovaginal receiver coil is used. Imaging of pelvic lymph nodes is still not reliable.

7. CT scanning is of limited value in assessing the pelvic organs and should probably not be used if MRI is available.

8. Radionuclide imaging can be of value in identifying and locating ovarian carcinoma.

9. Angiographic embolization is probably the treatment of first choice for postoperative pelvic haemorrhage.

10. Negative lymph nodes on FDG-PET are not a justification for omitting retroperitoneal lymph node dissection for the precise surgical staging of gynaecological cancers.

References

Akin O, Mironov S, Pandit-Taskar N, Hann LE 2007 Imaging of uterine cancer. Radiologic Clinics of North America 45: 167–182.

Alcazar JL, Galvan R 2009 Three-dimensional power Doppler ultrasound scanning for the prediction of endometrial cancer in women with postmenopausal bleeding and thickened endometrium. American Journal of Obstetrics and Gynecology 200: 44–46.

Ascher SM, Arnold LL, Patt RH et al 1994 Adenomyosis: prospective comparison of MR imaging and transvaginal sonography. Radiology 190: 803–806.

Badgwell D, Bast RC Jr 2007 Early detection of ovarian cancer. Disease Markers 23: 397–410.

Baerwald AR, Adams GP, Pierson RA 2005 Form and function of the corpus luteum during the human menstrual cycle. Ultrasound in Obstetrics and Gynecology 25: 498–507.

Bennett CC, Richards DS 2000 Patient acceptance of endovaginal ultrasound. Ultrasound in Obstetrics and Gynecology 15: 52–55.

Berretta R, Merisio C, Piantelli G et al 2008 Preoperative transvaginal ultrasonography and intraoperative gross examination for assessing myometrial invasion by endometrial cancer. Journal of Ultrasound in Medicine 27: 349–355.

Bourne TH, Campbell S, Steer CV, Royston P, Whitehead MI, Collins WP 1991 Detection of endometrial cancer by transvaginal ultrasonography with color flow imaging and blood flow analysis: a preliminary report. Gynecologic Oncology 40: 253–259.

Brinkman JF, Wladimiroff J 2000 A software tool for fetal blood flow analysis. Biomedical Instrumentation and Technology 34: 55–60.

Brosens I, Puttemans P, Campo R, Gordts S, Kinkel K 2004 Diagnosis of endometriosis: pelvic endoscopy and imaging techniques. Best Practice and Research Clinical Obstetrics and Gynaecology 18: 285–303.

Burghardt E, Hofmann HM, Ebner F, Haas J, Tamussino K, Justich E 1989 Magnetic resonance imaging in cervical cancer: a basis for objective classification. Gynecologic Oncology 33: 61–67.

Burghardt E, Baltzer J, Tulusan AH, Haas J 1992 Results of surgical treatment of 1028 cervical cancers studied with volumetry. Cancer 70: 648–655.

Byun JY, Kim SE, Choi BG, Ko GY, Jung SE, Choi KH 1999 Diffuse and focal adenomyosis: MR imaging findings. Radiographics 19: S161–S170.

Cabrita S, Rodrigues H, Abreu R et al 2008 Magnetic resonance imaging in the preoperative staging of endometrial carcinoma. European Journal of Gynaecological Oncology 29: 135–137.

Campbell S, Bhan V, Royston P, Whitehead MI, Collins WP 1989 Transabdominal ultrasound screening for early ovarian cancer. BMJ (Clinical Research Ed.) 299: 1363–1367.

Charles-Edwards EM, Messiou C, Morgan VA et al 2008 Diffusion-weighted imaging in cervical cancer with an endovaginal technique: potential value for improving tumor detection in stage Ia and Ib1 disease. Radiology 249: 541–550.

Choi YL, Kim HS, Ahn G 2000 Immunoexpression of inhibin alpha subunit, inhibin/activin betaA subunit and CD99 in ovarian tumors. Archives of Pathology and Laboratory Medicine 124: 563–569.

Chung HH, Kang SB, Cho JY et al 2007 Accuracy of MR imaging for the prediction of myometrial invasion of endometrial carcinoma. Gynecologic Oncology 104: 654–659.

Collins CD, Jackson JE 1995 Pelvic arterial embolization following hysterectomy and bilateral internal iliac artery ligation for intractable primary post partum haemorrhage. Clinical Radiology 50: 710–713.

Del Frate C, Girometti R, Pittino M, Del Frate G, Bazzocchi M, Zuiani C 2006 Deep retroperitoneal pelvic endometriosis: MR imaging appearance with laparoscopic correlation. Radiographics 26: 1705–1718.

deSouza NM, Brosens JJ, Schwieso JE, Paraschos T, Winston RM 1995 The potential value of magnetic resonance imaging in infertility. Clinical Radiology 50: 75–79.

deSouza NM, Scoones D, Krausz T, Gilderdale DJ, Soutter WP 1996 High-resolution MR imaging of stage I cervical neoplasia with a dedicated transvaginal coil: MR features and correlation of imaging and pathologic findings. AJR American Journal of Roentgenology 166: 553–559.

deSouza NM, McIndoe GA, Soutter WP et al 1998 Value of magnetic resonance imaging with an endovaginal receiver coil in the pre-operative assessment of stage I and IIa cervical neoplasia. BJOG: an International Journal of Obstetrics and Gynaecology 105: 500–507.

Dueholm M, Lundorf E 2007 Transvaginal ultrasound or MRI for diagnosis of adenomyosis. Current Opinion in Obstetrics and Gynecology 19: 505–512.

Dumontier I, Roseau G, Vincent B et al 2000 [Comparison of endoscopic ultrasound and magnetic resonance imaging in severe pelvic endometriosis]. Gastroenterologie Clinique et Biologique 24: 1197–1204.

Fleischer AC, Lyshchik A, Jones HW Jr et al 2008 Contrast-enhanced transvaginal sonography of benign versus malignant ovarian masses: preliminary findings. Journal of Ultrasound in Medicine 27: 1011–1018.

Forstner R 2007 Radiological staging of ovarian cancer: imaging findings and contribution of CT and MRI. European Radiology 17: 3223–3235.

Fotopoulou C, Sehouli J, Schefold JC et al 2008 Preoperative transvaginal ultrasound (TVS) in the description of pelvic tumor spread in endometrial cancer: results of a prospective study. Anticancer Research 28: 2453–2458.

Ganeshan A, Upponi S, Hon LQ, Uthappa MC, Warakaulle DR, Uberoi R 2007 Chronic pelvic pain due to pelvic congestion syndrome: the role of diagnostic and interventional radiology. Cardiovascular and Interventional Radiology 30: 1105–1111.

Gu P, Pan LL, Wu SQ, Sun L, Huang G 2009 CA 125, PET alone, PET-CT, CT and MRI in diagnosing recurrent ovarian carcinoma. A systematic review and meta-analysis. European Journal of Radiology 71: 164–174.

Haag T, Manhes H 1999 [Chronic varicose pelvic veins]. Journal des Maladies Vasculaires 24: 267–274.

Hardesty LA, Sumkin JH, Hakim C, Johns C, Nath M 2001 The ability of helical CT to preoperatively stage endometrial carcinoma. AJR American Journal of Roentgenology 176: 603–606.

Hauth EA, Jaeger HJ, Libera H, Lange S, Forsting M 2007 MR imaging of the uterus and cervix in healthy women: determination of normal values. European Radiology 17: 734–742.

Hawighorst H, Knapstein PG, Knopp MV, Vaupel P, van Kaick G 1999 Cervical carcinoma: standard and pharmacokinetic analysis of time-intensity curves for assessment of tumor angiogenesis and patient survival. Magma (New York, NY) 8: 55–62.

Hricak H, Alpers C, Crooks LE, Sheldon PE 1983 Magnetic resonance imaging of the female pelvis: initial experience. AJR American Journal of Roentgenology 141: 1119–1128.

Hricak H, Finck S, Honda G, Goranson H 1992 MR imaging in the evaluation of benign uterine masses: value of gadopentetate dimeglumine-enhanced T1-weighted images. AJR American Journal of Roentgenology 158: 1043–1050.

Hricak H, Swift PS, Campos Z, Quivey JM, Gildengorin V, Goranson H 1993 Irradiation of the cervix uteri: value of unenhanced and contrast-enhanced MR imaging. Radiology 189: 381–388.

Kalofonos HP, Karamouzis MV, Epenetos AA 2001 Radioimmunoscintigraphy in patients with ovarian cancer. Acta Oncology 40: 549–557.

Kim CK, Park BK, Choi JY, Kim BG, Han H 2007 Detection of recurrent ovarian cancer at MRI: comparison with integrated PET/CT. Journal of Computer Assisted Tomography 31: 868–875.

Kim SH, Choi BI, Han JK et al 1993 Preoperative staging of uterine cervical carcinoma: comparison of CT and MRI in 99 patients. Journal of Computer Assisted Tomography 17: 633–640.

Kinkel K, Chapron C, Balleyguier C, Fritel X, Dubuisson JB, Moreau JF 1999 Magnetic resonance imaging characteristics of deep endometriosis. Human Reproduction 14: 1080–1086.

Kinkel K, Forstner R, Danza FM et al 2009 Staging of endometrial cancer with MRI: Guidelines of the European Society of Urogenital Imaging. European Radiology 19: 1565–1574.

Kitajima K, Murakami K, Yamasaki E, Domeki Y, Kaji Y, Sugimura K 2008 Performance of FDG-PET/CT for diagnosis of recurrent uterine cervical cancer. European Radiology 18: 2040–2047.

Koyama T, Tamai K, Togashi K 2007 Staging of carcinoma of the uterine cervix and endometrium. European Radiology 17: 2009–2019.

Kunz G, Beil D, Huppert P, Leyendecker G 2000 Structural abnormalities of the uterine wall in women with endometriosis and infertility visualized by vaginal sonography and magnetic resonance imaging. Human Reproduction 15: 76–82.

Kurjak A 2000 Ultrasound scanning — Prof. Ian Donald (1910–1987). European Journal of Obstetrics, Gynecology and Reproductive Biology 90: 187–189.

Kyriazi S, Morgan VA, Collins DJ, deSouza NM 2009 Optimising diffusion-weighted imaging in the abdomen and pelvis: comparison of image quality between monopolar and bipolar single-shot spin-echo echo-planar sequences. European Journal of Radiology; in press.

Lam WW, So NM, Yang WT, Metreweli C 2000 Detection of parametrial invasion in cervical carcinoma: role of short tau inversion recovery sequence. Clinical Radiology 55: 702–707.

Liddle AD, Davies AH 2007 Pelvic congestion syndrome: chronic pelvic pain caused by ovarian and internal iliac varices. Phlebology 22: 100–104.

Loft A, Berthelsen AK, Roed H et al 2007 The diagnostic value of PET/CT scanning in patients with cervical cancer: a prospective study. Gynecologic Oncology 106: 29–34.

McCluggage WG 2000 Recent advances in immunohistochemistry in the diagnosis of ovarian neoplasms. Journal of Clinical Pathology 53: 327–334.

Menon U, Jacobs IJ 2000 Recent developments in ovarian cancer screening. Current Opinion in Obstetrics and Gynecology 12: 39–42.

Menon U, Talaat A, Rosenthal AN et al 2000 Performance of ultrasound as a second line test to serum CA125 in ovarian cancer screening. BJOG: an International Journal of Obstetrics and Gynaecology 107: 165–169.

National British Radiological Protection Board 1984 Revised guidelines on acceptable limits of exposure during nuclear magnetic clinical imaging. British Journal of Radiology 56: 974–977.

Ozsarlak O, Tjalma W, Schepens E et al 2003 The correlation of preoperative CT, MR imaging, and clinical staging (FIGO) with histopathology findings in primary cervical carcinoma. European Radiology 13: 2338–2345.

Palomba S, Russo T, Orio F Jr, Falbo A, Tolino A, Zullo F 2008 Perifollicular vascularity assessment for selecting the best oocytes for in vitro fertilization programs in older patients. Fertility and Sterility 90: 1305–1309.

Park JY, Kim EN, Kim DY et al 2008 Comparison of the validity of magnetic resonance imaging and positron emission tomography/computed tomography in the preoperative evaluation of patients with uterine corpus cancer. Gynecologic Oncology 108: 486–492.

Partridge E, Kreimer AR, Greenlee RT et al 2009 Results from four rounds of ovarian cancer screening in a randomized trial. Obstetrics and Gynecology 113: 775–782.

Peppercorn PD, Jeyarajah AR, Woolas R et al 1999 Role of MR imaging in the selection of patients with early cervical carcinoma for fertility-preserving surgery: initial experience. Radiology 212: 395–399.

Popowski Y, Hiltbrand E, Joliat D, Rouzaud M 2000 Open magnetic resonance imaging using titanium-zirconium needles: improved accuracy for interstitial brachytherapy implants? International Journal of Radiation Oncology, Biology, Physics 47: 759–765.

Postema S, Pattynama PM, van Rijswijk CS, Trimbos JB 1999 Cervical carcinoma: can dynamic contrast enhanced imaging help predict tumour aggressiveness? Radiology 213: 617–618.

Powell MC, Womack C, Buckley J, Worthington BS, Symonds EM 1986 Pre-operative magnetic resonance imaging of stage 1 endometrial adenocarcinoma. BJOG: an International Journal of Obstetrics and Gynaecology 93: 353–360.

Randall JM, Fisk NM, McTavish A, Templeton AA 1989 Transvaginal ultrasonic assessment of endometrial growth in spontaneous and hyperstimulated menstrual cycles. BJOG: an International Journal of Obstetrics and Gynaecology 96: 954–959.

Reinhardt MJ, Ehritt-Braun C, Vogelgesang D et al 2001 Metastatic lymph nodes in patients with cervical cancer: detection with MR imaging and FDG PET. Radiology 218: 776–782.

Reinhold C, Tafazoli F, Mehio A et al 1999 Uterine adenomyosis: endovaginal US and MR imaging features with histopathologic correlation. Radiographics 19: S147–S160.

Rockall AG, Sohaib SA, Harisinghani MG et al 2005 Diagnostic performance of nanoparticle-enhanced magnetic resonance imaging in the diagnosis of lymph node metastases in patients with endometrial and cervical cancer. Journal of Clinical Oncology 23: 2813–2821.

Sala E, Wakely S, Senior E, Lomas D 2007 MRI of malignant neoplasms of the uterine corpus and cervix. AJR American Journal of Roentgenology 188: 1577–1587.

Sala E, Crawford R, Senior E et al 2009 Added value of dynamic contrast-enhanced magnetic resonance imaging in predicting advanced stage disease in patients with endometrial carcinoma. International Journal of Gynecological Cancer 19: 141–146.

Sanjuan A, Escaramis G, Ayuso JR et al 2008 Role of magnetic resonance imaging and cause of pitfalls in detecting myometrial invasion and cervical involvement in endometrial cancer. Archives of Gynecology and Obstetrics 278: 535–539.

Sato S, Yokoyama Y, Sakamoto T, Futagami M, Saito Y 2000 Usefulness of mass screening for ovarian carcinoma using transvaginal ultrasonography. Cancer 89: 582–588.

Savelli L, Testa AC, Ferrandina G et al 2004 Pelvic relapses of uterine neoplasms: transvaginal sonographic and Doppler features. Gynecologic Oncology 93: 441–445.

Sebire NJ, Seckl MJ 2008 Gestational trophoblastic disease: current management of hydatidiform mole. BMJ (Clinical Research Ed.) 337: a1193.

Sironi S, Colombo E, Villa G et al 1992 Myometrial invasion by endometrial carcinoma: assessment with plain and gadolinium-enhanced MR imaging. Radiology 185: 207–212.

Sironi S, Bellomi M, Villa G, Rossi S, Del Maschio A 2002 Clinical stage I carcinoma of the uterine cervix value of preoperative magnetic resonance imaging in assessing parametrial invasion. Tumori 88: 291–295.

Sok D, Clarizia LJ, Farris LR, McDonald MJ 2009 Novel fluoroimmunoassay for ovarian cancer biomarker CA-125. Analytical and Bioanalytical Chemistry 393: 1521–1523.

Soussan M, Wartski M, Cherel P et al 2008 Impact of FDG PET-CT imaging on the decision making in the biologic suspicion of ovarian carcinoma recurrence. Gynecologic Oncology 108: 160–165.

Soutter WP, Hanoch J, D'Arcy T, Dina R, McIndoe GA, deSouza NM 2004 Pretreatment tumour volume measurement on high-resolution magnetic resonance imaging as a predictor of survival in cervical cancer. BJOG: an International Journal of Obstetrics and Gynecology 111: 741–747.

Subak LL, Hricak H, Powell CB, Azizi L, Stern JL 1995 Cervical carcinoma: computed tomography and magnetic resonance imaging for preoperative staging. Obstetrics and Gynecology 86: 43–50.

Suzuki R, Miyagi E, Takahashi N et al 2007 Validity of positron emission tomography using fluoro-2-deoxyglucose for the preoperative evaluation of endometrial cancer. International Journal of Gynecological Cancer 17: 890–896.

Tempany CM, Zou KH, Silverman SG, Brown DL, Kurtz AB, McNeil BJ 2000 Staging of advanced ovarian cancer: comparison of imaging modalities — report from the Radiological Diagnostic Oncology Group. Radiology 215: 761–767.

Timmerman D, Bourne TH, Tailor A et al 1999 A comparison of methods for preoperative discrimination between malignant and benign adnexal masses: the development of a new logistic regression model. American Journal of Obstetrics and Gynecology 181: 57–65.

van den Brule FA, Wery O, Huveneers J, Gaspard UJ 1998 [Contrast hysterosonography: an efficient means of investigation in gynecology. Review of the literature]. Journal de Gynecologie, Obstetrique et Biologie de la Reproduction (Paris) 27: 655–664.

Van Voorhis BJ 2008 Ultrasound assessment of the uterus and fallopian tube in infertile women. Seminars in Reproductive Medicine 26: 232–240.

Varras M 2004 Benefits and limitations of ultrasonographic evaluation of uterine adnexal lesions in early detection of ovarian cancer. Clinical and Experimental Obstetrics and Gynecology 31: 85–98.

Wade RV 1999 Images, imagination and ideas: a perspective on the impact of ultrasonography on the practice of obstetrics and gynecology. Presidential address. American Journal of Obstetrics and Gynecology 181: 235–239.

Weber G, Merz E, Bahlmann F, Rosch B 1998 Evaluation of different transvaginal sonographic diagnostic parameters in women with postmenopausal bleeding. Ultrasound in Obstetrics and Gynecology 12: 265–270.

Whitten CR, deSouza NM 2006 Magnetic resonance imaging of uterine malignancies. Topics in Magnetic Resonance Imaging 17: 365–377.

Williams AD, Cousins C, Soutter WP et al 2001 Detection of pelvic lymph node metastases in gynecologic malignancy: a comparison of CT, MR imaging, and positron emission tomography. AJR American Journal of Roentgenology 177: 343–348.

Yen TC, See LC, Lai CH et al 2008 Standardized uptake value in para-aortic lymph nodes is a significant prognostic factor in patients with primary advanced squamous cervical cancer. European Journal of Nuclear Medicine and Molecular Imaging 35: 493–501.

CHAPTER 6

One-stop gynaecology: the role of ultrasound in the acute gynaecological patient

Kevin Jones and Tom Bourne

Chapter Contents

INTRODUCTION	80	CLINICAL CONDITIONS	83
RESOURCES FOR SERVICES	81	CONCLUSION	90
THE EMERGENCY GYNAECOLOGICAL UNIT	81	KEY POINTS	90
ULTRASOUND OVERVIEW	82		

Introduction

Acute gynaecological symptoms such as pelvic pain and bleeding occur in pregnant women who have miscarriages, ectopic pregnancies and pregnancies of unknown location, or in women who are not pregnant with ovarian cyst accidents or acute pelvic inflammatory disease. The investigation of the acute gynaecological patient is moving away from the accident and emergency department and operating theatre, and into dedicated emergency gynaecology units (EGUs) located in an outpatient setting (Jones and Pearce 2009). EGUs offer an efficient way of organizing multidisciplinary services for women presenting with acute gynaecological symptoms. These changes have been driven by the demands of the patient and clinician to provide a rapid, accurate diagnosis, with the minimum of investigations and invasive procedures. They are underpinned by national standards and guidelines (Department of Health 2003, Royal College of Obstetricians and Gynaecologists 2006). Furthermore, changing from traditional care pathways to more cost-effective, patient-centred approaches to medical practice lies at the heart of modern health service management (Department of Health 2000, Jones 2008).

In the UK, the majority of gynaecological ultrasound scanning has traditionally been undertaken by radiographers and radiologists in a separate department on a separate day. Transvaginal ultrasonography (TVUS) is a pivotal investigation for the assessment of acute gynaecological patients. Therefore, in order to deliver modern acute gynaecological services, gynaecologists will have to learn these new skills (Jones 2005). TVUS probes, providing high-resolution images of the pelvic organs, have an established role in the characterization of adnexal masses, providing reliable and reproducible information regarding cyst type and probability of malignancy (Granberg et al 1989, 1990, Tailor et al

1997, Timmerman et al 1999a), particularly when they are used in combination with tumour markers (Moore et al 2008). They have superiority over transabdominal probes because of the higher resolution of pelvic anatomy. There is also no need for a full bladder, improving patient acceptability.

TVUS is a pivotal investigation in the delivery of an 'Ambulatory Gynaecology Service' (Jones 2008). This is a more comprehensive term which would include the assessment of patients with non-acute gynaecological symptoms such as menstrual disorders, postmenopausal bleeding and chronic pelvic pain. The discussion of these conditions falls outside the scope of this chapter.

The accurate identification of pathology on ultrasound will enable the clinician to plan the patient's management effectively. The ultrasound diagnosis may determine if the patient is suitable for minimal access surgery or they may need a laparotomy and a multidisciplinary oncology team. In this way, preoperative ultrasound assessment of the patient will improve patient counselling and satisfaction with treatment.

This chapter deals with assessment of the patient presenting with acute symptoms, in whom gynaecological pathology is suspected. By adopting a problem-orientated approach, the aim is to provide a series of reproducible pathways allowing effective investigation of these patients. TVUS is central to all these diagnostic pathways but it should be regarded as an extension of the clinical examination; a normal scan will not exclude all underlying gynaecological conditions. The first part of this chapter will explore the place of TVUS in the differential diagnosis of acute pain and bleeding in early pregnancy. The second part of the chapter will give an overview of the role of pelvic ultrasound in the evaluation of acute pelvic pain and vaginal bleeding in women with a negative pregnancy test.

DOI: 10.1016/B978-0-7020-3120-5.00006-0

Resources for Services

Ultrasound machine

Most gynaecology units will already have an ultrasound machine that can be used within a clinic setting. Minimum requirements are a transvaginal probe (6–7.5 MHz), a 3.5 MHz abdominal transducer and facilities for capturing images, either as a hard copy or digitally. A portable machine can be a wise investment if it is to be shared, for example, with the delivery suite, or to allow for ultrasound-guided procedures in the operating theatre. The ultrasound machine should not be more than 5 years old (Royal College of Radiologists/Royal College of Obstetricians and Gynaecologists 1995).

Reducing the risk of infection transmission

TVUS is a relatively non-invasive procedure. There is, however, a moderate risk of transmission of infection as the probe comes into contact with mucous membranes. The risk of infection is reduced by the use of an appropriate cover for the transducer. It is estimated that up to 7% of covers will sustain perforations, and contamination of the probe may also occur on removing the cover after use (Jimenez and Duff 1997). As a result, appropriate cleaning of the transducer must occur between patients. Sterilization of the probe is not practical, and disinfection using a germicidal (e.g. 70% alcohol) cloth or spray, after first wiping off the gel, is effective. The probe is then left to air dry for at least 5 min. Basic hygiene measures, such as washing hands after each case and ensuring that contaminated gloves do not come into contact with the ultrasound machine, must be used to minimize cross-infection. There is no need for the routine use of antibiotics during ultrasound scanning.

Computer database systems

A number of commercial database systems exist for the storage of data, including digital images. This allows a written report to be generated immediately for the referring physician and patient, and easy access to previous images for comparison, for example after treatment of conservative management of ovarian cysts.

Resuscitation equipment

All gynaecological clinics should have adequate resuscitation equipment in good order. The clinic staff should have up-to-date training in its appropriate use.

Analgesia

TVUS is a well-tolerated procedure, even in women who present with acute pelvic pain. It does not require the routine use of analgesia. Basama et al (2004) demonstrated that TVUS was considered acceptable, and not painful, embarrassing or stressful in a study of 425 women undergoing TVUS in an emergency setting.

Interventional radiology in acute gynaecology

Gynaecologists have been slow to use interventional radiological techniques outside the setting of the assisted conception unit. However, angiographic embolization has now become accepted as the treatment of choice for potentially life-threatening obstetric and gynaecological haemorrhage, and selected interventional radiological techniques can be carried out in the outpatient setting with minimal morbidity and complication rates. It is particularly useful in patients in whom surgery is relatively contraindicated; for example, extensive previous abdominal surgery or during pregnancy.

Ultrasound-guided ovarian cyst aspiration

It is now possible to aspirate ovarian cysts transvaginally. A TVUS probe with a biopsy guide attached is placed in the vagina and the ovarian lesion is targeted. Under ultrasound control, a needle is then passed through the transvaginal probe and fluid is aspirated from the cyst or collection. The size of the needle is adjusted according to the predicted viscosity of the fluid. When serous-type fluid is being aspirated, an 18- or 20-gauge needle will suffice. If the ovarian cyst is easily accessible and thin walled, it may not be necessary to administer intravenous sedation to cover the procedure. However, if intravenous sedation is needed, a combination of midazolam (Hypnovel®, Roche, Welwyn Garden City, UK), fentanyl and metoclopramide (Maxolon®, Shire, Basingstoke, UK) titrated in small doses is usually sufficient.

It is important that the ovarian cysts are unilocular and thin walled if the technique is going to be successful and safe. Subtle, superficial, internal mural nodules or small papillary excrescences should be searched for meticulously because these features may indicate a malignant lesion, in particular a borderline tumour. With careful attention to ultrasound surveillance, cyst aspiration can be performed safely (Caspi et al 1996, Troiano and Taylor 1998). In 33–50% of cases, cyst aspiration will constitute definitive therapy. In other cases, cysts will recur and it is important to remember that cytology alone is not sufficiently accurate to exclude malignancy. Cyst recurrence after drainage is higher than if the capsule is removed (Balat et al 1996), but cyst fluid cytology is not always representative of the cyst wall pathology (Dietrich et al 1999).

Haemorrhagic cysts that do not resolve spontaneously or those that are symptomatic may be aspirated, usually via an 18- or 20-gauge needle, resulting in complete relief of symptoms.

Cyst aspiration in pregnant women is also feasible, and this technique is useful for functional cysts that become large and symptomatic (Khaw and Walker 1990). Cyst aspiration decreases the risk of rupture or torsion. Cysts that persist into later pregnancy are more likely to be serous or mucinous, and may be malignant. However, in some cases, it may be useful to aspirate the cyst and to remove it post partum. Such treatment may be warranted after careful assessment because surgical treatment for cysts in pregnancy is not without risk, with reported miscarriage rates between 2% and 35%.

The Emergency Gynaecological Unit

The provision of an EGU is now recognized as a gold standard service (Royal College of Obstetricians and Gynaecologists 2006). It provides an easily accessible outpatient area with facilities for ultrasound-based assessment of pregnancy duration, viability and location, This allows the clinician to provide informed management and counselling of the patient in a setting which maximizes her privacy and comfort. The EGU should have a dedicated area for the triage, assessment and initial management of patients presenting with acute gynaecological disorders, including early pregnancy complications. There should be a separate area where the patient can change, a designated waiting area with toilet facility, and bed/trolley spaces to accommodate women who need to recline. An initial assessment of the clinical condition can be made and recorded on a preformed history sheet. The cost benefits of the EPU are well established (Bigrigg and Read 1991) as admission can be avoided in approximately 40% of patients, with a further 20% requiring a shorter stay. Ideally, there should be a dedicated unit for the assessment and investigation of women with suspected complications of early pregnancy. This will be centred around an ultrasound scanning room, run by dedicated ultrasound practitioners. There should be a private area in which the patient can change and also a separate counselling room with access to a counselling service and outside line telephone.

Referral to the EPU may be by prior arrangement with the general practitioner or other consultant, or, ideally, a 'walk-in' self-referral system can operate. The latter will provide the patient with the means to contact a unit directly when problems arise, although it will make clinics busy. Again, the history can be collected on a proforma. This will highlight relevant gynaecological and obstetric history for the clinician, including factors predisposing to ectopic pregnancy or women in whom recurrent miscarriages have been identified, and will also facilitate audit and research. A number of computer databases now exist which aid data collection and facilitate reporting. This means that the patient can leave the clinic with a detailed report and follow-up plan, and a report can be distributed immediately to the referring clinician.

Many of the women who attend as gynaecological emergencies present with pelvic pain with or without vaginal bleeding. The differential diagnosis should be whether or not the symptoms have a gynaecological cause or some other underlying pathology, such as a gastrointestinal (e.g. constipation, appendicitis, diverticulities) or urological (e.g. urinary tract infection, stone) cause. If the symptoms are thought to be gynaecological in nature, the next decision is whether or not the woman is pregnant. If she is pregnant, pregnancy location and viability must be established. If the symptoms are not pregnancy related, are they chronic (>6 months' duration) or acute? If they are acute, does she have an ovarian cyst accident (e.g. haemorrhage, rupture, torsion) or acute pelvic inflammatory disease?

Availability of rapid serum β-human chorionic gonadotrophin (β-hCG) assays will vary within units, but the judicious use and follow-up of serum changes in β-hCG is essential for a diagnosis where the pregnancy location is not readily identified. This may be achieved in a number of ways, but typically will be dependent upon a dedicated staff member to record and interpret results either via a computer database or log book. The patient is either contacted with further follow-up/intervention plans or the patient contacts the unit herself for these results.

Fortunately, the majority of women with pain or bleeding in early pregnancy will present subacutely; in all cases, however, an initial assessment of haemodynamic compromise must be made. Blood pressure, pulse, temperature and pulse oximetry should be recorded. Facilities for obtaining venous access and commencing intravenous volume replacement should be available.

Anti-D immunoglobulin use

Current guidelines (Royal College of Obstetricians and Gynaecologists 2000 & 2006) for the use of rhesus immunoprophylaxis in early pregnancy recommend that anti-D immunoglobulin should be given to all non-sensitized rhesus-D-negative women who have:

- an ectopic pregnancy;
- a therapeutic termination of pregnancy (surgical or medical);
- a threatened or spontaneous miscarriage after 12 weeks' gestation (note: where there is heavy, recurrent or painful bleeding prior to 12 weeks' gestation, anti-D immunoglobulin prophylaxis is also recommended); or
- surgical evacuation of retained products of conception prior to 12 weeks' gestation.

Psychological aspects

Women, and their partners, who are diagnosed with early pregnancy failure should be offered follow-up to allow for appropriate support and counselling. This will facilitate early referral to formal counselling services when necessary.

Ultrasound Overview

TVUS should be regarded as an extension of a bimanual examination rather than a replacement. A recent prospective comparative trial of endovaginal sonographic bimanual examination versus traditional digital bimanual examination in non-pregnant women with lower abdominal pain has been reported (Tayal et al 2008). The study clearly demonstrated that vaginal examinations combined with TVUS improved confidence in key findings, such as ovarian and uterine size or position irrespective of the patient's body mass index. The advantages of TVUS over the transabdominal approach are well documented (Gonzalez et al 1988, Mendelson et al 1988). The placement of the ultrasound probe closer to the pelvic organs means that higher frequency ultrasound transducers (6–7.5 MHz) can be used, which produce high-resolution images. TVUS assessment of ovarian volume and morphology correlates closely with subsequent operative findings at laparotomy (Rodriguez et al 1988).

No single ultrasound measurement of the different anatomical features in the first trimester has been shown to have a high predictive value for determining early pregnancy outcome, and Doppler studies are not helpful either (Jauniaux et al 2005). Despite this, high-resolution TVUS has transformed understanding of the pathophysiology and management of early pregnancy failure. The ultrasound findings in both a normal pregnancy and a failing pregnancy are well described (Dogra et al 2005). The intrauterine gestation sac can be visualized from approximately 4 weeks after the last menstrual period using a transvaginal transducer, which is approximately 2 weeks earlier than if using the transabdominal approach (Fossam et al 1988). This is dependent upon a regular 28-day cycle, and hence a more accurate approach to confirming pregnancy viability or failure is dependent upon either changes with time or the presence or absence of fetal cardiac activity. The diameter of the gestational sac increases at approximately 1 mm/day in early pregnancy (Nyberg et al 1985), and can be differentiated from the 'pseudosac' of ectopic pregnancy by its thick, echogenic rind surrounding the echo-lucent central chorionic sac and eccentric location to the endometrial midline. The presence of a normal intrauterine gestation sac is associated with β-hCG levels of >1000 IU. Detection at levels greater than this is dependent upon a number of factors, including type of probe and ultrasound machine used, the presence of leiomyomas, operator variations and multiple gestations (Nyberg et al 1985, Bernaschek et al 1988). The absence of a gestation sac should prompt the operator to look for an extrauterine gestation (including a close examination of the cornua and cervix as well as the adnexa). Visualization of the yolk sac is regarded as definitive evidence of an intrauterine pregnancy. The yolk sac can be visualized from 5 weeks' gestation (Figure 6.1), and the early embryonic pole from approximately 6 weeks. First recognized as a thickening along the yolk sac, it is linear to begin with, subsequently becoming curved in nature. The embryonic growth rate is 1 mm/day. Cardiac activity starts at approximately 5 weeks after the last menstrual period. Cardiac activity not detected in embryos of more than 4 mm is associated with embryonic demise (Brown et al 1990, Levi et al 1990, Goldstein 1992). However, a repeat scan to confirm diagnosis is always indicated. Embryonic bradycardia can be associated with poor outcome (Doubilet et al 1999), and a follow-up scan is warranted to confirm viability.

TVUS has an established role in the evaluation of adnexal masses. It provides an accurate assessment of ovarian morphology (Granberg et al 1989, 1990, Timmerman et al 1999b) and is a significant contributor to mathematical models being developed to assess ovarian tumours (Tailor et al 1997, Timmerman et al 1999a,c). There are several types of ovarian cyst that can be assessed using the recogni-

tion of characteristic morphological patterns (Jermy et al 2001). Endometriomas and benign cystic teratomas are two examples, accounting for over two-thirds of persistent adnexal masses in premenopausal women (Koonings et al 1989). These lesions can be particularly difficult to score using morphological scoring systems, and as angiogenesis is ubiquitous throughout the ovarian cycle, colour Doppler is of limited value (Alcazar et al 1997).

Clinical Conditions

Bleeding and/or pain with a positive pregnancy test

Sensitive urinary pregnancy testing kits, based on immunological assays, are able to detect β-hCG levels of between 20 and 50 IU with 99% accuracy. This has meant that an increasingly large number of women will present with bleeding and/or pain in early pregnancy. It has been estimated that approximately 30% of women will complain of pain or bleeding during early pregnancy, and approximately 15% of clinically recognizable pregnancies will result in miscarriage, the majority before the 13th week (Prendiville 1997). Due to the large volume of work in such a highly sensitive area of gynaecology, an integrated approach to diagnosis and management of women presenting with bleeding and/or pelvic pain during the first trimester is required.

With the judicious use of ultrasound, clinicians have the ability to alleviate anxiety concerning early pregnancy complications by accurately dating early pregnancy, confirming viability, diagnosing pregnancy failure, and either directly or indirectly confirming extrauterine gestation. To do this safely, knowledge of early pregnancy development, both ultrasonographically and biochemically, is pivotal.

Miscarriage

Once the diagnosis of intrauterine pregnancy has been established, the potential viability of the pregnancy will need to be addressed. The clinical value of the normal developmental timespan of the early embryonic and extraembryonic structures is its application in the diagnosis of pregnancy failure. What becomes more relevant is not the earliest point at which a structure can be seen (threshold), but the point at which a structure is always seen in a normally developing intrauterine pregnancy (discriminatory level), so its absence is diagnostic of pregnancy failure. Once an ectopic pregnancy has been excluded, all intrauterine pregnancies should be given the benefit of the doubt and serial scans should be performed to confirm a diagnosis. However, cardiac activity should always be visualized in an embryo measuring 6 mm or more (Figure 6.2).

Knowledge of early pregnancy anatomical landmarks allows one to follow fetal development within a normal pregnancy, and to establish safe guidelines in the diagnosis of a pathological pregnancy.

Terminology

- Missed miscarriage (early fetal demise): crown–rump length of at least 6 mm with no cardiac activity or no change in size on weekly serial scanning.

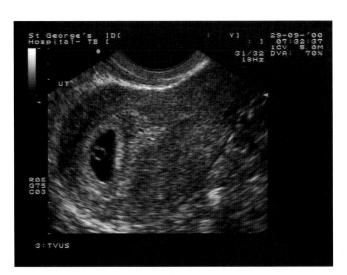

Figure 6.1 Intrauterine gestation and yolk sac: 5 weeks' gestation.

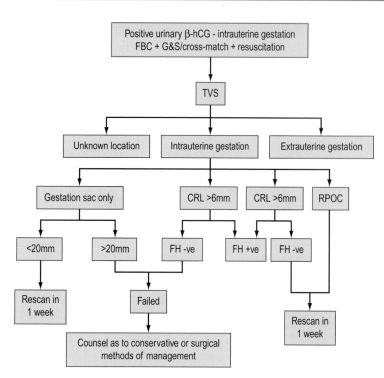

Figure 6.2 Assessment of viability in early pregnancy. β-hCG, β-human chorionic gonadotrophin; FBC, full blood count; TVS, transvaginal sonography; CRL, crown–rump length; RPOC, retained products of conception; G&S, groups and save; FH, fetal heart.

- Blighted ovum (early embryonic demise): mean diameter of gestational sac of at least 20 mm with no embryonic/extraembryonic structures present.
- Incomplete miscarriage: disrupted endometrial echo measuring >15 mm in the anteroposterior plane (Figure 6.3).
- Complete miscarriage: endometrial thickness of <15 mm measured in the anteroposterior plane associated with the cessation of heavy bleeding and pain.

Trouble shooting

- In practice, the presence of an intrauterine gestation usually excludes an ectopic pregnancy.
- Once ectopic pregnancy is excluded, early pregnancies should be given the benefit of the doubt; serial scans are of more value than serial β-hCG values.
- Cardiac activity should be seen with a crown–rump length of 6 mm or greater.
- A fetal pole/yolk sac should be seen with a gestation sac with a mean diameter of 20 mm.

Ectopic pregnancy

The exclusion of an ectopic gestation remains a primary goal for the clinician assessing a patient presenting with pain and/or bleeding in early pregnancy. Traditionally, the presence of an empty uterus with a positive urinary pregnancy test has meant hospital admission with either laparoscopy or follow-up scans until a diagnosis is made. However, the combined use of high-resolution vaginal probes and serum β-hCG assays has meant that patients with symptoms and clinical findings suggestive of an ectopic gestation will fall into one of three categories, as follows:

- an intrauterine pregnancy will be diagnosed on scan: to all extents and purposes, this will exclude an

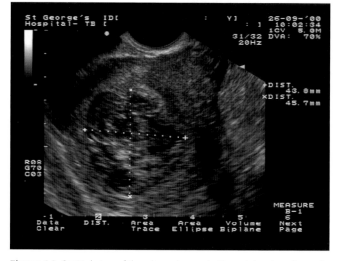

Figure 6.3 Sagittal view of the uterus demonstrating retained products of conception.

extrauterine location. The frequency of heterotopic pregnancy in spontaneous conceptions is estimated at between 1 : 10,000 and 1 : 50,000, but is as high as 1 : 100 in assisted conceptions (Ludwig et al 1999), and should be suspected if there are persistent symptoms;
- an extrauterine gestation or highly predictive features (e.g. haemoperitoneum) will be visualized by ultrasound (Figures 6.4–6.6); or
- no evidence of intra- or extrauterine gestation will be found on scan alone; a pregnancy of unknown location.

Further management of the patient will be dependent upon her clinical status. Within the authors' unit, there has been a significant reduction in patients presenting with acute haemodynamic compromise due to a ruptured ectopic

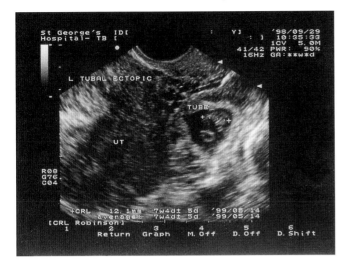

Figure 6.4 Sagittal section of the left adnexa demonstrating a tubal ectopic pregnancy. The crown–rump length is marked (12.1 mm).

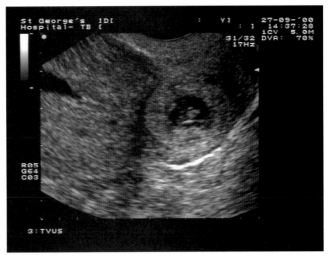

Figure 6.6 Sagittal view of the cervix containing a gestational sac, fetal pole and yolk sac. The proximal portion of the endometrial cavity contains free fluid and can be seen on the left side of the image.

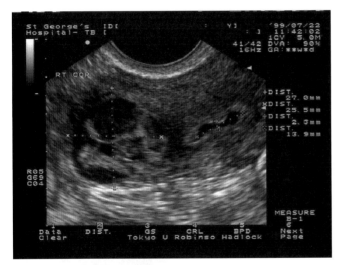

Figure 6.5 Cornual ectopic pregnancy. The gestation sac is seen separately from the endometrial echo.

pregnancy since the EPU was established. This has meant that more conservative methods of treatment can be used, whether surgical (laparoscopic salpingectomy, salpingotomy), medical (methotrexate) or expectant (Figure 6.7).

All non-surgical methods of treating ectopic gestations will need intensive follow-up to ensure resolution of symptoms and β-hCG values. Patient compliance is central to these patients being treated on an outpatient basis, along with a dedicated EPU service (see Chapter 25, Ectopic pregnancy, for more information).

Pregnancy of unknown location

A proportion of women presenting with complications of early pregnancy will have no sonographic features of extra- or intrauterine pregnancy. This group will include patients who have a very early, continuing, intrauterine pregnancy, those who have an ectopic gestation and those who have a failing pregnancy, whether intra- or extrauterine. Rarely, a

false-positive result may be due to a placental site tumour, for example of the ovary. Figure 6.8 demonstrates a suggested follow-up regime for women who fall into this category. Again, a coordinated EPU and rapid β-hCG assay service are essential.

Coexistent pathology

The prevalence of ovarian pathology in early pregnancy is high; one advantage of TVUS is the ability to visualize the adnexa clearly in early pregnancy. The majority of adnexal pathology will be functional in nature, typically corpus luteal, and will spontaneously resolve as the pregnancy enters the second trimester. Whether or not surgical intervention is indicated for persistent, symptomatic cysts will be dictated on an individual basis, and the role of cyst aspiration and laparoscopic surgical techniques can be maximized when there is clear ultrasound definition of cyst type.

Those patients managed expectantly should be rescanned 6 weeks post partum to ensure cyst resolution or to arrange surgical intervention if there is persistence of the cyst.

Postnatal assessment

Few studies have targeted the normal ultrasound parameters of the uterus and ovaries in the postnatal period. The sonographic appearances of retained products of conception are variable (Carlan et al 1997, Hertzberg and Bowie 1991). One study evaluating the appearance of the uterine cavity revealed an echogenic mass in 51% of women with normal postpartum bleeding at 7 days post partum (Edwards and Ellwood 2000). Sonohysterography has been shown to enhance the ability of TVUS to diagnose retained products of conception (Wolman et al 2000), although in the presence of suspected pelvic infection, this procedure should not be performed. Management should be based primarily on clinical findings, with sonographic evaluation of the uterus and endometrium reserved for those cases with persistent symptoms. Rarely, arteriovenous malformations can cause protracted, heavy bleeding in the puerperium. If suspected, colour Doppler

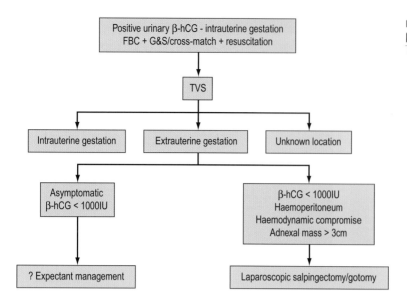

Figure 6.7 Assessment of an extrauterine pregnancy. β-hCG, β-human chorionic gonadotrophin; FBC, full blood count; TVS, transvaginal sonography; G&S, group and save.

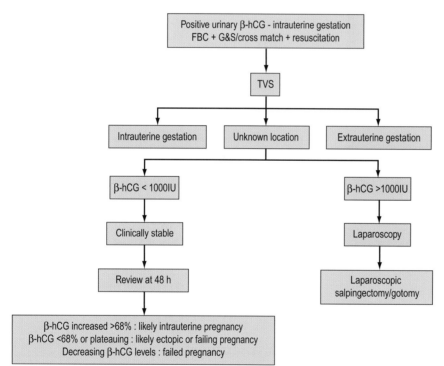

Figure 6.8 Assessment of pregnancy of unknown location. β-hCG, β-human chorionic gonadotrophin; FBC, full blood count; TVS, transvaginal sonography; G&S, group and save.

assessment of the uterine vasculature will aid their diagnosis, prior to arteriography and embolization. If surgical evacuation of retained products of conception is performed in the immediate postnatal period, the recognized higher morbidity associated with the procedure can be reduced by evacuating the uterus under sonographic guidance (Kohlenberg and Casper 1996).

Pelvic pain and a negative pregnancy test

TVUS undoubtedly has a pivotal role in the assessment of early pregnancy complications. Its role in those patients who are not pregnant, however, is more subtle and, rather than

being central to diagnosis, works in parallel with clinical findings and history, serum analyses, urinalysis and other radiological investigations. The role of ultrasound in the patient with acute pelvic pain and the patient with acute vaginal bleeding will be discussed below.

The premenopausal patient

The importance of a complete clinical history and examination cannot be overemphasized, especially with the use of pelvic ultrasound. The premenopausal ovary and endometrium, as visualized with the transvaginal probe, are dynamic structures, exhibiting cyclical changes in morphology and volume throughout the cycle. A knowledge of the normal variations that can be exhibited is important, as the most common ovarian pathology is the functional cyst.

The presence of adnexal pathology in the patient presenting with pelvic pain may be a coincidence, and gentle use of the transvaginal probe to map the pain within the pelvis will help to indicate the structures giving rise to the pain. The overwhelming advantages of the transvaginal approach in the assessment of pelvic pain are not only the excellent diagnostic capabilities, but also that, in the presence of an acute abdomen, especially in women with pelvic inflammatory disease, this route is tolerated much better than a transabdominal approach with a full bladder.

Pelvic pain in association with a pelvic mass

In those patients presenting with pelvic pain in whom there is evidence of a pelvic mass on ultrasound, an assessment needs to be made not only of pain severity and type, but also the nature of the mass. TVUS has a proven track record in experienced hands in the differentiation of uterine myomas from adnexal masses, and also in the characterization of adnexal masses.

The prevalence of adnexal pathology among premenopausal women is high and the overwhelming majority of these lesions will be benign in nature. A large proportion of benign ovarian cysts will be functional and, if symptoms settle, may be managed expectantly.

A careful history and a clear knowledge of the day of the menstrual cycle will prompt the sonographer to the most likely cause of the pain. For example, acute-onset, midcycle pain may be indicative of a follicular or corpus luteal cyst accident. Haemorrhage into a corpus luteal cyst has characteristic sonographic findings (Figure 6.9). The condition tends to be self-limiting and often responds to non-steroidal anti-inflammatory analgesia. Surgery should be avoided if possible.

Although usually self-limiting, the cyclical occurrence of haemorrhagic corpus luteal cyst can be a source of persistent morbidity; if there are no contraindications, use of the combined oral contraceptive to suppress ovulation is beneficial. This is also indicated for women who have clotting factor deficiencies, such as von Willebrand's disease. They may present with an acute abdomen, secondary to a haemoperitoneum, as a result of ovulation or corpus luteal haemorrhage or rupture.

Women with a history suggestive of endometriosis presenting with acute pain may have sonographic evidence of an endometrioma (Figure 6.10). These rarely undergo torsion, as they are often fixed within the pelvis, but may undergo rupture or acute haemorrhage within the cyst. Rarely, they can become infected. Recent cyst rupture may be suggested by the presence of resolving clinical symptoms, with free fluid present in the pouch of Douglas, often with a collapsing irregular cyst wall.

A suggested follow-up regime for women diagnosed with a pelvic mass is shown in Figure 6.11. Intervention will be dictated by the resolution, or not, of the patient's symptoms. If the symptoms resolve and there are no sonographic features of malignancy on the ultrasound, a repeat scan at 6 weeks should be performed to confirm cyst resolution.

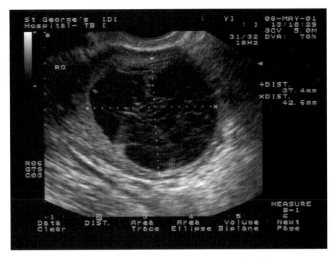

Figure 6.9 Haemorrhagic corpus luteal cyst. Fine strands of fibrin are seen within the cyst contents.

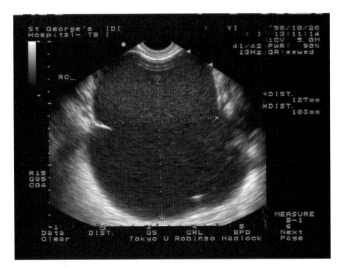

Figure 6.10 Large ovarian endometrioma: characteristic 'ground-glass' appearance of the cyst contents.

Ovarian torsion is unusual with adnexal masses <5 cm (Nicholas and Julian 1985). However, there are no pathognomonic features specific to adnexal torsion, and a high degree of clinical suspicion is essential. The clinical history is of acute-onset, constant pain that does not respond to analgesia, often with nausea and vomiting and systemic upset. Of the persistent adnexal masses in premenopausal women, benign cystic teratomas (Figure 6.12) are more likely to undergo torsion than endometriomas. The central feature of ovarian torsion is the cessation of vascular supply. Colour Doppler has therefore been used to interrogate the adnexal mass suspected of undergoing torsion. It is likely, however, that even if flow can be visualized within the mass, despite clinical symptoms and signs of ovarian torsion, ovarian blood flow may still be compromised, as demonstrated by surgically proven ovarian torsion despite the detection of blood flow within the mass (Rasado et al 1992).

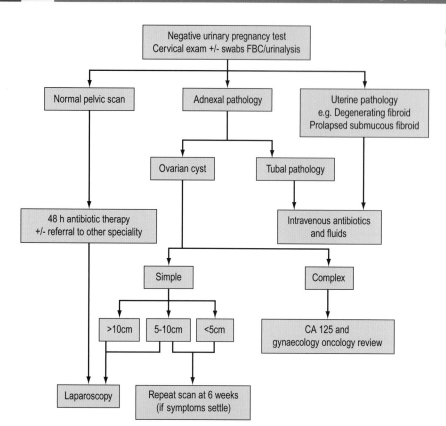

Figure 6.11 Assessment of pelvic mass. FBC, full blood count.

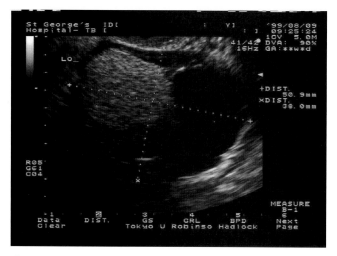

Figure 6.12 Benign cystic teratoma: acoustic shadowing is demonstrated.

Uterine leiomyomas

These may undergo torsion if pedunculated in nature, may prolapse through the cervix or may undergo degeneration, especially during pregnancy. In fibroid degeneration, the patient is often systemically unwell, with pyrexia, leucocytosis and generalized abdominal tenderness.

The ultrasound characteristics of leiomyomas are well documented and cystic areas can be visualized within the fibroid if it is degenerating. Advances in the management of uterine myomas have resulted in a need to provide accurate pretreatment information concerning their size, quantity and location. This is especially true with the increasing use of minimally invasive techniques of fibroid resection. The

ultrasound appearances of myomas are varied. Before the menopause, they tend to be a well-defined heterogeneous or hypoechoic uterine mass. TVUS is used in conjunction with abdominal scanning to ensure that pedunculated subserosal fibroids are not missed.

Tubal pathology

Acute pelvic inflammatory disease, with hydrosalpinx, pyosalpinx or frank tubo-ovarian abscesses, tends to present with systemic upset, leucocytosis, unilateral progressing to bilateral pelvic pain, menstrual disturbances and vaginal discharge. The differentials will therefore include adnexal torsion, acute fibroid degeneration, urinary tract infection and appendicitis.

Acute inflammatory processes within the fallopian tubes tend to produce thick-walled, cystic structures, tender to the touch of the probe (Figure 6.13). However, a chronic hydrosalpinx will have the appearance of a thin-walled structure, not obviously tender on probing and often detected coincidentally (Timor-Tritsch et al 1998).

Acute urinary retention

A full bladder may sometimes be confused with an ovarian cyst. If there is any doubt and the patient is unable to void urine, a catheter should be passed to ensure the bladder is empty. Occasionally, a blood clot may be visible within the bladder.

Pelvic pain with no mass on scan

In the absence of pathology on scan, blood should be taken for leucocytosis and culture. Urinalysis should be performed

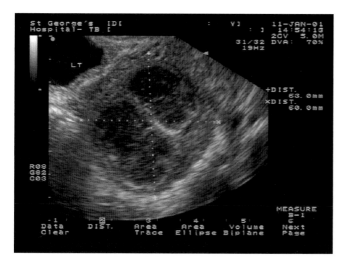

Figure 6.13 Tubo-ovarian abscess: an irregular, thick-walled multiloculated structure.

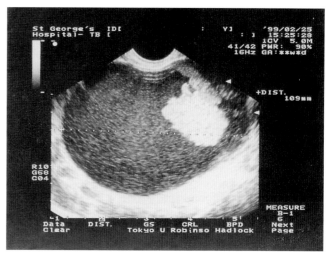

Figure 6.14 Ovarian endometroid adenocarcinoma: Stage Ia. Note the large papillary projection from the cyst wall.

and a complete infection screen, including endocervical and high vaginal swabs. Contact tracing should be performed via the genitourinary clinic. A transvaginal scan may reveal evidence of adhesions and loculated fluid, which may be indicative of previous pelvic or abdominal pathology.

Non-gynaecological pathology

It is often not possible to make a diagnosis based on clinical, ultrasound and serum findings alone. Medical, surgical and urological opinions should be sought where indicated, with early recourse to laparoscopy in those patients who have persistent or worsening symptoms.

The postmenopausal patient

Characterization of any adnexal mass is important within this age group as the risk of a mass being malignant is high (Figure 6.14). Unilocular cysts may be found in up to 20% of asymptomatic postmenopausal women. Numerous studies have shown that simple, unilocular cysts measuring <5 cm in diameter are associated with a very low risk of malignancy (Kroon and Andolf 1995). Blood should be taken for tumour markers and emergency laparotomy should be avoided if at all possible, to allow for adequate oncological work-up of the patient if indicated. Urinary retention must be excluded. Other chronic surgical and medical conditions are more predominant in the older age group, such as diverticulitis, constipation and urinary tract infections. Early recourse to advice from other specialties should be considered in women with pelvic or abdominal pain.

Acute bleeding and a negative pregnancy test

This is most effectively divided into problems occurring in the premenopausal and postmenopausal patient, as the aetiology can be very different. A full history and clinical examination is essential, along with resuscitation of the patient.

The investigation of abnormal uterine bleeding will centre on an assessment of the endometrium (Figure 6.15). Undirected endometrial sampling alone has no role in the evalu-

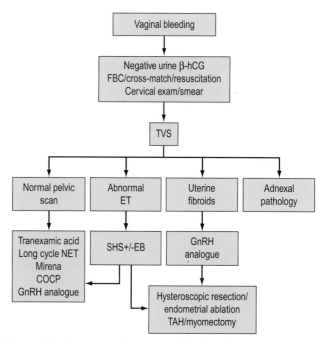

Figure 6.15 Assessment of acute vaginal bleeding. β-hCG, β-human chorionic gonadotrophin; FBC, full blood count; TVS, transvaginal sonography; COCP, combined oral contraceptive pill; GnRH, gonadotrophin-releasing hormone; TAH, total abdominal hysterectomy; NET, norethisterone acetate; EB, endometrial biopsy; ET, endometrial thickening; SHS, Saline Hysteroscopy Study.

ation of abnormal uterine bleeding. It will miss focal lesions, such as polyps and fibroids. Whilst TVUS remains a cost-effective, non-invasive, well-tolerated technique for examining the pelvic organs, it is less specific than hysteroscopy when differentiating between endometrial polyps, myomas, carcinoma and hyperplasia. The addition of a negative contrast medium, such as saline, into the uterine cavity addresses this problem. An overwhelming quantity of data has shown that high-resolution TVUS with saline instillation is as predictive as hysteroscopy in the detection of endometrial pathology.

The premenopausal patient

The main differentials within this group are genital tract disease, systemic disease and iatrogenic causes. When all these have been excluded, a diagnosis of dysfunctional uterine bleeding can be made. History, clinical examination and pelvic ultrasound will help to elucidate the cause. Disease of the genital tract in this age group will focus on benign rather than malignant conditions. Benign pelvic conditions will include fibroids, endometrial and cervical polyps, cervicitis, adenomyosis and endometriosis, along with pelvic infection and foreign bodies. Systemic problems contributing to abnormal uterine bleeding will include coagulation disorders, chronic liver and renal disease, and thyroid dysfunction. Iatrogenic causes will include anticoagulant therapy, intrauterine contraceptive devices and hormonal preparations. There needs to be heightened suspicion of an underlying systemic disease in younger patients presenting with heavy vaginal bleeding, as up to 20% (Kadir et al 1998) may have a coagulopathy. Screening for a coagulopathy is also advised in women with abnormal vaginal bleeding who fail medical or surgical therapy. The endometrial thickness on ultrasound will dictate the need for endometrial sampling, as will the patient's history.

The primary goal with acute uterine bleeding will be to ensure cessation of bleeding, usually with a combination of therapies, such as antifibrinolytics, high-dose progestogens, gonadotrophin-releasing hormone analogues or the Mirena intrauterine system, until definitive management can be effected. Occasionally, urgent examination under anaesthesia with the introduction of a uterine cavity balloon is indicated to stop the bleeding. Interventional radiology with uterine artery embolization may have a role in acute management.

The postmenopausal patient

Abnormal vaginal bleeding in this age group should be attributed to malignancy until proven otherwise. Malignant tumours of the endometrium, cervix, vagina and vulva may all present with vaginal bleeding, as can ovarian tumours, such as granulosa cell tumours. It is wise to confirm that the bleeding is genital tract in origin, as occasionally haematuria and rectal bleeding may present as suspected postmenopausal vaginal bleeding.

Conclusion

The National Service Framework for Children, Young People and Maternity Services (Department of Health 2003) is clear in its aim of providing patient-centred care with the identification and appropriate management of relevant social, medical and psychiatric problems, with a one-stop assessment, diagnosis and management ethos as set out in the NHS Plan (Department of Health 2000). EGUs are excellent examples of how this aspiration can be translated into clinical practice. TVUS plays a pivotal role in assessment of the acute gynaecological patient; as such, it is the core investigating modality in the EGU. It complements a full clinical examination, affording a 'view' of the pelvic structures. Its integration into the gynaecology emergency service facilitates more rapid diagnosis in a number of gynaecological conditions. It also helps to exclude gynaecological pathology, ensuring prompt referral to other specialties and multidisciplinary teams. Central to its appropriate use will be training and supervision, with up-to-date protocols and regular audit, and awareness of the limitations of personnel and the equipment.

KEY POINTS

1. A normal pelvic scan will not exclude all underlying gynaecological conditions.
2. Visualization of an intrauterine gestation will generally exclude an ectopic pregnancy.
3. Once an ectopic pregnancy has been excluded, early pregnancies should be given the benefit of the doubt.
4. Fetal heart activity should be seen with a crown–rump length of 6 mm or greater.
5. The sonographic appearances of retained products of conception in the immediate postnatal period are variable; management should be based primarily on clinical findings.
6. There are no pathognomonic features specific to adnexal torsion; a high degree of clinical suspicion is paramount.
7. Undirected endometrial sampling alone has no role in the evaluation of abnormal uterine bleeding.
8. Transvaginal saline sonohysterography is as predictive as hysteroscopy in the detection of endometrial pathology.
9. Up to 20% of young women presenting with heavy vaginal bleeding may have a coagulopathy.

References

Balat O, Sarac K, Sonmez S 1996 Ultrasound guided aspiration of benign ovarian cysts: an alterntive to surgery. European Journal of Radiology 22: 136–137.

Basama FM, Crosfill F, Price A 2004 Women's perception of transvaginal sonography in the first trimester in an early pregnancy assessment unit. Archives of Gynaecology and Obstetrics 269: 117–120.

Bernaschek G, Rudelstorfer R, Csascsich P 1988 Vaginal sonography versus serum human chorionic gonadotrophin in early detection of pregnancy. American Journal of Obstetrics and Gynecology 158: 608–612.

Bigrigg MA, Read MD 1991 Management of women referred to early pregnancy assessment unit: care and cost effectiveness. British Medical Journal 302: 577–579.

Brown DL, Emerson DS, Felker RE 1990 Diagnosis of embryonic demise by endovaginal sonography. Journal of Ultrasound in Medicine 9: 711–716.

Caspi B, Goldchmit R, Zalel Y, Appelman Z, Insler V 1996 Sonographically guided aspiration of ovarian cyst with simple appearance. Journal of Ultrasound in Medicine 15: 297–300.

Carlan SI, Scott WT, Pollack R, Harris K 1997 Appearance of the uterus by ultrasound immediately after placental delivery with pathologic correlation. Journal of Clinical Ultrasound 25: 301–308.

Department of Health 2000 The NHS Plan. A Plan for Investment, a Plan for Reform. HMSO, London.

Department of Health 2003 The National Service Framework for Children, Young People and Maternity Services. HMSO, London.

Dietrich M, Osmers RG, Grobe G et al 1999 Limitations of the evaluation of adnexal masses by its macroscopic aspects, cytology and biopsy. European Journal of Gynaecology and Reproduction Biology 82: 57–62.

Doubilet PM, Benson CB, Cow JS 1999 Long-term prognosis of pregnancies complicated by slow embryonic heart rates in the early first trimester. Journal of Ultrasound Medicine 18: 537–541.

Dogra V, Paspulati RM, Bhatt S 2005 First trimester bleeding evaluation. Ultrasound Quarterly 21: 149–154.

Edwards A, Ellwood DA 2000 Ultrasonographic evaluation of the postpartum uterus. Ultrasound in Obstetrics and Gynecology 16: 640–643.

Fernandez H, Yves Vincent SC, Pauthier S, Audibert F, Frydman R 1998 Randomised trial of conservative laparoscopic treatment and methotrexate administration in ectopic pregnancy and subsequent fertility. Human Reproduction 13: 3239–3243.

Fossam GT, Davajan V, Kletzky OA 1988 Early detection of pregnancy with transvaginal ultrasound. Fertility and Sterility 49: 788–791.

Goldstein SR 1992 Significance of cardiac activity on endovaginal ultrasound in very early embryos. Obstetrics and Gynecology 80: 670–672.

Gonzalez CJ, Curson R, Parson J 1988 Transabdominal versus transvaginal ultrasound scanning of ovarian follicles: are they comparable. Fertility and Sterility 50: 657–659.

Granberg S, Wikland M, Jansson I 1989 Macroscopic characterisation of ovarian tumors and the relation to the histological diagnosis: criteria to be used for ultrasound evaluation. Gynecologic Oncology 35: 139–144.

Granberg S, Norström A, Wikland M 1990 Tumors in the lower pelvis as imaged by transvaginal sonography. Gynecologic Oncology 37: 224–229.

Hafner T, Aslam N, Ross JA, Zosmer N, Jurkovic D 1999 The effectiveness of non-surgical management of early interstitial pregnancy: a report of ten cases and review of the literature. Ultrasound in Obstetrics and Gynecology 13: 131–136.

Hertzberg BS, Bowie JD 1991 Ultrasound of the postpartum uterus. Prediction of retained placental tissue. Journal of Ultrasound in Medicine 10: 451–456.

Jauniaux E, Johns J, Burton GJ 2005 The role of ultrasound imaging in diagnosing and investigating early pregnancy failure. Ultrasound in Obstetrics and Gynaecology 25: 613–624.

Jermy K, Luise C, Bourne T 2001 The characterization of common ovarian cysts in premenopausal women. Ultrasound in Obstetrics and Gynecology 17: 140–144.

Jimenez R, Duff P 1997 Sheathing of the endovaginal probe: is it adequate? Infectious Diseases in Obstetrics and Gynecology 1: 37–39.

Jones KD 2005 Gynaecological training in a consultant delivered service: a European perspective. The Obstetrician and Gynaecologist 7: 126–128.

Jones KD (ed) 2008 Ambulatory Gynaecology: a New Concept in Healthcare for Women. RCOG Press, London, Chapter 1, pp 1–11.

Jones K, Pearce C 2009 Organizing an acute gynaecology service: equipment and set up. Best Practice and Research Clinical Obstetrics and Gynaecology 23: 425–426.

Khaw KT, Walker WJ 1990 Ultrasound guided fine needle aspiration of ovarian cysts: diagnosis and treatment in pregnant and non-pregnant women. Clinical Radiology 141: 105–108.

Kadir RA, Economides DL, Sabin CA, Owens D, Lee CA 1998 Frequency of inherited bleeding disorders in women with menorrhagia. The Lancet 351: 485–489.

Kohlenberg CF, Casper GR 1996 The use of intraoperative ultrasound in the management of a perforated uterus with retained products of conception. Australia and New Zealand Journal of Obstetrics and Gynaecology 36: 482–484.

Koonings PP, Campbell K, Mishell D, Grimes D 1989 Relative frequency of ovarian neoplasms: a 10 year review. Obstetrics and Gynecology 74: 921–925.

Kroon E, Andolf E 1995 Diagnosis and follow-up of simple ovarian cysts detected by ultrasound in postmenopausal women. Obstetrics and Gynecology 85: 211–214.

Levi CS, Lyons EA, Zheng HX 1990 Endovaginal US: demonstration of cardiac activity in embryos of less than 5 mm in crown rump length. Radiology 176: 71–74.

Ludwig M, Kaisi M, Bauer O, Diedrich K 1999 Heterotopic pregnancy in a spontaneous cycle: do not forget about it! European Journal of Obstetrics, Gynecology and Reproductive Biology 87: 91–93.

Mendelson EB, Bohm-Velez M, Joseph N, Neiman HL 1988 Endometrial abnormalities: evaluation with transvaginal sonography. American Journal of Radiology 150: 139–142.

Moore RG, Brown AK, Miller CM et al 2008 The use of multiple novel serum tumor markers for the detection of ovarian carcinoma in patients with a pelvic mass. Gynecologic Oncology 108: 402–408.

Nicholas D, Julian P 1985 Torsion of the adnexa. Clinical Obstetrics and Gynecology 28: 375–380.

Nyberg DA, Filly RA, Mahony BS 1985 Early gestation: correlation of hCG levels and sonographic identification. AJR American Journal of Roentgenology 144: 951–954.

Prendiville WJ 1997 Miscarriage: epidemiological aspects. In: Grudzinskas JG, O'Brien PMS (eds) Problems in Early Pregnancy: Advances in Diagnosis and Management. RCOG Press, London.

Rasado W, Trambert M, Gosink B, Pretorius D 1992 Adnexal torsion: diagnosis by using Doppler sonography. American Journal of Radiology 159: 1251–1253.

Rodriguez MH, Platt LD, Medearis AL, Lacarra M, Lobo RA 1988 The use of transvaginal ultrasonography for evaluation of postmenopausal ovarian size and morphology. American Journal of Obstetrics and Gynecology 159: 810–814.

Royal College of Obstetricians and Gynaecologists 2000 Clinical Guideline Number 22. Anti-D Immunoglobulin for Rh Prophylaxis RCOG, London.

Royal College of Obstetricians and Gynaecologists 2006 Clinical Green Top Guidelines. The Management of Early Pregnancy Loss. RCOG Press, London.

Royal College of Radiologists/Royal College of Obstetricians and Gynaecologists 1995 Guidance on Ultrasound Procedures in Early Pregnancy. RCR/RCOG, London.

Tayal VS, Crean CA, Norton HJ et al 2008 Prospective comparative trial of endovaginal sonographic bimanual examination versus traditional digital bimanual examination in non pregnant women with lower abdominal pain with regard to body mass index classification. Journal of Ultrasound in Medicine 27: 1171–1177.

Tailor A, Jurkovic D, Bourne T, Collins W, Campbell S 1997 Sonographic prediction of malignancy in adnexal masses using multivariate logistic regression analysis. Ultrasound in Obstetrics and Gynecology 10: 41–47.

Timmerman D, Bourne TH, Tailor A et al 1999a A comparison of methods for the pre-operative discrimination between benign and malignant adnexal masses: the development of a new logistic regression model. American Journal of Obstetrics and Gynecology 181: 57–65.

Timmerman T, Schwärzler P, Collins W et al 1999b Subjective assessment of adnexal masses using ultrasonography: an analysis of interobserver variability and experience. Ultrasound in Obstetrics and Gynecology 13: 11–16.

Timmerman D, Verrelst H, Bourne T et al 1999c Artificial neural network models for the pre-operative discrimination between malignant and benign adnexal masses. Ultrasound in Obstetrics and Gynecology 13: 17–25.

Timor-Tritsch IE, Lerner JP, Monteagudo A, Murphy KE, Heller DS 1998 Transvaginal sonographic markers of tubal inflammatory disease. Ultrasound in Obstetrics and Gynecology 12: 56–66.

Troiano RN, Taylor KJ 1998 Sonographically guided therapeutic aspiration of benign-appearing ovarian cysts and endometriomas. AJR American Journal of Roentgenology 171: 1601–1605.

Wolman I, Gordon D, Yaron Y, Kupferminc M, Lessing JB, Jaffa AJ 2000 Transvaginal sonohysterography for the evaluation and treatment of retained products of conception. Gynecology and Obstetrics Investigation 50: 73–76.

CHAPTER 7

Preoperative care

Kate P. Stewart and Saad A. Amer

Chapter Contents

INTRODUCTION	93	PREOPERATIVE ASSESSMENT	96
CHOOSING THE OPERATION	93	PREOPERATIVE PREPARATION	99
CONSENT	93	KEY POINTS	103

Introduction

Approximately three million operations are performed each year in the UK National Health Service (NHS). Good preoperative care is the key to a successful outcome of these operations. This includes four main aspects: choosing the most appropriate operation, counselling and obtaining consent, preoperative assessment and preoperative preparation. The aim of this care is to optimize the patient's preoperative condition to achieve the best outcome from surgery and to minimize morbidity. Another important objective of preoperative care is to alleviate the patient's fear and anxiety whilst waiting for her surgery. Good preoperative care will also help to avoid delays and cancellations of surgery, thereby maximizing the patient's satisfaction during her journey through the hospital system. Although preoperative care is a patient-centred procedure, it should also involve preparation of the patient's family as well as members of the multidisciplinary teams involved with the care of the patient. Details of the intended operative procedure as well as any social or health concerns should be communicated with the relevant hospital teams.

Choosing the Operation

Choosing the optimum surgical procedure is a crucial first step in the preoperative care of patients. All management options should be carefully considered after full and thorough assessment of the patient's gynaecological as well as other coexisting medical conditions. All treatment options should be explored including no treatment, non-surgical alternatives or more conservative surgery. For example, a patient requesting sterilization should be informed about reversible long-term contraception, and she and her partner should be informed about vasectomy. Likewise, a patient requesting hysterectomy for menorrhagia should be informed of the reversible progestogen-releasing intrauterine system or less invasive endometrial ablation. It is the clinician's duty to make the patient fully aware of all her options. All the pros and cons and implications of various treatments as well as no treatment should be fully explained to patients. The final decision on the optimum treatment should be mutually agreed between the surgeon and the patient, taking into consideration her wishes and social circumstances (General Medical Council 2008). Quite often, patients do not remember all the information given to them verbally during their consultation. It is therefore important to hand them printed leaflets containing more detailed information on their intended procedure, as well as other relevant treatments. These should also be available in languages other than English depending on the local demographics. With the availability of information on the Internet, patients are very likely to read up on their intended procedures from various unknown Internet sources. Clinicians should therefore direct their patients towards trusted websites offering unbiased information, such as that of the Royal College of Obstetricians and Gynaecologists which provides specific information leaflets for patients.

Consent

Valid consent

It is a legal requirement and an ethical principle to obtain valid consent before starting any treatment or investigation. Although verbal consent is acceptable for most investigations and medical treatments, it is necessary to obtain written and signed consent before any surgical intervention under anaesthesia, with the exception of some emergency situations. For consent to be valid, it must be given voluntarily by an appropriately informed person (either the patient or someone with parental responsibility if the patient is under 16 years of age) who has the capacity to consent to the intervention. The woman must be informed regarding the nature of her condition. Written information should be given, especially as patients are often admitted on the day of surgery and have less time to ask questions. As discussed above, the patient must also be aware of

DOI: 10.1016/B978-0-7020-3120-5.00007-2

the alternatives to surgery and the option of no treatment. The Royal College of Obstetricians and Gynaecologists, the General Medical Council and the Department of Health all place importance and have provided guidance on valid consent (Department of Health 2001, General Medical Council 2008, Royal College of Obstetricians and Gynaecologists 2008a).

Consent and operative risks

Patients should be informed of frequent and established serious adverse outcomes related to the procedure. The likelihood of complications associated with the intended surgical procedure should be presented in a fashion comprehensible to the patient. The discussion should include all possible intraoperative risks as well as short- and long-term postoperative complications. Table 7.1 summarizes the risks associated with common gynaecological operations as detailed by the Royal College of Obstetricians and Gynaecologists (2004a–c, 2008a–d).

Consent for additional procedures

It is always good practice to discuss, and include in the consent, any possible additional procedures that may be required during the intended operation. Generally, any additional surgical treatment which has not previously been discussed with the woman should not be performed, even if this means a second operation (Royal College of Obstetricians and Gynaecologists 2008a). One must not exceed the scope of authority given by the woman, except in a life-threatening emergency. There are three different situations where an additional procedure may be necessary during the course of an elective surgery. Firstly, when a minor pathology related to the patient's symptoms is detected such as endometriosis or adhesions in women undergoing laparoscopy for pelvic pain or infertility. In this situation, treatment can be performed if the patient has been made aware of this possibility and has consented for additional minor treatment. The second situation arises when a more complex disease is detected such as a pelvic mass, suspicious looking ovary, severe endometriosis or severe adhesions. Surgery in these situations should be deferred to a second operation after adequate counselling of the patient. In particular, oophorectomy for unexpected disease detected at surgery should not normally be performed without previous consent. The third situation involves intraoperative complications such as injury to the bowel or urinary tract that could lead to serious consequences if left untreated. Corrective surgery must proceed in these cases, and full explanation should be given as soon as practical following surgery.

Who should obtain the consent?

It is the responsibility of the clinician undertaking the surgical procedure to obtain consent. However, if this is not possible, it may be delegated to another doctor who is adequately trained and has sufficient knowledge of the procedure to be performed (General Medical Council 2008). The consent, however, remains the responsibility of the surgeon performing the operation. The clinician obtaining the consent should see the patient on her own first, for at least part of the consultation. She should then be allowed the company of a trusted friend or relative for support if she wishes. If consent is taken on the day of surgery, enough time should be allowed for discussion (Royal College of Obstetricians and Gynaecologists 2008a).

Additional consents

- Fertility treatment using assisted reproduction technology (e.g. oocyte retrieval under general anaesthetic) requires specific consent forms according to the regulations set by the Human Fertilisation and Embryology Authority.
- If images or video records are going to be taken during surgery, consent should be obtained for this and the use specified; for example, for teaching or educational purposes (Royal College of Obstetricians and Gynaecologists 2008a).
- Consent for the presence of medical students during consultations and in the operating theatre as an observer or assistant should be obtained. If the medical student has consent for vaginal examination while the woman is anaesthetized, this should be in writing.
- It is not required to have consent for taking tissue samples unless it is intended for research purposes. Women should be advised that blocks or slides of tissue taken for histological examination might be kept as part of the medical record whilst the rest of the sample is destroyed.

Duration of consent

The consent will remain valid indefinitely unless withdrawn. However, if new information is available between the consent and the procedure (e.g. new evidence of risk or new treatment options), the doctor should inform the patient and reconfirm the consent. It is also wise to refresh the consent form if there is a significant amount of time between consent and the intervention (Department of Health 2001).

Consent of special groups of patients

Jehovah's Witnesses

Jehovah's Witnesses are an Adventist sect of Christianity founded in the USA in the late 19th Century. They believe that accepting a blood transfusion, even autologous blood transfusions in which one's own blood is stored for later transfusion, is a sin. This includes red blood cells, white blood cells, platelets and plasma. Jehovah's Witnesses are aware of the possible risk to life in refusing blood transfusion and they take full responsibility for this. It is important to respect their wishes and to consider alternative measures to blood transfusion. There are special consent forms for Jehovah's Witnesses' refusal of blood products, stating clearly that this may result in the death of the patient. They also specify what blood fractions they might accept (e.g. interferons, interleukins, albumin, clotting factors or erythropoietin) as well as any blood salvage procedures, such as cell saver that recycles and cleans blood from a patient and redirects it to the patient's body. More information can be found on the official website of Jehovah's Witnesses (www.watchtower.org).

Table 7.1 Risks and benefits of common gynaecological procedures

Procedure	Diagnostic hysteroscopy	Diagnostic laparoscopy	Laparoscopic sterilization	Abdominal hysterectomy for menorrhagia	Pelvic floor repair and vaginal hysterectomy for prolapse
Benefit	Identify the cause of symptoms	Identify the cause of symptoms	Permanently prevent pregnancy	Stop menstruation	Improve/resolve prolapse symptoms
Serious risks	• Risk: 2 in 1000 • Damage to uterus • Damage to bowel or bladder • Damage to major blood vessels • Failure to gain entry to uterine cavity • Infertility (rare) • Death: 3–8 in 100,000 due to complications	• Risk: 2 in 1000 • Damage to bowel* or bladder • Damage to uterus • Damage to major blood vessels • Failure to gain entry to abdominal cavity • Hernia at site of entry • Death: 3–8 in 100,000 die due to complications	• Unplanned pregnancy: lifetime failure rate 1 in 200 • Possibility of ectopic pregnancy if failure occurs • Failure to gain entry to abdominal cavity • Uterine perforation • Injuries to the bowel, bladder or blood vessels are serious but infrequent: 3 in 1000 • Death: 1 in 12,000 die as a result of complications	• Complication rate 2% • Damage to bladder and/or ureter (0.7%) • Long-term disturbance to bladder function • Damage to bowel (0.04%) • Haemorrhage requiring blood transfusion (1.5%) • Return to theatre for additional stitches (0.6%) • Pelvic abscess/infection (0.2%) • Venous thrombosis or pulmonary embolism (0.4%) • Death: 1 in 4000	• Damage to bladder or ureter • Damage to bowel • Excessive bleeding requiring transfusion or return to theatre • Long-term disturbance to bladder function • Pelvic abscess • Venous thrombosis and embolism • Dyspareunia • Recurrence of prolapse
Frequent risks	• Infection • Bleeding	• Bruising • Shoulder-tip pain • Wound gaping • Wound infection	• Bruising • Shoulder-tip pain	• Wound infection and bruising • Frequency of micturition • Delayed wound healing • Keloid formation • Early menopause: evidence is inconclusive	• Urinary retention • Vaginal bleeding • Frequency of micturition • Infection • Pain
Other procedures which may be necessary	• Laparoscopy • Laparotomy	• Laparotomy • Repair of damage to bowel, bladder, uterus or blood vessels • Blood transfusion	• Laparotomy • Repair of damage to bowel, bladder or blood vessels	• Blood transfusion (1.5%) • Repair to bladder, bowel or major blood vessel • Oophorectomy for unsuspected disease†	• Blood transfusion (2%) • Repair of bladder or bowel • Laparotomy and conversion to abdominal approach

*Up to 15% of bowel injuries are not diagnosed at the time of laparoscopy.
†Must be discussed prior to surgery.

Adults without capacity

The Mental Capacity Act 2005

Clinicians should work on the assumption that every adult has the capacity to make decisions about her care. The patient should only be regarded as lacking capacity if she is considered unable to comprehend and retain information in order to make a decision after all practical steps to help her do so have been taken without success. A woman is entitled to make a decision based on her own religious beliefs or values as long as she understands what is entailed in her decision, even if it is the clinician's belief that this is not in her best interests. Likewise, a woman should not be thought to lack capacity because she has previously made an unwise decision. The capacity of people with a learning disability, mental illness or apparent inability to communicate should not be underestimated. Capacity may also be temporarily affected by factors such as confusion, pain, fatigue, medication or shock.

Within the English legal system, no one is able to give consent to treatment of adults unable to give consent for themselves. The key principle in care of an incapable adult is that the treatment should be in their best interests. It is lawful to carry out a procedure that is in the best interests of the patient. One cannot sign the consent form on their behalf; rather, one should document in the medical notes why the patient cannot consent for the procedure and why it is in their best interests. This is not confined to the best medical interests; it is to preserve life, health or well-being of the patient. This also covers procedures such as washing and dressing.

It is good practice to involve those close to the patient in order to find out about the patient's values and preferences prior to the loss of capacity. In addition, patients should be encouraged and supported, as far as they are able, to be involved in decisions about their care.

Certain procedures such as sterilization, management of menorrhagia and abortion do occasionally arise in women with severe learning disabilities who lack capacity to consent. They give special concern about the best interests and human rights of the person who lacks capacity. They can be referred to court if there is any doubt that the procedure is the most appropriate therapeutic recourse. The least invasive and reversible option should always be favoured (Department of Health 2001).

Children and young people

People aged 16 years and over are entitled to consent to their own medical treatment using the same criteria for competency as for adults. It is not legally necessary to obtain consent from the person with parental responsibility in addition.

Girls aged less than 16 years must be assessed as 'Gillick competent' to consent for their procedure. This is named after the case of Gillick vs West Norfolk and Wisbeth AHA 1986. Mrs Gillick challenged the lawfulness of Department of Health guidance that doctors could provide contraceptive advice and treatment to girls under the age of 16 years without parental consent or knowledge. The House of Lords held that a doctor could give contraceptive advice and treatment to a young person under the age of 16 years if:

- she had sufficient maturity and intelligence to understand the nature and implications of the proposed treatment;
- she could not be persuaded to tell her parents or to allow her doctor to tell them;
- she was very likely to begin or continue having sexual intercourse with or without contraceptive treatment;
- her physical or mental health was likely to suffer unless she received the advice or treatment; and
- the advice or treatment was in the young person's best interests.

This case was specifically about contraceptive advice and treatment, but the case of Axon vs Secretary of State for Health (2006) makes it clear that the principles also apply to decisions about treatment and care for sexually transmitted infections and abortion. Thus, if a child is 'Gillick competent' and is able to give voluntary consent after receiving appropriate information, the consent is valid. It is not legally necessary to obtain agreement of an additional person with parental responsibility. It is, however, good practice to encourage them to inform their parents, unless it is clearly not in the child's best interest to do so. It is important to ensure that the consent is voluntary and to be aware of undue influences by parents, carers or sexual partner.

Conversely, if a child assessed as 'Gillick competent' refuses treatment, the person with parental responsibility can over-rule this decision if it is in the best interests of the child. Consideration should be given to applying for a court ruling for this intervention. For parents to be in a position to over-rule a competent child's refusal, they must be provided with sufficient information about the child's condition. This may be in breach of confidence on the part of the doctor treating the child, but may be justifiable in view of the child's best interests. The child should still be as involved as possible in making decisions about their care.

Finally, refusal of treatment by a competent child and persons with parental responsibility for a child can be over-ruled by a court if this is in the best interests of child (Department of Health 2001).

Preoperative Assessment

The purpose of preoperative assessment is to achieve an accurate diagnosis and to assess the patient's fitness for surgery (risk assessment).

Accurate diagnosis

A thorough clinical examination aided by specific investigations (as necessary) is essential in patients undergoing gynaecological surgery to confirm the diagnosis and to ensure correctness of the planned operation. Special attention should be paid to the extent and complexity of the disease, and the involvement of other organs. For example, patients with complex endometriosis should be assessed for possible involvement of the bowel, bladder or ureter with this disease. Patients undergoing pelvic surgery for stress incontinence should be considered for urodynamic studies if detrusor instability is suspected, if they have had previous surgery for stress incontinence or if they have substantial voiding dysfunction.

Although the diagnosis is usually established during the initial consultations in the outpatient clinic, it is important to reassess the patient closer to or on the day of surgery to detect any changes in her gynaecological condition that may require alteration or even cancellation of the planned surgery. A common example of this is the disappearance of an ovarian cyst prior to ovarian cystectomy. Another example is the enlargement of a leiomyoma to an extent that may necessitate a change in the planned route of surgery. In these cases, a repeat preoperative pelvic ultrasound scan close to the day of surgery should be considered.

Risk assessment

One should start with a thorough assessment of the patient's risk by way of a full medical and surgical history followed by general examination. This will determine which patients require further investigations. Routine preoperative testing of healthy individuals is of little benefit. Guidelines from the National Institute for Health and Clinical Excellence (2003) conclude that no routine laboratory testing or screening is necessary for preoperative evaluation unless there is a relevant clinical indication. Preoperative testing is a substantial drain on NHS resources, and substantial savings can be achieved by eliminating unnecessary investigations (Munro et al 1997). False-positive results may also cause unnecessary anxiety and result in additional investigations causing a delay in surgery. The indications and aims of common preoperative tests are shown in Table 7.2.

Purpose of preoperative risk assessment

- Estimation of physiological reserve (i.e. fitness for surgery).
- Planning perioperative care of patient's care:
  - Day case or inpatient
  - Postoperative recovery bed required in high-dependency unit/intensive care unit.
- Inform doctors and patient of change in risk.
- Opportunistic screening.
- To determine anaesthetic technique.
- To diagnose and correct physiological abnormalities (e.g. anaemia, hypertension, previously undiagnosed arrhythmias).
- To anticipate requirement for crossmatched blood.

Tests should be performed in adequate time to allow for counselling and arrangement of further investigations and/or management as necessary. This should minimize cancellations. Patients should be counselled and their consent obtained before performing all preoperative investigations.

Abnormal findings of preoperative investigations increase with patient's age and American Society of Anesthesiologists' grade. These results may change the management plan of the patient by way of altering, delaying or cancelling surgery. They may also necessitate onward referral to an appropriate speciality or to the anaesthetist. Preoperative correction of abnormalities is important to minimize risk to the patient. For example, anaemia predisposes to intraoperative hypoxia and delayed wound healing. Both anaemia and hypertension cause increased cardiac workload and risk of myocardial infarction.

Assessing patients' suitability for day surgery

Day surgery was devised as a way to increase the capacity of the NHS by the Department of Health in order to meet demands. Patients enjoy it, where appropriate, as a safe, efficient and effective care that provides the least disruption to their lives. Unless the patient requests inpatient treatment or is not found to be suitable, the operation should take place as a day case. The patient's suitability for surgery as a day case will depend on the assessment of their general medical status and fitness for anaesthetic. One should also take account of their home circumstances. Living alone is not a contraindication for day surgery, but they should be encouraged to have a carer to stay with them until they are able to care for themselves. If a patient is not able to go home, they should be assured that they will be cared for overnight.

Gynaecological procedures for day surgery (Department of Health 2002)

- Hysteroscopy (diagnostic and/or therapeutic).
- Transcervical resection of endometrium.
- Laparoscopy (diagnostic and/or therapeutic).
- Termination of pregnancy.

It is also recommended that mixing day-case and inpatient procedures on the same list increases the risk of cancellation of minor cases and hence decreases efficiency.

Assessing patients with allergies

Recognition of patients' allergies to certain medicines or any medical materials such as latex or plaster is of utmost importance. Exposure to such allergens could potentially result in fatal anaphylaxis. Awareness of patients' allergies will also determine theatre location in the case of latex allergy and is important for planning resources. However, it is important to ensure that an allergy is a true allergy rather than a side-effect. For example, a patient may be mistakenly labelled as allergic to penicillin when she has developed diarrhoea or vomiting as a side-effect following penicillin administration. Some allergens, such as penicillin and latex, can be confirmed by specific hypersensitivity tests. However, it can be difficult to confirm or exclude if a patient had a true hypersensitivity reaction to a certain agent. This lack of certainty can be problematic when the patient needs the specific drug or a related drug again and there is no easy substitute. In this case, it may be wise to consult an immunologist before the use of the suspected allergen.

Risk assessment of obese patients

The prevalence of obesity is increasing in the Western world. Obesity is defined as a body mass index (BMI) of more than 30 kg/m^2 and morbid obesity is defined as a BMI of more than 40 kg/m^2. Although absolute BMI should not be used as a sole indicator for suitability for surgery or its location, it is the most useful currently available measure of risk. People who are mildly obese pose few additional problems, but those who are morbidly obese have increased health risks associated with surgery. Table 7.3 summarizes common comorbidities in obese patients. They require extra time and early communication before surgery regarding scheduling of surgery, provision for sufficient operative time, resources

Table 7.2 Indications for preoperative tests

Test	Aim	Indication	Further management
Chest X-ray	Assess signs of cardiopulmonary disease	• Clinical indication (e.g. history of chest disease or recent chest symptoms) • Age >75 years • Age >60 years with another risk factor (e.g. smoking)	Assessment by anaesthetist and speciality if appropriate
Electrocardiogram	Identify silent myocardial infarction or arrhythmia	• Age >60 years • Age >40 years if clinical indication	Correction of arrhythmia
Full blood count	Identify occult anaemia	• Main factor is extent of planned surgery • Age >60 years as may have occult blood loss	Correction of anaemia. Blood cross-matched. Identify cause of anaemia
Coagulation	Identify clotting abnormality	• Always require a specific indication such as: 　• anticoagulant therapy 　• abnormal liver function tests 　• thrombocytopenia 　• malabsorption 　• cancer surgery	Liaise with haematology and blood transfusion service
Renal function	Identify renal failure. Avoid acute renal failure following major surgery	• Age • Diabetes mellitus • Hypertension • Medications (e.g. steroids, diuretics, non-steroidal anti-inflammatory drugs) • Renal disease	Close postoperative monitoring of urine output, change in medication or further renal assessment
Random blood sugar	Identify undiagnosed diabetes	• No consensus on definite indication • Opportunistic screening in those with renal disease	Fasting blood sugar for diagnosis of diabetes and referral to diabetes service
Urine pregnancy tests	Identify pregnant women – interpreted with last menstrual period. Tests should always be done with the patient's consent	• All women with a possibility of pregnancy, e.g.: 　• irregular menstrual cycles 　• delayed menses 　• uncertain last menstrual period	In the case of positive pregnancy tests, elective surgery is almost always cancelled due to the risk of fetal injury or loss
Urinalysis	Screen for infection	• All patients undergoing urogenital procedures and before major surgery	Treat infection to reduce morbidity
Sickle cell screening	Screen for haemoglobinopathy	• Women of African, Caribbean, Middle Eastern, Mediterranean or Asian background • Family history of sickle gene	Ideally, test should be done well in advance to allow counselling
Pulmonary function test	Assess respiratory function (expert clinical assessment may be more appropriate)	• Respiratory disease with ASA >2 and planned major surgery	

ASA, American Society of Anesthesiologists.

and personnel (Association of Anaesthetists of Great Britain and Ireland 2007).

Preoperative assessment is the key component in assessment and management of risk in the obese patient. All patients should have their height and weight measured and BMI calculated. Special attention should be paid to the patient's exercise tolerance and comorbidities placing obese patients at increased risk such as cardiac, respiratory and metabolic disease. Consideration could also be given to the treatment of sleep apnoea if present. Preoperative assessment should ideally be performed in a multidisciplinary setting with ready access to imaging, laboratory and specialist services to minimize hospital visits. The patient's size in itself may limit the quality of investigations ordered. The quality of electrocardiograms, chest X-rays and transthoracic echocardiograms is reduced and patients may not fit in the computed tomography or magnetic resonance imaging machine. Ideally, a consultant anaesthetist with an interest in the management of obese patients should be available.

Table 7.3 Comorbidities in obese patients

Respiratory	• Reduced functional residual capacity • Airway closure and desaturation when supine • Difficult intubation due to nuchal fat pad and deposition of fat into soft tissues of neck • Increased acid reflux • Sleep apnoea and obesity hypoventilation syndrome
Cardiac	• Hypertension • Hyperlipidaemia • Ischaemic heart disease • Heart failure

Metabolic diseases	• Increased incidence of diabetes mellitus
	• Complications of diabetes mellitus
	  • Cardiac and renal disease
	  • Autonomic dysfunction

Box 7.1 Patient-related risk factors for VTE

- Age >60 years
- Obesity (BMI >30 kg/m^2)
- Personal or family history of VTE
- Pregnancy or puerperium
- Use of oral contraceptives or hormone replacement therapy
- Varicose veins with associated phlebitis
- Thrombophilia including:
  - factor V Leiden
  - prothrombin mutation (G20210A, 5'UTR)
  - deficiencies of protein C, protein S and antithrombin
- Antiphospholipid syndrome
- Severe infection
- Acute medical illness
- Active cancer or cancer treatment
- Active heart or respiratory failure
- Behçet's disease
- Central venous catheter *in situ*
- Continuous travel of more than 3 h approximately 4 weeks before or after surgery
- Immobility (e.g. paralysis or limb in plaster)
- Inflammatory bowel disease (e.g. Crohn's disease or ulcerative colitis)
- Nephrotic syndrome
- Recent myocardial infarction or stroke

In order to reduce perioperative risk for obese patients, one should ensure correct case selection by preoperative assessment. This can ensure correct allocation to day-case or inpatient lists, preoperative counselling for smoking cessation and dietary advice, as well as thromboprophylaxis.

An equipment suitable for the morbidly obese patient should be made available. Trolleys, beds and operating tables have a maximum weight-bearing load, usually around 150 kg. Equipment suitable for the morbidly obese patient can carry heavier loads, is wider and can sometimes have a 'tilt-to-standing' mode to reduce manual handling. One should also ensure that large gowns, compression stockings and blood pressure cuffs are available.

Obese patients are at significantly increased risk of venous and pulmonary thromboembolism. All obese patients should be considered for mechanical and pharmacological thromboprophylaxis. With full consideration of assessment and explanation of potential risks, the patient may wish to reconsider whether or not to proceed with surgery or to postpone it until weight reduction has been achieved.

Preoperative Preparation

Thromboprophylaxis

Venous thromboembolism (VTE) kills 25,000 people per year in England. This is more than breast cancer or road traffic accidents. The incidence of deep venous thrombosis (DVT) in gynaecological surgery with no prophylaxis is 16% and the incidence of symptomatic pulmonary embolism (PE) is 1%. VTE usually occurs 1–2 weeks following surgery. DVT is commonly asymptomatic but may result in sudden death from PE or long-term morbidity secondary to venous insufficiency and post-thrombotic syndrome (National Institute for Health and Clinical Excellence 2007).

In order to minimize the risk of VTE in patients undergoing surgery, each patient should be assessed carefully for individual risk factors. Box 7.1 details patient-related risk factors for VTE.

Patients should be given verbal and written information on the risks of VTE and the effectiveness of prophylaxis before surgery. Patients on the combined oral contraceptive pill (COCP) who are undergoing major surgery with subsequent immobilization should be advised to stop the COCP 4 weeks prior to their operation.

Ample hydration and early mobilization

All patients should be given general advice before surgery to help decrease the risk of VTE, including ample hydration and early mobilization. In patients with restricted mobility, leg exercises by physiotherapy should be arranged. Although studies have shown smoking to be a risk factor for VTE in the general population, it does not appear to be so in patients undergoing surgery.

The National Institute for Health and Clinical Excellence (2007) has recommended thromboprophylaxis regimens for gynaecological surgery. Mechanical prophylaxis should be used in all patients with no risk factors for VTE. Pharmacological prophylaxis should be considered in the presence of any risk factors for VTE.

Mechanical prophylaxis

Mechanical prophylaxis includes compression stockings, intermittent pneumatic compression, electrical stimulation and foot impulse devices. There is no difference in the effectiveness of different types of mechanical prophylaxis. They appear to have a similar effect whether used alone or in conjunction with a pharmacological method. All patients should be offered thigh-length graduated compression stockings unless contraindicated (e.g. in peripheral arterial disease and diabetic neuropathy). They should be shown how to wear the stockings correctly and should be monitored and assisted as necessary. The stockings should be equivalent to Sigel profile (i.e. 18 mmHg at the ankle, 14 mmHg mid calf and 8 mmHg on the upper thigh). Knee stockings may be used instead of thigh-length stocking if there are fit or compliance issues. Patients should be encouraged to wear the stockings from the time of admission until they return to their normal mobility, as immobility is a risk factor for VTE. Intermittent pneumatic compression or foot impulse devices may be used as alternatives or in addition to graduated compression/antiembolism stockings while patients are in hospital.

Pharmacological prophylaxis

Pharmacological prophylaxis should be considered in patients undergoing surgery in the presence of any additional risk factors, as summarized in Box 7.1. Low-molecular-weight heparin (LMWH) should be offered in preference to unfractionated heparin. Fondaparinux can be offered as an alternative, within its licensed indications.

Heparin is composed of a mix of mucopolysaccharides of differing chain length and molecular size, hence the term 'unfractionated heparin'. It produces its major anticoagulant effect by binding to antithrombin (AT) and coagulation enzyme, thereby inactivating thrombin and activated factor X (Xa). For inhibition of thrombin, heparin must bind to both the coagulation enzyme and AT, whereas binding to the enzyme is not required for inhibition of factor Xa. LMWH is derived from heparin by chemical or enzymatic depolymerization to yield fragments approximately one-third the size of heparin. Compared with unfractionated heparin, LMWH has reduced ability to inactivate thrombin, but almost the same ability to inactivate factor Xa. The smaller fragments of LMWH cannot bind simultaneously to AT and coagulation enzyme, hence its inability to inhibit thrombin.

The main advantage of LMWH is its reduced binding to plasma proteins and cells, resulting in a more predictable dose–response relationship, a longer plasma half-life and a lower risk of thrombocytopenia and osteopenia compared with unfractionated heparin. Both decrease the risk of DVT and PE but increase the risk of bleeding.

Fondaparinux is a synthetic pentasaccharide based on the AT binding region of heparin in the body. Hence it is a catalyst for AT inhibition of factor Xa. However, it does not inhibit thrombin directly, because this requires a minimum of 13 additional saccharide units which are present in unfractionated heparin and LMWH. It is therefore a specific, indirect inhibitor of factor Xa through its potentiation of AT. Like LMWH, it is administered subcutaneously on a once-daily dosing regimen. It is more effective than LMWH at reducing the risk of DVT, but has not been shown to reduce the risk of PE and is associated with larger bleeds.

The timing of administering the LMWH should be planned carefully if regional anaesthesia is being employed, with a view to reducing the risk of haematoma formation. Regional anaesthesia should be used where appropriate as this decreases the risk of VTE compared with general anaesthesia. The available evidence is limited regarding whether LMWH can be safely given before surgery or if it should be delayed until after surgery.

Antibiotic prophylaxis

Surgical infections include infections of surgical wounds or tissues involved in the operation, occurring within 30 days of surgery. They prolong hospital stay and are an important outcome measure for surgical procedures. Surgical infections are caused by direct contact from surgical instruments or hands, from air contaminated with bacteria or by the patient's endogenous flora of the operation site. Additional risk factors for surgical site infections are shown in Table 7.4. The most causative organisms are *Staphylococcus aureus*, *Streptococcus pyogenes* and enterococci.

The goal of prophylactic antibiotics is to reduce the total number of bacteria contaminating the operative site and to inhibit their growth. This can be achieved by maintaining adequate tissue levels of antibiotics for the duration of the operation. Reduction of the contaminating bacteria allows the patient's natural defence mechanisms to eradicate the remaining organisms. In addition to prophylactic antibiotics, surgeons should remember that meticulous surgical techniques are also crucial in preventing infections.

The main drawback of using prophylactic antibiotics is increasing the prevalence of antibiotic-resistant bacteria that can predispose to infections such as *Clostridium difficile*. The prevalence of antibiotic resistance is related to the proportion of the population receiving antibiotics and the total antibiotic exposure. Antibiotic prophylaxis use should therefore be restricted to procedures where there is proven benefit.

Prophylactic antibiotics should ideally be given intravenously at anaesthetic induction or no more than 30 min before. This should ensure the maximum blood concentration at the time of skin incision and entry to the genitourinary tract when blood contamination occurs. If given too early, antibiotics could increase the resistance among colonizing organisms. On the other hand, late administration of prophylactic antibiotics will reduce their efficacy, especially if given more than 3 h after the start of the procedure. A single-dose prophylactic antibiotic is effective. Multiple doses may be necessary when surgery is prolonged and where there is a major blood loss of more than 1.5 l requir-

Table 7.4 Risk factors for surgical site infections

Patient related	Operation related
Extremes of age	Length of operation
Poor nutritional state	Skin antisepsis
Obesity	Preoperative skin shaving
Diabetes mellitus	Inadequate sterilization of equipment
Smoking	Poor surgical technique and tissue handling
Coexisting infection	
Bacterial colonization (e.g. methicillin-resistant *Staphylococcus aureus*)	
Immunosuppression	
Prolonged hospital stay	

ing fluid resuscitation, which results in reduction of the antibiotic concentration. Prolonged use of prophylactic antibiotics for more than 24 h should be avoided as it could result in an increase in resistant organisms (Scottish Intercollegiate Guidelines Network 2008).

A system of classification for operative wounds based on the degree of microbial contamination was developed by the US National Research Council group in 1964 (Berard and Gandon 1964, Culver et al 1991). Four wound classes with an increasing risk of surgical site infection were described: clean, clean-contaminated, contaminated and dirty (Table 7.5). Most gynaecological procedures fall into the 'clean-contaminated' category. Hence, prophylactic antibiotics are highly recommended for certain procedures. However, the final decision rests with the surgeon who should assess the risks and benefits for that patient. There is good research evidence supporting the use of prophylactic antibiotics for vaginal and abdominal hysterectomy with a significant reduction in the incidence of febrile morbidity, pelvic infection and wound infection.

Methicillin-resistant *S. aureus* (MRSA) may be a risk factor for surgical site infection. Those known to be carriers should receive MRSA eradication therapy prior to surgery, and most units now screen patients before surgery.

Urine and respiratory infection

Prophylactic antibiotics are not recommended for the sole prevention of respiratory or urinary tract infections. Although meta-analyses do show a significant reduction in the incidence of urinary tract infection, the results for respiratory tract infection are equivocal. Patients at higher risk of a urinary tract infection (e.g. elderly women and those with indwelling catheters) are more likely to develop bacterial resistance and *C. difficile* due to prophylactic antibiotics (Scottish Intercollegiate Guidelines Network 2008).

Antibiotic prophylaxis against infective endocarditis

Infective endocarditis is a rare condition affecting less than one in 10,000 cases, but with significant morbidity and mortality of up to 20% (National Institute for Health and Clinical Excellence 2008). It is inflammation of the myocardium, which occurs following bacteraemia in a patient with a pre-disposing cardiac condition. Pathogens are likely to be commensal organisms, the most common being *Streptococcus viridans*, *S. aureus* and enterococci (Gould et al 2006). Up to 75% of cases of infective endocarditis occur without a preceding interventional or dental procedure to account for bacteraemia. Furthermore, there is no consistent association between having an interventional procedure and infective endocarditis. Antibiotic prophylaxis has been shown to reduce the incidence of bacteraemia following an interventional procedure, but does not eliminate it (Bhattacharya et al 1995). The clinical effectiveness of prophylactic antibiotics remains to be proven.

There is not enough evidence in the literature to show an increased risk of infective endocarditis in women undergoing genitourinary procedures. The large number of gynaecological procedures undertaken would mean that the risks of antibiotic prophylaxis against infective endocarditis (e.g. anaphylaxis and bacterial resistance) might outweigh the benefit. The British Society for Antimicrobial Chemotherapy states that there are no good epidemiological data on the impact of bacteraemia from non-dental procedures on the risk of developing infective endocarditis (Gould et al 2006). Likewise, the current guidelines of the National Institute for Health and Clinical Excellence (2008) suggest that antibiotic prophylaxis is not recommended for people undergoing genitourinary tract procedures.

Weight loss

As discussed above, obesity is a major risk factor and is associated with an increase in the incidence of most surgical complications in gynaecological patients. In addition, obesity increases the technical difficulty and prolongs surgery. Obese women should therefore be strongly encouraged to reduce their weight before their planned surgery. However, preoperative weight loss must be controlled and preferably supervised as obese patients often have poor nutritional status, despite their excess weight. A very low calorie diet can be dangerous and may cause cardiac arrhythmias or even sudden death. Women who have undergone bariatric surgery could develop malabsorption. A supervised exercise programme may be best to help with weight loss, exercise tolerance and glucose tolerance (Association of Anaesthetists of Great Britain and Ireland 2007).

Table 7.5 Wound classification and risk of infection

Classification	Description	Infective risk
Clean	• Uninfected operative wound • No acute inflammation • No entry to genitourinary, alimentary or respiratory tracts • No break in aseptic technique	<2%
Clean-contaminated	• Opening to genitourinary, alimentary or respiratory tracts but no significant spillage of contents • No evidence of infection or major break in aseptic technique	<10%
Contaminated	• Opening to internal organs with inflammation or spillage of contents • Major break in aseptic technique	15–20%
Dirty	• Purulent inflammation present • Intraperitoneal abscess formation or visceral perforation	40%

Smoking cessation

Smokers have a substantially increased risk of intra- and postoperative complications. They are three to six times more likely to have intraoperative pulmonary complications and postoperative wound infections. Preoperative assessment is a good opportunity to offer smoking cessation intervention, as the patient may be more motivated. This approach has been shown to be effective in reducing preoperative smoking. However, whether or not smoking cessation of such short duration would lead to decreased operative complication rates remains to be determined (Møller and Villebro 2005).

Bowel preparation

Bowel preparation may be considered before gynaecological operations in patients with complex pelvic diseases involving the bowel, such as severe endometriosis, extensive adhesions or malignancy. In such cases, bowel preparation may be necessary if bowel surgery is anticipated or to provide better access for the surgeon. However, a large randomized trial investigating the value of preoperative bowel preparation in patients undergoing bowel resection and anastomosis showed no significant difference in the rate of anastomosis breakdown in women who received mechanical bowel preparation compared with those who did not (Contant et al 2007). However, patients experiencing anastomotic breakdown were less likely to develop an abscess if they had bowel preparation.

Bowel preparation has not been shown to improve the view of the operating field during laparoscopy. Furthermore, it may add to the patient's inconvenience and discomfort during her preoperative hospital stay (Muzzi et al 2006, Lijoi et al 2009).

Additional medications prior to gynaecological surgery

Gonadotrophin-releasing hormone analogues

Gonadotrophin-releasing hormone (GnRH) analogues can be used before fibroid surgery and endometrial ablation. GnRH analogues taken for 3–4 months prior to fibroid surgery (myomectomy or hysterectomy) have been shown to decrease uterine and fibroid size, and to improve menhorrhagia after surgery; and to reduce intraoperative blood loss, thereby improving pre- and postoperative haemoglobin levels. In reducing the fibroid size, GnRH analogues can also decrease the rate of vertical abdominal incisions, and reduce the operating time and hospital stay. However, these benefits of GnRH analogues should be balanced against their associated side-effects such as menopausal symptoms (Lethaby et al 2002).

GnRH analogues may also be of value in women undergoing endometrial ablation or resection to help thin out the endometrium. An alternative approach is to perform the procedure shortly after cessation of menstruation when the endometrium is at its thinnest. GnRH analogues are associated with shorter surgery time and increased rate of postoperative amenorrhoea with endometrial resection. However, this benefit does not seem to last in the long term

and does not extend to second-generation ablation treatments (Sowter et al 2002)

Misoprostol

Misoprostol is the most commonly used cervical priming agent worldwide. The most common use is in first-trimester abortion or for surgical management of miscarriage. It is effective in cervical softening and dilatation before surgery. However, there is not enough evidence to conclude that misoprostol is necessary to reduce complications such as cervical laceration. An alternative is Laminaria, although this requires administration to the endocervix via a speculum. Misoprostol can be administered vaginally and sublingually with similar effect, although the sublingual route has more side-effects. It can also be given orally but needs to be administered up to 12 h before surgery (Allen and Goldberg 2007).

Pre-existing medications

Anticoagulants

Patients already on prophylactic anticoagulants due to a previous VTE should stop treatment 5 days before surgery. Heparin and oral anticoagulants should be restarted soon after surgery. If possible, surgery should be postponed beyond 3 months of the previous event. If surgery cannot be delayed, oral agents should be converted to intravenous heparin and should continue following surgery until oral agents can be restarted. Vena caval filters should be considered if the patient has had a VTE within the past month and anticoagulation is contraindicated.

Hypoglycaemic agents

Patients whose diabetes is controlled by diet alone do not usually need any special preoperative measures, providing that dietary control is adequate.

Patients on oral hypoglyacemic agents should discontinue their medication on the day of surgery. Blood glucose should be monitored and, if the levels increase above 13 mmol/l, small doses of soluble insulin could be given. After surgery, metformin therapy should be temporarily suspended (except in minor procedures not associated with restricted intake of food and fluids) until the patient's oral intake has resumed. This is important to reduce the risk of lactic acidosis.

Patients undergoing major surgery requiring prolonged postoperative fasting should be put on an approved protocol of intravenous insulin and glucose infusion before surgery. The dose is determined by regular blood glucose testing. Following surgery, patients can resume their regular treatment when they have resumed their oral intake.

One should utilize the expertise of the multidisciplinary diabetes team and the experience of the patient herself in maintaining tight glucose control.

Oral contraception

Hormonal methods of contraception are used in 29% of women of reproductive age in the UK, with 18% using the COCP. The background risk of VTE is five per 100,000 women per year. This is increased by a factor of three in users of second-generation COCPs (containing levonorgestrel or

Table 7.6 World Health Organization eligibility criteria for contraceptive use in surgery

Contraceptive	Type of surgery	Recommendation
Combined oral contraceptive pill	Minor surgery Major surgery without immobilization Major surgery with prolonged immobilization	Unrestricted use Benefits outweighs risk Unacceptable risk
Progestogen-only pill	All surgery	Benefits outweigh risk

norethisterone) and by a factor of five in users of third-generation COCPs (containing desogestrel or gestodene). The absolute risk remains low with an incidence of 15–25 VTE per 100,000. This risk is increased in the first 4 months of use and falls to levels of non-users within 3 months. There is no evidence that progestogen-only pills increase the risk of VTE.

The Royal College of Obstetricians and Gynaecologists advises that the COCP should ideally be discontinued at least 4 weeks prior to major surgery where immobilization is expected. Discontinuation of the COCP has been shown to reduce the postoperative VTE rate from 1% to 0.5%. This small absolute risk reduction must be balanced against the risks of discontinuing an effective contraception with the risk of unplanned pregnancy (Royal College of Obstetricians and Gynaecologists 2004a). Table 7.6 shows the World Health Organization's recommendations for contraceptive use in surgery.

KEY POINTS

1. The most appropriate treatment option must be chosen for each patient.
2. The most appropriate treatment location must be chosen for each patient.
3. Preoperative risk assessment is essential to minimize morbidity and make theatre lists as efficient as possible.
4. Consent must always be obtained from a fully informed person with capacity to make a voluntary decision about their care.
5. Children must be 'Gillick competent' to consent to treatment.
6. Obesity is a major risk factor and requires more input before and after surgery.
7. VTE must be taken seriously and compression stockings should be used for all surgical patients. LMWH should be used if there are any additional risk factors.
8. Complete preoperative care requires a team approach with input from the surgical team, anaesthetist and the patient themselves to achieve the best outcome.

References

Allen RH, Goldberg AB 2007 Cervical dilation before first-trimester surgical abortion (<14 weeks gestation). Contraception 76: 139–156.

Association of Anaesthetists of Great Britain and Ireland 2007 Perioperative Management of the Morbidly Obese Patient. AAGBI, London.

Berard F, Gandon J 1964 Postoperative wound infections: the influence of ultraviolet irradiation of the operating room and of various other factors. Annals of Surgery 160 (Suppl 1): 1–192.

Bhattacharya S, Parkin DE, Reid TMS et al 1995 A prospective randomised study of the effects of prophylactic antibiotics on the incidence of bacteraemia following hysteroscopic surgery. European Journal of Obstetrics and Gynecology 63: 37–40.

Contant CM, Hop WC, Van't Sant HP et al 2007 Mechanical bowel preparation for elective colorectal surgery: a multicentre randomized trial. The Lancet 370: 2112–2117.

Culver DH, Horan TC, Gaines RP et al 1991 Surgical wound infection rates by wound class, operative procedure and patient risk. National Nosocomial Infections Surveillance system. American Journal of Medicine 91: 152S–157S.

Department of Health 2001 Reference Guide to Consent for Examination or treatment. DoH, London.

Department of Health 2002 Day Surgery Operational Guide — Waiting, Booking and Choice. DoH, London.

General Medical Council 2008 Consent: Patients and Doctors Making Decisions Together. GMC, London.

Gould FK, Elliott TSJ, Foweraker J et al 2006 Guidelines for the prevention of endocarditis: report of the Working Party of the British Society for Antimicrobial Chemotherapy. Journal of Antimicrobial Chemotherapy 58: 896–898.

Lethaby A, Vollenhoven B, Sowter M 2002 Efficacy of pre-operative gonadotrophin hormone releasing analogues for women with uterine fibroids undergoing hysterectomy or myomectomy: a systematic review. BJOG: an International Journal of Obstetrics and Gynaecology 109: 1097–1108.

Lijoi D, Ferrero S, Mistrangelo E et al 2009 Bowel preparation before laparoscopic gynaecological surgery in benign conditions using a 1-week low fibre diet: a surgeon blind, randomized and controlled trial. Archives of Gynecology and Obstetrics 280: 713–718.

Møller AM, Villebro N 2005 Interventions for pre-operative smoking cessation. Cochrane Database of Systematic Reviews 3: CD002294.

Munro J, Booth A, Nicholl J 1997 Routine pre-operative testing: a systematic review of the evidence. Health Technology Assessment 1: i–iv; 1–62.

Muzzi L, Bellati F, Zullo MA et al 2006 Mechanical bowel preparation before gynaecologic laparoscopy: a randomized, single-blind controlled trial. Fertility and Sterility 85: 689–693.

National Institute for Health and Clinical Excellence, developed by the National Collaborating Centre for Acute Care 2003 The Use of Routine Pre-operative Tests for Elective Surgery. NICE, London.

National Institute for Health and Clinical Excellence 2007 Clinical Guidance Clinical

Guideline 46. Venous Thromboembolism: Reducing the Risk of Venous Thromboembolism (Deep Vein Thrombosis and Pulmonary Embolism) in Inpatients Undergoing Surgery. National Collaborating Centre for Acute Care, London.

National Institute for Health and Clinical Excellence 2008 Clinical Guideline 64. Prophylaxis Against Infective Endocarditis. Antimicrobial Prophylaxis Against Infective Endocarditis in Adults and Children Undergoing Interventional Procedures. NICE, London.

Royal College of Obstetricians and Gynaecologists 2004a Guideline Number 40. Venous Thromboembolism and Hormonal Contraception. RCOG, London.

Royal College of Obstetricians and Gynaecologists 2004b Consent Advice Number 4. Abdominal Hysterectomy for Heavy Periods. RCOG, London.

Royal College of Obstetricians and Gynaecologists 2004c Consent Advice Number 5. Pelvic Floor Repair and Vaginal Hysterectomy for Prolapse. RCOG, London.

Royal College of Obstetricians and Gynaecologists 2008a Clinical Governance Advice Number 6. Obtaining Valid Consent. RCOG, London.

Royal College of Obstetricians and Gynaecologists 2008b Consent Advice Number 1. Diagnostic Hysteroscopy Under General Anaesthesia. RCOG, London.

Royal College of Obstetricians and Gynaecologists 2008c Consent Advice Number 2. Laparoscopy. RCOG, London.

Royal College of Obstetricians and Gynaecologists 2008d Consent Advice Number 3. Laparoscopic Tubal Occlusion. RCOG, London.

Scottish Intercollegiate Guidelines Network 2008 Guideline Number 104. Antibiotic Prophylaxis in Surgery. SIGN, Edinburgh.

Sowter MC, Lethaby A, Singala AA 2002 Pre-operative endometrial thinning agents before endometrial destruction for heavy menstrual bleeding. Cochrane Database of Systematic Reviews 2: CD001124.

CHAPTER 8

Principles of surgery and management of intraoperative complications

Angus McIndoe

Chapter Contents

INTRODUCTION	105	BOWEL DAMAGE	112
THE ROUTE	105	VASCULAR DAMAGE	112
OPENING AND CLOSING THE ABDOMEN	105	UTERINE PERFORATION AND FALSE PASSAGE	114
URETERIC DAMAGE	107	LAPAROSCOPY	114
BLADDER DAMAGE	109	KEY POINTS	115

Introduction

In major surgery, occasional damage to vital structures is unavoidable, but with good training, appropriate experience and careful application, such damage should be rare. Timely recognition of potential problems has a major impact on the long-term outcome for patients. The request for appropriate assistance from a more experienced colleague, either within the specialty or from another specialty, and early repair, preferably during the original operation, can make the difference between complete and rapid recovery and long-term morbidity and further surgery.

To minimize complications, a surgical technique should be developed that involves careful and accurate identification of tissue planes, preferably with sharp dissection, with the aim of causing the minimum of damage to tissues and structures that are to be preserved. A gentle approach should be used and tissues handled in such a way as to maintain optimum viability.

One should operate under direct vision at all times. The temptation to push an instrument deep into a plane of dissection should be avoided, since inadvertent damage may be caused and bleeding down a deep hole is more difficult to control. Sufficient time should be allowed for each operation, and surgery should not be hurried. Particularly when in training, greater speed will develop by a methodical attention to detail of technique rather than by hurrying individual cases, and outcome is always more important than operative time.

Every case undertaken should be seen as an opportunity to improve technique. Straightforward cases are particularly useful for the practice of sharp dissection to the correct tissue planes. When tissue planes are more difficult to identify, this practice will be invaluable.

One should aim to keep the operation under control at all times; it is much better to spend a little time controlling bleeding, so that the operation can proceed unhurriedly and with good visibility, than to rush on hoping to stop the bleeding as the operation progresses.

This chapter will discuss the common intraoperative complications, and the aspects of technique that reduce the likelihood of these complications occurring. The chapter will also highlight the range of methods used to repair damage, although for the most part, detailed descriptions are not appropriate in a textbook of this type.

The Route

The provisional decision whether to use an abdominal or a vaginal approach for hysterectomy should be made before theatre, but the final assessment of suitability for vaginal hysterectomy is performed under anaesthesia. Each surgeon has personal criteria for attempting vaginal hysterectomy that are based upon training and experience. While some advocate the vaginal removal of large fibroid uteri, most gynaecologists adopt a more cautious approach. Some have also described the removal of normal-sized ovaries, with or without the fallopian tubes, by a vaginal approach, but this requires both special training and instruments. In the event of difficulty, the surgeon should not hesitate to change to an abdominal approach.

Opening and Closing the Abdomen

The layers of the anterior abdominal wall include skin, subcutaneous fat, rectus sheath and oblique abdominal muscles, transversalis fascia and peritoneum. Within these structures

DOI: 10.1016/B978-0-7020-3120-5.00008-4

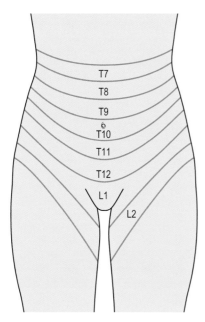

Figure 8.1 Dermatomes.

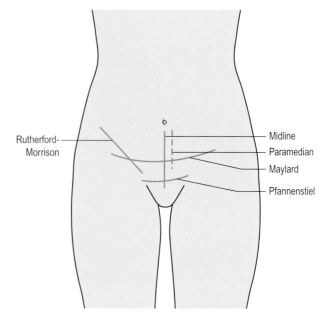

Figure 8.2 Abdominal incisions.

lie segmental arteries, veins and nerves that supply the dermatomes and myotomes, and also the epigastric vessels (Figure 8.1). Abdominal incisions have been developed that preserve function as well as possible and which heal rapidly with good strength. Commonly used incisions are shown in Figure 8.2.

It should not be forgotten that inappropriate wound closure technique can increase the risk of pulmonary complications and death (Niggebrugge et al 1999). While some surgeons prefer to use electrocautery rather than a cold scalpel to open the wound, there seems to be no difference in the early or late complications in midline incisions (Franchi et al 2001).

Incisions

The vertical midline incision avoids all major nerves, vessels and muscles by dividing the rectus sheath. It gives good access to the whole of the abdomen except the subdiaphragmatic areas, and is a very fast incision to make. Its principal drawback is that it heals slowly and suffers from a high incidence of wound dehiscence and incisional hernia. The development of improved sutures and technique has dramatically reduced these complications. A midline incision should always be closed using the 'mass closure' technique. This involves 1-cm-deep bites of the rectus muscle and peritoneum in a continuous closure, with sutures placed 1 cm apart. The suture material used does not affect the rates of dehiscence or infection, but incisional hernia is more common if braided absorbable material is used (Rucinski et al 2001). The same meta-analysis showed that incision pain and suture sinus formation are more common after non-absorbable material is inserted. Absorbable monofilament used in a continuous mass closure gave the best results.

The paramedian incision is only included for historical interest. The layered closure that was used improved strength when catgut sutures were employed, and reduced the incidence of dehiscence. It is inferior to the mass closure technique described above, and does not provide improved access to either side of the abdomen.

The majority of gynaecological surgery is performed through a transverse incision, usually a Pfannenstiel incision. By dividing each layer in a different direction, the function is well preserved. Even the muscle-cutting variants of the transverse incision heal more rapidly than vertical incisions. The cosmetic result is superior and, if correctly placed, access to the pelvis is good, although access to the pelvic brim is limited. This incision is difficult to extend if improved abdominal access is required.

The Maylard incision involves dividing all layers in the line of the skin incision and also divides the inferior epigastric vessels. The rectus sheath is not separated from the muscle and closure is in layers, leaving the muscle to be drawn together by the sheath. This incision provides improved access to the pelvic side wall when compared with the Pfannenstiel incision, and is useful for oncological surgery. Many centres now use this incision or a Pfannenstiel incision for radical hysterectomy (Orr et al 1995, Scribner et al 2001).

The Cherney incision is similar to the Pfannenstiel incision but the rectus muscles are divided 1 cm from their insertion into the symphysis pubis. The incision is closed in layers, but the muscle is repaired using a continuous suture in the membranous distal portion of the muscle. This incision can also be useful in oncological surgery or, if placed lower, is useful for complex urogynaecological procedures.

The Rutherford–Morrison incision involves dividing all layers in the line of the incision and is particularly useful for approaching ovarian masses in the second half of pregnancy. The incision is closed in layers and heals well.

Drains

Drains are used either therapeutically, to remove pus, infected material and products from an abscess, or to prevent accumulation of blood, pus, urine, lymph, bile or intestinal secretions. There is little evidence to support the use of pro-phylactic drains. In abdominal incisions, drains have been used in an attempt to reduce the incidence of haematoma and wound infection. Unfortunately, they tend to introduce organisms into an otherwise clean area and increase the incidence of wound infection (Cruise and Foord 1973). In addition, pelvic drains do not reduce infection following radical pelvic surgery (Orr et al 1987). Careful attention to haemostasis is preferable and drains should be avoided in most closures.

Closure of peritoneum

This practice has been questioned recently. Research in animal models has suggested that closure of the peritoneum increases rather than decreases peritoneal adhesions. Human studies support this finding, showing that closure of the pelvic peritoneum does not reduce the incidence of post-operative adhesions or obstruction (Table 8.1; Tulandi et al 1988). The peritoneum spreads rapidly across any raw areas left after surgery, although devascularized tissue, such as pedicles, are a focus for adhesion formation. Practice still varies with regard to peritoneal closure, although it probably results in increased adhesion formation (Royal College of Obstetricians and Gynaecologists 1998). However, if a suction drain is used in the wound, the peritoneum must be closed to avoid drawing the bowel into the wound.

Ureteric Damage

Ureters are the organs most respected by gynaecologists. They lie close to the genital tract and repair of a damaged ureter is technically demanding, with results that are not always satisfactory. By recognizing when and where the ureters are at greatest risk and by adopting a safe technique, the risk of damage to the ureter should be minimized.

Anatomical relations

The urinary and genital tracts are closely related in embryo-logical development, and their anatomy and physiology, not surprisingly, are intertwined. The ureter develops from a bud on the posterolateral border of the mesonephric duct near the cloaca, which elongates and eventually fuses with the developing kidney. The ventral portion of the cloaca devel-ops into the urethra, bladder and lower portion of the vagina.

The ureters enter the pelvis by crossing the common iliac arteries in the region of their bifurcation. They descend on the pelvic side wall, medial to the branches of the internal iliac arteries and lateral to the ovarian fossae. From there, they run on the anterior surface of the levator ani muscles lateral to the uterosacral ligaments to pass beneath the uterine arteries, 1–1.5 cm lateral to the cervix and vagina. The ureters then swing medially around the vagina, to enter the bladder 2–3 cm below the anterior vaginal fornix.

The ureter is accompanied by a plexus of freely anasto-mosing fine vessels running in the loose tissue surrrounding it. The blood supply in the upper portion is derived from the renal and ovarian vessels; in the middle third from branches of the aorta, common iliac and internal iliac arter-ies; and in the lower part from branches of the uterine, vaginal, middle haemorrhoidal and vesical arteries. The ureter may be mobilized extensively provided this plexus of vessels is preserved.

The ureter is at risk during gynaecological surgery in four regions: at the pelvic brim where it can be confused with the infundibulopelvic ligament; lateral to the ovarian fossa where it can be adherent to an ovarian mass; in the ureteric tunnel beneath the uterine artery; and anterior to the vagina where it runs into the bladder.

The ureter at the pelvic brim and ovarian fossa

At the pelvic brim, the infundibulopelvic ligament with the ovarian vessels also crosses the iliac vascular bundle, usually 1–2 cm distal to the bifurcation of the common iliac artery and the ureter (Figure 8.3). At this point, the ureter and the ovarian vessels are running in parallel in a similar plane and may be confused if care is not taken. Occasionally, the ureter may be duplex. Where the ureter runs lateral to the ovary, it will almost inevitably be associated with any inflammatory or malignant mass. Happily, it will lie on the lateral aspect of the mass where it can be identified and dissected free, usually without difficulty, although in patients with endome-triosis, the ureter may be fixed in dense fibrosis.

The key to the safe identification of the ureter on the pelvic side wall is to open the peritoneum and dissect in the retro-peritoneal space. This is most easily done by dividing the round ligament between two clips, dividing the peritoneum in a cranial direction 1.5 cm lateral to the ovarian vessels and in a caudal direction down towards the uterovesical fold. The loose areolar tissue then encountered should be separated by blunt dissection with careful diathermy of any small vessels. The ureter will lie on the lateral aspect of the leaf of peritoneum reflected by this manoeuvre. At this stage, the infundibulopelvic ligament can be safely divided with the ureter under direct vision. If the anatomy of the pelvic side wall has been distorted, this technique will almost always allow the ureter to be identified and followed within the pelvis. If an ovarian mass is present, the ureter may be dissected free from the mass in this retroperitoneal plane.

The lower ureter

The third position where the ureter is at risk is in the ureteric tunnel, where the ureter crosses beneath the uterine artery but superior to the cardinal ligament and approximately 1–1.5 cm lateral to the angle of the vagina (Figure 8.4). It is possible to palpate the ureter in this position by gripping the paracervical tissue between one finger in the pouch

Table 8.1 The effect of peritoneal closure on wound infection and adhesion formation.

	Closed (%)	Not Closed (%)
Wound infection	3.6	2.4
Adhesions	22.2	15.8
Obstruction	1.6	0

Source: From Tulandi T, Hum HS, Gelfand MM 1988 Closure of laparotomy incisions with or without peritoneal suturing and second look laparoscopy. American Journal of Obstetrics and Gynecology 158:536, with permission of Elsevier.

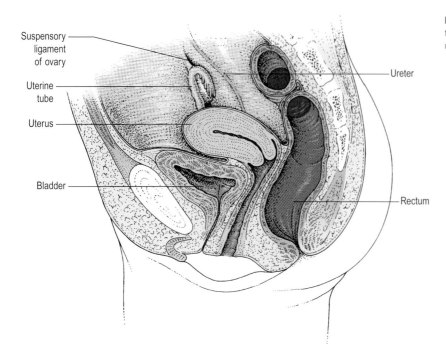

Suspensory ligament of ovary

Uterine tube

Uterus

Bladder

Ureter

Rectum

Figure 8.3 Relationship of ureter to ovarian vessels in the infundibulopelvic ligament. Note how close the ureter lies to the ovarian vessels at the pelvic brim.

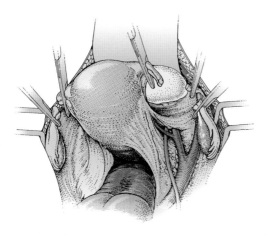

Figure 8.4 Relationship of ureter to the uterine artery. This diagram shows the dissection performed for a radical hysterectomy, but illustrates the close relationship between the ureter and the uterine artery.

of Douglas and the thumb placed laterally in front of the uterine pedicle. The ureter, which is felt as a firm cord running across the cardinal ligament, is surprisingly far lateral to the cervix if the bladder has been properly reflected and the anatomy is normal. However, adhesions, fibrosis or inadequate dissection may disrupt these relationships, causing the ureter to remain fixed near the lateral margin of the cervix.

Damage to the ureter in this site is prevented by carefully reflecting the bladder and by not taking a large pedicle that includes both the uterine artery and the paracervical tissue. The author prefers to take the uterine artery relatively high, at the level of the internal os, which allows the parametrium to fall laterally, taking the ureter with it. The ureter can then be palpated again and a second pedicle taken medial to the first, to include the cardinal ligament.

In most cases, damage to the ureter occurs at this site because the pedicle slips or the original ligature is not ade-

quate. This can be avoided by preparing the pedicle carefully before clamping it. Modern clamps, such as Roget's or Zeppelin's parametrial clamps, rarely slip, and ties should be placed accurately. If bleeding does occur, the ureter should be palpated again after replacing the clamp to ensure that it has not been included.

The ureter is occasionally damaged in its course across the anterior surface of the vagina. This may occur when taking a cuff of vagina, during a vaginal hysterectomy or colposuspension. When dissecting the upper vagina, it is important to keep in the correct plane close to the vaginal wall. Stitches placed either vaginally or abdominally in this area must be in tissue that has been accurately identified.

Repairing ureteric damage

If a ureter is damaged, the presence of the contralateral kidney should be checked. If the ureter has not been cut across but merely crushed or ligated in error, and this is recognized on the table, it is acceptable to remove the ligature and insert a stent into the ureter in the hope that a stenosis will not result. If the ureter is divided, repair will be necessary. In the past, gynaecologists have resorted to simply tying off the divided ureter but this is rarely justifiable now.

Repair of the ureter is technically demanding and may lead to long-term complications. It is not appropriate for a gynaecologist without urological training or extensive urological experience to undertake this. In principle, an end-to-end anastomosis can be performed for ureteric damage at the pelvic brim or above. The ureter is mobilized so that the ends can be brought together without tension. They are spatulated and the anastomosis performed using fine interrupted sutures over a Silastic stent (Figure 8.5). This is removed several weeks later. An alternative for damage at this level is to perform a uretero-ureteric anastomosis.

If the damage has occurred at the level of the ureteric tunnel or lower, the safest method of repair is to reimplant

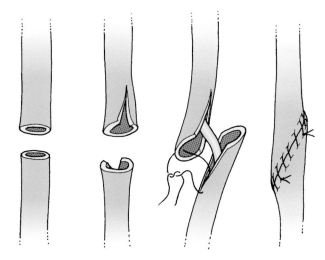

Figure 8.5 Reanastomosis of a divided ureter. A cleanly cut ureter may be reanastomosed by spatulating the ends and repairing it with fine sutures over a suitable splint. The splint is withdrawn from the bladder at a later date.

Reproduced with permission from Blandey J 1986 Operative Urology, 2nd edn. Blackwell Science, Oxford.

the ureter into the bladder. The bladder is opened between stay sutures. A submucosal tunnel is fashioned, taking care to avoid the other ureter. The distal end of the ureter is brought through the tunnel and, after spatulating the end, is sutured to the bladder mucosa. A couple of sutures into the serosal surface anchor the ureter to the outer layer of the bladder (Figure 8.6).

When damage has occurred higher on the pelvic side wall, the bladder can be elevated to the cut end of the ureter to allow reimplantation without tension, using either a psoas hitch or a Boari flap. In the former, an appropriate part of the bladder is elevated towards the end of the ureter. To facilitate this, the cystotomy is performed across the direction of elevation and is closed in the opposite direction to elongate the bladder. In addition, the contralateral superior vesical pedicle may be divided. The ureter is reimplanted as described previously and the bladder is fixed to the psoas muscle to relieve any tension. This technique will allow a ureter divided at any level in the pelvis up to the pelvic brim to be safely reimplanted (Figure 8.7).

The Boari flap is an alternative to the psoas hitch. A flap of bladder is elevated, the ureter is reimplanted into this and the flap is closed as a tube (Figure 8.8). This allows good elevation of the bladder at the expense of reduced bladder capacity.

Alternatively, a uretero-ureteric anastomosis to the opposite ureter can be performed. This has the disadvantage that both ureters may be compromised but may be the only method if access to the bladder is difficult.

Bladder Damage

Anatomical relations

The bladder, like the ureters, is intimately related to the genital tract by virtue of its embryological development.

Repair of the bladder, however, is more straightforward and the results are very good. It is an extraperitoneal organ that is located behind the symphysis pubis and rests on the anterior part of the levator diaphragm, the anterior vaginal wall and the cervix. The trigone is at the level of the upper vagina, with the base of the bladder related to the anterior vaginal fornix and cervix. When full, the bladder rises out of the pelvis towards the level of the umbilicus and presents a hazard during abdominal incision. The bladder is also at risk in this position if it is adherent after previous surgery or during caesarean section in labour, when the lower segment of the uterus is lifted out of the pelvis, elevating the bladder with it.

Avoiding damage

The bladder must always be emptied prior to pelvic surgery and the peritoneum should be opened superiorly, away from the bladder, when making a transverse incision. It can be palpated as a thickening in the peritoneum, and if there is any doubt about its position, careful dissection should allow the detrusor muscle to be recognized before the mucosa is opened. Opening the peritoneum by blunt dissection with fingers will not necessarily protect the bladder, as it is possible to dissect bluntly into it. Similarly, the technique of tearing the parietal peritoneum open by 'stretching' the wound once the abdominal cavity has been opened can lead to damage to the top of the bladder, particularly after previous surgery.

An essential part of any hysterectomy is separation of the bladder from the cervix and upper vagina. This plane can be found after division of the uterovesical fold of peritoneum merely by pushing caudally with a swab applied firmly to the anterior surface of the cervix cranial to the bladder. This is very quick but inevitably leaves a few small bleeding points on the back of the bladder that may be difficult to find. In addition, the bladder is occasionally damaged by this manoeuvre, particularly after previous surgery.

An alternative approach is to use a combination of sharp and blunt dissection. After dividing the uterovesical fold of peritoneum, the scissors are held slightly opened to begin separation in this plane by pushing the bladder off the cervix. Small blood vessels can be recognized and diathermied before cutting, to maintain haemostasis at all times. Once the correct plane has been identified in the midline, the dissection is extended laterally to mobilize the ureters and can be continued as far as necessary down the vagina. Although a little more time consuming, this technique is safe and can be used on simple cases to gain experience for more difficult situations.

When performing the operation vaginally, the same plane needs to be defined and dissected. If the plane does not develop easily, it is important to use sharp dissection, as merely pushing on the bladder may tear a hole. A sound in the bladder may help to define the correct plane. Alternatively, a finger over the fundus of the uterus or over the broad ligament to the side, once the pouch of Douglas is opened, can define the uterovesical fold of peritoneum and clarify the correct plane for dissection.

The bladder can also be damaged during closure of the vaginal vault, particularly if it has not been sufficiently

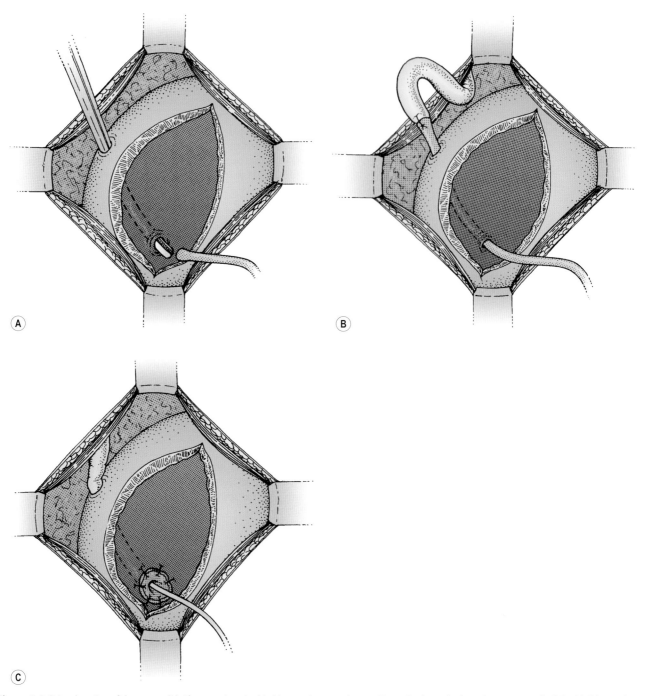

Figure 8.6 Reimplanation of the ureter. (A) After opening the bladder, a submucosal tunnel is made along the lateral posterior wall of the bladder. A thin rubber tube is slipped over the ends of the scissors. (B) The ureter is drawn through the tunnel with the rubber tube. (C) The end of the ureter is spatulated and sutured to the bladder mucosa with fine sutures. An indwelling stent may be left in place, although this is not usually necessary.
Reproduced with permission from Blandey J 1986 Operative Urology, 2nd edn. Blackwell Science, Oxford.

mobilized. Sutures may be placed through the detrusor muscle or even into the bladder itself, although this rarely causes problems (Meeks et al 1997). However, if this is recognized at the time of surgery, such stitches should be removed and the bladder mobilized to allow closure of the vault without including the bladder. If damage to the bladder has occurred, this should be repaired and the bladder drained as discussed below.

Repair of the bladder

Should a hole be made in the bladder, this can be repaired after the dissection of the bladder is complete. A stay stitch is usually placed at either end of the hole, and the incision is repaired in two layers using either chromic catgut or Vicryl. Care should be taken that the ureters are well away from the sutures, and, if there is any doubt, ureteral stents should be

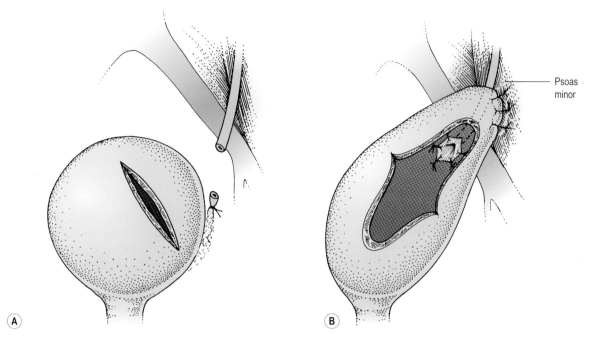

Psoas
minor

(A)

(B)

Figure 8.7 The psoas hitch procedure. (A) The bladder is incised in the transverse axis. (B) The bladder is fixed to the psoas minor tendon to relieve tension and the ureter is reimplanted as described. The bladder is closed in the longitudinal axis.
Reproduced with permission from Blandey J 1986 Operative Urology, 2nd edn. Blackwell Science, Oxford.

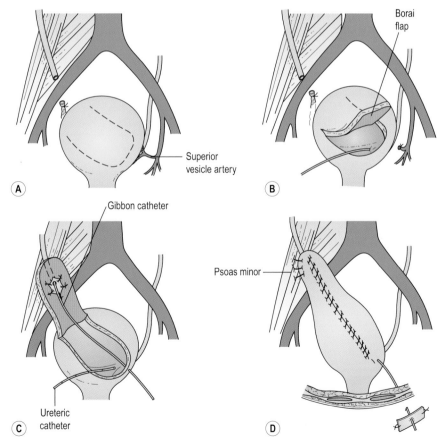

Borai
flap

Superior
vesicle artery

(A)

(B)

Gibbon catheter

Psoas minor

Ureteric
catheter

(C)

(D)

Figure 8.8 Boari flap. (A) The superior vesical artery on the opposite side is divided. (B) The Boari flap is fashioned. A stent in the contralateral ureter may be helpful. (C) The ureter is reimplanted through a submucosal tunnel in the flap. (D) The Boari flap is closed and fixed to the psoas muscle to relieve tension. *Reproduced with permission from Blandey J 1986 Operative Urology, 2nd edn. Blackwell Science, Oxford.*

inserted. After repair, the bladder is drained with an indwelling catheter for 7–10 days. Provided the bladder is well mobilized and repaired without tension, an excellent result should be achieved.

Repair of the bladder is less likely to be successful after radical radiotherapy, and a high incidence of fistulae is seen in this situation. An additional blood supply is provided by interposing a flap of omentum.

Bowel Damage

Inadvertent damage to the bowel should be unusual, unless adhesions are present. The occasions when damage is most likely to occur are during opening of the peritoneal cavity or when dissecting dense intra-abdominal adhesions. In addition, the rectum lies close to the uterosacral ligaments and posterior wall of the vagina, and may be at risk during extensive pelvic dissection for cervical or vaginal carcinoma.

When reopening a previous incision, it is preferable to enter the peritoneal cavity away from the previous closure. If that is not possible, great caution should be used when approaching the peritoneum. Very occasionally, the peritoneal cavity is almost obliterated and it may be neccessary to dissect extraperitoneally around the adhesions to enter the peritoneal cavity.

When dense intraperitoneal adhesions are encountered, the adhesions can usually be divided safely with care and patience. Occasionally, the bowel is so matted together that resection of a small portion may be necessary. Particular care must be used in a patient who has been treated with radio-

therapy, as the bowel is more friable and often densely adherent.

When dividing the uterosacral ligaments close to the pelvic side wall during a radical hysterectomy, the rectum is at risk of being included in the clamps. The rectovaginal space must be opened widely and the rectum dissected free. Care is necessary when entering this space to avoid direct damage to the rectum.

Repair of bowel

Repair of damaged bowel may involve primary closure of a small hole or may be facilitated by the excision of a portion of unhealthy bowel and reanastomosis (Figure 8.9). Consideration should be given to a defunctioning colostomy proximal to anastomosis of large bowel, particularly if the blood supply to the bowel wall is compromised in any way. Factors that have a bearing on this decision are previous radiotherapy, bowel obstruction, gross infection of the operative field or other medical factors such as diabetes, steroid therapy, malignancy and advanced age. If no adverse factors are present, a colostomy may not be necessary. Small bowel usually heals without the need for defunctioning. If there is any doubt about the safety of a repair, a surgeon who specializes in bowel should be involved to help with the repair.

Vascular Damage

Bleeding may occur at any stage of gynaecological surgery, especially if the anatomy is distorted or small tributaries are

Figure 8.9 Small bowel repair. (A) Suture of small intestine with continuous all-layers suture. (B) Connell inverting suture. (C) Full-thickness sutures reinforced with inverting Lembert suture. (D) Purse-string suture of small intestinal perforation.

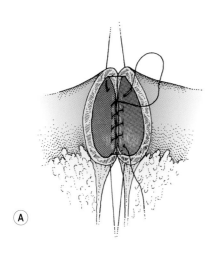

(A)

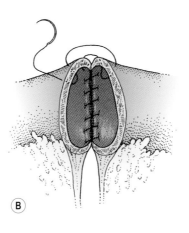

(B)

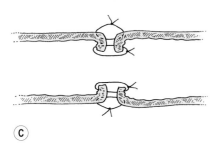

(C)

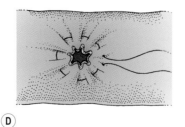

(D)

increased in size, providing collateral supply to fibroids or tumours. Careful and accurate surgical technique will avoid most, but not all, haemorrhagic complications.

Careful, gentle packing of the bowel out of the pelvis reduces the risk of haemorrhage by maximizing exposure of the operative field. While the bowel must be kept out of the pelvis as much as possible, the packs should not compress the inferior vena cava and obstruct the flow of blood out of the pelvis. Excessively tight packing results in distended pelvic veins and excessive venous bleeding. In the same way, a modest head-down tilt lowers the venous pressure in the pelvis and reduces blood loss.

Bleeding may occur from the main uterine or ovarian vessels while they are being identified, clamped and ligated. Using the technique of pelvic dissection described previously, the ovarian vessels can usually be identified and ligated without difficulty. However, the ovarian vein is particularly delicate and easily torn. A tie around the whole pedicle is preferable to transfixion, as the latter risks haematoma formation proximal to the tie. The proximity of the ureter to these vessels at the pelvic brim is an added problem when endometriosis, inflammatory disease, adhesions or tumours distort the anatomy. In contrast, the uterine artery is divided lateral to the uterus as a plexus of vessels in relatively tough tissue and sutures must be inserted. Care must be taken to include all branches in the ligature. The paracervical tissue and vaginal angle are also rich with arterial tributaries, and similar considerations apply. A figure-of-eight suture in the angle of the vagina is useful to ensure that the heel of the pedicle that contains these vessels does not slip out of the ligature. These pedicles should be adjacent to each other with no space between as haemorrhage can occur later, even if the area looks dry at the completion of the procedure.

Small bleeding points on peritoneum or bladder can be diathermied, but slight oozing from a pedicle signals inaccurate technique and should be corrected by oversewing the pedicle and the adjacent pedicle if necessary. The position of the ureter can be identified by palpation of the cardinal ligament lateral to the pedicle prior to the insertion of further sutures.

If bleeding from these vessels occurs, it will usually be controlled temporarily with pressure while appropriate instruments and ligatures are readied. The swab can then be removed gradually, exposing more of the field bit by bit until the bleeding point is revealed. Suction may be needed to keep the operative field clear. The location of the ureter must be determined by palpation or inspection before attending to the bleeding vessel. It is usually best to stop the bleeding by grasping the vessel gently with fine, long-handled artery forceps. A suture may then be inserted.

Damage to the large iliac vessels usually only occurs during surgery for cancer when lymph nodes or tumour are being removed from the surface of the vessels. However, deeply infiltrating endometriosis may become adherent to the internal iliac vessels, and any retroperitoneal tumour or postoperative adhesions may distort the anatomy so that the iliac vessels are exposed to trauma.

If the blood supply to the leg is compromised by damage to the external or common iliac vessels, serious morbidity can result and it is vital that repair is carried out to the highest standard. Usually, a vascular surgeon should be involved.

The internal iliac vessels may be safely ligated if damage occurs, but bleeding from the thin-walled veins on the pelvic side wall can be very difficult to control. Initially, bleeding should be controlled by direct pressure, either by a well-placed finger or using a swab. This allows time to assemble the necessary instruments, a fine sucker and fine sutures on small needles to repair the laceration or ligate the vessel, and also a chance to take a deep breath so that the subsequent suturing is not carried out in a panic. Great care should be taken, as rough handling of the vessels can make the situation worse. If in doubt, more experienced help should be obtained.

In most cases, tears in the common and external iliac veins can be repaired by suturing with fine Vicryl. Damage to the arteries is usually less of a problem because the muscular vessel wall constricts and contains the haemorrhage. Local pressure, sometimes supplemented by sutures, usually gives a very satisfactory result. The real danger comes from damage to the internal iliac veins and their branches, or ragged tears removing parts of the wall of the external or common iliac veins. The deeply placed veins retract into the muscle on the pelvic side wall where they become relatively inaccessible. Deeply placed mattress sutures are required to control the haemorrhage. Unfortunately, such sutures may involve one of the large pelvic nerves. This will only become apparent after the operation when the patient wakes up. It may prove impossible to control bleeding from these veins completely. The often-quoted technique of tying off the internal iliac artery in cases of troublesome bleeding is not without its own hazards. The origin of the artery lies over the bifurcation of the common iliac vein, and great care is needed to avoid damaging the internal iliac vein while dissecting behind the artery to pass the ligature. This technique is often less effective than might be hoped in controlling pelvic haemorrhage because such bleeding is often venous. Firm packing may prove to be the only alternative.

More common than either of the two dramatic scenarios above but equally dangerous is a steady ooze from many small venules and arterioles. This usually follows an extensive dissection such as may be required to remove an endometrioma or to mobilize an adherent bladder. This often happens at the end of a long operation during which there has been a slow but steady blood loss that, because it has not been particularly dramatic, has not been replaced fully. A consumptive coagulopathy results as the clotting factors are exhausted. The first step therefore is to hold a hot pack firmly on the bleeding area for 10 min. The second is to commence the prompt replacement of blood and clotting factors. When the pack is removed gently, all may be well or no more than two or three bleeders may persist. These may be controlled with judicious use of diathermy. If there is still significant generalized blood loss not obviously coming from a single significant vessel, a hot pack should be reinserted and kept firmly in place until the blood volume and clotting factors have been replaced adequately. This may take more than 1 h, during which it is often helpful for the surgical team to take a break. If necessary, the abdomen may be closed with the packs in place. Antibiotics are given and the packs removed gently the following day.

Uterine Perforation and False Passage

During dilatation of the cervix, pushing an instrument through the substance of the cervix rather than following the canal may create a false passage. Instruments may also be pushed through the fundus of the uterus into the peritoneal cavity.

When learning to dilate the cervix, one must develop a gentleness of touch that combines pressure with sensitivity or 'feel' for the tissues. It is important to avoid using force with instruments, but rather to feel for the path of least resistance. Due to the barrel-shaped contour of the endocervical canal, an exploring instrument can deviate from the axis of the cervix and not engage the internal os. The size of instrument chosen for this exploration is important, as a fine probe will create its own passage more easily and therefore less pressure should be used. It is said that right-handed people are more likely to perforate towards the right side of the cervical canal, although a false passage can be created in any direction. It then becomes very difficult to identify the true cervical canal and gain access to the uterine cavity.

If a false passage is suspected, one helpful manoeuvre is to perform a bimanual examination with the vulsellum attached and sound still within the passage. It is often possible to feel where the sound is in relation to the axis of the cervix and in which direction the true passage is likely to be found.

When a false passage has been created, provided damage to other organs is not suspected and the patient is not pregnant, the situation can usually be managed conservatively. In most cases, it is best to desist from further attempts at dilatation. In the pregnant patient, however, significant haemorrhage may occur, particularly following lateral perforation into the broad ligament and damage to the uterine vessels. If vaginal bleeding continues or the patient's general condition deteriorates, laparotomy will be necessary. The broad ligament will be full of blood if the uterine vessels have been damaged, and hysterectomy may be necessary to control the blood loss, although ligation of the uterine artery and repair of the perforation may be an option. In some cases, bleeding into the retroperitoneal space may not become apparent for several hours. Careful postoperative observation is necessary to detect this at an early stage.

The consequences of fundal perforation depend on whether the patient is pregnant and what instrument has created the perforation. In a non-pregnant uterus, a dilator through the fundus is very unlikely to cause any problems. It is likely that most perforations go unrecognized by the surgeon. The patient should be observed for a period after recovery but is unlikely to need further intervention. In a pregnant patient, perforation is said to be more likely to cause haemorrhage but, in general, a simple perforation can be managed conservatively. The temptation to 'confirm' the perforation by repeatedly reintroducing instruments into the uterus should be avoided as this may make matters worse.

If there is significant risk of damage to intra-abdominal organs, a laparotomy is indicated because laparoscopy cannot be relied upon to exclude damage to bowel. For example, if a suction catheter has been inserted through a perforation with suction connected, laparotomy and careful examination of the bowel are mandatory.

Laparoscopy

The incidence of complications in laparoscopic surgery relates very closely to the experience of the surgeon and the training they have received. Gynaecologists have built up extensive experience in the specialty with simple procedures over the last generation. Most senior house officers and junior registrars are trained in diagnostic laparoscopy as one of their earliest procedures. Nevertheless, adoption of the more advanced operative techniques has been slow, and experience in these areas is still very limited. If a high incidence of complications is to be avoided, it is essential that individual surgeons are well trained in the procedures they undertake. General complications of laparoscopy will be discussed but consideration of complications encountered in advanced laparoscopic surgery is outside the scope of this chapter (see Chapter 4, Laparoscopy, for more information).

Damage to bowel

Blind insertion of the Veress needle and first trocar may lead to perforation of intra-abdominal and retroperitoneal structures. Bowel is rarely damaged unless it is adherent to the anterior abdominal wall, but great care must be taken if the patient has had a previous operation or intra-abdominal sepsis. In these cases, the initial trocar may be placed away from the site of the previous incision in an attempt to avoid fixed bowel. Alternatively, the abdomen may be entered using an open minilaparotomy technique and then the incision sealed around a blunt-ended trocar. Difficulty may be encountered in maintaining a good seal using this technique, but specially designed trocars reduce this problem. A new device is available that incises the tissue in front of a blunt-ended trocar 1 mm at a time, and allows visualization of the end of the instrument as it is being inserted. This may prove to be useful in the small number of cases where difficulty is anticipated.

A surgeon experienced in laparoscopic suturing may repair minor damage to the bowel endoscopically. In most cases, it is much safer to perform a laparotomy to allow careful inspection of the whole bowel and open repair of any damage. As it can be difficult to find the hole in the bowel subsequently, it is wise to leave the offending instrument in place until the abdomen is open.

Damage to blood vessels

When inserting the Veress needle and the first trocar, it is vital that these instruments are kept away from the major vessels. The position of the sacral promontory can be palpated and the instruments angled in such a way that they pass below the promontory and into the free space in the midline of the pelvis. While damage to a major blood vessel may be all too obvious, the bleeding may be predominantly retroperitoneal and difficult to see laparoscopically. If the patient's blood pressure has dropped and pulse rate risen sufficiently to suggest the possibility of vascular damage, a laparotomy should be performed immediately. If the abdomen has to be opened in a hurry, one technique is to lift the laparoscope up to the anterior abdominal wall and cut down on to it, allowing immediate access.

Blood vessels in the abdominal wall may also be damaged. To reduce this risk, the abdominal wall is usually transilluminated to visualize vessels prior to insertion of the secondary trocars. The location of the inferior epigastric vessels should be recognized, as they will bleed profusely and this may be difficult to control. Minor bleeding around a trocar may be controlled either by leaving the trocar in place to tamponade the vessel, or by inserting a Foley catheter through the trocar, inflating the balloon with 30–50 ml of saline and withdrawing the trocar and balloon to apply pressure to the bleeding point. If the vessel requires suturing, this is facilitated by a long J-shaped needle.

Diathermy damage

Problems with laparoscopic use of diathermy stem either from the heat generated at the site of tissue destruction or from current finding an alternative path to earth through an adjacent organ. Tissue coagulated by diathermy becomes very hot and may retain its heat for several minutes. This heat will spread to underlying structures and adjacent organs, and may cause damage. Diathermied tissue must be allowed to cool before coming into contact with adjacent structures. A further problem is the rising impedance in desiccated, diathermied tissue. This may result in the current arcing to a nearby organ that offers a low-resistance path to earth. In a similar way, current may arc to nearby organs if the current is activated before the electrode is in contact with the tissue to be treated.

KEY POINTS

1. Accurate identification of tissue planes and careful dissection will reduce intraoperative complications.
2. The ureter should always be identified on the pelvic side wall before the infundibulopelvic ligament is divided.
3. The ureter should be identified and freed from ovarian masses by opening the retroperitoneal space.
4. If the ureter is damaged, repair should usually be undertaken by a urologist.
5. The bladder may be repaired using two layers of absorbable sutures. One should ensure that the ureters are not included in this repair.
6. Repair of bowel or great vessels, apart from minor damage, should usually be undertaken by a specialist surgeon.
7. Uterine perforation may often be managed conservatively.
8. Repair of laparoscopic damage to bowel will usually require a laparotomy.
9. If laparoscopic damage to major pelvic vessels is suspected, a laparotomy must be performed without delay.
10. Diathermy should only be applied when the electrodes are securely applied to the target tissue, and the target and surrounding tissues are in clear view.

References

Cruise PJE, Foord R 1973 A 5 year prospective study of 23,649 surgical wounds. Archives of Surgery 107: 206.

Franchi M, Ghezzi F, Benedetti-Panici PL et al 2001 A multicentre collaborative study on the use of cold scalpel and electrocautery for midline abdominal incision. Amerian Journal of Surgery 181: 128–132.

Meeks GR, Sams JO 4th, Field KW, Fulp KW, Margolis MT 1997 Formation of vesicovaginal fistula: the role of suture placement into the bladder during closure of the vaginal cuff after transabdominal hysterectomy. American Journal of Obstetrics and Gynecology 177: 1298–1303.

Niggebrugge AHP, Trimbos JB, Hermans J, Steup W-H, Van De Velde CJH 1999 Influence of abdominal-wound closure technique on complications after surgery: a randomised study. The Lancet 353: 1563–1567.

Orr JW Jr, Garter JE, Kilgore LC et al 1987 Closed suction pelvic drainage following radical pelvic surgery. American Journal of Obstetrics and Gynecology 155: 867.

Orr JW Jr, Orr PJ, Bolen DD, Holimon JL 1995 Radical hysterectomy: does the type of incision matter? American Journal of Obstetrics and Gynecology 173: 399–405.

Royal College of Obstetrics and Gynaecologists 1998 Peritoneal Closure. Guideline No. 15. RCOG, London.

Rucinski J, Margolis M, Panagopoulos G, Wise L 2001 Closure of the abdominal midline fascia: meta-analysis delineates the optimal technique. American Surgeon 67: 421–462.

Scribner DR Jr, Kamelle SA, Gould N et al 2001 A retrospective analysis of radical hysterectomies done for cervical cancer: is there a role for the Pfannenstiel incision? Gynecological Oncology 81: 481–484.

Tulandi T, Hum HS, Gelfand MM 1988 Closure of laparotomy incisions with or without peritoneal suturing and second look laparoscopy. American Journal of Obstetrics and Gynecology 158: 536.

CHAPTER 9

Postoperative care

Saad A. Amer

Chapter Contents

INTRODUCTION	116	KEY POINTS	126
ROUTINE POSTOPERATIVE CARE	116		
RECOGNITION AND MANAGEMENT OF POSTOPERATIVE COMPLICATIONS	120		

Introduction

The postoperative period is the span of time from the end of a surgical procedure until resumption of normal life activity. The duration of this period varies according to the nature of the procedure and the fitness of the patient. It is characterized by restoration of normal physiological functions, healing of tissues from the surgical trauma and a gradual return of physical strength. In the first few hours whilst the patient is recovering from the anaesthetic, she gradually regains her respiratory, cardiovascular and neurological functions, and establishes homeostasis. Recovery of the gastrointestinal tract and mobilization occur in the first 1–3 days after uncomplicated surgery. Healing of tissues and return of full physical strength continue for a variable length of time (1–6 weeks) after discharge from hospital. Although most of the complications from surgery occur in the early postoperative phase, they can still arise after discharge from hospital. Measures should therefore be put in place in collaboration with the general practitioner/primary care doctor and community nurse to support the patient whilst at home and to ensure recognition of any late adverse event.

The last decade has witnessed a dramatic change in the postoperative care of the gynaecological patient. Whilst it was previously routine for women to remain in hospital with bed rest for up to 2 weeks following a hysterectomy, most units nowadays discharge these patients after 3 days. More recently, a growing number of gynaecological units routinely perform laparoscopic hysterectomies as day cases. These changes have been driven by a number of factors, including a realization of the risks associated with prolonged immobilization and hospital stay, such as infective and thromboembolic complications. In addition to these clinical reasons, pressures on hospital beds and funding have driven down length of stay.

Good postoperative care will lead to a smooth and quick recovery from surgery with reduction of complications and a shorter hospital stay. There are three main objectives of postoperative care:

- supporting the patient during restoration of physiological functions;
- promoting healing of tissues; and
- recognizing and managing complications.

Postoperative care should be tailored to each individual's circumstances with attention to the particular needs of every patient. Standardization of care can be developed, but should be applied with a degree of flexibility to allow the individualization of care.

Postoperative care should be provided by well-trained and skilled nursing staff with input from the surgical team as well as members of a multidisciplinary team including physiotherapists, dieticians, pharmacists and microbiologists. Other specialist postoperative management should be provided as necessary, such as wound care and rehabilitation.

Routine Postoperative Care

Fluid and electrolyte balance

Patients undergoing gynaecological surgery, excluding minor and day-case procedures, require intravenous (IV) fluid administration until oral fluid intake is fully resumed. The daily requirement of fluid should be calculated accurately and the patient should be monitored carefully to ensure adequate hydration. This is important to avoid fluid overload (which could lead to pulmonary oedema) or dehydration (which could result in renal tubular necrosis). When calculating the fluid intake, one should consider the normal fluid requirement (approximately 2.5 l/24 h), intraoperative blood loss and insensible losses (e.g. due to raised temperature). Other factors to be considered when calculating fluid intake include preoperative depletion of fluids, long operative procedures, pyrexia, fluid loss through drains,

DOI: 10.1016/B978-0-7020-3120-5.00009-6

excessive vomiting, bowel distension, oral fluid intake, extravascular fluid accumulation (third space) and previous fluid replacement.

Urine output monitoring should be used to determine the status of the intravascular volume and total body water. The normal urine output is 30 ml/h. Patients voiding less than 17 ml/h are oliguric. Other clinical signs of dehydration include mucous membrane dryness, slow skin turgor, tachycardia and raised temperature. Patients should also be monitored for features of fluid overload such as jugular venous distension, mucous membrane turgor, pulmonary rales, third heart sound and pitting oedema. Central venous pressure monitoring should be considered when there is difficulty assessing intravascular volumes. Invasive direct measures of cardiac output that enable accurate measurement of intravascular filling (e.g. measurements of pulmonary wedge pressures and transoesophageal echo) are rarely required after gynaecological surgery.

Oliguria can be prerenal, renal or postrenal. Postoperative oliguria is most commonly prerenal and is caused by insufficient fluid replacement. This can be confirmed by a fluid challenge with the infusion of 250 ml of a colloid such as gelofusin over 15 min. Improvement of urine output after this fluid challenge confirms prerenal oliguria, which can be corrected by increasing the rate of IV fluid administration. If there is no improvement in urine output with the fluid challenge, the patient should be assessed for evidence of pulmonary oedema and renal impairment (due to tubular necrosis). In the elderly or those with known cardiac disease, fluid challenges should be given with caution as this may exacerbate pulmonary oedema.

If prerenal and renal causes of oliguria have been excluded, a postrenal aetiology such as ureteric obstruction should be considered. Diagnosis can be made with renal ultrasound. If this is inconclusive, ureteric catheters can be used for diagnosis and treatment.

The majority of gynaecological patients undergoing surgery are healthy and usually resume their diet within 24–48 h. Postoperative monitoring of electrolytes is therefore not required routinely in these patients. However, electrolyte imbalance may occur under certain circumstances such as persistent vomiting, prolonged IV fluid administration, and after surgery involving extensive tissue damage or excessive drainage from the surgical site. In addition, patients with renal impairment, diabetes or those receiving certain medications (e.g. potassium-sparing diuretics) are at increased risk of electrolyte disturbances. These patients should be monitored for electrolyte imbalance and treated promptly for any abnormality. Both hypo- and hyperkalaemia can result in cardiac arrhythmias and therefore require assessment by electrocardiogram (ECG). Hypokalaemia usually results from delayed oral intake or excessive vomiting. It can be corrected by increasing the potassium content of the IV fluid (20 mEq KCl/l). Hyperkalaemia can occur in patients undergoing extensive surgery due to shift of potassium from traumatized cells into the extracellular space. Moderate or severe hyperkalaemia (potassium level >6 mEq/l) is a medical emergency; if not corrected promptly, it can lead to severe cardiac arrhythmias and death. An input from the medical team should therefore be sought. It can be corrected by IV administration of glucose and insulin to promote potassium shift into the cells. Calcium gluconate is also given to protect the heart from dysrhythmias. Hyponatraemia is usually secondary to excessive fluid administration or absorption of excessive amounts of irrigating fluid during hysteroscopic surgery, and hypernatraemia is secondary to dehydration.

Bladder care

In women undergoing major gynaecological surgery, a urinary catheter is usually inserted just before the operation to keep the bladder empty throughout the procedure. This helps to minimize the risk of bladder injury and allows good access to the surgical field. Post operatively, the catheter is kept in place during the acute recovery phase for the patient's comfort, to allow monitoring of urine output and to avoid urinary retention due to the general anaesthetic or pain. The catheter should be removed as soon as the patient is able to mobilize and void comfortably. Early removal of the catheter is important as prolonged catheterization may be associated with an increased risk of urinary tract infection (Schiøtz and Tanbo 2006). In patients who sustained a bladder injury during surgery, the catheter should be kept for 7–10 days to allow full healing of the bladder wall, and many gynaecologists would perform a systogram prior to removing the catheter.

Postoperative voiding difficulty is a common problem in gynaecological surgery, especially following bladder neck operations, and can be due to spasm, oedema or tenderness of paraurethral tissue. It is also common following radical hysterectomy due to extensive perivesical dissection that interferes with the nerve and blood supply to the bladder. Other contributing factors include cystitis and psychogenic factors. Failure to pass urine could also occur as a result of regional anaesthesia (which may cause bladder overdistension and atony) and abdominal pain, which may inhibit the initial voluntary phase of voiding. Following bladder neck surgery, most voiding difficulty resolves within 1 or 2 weeks of surgery, but up to 20% of women can continue with this problem for an extended period (up to 6 months) before being able to void normally (Smith and Cardozo 1997).

If the patient does not pass urine for 4–6 h after catheter removal, residual urine volume should be measured after micturition using a bladder ultrasound scan. This should also be performed in women undergoing bladder neck surgery or radical hysterectomy. Voiding difficulty is diagnosed if the residual volume is consistently greater than 100 ml. If this problem persists after several voiding attempts, a catheter should be inserted for 24 h. The catheter is then removed and further residual volume measurements are carried out. If still high, the patient should be allowed home with an indwelling catheter for 7–10 days. Failing this, the catheter could be left in the bladder for a longer period. Eventually, if voiding difficulty persists, the patient should be trained to perform intermittent self-catheterization.

A suprapubic catheter should be considered during surgery in patients expected to have postoperative voiding difficulty. This allows easier and more accurate measurement of residual volumes. The catheter is clamped and the patient is asked to void urine. This is followed by measurement of residual urine passing through the suprapubic catheter. Another advantage of this catheter is the reduced risk of urinary tract infections compared with the urethral catheter.

Drains

Although not necessary in the majority of routine gynaecological procedures, drains can be helpful in certain cases. The main indication for placing a drain during gynaecological surgery is surface oozing following extensive pelvic surgery such as adhesiolysis, treatment of extensive endometriosis or complicated hysterectomy. Drainage in these cases is necessary to prevent haematoma formation and to allow early recognition of significant postoperative internal haemorrhage. However, the drain should not be used as a substitute for meticulous intraoperative haemostasis. Other indications for pelvic drainage include pelvic infection (e.g. tubo-ovarian abscess) and clotting disorders, which could result in persistent postoperative oozing.

Intraperitoneal (pelvic) drains have been associated with an increased incidence of infection, and should only be used when the benefits outweigh the risks. Evidence from recent randomized trials and systematic reviews is against the routine use of drains. A recent large randomized trial of drains compared with no drains following radical hysterectomy and pelvic lymph node dissection concluded that drains can be safely omitted in the absence of excessive bleeding during surgery or oozing at the end of surgery (Franchi et al 2007). A systematic review evaluating the value of routine suction drains after retroperitoneal lymphadenectomy in gynaecological tumours concluded that the prophylactic use of continuous suction drains is associated with a significant increase in morbidity and should be avoided (Bacha et al 2009). On the other hand, drainage of surgical wounds (especially clean-contaminated wounds) using a closed-suction system has been used prophylactically to reduce wound infection (Panici et al 2003).

There are two main types of drains: passive (non-suction) and active (suction). Passive drains, which drain by overflow assisted by gravity, are preferred for the peritoneal cavity, where soft tissue can block the fenestrations of suction drains. Passive drains should not be brought out through the incision, to avoid the risk of wound infection. Suction drains are sealed systems with a vacuum to drain a potential space created by surgery such as the subcutaneous or subfascial space. They are also used to drain lymphatic fluid from the groins after lymphadenectomy.

Early removal of drains is recommended to avoid infection and aid mobilization. The precise timing for removal of a drain should be determined on an individual basis and depends on the reasons for its insertion. Drains that were placed prophylactically to avoid the accumulation of blood, pus or lymph can usually be removed when drainage is <100 ml in 24 h, usually by 2 or 3 days after surgery. Drains placed for drainage of an abscess should be managed according to the resolution of the condition.

Postoperative pain management

Effective relief of postoperative pain is of paramount importance as it offers significant psychological and physiological benefits to the recovering patient. Not only does it mean a smooth postoperative course with earlier discharge from hospital, but it also helps to reduce the incidence of complications (Nagaratnam et al 2007). In addition, there is evidence that good pain relief can reduce the onset of chronic pain syndromes. Inadequate pain management could lead to reduced deep breathing, causing impaired oxygenation. It can also cause inability to cough and clear lung secretions which may lead to lung atelectasis. Pain reduces a patient's mobility, leading to slower recovery and increased risk of morbidities such as deep vein thrombosis (DVT). The benefits of good postoperative pain management are summarized in Table 9.1.

The first step in achieving good pain control is preoperative prediction and accurate postoperative assessment of the degree of pain. Such pain is subjective and can vary greatly in severity between patients from almost no pain to very severe pain. There are two main factors determining the degree of postoperative pain: firstly, the nature, extent and site of the surgery; and secondly, factors related to the patient including fear, anxiety and pain threshold. A previous experience of postoperative pain may also infuence the patient's expectation and perception of pain. It is therefore important to plan postoperative pain management through consultation between the surgeon and the anaesthetist based on the predicted pain severity. It is also important to explain to the patient the expected degree of pain and the steps that will be taken to ensure effective pain relief afterwards. It is usually helpful to establish the patient's expectations of pain before surgery. This approach has been shown to minimize the patient's fear and anxiety from pain and to reduce the requirement for postoperative analgesia (Karanikolas and Swarm 2000).

Methods of assessment

After surgery, pain can be assessed using one of several methods such as the visual analogue scale (VAS) or the verbal response score (VRS). With the VAS, the patient chooses a number between 0 and 10 to represent her pain. Zero indicates no pain and 10 means pain as severe as can be imagined. The VRS utilizes a simple five-point scale which either correlates pain severity to words (no pain, mild, moderate, severe, excruciating) or to a number (0–4). The pain should be assessed at regular intervals, preferably charted in graphical form and should form part of the routine postoperative observation.

Table 9.1 Benefits of effective postoperative pain relief

Improved recovery	Patient satisfaction
	Wound healing
	Early mobilization
	Early hospital discharge
Reduced morbidities	Respiratory complications
	Tachycardia and dysrhythmias
	Thromboembolic events
	Acute coronary syndromes
	Chronic pain syndrome

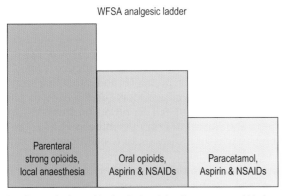

WFSA analgesic ladder

Parenteral strong opioids, local anaesthesia

Oral opioids, Aspirin & NSAIDs

Paracetamol, Aspirin & NSAIDs

Local anaesthesia = epidural, spinal, peripheral nerve or wound block.
NSAID = nonsteroidal anti-inflammatory drug.

Figure 9.1 The World Federation of Societies of Anaesthesiologists' analgesic ladder. Local anaesthesia indicates epidural, spinal or peripheral nerve or wound block. NSAID, non-steroidal anti-inflammatory drug.
Source: Charlton JE (1997) The management of postoperative pain. Update in Anesthesia 7: 2–17 (www.anaesthesiologists.org).

The analgesic ladder

The World Federation of Societies of Anaesthesiologists' analgesic ladder, which has been developed to treat acute pain, can be utilized for postoperative pain (Charlton 1997; Figure 9.1). In women undergoing major gynaecological surgery, the initial pain can be expected to be severe and may need injections of strong opioids [e.g. morphine, preferably by a patient-controlled analgesia (PCA) system], which can be combined with local anaesthesia. As pain decreases with time, analgesia can be stepped down and parenteral opioids can be gradually replaced by the oral route. Strong oral opioids (e.g. oromorph) can be given, to be gradually replaced with a combination of peripherally acting agents (e.g. paracetamol and non-steroidal anti-inflammatory drugs) and weak opioids (e.g. codeine phosphate). The final step is when the pain can be controlled by peripherally acting agents alone.

Opioid analgesia

PCA is an effective way of providing opioid analgesia where the patient titrates the dose to her need by pressing a button that delivers a small bolus (e.g. 1 mg morphine). The PCA system is preset by the anaesthetist to a minimum interval between boluses to prevent overdosage. It is therefore safe and offers high patient satisfaction. Continuous epidural analgesia provides great pain relief for up to 72 h and is more effective than PCA. In addition, it is associated with improved pulmonary function, short convalescence and a lower incidence of morbidities such as pulmonary complications, venous thromboembolism, gastrointestinal side-effects and central venous system depression. It is usually sited by the anaesthetist in theatre and left in for a few days after surgery. Its routine use may be limited by insufficient trained nursing staff to manage it and to treat potential side-effects.

Wound care

Good wound care will promote healing and minimize complications such as infection, haematoma formation or dehiscence. Wound care begins during surgery with careful handling of tissues, avoidance of cautery for skin incision, meticulous haemostasis, good closure techniques and avoidance of excessive traction on the skin edges (Boesch and Umek 2009). At the end of surgery, a wound dressing is applied, mainly to cover the fresh wound to prevent seepage of serum or blood, but this does not have any protective effect against infection. It should be removed on the first postoperative day when the wound has become dry. Any serous or serosanguinous discharge can be squeezed out by gentle pressure on the wound edges. Patients can be allowed a shower, but should keep the wound dry and clean. Sutures and staples can be removed from transverse wounds after 4–5 days, but vertical wounds usually require 7–10 days to heal.

Wound infection

Wound infection occurs in 3–5% of clean wounds and 10–20% of clean-contaminated wounds in the absence of antibiotic prophylaxis. It usually presents by the fifth postoperative day as erythema, induration and pain in the area surrounding the incision, and may be associated with pyrexia. A wound swab should be taken for culture, and broad-spectrum antibiotics should be given. If the infection progresses to pus formation under the suture line, this should be drained. Usually, at this stage, the wound separates either partially or completely, allowing drainage. However, if the wound remains intact or if the separation is only small, the wound should be opened (in theatre if necessary) to allow drainage. If there is a significant delay in healing with development of devitalized tissue, the wound should be opened in theatre, explored, debrided and packed with gauze, followed by twice-daily dressing changes. At this stage, the tissue viability team and microbiologists should be involved in the care of this chronically infected wound to ensure that the most appropriate dressings and treatments are given. Negative pressure wound therapy may be considered in these wounds to promote the production of granulation tissue and encourage neovascularization (Walsh et al 2009).

Necrotizing fasciitis

Necrotizing fasciitis is a rare but life-threatening and rapidly progressive infection of the superficial fascia and subcutaneous tissues (Addison et al 1984). It often occurs in diabetic and immunosuppressed patients, but can also affect women with other chronic illnesses. It is characterized by dusky and friable subcutaneous tissue with serous drainage from a small wound that may be separate from the original incision wound. It can also occur on the vulva or perineum, often not related to surgery. There is extensive tissue necrosis and a moderate or severe systemic toxic reaction. Very radical excision is essential with antibiotics and supportive therapy.

Postoperative feeding

Traditionally and for many years, postoperative oral intake of fluid and food has been delayed until the recovery of bowel function (return of bowel sounds and passage of flatus) from the temporary postoperative ileus. This was believed to be necessary to avoid vomiting and severe paralytic ileus. However, this practice has not been supported by good scientific evidence. A recent systematic review of early (<24 h) compared with delayed oral intake after major abdominal gynaecological surgery has provided evidence in favour of early oral intake. The study has shown early postoperative feeding to be safe and associated with a reduced length of hospital stay, but with an increase in the incidence of nausea (Charoenkwan et al 2007). Early feeding was not associated with an increase in complications such as ileus, vomiting or abdominal distension. However, the authors concluded that the timing of postoperative feeding should be individualized according to each patient's circumstances. In patients undergoing benign gynaecological procedures without significant insult to the gastrointestinal tract, early postoperative oral intake should be encouraged. On the other hand, feeding should be delayed in women at high risk of paralytic ileus (e.g. following extensive and prolonged procedures with excessive handling of the bowel).

Mobilization and physiotherapy

The benefits of early postoperative mobilization have been established since the 1940s (Brieger 1983). It reduces the muscle loss associated with inactivity, hastens recovery and reduces the incidence of pulmonary complications. Other benefits include a reduction in the risk of thromboembolic disease and respiratory infection. Mobilization involving an upright position appears to be of greatest benefit in the early postoperative period, with evidence of improvements in pulmonary function (Nielsen et al 2003), prevention of functional decline and possibly a positive effect on depression and anxiety (Brooks-Brunn 1995). Early involvement of skilled physiotherapists is essential to facilitate early mobilization and to deal with the problems arising from prolonged postoperative recovery. In particular, physiotherapists play an important role in the prevention and treatment of respiratory infection.

Recognition and Management of Postoperative Complications

Haemorrhage

Primary haemorrhage occurs in the immediate postoperative period and is usually a result of inadequate intraoperative haemostasis or slipped ligatures due to poor surgical technique. Patients undergoing complex gynaecological procedures such as treatment of endometriosis, division of extensive adhesions or myomectomy are at increased risk of primary postoperative haemorrhage. Secondary haemorrhage is delayed and usually has an infective aetiology. It is more commonly associated with vaginal procedures.

All patients undergoing major gynaecological surgery should be monitored closely for signs of internal haemorrhage in the immediate postoperative period. This can be achieved with regular observations of the pulse, blood pressure, urine output and abdominal distension. It is important to bear in mind that most gynaecological patients who are young and fit compensate very well for hypovolaemia, sustaining a normal blood pressure until late stages when the compensatory mechanisms fail with sudden collapse. It is therefore important, especially in high-risk patients, to watch for the early signs of hypovolaemia including tachycardia, peripheral vasoconstriction (manifested by cold hands and feet) and signs of anaemia (pallor and low haemoglobin). Although oliguria is another sign of hypovolaemia, it often occurs due to dehydration rather than haemorrhage. In cases of major and rapid haemorrhage, which is beyond the compensatory mechanisms, the patient will experience a rapid fall in blood pressure. In women with intra-abdominal drains, the volume of blood draining could be used as an indication of the severity of blood loss. However, lack of significant drainage does not exclude massive intra-abdominal bleeding, especially when a small drain is used which could get blocked. When there is uncertainty with the diagnosis, an abdominal ultrasound scan, if one is readily available, may aid the diagnosis by confirming intra-abdominal blood collection. The scan can also help in establishing the severity of the condition by estimating the amount of intra-abdominal blood. However, the diagnosis should be primarily based on clinical assessment of the patient.

When internal haemorrhage is suspected, whole blood should be immediately cross-matched and transfused as soon as available. In the mean time, hypovolaemia should be corrected by a colloid or crystalloid intravenous fluid until blood becomes available. The debate over the value of colloid vs crystalloid preparations for volume replacement remains unresolved. A recent Cochrane systematic review by Perel and Roberts (2007) concluded that the continued use of colloids in favour of crystalloids is not supported by evidence from randomized controlled trials and does not improve the outcome of treatment. An urgent full blood count and coagulation screen should be arranged. The coagulation status should be monitored repeatedly during the resuscitation of the patient due to the risk of consumptive coagulopathy. A haematologist should be consulted if there is any abnormality with the clotting system. The next step is for the surgeon to decide whether or not the patient should be taken back to theatre for exploration and achievement of haemostasis. Timing in these cases is critical as any delay in decision could have fatal consequences if the patient enters a state of irreversible shock or disseminated intravascular coagulopathy. On the other hand, rushing the patient back to theatre when conservative management may have been enough will unnecessarily subject the patient to the risks of repeated anaesthetic and surgery. More often, the bleeding is due to generalized ooze, and adequate haemostasis will be difficult to achieve surgically. In some cases, therefore, it may be better to continue the transfusion and correct any coagulation defect rather than to re-explore.

If a decision is made for surgical exploration, the patient should be taken to theatre after initial resuscitation. Patients bleeding vaginally after a hysterectomy could be examined vaginally under anaesthesia. The vault can be reopened and, if a bleeder is identified (usually vaginal branch of uterine artery in one of the angles), it can be secured with a suture. Once haemostasis has been achieved, the vaginal vault can be reclosed and a pack inserted if necessary. In all other cases, a relaparotomy should be performed and all the pedicles should be examined carefully. More recently, laparoscopy has been used successfully for exploration and establishment of haemostasis in patients with postoperative haemorrhage (Sobolev et al 2005). Intra-abdominal bleeding frequently originates from ovarian vessels. These must be identified clearly and separated from the ureter before the application of diathermy or a ligature. Sometimes, it can be difficult to localize the bleeding point and it may be venous rather than arterial. In these situations, compression with large packs for a few minutes can be effective, or will at least reduce the general ooze, allowing the main bleeding sites to be visualized clearly and dealt with. It is always important to ensure safety of the ureter by palpation or dissection before suturing. If effective haemostasis cannot be achieved, bilateral internal iliac artery ligation or angiographic embolization of bleeding vessels should be considered provided that expertise is available. Failure of haemostasis could be due to coagulopathy, which should be corrected promptly with input from the haematologist. Fresh frozen plasma, which contains all the protein constituents of plasma including the coagulation factors, is used to replace these factors in consumptive coagulopathy. Cryoprecipitate contains a high concentration of fibrinogen that may be required in massive blood transfusion. If haemostasis is impossible, the bleeding site could be compressed with several large packs, followed by closure of the abdomen. The packs should be removed under general anaesthetic after 24–48 h.

Haematoma formation

Vault

Vault haematoma following hysterectomy is relatively common, affecting approximately 20–30% of patients. In most cases, the haematoma is asymptomatic and is only detected on pelvic ultrasound scan. Frequent presentations include lower abdominal pain, low-grade temperature or vaginal discharge. Haematomas are usually self-limiting and will either resolve or discharge via the vaginal vault in the second week following surgery. Infected vault haematomas do not usually contaminate the peritoneal cavity, and generalized peritonitis is rare in these cases. The majority of haematomas can be managed conservatively until they subside. Prophylactic antibiotics can be given to minimize the risk of abscess formation. A large vault haematoma may require drainage, especially if there is evidence of sepsis or if conservative management fails. Drainage is usually performed in theatre under general anaesthetic via a vaginal approach. If interrupted sutures have been used, the removal of one or two may be sufficient to introduce a finger into the gap. Continuous vault sutures will need to be replaced completely when divided to enter the vault. With bimanual compression, the organized clot can be expelled but the blind use of instruments should be avoided. A large bore drain may be required at the end of the procedure to ensure complete drainage.

Wound

Abdominal wound haematomas are also common following open abdominal surgery. They usually cause swelling and bruising around the wound, associated with significant pain. Like the vault haematomas, they are self-limiting and will resolve with time. Management is usually conservative with reassurance of the patient. Large haematomas may require drainage, especially if there is evidence of infection or if they are associated with severe pain. This is usually carried out in theatre with opening of all or part of the incision. If a subfascial haematoma is suspected, the rectus sheath should also be opened.

Infection and pyrexia

In recent years, hospital-acquired infection has received a great deal of attention from the health authorities. The Department of Health has taken several measures to reduce the transmission of hospital infection, especially against the so-called 'hospital super bugs' (e.g. meticillin-resistant *Staphylococcus aureus* and *Clostridium difficile*). Most hospitals in the UK now have a dedicated infection control team led by a microbiologist who monitors the rates of hospital infections and develops local protocols on the use of antibiotics to minimize bacterial resistance. All hospital staff working in clinical areas receive regular infection control training. The main emphasis of infection control policies is on proper hand hygiene and maintenance of a clean patient environment.

Most major gynaecological procedures (e.g. abdominal and vaginal hysterectomy) fall into the clean-contaminated category (see Chapter 7) and are associated with an infection rate of 10–20% in the absence of antibiotic prophylaxis. In a meta-analysis of 25 randomized controlled trials, involving a total of 3604 women, antibiotic prophylaxis was found to reduce the incidence of infection after total abdominal hysterectomy from 21% to 9% (Mittendorf et al 1993). On the other hand, clean wounds which are performed under complete aseptic conditions are associated with infection rates of 1–5% without prophylaxis. Clean procedures include most adnexal surgeries, laparoscopic procedures and subtotal hysterectomy. Antibiotic prophylaxis does not decrease infection rates following these procedures and should not be given.

Postoperative fever occurring within the first 48 h is not usually caused by an infective process, but may be associated with haematoma formation or pulmonary atelectasis. Later development of pyrexia (after 72 h) is more likely to be infective in origin. The most common site of postoperative infection is the urinary tract (day 3), followed by wound infections (day 5) and collections. Non-infective causes of pyrexia such as DVT should also be considered in the differential diagnosis. Urinary tract infections are not usually associated with urinary symptoms; when suspected, this should be confirmed with urine microscopy and culture. The incidence of urinary tract infection is not changed by the use of prophylactic antibiotics (Brown et al 1988), and is mainly increased with the use of perioperative catheterization. Wound infection usually becomes manifest on the fifth postoperative day (see above). Swinging pyrexia, which persists despite intensive antibiotic therapy, may indicate an infected collection (e.g. pelvic abscess). An ultrasound or computed tomography (CT) scan of the pelvis and abdomen should be performed in these cases to detect any collection. If identified, infected collections not responding to antibiotics may need surgical evacuation. This could be carried out either via a vaginal route (especially after vaginal hysterectomy) or through a laparotomy.

Sepsis is a systemic response to infection which, in severe cases, can lead to septic shock manifested by hypotension and multiple organ failure (Wheeler and Bernard 1999). This requires prompt resuscitation (in an intensive care unit) and aggressive eradication of the source of infection with broad-spectrum antibiotics and surgery if appropriate (Tamussino 2002).

Venous thromboembolism

In the absence of thromboprophylaxis, patients undergoing major (>30 min) general and gynaecological surgery have a significant risk of both asymptomatic (approximately 30%) and symptomatic (approximately 8%) venous thromboembolism (Table 9.2). The risk increases with the number of risk factors (Scottish Intercollegiate Guidelines Network 2002). Women in the high-risk category should be counselled carefully before surgery, and referred to a haematology clinic for risk assessment and advice on perioperative management. The risk factors and thromboprophylaxis have been discussed in Chapter 7.

Diagnosis of deep vein thrombosis

It is always good practice to have a high index of suspicion for DVT following major gynaecological surgery, especially in high-risk patients. The majority of patients with DVT are asymptomatic and could go unrecognized until complicated with life-threatening pulmonary embolism (PE). The calf is the most common site for DVT and usually manifests with swelling, erythema and pain. Examination usually reveals low-grade pyrexia with a swollen, tender and warm calf. Patients with these manifestations should be treated as having DVT until proved otherwise. Diagnosis can be confirmed with Doppler ultrasound on the leg veins. Intravenous venography may be necessary in some cases, but is associated with risk of embolism. Ultrasonography has an average sensitivity and specificity of 97% for proximal DVT. If there is high probability of a DVT but a negative leg Doppler ultrasound, anticoagulation treatment should continue and Doppler studies should be repeated in 1 week.

Diagnosis of pulmonary embolism

Clinically, the 'classic' presentation of PE is an abrupt onset of pleuritic chest pain, shortness of breath and hypoxia.

Table 9.2 Risks of venous thromboembolism following general and gynaecological surgery in the absence of thromboprophylaxis

Type of venous thromboembolism	Risk (%)
Asymptomatic DVT	25
Asymptomatic proximal DVT	7
Symptomatic DVT	6
Symptomatic non-fatal PE	1–2
Fatal PE	0.5

Source: Scottish Intercollegiate Guidelines Network 2002 Prophylaxis of Venous Thromboembolism. SIGN, Edinburgh.
DVT, deep vein thrombosis; PE, pulmonary embolism.

Other less frequent symptoms include haemoptysis and dyspnoea. However, many patients with PE are either completely asymptomatic or have vague and non-specific symptoms such as back pain, shoulder pain, upper abdominal pain, syncope, painful respiration, high fever, productive cough, hiccoughs and wheezing. Therefore, a high level of suspicion should be practised in any postoperative patient presenting with any chest symptoms, especially if no other cause has been found for these symptoms. The main physical signs in patients with PE include tachypnoea, tachycardia, low-grade fever, rales and accentuated second heart sound. Each hospital should develop its protocol for the diagnosis of PE.

Screening for pulmonary embolism

The partial pressue of oxygen (PO_2) in arterial blood should be tested, although this test has little predictive value in patients clinically suspected to have PE. Another screening test is measuring the D-dimer, although it is likely to be raised in the postoperative period. A negative D-dimer in patients with mild-to-moderate clinical suspicion rules out venous thromboembolism. If the result is positive and/or if there is a high probability of PE, diagnostic imaging should be carried out. Other screening tests include ECG and a chest X-ray. The most common ECG findings in PE are tachycardia and non-specific ST–T wave abnormalities. Other findings include S1Q3T3, peaked P waves (p pulmonal), right axis deviation, right bundle-branch block or atrial fibrillation. ECG abnormalities are only present in approximately 20% of cases of PE. ECG is therefore a good positive test in PE (i.e. a positive ECG may be suggestive of PE, but a negative result does not exclude it). Chest X-ray should be performed to exclude other causes for chest symptoms (e.g. pneumothorax, pneumonia). Findings will usually be normal at presentation, although they may rarely show the Westermark sign (i.e. dilatation of the pulmonary vessels proximal to an embolism along with collapse of distal vessels). Over time, chest X-ray may show atelectasis or focal infiltrates, with a picture very similar to infectious pneumonia.

Definitive diagnosis of pulmonary embolism

Definitive diagnosis is by contrast pulmonary angiography. However, due to the invasive nature of this technique, other imaging modalities are more commonly used. Spiral CT scan has recently been shown to be comparable in accuracy to pulmonary angiography, and is now accepted as the preferred primary diagnostic tool. If this is not available, ventilation/perfusion scan (V/Q scan) can be used instead. If V/Q scan shows low probability, bilateral leg Doppler ultrasound studies should be performed. If both are negative with low clinical suspicion, PE can be ruled out. If, however, there is continuing clinical suspicion despite negative V/Q scan and leg Doppler studies, further imaging should be considered such as spiral CT scan, magnetic resonance imaging or angiography.

Treatment of venous thromboembolism

Confirmed or clinically suspected venous thromboembolism awaiting diagnostic confirmation requires immediate treatment with either low-molecular-weight heparin (LMWH) or unfractionated heparin (UFH). If the diagnosis is confirmed by spiral CT, treatment should continue. If a V/Q scan suggests a high or medium probability of PE, therapeutic anticoagulation should be continued. If the V/Q scan suggests a low probability of PE and ultrasound studies of the legs are positive, therapeutic anticoagulation should be continued. Where the V/Q scan suggests a low probability of PE and ultrasound studies of the legs are negative, anticoagulation can be discontinued if clinical suspicion is low.

LMWHs are the preferred initial treatment of choice. They are more effective than UFH with lower mortality and fewer haemorrhagic complications in the initial treatment of DVT, and are as effective as UFH in the initial management of PE. Systematic reviews have confirmed LMWH as a safe alternative to UFH with the advantage of a fixed-dose regimen reducing the need for monitoring. Long-term use of LMWH is associated with a lower risk of heparin-induced thrombocytopenia, osteoporosis and bone fractures than UFH. However, intravenous UFH remains the preferred treatment in massive PE because of its rapid effect and extensive experience of its use.

LMWH should be commenced and converted to oral anticoagulants once the patient is in the stable postoperative period and the risk of bleeding has reduced. The LMWH should be continued until an international normalized ratio of 2.0–3.0 is achieved. The haematology and anticoagulation clinic should be informed to continue the treatment on discharge and to perform other investigations as necessary.

Life-threatening massive PE requires an immediate multidisciplinary approach involving a senior anaesthetist, haematologist, physician, gynaecologist and intensivist. Cardiopulmonary resuscitation, thrombolytic therapy, percutaneous catheter thrombus fragmentation or surgical embolectomy may be needed in some cases.

Urinary tract injuries

Bladder

Bladder injury is the most common visceral injury in gynaecological surgery. The risk is increased in women with previous surgery, particularly caesarean section and anterior wall myomectomy, where the bladder becomes firmly adherent to the cervix and upper vagina. The damage usually occurs during dissection of the bladder from the cervix, even when applying gentle and blunt methods. The dome of the bladder is the usual site of injury. Intraoperative recognition of the injury is crucial in order to avoid long-term consequences such as fistula formation, which can be difficult to treat. Primary injuries are usually recognized at the time of surgery, although they can easily be missed. In women at high risk of bladder damage, it is usually good practice to exercise a high level of suspicion. Careful inspection of the bladder will usually reveal the injury. If still in doubt, a methylene blue test could be used to check for any bladder tears. A Foley catheter is inserted in the bladder (transurethrally) and methylene blue dye in saline solution is injected through the catheter to fill the bladder. The bladder is then observed as it distends for any leakage of the dye. If a defect is detected, it should be repaired in two layers with absorbable suture material. This can usually be performed by the gynaecologist. In cases of extensive bladder damage or lacerations, an urologist should be involved with this repair. Following surgery, the bladder should be drained continuously for 10–14 days. It will also be advisable to arrange a cystogram before removal of the catheter to ensure complete healing. An unrepaired bladder injury will result in vesicovaginal fistula, which usually presents in the first postoperative week. Fistulae presenting later may be the end result of a pelvic haematoma or vascular necrosis of the bladder wall.

Ureter

Ureteric damage is less common than bladder injury during gynaecological surgery, with an incidence that varies between 0.5% and 2.5% depending on the underlying pathology. The risk is particularly increased in patients with extensive endometriosis and/or adhesions, which could distort the course of the ureter. The incidence of ureteric damage is also increased in women who received pelvic radiotherapy prior to their surgery. The irradiated tissue is more difficult to dissect and takes longer to heal. The ureteric damage can either occur as a result of direct trauma to the ureter with sharp instruments at the time of surgery, or indirect damage due to delayed avascular necrosis resulting from excessive dissection of the ureter with damage of its blood supply. Delayed ureteric necrosis and damage could also result from thermal injury during the use of electrosurgery. Another form of ureteric damage results from ureteric obstruction due to involvement of the ureter in a suture. Intraoperative recognition of direct ureteric injury can be difficult and requires a significant amount of experience. It is always good practice to suspect ureteric injury in high-risk patients. Careful inspection of the ureter from the pelvic brim downwards will help to detect direct injuries. Common sites of damage are at the angle of the vagina and near the pelvic brim. If in doubt, a ureteric stent should be inserted by the urologist. Repair of ureteric damage should only be undertaken by a urologist. Injury near the brim of the pelvis is managed by end-to-side anastomosis or, more commonly, by end-to-end anastomosis to the opposite ureter. Damage near to the bladder is better repaired with ureteric reimplantation into the bladder using either a psoas hitch or bladder flap. Unrecognized ureteric injury will result in extravasation of urine, which collects in the pelvis causing pelvic discomfort and pyrexia. Urine may also leak from an abdominal or vaginal incision. Ureteric obstruction may cause loin pain and pyrexia in the postoperative period. It may also go completely unrecognized, and be discovered many years later as an incidental finding. Percutaneous nephrostomy may be required if hydronephrosis develops. Cystoscopy and retrograde insertion of ureteric stents is an alternative but often less satisfactory approach.

If a fistula is suspected in the immediate postoperative phase, a urinary catheter should be inserted immediately to assess urine output. A three-swab test will help to identify vesicovaginal fistula, but urine leakage around the catheter may be misleading. Other tests that may help to establish the diagnosis include ingestion of indigo carmine with later vaginal inspection to determine whether a fistula is present. Intravenous urography will help in locating the site of damage, but small fistulae may be difficult to see.

Spontaneous healing of a damaged bladder is dependent upon the extent of the urinary leakage. A small leakage usually heals in approximately 7–10 days and can therefore be managed conservatively. If this fails or if the leakage is more significant, surgical repair of the defect should be undertaken by a urologist.

Bowel complications

Bowel obstruction

Mechanical bowel obstruction caused by adhesions or twisting of a loop of bowel is rare in gynaecological surgery. It usually occurs approximately 1 week after surgery and presents with persistent vomiting and abdominal pain with absence of passage of flatus or faeces. Signs include abdominal distension and tenderness with tinkling bowel sounds. An abdominal X-ray would show dilated loops of bowel. It usually settles within 48–72 h with nasogastric aspiration plus IV fluids. If there is no improvement, contrast imaging should be performed to identify the site of obstruction for surgical correction. The presence of clinical evidence of peritonitis requires immediate surgery.

Paralytic ileus

Abdominal gynaecological surgery is usually followed by a physiological ileus due to manipulation of the bowel. The small bowel typically regains function within hours. The stomach regains activity in 1–2 days and the colon regains activity in 3–5 days (Cameron 2001). Postoperative adynamic ileus or paralytic ileus is defined as gut ileus persisting beyond 3 days following surgery (Livingston and Passaro 1990). Paralytic ileus is uncommon following benign gynaecological procedures as they are not usually associated with significant insult to the bowel.

Paralytic ileus manifests with abdominal distension, nausea and vomiting with delayed passage of flatus or faeces. A distinguishing feature is absent or hypoactive bowel sounds, unlike the high-pitched sound of mechanical obstruction. The abdomen of ileus reveals no discernible peristalsis or succession splash. An abdominal X-ray will reveal dilated loops of bowel.

The majority of patients will improve with conservative management by resting of the bowel, IV fluids and nasogastric tube drainage. Electrolyte imbalance, especially hypocalcaemia, should be corrected. Unresolved cases should be investigated for potentiating factors such as intraperitoneal abscess or retroperitoneal haematoma, which should be drained under radiological control (Gerzof et al 1981).

Bowel injury

Fortunately, inadvertent bowel injury is uncommon during benign gynaecological surgery with an incidence of 0.3–0.8%, with the majority (70%) being minor lacerations (Dicker et al 1982). The small bowel is the site of injury in approximately 75% of cases. Abdominal rather than vaginal or laparoscopic surgery is associated with a higher rate of damage. The incidence of bowel damage during laparoscopic surgery is 0.5% (Garry and Phillips 1995). The site, extent and timing of presentation of bowel injury will determine the presentation, management and outcome. Postoperative large bowel leak is a serious and life-threatening complication. Risk factors for bowel injury include adhesions, endometriosis, sepsis, obesity, and previous pelvic or abdominal radiotherapy.

Intraoperative detection of bowel injury

There are three main types of bowel injury: direct trauma with sharp instruments, thermal injury with electrosurgery, and devascularization with subsequent necrosis due to extensive dissection. The former injury results in intraoperative perforation or laceration. This is not always easy to recognize and requires a significant amount of experience. The damage may be detected if it occurs on a visible bowel surface or when there is an obvious leak of bowel contents (e.g. faeces). However, in a significant proportion of patients, neither of these is obvious and the damage can easily be missed. Small bowel contents are not usually easy to notice, which leads to 60% of small bowel injuries being missed (Hill 1994). To minimize the possibility of missing bowel damage, it is important to have a high level of suspicion, especially in difficult or high-risk cases. Consideration should be given to asking a colorectal surgeon to explore the bowel for suspected damage. In patients suspected to have bowel injury during extensive laparoscopic surgery in the cul-de-sac, a 30 cc Foley catheter could be inserted into the rectum. With clamping the bowel above the site of dissection, the pelvis is filled with physiological solution and air injected through the Foley catheter by a 100 cc syringe. The appearance of bubbles in the solution will indicate perforation. Alternatively, a 50% betadine solution could be injected and the bowel observed for trailers of betadine leakage.

Delayed presentation of bowel injury

Indirect bowel injuries cannot be appreciated during surgery and usually present several days later. It is therefore important that patients at high risk should be watched carefully in the first few postoperative days for signs of bowel injury. Patients undergoing day-case surgery present a major concern as they may develop bowel injury at home, which could potentially be fatal if not diagnosed early. It is therefore important to warn all day-case patients about early signs of bowel damage, and advise them to return to the hospital immediately rather than seeking help from their family doctors.

In women who sustain a direct trauma to the bowel that was missed during surgery, symptoms of bowel leak will present 48–72 h later. On the other hand, thermal bowel damage or delayed necrosis due to devascularization may not manifest itself until 6–8 days after surgery.

Minor laceration or Veress needle puncture

Most of these injuries heal without any consequences except if there is an obstruction distal to the injury. This may result in leak from the bowel a few days after surgery.

Large bowel leak

Large bowel leak is a serious and life-threatening complication, especially if there is delay in the diagnosis. The early symptoms of abdominal pain and distension associated with nausea and vomiting could be mistaken for postoperative symptoms. The diagnosis may not be apparent until septic shock and collapse supervene. Large bowel leak usually presents with generalized peritonitis, giving widespread peritonism and guarding with absent bowel sounds and marked deterioration of the patient's general well-being. In some cases, leaking may be localized with abscess formation, giving rise to swinging temperature which does not respond to antibiotics, vomiting and abdominal distension. Abdominal X-ray reveals gas under the diaphragm or distended loops of small bowel, although plain films are not usually helpful. It is important to ask a colorectal surgeon to review the patient at an early stage if bowel injury is suspected. An early resort to laparotomy and exploration may be crucial to achieve a good outcome.

Small bowel leak

The early symptoms of small bowel leak are less pronounced than those of the large bowel. Abdominal pain and distension associated with vomiting are the main early features. Initially, bowel sounds may still be present with passage of flatus and stool per rectum. With time, symptoms will worsen with localized signs of tenderness and development of a pelvic mass.

Faecal fistula

Rarely, a rectovaginal faecal fistula may develop following a difficult hysterectomy in patients with severe endometriosis with obliteration of the pouch of Douglas. If the large bowel leak is close to the vault, it can discharge through the vault resulting in a fistula. This is usually easily diagnosed with a speculum on vaginal examination, although a small fistula may be difficult to see.

Management of bowel injury

If the damage is recognized during surgery, a bowel surgeon should be summoned to theatre to manage the damage. Depending on the site and extent of the damage, the treatment will either be oversewing the injury, local resection and reanastomosis, or resection with a temporary defunctioning colostomy.

In patients with delayed presentation of bowel injury, laparotomy through a midline incision should be undertaken. If the leak is from the large bowel, diversion proximal to the leak may be required. A small bowel leak may be treated with resection and reanastomosis. Most of these patients are usually generally unwell and should receive postoperative care in an intensive care unit.

A rectovaginal fistula can be treated with resection of the affected bowel segment with closure of the rectal stump and colostomy (Hartmann's procedure). A small rectovaginal fistula can be managed conservatively with a defunctioning colostomy.

Pulmonary complications

Postoperative pulmonary complications after abdominal surgery include chest infection, atelectasis, pulmonary oedema and pulmonary embolism. Atelectasis is the most common pulmonary complication, and has been estimated to occur in 20% of patients having upper abdominal surgery and 10% of patients having lower abdominal surgery (Bartlett 1980).

Risk factors for postoperative pulmonary complications include smoking, old age, obesity, upper respiratory tract infection, positive cough test (recurrent coughing after deep inspiration and initial cough), perioperative nasogastric tube and long duration of anaesthesia (McAlister et al 2005, Pappachen et al 2006). Arterial blood gas analysis will determine the severity of the problem. Initial treatment is a higher concentration of oxygen supplied via an oxygen mask. Consideration of assisted ventilation should be made in patients unable to maintain saturation >90% or with PO_2 <8.0 kPa with referral to a critical care specialist.

Cardiovascular complications

Any patient receiving a general anaesthetic is at increased risk of developing myocardial ischaemia, especially if there is underlying heart disease. Obtaining a good medical history of cardiac disease is very important in predicting cardiac complications. Elective surgery should be delayed in patients with a history of myocardial infarction within the preceding 6 months (Doshani and Shafi 2003).

Cardiac complications include arrhythmias or myocardial infarction, which can present in the immediate postoperative period. Prolonged arrhythmias may lead to hypotension and exacerbate the effects of hypovolaemia secondary to surgery, resulting in further deterioration of tissue perfusion. Cardiac function may be further compromised by acidosis, hypoxaemia and fluid overload as a consequence of excessive fluid replacement to correct hypovolaemia.

Patients experiencing chest pain after surgery should be investigated for a cardiac cause. It is important to remember that chest pain may be masked by strong postoperative analgesia. Other important signs to raise the possibility of cardiac complications include unexplained tachycardia and hypotension, the presence of a new murmur or evidence of pulmonary oedema. These findings may indicate myocardial infarction and should be investigated with serial cardiac enzymes and ECG. Patients presenting with arrhythmias should be investigated for an underlying cause such as sepsis, hypovolaemia, pyrexia, electrolyte imbalance or drug toxicity. Referral to a cardiologist should be arranged when a cardiac problem is suspected. Thrombolytic therapy is contraindicated within 5 days of surgery.

KEY POINTS

1. Careful preoperative assessment and medical optimization prior to surgery improve postoperative care.

2. Appropriate choice of operation performed by those appropriately trained is the most important factor in minimizing postoperative complications.

3. Whilst most gynaecological procedures do not induce major fluid and electrolyte problems, gynaecologists need to be aware that certain circumstances could lead to electrolyte imbalance such as ileus and persistent vomiting.

4. Be alert to potential hyponatraemia if there are significant deficits of fluid following hysteroscopic procedures.

5. Effective postoperative analgesia using patient-based methods allows early mobilization and reduces respiratory complications.

6. Atelectasis and urinary tract infection are the most common causes of postoperative pyrexia.

7. Pelvic haematomas are common after hysterectomy and may be the cause of postoperative pyrexia or unexpected anaemia.

8. There is a significant risk of DVT after major gynaecological procedures, and each patient must be given appropriate prophylaxis relevant to risk status.

9. The majority of DVTs which precede PE are not recognized clinically, so be vigilant to detect potential DVTs.

10. If postoperative complications occur, it is the responsibility of the operating gynaecologist to liaise with the appropriate specialty and ensure that the patient is investigated and treated promptly.

11. Gynaecology patients are most often young and fit before surgery, and thus may not reveal signs of internal haemorrhage until the late stages and then quickly decompensate.

12. Early recognition of bowel and urinary tract damage reduces the risk of serious morbidity.

13. Damage to bowel and urinary tract should only be repaired by experienced practitioners.

14. Local audit will identify areas of concern in surgical technique and infection control.

References

Addison WA, Livengood CH, Hill GB, Sutton GP, Fortier KJ 1984 Necrotizing fasciitis of vulvar origin in diabetic patients. Obstetrics and Gynecology 63: 473–479.

Bacha OM, Plante M, Kirschnick LS, Edelweiss MI 2009 Evaluation of morbidity of suction drains after retroperitoneal lymphadenectomy in gynecological tumors: a systematic literature review. International Journal of Gynecological Cancer 19: 202–207.

Bartlett RH 1980 Pulmonary pathophysiology in surgical patients. Surgical Clinics of North America 60: 1132.

Boesch CE, Umek W 2009 Effects of wound closure on wound healing in gynecologic surgery: a systematic literature review. Journal of Reproductive Medicine 54: 139–144.

Brieger GH 1983 Early ambulation. A study in the history of surgery. Annals of Surgery 197: 443–449.

Brooks-Brunn JA 1995 Postoperative atelectasis and pneumonia: risk factors. American Journal of Critical Care 4: 340–349.

Brown EM, Depares J, Robertson AA et al 1988 Amoxycillin-clavulanic acid (Augmentin) versus metronidazole as prophylaxis in hysterectomy: a prospective, randomised clinical trial. BJOG: an International Journal of Obstetrics and Gynaecology 95: 286–293.

Cameron JL (ed) 2001 Current Surgical Therapy, 7th edn. Mosby, Chicago.

Charlton JE 1997 The management of postoperative pain. Update in Anesthesia 7: 2–17.

Charoenkwan K, Phillipson G, Vutyavanich T 2007 Early versus delayed (traditional) oral fluids and food for reducing complications after major abdominal gynaecologic surgery. Cochrane Database of Systematic Reviews 4: CD004508.

Dicker RC, Greenspan JR, Strauss LT et al 1982 Complications of abdominal and vaginal hysterectomy among women of reproductive age in the United States. The Collaborative Review of Sterilisation. American Journal of Obstetrics and Gynecology 144: 841–848.

Doshani A, Shafi M 2003 Pre- and post-operative care in gynaecology. Current Obstetrics and Gynaecology 13: 151–158.

Franchi M, Trimbos JB, Zanaboni F et al 2007 Randomised trial of drains versus no drains following radical hysterectomy and pelvic lymph node dissection: a European Organisation for Research and Treatment of Cancer–Gynaecological Cancer Group (EORTC-GCG) study in 234 patients. European Journal of Cancer 43: 1265–1268.

Garry R, Phillips R 1995 How safe is the laparoscopic approach to hysterectomy. Gynaecological Endoscopy 105: 77–80.

Gerzof SG, Robbins AH, Johnson WC 1981 Percutaneous catheter drainage of abdominal abscesses. New England Journal of Medicine 305: 193–197.

Hill DJ 1994 Complications of the laparoscopic approach. Baillières Clinical Obstetrics and Gynaecology 8: 865–879.

Karanikolas M, Swarm RA 2000 Current trends in perioperative pain management. Anesthesiology Clinics of North America 18: 575–599.

Livingston EH, Passaro EP Jr 1990 Postoperative ileus. Digestive Diseases and Science 35: 121–132.

McAlister FA, Bertsch K, Man J, Bradley J, Jacka M 2005 Incidence and risk factors for pulmonary complications after nonthoracic surgery. American Journal of Respiratory and Critical Care Medicine 171: 514–517.

Mittendorf R, Aronson MP, Berry RE et al 1993 Avoiding serious infections associated with abdominal hysterectomy: a meta-analysis of antibiotic prophylaxis. American Journal of Obstetrics and Gynecology 169: 1119–1124.

Nagaratnam M, Sutton H, Stephens R 2007 Prescribing analgesia for the surgical patient. British Journal of Hospital Medicine 68: M7, M10.

Nielsen KG, Holte K, Kehlet H 2003 Effects of posture on postoperative pulmonary function. Acta Anaesthesiologica Scandinavica 47: 1270–1275.

Panici PB, Zullo MA, Casalino B, Angioli R, Muzii L 2003 Subcutaneous drainage versus no drainage after minilaparotomy in gynecologic benign conditions: a randomized study. American Journal of Obstetrics and Gynecology 188: 71–75.

Pappachen S, Smith PR, Shah S, Brito V, Bader F, Khoury B 2006 Postoperative pulmonary complications after gynecologic surgery. International Journal of Gynecology and Obstetrics 93: 74–76.

Perel P, Roberts I 2007 Colloids versus crystalloids for fluid resuscitation in critically ill patients. Cochrane Database of Systematic Reviews 17: CD000567.

Schiøtz HA, Tanbo TG 2006 Postoperative voiding, bacteriuria and urinary tract infection with Foley catheterization after gynecological surgery. Acta Obstetricia et Gynecologica 85: 476–481.

Scottish Intercollegiate Guidelines Network 2002 Prophylaxis of Venous Thromboembolism. SIGN, Edinburgh.

Smith RN, Cardozo L 1997 Early voiding difficulty after colposuspension. British Journal of Urology 80: 911–914.

Sobolev VE, Dudanov IP, Alontseva NN, Bogdanova VS 2005 [The role of laparoscopy in the diagnosis and treatment of early postoperative complications]. Vestn Khir Im I I Grek 164: 95–99.

Tamussino K 2002 Postoperative infection. Clinical Obstetrics and Gynecology 45: 562–573.

Walsh C, Scaife C, Hopf H 2009 Prevention and management of surgical site infections in morbidly obese women. Obstetrics and Gynecology 113: 411–415.

Wheeler AP, Bernard GR 1999 Treating patients with severe sepsis. New England Journal of Medicine 340: 207–214.

CHAPTER 10

Hormones: their action and measurement in gynaecological practice

Scott McGill Nelson and Jurgis Gedis Grudzinskas

Chapter Contents			
INTRODUCTION	128	CLINICAL ASSAYS	138
HORMONES: TYPES AND ACTION	128	MEASUREMENT AND ACTION OF INDIVIDUAL HORMONES	139
REGULATION OF HORMONE SECRETION AND ACTION	129		
HORMONE RECEPTORS	131	KEY POINTS	142

Introduction

The term 'hormone', derived from the Greek word *hormaein* meaning to arouse or excite, was first used in 1905 by Sir Ernest Starling in his Croonian Lecture to the Royal College of Physicians. It is this ability to excite and modulate the behaviour of cells that is the fundamental defining characteristic of hormones.

Hormones are one of the important means by which cells communicate with each other. They ensure that the body's physiological systems are coordinated appropriately, and if this is impaired, as occurs with hormone deficiency or excess, function is compromised. Classically, hormones are synthesized by specialized cells, which may exist as distinct endocrine glands or be located as single cells within other organs, and secreted into the blood stream and transported through the circulation to a distant site of action (endocrine effect). However, autocrine or paracrine actions may also be prevalent and indeed modulate the function of the original endocrine cell type (Figure 10.1).

Hormones: Types and Action

There are three major groups of hormones according to biochemical structure and method of synthesis:

- peptides and proteins;
- amino acid derivatives; and
- steroids.

Peptide hormones

The majority of hormones are peptides and range in size from very small (thyrotrophin-releasing hormone has just three amino acids) to small [thyroid-stimulating hormone (TSH) has over 200 amino acids]. Some peptide hormones are secreted directly, but most are stored in granules, the release of which becomes a major control mechanism regulated potentially by another hormone as part of a cascade or by innervation.

Some peptide hormones have complex tertiary structures; for example, glycoproteins are composed of more than one peptide chain. Oxytocin and arginine vasopressin, two of the posterior pituitary hormones, have ring structures linked by disulphide bridges. Despite being remarkably similar in structure, they have very different physiological roles. The gonadotrophins, follicle-stimulating hormone (FSH) and luteinizing hormone (LH), TSH and human chorionic gonadotrophin (hCG) also have two chains (Figure 10.2). However, these α- and β-subunits are synthesized quite separately from separate genes. The α-subunit of each is shared; it is the distinctive β-subunit of each that confers biological specificity.

Amino acid derivatives

These hormones are small water-soluble compounds. Melatonin is derived from tryptophan, whereas the tyrosine derivatives include the thyroid hormones, the catecholamines, and dopamine from the hypothalamic–anterior pituitary unit and the central nervous system. The catecholamines of the adrenal medulla, ephedrine and norepinephrine, are identical to the sympathetic neurotransmitters and, like peptide hormones, they are stored in secretory granules prior to release.

Steroids

Steroid hormones are lipid-soluble molecules derived from modification of the four-carbon ring structure of cholesterol (Figure 10.3). Steroids can be classified according to the

DOI: 10.1016/B978-0-7020-3120-5.00010-2

number of carbon atoms they possess: C-21 (progestogens, cortisol, aldosterone), C-19 (androgens) and C-18 (oestrogens). The common names used for steroids also adhere to a loose convention. The suffix -ol indicates an important hydroxyl group, as in cholesterol or cortisol, whereas the suffix -one indicates an important ketone (e.g. testosterone). The extra presence of -di, as in diol (e.g. oestradiol) or dione (e.g. androstenedione), reflects two of these groups, respectively; -ene (androstenedione) within the name indicates a significant double bond in the steroid nucleus.

Regulation of Hormone Secretion and Action

Regulation and control of hormones is essential, and underpins not only the function of many endocrine systems but also their clinical investigation (Figure 10.4). Hormones utilize a variety of differential regulatory mechanisms.

Simple control

An elementary control system is one in which the signal itself is limited, either in magnitude or duration, so as to induce only a transient response. Refinement allows discrimination of a positive signal from background 'noise' to ensure that the target cell cannot or does not respond below a certain threshold level. An example of this is the pulsatile release of gonadotrophin-releasing hormone (GnRH) from the hypothalamus. Similarly, although uterine epithelial cells have receptors for oestrogen, androgen, glucocorticoid and progestogen, there is no progestational response because progesterone is not produced in the first half of the menstrual cycle.

Negative feedback

Negative feedback is the most common type of regulation used by biological systems. The hormone acts on the target cell to stimulate a response that inhibits the first hormone. An extension of this scenario exists for many of the hypothalamic–pituitary–end organ axes; for example, corticotrophin-releasing hormone from the hypothalamus stimulates the release of anterior pituitary adrenocorticotrophic hormone (ACTH) to increase peripheral cortisol production, which feeds back to the anterior pituitary and hypothalamus to reduce the original secretions.

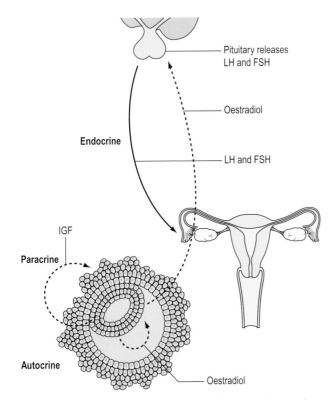

Figure 10.1 Example of endocrine, paracrine and autocrine hormonal communication. LH, luteinizing hormone; FSH, follicle-stimulating hormone; IGF, insulin-like growth factor.

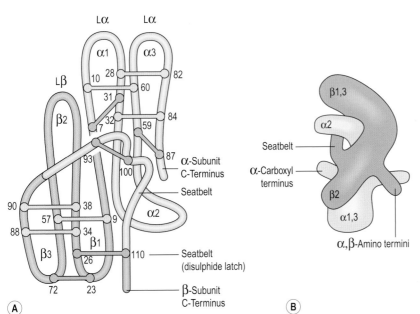

Figure 10.2 (A) Assembly of α and β subunits to form human chorionic gonadotrophin (hCG) dimer. Thick blue line, hCGα polypeptide chains; thick purple line, hCGβ polypeptide chains; numbers, amino acid numbers; Lα, loops of hCGα; Lβ, loops of hCGβ; pink bars, cystine knots on α and β subunits; thick green line of hCGβ, seatbelt region; thick green lines, seatbelt disulphide bonds; thin green line, small loop disulphide bond of β-seatbelt; blue lines, other disulphide bonds. (B) Spatial representation of α:β assembly in which the hCGα carboxyl terminal extension penetrates the hCGβ and is locked by the β-seatbelt portion.
(A) From Xing Y, Williams C, Campbell RK, Cook S, Knoppers M, Addona T, Altarocca V, Moyle WR. Threading of a glycosylated protein loop through a protein hole: implications for combination of human chorionic gonadotropin subunits. Protein Sci (2001) 10:226–235, Wiley. (B) From de Medeiros SF, Norman RJ. Human choriogonadotrophin protein core and sugar branches heterogeneity: basic and clinical insights. Hum Reprod Update. 2009 Jan-Feb;15(1):69–95. Epub 2008 Oct 22.

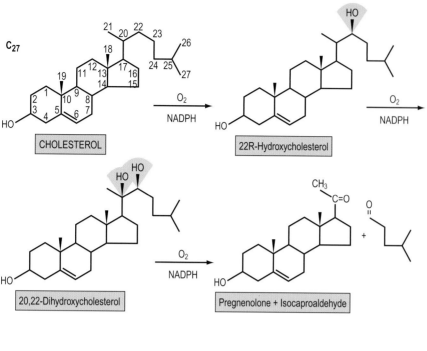

Figure 10.3 Enzymatic reaction catalysed by CYP11A; the first step in steroid hormone synthesis. CYP11A catalyses three sequential oxidation reactions followed by cleavage of the six carbon side chains to form pregnenolone. Each oxidation reaction requires one molecule of oxygen and one molecule of NADPH, and uses the mitochondrial electron transfer system.

Source: Reproduced from Payne and Hales; Overview of Steroidogenic Enzymes in the Pathway from Cholesterol to Active Steroid Hormones, (2004) Endocrine Reviews 25(6):947–970.

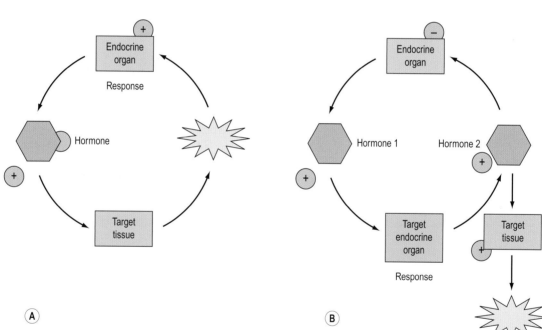

Figure 10.4 Two simplified models of hormone synthesis, action and feedback. (A) The endocrine organ releases a hormone which acts on the target tissue to stimulate (+) or inhibit (−) a response. The response may feedback either to inhibit or stimulate the endocrine organ to decrease or increase the supply of the hormone, respectively. (B) The endocrine organ produces hormone 1, which acts on a second endocrine gland to release hormone 2. In turn, hormone 2 acts dually on the target tissue to induce a response and feeds back negatively on to the original endocrine organ to regulate release of hormone 1. This model is illustrative of the axes between the anterior pituitary and its peripheral endocrine targets.

Positive feedback

Under certain circumstances, hormones feedback to the pituitary to enhance, rather than inhibit, secretion of the primary hormone. For example, the action of oestrogen on the pituitary gland to induce the ovulatory surge of LH and FSH; or during childbirth, stretch receptors in the myometrium send neurological signals to the brain to stimulate oxytocin release. The role of oxytocin in the suckling–milk ejection reflex is similar; a positive feedback loop that is only broken by cessation of the baby's feeding.

Inhibitory control

The secretion of some hormones is under inhibitory as well as stimulatory control. Dopamine prevents the secretion of prolactin, such that if dopamine secretion is diminished, prolactin secretion will increase. This complexity from dual inhibitory and secretory control allows more precise regulation of hormone secretion.

Endocrine rhythms

Many of the body's activities show periodic or cyclical changes and may either be circadian (24-h cycle, e.g. cortisol), ultradian (<24-h cycle, e.g. GnRH) or infradian (>24-h cycle, e.g. menstrual cycle). Control of these rhythms commonly comes from the nervous system, and although some are independent of the environment, others are coordinated and entrained by external cues, such as the 24-h light/dark cycle that becomes temporarily disrupted in jetlag. Cortisol secretion is maximal between 0400 h and 0800 h as we awaken, and minimal as we go to bed. In contrast, growth hormone (GH) and prolactin are secreted maximally 1 h after going to sleep. Clinically, knowledge of endocrine rhythms is important as analyses of hormones must take daily variation into account.

Availability of the hormone to a cell

A hormone can be present in the blood stream but unavailable to the target cell. A hormone circulating in the blood stream, not attached to a binding protein, readily enters cells by simple diffusion. However, most of the steroid hormones circulate bound to protein carriers, such as sex-hormone-binding globulin (SHBG), because their cholesterol origin makes them hydrophobic (King 1988). Consequently, they are generally unavailable, and alterations in the amount of circulating binding globulins can modulate the biological activities of each of their respective hormones. For example, approximately 40% of circulating oestrogen is bound to SHBG, and the remainder is bound to albumin and membrane proteins (Hovarth 1992). As testosterone is largely (80%) bound to SHBG and 19% is loosely bound to albumin, its androgenicity is mainly dependent upon the unbound fraction and partly upon the fraction associated with albumin. SHBG production in the liver is decreased by androgens, hence the binding capacity in men is lower than in normal women. In a hirsute woman, the SHBG level is depressed by the excess androgen, and the percentage of free and therefore active testosterone is elevated (Nestler et al 1991).

Tissue distribution

The tissue distribution of hormone receptors also determines the scope of hormone action, and the presence or absence of a given receptor determines whether a cell will respond to a given class of steroids. For example, the TSH receptor is limited to the thyroid and therefore TSH action is restricted to the thyroid. A hormone can also modify its own and/or another steroid hormone's activity by regulating the concentration of receptors in a cell. This has the biological effect of increasing tissue response to the hormone if the receptor number is increased, and vice versa if the receptor number is decreased. Oestrogen, for example, increases target tissue responsiveness to itself by increasing the concentration of FSH receptors in granulosa cells (Hillier 1994). This process is important in the selection and maintenance of the dominant ovarian follicle in the menstrual cycle. In order to respond to the ovulatory surge and become a 'successful' corpus luteum, the granulosa cells must acquire LH receptors. FSH induces LH receptor development on the granulosa cells of large antral follicles with oestrogen acting as chief coordinator. Progesterone, on the other hand, limits the tissue response to oestrogen by reducing, over time, the concentration of oestrogen receptors, hence its use in the prevention of endometrial hyperplasia and carcinoma (Studd and Wadsworth 2000).

Hormone Receptors

The clinical effects of hormones are mediated through the interaction of a hormone with its receptors. There are two principal superfamilies of hormone receptors. This broad classification is based on their cellular location and their characteristic features (Figure 10.5).

Cell surface receptors

Cell surface receptors are composed of three components, each with structural features, which reflect its location and function (Figure 10.6). The hormone acts as a ligand, with a ligand-binding pocket in the extracellular domain of the receptor being comparatively rich in cysteine residues that form internal disulphide bonds and repeated loops to ensure correct folding. This extracellular domain may also be cleaved for some hormones, and function as a binding protein in the circulation, thus limiting bioavailability (e.g. GH). The α-helical membrane-spanning domain is rich in the hydrophobic and uncharged amino acids, enabling it to be secured with the lipid bilayer. The C-terminal cytoplasmic domain either contains, or links to, separate catalytic systems which initiate the intracellular signals after hormone binding.

Stage 1. Availability of the receptor (up- and downregulation)

The cell's mechanism for sensing the low concentration of circulating trophic hormone is to have an extremely large number of receptors but to require only a very small percentage (as little as 1%) to be occupied by the hormone for its action to be evident (Sairam and Bhargavi 1985). Positive and negative modulation of receptor numbers by hormones is known as up- and downregulation. The mechanism of upregulation is unclear, but prolactin and GnRH, for example, can increase the concentration of their own receptors in the cell membrane (Katt et al 1985).

In downregulation, an excess concentration of a trophic hormone, such as LH or GnRH, results in a loss of receptors on the cell membranes and therefore a decrease in biological response. This process occurs by internalization of the receptors, and is the main biological mechanism by which the activity of polypeptide hormones is limited (Ron-El et al 2000). Thus the formation of the hormone–receptor complex on the cell surface initiates the cellular response, and the internalization of the complex (with eventual degradation of the hormone) terminates the response. It therefore appears that the principal reason for the pulsatile secretion of trophic hormones is to avoid downregulation and to maintain

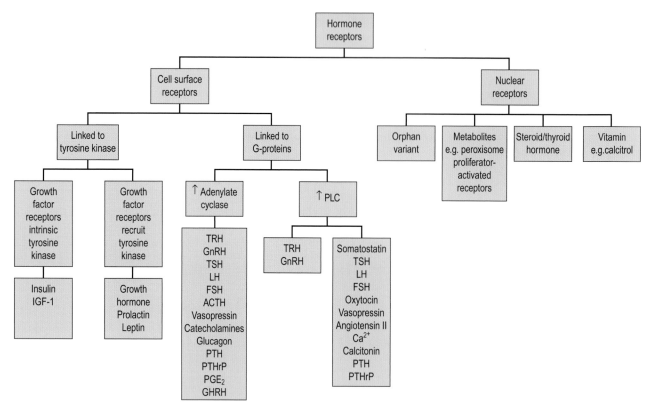

Figure 10.5 The different classes of hormone receptor. Some receptors can link to different G-proteins, which couple to either adenylate cyclase or phospholipase C (PLC). IGF-1, insulin-like growth factor-1; TRH, thyrotropin-releasing hormone; GnRH, gonadotrophin-releasing hormone; TSH, thyroid-stimulating hormone; LH, luteinizing hormone; FSH, follicle-stimulating hormone; ACTH, adrenocorticotrophic hormone; PTH, parathyroid hormone; PTHrP, parathyroid-hormone-related peptide; PGE_2, prostaglandin E_2; GHRH, growth-hormone-releasing hormone.

Adapted from Holt RIG, Hanley NA 2007. Essential Endocrinology and Diabetes, 5th edn. Blackwell Publishing, Massachusetts.

adequate receptor numbers. The pulse frequency, therefore, is a key factor in regulating receptor number.

It is believed that receptors are randomly inserted into the cell membrane after intracellular synthesis. They have two important sites — an external binding site, which is specific for a polypeptide hormone, and an internal site, which plays a role in the process of internalization (Kaplan 1981). When a hormone binds to the receptor and a high concentration of the hormone is present in the circulation, the hormone–receptor complex moves laterally in the cell membrane by a process called 'lateral migration' to a specialized area, the coated pit, the internal margin of which has a brush border (Goldstein et al 1979). Lateral migration, which takes minutes rather than seconds, thus concentrates hormone–receptor complexes in the coated pit, a process referred to as 'clustering' (Figure 10.7). When fully occupied, the coated pit invaginates, 'pinches off' and enters the cell as a vesicle. The coated vesicle is delivered to the lysosomes where it undergoes degradation, releasing the hormone receptors. The receptors may be recycled to the cell membranes and used again, or the receptor and hormone may be metabolized, thus decreasing the hormone's biological activity. This process is called 'receptor-mediated endocytosis' (Goldstein et al 1979; Figure 10.8).

As well as downregulation of polypeptide hormone receptors, the process of internalization can be utilized for other cellular metabolic events, including the transfer of vital substances into the cell, such as iron and vitamins. Hence, cell membrane receptors can be separated into two classes. Class I receptors are distributed in the cell membrane and transmit information to modify cell behaviour for these receptors. Internalization is a method for downregulation and recycling is not usually a feature. Hormones which utilize this category of receptor include FSH, LH, hCG, GnRH, TSH and insulin (Kaplan 1981). Class II receptors are located in the coated pits. Binding leads to internalization, which provides the cell with the required ligands or removes noxious agents from the biological fluid bathing the cell. These receptors are spared from degradation and can be recycled. Examples of this category include low-density lipoproteins, which supply cholesterol to steroid-producing cells (Parinaud et al 1987), and transfer of immunoglobulins across the placenta to provide fetal immunity.

Stage 2. Binding of the hormone to the receptor

Notably hormone–receptor systems demonstrate standard kinetics and are saturable and reversible (Figure 10.9). Consequently, the dissociation rate of the hormone and its receptor is an important component of the biological response, as the biological activity of the hormone is only maintained while the hormone–receptor complex is maintained. Hormones that are structurally similar may have

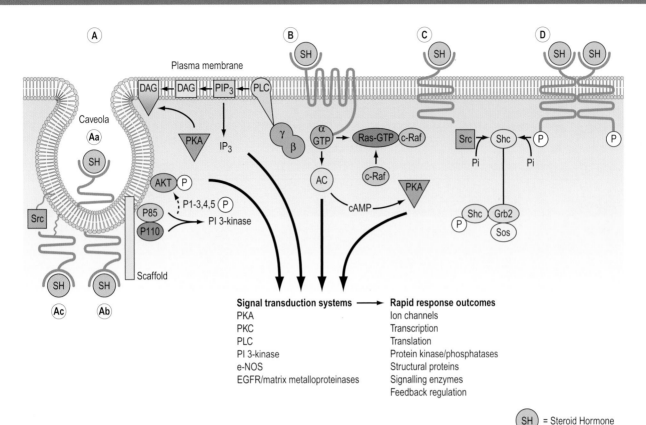

Figure 10.6 (A) Three classes of membrane receptor are shown, illustrating the classic nuclear steroid hormone receptor associated with a caveola. (Aa) The receptor is technically outside the cell and is associated with the outer surface of the plasma membrane in the flask of the caveola. (Ab) The receptor is tethered by a scaffolding protein to the plasma membrane on the inner surface of a caveola. (Ac) The receptor is tethered to the caveolae by a palmitic acid molecule that is esterified to a receptor Ser or Thr with the fatty acid side chain 'inserted' into the membrane (palmitoylation). (B) A G-protein coupled receptor with its ligand-binding domain on the outside of the cell and a seven-membrane-spanning peptide transition followed by an intracellular peptide domain that can bind G and proteins. (C) A single-membrane-spanning receptor with intrinsic kinase activity that might be functional as a monomer. (D) As for C except a homodimer. Caveolae are flask-shaped membrane invaginations present in the outer cell membrane of many cells; they are believed to serve as a 'platform' to accumulate or 'dock' signal-transduction-related molecules. The signal-transduction systems are listed as candidates for mediating rapid responses to steroid. The two ovals with Ras-GTP and c-Raf 'touching' are to suggest that c-Raf was recruited to the complex. AC, adenylyl cyclase; DAG, diacylglycerol; EGFR, epidermal growth factor receptor; e-NOS, endothelial nitric oxide synthase; IP₃, inositol triphosphate; MAP, mitogen-activated protein; PI 3-kinase, phosphatidylinositol 3 kinase; PIP₃, phosphatidylinositol triphosphate; PKA, protein kinase A; PKC, protein kinase C; PLC, phospholipase C. *Reproduced with permission from Norman et al.; Steroid-hormone rapid actions, membrane receptors and a conformational ensemble model, Nature Reviews Drug Discovery 3, 27–41 (January 2004).*

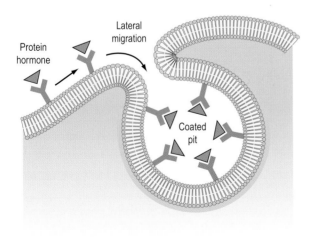

Figure 10.7 Structure of a coated pit, illustrating lateral migration.

some overlap in biological activity. For example, the similarity in structure between GH and prolactin means that GH has a lactogenic action whilst prolactin has some growth-promoting activity and stimulates somatomedin production.

The glycoprotein hormones (LH, FSH, TSH and hCG) share an identical α-chain and require another portion, the β-chain, to confer the specificity inherent in the relationship between hormones and their receptors. The β-subunits differ in both amino acid and carbohydrate content, and the chemical composition may be altered under certain conditions, thereby affecting the affinity of the hormone and its receptor (Willey 1999).

Stage 3. Signal transduction

On binding of a hormone to its cell surface receptor, protein phosphorylation and the generation of 'second messengers' mediates a cascade of cytoplasmic and cellular responses. This multistep cascade facilitates amplification of the cellular response to the hormone binding to a receptor, as many

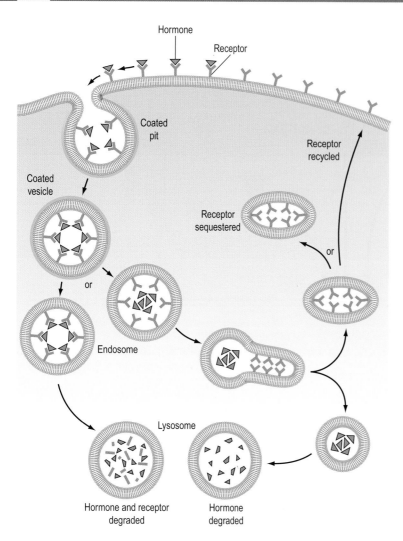

Figure 10.8 Possible routes of receptor and hormone during receptor-mediated endocytosis.

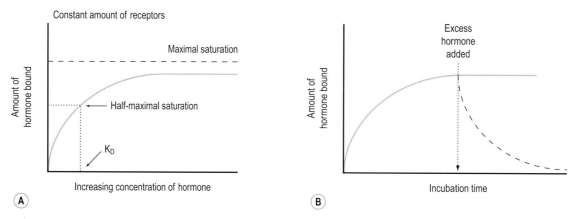

Figure 10.9 Pharmacokinetics of hormone receptors demonstrating that hormone–receptor systems are saturable and reversible. (A) Increasing amounts of hormone are incubated with a constant amount of receptor. The amount of bound hormone increases as more is added until the system becomes saturated. At this point, further addition of hormone fails to increase the amount bound to receptors. The concentration of hormone that is required for half-maximal saturation of the receptors is equal to the dissociation constant (K_D) of the hormone–receptor interaction. (B) Constant amounts of hormone and receptors are incubated together for different times. The amount of hormone bound increases with time until it reaches a plateau, when the bound and free hormone have reached a dynamic equilibrium. By adding further excess hormone, there is competition for the binding sites and the amount of the first hormone bound decreases with time (dashed line).

Adapted from Holt RIG, Hanley NA 2007. Essential Endocrinology and Diabetes, 5th edn. Blackwell Publishing, Massachusetts.

second messenger molecules are produced for each hormone–receptor complex. The cell surface receptors may be classified into two groups according to the second messenger and signalling cascades that are stimulated: (1) tyrosine kinase receptors and (2) G-protein coupled receptors (Figure 10.5).

Tyrosine kinase receptors

Initial phosphorylation of proteins is a key molecular switch, and approximately 10% of proteins are phosphorylated at any given time in a mammalian cell. Phosphorylation occurs when the polar hydroxyl group of serine, threonine or tyrosine has a phosphate group added from an ATP molecule in a reaction catalysed by a 'kinase' enzyme. The phosphorylation induces a conformational change in the three-dimensional shape of the protein, and the phosphorylated protein may also act as a kinase and phosphorylate the next protein in the sequence, creating a phosphorylation cascade.

Phosphorylation of tyrosine kinase receptors can occur through: (i) intrinsic tyrosine kinase activity located in the cytosolic domain of the receptor; or (ii) separate tyrosine kinases recruited after receptor activation. By either mechanism, conformation change induced by phosphorylation creates 'docking' sites for other proteins. Frequently, this occurs via conserved motifs within the target protein known as 'SH2' or 'SH3' domains. These domains may be involved in the activation of downstream kinases, or they may play a more passive role, stabilizing signalling proteins within a phosphorylation cascade.

The subfamily of receptors which recruit tyrosine kinase activity includes those that bind GH, prolactin and leptin, and also includes those for numerous cytokines and erythropoietin. The basic receptor composition, with major homology between family members in the extracellular domain, is the same for the other membrane-spanning receptors (Figure 10.6). Notably, similar mechanisms govern GH and prolactin receptor binding and signal transduction. Two different sites on the hormone are capable of binding receptors. The hormone–receptor interaction of the first leads to the binding of the second to another receptor molecule. It is the close proximity of the two receptor molecules which leads to dimerization of their cytoplasmic regions and signal transduction. With the exception of the receptor for erythropoietin, other cytokine receptors tend to form heterodimers with diverse partner proteins.

Activation of these hormone receptors rapidly recruits members of the Janus family of tyrosine kinases. The four members of the family contain distinctive, tandem kinase domains at their carboxy terminals leading to their name 'Janus-associated kinase' (JAK1–4) after the two-faced Roman deity, Janus. GH and prolactin receptors tend to associate with JAK2 and it is probable that their dimerization brings together two JAK2 molecules that cross-phosphorylate each other. The major downstream substrates of JAK are the STAT family of proteins (hence the term 'JAK-STAT' signalling). The name 'STAT' comes from their dual function: (i) signal transduction, located in the cytoplasm; and (ii) nuclear activation of transcription. Both activities rely on phosphorylation by JAK, facilitated by SH2-mediated docking on to the hormone receptor. Phosphorylated STAT proteins dissociated from the occupied receptor–kinase complex and then themselves dimerize to gain access to the nucleus. There, they activate genes regulating proliferation of the differentiation status of the target cell. One of the major targets is insulin-like growth factor 1. JAK signalling does not focus exclusively on STAT. GH receptor occupancy also stimulates MAPK (mitogen-activated protein kinase) and PI 3-kinase pathways. This overlap may account for some of the rapid metabolic effects of GH.

G-protein coupled receptors

G-protein coupled receptors are the most common subset of cell surface receptors, with more than 140 types. The most striking structural feature of all these receptors lies in the transmembrane domain, which comprises hydrophobic helices which cross the lipid bilayer of the plasma membrane seven times before being coupled to guanine (G)-proteins at the inner surface of the cell membrane. This coupling leads to the generation of intracellular second messengers such as cyclic adenosine monophosphate (cAMP), diacylglycerol (DAG) and inositol triphosphate (IP_3) — the latter two arising from phosphatidylinositol (PI) metabolism.

Signalling of G-protein receptors is mediated by hydrolysis of GTP (guanosine triphosphate) to GDP (guanosine diphosphate) (Figure 10.10). In their resting state, the G-proteins exist in the cell membrane as heterotrimeric complexes with α-, β- and γ-subunits. In practice, the β- and γ-subunits associate with such affinity that the functional units are Gα and Gβ/γ. When the hormone binds to the receptor, this causes a conformational change in receptor structure, which in turn causes a conformational change in the α-subunit allowing it to dissociate from the heterotrimeric complex and bind to a downstream catalytic unit, either adenylate cyclase facilitating the generation of cAMP or phospholipase C (PLC) for the production of DAG/IP_3. The energy to activate these targets comes from the cleavage of phosphate from GTP, thereby regenerating Gα-GDP. This ensures that it is no longer associated with adenylate cyclase or PLC, thereby switching off the cascade and recycling the Gα-GDP back to the start.

Although there are over 20 isoforms of the Gα-subunit, allowing a wide variety of cellular responses, they can be grouped into four major subfamilies. However, more than half of G-protein coupled receptors can interact with different Gα-subunits and thus modulate contrasting, and sometimes conflicting, intracellular second messenger systems. In part, this promiscuity can be attributed to the degree of hormonal stimulation or activation of different receptor subtypes. For instance, at low concentrations, LH receptors associate with $G_s\alpha$ to activate adenylate cyclase, whereas higher concentrations recruit $G_q\alpha$ to activate PLC.

Second messenger pathways: cyclic adenosine monophosphate

Activation of membrane-bound adenylate cyclase catalyses the conversion of ATP to the potent second messenger cAMP. cAMP interacts with protein kinase A (PKA) to unmask its catalytic site, which phosphorylates serine and threonine residues on a transcription factor called 'cAMP response element binding protein' (CREB). CREB then translocates to the nucleus where it binds to a short

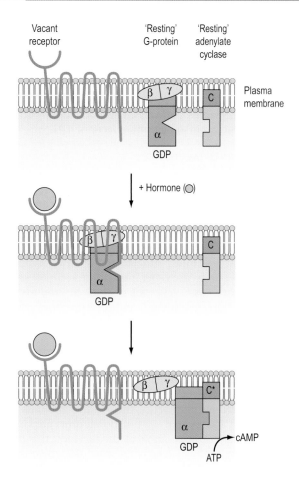

Figure 10.10 G-protein coupled receptors. The extracellular domain is ligand specific and hence less conserved across family members. The transmembrane domain has a characteristic heptahelical structure, most of which is embedded in the cell membrane and provides a hydrophobic core. Conserved cysteine residues can form a disulphide bridge between the second and third extracellular loops. The cytoplasmic domain links the receptor to the signal-transducing G-proteins and, in this example, is linked to membrane-bound adenylate cyclase. The activation of adenylate cyclase is shown c to C*.

Adapted from Holt RIG, Hanley NA 2007. Essential Endocrinology and Diabetes, 5th edn. Blackwell Publishing, Massachusetts.

which catalyses the conversion of PI 4,5-bisphosphate to DAG and IP_3. IP_3 stimulates the transient release of calcium from the endoplasmic reticulum to activate several calcium-sensitive enzymes, including the protein kinase, calmodulin and some isoforms of protein kinase C (PKC). Calcium ions also activate cytosolic guanylate cyclase, an enzyme that catalyses the formation of cyclic guanosine monophosphate.

The major target of DAG signalling is PKC, which activates phospholipase A2 to liberate arachidonate from phospholipids and generate potent eicosanoids, including thromboxanes, leucotrienes, lipoxins and prostaglandins. The latter are well-recognized paracrine and autocrine mediators capable of amplifying or prolonging a response to a hormone stimulus.

Nuclear receptors

The nuclear receptors are classified by their ligands, which are small lipophilic molecules that diffuse across the plasma membrane of target cells. The receptors, encoded by a single gene, typically bind DNA and function as transcription factors (Figure 10.11). Distinct polypeptide-encoding regions can be identified, for which evolutionary conservation can be as high as 60–90%. Many nuclear receptors exist for which no endogenous ligand has been identified, and these are termed 'orphan' nuclear receptors. In addition, some variant receptors have atypical DNA-binding domains and potentially function via indirect interaction with the genome.

The receptor family predominantly resides in the nucleus, although increasingly nuclear import and export appears to be an important regulatory mechanism, as has been long recognized for the glucocorticoid receptor. The receptors have their primary effect by regulating the expression of specific target genes. Consequently, this need for transcription and translation to elicit a biological effect means that cellular responses are relatively slow compared with cell surface receptor signalling. For example, high midcycle levels of oestradiol from the ovary lead to the increase in LH synthesis and secretion by the anterior pituitary that results in ovulation (Hillier 1994).

Target cell conversion of hormones destined for nuclear receptors

A further characteristic of several nuclear hormone receptors includes enzymatic modification of the ligand within the target cell. This converts the circulating hormone into a more, or less, potent metabolite prior to receptor binding. An extreme example of this is the inactivation of cortisol to cortisone by type 2 11β-hydroxysteroid dehydrogenase, which occurs in the placenta, thereby minimizing exposure of the fetus to maternal cortisol.

Hormone specificity of the receptor

This is the most important factor which determines specificity of action and occurs at two levels (King 1988). The presence or absence of a given receptor determines whether or not a cell will respond to a given class of steroids, whilst hormone specificity controls which particular compound is active. For example, the oestrogen receptor, which has the greatest specificity, binds oestradiol 10 times more efficiently

palindromic sequence in the promoter regions of cAMP-regulated genes. This signalling pathway regulates major metabolic pathways, including those for lipolysis, glycogenolysis and steroidogenesis.

The cAMP response is terminated by a large family of phosphodiesterases (PDEs), which can be activated by a variety of systems including phosphorylation of PKA in a negative feedback loop. PDEs rapidly hydrolyse cAMP to the inactive 5'AMP. In addition, activated PKA can phosphorylate serine and threonine residues of the G-protein coupled receptor to cause receptor desensitization.

Second messenger pathways: diacylglycerol and Ca^{2+}

Signalling by some hormones including GnRH and oxytocin is through recruitment of G-protein complexes containing the $G_q\alpha$-subunit. This activates membrane-associated PLC,

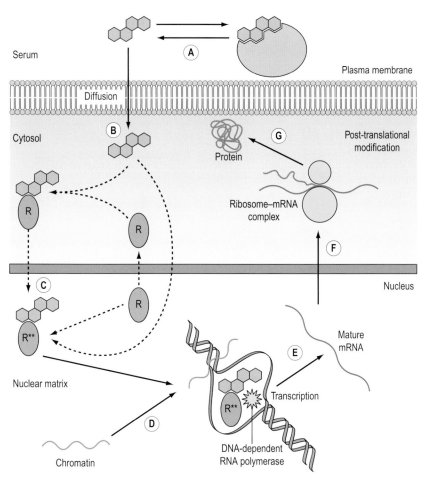

Figure 10.11 Steroid hormone action. Free steroid in equilibrium with that bound to protein (A) diffuses across the target cell membrane (B). Binding to its receptor may occur in the cytoplasm or in the cell nucleus. The activated hormone–receptor complex now present in the nucleus (C) binds to the hormone response element (HRE) of its largest target genes (D). This interaction promotes DNA-dependent RNA polymerase to start transcription (E) of mRNA. Post-transcriptional modification and splicing sees the mRNA exit the nucleus (F) for translation into protein on ribosomes. Post-translational modification provides the final protein (G).
Adapted from Holt RIG, Hanley NA 2007. Essential Endocrinology and Diabetes, 5th edn. Blackwell Publishing, Massachusetts.

than oestrone and about 1000 times more efficiently than the androgen, testosterone, whilst progesterone and cortisol are not recognized at all (Garcia and Rochefort 1977). This recognition specificity is a reflection of the different affinities that the receptor has for the different hormone structures. In biological terms, this means that oestradiol is more active than oestrone, whilst testosterone can have oestrogenic effects but only at pharmacological concentrations.

It is notable that the oestrogen receptor is not a single entity and that it is not restricted to the reproductive system. There are two receptors that can bind to oestrogen, the oestrogen receptor alpha (ERα) and the oestrogen receptor beta (ERβ). These receptors are functionally distinct, having different tissue distributions and different ligand activation, and as such play different roles in gene activation. Both ERα and ERβ interact with the same oestrogen ligand, oestradiol-17β, but they behave differently, sometimes even causing opposing effects. For example, ligand-bound ERα was found to activate transcription, while ligand-bound ERβ inhibited transcription from the AP1 site. They can respond to synthetic ligands in different ways as well; for instance, THC acts as an ERα agonist and as an ERβ antagonist. ERβ can act as a dominant inhibitor of ERα transcriptional activity in cells that express both receptors. Notably, the binding of oestradiol or selective oestrogen receptor modulators such as raloxifene (see below) to the receptor leads to oestrogen agonism and antagonism according to which receptor the ligand has bound to (see below) (Kearney and Purdie 2000).

Androgen, glucocorticoid, progestogen and mineralocorticoid receptors are less precise in their binding requirements than the oestrogen receptor (Beato and Klug 2000). For example, many progestogens, especially the synthetic ones, bind to both progestogen and androgen receptors when present in pharmacological concentrations. This dual specificity is reflected in the biological activities of the compounds. For example, the practice of giving synthetic progestogens to pregnant women to prevent miscarriage resulted in some of their offspring having clinical features associated with androgen exposure (Aarskog 1979). The androgenic side-effects of the synthetic progestogens used in the oral contraceptive pill are another example.

Nuclear localization, DNA binding and transcriptional activation

In their resting state, unbound steroid hormone receptors associate with heat-shock proteins, which obscure the DNA-binding domain so that they cannot bind the genome. On binding of steroid to the receptor, there is a conformational change and the heat-shock protein is dissociated, revealing two polypeptide loops stabilized by zinc ions, known as zinc fingers, facilitating dimerization and the binding of cofactors which will promote (coactivators) or inhibit (corepressors) the interaction of the receptor to its target genes. The receptors then affect gene expression by either binding directly to DNA target genes through specific hormone response elements, or by binding to other DNA-bound transcription factors such as AP1, SP1 or NF-κB. If the endpoint is transcriptional activation, binding of the hormone will result in recruitment of DNA-dependent RNA polymerase.

Clinical Assays

This section considers assay methodology for the endocrinological investigations commonly used in gynaecological practice. An understanding of basic methodology permits the clinician to have confidence in the selection of specific laboratory tests, and leads to a greater understanding of the assay for better interpretation of results (Chard 1987).

An assay determines the amount of a particular constituent of a mixture. The three types of analytical procedure commonly available in clinical practice are physiochemical assays, bioassays and binding assays.

Physicochemical assays

Some aspect of the physicochemical properties of a compound is utilized for its quantification. These are the assays used to measure some steroid hormones or intermediaries from their biosynthetic pathways. Techniques such as high-performance liquid chromatography or gas chromatography coupled with mass spectrometry are becoming increasingly used, and provide a definitive approach to the identification and quantification of hormones based on their physical characteristics.

Bioassays

Detection or quantification is dependent on the biological actions of the compound. There are two forms of endocrine bioassay. In-vivo bioassays investigate the biological potency of a hormone following its administration to an animal and quantification of a specific response. For example, human pregnancy could be diagnosed by the injection of maternal urine into the Black African Toad. If a high concentration of hCG was present in the urine, the toad would lay eggs. In-vitro bioassays measure biological effects when hormone is added to an isolated laboratory preparation of the target tissue. For example, in the bioassay of prolactin, when neural tumour cells grown in culture are exposed to prolactin, they replicate.

Binding assays

These assays involve the combination of the compound, for example, an antigen, with a binding substance, for example, an antibody, which is added in a fixed amount to the solution. The distribution of the antigen between the bound and free phases is directly related to the total amount of antigen present, and provides a means for quantifying the latter (Figure 10.12). Binding assays can be further subdivided into three groups: receptor assays, competitive protein-binding assays and immunoassays.

Receptor assays

A specific site on the surface of a tissue acts as the binding agent for a particular hormone; for example, oestrogen

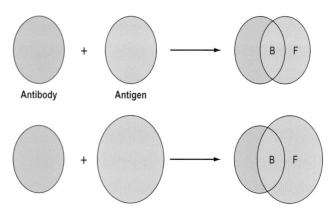

Figure 10.12 Distribution of free (F) and bound (B) antigen in the presence of a fixed amount of antibody.

receptors in breast tissue. The principles and designs are similar to immunoassays, with the hormone–receptor complex replacing the hormone–antibody complex. The hormone receptors and hence the assays derived from them have high affinity and hormone specificity, often generating favourable sensitivity, precision and sample capacity. They also bridge the gap between the bioassays and immunoassays.

Competitive protein-binding assays

A naturally occurring binding protein, such as SHBG, is used as the binder to quantify the amount of hormone present.

Immunoassays

A reaction, which reaches equilibrium, occurs between the hormone to be measured (antigen) and an antibody to monitor the reaction. A 'tracer' is attached to either the antigen or antibody to generate a quantitative signal. Non-isotopic tracers have superseded isotopic (radio-active) tracers, e.g. [125]I, and are typically based on enzymatic action such as fluorescence.

The basic binding reaction can be subdivided into two categories, based on whether the antibody is present in a limited concentration or whether it is present in excess. If varying concentrations of the labelled antigen react with an excess amount of antibody (Figure 10.13), it is termed an 'immunometric assay'. The principle of an immunometric assay is that a constant amount of antibody is added with increasing known amounts of the reference hormone. After incubation, the amount of hormone bound to the antibody is detected by adding, to all the tubes, an excess amount of a second labelled anti-hormone antibody. The second antibody is directed against a different antigenic site on the hormone from the first antibody. Thus, a triple complex is formed, with the hormone sandwiched between the two antibodies. The unbound fraction of the second antibody is removed, leaving the amount of triple complex to be determined by quantifying the bound label; for example, by measuring the radioactivity or fluorescence emitted. This emission is plotted against the increasing known amount of hormone standard to generate a calibration curve. To determine the standard curve with precision, against which patient samples can be interpolated, usually five to eight

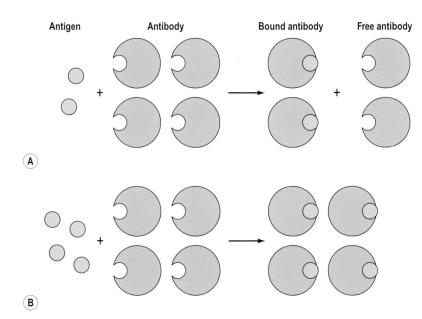

Antigen   Antibody   Bound antibody   Free antibody

(A)

(B)

Figure 10.13 (A) Immunometric assay with an excess of antibody. (B) Increasing concentrations of antigen give rise to a corresponding increase in bound antibody.

different concentrations are used. The immunometric assay is only suitable when the hormone to be measured is large enough to permit the discrete binding of two antibodies.

Enzymoimmunoassay, enzymoimmunometric assay and enzyme-labelled immunosorbent assay are currently the most widely used non-isotopic labels. Small quantities of antigen can be quantified by studying enzymatic substrate conversion that leads to a colour change. The colour formation can be a simple yes/no answer (Figure 10.14) as in a rapid pregnancy test, or the intensity of colour can be used to quantify the patient sample. The second marker antibody will not be bound, so following the wash step, it will not be present to react with its substrate.

Measurement and Action of Individual Hormones

In the interpretation of hormonal tests, it is important to be aware of local laboratory ranges and timing of the sample with respect to circadian and menstrual cycles, and also gestational age. The action of the individual hormones is discussed in further detail in the relevant chapters.

Anterior pituitary hormones

Follicle-stimulating hormone

Due to the marked fluctuations in FSH levels in a normal ovulatory cycle, timing of the blood sample in relation to ovulation is required to interpret results (Figure 10.15). The level can be as low as 0.5 IU/l at the luteal phase nadir and as high as 20 IU/l at the midcycle peak. However, values below 1 IU/l are associated with hypothalamic pituitary failure, and values of 20 IU/l or above indicate ovarian failure, as in the menopause.

In addition, FSH values within the wide range of normal can be associated with absent ovarian function if the production is below the threshold of follicular development for that patient; in other words, a normal result does not guarantee

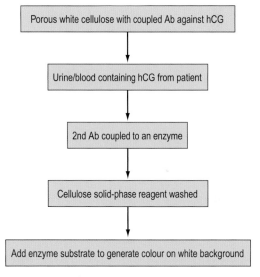

Porous white cellulose with coupled Ab against hCG

Urine/blood containing hCG from patient

2nd Ab coupled to an enzyme

Cellulose solid-phase reagent washed

Add enzyme substrate to generate colour on white background

Figure 10.14 Principle of rapid pregnancy test (tube test) using non-isotopic reagents. hCG, human chorionic gonadotrophin; Ab, antibody.

a normal endocrinological pattern in an individual patient. Fluctuating FSH levels mean that the investigation needs to be performed in the early follicular phase, particularly in a perimenopausal patient.

Luteinizing hormone

As for FSH, timing the sample in relation to the phase of the ovulatory cycle is vital (Figure 10.15). For example, the ovulatory surge is taken as above 20 IU/l. However, in polycystic ovary disease, a raised LH (13–25 IU/l) with normal FSH values is characteristic. Therefore, a raised LH in the early to midfollicular phase is of more significance than a midcycle raised LH. The LH level is within the normal range in a significant number of women with polycystic ovary disease, and the diagnosis requires the use of other tests. As the prospective timing of ovulation using the LH peak presents the

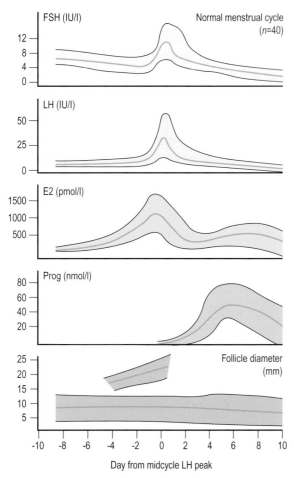

Figure 10.15 Serum concentrations (mean and 95 centiles) of follicle-stimulating hormone (FSH), luteinizing hormone (LH), oestradiol (E2) and progesterone (Prog) in relation to the size of the dominant follicle in 40 spontaneously ovulating women with regular cycles.

difficulty that the peak cannot be identified until the next value significantly lower than the peak is observed, clinical action is taken on the basis of the first definite rise in LH values (LH surge) rather than on the peak, which usually occurs a day later. This initial rise in LH underlies the mechanism of home ovulation kits using urine rather than blood samples.

Prolactin

Prolactin levels are influenced by the time of day when blood is collected and are increased by stress (including venepuncture). Transient rises can occur at ovulation. Therefore, a small elevation above the normal range can occur in normal women. Such a rise should be judged in the clinical setting. If a woman has a normal menstrual cycle, the result is unlikely to be significant. However, if she is amenorrhoeic, she should be investigated further.

Growth hormone

GH is secreted in short bursts, most of which occur in the first part of the night. These bursts are more frequent in children, so the results vary depending upon timing and age.

Secretion is also stimulated by stress and hypoglycaemia, and is inhibited by glucose and corticosteroids.

Thyroid-stimulating hormone

Normal levels of TSH range from 0.4 to 5 mmol/l. The measurement of tetraiodothyronine (T4) and TSH provides the most accurate assessment of thyroid functions. Levels also change across gestation, and specific pregnancy ranges are required to ensure adequate thyroxine replacement in women with hypothyroidism. When using thyroid hormone replacement therapy, both TSH and T4 should be measured because TSH alone cannot detect overdosage.

Thyroid hormones

Deficiency of the thyroid hormones triodothyronine (T3) and T4 leads to anovulation associated with increased gonadotrophin levels. Therefore, it is important to assess thyroid function in the work up of oligoamenorrhoea and prior to diagnosing premature ovarian failure

Circulating thyroid hormone is tightly bound to a group of proteins, chiefly thyroxine globulin. Oestrogen produces a rise in thyroxine-binding capacity and, therefore, thyroid function tests are affected by pregnancy and oestrogen-containing medications such as the contraceptive pill. Consequently, a raised thyroxine level does not mean that the free thyroxine concentration (the unbound and metabolically active hormone) is above the normal range. Due to the peripheral source of T3, its levels are not a direct reflection of thyroid secretion. In addition, T3 levels may be normal despite the presence of goitre with elevated TSH and depressed T4 concentrations, as T4 plays an instrumental role in TSH regulation. Therefore, measurement of free T4 and TSH provides the most accurate assessment of thyroid function. Measurement of T3 is important for the occasional case of hyperthyroidism due to excessive production of T3 with normal T4 levels (T3 toxicosis). Drugs taken orally for cholecystograms inhibit the peripheral conversion of T4 to T3, and can disrupt normal thyroid levels (giving elevated T4) for up to 30 days after administration.

Adrenal hormones

The adrenal cortex comprises three morphologically and functionally distinct regions. The outermost region (zona glomerulosa) secretes aldosterone. The zona fasciculata is the intermediate region and produces cortisol, which will be dealt with here. The zona reticularis encircles the medulla and synthesizes oestrogens and androgens.

Cortisol

Normal levels of cortisol in adults at 0900 h range from 300 to 700 nmol/l. If a 24-h urine collection is used, it is necessary to ensure that a complete collection has been obtained. The measurement of creatinine excretion will identify whether a collection is incomplete. As blood levels of cortisol vary greatly over a 24-h period, sample timing is important. Blood levels are highest in the morning and lowest in the evening. Most laboratories' normal values are based on sampling at 0900 h.

Dynamic testing of cortisol secretion by the adrenal glands is possible by means of a short synacthen test, whereby ACTH is administered intravenously after fasting, and the cortisol response measured in peripheral blood samples is quantified prior to ACTH administration and after 30 and 60 min.

Ovarian hormones

Oestradiol

Serum levels of oestradiol in spontaneous ovulation in relation to changes in FSH, LH, progesterone and the size of the dominant follicle are shown in Figure 10.15 (Macklon and Fauser 2000). There is a variation in oestradiol levels throughout the menstrual cycle. Results therefore need to be interpreted in relation to the timing of the sample in the cycle. Serum oestradiol levels in pregnancy range from 2 to 10 nmol/l in the first trimester and from 20 to 80 nmol/l in the third trimester. The major oestrogen in pregnancy is oestriol.

Progesterone

Variations throughout the menstrual cycle can lead to difficulties in interpretation if the result is taken at an unidentified time in the cycle, particularly if a single progesterone level is taken as a marker of ovulation (Figure 10.15). Normally, results taken 5–8 days prior to the next menstruation are suitable for the detection of ovulation, so the patient should be asked to keep a record of the timing of the blood sample and her next menstrual period. A result >30 nmol/l indicates ovulation, even if timing is not known. Levels in the mother during pregnancy increase in parallel with the growth of the placenta, being 30–45, 70–150 and 150–600 nmol/l in the first, second and third trimesters, respectively. Maternal progesterone levels are related to the weight of the fetus and placenta at term.

Inhibin

In the female, inhibin is synthesized predominantly by ovarian granulosa cells. Inhibin levels increase in the late follicular phase, acting synergistically with oestradiol to inhibit FSH synthesis and release, although this is predominantly over-ridden by the preovulatory LH and FSH surge (Bevan and Scanlan 1998). Inhibins A and B are dimeric proteins capable of suppressing FSH, with inhibin B being the principal form produced by the Sertoli cells in the testis which inhibits pituitary FSH secretion. Activins A, B and AB are dimeric proteins which share β-subunits with inhibin but stimulate FSH (Groome et al 2001).

Testosterone

Testosterone levels in females are lower than in males (females 0.5–3.0 nmol/l, males 9–35 nmol/l). The reverse is the case for SHBG (females 39–103 nmol/l, males 17–50 nmol/l). Testosterone arises from a variety of sources in the female. Approximately 50% is derived from peripheral conversion of androstenedione (secreted by the adrenal cortex), while the adrenal gland and ovary contribute approximately equal amounts (25%) to the circulating levels of testosterone, except at midcycle when the ovarian contribution increases by 10–15%. Approximately 80% of circulating testosterone is bound to SHBG.

Anti-Müllerian hormone

Anti-Müllerian hormone (AMH, Müllerian-inhibiting substance), a member of the transforming-growth factor-β family, has the primary role of regression of the Müllerian duct in the male fetus during early testis differentiation. However, expression of AMH persists after completion of the reproductive duct system in males, and furthermore commences in females, where it is produced by ovarian granulosa cells from early fetal life (Modi et al 2006). In females, AMH appears to have inhibitory effects upon the recruitment of primordial follicles (Durlinger et al 2002), and it may decrease the sensitivity of large preantral and small antral follicles to FSH (Figure 10.16) (Durlinger et al 2001). However, recent analyses of human follicles examining AMH receptor expression suggests that inhibitory effects at the earliest stages of development are unlikely (Rice et al 1997). Although AMH is initially observed in granulosa cells of primary follicles, maximal expression occurs in preantral and small antral follicles (Laven et al 2004, Weenen et al 2004). AMH expression declines as antral follicles increase in size, with nominal expression restricted to the granulosa cells of the cumulus (Weenen et al 2004). This loss of AMH expression during the FSH-dependent final stages of follicular growth, and the lack of expression by atretic follicles, suggests that basal levels of AMH may more accurately reflect the total developing follicular cohort, and consequently the potential ovarian response to FSH. Furthermore, AMH has been shown to be relatively stable across the menstrual cycle (La Marca et al 2010), consistent with its role reflecting the continuous, non-cyclic growth of small follicles in the ovary.

In harmony with the established relationship between age and declining ovarian reserve, AMH falls with increasing age (de Vet et al 2002). The clinical utility of AMH is its strong

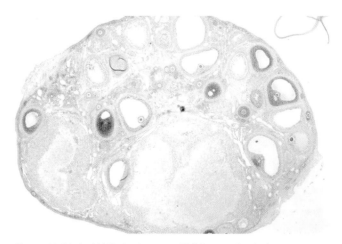

Figure 10.16 Anti-Müllerian hormone (AMH) expression in the ovary. Rhesus macque ovary stained for AMH by immunocytochemistry. Minimal expression in the primordial follicle, with increased expression by granulosa cells in the preantral and antral follicles. Ovarian stroma clearly negative. Image courtesy of Professor Hamish Fraser, MRC HRSU Edinburgh Scotland. MRC Medical Research Council, HRSU Human Reproduction Science Unit.

ability to predict ovarian response to FSH in cycles of assisted conception (Nelson et al 2007, 2009) and onset of the menopause (Sowers et al 2008).

Placenta

Human chorionic gonadotrophin

This is secreted by the blastocyst and appears in maternal blood shortly after implantation and then rises rapidly until 8 weeks' gestation. Levels show little change at 8–12 weeks' gestation, then decline to 18 weeks' gestation and remain fairly constant until term. There is some short-term variation in blood hCG levels but no circadian rhythm. At term, the levels in the female fetus are substantially higher than those in the male (Obiekwe and Chard 1983). The mechanisms which determine the levels of hCG in maternal blood are unknown.

A patient can continue to have a positive pregnancy test for at least 1 week after a miscarriage or therapeutic abortion due to the prolonged half-life of hCG; hCG may be detected up to 20 weeks later if sensitive assays are used. hCG measurements in blood and urine are used for the early detection of ectopic pregnancy, an increased risk of miscarriage, risk of embryos or fetuses with aneuploidy, prediction of pre-eclampsia or fetal growth restriction, and diagnosis or monitoring of trophoblast disease. The choice of assay for measurement of the prevalent form or proportion in relation to the intact hCG in any particular clinical setting is critical, as the complex cascade of enzymes involved in hCG secretion results in heterogeneous molecular forms (de Medeiros and Norman 2009). The synthesis of α- and β-subunits and their further glycosylation require different enzymes. After assembly, hCG reaches the cell surface and is secreted as a bioactive heterodimer. The hCG molecules are metabolized differently by the liver, ovary and kidney, but most of the hCG forms are excreted in the urine. It is clear that specific assays for intact hCG and its variants, α-hCG, β-hCG, hyperglycosylated hCG, nicked hCG and core fragment of β-hCG, have a wide spectrum of clinical implications (Cole 2009).

Pregnancy-associated plasma protein A

There is evidence that pregnancy-associated plasma protein A (PAPP-A) proteolyses insulin-like growth factor binding protein-4, thereby regulating local insulin-like growth factor availability. In addition, PAPP-A can no longer be regarded as 'pregnancy specific' (Boldt and Conover 2007). In pregnancy, PAPP-A can be detected in the maternal blood consistently from 6 to 8 weeks' gestation, with concentrations rising steadily throughout the pregnancy, but the mechanisms which regulate the synthesis of PAPP-A are not yet known. However, depressed serum levels of PAPP-A are seen in association with some fetal chromosomal abnormalities (trisomy 21, trisomy 18 and trisomy 13), Cornelia de Lange syndrome and ectopic pregnancy (El-Farra and Grudzinskas 1995, Kagan et al 2008). Maternal serum screening by maternal age, fetal nuchal translucency thickness, fetal heart rate, and maternal serum-free β-hCG and PAPP-A in the first trimester of pregnancy (11–13 weeks) will detect approximately 95% of pregnancies affected by trisomy 31, trisomy 18 and trisomy 13 (Kagan et al 2008). Serum PAPP-A levels are elevated in acute coronary syndromes and may be associated with adverse outcome (Schoos et al 2008).

Fetus

α-Fetoprotein

α-Fetoprotein (AFP) is synthesized by yolk sac, fetal liver and gastrointestinal tract. Its function is largely unknown; however, it is used as a marker in clinical practice for the identification of congenital abnormalities. Neural tube defects are associated with raised midtrimester levels of AFP, while Down's syndrome is associated with reduced midtrimester levels of AFP. The value of AFP varies with gestation and the number of fetuses present. The concentration of AFP in fetal serum rises rapidly to reach a peak at 12–14 weeks' gestation, at which time the levels are 2–3 g/l. Thereafter, it falls until term with a sharp drop at 32–34 weeks' gestation. In the mother, circulating AFP levels rise progressively to reach a peak at 32 weeks' gestation, and then decrease towards term.

The interpretation of normality of levels therefore depends upon gestation, and incorrect assessment of gestation could lead to an erroneous conclusion on the normality of the fetus. Levels are also raised in obstetric problems (threatened miscarriage, intrauterine growth restriction, perinatal death and antepartum haemorrhage) and some congenital abnormalities (exomphalos, nephrosis, Turner's syndrome, trisomy 13), but are depressed in trisomy 21 (Canick et al 2003). The introduction of more effective maternal serum markers and better-resolution fetal ultrasound has led to the diminished use of isolated AFP measurements.

KEY POINTS

1. Hormones are chemical messengers, classically distributed via the circulation, that elicit specific effects in target cells.
2. The three major types of hormones are peptides and the derivatives of amino acids and cholesterol.
3. Negative and positive feedback mechanisms operate to regulate hormone production.
4. Hormone action is mediated by binding to receptors and triggering intracellular responses.
5. The tissue distribution of the receptor determines where a hormone will exert its effect.
6. The two major subdivisions of hormone receptors are either cell surface or intracellular (usually nuclear).
7. Peptide hormones and catecholamines act on cell surface receptors.
8. Activation of cell surface receptors can generate fast responses in seconds or minutes.
9. Steroid and thyroid hormones act on intracellular, usually nuclear, receptors.
10. Activation of intracellular/nuclear receptors generates slower responses due to the need to produce protein from the expression of target genes.
11. Hormone potency is directly related to the length of time that the hormone–receptor complex occupies the nucleus.

12. Due to the amplification of hormone signals by the second messenger system, only 1% of cell receptors need to be occupied by the hormone for its action to be evident.

13. Downregulation by internalization of hormone receptors is a unique mechanism for limiting polypeptide hormone activity.

14. Agonists are substances that occupy cell receptors and stimulate natural physiological activity.

15. Antagonists are substances that occupy receptors without being internalized, hence blocking the cell function.

16. Endocrine investigations of ovarian function, with the sole exception of AMH, should be performed in the early follicular phase to guard against false results.

17. The choice of assay for specific measurement of the prevalent form or proportion in relation to the intact hormone in a particular clinical setting is critical, particularly for hCG and its variants.

References

Aarskog D 1979 Maternal progestin as a possible cause of hypospadias. New England Journal of Medicine 300: 75.

Beato M, Klug J 2000 Steroid hormone receptors: an update. Human Reproduction Update 6: 225–236.

Boldt HB, Conover CA 2007 Pregnancy-associated plasma protein-A (PAPP-A): a local regulator of IGF bioavailability through cleavage of IGFBPs. Growth Hormone and IGF Research 17: 10–18.

Canick JA, Kellner LH, Bombard AT 2003 Prenatal screening for open neural tube defects. Clinics in Laboratory Medicine 23: 385–394.

Chard T 1987 An Introduction to Radioimmunoassay and Related Techniques. Elsevier, Amsterdam.

Coccia ME, Rizzello F 2008 Ovarian reserve. Annals of the New York Academy of Sciences 1127: 27–30.

Cole L 2009 New discoveries on the biology and detection of human chorionic gonadotrophin. Reproductive Biology and Endocrinology 7: 8.

De Kretser DM, Menhardt A, Meehan T, Phillips DJ, O'Bryan K, Loveland A 2000 The roles of inhibin and related peptides in gonadal function. Molecular and Cellular Endocrinology 161: 43–46.

de Medeiros SF, Norman RJ 2009 Human choriogonadotrophin protein core and sugar branches heterogeneity: basic and clinical insights. Human Reproduction Update 15: 69–95.

de Vet A, Laven JS, de Jong FH, Themmen AP, Fauser BC 2002 Anti-Müllerian hormone serum levels: a putative marker for ovarian aging. Fertility and Sterility 77: 357–362.

Durlinger AL, Gruijters MJ, Kramer P et al 2001 Anti-Müllerian hormone attenuates the effects of FSH on follicle development in the mouse ovary. Endocrinology 142: 4891–4899.

Durlinger AL, Gruijters MJ, Kramer P et al 2002 Anti-Müllerian hormone inhibits initiation of primordial follicle growth in the mouse ovary. Endocrinology 143: 1076–1084.

El-Farra K, Grudzinskas JG 1995 Will PAPP-A be a biochemical marker for screening of Down's syndrome in the first trimester? Early Pregnancy 1: 4–12.

Garcia M, Rochefort H 1977 Androgens on the oestrogen receptor. II. Correlation between nuclear translocation and uterine protein synthesis. Steroids 29: 11.

Goldstein JL, Anderson RGW, Brown MS 1979 Coated pits, coated vesicles, and receptor-mediated endocytosis. Nature 279: 679.

Groome NP, Tsigou A, Cranfield M, Knight PG, Robertson DM 2001 Enzyme immunoassays for inhibin, activin and follistatin. Molecular and Cellular Endocrinology 180: 73–77.

Hillier SG 1994 Current concepts in the roles of follicle stimulating hormone and luteinising hormone in folliculogenesis. Human Reproduction 9: 188–191.

Holt RIG, Hanley NA 2007 Essential Endocrinology and Diabetes, 5th edn. Blackwell Publishing, Massachusetts, pp 3–52.

Hovarth PM 1992 Sex steroids: physiology and metabolism. In: Swarz DP (ed) Hormone Replacement Therapy. Williams and Wilkins, Baltimore, pp 1–10.

Kagan KO, Wright D, Valencia C, Maiz N, Nicolaides KH 2008 Screening for trisomies 21, 18 and 13 by maternal age, fetal nuchal translucency, fetal heart rate, free beta-hCG and pregnancy-associated plasma protein-A. Human Reproduction 23: 1968–1975.

Kaplan J 1981 Polypeptide-binding membrane receptors: analysis and classification. Science 212: 14.

Katt JA, Duncan JA, Herbon L et al 1985 The frequency of gonadotrophin-releasing hormone stimulation determines the number of pituitary gonadotrophin-releasing hormone receptors. Endocrinology 116: 2113.

La Marca A, Stabile G, Artenisio AC, Volpe A 2006 Serum anti-Müllerian hormone throughout the human menstrual cycle. Human Reproduction 21: 3103–3107.

La Marca A, Sighinolfi G, Radi D et al 2010 Anti-Mullerian hormone (AMH) as a predictive marker in assisted reproductive technology (ART). Human Reproduction Update 16(2): 113–130.

Laven JS, Mulders AG, Visser JA, Themmen AP, De Jong FH, Fauser BC 2004 Anti-Müllerian hormone serum concentrations in normoovulatory and anovulatory women of reproductive age. Journal of Clinical Endocrinology and Metabolism 89: 318–323.

Macklon NS, Fauser BCJM 2000 Regulation of follicle development and novel approaches to ovarian stimulation for IVF. Human Reproduction Update 6: 307–312.

Modi D, Bhartiya D, Puri C 2006 Developmental expression and cellular distribution of Müllerian inhibiting substance in the primate ovary. Reproduction 132: 443–453.

Nelson SM, Yates RW, Fleming R 2007 Serum anti-Müllerian hormone and FSH: prediction of live birth and extremes of response in stimulated cycles — implications for individualization of therapy. Human Reproduction 22: 2414–2421.

Nelson SM, Yates RW, Lyall H et al 2009 Anti-Müllerian hormone-based approach to controlled ovarian stimulation for assisted conception. Human Reproduction 2009 Jan 10 [Epub ahead of print].

Nestler JE, Powers LP, Matt DW 1991 A direct effect of hyperinsulinaemia on serum SHBG in obese women with PCOS. Journal of Clinical Endocrinology and Metabolism 72: 83–89.

Norman AW, Mizwicki MT, Norman DP 2004 Steroid-hormone rapid actions, membrane receptors and a conformational ensemble model. Nature Review Drug Discovery 3: 27–41.

Obiekwe BC, Chard T 1983 Placental proteins in late pregnancy: relation to fetal sex. Journal of Obstetrics and Gynaecology 3: 163.

Parinaud J, Perret B, Ribbes H et al 1987 High density lipoprotein and low density lipoprotein utilization by human granulosa cells for progesterone synthesis in serum-free culture: respective contributions of free and esterified cholesterol. Journal of Clinical Endocrinology and Metabolism 64: 409.

Payne AH, Hales DB 2004 Overview of steroidogenic enzymes in the pathway from cholesterol to active steroid hormones. Endocrine Reviews 25: 947–970.

Rasmussen H 1986 The calcium messenger system. New England Journal of Medicine 314: 1094.

Rice S, Ojha K, Whitehead S, Mason H 2007 Stage-specific expression of androgen receptor, follicle-stimulating hormone receptor, and anti-Müllerian hormone type II receptor in single, isolated, human preantral follicles: relevance to polycystic ovaries. Journal of Clinical Endocrinology and Metabolism 92: 1034–1040.

Rodbell M 1980 The role of hormone receptors and GTP-regulatory protein in membrane transduction. Nature 284: 17.

Rojas RJ, Asch RH 1985 Effects of luteinizing hormone-releasing hormone agonist and calcium upon adenyl cyclase activity of human corpus luteum membranes. Life Sciences 36: 841.

Ron-El R, Raziel A, Schachter M, Strassburger D, Kasterstein E, Friedler S 2000 Induction of ovulation after GNRH antagonists. Human Reproduction 6: 318–321.

Sairam MR, Bhargavi GN 1985 A role for glycosylation of the alpha subunit in transduction of biological signal in glycoprotein hormone. Science 229: 65.

Schoos M, Iversen K, Teisner A et al 2008 Release patterns of pregnancy-associated plasma protein A in patients with acute coronary syndromes assessed by an optimized monoclonal antibody assay. Scandinavian Journal of Clinical and Laboratory Investigation 14: 1–7.

Sowers MR, Eyvazzadeh AD, McConnell D et al 2008 Anti-Müllerian hormone and inhibin B in the definition of ovarian aging and the menopause transition. Journal of Clinical Endocrinology and Metabolism 93: 3478–3483.

Studd J, Wadsworth F 2000 Hormone replacement therapy. In: O'Brien PMS (ed) The Yearbook of Obstetrics and Gynaecology. RCOG Press, London, pp 374–391.

Weenen C, Laven JS, Von Bergh AR et al 2004 Anti-Müllerian hormone expression pattern in the human ovary: potential implications for initial and cyclic follicle recruitment. Molecular Human Reproduction 10: 77–83.

Willey KP 1999 An elusive role for glycosylation in the structure and function of reproductive hormones. Human Reproduction Update 5: 330–355.

CHAPTER 11

Biosynthesis of steroid hormones

Anthony E. Michael and Robert Abayasekara

Chapter Contents

INTRODUCTION	145		DEFECTS IN STEROID SYNTHESIS	152
PHYSIOLOGY	145		KEY POINTS	154
REGULATION OF STEROID SYNTHESIS	149			

Introduction

Steroid hormones are lipid molecules synthesized within the ovary, testis, placenta and adrenal cortex. Striking parallels exist in the organization of the biosynthetic pathways and the hormonal control of steroid production in each of these steroidogenic tissues. This chapter will outline the general principles of steroid hormone formation as regulated by trophic hormones, before considering detailed aspects of ovarian and adrenal biochemistry in health and disease. The chapter opens with a consideration of the general structures of steroid hormones, since relatively minor structural differences impact profoundly on the biological and clinical actions of each steroid hormone.

Physiology

The classification of steroid hormones

All steroid hormones are ultimately derived from the 27 carbon (C) substrate cholesterol and so share the same cyclohexaphenanthrene ring structure (Figures 11.1 and 11.2). Steroids are classified into five families dependent upon the number of carbon atoms and the chemical groups present at key carbon residues (Table 11.1). Those steroid hormones with 21 carbon atoms are collectively termed 'pregnenes', and this category of steroid hormones can be subdivided into three steroid families: progestins (e.g. progesterone), glucocorticoids (e.g. cortisol) and mineralocorticoids (e.g. aldosterone). While the progestins are secreted predominantly from the ovary, the glucocorticoids and mineralocorticoids are collectively termed 'corticosteroids', reflecting their origin in the cortex of the adrenal gland. The major structural difference between the three pregnene families is that while progestins possess a methyl group (CH_3) at position C21, both glucocorticoids and mineralocorticoids possess a C21 hydroxyl group (CH_2OH) (see Table 11.1 and Figure 11.2). Progestins can be metabolized to generate 19 carbon steroids, termed 'androgens' [dehydroepiandrosterone (DHEA), androstenedione and testosterone], which are secreted from both the testis and the adrenal cortex. Within the ovary, androgens are usually metabolized to generate the oestrogens (e.g. oestradiol-17β) with their characteristic 18 carbon structure (see Table 11.1 and Figure 11.2).

Within this classification scheme, there is a distinction to be made between Δ^5 and Δ^4 steroid hormones. Progestins and androgens of the Δ^5 series are characterized by possessing a hydroxyl group at position C3 and a C=C double bond between positions C5 and C6 in the steroid B-ring, as in cholesterol (Figure 11.1). In contrast, progestins and androgens of the Δ^4 series possess a ketone (C=O) at position C3 and have their C=C double bond between positions C4 and C5 in the A-ring of the steroid molecule (Figure 11.2). While this difference may seem a trivial biochemical detail, nothing could be further from the truth. The nature of the chemical group at position C3, together with the position of the C=C double bond, profoundly alters the conformation of the steroid molecule and, in so doing, influences the ability of the hormone to activate intracellular receptors. Hence, Δ^5 steroids, such as pregnenolone and DHEA, have low affinities for steroid receptors such that they can only exert limited biological actions. In contrast, the Δ^4 steroids, such as progesterone and testosterone, are potent activators of steroid receptors and so act as the dominant physiological hormones.

Origins and intracellular transport of cholesterol

An important issue in steroidogenesis is the provision of cholesterol, which can be derived from the following sources:

- circulating plasma lipoproteins;
- intracellular cholesteryl ester stores;
- cell membranes; and
- de-novo synthesis from acetate.

DOI: 10.1016/B978-0-7020-3120-5.00011-4

In both the ovary and adrenal cortex, plasma lipoproteins supply the majority of cholesterol for steroidogenesis and suppress intracellular cholesterol synthesis by inhibition of hydroxymethylglutaryl-coenzyme A reductase, the rate-determining enzyme for de-novo cholesterol synthesis.

Once inside the cell, cholesterol must be transported across the cytosol and into the mitochondria where the first and rate-determining reaction of steroid synthesis occurs: the catabolism of cholesterol to form pregnenolone (see below). The transport of cholesterol across the two mitochondrial membranes and interceding aqueous intermembrane space is now recognized as the true rate-limiting step for steroidogenesis, and so with this realization, it is this process which has been the focus of research into steroid biosynthesis over the past two decades. Although the understanding of the molecular mechanisms by which cholesterol passes from the outer leaflet of the outer mitochondrial membrane (OMM) to the inner leaflet of the inner mitochondrial membrane (IMM) is still far from complete, significant advances have been made over the past decade. In the mid 1990s, the importance of the steroidogenic acute regulatory (StAR) protein was first indicated when Clark and Stocco showed StAR to be a short half-life protein which is rapidly upregulated in steroidogenic cells following stimulation either by trophic hormones (e.g. gonadotrophins) or by the common second messenger, cyclic adenosine 3′,5′-monophosphate (cAMP) (Stocco and Clark 1996). Analysis of the StAR peptide sequence suggested that this protein gets

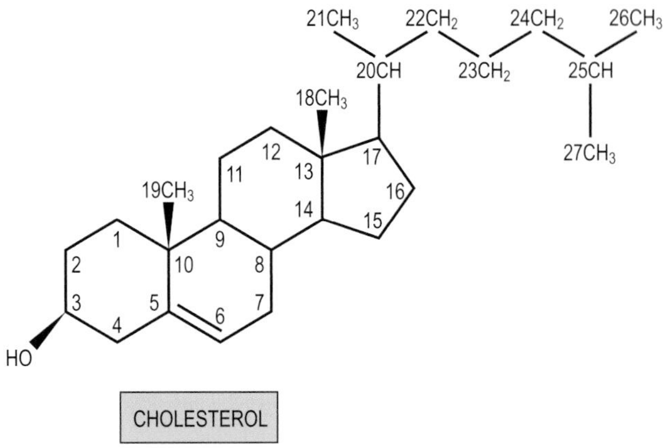

Figure 11.1 The cyclohexphenanthrene ring structure of cholesterol: the steroidogenic substrate.

Figure 11.2 Structures of the major physiological steroid in each steroid family.

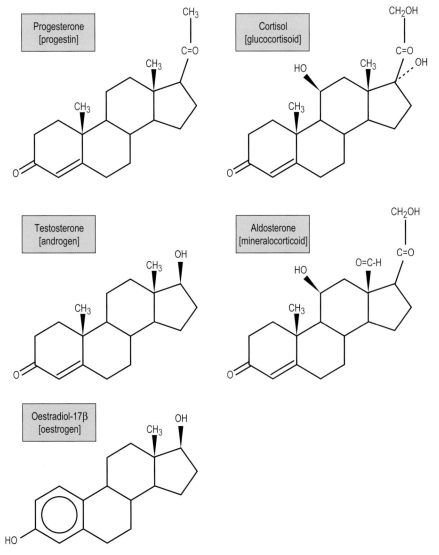

Table 11.1 Definitive structural features of the five major families of steroid hormones

		Steroid Family				
		Progestins	Glucocorticoids	Mineralocorticoids	Androgens	Oestrogens
No. of carbon atoms		21	21	21	19	18
Chemical group present at position	C21	CH_3	CH_2OH	CH_2OH	Absent	Absent
	C18	CH_3	CH_3	H–C=O (aldehyde)	CH_3	CH_3
	C17	D-ring side chain	D-ring side chain	D-ring side chain	17β-hydroxyl or ketone	17β-hydroxyl or ketone
	C11	Nil	11β-hydroxyl	11β-hydroxyl		
	C3	Ketone or 3β-hydroxyl	Ketone	Ketone	Ketone or 3β-hydroxyl	Planar hydroxyl group attached to aromatic A-ring

imported from the cytosol into the IMM, and it was postulated that the StAR protein might simply bind and transport cholesterol across the aqueous intermembrane space during the course of that import. However, subsequent site-directed mutagenesis studies revealed that the StAR protein could still drive cholesterol flux for steroidogenesis even when it was modified to prevent mitochondrial import, and it is now accepted that the StAR protein can act at the OMM to drive cholesterol passage from the outer leaflet of the OMM to the inner leaflet of the IMM without itself trafficking into the mitochondria (Miller 2007). This steroidogenic action of the StAR protein does, however, require: (i) that the StAR protein be phosphorylated on key serine residues by the cAMP-dependent protein kinase A (PKA); and (ii) that the phosphorylated form of the StAR protein interacts with the 18 kDa translocator protein (TSPO) expressed in the OMM (Figure 11.3) (Hauet et al 2005, Miller 2007). The TSPO protein, which was originally described as a peripheral benzodiazepine receptor (PBR), is very highly expressed in the OMM of steroidogenic cells. Recent studies have revealed that rather than reliance on a single protein to drive mitochondrial cholesterol uptake for steroidogenesis, this pivotal rate-limiting step involves a complex of proteins which includes the StAR and TSPO proteins in association with PBR-associated protein-7 (PAP7). By virtue of its structural interactions with both the TSPO protein and the PKAR1α regulatory subunit of PKA, PAP7 acts as a PKA-anchoring protein, localizing PKA to the OMM where it can phosphorylate the serine residues in the StAR protein to drive the StAR–TSPO interaction required to deliver cholesterol to the IMM for the first reaction in the steroidogenic pathway (Liu et al 2006, Miller 2007). While the StAR protein is not expressed in the placenta, this tissue does express a homologous protein, metastatic lymph node 64, which shares several functional and structural properties with the StAR protein, and is assumed to drive mitochondrial cholesterol uptake for placental steroidogenesis (Petrescu et al 2001).

Steroidogenic enzymes

Although the biochemical pathway of steroid hormone synthesis, summarized in Figure 11.4, can look like a bewildering railway map, the whole pathway becomes more straightforward on recognizing that the eight major steroidogenic enzymes can all be classified into just two enzyme families (the cytochrome P450 enzymes and the hydroxysteroid dehydrogenases), each with definitive functions. The steroidogenic cytochrome P450 (CYP) enzymes are members of a larger superfamily of CYP oxidase enzymes. Each CYP enzyme catalyses a hydroxylation reaction by serving as the terminal electron acceptor in an electron transport pathway which transfers electrons from a pyridine nucleotide cofactor, nicotinamide adenine dinucleotide phosphate, via two sequential flavoproteins (ferrodoxin reductase and ferrodoxin) on to atomic oxygen (Miller 2008). This allows the atomic oxygen to be inserted, by the CYP enzyme, into a hydrocarbon (C–H) bond thus generating a polar hydroxyl group (C–O–H) which renders the substrate molecule more water soluble/hydrophilic. The non-steroidogenic CYP enzymes include those hepatic oxidase enzymes responsible for the inactivation and clearance of a wide range of drugs. Each of the CYP enzymes within the steroidogenic pathway has traditionally been referred to by a variety of names that reflect their ability to catalyse hydroxylation of a steroid substrate at a specific carbon position. However, following the completion of the human genome (HUGO) project, all steroidogenic CYP enzymes have been assigned new systematic names which relate to the CYP gene that encodes the enzyme protein (Table 11.2).

In addition to their characteristic hydroxylase activities, some steroidogenic CYP enzymes also catalyse lyase reactions. Specifically, the CYP11A (cytochrome P450 cholesterol side chain cleavage) and CYP17 (cytochrome P450 17α-hydroxylase/C17,20-lyase) enzymes can each catalyse cleavage of the C–C bond weakened by the hydroxylation reactions. CYP11A acts in the IMM to catalyse the rate-limiting reaction in steroid synthesis: the conversion of cholesterol to pregnenolone. This crucial CYP enzyme hydroxylates two adjacent carbons (C20 and C22) in the D-ring side chain of cholesterol, facilitating cleavage between C20 and C22 to leave the Δ^5 21 carbon steroid, pregnenolone (Miller 2008). Similarly, CYP17 introduces a hydroxyl group at position C17 of either pregnenolone or progesterone, as a result of which the weakened C17–C20 bond breaks to generate either DHEA or androstenedione, respectively (Miller 2008) (see Figure 11.4). Other members of the CYP enzyme family

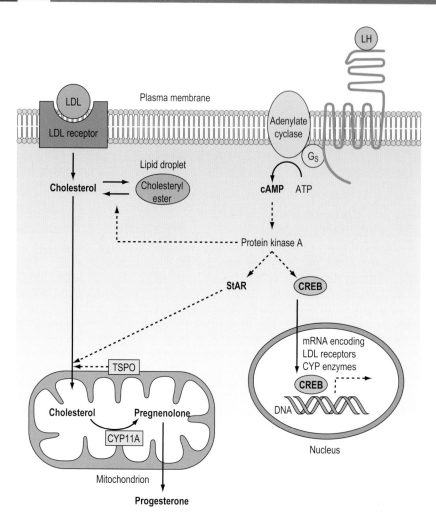

Figure 11.3 Cellular mechanisms for the acute and chronic steroidogenic responses to luteinizing hormone in a generalized ovarian cell. Open arrows indicate movement or metabolism; broken arrows indicate positive effects on downstream target proteins; see text for abbreviations.

simply catalyse introduction of oxygen to generate hydroxyl groups at specific carbon positions (see Table 11.2). The hydroxylations catalysed by CYP21 (21-hydroxylase) and CYP11B1 (11β-hydroxylase) are pivotal in the formation of corticosteroids by the adrenal cortex (Miller 2008). The hydroxyl group generated at position C18 by CYP11B2 (aldosterone synthase) undergoes rapid oxidation to form an aldehyde group (Curnow et al 1991), hence giving rise to the name 'aldosterone' (see Figure 11.2). Finally, CYP19 (aromatase) is the most complex member of the steroidogenic CYP enzyme family, catalysing a series of reactions that convert C19 androgens (androstenedione and testosterone) to their C18 oestrogen metabolites (oestrone and oestradiol, respectively). In this reaction sequence, the C19 methyl group is lost and the ketone at position C3 is reduced to a hydroxyl group (Miller 2008). This liberates electrons which are invested in the A-ring of the steroid to generate the aromatic phenol ring, the hallmark of oestrogens (see Figure 11.2) and a prerequisite for activation of the oestrogen receptor.

The second family of steroidogenic enzymes comprises the hydroxysteroid dehydrogenase (HSD) enzymes encoded by *HSD* genes (Penning 1997, Miller 2008). (As with the CYP enzymes, the HSD enzymes have all been renamed following the completion of the HUGO project, such that the systematic names for the 3βHSD and 17βHSD isoenzymes

have changed to HSD3B and HSD17B, respectively.) All of the HSD enzymes catalyse the interconversion of a hydroxyl group with a ketone to influence the affinity of the steroid hormone for its intracellular receptors (Penning 1997). Each HSD enzyme is specified by a number and a Greek letter; the number denotes the position of the carbon atom at which the enzyme acts, and the Greek letter indicates the orientation of the OH group relative to the steroid molecule (where α and β indicate bonds below and above the plane of the molecule, respectively).

There are two HSD enzymes of significance in steroid hormone production. The two cloned HSD3B isoenzymes convert the 3β-hydroxyl group of weak Δ⁵ steroids to a ketone, and also catalyse movement of the C=C double bond to generate the corresponding Δ⁴ steroid metabolite, thus increasing steroid potency (Penning 1997, Miller 2008). Hence, both the placental HSD3B1 enzyme and HSD3B2, expressed in the ovary, testis and adrenal gland, can convert weak Δ⁵ steroids, such as pregnenolone and DHEA, to the active Δ⁴ progestins and androgens, progesterone and androstenedione, respectively (see Figure 11.4). In contrast, the major HSD17B isoenzymes act at position C17 where they catalyse not oxidation but reduction, converting a ketone at C17 to a β-hydroxyl group. The significance of this reaction is attested to by the fact that androstenedione and oestrone (which have ketone groups

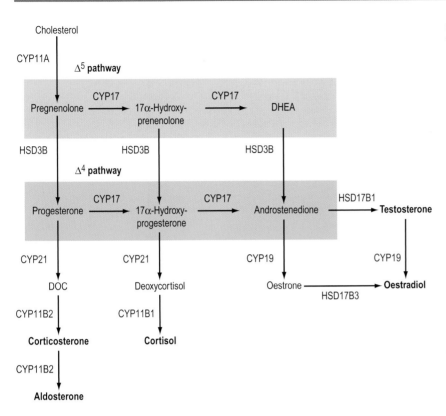

Figure 11.4 The general steroidogenic pathway. See text for abbreviations.

Table 11.2 The genetics and biochemistry of the steroidogenic cytochrome P450 (CYP) enzymes

Protein name			
Systematic name	Pseudonyms	Gene	Enzymatic reactions
CYP11A	P450$_{CSCC}$ / cholesterol side chain cleavage	*CYP11A*	Hydroxylation of C20 and C22 in cholesterol followed by cleavage of cholesterol side chain between C20 and C22 Converts cholesterol to pregnenolone
CYP11B1	P450$_{C11}$ / 11β-hydroxylase	*CYP11B1*	Hydroxylation of C11 (in β orientation)
CYP11B2	P450$_{C18}$ / aldosterone synthase	*CYP11B2*	Hydroxylation of C18 followed by oxidation to generate an aldehyde group at C18
CYP17	P450$_{C17}$ / 17α-hydroxylase; C17,20-lyase	*CYP17*	Hydroxylation of C17 (in α orientation) followed by cleavage of C17–C20 bond Converts progestins to androgens
CYP19	P450$_{AROM}$ / aromatase	*CYP19*	Generates an aromatic A-ring Converts androgens to oestrogens
CYP21	P450$_{C21}$ / 21-hydroxylase	*CYP21*	Hydroxylation of C21

at position C17) are relatively weak steroids, whereas their 17β-hydroxy-metabolites, testosterone and oestradiol-17β (see Figure 11.2), are the more potent androgen and oestrogen, respectively.

Regulation of Steroid Synthesis

In the ovary, testis and adrenal cortex, the synthesis of steroid hormones is regulated primarily by trophic hormones secreted from the anterior lobe of the pituitary gland, acting in conjunction with other endocrine, paracrine and auto-crine modulators of steroidogenesis. The anterior pituitary hormones, being hydrophilic, have to act via cell surface receptors coupled to signal transduction pathways that increase the expression and activities of steroidogenic enzymes. While several second messengers are generated in response to trophic hormones, the steroidogenic responses to these proteins are mediated primarily through the generation of cAMP with activation of PKA. In the acute response to endocrine stimulation, activation of PKA phosphorylates: (i) cholesteryl ester hydrolase (increasing mobilization of cholesterol from intracellular lipid droplets); and (ii) the StAR protein (thus promoting mitochondrial uptake of cholesterol for steroid biosynthesis) (Niswender 2002, Miller 2008). In addition, activation of the cAMP–PKA system rapidly upregulates expression of the StAR protein, apparently via the cAMP-response element modulator (CREM) protein interacting with a non-classical cAMP response element half-site in the promoter region of the *StAR* gene (Sugawara et al 2006). In the chronic steroidogenic response, PKA activates the cAMP response element binding (CREB) protein, and this transcription factor upregulates the expression of apolipoprotein B_{100} [low-density lipoprotein (LDL)] receptors (Golos et al 1986) together with several of the steroidogenic CYP enzymes (Simpson et at 1990, Sewer et al 2007, Miller 2008) (see Figure 11.3).

Endocrine control of ovarian steroid synthesis

There are subtle differences in the endocrine control of oestradiol-17β (hereafter, the -17β has been omitted from the term 'oestradiol') and progesterone synthesis in:

- the follicular phase of the ovarian cycle (which corresponds to the proliferative phase of the menstrual cycle);
- the luteal phase of the ovarian cycle (which corresponds to the secretory phase of the menstrual cycle); and
- the corpus luteum (CL) of early pregnancy.

In the developing ovarian follicle, the synthesis of oestradiol is dependent upon both luteinizing hormone (LH) and follicle-stimulating hormone (FSH) acting in concert (Hillier et al 1994). Within the theca cells, LH stimulates the synthesis of androstenedione. Until the mid-1990s, it was assumed that this weak androgen was metabolized to testosterone prior to secretion from the theca. However, molecular studies demonstrated that human theca cells do not express the HSD17B3 isoenzyme required to convert androstenedione to testosterone (Zhang et al 1996). Instead, androstenedione passes from the theca cell layer across the membrana propria into the follicular interior. Within the granulosa cells, CYP19 converts androstenedione to oestrone which is subsequently metabolized to oestradiol by the HSD17B1 enzyme. Hence, the synthesis of oestradiol in the ovarian follicle requires LH to stimulate androgen output from the theca cells, while FSH stimulates the expression of CYP19 in the granulosa cells (Hillier et al 1994) (Figure 11.5).

Clinical experience from assisted conception cycles has called into question this 'two cell–two gonadotrophin model' for follicular oestradiol biosynthesis. Prior to the development of highly purified and recombinant preparations of FSH, it had been assumed that the in-vivo oestradiol response to human menopausal gonadotrophin reflected the fact that this gonadotrophin exhibited both LH and FSH activities. However, even after effective suppression of pituitary gonadotrophin secretion using a gonadotrophin-releasing hormone (GnRH) analogue, follicular growth and oestradiol output can be stimulated by highly purified or recombinant FSH without the need for administration of exogenous LH (Schoot et al 1994). Although this finding prompted some researchers to question the need for LH to support ovarian oestradiol production, it has been contested that the low levels of endogenous LH remaining in patients following administration of a GnRH agonist/antagonist may

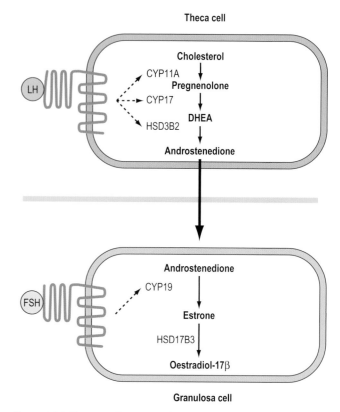

Figure 11.5 The two cell–two gonadotrophin model for follicular biosynthesis of oestradiol. See text for abbreviations.

still be adequate to stimulate synthesis of androgen precursor in the theca cells of ovarian follicles.

In the periovulatory phase of the ovarian cycle, oestradiol induces the expression of LH receptors within the luteinizing granulosa cells (Kessel et al 1985, Farookhi and Desjardins 1986). Hence, in the CL, both the granulosa- and theca-derived luteal cells express LH receptors (Rao et al 1978, Yeko et al 1989). Moreover, the luteinizing granulosa cells cease to express FSH receptors and so become unresponsive to FSH. In the luteal phase of the ovarian cycle, the majority of progesterone is synthesized within and secreted from the granulosa-derived cells of the CL under the endocrine stimulus of LH, acting via the cAMP second messenger system (Devoto et al 2002). Potential conversion of progesterone to androstenedione within the granulosa-derived luteal cells is restricted by the negligible expression of CYP17 (Sasano et al 1989). Molecular investigations have revealed that in the CL of women and non-human primates, oestradiol biosynthesis continues to require cooperation between two morphologically distinct cell populations. In the theca-derived luteal cells, cholesterol is converted to androstenedione by the sequential actions of CYP11A, CYP17 and HSD3B2. Androstenedione then diffuses into the neighbouring granulosa-derived luteal cells where it serves as a substrate for CYP19 in the synthesis of oestradiol (via oestrone) (Fisch et al 1989). Whereas expression of CYP19 in the follicular granulosa cells is reliant on FSH, expression of the same enzyme in luteinized granulosa cells is dependent upon LH (Devoto et al 2002). Hence, the CL employs a two cell–one gonadotrophin system for oestradiol biosynthesis, as opposed to the two cell–two gonadotrophin system evident in the preovulatory follicle.

In the event of conception, the steroidogenic activity of the CL must be sustained until the luteo–placental shift, at which point placental steroidogenesis supersedes ovarian steroid production. The functional rescue of the CL, in a phenomenon referred to as the 'maternal recognition of pregnancy', relies on the fact that human chorionic gonadotrophin (hCG) can stimulate steroid synthesis in luteal cells via the same receptors as LH (Rao et al 1978, Jia et al 1991). Indeed, while hCG has a longer plasma half-life than LH, the glycoprotein structures that dictate receptor specificity are identical in LH and hCG, such that both hormones can bind the LH receptor with similar affinities (Jia et al 1991). In-vitro studies indicate that, on binding to the LH receptor in primate granulosa-derived luteal cells, hCG and LH are equipotent in increasing both intracellular cAMP levels and progesterone synthesis (Molskness et al 1991, Abayasekara et al 1993).

In addition to the gonadotrophins, other hormones, including growth hormone (GH) and insulin, have been implicated in the endocrine regulation of ovarian steroidogenesis, acting in synergy with the pituitary gonadotrophins (Franks 1998, Devoto et al 2002). Both GH and insulin activate receptor tyrosine kinases which phosphorylate different protein targets to those in the cAMP–PKA signal transduction cascade. This ability to operate through different cell signalling pathways may explain, at the cellular level, how insulin and GH can synergize with the gonadotrophins in stimulating ovarian steroidogenesis.

Glucocorticoids can also participate in the endocrine control of ovarian steroid biosynthesis. In general, these adrenal steroids antagonize the effects of gonadotrophins and suppress the activities of steroidogenic enzymes in ovarian cells, which may contribute to the dysregulation of ovarian steroid production in syndromes of adrenal hyperactivity (including chronic stress, anorexia nervosa and Cushing's disease) (Michael and Cooke 1994).

Paracrine control of ovarian steroid synthesis

Within the ovary, a number of molecules exert paracrine/autocrine actions to modulate the steroidogenic response to the pituitary gonadotrophins. Recent interest has focused on such local actions of ovarian growth factors, some of which (e.g. vascular endothelial growth factor) influence ovarian activity (growth of ovarian follicles and development and maintenance of the CL) and steroid synthesis by mediating ovarian angiogenesis (Kaczmarek et al 2005). Others, such as the insulin-like growth factors (IGFs), act directly on follicular or luteal cells to synergize with LH or FSH in stimulating the activities of steroidogenic enzymes. For example, like insulin, IGFs I and II enhance the stimulation of theca cell androstenedione production by LH (Nahum et al 1995) and stimulate granulosa cell progesterone synthesis (Willis et al 1998). Members of the IGF family of growth factors provide the best example of how ovarian steroid production can be tightly controlled at the local level of the ovary. Not only are the paracrine/autocrine actions of IGFs dependent upon the local concentrations of each IGF and the appropriate plasma membrane receptors, but the effects of IGFs on ovarian steroidogenesis are further regulated by local concentrations

of IGF-binding proteins (IGF-BP1 to IGF-BP5 inclusive) (Giudice et al 1995).

Inhibin and activin, which were originally identified as major secretory products of the ovary and testis, are members of the transforming growth factor-β superfamily of growth factors (De Kretser and Robertson 1989, Hillier and Miro 1993). Within the developing ovarian follicle, inhibin and activin appear to act in concert to regulate the stimulation of androstenedione production in the theca cells and of CYP19 expression in the granulosa cells (Hsueh et al 1987, Hillier and Miro 1993).

Research in the 1990s clearly demonstrated that immune cells, particularly macrophages and lymphocytes, actively participate in the paracrine control of ovarian steroid synthesis (Chryssikopoulos 1997). At this juncture, it is relevant to note that cytokines released within the ovary from ovarian leucocytes can also modulate the effects of LH and FSH on ovarian steroidogenesis. For example, interleukin-1β can inhibit LH-stimulated androgen synthesis in cultured theca cells (Hurwitz et al 1991).

Finally, prostaglandins synthesized either within the ovary or in the uterus (transported to the ovary by countercurrent exchange from the uterine vein to ovarian artery) can also affect ovarian steroidogenesis. In general, prostaglandin (PG) E_2 stimulates steroid biosynthesis (apparently via the same cAMP–PKA pathway as LH), whereas $PGF_{2\alpha}$ can act in ovarian cells to antagonize LH action and thus inhibit progesterone synthesis in the CL (Michael et al 1994, Olofsson and Leung 1994). Indeed, it has been speculated that the local synthesis of $PGF_{2\alpha}$ within the CL may induce the functional regression of this transient ovarian gland at the end of the non-fertile menstrual cycle (Michael et al 1994, Olofsson and Leung 1994).

Endocrine control of adrenal steroid synthesis

In the same way as steroid biosynthesis by the ovary depends on LH and FSH from the gonadotroph cells of the anterior pituitary gland, the synthesis of corticosteroids by the cells of the adrenal cortex is dependent upon adrenocorticotrophic hormone (ACTH) secreted from the pituitary corticotroph cells. This hydrophilic protein hormone binds to cell surface receptors on adrenocortical cells to activate the cAMP–PKA signal transduction pathway (Schimmer 1995). Through increases in intracellular cAMP concentrations, ACTH stimulates cholesterol uptake (via LDL receptors), increases both the expression and activities of the CYP and HSD enzymes required to synthesize the adrenal steroid hormones (Simpson et al 1990, Sewer et al 2007), and crucially upregulates expression of the StAR protein which can then be activated by PKA-mediated phosphorylation (as in the ovary).

The adrenal cortex comprises three functional zones: the zona reticularis, zona fasciculata and zona glomerulosa. Cells in each adrenocortical zone express a different complement of steroidogenic enzymes and so synthesize different steroid products. Adrenal zona reticularis cells do not express HSD3B2 and so their major secreted product is DHEA: a 19 carbon, Δ^5 steroid (i.e. weak androgen) which tends to be secreted as DHEA sulphate (Endoh et al 1996). The major product secreted from cells in the zona fasciculata of the adrenal cortex is the glucocorticoid cortisol which exerts negative feedback at the hypothalamus and anterior pituitary gland to control subsequent endocrine input from ACTH. Hence, if the biosynthesis of cortisol is compromised or if a patient is glucocorticoid resistant (commonly due to a loss-of-function mutation in the glucocorticoid receptor), pituitary ACTH secretion becomes elevated and the ACTH induces increased proliferation of the adrenocortical cells; a condition termed 'congenital adrenal hyperplasia' (CAH; see below). The third and final zone of the adrenal cortex, the zona glomerulosa, expresses the CYP11B2 enzyme required for the conversion of corticosterone to aldosterone (Muller 1987). Hence, the major function of zona glomerulosa cells is the synthesis and secretion of the mineralocorticoid required to control sodium–potassium exchange in the kidney and colon. While the synthesis of DHEA(S) and cortisol is under the endocrine control of ACTH, the synthesis of aldosterone is regulated in a multifactorial manner, with the most important stimulus to secretion being altered electrolyte and fluid status (Muller 1987). A fall in plasma volume triggers an increase in the release of prorenin from the glomeruli of individual nephrons in the kidney. In the general circulation, the precursor protein prorenin is converted to the active enzyme renin which in turn metabolizes the plasma protein angiotensinogen to angiotensin I. Within the lungs, angiotensin-converting enzyme converts angiotensin I to angiotension II and it is the latter peptide which acts at the zona glomerulosa to increase the synthesis of aldosterone. Acting via mineralocorticoid receptors in the distal segments of renal nephrons and in the colon, aldosterone stimulates the uptake of sodium ions in exchange for potassium ions. Since the net influx of sodium ions exceeds the efflux of potassium ions, water is reclaimed from the lumen of the nephron or colon, thus increasing plasma volume and hence blood pressure to close this homeostatic loop. As aldosterone increases the loss of potassium from the body, the synthesis of aldosterone in zona glomerulosa cells can also be stimulated directly by a rise in the plasma potassium concentration (Muller 1987).

Defects in Steroid Synthesis

Genital virilization/female pseuohermaphroditism

Virilization of the external female genitalia (see Chapter 13) usually reflects a pathological increase in androgen secretion from either the adrenal zona reticularis or the ovary. The severity of clinical presentation, ranging from clitoromegaly with labial hypertrophy to male external genitalia (usually with hypospadias), depends upon the source and age of onset of the elevation in the plasma androgen concentration (hyperandrogenaemia).

Congenital adrenal hyperplasia

Increased adrenal androgen output (adrenal hyperandrogenism) is a hallmark of the common forms of CAH and usually reflects loss-of-function mutations in CYP21 or CYP11B1 which prevent cells of the zona fasciculata from synthesizing cortisol (Figures 11.6 and 11.7). The conse-

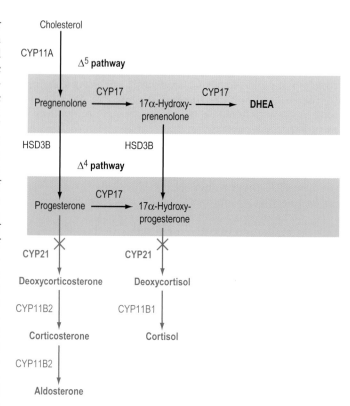

Figure 11.6 The adrenal steroidogenic pathway in 'salt-wasting' congenital adrenal hyperplasia; loss of function of CYP21. See text for abbreviations.

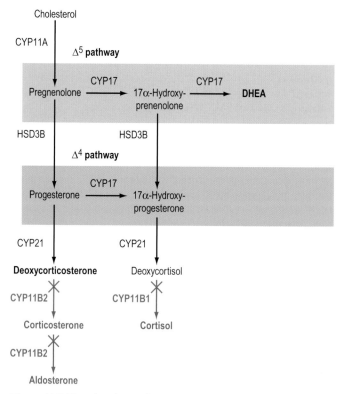

Figure 11.7 The adrenal steroidogenic pathway in 'salt-sparing' congenital adrenal hyperplasia; loss of function of CYP11B1. See text for abbreviations.

quent loss of negative feedback within the fetal hypothalamo–pituitary–adrenal axis causes an elevation in ACTH that stimulates adrenal hyperplasia with increased synthesis of DHEA in utero (White et al 1987). Although DHEA is only a weak androgen, this Δ^5 steroid can be metabolized to androstenedione and testosterone in peripheral tissue, such as subcutaneous adipose tissue. Within the genital skin fibroblasts, the sequential actions of the HSD3B, HSD17B and 5α-reductase enzymes convert DHEA to 5α-dihydrotestosterone (DHT) which causes virilization of the external genitalia. Under the action of DHT, the genital tubercle differentiates into a glans, the urethral folds fuse to form a phallus and the labioscrotal swellings fuse to form an empty scrotum (see Chapter 13). In addition to causing virilization of the external genitalia, adrenal hyperandrogenism will also manifest as development of male secondary sexual characteristics in a woman (see Chapter 26). Of these, the most notable tend to be male-pattern hair loss, hirsutism and increased body odour, symptoms commonly observed in women with polycystic ovary syndrome (PCOS) (see below and Chapter 18).

Although the effects of excessive DHEA production on the external genitalia and secondary sexual characteristics obviously affect a patient's future sexual identity and fertility, the other endocrine sequelae of CAH are of greater medical importance. In patients with complete loss of CYP21 activity (see Figure 11.6), the total absence of corticosteroids renders the patient unable to maintain normal glucose homeostasis (due to the loss of glucocorticoids) and to regulate sodium–potassium exchange in the kidney and colon (due to the loss of aldosterone). Hence, complete loss of CYP21 activity causes 'salt-wasting' CAH, alternatively referred to as 'simple virilizing' CAH (White et al 1987). In contrast, 'salt-sparing' CAH can result from either a partial loss of CYP21 activity or from a complete loss of CYP11B1 activity (White et al 1987, Nimkarn and New 2008) (see Figure 11.7). In either event, the absence of glucocorticoids presents as hypoglycaemia with depleted hepatic glycogen stores. However, in salt-sparing CAH, deoxycorticosterone (DOC), a weak mineralocorticoid, is able to exert some control over renal and colonic ion balance. Indeed, because the synthesis of DOC is outside the control of the renin–angiotensin axis, this steroid tends to hyperstimulate sodium resorption and loss of potassium, and because water movement follows the flux of sodium ions, the elevation of DOC usually results in the hypervolaemic syndrome of 'malignant hypertension' in patients with salt-sparing CAH.

Ovarian hyperandrogenism

Prior to puberty, the normal ovary synthesizes very low levels of steroid hormones. At and after puberty, LH stimulates androgen production by the follicular theca cells while FSH stimulates the metabolism of those androgens to oestrogens in the neighbouring granulosa cells. If this delicate biochemical system becomes disturbed, increased androgen production from the ovary (ovarian hyperandrogenism) can result in enlargement of the clitoris plus internal and external labia. As ovarian hyperandrogenism is usually (although not always) reliant on LH, virilization of the female external genitalia (as opposed to female pseudohermaphroditism) and the development of male secondary sexual characteris-

tics tend to be reported after the pubertal increase in gonadotrophin concentrations. An obvious exception to this generalization is observed in women presenting with hypergonadotrophic hypergonadism.

Essentially, there are three potential causes of ovarian hyperandrogenism:

- a disturbance in the LH:FSH ratio;
- stimulation of ovarian androgen synthesis by an agent other than a gonadotrophin; and
- decreased CYP19 activity.

In accordance with the two cell–two gonadotrophin model of oestradiol biosynthesis, alterations to the LH:FSH ratio, as reported in patients with PCOS and in menopausal women, can cause an imbalance between LH-stimulated androgen synthesis in the theca cells and the FSH-dependent aromatization of androstenedione in the granulosa cells. When LH is inappropriately elevated and/or FSH is suppressed, the synthesis of androstenedione in the theca can exceed the capacity of CYP19 to metabolize the thecal androgen substrate, such that there is net secretion of androgen from the ovary into the general circulation.

As noted earlier in this chapter, insulin and IGFs can also stimulate thecal androgen production, significantly enhancing the steroidogenic response of theca cells to LH (Nahum et al 1995). By definition, PCOS is characterized by elevated plasma concentrations of insulin (hyperinsulinaemia) accompanied by clinical signs of hyperandrogenism (see Chapter 18). A number of studies have indicated that the hyperinsulinaemia reported in women with PCOS reflects resistance to the cellular actions of insulin in peripheral tissues (muscle and adipose tissue) (Dunaif et al 1989). However, the ability of insulin to stimulate ovarian steroidogenesis appears to be preserved in PCOS patients (Ben-Shlomo 2003), such that in PCOS, the elevated concentrations of insulin may act in concert with LH to stimulate excess ovarian androgen production.

Mutations in the *CYP19* gene

A final mechanism for disturbing the delicate biochemical balance between the theca and granulosa cell compartments of the ovarian follicle is to decrease the capacity of the granulosa cells to metabolize thecal androstenedione substrate. The simplest mechanism to explain such a distortion in the steroidogenic pathway would be a complete loss-of-function mutation in the *CYP19* gene that encodes the aromatase enzyme. Due to the requirements for oestradiol and oestriol in pregnancy, fetuses affected by complete loss of function in CYP19 are usually miscarried. However, a few patients with severely limited CYP19 activity have been reported. In such patients, failure of the granulosa cells to metabolize any androgen precursor results in profound ovarian hyperandrogenism with progressive clitoromegaly and accelerated linear growth (MacGillivray et al 1998). Interestingly, affected girls do not show the usual cessation of linear growth at puberty, despite having plasma testosterone concentrations far in excess of the reference range for normal adolescent boys. These patients have revealed the crucial role for the CYP19 enzyme in the fusion of the epiphyses in the long bones; in both sexes; closure of the epiphyseal plates requires testosterone to be aromatized within the bone to oestradiol, such that women with defective CYP19 activity require administration of exogenous oestrogen to halt their linear growth (MacGillivray et al 1998).

Although mutations in CYP19 are rare, there are other disease states in which the capacity of granulosa cells to aromatize androgens is limited to the extent that ovarian hyperandrogenism ensues. For example, loss-of-function mutations in the FSH receptor, which have been associated with hypergonadotrophic ovarian dysgenesis, can prevent FSH from upregulating CYP19 expression in the granulosa cells despite a normal plasma LH:FSH ratio (Tapanainen et al 1998). Alternatively, glucocorticoids can inhibit the expression and activity of CYP19 in cultured granulosa cells (Hsueh and Erickson 1978, Fitzpatrick and Richards 1991), an observation that explains, in part, the association between adrenal hyperactivity and dysregulation of ovarian steroid synthesis in conditions such as anorexia nervosa and other chronic stress syndromes.

KEY POINTS

1. Steroid hormones are all synthesized from cholesterol, derived predominantly from plasma lipoproteins.

2. Each steroid hormone can be classified into one of five families, the names of which reflect their biological functions.

3. The biosynthesis of steroid hormones involves just two families of steroidogenic enzymes: CYP enzymes and HSD enzymes.

4. Steroid synthesis is controlled by trophic hormones which increase the expression and activities of steroidogenic enzymes and the StAR protein.

5. The endocrine actions of the gonadotrophins and ACTH are moderated by paracrine agents arising within the ovary and adrenal cortex, respectively.

6. In addition to compromising fertility, defects in the synthesis of ovarian and adrenal steroid hormones can dramatically alter the development of the external genitalia and the secondary sexual characteristics of a patient.

References

Abayasekara DRE, Michael AE, Webley GE, Flint APF 1993 Mode of action of prostaglandin F2α in human luteinized granulosa cells: role of protein kinase C. Molecular and Cellular Endocrinology 97: 81–91.

Ben-Shlomo I 2003 The polycystic ovary syndrome: what does insulin resistance have to do with it? Reproductive Biomedicine Online 6: 36–42.

Chryssikopoulos A 1997 The relationship between the immune and endocrine systems. Annals of the New York Academy of Sciences 816: 83–93.

Curnow KM, Tusie-Luna M-T, Pascoe L et al 1991 The product of the CYP11B2 gene is required for aldosterone biosynthesis in the human adrenal cortex. Molecular Endocrinology 5: 1513–1522.

De Kretser DM, Robertson DM 1989 The isolation and physiology of inhibin and related proteins. Biology of Reproduction 40: 33–47.

Devoto L, Kohen P, Vega M et al 2002 Control of human luteal steroidogenesis. Molecular and Cellular Endocrinology 186: 137–141.

Dunaif A, Segal KR, Futterweit W, Dobrjansky A 1989 Profound peripheral insulin resistance, independent of obesity, in polycystic ovary syndrome. Diabetes 38: 1165–1174.

Endoh A, Kristiansen SB, Casson PR, Buster JE, Hornsby PJ 1996 The zona reticularis is the site of dehydroepiandrosterone and dehydroepiandrosterone sulfate in the adult human adrenal cortex resulting from its low expression of 3β-hydroxysteroid dehydrogenase. Journal of Clinical Endocrinology and Metabolism 81: 3558–3565.

Farookhi R, Desjardins J 1986 Luteinizing hormone receptor induction in dispersed granulosa cells requires estrogen. Molecular and Cellular Endocrinology 47: 13–24.

Fisch B, Margara RA, Winston RML, Hillier SG 1989 Cellular basis of luteal steroidogenesis in the human ovary. Journal of Endocrinology 122: 303–311.

Fitzpatrick SL, Richards JS 1991 Regulation of cytochrome P450 aromatase messenger ribonucleic acid and activity by steroids and gonadotropins in rat granulosa cells. Endocrinology 129: 1452–1462.

Franks S 1998 Growth hormone and ovarian function. Baillière's Clinics in Endocrinology and Metabolism 12: 331–340.

Giudice LC, van Dessel HJ, Cataldo NA, Chandrasekher YA, Yap O, Fauser BC 1995 Circulating and ovarian IGF binding proteins: potential role in normo-ovulatory cycles and in polycystic ovarian syndrome. Progress in Growth Factor Research 6: 397–408.

Golos TG, August AM, Strauss III JF 1986 Expression of low density lipoprotein receptor in cultured human granulosa cells: regulation by human chorionic gonadotropin, cyclic AMP and sterol. Journal of Lipid Research 27: 1089–1096.

Hauet T, Yao ZX, Bose HS et al 2005 Peripheral-type benzodiazepine receptor-mediated action of steroidogenic acute regulatory protein on cholesterol entry into Leydig cell mitochondria. Molecular Endocrinology 19: 540–554.

Hillier SG, Miro F 1993 Inhibin, activin and follistatin. Potential roles in ovarian physiology. Annals of the New York Academy of Sciences 687: 29–38.

Hillier SG, Whitelaw PF, Smyth CD 1994 Follicular oestrogen synthesis: the 'two-cell, two-gonadotrophin' model revisited. Molecular and Cellular Endocrinology 100: 51–54.

Hsueh AJW, Erickson GF 1978 Glucocorticoid inhibition of FSH-induced estrogen production in cultured rat granulosa cells. Steroids 32: 639–648.

Hsueh AJW, Dahl KD, Vaughan J et al 1987 Heterodimers and homodimers of inhibin subunits have different paracrine action in the modulation of luteinizing hormone-stimulated androgen biosynthesis. Proceedings of the National Academy of Sciences USA 84: 5082–5086.

Hurwitz A, Payne DW, Packman JN et al 1991 Cytokine-mediated regulation of ovarian function: interleukin-1 inhibits gonadotropin-induced androgen biosynthesis. Endocrinology 129: 1250–1256.

Jia X-C, Oikawa M, Bo M et al 1991 Expression of human luteinizing hormone (LH) receptor: interaction with LH and chorionic gonadotropin from human but not equine, rat and ovine species. Molecular Endocrinology 5: 759–768.

Kaczmarek MM, Schams D, Ziecik A 2005 Role of vascular endothelial growth factor in ovarian physiology — an overview. Reproductive Biology 5: 111–136.

Kessel B, Liu YX, Jia XC, Hsueh AJW 1985 Autocrine role for estrogens in the augmentation of luteinizing hormone receptor formation in cultured rat granulosa cells. Biology of Reproduction 32: 1038–1050.

Liu J, Rone MB, Papadopoulos V 2006 Protein–protein interactions mediate mitochondrial cholesterol transport and steroid biosynthesis. Journal of Biological Chemistry 281: 38879–38893.

MacGillivray MH, Morishima A, Conte F, Grumbach M, Smith EP 1998 Pediatric endocrinology update: an overview. The essential roles of estrogens in pubertal growth, epiphyseal fusion and bone turnover: lessons from mutations in genes for aromatase and estrogen receptor. Hormone Research 49 (Suppl 1): 2–8.

Michael AE, Cooke BA 1994 A working hypothesis for the regulation of steroidogenesis and germ cell development in the gonads by glucocorticoids and 11β-hydroxysteroid dehydrogenase (11βHSD). Molecular and Cellular Endocrinology 100: 55–63.

Michael AE, Abayasekara DRE, Webley GE 1994 Cellular mechanisms of luteolysis. Molecular and Cellular Endocrinology 99: R1–R9.

Miller WL 2007 Mechanisms of StAR's regulation of mitochondrial cholesterol transport. Molecular and Cellular Enodcrinology 265/266: 46–50.

Miller WL 2008 Steroidogenic enzymes. Endocrine Development 13: 1–18.

Molskness TA, Zelinski-Wooten MB, Hild-Petito SA, Stouffer RL 1991 Comparison of the steroidogeneic response of luteinized granulosa cells from rhesus monkeys to luteinizing hormone and chorionic gonadotropin. Biology of Reproduction 45: 273–281.

Muller J 1987 Regulation of aldosterone biosynthesis. Monographs on Endocrinology 29. Springer-Verlag, Berlin.

Nahum R, Thong KJ, Hillier SG 1995 Metabolic regulation of androgen production by human thecal cells in vitro. Human Reproduction 10: 75–81.

Nimkarn S, New MI 2008 Steroid 11β-hydroxylase deficiency congenital adrenal hyperplasia. Trends in Endocrinology and Metabolism 19: 96–99.

Niswender GD 2002 Molecular control of luteal secretion of progesterone. Reproduction 123: 333–339.

Olofsson J, Leung PCK 1994 Auto/paracrine role of prostaglandins in corpus luteum function. Molecular and Cellular Endocrinology 100: 87–91.

Penning TM 1997 Molecular endocrinology of hydroxysteroid dehydrogenases. Endocrine Reviews 18: 281–305.

Petrescu AD, Gallegos AM, Okamura Y, Strauss JF, Schroeder F 2001 Steroidogenic acute regulatory protein binds cholesterol and modulates mitochondrial membrane sterol domain dynamics. Journal of Biological Chemistry 276: 36970–36982.

Rao CV, Sanfilippo J, Carman Jr FR 1978 Gonadotropin receptors in human corpora lutea of term pregnancies. American Journal of Obstetrics and Gynecology 132: 581–583.

Sasano H, Okanoto M, Mason JI et al 1989 Immunolocalization of aromatase, 17α-hydroxylase and side-chain-cleavage cytochromes P-450 in the human ovary. Journal of Reproduction and Fertility 85: 163–169.

Schimmer BP 1995 The 1994 Upjohn Award Lecture. Molecular and genetic approaches to the study of signal transduction in the adrenal cortex. Canadian Journal of Physiology and Pharmacology 73: 1097–1107.

Schoot DC, Harlin J, Shoham Z et al 1994 Recombinant human follicle-stimulating hormone and ovarian response in gonadotrophin-deficient women. Human Reproduction 9: 1237–1242.

Sewer MB, Dammer EB, Jagarlapudi S 2007 Transcriptional regulation of adrenocortical steroidogenic gene expression. Drug Metabolism Reviews 39: 371–388.

Simpson ER, Lund J, Ahlgren R, Waterman MR 1990 Regulation by cyclic cAMP of the genes encoding steroidogenic enzymes: when the light finally shines. Molecular and Cellular Endocrinology 70: C25–C28.

Stocco DM, Clark BJ 1996 Regulation of the acute production of steroids in steroidogenic cells. Endocrine Reviews 17: 221–244.

Sugawara T, Sakuragi N, Minakami H 2006 CREM confers cAMP responsiveness in human steroidogenic acute regulatory protein expression in NCI-H295R cells rather than SF-1/Ad4BP. Journal of Endocrinology 191: 327–337.

Tapanainen JS, Vaskivuo T, Aittomaki K, Huhtaniemi IT 1998 Inactivating FSH receptor mutations and gonadal dysfunction. Molecular and Cellular Endocrinology 145: 129–135.

White PC, New MI, Dupont B 1987 Congenital adrenal hyperplasia. New England Journal of Medicine 316: 1519–1524.

Willis DS, Mason HD, Watson H, Franks S 1998 Developmentally regulated responses of human granulosa cells to insulin-like growth factors (IGFs): IGF-1 and IGF-II action mediated via the type-1 IGF receptor. Journal of Clinical Endocrinology and Metabolism 83: 1256–1259.

Yeko TR, Khan-Dawood FS, Dawood MY 1989 Human corpus luteum: luteinizing hormone and chorionic gonadotropin receptors during the menstrual cycle. Journal of Clinical Endocrinology and Metabolism 68: 529–534.

Zhang Y, Word RA, Fesmire S, Carr BR, Rainey WE 1996 Human ovarian expression of 17β-hydroxysteroid dehydrogenase types 1, 2 and 3. Journal of Clinical Endocrinology and Metabolism 81: 3594–3598.

CHAPTER 12

Principles and new developments in molecular biology

Raheela Khan

Chapter Contents

INTRODUCTION	156	POST-TRANSCRIPTIONAL REPRESSION AND REGULATION	162
GLOBAL SCREENING AND ANALYSIS	156	APPLICATIONS TO REPRODUCTIVE BIOLOGY	163
PRACTICAL ASPECTS AND ANALYSIS	157	CONCLUSIONS	163
VALIDATION OF MICROARRAY DATA	159	KEY POINTS	164
GENOME-WIDE ASSOCIATION STUDIES	161		

Introduction

Expedited by completion of the draft version of the Human Genome Project in 2001 (Lander et al 2001, Venter et al 2001), the last decade has witnessed unprecedented advances in experimental methods in an ambitious effort to link genomics with whole-organism physiology and pathophysiology. The genome amongst individuals is 99.9% homologous, with diversity of function generated through postgenomic regulation at the mRNA and protein level. Detailed analysis of the human genome shows it to consist of approximately 3.1 billion base pairs (Little 2005). Of the genes, approximately 24,000, far fewer than the number expected, encode proteins with phenotypic diversity generated by multiple splice variants. It is estimated that over 800 additional genes are transcribed into small microRNAs (miRNA), although significantly more encode non-coding RNA (Little 2005). Clearly, the draft sequence has provided tantalising insight into the mysterious organization and complexity of the human genome that will be gradually unravelled for years to come.

New developments and refinement of large-scale, high-throughput investigations, often referred to as '-omic technologies', seem set to transform medicine. This is likely to be achieved through improved prediction, detection, diagnosis and treatment of disease, as well as better monitoring of the healthy state. There have also been crucial advances in the generation of new insight into our understanding of the regulation of global gene expression. Specifically, the central dogma which describes forward flow of information of DNA–RNA–protein, initially overturned by the discovery of the enzyme reverse transcriptase (which converts RNA to DNA), is matched by exciting developments in the field of RNA biology. The context of these developments and application of this new technology to gynaecology is presented herein with key examples from the literature.

Global Screening and Analysis

Traditionally, pursuit of scientific enquiry has been hypothesis-driven, which by its nature deconstructs complex biological systems into manageable 'bite-sized' studies with a very specific research question. In our wider quest to understand systems biology and networks, a reductionist approach is ill suited to investigating the integrative nature of whole-organism physiology, specifically the interactions between genes, protein and function. Given the immense volume of sequence data generated by the Human Genome Project, an escalation in research targeted towards population-based, high-throughput screening of gene expression has since been observed. The emphasis on networks, rapid advances in -omic technologies and high-dimensional biology has produced unparalleled insight into the relationships between the genome, transcriptome, proteome and, more recently, the metabolome. These innovative approaches have also necessitated unprecedented dependence on the discipline of bioinformatics. Table 12.1 lists key websites that are the backbone of such investigations requiring information on gene and protein sequences, gene annotation, sequence homology, microarray analysis etc. Many of these are freely available, with two of the most comprehensive and popular sources of sequence information being the National Center for Biotechnological Information (NCBI) and Ensembl.

Microarray technology

Gene sequence data in isolation provide little information on protein function. 'Functional genomics', the term used to describe the relationship between genes and physiological mechanisms on a global rather than individual basis, has evolved to probe these interactions. In particular, pioneering research using genechip technology enabling

DOI: 10.1016/B978-0-7020-3120-5.00012-6

simultaneous global gene expression of thousand of genes (Schena et al 1995, Brown and Botstein 1999) has been at the forefront of functional genomics, and is the mainstay of high-throughput assays. It is a powerful means of identifying subsets of genes that are either up- or down-regulated in a particular research scenario (Duggan et al 1999, Hegde et al 2000). Specifically, gene expression may be compared: (1) in different tissues/cells, (2) under developmental regulation (fetal versus adult) and on ageing, (3) in normal and disease states, and (4) in response to, for example, drug treatments, environmental cues etc.

Practical Aspects and Analysis

Microarrays

The success of DNA microarray technology exploits the complementarity of Watson–Crick base pairing that underlies hybridization of sample cDNA to either short oligonucleotide or cDNA sequences immobilized in a grid-like fashion on a solid substrate (Duggan et al 1999, Hegde et al 2000). Typically, a glass slide, nylon membrane or

Table 12.1 Commonly used web-based tools and databases for genome analysis

Function/ institute	Software	URL (http://...)
Nucleotide/protein sequence data	NCBI	www.ncbi.nlm.nih.gov
European Bioinformatics Institute	EMBL	www.ebi.ac.uk
Expert protein analysis system	Expasy	www.expasy.ch
Human and other genome sequences	Ensembl	www.ensembl.org
Human genome sequence data	NCBI	www.ncni.nlm.nih.gov/genome
Basic local alignment search tool	BLAST	www.ncbi.nlm.nih.gov/blast
ESTs, full-length clones, libraries	IMAGE	www.geneservice.co.uk/products/image/index.jsp
Human gene expression	HuGE	www.HugeIndex.org
Online Mendelian inheritance in man	OMIM	www.ncbi.nlm.nih.gov/omim
Haplotype map project	HapMap	www.hapmap.org
Microarray gene expression data	MGED	www.mged.org
Stanford microarray database	SMD	smd.stanford.edu/
Microarray manufacture	Affymetrix	www.affymetrix.org, www.dnachip.org/
Primer design	Primer 3	primer3.sourceforge.net/

EST, expressed sequence tag.

silicon wafer is the preferred format, although bead-based arrays are also available. For cDNA arrays, probe sequences principally derive from the IMAGE (Integrated Molecular Analysis of Genomes and their Expression) clone library arising from the Human Genome Project. These arrays include known genes whose function is as yet unknown, and expressed sequence tags whose full sequence and function are yet to be determined. High-density oligonucleotide arrays, such as those provided by Affymetrix, may be fabricated *in situ* by solid-phase chemical synthesis combined with photolithography. The sequences on Affymetric chips derive from 'refseq' — the definitive version of the gene sequence — contained within the NCBI suite of programs (Table 12.1). Currently, the latest arrays from Affymetrix offer unparalleled whole-genome analysis with over 700,000 probes representing over 28,000 human genes on a single array. Despite the diversity of microarrays available, some may not include the gene of interest to the specific research group, leading to the loss of key information in the study of gene pathways. An alternative strategy is to manufacture tailored arrays that include a smaller set of known genes of interest.

Once a research question has been formulated, the basic steps in a DNA microarray experiment, illustrated in Figure 12.1, commence with extraction and reverse transcription of total RNA or mRNA into cDNA from samples under investigation. Sample cDNA is then labelled either with radioactive or fluorescent probes and hybridized to the array. The main advantage of radioactive over fluorescent labelling is the enhanced sensitivity of the former. A currently popular approach involves differential labelling of test and control sample cDNA with the fluorophores Cy3 and Cy5. Following stringent washing to remove non-specific binding, image analysis of the emitted signal is performed either by quantitative phosphorimaging of radioactively labelled samples or by powerful laser scanning of fluorescence. These raw data are subsequently processed to generate scatter plots that offer a quick and easy means of surveying unaltered, up- or downregulated genes. A gene expression matrix, consisting of data organized in rows and columns reflecting the output of each individual gene in a particular sample, allows the data to be ranked and probabilities determined in order to identify individual fold changes in gene expression as a result of a biological effect. Typically, more than a two-fold change in transcript expression is taken to indicate biological relevance.

Inherent in these methods is the technical variation arising from a number of sources including RNA quality, variable probe labelling, high background etc. Distinguishing between real experimental changes and those due to technical variation is achieved by some form of normalization designed to remove bias and to ensure that the results obtained are an accurate depiction of a true biological effect. Normalization generally requires subtraction of background intensity from the signal of each gene. Other forms of normalization include comparison of gene expression against a known set of reference (housekeeping) genes included on the array that demonstrate constant expression irrespective of tissue type and conditions. The Human Gene Expression database (Table 12.1) is a useful source of information of such genes expressed in a variety of tissues.

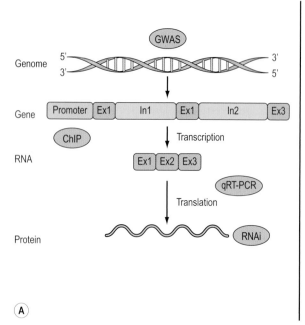

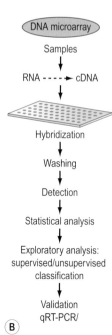

Figure 12.1 (A) Schematic illustration showing the transition from genome to protein. The structure of a gene contains introns (In) and exons (Ex). Techniques used in investigating aspects of molecular function are highlighted in the context of the entity targeted. Thus, GWAS for genome-wide association studies, ChIP (chromatin immunoprecipitation) for studying gene–protein interactions through the promoter region, and qRT-PCR (quantitative reverse transcriptase polymerase chain reaction) for transcript analysis using cDNA reverse transcribed from RNA and RNA interference for post-transcriptional silencing. (B) The steps involved in carrying out a DNA microarray experiment.

Statistical analysis

Once microarray data have been collected, standard methods used to determine real as opposed to chance changes in gene expression levels may be analysed using parametric or non-parametric techniques. In the former case, the *t*-test uses a measure of within-treatment error that results in finding genes that only have a large change in expression levels relative to the within-treatment variance. This is usually resolved by undertaking a suitable number of experiments to reduce the variance, but is not so easy with array data where experiments are expensive.

An alternative approach is to use fold change, in which the within-treatment variance is ignored. The problem with this is that variances do matter and vary between genes and treatments. Moreover, fold change may stem from an initially low level of expression, possibly reducing the biological significance of the change. A method of improving the power of the *t*-test is to use a Bayesian statistical approach that uses prior knowledge of within-treatment measurement (Baldi et al 1998). In the case of arrays, this is achieved by assuming that genes with similar expression levels have similar measurement errors (Baldi and Long 2001). In addition, the data are not viewed in isolation but in the context of known biological interactions.

Given the caveats that apply to the use of the *t*-test for statistical analysis of array data, an alternative method used to derive probability values that has been applied to microarray data is the use of permutation tests. Unlike the *t*-test, permutation tests do not require data to be normally distributed nor variances to be equal, and are therefore more likely to detect real changes in expression. Tusher et al (2001) have developed a method that uses permutation tests known as 'Significance Analysis of Microarrays' (SAM), where each gene is assigned a score taking into account its expression and standard deviation. The uptake of the SAM method has been greatly facilitated by the availability of an Excel plug-in. It also provides information on the false discovery rate, which corrects for false-positive results in order to eliminate random changes in gene expression.

Exploratory data analysis and data models

Since the aim of most microarray experiments is to identify differential gene expression compared with a control sample/condition, some means of organizing genes into meaningful subsets forms part of exploratory analysis. For example, a comparison between normal and endometriotic tissue may unveil changes in multiple genes involved in inflammation or cell adhesion. Similarly, treating a cell line with steroids may lead to a downregulation of genes encoding inflammatory cytokines. Exploratory analysis investigates such relationships using unsupervised or supervised classification to identify patterns of gene expression based on similarity measurements, yet providing little or no information on the statistical significance of the findings. Supervised classification is distinct from unsupervised methods since it involves making prior assumptions about the data sets but may introduce bias (Shipp et al 2002).

Broadly speaking, unsupervised methods that include cluster analysis (Kerr and Churchill 2007) or principal components analysis (Hilsenbeck et al 1999) identify groups of genes that change and cluster them into cognate groups. One of the shortfalls of this approach is that genes that do show changes with expression but have no perceived function may be overlooked. This is more so when one considers that it is likely that several genes may be implicated in a physiological response. A further problem is in identifying the best model within which to place the individual gene expression changes. Genes may be clustered using hierarchical clustering (Eisen et al 1998), two-way clustering (Alon et al 1999), k-mean clustering, principal components analysis (Tavazoie et al 1999) and self-organizing maps (Tamayo et al 1999). It is also preferable to determine the validity of applying particular clustering algorithms to one's data by carrying out bootstrap or jack knife analysis (Reimers 2005). Detailed mathematical arguments relating to supervised and unsupervised methods are beyond the scope of this chapter; readers are referred to the preceding references and the following sources for further information: Reimers (2005), D'Haeseleer (2005), Thalamuthu et al (2006) and Kerr et al (2008).

Limitations of microarrays

Although the use of microarrays has dramatically altered the field of molecular biology, it is no easy task to compare data across groups and arrays due to the variation in arrays used, normalization protocols employed, and statistical analyses and exploratory models applied. In an attempt to reach a consensus on sharing and storing array data, Brazma et al (2001) have launched Minimum Information About A Microarray Experiment (MIAME) as a mechanism for recording detailed relevant information on the execution and analysis of array experiments made publicly available for use by independent researchers.

Despite their undoubted utility in the laboratory, the limitations of DNA microarray methods are listed below.

- They do not detect mRNA but cDNA. The relationship between expression of mRNA and cDNA is complex and governed by several factors. Thus, cDNA levels may not mirror mRNA expression precisely.
- There is currently no method that allows reliable measurement of RNA.
- Arrays provide information on changes in hybridization signals for thousands of genes that cannot be performed in large replicates.
- Sources of error may arise from poor sample, RNA quality, probe labelling or background noise.
- It is not practicable to assess the identity of the DNA on the array, and errors relating to gene annotation, although rare, do occur.
- Having performed such studies at significant cost and effort, comparing microarray data is difficult and some agreement on standardizing experimental design in order to make valid comparisons has been proposed.

DNA microarrays remain a popular experimental tool, such that the technology has now extended to array-based global analysis of miRNAs, DNA methylation, genome-wide scanning and proteins. A further modification of this method for analysing histone modifications and gene-promoter sequence binding is based on chromatin immunoprecipitation (ChIP), which utilizes formaldehyde fixation to provide a snapshot of protein–DNA molecular interactions *in situ* (Wathelet et al 1998). This method has advantages over traditional in-vitro methods used to study transcription factors (i.e. electrophoretic mobility shift assays) and gene reporter studies that employ synthetic segments of promoter DNA that do not form chromatin with a structure reflective of that in native chromosomal DNA. ChIP-on-ChIP is an array-based method that allows mass screening of gene promoters involved in transcription and repression of genes (Collas 2009), and is a valuable addition to the armoury employed in studying gene regulation.

Validation of Microarray Data

All biological processes are ultimately regulated by the repertoire of genes that are expressed in a cell at a given time.

The cellular response to physiological and pathophysiological stimuli will also depend on changes in this profile. Array hybridization (and other techniques) is designed to identify the transcripts in a cell and to estimate their relative abundance. Thus, the array itself is a form of quantitative assessment. However, since array studies are often performed on relatively few specimens, additional quantitative methods are frequently required to investigate small numbers of genes in multiple samples. This is often termed 'array verification'. As array technology and the associated data-processing methods become more robust, use of this verification will decrease. Nonetheless, some verification is prudent and is most readily achieved using a polymerase chain reaction (PCR)-based approach.

Quantitative polymerase chain reaction

The sensitivity of the PCR has been instrumental in the elucidation of gene expression profiles at a cell and tissue level. Most readers will be familiar with the basis of the PCR which uses Taq polymerase, a thermostable enzyme isolated from the bacterium *Thermus aquaticus*, to exponentially amplify gene expression. Taq DNA polymerase has intrinsic 5′–3′exonuclease activity, optimal at approximately 72°C, and amplifies at a rate of 30–70 bases per second. The technique uses either template DNA or RNA from various sources (ex-vivo tissue biopsies, cell lines, blood, cloned DNA, microbial DNA) to compare expression of product (amplicon) under varied experimental conditions as decribed earlier. Quantitative PCR (qPCR) has rapidly supplanted conventional 'endpoint' PCR (Higuchi et al 1992, Wittwer et al 1997, Kubista et al 2006). It represents a major refinement where assay throughput has been greatly improved with 96- or 384-well plate formats, fluorescence detection and the commercial availability of ready prepared 'master mixes' that only require the addition of cDNA to amplify the relevant gene. The process of amplification essentially involves continual cycling between denaturation of double-stranded DNA to generate two single-template strands that undergo annealing to target primers, followed by strand extension and a consequent increase in product copy number.

Unlike DNA-PCR, which is relatively reliable and easily quantifiable, quantitative reverse transcriptase PCR (qRT-PCR), which requires the conversion of total RNA to cDNA with the enzyme reverse transcriptase (RT step), is a recognized error-prone reaction. RNA is significantly more labile than DNA, requiring careful handling. The crucial RT step is the source of much of the inaccuracy in quantification of gene expression due to inherent variability in, for example, the rate of reverse transcription and the choice of either oligo (dT)-18 or random hexamers for the priming of cDNA. The former produces a more accurate transcript profile which reflects the mRNA gene pool of the sample, with transcription requiring full-length, unfragmented, high-quality mRNA. Random hexamers prime cDNA from multiple points along the same transcript, thereby producing possibly more than one cDNA transcript per original target sequence, and also amplify ribosomal RNA. The choice of whether to use random hexamers, oligo-dT primers or a combination of both is a matter for the investigator. All RT reactions should be run in parallel with 'no RT' controls, that are duplicates of the original RNA reaction but with RT omitted in order to determine possible contamination with genomic DNA that would lead to false-positive results.

The heterogeneous nature of tissue samples is an additional complication, and it is advisable that, wherever possible, laser capture microdissection should be utilized in order to determine gene expression in specific cell types which will be more meaningful in interpreting association of gene expression with phenotype. Fortunately, this is relatively straightforward using techniques such as confocal immunofluorescence, immunohistochemistry and in-situ hybridization to determine a site of expression of the target protein or gene.

Primer design is a critical step in a PCR reaction. The current trend, however, is to purchase primers using software, in many cases provided by companies with expertise in qPCR. At a cost, these companies will also design primers on request, supplied as part of an assay kit where all reagents are optimized for the primers. The main disadvantage in ordering primers via this route is the lack of disclosure on information regarding the primer sequence, thus making it difficult to know exactly where the primer is annealing. Many freely available primer design tools are available on the internet.

Fluorescence chemistry in quantitative reverse transcriptase polymerase chain reaction

The two most widely used forms of fluorescence detection for qPCR are as follows.

- DNA-binding dyes: SYBR green was the first available fluorescent probe to be used in qPCR and qRT-PCR as it is easily incorporated into a normal reaction mix. It acts by intercalating with double-stranded DNA, thus generating approximately 1000-fold increased fluorescence intensity compared with unbound dye. Shortcomings of this method include its indiscriminate binding to any form of double-stranded DNA,

including both the amplicon as well as primer-dimers. However, melt-curve analysis that enables distinction between specific and non-specific amplification based on knowledge of the desired amplicon is easily performed as part of the reaction. Figure 12.2 illustrates qRT-PCR undertaken using human endometrial cDNA and SYBR green chemistry.

- Hydrolysis probes using Taqman chemistry, the most popular of the fluorescence approaches, are based on the incorporation of an oligonucleotide probe which hybridizes to the DNA circumscribed by the two PCR primers. The probe is typically labelled with a fluorophore at its 5' end and a quencher at the 3' end. The 5'–3' exonuclease activity of Taq polymerase as it progresses along the template digests a portion of the probe, sequentially removing each fluorescent dye molecule, finally achieving spatial separation from the dye at the other end of the probe. When these dyes are close together, their fluorescence is quenched [by fluorescence resonance energy transfer (FRET)]. Upon separation, this effect is lost and fluorescence is emitted. Since the product from one cycle is the template for the next, the amount of probe hybridized and therefore digested during each cycle increases. This leads to an increase in the emitted fluorescence which is proportional to the amount of initial template present. The Taqman probe method does not lend itself to melt-curve analysis. More sensitive FRET-based detection methods are available that do permit melt-curve analysis, but their use is limited by the expense in using this chemistry.

Data analysis and interpretation in quantitative polymerase chain reaction

Quantification of the qRT-PCR assay is most accurately determined during the exponential phase of the reaction when amplification products are being generated at a steady

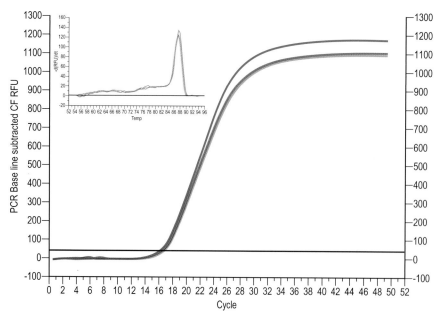

Figure 12.2 Quantitative reverse transcriptase polymerase chain reaction (PCR) of the adhesion molecule E-cadherin in human endometrium using the SYBR® green method. All three samples are characterized by a C_t of 17. Inset illustrates a melt curve showing a single peak produced during the amplification, indicating the formation of a specific amplicon. CF RFU, curve fit relative fluorescence units.
Source: Patel S, Shaw RW, Khan RN (unpublished data).

optimum rate, approximately 10–20 cycles into the reaction. The software creates an amplification plot with the measured fluorescence signal plotted against the cycle number. The single most important readout of the qRT-PCR is the C_t, and this is the first fluorescence signal that occurs above the threshold limit for fluorescence detection. Differences in C_t values are used to calculate the relative abundance of template between samples, as the C_t value is directly proportional to the amount of template at the start. A crucial factor in qPCR is the amplification efficiency, calculated from the slope of the calibration curve (see below) which should be close to 100% (Higuchi et al 1992).

Quantification in qPCR is carried out by one of two methods: absolute or relative. Both methods have advantages and disadvantages, and the decision regarding which one to use is one of personal choice.

Absolute quantification

This is a method by which known concentrations of nucleic acids are used to generate a standard curve from which unknown mRNA expression levels for target genes may be determined. For the method, known concentrations of cDNA or copy number are used in a calibration curve to create a standard curve with C_t plotted against log concentration or copy number cDNA. The data in Figure 12.2 illustrate an amplification curve showing E-cadherin expression in human endometrium.

Relative quantification

Also known as the delta delta C_t ($\Delta\Delta C_t$) method, this uses a simpler approach in that there is no requirement for a standard curve and all quantification is based on C_t values expressed relative to a housekeeping or reference gene (Pfaffl 2001). However, this method is only effective if the reference gene of choice is constant in expression between samples or treatment. The amplification efficiencies of both the target and reference genes should be equal. Despite this, it remains a widely used method.

Normalization

As with microarray data, normalization is an essential step in qRT-PCR and is typically performed in relation to a reference gene. As reference genes are known to vary in many different cell types under various conditions, it is good practice to probe samples for more than one single reference gene (Vandesompele et al 2002). A new standard for determining an appropriate reference gene is derived from the GeNorm programme, which takes actual C_t values from a sample for a number of tested reference genes that are stated in the paper and uses an algorithm to assign an M value to determine the most appropriate stable reference gene from those tested (Vandesompele et al 2002).

It is essential that qPCR and RT-qPCR studies are reported accurately. The varied format currently adopted by researchers does not lend itself to critical appraisal and does not permit comparisons to be made easily. As with microarrays, guidelines on the minimum information for publication of quantitative real-time PCR experiments have been developed (Bustin et al 2009). Researchers undertaking qPCR/ qRT-PCR are encouraged to comply with the recommendations made in this article.

Genome-Wide Association Studies

Mapping of single nucleotide polymorphisms and links to complex diseases

The abundance of sequence data produced by the Human Genome Project has made possible the use of microarrays in elucidating genomic variations that predict susceptibility to common diseases that include diabetes and cardiovascular disease (Wellcome Trust Case Control Consortium 2007). Thus, genome-wide association studies (GWAS) utilize large-scale, high-throughput methods to perform unbiased parallel genomic analysis of an unprecedented number of biological samples. The expectation is that this approach will be incorporated into personalized medicine or pharmacogenomics where responses to treatment will be predicated on an individual's genotype.

GWAS is based on the principle that predisposition to common diseases is attributable to a small number of genetic variations, and that large-scale screening of populations or families will identify sequence patterns predictive of disease (Nica and Dermitzakis 2008). Most complex diseases are a consequence of a composite, non-Mendelian inheritance of multiple genes. The most common source of genetic variation within the human genome is the single nucleotide polymorphism (SNP), where the replacement of one nucleotide with another at a related locus potentially alters the downstream protein product encoded. SNPs, approximately 12 million of which reside within the human genome, are the preferred genetic markers due to their abundance, occurring approximately once every 1000 base pairs. Access to the HapMap database — a repository cataloguing the genetic variation in ethnically distinct populations and their link to health and disease (Frazer et al 2007) — has been instrumental in the launch of GWAS studies. Not all SNPs cause disease (Stranger and Dermitzakis 2006) and, interestingly, experimental evidence indicates that SNPs account for only a small proportion of the phenotypic variance, implying association with other non-genetic factors, particularly gene–environment interactions.

The availability of arrays that contain millions of cDNA fragments allows an individual's genotype to be queried for up to 2 million known genetic variants. The design of GWAS may take the form of:

- a case–control study, in which individuals with disease are compared with a disease-free control group;
- a cohort design where a large number of individuals are recruited from a similar sample then categorized according to genetic variants; or
- the trio design, which attempts to survey an afflicted individual and his/her parents. This latter approach is best suited to Mendelian inheritance of disease (Pearson and Manolio 2008).

Pertinent to female health, the Womens' Genome Health Study, a full-cohort prospective GWAS, was commenced recently (Ridker et al 2008). The goal of this project is to produce a fully searchable database of SNPs for women in order to identify polymorphism patterns that predict disease in otherwise healthy women. The Women's Genome Health Study will use the same study population of well-characterized healthy women initially recruited to the Women's Health Study. These women have already undergone 12 years of monitoring for major health events that include, amongst several others, cardiovascular disease, cancer, diabetes and osteoporosis. Significantly, this study has collated an extensive amount of epidemiological information along with baseline blood samples for several disease biomarkers and DNA for genotyping, as well as dietary and behavioural data that will allow gene–environment and gene–gene interactions to be examined.

Post-Transcriptional Repression and Regulation

The role of microRNA and short, interfering RNA

Probably the single most important discovery in cell biology in recent years relates to that of small non-coding RNA molecules, specifically short, interfering RNA (siRNA) and miRNA (Figure 12.3). The landmark paper describing RNA interference (RNAi), where Fire et al (1998) used double-stranded RNA to silence gene expression in *Caenorhabditis elegans*, has caused a paradigm shift in our interpretation of post-transcriptional regulation. It is estimated that over half of the genes encoding proteins in the human are likely to be regulated by miRNAs, providing a compelling case for further research in this field.

Both miRNA and siRNA are produced endogenously in the nucleus, although siRNA was initially thought to have a solely exogenous origin, deriving principally from viruses. siRNA has since been demonstrated in native cells where it has been termed 'endo-siRNA'. Interestingly, biogenesis of both siRNA and miRNA proceeds by a similar mechanism, described below, which evokes silencing in association with

the Argonaute (Ago) superfamily of proteins (Meister et al 2005, Tomari and Zamore 2005).

miRNAs, in their fully-processed mature form, are short (18–24), single-stranded segments of RNA that bind to the 3' UTR region of mRNA to induce transcriptional silencing (Carthew and Sontheimer 2009). They are produced in the nucleus from DNA by the action of RNA polymerase II to generate a long (hundreds to thousands of nucleotides), double-stranded precursor, primary RNA or pri-miRNA. The latter is spliced in the nucleus into pre-miRNA (70 nucleotides in length) by the enzyme 'Drosha' (Lee et al 2002), then exported to the cytoplasm by an accessory protein, exportin 5. Further processing of pre-miRNA by the enzyme 'Dicer' yields a miRNA duplex of approximately 22 nucleotides and a two-nucleotide overhang at the 3' end (Yi et al 2003, Gregory et al 2005). Entry of this duplex into the RNA-induced silencing complex induces the association of one strand (the guide strand) with Ago where it is unwound and post-transcriptional repression of target mRNA ensues (see Figure 12.2). The other 'passenger' strand is degraded. It is interesting that perfect complementary base pairing between miRNA-mRNA results in degradation of the target mRNA, while a slight mismatch of base pairing induces silencing and translational repression (Tomari and Zamore 2005). Whilst the specific mechanisms that determine whether target mRNA is degraded or repressed remain an active area of research, imperfect base pairing has evolved as an ingenious mechanism that explains the multiplicity of targets for miRNA clusters. It should be borne in mind that some miRNA species only have one target.

Apart from their roles in development and stem cell differentiation, miRNAs appear to play a key role in both oncogenesis and tumour suppression. miRNAs involved in oncogenesis involve the mIR-17-92 cluster implicated in a mouse model of lymphoma (He et al 2005). Intriguingly, circulating miRNAs have been detected in blood and serum of cancer patients (Lawrie 2008), thus presenting an opportunity to harness miRNAs for diagnostic, prognostic and therapeutic purposes in the management of a wide range of malignancies.

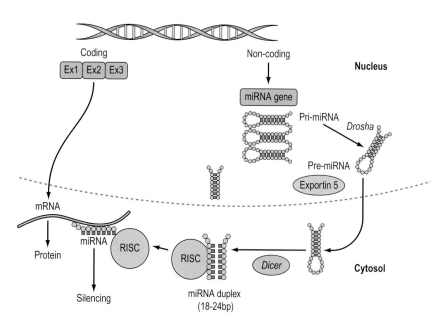

Figure 12.3 Post-transcriptional regulation of microRNA. Pri-miRNA, produced from the action of RNA polymerase II on the miRNA gene, is cleaved by the enzyme Drosha into a pre-miRNA transcript ~70 nucleotides long. Pre-miRNA exits the nucleus after associating with exportin 5, a nuclear transporter. In the cytosol, a ribonuclease III known as Dicer processes the pre-miRNA into a ~22 nucleotide duplex. The mature strand of the duplex then preferentially enters the RNA-induced silencing complex (RISC) to attach to newly formed RNA to elicit silencing. The shaded part of the figure illustrates the conventional sequence whereby mRNA is translated into protein.

The emergence of RNAi (Fire et al 1998) and the early success of siRNA in achieving targeted protein knockdown has overcome several obstacles. In practical applications, siRNA has been replaced with short hairpin RNA (shRNA), where the two individual strands of shRNA are linked by a short loop sequence of approximately eight nucleotides. shRNA mimics this short hairpin loop found in most native RNA species, therefore replicating function more faithfully than siRNA. Although siRNA technology holds great promise, one of the problems with its use was the observation that binding of the guide strand to large numbers of genes resulted in altered expression of a host of miRNA species; a phenomenon known as 'off-targeting'. While this has been largely overcome through improved design of siRNA, another problem surfaced with the finding that shRNA-expressing vectors were dose-dependently linked to increased mortality in experimental animals, indicating overloading of the siRNA pathway. In addition, this study also challenged the notion that siRNA species lack immunogenicity since an immune response that involved Toll-like receptors — the pattern recognition family of Toll-like receptors — could be elicited (Grimm 2009). Despite these concerns, the experimental and potential therapeutic advantages of siRNAs provide a compelling case for their translation to the clinical arena.

Applications to Reproductive Biology

Significant milestones in reproductive biology that have transformed lifestyles include the development of the oral contraceptive pill, hormone replacement therapy and in-vitro fertilization. The power of gene cloning, as exemplified by the case of 'Dolly the sheep', has helped to launch the field of regenerative medicine and stem cell biology. Science has made many other, less well-known breakthroughs that have contributed to improving female health. Despite this, effective pharmacological therapies for the treatment of endometriosis, infertility, recurrent miscarriage and polycystic ovary syndrome (PCOS) remain elusive. Indeed, our understanding of the main female reproductive disorders is limited due to a paucity of research funding compared with diseases such as diabetes, cardiovascular disease and cancer. Microarrays in conjunction with new developments in our understanding of transcriptional regulation may elucidate temporal, tissue- and cell-specific gene signatures. Moreover, given the similarities between PCOS and diabetes, a GWAS approach to this condition may identify common genetic variations that might inform or predict development of PCOS. High-throughput technologies will undoubtedly provide new approaches to knowledge, diagnosis and therapeutics in all areas of reproductive biology.

Implantation/fertility

One of the most intractable problems facing reproductive medicine is failed implantation, whether this arises in natural cycles or in assisted reproduction. Transcript profiling studies, summarized in a recent review (Sherwin et al 2006), have sought to define endometrial function and receptivity. More recently, functional genomics has provided new information on molecular phenotyping of normo-ovulatory women (Talbi et al 2006). The authors convincingly demonstrated that microarray methods are as effective as histological methods in dating the endometrium. By using k-means clustering, a unique molecular signature associated with early proliferative, early secretory, mid-secretory and late secretory phase endometrium was also identified. Whilst studies of miRNA in the female reproductive tract are in their infancy, deletion of 'Dicer', an enzyme involved in miRNA processing, causes multiple reproductive defects that include reduced ovulation rates, loss of embryo integrity and oviductal cysts (Luense et al 2009). Investigations in humans on the role of 'Dicer' may uncover a common function of this enzyme in fertility. Given the ubiquity of RNA silencing, it is likely that developments in understanding failed implantation and subfertility will involve further forays into the field of miRNAs.

Endometriosis

The surgical and medical treatment of endometriosis remains a major area of clinical interest. Current medical strategies seek to induce a pseudomenopause or pseudopregnancy. Newer approaches include the use of aromatase inhibitors, gonadotrophin-releasing hormone antagonists, selective oestrogen modulators and antiprogestins. Alternatively, it might be possible to find new response genes or miRNAs that are differentially expressed in endometriotic lesions compared with eutopic endometrium. A recent investigation showed differential expression of 22 miRNAs in ectopic versus eutopic endometrium (Ohlsson Teague et al 2009). The target pathways appear to involve the *c-jun* and protein kinase B signalling pathways. On this basis, new therapeutic strategies targeting these cascades or the miRNAs implicated offer new direction in the future treatment of endometriosis.

Ovarian cancer

Ovarian epithelial tumours are of several histological subtypes, broadly being divided into serous and mucinous and by the degree of differentiation. A downregulation of miR-21 and several of the let-7 family of miRNAs in ovarian tumours has been reported, while miR-221 expression was raised (Dahiya et al 2008). A recent investigation has also identified that the mRNA for key enzymes 'Drosha' and 'Dicer' that catalyse miRNA biogenesis is reduced by 51% and 60%, respectively, in invasive ovarian cancer. Furthermore, high levels of 'Dicer' and 'Drosha' correlated with increased patient survival (Merritt et al 2008). A study of six types of cancer including ovarian demonstrated that miRNA profiling in tiny volumes (<1 ml) of serum could clearly distinguish between normal donors and cancer patients (Lodes et al 2009). These findings raise the prospect of using less-invasive serum-based assays in ovarian cancer detection and progression.

Conclusions

Whilst the discovery of genes not previously thought to be involved in basic processes of reproduction is clearly important, it is still a long way to understanding their function and even further to developing new treatments. An additional opportunity provided by the new technology is to approach the question of biological function from a slightly different angle. Seldom does one gene exert an overarching effect on cellular function. Rather, the cell acts in response to many genes. Similarly with a tissue, the gene profile of a whole tissue will reflect cell type and the overall state of the many different cells that constitute the tissue. An alternative way of viewing these abundant data is to try to ask questions about the whole data set. In this system, complex patterns of gene expression are sought without making prior judgements about which genes are important or are most likely to be differentially expressed.

It is difficult to imagine new developments in technology that exceed the enormous power and potential of microarrays. However, we are poised at the threshold of a new era of next generation or deep sequencing methods. These platforms offer unparalleled supremacy which will, for the first time, enable comprehensive, integrative interrogation of sequences directly allied to -omics. Deep sequencing surpasses even the power of the newer arrays, while the sheer volume of data produced will require considerably enhanced statistical and computing power.

Microarray techniques have developed beyond cDNA to offer arrays for proteins, phosphoproteins, miRNAs, DNA methylation etc. which will allow a comprehensive interrogation of physiology at several levels. miRNAs have emerged as key players in cancer, with specific miRNAs and miRNA clusters contributing to tumorigenesis and cancer progression. There has been increased research activity into epigenetic mechanisms; the study of gene interactions with the environment. The advent of new knowledge and development of powerful new high-throughput methods is set to dramatically alter the face of medicine, and the era of pharmacogenomics is beckoning. Our hope is that the treatment of diseases that have afflicted women for years will improve significantly as a consequence of the great strides to be expected through RNAi, GWAS and deep sequencing for the improvement of female health globally.

KEY POINTS

1. Mapping of the human genome will define the finite nature of the human condition.

2. The introduction of DNA gene expression microarrays has led scientists to study genome-wide expression profiles, but creates its own difficulties in interpretation.

3. Such techniques allow the study of changes in expression of individual genes as a result of a biological effect. However, in many instances, interactions of several genes are required to induce a protein interaction, or one gene may affect more than one cellular function.

4. High-density arrays initially utilizing large numbers of cDNA fragments or synthesized oligonucleotide arrays have been modified for array-based investigations of miRNAs, DNA methylation, gene promoters, and metabolomic and proteomic expression.

5. The PCR is widely used in order to validate findings from microarrays as it can amplify the signal of interest and make detection of change more apparent. qPCR is the gold standard for DNA array verification.

6. The discovery of small, non-coding miRNAs and siRNAs along with the application of RNAi herald a new era investigating post-transcriptional regulation.

7. GWAS will provide unparalleled insight into genetic variation underpinning complex diseases

8. Deep sequencing platforms with unsurpassed power to date will generate new knowledge on the interactions between genes, RNA and proteins.

9. '-omic' technologies provide powerful and comprehensive tools for understanding reproductive biology. Careful application of the methodology will lead to new insights into disease causation and, potentially, new treatment options.

References

Alon U, Barkai N, Notterman DA et al 1999 Broad patterns of gene expression revealed by clustering analysis of tumor and normal colon tissues probed by oligonucleotide arrays. Proceeding of the National Academy of Sciences of the United States of America 96: 6745–6750.

Baldi P, Vanier MC, Bower JM 1998 On the use of Bayesian methods for evaluating compartmental neural models. Journal of Computational Neuroscience 5: 285–314.

Baldi P, Long AD 2001 A Bayesian framework for the analysis of microarray expression data: regularized t test and statistical inferences of gene changes. Bioinformatics 17: 509–519.

Brazma A, Hingamp P, Quackenbush J et al 2001 Minimum information about a microarray experiment (MIAME) — toward standards for microarray data. Nature Genetics 29: 365–371.

Brown PO, Botstein D 1999 Exploring the new world of the genome with DNA microarrays. Nature Genetics 21: 33–37.

Bustin SA, Benes V, Garson JA et al 2009 The MIQE guidelines: minimum information for publication of quantitative real-time PCR experiments. Clinical Chemistry 55: 611–622.

Carthew RW, Sontheimer EJ 2009 Origins and mechanisms of miRNAs and siRNAs. Cell 136: 642–655.

Collas P 2009 The state-of-the-art of chromatin immunoprecipitation. Methods in Molecular Biology 567: 1–25.

D'Haeseleer P 2005 How does gene expression clustering work? Nature Biotechnology 23: 1499–1501.

Dahiya N, Sherman-Baust CA, Wang TL et al 2008 MicroRNA expression and identification of putative miRNA targets in ovarian cancer. PLoS ONE 3: e2436.

Duggan DJ, Bittner M, Chen Y, Meltzer P, Trent JM 1999 Expression profiling using cDNA microarrays. Nature Genetics 21: 10–14.

Eisen MB, Spellman PT, Brown PO, Botstein D 1998 Cluster analysis and display of genome-wide expression patterns. Proceedings of the National Academy of Sciences of the United States of America 95: 14863–14868.

Fire A, Xu S, Montgomery MK, Kostas SA, Driver SE, Mello CC 1998 Potent and specific genetic interference by double-stranded RNA in *Caenorhabditis elegans*. Nature 391: 806–811.

Frazer KA, Ballinger DG, Cox DR et al 2007 A second generation human haplotype map of over 3.1 million SNPs. Nature 449: 851–861.

Gregory RI, Chendrimada TP, Cooch N, Shiekhattar R 2005 Human RISC couples microRNA biogenesis and posttranscriptional gene silencing. Cell 123: 631–640.

Grimm D 2009 Small silencing RNAs: state-of-the-art. Advanced Drug Delivery Reviews 61: 672–703.

He L, Thomson JM, Hemann MT et al 2005 A microRNA polycistron as a potential human oncogene. Nature 435: 828–833.

Hegde P, Qi R, Abernathy K et al 2000 A concise guide to cDNA microarray analysis. Biotechniques 29: 548–550.

Higuchi R, Dollinger G, Walsh PS, Griffith R 1992 Simultaneous amplification and detection of specific DNA sequences. Biotechnology 10: 413–417.

Hilsenbeck SG, Friedrichs WE, Schiff R et al 1999 Statistical analysis of array expression data as applied to the problem of tamoxifen resistance. Journal of the National Cancer Institute 91: 453–459.

Kerr MK, Churchill GA 2007 Statistical design and the analysis of gene expression microarray data. Genetical Research 89: 509–514.

Kerr G, Ruskin HJ, Crane M, Doolan P 2008 Techniques for clustering gene expression data. Computers in Biology and Medicine 38: 283–293.

Kubista M, Andrade JM, Bengtsson M et al 2006 The real-time polymerase chain reaction. Molecular Aspects of Medicine 27: 95–125.

Lander ES, Linton LM, Birren B et al 2001 Initial sequencing and analysis of the human genome. Nature 409: 860–921.

Lawrie CH 2008 MicroRNA expression in lymphoid malignancies: new hope for diagnosis and therapy? Journal of Cellular and Molecular Medicine 12: 1432–1444.

Lee Y, Jeon K, Lee JT, Kim S, Kim VN 2002 MicroRNA maturation: stepwise processing and subcellular localization. The EMBO Journal 21: 4663–4670.

Little PF 2005 Structure and function of the human genome. Genome Research 15: 1759–1766.

Lodes MJ, Caraballo M, Suciu D, Munro S, Kumar A, Anderson B 2009 Detection of cancer with serum miRNAs on an oligonucleotide microarray. PLoS ONE 4: e6229.

Luense LJ, Carletti MZ, Christenson LK 2009 Role of Dicer in female fertility. Trends in Endocrinology and Metabolism 20: 265–272.

Meister G, Landthaler M, Peters L et al 2005 Identification of novel argonaute-associated proteins. Current Biology 15: 2149–2155.

Merritt WM, Lin YG, Han LY et al 2008 Dicer, Drosha, and outcomes in patients with ovarian cancer. New England Journal of Medicine 359: 2641–2650.

Nica AC, Dermitzakis ET 2008 Using gene expression to investigate the genetic basis of complex disorders. Human Molecular Genetics 17: R129–R134.

Ohlsson Teague EM, Van der Hoek KH, Van der Hoek MB et al 2009 MicroRNA-regulated pathways associated with endometriosis. Molecular Endocrinology 23: 265–275.

Pearson TA, Manolio TA 2008 How to interpret a genome-wide association study. Journal of the American Medical Association 299: 1335–1344.

Pfaffl MW 2001 A new mathematical model for relative quantification in real-time RT-PCR. Nucleic Acids Research 29: e45.

Reimers M 2005 Statistical analysis of microarray data. Addiction Biology 10: 23–35.

Ridker PM, Chasman DI, Zee RY et al 2008 Rationale, design, and methodology of the Women's Genome Health Study: a genome-wide association study of more than 25,000 initially healthy american women. Clinical Chemistry 54: 249–255.

Schena M, Shalon D, Davis RW, Brown PO 1995 Quantitative monitoring of gene expression patterns with a complementary DNA microarray. Science 270: 467–470.

Sherwin R, Catalano R, Sharkey A 2006 Large-scale gene expression studies of the endometrium: what have we learnt? Reproduction 132: 1–10.

Shipp MA, Ross KN, Tamayo P et al 2002 Diffuse large B-cell lymphoma outcome prediction by gene-expression profiling and supervised machine learning. Nature Medicine 8: 68–74.

Stranger BE, Dermitzakis ET 2006 From DNA to RNA to disease and back: the 'central dogma' of regulatory disease variation. Human Genomics 2: 383–390.

Talbi S, Hamilton AE, Vo KC et al 2006 Molecular phenotyping of human endometrium distinguishes menstrual cycle phases and underlying biological processes in normo-ovulatory women. Endocrinology 147: 1097–1121.

Tamayo P, Slonim D, Mesirov J et al 1999 Interpreting patterns of gene expression with self-organizing maps: methods and application to hematopoietic differentiation. Proceedings of the National Academy of Sciences of the United States of America 96: 2907–2912.

Tavazoie S, Hughes JD, Campbell MJ, Cho RJ, Church GM 1999 Systematic determination of genetic network architecture. Nature Genetics 22: 281–285.

Thalamuthu A, Mukhopadhyay I, Zheng X, Tseng GC 2006 Evaluation and comparison of gene clustering methods in microarray analysis. Bioinformatics 22: 2405–2412.

Tomari Y, Zamore PD 2005 Perspective: machines for RNAi. Genes and Development 19: 517–529.

Tusher VG, Tibshirani R, Chu G 2001 Significance analysis of microarrays applied to the ionizing radiation response. Proceedings of the National Academy of Sciences of the United States of America 98: 5116–5121.

Vandesompele J, De Preter K, Pattyn F et al 2002 Accurate normalization of real-time quantitative RT-PCR data by geometric averaging of multiple internal control genes. Genome Biology 3: RESEARCH0034.11.

Venter JC, Adams MD, Myers EW et al 2001 The sequence of the human genome. Science 291: 1304–1351.

Wathelet MG, Lin CH, Parekh BS, Ronco LV, Howley PM, Maniatis T 1998 Virus infection induces the assembly of coordinately activated transcription factors on the IFN-beta enhancer in vivo. Molecular Cell 1: 507–518.

Wellcome Trust Case Control Consortium 2007 Genome-wide association study of 14,000 cases of seven common diseases and 3,000 shared controls. Nature 447: 661–678.

Wittwer CT, Herrmann MG, Moss AA, Rasmussen RP 1997 Continuous fluorescence monitoring of rapid cycle DNA amplification. Biotechniques 22: 130–131, 134–138.

Yi R, Qin Y, Macara IG, Cullen BR 2003 Exportin-5 mediates the nuclear export of pre-microRNAs and short hairpin RNAs. Genes and Development 17: 3011–3016.

Sexual differentiation: normal and abnormal

D. Keith Edmonds

Chapter Contents

INTRODUCTION	166	ANOMALOUS VAGINAL DEVELOPMENT	174
NORMAL EMBRYOLOGICAL DEVELOPMENT OF THE REPRODUCTIVE SYSTEM	166	MALFORMATIONS OF THE UTERUS	177
INTERSEX DISORDERS	169	KEY POINTS	179
46XY DISORDERS OF SEXUAL DEVELOPMENT	172		

Introduction

Sexual differentiation and its control are fundamental to the continuation of most species. The understanding of this process has advanced greatly in recent years, but before abnormalities of these disorders can be discussed, an understanding of normal sexual development is important. At fertilization, the haploid gametes unite and the conceptus contains 46 chromosomes with 22 autosomes derived from each of the gametes (i.e. sperm and ovum). The ovum donates one X chromosome and the sperm donates either one X or one Y chromosome; the axiom of mammalian reproduction is that a 46XX embryo will differentiate into a female, and a 46XY embryo becomes a male. It is, however, the presence or absence of the Y chromosome which determines whether the undifferentiated gonad becomes a testis or an ovary, and therefore the development of a male or female of the species.

Normal Embryological Development of the Reproductive System

Although chromosomal sex is determined at the time of fertilization, gonadal sex results from the differentiation of the indifferent undifferentiated gonad which becomes either a testis or an ovary. This begins during the fifth week of embryological development; at this time, an area of coelemic epithelium develops on the medial aspect of the urogenital ridge, and proliferation leads to the establishment of the gonadal ridge. Epithelial cords then grow into the mesenchyme (primary sex cords), and the gonad now possesses an outer cortex and an inner medulla. In XY individuals, the medulla becomes the testis and the cortex regresses. In embryos with an XX complement, the cortex differentiates to become an ovary and the medulla regresses. The primor-

dial germ cells develop by the fourth week in the endodermal cells of the yolk sac, and during the fifth week, they migrate along the dorsal mesentery of the hindgut to the gonadal ridges, eventually becoming incorporated into the mesenchyme and the primary sex cords by the end of the sixth week (Figure 13.1).

Development of the testis

The primary sex cords become concentrated on the medulla of the gonad and proliferate, and their ends anastomose to form the rete testis. The sex cords become isolated by the development of a capsule called the 'tunica albuginea' and the developing sex cords become the seminiferous tubules. Mesenchyme grows between the tubes to separate them (Leydig cells). The seminiferous tubules are composed of two layers of cells: supporting cells (Sertoli cells) derived from the germinal epithelium, and spermatogonia derived from the primordial germ cells (Figure 13.1).

Development of the ovary

The development of the ovary is much slower than that of the testis, and the ovary is not evident until the 10th week. Now, the primary sex cords regress and finally disappear. Around 12 weeks, secondary sex cords arise from the germinal epithelium, and the primordial germ cells become incorporated into these cortical cords. At 16 weeks, these cortical cords break up to form isolated groups of cells called 'primordial follicles'; each cell contains an oogonium derived from a primordial germ cell, surrounded by follicular cells arising from the cortical cords. These oogonia undergo rapid mitosis to increase the numbers to thousands of germ cells called 'primary oocytes'. Each oocyte is surrounded by a layer of follicular cells, the structure being called a 'primary follicle'. The surrounding mesenchyme becomes the stroma.

DOI: 10.1016/B978-0-7020-3120-5.00013-8

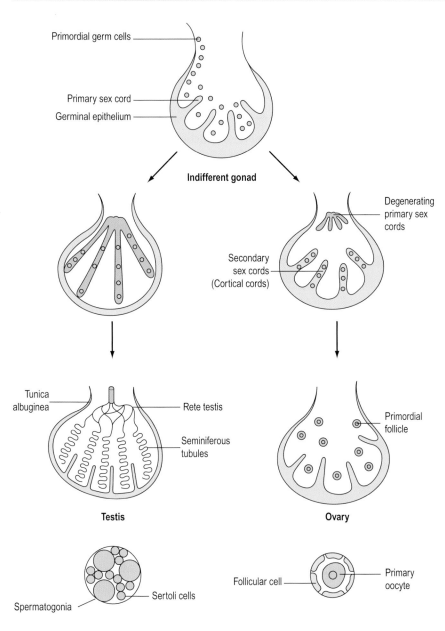

Figure 13.1 Normal gonadal differentiation.

Genetic control of gonadal development
(Figure 13.2)

The pathway which controls the genetic interaction which transforms intermediate mesoderm to the bipotential gonad is beginning to be understood. It is now possible to identify with certainty two genes that are associated with this process. These two genes are Wilms' tumour gene (*WT1*) and *FTZ1*. *WT1* has been found on chromosome 11, p13 and regulates DNA transcriptase (Hastie 1994, Dong et al 1997). *FTZ1* produces steroidogenic factor 1 (*SF-1*), and this has been found to be required for differentiation to the bipotential gonad (Wilhelm et al 2007).

As the presence of a Y chromosome is essential for testicular differentiation, the localization of testicular-determining factor (TDF) which was localized at the short arm of the Y chromosome using cloning and DNA sequencing tech-

niques, and the gene determining TDF was sequenced and designated *SRY* (sex-determining region Y gene) (Guellaen et al 1984, Behlke et al 1993). The second gene which is involved in the differentiation of the testis is known as *SOX9*, and this gene coexists with the *SRY* gene in its homeobox and is a regulator of DNA transcription. *SOX9* gene expression is increased in male gonadal differentiation and decreased in female gonadal differentiation. *SOX9* has also recently been shown to be a regulator of type II collagen which is involved in the formation of cartilage (Lefebvre et al 1997). The *DAX1* gene is responsible for development of the receptor on the surface of the undifferentiated gonad, which allows *SRY* and *SOX9* to differentiate the gonad to become a testis. Following the development of Leydig cells and Sertoli cells, *SF-1* is involved in the control of steroid hydroxylases, and P450 aromatase causes an increase in the synthesis of testosterone and a reduction in the conversion

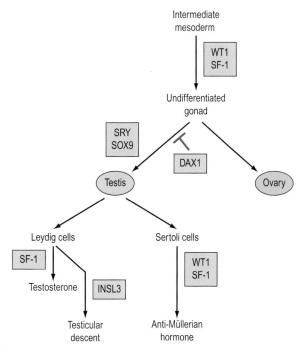

Figure 13.2 Diagram showing genetic control of gonadal development.

Box 13.1 Non-mosaic sex chromosome aneuploidy

- Kleinfelter's syndrome — infertile male
  47XXY
  48XXYY
  48XXXY
- 47XYY syndrome — fertile male
- Turner's syndrome
  45X — ovarian dysgenesis
- 47XXX syndrome — subfertile female

---

of androgens to oestrogens, leading to a contribution to testicular regulation (Ogata 2008). In combination with ST1, it is also responsible for Sertoli cells producing anti-Müllerian hormone. Following differentiation, Leydig cells produce insulin-like 3 (*INSL3*) gene, expression of which leads to testicular descent and shortening of the gubernaculums (Foresta and Ferlin 2004).

The genes involved in ovarian differentiation are much more difficult to define, although *DAX1* expression continues during ovarian differentiation. Therefore, it is suggested that *DAX1* antagonizes the actions of the *SRY* gene (Swain et al 1998).

Sex chromosome anomalies

Variations may occur in the number or the structure of chromosomes in a mosaic or a non-mosaic form. The non-mosiac forms are summarized in Box 13.1.

Aneuploidy

Aneuploidy may result from the non-disjunction of either miotic division or in either parent or in an early cleavage of the zygote. Some are more common in the offsprig of older women (e.g. 47XX and 47XXY), and the non-disjunction is presumed to arise mainly in the maternal miosis. The occurrence of 45X does not seem to be related to maternal age.

Although there are a wide range of clinical effects, some generalizations can be made:

- if there is a Y chromosome, the phenotype is usually male;
- if the number of sex chromosomes increases beyond three, there is a strong tendency to some degree of mental retardation;
- an additional Y chromosome tends to increase height;
- provided there is at least one Y chromosome, one or more extra chromosomes result in hypogonadism; and
- in each somatic cell, only one X chromosome is active; others are inactivated.

Kleinfelter's syndrome and XYY syndrome occur in approximately one in 700 newborn males, the clinical features of which are well recognized. These include hypogonadism, infertility, increased risk of testicular cancer, gynaecomastia, increased risk of male breast cancer, and sparse facial and body hair.

Turner's syndrome results from a chromosome constitution of a missing X chromosome. The overall incidence of this condition is approximately one in 2500 female births, but many of these have a mosaic pattern with a chromosome constitution of 46XX/45X. Small stature is invariable and gonadal failure is usual. There are other somatic features such as web neck, low hairline, cubitus valgus, pigmented naevi and cardiovascular anomalies, particularly coarctation of the aorta. These individuals do not have systematic impairment of the intellect, but they have some impairment of spacial ability.

XXX syndrome arises in approximately one in 1200 live female births, and no consistent clinical syndrome is associated with this.

Mosaicism

This is more common for sex chromosomes than for autosomes and arises when two cell lines arise from a single zygote due to non-disjunction in an early mitosis. The most common are 46XX and 46XY accompanied by a 45X cell line. The clinical effects are wide ranging depending on the balance of the mosaicism.

Structural abnormalities of X chromosomes

Apart from the number of X chromosomes in mosaicism, there are a number of possible variations within the X chromosome in the female. The X chromosome carries a large number of genes, not all of which have been delineated but some of which are responsible for metabolic and development disorders, and the gene map for the X chromosome is constantly being updated. If there is one normal X chromosome and the other is abnormal, inactivation of the abnormal X chromosome usually occurs in the somatic cells and this tends to diminish the effect of the abnormality, except in the ovary. Although only one X chromosome is sufficient for early ovarian development, germ cell maintenance requires several loci on the second X chromosome and on autosomes (Figure 13.3) (Simpson 1999).

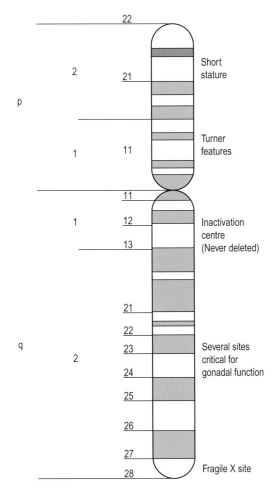

Figure 13.3 Diagram of banded chromatid of X chromosome indicating the main numerical locations, on the left. On the right, phenotypic effects of some sites affected by deletions or variations are noted (based on data in Therman and Susman 1993 and Simpson 1999).

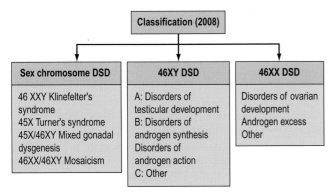

Figure 13.4 2008 classification of inter-sex disorders. DSD, disorders of sexual development.

Intersex Disorders

Intersex disorders are best classified into three groups (see Figure 13.4). This classification was suggested by Hughes (2008) as a new simple classification which includes all disorders of intersex.

Female (46XX) disorders of sexual development

Definition

This group of disorders comprises conditions in which masculinization of the external genitalia occurs in patients with a normal 46XX karyotype. The degree of masculinization is variable, ranging from mild clitoromegaly to complete fusion of the labial folds with a penile urethra.

Pathophysiology

The abnormalities occur when a female fetus is exposed to elevated levels of androgens. As the differentiation of the external genitalia to male or female depends on the conversion of testosterone to dihydrotestosterone (DHT) in the tissues of the cloaca, the presence of DHT leads to male-type development. If the female fetus is exposed to low levels of androgen, partial masculinization may occur, leading to ambiguous genitalia; however, if the levels are sufficiently high, complete male external genital development may occur, although the testes are naturally absent. If androgen exposure is delayed until after 12 weeks, virilization is limited to clitoral enlargement with no effect on the already differentiated labia. Androgens have no effect on internal sexual development, and therefore the ovaries, uterus and upper vagina are normally formed and functional.

Aetiology

The causes of androgenization are due to excessive androgens either:

- arising in a fetus (e.g. congenital adrenal hyperplasia);
- arising in the mother (e.g. androgen-secreting tumour); or
- ingested by the mother (e.g. progestogens, danazol).

There are also cases which are associated with other congenital abnormalities or which are idiopathic.

Congenital adrenal hyperplasia

Pathophysiology

This is the most common cause of female pseudohermaphroditism and is an autosomal-recessive disorder resulting in enzyme deficiency in the biosynthesis of cortisol in the adrenal gland. Cortisol production occurs in the zona fasciculata and zona reticularis (Figure 13.5), and is controlled by adrenocorticotrophic hormone (ACTH) secreted by the pituitary gland. Adrenal androgen production occurs in the same area and is influenced by ACTH. A deficiency in any enzyme in the pathway results in decreased production of cortisol with resultant elevated levels of ACTH. This leads to increased steroid production by the adrenal reticularis and consequent hyperplasia. The stimulation by ACTH elevates the levels of circulating androgens, and this results in virilization of the female fetus.

There are three adrenal enzyme deficiencies which result in masculinization: 21-hydroxylase, 11-hydroxylase and 3β-dehydrogenase deficiency.

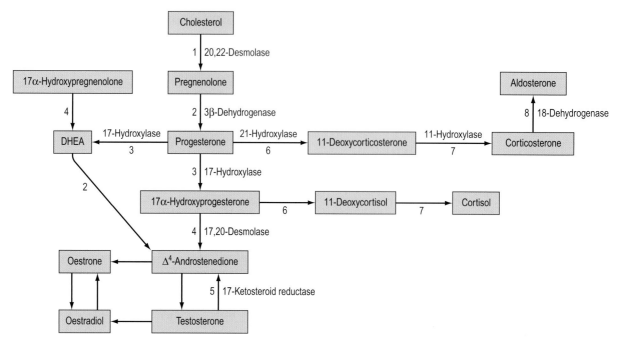

Figure 13.5 Adrenal synthesis of steroids.

21-Hydroxylase deficiency

This accounts for 90% of all cases of congenital adrenal hyperplasia. The deficiency results in an increase in progesterone and 17α-hydroxyprogesterone, and this substrate is therefore converted to androstenedione and subsequently to testosterone. Failure of 21-hydroxylase to convert progesterone to 11-deoxycorticosterone may result in aldosterone deficiency; this occurs in approximately two-thirds of cases and is the so-called 'salt-losing' type of congenital adrenal hyperplasia.

Aetiology

Deficiency of 21-hydroxylase is an autosomal-recessive disorder. The link between human leukocyte antigen (HLA) type and 21-hydroxylase deficiency was established by Dupont et al (1977), and this allowed mapping of the gene which was located on the short arm of chromosome 6. It is located between the HLA-B and HLA-DR loci, and subgroups of HLA-B have been closely linked to congenital adrenal hyperplasia type: HLA-BW47 is linked to salt-losing congenital adrenal hyperplasia and HLA-BW51 is linked to the simple virilizing form. Studies by Donohoue et al (1986) have shown that there are two 21-hydroxylase genes: *21-OHA* and *21-OHB*. Only one is active (*21-OHB*) and they both lie between the fourth components of complement C4A and C4B. A variety of mutations have been reported, including gene deletions of *21-OHB*, gene conversions and point mutations.

Epidemiology

The incidence of 21-hydroxylase deficiency is between one in 5000 and one in 15,000, based on neonatal screening programmes (Cacciari et al 1983), although a higher incidence (one in 700) has been reported in specific populations of Eskimos (Pang et al 1982). The incidence of the non-classic form of the disease, when androgenization fails to appear before late childhood or puberty, is much more common; approximately one in 300 in the White population and one in 30 in European Jews (Pang et al 1988).

Presentation

Affected females are born with an enlarged clitoris, fused labioscrotal folds and a urogenital sinus which may become a phallic urethra. There is often great variation in the degree of masculinization of the external genitalia; this is classified according to Prader (1958).

The internal genitalia develop normally as they are not influenced by androgens.

In salt-losing congenital adrenal hyperplasia, the infants develop dehydration, hypotension and hyponatraemia between 7 and 28 days of age, known as a 'salt-losing crisis'. Non-salt-losing congenital adrenal hyperplasia tends to cause less severe masculinization than the salt-losing type. In general, all children born with ambiguous genitalia, including cryptorchidism and hypospadias, should be screened for congenital adrenal hyperplasia. Without treatment, severe salt-losing disease is fatal.

When an infant is born with ambiguous genitalia, the management of the parents is very important. It is helpful to reassure them that the infant is healthy and that there is a developmental anomaly of the genitalia. If the initial examination of the child fails to identify palpable gonads, it is most likely that the child is female and the parents should be informed as such; the likelihood of congenital adrenal hyperplasia may be raised. The diagnosis must then be made with as much haste as possible to alleviate parental anxiety.

Investigation

The initial investigations are karyotyping, pelvic ultrasound and endocrine studies. The karyotype may be performed on a sample of cord blood or on a venous sample, and rapid results obtained. Pelvic ultrasound to discover the presence of a uterus and vagina will confirm the diagnosis. The specific diagnosis is made by measuring 17α-hydroxyprogesterone in serum, although a 24-h urinary estimate of 17-ketosteroids will also confirm the diagnosis.

Treatment

This is divided into four parts.

Acute salt-losing crisis

This involves correcting the electrolyte imbalance and replacing the cortisol deficiency with deoxycorticosterone acetate (DOCA), 1 mg/24 h. For the majority of cases, 9α-fludrocortisol is used at a dose of 0.1–0.2 mg/day added to the oral feed, and the dosage of DOCA or fludrocortisol is adjusted against the electrolyte levels.

Long-term cortisol replacement therapy

Although previous reports suggested that mineralocorticoid therapy could be discontinued after infancy (Newns 1974), more recent data suggest that it is essential to continue therapy for life (Hughes et al 1979).

Surgical correction

Once the sex of rearing has been established as female, some attempt to feminize the genitalia may be made, usually within the first 18 months of life. If the clitoris is enlarged, a reduction clitoridectomy can be performed and the perineal region modified (Edmonds 1989). There are major surgical problems associated with severe virilization in congenital adrenal hyperplasia. The urogenital sinus has been formed by labial fold fusion and the folds are usually thin, but may be thick with associated narrowing of the lower vagina, especially in salt-losers. If the labial folds are thin, division by a simple posterior incision may be performed around 3 or 4 years of age. However, thick perineal tissue should be left until after puberty, and no attempt at surgery should be made until the girl is physically and mentally sexually mature. The operation, when it is performed, involves a flap vaginoplasty with a pedicle graft of labia used to recreate the vagina. Alternatively, a Williams vaginoplasty may be used.

Mulaikal et al (1987) reviewed the fertility rates in 80 women with 21-hydroxylase deficiency; of 25 with the simple form who attempted pregnancy, 15 were successful, whereas only one of the salt-losers who tried to become pregnant succeeded. There is no doubt that a major reason for the failure of the salt-losing group is the disappointing results of surgery and subsequent lack of adequate sexual function.

Psychological support

As the child grows, long-term psychological guidance and support will be required for the parents initially and then the child.

Prenatal diagnosis

If the parents are heterozygous carriers of 21-hydroxylase deficiency, the fetus has a one in four chance of being affected. Thus, prenatal diagnosis is important, either by amniocentesis to measure levels of 17-hydroxyprogesterone in amniotic fluid, HLA typing of amniotic cells, or chorionic villus sampling and the use of specific DNA probes. Once the diagnosis has been made, the option is available to treat the pregnant woman with oral dexamethasone, which crosses the placenta and suppresses the secretion of ACTH and thus the circulating androgen levels.

11-Hydroxylase deficiency

This is the hypertensive form of congenital adrenal hyperplasia which accounts for approximately 5–8% of all cases (Zachmann et al 1983). The absence of 11-hydroxylase leads to elevated levels of 11-deoxycorticosterone (DOC), and although this means a decreased amount of aldosterone, DOC has salt-retaining properties, leading to hypertension. Androstenedione levels are also elevated and this can result in ambiguous genitalia.

The diagnosis is made by measuring elevated levels of urinary 17-hydroxycorticosteroids and raised serum androstenedione. Treatment is similar to 21-hydroxylase deficiency, with glucocorticoid replacement therapy.

The genetics, however, are rather different. There is no HLA association with 11-hydroxylase deficiency, but the use of a DNA probe has located the gene on the long arm of chromosome 8 (White et al 1985).

3β-Dehydrogenase deficiency

This rare form of congenital adrenal hyperplasia results in a block of steroidogenesis very early in the pathway, giving rise to severe salt-losing adrenal hyperplasia. The androgen most elevated is dehydroepiandrosterone, an androgen which causes mild virilization. The diagnosis rests on the measurement of elevated dehydroepiandrosterone. The gene encoding 3β-dehydrogenase has not yet been cloned but it is not linked to HLA.

Androgen-secreting tumours

Androgen-secreting tumours are rare in pregnancy, but may arise in the ovary or the adrenal gland. They cause fetal virilization. When they occur in the non-pregnant woman, anovulation is induced.

Ovary

A number of androgen-secreting tumours have been reported, including luteoma (Hensleigh and Woodruff 1978, Cohen et al 1982), polycystic ovaries (Fayez et al 1974), mucinous cystadenoma (Novak et al 1970, Post et al 1978), arrhenoblastoma (Barkan et al 1984) and Krukenberg tumours (Connor et al 1968, Forest et al 1978). Not all female fetuses will be affected and there is no association with gestation and exposure. The fetus may be partly protected by the conversion of the maternally derived androgen to oestrogen in the placenta, and thus the degree of virilization is variable.

Adrenal gland

There are only two reports of adrenal adenomas causing fetal masculinization (Murset et al 1970, Fuller et al 1983). These tumours may be responsive to human chorionic gonadotrophin, and thus levels of androgen may be higher in pregnancy than in the non-pregnant state, leading to androgenization of the fetus.

Drugs

The association between the use of progestogens and masculinization of the female fetus has received much publicity, but the only progestogen proven to have such an effect is 17-ethinyl testosterone (Ishizuka et al 1962). These infants had clitoromegaly and, in some cases, labioscrotal fusion, but the risk is very small (one in 50). Gestogens which are derived from testosterone should be avoided in the pregnant woman. There have been two case reports of androgenization of female fetuses from exposure to danazol during pregnancy (Castro-Magana et al 1981, Duck and Katamaya 1981), and both babies were born with external genitalia similar to those with adrenogenital syndrome.

Associated multiple congenital abnormalities

Female intersex has been described in association with a number of multiple abnormality states, most commonly those in association with the urinary and gastrointestinal tracts. It has also been described in association with VATER (Vertebrae, Anus, Trachea, Oesophagus and Renal) syndrome (Say and Carpentier 1979).

The management of these children with masculinized genitalia is to ensure the assignation of a sex of rearing, and to modify the genitalia appropriately. In all of these rare cases, the female role has been chosen and reduction clitoroplasty performed.

46XY Disorders of Sexual Development

The normal differentiation of the gonad to become a testis has been described above, and its subsequent secretion of testosterone leads to development of the Wolffian duct and the urogenital sinus to produce the normal male internal and external genitalia. Testosterone is the predominant male sex hormone secreted by the testis, but two other processes are necessary for normal development: the conversion of testosterone to DHT by 5α-reductase, and the presence of androgen receptors in the target cell which bind with the DHT or testosterone and produce appropriate nuclear function. Thus, a normal male genotype (i.e. XY) with a female phenotype will occur if there is:

- failure of testicular development;
- error(s) in testosterone biosynthesis; or
- androgen insensitivity at the target site.

Failure of testicular development

This group of disorders includes true gonadal dysgenesis, Leydig cell hypoplasia and the persistent Müllerian duct syndrome.

True gonadal dysgenesis

True gonadal dysgenesis is characterized by streak gonads, normal Müllerian structures and normal external female genitalia. It has been suggested that the streak gonads in these individuals were originally ovaries which contained oogonia which then subsequently underwent massive atresia, in a similar fashion to Turner's syndrome. The karyo-type is either 46XY or 46XX, and these patients usually present in their teenage years with failure of pubertal development.

46XY partial gonadal dysgenesis

In this condition, the infants are born with ambiguous genitalia, which results from the partially dysgenetic development of the testis. The dysgenetic gonads have various histological arrangements, with poor seminiferous tubules. However, some androgen can be produced by these testes, which results in partial androgenization of the external genitalia, leading to the genital ambiguity. These children have a high risk of gonadal tumours, especially gonadoblastoma, and in these circumstances, the gonads should be removed early to prevent this development.

Leydig cell hypoplasia

Leydig cell hypoplasia is an uncommon condition of which the aetiology remains speculative. The role of fetal luteinizing hormone in normal testicular development is unknown, but it may be necessary for maturation of the interstitial cells into Leydig cells. Failure of luteinizing hormone production in the first trimester will result in Leydig cell hypoplasia and male pseudohermaphroditism (or an autosomal-recessive disorder resulting in absent luteinizing hormone receptors will cause absence of Leydig cells). This manifests as ambiguous genitalia, in both circumstances due to some androgen production by Sertoli cells. Clinically, Leydig cell hypoplasia usually presents as a phenotypical female with primary amenorrhoea and sexual infantilism, but ambiguity at birth may result in diagnosis in infancy.

46XY true hermaphroditism

These individuals have the presence of both testicular and ovarian tissue with a 46XY karyotype. It has been suggested that mutation of the *SRY* gene may be the aetiology of this (Berkovitz and Seeherunvong 1998).

46XX sex reversal

This nomenclature is used to describe the situation in which testicular tissue develops in someone with a 46XX karyotype. If testicular development is normal, they are referred to as '46XX males', but when testicular determination is incomplete, they are referred to as '46XX true hermaphrodites'. In 46XX males, the external genitalia are usually normal or a small percentage may have hypospadias. Clinically, they do not present until puberty, when this is delayed due to failure to be able to produce testosterone and due to the degeneration of seminiferous tubules and Leydig cell hyperplasia, which seems to occur just prior to puberty. It seems that in the majority of these individuals, the sex reversal is related to the translocation of Y chromosome sequences, including the *SRY* gene from the paternal Y chromosome to the paternal X chromosome (Tomomasa et al 1999). However, one-third of individuals are not found to have Y chromosome sequences in their DNA, and this means that there must be a mutation in the genomic DNA which permits testicular determination to occur in the absence of TDF. These gene defects remain to be explained.

Errors in testosterone biosynthesis

This type of disorder accounts for only 4% of XY females, and results from deficiency of an enzyme involved in testosterone synthesis (see Figure 13.5).

20,22-Desmolase deficiency

Absence of this enzyme results in failure to convert cholesterol to pregnenolone, and a failure of subsequent steroid production. Most of the reported cases have died in early childhood due to adrenal insufficiency, but the XY individuals are all partially virilized with a small blind vaginal pouch. It is considered to be an autosomal-recessive disorder.

3β-Hydroxysteroid dehydrogenase deficiency

This is a rare disorder which affects both adrenal and gonadal function and is again autosomally recessive. The deficiency may be complete or incomplete, and thus the degree of virilization is variable, with various degrees of hypospadias or a small blind vagina with normal internal male genitalia and absent Müllerian structures. Those individuals who have survived and reached puberty have developed gynaecomastia, presumably because the absence of testosterone during fetal life has allowed breast bud development. The diagnosis is made by elevated levels of pregnenolone and 17-hydroxypregnenolone, and low levels of corticosteroids and testosterone.

17α-Hydroxylase deficiency

This syndrome produces a phenotype in XY individuals varying from normal female external genitalia and a blind vaginal pouch to hypospadias with a small phallus. The diagnosis is usually only made in adulthood with failure to develop secondary sexual characteristics. The impaired adrenal production of cortisol is not associated with clinical symptoms as the elevated levels of corticosterone compensate. The gonads should be removed if the patient is assigned a female gender and hormone replacement therapy instituted.

17,20-Desmolase deficiency

This enzyme defect primarily affects testosterone production and there is no adrenal insufficiency. The clinical findings range from normal female to undervirilized male genitalia, and the endocrine findings are of very low serum levels of testosterone with normal corticosteroids. Again, diagnosis may not be made until failure of pubertal development.

17-Ketosteroid reductase deficiency

This enzyme is responsible for the reversible conversion of androstenedione to testosterone and oestrone to oestradiol. These patients almost always present at birth with female external genitalia and testes in the inguinal canal, and undergo masculinization at puberty. Those individuals to be raised as females should have their gonads removed before puberty and oestrogen therapy started at puberty.

Androgen insensitivity at the target site (Table 13.1)

In this group of patients, testicular function is normal and circulating levels of androgen are consistent with normal male development. The majority of patients present at puberty with primary amenorrhoea, but some will present with ambiguous genitalia. The defect may be 5α-reductase deficiency or complete or partial androgen insensitivity.

5α-Reductase deficiency

This results in failure of the conversion of testosterone to DHT in target tissues and thus a failure of masculinization of the site. In infancy, there is usually a small phallus, some degree of hypospadias, a bifid scrotum and a blind vaginal pouch. The testes are found either in the inguinal canal or in the labioscrotal folds, and Müllerian structures are absent. At puberty, elevated levels of androgen lead to masculinization, including an increase in phallic growth, although this remains smaller than normal. Seminal production has been reported (Petersen et al 1977).

It is an autosomal-recessive trait and the resulting enzyme defect gives predictable hormone profiles with normal levels of testosterone but low levels of DHT. The diagnosis is important in individuals born with ambiguous genitalia in order to assign the sex of rearing, and this should be based on the potential for normal sexual function in adult life. The gonads should be removed if the sex of rearing is to be female, and oestrogen replacement therapy is instituted at puberty.

Complete androgen insensitivity

This is an X-linked recessive disorder characterized by the clinical features of normal female external genitalia, a blind

Table 13.1 Types of androgen insensitivity and their abnormalities

Defect	External genitalia	Internal genitalia	Gonad	Phenotype at puberty
5α-Reductase deficiency	Female or ambiguous	Male	Testis	Masculine
Complete androgen insensitivity	Female	Male	Testis	Infantile and breast growth
Partial androgen insensitivity	Ambiguous	Male	Testis	Partial masculine and breast growth

vaginal pouch, and absent Müllerian and Wolffian structures. The testes are found either in the labial folds, the inguinal canal or may be intra-abdominal.

These patients may lack the androgen receptor and may be shown to lack the gene located on the X chromosome between Xp11 and Xq13. Work by Brown et al (1982), however, suggests that there may be a variety of defects, ranging from absence of receptors to presence of a normal number of receptors which are inactive. The exact mechanism of the defects in patients with androgen receptors awaits definition.

The hormonal levels of testosterone which are elevated above normal due to increased luteinizing hormone production and the associated increase in testicular oestradiol and peripheral conversion of androgens to oestradiol promotes some breast development. Pubic hair growth depends on the degree of insensitivity but is usually rather scanty.

Patients either present with a hernial mass or with primary amenorrhoea despite secondary sexual characteristics; karyotyping makes the diagnosis. The gonads should be removed because of the malignant potential. The vagina may be of variable length and may be adequate, but those with a short vaginal pouch may need manual dilatation.

Partial androgen insensitivity

This is a complex condition which has been found to be due to a reduced binding affinity of DHT to the receptor or because the receptor binds the DHT but there are defects in the transcription to the nucleus. It is an X-linked recessive disorder and the partial expression means inevitable ambiguous genitalia with a blind vaginal pouch and phallic enlargement. The penis can be normal. The Wolffian ducts can be rudimentary or normal, but the testes are azoospermic. The most common presentation in infancy is hypospadias, with the urethra opening at the base of the phallus, and there may be cryptorchidism. At puberty, male secondary sexual characteristics develop poorly, but there is usually gynaecomastia. The management is dependent on the degree of ambiguity and subsequent choice of sex of rearing, with gonadectomy and hormone replacement therapy for those assigned a female role.

Anomalous Vaginal Development

When the vagina does not develop normally, a number of abnormalities have been described. The vagina may be partially maldeveloped, leading to a vaginal obstruction which may be complete or incomplete, or there may be total maldevelopment of the Müllerian ducts leading to various disorders.

Classification

Vaginal anomalies may be categorized as follows:

- congenital absence of the Müllerian ducts (the Mayer–Rokitansky–Kuster–Hauser syndrome);
- disorders of vertical fusion; and
- failure of lateral fusion.

Aetiology

Three mechanisms explain most vaginal anomalies. They may be familial; for example, XY females who have a hereditary disorder as described previously. Congenital absence of the vagina has been very rarely reported in XX siblings (Jones and Mermut 1974), and also in monozygotic twins with only one child affected (Lischke et al 1973).

The case of a female-limited autosomal-dominant trait was first reported by Shokeir (1978) who studied 16 Saskatchewan families in which there was a proband with vaginal agenesis. However, Carson et al (1983), in a study of 23 probands, disputed Shokeir's theory. The previous evidence with regard to monozygotic twins also makes this mode of inheritance unlikely. Polygenic or multifactorial inheritance does, however, offer some explanation that families may exhibit the trait as reported. The recurrent risk of a polygenic multifactorial trait in first-degree relatives is reported to be between 1% and 5%.

Finally, it is possible that Müllerian duct defects could be secondary to teratogens or other environmental factors, but no definite association has been demonstrated.

Epidemiology

The incidence of vaginal malformations has been variously estimated at between one in 4000 and one in 10,000 female births (Evans et al 1981). The infrequency of this anomaly makes accurate estimates of the true incidence very difficult to obtain, but when considered as a cause of primary amenorrhoea, vaginal malformation ranks second to gonadal dysgenesis.

Pathophysiology

The pathophysiology of vaginal absence may be either as a result of failure of the vaginal plate to form or failure of cavitation. Absence of the uterus and fallopian tubes indicates total failure of Müllerian duct development, but in the Rokitansky syndrome, the uterus is often present, although rudimentary, and therefore it must be failure of vaginal plate formation and subsequent vaginal development which leads to the absent vagina. Vertical fusion defects (Figure 13.6) may result from failure of fusion of the Müllerian system with the urogenital sinus, or may be due to incomplete canalization of the vagina. Disorders of lateral fusion are due to the failure of the Müllerian ducts to unite, and may create a duplicated uterovaginal septum which may be obstructive or non-obstructive, depending on the mode of development (Figure 13.7).

Presentation

Vaginal atresia

Vaginal atresia presents at puberty with complicated or uncomplicated primary amenorrhoea. In the majority who have an absent or rudimentary uterus, uncomplicated primary amenorrhoea is the presenting symptom, but those women who have a functional uterus may develop an associated haematometra and present with cyclical abdominal pain. If a haematometra does develop, there will be uterine distension and an abdominal mass may be palpable, but more commonly, it is felt on rectal examination.

Vertical fusion defects

Here, the transverse vaginal septum prevents loss of menstrual blood and therefore cryptomenorrhoea results. Most patients present as teenagers with cyclical abdominal pain, and a haematocolpos will be palpable within the pelvis on rectal examination. The patient may also present with associated pressure symptoms of urinary frequency and/or reten-

tion. The incidence of vertical fusion defects is reported as 46% high, 35% mid and 19% low septae in the vagina (Rock et al 1982).

Disorders of lateral fusion

These patients usually present with the incidental finding of a vaginal septum which is usually asymptomatic. It may first be diagnosed during pregnancy, at which time excision will be necessary to ensure a vaginal delivery. However, these patients may present with dyspareunia caused by the septum, and in most cases, one vagina is larger than the other and intercourse may have occurred partially successfully in the larger side. In the unilateral vaginal obstruction group, presentation is usually with abdominal pain and the associated symptoms of a haematometra and haematocolpos. The confusing clinical sign is the associated menstruation from the other side, and the diagnosis may be missed if careful examination is not performed in these teenagers.

Investigation

Vaginal atresia

A patient presenting with a clinically absent vagina and no cyclical abdominal pain requires an ultrasound examination of the pelvis to determine the presence or absence of a uterus and/or a haematometra. Laparoscopy in these patients is unnecessary. Some 15% of patients with the Rokitansky syndrome suffer major defects of the urinary system, including congenital absence of a kidney; 40% of patients also have trivial urinary abnormalities (d'Alberton et al 1981). It is therefore important to perform an intravenous urogram in order to establish any abnormalities in the renal system or the presence of a pelvic kidney, which may alert the surgeon to take extra care if abdominal surgery becomes necessary.

Anomalies of the bony skeleton occur in approximately 12% of patients. These include abnormalities of the lumbar spine, the cervical vertebrae and the limbs. However, it

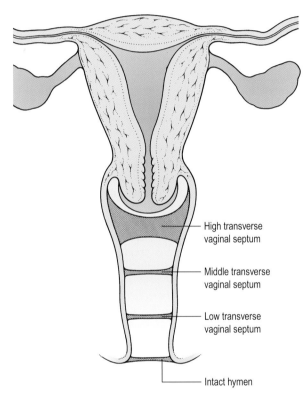

High transverse
vaginal septum

Middle transverse
vaginal septum

Low transverse
vaginal septum

Intact hymen

Figure 13.6 Disorders of vertical fusion.

Figure 13.7 Lateral fusion defects.

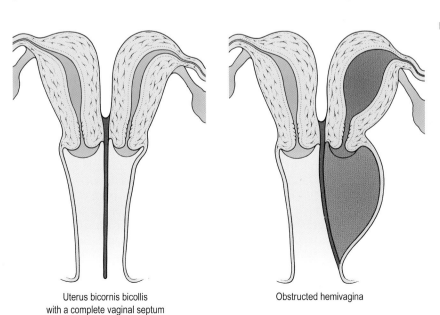

Uterus bicornis bicollis
with a complete vaginal septum

Obstructed hemivagina

may be that the incidence of bony abnormalities is higher than this, as investigation of the skeletal system is rarely performed.

Transverse vaginal septum

Investigations in these patients are limited to ultrasound assessment of the uterus for the detection of a haematometra and haematocolpos, and this may also be used to assess the level of the septal defect. Again, investigation of the urinary tract is pertinent.

Lateral fusion defects

Investigations in this group are only important if there is an obstructed outflow problem, and should follow those outlined for vertical fusion defects.

Treatment

Vaginal atresia

The patient with Müllerian agenesis requires careful psychological counselling and associated therapy. The psychological impact of being informed of an absent vagina comes as an immense shock to both patient and parents. It is almost always followed by a period of depression in which many patients question their femininity and look upon themselves as abnormal females. They very much doubt their ability to enter a heterosexual relationship which will be lasting, and feel worthless both sexually and certainly as regards being a reproductive partner. In some patients, the depression can be very profound and suicide may be threatened. There is also great maternal anxiety over the aetiology, as most mothers feel that they are responsible for the abnormality. Reassurance of the mother is as important as that of the daughter in the management of the patient.

Occasionally, cultural problems arise which make management much more difficult, especially in ethnic groups where the ability to procreate is fundamental to marriage and social acceptance. These patients and their parents can be very difficult to console and often refuse to accept the situation, questioning the diagnosis of their sterility over a number of years. The immediate reaction of most patients is to request surgical correction of the abnormality to return them to 'normal'. Unfortunately, opting for surgical treatment without adequate psychological and physical preparation inevitably leads to disaster. The author recommends a minimum of 6 months of preparation before any surgical procedure is performed, and during this time, psychological support can be implemented for the patient and her parents. There are two major areas of support required: first, the correction of the loss of esteem and inevitable depression; repeated counselling sessions by trained personnel are required if these symptoms are to be overcome. The second problem involves the psychological aspect; again, prolonged counselling sessions will be required if an adequate and fulfilling sex life is going to be possible in the future. The sexual life achieved by well-managed patients can be excellent and has been reported to be comparable to that of the normal population (Raboch and Horejsi 1982, Poland and Evans 1985).

Management of the absent vagina with a non-functioning uterus

In a patient with an absent or rudimentary uterus, the creation of a vaginal passage may be non-surgical or surgical. The non-surgical technique involves the repeated use of graduated vaginal dilators over a period of 6–12 months. A vaginal dimple of at least 1 cm is necessary for this technique to succeed, and patients require support and encouragement during this time. Patients are instructed to begin with a small vaginal dilator which is pressed firmly against the vaginal dimple for a period of some 20 minutes twice a day. Pressure is exerted but pain should be avoided, and repeated use of these vaginal dilators will meet with success in approximately 90% of cases with appropriate selection (Broadbent et al 1984, Edmonds 2003). This technique was first described by Frank in 1938, and in view of its undoubted success, with no complications, this method must be attempted in all girls with an absent vagina and a 1 cm dimple before any surgical procedure is considered.

In girls with a vaginal dimple of less than 1 cm or those in whom Frank's procedure fails, vaginoplasty will be required. There are currently three techniques in popular usage: the McIndoe–Reed operation, the amnion vaginoplasty and the Williams vulvovaginoplasty.

The McIndoe–Reed procedure was first described in 1938 (McIndoe and Banister 1938) and involved the use of a split-thickness skin graft over a solid mould; this mould is placed in a surgically created space between the urethra and the rectum. This space is created digitally following a transverse incision in the vaginal dimple. Digital exploration of the space must be performed with great care as damage to the bladder or the rectum may occur. The space created must reach the peritoneum of the pouch of Douglas if an adequate length of a vagina is to be created. A split-thickness skin graft is then taken from a donor site and an appropriately sized mould is chosen. The skin graft is then fashioned over the mould with the external skin surface in apposition to the mould. The skin-covered mould is then placed in the neovaginal space, and the labia are sutured together to hold the mould in situ. McIndoe reported his own series of 105 patients in 1959 and had a satisfactory outcome in 80% of patients. Cali and Pratt (1968) reported on their series of 123 patients; 90% had good sexual function but 6% had major complications which were primarily fistulae, and subsequent reconstructive surgery was necessary in 8%. These complications resulted in modifications of the technique and the use of a soft material for the mould to prevent fistula formation due to pressure necrosis.

The search for an alternative material to line the neovagina and avoid the scarring of the donor skin site led to the use of amnion for the vaginoplasty procedure (Ashworth et al 1986). The technique involves the creation of a neovaginal space in the same way as described for the McIndoe–Reed procedure, but amnion obtained at the time of elective caesarean section is used to line the neovagina. The mesenchymal surface of the amnion is placed against the new vaginal surface to promote epithelialization, and the mould is kept *in situ* for 7 days and then replaced with a new amnion graft for a further 7 days. Subsequently, patients are encouraged to use dilators on a frequent basis to maintain the vaginal passage. Again, reported success of approximately 90% has been achieved by these authors.

The Williams vulvovaginoplasty (Williams 1976) has almost no place in the management of these disorders, and is much less frequently used than in the past. In patients in whom dissection of a neovagina is impossible but the labia majora are normal, this technique is valuable. The principle of the operation is to create a vaginal pouch from the full-thickness skin flaps created from the labia majora, which are united in the midline. Following surgery and adequate healing, the patient is taught to use vaginal dilators in the same way as described in the Frank technique. There is no doubt that this does allow the patient and her partner to enjoy a sex life with mutual orgasm, but the angle of the vagina is unnatural and unsatisfactory for some patients. Although the operation is simple to perform, the psychological problems of the distorted external genitalia can be considerable.

The absent vagina with a coexistent functional uterus

This situation presents major problems, as the release of menstrual blood and the relief of associated pain are the primary aims; the creation of a normal vagina is an equally important yet secondary role. The functional uterus may be normal and a cervix may be present or absent. This situation is very rare; an operation to create a neovagina in an attempt to reanastomose a uterus which has been drained of its haematometra is highly specialized and will not be discussed further.

Complications

Some 25% of women will have some degree of dyspareunia following a vaginoplasty (Smith 1983). This is most commonly due to scarring at the upper margin of the vagina, involving the peritoneum. Similar incidences of dyspareunia occur in nearly all series and it is difficult to know how best to avoid this. It seems to occur regardless of technique, but contraction of the upper part of the vagina is difficult to avoid. The artificial vagina created in these ways acquires all the characteristics of normal vaginal epithelium, and the exposure of the grafted epithelium to a new environment means that care has to be taken to ensure it remains healthy. Four cases of intraepithelial neoplasia in neovaginas have been reported (Jackson 1959, Duckler 1972, Rotmensch et al 1983, Imrie et al 1986).

Management of disorders of vertical fusion

In these abnormalities, the type of procedure is governed by the type of abnormality. In the obstructed hymen, the procedure is extremely simple and a cruciate incision through the hymen will release the accumulated menstrual blood and resolve the problem. In obstructing transverse vaginal septae in the lower and middle thirds, surgical removal of the septum can almost always be performed transvaginally, and a reanastomosis of the upper and lower vaginal segments may be performed. Great care must be taken to ensure that the excision is adequate or a vaginal stenosis at the site of the septum will remain a problem. The high vaginal septum is the most difficult abnormality to manage, and it is almost always necessary to perform a laparotomy in order to expose the haematometra. The passage of a probe through the uterine cavity and cervix into the short upper vagina allows a second vaginal surgeon to explore the vagina from below and excise the septum. The absent portion of vagina is usually so great that reanastomosis of the vaginal mucosa cannot be achieved, and either a soft mould is inserted and granulation allowed to occur, or an amnion-covered soft mould should be inserted to promote epithelialization. Vaginal dilatation following removal of the mould must be encouraged in order to prevent constriction of the new vaginal area.

Results

The results of surgery are extremely good when judged by sexual satisfaction. However, Rock et al (1982) reported pregnancy success following surgical correction of transverse vaginal septa, and noted that patients with a transverse vaginal septum had only a 47% pregnancy rate when the site of the septum was taken into account. If the obstruction was in the lower third, all patients achieved a pregnancy, compared with 43% in the middle third and 25% in the upper third. It is suggested that the difficulties in conceiving may be secondary to the development of endometriosis, and the higher the site of the septum, the more likely the development of this disorder may be. Thus prompt diagnosis and surgical correction are important in an attempt to preserve the maximum reproductive capacity in these patients.

Complications

Complications are primarily those of dyspareunia and failure of pregnancy, as described above.

Disorders of lateral fusion

The treatment of this condition depends on the abnormality in patients with a midline septum and no other abnormality; excision of the septum should be performed and care must be taken as these septa can be very thick and removal can be rather difficult. When resecting the septum, generous pedicles should be taken to ensure haemostasis, and the results are extremely good as the remaining tissue usually retracts and causes no problem. In patients in whom there is an incomplete vaginal obstruction, the septum needs to be removed and care must be taken to remove as much of it as possible. Failure to do this will result in healing of an ostium and repeat obstruction of the hemivagina. The results and outlook for these patients are extremely good.

Malformations of the Uterus

Classification and pathophysiology

There have been numerous classification systems for uterine malformations, varying from those based on embryological development to those based on obstetric performance. However, the most widely used classification is that of

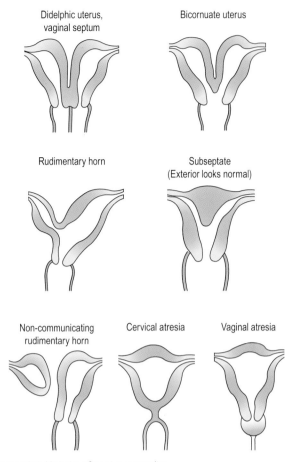

Didelphic uterus, vaginal septum

Bicornuate uterus

Rudimentary horn

Subseptate (Exterior looks normal)

Non-communicating rudimentary horn

Cervical atresia

Vaginal atresia

Figure 13.8 Varieties of uterine anomalies.

Buttram and Gibbons (1979), which is based upon the degree of failure of normal development. Six categories are described:

- Class I: Müllerian agenesis or hypoplasia;
- Class II: unicornuate uterus;
- Class III: uterus didelphis;
- Class IV: uterus bicornuate;
- Class V: septate uterus; and
- Class VI: diethylstilboestrol (DES) anomalies.

Many of these uterine malformations are shown in Figure 13.8.

A separate class of uterine malformations has been identified in the presence of communication between two separate uterocervical cavities.

The pathophysiology of failure of normal union of the Müllerian ducts is not clear. As proposed in the section on vaginal agenesis, the hypothesis of teratogens has been suggested but unsupported by evidence. It is most likely that this is a polygenic or multifactorial inheritance which slightly increases the risk of a uterovaginal abnormality arising in a family with no anomalies.

Incidence

The incidence of uterine anomalies is difficult to define as it depends entirely upon the interest of the investigator and the diligence with which investigation is pursued.

Obstetric series show an incidence of uterine abnormalities ranging from one in 100 to one in 1000 (Semmens 1962). In an infertile population, the incidence increases to approximately 3% (Sanfillippo et al 1978). It is likely that the incidence of uterine malformations is greatly overestimated, as no gynaecological or reproductive problems are ever experienced in the vast majority of patients.

Presentation

Abnormal uterine development may be symptomatic or asymptomatic. The most common clinical situations that will lead to a diagnosis of malformation of the uterus are recurrent pregnancy loss, primary infertility, urological abnormalities, menstrual disorders and DES exposure.

Recurrent pregnancy loss

Recurrent pregnancy wastage in the form of abortion or premature labour is a common way in which uterine anomalies will be discovered. The role of uterine anomalies in pregnancy wastage is discussed in Chapter 21 on female infertility and Chapter 23 on recurrent miscarriage.

Primary infertility

Uterine abnormalities may be discovered during investigation of an infertile woman. However, the relationship between infertility and uterine abnormalities remains controversial.

Urological abnormalities

Not uncommonly, urologists who discover malformations of the urinary system investigate the genital system and find abnormalities. Thompson and Lynn (1966) reported that 66% of patients with a maldevelopment of the renal tract had an associated Müllerian duct abnormality. However, only 13.5% of women with anomalous renal development had anomalous uterine development. In patients with a single kidney, the most common uterine abnormality is uterus didelphis with a vaginal septum which is associated with unilateral occlusion.

Menstrual disorders

Uterine abnormalities may be responsible for a number of menstrual disorders including oligomenorrhoea, dysmenorrhoea and menorrhagia. The specific menstrual symptoms will depend on the anomaly. In an interesting study by Sorensen (1981), investigating infertile women with oligomenorrhoea, 56% of patients were found to have mild uterine abnormalities. Sorensen suggested that this oligomenorrhoea might be due to poor vascularization or steroid receptor development in the malformed uterus. With regard to dysmenorrhoea, uterine abnormalities seem to be associated with a higher incidence of primary dysmenorrhoea, although this may also be associated with obstructed outflow problems. Rudimentary hemiuteri may also be the cause of dysmenorrhoea in some women.

Diethylstilboestrol exposure

The malformations associated with DES exposure have been well described (Kaufman et al 1980). These abnormalities include a classic T-shaped uterus with a widening of the interstitial and isthmic portions of the fallopian tubes and narrowing of the lower two-thirds of the uterus, as well as non-specific uterine abnormalities with changes of cavity seen on hysterosalpingography. These patients may present with impaired reproductive function, and pregnancy wastage may be as high as 50–60%. However, as DES exposure was terminated in 1970, almost all of these individuals will now have finished their reproductive performance.

Investigations and treatment

When uterine anomalies are suspected, a number of imaging techniques can be used to identify the abnormality. These include ultrasound, magnetic resonance imaging and hysterosalpingography. For a review, the reader is referred to Troiano and McCarthy (2004).

The value of treatment of uterine malformations is discussed in Chapter 21.

KEY POINTS

1. Gonadal differentiation into a testicle or ovary depends on the presence or absence of a Y chromosome.

2. The testis develops from the medulla whereas the ovary originates from the cortex or the primitive gonad.

3. Development of normal ovaries depends on the presence of two X chromosomes.

4. Deletion of either the short or long arms of the X chromosome may result in variable ovarian development or dysgenesis.

5. Development of the testis depends on TDF, which controls expression of the H-Y antigen, but other autosomally located genes are also involved.

6. Female intersex disorders denote external genital masculinization in patients with 46XX karyotype.

7. Differentiation of internal female sexual organs is not androgen dependent and, unlike the clitoris, the labia are only adversely affected if exposed to androgens before the 12th week of intrauterine life.

8. 21-Hydroxylase deficiency is an autosomal-recessive disorder and accounts for 90% of cases of congenital adrenal hyperplasia.

9. 21-Hydroxylase deficiency is the only adrenal enzymatic deficiency associated with the HLA gene located in chromosome 6.

10. Female fetus defeminization may follow maternal use of testosterone-related progestogens.

11. Prenatal diagnosis of congenital adrenal hyperplasia in heterozygous carriers is necessary, and treatment with dexamethasone prevents fetal infliction.

12. Successful pregnancy following resection of the vaginal septum is inversely related to the level of the septum in the vagina.

13. Intrauterine DES exposure may lead to a T-shaped uterus with impaired reproductive function.

14. Unilateral renal aplasia is frequently associated with failure of Müllerian duct development on the same side, since both are dependent on adequate development of the mesonephric system.

15. Where there is Müllerian agenesis, the urogenital sinus forms but does not lengthen, and the vagina is short although variable in length.

16. Virilizing features at puberty require thorough investigation and sensitive management.

References

Ashworth MF, Morton KE, Dewhurst CJ et al 1986 Vaginoplasty using amnion. Obstetrics and Gynecology 67: 443–444.

Barkan A, Cassorla F, Loriaux D, Marshall JC 1984 Pregnancy in a patient with virilising arrhenoblastoma. American Journal of Obstetrics and Gynecology 149: 909–910.

Behlke MA, Bogan JS, Beer-Romero P, Page DC 1993 Evidence that the SRY protein is encoded by a single exon on the human Y chromosome. Genomics 17: 736–739.

Berkovitz GD, Seeherunvong T 1998 Abnormalities of gonadal differentiation. Baillière's Clinical Endocrinology and Metabolism 12: 133–142.

Broadbent RT, Woolf RM, Herbertson R 1984 Non-operative construction of the vagina. Plastic and Reconstructive Surgery 73: 117–122.

Brown TR, Maes M, Rothwell SW, Migeon CJ 1982 Human complete androgen insensitivity with normal dihydrotestosterone receptor binding capacity in cultured genital skin biopsies. Journal of Clinical Endocrinology and Metabolism 55: 61–69.

Buttram VS, Gibbons WE 1979 Müllerian anomalies — a proposed classification. Fertility and Sterility 32: 40–48.

Cacciari E, Balsamo A, Cassio A et al 1983 Neonatal screening for congenital adrenal hyperplasia. Archives of Disease in Childhood 58: 803–806.

Cali RW, Pratt JH 1968 Congenital absence of the vagina. American Journal of Obstetrics and Gynecology 100: 752–754.

Carson SA, Simpson JL, Malinak LR et al 1983 Heritable aspects of uterine anomalies II. Genetic analysis of Müllerian aplasia. Fertility and Sterility 40: 86–91.

Castro-Magana M, Chervanky T, Collipp PJ, Ghavami-Maibadi Z, Angulo M, Stewart C 1981 Transient adrenogenital syndrome due to exposure to danazol in utero. American Journal of Diseases of Childhood 135: 1032–1034.

Cohen VA, Daughaday WH, Weldon V 1982 Fetal and maternal virilization association with pregnancy. American Journal of Diseases of Childhood 136: 353–356.

Connor TB, Ganis FM, Levin HS, Migeon CJ, Martin LG 1968 Gonadotrophin dependent Krukenberg tumour causing virilization during pregnancy. Journal of Clinical Endocrinology and Metabolism 28: 198–201.

D'Alberton A, Reschini E, Ferrari N, Candiani P 1981 Prevalence of urinary tract abnormalities in a large series of patients with uterovaginal atresia. Journal of Urology 126: 623–627.

Dong WF, Heng HH, Lowsky R 1997 Cloning, expression and chromosomal localisation to 11p12-13 of a human LIM homeobox gene, hLIM-1. DNA and Cell Biology 16: 671–678.

Donohoue PA, van Dop C, McLean RH et al 1986 Gene conversion in salt-losing congenital adrenal hyperplasia with absent complement C4B protein. Journal of Clinical Endocrinology and Metabolism 62: 995–1002.

Duck SC, Katamaya KP 1981 Danazol may cause female pseudohermaphroditism. Fertility and Sterility 35: 230–231.

Duckler L 1972 Squamous cell carcinoma developing in an artificial vagina. Obstetrics and Gynecology 40: 35.

Dupont B, Oberfield SE, Smithwick EM et al 1977 Close genetic linkage between HLA and congenital adrenal hyperplasia. The Lancet ii: 1309–1312.

Edmonds DK 1989 Intersexuality. In: Dewhurst's Practical Paediatric and Adolescent Gynaecology, 2nd edn. Butterworths, London.

Edmonds DK 2003 Congenital malformation of the genital tract. Best Practice and Research in Clinical Obstetrics and Gynaecology 17: 19–40.

Evans TN, Poland ML, Boving RL 1981 Vaginal malformations. American Journal of Obstetrics and Gynecology 141: 910–916.

Fayez JA, Bunch TR, Miller GL 1974 Virilization in pregnancy associated with polycystic ovary disease. Obstetrics and Gynecology 44: 511–521.

Forest MG, Orgiazzi J, Tranchant D, Mornex R, Bertrand J 1978 Approach to the mechanism of androgen production in a case of Krukenberg tumor responsible for virilization during pregnancy. Journal of Clinical Endocrinology and Metabolism 47: 428–434.

Foresta C, Ferlin A 2004 Role of INSL3 and LGR8 in cryptorchidism and testicular function. Reproductive Biomedicine Online 9: 294–298.

Frank RT 1938 The formation of an artificial vagina without operation. American Journal of Obstetrics and Gynecology 35: 1053–1055.

Fuller PJ, Pettigrew IG, Pike JW, Stockigt JR 1983 An adrenal adenoma causing virilization of mother and infant. Clinical Endocrinology 18: 143–153.

Guellaen G, Casanova M, Bishop C 1984 Human XX males with Y single copy DNA fragments. Nature 307: 172–173.

Hastie ND 1994 The genetics of Wilm's tumour. Annual Review of Genetics 28: 523–558.

Hensleigh PA, Woodruff DA 1978 Differential maternal fetal response to androgenizing luteoma or hyperreactio luteinalis. Obstetrical and Gynaecological Surgery 33: 262–271.

Hughes IA, Wilton A, Lole CA, Glay OP 1979 Continuing need for mineralocorticoid therapy in salt-losing congenital adrenal hyperplasia. Archives of Disease in Childhood 54: 350–358.

Hughes IA 2008 Disorders of sex development. A new definition and classification. Best Practice in Research in Clinical Endocrinology and Metabolism 22: 119–134.

Imrie JEA, Kennedy JH, Holmes JD et al 1986 Intraepithelial neoplasia arising in an artificial vagina. British Journal of Obstetrics and Gynaecology 93: 886–887.

Ishizuka SC, Kawashima Y, Nakanishi T et al 1962 Statistical observations on genital anomalies of newborns following the administration of progestins to their mothers. Journal of the Japanese Obstetrical and Gynaecological Society 9: 271–282.

Jackson GW 1959 Primary carcinoma of an artificial vagina. Obstetrics and Gynecology 14: 534.

Jones HW, Mermut S 1974 Familial occurrence of congenital absence of the vagina. Obstetrics and Gynecology 42: 38–40.

Kaufman RH, Adam E, Binder GL, Gerthoffer E 1980 Upper genital tract changes and pregnancy outcome in offspring exposed in utero to DES. American Journal of Obstetrics and Gynecology 137: 299–306.

Lefebvre V, Huang W, Harley VR 1997 SOX9 is a potent activator of the chondrocyte-specific enhancer of the proalpha1(II) collagen gene. Molecular Cellular and Biology 17: 2336–2246.

Lischke JH, Curtis CH, Lamb EJ 1973 Discordance of vaginal agenesis in monozygotic twins. Obstetrics and Gynecology 41: 902–922.

McIndoe AH 1959 Discussion on treatment of congenital absence of the vagina with emphasis on long term results. Proceedings of the Royal Society of Medicine 52: 952–953.

McIndoe AH, Banister JB 1938 An operation for the cure of congenital absence of the vagina. Journal of Obstetrics and Gynaecology of the British Commonwealth 45: 490–495.

Mulaikal RM, Migeon CJ, Rock JA 1987 Fertility rates in female patients with congenital adrenal hyperplasia due to 21-hydroxylase deficiency. New England Journal of Medicine 315: 178–181.

Murset G, Zachmann M, Prader A, Fischer J, Labhart A 1970 Male external genitalia of a girl caused by a virilizing adrenal tumour in the mother. Acta Endocrinologica 65: 627–638.

Newns GH 1974 Congenital adrenal hyperplasia. Archives of Disease in Childhood 49: 716–724.

Novak DJ, Lauchlan SC, McCauley JC 1970 Virilization during pregnancy: case report and review of literature. American Journal of Medicine 49: 281–286.

Ogata T 2008 Progress in analyzing disorders of sexual development. Sexual Development 2: 167–178.

Pang S, Murphey W, Levine LS et al 1982 A pilot newborn screening for congenital adrenal hyperplasia in Alaska. Journal of Clinical Endocrinology and Metabolism 55: 413–420.

Pang SY, Wallace MA, Hofman L et al 1988 Worldwide experience in newborn screening for congenital adrenal hyperplasia. Pediatrics 81: 866–874.

Petersen RE, Imperato-McGinley J, Gautier T, Sturla E 1977 Male pseudohermaphroditism due to 5α reductase deficiency. American Journal of Medicine 62: 170–191.

Poland ML, Evans TN 1985 Psychologic aspects of vaginal agenesis. Journal of Reproductive Medicine 30: 340–348.

Post WD, Steele HD, Gorwill H 1978 Mucinous cystadenoma and virilization during pregnancy. Canadian Medical Association Journal 118: 948–953.

Prader A 1958 Vollkommen männlichie aussere Genitalentwicklung und Salzverlustsyndrom bei Mädchen mit kongenitalem adrenogenitalem Syndrom. Helvetica Paediatrica Acta 13: 5–14.

Raboch J, Horejsi J 1982 Sexual life of women with Kuster–Rokitansky syndrome. Archives of Sexual Behavior 11: 215–219.

Rock JA, Zacur HA, Dlugi AM et al 1982 Pregnancy success following surgical correction of imperforate hymen and complete transverse vaginal septum. Obstetrics and Gynecology 59: 448–454.

Rotmensch J, Rosenheim N, Dillon M et al 1983 Carcinoma arising in a neovagina. Obstetrics and Gynecology 61: 534.

Sanfillippo JS, Yussman MA, Smith O 1978 Hysterosalpingography in the evaluation of infertility. Fertility and Sterility 30: 636–639.

Say B, Carpentier NJ 1979 Genital malformations in a child with VATER association. American Journal of Diseases of Childhood 133: 438–439.

Semmens JP 1962 Congenital anomalies of the female genital tract. Obstetrics and Gynecology 19: 328–333.

Shokeir MHK 1978 Aplasia of the Müllerian system. Evidence of probable sex limited autosomal dominant inheritance. Birth Defects 14: 147–151.

Simpson JL 1999 Genetics of human reproduction. Journal of Medical Genetics 89: 224–239.

Smith MR 1983 Vaginal aplasia: therapeutic options. American Journal of Obstetrics and Gynecology 146: 534–538.

Sorensen SS 1981 Minor Müllerian anomalies and oligomenorrhoea in infertile women. American Journal of Obstetrics and Gynecology 140: 636–640.

Swain A, Narvaez V, Burgoyne P 1998 Dax 1 antagonises SRY action in mammalian sex determination. Nature 391: 761–767.

Therman E, Susman M 1993 Abnormal human sex chromosome constitution. In: Human Chromosomes: Structure, Behavior and Effects, 3rd edn. Springer Verlag, New York, pp 220–227.

Thompson DP, Lynn HB 1966 Genital abnormalities associated with solitary kidney. Mayo Clinic Proceedings 41: 438–442.

Tomomasa H, Adachi Y, Iwabuchi M 1999 XX-male syndrome bearing the sex-determining region Y. Archives of Andrology 42: 89–96.

Troiano RN, McCarthy SM 2004 Müllerian duct anomalies: imaging and clinical issues. Radiology 233: 19–34.

White R, Leppert M, Bishop DT et al 1985 Construction of linkage maps with DNA markers for human chromosomes. Nature 313: 101–105.

Wilhelm D, Palmer S, Koopman P 2007 Sex determination and gonadal development in mammals. Physiology Review 87: 1–28.

Williams EA 1976 Uterovaginal agenesis. Annals of the Royal College of Surgeons of England 58: 266–277.

Zachmann M, Tassinari D, Prader A 1983 Clinical and biochemical variability of congenital adrenal hyperplasia due to 11-hydroxylase deficiency. Journal of Clinical Endocrinology and Metabolism 56: 222–229.

CHAPTER 14

Disorders of puberty

Adam Balen

Chapter Contents

INTRODUCTION	182	GYNAECOLOGICAL COMPLAINTS	193
PUBERTAL DEVELOPMENT	182	SUMMARY	194
PRECOCIOUS PUBERTY	187	KEY POINTS	194
DELAYED PUBERTY	189		
PRESENTATION OF CONGENITAL ANOMALIES OF THE GENITAL TRACT	191		

Introduction

Puberty and adolescence are recognized as periods involving marked endocrine changes which regulate growth and sexual development. Normal pubertal development is known to be centrally driven and dependent upon appropriate gonadotrophin and growth hormone (GH) secretion, and normal functioning of the hypothalamic–pituitary–gonadal axis. The mechanisms which control the precise timing of the onset of puberty, however, are still not clearly understood but are influenced by many factors including general health, nutrition, exercise, genetic influences and socio-economic conditions (Rees 1993). Most of the changes during puberty are gradual, although menarche is a single event that can be dated in girls. Normal puberty involves a fairly regular sequence of events between the ages of 10 and 16 years, and abnormal puberty can be defined as any disturbance in this. This chapter will provide an overview of the endocrine changes observed during normal pubertal development, and will describe the factors believed to influence the tempo of puberty and ovarian maturation before discussing some of the conditions that result in disordered pubertal development.

In broad terms, once a girl has passed menarche, she is potentially fertile and should be considered as a young woman. The degree of sexual and reproductive maturity is not always mirrored by emotional and psychological maturity, so consideration must be given to the particular needs of adolescent girls when they attend clinics and hospital with gynaecological problems.

It is recognized that adolescents have special needs. Adolescents with gynaecological problems have additional needs and often require a degree of privacy and sensitive handling. Many of the gynaecological problems encountered relate to intimate bodily functions at a time when the individual is maturing sexually and having to deal with issues that are embarrassing and may be considered taboo. Furthermore, consideration should be given to ethnic and cultural differences, and potential problems with communication, particularly as amongst the parents from ethnic minorities, it is often the father and not the mother who can speak English. As such, the need for interpreters and information written in different languages should be borne in mind.

During puberty and adolescence, the reasons why young women attend for consultation may be broadly subdivided as follows:

- sexual health: contraception, family planning, sexually transmitted disease;
- pregnancy: wanted and unwanted teenage pregnancy;
- gynaecological complaints: menstrual cycle dysfunction, pelvic pain, ovarian cysts and gynaecological pathology, which may occur at any stage during the reproductive years; and
- disorders of sexual development: complex and rare endocrine and developmental disorders of sexual differentiation and puberty, including intersex conditions.

This chapter will deal largely with the latter group, apart from when there is overlap with other chapters (see Chapters 13, 16 and 31).

Pubertal Development

Puberty represents a period of significant growth, hormonal change and the attainment of reproductive capacity. Its onset is marked by a significant increase in the amplitude of pulsatile release of gonadotrophin-releasing hormone (GnRH) by the hypothalamus (Mauras et al 1996). This usually occurs between the ages of 8 and 13.5 years in girls, and stimulates an increase in pituitary release of luteinizing hormone (LH) and follicle-stimulating hormone (FSH), which initially occurs as high-amplitude nocturnal pulses, although eventually both daytime and nocturnal pulsatile release are established (Delemarre et al 1991). FSH and LH, in turn, act upon the ovary to promote follicular development and sex steroid synthesis. As endocrine activity is initially nocturnal, there is no point in measuring gonadotrophin or sex steroid levels during the day.

In the female, this period is characterized clinically by accelerated linear growth, the development of breasts and pubic hair, and the eventual onset of menstruation (menarche) which occurs between the ages of 11 and 16 years in most women in the UK (Stark et al 1989). Menarche is often used as a marker of pubertal development as it is an easily identifiable event which can usually be dated with some accuracy. Adrenarche, the growth of pubic hair, is due to the secretion of adrenal androgens and precedes gonadarche by about 3 years. Thus, prepubertal children often have pubic hair, although, if pronounced, this should be investigated to exclude pathological causes (see below). Whilst androgen secretion is essential, oestrogen secretion facilitates pubic hair growth.

In tandem with the onset of pulsatile GnRH secretion, there is an increase in the amplitude of GH pulses released by the pituitary. Evidence suggests that this amplification of GH secretion may be regulated by the pubertal increase in levels of both androgenic and oestrogenic hormones (Mauras et al 1996, Caufriez 1997). In addition to this action, sex steroids have been shown to stimulate skeletal growth directly and thus augment the role of GH in promoting somatic growth and development (Giustina et al 1997). During the adolescent growth spurt, there is a greater gain in sitting height (mean 13.5 cm for girls, 15.4 cm for boys) than leg length (mean 11.5 cm for girls, 12.1 cm for boys) as the spurt for sitting height lasts longer (and is longer

in boys). At this time, there is a minimum rate of fat gain and maximum attainment of muscle bulk, with differential and opposite changes in boys and girls. Ossification of the skeleton, as measured in terms of 'bone age', is helpful in determining a child's progress through puberty and as a determinant of final stature.

Rising concentrations of GH are also believed to exert some effects on circulating insulin levels, although precise mechanisms are unclear. Some authors believe that GH induces peripheral insulin resistance which leads to compensatory increases in insulin secretion (Smith et al 1988, Nobels and Dewailly 1992). Increased levels of insulin during puberty may directly stimulate protein anabolism (Amiel et al 1991). Insulin also acts as a regulator of insulin-like growth factor-1 (IGF-1) through its effects on insulin-like growth factor binding protein-1 (IGFBP-1). IGF-1 is produced by hepatic cells under the influence of GH, and has actions which stimulate cellular growth and maturation. IGFBP-1 competes with IGF receptors to bind IGF-1, thus inhibiting cellular action of IGF-1. Studies have indicated that insulin acts to suppress production of IGFBP-1 and therefore increases circulating IGF-1 bioavailability (Holly et al 1989, Nobels and Dewailly 1992). Insulin has also been shown to be a regulator of free sex steroids through the control of sex-hormone-binding globulin (SHBG) production by the liver. Studies have shown that levels of SHBG decrease during puberty and that this fall parallels the rising levels of insulin (Holly et al 1989, Nobels and Dewailly 1992). The endocrine interactions involved in normal pubertal development are represented in a simplified diagram in Figure 14.1.

Tempo of pubertal development

Although the endocrine changes during puberty have become better understood, the exact 'trigger' which determines the onset of pulsatile GnRH release, and thus the initiation of

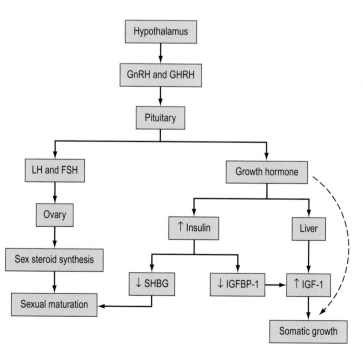

Figure 14.1 Schematic representation of the endocrine changes which regulate pubertal development. GnRH, gonadotrophin-releasing hormone; GHRH, growth-hormone-releasing hormone; LH, luteinizing hormone; FSH, follicle-stimulating hormone; SHBG, sex-hormone-binding globulin; IGFBP-1, insulin-like growth factor binding protein 1; IGF-1, insulin-like growth factor-1.

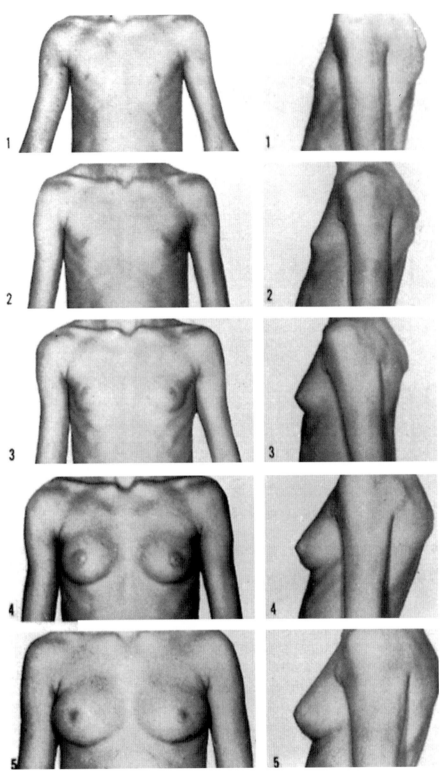

Figure 14.2 Stages of breast development at puberty. Stage 1: the infantile stage, which persists from the time the effect of maternal oestrogen on the breasts disappears, shortly after birth, until the pubertal changes begin. Stage 2: the bud stage. The breasts and papillae are elevated as a small mound and there is an increase in the diameter of the areola. This stage represents the first indication of pubertal change in the breast. Stage 3: the breasts and areola are further enlarged to create an appearance similar to that of a small adult breast, with a continuous rounded contour. Stage 4: the areola and papilla enlarge further to form a secondary mound projecting above the contour of the remainder of the breast. Stage 5: the typical adult breast with a smooth rounded contour. The secondary mound present in stage 4 has disappeared.

puberty, is still unclear. The question of which factors might regulate the onset of puberty and control the rate of pubertal development has prompted extensive research. The majority of studies examining young women have used age at menarche as the key marker of sexual maturity, and have attempted to elucidate which factors are involved in the timing of this event.

The first physical sign of puberty in girls is breast development, which occurs at an average age of 10–12.5 years (Figure 14.2). Age at onset of puberty is influenced by family history, race (earlier in Afro-Caribbeans) and nutrition (earlier in obese girls, with a secular trend to younger ages). Fifty percent of girls show signs of breast development by the age of 11 years, and investigations should be performed if there is no sign of breast development by the age of 14 years. In girls, the adolescent growth spurt occurs around 1 year after pubertal onset, while menarche occurs in the later stages of puberty at an average age of 12–15 years, at breast and pubic hair stage 4 (Figures 14.3 and 14.4; Marshall and Tanner 1969). Oestradiol concentration affects both the uterus and skeletal maturity. Most girls begin to menstruate when their bone age is between 13 and 14 years, and fewer than 20% are outside these limits. The appearance of axillary hair may antedate the rest of puberty by a few years and does not bear a constant relationship to the development of breasts as, again, it is androgens and not oestrogens that are most significant. The apocrine glands of the axilla and vulva begin to function at the time when axillary and pubic hair is appearing.

It has long been recognized that early maturing women have a tendency to be heavier for their height than their later maturing counterparts and, in contrast, that malnutrition and anorexia nervosa are associated with delayed menarche and amenorrhoea. These observed relationships between body weight and menarche led to the 'critical weight hypothesis' of Frisch and Revelle (1970), which hypothesized that attainment of a critical body weight led to metabolic changes which, in turn, triggered menarche. In further work, the investigators demonstrated that the ratio of lean body weight to fat decreased during the adolescent growth spurt in females from 5:1 to 3:1 at menarche, when the proportion of body fat was approximately 22% (Frisch 1990). They suggested that adipose tissue specifically was responsible for the development and maintenance of reproductive function, through its action as an extragonadal site for the conversion of androgens to oestrogens.

While few authors will dispute that nutrition and body weight play a role in pubertal development, the 'critical weight hypothesis' for menarche has not been supported by other studies. Cameron (1976) studied 36 British girls longitudinally, measuring weight and skinfold thickness at 3-month intervals for the 2 years before menarche to 2 years post menarche. He postulated that if a 'critical body fatness' was the true explanation for onset of menarche, he should expect to detect a reduction in the variability of his measurements at menarche compared with measurements taken before and after menarche, and this was not demonstrated in the study. In a much larger study, Garn et al (1983) analysed the triceps skinfold distributions of 2251 girls collected during three national surveys in the USA. Comparing premenarcheal and postmenarcheal girls, they confirmed that those who had attained menarche were, on average, fatter than premenarcheal girls. However, there was a marked overlap in skinfold thickness for both groups, and there was no evidence of a threshold level of fatness below which menarche did not occur. In a more recent study, de Ridder et al (1992) performed a longitudinal assessment of 68 premenarcheal school girls, including pubertal staging, skinfold measurements, waist–hip ratios and blood samples for the monitoring of gonadotrophins. They did not demonstrate a relationship between body fat mass and the age at onset of puberty or age at menarche, but did find that a greater body fat mass was related to a faster rate of pubertal development.

Although the studies above dispute the association of age at menarche with the achievement of a threshold weight or

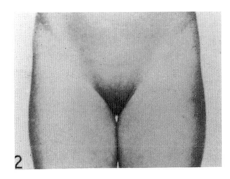

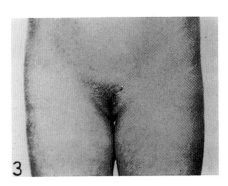

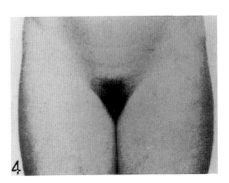

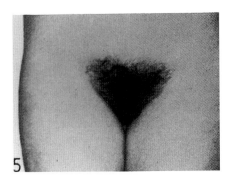

Figure 14.3 Stages of pubic hair development at puberty. Stage 2: sparse growth of slightly pigmented hairs on either the labia or the mons pubis. Stage 3: the hair is darker and coarser, and spreads sparsely over and on either side of the midline of the mons pubis. Stage 4: the hair is adult in character but covers a smaller area than in most adults and has not spread to the medial surface of the thighs. Stage 5: hair distributed as an inverse triangle and spreading to the medial surfaces of the thighs. It does not spread to the linea alba or elsewhere above the base of the triangle.

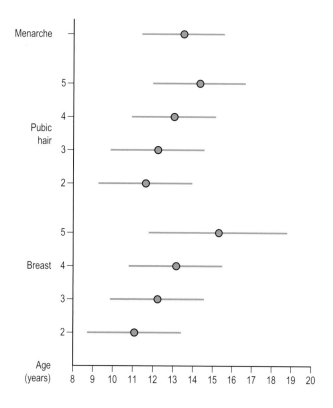

Figure 14.4 Timing of pubic hair and breast changes and menarche. Horizontal line represents mean ± 2 standard deviations.

body fat percentage, the association of earlier maturation in heavier girls still exists. Stark et al (1989) reported on data from 4427 girls who were part of the National Child Development Study cohort. Data relating to birth weight, age at menarche, and weights and heights measured at 7, 11 and 16 years were available. The authors reported that a larger proportion of girls with early menarche (before the age of 11 years) were heavier for their height at all ages when compared with those with late menarche (after 14 years). Interestingly, however, changes in relative weight in the years preceding menarche (ages 7–11 years) were not strongly associated with age at menarche, whereas being overweight at the age of 7 years was much more strongly associated with an early age at menarche. Birth weight was not related to age at menarche. The authors concluded that the increase in weight for height associated with early maturation actually begins well before the onset of puberty. These findings were replicated by Cooper et al (1996) who examined 1471 girls in the Medical Research Council National Survey of Health and Development. They found that girls who were heavier at 7 years of age experienced an earlier menarche; however, contrary to Stark et al, they found that birth weight was related to age at menarche and that girls with heavier birth weights experienced menarche at a later age.

Intense exercise, such as long-distance running, ballet, rowing, long-distance cycling and gymnastics, is associated with delayed menarche in young girls and with amenorrhoea in older women (Malina et al 1978, 1979, Frisch et al 1981, Baxter-Jones et al 1994). These 'endurance' sports are associated with lower body weight and percentage fat. The extent to which menarche is 'delayed' has been shown to be

related to the age at which participation in the sport begins and to the intensity of training (Frisch et al 1981). In view of the association between body weight and menarche described above, it is perhaps not surprising that girls participating in intense sporting activity experience a later age of menarche.

The influence of genetic factors on age at menarche is evident in the correlation demonstrated between mother–daughter and sister–sister pairs. Garn and Bailey (1978) analysed data from 550 mother–daughter pairs and reported a correlation of 0.25, which was adjusted to 0.23 once a correction was made for fatness. Similar correlation coefficients have been reported in other studies of mother–daughter pairs from European, African and American populations (Flug et al 1984, Benso et al 1989, Malina et al 1994, Cameron and Nagdee 1996). The strength of this 'genetic effect', however, must be interpreted carefully as the mothers' age at menarche was based on recall in most of these studies, and the accuracy of the estimation is therefore questionable. In addition, one must consider the effect of similarity in socio-economic status (and hence nutrition and fatness) that is likely to exist between mothers and daughters, and this in itself may contribute to similarity in menarcheal age.

The association between body weight and age at menarche has formed part of the basis for the explanation of the secular trend towards earlier menarche noted in the UK and other industrialized countries over the last century (Roberts et al 1971, Ostersehlt and Danker Hopf 1991). It has been generally accepted that this trend has reflected improvements in nutrition, health and environmental conditions. However, a recent plateau in this trend has been observed, and even reversal in some countries, which is at present unexplained (Dann and Roberts 1993, Tryggvadottir et al 1994, Veronesi and Gueresi 1994). It has been suggested that the recent decrease in menarcheal age is related to changes in social conditioning in developed countries. Promotion of very thin women as 'ideal' role models through media and fashion has contributed to an increase in dieting in adolescent girls. Increasing participation of women in endurance sports which have intense training regimens may also be a factor related to lower body weight in young girls.

These studies all indicate that pubertal development and body weight are intrinsically linked. However, the mechanism for this relationship has not been defined conclusively. Insulin has been suggested as a modulator of the tempo of pubertal development through the regulation of IGFBP-1 and SHBG (Smith et al 1988, Holly et al 1989, Nobels and Dewailly 1992). States of overnutrition and obesity are associated with increased serum concentrations of insulin (Parra et al 1971, Rosenbaum et al 1997). Therefore, if excessive nutritional intake persists during childhood, it is possible that hyperinsulinaemia may lead to lower levels of IGFBP-1 and reduced SHBG concentrations, thus enhancing IGF-1 and sex steroid bioavailability. The converse would be true in states of malnutrition, where low levels of insulin would allow for the development of increased IGFBP-1 and SHBG levels.

However, it is still unclear whether hyperinsulinaemia in childhood is a result of obesity or if it is the cause of obesity. The roles of genetic factors, which may determine insulin production and obesity risk in childhood, are also yet to be clearly explained. Recently, there has been much interest in the actions of the newly identified hormone leptin which is produced by adipose tissue (Sorensen et al 1996). Serum concentrations of leptin, a 167 amino acid product of white fat, have been shown to be related to body fat mass, and it is believed that leptin exerts its action on the hypothalamus to control calorie intake, decrease thermogenesis, increase levels of serum insulin and increase pulsatility of GnRH (Considine et al 1996, Sorensen et al 1996). With these actions, leptin may potentially have a role in the hormonal control of pubertal development, and some studies have shown that leptin levels do increase before the onset of puberty (Clayton et al 1997, Mantzoros et al 1997). It has been postulated that changes in circulating leptin levels may act as an initiator for the onset of puberty, and that this may explain the relationships between body fat and maturation observed by Frisch and Revelle (1970). This hypothesis is supported by the recent work of Clement et al (1998), who identified a homozygous mutation of the leptin receptor gene which results in early-onset morbid obesity and the absence of pubertal development in association with reduced GH secretion. These findings suggest that increased leptin levels associated with gains in fat mass may signal the hypothalamus to act as an important regulator of sexual maturation. It is possible that future research may clarify the role of leptin and leptin receptors in pubertal development, and may explain the variation in the timing of onset of puberty between individuals.

Ovarian and uterine development

Development of primordial follicles and secretion of oestrogens may be regarded as the final common path in the hormonal activity of puberty, and there is a close correlation between oestrogen levels and sexual maturation. The uterus grows in concordance with somatic growth, with differential increased growth of the corpus starting from approximately 7 years of age. However, the main differential increase of uterine size compared with somatic growth is only obvious after oestradiol secretion is measurably increased, and tends to occur between breast stages 3 and 4. Awareness of this comparatively late relative increase in uterine size has clinical relevance in the differentiation of arrested puberty and Müllerian agenesis, and also in the diagnosis of causes of precocious puberty. Blood oestrogen levels rise before and during puberty, and continue to do so for approximately 3 years after menarche before the normal adult follicular levels of oestrogen are seen. This gradual maturation is a reflection of the finding that many of the early cycles are anovulatory, and of the observation that the early postmenarcheal years are relatively infertile.

Ultrasound is the most suitable imaging technique for examination of the internal genitalia of girls as it is free from the risks of radiation and involves a quick, quiet and non-invasive procedure. Whilst higher resolution images can be obtained of the ovaries and uterus using transvaginal ultrasonography, only the transabdominal approach can be used in young girls and it may not always be possible to visualize both ovaries; furthermore, a full bladder is required. Nonetheless, transabdominal ultrasonography is an invaluable tool for the delineation of normal changes before and

through puberty, and also for the evaluation of paediatric disorders, such as pelvic masses and abnormal pubertal development. Ultrasonography can also be used in postmenarcheal girls to detect abnormal ovarian morphology and hence increase our understanding of common conditions such as polycystic ovary syndrome.

There are relatively few normal data on the maturation of the internal genitalia in girls, and a paper by Holm et al (1995) provides cross-sectional data of a large cohort of 166 school girls and medical students. It was demonstrated that uterine and ovarian volumes increase in size prepubertally, from as early as 6 years of age. Griffin et al (1995) demonstrated similar changes from the age of 4 years and, in their study of 153 girls, included subjects as young as 3 days. It was found that uterine shape changes constantly throughout childhood from a pear shape to a cylindrical shape and, finally, to the adult heart shape.

As girls go through puberty, the ovaries have been described as characteristically becoming multicystic due to low levels of FSH stimulating only partial folliculogenesis (Stanhope et al 1985). The multicystic appearance is also seen during resumption of ovarian activity after periods of quiescence; for example, in women who are recovering from weight-related amenorrhoea or those with hypogonadotrophic hypogonadism who are treated with pulsatile GnRH. The multicystic ovary differs from the polycystic ovary in that the cysts are larger (6–10 mm) and the stroma is of normal echogenicity. The morphological appearance of the polycystic ovary, on the other hand, requires the presence of at least 10 cysts (2–8 mm) per ovary in the presence of an echodense stroma (see Chapter 18).

Menarche

The first period occurs because there has been sufficient endometrial stimulation to result in a withdrawal bleed when there is a temporary fall in the oestrogen level. It can be associated with an ovulatory/corpus luteum sequence but this is not usual. The first menstruation simply indicates that a particular threshold has been reached in an already oscillating system, but is an obvious outward sign and of significance; menarche denotes an intact hypothalamic–pituitary–ovarian axis, functioning ovaries, the presence of a uterus and patency of the genital tract.

Menarche generally occurs within 2 years of the earliest sign of breast development and within 1 year of peak growth velocity and close to breast stage 4, usually between the ages of 10 and 16 years.

Precocious Puberty

Precocious onset of puberty is defined as occurring younger than 2 standard deviations before the average age, i.e. <8 years old in females (compared with <9 years in males). Thus, in many girls, early onset of puberty merely represents one end of the normal distribution. However, a number of pathological conditions may prematurely activate the GnRH–LH/FSH axis, resulting in the precocious onset of puberty. Furthermore, certain physical secondary sexual features (e.g. virilization without breast development) may occur in the absence of 'true puberty' (i.e.

Gonadotrophin dependent ('true' or 'central' precocious puberty)

- Idiopathic (family history, overweight/obese)
- Intracranial lesions (tumours, hydrocephalus, irradiation, trauma, encephalitis)
- Gonadotrophin-secreting tumours
- Congenital brain defects, third ventricle cysts, neurofibromatosis, hamartomas
- Hypothyroidism (autoimmune)

Variants

- Premature thelarche (and thelarche variant)
- Adrenarche

Gonadotrophin independent

- Congenital adrenal hyperplasia
- Cushing's disease
- Sex-steroid-secreting tumours (adrenal or ovarian), chorion epithelioma
- McCune–Albright syndrome
- Exogenous oestrogen ingestion/administration

absent hypothalamic–pituitary activation) due to abnormal peripheral secretion of sex steroids (Box 14.1).

True precocious puberty

The appearance of pubertal physical features follows the normal sequence ('consonance'), beginning with breast development. The diagnosis is made by the finding of elevated basal gonadotrophin levels and, after stimulation with i.v. GnRH, the serum LH concentration is higher than FSH. It is important to consider intracranial pathology and arrange imaging if indicated. Pelvic ultrasound will reveal the presence of multicystic ovaries and a uterus that is developing adult proportions. Bone age will be advanced.

Premature thelarche

Premature breast development in the absence of other signs of puberty may present at any age from infancy. Breast size may fluctuate and is often asymmetrical. Bone maturation, growth rate and final height are unaffected. The cause is unknown. The diagnosis is made by the finding of elevated FSH levels (but not LH), both basal and following GnRH stimulation. Ovarian ultrasound often reveals a single large, functional ovarian cyst. Serum oestradiol concentrations are usually low and bone age is unaffected. It is important to monitor carefully in order to exclude the onset of true precocious puberty.

Autoimmune hypothyroidism may also result in isolated breast development, although this is rarely seen before 5 years of age.

Thelarche variants

There appears to be a whole spectrum of presentations between premature thelarche and true precocious puberty.

Thus, some girls with early breast development also demonstrate increased height velocity and bone maturation, and ovarian ultrasound reveals a multicystic appearance (as distinct from polycystic, see Chapter 18).

Premature adrenarche

The normal onset of adrenal androgen secretion ('adrenarche') occurs 1–2 years prior to the onset of puberty. 'Premature' or 'exaggerated' adrenarche results in mild virilization (e.g. pubic hair and acne, but not clitoromegaly). The cause is unknown. The diagnosis is made by the finding of low serum gonadotrophin levels and mildly elevated adrenal androgen levels (dehydroepiandrosterone sulphate, androstenedione). It is important to exclude late-onset congenital adrenal hyperplasia (CAH) and androgen-secreting tumours.

Congenital adrenal hyperplasia

CAH due to deficiency of the enzyme 21-hydroxylase leads to cortisol deficiency, oversecretion of adrenocorticotrophic hormone (ACTH) due to loss of feedback inhibition, and excessive production of adrenal androgens (see Chapter 11). Inheritance is autosomal recessive. Classic CAH usually presents in the neonate with ambiguous genitalia and a salt-losing crisis (see Chapter 13), whilst non-classic or late-onset CAH presents in adolescence with moderate to severe virilization (pubic hair, hirsutism, acne and clitoromegaly) and rapid growth.

The diagnosis is made by the finding of raised levels of cortisol precursors, particularly 17-OH progesterone, both at baseline and post i.v. ACTH stimulation, in both plasma and urine. Gonadotrophin levels are suppressed. Bilateral adrenal hyperplasia may be seen on abdominal ultrasound. Management of CAH is by hydrocortisone replacement therapy, which suppresses ACTH and adrenal androgen secretion (the classic presentation may also require fludrocortisone to replace aldosterone secretion).

Androgenization of the female external genitalia may lead not only to clitoromegaly but also fusion of the labio-scrotal folds. There may, in addition, be a urethral fistula which may require careful repair at the time of an introitoplasty. Clitoral reduction should be undertaken with care to preserve the neurovascular bundle and sensation. Surgery may be undertaken during the neonatal period, and may be required again during adolescence. As with all surgery for intersex disorders, the precise timing is open to debate, as is the degree to which the patient, rather than her parents and doctors, is involved in the decision-making process.

Peripheral tumours

Sex-steroid-secreting tumours

Abnormal production of androgens ± oestrogens may arise from tumours of the adrenal glands (adenomas or carcinomas), ovaries (granulosa cell or theca cell neoplasia) or teratomas. Androgen-secreting tumours are usually associated with severe virilization in young girls (<6 years old). The diagnosis is made by the finding of excessively raised circulating plasma sex hormone levels. A 24-h urine collection for steroid profile often demonstrates excess levels of sex steroid metabolites. Gonadotrophin levels are suppressed and α-fetoprotein levels may be raised. These tumours are often palpable and an abdominal ultrasound scan will confirm the diagnosis.

Gonadotrophin-secreting tumours

Very rarely, a human chorionic gonadotrophin (hCG)-secreting hepatoblastoma, choriocarcinoma or dysgerminoma causes precocious puberty. Circulating levels of hCG are usually extremely high.

McCune–Albright syndrome

This sporadic condition results in spontaneous activation of gonadotrophin receptors and excessive sex steroid secretion independent of normal ligand binding. It is due to a somatic activating mutation of the G-protein α-subunit which also affects bones (polyostotic fibrous dysplasia), skin (café au lait spots) and potentially multiple other endocrinopathies (hyperthyroidism or hyperparathyroidism). All cells descended from the mutated embryonic cell line are affected, while cells descended from non-mutated cells develop into normal tissues. Thus, the phenotype is highly variable in physical distribution and severity. The diagnosis is made by clinical assessment, based on the presence of skin, bone and other lesions. Biopsy of affected skin may allow identification of the genetic mutation. Gonadotrophin levels are suppressed.

Management of precocious puberty

It is important to exclude severe diseases (e.g. CAH, cranial or peripheral tumours) which will require specific therapy. Following reduction in peripheral sex steroid levels, due to CAH or sex-steroid-secreting tumours, central precocious puberty may occur due to hypothalamic maturation (especially if the girl's bone age is already >11 years). Premature thelarche and thelarche variant need no treatment as there are no long-term consequences and, furthermore, treatment appears to be without effect.

Inhibition of puberty

Pituitary gonadotrophin secretion can be suppressed by constant high levels of a GnRH agonist, given by subcutaneous depot injection (e.g. leuprorelin acetate 3.5 mg monthly). Circulating sex steroid levels should become undetectable, and LH and FSH levels post i.v. LH-releasing hormone should return to prepubertal levels. The dose interval may need to be shortened to 3 weeks to fully suppress puberty. Following investigation and reassurance, however, many older girls and their parents are happy to avoid treatment. The aims of stopping puberty are:

- to avoid psychosocial problems arising from early sexual maturation; and
- to prevent reduction in final adult height due to premature bone maturation and early epiphyseal fusion. A wrist X-ray for estimation of bone age is essential in the investigation of precocious puberty, and may be used to predict final height when considering the need for treatment.

Androgen receptor blockade

Androgen receptor blocking agents, such as cyproterone acetate, finasteride or flutamide, may be used for symptomatic treatment of excess androgen production in girls with premature adrenarche.

Delayed Puberty

Delayed puberty is defined as the absence of onset of puberty by more than 2 standard deviations later than the average age, i.e. >14 years in females (compared with >16 years in males). Delayed puberty may be idiopathic/familial or due to a number of general conditions resulting in undernutrition. Absence of puberty may also be due to gonadal failure (elevated gonadotrophin levels) or impairment of gonadotrophin secretion. Occasionally, some girls enter puberty spontaneously but then fail to progress normally through puberty (Figure 14.5 and Box 14.2).

Constitutional delay of growth and puberty

Rates of skeletal and sexual maturation are closely linked, but vary widely between individuals and are influenced by family history and rate of early childhood weight gain. Although constitutional delay presents more commonly in males, this may merely reflect their higher level of concern. These girls are otherwise healthy. The diagnosis is made by exclusion, but often can only be confirmed retrospectively following spontaneous initiation of the hypothalamic–pituitary axis. It can be very difficult to distinguish hypogonadotrophic hypogonadism from constitutional delay in puberty, and therefore it is better to provide treatment and revisit the diagnosis at a later date. Appropriate investigations, after physical examination and measurement of weight

---

Box 14.2 Causes of delayed puberty

General

- Constitutional delay of growth and puberty
- Malabsorption (e.g. coeliac disease, inflammatory bowel disease)
- Underweight (due to severe dieting/anorexia nervosa, overexercise or competitive sports)
- Other chronic disease (asthma, cystic fibrosis, renal failure)

Gonadal failure (hypergonadotrophic hypogonadism; see Chapter 16)

- Turner's syndrome, gonadal dysgenesis and premature ovarian failure
- Post malignancy (following chemotherapy, local radiotherapy or surgical removal)
- Polyglandular autoimmune syndromes

Gonadotrophin deficiency

- Congenital hypogonadotrophic hypogonadism (± anosmia)
- Hypothalamic/pituitary lesions (tumours, post radiotherapy or surgery)
- Haemochromatosis/iron overload
- Rare inactivating mutations of genes encoding luteinizing hormone, follicle-stimulating hormone or their receptors

	2	3	4	5
Breast stage	2 (9.2 – 13.2)	3 (10.2 – 14.2)	4 (10.8 – 15.6)	5 (11.8 – 18.6)
Pubic hair stage	2 (9.3 – 13.7)	3 (10.0 – 14.4)	4 (10.7 – 15.1)	5 (12.2 – 16.5)
Menarche	(11.2 – 14.8)			
Peak height velocity	(10.2 – 13.6)			

Age 10 11 12 13 14 15

Figure 14.5 Timing of events in female puberty (95 percentiles for age in years).

and height, include assessment of serum concentrations of gonadotrophins, prolactin and thyroid function, and assessment of bone age (radial X-ray). Pelvic ultrasonography may be helpful, as is a karyotype if features of Turner's syndrome are suspected.

Turner's syndrome

Characteristic features of Turner's syndrome may not be obvious, particularly if due to chromosomal mosaicism, and karyotype should be investigated in all girls presenting with pubertal delay. Up to 25% of girls with Turner's syndrome enter puberty spontaneously; however, only 10% progress through puberty and only 1% develop ovulatory cycles. Thus, the chromosomal abnormality seems to result in premature ovarian exhaustion rather than a primary failure of ovarian development. Turner's syndrome is the most common cause of gonadal dysgenesis. In its most severe form, the XO genotype is associated with the classic Turner's features including short stature, webbing of the neck, cubitus valgus, widely spaced nipples, cardiac and renal abnormalities, and often autoimmune hypothyroidism. Spontaneous menstruation may occur (particularly when there is mosaicism), but premature ovarian failure (POF) usually ensues.

The clinical diagnosis is confirmed by the finding of a 45XO karyotype (at least 30 cells should be examined due to the possibility of mosaicism). Cytogenetic analysis should also be performed looking for the presence of Y fragments, which indicate an increased risk of gonadoblastoma, and thus the 'streak' gonads should be removed (usually laparoscopically). Serum gonadotrophin concentrations are elevated compared with adolescents of the same age, and may approach the menopausal range.

Management includes low-dose oestrogen therapy to promote breast development without further disturbing linear growth (Figure 14.6). Treatment with GH has also benefited some individuals. Cyclical oestrogen plus progestogen may be used as maintenance therapy. A regular withdrawal bleed is essential in order to prevent endometrial hyperplasia. Spontaneous conception has been reported in patients with Turner's syndrome, but is rare. However, the possibility of assisted conception and oocyte donation should be discussed at an early age.

Other causes of premature ovarian failure

POF, by definition, is the cessation of periods accompanied by raised gonadotrophin concentration prior to the age of

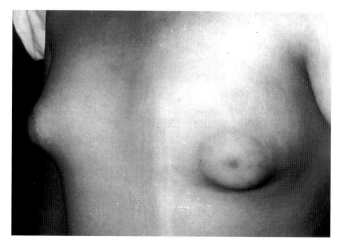

Figure 14.6 Breast development in Turner's syndrome following oestrogen administration. There is good areolar development but little breast tissue after several years of hormone replacement.

40 years. It may occur at any age. The exact incidence of this condition is unknown as many cases go unrecognized, but estimates vary between 1% and 5% of the female population (Coulam et al 1986). In approximately two-thirds of cases, the cause of ovarian failure cannot be identified (Conway et al 1996). It is unknown whether these cases are truly 'idiopathic' or due to as yet undiscovered genetic, immunological or environmental factors. A series of 323 women with POF attending an endocrinology clinic in London identified 23% with Turner's syndrome, 6% after chemotherapy, 4% with familial POF and 2% each who had pelvic surgery, pelvic irradiation, galactosaemia and 46XY gonadal dysgenesis (Conway et al 1996). Viral and bacterial infection may also lead to ovarian failure; thus, infections such as mumps, cytomegalovirus or human immunodeficiency virus in adult life can adversely affect long-term ovarian function, as can severe pelvic inflammatory disease.

Ovarian failure occurring before puberty is usually due to a chromosomal abnormality or a childhood malignancy that required chemotherapy or radiotherapy, from which, parenthetically, there are increasing numbers of survivors into adulthood with POF. The likelihood of developing ovarian failure after therapy for cancer is difficult to predict, but the age of the patient is a significant factor; the younger the patient, the greater the follicle pool and the better her chances of retaining ovarian function.

Adolescents who lose ovarian function soon after menarche are often found to have a Turner's mosaic (46XX/45X) or an X-chromosome trisomy (47XXX). There are many genes on the X chromosome that are essential for normal ovarian function. It would appear that two active X chromosomes are required during fetal life in order to lay down a normal follicle store. In fetuses with Turner's syndrome, normal numbers of oocytes appear on the genital ridge but accelerated atresia takes place during late fetal life. Thus, streak gonads occur and it is only the mosaic form of Turner's syndrome that permits any possibility of ovarian function. X mosaicisms are the most common chromosomal abnormality in reported series of POF, ranging from 5% to 40% (Anasti 1998). Other X chromosome anomalies may result in ovarian failure; for example, balanced translocations in the long arm of chromosome X between Xq13 and q26, which is a critical region for ovarian function.

There are a number of syndromes that are associated with POF, such as familial blepharophimosis, in which the abnormality is on chromosome 3. Galactosaemia is another rare example, in which a metabolic defect has a direct inhibitory effect on ovarian function, probably due to a build-up of galactose within the ovary that decreases the initial number of oogonia.

Polyglandular autoimmune syndromes

Antiovarian antibodies are occasionally detected in both type 1 (hypoparathyroidism, Addison's disease, mucocutaneous candidiasis) and type 2 (Addison's disease, hypothyroidism, type 1 diabetes) polyglandular autoimmune syndromes. Autoimmune ovarian failure may also occur in the absence of positive antibodies due to poor sensitivity of current assays.

Congenital hypogonadotrophic hypogonadism

Congenital hypogonadotrophic deficiency associated with complete or partial anosmia ± other midline defects and mental retardation (Kallman or DeMorsier syndrome) may be inherited in autosomal-dominant, -recessive or X-linked recessive patterns, suggesting that a number of mutated genes may be causative. Congenital hypogonadotrophism may also occur without anosmia in isolation or in panhypopituitarism. The diagnosis is made by a family history or related features of Kallman syndrome. Absent LH and FSH response to i.v. GnRH stimulation may be indistinguishable from constitutional delay of puberty, and retesting may be required after completing pubertal development with exogenous oestrogen.

Management of delayed puberty

Following exclusion of other diagnoses, many patients are happy to await spontaneous pubertal development. However, severe delay in pubertal onset may be a risk factor for decreased bone mineral density and osteoporosis. In subjects with hypergonadotrophic hypogonadism, puberty may be induced from any age; however, in Turner's syndrome, delay in induction to around 14 years of age possibly permits maximal response to GH therapy (see Box 14.3).

Box 14.3 Induction of puberty for girls with ovarian failure

Ethinyloestradiol
- 2 µg daily for 6 months
- 5 µg daily for 6 months
- 10 µg daily for 6 months
- 15 µg daily for 6 months
- 20 µg daily for 6 months
- 30 µg daily for 6 months

Menstruation may occur once a 15 µg preparation is being used. Once bleeding occurs, a cyclical oestrogen/progestogen preparation should be prescribed, usually in the form of the contraceptive pill.

Pubertal development

Oral oestrogen therapy should be commenced at a very low dose (e.g. ethinyloestradiol 2 µg daily) and gradually increased according to breast response and age. Oral progesterone should be added if breakthrough bleeding occurs or when ethinyloestradiol dose reaches 20 µg/day. Eventually, maintenance therapy is provided either with a combined oral contraceptive pill or a conventional, cyclical postmenopausal hormone replacement preparation.

Fertility

In gonadotrophin deficiency, ovulation and fertility may be achieved by ovulation induction using either pulsatile GnRH (for hypothalamic problems) or gonadotrophin therapy (for pituitary or hypothalamic disease). If the patient with hypogonadotrophic hypogonadism is particularly anxious about future fertility, a non-therapeutic trial of exogenous pulsatile GnRH administration, via a miniature portable infusion pump, confirms pituitary responsiveness. However, induction of ovulation can be achieved, bypassing the pituitary, by direct administration of human menopausal gonadotrophin (hMG). hMG is a more suitable choice than the more recently developed recombinant FSH preparations as it also contains LH which is necessary to stimulate oestrogen biosynthesis. Patients with POF may choose assisted conception with donated oocytes.

Presentation of Congenital Anomalies of the Genital Tract (see Chapter 13)

Disorders of sexual development may result in ambiguous genitalia or anomalies of the internal genital tract, and may be due to genetic defects, abnormalities of steroidogenesis, and dysynchrony during organogenesis. Age of presentation will depend upon the degree of dysfunction caused. Ambiguous genitalia occur in approximately 1:30,000 newborns. The rate with which other congenital anomalies present varies depending upon the population studied and the age at which the problem is likely to be noticed. Population-based statistics are still lacking for many conditions, largely because patients present to different specialists (e.g. gynaecologists, paediatric endocrinologists, urologists, etc.), and there are rarely clear pathways for communication between the different professional groups from which to create a comprehensive service for both provision of treatment and collection of data.

Patients require sensitive care by an expert multidisciplinary group that includes gynaecologists, paediatric endocrinologists, paediatric surgeons and urologists, plastic surgeons, psychologists, specialist nurses, geneticists and urologists. A network of support should be provided to the patient and her parents and family. The adolescent period is a particularly sensitive time as the individual becomes aware of her diagnosis and its impact on her sexuality, sexual function and fertility. It is particularly important to provide a seamless handover from paediatric to adult services at this time, and dedicated adolescent clinics may have an important role.

Müllerian duct abnormalities

In the absence of a Y chromosome, testis and testosterone, the Wolffian duct regresses after the sixth week of embryonic life. The Müllerian ducts then develop into the uterus and fallopian tubes, and fuse caudally with the urogenital sinus to form the vagina. Abnormalities in the process of fusion may be either medial or vertical, and result in primary amenorrhoea; complete or partial Müllerian agenesis may also occur. Renal developmental abnormalities are commonly seen in association with abnormalities of the genital tract, so assessment by intravenous urography is advisable before attempting corrective surgery.

Congenital absence of the vagina

Women with Mayer–Rokitansky–Kuster–Hauser syndrome (or Rokitansky syndrome) have a 46XX genotype and a normal female phenotype with spontaneous development of secondary sexual characteristics, as ovarian tissue is present and functions normally. The Müllerian ducts have failed to fuse and so there is vaginal agenesis. The incidence is about 1 : 5000 female births and may be associated with renal tract anomalies (15–40%) or anomalies of the skeletal system (10–20%). The external genitalia have a normal appearance but the vagina is short and blind ending, such that either surgery or gradual dilatation is necessary to achieve a capacity appropriate for normal sexual function. Hormone treatment is not required as ovarian oestrogen output is normal. Indeed, ovulation occurs and ovarian stimulation followed by oocyte retrieval can be performed in order to achieve a 'biological' pregnancy through the services of a surrogate mother.

The vaginal dimple can vary in length from just a slight depression between the labia to up to 5–6 cm. Vaginal dilators, made of plastic or glass, are used first to stretch the vaginal skin, and the patient is encouraged to apply pressure for 15 min twice daily with successive sizes of dilator. An adequately sized vagina is usually formed by 6 months but this may take longer, and long-term use of dilators may be required depending upon the frequency of sexual intercourse.

A number of surgical approaches have been employed to create a neovagina. The Vecchetti procedure uses the same principle of progressive dilatation, with the application of pressure from a plastic sphere in the vagina which is attached to two wires that have been passed from the top of the vagina through to the anterior wall of the abdomen, where they are attached to a traction device that is tightened daily. Plastic surgical techniques include:

- the McIndoe vaginoplasty, in which a split skin graft is placed over a mould which has been inserted into a space created where the vagina should be;
- tissue expansion vaginoplasty, in which expansion balloons are inserted into the labia and inflated with water over a period of 2 weeks in order to stretch the labial skinfolds sufficiently to be used to fashion a vagina;
- an artificial vagina created from bowel, a technique less favoured nowadays because of problems with persistent discharge; and
- the Williams vaginoplasty, in which the labia are used to create a pouch, also rarely used nowadays because of problems with a poor anatomical result and an awkward angle for intercourse.

The diagnosis of Rokitansky syndrome can usually be made without the need for a laparoscopy. Sometimes, however, an ultrasound scan will reveal the presence of a uterine remnant (anlagen) which is usually small and hardly ever of sufficient size to function normally. If there is active endometrial tissue within the uterine anlagan, the patient may experience cyclical pain and the anlagan should be excised (usually laparoscopically).

Fusion abnormalities of the vagina

Longitudinal fusion abnormalities may lead to a complete septum that may be associated with two complete uterine horns with two cervices, or a partial septum causing a unilateral obstruction. Excision is required to both prevent retention of uterine secretions and permit sexual intercourse. Transverse fusion abnormalities usually present with primary amenorrhoea and require careful assessment before surgery. The most common problem is an imperforate hymen in which cyclical lower abdominal pain combines with a visible haematocolpos and a bulging purple/blue hymen with menstrual secretions stretching the thin hymen. The surgery required is a simple incision which should be performed when the diagnosis is made to prevent excessive build-up of menstrual blood, which may lead to a haematometra and consequent increased risk of endometriosis (secondary to retrograde menstruation). A transverse vaginal septum due to failure of fusion or canalization between the Müllerian tubercle and sinovaginal bulb may present like an imperforate hymen, but is associated with a pink bulge at the introitus as the septum is thicker than the hymen. Greater care must be taken during surgery to prevent annular constriction rings, and the procedure should only be performed in dedicated centres by experienced surgeons. When there is a transverse septum, it has been found to be high in 46% of patients, in the middle of the vagina in 40%, and low in the remaining 14%. It is the patients in the last two groups who have higher pregnancy rates after surgery.

Müllerian/uterine anomalies

Uterine anomalies occur in 3–10% of the fertile female population and can be subdivided according to the nature of the abnormality. They been usefully classified by the American Society for Reproductive Medicine into six groups:

- segmental agenesis or hypoplasia, which may involve vagina, cervix, uterine corpus or fallopian tubes. Mayer–Rokitansky–Kuster–Hauser syndrome is included here;
- unicornuate uterus, with or without a rudimentary horn that may or may not contain endometrium and be connected to the main uterine cavity. On the affected side, the kidney and ureter are generally absent;
- uterus didelphis: due to partial or complete failure of lateral Müllerian duct fusion, leading to partial or complete duplication of the vagina, cervix and uterus;
- bicornuate uterus, with a single vagina and cervix and two uterine bodies, that may be completely separated or fused centrally with a partial septum;
- septate or arcuate uterus, with a septum that may be partial or complete; and
- diethylstilboestrol-related anomalies, which may demonstrate various shapes due to the effect of diethylstilboestrol.

These anomalies are often discovered by chance during coincidental investigations for infertility. The diagnosis is made by a combination of ultrasound, magnetic resonance imaging and X-ray hysterosalpingography (the latter during the course of an infertility work-up). Women with uterine anomalies are usually asymptomatic, unless there is obstruction to menstrual flow, when cyclical pain may be experienced. Whilst infertility per se is rarely caused by uterine anomalies, they may be associated with endometriosis if there is retrograde menstruation secondary to obstruction. Furthermore, recurrent miscarriage may be experienced by some women with uterine malformations.

Surgery is reserved for those cases where there is obstruction; for example, the removal of a rudimentary uterine horn or excision of a vaginal septum. The excision of a uterine septum has been shown to improve pregnancy outcome and should be performed by an experienced hysteroscopist. On the other hand, metroplasty (Strassman procedure) of the horns of a bicornuate uterus is seldom performed nowadays as its benefit has been questioned.

Androgen insensitivity syndrome

Girls who are phenotypically normal but have absent pubic and axillary hair in the presence of normal breast development are likely to have complete androgen insensitivity syndrome (formerly known as 'testicular feminization syndrome', a term that is no longer favoured). In this condition, the karyotype is 46XY and, whilst testes are present, there is an insensitivity to secreted androgens because of abnormalities in the androgen receptor. The incidence is approximately 1 : 60,000 'male' births and it is inherited as an X-linked trait (the androgen receptor is on the short arm of the X chromosome). Anti-Müllerian factors prevent the development of internal Müllerian structures, and the Wolffian structures also fail to develop because of the insensitivity to testosterone. The external genitalia appear female. In approximately 10% of cases, the defect is incomplete (partial androgen insensitivity syndrome); the external genitalia may be ambiguous at birth, with labioscrotal fusion, and virilization may sometimes occur before puberty.

After puberty, gonadal tissue should be removed to prevent malignant transformation (dysgerminoma), which occurs in approximately 5% of cases. Exogenous oestrogen should then be prescribed; cyclical treatment is not required because the uterus is absent. The syndrome may be diagnosed in infancy if a testis is found in either the labia or an inguinal hernia, in which case both testes should be removed at this time because of the potential risk of malignancy. Some cases, however, only present at puberty with primary amenorrhoea, and removal of abdominal/inguinal testes should then be performed.

Careful psychological assessment and counselling are obligatory to allow an understanding of the gonadal dysfunction and necessity for hormone treatment. It may be helpful to describe the gonads as internal sexual organs that have been incompletely formed and which are therefore prone to develop cancer if they are not removed. In general, a completely honest approach is favoured so that the individual is provided with full information about her condition, its origins and management. It is certainly the author's experience that the vast majority of patients desire a full explanation of their condition, and respond better to treatment if they are included in the decision-making processes. Patients with these problems should be referred to centres where there are specialists experienced in their management, so that a comprehensive team approach can be provided.

There are several uncommon intersex disorders which result in primary amenorrhoea, and while their management must be individualized, it will often broadly follow the above outline. Examples are male pseudohermaphroditism, caused by 5α-reductase deficiency, and female pseudohermaphroditism, caused by CAH (see above). In contrast to the androgen insensitivity syndrome, in these conditions, there is deficient or absent breast development, yet normal or increased pubic and axillary hair. 5α-reductase deficiency is an autosomal-recessive condition, diagnosed by the presence of undervirilization (which may change at puberty) and an elevated testosterone:dihydrotestoster-one ratio.

Cloacal anomalies

Cloacal anomalies may take a variety of forms depending upon the relative contribution of gastrointestinal, genital and renal tracts. The cloaca should be divided anteriorly into the urogenital sinus, and posteriorly into the rectum. Major surgery is often required during the neonatal period to provide anterior abdominal wall integrity and continence of faeces and urine. Several operations may be required, and the uterus and genitalia, if present, may be adversely affected such that, at puberty, there is obstruction to menstrual flow and also an increased rate of ovarian cyst formation, presumably due to ovarian entrapment restricting normal follicular growth and ovulation.

Gynaecological Complaints

Disorders of the menstrual cycle are common and often normal in adolescence, and will rarely require secondary level care unless there is underlying pathology. Most conditions will be dealt with in an outpatient setting and will seldom require a hospital stay. The adolescent female will require careful explanation of what is normal, what can be expected and how things may change. Provision should be made to see her either alone, with her mother or, as is often the case, with a close female friend. Adolescents need to be given autonomy and ownership of their condition in order to encourage attendance for follow-up appointments.

Menorrhagia

In a young woman with intractable menorrhagia, an assessment of blood clotting may be beneficial. Disorders of haemostasis such as von Willebrand's disease, deficiencies of factors V, VII, X and XI, and idiopathic thrombocytopenic purpura are thought to increase menstrual loss. Young girls with heavy periods in the years after the menarche are very unlikely to have any pelvic pathology. A very small number of young girls have persistent heavy irregular periods associated with anovular cycles, particularly those with polycystic ovary syndrome (see Chapter 18). In these cases, sustained unopposed oestrogen levels lead to endometrial hyperplasia which may ultimately progress to carcinoma.

Primary dysmenorrhoea

In general, primary dysmenorrhoea appears 6–12 months after the menarche when ovulatory cycles have become established. The early cycles after the menarche are usually anovular and tend to be painless. The pain usually consists of lower abdominal cramps and backache, and there may be associated gastrointestinal disturbances such as diarrhoea and vomiting. Symptoms occur predominantly during the first 2 days of menstruation. Primary dysmenorrhoea does not tend to be associated with excessive menstrual bleeding. Although excessive levels of prostaglandins, leukotrienes and vasopressin have been found in primary dysmenorrhoea, the primary stimulus for their production remains unknown. The clear involvement of prostaglandins in primary dysmenorrhoea has led to the use of prostaglandin synthetase inhibitors, such as mefenamic acid, naproxen, ibuprofen and aspirin, to treat the disorder. Ibuprofen is the preferred analgesic because of its favourable efficacy and safety profiles.

Summary

The endocrine changes during puberty are regulated by the hypothalamic–pituitary–ovarian axis which controls growth and gonadotrophin pulsatility. Insulin plays a pivotal role by its influence on IGFBP-1 and SHBG levels. Recent studies also indicate that the hormone leptin, which is secreted by fat cells and which acts on the hypothalamus to induce satiety, may influence energy metabolism and GnRH pulsatility. Body weight, nutrition, and genetic and socioeconomic factors may all play a role in the initiation and timing of puberty, but the precise mechanisms still remain unclear.

Anomalous pubertal development requires careful evaluation to exclude sinister causes. Once initial investigations have been performed, it is often reasonable to hold off medical therapies and observe the rate of change. Treatments are available to suppress precocious puberty and to initiate breast development and menstruation for girls with delayed puberty or ovarian failure, respectively.

Management of all intersex conditions requires the skills of a multidisciplinary team that includes paediatric surgeons, urologists (often paediatric and adult), plastic surgeons, endocrinologists, specialist nurses, psychologists and gynaecologists, whose role is to help coordinate the transition from childhood through adolescence and then womanhood, and help with issues relating to sexual function and sexual identity, endocrinology and fertility. It is during the difficult time of adolescence that the patient usually first realizes that there are serious problems, and it is often the specialist gynaecologist who helps her to understand the diagnosis and requirements for management. The support of a skilled nurse and clinical psychologist is invaluable at this time.

KEY POINTS

1. Puberty is a coherent process involving oestrogen production, increased somatic growth and the development of secondary sexual characteristics.

2. The essential hormonal event of puberty is the augmentation of pulsatile gonadotrophin secretion, which is affected by endocrine, nutritional and psychological factors.

3. Menarche occurs after sufficient endometrium has developed to result in a withdrawal bleed when the oestrogen level temporarily falls. It usually occurs within 2 years of the earliest sign of breast development.

4. Appropriate investigation of abnormal events surrounding puberty must be based upon detailed history and examination of the patient.

5. The most common cause of delayed puberty is ovarian failure. More than half of girls with delayed puberty have chromosome anomalies.

6. Serum gonadotrophin levels are important in distinguishing hypo- and hypergonadotrophic causes of delayed puberty.

7. Oestrogen and progesterone replacement are used in primary ovarian failure to induce pubertal growth and secondary sexual characteristics.

8. Precocious puberty, where breast development occurs before the age of 8 years, is most commonly due to constitutional early development.

9. Precocious puberty requires prompt investigation and treatment in order to avoid short stature from premature closure of the epiphyses.

10. Anorexia nervosa and acute weight loss are associated with amenorrhoea.

11. The psychological stress of pubertal disorders must be recognized and dealt with sympathetically in order to avoid excessive undermining of the patient's self-confidence.

12. Oocyte donation has been successfully used to allow patients with primary ovarian failure to achieve pregnancy and have their own children.

Acknowledgements

The author wishes to thank Dr Kathy Michelmore DPhil, Department of General Practice, Royal Victoria Hospital, Newcastle and Dr Ken Ong DPhil, Department of Paediatrics, Addenbrookes Hospital, Cambridge for help in preparing this chapter.

References

Amiel SA, Caprio S, Sherwin RS, Plewe G, Hymond MW, Tamborlane WV 1991 Insulin resistance of puberty: a defect restricted to peripheral glucose metabolism. Journal of Clinical Endocrinology and Metabolism 72: 277–282.

Anasti JN 1998 Premature ovarian failure: an update. Fertility and Sterility 70: 1–15.

Baxter Jones AD, Helms P, Baines Preece J, Preece M 1994 Menarche in intensively trained gymnasts, swimmers and tennis players. Annals of Human Biology 21: 407–415.

Benso L, Lorenzino C, Pastorin L, Barotto M, Signorile F, Mostert M 1989 The distribution of age at menarche in a random series of Turin girls followed longitudinally. Annals of Human Biology 16: 549–552.

Cameron N, Nagdee I 1996 Menarcheal age in two generations of South African Indians. Annals of Human Biology 23: 113–119.

Cameron N 1976 Weight and skinfold variation at menarche and the critical body weight hypothesis. Annals of Human Biology 3: 279–282.

Caufriez A 1997 The pubertal spurt: effects of sex steroids on growth hormone and insulin-like growth factor I. European Journal of Obstetrics, Gynecology and Reproductive Biology 71: 215–217.

Clayton PE, Gill MS, Hall CM, Tillmann V, Whatmore AJ, Price DA 1997 Serum leptin through childhood and adolescence. Clinical Endocrinology 46: 727–733.

Clement K, Vaisse C, Lahlou N et al 1998 A mutation in the human leptin receptor gene causes obesity and pituitary dysfunction. Nature 392: 398–401.

Considine RV, Sinha MK, Heiman ML et al 1996 Serum immunoreactive-leptin concentrations in normal-weight and obese humans. New England Journal of Medicine 334: 292–295.

Conway GS, Kaltas G, Patel A, Davies MC, Jacobs HS 1996 Characterization of idiopathic premature ovarian failure. Fertility and Sterility 65: 337–341.

Cooper C, Kuh D, Egger P, Wadsworth M, Barker D 1996 Childhood growth and age at menarche. British Journal of Obstetrics and Gynaecology 103: 814–817.

Coulam CB, Adamson SC, Annegers JF 1986 Incidence of premature ovarian failure. Obstetrics and Gynecology 67: 604–606.

Dann TC, Roberts DF 1993 Menarcheal age in University of Warwick young women. Journal of Biosocial Science 25: 531–538.

Delemarre HA, Wennink JM, Odink RJ 1991 Gonadotrophin and growth hormone secretion throughout puberty. Acta Paediatrica Scandinavica 372 (Suppl): 26–31.

de Ridder CM, Thijssen JH, Bruning PF, van den Brande JL, Zonderland ML, Erich WB 1992 Body fat mass, body fat distribution, and pubertal development: a longitudinal study of physical and hormonal sexual maturation of girls. Journal of Clinical Endocrinology and Metabolism 75: 442–446.

Flug D, Largo RH, Prader A 1984 Menstrual patterns in adolescent Swiss girls: a longitudinal study. Annals of Human Biology 11: 495–508.

Frisch RE 1990 The right weight: body fat, menarche and ovulation. Baillière's Clinical Obstetrics and Gynaecology 4: 419–439.

Frisch RE, Revelle R 1970 Height and weight at menarche and a hypothesis of critical body weights and adolescent events. Science 169: 397–399.

Frisch RE, Gotz Welbergen AV, McArthur JW et al 1981 Delayed menarche and amenorrhea of college athletes in relation to age of onset of training. JAMA: the Journal of the Anerican Medical Association 246: 1559–1563.

Garn SM, LaVelle M, Pilkington JJ 1983 Comparisons of fatness in premenarcheal and postmenarcheal girls of the same age. Journal of Pediatrics 103: 328–331.

Garn SM, Bailey SM 1978 Genetics of maturational processes. In: Falkner F, Tanner J (eds) Human Growth. Baillière Tindall, London.

Giustina A, Scalvini T, Tassi C et al 1997 Maturation of the regulation of growth hormone secretion in young males with hypogonadotropic hypogonadism pharmacologically exposed to progressive increments in serum testosterone. Journal of Clinical Endocrinology and Metabolism 82: 1210–1219.

Griffin IJ, Cole TJ, Duncan KA, Hollman AS, Donaldson MDC 1995 Pelvic ultrasound measurements in normal girls. Acta Paediatrica 84: 536–543.

Holly JM, Smith CP, Dunger DB et al 1989 Relationship between the pubertal fall in sex hormone binding globulin and insulin-like growth factor binding protein-I. A synchronized approach to pubertal development? Clinical Endocrinology 31: 277–284.

Holm K, Mosfeldt Laursen E, Brocks V, Muller J 1995 Pubertal maturation of the internal genitalia: an ultrasound evaluation of 166 healthy girls. Ultrasound in Obstetrics and Gynecology 6: 175–181.

Malina RM, Spirduso WW, Tate C, Baylor AM 1978 Age at menarche and selected menstrual characteristics in athletes at different competitive levels and in different sports. Medicine and Science in Sports 10: 218–222.

Malina RM, Bouchard C, Shoup RF, Demirjian A, Lariviere G 1979 Age at menarche, family size, and birth order in athletes at the Montreal Olympic Games, 1976. Medicine and Science in Sports 11: 354–358.

Malina RM, Ryan RC, Bonci CM 1994 Age at menarche in athletes and their mothers and sisters. Annals of Human Biology 21: 417–422.

Mantzoros CS, Flier JS, Rogol AD 1997 A longitudinal assessment of hormonal and physical alterations during normal puberty in boys. V. Rising leptin levels may signal the onset of puberty. Journal of Clinical Endocrinology and Metabolism 82: 1066–1070.

Mauras N, Rogol AD, Haymond MW, Veldhuis JD 1996 Sex steroids, growth hormone, insulin-like growth factor-1: neuroendocrine and metabolic regulation in puberty. Hormone Research 45: 74–80.

Marshall WA, Tanner JM 1969 Variations in the pattern of pubertal changes in girls. Archives of Disease in Childhood 44: 291–303.

Nobels F, Dewailly D 1992 Puberty and polycystic ovarian syndrome: the insulin/insulin-like growth factor I hypothesis. Fertility and Sterility 58: 655–666.

Ostersehlt D, Danker Hopf E 1991 Changes in age at menarche in Germany: evidence for a continuing decline. American Journal of Human Biology 3: 647–654.

Parra A, Schultz RB, Graystone JE, Cheek DB 1971 Correlative studies in obese children and adolescents concerning body composition and plasma insulin and growth hormone levels. Pediatric Research 5: 603–613.

Rees M 1993 Menarche when and why? The Lancet 342: 1375–1376.

Roberts DF, Rozner LM, Swan AV 1971 Age at menarche, physique and environment in industrial north east England. Acta Paediatrica Scandinavica 60: 158–164.

Rosenbaum M, Leibel RL, Hirsch J 1997 Obesity. New England Journal of Medicine 337: 396–407.

Stanhope R, Adams J, Jacobs HS, Brook CGD 1985 Ovarian ultrasound assessment in normal children, idiopathic precocious puberty and during low dose pulsatile GnRH therapy of hypogonadotrophic hypogonadism. Archives of Diseases in Childhood 60: 116–119.

Stark O, Peckham CS, Moynihan C 1989 Weight and age at menarche. Archives of Diseases in Childhood 64: 383–387.

Smith CP, Archibald HR, Thomas JM et al 1988 Basal and stimulated insulin levels rise with advancing puberty. Clinical Endocrinology 28: 7–14.

Sorensen TI, Echwald S, Holm JC 1996 Leptin in obesity. British Medical Journal 313: 953–954.

Tryggvadottir L, Tulinius H, Larusdottir M 1994 A decline and a halt in mean age at menarche in Iceland. Annals of Human Biology 21: 179–186.

Veronesi FM, Gueresi P 1994 Trend in menarcheal age and socioeconomic influence in Bologna (northern Italy). Annals of Human Biology 21: 187–196.

Further Reading

Balen A, Creighton S, Davies M et al (eds) 2002 The Multidisciplinary Approach to Paediatric and Adolescent Gynaecology. Cambridge University Press, Cambridge.

Sanfilippo JS 1994 Pediatric and Adolescent Gynaecology. WB Saunders, Philadelphia.

CHAPTER 15

Control of hypothalamic–pituitary–ovarian function

Robert W. Shaw

Chapter Contents

INTRODUCTION	197
ANATOMY OF THE HYPOTHALAMIC–PITUITARY AXIS	197
HYPOTHALAMIC REGULATION OF PITUITARY SECRETION	198
MODULATORY ROLE OF MONOAMINES, OTHER NEUROTRANSMITTERS AND SECOND MESSENGERS ON GnRH SECRETION	201
OTHER NEUROTRANSMITTERS AND SECOND MESSENGERS	204
MODULATORY EFFECT OF OVARIAN STEROIDS	205
SELF-PRIMING OF THE PITUITARY GONADOTROPH BY GnRH	206
PULSATILE NATURE OF GONADOTROPHIN RELEASE	207
INTEGRATIVE CONTROL OF THE HYPOTHALAMIC–PITUITARY UNIT DURING THE MENSTRUAL CYCLE	208
KEY POINTS	210

Introduction

For the regulation of reproductive function, there are two major sites of action within the brain: the hypothalamus and the pituitary gland. A full understanding of the complex mechanisms involved in the fine tuning of the release of follicle-stimulating hormone (FSH) and luteinizing hormone (LH) will allow the clinician to understand the effects of stress, diet, exercise and other diverse influences which can affect the pituitary–gonadal axis and result in disorders of ovulation.

The hypothalamus lies at the base of the brain between the anterior margin of the optic chiasma anteriorly and the posterior margin of the mammillary bodies posteriorly. Precise boundaries are difficult to define, but it extends from the hypothalamic sulcus above to the tuber cinereum below, which itself connects the hypothalamus with the pituitary gland via its extension distally into the pituitary stalk.

The hypothalamus is the important final pathway between the brain and the pituitary gland. Secretion of hormones from the anterior pituitary is under the control of hypothalamic-releasing or -inhibiting factors. In turn, the pituitary hormones regulate cellular growth and differentiation and functional activity in their separate target organs. Internal environmental maintenance results in multiple biochemical signals converging upon neurones within the hypothalamus, leading to release of the pituitary hormones which coordinate appropriate metabolic responses.

Anatomy of the Hypothalamic–Pituitary Axis

The portion of the hypothalamus of special interest in the control of reproductive function is the neurohypophysis, which can be divided into three regions:

- the infundibulum, which constitutes the floor of the third ventricle (often termed the 'median eminence') and parts of the wall of the third ventricle, which is continuous with
- the infundibular stem or pituitary stalk, which is continuous distally with
- the infundibular process or posterior pituitary gland (Figure 15.1).

The adenohypophysis consists of:

- the pars distalis or anterior lobe of the pituitary;
- the pars intermedia, the intermediate lobe; and
- the pars tuberalis, which is a thin layer of adenohypophyseal cells lying on the surface of the infundibular stem and infundibulum.

The anterior pituitary does not normally receive an arterial vasculature but receives blood through portal vessels. The arteries supplying the median eminence and infundibular stalk empty into a dense network of capillaries, which are heavily innervated and drain into the portal venous plexus. In the human, these are present on all sides of the infundibular stalk, particularly posteriorly. These lead to the anterior pituitary formed by vessels from the median eminence and upper stalk joined ventrally by the short portal vessels arising

DOI: 10.1016/B978-0-7020-3120-5.00015-1

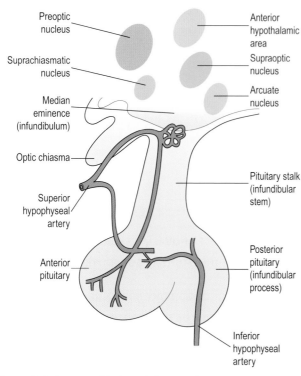

Figure 15.1 Anatomy of the hypothalamus and pituitary.

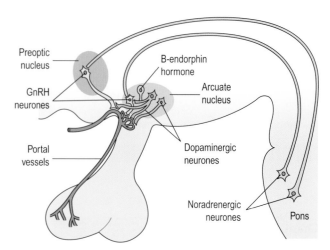

Figure 15.2 Representation of neurochemical interactions which are important in the control of gonadotrophin-releasing hormone (GnRH) secretion.

in the lower infundibular stalk. Some 80–90% of the blood supply to the anterior pituitary is provided by the long portal vessels; the remainder comes from the short portal veins. The sinusoids of the adenohypophysis thus receive blood that has first traversed capillaries residing in the neurohypophyseal complex, and this unique relationship provides the basis for the view that the hypothalamus regulates the secretion of adenohypophyseal hormones through neurohormonal mechanisms involving hypothalamic-releasing and -inhibiting factors.

In contrast, the neurohypophysis — posterior pituitary — is an extension of the hypothalamus and the neurosecretory neurones of the supraoptic and paraventricular nuclei. These neurones release vasopressin, oxytocin and their associated neurophysins.

Neural connections

There are numerous and extensive neural pathways connecting the hypothalamus with the rest of the brain. The majority of afferent hypothalamic nerve fibres run in the lateral hypothalamic areas, whilst efferent pathways are more medially placed. One important efferent connection is the supraopticohypophyseal nerve tract carrying fibres from the supraoptic and paraventricular nuclei to the infundibular process of the pituitary, whilst other fibres carry hypothalamic-releasing or -inhibiting factors from the medial and basal parts of the hypothalamus to the anterior pituitary (Figure 15.2).

Gonadotrophin-releasing hormone (GnRH)-secreting neurones appear in the medial olfactory placode and enter the brain with the nervus terminalis, a cranial nerve that projects from the nose to the septal preoptic nuclei in the

brain. By migration during embryogenesis, the cells, between 1000 and 3000 GnRH-producing neurones, predominantly settle in the arcuate nucleus of the hypothalamus (Schwanzel-Fukunda et al 1989). Failure of this migration has been shown to result in Kallmann's syndrome; a disorder associated with an absence of GnRH secretion and a defect of smell-anosmia (a failure of both olfactory axonal and GnRH neuronal migration from the olfactory placode). A 5–7-fold increased frequency of this condition is found in males, indicating that an X-linked transmission is the most common, although autosomal-dominant and autosomal-recessive modes of transmission have also been established (Waldstreicher et al 1996).

The mutations responsible for this syndrome result in the failure to produce a protein, homologous to members of the fibronectin family, responsible for cell adhesion and protease inhibition that is necessary for migration of these neurones (Bick et al 1992). GnRH neurones have cilia — as do olfactory epithelial cells in the nose — and the olfactory origin and structural similarity of these cells suggest an evolution from reproduction controlled by pheromones.

Hypothalamic Regulation of Pituitary Secretion

Considerable efforts have been made in the past 25 years to identify, characterize and synthesize the substances thought to be produced in the neural elements of the infundibulum. Several substances which can either stimulate or suppress the rate of release of one or more hormones from the pituitary gland have been found in the infundibular complex. These can be classified into hypophysiotrophic, neurohypophyseal and pituitary peptide hormones and are listed in Table 15.1. Other substances will probably be added to this list in the future.

Disorders of hypothalamic control of metabolic as well as reproductive hormones can influence the hypothalamic–pituitary–ovarian axis. For example, reproductive dysfunction may be associated with thyroid deficiency or excess,

Table 15.1 Hypothalamic and pituitary hormones

Hypothalamic hormones	
Gonadotrophin-releasing hormone	GnRH
Thyrotrophin-releasing hormone	TRH
Corticotrophin-releasing factor	CRF
Growth-hormone-releasing hormone	GHRH
Somatostatin	
Prolactin-inhibiting factor	PIF
Growth hormone secretagone receptor	Ghrelin
Posterior pituitary products	
Vasopressin	
Oxytocin	
Neurophysin I and II	
Anterior pituitary peptide hormones	
Adrenocorticotrophic hormone	ACTH
Prolactin	PRL
Luteinizing hormone	LH
Follicle-stimulating hormone	FSH
Growth hormone	GH
Thyroid-stimulating hormone	TSH

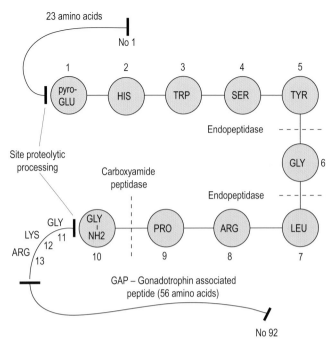

Figure 15.3 The structure of pre–pro-gonadotrophin-releasing hormone (GnRH). Highlighted is the decapeptide of the active molecule GnRH (molecular weight 1181). Sites of cleavage from the gonadotrophin-associated peptide are shown, as well as the main sites of enzymatic degradation of GnRH by endo- and carboxyamide peptidases in the pituitary.

adrenocorticotropic hormone (ACTH) excess (Cushing's syndrome) or growth hormone excess (acromegaly).

Further discussion in this chapter will be restricted to the roles played by GnRH, prolactin, dopamine and other neurotransmitters controlling the rates of release and synthesis of the gonadotrophins.

GnRH

In 1971, Schally et al isolated pure preparations of porcine LH-releasing hormone (LHRH) from hypothalamic extracts. Subsequently, its structure was discovered and synthesis was achieved (Matsuo et al 1971a,b). The finding of FSH-releasing activity of this LHRH led to the hypothesis of a single hypothalamic-releasing hormone, GnRH, controlling secretion of both LH and FSH from the pituitary gland, with the suggestion that sex steroids might play a role in modulating the proportions of LH and FSH released. The amino acid sequence of GnRH is shown in Figure 15.3; it is a decapeptide secreted with a large pre- and postprecursor molecule.

GnRH neurone system

The GnRH neurone system has been mapped in detail using primarily immunocytochemical methods. The GnRH neurones are not grouped into specific nuclei but form a loose network in several anatomical divisions. However, GnRH neurone bodies are found principally in two areas: the pre-optic anterior hypothalamic area and the tuberal hypothala-

mus, particularly the arcuate nucleus and periventricular nucleus. Axons from GnRH neurones project to many sites in the brain; the most distinct tract is from the medial basal hypothalamus to the median eminence, where extensive plexuses of boutons are found on the primary portal vessels. GnRH, then, has ready and direct access to the anterior pituitary gonadotroph cells via the portal capillary plexus (see Figure 15.2). There are also numerous projections of GnRH-secreting neurones to the limbic system and the circumventricular organ, other than the median eminence. The role of these connections is currently unknown, but they may connect with other cells or GnRH may bind to different receptors (type II) which may modulate sexual behaviour or sexual arousal.

The GnRH terminals in the median eminence remain outside the blood–brain barrier and can therefore be exposed to chemical agents within the general circulation. The GnRH neurones themselves have receptors for a number of neurotransmitters, in common with other neurones, and release them in their contacts with other neurones. In addition, their activity and release of GnRH can be influenced by GnRH agonists and antagonists. Exposure to GnRH agonists causes a greater release of GnRH but at less frequent pulse intervals. Exposure to GnRH antagonists induces a slower and non-pulsatile release of GnRH. Hence, GnRH neurones have an internal feedback loop for control of GnRH release through receptors for their own secretory product.

It has been estimated that there may be as few as 2000–3000 GnRH neurones dispersed within the hypothalamus, located predominantly in the preoptic and mediobasal areas. Considerable reduction in number can occur without affecting the pulsatile release of gonadotrophins. The pulsatile nature of gonadotrophin release is dependent upon small numbers of GnRH neurones working in synergy; the so-called 'pulse generators'.

Regulation of gonadotrophin secretion by GnRH

The GnRH gene sequence was first isolated by Seeburg and Adelman in 1984. The GnRH decapeptide is derived from the post-translational processing of a larger precursor molecule that has been termed 'pre–pro-GnRH'. This appears to be a tripartite structure with a preceding 23-amino acid sequence joined to the decapeptide GnRH, which is then attached via a 3-amino acid sequence, glycine–lycine–arginine (GLY–LYS–ARG), to a 56-amino acid terminal peptide, which is termed the 'gonadotrophin-associated peptide' (GAP). The post-GnRH-decapeptide GLY–LYS–ARG 3-amino acid section is an important site for proteolytic processing. GAP itself is thought to have some prolactin-inhibiting properties (Figure 15.3). GnRH genes are encoded from a single gene located on the shorter arm of chromosome 8.

Using radioimmunoassays, GnRH has been demonstrated in the hypophyseal portal blood from a number of animal species (Carmel et al 1976). Electrical stimulation of the preoptic area of the brain in female rats on the day of pro-oestrus increases the GnRH concentration in portal blood, and the stimulus induces a marked release of LH from the anterior pituitary. In contrast, administration of antibodies against GnRH prevents this electrically stimulated LH release. These data provide evidence favouring a cause-and-effect relationship between GnRH release by the hypothalamus and LH release by the anterior pituitary.

It is now firmly established that GnRH can stimulate the secretion of both LH and FSH in animals and humans. Following intravenous administration of synthetic GnRH, a significant rise in serum LH, and sometimes FSH, will be seen within 5 min, reaching a peak within approximately 30 min, but FSH peaks are often delayed further. LH release has a linear log-dose relationship up to doses of 250 µg but no such relationship can be found for FSH.

In the female, the magnitude of gonadotrophin release, particularly LH, in individuals varies with the stage of the menstrual cycle, being greatest in the preovulatory phase, less marked in the luteal phase and least in the follicular phase of any individual cycle (Yen et al 1972, Shaw et al 1974) (Figure 15.4).

GnRH is thus the humoral link between the neural and endocrine components controlling LH and FSH release.

Mechanism of action of GnRH on pituitary cells

The first step in the action of GnRH on the pituitary gonadotroph is recognition of a specific receptor. GnRH receptor complexes often form clusters and become internalized, then undergo degradation in the lysosomes. The receptor fragments then pass back rapidly to the surface of the cell. This recycling process is causally related to upregulation of the receptor by GnRH. GnRH receptors tend to be of 60 kDa,

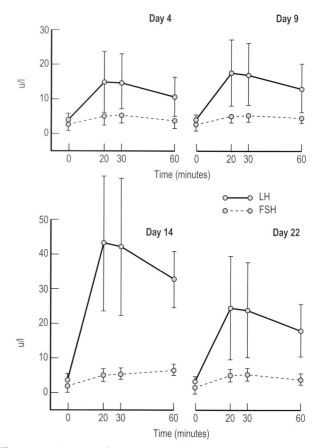

Figure 15.4 Luteinizing hormone (LH) and follicle-stimulating hormone (FSH) release following 100 mg gonadotrophin-releasing hormone at different phases of the same menstrual cycle in six normal women (mean ± SD).
From Shaw RW, Butt WR, London DR, Marshall JC 1974 Variation in response to synthetic luteinizing hormone-releasing hormone (LHRH) at different phases of the same menstrual cycle in normal women. Journal of Obstetrics and Gynaecology of the British Commonwealth 81:632–639.

to be glycoproteins and to have a transmembrane character of a complex nature with seven transmembrane domains. A negatively charged domain interacts predominantly with ARG in position 8 of the GnRH molecule.

The transmembrane domains have many formats which are common to humans and other species, and ligand-binding sites are fairly superficial within the receptor. In the human, the C-terminal tail is lost on the type 1 receptor (as found in the pituitary). Thus, once GnRH binds to the receptor, decoupling does not occur rapidly. This may be beneficial in allowing protracted LH release to occur.

Various GnRH agonists and antagonists have different binding ligands. An understanding of the site and mechanisms of binding to the GnRH receptor have allowed specific structural changes to be made to GnRH analogues to produce more potent pharmacological agents and to attempt to develop non-peptide antagonists.

Prolonged exposure to GnRH leads to suppression of LH release, called 'downregulation', which is associated with reduced numbers of GnRH receptors. This phenomenon is vitally important in understanding the mechanism of action of the GnRH analogues.

There are three principal positive actions of GnRH on gonadotrophin secretion:

- synthesis and storage (to reserve pool) of gonadotrophins;
- activation — movement of FSH and LH from the reserve pool to a pool for direct secretion — self-priming action; and
- immediate release (secretion) of gonadotrophins.

The binding of GnRH to its receptor induces a complex series of intracellular responses, which result in hormone secretion and biosynthesis of the α and β subunits of LH and FSH. In addition, dimerization of α and β subunits and the glycosylation processes are induced. The mechanism of action of GnRH is depicted in Figure 15.5. Within seconds of GnRH binding to and activating GnRH receptors on the pituitary gonadotrophs, intracellular free Ca^{2+} concentrations increase. This Ca^{2+} is initially mobilized from intracellular stores (e.g. endoplasmic reticulum) but also, to maintain sustained LH release, extracellular Ca^{2+} enters the gonadotroph through receptor-regulated voltage-dependent Ca^{2+} channels.

The initial mobilization of intracellular Ca^{2+} is induced by inositol triphosphate, released as a consequence of receptor activation of the membrane-bound phospholipase-C enzyme. Diacylglycerol is also released by the action of phospholipase-C and in turn activates the phosphorylating enzyme protein kinase C. The adenyl cyclase complex is also stimulated and cyclic adenosine monophosphate (cAMP) is generated. Ca^{2+}, protein kinase C and cAMP then interact to stimulate release of stored LH and FSH and subsequent biosynthesis (for review, see Clayton 1989).

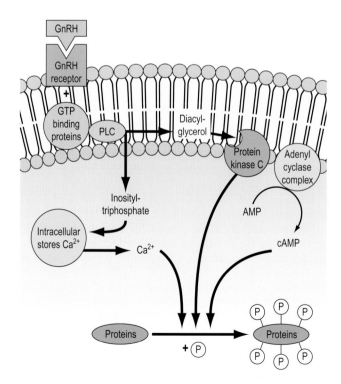

Figure 15.5 Schematic representation of gonadotrophin-releasing hormone (GnRH)-receptor signal activation. GTP, guanosine triphosphate; PLC, phospholipase-C enzyme, AMP, adenosine monophosphate; cAMP, cyclic AMP; P, phosphate group.

GnRH agonist analogues

The current generation of GnRH analogues in clinical use are predominantly agonists. GnRH is degraded by peptidases in the pituitary and hypothalamus which cleave the native decapeptide at the Gly^6-Leu^7 bond and at position 10. Substitution at position 6 with another amino acid renders the analogue less susceptible to enzymatic breakdown, resulting in a half-life 2.5–6 times longer than the native GnRH, whilst still allowing the analogue to bind to the pituitary gonadotroph GnRH receptor site. Several agonistic analogues are available for clinical use (see Table 15.2). Following an initial few days of increased secretion of LH and FSH after the first administration of a GnRH agonist, downregulation of the GnRH receptor is achieved with subsequently suppressed release of LH and FSH, and hence a reduced stimulus to the ovary resulting in failure of follicle growth and reduced ovarian steroidogenesis.

GnRH antagonist analogues

GnRH antagonists are characterized by multiple modification of the amino acid sequence of native GnRH; predominantly the pyroglutamic and glycine termini (position 1 and 10) and deletion and substitution of hydrophobic D amino acids at positions 2 and 3 (see Table 15.2).

GnRH antagonists bind to the GnRH receptor without affecting its internalization and initiating gonadotrophin synthesis and release. The GnRH antagonists have the advantage over agonists of immediately reducing circulating gonadotrophin levels with rapid reversal on withdrawal. However, to date, the compounds available are of relatively low bioactivity and hydrophobic, requiring repeated daily administration. Their clinical roles are mainly restricted to their use to prevent premature luteinization in assisted conception cycles.

The wide-ranging group of clinical conditions in which GnRH, GnRH agonists or GnRH antagonists have found application are listed in Box 15.1. These are discussed in greater depth in Chapters 22 and 32–34.

Modulatory Role of Monoamines, Other Neurotransmitters and Second Messengers on GnRH Secretion

Past studies indicated that LH release and ovulation were dependent upon drug-affected neural stimuli of both cholinergic and adrenergic origin. The infundibulum contains large stores of noradrenaline (norepinephrine), a lesser quantity of dopamine and a small amount of adrenaline (epinephrine) (Figure 15.6).

Dopamine and noradrenaline are synthesized in nerve terminals by decarboxylation of dihydroxyphenylalanine (DOPA), itself derived from hydroxylation of tyrosine.

Dopamine

The hypothalamic tuberoinfundibular dopaminergic pathway is formed by neurones, with cell bodies located in the arcuate nucleus and axons which project to the external layer of the median eminence in close juxtaposition to portal

Table 15.2 Gonadotrophin-releasing hormone (GnRH) and its agonists and antagonists: peptide structural modifications

Position	1	2	3	4	5	6	7	8	9	10
Native GnRH	pGlu	His	Trp	Ser	Tyr	Gly	Leu	Arg	Pro	Gly-NH$_2$
GnRH agonists										
Leuprolide						D-Leu				NH-Ethylamide
Buserelin						D-Ser (tertiary butanol)				NH-Ethylamide
Nafarelin						D-Naphthylalanine (2)				
Histrelin						D-His (tertiary benzyl)				NH-Ethylamide
Goserelin						D-Ser (tertiary butanol)				Aza-Gly
Deslorelin						D-Trp				NH-Ethylamide
Tryptorelin						D-Trp				
GnRH antagonists										
Abarelix	D-Ala	D-Phe	D-Ala			D-Cit				D-Ala
Cetrorelix	D-Nal	D-Phe	D-Pal			D-Cit				D-Ala
Ganirelix	D-Nal	D-Phe	D-Pal			D-hArg	hArg			D-Ala

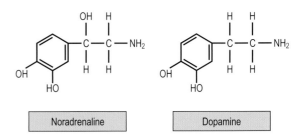

Box 15.1 Clinical applications of GnRH and its agonists and antagonists

Activation of pituitary-gonadal function (GnRH)
- Delayed puberty
- Ovulation induction
  - Functional hypothalamic amenorrhoea
  - Kallmann's syndrome

Pituitary-gonadal inhibition (agonists/antagonists)
- Precocious puberty
- Hormone-dependent disorders
  - Endometriosis
  - Uterine leiomyoma
  - Adenomyosis
  - Breast cancer
- Suppression of ovarian function
  - Polycystic ovary syndrome
  - In-vitro fertilization
  - Contraception
  - Premenstrual syndrome
  - Dysfunctional uterine bleeding

Figure 15.6 Chemical structure of biogenic amines.

vessels. The coexistence of dopamine- and GnRH-containing axons in the same region of the median eminence suggests the possibility of dopaminergic involvement in the control of gonadotrophin secretion.

The addition of dopamine to pituitaries coincubated with hypothalamic fragments increases the release of LH, while the addition of phentolamine, an α-receptor blocker, prevents dopamine-induced LH release. These early in-vitro experiments suggested that the hormonal background was capable of modifying the response to dopamine, since it seemed ineffective in ovariectomized animals or during oestrus or dioestrus day 1 of the oestrous cycle. Dopamine was more effective at pro-oestrus or in oestrogen- and

progesterone-primed rats (McCann et al 1974, Ojeda and McCann 1978).

In humans, the inhibitory role of dopamine and its agonists on LH, as well as that of prolactin release, has been demonstrated (LeBlanc et al 1976, Lachelin et al 1977). Elevated levels of prolactin can also stimulate dopamine turnover in the hypothalamus, and it is postulated that the stimulated dopamine secretion alters GnRH secretion and hence reduces FSH and LH release in situations of hyperprolactinaemia. Hence, dopamine in the human may principally have an inhibitory effect on GnRH secretion.

The contradictory roles played by dopamine in GnRH release are, in all likelihood, the consequence of more than one action of dopamine on the GnRH-secreting neurone. The steroid environment appears to modify the components involved in the dopaminergic control of GnRH secretion, with oestrogen appearing to affect the population of excitatory or inhibitory dopamine receptors, and suggesting that the feedback control of GnRH output by oestrogen is partly exerted at a hypothalamic level by reducing dopamine neuronal activity.

Noradrenaline

Most experimental evidence supports a stimulatory role for noradrenaline in the control of gonadotrophin release.

Turnover of hypothalamic noradrenaline is increased during the preovulatory surge of gonadotrophins at pro-oestrus, and noradrenaline synthesis in the anterior hypothalamus is enhanced in ovariectomized rats. These effects on GnRH secretion appear to be mediated by α receptors, since phenoxybenzamine, an α blocker, suppresses the postcastration rise in gonadotrophins in male rats, and phentolamine blocks the pulsatile release of LH in ovariectomized monkeys (for review, see McCann and Ojeda 1976).

Selective blockade of noradrenaline synthesis prevents the preovulatory LH surge and that induced by gonadal steroids; the above data suggest that noradrenergic terminals in the preoptic or anterior hypothalamic area synapse with GnRH neurones involved in the control of the preovulatory surge of gonadotrophins.

Most of the cell bodies that synthesize noradrenaline are located in the mesencephalon and lower brainstem, and these cells also synthesize serotonin. The axons from these cells ascend into the medial forebrain bundle to terminate in various brain structures including the hypothalamus. The probable mode of action of catecholamines is to influence the frequency of GnRH release (see Figure 15.7).

Serotonin

High concentrations of serotonin are found in the median eminence, with most of the serotonin-containing neurones originating from the raphe nucleus in the midbrain–pons area. Present evidence shows that serotonin plays a predominantly inhibitory role in gonadotrophin release (see McCann and Ojeda 1976).

Neuropeptide Y

Gonadal steroids regulate the secretion and gene expression of neuropeptide Y in hypothalamic neurones (Sahu et al 1992). Neuropeptide Y stimulates pulsatile release of GnRH and potentiates gonadotrophin response to GnRH (Pau et al 1995). In the absence of oestrogens, neuropeptide Y inhibits gonadotrophin secretion, and increased amounts of neuropeptide Y are found in cases of under-nutrition and the cerebrospinal fluid of women with anexoria and bulimia nervosa. These findings explain a link between under-nutrition and suppressed LH and FSH secretion in those conditions.

Endogenous opioids

Endogenous opioids play a central role in the neural control of gonadotrophin secretion by way of an inhibitory effect on hypothalamic GnRH secretion. These are a fascinating group of peptides, with 'endorphins' being the name coined to denote a substance with morphine-like action, of endogenous origin, in the brain. Endorphin production is regulated by gene transcription, and since these are precursor peptides, all opioids are derived from three precursor peptides:

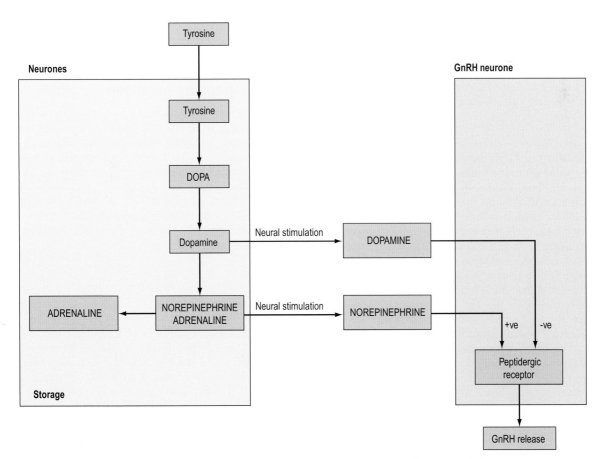

Figure 15.7 Opposing roles of dopamine and noradrenaline on the release of gonadotrophin-releasing hormone (GnRH).

- pro-opiomelanocortin is the source of endorphins;
- pro-enkephalin A and B are the source of enkephalins; and
- pro-dynorphin yields dynorphins.

A single injection of morphine, administered to oophorectomized monkeys, brings about immediate cessation of GnRH pulse generation (Yen et al 1985). Hypothalamic opioidergic neurones are found in the arcuate nucleus of the medial basal hypothalamus, in close contact with GnRH neurones. The administration of an opioid antagonist, naloxone, produces an increased frequency and amplitude of GnRH and LH secretion. These changes are most marked in the luteal phase of the cycle, and it is thought that the negative feedback of oestrogen may partly be effected through opioid-induced inhibition of GnRH secretion (Ropert et al 1981), as is the negative feedback of progesterone on GnRH secretion.

Changes in opioid tone seem to mediate the hypogonadotrophic state seen in hyperprolactinaemia, exercise and other causes of hypothalamic amenorrhoea. Treatment of patients with hypothalamic amenorrhoea (who have suppressed GnRH pulsatile secretion) with naltrexone — an opioid receptor blocker — allows return of pulsatile LH and FSH secretion and return of ovulation (Wildt et al 1993).

Corticotrophin-releasing hormone

Experimental studies indicate that corticotrophin-releasing hormone inhibits hypothalamic GnRH secretion both directly and by augmenting endogenous opioid secretion. Corticotrophin-releasing hormone infusions inhibit gonadotrophin release in primates (Xiao et al 1989), and suppress the electrophysiological activity of the GnRH pulse generator (Knobil 1989). Women with hypothalamic amenorrhoea have increased levels of cortisol in their circulation, suggesting that this is the mechanism by which stress influences the hypothalamic–pituitary–ovarian axis.

Leptin

Leptin, identified in 1994, is a 167-amino acid protein transcribed by the *ob* gene. The human leptin gene is on chromosome 7q31, and leptin is mainly produced in white adipose tissue with a small amount from brown adipose tissue. In humans, leptin concentrations increase with the onset of puberty, and low levels may contribute to the amenorrhoea seen in anorexia nervosa. Leptin only acts in the hypothalamus where it can produce rapid synaptic modulatory effects and increase GnRH release from the medial basal hypothalamus. Nocturnal changes in LH pulse parameters are associated temporarily with the rise in plasma leptin at night. These fluctuations in leptin are synchronized with serum LH changes. Leptin's predominant role is to act as an adipostat, having the capacity to improve glucose homeostasis and to stimulate energy utilization by increasing thermogenic activity and capacity.

Prolactin

Prolactin gene expression occurs on the lactotrophes of the anterior pituitary gland, in the myometrium and decidualized endometrium. Differences in mRNA in these sites indicate that there are differences in prolactin gene regulation, and only that secreted by the pituitary gland is likely to be relevant in feedback on the hypothalamic–pituitary–ovarian axis. Transcription of the prolactin gene is regulated by a transcription factor which binds to the 5′ promoter region, and this is also involved in growth hormone and TSH secretion. The main function of prolactin is in lactogenesis, and the secretion of prolactin is under the inhibitory control of hypothalamic dopamine released into the portal circulation. In addition to direct inhibition of prolactin gene expression, dopamine binding to the D_2 receptor inhibits lactotrophe development and growth.

Several factors exert a stimulatory effect on prolactin secretion, particularly thyrotrophin-releasing hormine, vasoactive intestinal peptide and oestrogen, whilst endogenous opioids inhibit release, probably by modulating the dopaminergic neurones.

Elevated circulating levels of prolactin result in reduced pulse amplitude and frequency of gonadotrophin release with resultant anovulation during lactation and in conditions which cause hyperprolactinaemia.

Other Neurotransmitters and Second Messengers

Other neurotransmitters may play a less important role in the regulation of GnRH neurones. Acetylcholine and γ-aminobutyric acid stimulate LH release. Both these agents are far more common as neurotransmitting agents than dopamine or noradrenaline in central nervous system nerve terminals in general, but their importance in GnRH neuronal activity seems to be less than that of dopamine and noradrenaline.

The intrapituitary paracrine–autocrine system

Growth factors and cytokines provide a paracrine–autocrine system which regulates cell development and replication, and pituitary hormone synthesis and secretion. As with other organs in the body, the pituitary contains epidermal growth factors, fibroblast growth factors, insulin-like growth factors, interleukins, activin, inhibin, endothelin and many others. Interactions between all of these substances constitute a complex interplay, but one group of compounds are better understood — those of the activin-inhibin and follistatin substances (see Figure 15.8).

Inhibin

Inhibin is secreted by granulosa cells in the ovary and selectively inhibits FSH but not LH secretion. Inhibin consists of two peptides — the α and β subunits — linked by a disulphide bond. Two forms of inhibin have been purified — inhibin A and inhibin B with identical α subunits but separate, although similar, β subunits. Messenger RNA for the α and β subunits is found in granulosa cells but also in pituitary gonadotrophes. Whilst inhibin predominantly suppresses FSH secretion, limiting the numbers of follicles recruited at the start of a cycle, cells actively synthesizing LH respond to inhibin by increasing GnRH receptor numbers. Inhibin A reaches peak levels in the luteal phase

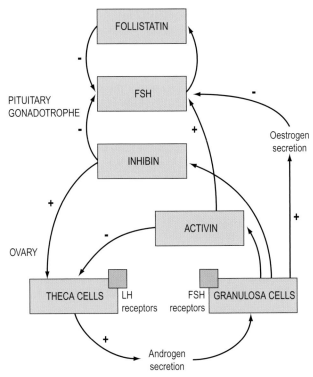

Figure 15.8 Paracrine and autocrine control of follicle-stimulating hormone (FSH) and release and function. LH, luteinizing hormone.

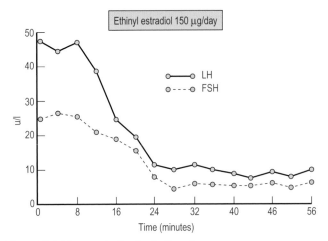

Figure 15.9 The negative feedback effect of oestrogen on serum luteinizing hormone (LH) and follicle-stimulating hormone (FSH) in a postmenopausal woman.
Source: Shaw 1975, unpublished data.

and falls in concentration as the corpus luteum undergoes luteolysis.

Activin

Activin is produced by granulosa cells but is also present in pituitary gonadotropes. It contains two subunits identical to the β subunits of inhibin A and B, but some variants of the β subunits have also been identified, although their role and function are not thought to be important. Activin augments the secretion of FSH and inhibits prolactin, ACTH and growth hormone response (Corrigan et al 1991, Blumenfeld 2001). Activin increases pituitary responsiveness to GnRH by enhancing GnRH receptor formation, and its effects are blocked by inhibin and follistatin.

Follistatin

This is a peptide secreted by a variety of pituitary cells including gonadotrophes. It inhibits FSH synthesis and secretion, and the FSH response to GnRH by binding to activin and thus decreasing the activity of activin (Besecke et al 1997).

Overview of GnRH secretion

GnRH thus stimulates gonadotrophin synthesis and secretion as well as activin-enhancing and follistatin-suppressing GnRH activity. Numerous other neurotransmitters and ovarian steroids also interplay in altering and modifying pituitary responsiveness to GnRH, which results in the various changes on pulse amplitude and frequency observed throughout the menstrual cycle.

Modulatory Effect of Ovarian Steroids

Negative feedback

Negative feedback control or inhibition of pituitary LH and FSH release has been postulated since 1932, when Moore and Price considered that the ovary and adenohypophysis were linked in a rigid system of hormonal interactions. The quantitative relationship between ovarian steroids and gonadotrophin release can be demonstrated by disturbing the negative feedback loop by oophorectomy which produces, over a period of days, an increase in circulating LH and FSH; this reaches a plateau at approximately 3 weeks with levels which are some 10 times higher than preoperative values. Alternatively, the administration of exogenous oestrogens to oophorectomized or postmenopausal women will result in rapid suppression of elevated circulating gonadotrophin levels (Figure 15.9).

The negative feedback changes result from both a direct pituitary site of action of oestradiol, with a decrease in sensitivity of the gonadotroph to GnRH (McCann et al 1974), and an action within the hypothalamus and a decrease in GnRH secretion, possibly via increased inhibitory dopaminergic and opiate activity.

The threshold for the negative feedback action of oestrogen is set to bring about suppression of gonadotrophin release with relatively small increases in oestradiol-17β in the normal female. This negative feedback loop is the main factor which maintains the relatively low basal concentrations of plasma LH and FSH in the normal female. Circulating levels of oestradiol-17β within the range of 100–200 pmol/l will suppress the early follicular phase gonadotrophin rise which initiates follicular development.

A negative feedback effect of progesterone on gonadotrophin secretion is now well established. Whilst progesterone, even in large doses, has little effect on baseline LH release, it can suppress the ovulatory surge of LH, as demonstrated in human females administered synthetic progestogens (Larsson-Cohn et al 1972), and oestrogen-induced positive feedback surges cannot be produced during the luteal phase in women (Shaw 1975). The principal negative feedback action of progesterone is thus upon the midcycle gonadotrophin surge, and it may be responsible for its short 24-h duration. It also seems likely that progesterone is an important factor in the reduced frequency of gonadotrophin pulses observed during the luteal phase of the cycle compared with their frequency in the follicular phase (see below).

Positive feedback

The fact that oestrogen may stimulate (positive feedback) rather than inhibit gonadotrophin release under certain circumstances was first proposed by Hohlweg and Junkmann (1932). Their proposal has since been substantiated by numerous experimental reports in animals and humans. Under physiological conditions, the positive feedback only operates in females; it is brought about by oestrogen and appears to be an essential component in producing the midcycle ovulatory surge of gonadotrophins. Administration of oestradiol-17β to females during the early or midfollicular phase of the cycle will induce a surge of gonadotrophins (Yen et al 1974, Shaw 1975) (Figure 15.10), but treatment with the same doses of oestrogen during the midfollicular phase induces a far greater release of LH than during the early follicular phase (Yen et al 1974). Studies on the dynamics of this positive feedback response to oestrogen, observed in greatest detail in the rhesus monkey, demonstrate an activation delay of some 32–48 h from the commencement of oestrogen administration until the onset of the positive-feedback-induced gonadotrophin surge, a minimum threshold level to be exceeded and a strength-duration aspect of the stimulus (Karsch et al 1973).

Oestrogen elicits gonadotrophin release by increasing pituitary responsiveness to GnRH and possibly by stimulating increased GnRH secretion by the hypothalamus. In the normally menstruating female, oestrogen pretreatment produces an initial suppressive action on pituitary responsiveness (Shaw et al 1975a) followed by a later augmenting action which is both concentration and duration dependent (Shaw et al 1975a, Young and Jaffe 1976). The augmenting effect of oestrogen on GnRH pituitary responsiveness is demonstrated in Figure 15.11.

These data and others suggest that the midcycle oestrogen-induced surge of gonadotrophins may occur without the need for any increased output of hypothalamic GnRH, and indeed, this occurs in patients with endogenous GnRH deficiency receiving pulsatile GnRH treatment at a constant rate.

Progesterone by itself does not appear to exert a positive feedback effect. However, when administered to females in whom the pituitary has undergone either endogenously induced or exogenously administered oestrogen priming, progesterone can induce increased pituitary responsiveness to GnRH (Shaw et al 1975b; Figure 15.12). Since circulating progesterone levels are increasing significantly during the periovulatory period, this action may be of importance in determining the magnitude and duration of the midcycle gonadotrophin surge.

Self-Priming of the Pituitary Gonadotroph by GnRH

Results from in-vitro experiments with pituitary cells in culture indicate that GnRH is not only involved in the release of stored LH and FSH, but is of importance in maintaining the synthesis of gonadotrophins within the gonadotroph. Hence repeated exposure to GnRH of the gonadotrophin-producing cells seems essential for the maintenance of adequate pituitary stores.

Rommler and Hammerstein (1974) first demonstrated that the response to a second injection of GnRH was greater than the initial response in females, when they were retested

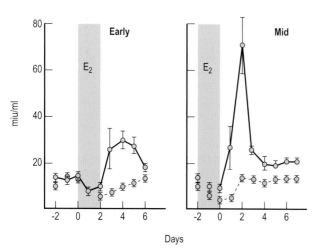

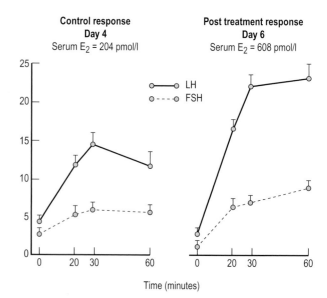

Figure 15.10 The positive feedback effect of exogenous oestrogen (E₂ = 200 μg ethinyl oestradiol/day) on gonadotrophin release; qualitative differences in the early and midfollicular phase of the cycle. ●, luteinizing hormone; ○, follicle-stimulating hormone.

Reproduced with permission from: Yen SSC, van den Berg G, Tsai CC, Siler T 1974 Causal relationship between the hormonal variables in the menstrual cycle. In: Ferin M et al (eds) Biorhythms and Human Reproduction. John Wiley, New York, pp 219–238.

Figure 15.11 Oestrogen augmentation of pituitary response to 100 mg gonadotrophin-releasing hormone bolus in four women receiving 2.5 mg oestradiol benzoate IM, 2 h after initial control response on day 4 of cycle and retested 48 h later on day 6 of cycle.

Source: Shaw RW 1975 A Study of Hypothalamic–Pituitary–Gonadal Relationships in the Female. MD Thesis, Birmingham University, Birmingham.

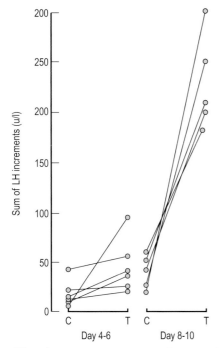

Figure 15.12 Effect of progesterone pretreatment (12.5 mg IM) on luteinizing hormone (LH) response to 100 mg gonadotrophin-releasing hormone IV during the early and midfollicular phases of the cycle, showing the increased priming effect of oestrogen. C, control; T, after progesterone.
From Shaw RW, Butt WR, London DR 1975b The effect of progesterone on FSH and LH response to LH-RH in normal women. Clinical Endocrinology 4:543–550.

1–4 h following the first exposure. This response has been termed 'self-priming'.

Wang et al (1976) published more intensive studies, carried out throughout the menstrual cycle, and were able to demonstrate that self-priming had a definite cycle relationship which was greatest in the late follicular phase and around midcycle (i.e. at times of increased circulating oestrogen levels), and that oestrogen preferentially induces LH rather than FSH release (Figure 15.13).

This self-priming effect of GnRH is of importance in understanding the physiological control mechanism of gonadotrophin release. It suggests that there are two pools of gonadotrophins, one readily releasable by initial exposure to GnRH and a second reserve pool. The exposure of this larger reserve pool to GnRH allows it to be more readily released by a subsequent exposure to GnRH, and is suggestive of a transfer of gonadotrophins from one pool to the other. The stage of the cycle, i.e. the prevailing environment of endogenous sex steroids, which are the modulators, and the degree of GnRH stimulation which is the prime controller, together influence these transfer capabilities and sensitivity of the pituitary in its response to GnRH.

Pulsatile Nature of Gonadotrophin Release

The pulsatile nature of hypothalamic GnRH release is now known to determine episodic pituitary gonadotrophin secretion.

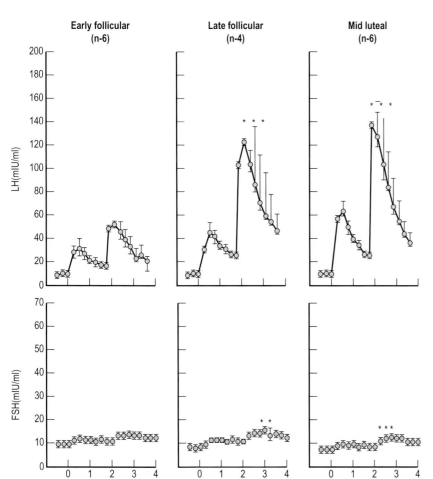

Figure 15.13 Self-priming effect of bolus injection of gonadotrophin-releasing hormone. Differing responses at different phases of the menstrual cycle. LH, luteinizing hormone; FSH, follicle-stimulating hormone.
From Wang CF, Lusley BL, Lein A, Yen SSC 1976 The functional changes of the pituitary gonadotrophs during the menstrual cycle. Journal of Clinical Endocrinology and Metabolism 42:718–724.

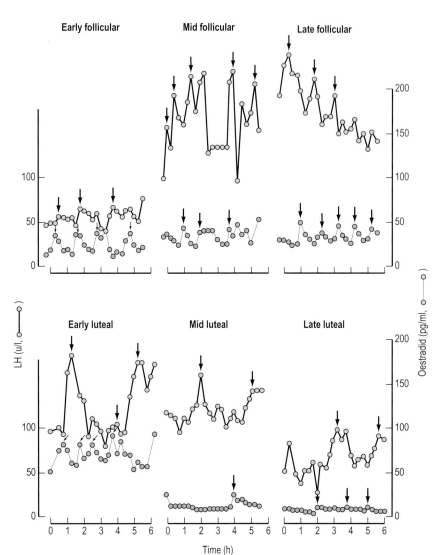

Figure 15.14 Concentrations of luteinizing hormone (LH) and oestradiol at different phases of the menstrual cycle, demonstrating different pulse frequency and amplitude.
From Backstrom CT, McNeilly AS, Leak RM, Baird DT 1982 Pulsatile secretion of LH. FSH, prolactin, ooestradiol and progesterone during the human menstrual cycle. Clinical Endocrinology 17:29–42.

This pulsatile pattern of GnRH concentration has been reported in the pituitary stalk effluent of the rhesus monkey (Carmel et al 1976). This suggests that the pulsatile pattern of gonadotrophin release from the anterior pituitary is probably causally related to the periodic increase in the hypothalamic GnRH system.

Further support for this hypothesis is obtained from the facts that antisera to GnRH abolish the pulsatile release of gonadotrophins, and that pulsatile LH release can only be reinstated by pulsed delivery of GnRH and not by constant infusion.

Comparison of the pulsatile pattern of gonadotrophin release at different phases of the menstrual cycle demonstrates profound modulation by ovarian steroids (Figure 15.14).

In hypogonadal subjects, pulses exhibit high amplitude and high frequency with reversal of the LH:FSH ratio. However, the higher circulating level of FSH is probably not due to a higher FSH secretory rate but rather to an accumulation related to its slower clearance rate (longer half-life).

In females with normal cycles, a characteristic low-amplitude, high-frequency pulse pattern is observed during the follicular phase. This suggests that oestrogen appears to be most effective in reducing the amplitude of gonadotrophin pulses, more markedly in FSH than LH. In contrast, the pulse pattern during the luteal phase is one of high amplitude and low frequency, probably modified by progesterone effects, on the catecholaminergic and GnRH neurone systems (Figure 15.14).

Integrative Control of the Hypothalamic–Pituitary Unit during the Menstrual Cycle

How can the complex inter-related changes in ovarian steroids and pituitary gonadotrophins that occur within each menstrual cycle be explained on the basis of our present understanding of the control of the hypothalamic pituitary unit (see Figure 15.15 for overview).

LH and FSH are released from the anterior pituitary in an episodic, pulsatile manner, and the available evidence supports a hypothalamic mechanism for this pulsatile release. Both oestradiol-17β and progesterone can induce a positive feedback release of gonadotrophins, in many

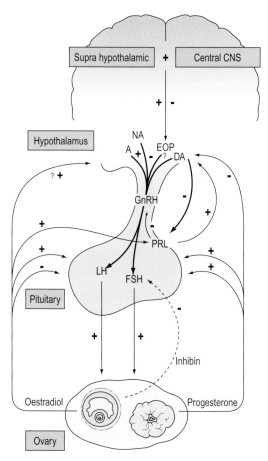

Figure 15.15 Feedback control mechanisms in the hypothalamic–pituitary–ovarian axis. CNS, central nervous system; NA, noradrenaline; A, adrenaline; EOP, endogenous opioids; PRL, prolactin; DA, dopamine; GnRH, gonadotrophin-releasing hormone; LH, luteinizing hormone; FSH, follicle-stimulating hormone.

Follicular phase

In the early follicular phase, both the immediately releasable and the reserve pool of gonadotrophins are at a minimum. The increased FSH release, responsible for initiating follicle development, must indicate an increased output of GnRH, with the lowering of negative feedback action in the presence of low levels of oestrogen and progestogen. As follicles develop, oestrogen levels rise and the negative feedback action of oestrogen on GnRH increases, suppressing FSH levels. Increasing levels of inhibin from the rapidly dividing granulosa cells of the dominant follicle further suppress FSH secretion at a pituitary level.

With these progressive increases in oestradiol throughout the midfollicular phase, the quantitative estimates of the primary, immediately releasable, pool of gonadotrophins increase slightly, whilst the reserve pool increases greatly, thus demonstrating the augmentation action of oestradiol primarily upon the reserve pool. Since there is no marked increase in circulating gonadotrophin levels during this phase, secretion of GnRH must be minimal or else there is evidence of impedance of GnRH sensitivity by oestrogen.

Mechanism for preovulatory gonadotrophin surge

During the late follicular phase, there is an increase in the amount of oestradiol secreted by the ovary. Under this influence, the sensitivity of the gonadotroph to GnRH eventually reaches a phase when GnRH can exert its full self-priming action. The consequence is the transference of gonadotrophins from the secondary reserve pool to the releasable pool. The increased pituitary responsiveness to GnRH may be further enhanced by the slight progesterone rise which can affect its action on a fully oestrogen-primed anterior pituitary. These changes culminate in the production of the ovulatory gonadotrophin surge. It is possible that these events could occur even if the gonadotrophs were exposed to a constant level of GnRH. However, an increased secretion of GnRH, as reported in rhesus monkeys and rats (Sarker et al 1976), at midcycle, which would act synergistically with the changes in pituitary sensitivity, also seems likely in the human.

The LH and FSH surges begin abruptly (LH levels doubling over 2 h) and are temporarily associated with attainment of peak oestradiol-17β levels. The mean duration of the LH surge is 48 h, with an ascending limb of 14 h which is accompanied by a decline in oestradiol-17β and 17-hydroxyprogesterone concentrations but a sustained rise in inhibin levels.

The ascending limb of LH is followed by a peak plateau of gonadotrophin levels lasting some 14 h and a transient levelling of progesterone concentrations. The descending limb is long, lasting approximately 20 h, and accompanying this is a second rise in progesterone, a further decline in oestradiol-17β and 17-hydroxyprogesterone, and a rise in inhibin levels.

The concentration of inhibin during the periovulatory interval is not correlated with oestradiol-17β or progesterone changes. It may merely reflect the release from follicular fluid of stored inhibin.

respects comparable to that seen at midcycle, but progesterone can only produce its effect on a previously oestrogen-primed pituitary gland. There is presumptive evidence that these positive feedback stimuli also involve a direct pituitary action, with alteration in sensitivity to GnRH preceding an induced increase in hypothalamic release of GnRH.

The pattern of gonadotrophin release from the pituitary in response to repeated pulses of submaximal dose of GnRH or constant low-dose infusion over several hours suggests the presence of two functionally related pools of gonadotrophins. The first primary pool is immediately releasable, while the secondary pool requires a continued stimulus input and represents the effect of GnRH on synthesis and storage of gonadotrophins within the pituitary cell. The sizes or activity of these two pools represent pituitary sensitivity and reserve, respectively, which vary throughout the cycle and are regulated by the feedback action of ovarian steroids and by the self-priming action of GnRH itself. Oestradiol preferentially induces the augmentation of reserve and impedes sensitivity to GnRH, with a differential effect apparent for LH release. This oestradiol effect is both dose and time related.

Ovulation occurs 1–2 h before the final phase of progesterone rise or 35–44 h from the onset of the LH surge.

Luteal phase

The significantly lower basal gonadotrophin secretion in the face of high pituitary capacity during the midluteal phase suggests that endogenous GnRH should be very low.

A progressive decrease in sensitivity and reserve characterizes pituitary function during the late luteal phase and into the early follicular phase of the next cycle. This is probably due to a progressive decline in oestrogen and progesterone on which sensitivity and reserve are dependent. The role played by the proposed ovarian inhibin on preferentially controlling FSH secretion has still to be completely determined.

It is therefore apparent that the functional state of the pituitary gonadotroph as a target cell is ultimately determined by the modulating effect of ovarian steroid hormones via their influence on the gonadotroph's sensitivity and reserves, and upon the hypophysiotrophic effect of GnRH.

With such a complex inter-related control mechanism, it is perhaps not surprising that many drugs which affect neurotransmitters, ill health or associated endocrine disorders can disrupt normal hypothalamic–pituitary–ovarian function, resulting in disordered follicular growth and suppression of ovulation and in severe cases cause amenorrhoea.

KEY POINTS

1. The unique portal blood supply to the pituitary gland provides the basis of hypothalamic regulation of the pituitary secretion. It also explains the vulnerability of the gland to hypotension.

2. GnRH, secreted by neurones of the hypothalamus into the portal system, controls the release of both FSH and LH, with ovarian sex steroids playing a role in modulating the proportions of each hormone secreted.

3. The final step in the release of stored LH and FSH, and subsequent induction of further biosynthesis of both hormones following GnRH stimulation, involves Ca^{2+}, protein kinase C and cAMP.

4. The control of GnRH secretion is highly complex and depends upon a number of inhibitory (dopamine, endorphins) and excitatory (noradrenaline, prostaglandins) neurotransmitters, and is modulated by various other substances such as activin, inhibin and follistatin.

5. The response of the pituitary gland to exogenous GnRH depends upon the ovarian sex steroid environment prevailing and the degree of GnRH stimulation. Prolonged exposure to GnRH produces downregulation of LH release, which is used pharmacologically to induce a state of hypogonadotrophic hypogonadism to treat many ovarian-steroid-hormone-dependent disorders.

References

Backstrom CT, McNeilly AS, Leak RM, Baird DT 1982 Pulsatile secretion of LH, FSH, prolactin, oestradiol and progesterone during the human menstrual cycle. Clinical Endocrinology 17: 29–42.

Besecke LM, Guendner MJ, Sluss PA et al 1997 Pituitary follistatin regulates activin mediated production of follicle-stimulating hormone during the rat estrous cycle. Endocrinology 132: 2841–2848.

Bick D, Franco B, Sherins RJ et al 1992 Brief report: intragenic deletion of the KALIG-1 gene in Kallmann's syndrome. New England Journal of Medicine 326: 1752–1755.

Blumenfeld Z 2001 Response of human fetal pituitary cells to activin, inhibin, hypophysiotrophe and neuroregulatory factors in-vitro. Early Pregnancy 5: 41–42.

Carmel PD, Araki S, Ferin M 1976 Prolonged stalk portal blood collection in rhesus monkeys. Pulsatile release of gonadotrophin-releasing hormone (GnRH). Endocrinology 99: 243–248.

Clayton RN 1989 Cellular actions of gonadotrophin-releasing hormone: the receptor and beyond. In: Shaw RW, Marshall JC (eds) LHRH and its Analogues — their Use in Gynaecological Practice. Wright, London, pp 19–34.

Corrigan AZ, Bilezikjian LM, Carroll RS et al 1991 Evidence for an autocrine role of activin B within rat anterior pituitary cultures. Endocrinology 128: 1682–1684.

Hohlweg W, Junkmann K 1932 Die hormonal-nervosae Regulierung der Funktion des Hypophysenvorderlappens. Klinische Wochenschrift 11: 321–323.

Karsch FJ, Weick RF, Butler WR et al 1973 Induced LH surges in the rhesus monkey: strength-duration characteristics of the oestrogen stimulus. Endocrinology 92: 1740–1747.

Knobil E 1989 The electrophysiology of the GnRH pulse generator. Journal of Steroid Biochemistry 33: 669–671.

Lachelin GCL, LeBlanc H, Yen SSC 1977 The inhibitory effect of dopamine agonists on LH release in women. Journal of Clinical Endocrinology and Metabolism 44: 728–732.

Larsson-Cohn V, Johansson EDB, Wide L, Gemzell C 1972 Effects of continuous daily administration of 0.1 mg of norethindrone on the plasma levels of progesterone and on the urinary excretion of luteinizing hormone and total oestrogens. Acta Endocrinologica (Copenhagen) 71: 551–556.

LeBlanc H, Lachelin GCL, Abu-Fadil S, Yen SSC 1976 Effects of dopamine infusion on pituitary hormone secretion in humans. Journal of Clinical Endocrinology and Metabolism 43: 668–674.

Matsuo H, Arimura A, Nair RMG, Schally AV 1971a Synthesis of the porcine LH- and FSH releasing hormone by the solid phase method. Biochemical and Biophysical Research Communications 45: 822–827.

Matsuo H, Baba Y, Nair RMG, Anmura A, Schally AV 1971b Structure of porcine LH- and FSH-releasing hormone. I The proposed amino acid sequence. Biochemical and Biophysical Research Communications 43: 1334–1339.

McCann SM, Ojeda SR 1976 Synaptic transmitters involved in the release of hypothalamic releasing and inhibiting hormones. In: Ehrenpreis S, Kopin IJ (eds) Reviews of Neuroscience, Vol 2. Raven Press, New York, pp 91–110.

McCann SM, Ojeda SR, Fawcett CP, Krulich L 1974 Catecholaminergic control of gonadotrophin and prolactin secretion with particular reference to the possible participation of dopamine. Advances in Neurology 5: 435–445.

Moore CR, Price D 1932 Gonad hormone function and the reciprocal influence between gonads and hypophysis. American Journal of Anatomy 50: 13–72.

Ojeda SR, McCann SM 1978 Control of LH and FSH release by LHRH: influence of putative neurotransmitters. Clinics in Obstetrics and Gynaecology 5: 283–303.

Pau KF, Berria M, Hess DL, Spies HG 1995 Hypothalamic site-dependent effects of neuropeptide Y on gonadotropin-releasing hormone secretion in the rhesus macaques. Journal of Neuroendocrinology 7: 63–67.

Rommler A, Hammerstein J 1974 Time-dependent alterations in pituitary responsiveness caused by LH-RH stimulations in man. Acta Endocrinologica (Copenhagen) 21 (Suppl): 184.

Ropert JR, Quigley ME, Yen SSC 1981 Endogenous opiates modulate pulsatile LH release in humans. Journal of Clinical Endocrinology and Metabolism 52: 584–585.

Sahu A, Phelps CP, White JD, Crowley WR, Kalra SP, Kalra PS 1992 Steroidal regulation of neuropeptide Y release and gene expression. Endocrinology 130: 3331–3336.

Sarker DK, Chiappa SA, Fink G 1976 Gonadotrophin releasing hormone surge in proestrus rats. Nature 264: 461–463.

Schally AV, Arimura A, Kastin A 1971 Gonadotrophin releasing hormone — one polypeptide regulates secretion of LH and FSH. Science 173: 1036–1038.

Schwanzel-Fukunda M, Bick D, Pfaff DW 1989 Luteinizing hormone-releasing hormone (LHRH) — expressing cells do not migrate normally in an inherited hypogonadal (Kallmann) syndrome. Molecular Brain Research 6: 311–315.

Schwanzel-Fukunda M, Pfaff DW 1989 Origin of luteinizing hormone releasing hormone neurons. Nature 338: 161.

Seeburg PH, Adelman JP 1984 Characterisation of cDNA for precursor of human luteinizing hormone-releasing hormone. Nature 311: 666–669.

Shaw RW 1975 A Study of Hypothalamic–Pituitary–Gonadal Relationships in the Female. MD Thesis, Birmingham University, Birmingham.

Shaw RW, Butt WR, London DR, Marshall JC 1974 Variation in response to synthetic luteinizing hormone-releasing hormone (LHRH) at different phases of the same menstrual cycle in normal women. Journal of Obstetrics and Gynaecology of the British Commonwealth 81: 632–639.

Shaw RW, Butt WR, London DR 1975a Effect of oestrogen pretreatment on subsequent response to luteinizing hormone-releasing hormone (LH-RH) in normal women. Clinical Endocrinology 4: 297–304.

Shaw RW, Butt WR, London DR 1975b The effect of progesterone on FSH and LH response to LH-RH in normal women. Clinical Endocrinology 4: 543–550.

Waldstreicher J, Seminara SB, Jameson JL et al 1996 The genetic and clinical heterogeneity of gonadotropin-releasing hormone deficiency in the human. Journal of Clinical Endocrinology and Metabolism 81: 4388.

Wang CF, Lusley BL, Lein A, Yen SSC 1976 The functional changes of the pituitary gonadotrophs during the menstrual cycle. Journal of Clinical Endocrinology and Metabolism 42: 718–724.

Wildt L, Leyendecker G, Sir-Petermann T, Waibel-Treber S 1993 Treatment with naltrexone and hypothalamic ovarian failure: induction of ovulation and pregnancy. Human Reproduction 8: 350–358.

Xiao E, Luckhaus J, Niemann W et al 1989 Acute inhibition of gonadotrophin secretion by corticotrophin-releasing hormone in the primate. Are adrenal glands involved? Endocrinology 124: 1632–1639.

Yen SSC, van den Berg G, Rebar R, Ehara Y 1972 Variations of pituitary responsiveness to synthetic LRF during different phases of the menstrual cycle. Journal of Clinical Endocrinology and Metabolism 35: 931–934.

Yen SSC, van den Berg G, Tsai CC, Siler T 1974 Causal relationship between the hormonal variables in the menstrual cycle. In: Ferin M et al (eds) Biorhythms and Human Reproduction. John Wiley, New York, pp 219–238.

Yen SSC, Quigley ME, Reid RL, Cetel NS 1985 Neuroendocrinology of opioid peptides and their role in the control of gonadotrophin and prolactin secretion. American Journal of Obstetrics and Gynecology 152: 485–493.

Young JR, Jaffe RB 1976 Strength duration characteristics of estrogen effects on gonadotrophin response to gonadotrophin-releasing hormone in women. II Effects of varying concentrations of oestradiol. Journal of Clinical Endocrinology and Metabolism 42: 432–442.

CHAPTER 16

Amenorrhoea, oligomenorrhoea and hypothalamic–pituitary dysfunction

Hilary O.D. Critchley, Andrew Horne and Kirsty Munro

Chapter Contents

INTRODUCTION	212	THERAPEUTIC ISSUES	225
DEFINITIONS	212	FERTILITY ISSUES	226
CAUSES OF AMENORRHOEA	213	CONTRACEPTIVE ADVICE	226
DIAGNOSIS AND MANAGEMENT OF OLIGOMENORRHOEA AND AMENORRHOEA	223	KEY POINTS	227

Introduction

Amenorrhoea and oligomenorrhoea are symptoms of ovarian and reproductive dysfunction. Patients thus commonly present to the gynaecologist with complaints of problematic menstruation or fertility delay. This chapter provides an overview of the current understanding and general management of the associated disorders of the hypothalamic–pituitary–ovarian (HPO) axis that result in amenorrhoea and oligomenorrhoea. These symptoms are also features of the polycystic ovary syndrome (PCOS), and a detailed description of the symptoms, diagnosis and management of PCOS is provided in Chapter 18.

Definitions

Normal menstruation

Regular monthly menstruation is a phenomenon of modern society. Furthermore, the availability of effective contraception has enabled couples to choose both the size and timing of their desired family. The classic data (derived from 22,754 calendar years of experience) from the studies of Treloar et al (1967) demonstrated that each woman has her own central trend and variation in menstrual cycle length, both of which change with age (Figure 16.1). The first (and last) few years of menstrual life are marked by a variable pattern of mixed short and long intervals, with a characteristic transition into and out of the more regular pattern of middle life (Figure 16.2). The length, regularity and frequency of normal menstrual cycles have been described in both population and observational studies (Harlow and Ephross 1995, Fraser and Inceboz 2000). Mean menstrual cycle length between the ages of 20 and 34 years varies between 28 and 30.7 days

(range 19.7–43.5 between the 5th and 95th centiles). Physiologically regular menses indicate cyclical ovarian activity, in turn dependent upon an intact HPO axis. Aberrations in menstrual pattern are thus an indication of disorder of ovarian function. The average age of the menarche is 12.8 years, but this has been gradually decreasing. Factors such as ethnic origin, socio-economic status and nutrition can affect age of menarche. With obesity presently such a prominent problem, it is interesting to note that there is a relationship between age of menarche and body mass index (BMI), with early menarche associated with raised BMI (Golden and Carlson 2008).

Amenorrhoea

Amenorrhoea is complete absence or cessation of menstrual bleeding for more than 6 months (not due to pregnancy). Primary amenorrhoea is defined as no spontaneous onset of menstruation by the age of 16 years. Secondary amenorrhoea is defined as the absence of menstruation for 6 months or longer if the patient has previously experienced regular menses, and for 12 months or more when a patient has oligomenorrhoea. The menopause is a retrospective diagnosis, defined as 12 months of amenorrhoea. If there is any clinical confusion, serum follicle-stimulating hormone (FSH) may be checked (>30 U/l on two separate occasions, 6 months apart).

Oligomenorrhoea

Oligomenorrhoea is a reduction in the frequency of menstruation where menstrual intervals may vary between 6 weeks and 6 months. It is important to note, however, that regular menstrual cycles every 6 weeks are usually indistinguishable from normal shorter interval cycles in terms of follicular growth and hormone production. Oligomenorrhoea may therefore include a spectrum of conditions ranging from virtual normality at one end to the same causes as amenorrhoea at the other. The main difference appears to be in the frequency of polycystic ovaries, which ultrasound and endocrine studies show to account for approximately 90% of cases of oligomenorrhoea and 33% of cases of amenorrhoea.

Causes of Amenorrhoea

Causes of amenorrhoea are classified according to a systematic endocrine approach and are listed in Box 16.1 (Baird 1997). Disorders in other endocrine systems, such as thyroid disease and adrenal disease, may result in amenorrhoea.

Physiological amenorrhoea

Amenorrhoea is physiological at certain critical times in a woman's life, these being prepuberty, during pregnancy and lactation, and in the postmenopausal period. Amenorrhoea, if not physiological, has an estimated prevalence in the female population of reproductive age of 1.8–3% (Pet-

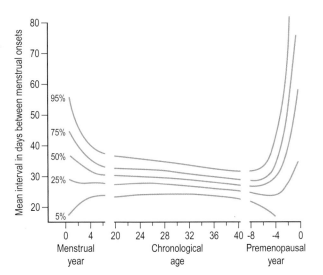

Figure 16.1 Distribution of menstrual intervals during three zones of experience: postmenarcheal, age 20–40 years and premenopausal.
Reproduced with permission from Treloar AE, Boynton RE, Behn BG, Brown BW 1967 Variation of the human menstrual cycle through reproductive life. International Journal of Fertility 12:77–126.

tersson et al 1973). Amenorrhoea may be either primary or secondary. The prevalence of secondary amenorrhoea is in the order of 2–5% (Singh 1981). The aetiology of primary and secondary amenorrhoea may be similar. Causes of primary amenorrhoea are listed in Box 16.2. In practice, investigation of primary amenorrhoea is usually initiated by the age of 14 years if there is evidence of delayed puberty (absent secondary sexual characteristics and absent menses), or no menstruation within 4 years of the onset of adrenarche and thelarche (Zreik and Olive 1998). The diagnosis of cause of primary amenorrhoea may be categorized depending on whether or not the uterus is present, and whether or not there is breast development. Zreik and Olive (1998) described a very useful scheme to aid diagnosis of primary amenorrhoea (Figure 16.3).

Anatomical causes

Anatomical abnormalities of the genital tract account for approximately 1% of cases of amenorrhoea. The anatomical causes of amenorrhoea are summarized in Box 16.3. In girls with breast development but evidence of an absent uterus, two disorders need to be considered. First, congenital absence of the uterus (Müllerian agenesis, Mayer–Rokitansky–Kuster–Hauser syndrome) is due to an early development failure of the Müllerian system. Affected girls have a normal XX karyotype, normal ovaries and secondary sexual characteristics. The vagina is absent or hypoplastic. Magnetic resonance imaging is a useful adjunct diagnostic test for establishment of the diagnosis, thereby avoiding laparoscopy. Since anomalies of the Wolffian duct system may be present in these patients, an intravenous urogram is an important investigation for this condition. The second disorder to consider is testicular feminization or androgen insensitivity, an X-linked inherited disorder. Patients have a 46XY karyotype, a female phenotype and undescended testes. The uterus is absent and there is a short, blind vaginal pouch. The X-linked androgen receptor is essential for androgen action, leading to normal primary male sexual development prior to birth (masculinization). Thus, androgen receptor dysfunction in XY individuals results in androgen insensitivity syndrome. Diagnosis of this syndrome is established on clinical findings, endocrine investigations and, if possible, family history. There are three phenotypes: complete androgen insensitivity syndrome (CAIS), partial androgen insensitivity syndrome (PAIS) and mixed androgen insensitivity syndrome (MAIS). CAIS is most often diagnosed on clinical findings and laboratory investigations,

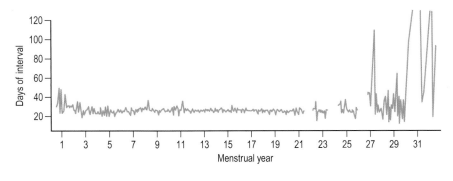

Figure 16.2 Example of a complete history of menstrual intervals from menarche to menopause.
Reproduced with permission from Treloar AE, Boynton RE, Behn BG, Brown BW 1967 International Journal of Fertility 12: 77–126.

Box 16.1 Classification of causes of amenorrhoea

Physiological

Prepuberty
Pregnancy
Lactation
Postmenopause

Pathological

Local genital causes
Congenital
  Testicular feminization
  Congenital absence of the uterus
  Imperforate hymen
Acquired
  Asherman's syndrome

Hypothalamic

Congenital
  Kallman's syndrome
Acquired
  Weight loss
  Extreme exercise
  Craniopharyngioma

Pituitary

Tumour
  Prolactinoma
Infarction
  Sheehan's syndrome
Iatrogenic damage
  Surgery
  Radiotherapy

Ovarian

Congenital
  Gonadotrophin receptor defect
  Resistant ovary syndrome
  Ovarian dysgenesis
Acquired
  Irradiation
  Chemotherapy
  Surgical
  Autoimmune disease
  Polycystic ovary syndrome

Adapted from Baird, Amenorrhoea. Lancet 350:275–279. © The Lancet Ltd 1997.

Box 16.2 Causes of primary amenorrhoea

Delayed puberty

Familial
Nutritional
Delayed adrenarche

Structural congenital abnormalities

Imperforate hymen (cryptomenorrhoea)
Absent uterus ± vagina

Chromosomal abnormalities

XO (Turner's syndrome)
XO/XY mosaics
XY (testicular feminization)

Endocrine causes

Hyperprolactinaemia
Ovarian failure
Gonadotrophin deficiency (hypogonadotrophic hypogonadism)
Polycystic ovary syndrome (hyperandrogenism)
Thyroid dysfunction (hypothyroidism)
Tumours

---

cases) of phenotypic features, androgen receptor binding, and mutational analysis of cases of intersex and ambiguous genitalia has been established (Ahmed et al 2000). All cases of PAIS presented within the first month of life. The median age for presentation of individuals with CAIS was 1 year. The gonads were removed before puberty in 66% of cases with CAIS, and after puberty in 29% of cases. The indication for gonadal removal is the high incidence of neoplasia (5%).

A further anatomical cause of primary amenorrhoea is the presence of an imperforate hymen that obstructs the outflow of menses. Girls commonly present with cyclical pelvic pain and a delayed menarche. Secondary amenorrhoea can result from anatomical abnormalities; the endometrium may be destroyed as a result of infection (e.g. pelvic tuberculosis) or iatrogenically, as a result of an endometrial ablation procedure. Complications of uterine curettage can also result in amenorrhoea. An example of this is Asherman's syndrome (Asherman 1948), which is defined by the presence of intrauterine permanent adhesions, obliterating the uterine cavity either partially or completely. The main cause of this syndrome is the procedure of endometrial curettage required to treat secondary postpartum haemorrhage due to retained placental products. It has also been suggested that missed miscarriages are an important risk factor for the development of adhesions.

Hypothalamic–pituitary dysfunction (endocrine causes)

The hypothalamic–pituitary axis is regulated at two levels. At a higher level, gonadotrophin-releasing hormone (GnRH) neurones within the hypothalamus are stimulated by afferent inputs from the central nervous system. Furthermore, there is endocrine control of GnRH synthesis and secretion

and PAIS and MAIS usually require a family history consistent with X-linked inheritance (Gottlieb et al 1999). Androgen insensitivity may be caused by several mutations of the androgen receptor (Gottlieb et al 1999), resulting in a lack of androgenization during sexual differentiation (Imperato-McGinley 1995). Development of the uterus and upper vagina is inhibited, as the secretion of anti-Müllerian hormone (AMH) by the testes is normal in these patients. Recently, due to nationwide cooperation between paediatric endocrinologists in the UK, an extensive database (278

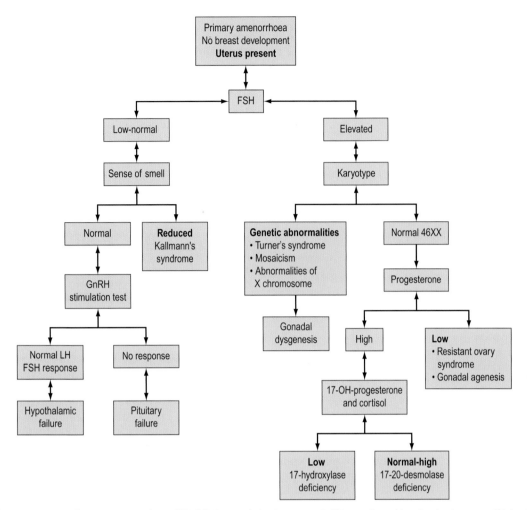

Figure 16.3 The investigation of primary amenorrhoea. FSH, follicle-stimulating hormone; GnRH, gonadotrophin-releasing hormone; LH, luteinizing hormone.

Zreik TG, Olive, DL. Amenorrhea. IN: IS Fraser and SK Smith (eds), Clinical Disorders of the Endometrium and Menstrual Cycle. Oxford University Press, Oxford, UK, pp 229–238, 1998.

Box 16.3 Anatomical causes of amenorrhoea

Developmental defects

Absent ovaries (extremely rare)

Absent uterus (with or without absent vagina)

Imperforate hymen (lower vaginal aplasia)

Developmental defects of endocrine origin

Androgen-resistant syndrome (testicular feminization) in male pseudohermaphrodites (genetic and gonadal males) including inhibition of uterovaginal development

Acquired conditions

Endometrial fibrosis

    Traumatic (Asherman's syndrome)

    Infective (pelvic tuberculosis)

Cervical stenosis

    Surgical trauma (e.g. endometrial ablation)

    Infective

Vaginal stenosis (extremely rare)

    Chemical inflammation

---

by means of gonadal feedback mechanisms and GnRH itself. At a lower level, the output of FSH and luteinizing hormone (LH) by the gonadotropes in the anterior pituitary reflects GnRH activity. Gonadotrophin synthesis and secretion are, in turn, influenced by endocrine feedback from the ovaries as well as paracrine mechanisms and other extrinsic factors. Endocrine causes of oligomenorrhoea and amenorrhoea include disorders of the HPO axis that are summarized in Box 16.4. Disturbances in menstrual pattern will be the consequence of either a structural or functional defect in the tightly controlled feedback system involving the hypothalamus, anterior pituitary and ovary (Baird 1997; Figure 16.4). If the uterus is present and there is no breast development, absence of menstruation may be due to failure of secretion of GnRH or to failure of pituitary or gonadal function (see Figures 16.3 and 16.4). Hypothalamic amenorrhoea suggests an intact HPO axis.

Kallman's syndrome

Kallman's syndrome, occurring in 1:50,000 girls (Kallman et al 1944), has the associated symptom of anosmia and is an inherited autosomal-dominant or X-linked autosomal-recessive anomaly. The impairment of olfactory sensation is often subtle. Women with this condition typically present with primary amenorrhoea and poor development of secondary sexual characteristics. If untreated, infertility results. The gonadotrophin deficiency is due to an inability to activate pulsatile GnRH secretion (Leiblich et al 1982). Five Kallman's syndrome genes have been identified to date. The syndrome appears to result from insufficient cell signalling through fibroblast growth factor receptor 1 (FGFR1), in which integrins play a role in signalling, and the prokineticin receptor 2, a G-protein coupled receptor essential for normal development of the olfactory bulbs and sexual maturation (Abreu et al 2008). Some cases are due to a mutation in the *KAL* gene situated on the p22.3 region of the X chromosome (tip of the short arm) that codes for an adhesion-molecule-like X chromosome (Legouis et al 1991). This protein has homology with fibronectin and plays a role in the migration of GnRH-like neurones from the nasal pit to the hypothalamus (Rugarli and Ballabio 1993). *KAL1* gene mutations account for 33–70% of cases of the X-linked form of Kallman's syndrome. Ovulation induction can achieve pregnancy for these women, but requires both exogenous FSH and LH to successfully stimulate follicular maturation and ovarian steroidogenesis.

Hypogonadotrophic hypogonadism

Female hypogonadism refers to deficient or abnormal function of the HPO axis that clinically presents with menstrual cycle disturbances. Female hypogonadism can be due to a congenital or acquired cause, and the defect can be at the level of the hypothalamus, pituitary or ovary. It is characterized by reduced secretion of FSH (although this can be normal) and LH. There is a consequent failure of follicular development and oestradiol production by the ovaries. A hypo-oestrogenic state thus prevails. If the situation is present before puberty, the girl will present with primary amenorrhoea and a lack of secondary sexual features. Usually, no organic lesion is identified in the hypothalamus or anterior pituitary, and the situation is considered to be idiopathic. Mutations in three genes account for 15–20% of all cases of idiopathic hypogonadotrophic hypogonadism: *KAL1*, *GNRHR* and *FGFR1*. Nearly all mutations are point mutations (Pederson-White et al 2008). Severe weight loss, psychological stress and chronic debilitating disease are all associated with a cessation of hypothalamic function, and are conditions that will be addressed later.

Hypothalamic and pituitary lesions

The most likely hypothalamic lesion to present to a gynaecologist is a craniopharyngioma. Compression of the hypothalamus will suppress GnRH secretion and interrupt portal flow of GnRH in the pituitary stalk. The peripubertal period is the most common age for presentation. The lesions are cystic and often calcified, and are readily recognizable on a lateral skull radiograph or with imaging techniques, such as magnetic resonance imaging. Other tumours which may affect hypothalamic–pituitary function are gliomas (which may arise from the optic tract), meningiomas, endodermal sinus tumour (yolk sac carcinoma), which secretes α-fetoprotein, and congenital hamartomas composed of GnRH neurosecretory cells which can lead to precocious puberty (Yen 1999). Congenital absence of the anterior pituitary gland along with other midline structural defects is extremely rare. Primary deficiency of pituitary hormone secretion is also very uncommon. Growth hormone deficiency may occur in isolation or with panhypopituitary dwarfism. Pituitary failure may be secondary to other organic disease, such as pituitary adenoma, mumps, encephalitis, infarction (Sheehan's syndrome, secondary to major obstetric haemorrhage) and irradiation. Pituitary cells are relatively resistant to irradiation compared with other brain tissues that are more radiosensitive. Disturbance of pituitary function may therefore be indirectly due to hypothalamic damage. Subjects with gonadal failure are oestrogen deficient and have elevated gonadotrophins (hypergonadotrophic hypogonadism). Causes of gonadal failure are listed in Box 16.5 and will be addressed in detail later. One of the most common chromosomal causes of primary amenorrhoea is Turner's syndrome. Enzyme-deficiency states associated with primary amenorrhoea include galactosaemia and 17-hydroxylase deficiency.

Central nervous system–hypothalamic disturbance

The modulating influence of extrahypothalamic brain centres on the pulsatile nature of hypothalamic GnRH secretion is addressed in Chapter 15. Psychological disorders account for approximately one-third of cases of amenorrhoea due to central nervous system–hypothalamic disturbance. Functional disorders of the hypothalamic–pituitary axis that cause amenorrhoea result from weight loss, extreme exercise and psychological stress. In each of these situations, there is

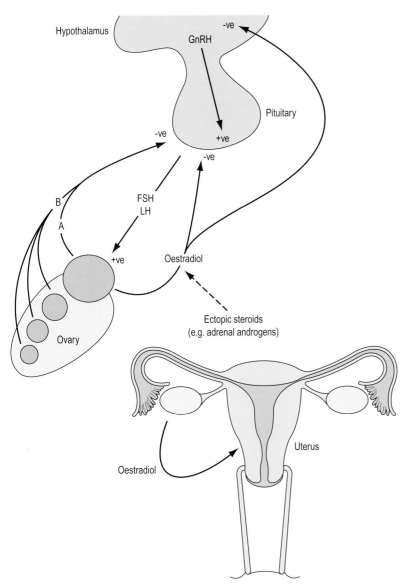

Figure 16.4 The hypothalamic–pituitary–ovarian–uterine axis. GnRH, gonadotrophin-releasing hormone; FSH, follicle-stimulating hormone; LH, luteinizing hormone; A, inhibin B; B, Antimullerian hormone. *Adapted with permission from Baird DT 1997 The Lancet 350: 275–279. ©The Lancet Ltd 1997.*

a decrease in GnRH neuronal activity in the hypothalamus with a subsequent decrease in gonadotrophin secretion (FSH and LH). Ovarian follicular development and ovulation fail to occur if LH pulsatility is less frequent than every 2 h (Baird 1997).

Weight-related amenorrhoea

Marked weight loss, such as that occurring with anorexia nervosa, may result in amenorrhoea. However, menstrual irregularity is an associated feature of all eating disorders rather than being restricted to anorexia nervosa alone. The amount of weight loss that may result in cessation of menstruation varies from a few kilograms in an adolescent who is dieting to a loss of up to 50% of body weight in women with anorexia nervosa (Warren 1995). Regular menses are unlikely to occur in subjects with BMI <19 kg/m^2 (Balen et al 1995). It has been reported that nearly one-fifth of the body mass should be adipose tissue for ovulatory cycles to be sustained (Frisch 1984). The rate of loss of weight

seems to be important, and rapid loss is frequently associated with psychological disturbance. The chronic hypo-oestrogenic state that becomes established in long-standing amenorrhoea carries significant risk of premature osteoporosis and cardiovascular disease. Irregular cycles and anovulation are also common in PCOS and may be due to the commonly associated raised BMI. The insulin resistance with PCOS which is exacerbated by an increase in BMI affects the intraovarian response to gonadotrophins (Greer et al 1980).

Exercise-related amenorrhoea

Irregularities of menstrual pattern are reported in association with many competitive sporting activities. There is typically a progressive failure of regular menses with anovulatory cycles and amenorrhoea and, in prepubertal girls, a delayed menarche. Usually, the degree of menstrual aberration reflects the intensity and length of sporting activity (Yen 1999). Secondary amenorrhoea and oligomenorrhoea are

Box 16.5 Aetiological classification of premature ovarian failure

Genetic
Gonadal dysgenesis
    X chromosome deletion (XO; Turner's syndrome)
    Normal XX complement (pure gonadal dysgenesis)

Metabolic disorders
Galactosaemia
17-hydroxylase deficiency

Immunological deficiency

Autoimmune diseases

Infections
Pelvic tuberculosis
Mumps

Environmental causes
Cigarette smoking

Iatrogenic
Surgery
Chemotherapy
Irradiation

Idiopathic

also common in professional dancers (Warren et al 1986). Women with hypothalamic amenorrhoea associated with an excessive exercise habit, weight loss and stress have hypercortisolism, on account of raised corticotrophin-releasing hormone (CRH) and adrenocorticotrophic hormone. Consequently, there is likely to be disruption of reproductive function as CRH directly inhibits GnRH secretion, possibly via increased endogenous opioid secretion (Speroff et al 1999a). A detailed study was reported by Laughlin and Yen (1996) which addressed the interactions between energy balance and regulators of metabolic fuel and the association with reduced LH pulsatility in women with exercise-induced menstrual dysfunction. Notable differences were observed in nutritional intake, insulin/glucose dynamics, the somatotrophic axis and LH pulsatility with both degree of exercise and menstrual pattern. Those athletes who were amenorrhoeic demonstrated an increase in insulin sensitivity and a reduced hypoglycaemic effect of insulin-like growth factor 1 (IGF-1), along with raised growth hormone and cortisol concentrations. The authors suggest that there is a cascade of glucoregulatory adaptations designed to redistribute metabolic fuel and thereby conserve protein. Furthermore, the reduced GnRH/LH pulse generator activity is in response to both a reduced stimulatory effect of IGF-1 (due to increased IGF-binding protein 1) and central negative effects of corticotrophin-releasing factor. The outlook for women with stress-/exercise-related amenorrhoea is very good if recognized early. Most women see a return of ovulatory cycles with weight gain or reduction in levels of stress or exercise habit (Speroff et al 1999a). Hormone replacement may be indicated for women with long-standing hypothalamic amenorrhoea as there will be a risk of bone loss and cardiovascular changes.

Metabolic hormones regulating reproductive function

Kisspeptins, and their cognate receptor gpr-54, were first found to regulate the hypothalamic–pituitary–gonadal axis in 2003, when two groups demonstrated that mutations in gpr-54 cause idiopathic hypogonadotropic hypogonadism characterized by delayed or absent puberty (Roseweir and Millar 2009). KiSS1 neurones have recently been suggested to mediate leptin's effect on the reproductive system by encoding hypothalamic neuropeptides. Leptin is the primary product of the *ob* gene and is a 167 amino acid peptide made exclusively in adipose tissue; it acts on the hypothalamus. It is likely that leptin plays a central role in energy production, reproduction and weight, and it has been proposed as a mediator between adipose tissue and the gonads (Matkovic et al 1997). In both eating disorders and excessive exercise, amenorrhoea results from an adaptive response to an energy deficit, partially mediated by leptin. A critical blood leptin level has been reported as necessary to trigger reproductive function in women, suggesting a threshold effect. In this context, severe weight loss is known to result in subnormal gonadotrophin concentrations. Leptin receptors have been identified in the hypothalamus, and leptin inhibits neuropeptide Y (NPY) synthesis and release. A link between leptin and GnRH neurones is, in part, mediated by NPY. Secondary leptin deficiency can present as weight-related amenorrhoea in women (Conway and Jacobs 1997). Speroff et al (1999a) noted that CRH is elevated in stress- and, particularly, weight-loss-related amenorrhoea. It has been proposed that the decrease in leptin and increase in NPY described in stress-related weight loss are inadequate to suppress the stress-induced increase in CRH. Moreover, the increase in CRH and resulting hypercortisolism exacerbate the increase in metabolism and weight loss. Research leading to a better understanding of the metabolic regulation of reproductive function has implications for the prevention and management of reproductive dysfunction and its associated comorbidities.

Neurological and psychiatric disorders

Epilepsy, bipolar disorder and migraines are common disorders which can be associated with disturbances in menstrual function in adolescent girls. With epilepsy, it is thought that both the disease itself and the treatment medications contribute to the aetiology of the menstrual abnormality by disturbing the HPO axis. Many antipsychotic drugs are also dopamine antagonists, and can cause prolactin levels to increase up to 10-fold, again resulting in inhibition of the HPO axis (see Box 16.6).

Chronic illness

A variety of mechanisms in chronic illness can result in pubertal delay and cessation of menses. These include

Box 16.6 Pharmacological agents associated with hyperprolactinaemia

Phenothiazines

Perphenazine

Chlorpromazine

Thioridazine

Trifluoperazine

Prochlorperazine

Butyrophenones

Haloperidol

Pimozide (Orap)

Bezamides

Metoclopramide

Clebopride

Cimetidine

Rauwolfia alkaloids

Reserpine

Methyldopa

changes in nutrition, behaviour, metabolism, hormone balance, associated stress and medications.

Idiopathic delayed puberty

The limiting factor for increasing amounts of gonadotrophin secretion as normal puberty approaches is hypothalamic GnRH release (Yen 1999). Delayed puberty may be recognized by the age of 14 years if breast development is still absent. Most cases are due to idiopathic hypothalamic failure and usually resolve spontaneously. There may often be a family history of late puberty. Enquiry should seek any history of impaired olfaction, marked weight loss, extremes of exercise and ill health. Other causes of amenorrhoea with oestrogen deficiency should be excluded with a lateral skull radiograph/hypothalamic–pituitary imaging (non-endocrine tumours, e.g. craniopharyngioma), and serum prolactin (prolactinoma) and FSH measurements (ovarian dysgenesis). If the diagnosis is idiopathic delayed puberty, it remains difficult to distinguish whether the failure is purely delayed or permanent, and thus treatment should commence without delay. Once the patient's secondary sexual characteristics are mature, treatment may be periodically interrupted to establish whether there is spontaneous HPO activity.

Hyperprolactinaemia

In girls with primary amenorrhoea with normal breast development and a uterus, hyperprolactinaemia must be considered. Approximately 15–20% of women with secondary amenorrhoea have elevated serum prolactin concentrations (Jacobs et al 1976). Unlike the other trophic hormones secreted by the anterior pituitary, prolactin secretion is regulated primarily by inhibition from the hypothalamus by dopamine. Prolactin secretion is not subject directly or indirectly to negative feedback by peripheral hormones. Regulation of secretion is via a short-loop feedback on hypothalamic dopamine by means of a countercurrent flow in the hypophyseal portal system (as well as inhibition of GnRH pulsatile secretion). Prolactin secretion is stimulated by peripheral oestrogen, and this is derived from the placenta in pregnancy.

Circulating concentrations of prolactin rise during pregnancy; at term, the levels are four to 20 times higher than those in non-pregnant women. After delivery, prolactin levels decline in non-lactating women over a 15–20-day period. In lactating women, circulating levels of prolactin are maintained by suckling, and hyperprolactinaemia may last for up to 2 years. During breastfeeding, there is an increase in the sensitivity of the HPO axis to the negative feedback effect of oestradiol (Illingworth et al 1995). The duration and causes of this period of hypersensitivity to oestrogen are unknown. Data are available to support the concept that the suckling-induced suppression of the GnRH system during lactation is associated with enhancement of the negative effects of oestradiol on the hypothalamic GnRH system (Perheentupa et al 2000). Pathological hyperprolactinaemia is associated with amenorrhoea. There is no ovarian function, reduced or absent pulsatility of LH secretion, and an absence of positive feedback response to oestrogen. Treatment of raised prolactin concentrations restores ovulation in 80–90% of women (Randeva et al 2000), and normal cyclical activity returns once prolactin levels are reduced. Pathological hyperprolactinaemia may be induced by drugs that inhibit dopamine action or production. A list of potential compounds is given in Box 16.6. Pharmacological agents account for 1–2% of cases (see Box 16.6). The most common causes of hyperprolactinaemia are pituitary prolactinomas (40–50% of cases) and idiopathic hypersecretion. Primary hypothyroidism will be the coincident diagnosis in 3–5% of cases. Rare causes are ectopic production from a distant extrapituitary tumour, and chronic renal failure may be associated with hyperprolactinaemia, due to both decreased excretion of the hormone and central mechanisms affecting dopamine secretion. Only about half of patients who present with hyperprolactinaemia describe galactorrhoea. Moreover, only about half of the women who report galactorrhoea have raised prolactin levels (Baird 1997). Serum prolactin measurements are essential. Usually, a second sample is required if the first is raised. A common problem is the misinterpretation of the upper normal limit of a geometric (skewed) distribution of normal values. The upper limit is taken at approximately 800 mU/l. The functional relevance of borderline hyperprolactinaemia is unclear. It is most important to consider the prolactin concentration in the context of the associated ovulatory disorder. Significant hyperprolactinaemia is usually associated with oligomenorrhoea or amenorrhoea. Mild hyperprolactinaemia is identified with some cases of PCOS. The phenomenon is likely to be the consequence of excess oestrogenic stimulation. Conversely, prolactin levels are low in hypothalamic amenorrhoea and are likely to be due to lack of oestrogenic stimulation. Thyroid-releasing hormone stimulates prolactin. This can be raised in hypothyroidism, so thyroid function tests should be checked in hyperprolactinaemia. In addition, serotonin can increase prolactin with resulting possible effects from the use of drugs such as selective serotonin reuptake inhibitors.

The mechanism by which hyperprolactinaemia interferes with ovarian function is not clearly defined. It has been suggested that in hyperprolactinaemia, endogenous opioids may have an inhibitory effect on hypothalamic GnRH-secreting neurones (Grossman et al 1982). However, this is not a consistent observation, and prolactin may, in fact, have a direct effect on hypothalamic activity. Although serum levels of prolactin in women with idiopathic hyperprolactinaemia or with pituitary tumours may normalize after treatment with a dopamine agonist (or after pituitary surgery), there are many issues about treatment and long-term follow-up that remain unresolved. Recently published guidelines have advised that the minimal length of dopamine agonist therapy should be 1 year (Casanueva et al 2006). A recent report indicates that dopamine agonists can be safely withdrawn in patients with long-term normalization of prolactin levels and no evidence of tumour on magnetic resonance imaging (Colao et al 2003). The natural history of hyperprolactinaemia is not known. Interestingly, as many as 10% of patients may have a spontaneous remission (Glasier et al 1987). In a longitudinal prospective 3–7 year study of 30 women with untreated hyperprolactinaemia, with annual clinical, radiographic and hormonal evaluation, progression of the disease was observed to be unlikely; in fact, some women showed clinical and radiographic improvement (Schlechte et al 1989).

Ovarian failure

It is well established that the number of follicles in the human ovary declines steadily from midlife onwards. The onset of menopause is prompted by the number of ovarian follicles falling below a critical number as the consequence of the programmed disappearance of a limited store of follicles. The process is irreversible as oogonal stem cells disappear after birth. The loss of follicles is age dependent, and the rate of disappearance increases with age. There is a reported acceleration of loss from the age of 37.5 years (Faddy et al 1992). In this context, Richardson et al (1987) observed that entry into the perimenopausal phase of life was associated with a marked decline in follicle reserve, and that the reserve of follicles was nearly exhausted as menopause approached.

Premature ovarian failure (POF), or more appropriately primary ovarian insufficiency, is defined as the triad of amenorrhoea, oestrogen deficiency and elevated concentrations of FSH and LH in women less than 40 years old. It also includes women with primary amenorrhoea; that is, those who have no known prior ovarian function. Secondary ovarian failure occurs in women who have previously menstruated. The causes of both are similar. In patients diagnosed with POF, particularly with a recent diagnosis or a fluctuating FSH, there has been a reported pregnancy rate of 5–10% (van Kasteran and Schoemaker 1999). For those less fortunate, oocyte donation is a possible alternative.

The age that best separates 'premature' from 'normal' menopause is arbitrary. The definition of POF assumes that those patients with the disorder constitute a group with specific characteristics that distinguish them from patients with normal menopause (Alper et al 1986). Forty years is the preferred age for definition for practical purposes. Many women with POF at 40 years or younger are concerned with fertility. If one were to define abnormality as those values greater than, or less than, two standard deviations (SD) from the mean (where 95% of the observations of a normally distributed variable are found), then 40 years is also an appropriate age. If the age of menopause is assumed to be a normally distributed variable, Walsh (1978) reported the mean age of menopause as 50.4 years (SD 3.72 years), and 2.5% of women reach menopause at 43 years of age or younger. There are no unique features that unequivocally establish the diagnosis of POF. Indeed, the diagnosis of POF is often delayed, even with the classic symptoms of menopause. At least 4 months with missing or irregular periods may indicate carrying out a serum FSH which, if elevated in the menopausal range on at least two occasions a few weeks apart, is a useful diagnostic test; ultrasound and ovarian biopsy have no role. A delay in diagnosis may result in preventable bone loss (Neale 2009). Ovarian failure itself is an irreversible pathological process with major implications for the patient (in particular, reduced bone mineral density, increased cardiovascular risk and infertility), and thus its diagnosis is an important responsibility for the gynaecologist.

The incidence of POF is not precisely known. Calculations based on the incidence of permanent secondary amenorrhoea suggest 2–3% (Bachmann and Kemmann 1982). Coulam et al (1986) reported POF in 1–3% of the general population. These latter authors conducted a detailed assessment of age-specific incidence rates of natural menopause for a cohort of 1858 women during a 4-year period, and identified a 1% risk at 40 years of age. The incidence at 30 years of age is 0.1% and decreases as age decreases (Anasti 1998). As such, the condition is not rare.

Advances in modern molecular biology have enabled major contributions to be made to understanding the aetiology of POF; however, despite this, only one-third of women have an identifiable pathology (Conway 1997). POF indicates absent ovarian function; it is not a disease but a clinical state and is often a fluctuating condition. Ovarian failure may be primary or secondary, and the chromosomes of the patient may be normal or abnormal. Common causes of POF are summarized in Box 16.5. Genetic disorders are the most common identifiable causes. Chromosomal anomalies are found in women with primary amenorrhoea and ovarian dysgenesis. In Turner's syndrome, there is an X chromosome deletion. Typically, these patients have streak ovaries, are of short stature and have a characteristic phenotype, including one or some of the following features: neck webbing, widely spaced nipples, increased carrying angle and coarctation of the aorta. Approximately two-thirds of Turner's patients have the total loss of one X chromosome, and the rest either exhibit a structural abnormality in one X chromosome or display mosaicism with an abnormal X chromosome (Speroff et al 1999b). Menstrual function and pregnancy are possible among patients with XO mosaicism. In Turner's girls, 10–20% experience spontaneous puberty and 2–5% experience spontaneous menstruation (Pasquino et al 1997). Girls with ovarian dysgenesis may be grouped according to their karyotype (Speroff et al 1999c). Fifty percent of girls will have Turner's syndrome and 25% will be mosaics (45X/46XX). Patients may have gonadal dysgenesis and a normal XX chromosome complement (25%). This is pure gonadal dysgenesis and the girls invariably have streak ovaries (Sohval 1965), diagnosis of the latter only being made after direct visualization, usually at laparoscopy. In XY gonadal dysgenesis, the testis fails to develop due to loss or mutation of the sex-determining region of the Y chromosome (Tdy or SRY). The testis-determining gene, Tdy, is situated on the short arm of the Y chromosome, and the gene responsible for the H-Y antigen is on the long arm (Goodfellow and Lovell-Badge 1993). If an XY karyotype is detected, the gonadal streaks should be removed since there is a risk of neoplastic transformation. Recent attention has focused on other genetic determinants of POF. Gonadotrophin resistance as a consequence of an FSH receptor mutation has been described (Aittomaki et al 1995). It has been known for some time that fragile X mental retardation 1 gene (FMR1) is characterized by a dynamic CGG repeat expansion in the 5′ untranslated region. Female carriers of the FMR1 premutation allele are at risk of passing the FMR full mutation (>200 repeats) to their offspring, resulting in mental retardation known as fragile X (De Caro et al 2008). This is the most common inherited form of mental retardation. Women who carry one X chromosome with a fragile X premutation display an increased prevalence of POF (Conway et al 1995). This is estimated to be approximately 15–24% compared with the incidence of 1% in the general population. The US National Society of Genetic Counselors does not currently recommend routine testing of minors for the FMR1 premutation allele. There is ongoing discussion regarding the most appropriate terminology to describe the reproductive abnormalities associated with the FMR1 mutation, sometimes known as fragile X-associated primary ovarian insufficiency.

It is felt that the term 'primary ovarian insufficiency' may be preferable to 'POF' as it better describes what is, in fact, a spectrum of ovarian changes rather than what is sometimes not complete dysfunction of the ovary. Family history remains a predictor of early menopause. In a case–control study of 344 cases of early menopause, a family history of earlier menopause (before 46 years) was associated with an increased risk of early menopause, with the link being strongest in women with a history of menopause before 40 years of age (Cramer et al 1995). Within the last few years, a mutation in the FOXL2 gene, located on chromosome 3 and essential for proper reproductive function in females, has been implicated in POF (Crisponi et al 2001). The authors indicate that this is the first human gene to be identified that may play a role in the maintenance of ovarian follicles. Those carrying mutations in FOXL2 display blepharophimosis/ptosis/epicanthus inversus syndrome, an autosomal-dominant disease associated with eyelid defects and POF. It is quite remarkable that FOXL2 encodes a protein important to both eye and ovarian development. FOXL2 mutations and other gene mutations will only account for a small fraction of cases of POF, but the identification of genes regulated by FOXL2 will contribute to understanding of the biochemical pathways that may be aberrant in POF, and hence potentially offer novel treatments for female infertility in the future. Another gene thought to be related to POF is BMP15. Recent studies have demonstrated heterozygous BMP15 missense mutations in women with POF. Patients with galactosaemia treated in early life with a galactose-free diet exhibit a high frequency of ovarian failure. Affected individuals have mutations of the galactose 1-phosphate uridyltransferase gene (Kaufman et al 1981). The associated feature of ovarian failure is considered to be a consequence of accumulated galactose disturbing the migration of the germ cells from the urogenital ridge to the gonad in fetal life. There is an association between autoimmune disease and ovarian failure, and between 10% and 20% of women with POF have intercurrent autoimmune conditions (Conway et al 1996). These include Addison's disease, hypothyroidism, pernicious anaemia, Hashimoto's disease, idiopathic thrombocytopenia, rheumatoid arthritis with vitiligo, alopecia areata, Cushing's disease, autoimmune haemolytic anaemia and myaesthenia gravis. Among patients in whom the aetiology of POF is obscure, there are other lines of evidence to suggest autoimmune mechanisms. Circulating antibodies to ovarian tissue have been demonstrated in the sera of women with POF. Organ-specific autoimmunity may be directed against the intracellular enzymes involved in hormone production. 3-β-hydroxysteroid dehydrogenase (3-β-HSD) has been identified as an autoantigen in one-fifth of women with POF. This observation now offers a potential marker for autoimmune ovarian damage, although the presence of anti-3-β-HSD antibodies may be the consequence of ovarian inflammation rather than the causal antigen (Arif et al 1996). Infections associated with loss of ovarian function are mumps and pelvic tuberculosis. Environmental factors contributing to an early menopause include cigarette smoking. As a consequence of the improved survival for patients with certain neoplastic conditions treated with radiotherapy and chemotherapy, an increasing number of survivors are facing the absence of ovarian function. Irradiation is known to induce POF and was once a method of castration. The reproductive system is one of the major sites of secondary effects of anticancer treatment (Ogilvy-Stuart and Shalet 1993). Different therapeutic insults will be associated with different risks for early menopause. It is important to have accurate information on the gonadotoxicity of different cancer treatment regimens to improve patient information and optimize approaches for fertility preservation. For survivors of treatment for cancer, treatment with radiotherapy below the diaphragm and alkylating agent chemotherapy, the average age at menopause was approximately 31 years. Other modes of treatment conferred an excess risk of ovarian failure, although not as great (Byrne 1999; Figure 16.5).

Anderson and Cameron (2007) detected changes in the ultrasound markers of the ovarian reserve (OR), with decreases in both ovarian volume and antral follicle count during chemotherapy. Anderson and Cameron (2007) assessed the OR markers in premenopausal women to investigate and compare the effects of chemotherapy and long-term gonadotrophin withdrawal on ovarian function, and detected changes in ultrasound markers of the OR, with decreases in both ovarian volume and antral follicle count during chemotherapy. These data confirm the value of AMH

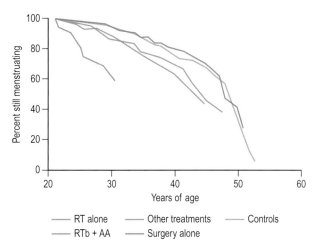

Figure 16.5 Menopause in childhood cancer survivors and controls expressed as the proportion still menstruating. RTb + AA, radiation therapy below the diaphragm plus alkylating agents; RT alone, radiation therapy alone.
Reproduced with permission from Byrne J, Fears TR, Gail MH et al 1992 Early menopause in long-term survivors of cancer during adolescence. American Journal of Obstetrics and Gynecology 166:788–793.

concentration as an early indicator of ovarian ageing, including assessment of chemotherapy-induced ovarian follicle loss. FSH and AMH concentration measurements may be useful for the comparison of ovarian toxicity of different chemotherapy regimens. Adverse effects on female reproductive function may be mediated through effects at one or more levels of the HPO axis (Wallace et al 1989) or at the uterus (Critchley et al 1992). Commonly, anticancer treatment (chemotherapy, particularly alkylating agents, and scatter radiation to the ovary) affects the ovary as a consequence of depletion of the stock of primordial follicles, thereby advancing or inducing menopause (Critchley and Wallace 2005). Effects on the hypothalamus and pituitary may be subtle. High-dose cranial irradiation is known to have direct damaging effects, but the effects of the lower doses used in the management of childhood leukaemia are, as yet, uncertain. Data concerning ovarian function after treatment of standard risk leukaemia have been reassuring (Wallace et al 1993). A recent study by Bath et al (2001) examined HPO function in 12 women in first remission from childhood acute lymphoblastic leukaemia. This study revealed a high prevalence of short luteal phases (<11 days) among these women compared with a normal control group. A reduced LH excretion (probably secondary to cranial irradiation) and ovarian oestrogen production (probably reflecting a reduction in gonadotrophic stimulus) were observed in the women with acute lymphoblastic leukaemia. Such disturbances in LH secretion may have an effect on reproductive potential (Box 16.7).

Ovarian reserve

The OR, a term that has evolved in the era of assisted reproductive technology, refers to the residual oocyte-granulosa cell repertoire. An improved ascertainment of OR status may help to optimize the planned therapeutic intervention, and

thus minimize the emotional and financial strain placed upon couples seeking fertility treatment. A spectrum of markers prognostic of the OR are validated to varying degrees in the infertile population. These include biochemical markers (FSH, prostaglandin E2, inhibin B, AMH and FSH:LH ratio) and ovarian morphometeric markers (ovarian volume, antral follicle count and mean ovarian diameter) assessed in the early follicular phase (basal) of the menstrual cycle (Bowen et al 2007).

Raised follicle-stimulating hormone (FSH) is important as it is the first measurable parameter that changes in reproductive ageing. Pituitary FSH production is co-regulated by inhibin and oestradiol, acting via negative endocrine feedback (Muttukrishna et al 2000). Anti-Mullerian hormone (AMH) has recently been suggested as a more accurate indicator of the presence of ovarian follicles (Durlinger et al 2002). Since there is no change in AMH levels in response to gonadotrophins, AMH can be measured throughout the cycle in contrast to the other parameters, which can only be determined during the early follicular phase: an advantage for both patients and clinicians. It reflects earlier stages of follicle development than inhibin B and oestradiol, and thus is believed to more closely approximate the number of primordial follicles in the ovary. Inhibin B is a product of the granulosa cells. It has recently been shown that the value of inhibin B as a measure of the OR is greatly increased following administration of a single dose of FSH to stimulate granulosa cell function in small healthy follicles.

A nationwide prospective cohort study in the Netherlands concluded that, compared with inhibin B and antral follicle count, AMH was more consistently correlated with the clinical degree of follicle pool depletion in young women presenting with elevated FSH levels (Knauff et al 2009). AMH may provide a more accurate assessment of the follicle pool in young hypergonadotropic patients, especially in the clinically challenging subgroups of patients with elevated FSH and regular menses (i.e. incipient ovarian failure), and in hypergonadotropic women with cycle disturbances not fulfilling the diagnostic criteria for POF (i.e. transitional ovarian failure). Ultrasound measurement of both ovarian volume and antral follicle count (the number of small follicles present) is also of value.

Assessment of the OR by measuring the ellipsoid ovarian volume via transvaginal ultrasound is cumbersome and time consuming as it requires an additional third-dimensional measurement, not routinely taken in clinical practice.

Whilst all individual ovarian parameters (width, length or an average of the two) reliably reflect the OR in premenopausal infertile women, the mean ovarian width (as determined by ultrasound) exhibits a more robust relationship with OR status compared with ovarian length or the average of the two dimensions (Fratarelli et al 2002).

Endocrine disorders arising outside the HPO axis leading to chronic anovulation

Other endocrine disorders may interfere with the normal feedback loops of the HPO axis, thereby causing a disturbance in cyclical ovarian activity and manifesting as amenorrhoea or oligomenorrhoea (Baird 1997). Thyroid disease may cause amenorrhoea and oligomenorrhoea. There is an increase in circulating concentrations of oestrogen and testosterone in hyperthyroidism as levels of sex-hormone-binding globulin increase. In hypothyroidism, there may be associated raised levels of prolactin due to stimulation with thyrotrophic-releasing hormone. In adrenal disease, the excessive secretion of sex steroids leads to amenorrhoea, as gonadotrophin secretion will be suppressed.

Diagnosis and Management of Oligomenorrhoea and Amenorrhoea

The successful management of oligomenorrhoea and amenorrhoea is dependent upon the correct diagnosis and an assessment of the requirements of the patient. Patients will articulate different needs which may include advice about future fertility prospects, fertility control, symptoms of hirsutism, delayed secondary sexual development, protection from osteoporosis and endometrial protection from unopposed oestrogen action. A thorough history and clinical examination (as appropriate) are of paramount importance in establishing the diagnosis of an endocrine disorder, complemented with an appropriate examination and conduct of straightforward endocrine investigations. Since the withdrawal of sex steroids results in endometrial bleeding, a detailed menstrual history will be extremely valuable in the determination of endogenous ovarian activity. Provided that the patient has not been administered exogenous hormone preparations, a report of only light menstrual bleeding will indicate sufficient ovarian production of oestrogen to produce endometrial proliferation. Hence if a history is given of oligomenorrhoea, there must be some capacity for ovarian activity. It is essential to exclude an anatomical cause of amenorrhoea. The bimanual assessment of a young woman who has never been sexually active is inappropriate. The examination of secondary sexual characteristics (breast development) and the external genitalia of an adolescent should be performed in the presence of the patient's parent. Indeed, a deferred examination separate from the initial consultation may be most appropriate, thereby providing an opportunity for confidence to be established in the subsequent doctor–patient relationship. Modern imaging techniques, particularly transabdominal ultrasound, are valuable non-invasive modes of establishing information about reproductive anatomy. In the context of a history of amenorrhoea, an enquiry about experience of hot flushes may elicit a diagnosis of ovarian failure. A detailed drug history (see Box 16.6) and information about diet, exercise habit and weight change are essential. Furthermore, enquiry about life events producing psychological stress should be made. Signs of hyperandrogenism may be evident, such as hirsutism, acne and balding. Enquiry about the presence of galactorrhoea should be made. A distinction is required between hyperandrogenism and virilization, and acanthosis nigricans is a feature of severe insulin resistance. An assessment of the development of secondary sexual characteristics and BMI is important. Baseline endocrine investigations should include the exclusion of pregnancy (most common cause of secondary amenorrhoea), measurement of serum gonadotrophin (FSH and LH), oestradiol and prolactin concentrations, and markers of thyroid function (thyroxine and/or thyroid-stimulating hormone) if there are clinical signs of thyroid disease or any signs of hyperprolactinaemia. It is also possible to assess endogenous ovarian activity over the cycle with once- or twice-weekly serial measurements of oestradiol and progesterone concentrations in serum (or plasma) or their metabolites in urine. Serum androgens (testosterone) should be measured in subjects with hirsutism or androgenization. The possible use of transabdominal (and, where appropriate, transvaginal) ultrasound as mentioned above may be a useful adjunct to clinical examination. These baseline endocrine investigations will permit the categorization of patients into essentially one of four diagnostic groups: hypergonadotrophic hypogonadism, hyperprolactinaemia, hypogonadotrophic hypogonadism and normogonadotrophic anovulation (Baird 1997; Figure 16.6).

Ovarian failure

The endocrine status in ovarian failure (or, rarely, resistant ovary syndrome) is identified by the demonstration of a raised serum FSH concentration (>30 IU/l) and a low serum oestradiol level (<60 pmol/l). In cases of primary amenorrhoea and thus primary ovarian failure, a chromosomal analysis will permit the identification of women with testicular dysgenesis. It is important that women have their residual gonadal tissue removed on account of the risk of neoplastic change. Sex steroid replacement therapy with cyclic oestrogen and progestogen should be started without delay, particularly in girls with primary ovarian failure, in the latter group to induce secondary sexual characteristics and among all affected patients in order to prevent premature bone loss. This should be continued until the age of 50–54 years.

Hyperprolactinaemia

Although the true prevalence of hyperprolactinemia is difficult to establish, it is estimated that among women presenting with reproductive disorders, approximately 15% with anovulation and 43% with anovulation and galactorrhea have hyperprolactinemia. Hyperprolactinaemia (raised serum prolactin) is diagnosed when concentrations of prolactin are outwith the normal range (up to 500 mU/l). It should be noted that serum prolactin levels may be transiently and moderately raised (>700 mU/l) at times of stress. A persistent, albeit moderate, elevation of prolactin will be recorded in the presence of hypothyroidism, and is a common feature among women with PCOS. In the latter group, levels as high as 2500 mU/l have been reported (Baird 1997, Balen 2000). Thyroid disease may be excluded with estimation of serum thyrotrophin concentrations. Patients with PCOS-related hyperprolactinaemia may be distinguished from women with unrelated hyperprolactinaemia and polycystic ovaries on ultrasound by means of a progestogen challenge test (Lunenfeld and Insler 1974),

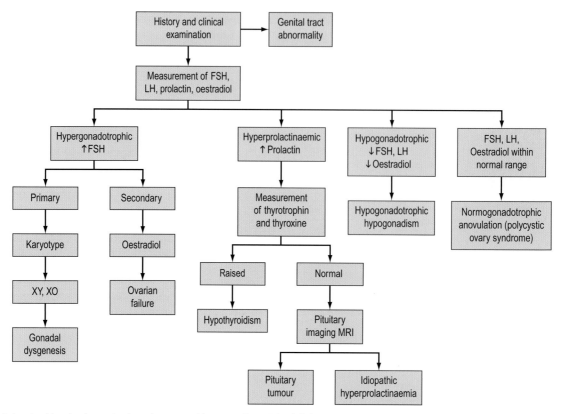

Figure 16.6 An algorithm for the evaluation of women with amenorrhoea. FSH, follicle-stimulating hormone; LH, luteinizing hormone; MRI, magnetic resonance imaging.

Reproduced with permission from Baird DT 1997 The Lancet 350: 275–279. © The Lancet Ltd 1997.

which will induce a withdrawal bleed from an oestrogen-primed endometrium. Serum prolactin measurements >1500 mU/l will require more detailed investigations. Imaging of the pituitary fossa is best undertaken with either magnetic resonance imaging or computed tomography. Serum prolactin concentrations >5000 mU/l are associated with macroprolactinomas (>1 cm diameter). Diagnostic imaging will detect the presence of a hypothalamic tumour or a non-functioning pituitary tumour causing compression of the hypothalamus or a pituitary microadenoma (Figures 16.7 and 16.8).

Hypogonadotrophic hypogonadism

Hypogonadotrophic hypogonadism is characterized by reduced FSH and LH secretion, and consequent absence of follicular development and oestradiol production. Before puberty, the situation will manifest as primary amenorrhoea and lack of development of secondary sexual characteristics. Usually, however, no organic disease is identified in the hypothalamus or anterior pituitary gland. On rare occasions, it may be necessary to distinguish hypothalamic causes from pituitary causes with a GnRH stimulation test (100 μg s.c.) following 1 week of ethinyl oestradiol orally at a dose of 5–10 μg/day. The administration of this supraphysiological dose of GnRH assesses the responsiveness and capacity of the pituitary to secrete gonadotrophins (Yen et al 1973). A better index of 'pituitary reserve' is

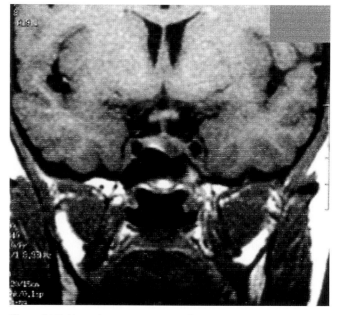

Figure 16.7 Magnetic resonance image of a pituitary microadenoma (coronal T1 non-contrast image) demonstrating a focal rounded area of low signal in the left half of the gland measuring 7 mm. The lesion distorts both the superior and inferior margins of the pituitary gland. The pituitary infundibulum is midline with no evidence of extension into the suprasellar cistern.

Image courtesy of Dr Dilip Patel, Edinburgh Royal Infirmary.

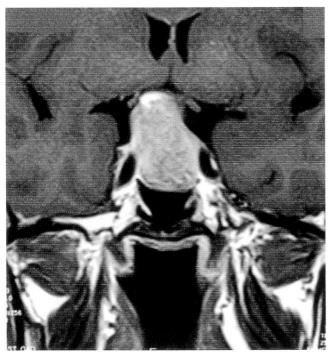

Figure 16.8 Magnetic resonance image of a pituitary macroadenoma (coronal T1 postcontrast image) demonstrating a large contrast-enhancing mass arising from the pituitary fossa (which is enlarged) and extending into the suprasellar cistern and compressing the optic chiasm.
Image courtesy of Dr Dilip Patel, Edinburgh Royal Infirmary.

provided by assessment of the response to repeated physiological doses of GnRH (5–10 µg) at 2–3-h intervals (rather than a single supraphysiological injection). This assessment of pituitary secretory capacity correlates better with the degree of spontaneous secretion, as indicated by the amplitude and frequency of LH pulses. Raised FSH and LH concentrations in response to GnRH stimulation may indicate hypothalamic failure. Such patients require imaging to exclude a craniopharyngioma and consideration of Kallman's syndrome.

Normogonadotrophic anovulation

Normogonadotrophic anovulation occurs in one-third of women with secondary amenorrhoea who display normal gonadotrophin concentrations. Women with PCOS should be considered in this category, and their diagnosis and treatment are discussed in depth in Chapter 18.

Therapeutic Issues

Oestrogen deficiency

In addition to a thorough explanation to patients about the diagnosis and its consequences, women with ovarian failure require sex steroid replacement therapy with cyclic oestrogen and progestogen. Lack of oestrogen after the normal age of menopause has an adverse effect on bone and blood vessel health. Premenopausal levels of oestradiol in women with normal ovarian function protect the female

skeleton from demineralization (Howell and Shalet 1999). The cardiovascular protective effects of oestrogen are well documented in older women who have had endogenous protection for many years before the menopause (Mendelsohn and Karas 1999). In Turner's syndrome, there is evidence to suggest that women do not achieve peak bone mass and have a higher rate of fractures (Davies et al 1995). In girls with Turner's syndrome, the rate of bone mineral acquisition on the oral contraceptive pill is less than is seen in normal adolescents, with a 25% reduction in bone mineral content from that predicted for age, height, weight and bone size. It is possible that this may be a reflection of suboptimal oestrogen replacement. Research to date has delivered well-evaluated hormone replacement regimens for older women designed to mitigate the adverse effects of lack of oestrogen and taken for somewhere in the order of 10 years. Some women seek alternatives to conventional hormone replacement therapy (HRT) which can include antidepressants (e.g. serotonin) and herbal preparations. A recent systematic review looking at black cohosh as a treatment for menopausal symptoms concluded that the efficacy was uncertain and that further trials are warranted (Borrelli and Ernst 2008). Currently, younger women with a premature menopause are offered combined sex steroid replacement in the convenient form of the combined oral contraceptive pill or HRT, which should be continued at least until the average age of natural menopause (52 years in the UK). This view is endorsed by regulatory bodies such as the Committee on Safety of Medicines (now the Commission on Human Medicines) in the UK (Pitkin et al 2007). These preparations are not designed to achieve physiological replacement of oestrogen or progesterone, either in dosage or biochemical structure. The optimal mode and formulation of sex steroid replacement have not yet been established for young women with ovarian failure. The well-documented risks with HRT relate to the postmenopausal age category and not those with premature menopause. Indeed, recent guidelines from the British Menopause Society (2008) confirm that there is no increase in the risk of breast cancer or cardiovascular disease with the use of HRT for patients with premature menopause. There may also be a need for topical oestrogen in the form of vaginal cream or pessary. In addition, testosterone replacement may need to be considered where there are marked symptoms of reduced libido; this is delivered in a patch. Patients should be warned about possible side-effects of excess hair growth and acne. A recent randomized, double-blind, placebo-controlled trial showed transdermal testosterone therapy to be very effective (Shifren et al 2006). Early menopause is a risk factor for osteoporosis, so women with an early menopause should have bone density testing performed within 10 years of menopause so that osteopenia or osteoporosis will be diagnosed early and appropriate antiresorptive therapy initiated.

Management of hyperprolactinaemia

The management of women with hyperprolactinaemia has to take into account the individual's desire or otherwise for pregnancy, her oestrogen status, and the presence/absence and size of a pituitary tumour. Women who describe regular menses and who are found to have raised prolactin concentrations do not require treatment unless their menstrual cycles are anovulatory and they wish for pregnancy (Soule and Jacobs 1995). Dopaminergic agents are recommended as the primary therapy for prolactin-secreting adenomas and idiopathic hyperprolactinaemia (Webster et al 1994). The effects induced by dopamine agonists are suppressive but not tumoricidal. Thus, the therapeutic effect is only maintained for as long as the drug is administered. Consequently, in most cases, treatment has to be continued life-long with a few exceptions, in whom normoprolactinemia persists even after discontinuation of dopamine agonists. Surgery (trans-sphenoidal adenectomy) is usually reserved for dopamine-resistant conditions, intolerable side-effects of therapy and where there is failure to adequately shrink a macroadenoma (Balen 2000). Dopamine agonists include bromocriptine and cabergoline, the latter being better tolerated than the former, which may be explained in part by the longer half-life which results in fewer changes in drug concentration in the blood. There have been recent guidelines from the European Medicines Agency (2008) regarding the use of dopamine agonists and the risk of cardiac fibrosis. Prescribing recommendations include avoiding using such drugs in any patient with a history of cardiac fibrosis, monitoring for signs of fibrosis throughout treatment by blood tests or chest X-rays, and ensuring adherence to a daily maximum dose of 30 mg bromocriptine. The fall in circulating prolactin concentrations with therapy is accompanied by an increase in frequency of LH pulses. The return of menstruation is usually associated with anovulatory cycles. Since normal ovarian cycles have usually returned by 6 months, it may be necessary to provide contraception unless immediate fertility is desired. A tumour >1 cm in diameter should be surgically removed or reduced in size by dopaminergic therapy prior to pregnancy, since there is a small risk of tumour enlargement during pregnancy. Once pregnancy is diagnosed, dopaminergic therapy should be discontinued. There is no evidence to indicate that bromocriptine is teratogenic. Bromocriptine therapy should be recommended if there was evidence of tumour enlargement during the pregnancy. Should hyperprolactinaemia be a consequence of drug administration itself (see Box 16.6), cessation of the offending preparation should be recommended after due consultation with other health professionals involved in the patient's care. If continuation of a psychotrophic preparation is essential for the patient's good health (e.g. in the case of schizophrenia), administration of a low-dose oral contraceptive preparation, in addition to continuation of the required dopaminergic therapy, will provide protection against coincident symptoms of oestrogen deficiency. Serum concentrations of prolactin should continue to be monitored. Surgical intervention is necessary for non-functioning tumours. These tumours are detected by a combination of imaging and a serum prolactin concentration <3000 milliunits/l (Balen 2000). A suprasellar extension of the tumour will also be an indication for surgery when dopaminergic therapy has failed to produce regression, or there is a wish for pregnancy. Surgery may carry a risk of hypopituitarism and, if present, usually manifests promptly following surgery. Pituitary irradiation (although not common) has a risk of incipient hypopituitarism and therefore necessitates long-term surveillance (Soule and Jacobs 1995).

Fertility Issues

There may be reasonable optimism about future fertility prospects for women with amenorrhoea, provided that they do not have POF. Women with oligomenorrhoea, however, have a slightly reduced chance overall (Hull et al 1982). In women with normal gonadotrophin concentrations, it is relatively easy to restore fertility with induction of ovulation with an antioestrogen preparation such as clomiphene citrate. Some women will also require administration of human chorionic gonadotrophin to induce ovulation, despite a response to clomiphene in terms of follicular development. Patients with low gonadotrophin concentrations will require ovulation induction with gonadotrophins or pulsatile GnRH therapy. Detail about ovulation induction regimes is addressed in Chapter 17. The assessment of oestrogen status is a useful index of likely responsiveness to ovulation induction agents, such as clomiphene citrate. Furthermore, it identifies the requirement for long-term hormone replacement, where there is a risk of osteoporosis due to oestrogen deficiency, or for endometrial protection with a progestogen, where there is continuous unopposed oestrogen stimulation. The progestogen challenge test utilizes the endometrial response to administration and withdrawal of progestogen. The oestrogen-primed endometrium will exhibit a withdrawal bleed some 24–48 h following cessation of progestogen administration. An alternative mode of assessment of oestrogen status is the measurement of endometrial thickness with ultrasound. The restoration of fertility may be possible in young women with ovarian failure with HRT and assisted reproduction which includes the use of donor oocytes and embryo transfer. More controversial is the use of assisted reproductive technology and surrogacy for the fulfilment of family desires among women who have congenital absence of the uterus or who have undergone hysterectomy for cancer at a young age (Brinsden et al 2000).

Contraceptive Advice

It is inevitable that young women with oligomenorrhoea or amenorrhoea will have concerns about contraceptive requirements and perceived influences on future fertility potential. Furthermore, contraception may be required after ovulation induction therapy. The usual range of contraceptive options should be considered. Copper intrauterine contraceptive devices (IUCD) are often avoided in nulliparous patients. Women with oligomenorrhoea or amenorrhoea are likely to have a degree of oestrogen deficiency with a small uterus. In these women, even those who are parous, insertion and containment of the IUCD may be problematic. There is no evidence that combined oestrogen/progestogen contraceptive preparations contribute to subsequent amenorrhoea or subfertility. Indeed, there are positive benefits for the use of such preparations. Protection against unopposed oestrogen stimulation of the endometrium in women with chronic anovulation is provided by use of the combined pill or administration of cyclic progestogens.

KEY POINTS

1. Physiologically regular menses are an indication of cyclical ovarian activity, in turn dependent upon an intact HPO axis. Amenorrhoea and oligomenorrhoea are symptoms of ovarian and reproductive dysfunction.

2. Amenorrhoea is physiological at certain critical times in a woman's life, these being prepuberty, during pregnancy and lactation, and in the postmenopausal period. Pathological amenorrhoea may be primary or secondary, and there may be common aetiology.

3. The hypothalamic–pituitary axis is regulated at two levels. At a higher level, GnRH neurones within the hypothalamus are stimulated by afferent inputs from the central nervous system. At a lower level, the output of FSH and LH from the anterior pituitary reflects GnRH activity. Gonadotrophin synthesis, in turn, is influenced by endocrine feedback from the ovaries as well as paracrine mechanisms and other extrinsic factors. Disturbances in menstrual pattern will be the consequence of either a structural or a functional defect in the tightly controlled feedback system involving the hypothalamus, pituitary and ovary.

4. Baseline endocrine investigations will permit the categorization of patients into essentially one of four diagnostic groups: hypergonadotrophic hypogonadism, hyperprolactinaemia, hypogonadotrophic hypogonadism and normogonadotrophic anovulation.

5. The number of follicles in the human ovary declines steadily from midlife onwards. POF is the triad of amenorrhoea and elevated FSH and LH in women less than 40 years of age (hypergonadotrophic hypogonadism). Subjects with gonadal failure are oestrogen deficient. One of the most common chromosomal causes of primary ovarian failure (and primary amenorrhoea) is Turner's syndrome. Women with ovarian failure require sex steroid replacement therapy with cyclic oestrogen and progestogen. Oestrogen deficiency has an adverse effect on bone (osteoporosis) and blood vessel health. OR can be measured (or at least estimated) by measuring FSH, prostaglandin E2, inhibin B, AMH, FSH:LH ratio and ovarian morphometeric markers (ovarian volume, antral follicle count and mean ovarian diameter).

6. Hyperprolactinaemia is diagnosed when prolactin concentrations are outwith the normal range. Serum levels may be transiently raised at times of stress. Serum prolactin measurements >1500 milliunits/l require diagnostic imaging of the pituitary fossa. Approximately 15–20% of women with secondary amenorrhoea display elevated serum prolactin concentrations. In 1–2% of cases, the hyperprolactinaemia is induced by drugs that inhibit dopamine action or production. Only half of women who present with hyperprolactinaemia describe galactorrhoea. It is most important to consider the prolactin concentration in the context of the associated ovulatory disorder. Significant hyperprolactinaemia is usually associated with oligomenorrhoea or amenorrhoea.

7. Hypothalamic hypogonadism is characterized by reduced FSH and LH secretion, and an absence of follicular development and oestradiol production. As a rule, no organic disease is identified in the hypothalamus or anterior pituitary gland.

8. Severe weight loss, stress and excessive exercise habit are all associated with cessation of hypothalamic function. In each of these situations, there is a decrease in GnRH neuronal activity in the hypothalamus with a consequent decrease in gonadotrophin secretion. Thus, ovarian follicular development and ovulation fail to occur and a hypo-oestrogenic state develops. A chronic hypo-oestrogenic state will carry significant risk of premature osteoporosis and cardiovascular disease.

9. Other endocrine disorders, such as thyroid and adrenal disease, may interfere with the normal feedback loops of the HPO axis, cause disturbance of cyclical ovarian activity and thus lead to oligomenorrhoea or amenorrhoea.

10. Successful management of amenorrhoea and oligomenorrhoea is dependent upon the correct diagnosis and assessment of the needs of the patient. Each woman will have different requirements, which may include advice on future fertility prospects, fertility control, symptoms of hirsutism, delayed secondary sexual development, risk of osteoporosis and endometrial protection from unopposed oestrogen action.

11. There may be reasonable optimism about future fertility prospects for women with amenorrhoea, provided that they do not have POF. Women with oligomenorrhoea have a slightly reduced chance overall. The mainstay of management is ovulation induction. The restoration of fertility is possible in young women with POF with hormone replacement and assisted reproductive technology that includes the use of donor oocytes and embryo transfer.

Acknowledgements

The material in this chapter contains contributions from previous editions and the authors are grateful to previous authors for the work done. The authors wish to thank Dr Colin Duncan, University of Edinburgh, for helpful comments on the manuscript content and Mrs Sheila Milne for secretarial assistance.

References

Abreu AP, Trarbach EB, de Castro M et al 2008 Loss-of-function mutations in the genes encoding prokineticin-2 or prokineticin receptor-2 cause autosomal recessive Kallmann syndrome. Journal of Clinical Endocrinology and Metabolism 93: 4113–4118.

Ahmed SF, Cheng A, Dovey L et al 2000 Phenotypic features, androgen receptor binding, and mutational analysis in 278 clinical cases reported as androgen insensitivity syndrome. Journal of Clinical Endocrinology and Metabolism 85: 658–665.

Aittomaki K, Lucena JL, Pakarinen P et al 1995 Mutation in the follicle-stimulating hormone receptor gene causes hereditary hypergonadotrophic ovarian failure. Cell 82: 959–968.

Alper MM, Garner PR, Seibel MM 1986 Premature ovarian failure: current concepts. Journal of Reproductive Medicine 31: 699–708.

Anasti JN 1998 Premature ovarian failure: an update. Fertility and Sterility 70: 1–15.

Anderson RA, Cameron DA 2007 Assessment of the effect of chemotherapy on ovarian function in women with breast cancer. Journal of Clinical Oncology 25: 1630–1631.

Arif S, Vallian S, Farazneh F et al 1996 Identification of 3 beta-hydroxysteroid dehydrogenase as novel target of steroid cell autoantibodies: association of autoantibodies with endocrine autoimmune disease. Journal of Clinical Endocrinology and Metabolism 81: 4439–4445.

Asherman JG 1948 Amenorrhoea traumatica (atretica). Journal of Obstetrics and Gynaecology of the British Empire 55: 23–30.

Bachmann GA, Kemmann E 1982 Prevalence of oligomenorrhoea and amenorrhoea in a college population. American Journal of Obstetrics and Gynecology 144: 98–102.

Baird DT 1997 Amenorrhoea. The Lancet 350: 275–279.

Balen AH 2000 Amenorrhoea, oligomenorrhoea and polycystic ovarian syndrome. In: O'Brien S, Cameron I, Maclean A (eds) Disorders of the Menstrual Cycle. RCOG Press, London.

Balen AH, Conway GS, Kaltsas G et al 1995 Polycystic ovary syndrome: the spectrum of the disorder in 1741 patients. Human Reproduction 10: 2017–2111.

Bath LE, Anderson RA, Critchley HO, Kelnar CJ, Wallace WH 2001 Hypothalamic–pituitary–ovarian dysfunction after pre-pubertal chemotherapy and cranial irradiation for acute leukaemia. Human Reproduction 16: 1838–1844.

Borrelli F, Ernst E 2008 Black cohosh (*Cimicifuga racemosa*) for menopausal symptoms: a systematic review of its efficacy. Pharmacological Research 58: 8–14.

Bowen S, Norian J, Santoro N, Pal L 2007 Simple tools for assessment of ovarian reserve (OR): individual ovarian dimensions are reliable predictors of OR. Fertility and Sterility 88: 390–395.

Brinsden PR, Appleton TC, Murray E, Hussein M, Akagbosu F, Marcus SF 2000 Treatment by in vitro fertilisation with surrogacy: experience of one British centre. BMJ (Clinical Research Ed.) 320: 924–928.

British Menopause Society 2008 Premature Menopause. Available at: http://www.thebms.org.uk/factdetail.php?id=1

Byrne J 1999 Infertility and premature menopause in childhood cancer survivors. Medical and Pediatric Oncology 33: 24–28.

Byrne J, Fears TR, Gail MH et al 1992 Early menopause in long-term survivors of cancer during adolescence. American Journal of Obstetrics and Gynecology 166: 788–793.

Casanueva F, Molitch M, Schlechte JA et al 2006 Guidelines of the Pituitary Society for the diagnosis and management of prolactinomas. Clinical Endocrinology 65: 265–273.

Colao A, Di Sarno A, Cappabianca P, Di Somma C, Pivonello R, Lombardi G 2003 Withdrawal of long-term cabergoline therapy for tumoural and nontumoural hyperprolactinaemia. New England Journal of Medicine 349: 2023–2033.

Conway GS 1997 Premature ovarian failure. Current Opinion in Obstetrics and Gynecology 9: 202–206.

Conway GS, Hettiarachchi S, Murray A, Jacobs PA 1995 Fragile X permutations in familial premature ovarian failure. The Lancet 346: 309–310.

Conway GS, Kaltsas G, Patel A, Davies MC, Jacobs HS 1996 Characteristics of idiopathic premature ovarian failure. Fertility and Sterility 65: 337–341.

Conway GS, Jacobs HS 1997 Leptin: a hormone of reproduction. Human Reproduction 12: 633–635.

Coulam CB, Adamson SC, Annegers JF 1986 Incidence of premature ovarian failure. Obstetrics and Gynecology 67: 604–606.

Cramer DW, Xu H, Harlow BL 1995 Family history as predictor of early menopause. Fertility and Sterility 64: 740–745.

Crisponi L, Deiana M, Loi A et al 2001 The putative forkhead transcription factor FOXL2 is mutated in blepharophimosis/ptosis/epicanthus inversus syndrome. Nature Genetics 27: 159–166.

Critchley HO, Wallace WH, Shalet SM, Mamtora H, Higginson J, Anderson DC 1992 Abdominal irradiation in childhood: the potential for pregnancy. BJOG: an International Journal of Obstetrics and Gynaecology 99: 392–394.

Critchley HO, Wallace WH 2005 Impact of cancer treatment on uterine function. Journal of the National Cancer Institute Monographs 34: 64–68.

Davies MC, Gulekli B, Jacobs HS 1995 Osteoporosis in Turner's syndrome and other forms of primary amenorrhoea. Clinical Endocrinology (Oxford) 43: 741–746.

De Caro JJ, Dominguez C, Sherman SL 2008 Reproductive health of adolescent girls who carry the FMR1 premutation: expected phenotype based on current knowledge of fragile x-associated primary ovarian insufficiency. Annals of the New York Academy of Sciences 1135: 99–111.

Durlinger AL, Visser JA, Themmen AP 2002 Regulation of ovarian function: the role of anti-Müllerian hormone. Reproduction 124: 601–609.

European Medicines Agency 2008 Questions and Answers on the Review of Ergot-derived Dopamine Agonists. Available at: http://www.emea.europa.eu/pdfs/general/direct/pr/31905408en.pdf

Faddy MJ, Gosden RG, Gougeon A, Richarson SJ, Nelson JF 1992 Accelerated disappearance of ovarian follicles in mid-life: implications for forecasting menopause. Human Reproduction 7: 1342–1346.

Fraser IS, Inceboz US 2000 Defining disturbances of the menstrual cycle In: O'Brien S, Cameron I, Maclean A (eds) Disorders of the Menstrual Cycle. RCOG Press, London.

Frattarelli JL, Levi AJ, Miller BT 2002 A prospective novel method of determining ovarian size during in vitro fertilization cycles. Journal of Assisted Reproduction and Genetics 19: 39–41.

Frisch RE 1984 Body fat, puberty and fertility. Biological Reviews of the Cambridge Philosophical Society 59: 161–188.

Glasier AF, Hendry RA, Seth J, Baird DT 1987 Does treatment with bromocriptine influence the course of hyperprolactinaemia? Clinical Reproduction and Fertility 5: 359–366.

Golden NH, Carlson JL 2008 The pathophysiology of amenorrhoea in the adolescent. Annals of the New York Academy of Sciences 1135: 163–178.

Goodfellow PN, Lovell-Badge R 1993 SRY and sex determination in mammals. Annual Review of Genetics 27: 71–92.

Gottlieb B, Pinsky L, Beitel LK, Trifiro M 1999 Androgen insensitivity. American Journal of Medical Genetics 89: 210–217.

Greer ME, Moraczewski T, Rakoff JS 1980 Prevalence of hyperprolactinemia in anovulatory women. Obstetrics and Gynaecology 56: 65–69.

Grossman A, Moult PJ, McIntyre H et al 1982 Opiate mediation of amenorrhoea in hyperprolactinaemia and in weight loss related amenorrhoea. Clinical Endocrinology (Oxford) 17: 379–388.

Harlow SD, Ephross SA 1995 Epidemiology of menstruation and its relevance to women's health. Epidemiologic Reviews 17: 265–286.

Howell SJ, Shalet SM 1999 Aetiology-specific effect of premature ovarian failure on bone mass — is residual ovarian function important? Clinical Endocrinology (Oxford) 51: 531–534.

Hull MG, Savage PE, Bromham DR 1982 Anovulatory and ovulatory infertility: results with simplied management. BMJ (Clinical Research Ed.) 284: 1681–1685.

Illingworth PJ, Seaton JEV, McKinlay C, Reid-Thomas V, McNeilly AS 1995 Low dose transdermal oestradiol suppresses gonadotrophin secretion in breast-feeding women. Human Reproduction 10: 1671–1677.

Imperato-McGinley J 1995 Male pseudohermaphroditism. In: Adashi EY, Rock JA, Rosenwalks Z (eds) Reproductive Endocrinology, Surgery and Technology, vol. 1. Oxford University Press, Philadelphia.

Jacobs HS, Franks S, Murray MA, Hull MG, Steele SJ, Nabarro JDN 1976 Clinical and endocrine features of hyperprolactinemic amenorrhoea. Clinical Endocrinology (Oxford) 5: 439–454.

Kallman F, Schonfield WA, Barrera SE 1944 The genetic aspects of primary eunuchoidism. American Journal of Mental Deficiency 48: 203–236.

Kaufman FR, Kogut MD, Donnell GN, Goebelsmann U, March, C, Koch R 1981 Hypergonadotropic hypogonadism in female patients with galactosemia. New England Journal of Medicine 304: 994–998.

Knauff EA, Eijkemans MJ, Lambalk CB et al 2009 Anti-Müllerian hormone, inhibin B, and antral follicle count in young women with ovarian failure. Journal of Clinical Endocrinology and Metabolism 94: 786–792.

Laughlin GA, Yen SS 1996 Nutritional and endocrine–metabolic aberrations in amenorrheic athletes. Journal of Clinical Endocrinology and Metabolism 81: 4301–4309.

Legouis R, Hardelin JP, Levilliers J et al 1991 The candidate gene for the X-linked Kallman syndrome encodes a protein related to adhesion molecules. Cell 67: 423–435.

Leiblich JM, Rogol AD, White BJ, Rosen SW 1982 Syndrome of anosmia with hypogonadotropic hypogonadism (Kallman's syndrome): clinical and laboratory studies in 23 cases. American Journal of Medicine 73: 506–519.

Lunenfeld B, Insler V 1974 Classification of amenorrhoea states and their treatment by ovulation induction. Clinical Endocrinology (Oxford) 3: 223–237.

Matkovic V, Ilich JZ, Skugor M et al 1997 Leptin is inversely related to age at menarche in human females. Journal of Clinical Endocrinology and Metabolism 82: 3239–3245.

Mendelsohn ME, Karas RH 1999 The protective effects of estrogen on the cardiovascular system. New England Journal of Medicine 340: 1801–1811.

Muttukrishna S, Child T, Lockwood GM, Groome NP, Barlow DH, Ledger WL 2000 Serum concentrations of dimeric inhibins, activin A, gonadotrophins and ovarian steroids during the menstrual cycle in older women. Human Reproduction 15: 549–556.

Neale T 2009 Missed menstrual cycles in young women may signal ovarian insufficiency. New England Journal of Medicine 360: 606–614.

Ogilvy-Stuart AL, Shalet SM 1993 Effect of radiation on the human reproductive system. Environmental Health Perspectives 101 (Suppl 2): 109–116.

Pasquino AM, Passeri F, Pucarelli I, Segni M, Municchi G 1997 Spontaneous pubertal development in Turner's syndrome. Italian Study Group for Turner's Syndrome. Journal of Clinical Endocrinology and Metabolism 82: 1810–1813.

Pederson-White JR, Chorich LP, Bick DP, Sherins RJ, Layman LC 2008 The prevalence of intragenic deletions in patients with idiopathic hypogonadotrophic hypogonadsim and Kallmann syndrome. Molecular Human Reproduction 14: 367–370.

Perheentupa A, Critchley HO, Illingworth PJ, McNeilly AS 2000 Enhanced sensitivity to steroid-negative feedback during breast-feeding: low dose estradiol (transdermal estradiol supplementation) suppresses gonadotropins and ovarian activity assessed by inhibin B. Journal of Clinical Endocrinology and Metabolism 85: 4280–4286.

Pettersson F, Fries H, Nillius SJ 1973 Epidemiology of secondary amenorrhoea. I. Incidence and prevalence rates. American Journal of Obstetrics and Gynecology 117: 80–86.

Pitkin J, Rees MC, Gray S et al 2007 Management of premature menopause. Menopause International 13: 44–45.

Randeva HS, Davis M, Prelevic GM 2000 Prolactinoma and pregnancy. BJOG: an International Journal of Obstetrics and Gynaecology 107: 1064–1068.

Richardson SJ, Senikas V, Nelson JF 1987 Follicular depletion during the menopausal transition: evidence for accelerated loss and ultimate exhaustion. Journal of Clinical Endocrinology and Metabolism 65: 1231–1237.

Roseweir AK, Millar RP 2009 The role of kisspeptin in the role of gonadotrophin secretion. Human Reproduction Update 15: 203–212.

Rugarli EI, Ballabio A 1993 Kallman syndrome from genetics to neurobiology. JAMA: the Journal of the American Medical Association 270: 2713–2716.

Schlechte J, Dolan K, Sherman B, Chapler F, Luciano A 1989 The natural history of untreated hyperprolactinemia: a prospective analysis. Journal of Clinical Endocrinology and Metabolism 68: 412–418.

Shifren JL, Davis SR, Moreau M et al 2006 Testosterone patch for the treatment of hypoactive sexual desire disorder in naturally menopausal women: results from the INTIMATE NM1 Study. Menopause 13: 770–779.

Singh KB 1981 Menstrual disorders in college students. American Journal of Obstetrics and Gynecology 140: 299–302.

Sohval AR 1965 The syndrome of pure gonadal dysgenesis. American Journal of Medicine 38: 615–625.

Soule SG, Jacobs HS 1995 Prolactinomas: present day management. BJOG: an International Journal of Obstetrics and Gynaecology 102: 178–181.

Speroff L, Glass RH, Kase NG 1999a Amenorrhoea. In: Speroff L, Glass RH, Kase NG (eds) Clinical Gynecologic Endocrinology and Infertility, 6th edn. Lippincott, Williams and Wilkins, Baltimore.

Speroff L, Glass RH, Kase NG 1999b Amenorrhoea. In: Speroff L, Glass RH, Kase NG (eds) Clinical Gynecologic Endocrinology and Infertility, 6th edn. Lippincott, Williams and Wilkins, Baltimore.

Speroff L, Glass RH, Kase NG 1999c Normal and abnormal sexual development. In: Speroff L, Glass RH, Kase NG (eds) Clinical Gynecologic Endocrinology and Infertility, 6th edn. Lippincott, Williams and Wilkins, Baltimore.

Treloar AE, Boynton RE, Behn BG, Brown BW 1967 Variation of the human menstrual cycle through reproductive life. International Journal of Fertility 12: 77–126.

van Kasteren YM, Schoemaker J 1999 Premature ovarian failure: a systematic review on therapeutic interventions to restore ovarian function and achieve pregnancy. Human Reproduction Update 5: 483–492.

Wallace WH, Shalet SM, Crowne EC, Morris-Jones PH, Gattameneni HR 1989 Ovarian failure following abdominal irradiation in childhood: natural history and prognosis. Clinical Oncology (Royal College of Radiologists) 1: 75–79.

Wallace WH, Shalet SM, Tetlow LJ, Morris-Jones PH 1993 Ovarian function following the treatment of childhood acute lymphoblastic leukaemia. Medical and Pediatric Oncology 21: 333–339.

Walsh RJ 1978 The age of the menopause of Australian women. Medical Journal of Australia 2: 181–182, 215.

Warren MP 1995 Anorexia nervosa. In: de Groot LJ (ed) Endocrinology, 3rd edn. WB Saunders, Philadelphia.

Warren MP, Brooks-Gunn J, Hamilton LH, Warren LF, Hamilton WG 1986 Scoliosis and fractures in young ballet dancers: relation to delayed menarche and secondary amenorrhoea. New England Journal of Medicine 314: 1348–1353.

Webster J, Piscitelli G, Polli A, Ferrari CI, Ismail I, Scanlon MF 1994 A comparison of cabergoline and bromocriptine in the treatment of hyperprolactinaemic amenorrhoea. New England Journal of Medicine 331: 904–909.

Yen SS, Rebar R, Vandenberg G, Ehara Y, Siler T 1973 Pituitary gonadotrophin responsiveness to synthetic LRF in subjects with normal and abnormal hypothalamic–pituitary–gonadal axis. Journal of Reproduction and Fertility 20 (Suppl): 137–161.

Yen SSC 1999 Chronic anovulation due to CNS–hypothalamic–pituitary dysfunction. In: Yen SSC, Jaffe RB, Barbieri RL (eds) Reproductive Endocrinology, Physiology, Pathophysiology, and Clinical Management, 4th edn. WB Saunders, Philadelphia.

Zreik TG, Olive D 1998 Amenorrhoea. In: O'Brien S, Cameron I, Maclean A (eds) Disorders of the Menstrual Cycle. RCOG Press, London.

CHAPTER 17

Ovulation induction

Maria Vogiatzi and Robert W. Shaw

Chapter Contents

INTRODUCTION	231		PULSATILE GONADOTROPHIN-RELEASING HORMONE	239
PRINCIPLES OF OVULATION	231		GONADOTROPHINS	240
OVULATION DISORDERS	232		WEIGHT REDUCTION	242
DIAGNOSIS AND TREATMENT	234		SURGICAL MANAGEMENT: LAPAROSCOPIC OVARIAN DRILLING	243
MEDICAL INDUCTION OF OVULATION	236		RISKS OF INDUCTION OF OVULATION	244
ANTIOESTROGENS	236		CONCLUSIONS	248
DOPAMINE AGONISTS	238		KEY POINTS	248
INSULIN-SENSITIZING AGENTS	239			

Introduction

The aim of ovulation induction is to achieve development of a single follicle and subsequent ovulation in anovulatory infertile women. The ability to induce ovulation is possible in most women, with excellent conception rates. Anovulation accounts for 20–25% of the causes of infertility, and clinicians who manage infertile couples ought to have a sound understanding of the control of follicular development in a normal cycle (see Chapter 15), causes of anovulation (see Chapter 16), appropriate investigations and different treatment options, including their indications and risks. This chapter will briefly review the physiology of ovulation, including the basic principles of ovulation induction, and describe treatment strategies based on the underlying cause of the anovulation.

Principles of Ovulation

The ovary has two main functions: the cyclic release of haploid oocytes for fertilization by spermatozoa, and the production of steroid hormones (mainly oestrogen and progesterone). Both activities occur from puberty, when full sexual maturation has taken place, until the menopause, controlled by a sequence of hypothalamic–pituitary–ovarian interactions which, in turn, are synchronized by the endocrine, paracrine and autocrine secretory products of the ovary.

Follicular development: recruitment, selection and dominance

The primordial follicle constitutes the fundamental functional unit of the ovary. The primordial follicles contain oocytes that enter meiosis and are arrested in the diplotene stage of meiotic prophase to become primary oocytes. They can stay in this arrested phase for up to 50 years. Regular recruitment of primordial follicles occurs from puberty. The following stages of follicular development have been identified en route to ovulation: first, the primordial follicle becomes a primary or preantral follicle, then a secondary or antral follicle and finally a preovulatory follicle. The duration of each stage varies, with the primary to preantral stage being the longest and the preovulatory stage being the shortest.

In humans, approximately 15–20 early antral follicles are recruited for development at the start of each menstrual cycle. Of these 15–20 follicles, one usually emerges as dominant and is competent to ovulate. It takes approximately 85 days for a primordial follicle to reach the preovulatory stage. This follicular growth and development is regulated by gonadotrophins, and it is acknowledged that a lack of gonadotrophins leads to apoptotic death of the oocyte with subsequent accumulation of leukocytes and macrophages, as well as formation of fibrous scar tissue. This process is called 'atresia'.

The follicle destined to ovulate is recruited from these preantral follicles in the first days of the menstrual cycle. An

DOI: 10.1016/B978-0-7020-3120-5.00017-5

increase in follicle-stimulating hormone (FSH) is the critical feature in rescuing a cohort of follicles from atresia, eventually allowing a dominant follicle to emerge and proceed to ovulation. Maintenance of this increase in FSH for a critical duration of time over 4–6 days is essential.

The first signs of follicular development consist of an increase in the size of the oocyte and a change in the shape of the granulosa cells as they become more cuboidal. Small gap junctions also appear between the oocyte and the granulosa cells. The stromal cells differentiate into two layers: the theca interna and the theca externa. The granulosa layer is separated from the stromal cells by a basement membrane called the 'basal lamina'.

As the oocyte enlarges, it enters the preantral stage. During this phase, there is further granulosa cell proliferation and growth. This is initiated by FSH. FSH also induces steroidogenesis in the granulosa cells and, in particular, oestrogen production. The oocyte is surrounded by a membrane called the 'zona pellucida'. Under the synergistic effect of oestrogen and FSH, there is an increase in the production of follicular fluid. This leads to the formation of a cavity, called the 'antrum', and the follicle is now described as the antral follicle. The granulosa cells form the cumulus oophorus.

Only the cells of the theca interna possess receptors for luteinizing hormone (LH), whereas the granulosa cells bind FSH. Under the influence of gonadotrophins, the antral follicles produce steroids. The main oestrogens produced are oestradiol-17β and oestrone. In addition to this, antral follicles produce 30–70% of the circulating androgens, mainly androstenedione and testosterone. In particular, it is the thecal cells that produce androgens from acetate and cholesterol, and this action is stimulated by LH. On the other hand, the granulosa cells cannot produce androgens, but aromatize them to oestrogens; this process of aromatization is stimulated by FSH.

Follicular growth starts with the regression of the corpus luteum at the end of the previous cycle. As the levels of steroid hormones and inhibin drop, their inhibitory effect on FSH is abolished and FSH levels rise. This increase starts approximately 2 days prior to menstruation. As the follicles grow, the production of oestradiol and inhibin increases and FSH levels subsequently fall. The dominant follicle will be selected from day 5–7 of the menstrual cycle. The selection of a single dominant follicle appears to be the result of two oestrogen actions: a positive influence of oestrogen on FSH action within the maturing follicle, and a negative feedback mechanism on FSH at the hypothalamic–pituitary level. This latter action leads to a decline in gonadotrophin levels and ultimately to atresia of the less-developed follicles. Local paracrine–autocrine factors are also involved in this process, such as tumour necrosis factor and anti-Müllerian hormone. The dominant follicle is not affected by this decline in FSH levels, as it is more sensitive to FSH. Provided that a critical exposure of FSH was initially sustained, the dominant follicle continues to grow. In turn, FSH induces the development of LH receptors on the granulosa cells. Thus, LH plays a crucial role in the late stages of follicular development (Figure 17.1).

As the dominant follicle grows, it produces oestradiol. This explains the significant rise in oestradiol levels observed in the late follicular phase. High levels of oestradiol exert a positive feedback effect on LH secretion and enhance the follicle's sensitivity to FSH. LH enhances androgen production in the theca cells, which leads to further oestrogen secretion by the granulosa cells via the process of aromatization. At midcycle, oestradiol levels reach a peak; this induces the LH surge, resumption of meiosis in the oocyte, luteinization of the granulosa cells and synthesis of prostaglandins. The prostaglandins stimulate the release of proteolytic enzymes within the follicular wall, which lead to ovulation (release of oocyte) 34–36 h after the LH surge commences.

Ovulation Disorders

Assessing ovulation

The choice of treatment to induce ovulation depends on reaching the correct diagnosis of the cause of anovulation. A thorough medical history and physical examination are the preliminary steps, and further investigations should be undertaken as indicated. It is highly recommended that these investigations should be conducted in a specialist centre, where there is access to skilled ultrasonography, radiology and a specialist endocrine laboratory. These tests will help the clinician to diagnose the cause of anovulation and exclude any important underlying pathology. Thyroid disease, hyperprolactinaemia, pituitary and ovarian tumours, polycystic ovary syndrome (PCOS), adrenal disease, extremes of weight and eating disorders are all associated with ovulation dysfunction. Early diagnosis is essential, as treatment of the underlying cause is more likely to succeed and prevent any long-term health consequences.

Classification

Ovulation disorders can be classified according to the anatomical site where the hypothalamic–pituitary–ovarian axis

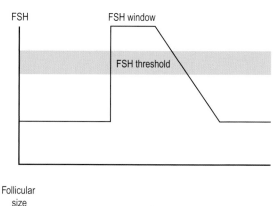

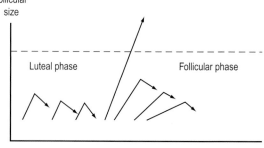

Figure 17.1 Follicle-stimulating hormone (FSH) threshold and window.

is deficient. The World Health Organization (WHO) classifies ovulation disorders into three groups, as follows.

- Group I: hypothalamic–pituitary failure. This group includes women with hypothalamic amenorrhoea or hypogonadotrophic hypogonadism. This includes anovulation related to stress, exercise, weight loss, anorexia nervosa, Kallmann's syndrome and isolated (idiopathic) gonadotrophin deficiency. It does not include women with hypothalamic or pituitary tumours. This group of women have low serum FSH, LH and oestrogen levels, but normal prolactin.
- Group II: hypothalamic–pituitary dysfunction. This group includes women with amenorrhoea or oligomenorrhoea, with or without hyperandrogenism. This group predominantly comprises women with PCOS. Characteristically, these women exhibit normal FSH, oestrogen and prolactin levels, and variable changes in serum LH and testosterone.
- Group III: ovarian failure. This category includes women with amenorrhoea and elevated serum FSH and LH.
- Hyperprolactinaemic anovulation is considered a separate entity.

History

The majority of women of reproductive age have regular cycles ranging from 25 to 35 days. Usually, the presence of such cycles indicates ovulation.

Nevertheless, irregular, erratic or infrequent menses are suggestive of anovulation. Therefore, a detailed menstrual history should be taken. Amenorrhoea (absence of menstruation for 6 months), oligomenorrhoea (menses occurring less frequently than 6 weeks) and polymenorrhoea (menses occurring more frequently than 21 days) are associated with anovulation.

In addition, galactorrhoea, hot flushes and symptoms suggestive of thyroid disease could indicate an underlying ovulation dysfunction.

A careful gynaecological, medical, surgical and family history should be elicited. In particular, other causes of infertility should be excluded. A previous history of pelvic inflammatory disease, use of an intrauterine device, previous ectopic pregnancy or previous pelvic surgery is suggestive of tubal/ovarian pathology. In addition to this, any previous fertility investigations and therapies should be noted, and the absence of a contributory male factor should be confirmed.

Physical examination

The height and weight of the woman are of particular importance. Any deviation from normal should be noted, as this could be directly related to the underlying cause of anovulation (e.g. obesity and PCOS, short stature and Turner's syndrome etc.). A more sensitive indicator is the body mass index (BMI), which is calculated from weight in kg/height in m^2. The range for BMI is as follows.

- Underweight: <18.5
- Normal: 18.5–24.9
- Overweight: 25.0–29.9
- Obesity: 30.0–39.9
- Extreme obesity: ≥40

A general physical examination should be performed. This will include examination of the thyroid gland, breasts, facial and body hair. A thorough gynaecological examination must also be undertaken.

Investigations

Assessing ovulation is one of the primary investigations of infertility. Nevertheless, other factors should be evaluated. As 30–40% of cases of infertility are due to a male factor, a semen analysis should be requested early in the course of the investigations. Moreover, the female partner should have a test to assess tubal patency, such as a hysterosalpingogram, a diagnostic laparoscopy and dye test, or a hystero-ultrasonography (hycosy).

A serum progesterone measurement is the simplest and most reliable test to evaluate ovulatory function. The measurement of serum progesterone level should be performed in the midluteal phase (i.e. 7 days before the expected onset of the next period). Typically, in a 28-day cycle, the test is conducted on the 21st day of the menstrual cycle. Nevertheless, in women with prolonged, irregular cycles, serum progesterone is measured later in the cycle (i.e. on day 28 of a 35-day cycle) and is repeated weekly thereafter until the next menstruation. A mistimed blood sample is the most common cause of an abnormal result; thus, the first day of the next menstrual cycle should be recorded, and the midluteal phase will be calculated based on that to evaluate whether the test was appropriately timed.

Serum progesterone levels above 30 nmol/l are suggestive of ovulation. Any abnormal result indicates the need for further hormonal investigations. These will include measurement of serum FSH, LH and prolactin and thyroid function tests. Serum FSH and LH should be performed on day 2–5 of the cycle to avoid confusion with the normal, mid-cycle surge. In amenorrhoeic women or women with very infrequent cycles, the measurement of gonadotrophins can be done at any time and their interpretation will be based on the timing of their next menstruation. Both prolactin and thyroid function tests can be done at any time during the cycle.

The normal reference value for prolactin may vary between different laboratories. Usually, levels above 600 mIU/ml are considered abnormal. Raised prolactin concentrations should be confirmed by a repeat measurement. The evaluation of hyperprolactinaemia should include pituitary/hypothalamic imaging, such as radiography, computed tomography or magnetic resonance imaging. The pituitary imaging is essential to exclude a prolactin-producing adenoma or an empty sella. Moreover, as primary hypothyroidism can lead to secondary hyperprolactinaemia, thyroid function tests are indicated in the presence of hyperprolactinaemia and a careful drug history to exclude a pharmacological cause.

In the presence of low gonadotrophin levels, pituitary/hypothalamic imaging is indicated in order to exclude a space-occupying lesion, as well as a full pituitary hormone secretion assessment.

In the case of PCOS, the hormonal investigations should include serum androgens (testosterone, free testosterone, androstenedione and dehydroepiandrosterone sulphate), as they are often elevated, and baseline 17OH-progesterone. Depending on the results, adrenocorticotrophic hormone concentrations may be measured to exclude adrenal pathology. If PCOS is suspected, a transvaginal ultrasound should be performed to assess the ovaries and look for the characteristic peripheral follicles ('necklace sign'). The criteria used for the ultrasonographic diagnosis of PCOS include the presence of more than 10 follicles with a diameter of 2–10 mm and increased density of the ovarian stroma (Adams et al 1986).

If premature ovarian failure is diagnosed, further investigations should include chromosome analysis and autoantibody screening.

Basal body temperature (BBT) charts have also been used for assessing ovulation, as ovulatory cycles have been associated with a classic biphasic BBT pattern. The woman is asked to record her temperature every morning, before getting out of bed. Usually, the temperature shows a rise after ovulation. Chaotic BBT recordings are suggestive of anovulation. Nevertheless, the BBT may not appear clearly biphasic in some patients with ovulatory cycles. Therefore, BBT charts are not considered reliable to predict ovulation, and their use is not recommended alone without serum progesterone measurements.

Diagnosis and Treatment

Based on the results of the above investigations, the causes of anovulation can be divided into four main categories (see Box 17.1).

Box 17.1 Classification of ovulation disorders

Intrinsic ovarian failure
- Genetic
- Autoimmune
- Others (e.g. chemotherapy and radiotherapy)

Secondary ovarian dysfunction

Disorders of gonadotrophin regulation

Specific
- Hyperprolactinaemia
- Kallmann's syndrome (WHO Group I)

Functional (WHO Group II)
- Weight loss
- Exercise
- Drugs
- Idopathic

Gonadotrophin deficiency (WHO Group I)
- Pituitary tumour
- Pituitary necrosis or thrombosis

Disorders of gonadotrophin action (WHO Group II)
- Polycystic ovary syndrome

Hyperprolactinaemia

Causes of hyperprolactinaemia include:

- prolactin-producing adenomas (microadenomas <1 cm, macroadenomas >1 cm);
- any masses that apply pressure on the pituitary stalk and therefore block the inhibitory effect of the hypothalamus;
- primary hypothyroidism;
- drugs that inhibit central dopaminergic activity, such as oestrogen (combined oral contraceptive), dopamine receptor antagonists (metoclopramide, phenothiazines), opioids and dopamine-depleting agents (reserpine, methyldopa);
- chronic renal failure; and
- ectopic prolactin secretion by an extrapituitary tumour.

High levels of prolactin interfere with the pulsatile secretion of gonadotrophin-releasing hormone (GnRH) and subsequently impair normal ovarian function. Therefore, women with hyperprolactinaemia may present with menstrual irregularities, anovulation and galactorrhoea.

In the case of microprolactinomas, the mainstay of therapy is the administration of dopamine agonists, such as bromocriptine and cabergoline. Surgical treatment, in the form of trans-sphenoidal pituitary adenomectomy, is indicated for macroprolactinomas but is associated with risks including panhypopituitarism and cerebrospinal fluid leakage.

Non-prolactin-secreting tumours are treated surgically in combination with radiotherapy.

Primary hypothyroidism causing hyperprolactinaemia is treated with thyroid replacement therapy.

Hypergonadotrophic hypogonadism

Hypergonadotrophic hypogonadism or premature ovarian failure is defined as menopause occurring before the age of 40 years. It may be due to various causes:

- chromosomal abnormalities (e.g. mosaic Turner's syndrome);
- autoimmune disease: autoantibodies are detected against ovarian cells, gonadotrophin receptors and/or the oocytes. Often, premature ovarian failure occurs in association with other autoimmune disorders, such as diabetes mellitus, hypothyroidism and Addison's disease;
- infection (e.g. mumps oophoritis);
- previous surgery, radiotherapy or chemotherapy; or
- idiopathic.

The only treatment option for patients with premature ovarian failure is in-vitro fertilization (IVF) with donor eggs. In terms of their long-term management, they should be offered hormone replacement therapy to protect their skeleton and cardiovascular system from the effects of hypo-oestrogenism.

Hypogonadotrophic hypogonadism

Hypogonadotrophic hypogonadism is a state of gonadal dysfunction, characterized by hypo-oestrogenaemia, anovulation and amenorrhoea, due to anatomical and/or functional disorders of the hypothalamus/pituitary gland. In hypogonadotrophic hypogonadism, there is a deficient secretion of GnRH and/or FSH and LH. Patients present with primary or secondary amenorrhoea and infertility.

Its causes can be either congenital or acquired. Kallman's syndrome is one of the congenital causes. It consists of isolated gonadotrophin deficiency and anosmia. The syndrome is usually sporadic but it can also be inherited (see Chapter 16).

Acquired causes of hypogonadotrophic hypogonadism include:

- central nervous system tumours, i.e. space-occupying lesions around the hypothalamus or the pituitary that disrupt gonadotrophin secretion. The most common of these tumours is craniopharyngioma;
- Sheehan's syndrome, i.e. pituitary necrosis due to massive obstetric haemorrhage with hypovolaemic shock;
- postradiation hypothalamic dysfunction;
- isolated GnRH deficiency;
- inflammatory or infiltrative processes of the pituitary;
- pituitary infarction
- eating disorders (anorexia nervosa) with excessive weight loss;
- stress; and
- excessive exercise.

In patients with hypogonadotrophic hypogonadism, ovulation is restored with the administration of gonadotrophins. Pulsatile GnRH is only indicated in the presence of intact pituitary function.

If a central nervous system tumour is present, surgery is indicated.

Patients with anorexia nervosa may benefit from weight gain and psychotherapy. Nevertheless, in cases of persistent anovulation despite adequate weight gain, gonadotrophins or pulsatile GnRH can be considered.

Normogonadotrophic hypogonadism

This category includes women with anovulation with normal FSH, LH and prolactin levels. They may present with regular menses, oligomenorrhoea or even amenorrhoea. Predominantly, this group comprises women with PCOS. This is discussed in more detail in Chapter 18.

Other causes of normogonadotrophic hypogonadism and hyperandrogenism include:

- late-onset congenital adrenal hyperplasia;
- adrenal tumours; and
- androgen-producing ovarian tumours (see Chapter 26).

In the presence of PCOS, obese patients will benefit from weight loss. This will not only improve their response to ovulation induction, but may also lead to resumption of spontaneous ovulation. The pharmacologic agent most commonly used for ovulation induction in women with PCOS is clomiphene citrate (CC). If patients fail to respond to it, gonadotrophins or insulin-sensitizing agents may also be used. Laparoscopic ovarian drilling has also been used for PCOS patients unresponsive to CC.

A summary of investigations, classifications and treatments is shown in Figure 17.3, and an overview of assessments and treatments is given in the guidelines of the National Institute for Health and Clinical Excellence (2004).

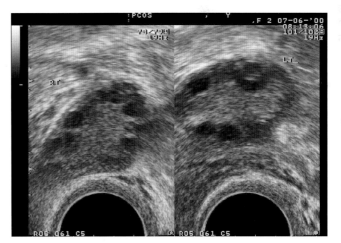

Figure 17.2 Ultrasound appearances of a polycystic ovary: longitudinal and transverse views.

Figure 17.3 Flowchart of diagnosis and treatment. FSH, follicle-stimulating hormone; LH, luteinizing hormone; TSH, thyroid-stimulating hormone; GnRH, gondotrophin-releasing hormone.

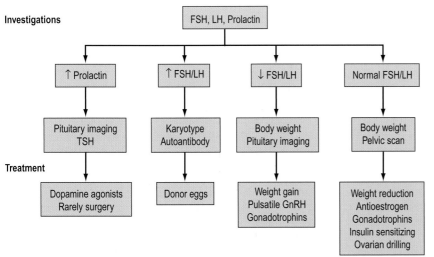

Medical Induction of Ovulation

Effective use of drugs used to induce ovulation comes from an indepth understanding of their mechanism of action.

Antioestrogens

Non-steroidal selective oestrogen receptor modulators, including CC and tamoxifen, are used for ovulation induction. It is thought that they bind with oestrogen receptors in the hypothalamus, leading to a perceived drop in the endogenous oestrogen levels. As a consequence, GnRH and endogenous gonadotrophin secretion is increased, leading to induction of ovulation. Figure 17.4 shows the structure of the drugs.

Clomiphene citrate

CC is the most commonly used ovulation induction agent, and most evidence on the efficacy of antioestrogens derives from its use, since its introduction in 1962.

Pharmacology/mechanism of action

CC is a non-steroidal triphenylethylene derivative with both oestrogenic and antioestrogenic properties; nevertheless, it mainly acts as an antioestrogen.

Indications for treatment

CC is the drug of choice for anovulatory infertile women with WHO Group II ovulation disorder, that is women with oligo- or amenorrhoea, with or without hyperandrogenism, and normal levels of prolactin, oestrogen and thyroid hormones. Typically, this group includes women with PCOS.

CC has also been tried for the treatment of unexplained infertility. Nonetheless, when CC treatment was compared with placebo or no treatment, there was no evidence that CC was more effective in this subgroup of infertile women (Hughes et al 2000).

Treatment regimens and monitoring

CC treatment is typically started with a daily dose of 50 mg, from day 2 of the cycle, for a total of 5 days. For amenorrhoeic women, treatment can be commenced at any time, provided pregnancy has been excluded or following a progestogen challenge test. Different regimens have also been tried, and overall CC treatment can safely be initiated anywhere between days 2 and 5 of the cycle for a total period of 5 days. Ovulation usually occurs 5–10 days after the course of treatment has been completed.

If ovulation is not induced with the initial dose of 50 mg, the dose of CC can be increased in 50-mg increments in subsequent cycles up to a maximum dose of 250 mg/day. Approximately 70% of anovulatory women treated with CC respond to a dose of 100–150 mg/day (Gysler et al 1982). In practice, doses of 250 mg are rarely used. Women who do not ovulate while taking a dose of 150 mg are considered

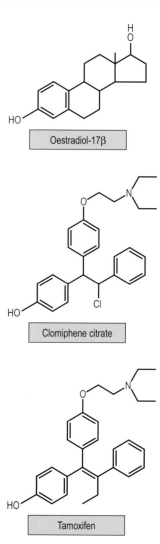

Figure 17.4 Structure of oestradiol and antioestrogen derivatives used in ovulation induction.

to be 'clomiphene-resistant' (Vandermolen et al 2001). The required CC dose is correlated to body weight, as there is a significant association between CC treatment failure and BMI greater than 27 kg/m². Women who are overweight should be advised that a 5% reduction in weight may improve endocrine and ovarian function, increase spontaneous conception rates and improve the response to CC treatment. Lower doses of 25–50 mg/day should be considered for those women who are exceptionally sensitive to treatment with CC.

Monitoring of CC treatment is recommended. Ovulation is confirmed either with serum progesterone measurements or with the use of transvaginal ultrasonography. Serum progesterone concentrations are measured during the luteal phase. Ultrasound monitoring should be offered at least during the first treatment cycle to ensure that the woman is on the lowest necessary dose to achieve ovulation (National Institute for Health and Clinical Excellence 2004). Monitoring will minimize the risk of multiple pregnancy and ovarian hyperstimulation syndrome (OHSS), and is essential in patients in whom ovulation does not seem to have been induced.

Results

Studies with CC have shown an ovulation rate of 60–85% and a pregnancy rate of 30–40%. The discrepancy between ovulation and fecundity rates has not been explained, but may be due to other coexisting fertility factors, such as endometriosis or tubal damage. Some argue that it may be associated with possible antioestrogenic effects that CC exhibits on the endometrium and cervical mucus (Milson et al 2002).

A systematic review of 12 randomized controlled trials supported the effectiveness of CC therapy for anovulatory infertile women (Beck et al 2005). Clomiphene was found to be effective in increasing pregnancy rate compared with placebo [fixed odds ratio (OR) 5.8, 95% confidence interval (CI) 1.6–21.5; number needed to treat (NNT) 5.9, 95% CI 3.6–16.7].

Cumulative conception rates continue to rise after six cycles of treatment, reaching a plateau after 12 cycles. However, prolonged treatment with CC may be associated with an increased risk of ovarian malignancy. Therefore, after completion of 12 cycles of treatment, alternative therapies ought to be considered (National Institute for Health and Clinical Excellence 2004). Factors associated with increased risk of CC treatment failure include increased maternal age, raised BMI and history of severe oligomenorrhoea (Milson et al 2002).

Side-effects

Side-effects with CC treatment are common, but usually mild and transient. Hot flushes and other vasomotor symptoms may occur in up to 10% of patients. Other symptoms include abdominal pain, nausea, vomiting, breast tenderness, headache, insomnia and hair loss. Rarely, visual disturbances (scotomata, blurred or doubled vision) may occur. In the latter case, CC should be discontinued and ophthalmology assessment arranged if symptoms do not cease.

Risks of treatment

With CC therapy, the risk of multiple gestation is approximately 2–13% (Venn and Lumley 1994). OHSS may occur in approximately 13% of cases, whereas severe OHSS is rare. Counselling of women undergoing ovulation induction with CC regarding the above risks is, therefore, essential.

The incidence of spontaneous miscarriage is 13–25% (Milson et al 2002). This figure is no different from the incidence of miscarriage in spontaneous conceptions. In addition to this, there is no evidence to indicate that CC treatment is associated with a higher incidence of congenital abnormalities.

Adjuvant treatment

A systematic review of 12 randomized controlled trials (Beck et al 2005) examined the concomitant administration of CC with other agents to infertile anovulatory women. The use of clomiphene in combination with tamoxifen did not provide any evidence of increased effect on pregnancy rate compared with clomiphene alone. The results were similar when CC plus ketoconazole was compared with CC alone, and CC plus bromocriptine was compared with CC alone.

However, clomiphene plus dexamethasone treatment resulted in a significant improvement in pregnancy rate (fixed OR 11.3, 95% CI 5.3–24.0; NNT 2.7, 95% CI 2.1–3.6) compared with clomiphene alone, as did clomiphene plus pretreatment with combined oral contraceptives (fixed OR 27.2, 95% CI 3.1–235.0; NNT 2.0, 95% CI 1.4–3.4).

Tamoxifen

Tamoxifen is a triphenylethylene derivative structurally similar to CC. It has been widely used in the treatment of breast cancer. In ovulation induction, tamoxifen is administered in doses of 20–80 mg/day, from day 2 to day 6 of the cycle. Tamoxifen, unlike CC, does not exhibit any antioestrogenic effects on the endometrium or vaginal mucosa. Therefore, it was thought that its use might be superior to CC.

Preliminary research has shown that tamoxifen has similar ovulation (44% with tamoxifen vs 45% with CC) and pregnancy rates (22% with tamoxifen vs 15% with CC) (Boostanfar 2001, Gerhard and Runnebaum 1979) compared with CC.

A meta-analysis, involving four trials, compared tamoxifen with CC in anovulatory women and showed that the two drugs were equally effective. Both drugs resulted in similar ovulation rates (OR 0.755, 95% CI 0.513–1.111). No benefit of tamoxifen over CC in achievement of pregnancy per cycle (OR 1.056, 95% CI 0.583–1.912) or per ovulatory cycle (OR 1.162, 95% CI 0.632–2.134) was demonstrated (Steiner et al 2005).

One randomized controlled trial showed that combination therapy of tamoxifen with CC did not improve pregnancy rates [8.6% with tamoxifen/CC vs 4.8% with CC alone; relative risk (RR) 1.80, 95% CI 0.20–16.21] (Suginami 1993).

In most units, tamoxifen is utilized as a second-line therapy in patients who experience side-effects on CC or who appear non-responsive.

Letrozole

Letrozole, an aromatase inhibitor, may be an alternative option for clomiphene-resistant anovulatory women. It has even been suggested that letrozole could be used as a first-line ovulation induction agent instead of CC. However, experience with this medication remains limited, and further research is needed to establish its role, utility and safety.

Pharmacology and mechanism of action

Aromatase inhibitors were initially introduced for the treatment of breast cancer. Aromatase is a cytochrome P-450 haemoprotein that catalyses the rate-limiting step in the production of oestrogens using androgens as a substrate. Letrozole is a highly potent, selective and reversible aromatase inhibitor (Bayar et al 2006). Letrozole inhibits peripheral oestrogen production and, therefore, stimulates endogenous FSH secretion. Moreover, the accumulated androgens may increase follicular sensitivity to FSH (Mitwally and Casper 2004). Its high oral bioavailability and short half-life make it a suitable agent for ovulation induction. One potential advantage of letrozole over CC is its lack of direct antioestrogenic effects on the cervical mucus, the endometrium, uterine blood flow and embryo development (Barroso et al 2006).

Results

In a Cochrane review, Cantineau et al (2007) identified five trials comparing aromatase inhibitors with antioestrogens used as ovulation induction agents in ovarian stimulation protocols for intrauterine insemination (IUI) in subfertile women. No benefits of letrozole use were identified. Other studies involving women with anovulation or unexplained infertility have shown comparable pregnancy rates between letrozole and CC (Barroso et al 2006, Bayar et al 2006, Davar et al 2006, Jee et al 2006). One study reported higher pregnancy rates in PCOS patients treated with letrozole (Atay et al 2006). Results from larger randomized controlled trials are needed to determine the role of letrozole in ovulation induction.

Dopamine Agonists

Pharmacology and mechanism of action

Prolactin secretion from the anterior pituitary is mainly regulated by the inhibitory control of dopamine. Therefore, drugs that exhibit a dopaminomimetic activity reduce prolactin serum concentrations and restore gonadal function in hyperprolactinaemic women, with or without a pituitary adenoma. If a prolactinoma is present, dopamine agonists may also reduce tumour size (see Chapter 16).

The two most commonly used dopamine agonists are bromocriptine and cabergoline. Both medications are ergot alkaloids that mimic dopamine's actions as they bind to dopamine receptors. Bromocriptine's serum concentrations peak 1–3 h after oral administration, but very little remains in the circulation after 14 h. Cabergoline is a longer-acting dopamine agonist with a higher affinity for the dopamine receptors than bromocriptine. A single dose of cabergoline inhibits prolactin secretion for 7 days.

A newer dopamine agonist licensed for the treatment of hyperprolactinaemia is quinagolide. Quinagolide is a non-ergot dopamine D_2 agonist. It has a longer biological half-life than bromocriptine.

Indications for treatment

Dopamine agonists are the treatment of choice for infertile women with hyperprolactinaemia. Nevertheless, if ovulation is not achieved despite establishment of euprolactinaemia, adjuvant therapy with CC or gonadotrophins must be considered.

It has been observed that approximately 30% of patients with PCOS show hyperprolactinaemia. In these patients, adjuvant therapy with dopamine agonists may be considered. The pathophysiology behind this remains unclear.

Regimen, monitoring and results

Bromocriptine is the most widely used preparation. Treatment starts at a low dose and is increased gradually. The initial dose should be low in order to minimize gastrointestinal and cardiovascular side-effects. Usually, therapy is initiated with 1.25 mg bromocriptine given at bedtime to suppress the nocturnal prolactin secretion. The dose is gradually increased until the dose required to maintain normal prolactin levels has been established. The usual daily dose is 7.5 mg in divided doses, increased if necessary to a maximum of 30 mg/day. Serum prolactin concentrations must be monitored regularly, and ovulation is monitored with serum progesterone concentrations. Ovulation is usually monofollicular, and ultrasound monitoring of follicle size and numbers is unnecessary if ovulation and regular menses are induced.

Women with a microprolactinoma who are planning to conceive should be prescribed bromocriptine. If pregnancy occurs, bromocriptine may be discontinued as the risk of tumour growth is very small (2%). Nevertheless, in the case of macroprolactinomas, the risk of growth is significant (25%) and treatment with bromocriptine should be continued throughout pregnancy (Balen 2004). Monitoring of these women is done clinically, based on symptoms such as headaches and visual disturbances, and will include visual field assessments and management jointly with an endocrinologist.

Cabergoline treatment is initiated at 500 µg/week, either as a single dose or as two divided doses on separate days. Prolactin levels must be monitored monthly and cabergoline dosage increased, if necessary, at monthly intervals. The usual therapeutic dose is 1 mg/week, ranging from 0.25 to 2 mg/week. The manufacturer advises discontinuation of the drug during pregnancy.

Quinagolide treatment should also be initiated at a low dose. Usually, it is commenced at 25 µg given at bedtime for 3 days. Then, it is increased at 3-day intervals in steps of 25 µg. The usual maintenance dose is 75–150 µg/day. The manufacturer advises discontinuation of the drug during pregnancy, unless medical reasons for continuing arise.

With the use of dopamine agonists, euprolactinaemia is achieved in approximately 60–85% of women. Regular menses are restored in 70–90% of cases and ovulation in 50–75%. If a prolactinoma is present, a decrease in tumour size is achieved in 70% of patients. Pregnancy rates of 30–70% have been reported overall.

Two large randomized controlled trials compared cabergoline with bromocriptine in women with hyperlactinaemic amenorrhoea. Cabergoline was found to be more effective than bromocriptine in achieving euprolactinaemia (83% and 93% with cabergoline vs 59% and 48% with bromocriptine). Moreover, cabergoline was more effective in restoring ovulation and increasing pregnancy rates (72% and 72% with cabergoline and 52% and 48% with bromocriptine) (Webster et al 1994, Pascal-Vigneron et al 1995). Nevertheless, consideration must be given to safety for use in pregnancy (National Institute for Health and Clinical Excellence 2004).

Side-effects

Side-effects of dopamine agonist treatment are common, but are usually mild and transient. Approximately 5% of patients will discontinue treatment for this reason. Side-effects are mainly gastrointestinal and cardiovascular. Gastrointestinal side-effects include nausea, vomiting and constipation. Other side-effects include drowsiness, orthostatic hypotension, headaches and nasal congestion. Side-effects can be minimized if treatment is initiated at a low dose and then gradually increased. Moreover, vaginal administration of the medication may help. The incidence of side-effects is lower with cabergoline than with bromocriptine.

With dopamine agonists, there is no increase in the risk of OHSS, multiple pregnancy or spontaneous miscarriage.

Insulin-Sensitizing Agents

PCOS is characterized by chronic anovulatory infertility and hyperandrogenism with clinical manifestations of oligo- or amenorrhoea, hirsutism and acne. Women with PCOS exhibit an increased prevalence of cardiovascular risk factors, including a higher incidence of obesity, insulin resistance and hyperinsulinaemia (Royal College of Obstetricians and Gynaecologists 2007). Increased insulin concentrations lead to hyperandrogenism and subsequently anovulation. In obese (BMI >30 kg/m^2) PCOS women, weight reduction alone may decrease hyperinsulinaemia and hyperandrogenism, and restore ovulation. Therefore, prior to commencing drug treatment, women should be advised to lose weight, as this would improve their chance of spontaneous ovulation and improve their response to ovulation induction.

Metformin

Insulin-sensitizing agents have been tried as ovulation induction drugs in PCOS patients. The most commonly used is metformin, a biguanide oral hypoglycaemic drug used for the treatment of type 2 diabetes mellitus. Metformin has been proven to reduce serum insulin and androgen concentrations, and improve ovulation rates and hirsutism (Lord et al 2003). Metformin has been used as an ovulation induction agent in many trials; nevertheless, these trials are characterized by heterogeneity in terms of dosage, timing and duration of treatment (Al-Inany and Johnson 2006).

A Cochrane review, including women with clomiphene-resistant PCOS and a mean BMI greater than 25 kg/m^2, concluded that metformin as a single agent did not increase pregnancy rates compared with placebo. Treatment with both metformin and CC did increase clinical pregnancy rates compared with CC alone (OR 4.88, 95% CI 2.46–9.67). Metformin as a single agent was, however, shown to induce ovulation compared with placebo (OR 3.88, 95% CI 2.25–6.69). Moreover, metformin in combination with CC was more effective at inducing ovulation compared with CC alone (OR 4.41, 95% CI 2.37–8.22) (Lord et al 2003).

Two large randomized controlled trials (Moll et al 2006, Legro et al 2007) concluded that metformin should not be used as a primary method for ovulation induction in PCOS patients. Moll et al (2006) compared the effect of CC plus metformin and CC plus placebo on ovulation induction in PCOS women. They concluded that there were no significant differences in ovulation, ongoing pregnancy or miscarriage rates. Nevertheless, a large proportion of women in the metformin group discontinued treatment because of side-effects. Legro et al (2007) compared CC plus placebo, metformin plus placebo and CC plus metformin. The livebirth rate was 22.5% in the CC group, 7.2% in the metformin group and 26.8% in the combination group. Conception rates were lower in the metformin group (21.7%) than in the CC group (39.5%) or the combination group (46%).

Therefore, infertile women with PCOS should not be offered metformin as a first-line agent, and CC remains the drug of choice. Nonetheless, PCOS patients who have not responded to CC and who have a BMI greater than 25 kg/m^2 should be offered combined metformin and CC treatment (National Institute for Health and Clinical Excellence 2004).

It must be noted that metformin has not been licensed in the UK for use in women who are not diabetic. Therefore, careful counselling of women is mandatory prior to commencing treatment with metformin.

Treatment with metformin is mainly associated with gastrointestinal side-effects, including nausea, vomiting, diarrhoea and abdominal cramps. Lactic acidosis is a rare event. No evidence of fetal toxicity or teratogenicity has been reported.

Other drugs

Other insulin-sensitizing agents tried in the management of anovulatory infertility include the thiazolidinedione hypoglycaemic drugs. Experience with these drugs in PCOS women is limited. Troglitazone was shown to be effective in inducing ovulation. Nevertheless, it was withdrawn from the market after reports of hepatotoxicity. Rosiglitazone and pioglitazone are newer drugs used for the treatment of type 2 diabetes mellitus. Regular monitoring of liver enzymes is recommended, as these drugs may also have hepatotoxic effects. These agents are 'class C' drugs with evidence of teratogenicity in animals (Lord et al 2003), and far more data are required in ovulation induction patients to determine their potential role and safety.

Pulsatile Gonadotrophin-Releasing Hormone

Pulsatile GnRH has been used for ovulation induction since 1980. It is the treatment of choice for women with hypogonadotrophic hypogonadism with an intact pituitary function (Braat et al 1991).

Mechanism of action

In patients with hypogonadotrophic hypogonadism, the administration of exogenous pulsatile GnRH restores normal pulsatile pituitary gonadotrophin secretion. Subsequently, follicular recruitment and growth proceed as in a normal menstrual cycle, leading to the development of a single dominant follicle (Martin et al 1993).

Regimen and monitoring

Pulsatile GnRH is administered via a portable mini-pump, either intravenously or subcutaneously. This pump must be worn continuously throughout the treatment. A 2.5–20.0 μg/bolus is administered via the pump at 60–90-min intervals. The treatment starts at a low dose (2.5–5.0 μg/pulse) and is gradually increased until ovulation is achieved. The intravenous route is preferred by some authors as it mimics the physiological spikes of the hormone and, therefore, is more physiological, requires lower doses and is more cost-effective than the subcutaneous route of administration.

Monitoring is performed with regular serum oestradiol measurements and pelvic ultrasound every 3–4 days. The luteal phase is supported either by continuing the same pulsatile GnRH regimen or with the administration of exogenous human chorionic gonadotrophin (hCG).

Results

Pulsatile GnRH is a highly effective method of ovulation induction. Ovulation rates and pregnancy rates per treatment cycle of 70–93% and 18–29% have been reported (Braat et al 1991, Martin et al 1993, Filicori et al 1994).

Nevertheless, ovulation induction with pulsatile GnRH has been less successful in women with PCOS, raised BMI and high serum LH, testosterone or insulin levels (Filicori et al 1994).

Twin pregnancy rates ranged between 3.8% and 13.5% (Braat et al 1991, Martin et al 1993, Filicori et al 1994). This risk is significantly lower than that associated with gonadotrophin treatment (approximately 15%) (Martin et al 1993). Higher order pregnancies are rarely seen with pulsatile GnRH therapy.

The risk of OHSS is very low when exogenous GnRH is used. In comparison with gonadotrophin ovulation induction, GnRH treatment is associated with a lower risk of multiple folliculogenesis and ovarian enlargement (Martin et al 1993).

Spontaneous miscarriage rates have been approximately 10–30%. These appear to be higher in PCOS patients (40%) and lower in women with hypogonadotrophic hypogonadism (20%) (Filicori et al 1994). It is believed that in PCOS women, pretreatment with GnRH analogues may improve outcomes and lower the incidence of multiple pregnancies. Nonetheless, a systematic review by Bayram et al (2004) found no evidence to support the use of pulsatile GnRH in clomiphene-resistant PCOS women.

Side-effects

Overall, exogenous pulsatile GnRH is simple to use, does not require expensive monitoring and is associated with lower risks of multiple pregnancy and OHSS in comparison with gonadotrophin treatment. Nevertheless, many women are reluctant to use this treatment as it requires maintenance of an indwelling cannula for a long period of time; moreover, cases of infection at the site of the cannula have been reported. These seem to be more serious with the intravenous route of administration, whilst the subcutaneous route is mainly associated with local inflammation at the site of needle insertion.

Gonadotrophins

Since the 1960s, exogenous gonadotrophins have been used for ovulation induction in women with WHO Group I and II anovulatory infertility. Gonadotrophins are considered highly effective in inducing ovulation in these groups of patients. Nevertheless, their use has been associated with risks of multiple pregnancy and ovarian hyperstimulation.

Preparations

A number of preparations of exogenous gonadotrophins exist but not all are still available in every country.

Urinary human menopausal gonadotrophin

Human menopausal gonadotrophin (hMG, Menotropin) derives from the urine of postmenopausal women. It contains equal amounts of FSH and LH (75 IU of each), as well as other urinary proteins (>95% of total protein content). The initial preparations were crude as they contained significant amounts of non-gonadotrophin proteins; moreover, they had to be administered intramuscularly. Newer hMG preparations are more purified, contain fewer proteins and can be administered subcutaneously.

Urinary follicle-stimulating hormone

Purified urinary FSH was first introduced in the 1980s (Urofollitropin). It was developed after removing LH by using monoclonal antibody technology (immunoaffinity chromatography). Purified urinary FSH contains 75 IU FSH and less than 1 IU LH. Still-significant amounts of non-gonadotrophin proteins were present and the preparation had to be given intramuscularly. Newer preparations are more highly purified, contain less than 0.001 IU LH and can be given subcutaneously, allowing self-administration.

Recombinant follicle-stimulating hormone

Recombinant FSH was developed by genetic engineering in 1988. Through recombinant DNA techniques, the genes responsible for expression of the α and β subunits of FSH were introduced to the genome of a Chinese hamster ovary cell line. These cells would then produce FSH. The synthesized FSH is purified using chromatography. In comparison with urinary FSH, recombinant FSH has the same structure of side chains, but contains more basic and less acidic isoforms. Its pharmacokinetic characteristics are similar to those of urinary FSH.

Recombinant luteinizing hormone

Recombinant LH was only introduced recently. Its production is based on the same principles of genetic engineering that apply to the synthesis of recombinant FSH. Its pharmacokinetics are similar to those of human pituitary LH.

Urinary human chorionic gonadotrophin

Urinary hCG is extracted from the placenta or the urine of pregnant women. It is used in gonadotrophin-stimulated cycles to be a surrogate for the LH surge and to trigger ovulation once a follicle reaches maturation. The preparation is administered either intramuscularly or subcutaneously.

Recombinant human chorionic gonadotrophin

Recombinant hCG is also available. Studies suggest that 250 μg recombinant hCG is equivalent to 5000–10,000 IU urinary hCG.

Thus far, research indicates that different gonadotrophin preparations are equally effective. When recombinant hCG was compared with urinary hCG, no differences in clinical outcomes (including ongoing pregnancy and livebirth rates, miscarriage and OHSS rates) were demonstrated (Al-Inany et al 2005). When recombinant FSH was compared with urinary hMG, no significant differences in pregnancy rates were observed (Nugent et al 2000).

Nevertheless, recombinant gonadotrophins have certain advantages in comparison with urinary products. They have high batch-to-batch consistency, unlimited supply, high purity and are associated with less risk of allergic reaction as they do not contain any non-gonadotrophin proteins. However, their increased cost is a major disadvantage. Thus, when deciding which preparation to use, factors such as patient safety, cost and drug availability must be taken into consideration (Table 17.1)

Indications

Ovulation induction with gonadotrophins is indicated for:

- women with WHO Group I anovulatory infertility (hypogonadotrophic hypogonadism);
- women with WHO Group II anovulatory infertility (including women with PCOS) who failed to ovulate on CC; and

Table 17.1 Preparations of gonadotrophins for ovulation induction

Formulation	Proprietary Name	Administered
Urinary		
Human menopausal gonadotrophin FSH 75 U and LH 75 U/ampoule	Merional Menopur	IM SC
Urofollitrophin FSH 75 U and LH <1 U/ampoule	Fostimon	IM/SC
Human chorionic gonadotrophin 5000 U/ampoule	Choragon Pregnyl	IM/SC
Recombinant		
Follitrophin α FSH 75 U/ampoule	Gonal-F	SC
Follitrophin β FSH 75 U or multiples in cartridges	Puregon	SC
Lutrophin α LH 75 U/ampoule	Luveris	SC
Follitrophin α with lutrophin α FSH 150 U and LH 75 U	Pergoveris	SC
Choriogonadotrophin α 6500 U ≡ 250 μg	Ovitrelle	SC

FSH, follicle-stimulating hormone; LH, luteinizing hormone; IM, intramuscular; SC, subcutaneous.

- women with unexplained infertility or ovulatory women undergoing IUI for unexplained or mild male factor infertility.

The choice of therapeutic regimen will depend on the underlying cause of infertility. Treatment must be tailored to the individual's needs.

Hypogonadotrophic hypogonadism

Women with hypogonadotrophic hypogonadism have extremely low levels of endogenous gonadotrophins. Therefore, both exogenous FSH and LH are required. FSH is essential for follicular growth and oocyte maturation, whereas LH is required for steroidogenesis, luteinization and ovulation. The treatment of choice for this group of patients is hMG, as it contains both FSH and LH (Shoham et al 1991). Nonetheless, the use of recombinant FSH and LH may be an alternative. The regimen used for these women is the 'step-up protocol'. The luteal phase is usually supported with the administration of hCG, as these patients have very low levels of LH.

Polycystic ovary syndrome

Clomiphene-resistant PCOS women may be candidates for treatment with gonadotrophins. In contrast to women with hypogonadotrophic hypogonadism, PCOS patients have FSH and LH levels which are normal or may be elevated. These patients are at increased risk of multiple pregnancy and OHSS. Therefore, relatively low doses of gonadotrophins are needed for ovulation induction. The protocols used for this category of patients are the 'chronic low-dose step-up protocol', the 'step-down' protocol and the 'sequential protocol'. Luteal phase support is not routinely required but, if needed, progesterone support is preferred.

A systematic review of 14 randomized controlled trials found that urinary hMG and urinary FSH had similar effectiveness in terms of pregnancy rates. However, the incidence of OHSS was reduced with FSH compared with hMG. No significant differences were reported between the use of subcutaneous pulsatile and intramuscular injection of gonadotrophins, daily or alternate-day administration, and 'step-up' or 'standard' regimens (Nugent et al 2000).

A Cochrane review including four randomized controlled trials concluded that when recombinant FSH was compared with urinary FSH, there were no significant differences in terms of ovulation, pregnancy, miscarriage, multiple pregnancy and OHSS rates. No significant differences were demonstrated between administering recombinant FSH as a chronic low dose or as a standard regimen (Bayram et al 2001). The reader is referred to the review by Amer (2007) for further information.

Ovulatory patients undergoing intrauterine insemination

Gonadotrophins have been used for superovulation induction in women with unexplained infertility or ovulatory women with age-related or mild male factor infertility undergoing IUI. In these women, both the step-up and step-down regimens have been applied. The purpose of gonadotrophin treatment is to induce multifollicular development

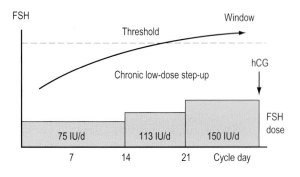

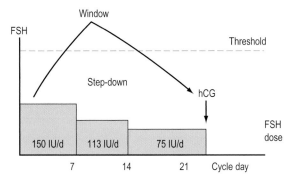

Figure 17.5 Chronic 'low-dose step-up' protocol vs 'step-down' protocol for gonadotrophin administration. FSH, follicle-stimulating hormone; hCG, human chorionic gonadotrophin.

('superovulation'). Careful monitoring is essential as the risks of OHSS and multiple pregnancy are high.

Regimens and monitoring

Varying regimens of administering exogenous gonadotrophins have been developed (see Figure 17.5).

Step-up protocol

The step-up protocol is used for women with hypogonadotrophic hypogonadism and for clomiphene-resistant PCOS patients.

Women with WHO Group I anovulation (hypogonadotrophic hypogonadism) are initially given a daily dose of 150 IU hMG. The dose is increased by 75 IU after 4–5 days depending on the response. This is assessed by serum oestradiol concentration and transvaginal ultrasonography. If an ovarian response is confirmed, the gonadotrophin dose is not altered. The frequency of monitoring may be intensified, depending on oestradiol levels and the size or number of the growing follicles. When one or two follicles reach a mean diameter of 18 mm, 5000–10,000 IU hCG is administered to trigger ovulation. Ovulation usually occurs after 36–48 h and couples are advised to have intercourse on the day of the injection and the day after. This regimen is also known as the 'regular-dose step-up protocol'.

In women with PCOS, the 'chronic low-dose step-up protocol' is preferred. Treatment is initiated with a low FSH dose (50–75 IU) continued for a longer period (14 days). Small increments are allowed (25–37.5 IU every 5–7 days) until a dominant follicle emerges.

Step-down protocol

In this regimen, treatment is initiated at higher doses of FSH and then gradually reduced. The purpose of this approach is to mimic the FSH fluctuations during the normal ovulatory cycle. Therapy is commenced at 150 IU/day on day 2 or 3 of the cycle. When a dominant follicle emerges, FSH is reduced by 37.5 IU/day. After 2–3 days, FSH is further decreased to 75 IU/day. This last dose is continued until hCG is administered to trigger ovulation.

Sequential protocol

Treatment is started with a 'step-up' protocol, followed by a 'step-down' regimen once a dominant follicle (≥14 mm) has emerged.

Concomitant use of gonadotrophin-releasing hormone agonist

Combined treatment with a GnRH agonist and gonadotrophins has been used in PCOS women undergoing IVF. In ovulation induction, pretreatment with a GnRH agonist may theoretically suppress endogenous LH levels. If this treatment is continued during gonadotrophin administration, premature luteinization may be prevented.

In a randomized clinical trial when GnRH agonists were used concomitantly with gonadotrophins, no significant differences were shown in ovulation or pregnancy rates compared with using gonadotrophins alone (Vegetti 1998). Moreover, Nugent et al (2000) found an increase in the incidence of OHSS when GnRH analogues were added to gonadotrophins. Therefore, the use of GnRH agonists is not recommended for PCOS women undergoing ovulation induction with gonadotrophins.

Results

In women with WHO Group I ovulation dysfunction, pregnancy rates of 25% per cycle and cumulative pregnancy rates of 90% after six cycles of treatment have been achieved (Amer 2007). Nevertheless, success rates were lower in PCOS women (5–25% and 30–60%, respectively).

Risks

Treatment with gonadotrophins is associated with an increased risk of multiple pregnancy and OHSS. These complications will be discussed in more detail later in this chapter.

When non-purified preparations are used, their administration may be associated with an increased risk of local reaction (at the injection site) or, on rare occasions, with a severe anaphylactic reaction. In this case, consideration should be given to switch to recombinant gonadotrophin preparations.

Weight Reduction

Obesity has been described as the new worldwide health epidemic. In the UK, obesity affects 24% of the adult female population. As the number of obese women is increasing, so is the prevalence of the disease among those who seek fertility treatment.

Obesity has been associated with a number of reproductive disorders. These include menstrual disorders, infertility, miscarriage and obstetric complications, both fetal and maternal. It appears that it is not only the increased amount of fat *per se*, but also the fat distribution that is related with these disorders. Thus, an increased waist:hip ratio has a more important effect on fertility than weight alone.

The exact mechanism through which obesity impairs ovarian function, and thus fertility, is largely unknown. It seems that obesity causes low sex-hormone-binding globulin concentrations, hyperandrogenaemia and hyperinsulinaemia. Adipose tissue affects gonadal function via the secretion of adipokines. These include leptin, adiponectin, ghrelin and resistin. The most investigated of all is leptin. Obese women have elevated serum and follicular fluid leptin concentrations. High leptin levels cause a reduction in insulin-induced steroidogenesis in granulosa and theca cells. Leptin also inhibits oestradiol production by the granulosa cells. On the other hand, adiponectin levels decrease in obesity, leading to insulin resistance. Thus, hyperinsulinaemia may be due to the effects of low adiponectin levels and increased resistin levels. The resulting hyperandrogenaemia is caused by the inhibition of sex-hormone-binding globulin and insulin-like growth factor binding protein-1.

As far as fertility is concerned, large retrospective studies have shown a link between obesity and anovulation. Anovulation seems to be the result of hyperandrogenaemia and increased levels of leptin. Obese anovulatory women may or may not have PCOS. It is unknown whether obesity leads to PCOS or vice versa.

The impact of obesity on assisted conception techniques has also been investigated. Regarding ovulation induction, it seems that obese women can be more resistant to CC than non-obese women. As far as IVF is concerned, the evidence from the literature is inconclusive. Although obese women appear to require higher doses of drugs for ovarian stimulation, have a lower chance of pregnancy following IVF and an increased miscarriage rate, it is not clear whether there is an effect of BMI on livebirth rates, cycle cancellation, oocyte recovery or ovarian hyperstimulation incidence (Maheshwari et al 2007).

In this group of patients, weight reduction improves biochemical indices and fertility rates. A 5–10% decrease in body weight will lead to a 30% reduction in body fat, which is sufficient to restore regular menstruation and ovulation. A prospective study was conducted by Clark et al (1995). This study looked at the effect of weight loss, with diet and exercise, on women with anovulation, clomiphene resistance and a BMI greater than 30. Weight reduction led to resumption of ovulation and subsequent pregnancy, as well as a reduction of testosterone levels and increased sex-hormone-binding globulin concentrations.

According to the guidelines of the British Fertility Society, it is advised that women with a BMI greater than 35 kg/m^2 should not receive fertility investigations or treatment until they reduce their BMI to less than 35 kg/m^2. Women who are trying to conceive should be advised to maintain a BMI in the range of 20–25 kg/m^2. Women with a BMI greater than 30 kg/m^2 should be encouraged to lose weight to a BMI less than 30 kg/m^2 before receiving fertility therapy either in the form of ovulation induction or as assisted reproduction technology.

Nevertheless, the management of obesity is difficult and requires a multidisciplinary approach. Women should be encouraged to adopt a healthy lifestyle. This would include modification of their dietary quality and change in physical activity. If this fails, pharmacotherapy ought to be considered and, ultimately, obesity surgery. If there is an underlying eating disorder, psychopathology should also be taken into consideration and appropriate referrals made.

Pharmacotherapy includes two main groups of drugs: peripherally acting and centrally acting drugs. The first category mainly infers to orlistat. This medication inhibits gastric and pancreatic lipase and, therefore, reduces fat absorption from the intestine. Orlistat has been shown to decrease testosterone levels in PCOS patients. Although it is generally well tolerated, it can cause gastrointestinal disturbances, which consequently lead to low patient compliance. Orlistat is not licensed for use in pregnancy. The second category of drugs includes sibutramine, which inhibits serotonin and noradrenaline reuptake. It can cause a greater reduction in insulin levels and insulin resistance compared with metformin. Another medication is remonabant, a selective cannabinoid-1 receptor blocker. Both sibutramine and remonabant are contraindicated in pregnancy.

As far as bariatric surgery is concerned, laparoscopic adjustable gastric banding remains the mainstream therapy. Nonetheless, further research is required in order to establish its role in improving fertility. After the procedure, contraception is required until the target weight is reached.

Surgical Management: Laparoscopic Ovarian Drilling

Surgical ovarian wedge resection, introduced in 1939, was the first established treatment for anovulatory PCOS patients. The procedure was performed via laparotomy, and 75% of each ovary was removed. It was speculated that by removing part of the hormone-producing ovarian tissue, androgen and inhibin levels would be reduced. This was followed by an increase in FSH levels and a decrease in LH, leading to spontaneous resumption of ovulation. Nevertheless, the response rate was variable and the procedure was abandoned largely because of the risk of postoperative adhesion formation. As soon as effective medical methods of ovulation became available, ovarian wedge resection became obsolete.

Nonetheless, ovulation induction with CC is not always successful and 20% of women are described as 'CC resistant'. CC-resistant patients can receive treatment with gonadotrophins, but these are relatively expensive, require intensive monitoring and are associated with increased risk of OHSS and multiple pregnancy. Laparoscopic ovarian drilling (LOD) has therefore been introduced as an alternative therapy for this group of patients.

LOD was first described by Gjonnaess in 1984. Both laparoscopic ovarian cautery and laser vaporization (using carbon dioxide, argon or neodymium:yttrium aluminium garnet lasers) have been used since. The aim is to create approximately 10 holes per ovary in the ovarian surface and stroma. The mechanism of action is thought to be similar to that of ovarian wedge resection. With LOD, androgen-producing ovarian tissue is destroyed. This subsequently causes a decline in the serum levels of androgens, inhibin and LH and an increase in FSH levels. Therefore, disturbances in the ovarian–pituitary feedback mechanism are corrected, leading to follicular recruitment, maturation and ovulation. A long-term cohort study has also shown that up to 20 years after LOD, there was persistence of ovulation and normalization of serum androgens and sex-hormone-binding globulin levels in 60% of the participants (Gjonnaess 1998, Amer et al 2002).

With the employment of LOD, spontaneous ovulation rates of 30–90% and pregnancy rates of 13–88% have been described. In the literature, most data derive from randomized controlled trials comparing ovarian drilling with ovulation induction using exogenous gonadotrophins. There is no evidence of a difference in livebirth outcomes following either LOD (after 6–12 months of follow-up) or three to six cycles of ovulation induction with gonadotrophins in CC-resistant women. Moreover, there was no evidence of a difference in clinical pregnancy rate, miscarriage rate, ovulation rate and quality of life. Nonetheless, multiple pregnancy rates were reduced after LOD (Farquhar et al 2007). Moreover, there appears to be no difference between LOD of one ovary vs drilling of both ovaries in terms of ovulation induction.

In CC-resistant women, LOD may improve clomiphene sensitivity, since when CC or gonadotrophins were added after ovarian drilling, higher pregnancy rates were reported.

Attempts have been made to identify predictors of success in women undergoing LOD, as 43% may not ovulate spontaneously after ovarian drilling. This seems to be related to factors such as the duration of infertility, BMI and free androgen index.

In summary, as there is no evidence of a difference in efficacy between LOD and gonadotrophin ovulation induction, LOD may be the treatment of choice as it is associated with a lower risk of multiple pregnancy and OHSS. Nevertheless, LOD carries risks such as pelvic infection, postoperative adhesion formation, risks of general anaesthesia and the theoretical risk of premature ovarian failure. All these should be taken into consideration before embarking on this procedure. Careful counselling and selection of patients is therefore mandatory. The operation should only be performed by fully trained laparoscopic surgeons. At the moment, the use of LOD is restricted to anovulatory women with a normal BMI. Its use is not recommended as an attempt to decrease the risk of developing diabetes mellitus or coronary artery disease. Long-term risks for women with PCOS (Royal College of Obstetricians and Gynaecologists 2007).

Risks of Induction of Ovulation

Ovarian hyperstimulation syndrome

OHSS is a rare, serious and potentially life-threatening complication of ovulation induction. It is a systemic disease resulting from vasoactive products released from hyperstimulated ovaries. It occurs during the luteal phase of the cycle or during early pregnancy. The incidence of mild OHSS in ovulation induction with CC is 13.5%, whereas moderate and severe forms have only been described sporadically. In IVF/intracytoplasmic sperm injection (ICSI) cycles, the incidence of mild, moderate and severe OHSS may be 33%, 3–6% and 0.1–2%, respectively (Delvigne and Rozenberg 2002). Only a few cases of OHSS have occurred in spontaneous cycles. The true incidence of mortality from OHSS is unknown; nevertheless, deaths are rare.

Pathophysiology

The pathophysiology of OHSS is characterized by an increased capillary permeability, leading to a shift of fluid from the intravascular to the extravascular space, with third-space fluid accumulation and intravascular dehydration. The exact mechanism remains unknown. It is believed that the increased vascular permeability is the result of vasoactive agents released by the hyperstimulated ovaries. Several agents have been proposed, including oestradiol, LH, prolactin, histamine, prostaglandins, prorenin (renin–angiotensin cascade), serotonin, interleukins and vascular endothelial growth factor.

In the initial stages of OHSS, there is an increase in the size of the ovaries and abdominal discomfort. In more severe forms, ovaries become cystic and there is abdominal distention with pain, nausea, vomiting and diarrhoea. This may be followed by ascites, pleural effusion and, on rare occasions, pericardial effusions. There is marked intravascular volume depletion with haemoconcentration that may lead to severe manifestations, including thromboembolism, severe hypoalbuminaemia, hypovolaemia, oliguria and electrolyte disturbances. Cases of acute respiratory distress syndrome have also been reported. Occasionally, liver impairment may occur.

Diagnosis/classification

The diagnosis of OHSS is based on clinical grounds. A history of ovulation induction accompanied by symptoms of abdominal pain, nausea and vomiting should raise the possibility of OHSS. Other conditions, such as ovarian cyst accidents (e.g. torsion, rupture, haemorrhage), pelvic inflammatory disease and ectopic pregnancy should be considered.

Different classification systems of OHSS have been proposed. The latest system was suggested by Marthur in 2005 and is shown in Table 17.2 as adopted by the Royal College of Obstetricians and Gynaecologists. Four categories of OHSS are noted: mild, moderate, severe and critical. As the management of the condition will be dictated by its severity, it is mandatory to assess each case properly and classify it according to Table 17.2.

Risk factors

Several risk factors of OHSS have been identified in an attempt to prevent this serious iatrogenic complication.

Age

Most studies have reported that women who developed OHSS were significantly younger than those who did not develop OHSS. Women under the age of 30 years are at

Table 17.2 Classification of severity of ovarian hyperstimulation syndrome (OHSS)

Grade	Symptoms
Mild	Abdominal bloating
	Mild abdominal pain
	Ovarian size usually <8 cm*
Moderate	Moderate abdominal pain
	Nausea ± vomiting
	Ultrasound evidence of ascites
	Ovarian size usually 8–12 cm*
Severe	Clinical ascites (occasionally hydrothorax)
	Oliguria
	Haemoconcentration haematocrit >45%
	Hypoproteinaemia
	Ovarian size usually >12 cm*
Critical	Tense ascites or large hydrothorax
	Haematocrit >55%
	White cell count >25,000/ml
	Oligo/anuria
	Thromboembolism
	Acute respiratory distress syndrome

*Ovarian size may not correlate with severity of OHSS in cases of assisted reproduction because of the effect of follicular aspiration.

higher risk. A possible explanation could be that ovaries of younger women are more responsive to gonadotrophins, as they contain a higher number of gonadotrophin receptors and a larger number of follicles responding to gonadotrophins.

Allergies

It has been observed that the prevalence of allergies is significantly increased in women who develop OHSS.

Polycystic ovary syndrome

PCOS patients are at high risk. In addition to this, women with 'isolated characteristics of PCO', such as PCO-like ultrasonographic images ('necklace sign'), an LH:FSH ratio greater than 2 or hyperandrogenism are also at increased risk.

Pregnancy

The risk of OHSS is two- to five-fold higher if pregnancy occurs, and may present as a late-onset variant.

Types of stimulatory drugs

Severe OHSS is only rarely associated with clomiphene ovulation induction, whereas moderate forms of the syndrome are encountered in 8% of cycles stimulated with clomiphene. The incidence is much higher when gonadotrophins are used. A study reported that the incidences of mild, moderate and severe OHSS following induction with gonadotrophins are 20%, 6–7% and 1–2%, respectively. GnRH agonists have also been associated with an increase in OHSS incidence. This may be due to inhibition of the spontaneous luteinization process linked with the LH peak.

On the other hand, the use of GnRH antagonists does not increase the risk of OHSS. Insulin-sensitizing agents do not seem to affect its incidence.

Response to ovulation stimulation

High levels of oestradiol, a large number of preovulatory follicles and the presence of large follicles have been associated with an increased risk of OHSS. Other potential predictors of OHSS may include inhibin A and B and vascular endothelial growth factor levels. Further research is required in order to evaluate their positive predictive value and possible future use.

Previous ovarian hyperstimulation syndrome

The risk of developing OHSS is increased in patients who have developed it previously, and altered stimulation protocols need to be utilized.

Prevention

Although several strategies have been developed, OHSS cannot be totally prevented. This mainly applies to late OHSS triggered by the rising serum hCG secreted in early pregnancy. Nevertheless, prevention and early recognition of OHSS are fundamental in ensuring patients' safety. Identification of any risk factors may reduce the risk of developing OHSS, as adaptations can be made to the ovulation regimen. Careful monitoring of the stimulation with the use of ultrasonography should be implemented, as it has a good predictive value in the occurrence of OHSS (Blankstein et al 1987). For instance, starting with a lower dose of gonadotrophin, reducing the dose when OHSS is suspected or even cancelling the cycle and withholding hCG injection may prevent OHSS. In the latter case, the couple should be advised to refrain from intercourse or to use barrier methods of contraception.

Management

OHSS is a rare disease and many healthcare professionals may be unfamiliar with the syndrome. Protocols for the management of OHSS should therefore be in place. Treatment is predominantly supportive, as OHSS resolves spontaneously. Usually, this takes 7 days in non-pregnant women and 10–20 days in pregnant women.

A physical examination, including body weight, abdominal girth measurements, abdominal and cardiorespiratory examination, and assessment of hydration, must be performed. A pelvic ultrasound will help to assess the size of the ovaries and check for ascites. Blood tests should include full blood count, urea and electrolytes, liver function tests and clotting screen. In case of dyspnoea, a chest X-ray or chest ultrasonography should be requested. If pericardial effusion is suspected, an electrocardiogram and echocardiogram will be essential.

Outpatient management

Women with mild OHSS and many with moderate OHSS may be managed as outpatients. Paracetamol and codeine are the analgesics of choice. Non-steroidal anti-inflammatory drugs are contraindicated, as they may compromise renal function. Women should be advised to drink to thirst and not to excess. A review is required every 2–3 days. Nevertheless, urgent reassessment is warranted if the woman develops severe abdominal pain, increasing abdominal

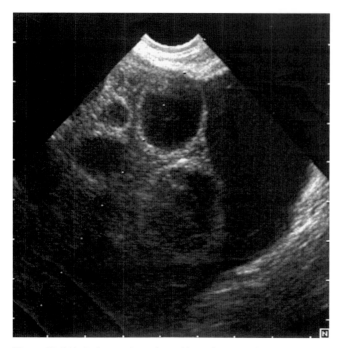

Figure 17.6 Vaginal scan of a patient with moderate ovarian hyperstimulation syndrome, showing enlarged ovary, luteal cysts and ascitic fluid.

distention, dyspnoea or has a subjective impression of decreasing urine output (Royal College of Obstetricians and Gynaecologists 2006).

Inpatient management

Women with severe OHSS and those with moderate OHSS whose symptoms cannot be controlled with oral medication should be admitted to hospital. Critical cases of OHSS may require admission to an intensive care unit for invasive monitoring (see Figure 17.6).

Monitoring of these patients should include:

- heart rate and blood pressure;
- abdominal girth and weight (measured daily);
- intake and output chart;
- daily haemoglobin, haematocrit and platelet count; and
- daily serum creatinine and electrolytes.

Measures of worsening OHSS include: increasing abdominal pain, oliguria (in particular, a persistent positive fluid balance or daily urine output <1000 ml/day), weight gain, increased girth circumference, worsening dyspnoea and haemoconcentration (as measured by raised haemoglobin, haematocrit or white cell count).

If pain is not adequately controlled with paracetamol, oral or parenteral opiates ought to be considered. Nausea is usually caused by the presence of ascites, and measures taken to reduce ascites also contribute to relief from nausea. The recommended antiemetics are those appropriate for early pregnancy, such as metoclopramide, cyclizine and prochlorperazine. The intravascular volume is maintained by encouraging women to drink to thirst. In cases of severe vomiting, intravenous crystalloids, such as normal saline, must be administered, aiming for a fluid intake of 2–3 l/day. In the case of haemoconcentration, more intensive hydration is needed; if the problem persists, colloid therapy needs to be considered. Colloids that have been used for this purpose include human albumin, dextran, Haemaccel, 6% hydroxyethylstarch and mannitol. Nevertheless, there is no evidence to recommend any specific fluid regimen. Diuretics should be avoided for fear of intravascular volume depletion. In cases of increasing abdominal distention or persistent oliguria, an ultrasound-guided paracentesis should be considered. Drainage of ascitic fluid provides rapid symptomatic relief from pain and dyspnoea, and is followed by a significant improvement in urine output. Intravenous colloid replacement should be considered in order to avoid cardiovascular collapse. Thromboprophylaxis should be given to all women with OHSS who are admitted. This will include full-length venous support stockings and subcutaneous prophylactic heparin. Surgical treatment is reserved for cases of suspected adnexal torsion.

Counselling

Women who undergo ovulation induction should be counselled carefully about the risks and possible symptoms of OHSS. A 24-h contact number and access to a clinician should be offered to these women.

In the case of OHSS, further counselling is needed to provide information and reassurance. For an overview of management of OHSS, the reader is referred to the guidelines of the Royal College of Obstetricians and Gynaecologists (2006).

Multiple pregnancy

In many developed countries, there has been a 30–50% increase in twin births since 1980. Triplet deliveries have increased three- to five-fold during this period. The incidence of multiple births in the UK has risen from 10–15/100,000 maternities before 1981 to 12.1/1000 maternities in 1991 and 14.9/1000 maternities in 2004 (Office for National Statistics 2006). The number of multiple pregnancies conceived is even higher, as spontaneous and iatrogenic fetoreductions are not included in birth statistics.

Multiple pregnancies are high risk as they carry risks for both the mother and the fetus. They are often complicated by preterm delivery, intrauterine growth restriction or a small-for-gestational-age fetus and their sequelae, pre-eclampsia and eclampsia, gestational diabetes, antepartum haemorrhage and assisted delivery. Multiple pregnancies are associated with high infant mortality and morbidity, and carry major long-term consequences for childhood and adult life, especially in terms of neurodevelopmental impairments. Moreover, twin and higher order pregnancies carry significant socioeconomic and psychological consequences for family life.

Approximately 20% of the increase in multiple births can be attributed to advanced maternal age, as it is known that older women are more likely to have a multiple pregnancy. The remainder is associated with ovulation induction and assisted reproductive technologies, such as IVF and ICSI. The exact numbers of higher order pregnancies resulting from ovarian stimulation, with or without IUI, are unknown as there are no national registers that record the outcome of controlled ovarian simulation (ESHRE Task Force on Ethics and Law 2003).

Nonetheless, ovarian simulation, with or without IUI, contributes significantly to the occurrence of multiple births. A study by Lynch et al (2001) showed that 20% of all multiple pregnancies were attributable to ovulation induction agents, which is considerably higher than the 14% attributable to IVF. Similarly, 34% of higher order pregnancies in the UK in 1989 resulted from ovulation induction (Levene et al 1992). Multiple pregnancies occurred in 2–13% of women with all causes of infertility taking CC, whereas women with clomiphene-resistant PCOS treated with gonadotrophins have a multiple pregnancy rate of 36%.

In view of these facts, it is mandatory to design prevention strategies to avoid multiple gestations. In the case of ovarian stimulation, judicious use of ovulation induction drugs and monitoring of the follicular size and number with ultrasonography are essential. In addition to this, ovulation induction ought to be carried out in specialist clinics so that careful monitoring is achieved. Furthermore, specific interventions may reduce the risk of multiple pregnancy. These include withholding the hCG injection and cancelling the cycle, selective aspiration of supernumerary follicles and conversion to IVF cycles. Women who undergo ovulation induction must be counselled regarding the risk of multiple pregnancy and its consequences.

In the event of multiple pregnancy, selective fetal reduction ought to be considered. Multifetal pregnancy reduction (MFPR) refers to 'the termination of one or more normal fetuses in a multifetal pregnancy in order to improve survival rates for the remaining fetuses and decrease maternal morbidity'. For higher order pregnancies, not performing a reduction will increase the risk of losing the pregnancy.

Three different techniques of MFPR have been described. The most commonly used is the transabdominal needle insertion of potassium chloride to the fetal thorax above the diaphragm. This procedure is usually performed at 10–12 weeks of gestation. The selection of the embryo is based on which one is easiest to reach. The second method is the transcervical mini-suction, done between 8 and 11 weeks. Loss of the entire pregnancy has been reported in 50% of cases managed with this technique. The third method consists of transvaginal aspiration of the embryo, usually done at 10–12 weeks (Evans et al 1998).

It is widely accepted that for any higher order multiple pregnancy, reduction to twins has the highest survival rate. Reduction to a singleton pregnancy is not accepted because of the risk of losing that pregnancy if there is a problem later. Women with significant medical disease, such as cardiac disease, or uterine malformations are exceptions to this rule, and reduction to a singleton pregnancy may be considered in such cases (Evans et al 1998).

Prevention of multiple pregnancies should be preferred to MFPR, since it is associated with the ethical dilemmas of abortion. Moreover, it is acknowledged that the original higher order pregnancy may have detrimental effects on the development of the remaining fetuses, in terms of risk of preterm delivery, even after the event of fetocide (ESHRE Task Force on Ethics and Law 2003).

Ovarian cancer

Ovarian cancer is the fourth most common cancer among women in England and Wales, and is the most common cause of gynaecological cancer death. The possibility of a link between ovulation and ovarian oncogenesis led to concerns that fertility treatments may increase the risk of developing ovarian cancer. In particular, the possible association between drugs used for ovulation induction and the risk of ovarian cancer has been the subject of much debate. Concerns have been raised about the effects of multiple ovulations and trauma to the ovarian epithelium (Fathalla 1971), as well as the high levels of gonadotrophins reached during fertility treatment. It has been speculated that the latter may lead to the production of intraovarian carcinogens and malignant transformation (Daly 1992).

A causal relationship between fertility treatment and ovarian cancer was supported by some anecdotal case reports and epidemiological studies. However, other studies showed conflicting results.

A collaborative analysis on data from 12 case–control studies of ovarian cancer conducted in the USA (Whittemore et al 1992) showed that the risk was increased among women who had used fertility drugs (OR 2.8, 95% CI 1.3–6.1) compared with women without a clinical history of infertility. On the other hand, infertile women who had not used fertility drugs experienced no increase in risk (OR 0.91, 95% CI 0.66–1.3). The above risk was higher among nulligravid women than among gravid women. Nevertheless, the information available on specific fertility medication was too incomplete to draw any conclusions.

A case–control study found that women taking clomiphene had a higher risk of developing the disease compared with women who were not taking clomiphene (RR 2.3, 95% CI 0.5–11.4). Prolonged use of clomiphene (12 months or more) was associated with a higher risk of ovarian cancer (RR 11.1, 95% CI 1.5–82.3). Nonetheless, treatment with the drug for less than 1 year was not associated with increased risk (Rossing et al 1994).

On the other hand, several reviews have reported insufficient evidence to support a direct causal relationship between fertility drug treatment and ovarian cancer (Nugent et al 1998, Klip et al 2000).

A UK epidemiological report of cancer incidence among women who had ovarian stimulation treatment found no evidence of a link between infertility treatment and ovarian cancer. This cohort study included 5556 women of whom 75% received ovulation induction drug treatment. The incidence rates of ovarian carcinoma were not significantly different from expectation based on national cancer rates (Doyle et al 2002).

It is acknowledged that nulliparous women who have not received any fertility treatment have almost double the risk of ovarian malignancy. Therefore, the association between nulliparity, infertility and ovarian cancer needs to be considered, as infertility appears to be an independent risk factor for ovarian malignancy. This link may be the reason behind the conflicting results of research.

In view of the above controversial evidence, women who receive ovulation induction therapy should be monitored closely and the number of treatment cycles should be shortened. It is accepted that ovulation induction with clomiphene is not associated with increased risk of ovarian malignancy, provided it is not used for more than 12 cycles. Its administration should be confined to the lowest effective dose. Gonadotrophins should be used for the lowest number of cycles and at the lowest effective doses possible.

Women who undergo fertility treatment ought to be counselled regarding the possible association between medical ovulation induction and ovarian cancer, and their informed consent should be sought (National Institute for Health and Clinical Excellence 2004). A survey of women attending a fertility clinic reported that the majority (67%) of women were aware of the potential link between fertility treatment and ovarian cancer. Moreover, 79% of participants were willing to accept this potential increased risk (Rosen et al 1997).

Other cancers

There is no current evidence to support a link between ovulation induction therapy and other cancers, such as breast, cervical, endometrial, colorectal and thyroid cancer and melanoma (Klip et al 2000).

Prion disease

It is common knowledge that products derived from or containing materials of human or bovine origin carry the theoretical risk of transmitting prion disease. This risk could apply to gonadotrophins of pituitary or urinary extraction origin. Nevertheless, to date, there has been no evidence of transmission of prion disease by any gonadotrophin (National Institute for Health and Clinical Excellence 2004). As a precaution, the Committee on Safety of Medicines recommended that no human urine used in the production of medicines should be sourced from a country with one or more indigenous cases of variant Creutzfeldt–Jakob disease.

Conclusions

Successful induction of ovulation can usually be achieved in the majority of women with anovulation, and high pregnancy rates can be obtained provided that no other fertility factors are present. Appropriate initial investigation will determine the underlying cause and direct the clinician to the most appropriate treatment to correct anovulation.

KEY POINTS

1. The cohort of growing follicles undergoes a process of recruitment, selection, dominance and growth which takes approximately 85 days.

2. Understanding the concept of the FSH threshold and window is essential to achieve the goal of ovulation induction (i.e. development of a single follicle and subsequent ovulation in anovulatory women).

3. In developed countries, 20–25% of patients who present with infertility suffer from ovulation disorders.

4. Appropriate investigation of the hypothalamic–pituitary–ovarian axis, thyroid and adrenal function are necessary to categorize patients accurately and choose an appropriate method of ovulation induction.

5. Anovulatory patients should be fully informed of the success of each method, the monitoring required and the possible associated risks prior to initiating the treatment. Simple treatment associated with low complication rates and lower costs should be tried first.

6. Each unit offering ovulation induction treatment should be equipped with skilful ultrasonography and specialist endocrine laboratory services. Local protocols should be available to reduce or prevent the risk of multiple pregnancy and OHSS.

7. Pulsatile GnRH treatment should be the treatment of choice for anovulatory patients suffering from hypogonadotrophic hypogonadism with low levels of endogenous oestradiol because of reduced risks compared with gonadotrophin treatment.

8. Careful monitoring of ovarian response with ultrasound and serum oestradiol measurements is required in every patient administered gonadotrophin therapy.

9. Treatment of patients with PCOS with anovulation remains a challenge. If they are overweight (BMI ≥30), weight loss should be the first approach.

10. Laparoscopic drilling in clomiphene-resistant PCOS patients should be considered before administering gonadotrophins to avoid the risk of OHSS and multiple pregnancies.

11. The place of metformin and letrozole alone to induce ovulation in patients with PCOS is yet to be clarified from appropriate randomized controlled trials.

12. Risk factors for OHSS have been identified. If patients fall within these categories, very careful and prudent administration of gonadotrophins is required, particularly when more than one risk factor exists.

13. Cancellation of the cycle or conversion to an IVF cycle is recommended if too many follicles are recruited and reach maturity during ovulation induction cycles.

14. The association between ovarian cancer risk and gonadotrophin-stimulated cycles or prolonged clomiphene use remains unclear. The use of the lowest dose of either group of drugs which achieves ovulation is recommended.

References

Adams J, Polson DW, Franks S 1986 Prevalence of polycystic ovaries in women with anovulation and idiopathic hirsutism. British Medical Journal 293: 355–359.

Al-Inany HG, Aboulghar M, Mansour R, Proctor M 2005 Recombinant versus urinary human chorionic gonadotrophin for ovulation induction in assisted conception. Cochrane Database of Systematic Reviews 2: CD003719.

Al-Inany H, Johnson N 2006 Drugs for anovulatory infertility in polycystic ovary syndrome. BMJ (Clinical Research Ed.) 332: 1461–1462.

Amer SA 2007 Gonadotrophin induction of ovulation. Obstetrics, Gynaecology and Reproductive Medicine 17: 205–210.

Amer SA, Banu Z, Li TC, Cooke ID 2002 Long-term follow-up of patients with polycystic ovary syndrome after laparoscopic ovarian drilling: endocrine and ultrasonographic outcomes. Human Reproduction 17: 2851–2857.

Atay V, Cam C, Muhcu M, Cam M, Karateke A 2006 Comparison of letrozole and clomiphene citrate in women with polycystic ovaries undergoing ovarian stimulation. Journal of International Medical Research 34: 73–76.

Balen A 2004 Ovulation induction. Current Obstetrics and Gynaecology 14: 261–268.

Barroso G, Menocal G, Felix H, Rojas-Ruiz JC, Aswan M, Oehninger S 2006 Comparison of the efficacy of the aromatase inhibitor letrozole and clomiphene citrate as adjuvants to recombinant follicle-stimulating hormone in controlled ovarian hyperstimulation: a prospective, randomized, blinded clinical trial. Fertility and Sterility 86: 1428–1431.

Bayar U, Tanriverdi HA, Barut A, Ayoplu F, Ozcan O, Kaya E 2006 Letrozole vs. clomiphene citrate in patients with ovulatory infertility. Fertility and Sterility 85:1045–1048.

Bayram N, van Wely M, van Der Veen F 2001 Recombinant FSH versus urinary gonadotrophins or recombinant FSH for ovulation induction in subfertility associated with polycystic ovary syndrome. Cochrane Database of Systematic Reviews 2: CD002121.

Bayram N, van Wely M, Vanderkerckhove P, Lilford R, van der Veen F 2004 Pulsatile luteinizing hormone releasing hormone for ovulation induction in subfertility associated with polycystic ovary syndrome. Cochrane Database of Systematic Reviews 1: CD000412.

Beck JI, Boothroyd C, Proctor M, Farquhar C, Hughes E 2005 Oral anti-oestrogens and medical adjuncts for subfertility associated with anovulation. Cochrane Database of Systematic Reviews 1: CD002249.

Blankstein J, Shalev J, Saadon T et al 1987 Ovarian hyperstimulation syndrome: prediction by number and size of preovulatory ovarian follicles. Fertility and Sterility 47: 597–602.

Boostanfar R 2001 A prospective randomized trial comparing clomiphene citrate with tamoxifen citrate for ovulation induction. Fertility and Sterility 75: 1024–1026.

Braat DD, Schoemaker R, Schoemaker J 1991 Life table analysis of fecundity in intravenously gonadotropin-releasing hormone-treated patients with normogonadotropic and hypogonadotropic amenorrhoea. Fertility and Sterility 55: 266–271.

Cantineau AEP, Cohlen BJ, Heineman MJ 2007 Ovarian stimulation protocols (anti-oestrogens, gonadotrophins with and without GnRH agonists/antagonists) for intrauterine insemination (IUI) in women with subfertility. Cochrane Database of Systematic Reviews 2: CD005356.

Clark AM, Ledger W, Galletly C et al 1995 Weight loss results in significant improvement in pregnancy and ovulation rates in anovulatory obese women. Human Reproduction 10: 2705–2712.

Daly MB 1992 The epidemiology of ovarian cancer. Hematology/Oncology Clinics of North America 6: 729–738.

Davar R, Asgharnia M, Tayebi N, Aflatoonian A 2006 Comparison of the use of letrozole and clomiphene citrate in regularly ovulating women undergoing intrauterine insemination. Middle East Fertility Society Journal 11: 113–118.

Delvigne A, Rozenberg S 2002 Epidemiology and prevention of ovarian hyperstimulation syndrome (OHSS): a review. Human Reproduction Update 8: 559–577.

Doyle P, Maconochie N, Beral V, Swerdlow AS, Tan SL 2002 Cancer incidence following treatment for infertility at a clinic in the UK. Human Reproduction 17: 2209–2213.

ESHRE Task Force on Ethics and Law 2003 Ethical issues related to multiple pregnancies in medically assisted procreation. Human Reproduction 18: 1976–1979.

Evans MI, Kramer RL, Yaron Y, Drugan A, Johnson MP 1998 What are the ethical and technical problems associated with multifetal pregnancy reduction? Clinical Obstetrics and Gynecology 41: 46–54.

Farquhar C, Lilford RJ, Marjoribanks J, Vandekerckhove P 2007 Laparoscopic 'drilling' by diathermy or laser for ovulation induction in anovulatory polycystic ovary syndrome. Cochrane Database of Systematic Reviews 3: CD001122.

Fathalla MF 1971 Incessant ovulation — a factor in ovarian neoplasia. The Lancet ii: 163.

Filicori M , Flamigni C, Cognigni P et al 1994 Treatment of anovulation with pulsatile gonadotrophin-releasing hormone: prognostic factors and clinical results in 600 cycles. Journal of Clinical Endocrinology and Metabolism 79: 1215–1220.

George K, Nair R, Tharyan P 2008 Ovulation triggers in anovulatory women undergoing ovulation induction. Cochrane Database of Systematic Reviews 3: CD006900.

Gerhard I, Runnebaum B 1979 Comparison between tamoxifen and clomiphene therapy in women with anovulation. Archives of Gynecology 227: 279–288.

Gjonnaess H 1998 Late endocrine effects of ovarian electrocautery in women with polycystic ovary syndrome. Fertility and Sterility 69: 697–701.

Gysler M, March CM, Mishell DR Jr, Bailey EJ 1982 A decade's experience with an individualized clomiphene treatment regimen including its effect on the postcoital test. Fertility and Sterility 37: 161–167.

Hughes E, Collins J, Vandekerckhove P 2000 Clomiphene citrate for unexplained subfertility in women. Cochrane Database of Systematic Reviews 2: CD000057.

Update in Cochrane Database of Systematic Reviews 2000; 3: CD000057.

Jee BC, Ku SY, Suh CS, Kim KC, Lee WD, Kim SH 2006 Use of letrozole versus clomiphene citrate combined with gonadotropins in intrauterine insemination cycles: a pilot study. Fertility and Sterility 85: 1774–1777.

Klip H, Burger CW, Kenemans P, van Leeuwen FE 2000 Cancer risk associated with subfertility and ovulation induction: a review. Cancer Causes and Control 11: 319–344.

Legro RS, Barnhart HX, Schlaff WD et al 2007 Clomiphene, metformin, or both for infertility in the polycystic ovary syndrome. New England Journal of Medicine 356: 551–566.

Levene MI, Wild J, Steer P 1992 Higher multiple births and the modern management of infertility in Britain. The British Association of Perinatal Medicine. BJOG: an International Journal of Obstetrics and Gynaecology 99: 607–613.

Lord JM, Flight IH, Norman RJ 2003 Insulin-sensitising drugs (metformin, troglitazone, rosiglitazone, pioglitazone, D-chiro-inositol) for polycystic ovary syndrome. Cochrane Database of Systematic Reviews 3: CD003053.

Lynch A, McDuffie R, Murphy J et al 2001 Assisted reproductive interventions and multiple birth. Obstetrics and Gynecology 97: 195–200.

Maheshwari A, Stofberg L, Bhattacharya S 2007 Effect of overweight on assisted reproductive technology — a systematic review, Human Reproduction Update 13: 433–444.

Martin KA, Hall JE, Adams JM, Crowley JNWF 1993 Comparison of exogenous gonadotropins and pulsatile gonadotropin-releasing hormone for induction of ovulation in hypogonadotropic amenorrhoea. Journal of Clinical Endocrinology and Metabolism 77: 125–129.

Milson SR, Gibson G, Buckingham K, Gunn AJ 2002 Factors associated with pregnancy or miscarriage after clomiphene therapy in WHO Group II anovulatory women. Australian and New Zealand Journal of Obstetrics and Gynaecology 42: 170–175.

Mitwally MF, Casper RF 2004 Aromatase inhibition reduces the dose of gonadotrophin required for controlled ovarian hyperstimulation. Journal of the Society for Gynecologic Investigation 11: 406–415.

Moll E, Bossuyt PMM, Korevaar JC, Lambalk CB, van der Veen F 2006 Effect of clomiphene citrate plus metformin and clomiphene citrate plus placebo on induction of ovulation in women with newly diagnosed polycystic ovary syndrome: randomised double blind clinical trial. BMJ (Clinical Research Ed.) 332: 1485–1488.

National Institute for Health and Clinical Excellence 2004 Clinical Guideline 11. Fertility: Assessment and Treatment for People with Fertility Problems. NICE, London.

Nugent D, Salha O, Balen AH, Rutherford AJ 1998 Ovarian neoplasia and subfertility treatments. BJOG: an International Journal of Obstetrics and Gynaecology 105: 584–591.

Nugent D, Vandekerckhove P, Hughes E, Arnot M, Lilford R 2000 Gonadotrophin therapy for ovulation induction in subfertility associated with polycystic ovary syndrome. Cochrane Database of Systematic Reviews 4: CD000410.

Office for National Statistics 2006 Population Censuses and Surveys. Birth Statistics. Births: 1938–2004, Maternities with Multiple Births. HMSO.

Pascal-Vigneron V, Weryha G, Bosc M, Leclere J 1995 [Hyperprolactinemic amenorrhea: treatment with cabergoline versus bromocriptine. Results of a national multicenter randomized double-blind study]. Presse Medicale 24: 753–757.

Royal College of Obstetricians and Gynaecologists 2006 The Management of Ovarian Hyperstimulation Syndrome. Green-top Guideline No. 5. RCOG, London.

Royal College of Obstetricians and Gynaecologists 2007 Long-term Consequences of Polycystic Ovary Syndrome. Green-top Guideline No. 33. RCOG, London.

Rosen B, Irvine J, Ritvo P et al 1997 The feasibility of assessing women's perceptions of the risks and benefits of fertility drug therapy in relation to ovarian cancer risk. Fertility and Sterility 68: 90–94.

Rossing MA, Daling JR, Weiss NS, Moore DE, Self SG 1994 Ovarian tumors in a cohort of infertile women. New England Journal of Medicine 331: 771–776.

Shoham Z, Balen A, Patel A, Jacobs HS 1991 Results of ovulation induction using human menopausal gonadotropin or purified follicle stimulating hormone in hypogonadotropic hypogonadism patients. Fertility and Sterility 56: 1048–1053.

Steiner AZ, Terplan M, Paulson RJ 2005 Comparison of tamoxifen and clomiphene citrate for ovulation induction: a meta-analysis. Human Reproduction 20: 1511–1515.

Suginami H 1993 A clomiphene citrate and tamoxifen citrate combination therapy: a novel therapy for ovulation induction. Fertility and Sterility 59: 976–979.

Vandermolen DT, Ratts VS, Evans WS, Stovall DW, Kauma SW, Nestler JE 2001 Metformin increases the ovulatory rate and pregnancy rate from clomiphene citrate in patients with polycystic ovary syndrome who are resistant to clomiphene citrate alone. Fertility and Sterility 75: 310–315.

Vegetti W 1998 Ovarian stimulation with low-dose pure follicle-stimulating hormone in polycystic ovarian syndrome anovulatory patients: effect of long-term pretreatment with gonadotrophin-releasing hormone analogue. Gynecologic and Obstetric Investigation 45: 186–189.

Venn A, Lumley J 1994 Clomiphene citrate and pregnancy outcome. Australian and New Zealand Journal of Obstetrics and Gynaecology 34: 56–66.

Webster J, Piscitelli G, Polli A, Ferrari CI, Ismail I, Scanlon MF 1994 A comparison of cabergoline and bromocriptine in the treatment of hyperprolactinemic amenorrhea. Cabergoline Comparative Study Group. New England Journal of Medicine 331: 904–909.

Whittemore AS, Harris R, Itnyre J 1992 Characteristics relating to ovarian cancer risk: collaborative analysis of 12 US case–control studies. II. Invasive epithelial ovarian cancers in white women. Collaborative Ovarian Cancer Group. American Journal of Epidemiology 136: 1184–1203.

CHAPTER 18

Polycystic ovary syndrome

Adam Balen

Chapter Contents

INTRODUCTION	251	MANAGEMENT OF NON-FERTILITY ASPECTS OF POLYCYSTIC OVARIES	258
PATHOGENESIS	251	OVULATION INDUCTION	260
INVESTIGATIONS	253	CONCLUSIONS	263
HETEROGENEITY OF PCOS	255	KEY POINTS	263
HEALTH CONSEQUENCES	256		

Introduction

Polycystic ovary syndrome (PCOS) is the most common endocrine disturbance affecting women, and is a heterogeneous collection of signs and symptoms that, gathered together, form a spectrum of a disorder with a mild presentation in some women, and a severe disturbance of reproductive, endocrine and metabolic function in other women (Balen et al 1995). The pathophysiology of PCOS appears to be multifactorial. The definition of PCOS has been much debated. Key features include menstrual cycle disturbance, hyperandrogenism and obesity. There are many extraovarian aspects to the pathophysiology of PCOS, yet ovarian dysfunction is central. The international consensus definition of PCOS is the presence of two out of the following three criteria: (i) oligo-ovulation and/or anovulation; (ii) hyperandrogenism (clinical and/or biochemical); and (iii) polycystic ovaries, with the exclusion of other aetiologies of menstrual disturbance or hyperandrogenism (Fauser et al 2004). There is considerable heterogeneity of symptoms and signs amongst women with PCOS, and for an individual, these may change over time. Polycystic ovaries can exist without clinical signs of PCOS, expression of which may be precipitated by various factors, most predominantly an increase in body weight.

The morphology of the polycystic ovary is an ovary with 12 or more follicles measuring 2–9 mm in diameter and/or increased ovarian volume (>10 cm^3) (Balen et al 2003) (Figures 18.1–18.5). Polycystic ovaries are commonly detected by pelvic ultrasound, with estimates of prevalence in the general population being in the order of 20–33% (Michelmore et al 1999). However, not all women with polycystic ovaries demonstrate the clinical and biochemical features which define PCOS. These include menstrual cycle disturbances, hirsutism, acne, alopecia and abnormalities of biochemical profiles, including elevated serum concentrations of luteinizing hormone (LH), testosterone and androstenedione. Obesity and hyperinsulinaemia are associated features, although only 40–50% of women with PCOS are overweight (Balen and Michelmore 2002). Presentation of PCOS is so varied that one, all or any combination of the above features may be present in association with an ultrasound picture of polycystic ovaries (Table 18.1).

Pathogenesis

The pathogenesis of polycystic ovaries and PCOS is still being elucidated, but the heterogeneity of presentation of PCOS suggests that a single cause is unlikely. Some genetic studies have identified a link between PCOS and disordered insulin metabolism, and indicate that PCOS may be the presentation of a complex genetic trait disorder (Franks et al 2001). PCOS runs in families, with approximately half of first-degree relatives (i.e. sisters, mothers and daughters) also being affected; incidentally, male relatives also show an increased rate of metabolic problems. The features of obesity, hyperinsulinaemia and hyperandrogenaemia, which are commonly seen in PCOS, are also known to be factors which confer an increased risk of cardiovascular disease and type 2 diabetes (Rajkowha et al 2000). There are studies which indicate that women with PCOS have an increased risk for these diseases which pose long-term risks for health.

PCOS appears to have its origins during adolescence and is thought to be associated with increased weight gain during puberty. However, the polycystic ovary gene(s) has not yet been identified, and the effects of environmental influences such as weight changes and circulating hormone concentrations, and the age at which these occur, are still being unravelled. Prior to puberty, there appears to be two periods of increased ovarian growth. The first is at adrenarche in response to increased concentrations of circulating

Table 18.1 The spectrum of clinical manifestations of polycystic ovary syndrome

Symptoms	Serum endocrinology	Possible late sequelae
Obesity	↑ Androgens (testosterone and androstenedione)	Diabetes mellitus Dyslipidaemia
Menstrual disturbance	↑ Luteinizing hormone	Hypertension
Infertility	↑ Fasting insulin ↑ Prolactin	Cardiovascular disease
Hyperandrogenism	↓ Sex-hormone-binding globulin ↑ Oestradiol, oestrone	Endometrial carcinoma Breast cancer
Asymptomatic		

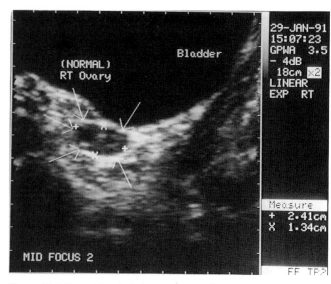

Figure 18.1 Transabdominal ultrasound scan of a normal ovary.

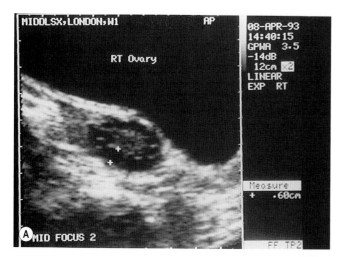

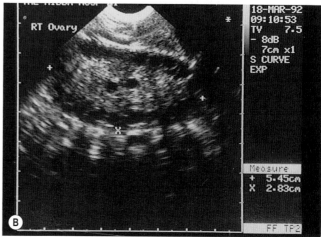

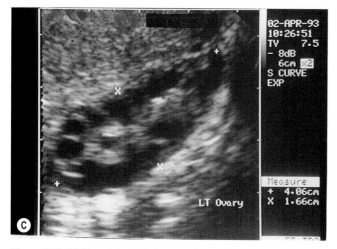

Figure 18.2 (A) Transabdominal ultrasound scan of a polycystic ovary. (B,C) Transabdominal ultrasound scans of a polycystic ovary.

androgens, and the second is just before and during puberty due to rising gonadotrophin levels, and the actions of growth hormone, insulin-like growth factor-1 (IGF-1) and insulin on the ovary. Sampaolo et al (1994) reported a study of 49 obese girls at different stages of puberty, com-paring their pelvic ultrasound features and endocrine pro-files with 35 age- and pubertal-stage-matched controls. They found that obesity was associated with a significant increase in uterine and ovarian volume. They also found that obese postmenarcheal girls with polycystic ovaries had larger

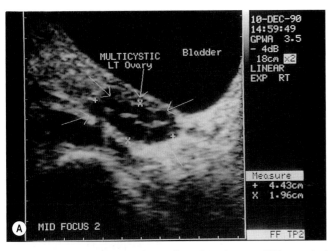

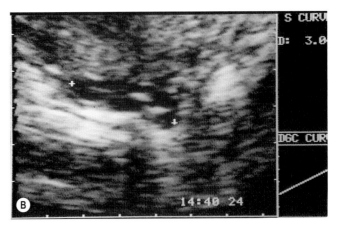

Figure 18.3 (A) Transabdominal scan of a multicystic ovary. (B) Transvaginal ultrasound scan of a multicystic ovary.

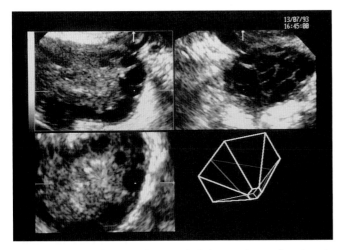

Figure 18.4 Three-dimensional transvaginal ultrasound scan of a polycystic ovary.
Courtesy of Dr A. Kyei-Mensah.

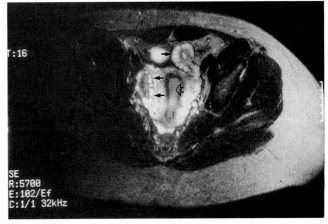

Figure 18.5 Magnetic resonance imaging of a pelvis, demonstrating two polycystic ovaries (closed arrows) and a hyperplastic endometrium (open arrow).

uterine and ovarian volumes than obese postmenarcheal girls with normal ovaries. Sampaolo et al concluded that obesity leads to hyperinsulinism, which causes both hyperandrogenaemia and raised IGF-1 levels, which augments the ovarian response to gonadotrophins. This implies that obesity may be important in the pathogenesis of polycystic ovaries, but further study is required to evaluate this. It is known that obesity is not a prerequisite for PCOS. After menarche, it is common for the menstrual cycle to be erratic for several months. If the irregularity persists beyond 2 years, there is a high chance that the adolescent girl has PCOS.

Investigations

The investigation of PCOS requires the exclusion of specific underlying diseases of the hypothalamic–pituitary–ovarian axis and the adrenal glands in order to exclude endocrine causes of menstrual cycle disturbance (e.g. hyperprolactinaemia, thyroid disease, hypothalamic dysfunction, ovarian failure), and other causes of androgen excess such as congenital adrenal hyperplasia (CAH), Cushing's syndrome or androgen-secreting tumours of the ovary or adrenal gland.

Endocrine profile

An endocrine profile is best taken during a menstrual bleed, although it may need to be taken at random in an oligomenorrhoeic or amenorrhoeic woman. Follicle-stimulating hormone (FSH), LH, oestradiol, testosterone, prolactin and thyroid function should be measured. If the patient wishes to conceive, it is necessary to ascertain whether ovulation is occurring. Patients with anovulatory infertility will have oligomenorrhoea or amenorrhoea and a low luteal-phase progesterone. A progesterone concentration of more than 30 nmol/l suggests ovulation, but it can be difficult to know when to take the blood if the patient has an erratic cycle, and impossible if she is amenorrhoeic. If the progesterone concentration is 15–30 nmol/l, the timing may have been incorrect. It is then necessary to check the timing of the blood test to subsequent menstruation, and repeat the test

Table 18.2 Hormonal patterns in different causes of menstrual irregularity

Follicle-stimulating hormone	Luteinizing hormone	Oestradiol	Diagnosis
Normal	Elevated	Usually normal	Polycystic ovary syndrome
Normal	Low	Low	Weight-related amenorrhoea
Low	Low	Low	Hypogonadotrophic hypogonadism, functional or organic
Elevated	Elevated	Low	If oligomenorrhoeic or amenorrhoeic: ovarian failure
Elevated	Elevated	High	If mid-cycle, think of mid-cycle surge

in the following cycle (sometimes two progesterone measurements in the same cycle are helpful). The optimal way to assess ovulation in women with irregular cycles is by a combination of serial ultrasound scans and serum endocrine measurements (FSH and LH in the follicular phase, progesterone in the luteal phase).

Women with PCOS usually have a normal serum FSH concentration (Table 18.2). LH is the second gonadotrophin which, like FSH, is released by the gonadotrophs in the anterior pituitary gland, under the influence of pulsatile release of gonadotrophin-releasing hormone (GnRH). The differential control of FSH and LH secretion relies upon the need for priming of the pituitary by oestradiol before it will become responsive to GnRH and release LH. FSH secretion, on the other hand, is under tonic inhibitory control by inhibin acting in a negative feedback loop from the ovaries. Therefore, in times of oestrogen deficiency, such as weight-related amenorrhoea, LH concentrations in the circulation are lower than FSH, whilst the mid-cycle surge that is primed by rising oestradiol secretion from the ovary results in a greater release of LH than FSH.

An elevated serum concentration of LH in the follicular phase of the cycle suggests that the patient has PCOS, usually associated with a concentration of more than 10 IU/l in the early to mid-follicular phase of the cycle. In a series of over 1700 women with PCOS, approximately 40% of patients were found to have an elevated serum concentration of LH, which was associated with a significantly higher risk of infertility than in those with normal LH levels (Balen et al 1995). Other causes of an elevated LH serum concentration are the mid-cycle surge and ovarian failure (Table 18.2).

LH stimulates ovarian production of androgens, and LH is most commonly elevated in slim women with PCOS. In overweight women, hypersecretion of insulin is the main cause of androgen secretion by the ovaries.

The normal female range for total serum testosterone is 0.5–3.5 nmol/l. The most usual cause of an elevated serum testosterone level is PCOS. Most women with PCOS, however, have a normal total serum testosterone concentration. Measurement of the sex-hormone-binding globulin (SHBG) concentration (normal range 16–119 nmol/l) will permit calculation of the 'free androgen index' [(testosterone × 100)/SHBG], which should be less than 5. Women who are obese have high circulating levels of insulin which reduces synthesis of SHBG by the liver, so the free androgen index is often elevated when total testosterone is in the normal range.

If the serum testosterone concentration is greater than 5 nmol/l, it is necessary to exclude other causes of hyperandrogenaemia, such as late-onset CAH, Cushing's syndrome and androgen-secreting tumours. Women with the most common form of CAH (21-hydroxylase deficiency) will have an elevated serum 17-hydroxyprogesterone concentration (17-OHP >20 nmol/l) and an exaggerated response to an intravenous bolus of adrenocorticotrophic hormone (250 mg tetracosactrin will cause an elevation of 17-OHP, usually between 65 and 470 nmol/l).

Features of hyperandrogenism

Signs of hyperandrogenism (acne, hirsutism, balding) are suggestive of PCOS, although biochemical screening helps to differentiate other causes of androgen excess. Hirsutism can be graded and given a 'Ferriman Gallwey score'. It is useful to monitor the progress of hirsutism, or its response to treatment, by making serial records, either using a chart or by taking photographs of affected areas of the body. It is important to distinguish between hyperandrogenism and virilization, which is associated with high circulating androgen levels and causes deepening of the voice, increase in muscle bulk, breast atrophy and cliteromegaly. Virilization suggests a more profound disturbance of androgen secretion than usually seen with PCOS, and indicates the need to exclude CAH, Cushing's syndrome and androgen-secreting tumours.

Hyperinsulinaemia

The association between insulin resistance, compensatory hyperinsulinaemia and hyperandrogenism has provided insight into the pathogenesis of PCOS. The cellular and molecular mechanisms of insulin resistance in PCOS have been investigated extensively, and it is evident that the major defect is a decrease in insulin sensitivity secondary to a post-binding abnormality in insulin-receptor-mediated signal transduction, with a less substantial, but significant, decrease in insulin responsiveness (Dunaif 1997). It appears that decreased insulin sensitivity in PCOS is potentially an intrinsic defect in genetically susceptible women, since it is independent of obesity, metabolic abnormalities, body fat topography and sex hormone levels.

Although the insulin resistance may occur irrespective of body mass index (BMI), the common association between PCOS and obesity has a synergistic deleterious impact on glucose homeostasis, and can worsen both hyperandrogenism and anovulation. An assessment of BMI alone is not thought to provide a reliable prediction of cardiovascular risk. It has been reported that the association between BMI and coronary heart disease almost disappeared after correction for dyslipidaemia, hyperglycaemia and hypertension. Some women have profound metabolic abnormalities in the presence of a normal BMI, and others have few risk factors with an elevated BMI. It has been suggested that rather than BMI itself, it is the distribution of fat that is important, with android obesity being more of a risk factor than gynaecoid obesity. Hence the value of measuring the waist:hip ratio or waist circumference, which detect abdominal visceral fat rather than subcutaneous fat. It is the visceral fat which is metabolically active and, when increased, results in increased rates of insulin resistance, type 2 diabetes, dyslipidaemia, hypertension and left ventricular enlargement. There is a closer link between waist circumference and visceral fat mass, as assessed by computer tomography, than waist:hip ratio or BMI (Lord and Wilkin 2002). Waist circumference should ideally be less than 79 cm, whilst a measurement of greater than 87 cm carries a significant risk. Exercise has a significant effect on reducing visceral fat and reducing cardiovascular risk; indeed, a 10% reduction in body weight may equate to a 30% reduction in visceral fat.

Insulin acts through multiple sites to increase endogenous androgen levels. Increased peripheral insulin resistance results in a higher serum insulin concentration. Excess insulin binds to IGF-1 receptors which enhances androgen production by theca cells in response to LH stimulation. Hyperinsulinaemia also decreases the synthesis of SHBG by the liver. Therefore, there is an increase in the serum free testosterone concentration, and consequent peripheral androgen action. Intraovarian androgen excess is responsible for anovulation by acting directly on the ovary, promoting the process of follicular atresia. This latter process is characterized by apoptosis of granulosa cells. As a consequence, there is an increasingly larger stromal compartment, which retains LH responsiveness and continues to secrete androgens. Hyperinsulinaemia also stimulates trophic changes in the skin that results in acanthosis nigricans in the skin creases (Figure 18.6).

Insulin resistance is defined as a reduced glucose response to a given amount of insulin and may occur secondary to resistance at the insulin receptor, decreased hepatic clearance of insulin and/or increased pancreatic sensitivity. Both obese and non-obese women with PCOS are more insulin resistant and hyperinsulinaemic than age- and weight-matched women with normal ovaries. Thus, there appear to be factors in women with PCOS which promote insulin resistance and that are independent of obesity.

Insulin resistance can be measured by a number of expensive and complex tests, but it is not necessary to measure it routinely in clinical practice; it is more important to check for impaired glucose tolerance. Simple screening tests for risk of impaired glucose tolerance (IGT) include an assessment of BMI and waist circumference. If the fasting blood glucose is less than 5.2 mmmol/l, the risk of impaired glucose tolerance is low. The 2-h standard 75 g oral glucose tolerance test may be conducted in those at high risk (BMI >30 kg/m² in Caucasian women and >25 kg/m² in women from South Asia, who have a greater degree of insulin resistance at a lower body weight) (Table 18.3).

Heterogeneity of PCOS

A few years ago, the author reported a large series of women with polycystic ovaries detected by ultrasound scan

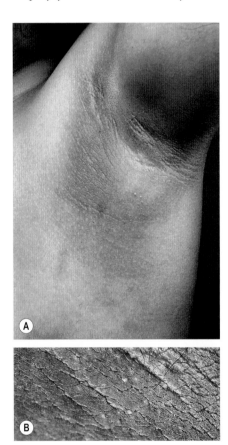

Figure 18.6 Acanthosis nigricans as seen typically in the axilla or skin of the neck in women with insulin resistance. (A) Axilla. (B) Close-up, demonstrating hypertrophic and pigmented skin.

Table 18.3 Definitions of glucose tolerance after a 75 g glucose tolerance test

	Diabetes mellitus	**Impaired glucose tolerance**	**Impaired fasting glycaemia**
Fasting glucose (mmol/l)	≧7.0	<7.0	≧6.1 and <7.0
2-h glucose (mmol/l)	≧11.1	≧7.8	<7.8
Action	Refer to diabetic clinic	Dietary advice. Check fasting glucose annually	Dietary advice. Check fasting glucose annually

(Balen et al 1995). All of the 1871 patients had at least one symptom of PCOS. Thirty-eight percent of the women were overweight (BMI >25 kg/m^2). Obesity was significantly associated with an increased risk of hirsutism, menstrual cycle disturbance and an elevated serum testosterone concentration. Obesity was also associated with an increased rate of infertility. Twenty-six percent of patients with primary infertility and 14% of patients with secondary infertility had a BMI of more than 30 kg/m^2. Approximately 30% of the patients had a regular menstrual cycle, 50% had oligomenorrhoea and 20% had amenorrhoea. In this study, the classical endocrine features of raised serum LH and testosterone were found in 40% and 30% of patients, respectively. Ovarian volume was significantly correlated with serum LH and testosterone concentrations. Other studies have reported correlation between markers of insulin resistance and ovarian volume and ovarian stromal echogenicity, which in turn have been correlated with androgen production.

National and racial differences in expression

Approximately 75–80% of women with polycystic ovaries have signs or symptoms of PCOS. Thus, in the UK, where it has been reported that up to 33% of women have polycystic ovaries (Michelmore et al 1999), 20–25% of women may have a degree of PCOS, albeit mild in many cases. There are large national and ethnic variations in the expression of PCOS, with women from the Far East having little in the way of hirsutism, whilst those with dark hair from Mediterranean and Middle Eastern or South Asian countries have a greater degree of expression. The highest reported prevalence of polycystic ovaries has been 52% among South Asian immigrants in Britain, of whom 49% had menstrual irregularity (Rodin et al 1998). It was also shown that South Asian women with polycystic ovaries had a comparable degree of insulin resistance to controls with established type 2 diabetes. Generally, there has been a paucity of data of the prevalence of PCOS among women of South Asian origin, both among migrant and native groups. Type 2 diabetes and insulin resistance have a high prevalence among indigenous populations in South Asia, with a rising prevalence among women. Insulin resistance and hyperinsulinaemia are common antecedents of type 2 diabetes, with a high prevalence in South Asians. Type 2 diabetes also has a familial basis, inherited as a complex genetic trait that interacts with environmental factors, chiefly nutrition, commencing from fetal life. It has been shown that ethnic variations in the overt features of PCOS (symptoms of hyperandrogenism, menstrual irregularity and obesity) in women of South Asian descent are linked to the higher prevalence and degree of insulin resistance in South Asians. It has also been shown that South Asians with anovulatory PCOS have greater insulin resistance and more severe symptoms of PCOS than anovular White Caucasians with PCOS (Wijeyaratne et al 2002).

The question remains as to whether differences in expression of PCOS are due to dietary and lifestyle factors or to genetic variations in hormone actions, such as polymorphisms in gonadotrophin subunits or receptor function (affecting the expression of androgens, gonadotrophins or insulin). A full discussion of the genetics of PCOS is beyond the scope of this chapter, and there are a number of candidate genes that have been proposed (see Franks et al 2001). It may be that some families or racial groups have genetic differences that affect the expression or presentation of PCOS.

Health Consequences

Ischaemic heart disease

Obesity and metabolic abnormalities are recognized risk factors for the development of ischaemic heart disease (IHD) in the general population, and these are also recognized features of PCOS. In Europe, IHD accounts for 18% of deaths in men and 14% of deaths in women. In men, the incidence of IHD increases after the age of 35 years, while in women, an increased incidence is noted after the age of 55 years. The questions are whether women with PCOS are at increased risk of IHD, and whether this will occur at an earlier age than in women with normal ovaries. The basis for the idea that women with PCOS are at greater risk for cardiovascular disease is that these women are more insulin resistant than weight-matched controls, and that the metabolic disturbances associated with insulin resistance are known to increase cardiovascular risk in other populations.

Insulin resistance

In the general population, cardiovascular risk factors include insulin resistance, obesity (especially an increase in waist circumference), glucose intolerance, diabetes, hypertension and dyslipidaemia (particularly raised serum triglycerides). Insulin sensitivity varies depending upon menstrual pattern. Women with PCOS who are oligomenorrhoeic are more likely to be insulin resistant than those with regular cycles, irrespective of their BMI. Women with PCOS have a defect in insulin signalling at the insulin receptor, which causes insulin resistance. The sex-steroid-induced increase in growth hormone that initiates the adolescent growth spurt also leads to insulin resistance, and explains the timing of onset of symptoms in those prone to develop PCOS. The presence of obesity and/or type 2 diabetes worsens the degree of insulin resistance.

Insulin resistance is restricted to the extrasplanchnic actions of insulin on glucose dispersal. The liver is not affected [hence the decrease in SHBG and high-density lipoproteins (HDLs)], and neither is the ovary (hence the menstrual problems and hypersecretion of androgens) nor the skin (hence the development of acanthosis nigricans). Insulin resistance causes compensatory hypersecretion of insulin, particularly in response to glucose, so euglycaemia is usually maintained at the expense of hyperinsulinaemia.

It is reported that up to 20% of slim women and 40% of obese women with PCOS demonstrate impaired glucose tolerance. Insulin resistance combined with abdominal obesity is thought to account for the higher prevalence of type 2 diabetes in PCOS. There is a concomitant increased risk of gestational diabetes.

Dyslipidaemic women with PCOS have high concentrations of serum triglycerides and suppressed HDL levels, particularly a lower HDL$_2$ subfraction. HDLs play an important role in lipid metabolism and are the most important lipid parameter in predicting cardiovascular risk in women. HDLs perform the task of 'reverse cholesterol transport'. That is, they remove excess lipids from the circulation and tissues to transport them to the liver for excretion, or transfer them to other lipoprotein particles.

In a large retrospective study, Pierpoint et al (1998) reported the mortality rate in 1028 women diagnosed with PCOS between 1930 and 1979. All of the women were over 45 years of age and 770 women had been treated by wedge resection of the ovaries. In total, 786 women were traced; the mean age at diagnosis was 26.4 years and the average duration of follow-up was 30 years. There were 59 deaths, of which 15 were from circulatory disease. Of these 15 deaths, 13 were from IHD. There were six deaths from diabetes as an underlying or contributory cause, compared with the expected 1.7 deaths. The standardized mortality rate (SMR), both overall and for cardiovascular disease, was not higher in the women with PCOS compared with the national mortality rates in women, although the observed proportion of women with diabetes as a contributory or underlying factor leading to death was significantly higher than expected [odds ratio 3.6, 95% confidence interval (CI) 1.5–8.4]. Thus, despite surrogate markers for cardiovascular disease, Pierpoint et al (1998) found no increased rate of death from cardiovascular disease. A follow-up report from the same study, however, did demonstrate an increased, although non-significant, risk of death due to diabetes [after adjustment for BMI, the odds ratio was 2.2 (95% CI 0.9–5.2) for diabetes (Wild et al 2000)]. There was still no increase in long-term coronary heart disease mortality in the PCOS group, although there was evidence of increased stroke-related mortality, even after adjustment for BMI.

Homocysteine

A moderately increased total plasma homocysteine (Hcy) concentration is associated with an increased risk of atherosclerosis. Hcy is an essential intermediate in the transfer of activated methyl groups from tetrahydrofolate to S-adenosylmethionine, in the synthesis of cysteine from methionine, and in the production of homocysteine thiolactone. An abnormal elevation of Hcy in plasma and urine is caused by an imbalance between Hcy production and metabolism, which can be of demographic, genetic, nutritional or metabolic aetiology, and is associated with premature vascular disease. Mild hyperhomocysteinaemia has been demonstrated to induce sustained injury to the arterial endothelial cells that accelerate the development of thrombosis and atherosclerosis. Normal concentrations of total plasma Hcy are in the range of 5–16 µmol/l, although 10 µmol/l is considered to be the desirable upper limit; there is an age-related rise and lower concentrations are found in women. There have been reports of elevated plasma Hcy in Caucasian women with PCOS, and this may be greater in the South Asian population (Rendeva et al 2002). Weight reduction and regular physical exercise are recognized interventions that help to reduce insulin resistance and the metabolic syndrome.

Endometrial cancer

Endometrial adenocarcinoma is the second most common female genital malignancy, but only 4% of cases occur in women under 40 years of age. The risk of developing endometrial cancer has been shown to be adversely influenced by a number of factors including obesity, long-term use of unopposed oestrogens, nulliparity and infertility. The relative risk of endometrial cancer is 1.6 in women with a menarche before the age of 12 years, and 2.4 in women who have their menopause after the age of 52 years (Elwood et al 1977). Women with endometrial carcinoma have had fewer births compared with controls, and it has also been demonstrated that infertility per se gives a relative risk of 2. Hypertension and type 2 diabetes have long been linked to endometrial cancer, with relative risks of 2.1 and 2.8, respectively; these conditions are now known to be associated with PCOS.

A study by Coulam et al (1983) examined the risk of developing endometrial carcinoma in a group of 1270 patients who were diagnosed with chronic anovulation syndrome. The defining characteristics of this group included pathological or macroscopic evidence of the Stein–Leventhal syndrome, or a clinical diagnosis of chronic anovulation. This study identified the excess risk of endometrial cancer to be 3.1 (95% CI 1.1–7.3), and proposed that this might be due to abnormal levels of unopposed oestrogen. However, the true risk of endometrial carcinoma in women with PCOS is difficult to ascertain.

Endometrial hyperplasia

Endometrial hyperplasia may be a precursor to adenocarcinoma, with cystic glandular hyperplasia progressing in perhaps 0.4% of cases and adenomatous hyperplasia in up to 18% of cases over 2–10 years. Precise estimation of the rate of progression is impossible to determine. Some authors have reported conservative management of endometrial adenocarcinoma in women with PCOS, with a combination of curettage and high-dose progestogens. The rationale is that cancer of the endometrium often presents at an early stage, is well differentiated, has a low risk of metastasis, and therefore is not perceived as being life threatening, while poorly differentiated adenocarcinoma in a young woman has a worse prognosis and warrants hysterectomy. In general, however, the literature on women with PCOS and endometrial hyperplasia or adenocarcinoma suggests that this group has a poor prognosis for fertility. This may be because of the factors that predispose to the endometrial pathology — chronic anovulation often combined with severe obesity — or secondary to the endometrial pathology disrupting potential embryonic implantation. Thus, a more traditional and radical surgical approach (i.e. hysterectomy) is suggested as the safest way to prevent progression of the cancer (Balen 2001).

Although the degree of risk has not been clearly defined, it is generally accepted that for women with PCOS who experience amenorrhoea or oligomenorrhoea, the induction of artificial withdrawal bleeds to prevent endometrial hyperplasia is prudent management. Indeed, the author considers it important that women with PCOS should shed their endometrium at least every 3 months. For those women with oligomenorrhoea or amenorrhoea who do not wish to use cyclical hormone therapy, an ultrasound scan is recommended to measure endometrial thickness and morphology every 6–12 months (depending upon menstrual history). An endometrial thickness of more than 10 mm in an amenorrhoeic woman warrants an artificially induced bleed, which should be followed by a repeat ultrasound scan and endometrial biopsy if the endometrium has not been shed. Another option is to consider a progestogen-secreting intrauterine system, such as the Mirena.

Breast cancer

Obesity, hyperandrogenism and infertility occur frequently in PCOS, and are features known to be associated with the development of breast cancer. However, studies examining the relationship between PCOS and breast carcinoma have not always identified a significantly increased risk. The study by Coulam et al (1983) calculated a relative risk of 1.5 (95% CI 0.75–2.55) for breast cancer in their group of women with chronic anovulation, which was not statistically significant. After stratification by age, however, the relative risk was found to be 3.6 (95% CI 1.2–8.3) in the postmenopausal age group. More recently, Pierpoint et al (1998) reported SMRs calculated for patients with PCOS compared with the normal population. The SMR for all neoplasms was 0.91 (95% CI 0.60–1.32) and the SMR for breast cancer was 1.48 (95% CI 0.79–2.54). In fact, breast cancer was the leading cause of death in this cohort.

Ovarian cancer

In recent years, there has been much debate about the risk of ovarian cancer in women with infertility, particularly in relation to the use of drugs to induce superovulation for assisted conception procedures. Inherently, the risk of ovarian cancer appears to be increased in women who have multiple ovulations; that is, those who are nulliparous (possibly because of infertility) with an early menarche and late menopause. Thus, it may be that inducing multiple ovulations in women with infertility will increase their risk; a hypothesis that is by no means proven. Women with PCOS who are oligo-ovulatory or anovulatory might therefore be expected to be at low risk of developing ovarian cancer if it is lifetime number of ovulations rather than pregnancies that is critical. Ovulation induction to correct anovulatory infertility aims to induce unifollicular ovulation and so, in theory, should increase the risk of a woman with PCOS compared with that of a normal ovulating woman. The polycystic ovary, however, is notoriously sensitive to stimulation and it is only in recent years, with the development of high-resolution transvaginal ultrasonography, that the rate of unifollicular ovulation has attained acceptable levels. The use of clomiphene citrate and gonadotrophin therapy for ovulation induction in the 1960s, 1970s and 1980s resulted in many more multiple ovulations (and indeed multiple pregnancies) than in recent times, and might therefore present with an increased rate of ovarian cancer when these women reach their 60s, the age of greatest incidence.

A few studies have addressed the possibility of an association between polycystic ovaries and ovarian cancer. The results are conflicting, and generalizability is limited due to problems with the study designs. In the large UK study of Pierpoint et al (1998), the SMR for ovarian cancer was 0.39 (95% CI 0.01–2.17).

Management of Non-Fertility Aspects of Polycystic Ovaries

Psychological support and quality of life

The symptoms typically associated with the condition have also been shown to lead to a significant reduction in health-related quality of life (Jones et al 2004). Health-related quality of life is a multidimensional, dynamic concept that encompasses physical, psychological and social aspects that are associated with a particular disease or its treatment. Therefore, any management of the woman with PCOS needs to consider and understand the negative impact that this condition may have upon these psychosocial parameters. For example, although the management of hirsuitism may be considered as a purely cosmetic issue, excessive facial hair has been shown to be one of the major causes of marked psychological stress in women with PCOS, often caused by embarrassment about the excessive hair growth. Infertility and weight issues have also been found to affect other social and psychological parameters. Infertility can cause tensions within the family, altered self-perception and problems at work. Whilst obesity worsens the symptoms, the metabolic scenario conspires against weight loss; many women experience frustration in attempts to lose weight and suffer from low-esteem and poor body image.

Obesity

The management of women with PCOS should be focused on the patient's particular problems. Obesity worsens both symptomatology and the endocrine profile, so obese women (BMI >30 kg/m^2) should be encouraged to lose weight by a combination of calorie restriction and exercise. Weight loss improves the endocrine profile, the likelihood of ovulation and the likelihood of a healthy pregnancy.

Metformin

Insulin-sensitizing agents such as metformin became popular for the management of PCOS as it was thought that they might act directly at the pathogenesis of the syndrome and help to correct both metabolic and endocrine problems. Early studies suggested an improvement in reproductive function and menstrual cycle regulation, and the possibility of benefits to health of long-term use, including deferring the onset of type 2 diabetes. However, the results of large prospective, randomized studies have failed to demonstrate benefit; weight loss is not achieved by the therapy, and whilst some biochemical parameters may improve, this does not translate into a significant benefit in outcomes. Therefore, at present, the role of insulin-sensitizing and insulin-lowering drugs, such as metformin and the thiazolidinediones, is uncertain in the management of PCOS.

Diet

Much has been written about diet and PCOS. The right diet for an individual is one that is practical, sustainable and compatible with her lifestyle. There does not appear to be a particular diet that is most appropriate for women with

PCOS. It is sensible to reduce glycaemic load by lowering sugar content in favour of more complex carbohydrates, and to avoid fatty foods. Meal replacement therapy or low calorie diets may be appropriate; it is often helpful to refer to a dietitian, if available. An increase in physical activity is essential, preferably as part of the daily routine. Thirty minutes of brisk exercise per day is encouraged to maintain health; but to lose weight, or sustain weight loss, 60–90 min/day is advised. Concurrent behavioural therapy improves the chances of success of any method of weight loss.

Antiobesity drugs

These may help with weight loss, and both orlistat and sibutramine have been shown to be effective in PCOS in small studies. Orlistat is a pancreatic lipase inhibitor which prevents absorption of approximately 30% of dietary fat, whereas sibutramine is a centrally acting serotonin and noradrenaline reuptake inhibitor which enhances satiety. Both agents can also improve insulin sensitivity and are currently licensed for individuals with a BMI of more than 30 kg/m^2, or lower if comorbidities such as type 2 diabetes are present. Both agents have been shown to improve insulin resistance, lipid profile and glycaemic control, and orlistat has been shown to reduce blood pressure and testosterone. Orlistat and sibutramine are increasingly being used in primary care as an adjunct to diet and lifestyle advice; both require monitoring for efficacy, and sibutramine requires monitoring for possible increases in blood pressure. New agents in development for obesity may also have a role to play in PCOS.

Bariatric surgery

This is being used increasingly because of the global epidemic of obesity, and it certainly has a role in the management of obese women with PCOS. It is recommended by some that anyone with a BMI of more than 35 kg/m^2 should be referred for consideration of bariatric surgery. If there are comorbidities, such as diabetes, the BMI cut-off for surgery is less than 30–35 kg/m^2.

Menstrual irregularity

The simplest way to control the menstrual cycle is the use of a low-dose combined oral contraceptive preparation (COCP). This will result in an artificial cycle and regular shedding of the endometrium. It is also important, once again, to encourage weight loss. As women with PCOS are thought to be at increased risk of cardiovascular disease, a 'lipid friendly' combined contraceptive pill should be used. The third-generation oral contraceptives are lipid friendly but present the potential disadvantage of venous thromboembolism, particularly in overweight women. Dianette® is a COCP that has antiandrogenic properties and will have additional benefits for women with hyperandrogenism, and Yasmin® contains a newer antiandrogen, drosperinone, which is a derivative of spironolactone. Alternatives to the COCP include a progestogen, for example medroxyprogesterone acetate (Provera) or dydrogesterone (Duphaston), for 12 days every 1–3 months to induce a withdrawal bleed, or simply the insertion of a Mirena intrauterine system.

In women with anovulatory cycles, the action of oestradiol on the endometrium is unopposed because of the lack of cyclical progesterone secretion. This may result in episodes of irregular uterine bleeding and, in the long term, endometrial hyperplasia and even endometrial cancer (see above). An ultrasound assessment of endometrial thickness provides a bioassay for oestradiol production by the ovaries and conversion of androgens in the peripheral fat. If the endometrium is thicker than 10 mm, a withdrawal bleed should be induced; if the endometrium fails to shed, endometrial sampling is required to exclude endometrial hyperplasia or malignancy.

Hyperandrogenism and hirsutism

The bioavailability of testosterone is affected by the serum concentration of SHBG. High levels of insulin lower the production of SHBG and therefore increase the free fraction of androgen. Elevated serum androgen concentrations stimulate peripheral androgen receptors, resulting in an increase in 5-α reductase activity, directly increasing the conversion of testosterone to the more potent metabolite, dihydrotestosterone. Symptoms of hyperandrogenism include hirsutism and acne, which are both distressing conditions. Hirsutism is characterized by terminal hair growth in a male pattern of distribution, including chin, upper lip, chest, upper and lower back, upper and lower abdomen, upper arm, thigh and buttocks. A standardized scoring system, such as the modified Ferriman and Gallwey score, should be used to evaluate the degree of hirsutism before and during treatments (Figure 18.7).

Treatment options include cosmetic and medical therapies. As drug therapies may take 6–9 months or longer before any improvement in hirsutism is perceived, physical treatments including electrolysis, waxing and bleaching may be helpful whilst waiting for medical treatments to work. For many years, the most 'permanent' physical treatment for unwanted hair has been electrolysis. It is time consuming, painful and expensive, and should be performed by an expert practitioner. Regrowth is not uncommon and there is no really permanent cosmetic treatment, but the last few years have seen much development in the use of laser and photothermolysis techniques. There are many different types of laser in production and each requires evaluation of dose intensity, effectiveness and safety. The technique is promising, being faster and more effective than shaving, waxing or chemical depilation. Repeated treatments are required for a near-permanent effect because only those hair follicles in the growing phase are obliterated at each treatment. Hair growth occurs in three cycles so 6–9 months of regular treatments are typical. Patients should be appropriately selected (dark hair on fair skin is best), and warned that complete hair removal cannot be guaranteed and some scarring may occur. At present, it is not widely available and is still an expensive option.

Vaniqa (eflornithine) has recently been developed as a topical treatment for hirsutism. It works by inhibiting the enzyme ornithine decarboxylase in hair follicles, and may be a useful therapy for those who wish to avoid hormonal treatments, but may also be used in conjunction with hormonal therapy.

Medical regimens should stop further progression of hirsutism and decrease the rate of hair growth. Therapy for acne should aim to lower sebum excretion, alter follicular

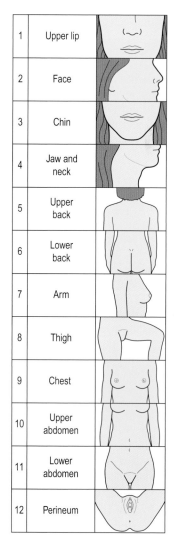

1	Upper lip
2	Face
3	Chin
4	Jaw and neck
5	Upper back
6	Lower back
7	Arm
8	Thigh
9	Chest
10	Upper abdomen
11	Lower abdomen
12	Perineum

Figure 18.7 Ferriman and Gallwey score. Each area is given a score from 1 to 4 (1 = mild, 2 = moderate, 3 = complete light coverage, 4 = heavy coverage).

cell desquamation, reduce propionibacteria and reduce inflammation.

If using antiandrogen therapy, adequate contraception is important in women of reproductive age as transplacental passage of antiandrogens may disturb the genital development of a male fetus.

The best pharmacological treatment of proven effectiveness is a combination of the synthetic progestogen cyproterone acetate, which is antigonadotrophic and antiandrogenic, with ethinyl oestradiol. Dianette contains ethinyloestradiol (35 μg) in combination with cyproterone, although at a lower dose (2 mg). Dianette is licensed for moderate to severe hirsutism and severe acne. The antiandrogen effect reduces sebum excretion in 2–3 months and results in clinical improvement in acne in 4–6 months.

Oestrogens lower circulating androgens by a combination of a slight inhibition of gonadotrophin secretion and gonadotrophin-sensitive ovarian steroid production, and by an increase in hepatic production of SHBG resulting in lower free testosterone. Cyproterone acetate can rarely cause liver damage and liver function should be checked regularly

(after 6 months and then annually). There is conflicting data about a possible increased risk of thromboembolism, although there are many women who take Dianette on a long-term basis without any ill effects.

Spironolactone is a weak diuretic with antiandrogenic properties, and may be used at a daily dose of 25–100 mg in women with either hirsutism and/or acne in whom the COCP is contraindicated. Drosperinone is a derivative of spironolactone and contained in the new COCP, Yasmin, which also appears to be effective for women with PCOS. Other antiandrogens such as ketoconazole, finasteride and flutamide have been tried, but are not widely used in the UK for the treatment of hirsutism in women due to their adverse and potentially serious side-effects. Furthermore, they are no more effective than cyproterone acetate.

Topical antiacne agents can be safely and successfully combined with systemic antiandrogen therapy in an attempt to target as many aetiological factors as possible. However, these topical treatments alone have little effect on sebum production, so are not generally successful when utilized alone in acne associated with PCOS. Topical retinoids impact on the microcomedo which is the precursor to non-inflammatory and inflammatory acne lesions. They also have direct comedolytic and anti-inflammatory activity. These agents are useful adjuvant therapies in combination with antiandrogen treatments, and can be used as maintenance treatment after discontinuation of systemic therapy. Topical antimicrobials (benzoyl peroxide/antibiotics) have good anti-inflammatory activity and should help to reduce inflammatory lesions when used alongside antiandrogen treatment.

Oral isotretinoin, a hospital-only prescribed medication, is the single systemic therapy that targets the four main aetiological factors implicated in acne. However, it is currently only licensed for severe acne that has not responded to alternative therapies. A recent European Directive concerning isotretinoin has enforced a strict pregnancy prevention programme due to the high risk of teratogenecity with this drug. COCPs can be used safely alongside oral isotretinoin and are recommended by the European Directive. Although clinical clearance of acne lesions with oral isotretinoin is very likely, relapse rates post therapy are higher than average when acne is associated with PCOS.

Ovulation Induction

Ovulation induction has traditionally involved the use of clomiphene citrate and then gonadotrophin therapy or laparoscopic ovarian surgery in those who are clomiphene resistant. The principles of management of anovulatory infertility are firstly to optimize health before commencing therapy, for example weight loss for those who are overweight, and then induce regular unifollicular ovulation, while minimizing the risks of ovarian hyperstimualtion syndrome (OHSS) and multiple pregnancy (see Chapter 17, Ovulation induction, for more information).

Obesity reduces fertility, and increases the risk of miscarriage, some congenital anomalies and pregnancy-related complications, e.g. pre-eclampsia, gestational diabetes, problems during delivery, and maternal and fetal mortality (Balen et al 2006). Monitoring treatment is also harder in obese women because their ovaries are more difficult to see on ultrasound scans, thus raising the risk of missing multiple ovulation and multiple pregnancy. National guidelines in the UK for managing overweight women with PCOS advise weight loss, preferably to a BMI of less than 30 kg/m², before commencing drugs for ovarian stimulation (Balen and Anderson 2007).

Obese women (BMI >30 kg/m²) should therefore be encouraged to lose weight. Clark et al (1995) investigated the effects of a weight loss and exercise programme on women with anovulatory infertility, clomiphene resistance and a BMI of more than 30 kg/m². The emphasis of the study was a realistic exercise schedule combined with positive reinforcement of a suitable eating programme over a 6-month period. Weight loss had a significant effect on endocrine function, ovulation and subsequent pregnancy.

Clomiphene citrate

Antioestrogen therapy with clomiphene citrate or tamoxifen has traditionally been used as first-line therapy for anovulatory PCOS. A recent meta-analysis confirmed that clomiphene is effective in increasing pregnancy rates when compared with placebo as first-line therapy (fixed odds ratio 5.8, 95% CI 1.6–21.5; number needed to treat 5.9, 95% CI 3.6–16.7) (Beck et al 2005). Antioestrogen therapy is usually commenced on day 2 of the cycle and given for 5 days. If the patient has oligomenorrhoea or amenorrhoea, it is necessary to exclude pregnancy and then induce a withdrawal bleed with a short course of a progestogen, such as medroxyprogesterone acetate 5–20 mg/day for 5–10 days. The starting dose of clomiphene citrate is 50 mg/day for 5 days beginning on days 3–5 of the menstrual cycle. The dose of clomiphene citrate should only be increased if there is no response after three cycles, as of those women who will respond to 50 mg/day, only two-thirds will do so in the first cycle. Doses of 150 mg/day or more do not appear to be of benefit. If there is an over-response to 50 mg/day, as in some women with PCOS, the dose can be decreased to 25 mg/day.

Clomiphene citrate may cause an exaggeration in the hypersecretion of LH and have antioestrogenic effects on the endometrium and cervical mucus. All women who are prescribed clomiphene citrate should be carefully monitored with a combination of endocrine and ultrasonographic assessment of follicular growth and ovulation because of the risk of multiple pregnancies, which is approximately 10% (Figures 18.8 and 18.9). Clomiphene therapy should therefore be prescribed and managed by specialists in reproductive medicine.

Aromatase inhibitors

Aromatase inhibitors have been proposed as an alternative treatment to clomiphene citrate therapy, as the discrepancy between ovulation and pregnancy rates with clomiphene citrate has been attributed to its antioestrogenic action and oestrogen receptor depletion. The aromatase inhibitors suppress oestrogen production and thereby mimic the central reduction of negative feedback through which clomiphene citrate works. Letrozole, the most widely used antiaromatase for this indication, has been shown to be effective, in early trials, in inducing ovulation and pregnancy in women with

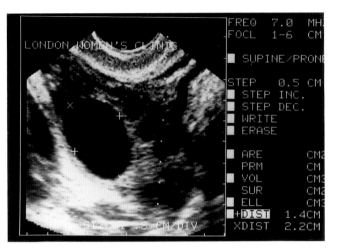

Figure 18.8 Stimulation of a single mature follicle in a polycystic ovary (transvaginal ultrasound scan).

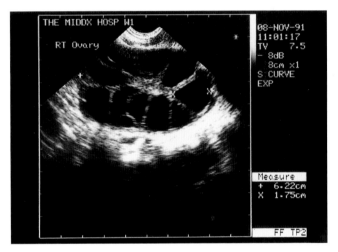

Figure 18.9 Transvaginal ultrasound scan of an overstimulated polycystic ovary. Both ovaries are likely to have this appearance, and the treatment must be discontinued to minimize the risk of multiple pregnancy and ovarian hyperstimulation syndrome.

anovulatory PCOS. Anastrozole is a possible alternative. Evidence from larger trials is still awaited, but some encouragement may be taken from the solidity of the working hypothesis and the success of the preliminary results.

Gonadotrophins

Gonadotrophin therapy is indicated for women with anovulatory PCOS who have been treated with antioestrogens if they have failed to ovulate or if they have a response to clomiphene that is likely to reduce their chance of conception (e.g. persistent hypersecretion of LH or antioestrogenic effect on cervical mucus).

In order to prevent the risks of overstimulation and multiple pregnancy, the traditional standard step-up regimens (when 75–150 IU is increased by 75 IU every 3–5 days) have been replaced by low-dose step-up regimens. The low-dose step-up regimen employs a starting dose of 25–50 IU, which is only increased after 14 days if there is no response, and then by only half an ampoule every 7 days. Treatment cycles using this approach can be quite long (up to 28–35 days), but the risk of multiple follicular growth is lower than with conventional step-up regimens (Tarlatzis et al 2008) (see Chapter 17, Ovulation induction, for more information).

It can be extremely difficult to predict the response to stimulation of a woman with polycystic ovaries; indeed, this is the greatest therapeutic challenge in all ovulation induction therapies. The polycystic ovary is characteristically quiescent, at least when viewed by ultrasound, before often exhibiting an explosive response to stimulation. It can be very challenging to stimulate the development of a single dominant follicle, and while attempts have been made to predict a multifollicular response by looking at mid-follicular endocrine profiles and numbers of small follicles, it is more difficult to do so prior to commencing ovarian stimulation and hence determine the required starting dose of gonadotrophin. In order to prevent the risks of OHSS and multiple pregnancy, however, the cycle should be cancelled on day 8 of stimulation if there are more than five to seven follicles ≥8 mm. Ovulation is triggered with a single injection of human chorionic gonadotrophin (hCG) 5000 units (i.m. or s.c.). The inclusion criterion for hCG administration should be the development of at least one follicle with a largest diameter of at least 17 mm. In order to reduce the risk of multiple pregnancy and OHSS, the exclusion criterion for hCG administration is the development of a total of three or more follicles larger than 14 mm in diameter. In overstimulated cycles, hCG is withheld and the patient is counselled about the risks and advised to refrain from sexual intercourse.

Insulin-sensitizing agents

It is logical to assume that therapy that achieves a fall in serum insulin concentrations should improve the symptoms of PCOS. The biguanide metformin inhibits the production of hepatic glucose, thereby decreasing insulin secretion, and also enhances insulin sensitivity at the cellular level. Early studies involved a small number of participants and were encouraging, whereas more recent large studies looking at the use of metformin either alone or combined with clomiphene citrate have failed to demonstrate significant benefit with respect to weight reduction, improved menstrual cycle function or livebirth rates (Moll et al 2006, Tang et al 2006, Legro et al 2007).

In summary, although the initial studies appeared promising, subsequent large randomized-controlled trials have not demonstrated the anticipated beneficial effects of metformin as a first-line therapy for treatment of the anovulatory patient with PCOS. The study authors concur that the primary aim for overweight women with PCOS is to make lifestyle changes with a combination of diet and exercise in order to lose weight and to improve ovarian function. In conclusion, the position of metformin in the management of PCOS is by no means clear and, on the basis of current evidence, it is not the first-line treatment of choice (Tarlatzis et al 2008).

Surgical ovulation induction

An alternative to gonadotrophin therapy for clomiphene-resistant PCOS is laparoscopic ovarian surgery, which has replaced the more invasive and damaging technique of ovarian wedge resection. Laparoscopic ovarian surgery is free of the risks of multiple pregnancy and ovarian hyperstimulation, and does not require intensive ultrasound monitoring. Furthermore, ovarian diathermy appears to be as effective as routine gonadotrophin therapy in the treatment of clomiphene-insensitive PCOS. In addition, laparoscopic ovarian surgery is a useful therapy for anovulatory women with PCOS who fail to respond to clomiphene and who persistently hypersecrete LH, or who need a laparoscopic assessment of their pelvis, or who live too far away from the hospital to be able to attend for the intensive monitoring required in gonadotrophin therapy. Surgery does, of course, carry its own risks and must only be performed by fully trained laparoscopic surgeons.

Wedge resection of the ovaries resulted in significant adhesions (100% of cases) in some published series. The risk of adhesion formation is far less after laparoscopic ovarian diathermy (10–20% of cases), and the adhesions that do form are usually fine and of limited clinical significance. The author's technique involves instilling 200 ml Hartmann's solution or Adept® into the pouch of Douglas, which, by cooling the ovaries, prevents heat injury to adjacent tissues and reduces adhesion formation. It is suggested that a minimum amount of ovarian destruction should be employed. Furthermore, a combined approach may be suitable for some women, whereby low-dose diathermy is followed by low-dose ovarian stimulation.

An additional concern is the possibility of ovarian destruction leading to ovarian failure; an obvious disaster in a woman wishing to conceive. Cases of ovarian failure have been reported after both wedge resection and laparoscopic surgery. An unfortunate vogue has developed whereby women with polycystic ovaries who have over-responded to superovulation for in-vitro fertilization (IVF) are subjected to ovarian diathermy as a way of reducing the likelihood of subsequent OHSS. If one accepts that appropriately performed ovarian diathermy works by sensitizing the ovary to FSH, one could extrapolate that ovarian diathermy prior to superovulation for IVF should make the ovary more, and not less, likely to overstimulate. The amount of ovarian destruction that is required to reduce the chance of overstimulation is therefore likely to be considerable. Great caution is urged before proceeding with such an approach because of concerns about permanent ovarian atrophy.

After laparoscopic ovarian surgery, serum concentrations of LH and testosterone fall with restoration of ovarian activity. Whether or not patients respond to laparoscopic ovarian diathermy (LOD) appears to depend on their pretreatment characteristics, with patients with high basal LH concentrations having a better clinical and endocrine response. Ovarian diathermy appears to be as effective as routine gonadotrophin therapy in the treatment of clomiphene-citrate-insensitive PCOS, and the Cochrane Database concludes that whilst there is insufficient evidence to demonstrate a difference between 6–12 months follow-up after LOD and three to six cycles of ovulation induction with gonadotrophins, multiple pregnancy rates are considerably reduced with LOD (Farquhar et al 2002). The largest randomized controlled trial to date is a multicentre study performed in The Netherlands in which 168 patients, resistant to clomiphene citrate, were randomized to either LOD ($n = 83$) or ovulation induction with recombinant FSH (rFSH, $n = 65$)

Table 18.4 Indications for laparoscopic ovarian diathermy (LOD)

Anovulatory polycystic ovary syndrome
Clomiphene citrate resistance
Persistent hypersecretion of luteinizing hormone
Repeated over-response to clomiphene citrate or gonadotrophins
Patients who find it difficult to travel for regular scans
No value for therapy of long-term effects of polycystic ovary syndrome,
  e.g. hirsutism, obesity

Table 18.5 Strategy for ovulation induction in anovulatory polycystic ovary syndrome

Slim patient	Overweight patient (body mass index >30 kg/m^2)
1. Clomiphene citrate therapy	1. Lifestyle changes
2. LOD if luteinizing hormone elevated	2. Clomiphene citrate therapy
3. Gonadotrophin therapy or LOD if clomiphene citrate resistant	3. Gonadotrophin therapy or LOD if clomiphene citrate resistant
4. IVF if no pregnancy after nine to 12 ovulations	4. IVF if no pregnancy after nine to 12 ovulations

IVF, in-vitro fertilization; LOD, laparoscopic ovarian diathermy.

(Bayram et al 2004). The initial cumulative pregnancy rate after 6 months was 34% in the LOD arm vs 67% in the rFSH arm. Those who did not ovulate in response to LOD were first given clomiphene citrate and then rFSH, so by 12 months, the cumulative pregnancy rate was similar in each group at 67%. Thus, those treated with LOD took longer to conceive, and 54% required additional medical ovulation induction therapy.

Laparoscopic ovarian diathermy is associated with a low risk of multiple pregnancy and so does not need the same intensity of monitoring as the use of drugs to stimulate ovulation. Indications for LOD are listed in Table 18.4. A strategy for ovulation induction for women with PCOS is outlined in Table 18.5.

Conclusions

PCOS is one of the most common endocrine disorders. It may present, at one end of the spectrum, with the single finding of polycystic ovarian morphology as detected by pelvic ultrasound. At the other end of the spectrum, symptoms such as obesity, hyperandrogenism, menstrual cycle disturbance and infertility may occur either singly or in combination. Women with PCOS are characterized by the presence of insulin resistance, central obesity and dyslipidaemia, which appears to place them at higher risk of developing diabetes as well as cardiovascular disease. There are a number of environmental factors that may influence the expression of PCOS, in particular a tendency to insulin-resistant states induced by overeating and underexercising. A plausible hypothesis for the survival of PCOS in the population is that of the 'thrifty phenotype/genotype', whereby in times of famine, individuals who have a tendency to obesity preserve the population by maintaining fertility, while those of normal body weight fall below the threshold body weight for fertility. This may explain the greater prevalence of PCOS among South Asians in the UK, where there is relatively greater nutrition and thus the right environment to express PCOS. In addition, the 'thrifty phenotype' hypothesis suggests that in-utero insulin resistance results as an adaptation to impaired nutrition, and this persists through to adult life and is amplified by overnutrition (obesity).

PCOS is probably the same the world over, although without an agreed definition, one cannot say for sure that this is the case. There may be factors that affect expression and presentation, whether because of racial differences in the colour and distribution of hair (e.g. Japanese vs Mediterranean women) or variations in hormone production and receptor activity. Fundamentally, the underlying condition is likely to be the same. Management should be directed towards an individual's needs (whether cosmetic, reproductive or metabolic), and attention should be given to potential long-term sequelae.

Women with PCOS are characterized by the presence of insulin resistance, central obesity and dyslipidaemia, which appears to place them at higher risk of developing diabetes as well as cardiovascular disease. The retrospective long-term follow-up studies have confirmed the higher incidence of diabetes, although they have not shown a higher risk of mortality from IHD. Cross-sectional studies have demonstrated a significant association between PCOS and IHD. Prospective longitudinal studies confirming this risk are still awaited. There does seem to be sufficient biochemical evidence regarding the potential for long-term risks of cardiovascular disease and diabetes, which need to be addressed when counselling women with PCOS. Encouraging weight loss remains the most effective first-line therapeutic intervention in these women, albeit hard to achieve. Further longitudinal studies need to be performed to investigate the natural history of PCOS and its sequelae for the health of women.

KEY POINTS

1. PCOS is the most common endocrine disorder in women (approximate prevalence 20–25%).

2. PCOS is a heterogeneous condition. Diagnosis is made by finding two out of the following three criteria: (i) menstrual cycle disturbance, (ii) clinical or biochemical hyperandrogenism, and (iii) ultrasound detection of polycystic ovaries.

3. Management is symptom orientated.

4. If obese, weight loss improves symptoms and endocrinology and should be encouraged. A glucose tolerance test should be performed for women with a BMI of more than 30 kg/m^2.

5. Menstrual cycle control is achieved by cyclical oral contraceptives or progestogens.

6. Ovulation induction may be difficult and may require progression through various treatments, which should be monitored carefully to prevent multiple pregnancy.

7. Ovulation induction may be achieved with clomiphene citrate, gonadotrophin therapy or laparoscopic ovarian diathermy.

8. Hyperandrogenism is usually managed with an oral contraceptive containing ethinyloestradiol in combination with either cyproterone acetate or drospirenone. Alternatives include spironolactone, flutamide and finasteride, all of which have potential adverse effects.

9. Insulin-sensitizing agents (e.g. metformin) are not indicated in first-line management, and should usually only be prescribed if there is impaired glucose tolerance or frank diabetes.

References

Balen AH 2001 Polycystic ovary syndrome and cancer. Human Reproduction Update 7: 522–525.

Balen AH, Conway GS, Kaltsas G et al 1995 Polycystic ovary syndrome: the spectrum of the disorder in 1741 patients. Human Reproduction 10: 2107–2111.

Balen AH, Michelmore K 2002 What is polycystic ovary syndrome? Are national views important? Human Reproduction 17: 2219–2227.

Balen AH, Laven JSE, Tan SL, Dewailly D 2003 Ultrasound assessment of the polycystic ovary: international consensus definitions. Human Reproduction Update 9: 505–514.

Balen AH, Anderson R 2007 Impact of obesity on female reproductive health: British Fertility Society policy and practice guidelines. Human Fertility 10: 195–206.

Balen AH, Dresner M, Scott EM, Drife JO 2006 Should obese women with polycystic ovary syndrome (PCOS) receive treatment for infertility? BMJ (Clinical Research Ed.) 332: 434–435.

Bayram N, van Wely M, Kaaijk EM, Bossuyt PMM, van der Veen F 2004 Using an electrocautery strategy or recombinant FSH to induce ovulation in polycystic ovary syndrome: a randomised controlled trial. BMJ (Clinical Research Ed.) 328: 192–195.

Beck JI, Boothroyd C, Proctor M, Farquhar C, Hughes E 2005 Oral anti-oestrogens and medical adjuncts for subfertility associated with anovulation. Cochrane Database of Systematic Reviews 1:CD002249.

Clark AM, Ledger W, Galletly C et al 1995 Weight loss results in significant improvement in pregnancy and ovulation rates in anovulatory obese women. Human Reproduction 10: 2705–2712.

Coulam CB, Annegers JF, Kranz JS 1983 Chronic anovulation syndrome and associated neoplasia. Obstetrics and Gynecology 61: 403–407.

Dunaif A 1997 Insulin resistance and the polycystic ovary syndrome: mechanisms and implication for pathogenesis. Endocrine Review 18: 774–800.

Elwood JM, Cole P, Rothman KJ et al 1977 Epidemiology of endometrial cancer. Journal of the National Cancer Institute 59: 1055–1060.

Farquhar C, Vandekerckhove P, Lilford R 2002 Laparoscopic 'drilling' by diathermy or laser for ovulation induction in anovulatory polycystic ovary syndrome. Cochrane Database of Systematic Reviews 1.

Fauser B, Tarlatzis B, Chang J et al 2004 Revised 2003 consensus on diagnostic criteria and long-term health risks related to polycystic ovary syndrome (PCOS). Human Reproduction 19: 41–47.

Franks S, Gharani N, McCarthy M 2001 Candidate genes in polycystic ovary syndrome. Human Reproduction Update 7: 405–410.

Jones GL, Benes K, Clark TL et al 2004 The polycystic ovary syndrome health-related quality of life questionnaire (PCOSQ): a validation. Human Reproduction 19: 317–377.

Kousta E, White DM, Franks S 1997 Modern use of clomifene citrate in induction of ovulation. Human Reproduction Update 3: 359–365.

Legro RS, Barnhart HX, Schlaff WD et al 2007 Clomiphene, metformin, or both for infertility in the polycystic ovary syndrome. New England Journal of Medicine 356: 551–566.

Lord J, Wilkin T 2002 Polycystic ovary syndrome and fat distribution: the central issue? Human Fertility 5: 67–71.

Michelmore KF, Balen AH, Dunger DB, Vessey MP 1999 Polycystic ovaries and associated clinical and biochemical features in young women. Clinical Endocrinology 51: 779–786.

Moll E, Bossuyt PMM, Korevaar JC, Lambalk CB, van der Veen F 2006 Effect of clomifene citrate plus metformin and clomifene citrate plus placebo on induction of ovulation in women with newly diagnosed polycystic ovary syndrome: randomised double blind clinical trial. BMJ (Clinical Research Ed.) 332: 1485–1488.

Pierpoint T, McKeigue PM, Isaacs AJ, Wild SH, Jacobs HS 1998 Mortality of women with polycystic ovary syndrome at long-term follow-up. Journal of Clinical Epidemiology 51: 581–586.

Rajkowha M, Glass MR, Rutherford AJ, Michelmore K, Balen AH 2000 Polycystic ovary syndrome: a risk factor for cardiovascular disease? British Journal of Obstetrics and Gynaecology 107: 11–18.

Rendeva HS, Lewandowski KC, Drzewoski J et al 2002 Exercise decreases plasma total homocysteine in overweight young women with polycystic ovary syndrome. Journal of Clinical Endocrinology and Metabolism 87: 4496–4501.

Rodin DA, Bano G, Bland JM, Taylor K, Nussey SS 1998 Polycystic ovaries and associated metabolic abnormalities in Indian subcontinent Asian women. Clinical Endocrinology 49: 91–99.

Sampaolo P, Livien C, Montanari L, Paganelli A, Salesi A, Lorini R 1994 Precocious signs of polycystic ovaries in obese girls. Ultrasound Obstetrics and Gynaecology 4: 1–6.

Tang T, Glanville J, Hayden CJ, White D, Barth JH, Balen AH 2006 Combined life-style modification and metformin in obese patients with polycystic ovary syndrome (PCOS). A randomised, placebo-controlled, double-blind multi-centre study. Human Reproduction 21: 80–89.

Tarlatzis BC, Fauser BCJM, Chang J et al 2008 Consensus on infertility treatment related to polycystic ovary syndrome. Human Reproduction 23: 462–477.

Wijeyaratne CN, Balen AH, Barth J, Belchetz PE 2002 Polycystic ovary syndrome in south Asian women: a case control study. Clinical Endocrinology 57: 343–350.

Wild S, Pierpoint T, McKeigue P, Jacobs H 2000 Cardiovascular disease in women with polycystic ovary syndrome at long-term follow-up: a retrospective cohort study. Clinical Endocrinology 52: 595–600.

Further Reading

Balen AH, Conway G, Homberg R, Legro R 2005 Clinical Management of Polycystic Ovary Syndrome. Taylor and Francis, London, 234 pp.

CHAPTER 19

Fertilization to implantation

Hayden Homer and Alison Murdoch

Chapter Contents

INTRODUCTION	265		IMMUNE FACTORS IN IMPLANTATION	272
PRELUDE TO FERTILIZATION	265		CLINICAL AND SCIENTIFIC CORRELATES	273
FERTILIZATION	266		STEM CELL TECHNOLOGY	273
PREIMPLANTATION	268		CONCLUDING REMARKS	275
IMPLANTATION	270		KEY POINTS	275

Introduction

At fertilization, two gametes fuse to generate an embryo which subsequently initiates an elaborate developmental programme whilst negotiating its way to the uterine cavity, the site of implantation. Recent years have seen great strides in our understanding of the molecular minutiae underpinning these events. These advances have furthered insight into human reproductive failure, guided the refinement of treatment designed to alleviate subfertility, and contributed to the evolution of avant-garde scientific developments, most notably stem cell technology.

This chapter provides an overview of fertilization, preimplantation embryonic development and implantation, and their collaboration in reproduction. The chapter will begin by outlining the essential prerequisites for fertilization, and conclude with a bird's eye view of some of the clinical and scientific innovations that have been mined from an improved understanding of these elaborate processes.

Prelude to Fertilization

Sexual dimorphism in gametogenesis

Male gametes (spermatozoa) and female gametes (ova or eggs) possess half the normal chromosome complement. The merging of two gametes at fertilization restores the complete chromosome set in the embryo.

Spermatogenesis and oogenesis produce male and female gametes, respectively, and are characterized by a unique nuclear division, known as 'meiosis', which halves chromosome numbers. Notably however, the tempo of gametogenesis differs markedly between males and females. Spermatogenesis progresses uninterruptedly over approximately 60–70 days, whereas oogenesis often spans decades and is a discontinuous process punctuated by two arrest stages (Homer 2007).

With the exception of the relatively small amount of DNA associated with mitochondria which is exclusively oocyte-derived, spermatozoa and eggs have comparable stakes in the embryo's genetic blueprint. In stark contrast, male and female gametes make very different cytoplasmic contributions (Figure 19.1). Virtually all of the embryo's biosynthetic raw materials and organelles are derived from the egg, with the centriole being the only male cytoplasmic contribution. The fate of an embryo is therefore critically dependent upon stores built up in the oocyte during an extended growth phase lasting 2–3 months, resulting in a 100-fold increase in oocyte volume (Telfer and McLaughlin 2007). Consequently, any compromise to egg quality, such as is seen with advancing female age, has devastating consequences for embryonic and reproductive potential (Homer 2007). Accordingly, older women experience lower in-vitro fertilization (IVF) success rates, along with increased risks for miscarriage and chromosomally abnormal offspring.

In stark contrast to oogenesis which has embryonic sustenance as an over-riding concern, spermatogenesis aims to produce a lightweight and motile gamete capable of penetrating the oocyte. Spermatogenesis fulfils this objective by incorporating a remodelling phase known as 'spermiogenesis', the most remarkable cellular metamorphosis in the human body. Spermiogenesis strips the spermatid of almost all of its cytoplasm, makes the nucleus highly compact by integrating unique DNA-binding proteins called 'protamines' (Sassone-Corsi 2002), and fashions a propulsive tail with an adjacent fuel source in the mitochondria-laden mid-piece (Figures 19.2 and 19.3). A specialized lysosomal-like secretory granule known as the acrosome is also forged, forming a cap-like structure over the nuclear surface (Figures 19.2 and 19.3). The acrosome contains enzymes essential for

DOI: 10.1016/B978-0-7020-3120-5.00019-9

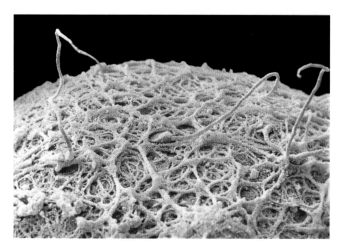

Figure 19.1 Colour-enhanced scanning electron micrograph of human sperm attempting to fertilize an egg. Note the marked difference in size between the spermatozoa and the egg. *Reproduced with permission from the Wellcome Trust.*

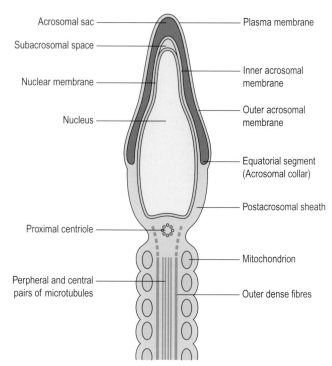

Figure 19.2 Human spermatozoon showing principal structures.

digesting a path through the egg's outer covering known as the 'zona pellucida'.

Maturation and capacitation

On release into the seminiferous tubule lumen, spermatozoa are immotile and lack fertilizing capacity, only acquiring these facets after maturation and capacitation.

Maturation occurs in the epididymis endowing spermatozoa with the potential for movement and fertilization. The molecular basis for maturation remains unresolved, but is known to depend upon androgens and exposure to the dynamic microenvironment created by the secretory and absorptive functions of the epididymal epithelium (Nixon et al 2007).

Capacitation enables spermatozoa to recognize their full fertilization potential and occurs within the female genital tract. It is characterized by cyclic adenosine monophosphate (cAMP)-dependent tyrosine phosphorylation of intracellular proteins, most of which are components of the sperm exocytotic and motility machinery (Nixon et al 2007). The capacitated spermatozoon is now distinguished by hyperactivated motility and a change in surface membrane properties, rendering it sensitive to signals encountered in the immediate vicinity of the ovulated egg.

Transport of gametes in the female genital tract

At coitus, sperm are deposited in the upper vagina and on the external cervical surface. In spite of coagulum formation, more than 99% of sperm are lost by leakage from the vagina, with only a small minority gaining access to the relative haven of the cervical crypts. From there, only about one in every million spermatozoa will successfully navigate the 16–20-cm journey to the tubal ampulla, propelled by innate motility and aided by currents created by tubal ciliary activity.

At the time of ovulation, the egg and its tunic of cumulus cells are directed by tubal fimbria and cilia into the tubal

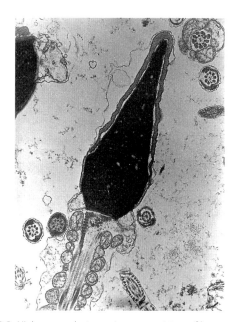

Figure 19.3 High-power electron microscopy picture of human spermatozoon, complementing the features shown schematically in Figure 19.2.

ostium and then towards the tubal ampulla (Figure 19.4). The cumulus–egg complex attracts sperm by releasing chemoattractants that stimulate sperm odorant receptors, thereby inducing cAMP-mediated sperm chemotaxis.

Fertilization

Fertilization commences with spermatozoal penetration of the oocyte's outer coverings, and concludes with syngamy,

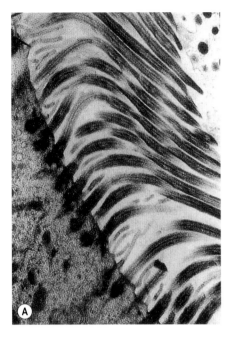
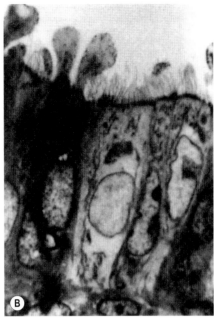

Figure 19.4 Electron microscopy pictures of (A) fimbrial cilia and (B) the postovulatory tubal mucosa demonstrating secretory and ciliated cells.
(A) Reproduced with permission from Mastroianni & Coutifaris, Reproductive physiology, Parthenon Pub. Group, 1990.

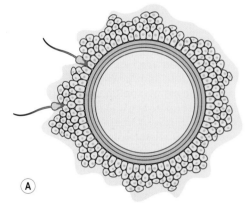
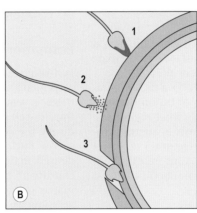
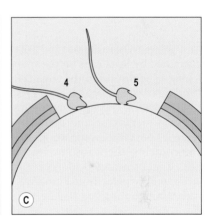

Figure 19.5 Stages of fertilization. (A) Acrosome intact spermatozoa penetrate the cumulus cells to reach the zona pellucida. (B) Spermatozoa then bind to the zona (1), undergo the acrosome reaction (2) and penetrate the zona (3) before entering the perivitelline space. (C) In the perivitelline space, the equatorial head region of the spermatozoa binds the egg plasma membrane (4), after which fusion occurs (5).
From Primakoff and Myles, Penetration, Adhesion, and Fusion in Mammalian Sperm-Egg Interaction, Science; 296; 2183–2185; 2002, Reprinted with permission from AAAS.

the amalgamation of male and female paternal genomes on the first mitotic spindle, altogether lasting approximately 18–21 h.

Cumulus penetration

The first obstacle encountered by any would-be suitor of the ovulated egg is a covering of cumulus cells embedded in an extracellular matrix comprised primarily of the glycosaminoglycan, hyaluronan (Figure 19.5A). Spermatozoa digest a path through the extracellular matrix via hyperactivated motility and a glycophosphatidyl inositol (GPI)-anchored surface hyaluronidase termed 'PH-20' (Primakoff and Myles 2002). Notably, eggs influence sperm penetration, albeit indirectly, by secreting factors such as growth differentiation factor-9 and bone morphogenic protein-15 which regulate cumulus integrity (Swain and Pool 2008).

Sperm–zona interaction

After cumulus penetration, sperm must engage and penetrate the zona pellucida (Figure 19.5B and C). The zona is secreted by the growing oocyte and, in humans, comprises four glycoproteins: ZP1, ZP2, ZP3 and ZP4 (Wassarman 2008). ZP3 in concert with O-linked oligosaccharides functions as the primary sperm receptor that preferentially binds the plasma membrane overlying the intact acrosome. ZP2 is postulated to serve as a secondary receptor that attaches to the inner acrosomal membrane of acrosome-reacted sperm. The zona is also important for mediating species specificity in gamete interaction, and for preventing polyspermy following the cortical reaction (discussed later).

The complementary spermatozoal ligand for ZP3 defies unequivocal identification at present. It appears that the coordinated action of several proteins such as GalTI-1

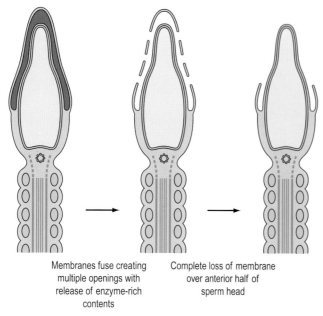

Membranes fuse creating multiple openings with release of enzyme-rich contents

Complete loss of membrane over anterior half of sperm head

Figure 19.6 Acrosome reaction.
From Wang and Dey; Roadmap to embryo implantation: clues from mouse models; Nature Reviews Genetics, 7;185–199,2006.

(β-1,4-galactosyltransferase) and SED1 that are recruited and constrained by lipid rafts on the sperm surface may mediate docking of sperm on to the zona (Nixon et al 2007).

Binding of sperm ligands with ZP3 induces a rise in intracellular calcium, triggering multiple sites of fusion between the sperm membrane and the outer acrosomal membrane (Figure 19.6). This culminates in exocytosis of sperm acrosome contents, the acrosome reaction (Figures 19.5B and 19.6). The proteases and glycosidases thus released, in concert with hyperactivated motility, enable sperm to digest a path through the zona (Figure 19.5B).

Sperm–egg binding and fusion

Having penetrated the zona, spermatozoa enter the perivitelline space between the egg membrane (oolemma) and the zona (Figure 19.5B). Here, further receptor–ligand interactions enable binding of equatorial sperm membrane and oolemma, followed by insertion of the sperm membrane into the opposing oocyte bilayer at fusion (Figure 19.5C).

Initial interest in interplay between oolemmal integrins (e.g. $\alpha6\beta1$) and sperm disintegrins (e.g. fertilin and cyritestin) as mediators of binding-fusion has dissipated due to lack of corroborative evidence from integrin/disintegrin knockout mouse models. Instead, focus is currently on alternative candidates such as sperm lysozyme-like protein and Izumo on sperm, and GPI-anchored proteins and the CD9 tetraspanin on eggs (Kaji et al 2000, Nixon et al 2007).

Egg activation

Sperm–egg fusion induces calcium oscillations in the egg emanating from the point of sperm entry. These calcium transients result from inositol triphosphate production brought about by a soluble sperm-specific factor known as 'phospholipase-Cζ' (Swann et al 2006). Calcium signals

induce the two principal events associated with egg activation: breaking the second meiotic arrest and the cortical reaction.

At the time of fusion, the egg is arrested in meiosis II. This state of suspended animation is dependent upon maturation-promoting factor that is itself sustained by an ooplasmic activity known as 'cytostatic factor' (Tunquist and Maller 2003). The recent characterization of two proteins, early mitotic inhibitor 2 and the calcineurin phosphatase, has elucidated the link between calcium and meiosis II resumption. Following fusion, the ensuing calcium surge induces calcium/calmodulin-dependent-kinase-II-dependent early mitotic inhibitor 2 destruction and transient calcineurin activation, together resulting in cytostatic factor and maturation-promoting factor inactivation and relief from meiosis II arrest (Mochida and Hunt 2007, Wu and Kornbluth 2008).

In response to rising intracellular calcium levels in the egg, specialized organelles known as 'cortical granules' migrate towards and fuse with the oolemma, thereby releasing their enzyme contents into the perivitelline space. This so-called cortical reaction serves to impose a block to polyspermy by a number of mechanisms. These include the cleavage of ZP3 oligosaccharides by β-hexosaminidase B thereby removing receptors for sperm binding, and ZP cross-linking making the zona impenetrable to sperm.

Formation of pronuclei and syngamy

Following fusion, the sperm nucleus enters the ooplasm accompanied by its centriole and flagellum. The male centriole is required for nucleating spindle microtubules and thus for cell division, the female equivalent having been lost during the oocyte's growth stage. On entering the ooplasm, sperm nuclear membranes dissolve and the highly condensed male chromatin undergoes decondensation as its constituent protamines are reduced by glutathione and ultimately replaced by histones present in the ooplasm.

Pronuclei formation in the resulting zygote involves the reformation of a nuclear envelope around each of the haploid parental genomes. The pronuclei migrate towards one another and their constituent chromosomes undergo replication in preparation for the first mitotic division of the embryo. Following DNA duplication, pronuclear membranes break down, and the maternal and paternal chromosomes come together for the first time on the first mitotic spindle at syngamy. Immediately thereafter, chromosomes move apart at anaphase, the cleavage furrow forms and the one-cell zygote becomes a two-cell embryo.

Preimplantation

Preimplantation development encompasses the period from fertilization to implantation. Key events occurring during this time include continued cell division, morphological refashioning and genetic reprogramming.

Timelines and key morphologic changes of embryonic development

During early embryonic divisions, increasing cell number is not accompanied by any appreciable increase in embryonic size, reflected by the continued presence of the zona (Figure 19.7). Instead, during this time, the cytoplasm inherited from the egg is merely redistributed to the accumulating blastomeres which get progressively smaller, again vividly illustrating the central role played by the egg in embryogenesis.

Around the eight-cell stage (3–4 days post ovulation), the embryo undergoes compaction whereby membrane surfaces between neighbouring embryonic cells (or blastomeres) become indistinct, leading to the formation of a morula by the 16-cell stage. Around this time, the embryo enters the uterine cavity to begin its rapport with the endometrium (Figure 19.7). Shortly thereafter, at the 32–64-cell stage (4–5 days post ovulation), the blastocyst is formed, characterized by the presence of a cavity or blastocoel and the presence of two cell types: an outer trophoectoderm (TE) or trophoblast which is the placental precursor, and an eccentrically placed inner cell mass (ICM) which is the progenitor of the embryo proper (Figure 19.7). As discussed in greater detail later, isolation and culture of cells from the inner cell mass at this stage results in the derivation of an embryonic stem (ES) cell line (see Figure 19.10C).

Oviductal transport and nutritional support

Tubal embryo transport is dependent upon coordinated oviductal smooth muscle activity mediated by the sympathetic nervous system. The emerging picture is that sympathetic tone requires fine-tuning by lipid mediators, known as 'endocannabinoids' (e.g. anandamide), acting via CB1 receptors. Human fallopian tubes were recently shown to express CB1, the levels of which peak during the luteal phase, likely reflecting control by progesterone (Horne et al 2008). The importance of endocannabinoid signalling is underlined by high rates of oviductal embryo retention in CB1-deficient mice (Wang et al 2004), and lowered tubal CB1 expression in women with ectopic pregnancies (Horne et al 2008).

The embryo's nutritional requirements change during early development. Thus, the early-cleavage-stage embryo is relatively metabolically quiescent and utilizes pyruvate as an energy source, whereas blastocysts demonstrate high metabolic activity and use glucose as their sole energy supply. In response to this, the oviduct is rich in pyruvate and non-essential amino acids, and low in glucose, whereas the uterine cavity is rich in glucose and essential amino acids (Watkins et al 2008).

Genetic aspects: embryonic reprogramming to embryonic genome activation

Underlying the overt structural changes described above are dramatic alterations in the regulation of gene expression. Under the influence of ooplasmic factors, the specialized gene expression programmes of both male and female gametes are largely erased to provide a *tabula rasa* on which to establish a well-orchestrated embryonic gene expression pattern required for preimplantation development (Niemann et al 2008).

This reprogramming is imposed by epigenetic modifications consisting of changes to DNA methylation status and to the histones on which the DNA is wound (Egli et al 2008). By altering the accessibility of DNA to the transcription machinery, epigenetic changes alter gene expression without altering the core genetic code. Epigenetic reprogramming is ultimately responsible for the acquisition of totipotency by early embryonic cells, conferring on them the capacity to form any cell type in the body, including extra-embryonic trophoblast.

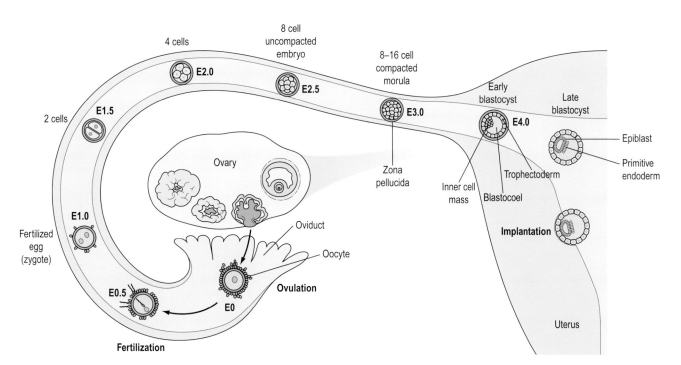

Figure 19.7 Timeline of preimplantation embryonic development during transit of the embryo through the fallopian tube and into the uterine cavity.
From Wang and Dey; Roadmap to embryo implantation: clues from mouse models; Nature Reviews Genetics, 7;185–199,2006.

One group of genes must, however, remain shielded from this global reprogramming effort. These are the imprinted genes for which it is critically important that a parent-of-origin-specific pattern of expression is retained (Swales and Spears 2005). Male and female imprints are laid down during gametogenesis, and must be sequestered away from the reprogramming route if proper embryonic development is to follow.

Until its own genome is fully activated, the early embryo is heavily reliant on maternal transcripts present in the egg for directing new protein synthesis integral to early development. As epigenetic marks are laid down, the embryonic genome becomes progressively activated. Synchronous with this embryonic genome activation (EGA) is the degradation of oocyte-derived transcripts, thereby marking a maternal-to-embryonic baton change in genetic control. The major EGA burst occurs at the four-cell stage in humans and at the two-cell stage in mice. Recent evidence from mice suggests that EGA occurs in three successive and overlapping waves comprising minor and major EGA and mid-preimplantation EGA (Wang and Dey 2006).

Expression of specific genes is required for segregation of the TE and ICM lineages at the morula-to-blastocyst transition. The current consensus is that Nanog and Oct4 are required for ICM specification and for suppressing the formation of extraembryonic lineages. On the other hand, Cdx2 is required for TE specification by ensuring the repression of Oct4 and Nanog in the TE (Wang and Dey 2006).

Implantation

Having entered the uterine cavity, the trophoectoderm of the free-living blastocyst engages in foreplay with the endometrial luminal epithelium in the hope of securing a reliable nutrient supply. Successful implantation is the culmination of a highly intricate molecular dialogue between an implantation-competent blastocyst and a receptive endometrium. The process of implantation is schematically shown in Figure 19.8, but involves a series of complex biological interactions between the embryo and endometrium to be successful.

Morphologic changes and the window of implantation

Implantation requires the simultaneous presence of an activated embryo and a receptive endometrium. The endometrium is only receptive during a restricted timeframe referred to as the 'implantation window'; prior to this window, the endometrium is prereceptive, whilst afterwards it is refractory and hostile to blastocyst survival. In humans, the receptive phase occurs approximately 5–9 days following ovulation, corresponding to days 20–24 of an idealized 28-day cycle (Diedrich et al 2007).

The principal regulators of uterine receptivity are oestrogen and progesterone acting via nuclear oestrogen receptors (ERα and ERβ) and progesterone receptors (PRα and PRβ). Endometrial expression of the homeobox gene, *HOXA-10*, rises dramatically at implantation and conveys progesterone responsiveness within the uterine stroma (Achache and Revel 2006). Oestrogen induces epithelial and stromal proliferation as well as PR expression. Progesterone, on the other hand, promotes stromal transformation or decidualization, glandular secretion and vascular remodelling. Bleb-like protrusions called 'pinopods' that extend beyond the epithelial microvilli tips are also under the influence of progesterone. Pinopods are preferential sites of embryo–endometrial interactions (see Figure 19.9C) and may serve

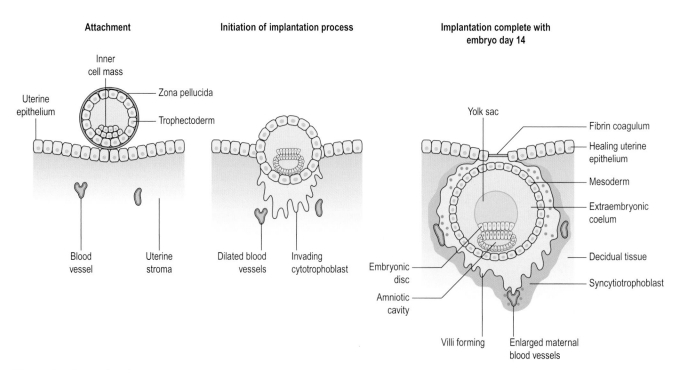

Figure 19.8 Stages of implantation.

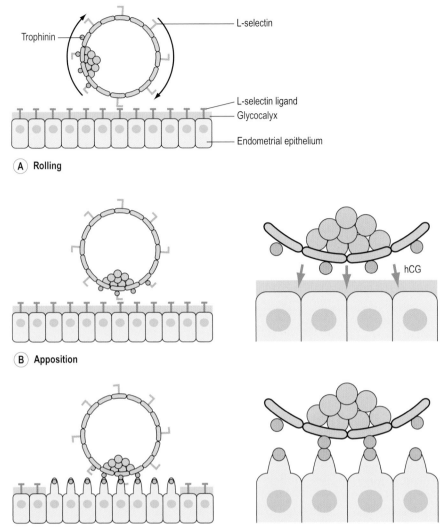

Figure 19.9 Schematic model of the roles of L-selectin and trophinin in human implantation. (A) The blastocyst expresses L-selectin and is proposed to 'roll' along the glycocalyx-covered endometrial surface epithelium. MUC1 in the glycocalyx prevents embryonic adhesion except in areas expressing L-selectin ligand. (B) Human chorionic gonadotrophin (hCG) secreted by the blastocyst induces localized expression of trophinin by the endometrial epithelium. (C) Trophinin is concentrated on pinopods which project above the glycocalyx layer. In order to facilitate adhesion, the glycocalyx adjacent to the embryo is attenuated, allowing for direct trophinin–trophinin interaction between pinopods and the trophoectoderm.

as morphological markers of uterine receptivity (Achache and Revel 2006).

The process of implantation is classified into three stages that form a continuum: apposition, adhesion and penetration. Thinning of the epithelial glycocalyx layer, retraction of long apical microvilli, and proteolytic digestion of the zona pellucida enable endometrial and trophoblastic microvilli to interdigitate. Shortly after attachment, the underlying stroma exhibits increased vascular permeability and oedema, alterations in intercellular matrix, sprouting of new capillaries and altered stromal cell morphology, collectively referred to as the 'primary decidualization reaction'. After 2–3 days, this reaction is more pervasive, giving rise to the secondary decidua as preparation of the major endometrial component of the placenta gets underway.

Within a few hours of attachment, penetration follows as trophoblastic processes erode the basal lamina. Implantation is described as interstitial in humans by virtue of the fact that the embryo invades the stroma deeply enough for the luminal epithelium to be reconstituted over it (Figure 19.8). Some trophoblastic cells fuse, forming the syncytiotrophoblast, whilst others retain their cellularity and serve

as a trophoblastic reservoir known as the 'cytotrophoblast' (Figure 19.8). Maternal blood vessels are eroded so that the syncytiotrophoblast is bathed in maternal blood. These initial steps form the basis for the establishment of the elaborate placental circulation, the details of which can be found in textbooks devoted to obstetrics.

Molecular cross-talk during implantation

Next, this chapter will describe some of implantation's bewildering molecular entourage. A recurring theme is that of reciprocal interactions between receptor–ligand pairs on the embryo and endometrium reminiscent of sperm–egg interplay during fertilization. Furthermore, it has become evident that the embryo is not merely a passive spectator, but actively directs many aspects of the implantation process.

Adhesion molecules and mucins

Members of the cell adhesion molecule (CAM) family, such as selectins, integrins and cadherins, positively regulate embryo–endometrial interaction (Achache and Revel 2006,

Guzeloglu-Kayisli et al 2007). Embryonic L-selectin interacts with luminal epithelial oligosaccharides (e.g. MECA-79), constituting an initial step in the attachment process (Genbacev et al 2003) (Figure 19.9A). The trophoectoderm expresses another adhesion molecule termed 'trophinin', which is also expressed on endometrial pinopods under the influence of human chorionic gonadotrophin (hCG) secreted by the blastocyst (Fukuda and Sugihara 2008) (Figure 19.9B and C). The ensuing trophinin–trophinin interaction is proposed to be a more potent bond than that mediated by L-selectin (Fukuda and Sugihara 2008) (Figure 19.9C). Although the L-selectin/trophonin system is crucial for human implantation, it appears to be dispensable in mice.

Attachment is further facilitated by integrins such as trophoblastic α1β1 and endometrial αVβ3 which bind to ligands such as osteopontin and oncofetal fibronectin on the luminal epithelium and trophoblast, respectively (Achache and Revel 2006). During the proliferative phase, high oestrogen levels acting via ERα inhibit αVβ3 expression, whilst secretory-phase progesterone has the opposite effect possibly via increased epidermal growth factor (EGF) in combination with downregulation of ERα levels. Interestingly, the embryo may upregulate β3 integrins via its interleukin-1 (IL-1) system, thereby actively participating in establishing endometrial receptivity. Calcium-regulated expression of E-cadherin mediated by progesterone and endometrial calcitonin is also thought to contribute to implantation.

In contrast to CAMs, glycoproteins known as 'mucins' (e.g. MUC1) extend beyond the glycocalyx and sterically inhibit adhesion (Achache and Revel 2006) (see Figure 19.9). Although data are contradictory, it is felt that under the influence of progesterone, MUC1 levels are locally reduced on pinopods, thereby unmasking CAMs to facilitate embryo–endometrial interaction. Local downregulation of MUC1 at the implantation site, possibly via blastocyst tumour necrosis factor-α-mediated increases in sheddase enzymes, lends further support for an active embryonic input.

Cytokines and growth factors

Leukaemia inhibitory factor (LIF) is a member of the cytokine family whose endometrial expression peaks during the mid- to late-secretory phase. Implantation fails in mutant mice lacking LIF (Stewart et al 1992), and patients suffering from infertility and recurrent implantation failure display suboptimal endometrial LIF expression (Hambartsoumian 1998), underscoring a pivotal role for LIF in implantation. Embryonic signals such as hCG and insulin-like growth factor (IGF) may regulate LIF expression. Conversely, LIF may interact with embryonic LIF receptors to mediate trophoblast growth and differentiation.

Three other cytokines, IL-1 (mentioned above), IL-6 and IL-11, peak in the endometrium during the luteal phase, and are also implicated in implantation.

Growth factors constitute another class of proimplantation mediators and include IGF, transforming growth factor-β and the EGF family, the latter embracing EGF itself, heparin-binding EGF-like growth factor (HB-EGF) and amphiregulin, amongst others (Achache and Revel 2006, Guzeloglu-Kayisli et al 2007). In mice, HB-EGF is the earliest molecular marker of implantation, found exclusively at the sites of active blastocysts (Wang and Dey 2006). HB-EGF derived from blastocysts induces endometrial HB-EGF expression in a paracrine manner, which in turn interacts with blastocyst receptors (ErbB1 and ErbB4). This HB-EGF autoinduction loop induces blastocyst activation, shedding of the zona pellucida and initiation of attachment. HB-EGF function is conserved as its expression in humans is maximal in the late secretory phase, and HB-EGF-expressing cells adhere to blastocyst ErbB4 (Chobotova et al 2002).

Matrix metalloproteinases and prostaglandins

Implantation is characterized by extensive tissue remodelling and vascular changes. Matrix metalloproteinases (e.g. MMP-9), in concert with tissue inhibitors of matrix metalloproteinases (e.g. TIMP-1), mediate controlled matrix degradation during invasion (Guzeloglu-Kayisli et al 2007).

Prostaglandins are members of the eicosanoid family that direct vascular events required for fully executing the implantation process (Achache and Revel 2006, Wang and Dey 2006). Prostaglandins are produced from membrane phospholipids under the consecutive action of phospholipase A_2 (PLA$_2$), cyclo-oxygenase (COX) and prostaglandin synthase enzymes. COX2-derived prostacyclin (PGI$_2$) is the primary prostaglandin produced at the implantation site, where it acts via the peroxisome-proliferator-activated receptor-δ receptor. Prostaglandin-deficient mice, due to lack of either PLA$_2$ or COX2, suffer higher rates of pregnancy failure resulting from delayed implantation. Furthermore, COX2-derived prostaglandins are also implicated in angiogenesis by differentially regulating vascular endothelial growth factor and angiopoietin signalling cascades. Evidence from mice intimates that prostaglandins are a focal downstream signalling target as LIF induces HB-EGF, which is in turn required for COX2 expression. In humans, COX expression is maximal during the menstrual and proliferative phases, and may be important for fine-tuning uterine receptivity during the window of implantation.

Immune Factors in Implantation

Immune tolerance

Although half of its genes are paternally derived, the implanting embryo is able to evade the maternal immune system during normal pregnancy (Trowsdale and Betz 2006). One aspect of immune tolerance is related to the unique expression of human leukocyte antigen (HLA) antigens on extravillous trophoblast cells which display HLA-C, HLA-E and HLA-G molecules, but not HLA-A or HLA-B which mediate allograft rejection. Other likely factors include trophoblastic expression of Fas ligand (CD95L) that promotes apoptosis of activated lymphocytes expressing Fas (CD95), as well as suppression of T-cell proliferation secondary to reduced levels of uterine tryptophan, and the systemic and decidual expansion of regulatory T-cells (CD4+CD25+Foxp3+ T-cells).

Uterine natural killer cells

A hallmark of decidualization is the presence of uterine natural killer cells (uNK cells; CD56$^{+bright}$/CD16$^-$) which represent 70% of the uterine lymphocyte population at the implantation site (Moffett-King 2002). The term 'killer' is misleading as there is no compelling evidence that uNK cells kill trophoblast cells; unlike their highly cytotoxic blood counterparts (CD56^{+dim}/CD16^{+}), uNK cells are of low cytotoxicity. On the contrary, it is currently felt that uNK cells may exert a beneficial effect in controlling trophoblast invasion, possibly mediated via interaction between uNK cell killer immunoglobulin receptor and trophoblastic HLA-C (Moffett and Loke 2006). Given the uncertain role of the uNK cell in human pregnancy and the equally uncertain relationship between blood and uNK cells, tenuous links between blood NK cell levels and risk of pregnancy failure remain of uncertain significance (Moffett et al 2004).

Clinical and Scientific Correlates

Assisted reproductive technology

The world recently celebrated the 30th birthday of Louise Brown, the first IVF baby. Since her birth on 25 July 1978, more than 4 million children have been born worldwide using this technology. As with natural pregnancy, the cornerstones for IVF success centre on good-quality embryos, a receptive endometrium and a productive embryo–endometrial rapport. Some of the advances, controversy and concerns surrounding this powerful technology are described below.

Embryo–endometrial synchronization

A greater appreciation of embryo development has translated into improved IVF success rates by altering parameters to mimic the in-vivo situation more closely. During natural conception, the cleavage-stage embryo (2–3 days post fertilization) is first geared towards interacting with the oviductal milieu, whilst the blastocyst-stage embryo (5–6 days post fertilization) is more temporally synchronized with the endometrium. In keeping with this, significantly better IVF implantation rates accrue after transferring blastocyst-stage embryos into the uterine cavity compared with transferring cleavage-stage embryos (Papanikolaou et al 2008). Culture of embryos to the blastocyst stage in the laboratory setting has become increasingly more achievable with the development of improved sequential embryo culture media. These media formulations have, in turn, arisen from a greater understanding of the evolving needs of the preimplantation embryo during its journey from the oviduct to the uterine cavity.

Embryonic aneuploidy and preimplantation genetic screening

One of the over-arching determinants of embryo quality is chromosome constitution. The presence of too few or too many chromosomes (aneuploidy) is a major contributor to IVF failure and miscarriage.

On this basis, preimplantation genetic screening (PGS) has been pursued to enable the selection of embryos having normal chromosome numbers (euploid). PGS differs from preimplantaion genetic diagnosis, which is applied to patients at high risk of transferring a defined genetic disorder. PGS most commonly involves the removal of one or two cells from the embryo and their subsequent analysis using fluorescence in-situ hybridization to probe for a panel of chromosomes (usually 13, 14, 15, 16, 18, 21, 22, X and Y).

Studies involving PGS have produced conflicting results. The only two completed randomized controlled trials to date did not provide any compelling evidence that PGS improves pregnancy outcomes (Anderson and Pickering 2008). The results of these studies present something of an enigma in so far as there is no *a priori* reason why a euploid embryo should not result in a better outcome than one that is aneuploid. It is only when better diagnostic techniques emerge that are less detrimental to the embryo and which give a more comprehensive readout of the embryo's entire chromosomal constitution (not just a nine-chromosome sample) that the role of PGS in assisted reproductive technology (ART) will be better informed.

IVF/ICSI: proceed with caution

Notwithstanding advances that more closely replicate 'physiological' conditions, there remain aspects of ART that are not normally encountered in spontaneous conception and which justifiably fuel considerable trepidation regarding their potential impact on resulting offspring.

Since its introduction over a decade and a half ago, intracytoplasmic sperm injection (ICSI) has become an established tool for overcoming male factor subfertility (Varghese et al 2007). However, ICSI bypasses many of the stringent natural selection mechanisms detailed previously that would normally preclude successful fertilization by defective spermatozoa. Thus, ICSI will ensure that infertility-related genetic traits such as Y-chromosome microdeletions in the azoospermia factor region are handed down to male offspring. Apart from propagating male infertility traits, it is unknown at present whether such genetic defects harbour any additional, more sinister, consequences. It is notable in this respect that there have been reports of increased rates (albeit small) of congenital abnormalities, especially of the genitourinary system, amongst ICSI-derived offspring. However, because the oldest child conceived through ICSI is still only a teenager, long-term studies are lacking and clarification on any such links, if indeed they do exist, remain outstanding.

Another area of concern is the potential effect of the artificial embryonic environment during IVF on the epigenome, in particular on imprinted genes (Watkins et al 2008).

Stem Cell Technology

The remarkable capacity of the oocyte to reprogramme gametic nuclei following fertilization has contributed to the birth of, arguably, the most exciting and promising scientific endeavour of our generation: somatic-cell nuclear transfer (SCNT) and the generation of embryonic stem cells (ES cells) (Hochedlinger and Jaenisch 2003).

Somatic-cell nuclear transfer

SCNT denotes the introduction of a donor somatic cell nucleus into an enucleated egg (Hochedlinger and Jaenisch

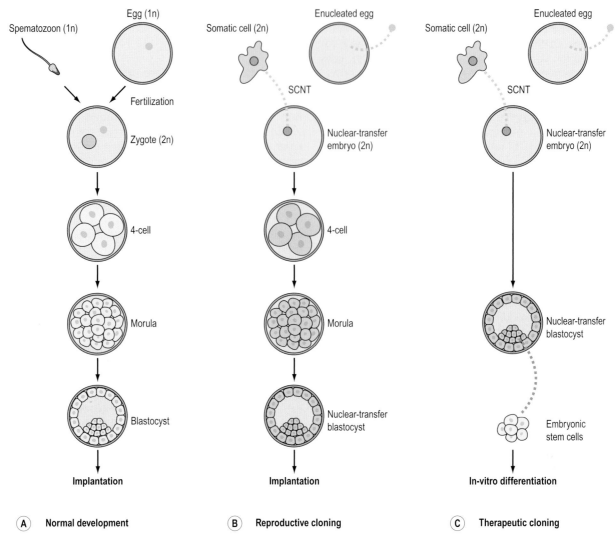

Figure 19.10 Schematic comparison of natural fertilization and embryonic development with reproductive and therapeutic cloning. (A) During normal fertilization and in-vitro fertilization, spermatozoa and eggs containing half the chromosome complement (1n) fuse to reconstitute the complete diploid chromosome set (2n) in the zygote. Subsequent embryonic development produces a morula followed by a blastocyst, at which stage implantation occurs. (B) During reproductive cloning, the diploid nucleus of an adult donor cell is introduced into an enucleated oocyte which can be activated to commence embryonic development to the blastocyst stage. Following transfer of such cloned blastocysts into surrogate mothers, a small proportion will implant and develop into an animal that is the clone of the animal from which the adult donor cell was derived. (C) The initial steps of therapeutic cloning are similar to reproductive cloning up until blastocyst development. At this stage, instead of transferring the blastocyst into a surrogate mother, cells from the inner cell mass are explanted in culture to yield a line of embryonic stem cells that can potentially differentiate in vitro into any type of cell for therapeutic purposes. SCNT, somatic-cell nuclear transfer.

2003) (Figure 19.10B). The transcriptional programme of the donor nucleus is erased by ooplasmic factors and reprogrammed towards an embryonic schedule of development. Once activated using an artificial stimulus, the egg containing the donor nucleus can then be coaxed into developing into a so-called 'cloned' blastocyst in the same way that an egg fertilized by a spermatozoon can develop into a blastocyst during IVF. Notably, unlike the IVF embryo which is a genetic composite of two gametic genomes, the SCNT embryo is genetically identical to that of (or a clone of) the donor somatic cell (Figure 19.10, compare A and B). The first cloned human blastocysts derived after SCNT with human ES cells (Stojkovic et al 2005) and adult fibroblasts (French et al 2008) have been reported recently.

'Reproductive cloning' and 'therapeutic cloning'

The blastocyst resulting from SCNT could be transferred into a recipient uterus with the aim of producing cloned offspring with the identical genetic composition of the donor nucleus (Figure 19.10B). Although highly inefficient, such 'reproductive cloning' has resulted in the birth of animals from 12 species, the first mammalian clone being 'Dolly the sheep' (Wilmut et al 1997). Importantly, however, human reproductive cloning is unanimously considered morally and ethically repugnant, and is legally prohibited in the UK by the Human Reproductive Cloning Act (2001) (Lovell-Badge 2008).

The overwhelming interest in this field does not surround 'reproductive cloning' but instead centres largely on 'therapeutic cloning'. For therapeutic cloning, cells from the inner cell mass of an SCNT blastocyst are explanted in culture to yield a line of pluripotent ES cells potentially capable of differentiating into any adult cell type (Hochedlinger and Jaenisch 2003) (Figure 19.10C). ES cell lines have recently been derived from primates following SCNT (Byrne et al 2007).

Regenerative medicine: the potential benefit of nuclear reprogramming

One of the ultimate goals of this technology is the laboratory generation of 'customized' patient-specific cells of any tissue type for use in regenerative therapies. For example, neurones engineered in a culture dish from ES cells might be made available for treating neurodegenerative diseases. Importantly, being autologous, such patient-specific cells circumvent immunocompatibility issues that severely limit the utility of more conventional tissue transplantation approaches.

Nuclear reprogramming technology also provides avenues for cell-based drug discovery and for more fundamental research into understanding embryonic development, the genetic basis for disease and the molecular circuitry underpinning cellular differentiation.

Alternative methods of nuclear reprogramming

One of the major obstacles to stem cell research is the dearth of human oocytes available for SCNT (Hall and Stojkovic 2006). One means for sidestepping this problem is the star-tling revelation that nuclear reprogramming could be effected by a cocktail of just four transcription factors (OCT4, SOX2, KLF4 and MYC) to produce so-called 'induced pluripotent stem' (iPS) cells (Okita et al 2007). This is a field that is progressing with unprecedented rapidity, driven by the goal of regenerative medicine. There are clear links between the nuclear reprogramming events that underpin the earliest events of embryo development and the molecular processes that are needed to reprogramme an adult nucleus. It is anticipated that our understanding of the latter may lead to explanations for many of the problems that occur during human fertilization and preimplantation development.

Concluding Remarks

Relentless scientific toil, largely undertaken in animal models like the mouse, has made us privy to many of the molecular forces driving critical stages in mammalian reproduction. However, it is becoming increasingly evident that humans exhibit unique signalling details that are not replicated in animal models (Diedrich et al 2007, Childs et al 2008, Fukuda and Sugihara 2008). It will therefore be important that greater inroads be made into the workings of the human system if clinical practice is to be better served. In the future, techniques such as gene expression profiling will lead to a better appreciation of the molecular signature defining a receptive human endometrium (Diedrich et al 2007). The growing emphasis on single embryo transfer during IVF as a means for reducing unacceptably high multiple pregnancy rates places greater burden on selecting the best quality embryos (Cutting et al 2008). In this regard, the application of metabolomics, proteomics and comparative genomic hybridization to embryo selection holds promise for 'sifting the wheat from the chaff'.

KEY POINTS

1. Gametogenesis produces spermatozoa and eggs via meiosis, which reshuffles genetic material and halves chromosome numbers. Fusion of gametes at fertilization restores the full diploid chromosome complement in the embryo.

2. In order to attain full fertilization potential, spermatozoa undergo maturation in the epididymis followed by capacitation in the female genital tract. The vast majority of the embryo's cytoplasm and its component organelles are derived from the egg, the quality of which is therefore a major determinant of embryo quality and hence reproductive performance.

3. At ovulation, the egg with its outer zona pellucida is surrounded by a covering of follicle-derived cumulus cells embedded in a glycoprotein matrix comprised predominantly of hyaluronan. Fertilization involves spermatozoal penetration of cumulus cells, interaction with and penetration of the zona pellucida, and binding and fusion between the spermatozoal and egg membranes.

4. Spermatozoa penetrate the cumulus cell covering by means of hyperactivated motility and a surface-anchored hyaluronidase. Having penetrated the cumulus covering, interaction of spermatozoal surface ligands with an egg receptor comprising zonal glycoproteins (ZP2 and ZP3) induces the acrosome reaction.

5. The acrosome is a lysosomal-like secretory granule that forms a cap-like structure over the spermatozoal nucleus. The acrosome reaction involves a calcium-mediated release of enzymes which, in concert with hyperactivated motility, enable a spermatozoon to penetrate the zona pellucida and enter the perivitelline space where fusion occurs.

6. At the time of fusion, a soluble sperm factor known as 'phospholipase-C' is introduced into the metaphase-arrested egg, resulting in calcium transients which break the egg's meiotic arrest and induce the cortical reaction so as to prevent polyspermy.

7. Nuclear envelopes assemble around the male and female genomes to form pronuclei in what is now referred to as a 'zygote'. Following DNA replication, pronuclear membranes break down, and male and female chromosomes intermingle for the first time on the first mitotic spindle at syngamy.

8. The embryo increases its cell numbers forming a morula (16 cells) by 3–4 days post ovulation and a blastocyst (32–64 cells) by 4–5 days post ovulation. The blastocyst is characterized by the presence of a fluid-filled cavity or blastocoel along with two cell types: an outer trophoectoderm which is the placental precursor, and the inner cell mass which gives rise to the embryo proper.

9. The ooplasm possesses a unique capacity to reprogramme nuclei into an embryonic pattern of gene expression. Maternal transcripts inherited from the egg direct protein synthesis in the early embryo until embryonic genome activation occurs.

10. Implantation proceeds through three stages (apposition, adhesion and penetration) and requires a receptive endometrium that is present during a limited interval known as the 'implantation window'. The principal mediators of receptivity are oestrogen which promotes epithelial and stromal proliferation, and progesterone which induces decidualization and glandular secretion.

11. A multitude of molecular factors are proposed to mediate implantation including CAMs (e.g. L-selectin and trophinin), cytokines (e.g. LIF), growth factors (e.g. HB-EGF), matrix metalloproteinases and prostaglandins (e.g. prostacyclin).

12. Maternal immune system tolerance to the embryo is mediated by factors such as a unique profile of trophoblastic HLA expression and an increase in decidual regulatory T-cells. The role of uterine and blood NK cells in pregnancy failure remains uncertain.

13. ART success rates have improved through a better appreciation of normal embryogenesis. One example is blastocyst-stage transfer, which has become possible by improvements in in-vitro embryo culture techniques.

14. Although IVF/ICSI has now become commonplace, it is important to remain cognisant of potential adverse effects, and to continue to monitor offspring born following this technology.

15. SCNT capitalizes on the ability of the ooplasm to reprogramme differentiated nuclei, and involves the transfer of an adult cell nucleus into an enucleated egg. Therapeutic cloning refers to the derivation of ES cells from SCNT embryos, and holds promise for generating replacement tissue in regenerative medicine.

16. The shortage of human oocytes remains a major stumbling block to ES cell technology, and has recently led to alternatives such as iPS cells and growing interest in admixed embryos.

References

Achache H, Revel A 2006 Endometrial receptivity markers, the journey to successful embryo implantation. Human Reproduction Update 12: 731–746.

Anderson RA, Pickering S 2008 The current status of preimplantation genetic screening: British Fertility Society policy and practice guidelines. Human Fertility (Cambridge, England) 11: 71–75.

Byrne JA, Pedersen DA, Clepper LL et al 2007 Producing primate embryonic stem cells by somatic cell nuclear transfer. Nature 450: 497–502.

Childs AJ, Saunders PT, Anderson RA 2008 Modelling germ cell development in vitro. Molecular Human Reproduction 14: 501–511.

Chobotova K, Spyropoulou I, Carver J et al 2002 Heparin-binding epidermal growth factor and its receptor ErbB4 mediate implantation of the human blastocyst. Mechanisms of Development 119: 137–144.

Cutting R, Morroll D, Roberts SA et al 2008 Elective single embryo transfer: guidelines for practice. British Fertility Society and Association of Clinical Embryologists. Human Fertility (Cambridge, England) 11: 131–146.

Diedrich K, Fauser BC, Devroey P, Griesinger G, Evian Annual Reproduction (EVAR) Workshop Group 2007 The role of the endometrium and embryo in human implantation. Human Reproduction Update 13: 365–377.

Egli D, Birkhoff G, Eggan K 2008 Mediators of reprogramming: transcription factors and transitions through mitosis. Nature Reviews. Molecular Cell Biology 9: 505–516.

French AJ, Adams CA, Anderson LS, Kitchen JR, Hughes MR, Wood SH 2008 Development of human cloned blastocysts following somatic cell nuclear transfer with adult fibroblasts. Stem Cells 26: 485–493.

Fukuda MN, Sugihara K 2008 An integrated view of L-selectin and trophinin function in human embryo implantation. Journal of Obstetrics and Gynaecology Research 34: 129–136.

Genbacev OD, Prakobphol A, Foulk RA et al 2003 Trophoblast L-selectin-mediated adhesion at the maternal–fetal interface. Science 299: 405–408.

Guzeloglu-Kayisli O, Basar M, Arici A 2007 Basic aspects of implantation. Reproductive Biomedicine Online 15: 728–739.

Hall VJ, Stojkovic M 2006 The status of human nuclear transfer. Stem Cell Reviews 2: 301–308.

Hambartsoumian E 1998 Endometrial leukemia inhibitory factor (LIF) as a possible cause of unexplained infertility and multiple failures of implantation. American Journal of Reproductive Immunology 39: 137–143.

Hochedlinger K, Jaenisch R 2003 Nuclear transplantation, embryonic stem cells, and the potential for cell therapy. New England Journal of Medicine 349: 275–286.

Homer HA 2007 Ageing, aneuploidy and meiosis: eggs in a race against time. In: Hillard T (ed) The Yearbook of Obstetrics and Gynaecology. RCOG Press London, pp 139–158.

Horne AW, Phillips JA, Kane N et al 2008 CB1 expression is attenuated in fallopian tube and decidua of women with ectopic pregnancy. PLoS ONE 3: e3969.

Kaji K, Oda S, Shikano T et al 2000 The gamete fusion process is defective in eggs of Cd9-deficient mice. Nature Genetics 24: 279–282.

Lovell-Badge R 2008 The regulation of human embryo and stem-cell research in the United Kingdom. Nature Reviews. Molecular Cell Biology 9: 998–1003.

Mastroianni L, Coutifaris C 1990 Reproductive Physiology, Vol. I. Parthenon, Carnforth.

Mochida S, Hunt T 2007 Calcineurin is required to release Xenopus egg extracts from meiotic M phase. Nature 449: 336–340.

Moffett A, Loke C 2006 Immunology of placentation in eutherian mammals. Nature Reviews. Immunology 6: 584–594.

Moffett A, Regan L, Braude P 2004 Natural killer cells, miscarriage, and infertility. BMJ (Clinical Research Ed.) 329: 1283–1285.

Moffett-King A 2002 Natural killer cells and pregnancy. Nature Reviews. Immunology 2: 656–663.

Niemann H, Tian XC, King WA, Lee RS 2008 Epigenetic reprogramming in embryonic and foetal development upon somatic cell nuclear transfer cloning. Reproduction 135: 151–163.

Nixon B, Aitken RJ, McLaughlin EA 2007 New insights into the molecular mechanisms of sperm–egg interaction. Cellular and Molecular Life Sciences 64: 1805–1823.

Okita K, Ichisaka T, Yamanaka S 2007 Generation of germline-competent induced pluripotent stem cells. Nature 448: 313–317.

Papanikolaou EG, Kolibianakis EM, Tournaye H et al 2008 Live birth rates after transfer of equal number of blastocysts or cleavage-stage embryos in IVF. A systematic review and meta-analysis. Human Reproduction 23: 91–99.

Primakoff P, Myles DG 2002 Penetration, adhesion, and fusion in mammalian sperm–egg interaction. Science 296: 2183–2185.

Sassone-Corsi P 2002 Unique chromatin remodeling and transcriptional regulation in spermatogenesis. Science 296: 2176–2178.

Stewart CL, Kaspar P, Brunet LJ et al 1992 Blastocyst implantation depends on maternal expression of leukaemia inhibitory factor. Nature 359: 76–79.

Stojkovic M, Stojkovic P, Leary C et al 2005 Derivation of a human blastocyst after heterologous nuclear transfer to donated oocytes. Reproductive Biomedicine Online 11: 226–231.

Swain JE, Pool TB 2008 ART failure: oocyte contributions to unsuccessful fertilization. Human Reproduction Update 14: 431–446.

Swales AK, Spears N 2005 Genomic imprinting and reproduction. Reproduction 130: 389–399.

Swann K, Saunders CM, Rogers NT, Lai FA 2006 PLCzeta(zeta): a sperm protein that triggers Ca2+ oscillations and egg activation in mammals. Seminars in Cell and Developmental Biology 17: 264–273.

Telfer EE, McLaughlin M 2007 Natural history of the mammalian oocyte. Reproductive Biomedicine Online 15: 288–295.

Trowsdale J, Betz AG 2006 Mother's little helpers: mechanisms of maternal–fetal tolerance. Nature Immunology 7: 241–246.

Tunquist BJ, Maller JL 2003 Under arrest: cytostatic factor (CSF)-mediated metaphase arrest in vertebrate eggs. Genes and Development 17: 683–710.

Varghese AC, Goldberg E, Agarwal A 2007 Current and future perspectives on intracytoplasmic sperm injection: a critical commentary. Reproductive Biomedicine Online 15: 719–727.

Wang H, Dey SK 2006 Roadmap to embryo implantation: clues from mouse models. Nature Reviews. Genetics 7: 185–199.

Wang H, Guo Y, Wang D et al 2004 Aberrant cannabinoid signaling impairs oviductal transport of embryos. Nature Medicine 10: 1074–1080.

Wassarman PM 2008 Zona pellucida glycoproteins. Journal of Biological Chemistry 283: 24285–24289.

Watkins AJ, Papenbrock T, Fleming TP 2008 The preimplantation embryo: handle with care. Seminars in Reproductive Medicine 26: 175–185.

Wilmut I, Schnieke AE, McWhir J, Kind AJ, Campbell KH 1997 Viable offspring derived from fetal and adult mammalian cells. Nature 385: 810–813.

Wu JQ, Kornbluth S 2008 Across the meiotic divide — CSF activity in the post-Emi2/XErp1 era. Journal of Cell Science 121: 3509–3514.

CHAPTER 20

Disorders and investigation of female reproduction

Mark Hamilton

Chapter Contents

INTRODUCTION	278	ENDOMETRIOSIS, FIBROIDS AND UTERINE FACTORS	287
EPIDEMIOLOGY	278	UNEXPLAINED INFERTILITY	288
INITIAL ASSESSMENT	279	INSIGHTS FROM ASSISTED CONCEPTION	289
APPROPRIATE INITIAL INVESTIGATIONS	281	CONCLUSIONS	289
DISORDERS OF OVULATION	281	KEY POINTS	290
TUBAL FACTOR INFERTILITY	283		

Introduction

The intention of this chapter is to provide an overview of a spectrum of disorders of female reproduction, including infertility, which may present to gynaecologists in clinical practice. Observations on epidemiological issues of importance are made, leading to a discussion of the initial assessment of infertile couples in the setting of primary care. A critique of the place of secondary investigations is provided, under the broad headings of disorders of ovulation, tubal factor infertility, endometriosis and uterine factors, and unexplained infertility. Insights into the pathogenesis of infertility brought about by assisted conception techniques are also examined. The need for integration of services in enabling efficient and accurate assessment of the infertile is emphasized throughout.

Epidemiology

Time to conception

A common definition employed in describing infertility is the inability of a couple to conceive following 12–24 months of exposure to pregnancy. The length of exposure time considered is determined by the observation that in the general population, which would include a proportion of couples with infertility, one would expect the chance of conception in any individual cycle to be 20%. Thus, by 1 year of exposure, approximately 85% of couples would have achieved conception, and once 2 years has elapsed, some 92% would have conceived (Evers 2002). Others have evaluated conception rates in truly fertile couples and found that the expectation of pregnancy at 3, 6, 9 and 12 months was 42%, 75%, 88% and 98%, respectively (Gnoth et al 2003). In practical terms, the failure to achieve pregnancy causes enormous

distress to those affected. For people with fertility problems, using a definition of 1 year to describe infertility is usual, and most will have sought medical advice or assistance by that time. Natural fertility rates decline in association with increasing female age, although in an ultimately fertile group of women, it is not certain that their monthly fecundability (percentage chance of conception) is any less than younger cohorts. It may be sensible to consider specialist referral of women over 35 years of age in advance of 1 year, although it is acknowledged that, in many instances, conception will occur naturally in these cases since it can be assumed that a proportion will not be infertile.

Prevalence

Estimates of the prevalence of infertility in the population will be influenced by the duration of infertility used in the definition and the population studied. The setting of prevalence studies, such as primary care (Snick et al 1997) or hospital clinics (Hull et al 1985), will influence the prevalence figures. Community-based data, which would give an accurate reflection of prevalence within the general population, are limited. It is not surprising, therefore, that existing studies suggest a range of lifetime prevalence of infertility extending from 6.6% to 32.6%. One population-based study in the North East of Scotland (Templeton et al 1990), which took account of conceptions resulting in miscarriage and ectopic pregnancy, found a prevalence of 14% using a 2-year definition.

A number of factors have been a matter of concern in recent years with respect to their potential impact on the prevalence of infertility, including the incidence of sexually transmitted infection such as *Chlamydia trachomatis* in the young (Macmillan and Templeton 1999). In addition, there have been suggestions that environmental factors may affect male fertility (Oliva et al 2001), and one should wonder

DOI: 10.1016/B978-0-7020-3120-5.00020-5

about the possible effects on female fertility of delayed child-bearing as determined by changes in lifestyle and working patterns. Despite these legitimate concerns, when the population-based study was repeated (Bhattacharya et al 2009), the observed prevalence of infertility had not increased in North East Scotland in the succeeding 20 years.

A lack of observed change in prevalence should not encourage complacency in respect of public health responsibilities. While opportunities to prevent infertility are limited, encouragement to the young to engage in safe sexual practices, limiting exposure to risk of sexually transmitted infection, is clearly important. For teenage girls, rubella immunization programmes should be in place and human papillomavirus vaccination programmes are now being established. Education of the public about the known decline in fertility which occurs with age, particularly in females over 35 years of age, is also important. In addition, the need for folic acid supplementation for women to reduce the risk of neural tube defects should be promoted, as well as the need to make certain lifestyle adjustments on issues such as the potential need to moderate levels of smoking and alcohol consumption, as well as achieving optimal weight. There is convincing evidence that smoking, active or passive, affects reproductive performance in women and men, as well as increasing the risk of small-for-gestational-age infants, stillbirth and infant mortality (National Collaborating Centre for Women's and Children's Health for the National Institute of Clinical Excellence 2004).

The requirement to take account of future reproductive needs in women is essential where abdominal or pelvic surgery is carried out, and careful technique should be employed to minimize the risk of pelvic adhesions. Where uterine instrumentation is considered, particularly in women under 25 years of age, the prevention of *Chlamydia* infection is receiving appropriate attention (Macmillan and Templeton 1999). Screening tests to detect the organism in first-void urine samples or cervical swabs using nucleic acid amplification techniques should be available routinely, and antibiotic treatment should be given for identified cases and potential contacts. Good lines of communication to sexual health and genitourinary medicine services will facilitate swift management.

Diagnostic categories

The management of people with infertility problems is largely dictated by the major diagnostic category in which they fit. Typical figures are shown in Table 20.1.

Diagnostic categories in most studies include male factors, disorders of ovulation, tubal factors, endometriosis and unexplained infertility. The distribution of causes, when analysed, will be affected by whether the female has been pregnant in the past (i.e. secondary infertility). This has an association with an increased risk of tubal factor infertility compared with those couples with primary infertility (i.e. where there has not been a pregnancy in the past) (see Chapter 21, Disorders of male reproduction, for more information). The possibility that male factors may contribute to a couple's infertility should not be ignored, even where the man has fathered a pregnancy in the past. It should be borne in mind that more than one factor may contribute to a couple's infertility, and each may require simultaneous manage-

Table 20.1 Diagnostic categories and distribution of couples with primary and secondary infertility

Diagnostic category	Infertility	
	Primary (%)	Secondary (%)
Male factor	25	20
Disorders of ovulation	20	15
Tubal factor	15	40
Endometriosis	10	5
Unexplained	30	20

ment; for example, ovulation induction for a woman who is not ovulating, in combination with donor insemination. Decisions to initiate active treatment will be influenced by the age of the female, the duration of infertility, and whether or not there has been a pregnancy in the past. Initiating intrusive and potentially harmful treatment should take account of natural expectations of pregnancy. In many instances, expectant management will be appropriate.

Initial Assessment

When to refer

The point at which any couple might seek assistance will be influenced by a number of factors, not least the degree of anxiety which couples feel in confronting seemingly relentless monthly disappointments. It should be borne in mind that libido and, consequently, coital frequency may be influenced by the experience of infertility and thus affect prognosis. While there is some evidence that sperm parameters may be adversely affected by very frequent ejaculation, the evidence suggests that fertility potential is unaffected. Bearing in mind that sperm can be expected to survive for up to 7 days within the female reproductive tract, couples should be advised to have intercourse every 2–3 days to optimize the chance of conception. The use of temperature charts or ovulation [luteinizing hormone (LH)] prediction kits to time intercourse should be discouraged.

It may be apparent to individuals that they may be at risk of a fertility problem, and advice may be sought at an early stage. For example, the male may have had a vasectomy, or undergone testicular surgery in childhood, e.g. orchidopexy; either partner may be a survivor of childhood cancer and have undergone chemotherapy; or the female may be aware of an association of absent or irregular periods with infertility. For some couples, a concern through the high profile which infertility now attracts in the media may have eroded their self-assurance about their fecundity.

In any circumstance, all people seeking advice about fertility should have prompt access to an integrated multi-disciplinary service that provides efficient and accurate assessment of their clinical situation. This should lead to individualized care founded on evidence-based principles of management. Care should be reinforced by access to adequate information and appropriate counselling services. At all times, the infertile should be treated with respect and supported in making informed choices about their clinical management.

Integrated care

Integrated care, by definition, must include the general practitioner (GP), whose role is of fundamental importance (Hamilton 1992). Infertility is a deeply personal problem and many individuals will prefer to discuss intimate matters with someone they know and trust. The counselling support that the GP can provide as preliminary assessment is made and investigations initiated is an excellent foundation for provision of care. Not infrequently, the male and female may be registered with different GPs. This can present difficulties. One should always consider that infertility is a problem affecting both parties, and each may contribute to the pathogenesis. Once referral is made to a specialist clinic, increasing the demands on couples' time, the intrusive nature of some of the investigations may add to the stress of the situation. Infertility, its investigation and treatment, can threaten domestic stability and it is often the GP, through longstanding knowledge of the couple and their families, who may be in the best position to provide support for those struggling to come to terms with continued disappointment.

All patients should be seen as couples in appropriate surroundings, and the facilities in the surgery should permit examination of both partners. Sufficient time, ideally 30 min, should be made available to permit adequate overall assessment of the problem.

Female assessment: history

Points requiring particular attention in the history and examination of the female are shown in Table 20.2.

Table 20.2 The initial assessment of female infertility: history and examination

Area of investigation	History	Area of investigation	Examination
Infertility	Duration of infertility Length and type of contraceptive use Fertility in previous relationships as well as in present liaison Previous investigation and treatment Subsequent fertility, if known, in any former partners Previous fertility investigations and treatment	General	Height, weight, body mass index Fat and hair distribution (Ferriman Galwey score to quantify hirsutism) Note presence or absence of acne and galactorrhoea
Medical	Menstrual history • Menarche • Cyclicity • Pain • Bouts of amenorrhoea • Menorrhagia • Intermenstrual bleeding Number of previous pregnancies including abortions, miscarriages and ectopic pregnancies Any associated sepsis Time to initiate previous pregnancies Past and present drug history, e.g. agents which cause hyperprolactinaemia, past cytotoxic treatment or radiotherapy	Abdominal	Check for abdominal masses or tenderness
Surgical	Previous abdominal or pelvic surgery in particular gynaecological procedures	Pelvis	Assess state of hymen Assess normality of clitoris and labia Assess vagina, looking for problems such as infection, vaginal septa, endometriotic deposits Check for presence of cervical polyps Assess accessibility of the cervix for insemination Record uterine size, position, mobility and tenderness. Perform cervical smear if appropriate
Occupational	Work patterns including separation from partner		
Sexual	Coital frequency and timing, including knowledge of the fertile period Dyspareunia Postcoital bleeding		

Appropriate Initial Investigations

Should couples present to the GP in advance of 1 year of infertility, it may be unnecessary to pursue vigorous investigation unless there is something obvious in either the history or examination. For the GP, it is advisable to ensure that the female is rubella immune and that she is taking folic acid supplementation (0.4 mg/day) to reduce the chance of the fetus developing a neural tube defect. If there is a past history of neural tube defect or the patient is taking antiepileptic medication, a higher dose (5 mg/day) is required.

Merely providing the couple with an outline of their excellent fertility potential over the next year may be all that is required to set their minds at rest. More urgency may be required where the female partner is over 35 years of age.

In the hospital setting, the infertile should have access to advice in a multidisciplinary fertility clinic. It may be helpful for the clinic to employ dedicated liaison staff to assist with the referral process.

The sequence of investigation will be the same regardless of whether the couple are seen for the first time in the GP surgery or the fertility clinic. An explanation of the steps in the process of investigation should be given to the couple at the outset. Three simple questions need to be answered:

- Are sperm available? (i.e. is there evidence of normal spermatogenesis and ejaculatory competence?)
- Are eggs available? (i.e. is the woman ovulating?)
- Can the gametes meet? (i.e. is there a pelvic problem in the female impairing normal gamete/embryo transport and is coital function adequate?)

The principles of investigation of the male will be discussed in detail in Chapter 21. Suffice it to say that semen analysis remains the cornerstone of assessment. In administrative terms, it is helpful if the analysis is done in a dedicated andrology laboratory which serves the fertility clinic, to which onward referral would be made if required.

Disorders of Ovulation

Disturbances in ovulation are the principal factor in approximately 20% of couples presenting to clinics with fertility difficulties. In women who have a regular monthly menstrual cycle (21–42 days), it is most likely that ovulation is occurring normally. The release of the egg from a mature follicle is dependent on the production of a surge of LH by the pituitary gland. This hormonal dynamic initiates the final steps in meiosis, required to allow the oocyte to reach maturity, thus permitting normal fertilization. LH causes the ovarian follicle to rupture and release the egg within; under its influence, the steroid biosynthetic capability of the ovary changes dramatically. Granulosa cells almost exclusively synthesize and release oestradiol in the follicular phase of the cycle, but produce both oestradiol and progesterone during the luteal phase of the cycle. The direct observation of follicular rupture to assess ovulation is not practical in a clinical sense, and thus the release of the oocyte is usually inferred through indirect methods, most often the measurement of progesterone in the putative luteal phase of the cycle.

Presumptive signs of ovulation

Similarly, clinical signs, in addition to regular menstruation, which suggest rather than prove that ovulation is occurring include the presence of Mittelschmerz (mid-cycle abdominal discomfort) or mid-cycle spotting induced through a transient fall in oestradiol coincidental to the LH surge. The production of mid-cycle mucus is oestrogen dependent, and a change in consistency and stretchability (Spinnbarkeit) occurs under the influence of progesterone. This is used in natural family planning techniques as a contraceptive method, but conversely may occasionally have a place in timing intercourse or artificial insemination in promoting fertility. Under the influence of progesterone, basal body temperature (BBT) may rise by 0.5–1.0 °C after ovulation. While for some, the finding of such a rise (through serial measurement taken each morning during the periovulatory phase of the cycle) is reassuring, the correlation with serum progesterone levels is poor; couples often find the confusion and uncertainty this brings to be stressful. For this reason, BBT monitoring is not recommended routinely in most clinics.

Measurement of serum progesterone

Serum progesterone levels in excess of 30 nmol/l 7 days after ovulation are usually taken as indicative of satisfactory ovulation, although lower levels are not incompatible with egg release and corpus luteum formation (Hull et al 1982, Wathen et al 1984). This is a retrospective measure of ovulation in so far as the peak level of progesterone is found after egg release. It is important to relate progesterone levels to the timing of subsequent menstruation. Samples will typically be checked on day 21 of a 28-day cycle. Serial checks will be required if the cycle is longer than this or is variable in length. Shorter cycle length will require an assessment earlier than day 21. Testing for LH is difficult in practice since the day of the LH surge cannot be predicted in advance with certainty. Urinary kits are available to detect LH and can be helpful in treatment cycles where the timing of artificial insemination is critical. Their use in detecting ovulation in routine investigation is not encouraged.

In the absence of any additional clues in history or examination to suggest an endocrine disturbance, assessment of ovulation through progesterone measurement will be sufficient on its own to confirm normal ovulatory function. However, if there is a history of irregular periods or amenorrhoea, especially if associated with galactorrhoea, hirsutism or obesity, additional endocrine investigations will be required. These include the measurement of follicle-stimulating hormone (FSH), LH, thyroid-stimulating hormone and prolactin, timing sampling to coincide with the early follicular phase of the cycle if the woman is having periods. If significant hirsutism or acne is present, the measurement of testosterone, sex-hormone-binding globulin and adrenal androgens, including androstenedione, dehydroepiandrosterone, dehydroepiandrosterone sulphate and 17-hydroxy progesterone (17-OHP), should be performed.

Ultrasound follicle tracking

Ovarian ultrasound to track follicular development, rupture and corpus luteum formation may be useful in ovulation induction treatment cycles; however, it is time consuming and intrusive, and thus is rarely used in the routine investigation of ovulation. Observation of cysts within the ovary in the luteal phase may be indicative of luteinized unruptured follicles. On occasions, these may be associated with subnormal production of progesterone, so-called 'luteal-phase deficiency'. It is uncertain whether or not these phenomena are important in the genesis of infertility, since luteal cysts and suboptimal progesterone profiles are not seen consistently in tracked cycles in individual patients. However, scanning in the early follicular phase is helpful in assessing ovarian morphology. A diagnosis of polycystic ovaries is made if there are at least 12 follicles of 2–9 mm diameter and/or the ovarian volume is greater than 10 cm³. Assessment of endometrial thickness within the uterus may be a useful indicator of the level of oestrogen exposure in women presenting with amenorrhoea, which can be of assistance in reaching a diagnosis.

Ovulation failure

The World Health Organization (WHO) classification of ovulatory dysfunction (Table 20.3) is a helpful system of categorizing disorders of ovulation based on the pathogenesis of the disorder.

WHO Type I ovulatory dysfunction may be due to a failure of the hypothalamus to produce gonadotrophin-releasing hormone (GnRH) which regulates the production of gonadotrophins by the pituitary gland. Typically, FSH and LH levels are low (<5 IU/l). Oestrogen levels are also low, and an ultrasound scan of the uterus will show a thin or absent endometrial stripe. The patient fails to menstruate after exposure to a short course of progestagen treatment.

A similar situation may arise in cases of hyperprolactinaemia, which may be associated with galactorrhoea as well as amenorrhoea. Normal pulsatile release of GnRH from the hypothalamus is compromised, and follicular growth ceases with resultant amenorrhoea. This may also occur in some instances of hypothyroidism, where high levels of thyrotrophin-releasing hormone can alter dopamine-mediated regulation of the anterior pituitary and cause hyperprolactinaemia. If hyperprolactinaemia is found, magnetic resonance imaging of the pituitary may identify a microadenoma or, occasionally, a larger pituitary tumour. Some drugs that block the effect of dopamine, such as phenothiazines, certain antipsychotics, metoclopramide and others, can cause hyperprolactinaemia.

Acquired GnRH deficiency may also arise in association with weight loss, as seen in anorexia nervosa and in individuals who undertake excessive exercise. Kallman's syndrome presents as hypothalamic amenorrhoea associated with anosmia, and results from a congenital absence of GnRH-releasing neurones in the hypothalamus. The syndrome is characterized by a lack of gonadotrophin secretion from the anterior pituitary and consequent hypogonadism. Pituitary failure may arise due to necrosis or thrombosis secondary to tumour formation. Rarely, massive obstetric haemorrhage and prolonged hypotension can lead to pituitary infarction (Sheehan's syndrome).

The most common ovulation disturbances (WHO Type II) are associated with disordered hypothalamic–pituitary–ovarian function. These women will have oestrogen levels in the normal range and many are overweight, presenting with infrequent or absent periods. A common finding is the presence of polycystic ovaries on ultrasound, seen in up to 90% of such cases. In contrast to WHO Type I patients, these women will usually menstruate after exposure to a short course of progestagen treatment. Ultrasound scanning should be timed to coincide with either a natural or progestagen-induced menstrual period. Where there is clinical or biochemical evidence of hyperandrogenism, this, together with menstrual irregularity and ovarian morphology, should be taken into account in reaching a diagnosis of polycystic ovary syndrome (PCOS). A consensus view on standardized criteria for the diagnosis of PCOS has helped in establishing a uniform approach, and facilitated easier comparison of clinical and research experience in different centres (Rotterdam ESHRE/ASRM-sponsored PCOS Consensus Workshop Group 2004a,b). It was agreed that the presence of any two of the following triad are sufficient to make the diagnosis: (i) oligo-ovulation and/or anovulation; (ii) polycystic ovaries on ultrasound; and (iii) clinical and/or biochemical hyperandrogenism.

Approximately 10–20% of patients with PCOS have an associated elevation in prolactin, but this is usually mild and not of clinical consequence. On occasions, ovulatory failure may result from 21-hydroxylase deficiency in the adrenal gland leading to elevated serum levels of 17-OHP, an androgenic steroid precursor of cortisol. High androgens disturb normal follicular growth, and patients may present with irregular or absent periods associated with signs of androgen excess including hirsutism, acne and enlargement of the clitoris. Other causes of hyperandrogenism, such as adrenal tumours and Cushing's syndrome, may need to be considered where adrenal androgen levels are found to be high.

Insulin resistance has been well described in women with PCOS, and it has been estimated that they have a three to seven times higher risk of developing type 2 diabetes in later life; regular screening may therefore be appropriate. Amen-

Table 20.3 The World Health Organization classification of ovulatory disorders

Group	Type of Disorder	%	Biochemical Characteristics
I	Hypothalamic pituitary failure (hypothalamic amenorrhoea or hypogonadotrophic hypogonadism)	10	Low basal gonadotrophins, normal prolactin, low oestrogen
II	Hypothalamic pituitary dysfunction	85	Gonadotrophins and oestrogen levels in the normal range
III	Ovarian failure	4–5	High gonadotrophins, low oestrogen

orrhoea in PCOS may also be associated with an increased lifetime risk of endometrial cancer. Progestagen-induced menstruation should thus be facilitated three to four times per year, particularly if increased endometrial thickness is seen on ultrasound.

Ovarian failure

In patients presenting with amenorrhoea and where initial biochemical screening and physical examination lead one to suspect ovarian failure (WHO Type III), the presence of a genetic disorder such as Turner's syndrome (45XO) or Turner mosaic (45XO/46XX) should be considered and a karyotype performed. Occasionally, deletions in one of the X chromosomes or defects in the *fragile X* gene may lead to ovarian failure, but agenesis of the ovaries (associated with primary amenorrhoea) and premature ovarian failure (presenting as secondary amenorrhoea before 40 years of age) is sometimes found in the presence of a normal karyotype. Acquired ovarian failure may occur as a result of previous medical treatment such as chemotherapy or radiotherapy for cancer. Autoimmune ovarian failure should be considered, and screening for antiovarian antibodies may be useful in reaching a diagnosis. If positive, the need to screen for other autoimmune disorders including hypothyroidism, adrenal insufficiency (Addison's disease), diabetes mellitus and pernicious anaemia should be considered (see Chapter 17, Ovulation induction, for more information).

Tubal Factor Infertility

Tubal pathology is a contributory factor in 15–30% of women presenting with infertility. Normal tubal function should permit gamete transport, fertilization and the subsequent passage of the embryo to the uterus such that implantation can take place at the appropriate stage in the menstrual cycle. The most common cause of tubal factor infertility is past pelvic infection through sexually transmitted infection, e.g. *Chlamydia trachomatis*, although previous pregnancy, both successful and failed, or past history of pelvic surgery or endometriosis can be implicated. Occasionally, a Müllerian developmental anomaly may be involved.

The following tests of pelvic anatomy are commonly performed in the diagnostic work-up of women with infertility: (i) X-ray hysterosalpingography (HSG); (ii) laparoscopy; and (iii) hysterosalpingo contrast sonography (HyCoSy).

If the duration of infertility is short (<1 year) and the history and examination findings do not suggest that a tubal factor is likely, examination of the pelvis may be deferred until the duration of infertility approaches 18 months. However, if there is a positive feature in the history, if the pelvic findings on bimanual examination are abnormal or if a screening test for *Chlamydia* is positive, an assessment should be arranged without delay.

X-ray hysterosalpingography

This is an outpatient examination and involves the instillation of either a water- or oil-soluble contrast medium through a cannula attached to the cervix. The fluid, being

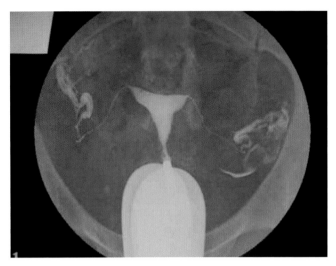

Figure 20.1 X-ray hysterosalpingography. This shows a normal uterine outline with passage of dye through tubes of normal calibre and spillage of dye into the pelvis.

radio-opaque, can be visualized under X-ray screening conditions. An assessment is made of the normality of the uterine cavity. Passage of dye to the side of the uterus permits an assessment of tubal anatomy (Figure 20.1). The diameter of the tube should be small through its interstitial, isthmic and ampullary portions, but the diameter increases slightly as the infundibulum is reached. Unimpaired passage of dye throughout the length of the tube and dispersal into the peritoneal cavity is suggestive of normal anatomy. If there is impaired flow or localization of spill distally, one should be suspicious of peritubal adhesions. The finding of a hydrosalpinx will be indicative of severe tubal damage. Sometimes, unilateral or bilateral tubal spasm occurs and a mistaken diagnosis of proximal tubal obstruction is made. An intravenous injection of glucagon can help to relax this, but if the finding persists, a cornual block is a possibility. It is important, particularly in women under 25 years of age, to consider the need for antibiotic prophylaxis since *Chlamydia* infection could be reactivated in susceptible women. Azithromycin or doxycycline is usually used.

HSG should not be carried out if the patient is menstruating. In addition, women should be advised to avoid conception in the cycle in which the procedure is carried out. If unprotected intercourse has occurred, the examination should be deferred.

The contrast medium used in HSG may contain iodine, and the possibility of allergic reactions should be borne in mind. Significant extravasation of oil-soluble contrast media within the pelvis may lead to lipogranuloma formation. There is some evidence that the use of an oil-soluble contrast medium (lipiodol) may enhance the chance of pregnancy in unexplained infertility (Johnson et al 2004), although it has not gained widespread popularity as a therapeutic choice.

Laparoscopy and dye hydrotubation

It is generally accepted that laparoscopy and dye hydrotubation is the gold standard of tubal assessment. In this procedure, which, like HSG, should avoid the time of menstruation and any chance of pregnancy, a coloured dye is injected through the cervix while carrying out a laparoscopic inspection of the pelvis (Figure 20.2). Failure of dye to pass through the tube is indicative of blockage (Figure 20.3).

Direct visualization of the pelvis permits identification of adhesions, fibroids, endometriosis, ovarian cysts and other pathology which may be relevant to infertility and would be missed at HSG. The likelihood of finding tubal disease is increased if the patient has a positive *Chlamydia* screening test (Coppus et al 2007). Immediate treatment of pathology is also possible at laparoscopy, which may be particularly relevant where endometriosis is found, provided that appropriate consent has been obtained.

The procedure should be carried out in a systematic fashion and a written record, together with photographs if possible, should be made of the findings. At least two ports are required to allow manipulation of pelvic structures to ensure thorough assessment. The bowel can sometimes obscure the view, and a probe to move this out of the way will often be helpful. Sometimes, a third port may be required if the surgeon wishes to treat minor adhesions or endometriosis, in order to allow the introduction of

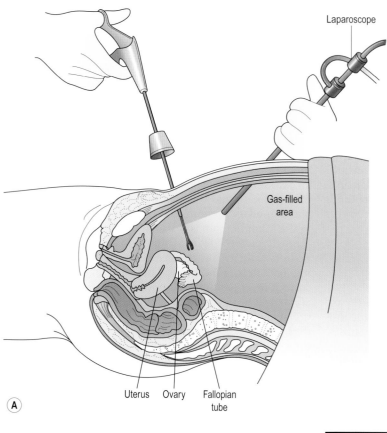

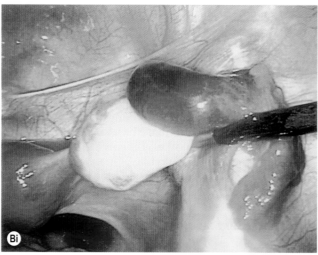

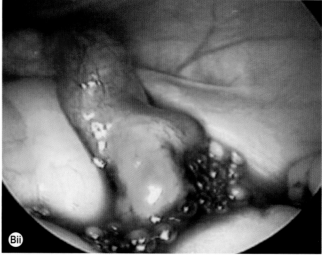

Figure 20.2 The technique of laparoscopy. (A) Instrumentation. This shows the uterine body with the right fallopian tube and the ovary. (Bi) Normal pelvis with spillage of dye from the fimbrial end of tube (Bii).

scissors or diathermy/laser instruments and suction/irrigation apparatus.

The use of a diagram, such as that produced by the American Society for Reproductive Medicine (ASRM), to record findings is often helpful in explaining to patients what has been seen and done, as well as providing a formal record of the findings, particularly if endometriosis is found (Figure 20.4).

General anaesthesia carries a small risk of reaction to the drugs used. In addition, the introduction of laparoscopic instruments presents a risk of injury to intra-abdominal structures such as the bowel, bladder and blood vessels. Patients who have undergone previous abdominal surgery, in particular those with a mid-line incision, are particularly at risk. The technique used in the introduction of instruments may need to be adapted to take account of this increased hazard. Alternatively, HSG may be preferred.

Hysterosalpingo contrast sonography

In the last two decades, HyCoSy has attracted some interest as an additional method for assessing tubal patency (Hamilton et al 1998). Carried out as an outpatient or office procedure, a small balloon catheter is inserted into the uterine

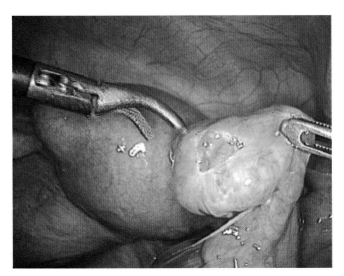

Figure 20.3 A blocked fallopian tube with hydrosalpinx formation. The distal end of the tube has been exposed, revealing terminal clubbing.

cavity through the cervix (Figure 20.5). A vaginal scan is performed while a suspension of an ultrasound contrast agent (Echovist) is injected through the catheter. Usually, only 2–5 ml of fluid will be required. The medium contains galactose granules, and if flow is seen through the length of the tube, it is likely to be patent. Hydrosalpinges can also be identified. Saline alone can be used if inspection of the uterine cavity alone is required, and good imaging of endometrial polyps can be obtained. The technique requires considerable ultrasound skill, and some patients find the instillation of the fluid uncomfortable. There is no evidence of therapeutic benefit through flushing with the medium used in HyCoSy (Lindborg et al 2009).

Hysteroscopy

Hysteroscopic examination of the uterine cavity may be carried out as an outpatient procedure, although if a laparoscopic assessment is being carried out, it is a simple affair to combine the two procedures. Either carbon dioxide or saline/glycine may be used to distend the cavity to permit adequate inspection. Uterine malformations, fibroids, endometrial polyps, adhesions and other conditions may be identified and treated using this technique, although it is controversial whether or not some of these findings contribute to infertility to any great degree.

Evaluation of diagnostic tests of tubal factor infertility

With HSG, one is interested to know whether the test identifies normal and abnormal tubes correctly compared with the gold standard, laparoscopy. The value of a test for tubal blockage (test positive) can therefore be described using a number of statistical descriptors, as shown in Table 20.4.

A meta-analysis evaluating HSG assessment of tubal patency using laparoscopy as the gold standard showed 65% sensitivity and 83% specificity (Swart et al 1995, Mol et al 1996). One can deduce from this that although HSG is of limited value in detecting tubal blockage because of its low sensitivity, its high specificity makes it a better test for identification of tubal patency. The negative predictive value (94%) of the test as a predictor of tubal patency is also high, suggesting that the finding of normal tubes on HSG is likely to be correct. However, a low positive predictive value of

Table 20.4 Hysterosalpingography as a diagnostic test of tubal patency: performance vs laparoscopy

Sensitivity	Does the test correctly identify all patients with blocked tubes?	True positives / True positives + false negatives	65%
Specificity	Does the test correctly identify all patients with patent tubes?	True negatives / True negatives + false positives	83%
Positive predictive value	The proportion of patients with positive test results (tubes blocked) who are correctly diagnosed	True positives / True positives + false positives	38%
Negative predictive value	The proportion of patients with negative test results (tubes patent) who are correctly assigned as normal	True negatives / True negatives + false negatives	94%

Data from Swart P, Mol BWJ, van der Veen F, van Beurden M, Redekop WK and Bossuyt PMM. The accuracy of hysterosalpingography in the diagnosis of tubal pathology, a meta-analysis. Fertility and Sterility 64 486–491 (1995).

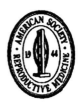

AMERICAN SOCIETY FOR REPRODUCTIVE MEDICINE
REVISED CLASSIFICATION OF ENDOMETRIOSIS

Patient's Name _____ Date _____

Stage I (Minimal) - 1-5	Laparoscopy _____ Laparotomy _____ Photography _____
Stage II (Mild) - 6-15	Recommended Treatment _____
Stage III (Moderate) - 16-40	
Stage IV (Severe) - >40	
Total _____	Prognosis _____

	ENDOMETRIOSIS	<1cm	1-3cm	>3cm
PERITONEUM	Superficial	1	2	4
	Deep	2	4	6
OVARY	R Superficial	1	2	4
	Deep	4	16	20
	L Superficial	1	2	4
	Deep	4	16	20

	POSTERIOR CULDESAC OBLITERATION	Partial		Complete	
		4		40	

	ADHESIONS	<1/3 Enclosure	1/3-2/3 Enclosure	>2/3 Enclosure
OVARY	R Filmy	1	2	4
	Dense	4	8	16
	L Filmy	1	2	4
	Dense	4	8	16
TUBE	R Filmy	1	2	4
	Dense	4*	8*	16
	L Filmy	1	2	4
	Dense	4*	8*	16

*If the fimbriated end of the fallopian tube is completely enclosed, change the point assignment to 16.

Denote appearance of superficial implant types as red [(R), red, red-pink, flamelike, vesicular blobs, clear vesicles], white [(W), opacifications, peritoneal defects, yellow-brown], or black [(B) black, hemosiderin deposits, blue]. Denote percent of total described as R___%, W___% and B___%. Total should equal 100%.

Additional Endometriosis: _____

Associated Pathology: _____

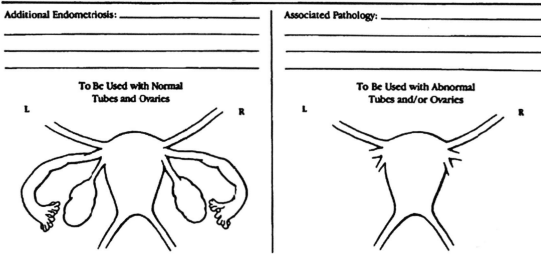

To Be Used with Normal Tubes and Ovaries

To Be Used with Abnormal Tubes and/or Ovaries

Figure 20.4 The revised American Society for Reproductive Medicine scoring system for endometriosis.
Revised classification of Endometriosis, American Society for Reproductive Medicine, Vol.47, No.8, May 1997.

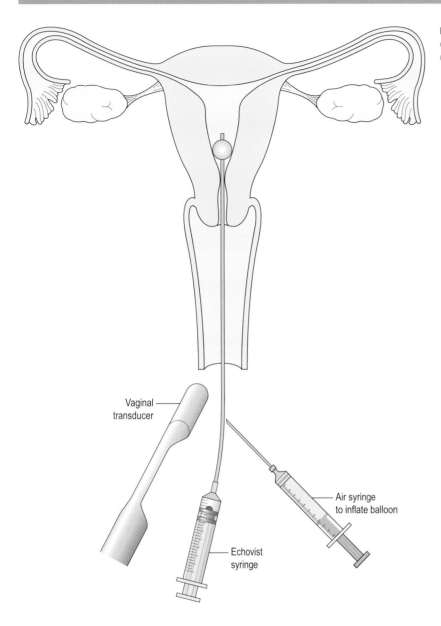

Figure 20.5 Equipment set-up for hysterosalpingo contrast sonography.
Copyright © Bayer Healthcare Pharmaceuticals.

Vaginal transducer

Air syringe to inflate balloon

Echovist syringe

38% of the test suggests that HSG is not a reliable indicator of tubal occlusion, and in the circumstances of an abnormal HSG result, it would be wise to consider a laparoscopic assessment to confirm or refute the findings (National Collaborating Centre for Women's and Children's Health for the National Institute of Clinical Excellence 2004).

HyCoSy also performs fairly well in detecting normality and hydrosalpinx formation; however, similar to HSG, it is less reliable in identifying tubal blockage (Hamilton et al 1998).

Endoscopic assessment of the tubal lumen to study mucosal appearance has not proved to be helpful in routine work-up of infertility. Falloposcopy achieves access to the tube per vaginam (Rimbach et al 2001). Salpingoscopy can be performed at laparoscopy or laparotomy where the tube is cannulated through the fimbria (de Bruyne et al 1997). Initially thought to be of potential use in selecting patients with healthy tubal epithelium who might be suitable for tubal surgery, neither of the techniques has gained much popularity and they are rarely used.

Endometriosis, Fibroids and Uterine Factors

Endometriosis

Endometriosis is a debilitating condition which has associations with infertility, particularly where there is anatomical distortion of the pelvis. Women who are susceptible to the condition may have genetic, immunological, hormonal or environmental factors contributing to the problem (Crosignani et al 2006). A family history of the condition should alert the gynaecologist to the possibility, particularly if the common symptoms of dysmenorrhoea and chronic pelvic pain are present. Pelvic examination may reveal a fixed, tender retroverted uterus, and on occasions, there may be endometriotic nodules presenting the vault of the vagina or the rectovaginal septum. A combined rectal and vaginal examination may be helpful if this is suspected. Laparoscopic visualization of endometriotic lesions is the cornerstone of diagnosis, although a histological confirmation of an excised lesion is strictly necessary to be absolutely certain.

The accuracy of the diagnosis therefore depends on the degree of skill and vigilance of the surgeon. If endometriosis is found at laparoscopy, it is helpful to stage the disease by reference to the ASRM guidelines (American Society for Reproductive Medicine 1996). There is some evidence that women with mild endometriosis have reduced fertility (Akande et al 2004), and that treatment, such as with diathermy, may improve the natural chances of conception in minimal/mild disease (Marcoux et al 1997). A suspicion of endometriosis may be raised if vaginal ultrasound examination of the pelvis is painful, or if a cyst with a hazy 'ground glass' appearance is seen in the ovary, suggestive of an endometrioma. Magnetic resonance imaging of the uterus may be helpful if one suspects adenomyosis. Biochemical assay of CA125, if raised, may be suggestive of endometriosis, although this is non-specific. Women with Müllerian abnormalities promoting retrograde menstruation are at greater risk of developing endometriosis.

Fibroids

Fibroids are among the most common benign tumours in women, with a reported prevalence of 3–8% in unselected women of reproductive age (Borgfeldt and Andolf 2000), although they occur with higher frequency in older women and in certain ethnic populations. Fibroids are often asymptomatic but an association with infertility is possible (Somigliana et al 2007), particularly where the tumour impinges on the cavity of the uterus (Khalaf et al 2006, Klatsky et al 2007). Abdominal palpation and vaginal examination may reveal a mass arising from the pelvis. Ultrasound examination is usually performed to confirm the diagnosis, and this has high sensitivity and specificity as a test. If the relationship between the fibroid and the uterine cavity is unclear from an initial ultrasound assessment, HyCoSy or HSG may be useful to distinguish submucosal from intramural lesions. Hysteroscopic evaluation of the degree of myometrial penetration by the fibroid is essential if surgical excision is contemplated (Di Spiezio Sardo et al 2008). Discrimination between adenomyosis and fibroids may be facilitated with the use of ultrasound where the absence of a tumour capsule and lacunae within the lesion may be suggestive of the former. Magnetic resonance imaging can also be of help.

Potential endometrial abnormalities

Undiagnosed uterine pathology as a cause of infertility, recurrent implantation failure (RIF) or recurrent miscarriage is an attractive concept. However, the evidence that disturbed endometrial receptivity is important in infertility is mixed. Endometrial assessment by timed sampling and histological dating is the most described method of assessing the normality of endometrial development. It is dependent on accurate timing of sampling endometrium relevant to the LH surge (Li et al 2002), and has been largely abandoned in routine practice, as has the concept of luteal-phase deficiency as a major cause of infertility. Ultrasound-measured endometrial thickness is a poor predictor of implantation potential in in-vitro fertilization (IVF) (Margalioth et al 2006), particularly where high-quality embryos are available. Disturbances in cytokine expression and action have

been postulated as a cause of RIF, but analysis of these factors remains a research tool rather than a clinical tool. The role of immunological causes and thrombophilia in infertility is also uncertain. Some early studies suggested an association between antiphospholipid syndrome and RIF, but this has not been confirmed in larger prospective studies. The role of natural killer cells in RIF is disputed (Rai et al 2005). For the moment, there is no convincing evidence for an association. An association between hereditary thrombophilia and RIF has also been described in some, but not all, studies, and screening for these disorders is still controversial (see Chapter 23, Sporadic and recurrent miscarriage, for more information).

Unexplained Infertility

Despite the use of investigation pathways as outlined above, it is debatable whether or not the basic tests of semen quality, ovulation and tubal patency are in any way accurate in predicting live birth (Taylor and Collins 1992). From the above discussion, it will also be clear that there is an ongoing, and relevant, debate concerning the existence of subtle disturbances in reproductive function in the female and their impact on fertility. While endometrial function is undoubtedly important in the genesis of conception, a number of other elements in the path to establishment of pregnancy have been considered as causes of infertility. Few are amenable to simple investigation. Possibilities are listed in Table 20.5.

Postcoital testing

An area of considerable interest over many years has been the assessment of sperm–cervical mucus interaction through the postcoital test (PCT). As the time of ovulation nears, cervical mucus secretion, under the influence of oestradiol, changes in quantity. After intercourse, sperm should swim freely within the mucus and transportation of sperm to the upper genital tract can take place. Cervical mucus–sperm hostility as a cause of infertility continues to be debated due to the methodological issues of concern in its use. The test is intrusive in so far as the couple are asked to have intercourse at a prescribed time, and then the female attends the clinic for a sample of mucus to be obtained from the cervix. The investigator examines the specimen to determine if there are motile sperm visible under light microscopy. In theory, the test could give an indication that intercourse has taken place, that timing is correct, that the mucus is receptive, and that sperm numbers and motility are adequate. In critically evaluating the usefulness of the PCT in clinical practice, many would argue that it lacks predictive power in its ability to identify those who will conceive naturally from those who will not (Oei et al 1995). Furthermore, there is no standardization of the methodology of the test; for example, timing of intercourse in relation to ovulation, timing of examination of sampled mucus relative to intercourse, and 'normal' sperm numbers and motility levels within examined mucus (Evers 2002). One study (Glazener et al 2000) found the PCT to be useful in predicting spontaneous conception in couples with otherwise unexplained infertility of a short duration (<3 years).

Table 20.5 Putative causes of unexplained infertility

Endocrine factors

Abnormal follicle growth
Suboptimal progesterone secretion (luteal-phase deficiency)
Luteinized unruptured follicle syndrome
Hypersecretion of luteinizing hormone
Ovulatory hyperprolactinaemia

Ovarian factors

Zona pellucida antibodies
Diminished ovarian reserve (ovarian ageing)

Uterine/endometrial factors

Congenital uterine abnormalities
Submucous fibroids
Abnormal uterine perfusion
Altered cytokine expression and action
Disturbed T-cell and natural killer cell function

Tubal factors

Disturbed tubal function, i.e. peristalsis, cilia
Suboptimal metabolic support of gametes and embryos
Altered immune activity

Peritoneal factors

Mild endometriosis
Occult infection
Altered immune activity

Genetic factors

Gamete and embryo aneuploidy
Poor embryo morphology, cleavage and blastocyst formation

Sperm–cervical mucus interaction

Altered cervical mucus production
Antisperm antibodies

Psychogenic factors

Inadequate coital function

However, a study which examined whether or not intra-uterine insemination improved the chance of conception, where a PCT was negative, only showed a marginal effect (Mol 2001).

Diagnostic category

Unexplained infertility presents a frustrating diagnosis for both clinician and patient. The range and accuracy of the tests which are used to investigate the infertile will influence the chance of a 'diagnostic label' being attached to the problem (Gleicher and Barad 2006). Whether such a label leads to help in forming a prognosis or formulating a treatment plan is debatable (Siristatidis and Bhattacharya 2007). In some instances, the finding of 'abnormality' occurs with similar frequency in both those who ultimately conceive naturally and those who remain infertile (Guzick et al 1994). In recent times, the age profile of patients attending fertility clinics has changed, with many women delaying childbearing for a variety of reasons. For many, age alone is a major

factor in determining prognosis, and age may also influence the probability of a diagnosis of unexplained infertility being made. It has been estimated that the chance of reaching a diagnosis of unexplained infertility is doubled if the female is over 35 years of age compared with females under 30 years of age (Maheshwari et al 2008). As discussed below, diminished ovarian reserve may, in theory, be a missed cause of infertility in otherwise unexplained infertility. For most clinics, female age, together with parity and the duration of infertility, are the three factors with the greatest bearing on prognosis.

Insights from Assisted Conception

The assisted conception population will usually include those who have prolonged infertility and, as such, is arguably not truly representative of the general infertility population. However, outcomes in those who access IVF treatment, although under very different conditions, may give some insight into what may be occurring in natural attempts to conceive, and afford help to couples in coming to terms with their infertility. Occasionally, poor fertilization outcomes may unmask functional problems regarding sperm or egg quality. Failed fertilization may be due to hardening of the zona pellucida, associated with ageing of the oocyte. Embryo quality, as judged by morphology and cleavage patterns, may be consistently suboptimal. The association with such findings and aneuploidy in embryos is well established. Women who fail to respond well to ovarian stimulation may have a qualitative or quantitative disturbance in follicular physiology. Tests of ovarian reserve to predict outcome have been widely used in those who are embarking on IVF treatment. Early-follicular-phase FSH, anti-Müllerian hormone, inhibin-B and ovarian-ultrasound-observed antral follicle count are the most popular measures. Dynamic tests of ovarian reserve have also been described using clomiphene or exogenous gonadotrophin stimulation. However, the predictive power of all these tests, relevant to a number of endpoints including eggs retrieved and clinical pregnancy, is poor, except at the extremes of ranges. For the moment, they should be regarded as unsuitable for routine evaluation of the infertile female (Maheshwari et al 2008).

Conclusions

Infertility is a major public health problem, causing significant distress to those directly involved, as well as family and friends. It is essential that the limited public resources are used prudently to maximize the quality of care provided. The preliminary assessment of the availability of eggs and sperm, together with a determination that the gametes can meet, should provide a diagnosis for the majority of couples. It should be possible to provide a prognosis, usually favourable, and where necessary, treatment can be initiated within a relatively short time. The importance of efficient mechanisms of referral and investigation cannot be overestimated. Regional integration of services, from GP to tertiary-level hospital settings, should be established to minimize delay for patients and avoid unnecessary repetition of investigations.

References

Akande VA, Hunt LP, Cahill D, Jenkins JM 2004 Difference in time to natural conception between women with unexplained infertility and infertile women with minor endometriosis. Human Reproduction 19: 96–103.

American Society for Reproductive Medicine 1996 Revised American Society for Reprductive Medicine classification of endometriosis 1996. Fertility and Sterility 67: 817–821.

Bhattacharya S, Porter M, Amalraj E, et al 2009 The epidemiology of infertility in the North East of Scotland. Human Reproduction 24: 3096–3107.

Borgfeldt C, Andolf E 2000 Transvaginal ultrasonographic findings in the uterus and the endometrium: low prevalence of leiomyoma in a random sample of women age 25–40 years. Acta Obstetricia et Gynecologica Scandinavica 79: 202–207.

Coppus SFPJ, Opmeer BC, Logan S, van der Veen F, Bhattacharya S, Mol BWJ 2007 The predictive value of medical history taking and *Chlamydia* IgG ELISA antibody testing (CAT) in the selection of subfertile women for diagnostic laparoscopy: a clinical prediction model approach. Human Reproduction 22: 1353–1358.

Crosignani PG, Olive D, Bergqvist A, Luciano A 2006 Advances in the management of endometriosis: an update for clinicians. Human Reproduction Update 12: 179–189.

de Bruyne F, Hucke J, Willers R 1997 The prognostic value of salpingoscopy. Human Reproduction 12: 266–271.

Di Spiezio Sardo A, Mazzon I, Bramante S et al 2008 Hysteroscopic myomectomy: a comprehensive review of surgical techniques. Human Reproduction Update 14: 101–119.

Evers JLH 2002 Female subfertility. The Lancet 360: 151–159.

Glazener CMA, Ford WCL, Hull MGR 2000 The prognostic power of the post-coital test for natural conception depends on the duration of infertility. Human Reproduction 15: 1953–1957.

Gleicher N, Barad D 2006 Unexplained infertility: does it really exist? Human Reproduction 21: 1951–1955.

Gnoth C, Frank-Hermann P, Freundl G, Godehardt D, Godehardt E 2003 Time to pregnancy: results of the German prospective study and impact on the management of infertility. Human Reproduction 18: 1959–1966.

Guzick DS, Grefenstette I, Baffone K et al 1994 Infertility evaluation in fertile women: a model for assessing the efficacy of infertility testing. Human Reproduction 9: 2306–2310.

Hamilton MPR 1992 The initial assessment of the infertile couple. Current Obstetrics and Gynaecology 2: 2–7.

Hamilton JA, Larson AJ, Lower AM, Hasnain S, Grudzinskas JG 1998 Evaluation of the performance of hysterosalpingo contrast sonography in 500 consecutive, unselected, infertile women. Human Reproduction 13: 1519–1526.

Hull MG, Savage PE, Bromham DR, Ismail AA, Morris AF 1982 The value of a single serum progesterone measurement in the mid-luteal phase as a criterion of a potentially fertile cycle ('ovulation') derived from treated and untreated conception cycles. Fertility and Sterility 37: 355–360.

Hull MGR, Glazener CMA, Kelly NJ et al 1985 Population study of causes, treatment and outcome of infertility. BMJ (Clinical Research Ed.) 291: 1693–1697.

Johnson NP, Farquhar CM, Hadden WE, Suckling J, Yu Y, Sadler L 2004 The FLUSH trial — Flushing with Lipiodol for unexplained (and endometriosis-related) subfertility by hysterosaplingograpgy: a randomized trial. Human Reproduction 19: 2043–2051.

Khalaf Y, Ross C, El-Toukhy T, Hart R, Seed P, Braude P 2006 The effect of small intramural uterine fibroids on the cumulative outcome of assisted conception. Human Reproduction 21: 2640–2644.

Klatsky PC, Lane DE, Ryan IP, Fujimoto VY 2007 The effect of fibroids without cavity involvement on ART outcomes independent of ovarian age. Human Reproduction 22: 521–526.

Li TC, Tuckerman EM, Laird SM 2002 Endometrial factors in recurrent miscarriage. Human Reproduction Update 8: 43–52.

Lindborg L, Thorburn J, Bergh C, Strandell A 2009 Influence of HyCoSy on spontaneous pregnancy: a randomised controlled trial. Human Reproduction 24: 1075–1079.

Macmillan S, Templeton A 1999 Screening for *Chlamydia trachomatis* in subfertile women. Human Reproduction 12: 3009–3012.

Maheshwari A, Fowler P, Bhattacharya S 2006 Assessment of ovarian reserve — should we perform tests of ovarian reserve routinely? Human Reproduction 21: 2729–2735.

Maheshwari A, Hamilton M, Bhattacharya S 2008 Effect of female age on the diagnostic categories of infertility. Human Reproduction 23: 538–542.

Marcoux S, Maheux R, Berube S 1997 Laparoscopic surgery in infertile women with minimal or mild endometriosis. New England Journal of Medicine 337: 217–222.

Margalioth EJ, Ben-Chetrit A, Gal M, Eldar-Geva T 2006 Investigation and treatment of repeated implantation failure after IVF-ET. Human Reproduction 21: 3036–3043.

Mol BW 2001 Diagnostic potential of the post-coital test. In: Heineman MJ (ed) Evidence Based Reproductive Medicine in Clinical Practice. American Society for Reproductive Medicine, Birmingham, pp 73–82.

Mol BWJ, Swart P, Bossuyt PMM, van Beurden M, van der Veen F 1996 Reproducibility of the interpretation of hysterosalpingography in the diagnosis of tubal pathology. Human Reproduction 11: 1204–1208.

National Collaborating Centre for Women's and Children's Health for the National Institute of Clinical Excellence 2004 Fertility: Assessment and Treatment for People with Fertility Problems. RCOG Press, London.

Oei SG, Helmerhorst FM, Keirse MJNC 1995 When is the post-coital test normal? A critical appraisal. Human Reproduction 10: 1711–1714.

Oliva A, Spira A, Multigner L 2001 Contribution of environmental factors to the risk of male infertility. Human Reproduction 16: 1768–1776.

Rai R, Sacks G, Trew G 2005 Natural killer cells and reproductive failure — theory, practice and prejudice. Human Reproduction 20: 1123–1126.

Rimbach S, Bastert G, Wallwiener D 2001 Technical results of falloposcopy for fertility diagnosis in a large multicentre study. Human Reproduction 16: 925–930.

Rotterdam ESHRE/ASRM-sponsored PCOS Consensus Workshop Group 2004a Revised 2003 consensus on diagnostic criteria and long-term health risks related to polycystic ovary syndrome (PCOS). Human Reproduction 1: 41–47.

Rotterdam ESHRE/ASRM-sponsored PCOS Consensus Workshop Group 2004b Revised 2003 consensus on diagnostic criteria and long-term health risks related to polycystic ovary syndrome. Fertility and Sterility 81: 19–25.

Siristatidis C, Bhattacharya S 2007 Unexplained infertility: does it really exist? Does it matter? Human Reproduction 22: 2084–2087.

Snick HKA, Snick TS, Evers JLH, Collins JA 1997 The spontaneous pregnancy prognosis is untreated subfertile couples: the Walcheren primary care study. Human Reproduction 12: 1582–1588.

Somigliana E, Vercellini P, Daguati R, Pasin R, de Giorgi O, Crosignani PG 2007 Fibroids and female reproduction: a critical analysis of the evidence. Human Reproduction Update 13: 465–476.

Swart P, Mol BWJ, van der Veen F, van Beurden M, Redekop WK, Bossuyt PMM 1995 The accuracy of hysterosalpingography in the diagnosis of tubal pathology, a meta-analysis. Fertility and Sterility 64: 486–491.

Taylor PJ, Collins JA 1992 Unexplained Infertility. Oxford University Press, Oxford.

Templeton A, Fraser C, Thompson B 1990 The epidemiology of infertility in Aberdeen. BMJ (Clinical Research Ed.) 301: 148–152.

Wathen NC, Perry L, Lilford RJ, Chard T 1984 Interpretation of single progesterone measurement in diagnosis of anovulation and defective luteal phase: observations on analysis of the normal range. BMJ (Clinical Research Ed.) 288: 7–9.

CHAPTER 21

Disorders of male reproduction

Richard A. Anderson and D. Stewart Irvine

Chapter Contents

INTRODUCTION	292		CLINICAL MANAGEMENT	302
HORMONAL CONTROL OF SPERMATOGENESIS	294		CHANGES IN MALE REPRODUCTIVE HEALTH	309
MALE INFERTILITY	297		KEY POINTS	310

Introduction

There has been rapid progress during the past 20 years in our understanding of male reproductive physiology, with wide-ranging contributions from cell and molecular biologists, urologists and endocrinologists, whose efforts have contributed to establishing the discipline of andrology. However, this specialty is not established in the UK, and men with reproductive disorders often present to the gynaecologist through the intermediary of their female partners. It is therefore important for gynaecologists to have some knowledge of male reproductive function and its disorders in order to recognize potential problems, as well as an understanding of the available diagnostic techniques and treatment options.

This chapter aims to provide the practising gynaecologist with an overview of clinical andrology with an emphasis on male infertility. A description of normal physiology is given as the foundation for explaining pathophysiological mechanisms and as a basis for formulating rational treatment where possible.

Physiology

The testis can be thought of as having two major interconnected functions in the adult: the production of testosterone, which maintains a wide range of physiological processes; and the production of spermatozoa and thereby fertility.

Spermatogenesis

Spermatogenesis takes place in several hundred tightly coiled seminiferous tubules arranged in lobules (Figure 21.1) (Dym 1977), which constitute some 80% of testicular volume in man. Testis volume therefore reflects spermatogenesis more than testosterone production. Each tubule resembles a loop draining at both ends into a network of tubules, the rete testis, and thence into the epididymis, a single but highly coiled tube which, in turn, drains into the unconvoluted and muscular-walled vas deferens.

The walls of the seminiferous tubules are composed of germ cells and Sertoli cells around a central lumen, surrounded by peritubular myoid cells and a basement membrane (Figure 21.2). Spermatogenesis is a continuous sequence of closely regulated events, highly organized in space and time, whereby cohorts of undifferentiated diploid germ cells (spermatogonia) multiply and, while maintaining the population of stem cell spermatogonia, are then transformed into haploid spermatozoa. The following events can be observed in the seminiferous epithelium during normal spermatogenesis.

- Mitotic division (at least four) of stem cells to form cohorts of spermatogonia which, at intervals of 16 days, differentiate into primary preleptotene spermatocytes to initiate meiosis.
- Meiotic reduction divisions of spermatocytes to form round spermatids.
- Continuous remodelling of Sertoli cells in order to direct the migration of germ cells from basal to luminal positions.
- Transformation (spermiogenesis) of large spherical spermatids into compact, virtually cytoplasm-free spermatozoa with condensed DNA in the head crowned by an apical acrosomal cap, and a tail capable of propulsive beating movements.
- Spermiation, whereby the spermatozoa are released from the Sertoli cell cytoplasm into the tubular lumen.

Cohorts of undifferentiated germ cells, joined to each other by cytoplasmic bridges, progress through these different steps in synchrony so that several generations of developing germ cells are usually observed at any one part of the seminiferous epithelium at any one time. The total time taken for a cohort of spermatogonia to develop into spermatozoa is 74 days, during which time at least three further generations of spermatogonia have also successively, at intervals of 16 days, initiated their development. In the human, spermatogenesis is arranged in a helical manner, so that cross-sections show more than one stage of spermatogenesis within individual seminiferous tubules. This

DOI: 10.1016/B978-0-7020-3120-5.00021-7

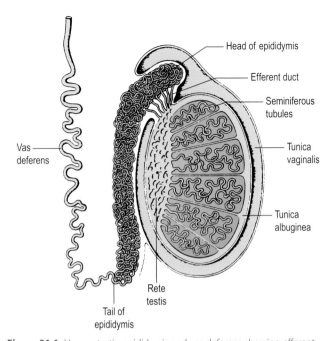

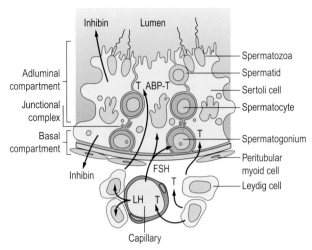

Figure 21.2 Diagrammatic representation of the anatomical and functional relationship between germ cells, Sertoli cells and Leydig cells. Note the division of the seminiferous epithelium into adluminal and basal compartments by the tight junctions between adjacent Sertoli cells and the bidirectional secretion of Sertoli cell products (e.g. inhibin) into the lumen and interstitial space. ABP-T, androgen-binding protein testosterone; FSH, follicle-stimulating hormone; LH, luteinizing hormone; T, testosterone.

Figure 21.1 Human testis, epididymis and vas deferens showing efferent ducts leading from the rete testis to the caput epididymis and the cauda epididymis, continuing to become the vas deferens.
From Dym M (1977). In Histology pp. 981 eds L Weiss and RO Greep, with permission of Elsevier.

organizational arrangement differs from that in many other species (e.g. rodents), in which spermatogenesis is arranged longitudinally and thus only one stage of spermatogenesis is seen in a cross-section of a tubule.

Sertoli cell function

Sertoli cells have extensive cytoplasm which spans the full height of the seminiferous epithelium from basement membrane to lumen (Figure 21.2). Where adjacent Sertoli cells come into contact with each other near the basement membrane, special occluding junctions are formed which divide the seminiferous epithelium into a basal (outer) compartment, which interacts with the systemic circulation, and an adluminal (inner) compartment enclosed by a functional permeability barrier, the blood–testis barrier (Figure 21.2). Spermatogonia divide by mitosis in the basal compartment, while the two reduction divisions of the spermatocytes and spermiogenesis are confined to the avascular microenvironment of the adluminal compartment created by the blood–testis barrier. The developing germ cells are therefore completely dependent on Sertoli cells for metabolic support. In response to appropriate trophic stimuli [of which follicle-stimulating hormone (FSH) and testosterone are the best described], Sertoli cells secrete a wide range of substances including growth factors and a distinctive tubular fluid high in potassium and low in protein which bathes the mature spermatozoa.

Sertoli cells contribute directly to the feedback regulation of pituitary gonadotrophin secretion. The existence of an endocrine product of the testis termed 'inhibin' was postulated for many decades. Inhibin B is a dimeric glycoprotein secreted by Sertoli cells which has a physiological role in the regulation of FSH secretion. Inhibin B concentrations reflect the functional activity of the seminiferous tubule and show a positive relationship with sperm production. Its production requires and reflects the interaction of the germ cell population with the Sertoli cells, and is absent in men with Sertoli cell only syndrome. The measurement of inhibin B may be of clinical value as a marker of the activity of the seminiferous epithelium (O'Connor and De Kretser 2004). Inhibin A, the product of the dominant follicle and the corpus luteum in women, is not present in the circulation in men.

Unlike the actively dividing germ cells, Sertoli cells do not proliferate in the adult testis. Spermatogenesis is a cyclical process which is critically dependent on changes in Sertoli cell function associated with the constantly changing combination of germ cells in contact with its cytoplasm. Changes in the germ cell complement in contact with any one Sertoli cell occur at a fixed sequence and interval. Thus, the synchronization of these repetitive cyclical changes in Sertoli cell function, associated with the variations in germ cell metabolic requirements as they divide and differentiate, has now become one of the central tenets of our conceptualization of normal spermatogenesis (Sharpe 1990). Although pituitary gonadotrophins provide obligatory trophic support for testicular function as a whole, the classic concept that luteinizing hormone (LH) stimulates Leydig cell steroidogenesis and FSH controls functions in the seminiferous tubules is far too simplistic in the light of our current understanding of spermatogenesis. There is now good evidence that the interstitial and tubular compartments are not functionally distinct, but that there is a close and complex interrelationship between them. Thus, testosterone from the interstitial Leydig cells stimulates Sertoli cell functions either directly or via the peritubular cells, as does Leydig-cell-derived insulin-like factor 3, itself critical for testicular descent (Ivell et al 2005). Altered tubular/Sertoli cell function, on the other hand, can induce changes in Leydig cell steroidogenesis, although the identity of the intercompartmental regulator(s) is unknown.

Testosterone is the only and probably the most important paracrine hormone clearly identified, and its presence in sufficient concentrations in the seminiferous tubules is an absolute requirement for spermatogenesis. How much testosterone is required and how it exerts its effects are just some of the fundamental questions that are still unanswered. Despite the large gaps in our existing knowledge, it is becoming increasingly accepted that local coordination of the multifarious functions in a variety of different cell types within the testis, orchestrated by the diverse functional capabilities of the Sertoli cells, holds the key to quantitatively normal spermatogenesis.

The Leydig cell

The adult human testis contains some 500 million Leydig cells clustered in the interstitial spaces adjacent to the seminiferous tubules. The biosynthesis of testosterone in Leydig cells is under the control of LH which binds to specific surface membrane receptors. Steroidogenesis is stimulated through a cyclic adenosine monophosphate (cAMP)–protein kinase C mechanism which mobilizes cholesterol substrate and promotes the conversion of cholesterol to pregnenolone by splitting the C21 side chain. The subsequent steps in the biosynthetic pathway involve the weakly androgenic intermediates dehydroepiandrosterone and androstenedione before testosterone, the principal secretory product, is obtained. Testosterone is secreted into the spermatic venous system, testicular lymphatics and tubular fluid.

Testosterone is the most important circulating androgen in the adult male, since most dihydrotestosterone is formed locally in androgen-responsive target tissues. When circulating in plasma, testosterone is bound to sex-hormone-binding globulin (SHBG) and albumin. The latter binds to all steroids with low affinity, while SHBG, a glycoprotein synthesized in the liver, has a high affinity but a low capacity for testosterone. In men, 60% of circulating testosterone is bound to SHBG, 38% is bound to albumin and 2% is free. Free and albumin-bound testosterone constitute the bioavailable fractions of circulating testosterone, but recent evidence suggests that SHBG-bound testosterone may also be extractable in some tissues, although the functional significance of this is unclear. The plasma concentration of SHBG is regulated by factors including steroid hormones, its synthesis being increased by oestrogens and reduced by testosterone. It is also related to body weight, being lower in the obese. These relationships are the same as in women.

Hormonal Control of Spermatogenesis

The hormonal control of spermatogenesis requires the actions of the pituitary gonadotrophins LH and FSH. There is general agreement that both LH and FSH are needed for the initiation of spermatogenesis during puberty. However, the specific roles and relative contributions of the two gonadotrophins in maintaining spermatogenesis are unclear (Liu et al 2002).

LH stimulates Leydig cell steroidogenesis, resulting in increased production of testosterone. Normal spermatogenesis is absolutely dependent on testosterone. Specific androgen receptors have not been demonstrated in germ cells, but are present in Sertoli and peritubular cells. This indicates that the actions of androgens in spermatogenesis are mediated by the somatic cells of the seminiferous tubules. The concentration of testosterone in the testis is 50 times higher than that in the peripheral circulation. There is thus an apparent gross overabundance of testosterone within the normal adult testis, the significance of which is uncertain. It is possible that some androgen-mediated functions in the testis are not mediated by classic androgen receptors. Steroids other than testosterone may also have important roles in the regulation of steroidogenesis. In particular, oestrogen receptors are widely distributed in the male reproductive tract, including the presence of oestrogen receptor β.

FSH initiates function in immature Sertoli cells, prior to the onset of spermatogenesis, by stimulating the formation of the blood–testis barrier and the secretion of tubular fluid and other specific secretory products via FSH receptors which activate intracellular cAMP. Once spermatogenesis is established in the adult testis, Sertoli cells become less responsive to FSH. Evidence for the non-essential role of FSH is provided by individuals with inactivating mutations of the FSH receptor. Such men have been documented to have complete spermatogenesis but with low sperm concentrations (Tapanainen et al 1997). However, it can be shown, in animals immunized against FSH and in experimentally induced hypogonadotrophic men given gonadotrophin replacement, that both testosterone (depending on LH) and FSH are required for quantitatively normal spermatogenesis in the adult (testosterone-replete) testis by determining the number of spermatogonia available by meiosis. However, testosterone on its own can maintain qualitatively normal spermatogenesis once it has been initiated (Matsumoto et al 1984). FSH therefore acts either by increasing spermatogonial mitosis or by decreasing the number of cells that degenerate at each cell division. Testosterone is essential for the subsequent stages from meiosis to spermiogenesis.

Hypothalamic–pituitary–testicular axis

The secretion of gonadotrophins from the anterior pituitary gland is controlled by gonadotrophin-releasing hormone (GnRH) released into the pituitary portal circulation from axon terminals in the hypothalamic median eminence. These neurosecretory neurones in the medial basal hypothalamus are responsive to a wide variety of sensory inputs as well as to gonadal negative feedback. GnRH stimulates the secretion of both LH and FSH. In the adult male, GnRH is released episodically into the pituitary portal circulation at a frequency of approximately every 140 min; each volley of GnRH elicits an immediate release of LH, producing the typical pulsatile pattern of LH in the systemic circulation (Figure 21.3; Wu et al 1989). Although also secreted episodically, FSH and testosterone pulses are not apparent in normal men because of the slower secretion of newly synthesized rather than stored hormone and the longer circulating half-lives. The intermittent mode of GnRH stimulation, within a narrow physiological range of frequency, is obligatory for sustaining the normal pattern of gonadotrophin secretion.

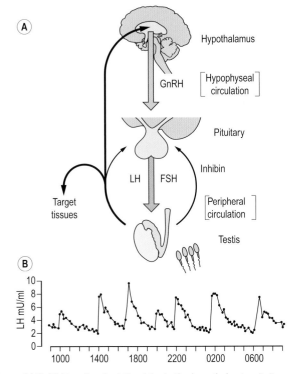

Figure 21.3 (A) Functional relationships in the hypothalamic–pituitary–testicular axis. Gonadotrophin-releasing hormone (GnRH) is secreted into the hypophyseal circulation in an episodic manner, represented by a luteinizing hormone (LH) pulse in the peripheral circulation. (B) Peripheral blood LH concentration sampled in an adult male at 10-min intervals for 24 h from 0900 to 0900 h.

Continuous or high-frequency GnRH stimulation paradoxically desensitizes the pituitary gonadotrophin response in men as in women, because of depletion of receptors and refractoriness of postreceptor response mechanisms. It has recently been demonstrated that the secretion of GnRH is dependent on the newly-described kisspeptin (also known as 'metastin'). Mutations of the kisspeptin receptor result in pubertal failure. Kisspeptin-containing neurones impinge directly on GnRH neurones in the hypothalamus, and there is emerging evidence that they also mediate effects of metabolic signals such as leptin on the reproductive axis (Seminara and Crowley 2008).

Testosterone exerts the major negative feedback action on gonadotrophin secretion. Its effect is predominantly to restrict the frequency of GnRH pulses from the hypothalamus to within the physiological range. Testosterone also acts on the pituitary to reduce the amplitude of the LH response to GnRH. It is now recognized that these inhibitory effects on GnRH and gonadotrophin secretion are, in part, mediated following conversion of testosterone to oestradiol by the enzyme P450 aromatase. This is demonstrated both by administration of aromatase inhibitors to normal men and by the finding that men with either mutant, non-functional oestrogen receptors or absent aromatase activity have markedly elevated gonadotrophin concentrations despite high-normal testosterone concentrations (Smith et al 1994, Morishima et al 1995). Interestingly, these men also showed marked osteoporosis, suggesting a distinct role for oestrogen in bone. Feedback inhibition of pituitary FSH synthesis is predominantly mediated by inhibin B and also by testoster-

one, particularly at high concentrations. The regulation of FSH secretion by inhibin in addition to testosterone results in the selective rise in FSH but not LH concentrations in men with various disorders of spermatogenesis.

The spermatozoon

The primary function of the spermatozoon is the delivery of a male pronucleus to the fertilized egg. The spermatozoon must conserve its DNA and transport it to the site of fertilization, where it must recognize and fuse with a receptive egg. The ejaculated spermatozoon must first escape from the seminal plasma in which it is deposited beside the cervix, and penetrate the barrier presented by cervical mucus. It must then travel through the uterus to the site of fertilization in the fallopian tube. During this journey, it must complete the process of functional maturation known as 'capacitation', an ordered series of events involving reorganization of cell surface components and changes in cellular metabolism and motility patterns, which are a prerequisite for successful fertilization. Having reached the oviduct, the male gamete must recognize the oocyte, penetrate the cumulus oophorus and bind to the zona pellucida. At this point, it must display a unique pattern of movement known as 'hyperactivated motility' and undergo the acrosome reaction. This process is initiated by a specific protein component of the zona pellucida (ZP3) and results in release of the contents of the acrosomal matrix, which include the serine protease acrosin and other hydrolytic enzymes including hyaluronidase. In addition, the acrosome reaction results in the generation of a fusogenic equatorial segment, which is the zone of fusion with the oocyte plasma membrane. For a review of sperm structure and function, the reader is referred to Grudzinskas (1995).

To enable it to undertake these complex functions, the human spermatozoon has developed a highly specialized morphology, with its various structural components tailored to specific functional attributes. The appearance of the spermatozoon was first described over 300 years ago by Anthony van Leeuwenhoek. In outline, the spermatozoon has a dense oval head capped by an acrosome and is propelled by a motile tail (Figure 21.4; Fawcett 1975). The head is made up largely of highly condensed nuclear chromatin constituting the haploid chromosome complement, complexed with highly basic proteins termed 'protamines'. It is covered in its anterior half by the acrosome, a membrane-enclosed sac of enzymes including acrosin and hyaluronidase. The area of the sperm head immediately behind the acrosome (the equatorial region) is important as it is this part which attaches to and fuses with the egg. The shape of the human sperm head is highly pleomorphic, making the morphological definition of a normal sperm head extremely challenging. Behind the head may be found a cytoplasmic droplet which consists of the remains of the residual cytoplasm left after the morphological remodelling of the cell during spermiogenesis.

The tail of flagellum is usually further divided into the midpiece, principal piece and terminal piece, joined to the head by the connecting piece. The motor apparatus of the tail is the axoneme which consists of a central pair (doublets) of microtubules of non-contractile tubulin protein enclosed in a sheath linked radially to nine outer pairs of

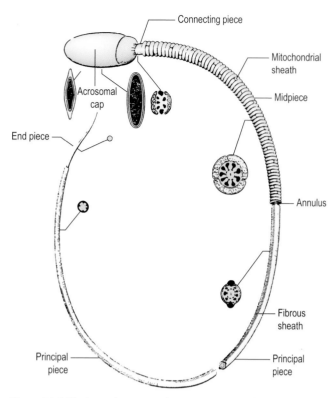

Figure 21.4 The internal structure of a spermatozoon with the cell membrane removed.

From Fawcett DW, The mammalian spermatozoon. Dev Biol; 44: 394–436, 1975; with permission of Elsevier.

microtubules. The axonemal complex is surrounded by columns of outer dense fibres, which are, in turn, covered by a helix of mitochondria in the midpiece and a fibrous sheath in the principal piece. The dense fibres and the fibrous sheath form the cytoskeleton of the flagellum. Through the hydrolysis of adenosine triphosphate, the dynein arms undergo a series of conformational changes resulting in adjacent doublets sliding over one another. Synchronized movement of groups of microtubules propagating waves of bending motions of the tail is the key to the various modes of coordinated sperm motility. Energy for sperm motility is provided by the sheath of mitochondria in the midpiece of the tail through a second messenger system, involving the calcium-mediated calmodulin-dependent conversion of adenosine triphosphate to cAMP and interaction with the adenosine triphosphatase of the dynein.

Sperm transport and maturation

Spermatozoa within the testis and male tract are quiescent and play little active role in their own transport along the tract. Moreover, they are functionally immature and the maturation process continues as they pass through the epididymis. Passage out of the seminiferous tubules and through the main testicular collecting duct, the rete testis, is due to the flow of secretions from Sertoli cells and rete epithelium and to the intrinsic smooth muscle contractions of the tubules. From the rete, the cells pass through the efferent ducts to the epididymis, a 3–4-m-long single coiled tube whose function is under androgen and neural (adrenergic)

control. It is typically subdivided into a caput or head region, a middle body or corpus, and a distal tail or cauda region which leads into the proximal vas deferens. The epididymal epithelium actively reabsorbs testicular fluid but also secretes a hyperosmolar fluid rich in glycerophosphorylcholine inositol and carnitine. The specific transport of these compounds across the epithelium creates a favourable fluid environment where progressive motility and fertilizing capacity of the spermatozoa are normally acquired. Some of these maturational changes are probably 'housekeeping' functions to ensure that the cell remains viable during its stay in the excurrent ducts, while others are associated with the development of fertilizing ability. In many animal species, spermatozoa retain fertility for several weeks in the cauda epididymis, which acts as a sperm reservoir prior to ejaculation. The human cauda epididymis, in contrast, has a relatively poor storage function, which diminishes further along the vas.

At ejaculation, spermatozoa pass along the vas and are mixed with the secretions of the accessory glands which form over 90% of the volume of the ejaculate. The seminal vesicles contribute the largest volume of alkaline fluid to the ejaculate, and are also the souce of seminal fructose, prostaglandins and coagulating proteins. Prostatic secretions contain proteolytic enzymes (which normally liquefy the coagulated proteins in semen within 20–30 min) and are rich in citric acid and zinc. Seminal plasma provides a support medium for transporting male gametes out of the body and for buffering the acidic pH of the vagina, so that a reservoir of functional sperm can be established after ejaculation. Just as testicular germ cells are subjected to constant attrition, ejaculated spermatozoa have to traverse the cervix, uterus and uterotubal junction before reaching the middle third of the oviduct, the site of fertilization. At each barrier, the sperm population is further reduced so that eventually only 200 or so of the most robust spermatozoa have the opportunity to fertilize the ovum. The number of functionally competent sperm is more important than the total number ejaculated.

The cervical canal is the first selective filtering barrier to meet the ejaculated sperm (Figure 21.5). This barrier is virtually complete except during midcycle, when oestrogenized cervical mucus glycoprotein fibrils form parallel chains called 'micelles' which permit spermatozoa with active progressive motility to swim through at a rate of 2–3 mm/min. Spermatozoa probably enter the uterine cavity from the internal os by virtue of their own motility, and appear in the uterine cavity approximately 90 min after insemination. The uterotubal junction is the second of the major physical barriers for spermatozoa. The mechanism for selectivity is not clear, but may depend on factors other than sperm motility since inert particles can pass through. Once the uterotubal junction has been successfully negotiated, a minority of sperm immediately traverse the oviduct to the ampulla; however, the majority congregate in the isthmus until ovulation has occurred. At this time, capacitated sperm showing hyperactivated movements of the tail gradually progress towards the fimbriated end, helped on by the muscular contraction of the oviduct wall and the flow of fluid in the oviduct. A maximum number of spermatozoa is present in the cervix 15–20 min following insemination and remains constant for 24 h, although a rapid decline has commenced

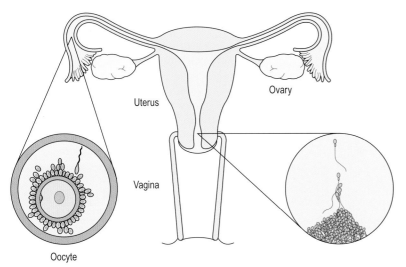

Uterus

Ovary

Vagina

Oocyte

Figure 21.5 Attributes of sperm function associated with fertility *in vivo*. The spermatozoon must escape from seminal plasma, penetrate and traverse the cervical mucus barrier, reach the site of fertilization, undergo capacitation, bind to and penetrate the zona pellucida, fuse with the plasma membrane of the egg, and undergo nuclear decondensation within the cytoplasm of the oocyte.

by 48 h. Some spermatozoa may remain motile at the site of fertilization for up to 3 days (Mortimer 1995).

Male reproductive ageing

Reproductive ageing in the male is not accompanied by such an overt and abrupt fall in gonadal function as occurs in women, but by a more gradual decline. These differences reflect the consequence of a finite pool of gametes compared with one that continually replicates from a stock of stem cells, and the clearer distinction between the endocrine and gametogenic functions of the gonads.

The decline in function of the endocrine output of the hypothalamo–pituitary–testicular axis with age is well established and results in a fall of approximately 50% in plasma testosterone concentrations (Vermeulen 1991). This has both central and peripheral components; thus, there is a relatively small increase in LH. The 'andropause' is increasingly the subject of investigation (Wu 2007), with large placebo-controlled studies of the effect of replacement under way. Changes in Sertoli cell function and spermatogenesis with ageing have received more limited investigation, but the data do suggest that there is indeed an age-related decline in function. Spermatogenesis, however, may be well maintained in elderly men.

Male Infertility

Definition and epidemiology

Infertility is commonly defined as the failure of conception after at least 12 months of unprotected intercourse (Rowe 1993), but such a definition serves to obscure the true complexity of the clinical situation. In reality, those couples who fail to achieve a pregnancy within 12–24 months include those who can be considered sterile (i.e. who will never achieve a spontaneous pregnancy) and those who are more properly termed 'subfertile' and who have reduced fecundability (probability of achieving a pregnancy within one menstrual cycle) and hence a prolonged time to pregnancy. Accurate assessment of the prevalence of infertility has always been difficult because of the scarcity of large-scale, population-based studies. Estimates suggest that some 14–17% of couples may be affected at some time in their reproductive lives (Hull et al 1985), with European data suggesting that as many as one in four couples who try may experience difficulties in conceiving (Schmidt 2006).

While infertility is relatively common, it is very difficult indeed to establish the relative contribution of the male partner, given the profound difficulties which exist in the accurate diagnosis of male infertility. Most studies which have attempted to evaluate the aetiology of infertility have used the conventional criteria of semen quality, promulgated by the World Health Organization (WHO) (World Health Organization 1999), to define the 'male factor'. Although of great importance and shortly to be updated, these criteria are of limited diagnostic value, and a significant proportion of men with normal conventional criteria of semen quality will be infertile because of defects in sperm function, while a significant number of men with abnormal semen quality will have normal sperm function. Very few studies on the epidemiology of male infertility have used functional, as opposed to descriptive, diagnostic criteria. Nevertheless, one common theme to emerge is that, using the available diagnostic techniques, male factor infertility is, in many studies, the most common single diagnostic category.

Pathophysiology

In the simplest terms, male infertility is a failure to fertilize the normal ovum arising from a deficiency of functionally competent sperm at the site of fertilization. Since less than 0.1% of ejaculated sperm actually reach the fallopian tube, it is defective sperm function rather than inadequate numbers of sperm ejaculated that constitutes the most important pathophysiological mechanism in male infertility. Specific lesions leading to defective sperm motility or transport and abnormal sperm–egg interaction are probably the key factors responsible for loss of fertilizing capacity in the gametes. In most instances, however, inadequate sperm function is usually but not invariably accompanied by reduced sperm production, suggesting that specific defects in spermatozoa commonly arise from disturbances in regulatory mechanisms which interfere with both germ cell multiplication and maturation in the seminiferous tubules. There is rarely any clinical evidence of systemic endocrine deficiency in men with male infertility. By inference, therefore, disturbances in paracrine regulation within the testis could lead to low sperm output (oligozoospermia), from an increased rate of degeneration in the differentiating spermatogonia at successive mitotic divisions, as well as abnormal spermiogenesis giving rise to spermatozoa with poor motility (asthenozoospermia) and/or abnormal morphology (teratozoospermia). Abnormal epididymal function may lead to defective sperm maturation, impairment of sperm transport or even cell death. Interruption of the transport of normal sperm may be due to mechanical barriers between the epididymis and fallopian tube or abnormal coitus and/or ejaculation.

Aetiology

Notwithstanding the difficulties in diagnosis outlined above, WHO has proposed a scheme for the diagnostic classification of the male partner of the infertile couple (Rowe 1993) (Box 21.1). This approach is of enormous value as a basis for standardization and for comparative multicentre studies. However, many of the male diagnostic categories are of a descriptive nature (e.g. idiopathic oligozoospermia) or of controversial clinical relevance (e.g. male accessory gland infection). Moreover, recent advances in our understanding of the causes of male infertility, particularly in the area of genetic problems (Hargreave 2000), mean that this classification is in need of review. The relative frequency of the major diagnostic categories is shown in Figure 21.6, using data taken from a WHO study of over 8500 couples from 33 centres in 25 countries (Comhaire et al 1987). It can be seen

---

Box 21.1 Diagnostic categories for the male partner of an infertile couple according to WHO

No demonstrable cause
Idiopathic oligozoospermia
Idiopathic asthenozoospermia
Idiopathic teratozoospermia
Idiopathic azoospermia
Obstructive azoospermia
Isolated seminal plasma
  abnormalities
Sexual or ejaculatory dysfunction

Systemic causes
Endocrine causes
Iatrogenic causes
Congenital abnormalities
Acquired testicular damage
Varicocoele
Immunological infertility
Male accessory gland infection

Source: Rowe PG 1993 WHO Manual for the Standardized Investigation and Diagnosis of the Infertile Couple. Cambridge University Press, Cambridge, UK.

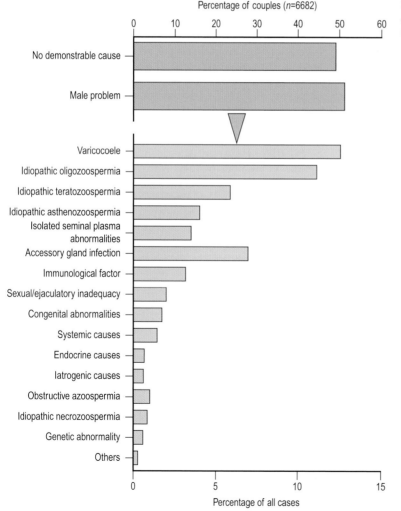

Figure 21.6 Aetiology of male factor infertility.
Adapted from Comhaire FH, de Kretser D and Farley TMM Towards more objectivity in diagnosis and management of male infertility. Results of a WHO Multicentre Study. International Journal of Andrology 1987; 10(S7): 1–53.

that the largest single male 'diagnostic' category was men with seminal abnormalities of unknown cause. Beyond this, varicocoele was a relatively common pathology, as was male accessory gland infection; however, systemic, iatrogenic and endocrine causes were very infrequent.

Genetic causes

Perhaps the most striking advances in our understanding of the aetiology of male infertility in the past decade have been in the area of genetics. Many of the 'systemic' disorders commonly associated with male infertility (see below) are now understood to have a genetic basis, and as our knowledge of the aetiology of disease expands, this will be increasingly the case. Traditionally, genetic causes of male infertility have been sought at the level of chromosomal abnormalities, with chromosomal abnormalities being detected in between 2.1% and 8.9% of men attending infertility clinics (Chandley 1994). The frequency of chromosomal abnormalities increased as sperm concentration declined, with abnormal karyotypes being found in 15% of azoospermic patients, 90% of whom had Klinefelter's syndrome (47XXY), which accounted for half of the entire chromosomally abnormal group. In oligozoospermic patients, the incidence of chromosome abnormalities was 4%. However, it has been recognized for some time that structural anomalies of the Y chromosome, resulting in deletion of the distal fluorescent heterochromatin in the long arm, are associated with severe abnormalities of spermatogenesis. More recent studies have defined a family of genes on the Y chromosome involved in spermatogenesis, and it has become clear that a little over 10% of cases of non-obstructive azoospermia may have deletions affecting these genes. A proportion of cases of very severe oligozoospermia may have a similar aetiology. Microdeletions have been found in three non-overlapping regions of the Y chromosome, AZF a-b-c. Several genes have been described and these include *RBM*, *DAZ*, *DFFRY*, *DBY* and *CDY*. The abnormality most commonly reported in the literature is a microdeletion in the AZFc region and encompassing the *DAZ* gene. However, there is no exact correlation between *DAZ* deletion and the presence or absence of spermatogenesis, but this may be because of an autosomal copy of the *DAZ* gene (Hargreave 2000). DNA fragmentation has also been identified as the cause of defective sperm function (Tarozzi et al 2007). The ability of microassisted fertilization to overcome severe deficits in spermatogenesis has reinforced the importance of understanding and investigating genetic causes of male subfertility, as these will now be transmitted to the next generation of males.

Cryptorchidism

Undescended testis is a good example of a condition present at birth, and presumed to have its origins in intrauterine life, which is significantly associated with an increased risk of impaired spermatogenesis in later life and with an increased risk of testicular cancer (Irvine 1997). The testis which is not in a low scrotal position by the age of 2 years is histologically abnormal; spontaneous descent rarely occurs after 1 year and there is little evidence that surgical orchidopexy for an undescended testis after 2 years of age improves fertility. For these reasons, treatment should ideally be undertaken between 1 and 2 years of age. Evidence suggests that fertility may also be impaired in boys with retractile testis who experience spontaneous descent during puberty. Apart from the association with infertility, cryptorchidism is a well-established risk factor for testicular cancer, the risk of which in a patient with a history of undescended testis, whether successfully treated or not, is four to 10 times higher than in the general population.

Orchitis

Symptomatic orchitis occurs as a complication in 27–30% of males over the age of 10–11 years who suffer from mumps. In 17% of cases, orchitis is bilateral and seminiferous tubular atrophy is a common sequela of mumps orchitis, although recovery of spermatogenesis even after persistent azoospermia for 1 year has been reported (Sandler 1954). The prevalence of infertility after mumps orchitis is unknown, but fertility should only be impaired significantly if the orchitis is bilateral and occurs after puberty.

Varicocoele

The subject of varicocoele has generated controversy amongst the andrological community since the Edinburgh urologist Selby Tulloch first reported the apparently beneficial effects of treatment (Tulloch 1952). The available evidence certainly suggests that varicocoele is a common pathology and that it is more common in men with lower sperm counts. The diagnosis of visible (grade 3) and palpable (grade 2) varicocoeles is not difficult when the patient is examined in a standing position. The detection of subclinical (grade 1) varicocoeles, where spermatic vein reflux can only be detected during the Valsalva manoeuvre, requires more experience and has been aided by the use of Doppler or scrotal thermography. Prevalence figures from 5% to 25% have been reported in surveys of apparently healthy men (Hargreave 1994). In contrast, amongst men attending infertility clinics, varicocoele affects some 11% of men with normal semen and 25% of men with abnormal semen (World Health Organization 1992). The difficulty has been in establishing with certainty whether or not varicocoele affects spermatogenesis and, most importantly, whether or not treatment of varicocoele improves fertility, and if so, in which groups of men. It seems clear that varicocoele is associated with abnormal semen quality, and while the mechanism of this relationship remains to be established with certainty, abnormal testicular temperature regulation is known to be associated with varicocoele and impairment in semen quality.

Whatever the pathophysiology, there is a body of evidence suggesting that varicocoele causes progressive testicular damage, further complicating an assessment of its role in the aetiology of male infertility. Substantial controversy exists, however, over the question of whether or not the correction of varicocoele improves fertility (Evers et al 2008). Most of the appropriately designed controlled studies suggest that treatment is clearly associated with an improvement in semen quality; however, when the achievement of pregnancy is used as the endpoint, some studies find treatment to be effective while some suggest that it is of no benefit.

Occupational and environmental factors

The actively dividing male germ cells are one of the most sensitive cell types in the body with regard to the toxic effects of radiation, cytotoxic drugs and an increasing number of chemicals. Indeed, male gonadal function may be one of the most sensitive indices of overexposure to potential toxins (in the workplace, environment, foods, cosmetics and medicines) (Sharpe 2000, Bonde and Storgaard 2002). Data on occupational hazards to male reproduction remain controversial. Exposure to heavy metals, such as cadmium, lead, arsenic and zinc, has been reported to impair spermatogenesis, although the data are conflicting. Certain pesticides and herbicides have more clearly been shown to be toxic to spermatogenesis, as have some organic chemicals. The best documented modern example is the pesticide dibromochloropropane, which was responsible for azoospermic infertility in half of the male workers in a factory. There would seem to be clear evidence that occupational or environmental exposure to heat will have adverse consequences for spermatogenesis and will prolong time to pregnancy (Thonneau et al 1996). Recreational drugs such as cigarettes, alcohol and cannabis have all been linked with lower semen quality, and there is conflicting evidence on whether or not dress habit has a significant effect.

Recent data have demonstrated that male reproductive health is deteriorating, with evidence of a secular decline in semen quality (Carlsen et al 1992, Auger et al 1995, Irvine 1996), an increase in the incidence of congenital malformation of the male reproductive tract and an increase in the incidence of testicular cancer; however, there is, as yet, no evidence that these changes are having an influence on the prevalence of male infertility.

Iatrogenic infertility

Many general medical disorders are associated with male infertility, either directly (e.g. Kartagener's syndrome), indirectly as a consequence of systemic disturbance (e.g. diabetes) or as a consequence of medical or surgical intervention on account of the primary disease. A number of pharmaceuticals can impair sperm production, the most common example in clinical practice today being sulphasalazine for the treatment of inflammatory bowel diseases. A number of other drugs are also associated with detrimental effects on spermatogenesis, including nitrofurantoin, anabolic steroids, sex steroids and anticonvulsants. Cytotoxic treatment regimes for Hodgkin's disease, lymphoma, leukaemia and other malignancies damage the differentiating spermatogonia, so that most patients become azoospermic after 8 weeks. The degree of stem cell killing governs whether there is recovery of spermatogenesis or not after treatment. This is dependent on the cumulative dose of the drug combination used. Long-term follow-up has shown that following six or more courses of MOPP (mustine, vincristine, procarbazine and prednisolone), over 85% of patients remained azoospermic and recovery is unlikely after 4 years. Similarly, radiation exposure of over 6 Gy destroys germ cells with no chance of recovery. While 1–4 Gy produces complete cessation of spermatogenesis with only some stem spermatogonia surviving, there may be recovery after 12–36 months. Spermatogenesis may continue to improve for several years, but even then it may not be complete.

Genital tract obstruction

The combination of azoospermia, normal testicular volume and normal FSH are the hallmarks of genital tract obstruction. The incidence and relative importance of individual causes of obstruction differ according to geographic locality. Postcongenital and postvasectomy obstructions are the most common, but in some parts of the world, infectious causes, particularly gonorrhoea and tuberculosis, are of greater importance.

The most common congenital abnormality is agenesis or malformations of the Wolffian-duct-derived structures: the corpus/cauda epididymis, vas deferens and seminal vesicles. Diagnosis is usually quite easy; the scrotal vasa are not palpable and the ejaculate consists of low volumes (>1 ml) of acidic non-coagulating prostatic fluid devoid of fructose and sperm. Congenital bilateral absence of the vas deferens is associated with *CFTR* mutations and is found in approximately 2% of men with obstructive azoospermia (Hargreave 2000). In recent years, increasing numbers of mutations of the *CFTR* gene have been characterized and more than 400 have been described. In general, the more mutations tested for, the higher the percentage of men found to have mutations. As such, in more recent publications, detection rates have been almost 70–80%.

Male accessory gland infection

The second most common diagnostic grouping in the WHO survey is also an area of considerable aetiological controversy. Infection in the lower genital tract can be a treatable cause of male infertility, and the incidence varies in different communities. Gram-negative enterococci, chlamydia and gonococcus are established pathogenic organisms which usually produce unequivocal clinical evidence of infection (adnexitis), such as painful ejaculation, pelvic or sacral pain, urethral discharge, haematospermia, dysuria, irregular tender epididymides and tender boggy prostate. This can be confirmed by semen culture and urethral swabs. Inflammation of the accessory glands and excurrent ducts may give rise to disturbed function, formation of sperm antibody and permanent structural damage with obstruction in the outflow tract.

Thus, whilst there is little doubt that overt sexually transmitted disease may damage male fertility and should be appropriately managed, there is much more doubt about the relevance of subclinical infection. The entity of asymptomatic prostatitis is poorly defined and there is little evidence to support a genuine role for occult infections in male infertility. There is thus no place for microbiological screening investigations unless there is clinical suspicion of adnexitis. Furthermore, the isolation of non-pathogenic organisms such as staphylococcus, streptococcus, diptheroids, *Ureaplasma urealyticum* and *Mycoplasma hominis*, which are commensals in the normal urethra, does not warrant the indiscriminate use of antibiotics in the hope of correcting any abnormalities in the semen parameters.

One possible consequence of seminal leucocytosis is the excessive generation of reactive oxygen species (ROS). There is good evidence linking the excessive generation of ROS with male infertility as an aetiological entity in its own right; prospective studies have shown that couples with elevated levels of ROS generation are less likely to conceive either spontaneously or in the context of in-vitro fertilization (IVF).

Immunological causes

Suspected immunological infertility was found in some 3% of couples in a WHO survey on the basis of the finding of 10% or more of motile spermatozoa coated with antibody using assays such as the Immunobead test or the mixed antiglobulin reaction. Whilst antisperm antibodies are found in perhaps one in six of the male partners of infertile couples, a prevalence which is higher than that for fertile controls, their effect on fertility is hard to determine. Some studies suggest that 'antibody-positive' couples conceive at a lower rate than those without immunological problems. Unfortunately, antibodies to sperm surface antigens are also found in fertile control populations, and current techniques do not permit the meaningful separation of cases with autoimmunity to biologically relevant epitopes (Paradisi et al 1995). Given the consensus view that assisted conception is the treatment of choice, this may not now be a clinically relevant issue.

Gonadotrophin deficiency

The clinical features of gonadotrophin deficiency depend on the cause and time of onset, in particular whether the man is pre- or postpubertal. The spectrum includes patients with complete congenital deficiency in GnRH, which results in total failure of testicular and secondary sexual development. Other patients have less severe or partial GnRH deficiency, so have larger (4–10 ml) but still underdeveloped testes with more evidence of germ cell activity; this may be described as the so-called 'fertile eunuch syndrome'. In three-quarters of these patients, anosmia or hyposmia and a variety of midline defects can be detected; this is the association known as 'Kallmann's syndrome'.

In contrast to these congenital varieties of isolated hypogonadotrophic hypogonadism, postnatally or postpubertally acquired gonadotrophin deficiency may arise from tumours, chronic inflammatory lesions, iron overload or injuries of the hypothalamus and pituitary, so that deficits in other pituitary hormones usually coexist. These patients have developed seminiferous tubules which have regressed through lack of trophic hormone support. Their testicular volumes are larger (10–15 ml) than in the former two groups.

Gonadotrophin treatment of these syndromes is discussed below. Androgen treatment is required by hypogonadal men for long-term replacement, and is generally given by injection of testosterone esters every 3–4 weeks, aiming to maintain plasma testosterone concentrations in the physiological range. This is made more difficult by the high peaks and low troughs following administration of these preparations; monitoring of dosage should take place immediately before subsequent injection (i.e. at the trough). Other preparations include the orally active testosterone undecanoate, transdermal patches, gels and subcutaneous testosterone pellets.

Undecanoate is largely confined to paediatric practice for pubertal induction as circulating concentrations tend to be low. Testosterone patches frequently cause skin irritation, although this is not a problem with the gels as these do not contain the enhancers necessary to promote absorption across the skin. New injectable esters are becoming available with a longer duration of action, with up to 3 months between administration (Srinivas-Shankar and Wu 2006). Testosterone will restore sexual interest and activity, and penile erections during and on waking from sleep. Other symptoms of testosterone deficiency include tiredness, irritability and loss of body hair. Testosterone will not induce or improve fertility, and there is no place for androgen treatment of men wishing to conceive.

Coital disorders

Inadequate coital technique (including the use of vaginal lubricants with spermicidal properties) and frequency and faulty timing of intercourse may contribute to continuing infertility, but are rarely the only aetiological factors in the infertile couple. Erectile and ejaculatory failure may be caused by psychosexual dysfunction, depression, spinal cord injuries, retroperitoneal and bladder neck surgery, diabetes mellitus, multiple sclerosis, vascular insufficiency, adrenergic blocking antihypertensive agents, psychotrophic drugs, alcohol abuse and chronic renal failure. Primary endocrine pathologies such as androgen deficiency, hyperprolactinaemia and hypothyroidism seldom present with infertility without diminished libido and clinical features specific to the hormonal disturbances. Retrograde ejaculation must be differentiated from aspermia or anejaculation by examination of postejaculatory urine for the presence of spermatozoa.

Idiopathic impairment of semen quality

Regrettably, this descriptive label continues to be required for a very substantial proportion of men attending infertility clinics. Failure of seminiferous tubular function to the extent of producing azoospermia or severe oligozoospermia (>5 million) is usually associated with small (under 15 ml) and soft testes and elevated FSH. Histologically, the tubules may show completely absent or reduced numbers of germ cells, narrow tubular diameter, and thickening and hyalinization of peritubular tissue. These changes are non-specific and are not always uniformly distributed throughout the testes. There is no evidence to support the contention that testosterone deficiency is the primary cause of defective spermatogenesis, nor that abnormalities in GnRH pulse frequency may be the underlying cause of idiopathic hypospermatogenesis. These patients usually remain infertile and there is no curative treatment available. Less severe degrees of oligozoospermia are commonly associated with abnormal morphology and reduced motility.

'Asthenozoospermia' is the descriptive term applied to impaired sperm motility. Absent or extremely low sperm motility of only 1–2% may result from absence of dynein arms, radial spokes or nexin bridges, and dysplasia of fibrous sheath. This is associated with similar defects in respiratory cilia and therefore, frequently, a history of chronic respiratory infection, bronchiectasis and sinusitis: the 'immotile cilia syndrome'. In addition, some of these patients have situs inversus (Kartagener's syndrome). Based on this classic but extremely rare example, it is now becoming clear that more common but less severe degrees of asthenozoospermia may also be associated with more subtle structural malformations in the axonemal complex, recognizable only with ultrastructural examination and functionally evident as suboptimal sperm movements.

'Teratozoospermia' is the term used to describe altered morphology. Surface morphology directly reflects the maturity and functional integrity of the spermatozoa so that morphological analysis of ejaculated sperm is an important means of assessing spermatogenesis in the testis. Indeed, some workers believe that sperm morphology is the best predictor of spontaneous fertility or the outcome of IVF (Kruger et al 1995). It has been reported that morphology in the individual spermatozoon is related to movement characteristics (swimming velocity, sperm head trajectories, flagellar beat frequency) and its ability to exhibit hyperactivation. Similarly, the ability to undergo the acrosome reaction has also been shown to be significantly higher in sperm with morphologically normal, compared with abnormal, sperm heads. Ultrastructural studies have also revealed a variety of structural malformations of the acrosome complex, the most extreme example being the round-headed sperm where the acrosome is completely missing, but lesser degrees of acrosomal defects are increasingly being identified. These attempts to relate specific functional defects to recognizable structural malformations in individual spermatozoa provide evidence that morphologically abnormal sperm are also functionally impaired.

Clinical Management

The essence of clinical management is to assess the prognosis (chances of conception per year or per cycle of assisted conception) and to advise the couple as to those treatment options that should improve the prognosis. This advice is based upon a sound knowledge of the causes of infertility and the treatment options available. In doing this, it is important to recognize that a number of general epidemiological factors will have a bearing on a couple's fertility. Examples of this include age, although the impact of male age is less certain. Similarly, a longer duration of infertility, even when allowing for age, results in a reduction in fertility. On the other hand, the occurrence of any previous pregnancy will enhance the outcome of treatment after IVF.

Recent advances in assisted conception technology have revolutionized the management of couples with male factor infertility, and have advanced our understanding of the aetiology of male infertility by drawing attention to the major contribution of genetic factors. Paradoxically, they have also encouraged a minimalist clinical approach to the diagnosis of men with fertility problems, given the limited range of effective therapeutic options. The dangers of this approach have been highlighted in the light of existing concerns over the safety of microassisted fertilization (Cummins and Jequier 1994).

Many clinicians endeavour to manage male infertility at a distance, a request for semen analysis preceding, even substituting for, taking a history from and performing a physical examination of the male partner. Those who take this attitude do their patients a disservice; they foster the idea that the male contribution to infertility is limited and while a semen analysis will only occasionally provide the clinician with a diagnosis, a careful history and examination may identify the cause of a couple's infertility. A number of significant features of the clinical history, together with their associated rates of azoospermia or abnormal semen quality, are shown in Table 21.1.

History

Infertility is, of course, the problem of a couple and must be managed as such, with the history being taken from both partners together. The duration of the present union and the duration of infertility complained of should be established at the outset, together with the history of any pregnancies for which the individual may have been responsible. In the patient's past medical history, areas which should receive special attention are a history of mumps virus infection, the age at which this occurred and whether or not there was an associated orchitis. As can be seen from Table 21.1, 84% of men with a history of bilateral mumps orchitis have abnormal semen and 22% are azoospermic. Diabetes mellitus and certain neurological diseases are known to be associated with ejaculatory disturbances, and

Table 21.1 Features in the clinical history with an influence on male fertility and their associated rates of azoospermia and abnormal semen quality

Feature	% of cases with azoospermia	% of cases with abnormal semen
Diabetes mellitus	16.7	60.0
Bronchiectasis	32.0	82.4
Higher fever	5.2	64.4
Long-term medication	12.3	52.9
Urinary tract infection	8.9	60.1
Sexually transmitted disease	7.6	50.4
Epididymitis	17.3	70.2
Testicular injury	12.6	56.9
Testicular torsion	18.2	88.9
Unilateral maldescent	20.8	65.7
Testicular maldescent (bilateral)	40.8	75.9
Mumps orchitis (bilateral)	22.0	84.4
Excessive alcohol consumption	9.6	51.8

From Comhaire FH, de Kretser D and Farley TMM Towards more objectivity in diagnosis and management of male infertility. Results of a WHO Multicentre Study. International Journal of Andrology 1987; 10(S7): 1–53.

a history of these or of any other systemic illness should be sought, as should a history of recent pyrexial illness as this may compromise spermatogenesis for many weeks. A history of respiratory disease should be sought carefully, including recurrent respiratory tract infections, sinusitis, bronchiectasis or cystic fibrosis, as these conditions can be associated with ciliary dysfunction and therefore with impaired sperm motility, as in Kartagener's syndrome, or with obstructive azoospermia, as in Young's syndrome. As many as 82% of men with a history of bronchiectasis have abnormal semen and 32% are azoospermic. Parasitic diseases, such as schistosomiasis and filiariasis, are rare but must be borne in mind as potential causes of excurrent duct obstruction and prostatovesiculitis.

Any symptomatology related to the urinary tract, such as dysuria, urethral discharge, frequency or haematuria, is of self-evident importance. Likewise, aspects of the specific reproductive history which are of importance include any history of testicular maldescent, injury, torsion or epididymo-orchitis, and any history of surgery which may have compromised the genital tract, such as herniorrhaphy, orchidopexy, drainage of hydrocoele, ligation of a varicocoele or bladder neck surgery. Other specific conditions may impair reproductive performance, and a group of patients now requiring infertility investigations are those who have survived treatment for testicular or lymphatic malignancy and who may suffer the consequences of chemotherapy, radiotherapy or retroperitoneal lymph node dissection. A history of drug ingestion, including sulphasalazine, cimetidine or nitrofurantoin, or of exposure to other toxins, including alcohol and tobacco, known to impair spermatogenesis is important, as is the occupational history in terms of exposure to toxic chemicals and hyperthermia. The sexual history should endeavour to cover the adequacy of erectile function and if there is doubt, the presence of early morning and masturbatory erections should be enquired into in order to differentiate organic from psychogenic impotence. The occurrence of intravaginal ejaculation should be established and again, if there is doubt, the occurrence of nocturnal or masturbatory ejaculation sought, in addition to which the characteristics of ejaculation such as associated pain, prematurity or delay should be established. A number of couples attending infertility clinics will be infertile as a consequence of sexual dysfunction, and a number of couples with sexual dysfunction will present to infertility clinics seeking primary help. Of course, any history of sexually transmitted disease and its outcome is of note, as is a history of drug abuse or of other factors exposing the patient to high risk of infection with human immunodeficiency virus, due to the problems which this poses for the couple in terms of the risks of transmission and pregnancy, and in terms of the problems presented to laboratory staff handling blood and semen samples.

Examination

The examination of the male partner should include a general medical examination covering height and weight, blood pressure and all of the major systems, including the respiratory system. The secondary sexual development of the patient must be assessed and signs of hypogonadism sought, including examination of the visual fields, to assess pituitary

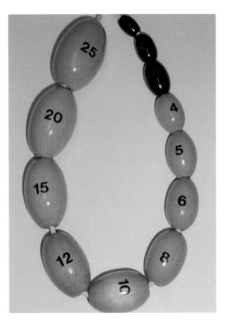

Figure 21.7 Prader orchidometer for the assessment of testicular volume.
From L Hagenäs, Normal och avvikande pubertet hos pojkar, Journal of the Norwegian Medical Association, 2008; 128:1284–8.

enlargement, and examination of the sense of smell to exclude Kallmann's syndrome if indicated. Gynaecomastia should be specifically examined for in this context. On examination of the abdomen, it is important to note the presence of scars or lymphadenopathy in the groins.

Turning to the urogenital examination, the penis is examined for evidence of phimosis, hypospadias, epispadias or the characteristic plaques of Peyronie's disease. The scrotum should be examined and the site of the testes determined, following which the testicular volume in millilitres should be determined with the aid of a Prader orchidometer (Figure 21.7) and their consistency evaluated. It is known that a clear relationship exists between testicular volume and sperm production. Any tenderness of the gonads should be noted and the epididymides carefully palpated from caput to cauda to exclude thickening, tenderness, cystic lesions, atrophy or absence of the epididymides. The vasa deferentia should next be palpated to establish that they are not congenitally absent and any thickening or induration should be noted. Scrotal swellings, such as hydrocoele or hernia, should be noted and the presence and grade of varicocoele should be established by asking the patient to perform Valsalva's manoeuvre. The inguinal regions should be inspected for hernia, scarring or the presence of lymphadenopathy. A rectal examination should be performed to assess the state of the prostate and seminal vesicles, although this seldom provides useful information and may be omitted unless ejaculatory duct obstruction or prostatovesiculitis is suspected.

Semen analysis

The conventional criteria of semen quality have changed little since van Leeuwenhoek first described spermatozoa in the human ejaculate in 1685. A standard semen analysis, performed according to clearly established guidelines promulgated by WHO (World Health Organization 1999) (Box 21.2), provides descriptive information concerning sperm number, motility and morphology, together with aspects of the physical characteristics of the ejaculate.

Sample collection and delivery

The sample should be collected after a minimum of 48 h and not longer than 7 days of sexual abstinence. Two semen samples should be collected for initial evaluation, not less than 7 days or more than 3 months apart. This is in order to take account of the effects of interejaculate variability and length of abstinence that are known to occur. The sample should be collected by masturbation into a clean wide-mouthed glass or plastic container and delivered to the laboratory within 1 h of collection, if it is not possible for the patient to produce the sample at the laboratory. The sample should be evaluated by inspection and should normally be grey-opalescent and homogeneous, liquefying within 60 min. Abnormalities of appearance or failure of liquefaction are noted, following which the semen volume is measured. Abnormally low volumes are commonly due to incomplete sample collection, but may be due to ejaculatory dysfunction. A normal sample has a volume of 2.0 ml or more. The consistency or 'viscosity' of the liquefied sample should be evaluated, and the pH of the sample should be in the range of 7.2–7.8.

Microscopic evaluation

Motility

One hundred spermatozoa are examined at ×400–600, preferably using phase contrast optics, and their motility is assessed and subjectively graded as rapid and linearly progressive motility (grade 4), slower and sluggish linear or non-linear movement (grade 3), non-progressive motility (grade 2) or immotile (grade 1). The percentage of spermatozoa in each category is scored, WHO criteria requiring 50% or more cells with grade 3 or 4 motility. Epithelial cells, spermatogenic cells and white blood cells may be seen, their concentration in a normal sample being less than 1×10^6/ml. If more are present, a specific stain should be

performed for peroxidase-positive white blood cells. The adherence of spermatozoa to each other (agglutination) is noted and reported on an arbitrary scale. If the percentage of immotile spermatozoa exceeds 60%, the proportion of live spermatozoa may be determined.

Sperm concentration

This should be determined accurately by diluting a portion of the semen sample with a diluent to immobilize the spermatozoa and then loading this diluted preparation into a standard haemocytometer, the number of spermatozoa being counted by standard techniques and the result expressed as the concentration of spermatozoa ($\times 10^6$/ml). This should be at least 20×10^6/ml.

Morphology

A smear slide of fresh semen is prepared, air dried, stained by the Giemsa, modified Papanicolaou or Bryan-Leishman methods and examined by light microscopy for the various morphological abnormalities which are described. The result is expressed as the percentage of spermatozoa which are morphologically normal.

In addition to the above, a number of supplementary procedures may be undertaken in the evaluation of human semen, including semen culture, and biochemical evaluation for quantitation of acid phosphatases, citric acid and zinc (as markers of prostatic function), fructose and prostaglandins (as markers of seminal vesicular function) and free L-carnitine (as a marker of epididymal function). WHO has issued a statement of the commonly accepted normal values for the parameters discussed above (Box 21.2), although making the point that it is preferable for each laboratory to establish its own normal ranges for each variable, by evaluating semen from individuals of proven fertility amongst its own local population. It is anticipated that a revised analysis of sperm norms will be published soon by WHO.

Antisperm antibodies

The mixed agglutination reaction uses sheep red blood cells coated with rabbit antibodies to specific classes of human immunoglobulins, which will attach to motile sperm carrying immunoglobulins of the same class on their surface membrane (Bronson et al 1984). This permits the detection of immunoglobulin gamma A, G or M on the surface of the sperm head or tail. The direct test uses washed sperm from the patient, and the presence of surface-bound antibody, indicated by particulate binding in over 10% of spermatozoa, is considered to be a positive result. It depends on the availability of sufficient numbers of motile sperm in the patient's fresh semen sample and is currently the standard screening test in most laboratories. The indirect test uses decomplemented patient serum or seminal plasma which is incubated with motile donor sperm, and is known as the 'tray agglutination test'. Antisperm antibodies will bind to donor sperm and their presence is detected by attachment of particles to the sperm surface. The indirect test is therefore more convenient for screening larger numbers of patients. A positive screening test, however, must be substantiated by investigations to assess the biological significance of sperm antibody.

Additional diagnostic tests on semen

Although of central importance in the evaluation of the male partner of an infertile couple, the conventional criteria of semen quality are of a purely descriptive nature and there is widespread agreement that this information is of limited value in providing an assessment of the ability of a given individual to achieve a pregnancy. In an attempt to overcome this problem, numerous additional tests of sperm function have evolved, including the study of human sperm movement characteristics, initially by time-exposure photomicrography and more recently by computer-assisted image analysis, the study of the penetration of human spermatozoa into cervical mucus and the zona-free hamster oocyte penetration test. This latter test examines a number of key aspects of human sperm function, including the ability of spermatozoa to capacitate, acrosome react and fuse with the vitelline membrane of the oocyte. More recently, biochemical tests, such as measurement of ROS production, have been developed. Although many of the advanced sperm function tests that have been described provide valuable diagnostic information in the hands of competent laboratories, they are typically difficult to perform and have poor predictive values when more widely applied. They are useful research tools and capable of identifying some of the specific causes of infertility. In clinical practice, IVF remains the best test of sperm function, and failed fertilization is probably best treated by intracytoplasmic sperm injection (ICSI).

Hormone measurements

The measurement of plasma FSH is useful in distinguishing primary from secondary testicular failure and in identifying patients with obstructive azoospermia. In the presence of azoospermia or oligozoospermia, an elevated FSH, particularly with reduced testicular volume, is presumptive evidence of severe and usually irreversible seminiferous tubular damage. Low or undetectable FSH (usually associated with low LH and testosterone, with clinical evidence of androgen deficiency) is suggestive of hypogonadotrophism. Conversely, azoospermia with normal FSH and normal testicular volume usually indicates the presence of bilateral genital tract obstruction. Occasional exceptions to these general rules occur from time to time, as azoospermic men with the Sertoli cell only syndrome may have normal FSH levels, while some men with high FSH may have normal spermatogenesis.

Testosterone and LH measurements are indicated in the assessment of the infertile male when there is clinical suspicion of androgen deficiency, sex steroid abuse or steroid-secreting lesions such as functioning adrenal/testicular tumours. In men presenting with infertility, testosterone is usually within the normal range although some degree of Leydig cell dysfunction, as evidenced by statistically lower testosterone and higher LH compared with normal, is not uncommon. This may identify those who may be considered for androgen replacement, although this has no bearing on fertility. High LH and testosterone should raise the possibility of abnormalities in androgen receptors, while low LH and testosterone suggest hypogonadotrophism.

Hyperprolactinaemia is not a frequent cause of male infertility, but prolactin measurement should be undertaken if there is clinical evidence of sexual dysfunction (particularly loss of interest in sex) or pituitary disease leading to secondary testicular failure. Oestradiol measurement is rarely indicated except in the presence of gynaecomastia, which is also a feature of Klinefelter's syndrome.

Dynamic tests of pituitary–testicular function such as GnRH, thyrotrophin-releasing hormone and human chorionic gonadotrophin stimulation generally do not add to the basal measurements described above. Bearing in mind the episodic nature of LH secretion, the diurnal variation in testosterone and the stress-related secretion of prolactin, it is usually sufficient to repeat their measurements in the morning, under resting conditions if necessary.

Chromosome analysis

Chromosome karyotyping should be carried out in patients with azoospermia or severe oligospermia with reduced testicular volumes and elevated FSH. Cytogenetic abnormalities, by far the most common being Klinefelter's syndrome, may be detected in approximately 10% of this group and are of importance if treatment by ICSI is being contemplated. Although still only research, screening for microdeletions on the Y chromosome is likely to enter routine clinical practice in the near future (Krausz and Degl'Innocenti 2006).

Testicular biopsy

With the use of plasma FSH to differentiate between primary testicular failure and obstructive lesions, the need for testicular biopsy in the investigation of male infertility has largely been superseded, although it clearly has a place in the surgical retrieval of sperm for ICSI. When genital tract obstruction is suspected, testicular biopsy is useful in confirming normal spermatogenesis and excluding spermatogenic arrest, but should only be undertaken under circumstances where sperm may be stored for subsequent use in assisted conception. When the clinical differentiation between spermatogenic failure and obstruction is uncertain (e.g. asymmetrical findings on examination between right and left testes or adnexae), scrotal exploration with testicular biopsy may be helpful, again with facilities for sperm storage to hand. Vasography during scrotal exploration is required to confirm the diagnosis of obstructed ejaculatory ducts. It is important to remember that even in primary testicular failure with small testes, elevated levels of FSH and a testicular biopsy showing Sertoli cell only syndrome, some areas of spermatogenesis may be present in the testis. There are many techniques for describing the appearances of a testicular biopsy, but the combination of words and a qualitative assessment, using Johnsen scoring (Johnsen 1970), is useful. In the Johnsen score, the histological features of spermatogenesis are scored from 1 to 10 (2, Sertoli cell only; 3, spermatogonia; 4, 5, spermatocytes; 6, 7, spermatids; 8, 9, 10, spermatozoa).

Treatment

The management of male infertility often remains a difficult and somewhat unsatisfactory experience for patients as well as doctors. Many patients present no recognizable or reversible aetiological factors for treatment, and the doctor frequently fails to appreciate that normal semen values do not relate to fertility. In recent years, there have been a number of advances which have made a significant impact on our therapeutic capabilities. It is important to improve semen quality and to treat those factors that impair fertility.

General measures

Although much has been written about the nature of general advice which should be given, objective evidence for its efficacy in improving fertility is sadly lacking (Bonde and Storgaard 2002). Commonly raised issues include avoidance of stress, a healthy diet and exercise. Recreational drugs such as cigarettes, excessive alcohol consumption and cannabis should certainly be withdrawn or reduced if possible. Occupational or social situations that may chronically elevate testicular temperature should be avoided. Medications that interfere with fertility, such as nitrofurantoin, anabolic steroids, sex steroids and anticonvulsants, should be avoided if possible. In patients with inflammatory bowel disease treated by sulphasalazine, changing treatment to 5-aminosalicylic acid removes the toxic agent, sulphapyridine, and leads to a rapid recovery of fertility without deterioration in disease activity. Although testicular function may improve in patients with chronic renal failure after successful transplantation, fertility impairment may be perpetuated by the continued use of immunosuppressive agents.

Medical treatment

Perhaps the most important point to stress is that empirical treatments for idiopathic oligozoospermia, such as antioestrogens, androgens, bromocriptine and kinin-enhancing drugs, have not been shown to be effective in the treatment of men with abnormalities of semen quality and they should not be used. Although free radicals undoubtedly have a role to play in male infertility (Aitken 1989), few centres measure them routinely and there is, as yet, no evidence that the antioxidant treatments which are used on an empirical basis are effective. Endocrine treatment is only effective in the presence of specific endocrine disturbances, which are rare.

Management of gonadotrophin deficiency

Patients with gonadotrophin deficiency due to acquired conditions and those with GnRH deficiency usually respond to human chorionic gonadotrophin (1000–3000 IU once or twice weekly) alone for 6–12 months (Burger 1982). During this time, the rise in testosterone will virilize the patient and the testes will usually increase in size. If there are no sperm in the ejaculate at the end of 6–12 months, FSH should be added, usually in the form of human menopausal gonadotrophin which contains both FSH and LH. This graded approach may take up to 2 years before one can ascertain if spermatogenesis is established or not. Longer-acting gonadotrophin preparations might be of clinical value in this context.

The treatment outcome of gonadotrophin induction of spermatogenesis is relatively successful, with up to 90% showing some degree of spermatogenesis. Up to 70% can be expected to achieve pregnancies (Büchter et al 1998, Liu et al 2002). Previous treatment with testosterone does not compromise the response to subsequent exogenous gonadotrophin, but there is a clear relationship between pretreatment testicular volume and duration of treatment required. Thus, spermatogenesis will generally be restored more quickly and with less frequent need for FSH in men with acquired gonadotrophin deficiency in adulthood (e.g. as a result of treatment for a pituitary tumour) than in those who have not gone through puberty spontaneously.

Management of genital tract infection

Infection of the male genital tract should be treated if present, but there is no evidence that this will improve fertility. Symptomatic urethritis responds to treatment with the appropriate antibiotics. Chronic infection of the male genital tract is more difficult to diagnose and the presence of pus cells in the semen only indicates an infection in some patients. An alkaline pH (>8.0) may occur in prostatitis due to decreased secretion of acid phosphatase by the prostate. Repeated growth on culture of the same organisms is probably of significance, as is the finding of organisms during a modified Stamey test (Meares and Stamey 1972), where the semen culture replaces the culture of expressed prostatic secretions. If treatment is felt to be warranted, the antibiotics chosen to treat prostatoseminal vesiculitis (such as doxycycline, erythromycins, cephalosporins or oflaxacin) should be secreted by the male accessory glands, and treatment should be continued for 4–12 weeks depending on the chronicity of the infection. In longer courses of treatment, it is customary to rotate the antibiotics, but overall the current tendency is towards a shorter duration (6 weeks) of treatment consisting of two antibiotics, each of which is taken for 3 weeks.

Management of antisperm antibodies

The presence of antisperm antibodies may be a cause of male factor infertility. The use of systemic corticosteroids for treatment of antisperm antibodies remains controversial and can only be recommended in the context of further research as the evidence of benefit is conflicting and there are potentially serious side-effects. Commonly, treatment by assisted conception is recommended.

Erectile failure

The inability of the man to obtain vaginal penetration may be overcome by various pharmacological approaches, and this is particularly useful in men with neurological problems or with performance anxiety. If intracavernous agents are used, the physician should be familiar with the technique and avoid the tragedy of a priapism. Papaverine was the drug of choice for many years but this has been superseded by alprostadil, a prostaglandin E_1 preparation, and more recently by oral sildenafil and other phosphodiesterase type 5 inhibitors (Hackett G, Kell P, Ralph D et al, British Society for Sexual Medicine 2008). In those men with organic impotence, the implantation of a penile prosthesis may provide a solution to the problem.

Ejaculatory failure

Absent emission or retrograde ejaculation due to sympathetic denervation may respond to sympathomimetic drugs. The first choice is desipramine (50 mg on alternate days) for its noradrenaline reuptake blocking action. Ephedrine 30 mg twice daily, brompheniramine maleate 8 mg twice daily or imipramine 25 mg three times daily may also be tried. It is always worth trying desipramine in those men with a diabetic autonomic neuropathy. Urine inhibits sperm motility and, for this reason, spermatozoa should be separated from the urine as soon as possible and used for artificial insemination or assisted conception. Surgical reconstruction of the bladder neck is rarely required.

Surgical treatments

Surgery on the male genital tract should only be carried out in centres where there are appropriate facilities and trained staff. Vasectomy reversal is an effective treatment for men who want to reverse their sterilization, and surgical correction of epididymal blockage can be considered in cases of obstructive azoospermia. Testicular biopsy should only be performed in the context of a tertiary service where there are facilities for sperm recovery and cryostorage.

Relief of obstruction

Obstructive lesions of the seminal tract should be suspected in azoospermia or severe oligozoospermia with normally sized testes and with normal plasma FSH levels. Where surgery is undertaken, it is convenient to explore and biopsy the testes, perform vasography and correct any obstruction that is identified under the same general anaesthetic. A fuller account of the indications, techniques and outcomes of surgical treatments of male infertility may be found elsewhere (Pryor et al 1997).

Epididymal obstruction

The results of reconstructive surgery on the epididymis are varied and depend upon the cause and duration of obstruction and the expertise of the surgeon. Congenital blockages have poor outcome, as do blockages resulting from tuberculous or chlamydial infections. The overall patency rate would appear to be approximately 10–15% of operations, as in many patients there is a great deal of scarring and the epididymis is filled with inspissated material. The best results are achieved when there is localized postgonococcal obstruction in the cauda epididymis. In these instances, sperm may appear in 50% of ejaculates after surgery. A microsurgical technique would appear to give a 10% improvement in patency rates. Spermatozoa acquire motility as they pass through the epididymis, and higher pregnancy rates occur when the blockage is in the distal part of the epididymis (Schoysman and Bedford 1986).

Vasal obstruction

Vasal obstruction is less common in infertility practice and is treated by vasovasostomy. Many techniques are described but an end-to-end one-layer anastomosis with 6-0 sutures is simple and effective. Vasal obstruction most commonly occurs following vasectomy, and after vasovasostomy, patency is to be expected in 80–90% of men with a conception rate of 40–50% in 1 year. Magnification is desirable and the use of an operating microscope for vasovasostomy is excellent training for the more difficult tubulovasostomy that is necessary in epididymal obstruction. The prognosis is worse for those men with a long interval between the vasectomy and reversal (Silber 1989), but time does not prohibit any attempt to operate. The age of the female partner is of importance with regard to conception rates.

Ejaculatory duct obstruction

This is an uncommon cause of obstruction and is readily diagnosed by a low volume of semen, azoospermia or extreme oligozoospermia, and an acid pH in a man with palpable vasa. Müllerian duct cysts are amenable to treatment (Pryor et al 1997), with sperm appearing in the ejaculate of 80% of men and conception in 33% of female partners. Other forms of ejaculatory duct obstruction do less well and are probably best treated by sperm retrieval.

Varicocoele treatment

As discussed above, this remains an area of considerable controversy. Varicocoele is a common finding amongst an infertility clinic population. In trying to interpret the available evidence and decide whether and when to treat, it is wise to remember the many other factors that have a considerable bearing on a couple's fertility. There is no evidence to suggest that treating varicocoele in the presence of normal semen quality is beneficial. Available evidence does suggest that treatment in men with oligozoospermia will improve semen quality, but evidence on whether this will result in pregnancy remains unclear, probably due to the heterogeneous populations studied. It is clear that any benefit is not substantial, and in many cases, particularly where the female partner is above 35 years of age, the duration of the couple's infertility is prolonged or the deficit in semen quality is severe, assisted conception techniques have more to offer.

Assisted conception and male infertility

Early developments in IVF focused on couples with female factor infertility and particularly women suffering from bilateral tubal occlusion. Conventional IVF rapidly became established as an effective treatment option for couples with tubal disease and with unexplained infertility, but it soon became apparent that it yielded generally poor pregnancy rates for couples with male factor infertility. Although there was much discussion in the literature on the fine tuning of the IVF procedure for couples with problems in the male partner, management options for couples with poor semen quality remained very limited until the breakthrough of effective microassisted fertilization in 1992 (Palermo et al 1992).

Micromanipulation techniques

Partial zona dissection was the first micromanipulation technique studied in animal models with clinical intent, and early reports in human practice of clinical pregnancies were encouraging, suggesting that monospermic fertilization and cleavage rates could be doubled by these approaches. However, concerns existed over the risk of polyspermy, along with doubts about appropriate case selection. Subzonal insemination (SUZI) involves the injection of spermatozoa into the privitelline space; again, initial reports of its use were encouraging, although other groups found the technique to be less successful. The developments in human microassisted fertilization culminated in ICSI, with the first human pregnancies resulting from this technique being described by the Brussels group (Palermo et al 1992). This approach involves injection of a single spermatozoon directly into the cytoplasm of the oocyte through the intact zona pellucida, and it very soon became apparent that this technique produced superior results to partial zona dissection or SUZI, with pregnancy rates of 22% per started cycle being reported (Van Steirteghem et al 1993, Abdalla et al 1995). Indeed, such has been the success of ICSI that some commentators suggest that it might be considered the treatment of choice for all cases where in-vitro conception is indicated.

A meta-analysis has concluded that for couples with normal semen, there is no evidence of any benefit, either in fertilization rates per retrieved oocyte or in pregnancy rates, between ICSI and conventional IVF. In contrast, for couples with borderline semen, ICSI results in higher fertilization rates than IVF, and couples with very poor semen will have better fertilization outcomes with ICSI than with SUZI or additional IVF (van Rumste et al 2000).

ICSI with epididymal spermatozoa

Initially, clinical ICSI was used in the treatment of couples in whom the male partner had substantially abnormal semen quality, but it was not long before the technology was applied to the significant numbers of men who present with no sperm in their ejaculates. Amongst men with obstructive azoospermia, attention focused on spermatozoa derived from the epididymis. The first pregnancies achieved with epididymal sperm were described using conventional IVF. However, fertilization rates were low, so whilst it was established that sperm from the epididymis had a degree of functional competence, this was limited (Liu et al 1994, Silber et al 1994).

As a consequence of the successful use of epididymal spermatozoa in ICSI, techniques have been described to facilitate the surgical retrieval of spermatozoa. The major approaches include microsurgical epididymal sperm aspiration (MESA) and percutaenous epididymal sperm aspiration (PESA). MESA involves a formal scrotal exploration, is commonly performed under general anaesthetic and hence is a significant surgical intervention. PESA is a widely used technique which is less invasive, can be performed under local anaesthesia and can be undertaken repeatedly. However, PESA provides less diagnostic information and the yield of spermatozoa may be lower (Girardi 1999).

ICSI with testicular spermatozoa

In contrast to the position in men with obstructive azoospermia, amongst men with non-obstructive azoospermia, attention naturally focuses on the testis as a site for sperm recovery. With the availability of ICSI, it has become clear that non-obstructive azoospermia is a very heterogeneous condition and that testicular histology is similarly heterogeneous, with foci of apparently normal spermatogenesis adjacent to seminiferous tubules devoid of germ cells. Surgical sperm recovery from men with non-obstructive azoospermia has become a routine part of clinical infertility practice, and as with the epididymis, cryopreservation of testis-derived spermatozoa has also become routine. A recent review concluded that surgical sperm recovery would be successful in some 48% of men with non-obstructive azoospermia. Undoubtedly one of the major problems confronting the process of surgical sperm recovery from men with non-obstructive azoospermia is the fact that there are currently

no good predictors of which patients will have sperm recovered successfully and which will not. Against this background, a number of groups have argued that surgical recovery of sperm from the testis coupled with cryopreservation should precede ovarian stimulation in the female partner.

For those men in whom mature spermatozoa cannot be recovered, there is currently interest in the possibility of using less mature cells, commonly elongating or round spermatids, to achieve fertilization. Work in animal models has suggested that this may be a viable approach and there are a number of clinical case reports in the literature. At the present time, however, uncertainties over the safety and efficacy of this approach confine its use to properly designed clinical trials.

ICSI has become well established as an effective form of treatment for couples with male factor infertility. In the last year for which data are available (2006), the UK's Human Fertilisation and Embryology Authority reported that 47% of 41,827 IVF cycles in the UK used ICSI. Given that ICSI is effective, is it also safe? The rapid development of microassisted conception techniques and the widespread use of ICSI in alleviating male infertility have raised concerns about the health of the offspring. ICSI, by directly injecting individual spermatozoa into a mature oocyte, bypasses the natural physiological processes of normal sperm selection, raising concerns over the potential risk of congenital malformations and genetic defects in children born after ICSI.

Without doubt, the most thorough and detailed follow-up studies of ICSI offspring have been those orchestrated by the Brussels group (Bonduelle et al 1999) who have undertaken a prospective follow-up study of 1987 children born after ICSI, aiming to compile data on karyotypes, congenital malformations, growth parameters and developmental milestones. It was found that 1.66% of karyotypes determined by prenatal diagnosis were abnormal *de novo* (nine each of autosomal and sex chromosomal aberrations) and 0.92% were inherited structural aberrations. Most of these were transmitted from the father. Forty-six major malformations (2.3%) were observed at birth. Seven malformations observed by prenatal ultrasound were terminated. Twenty-one (1.1%) stillbirths, including four with major malformations, occurred later than 20 weeks of pregnancy.

Several other large cohort studies have been reported, and as the database of ICSI offspring grows larger, the available evidence on the health of these offspring is generally reassuring (Leunens et al 2008). It is important, however, to appreciate the important role that genetic aetiology plays in the origins of much male subfertility and the ability of ICSI to promote the transgenerational transmission of genetic defects causing gametogenic failure. The significantly increased risk of chromosomal abnormalities in men with impaired semen quality is easily managed by the appropriate investigation and counselling which are required prior to treatment. It is less easy to be certain how to respond to the available evidence on microdeletions of the Y chromosome in men with severely impaired semen quality. The strength of the association between Y chromosome deletions and severely impaired semen quality is impressive, and it is increasingly suggested that these lesions may result in progression from oligozoospermia to azoospermia over time. It is also clear that these genetic deletions, if present, can be transmitted to offspring via ICSI. On the basis of this evidence, some authorities now advocate screening of men for Y chromosome microdeletions prior to ICSI, and advocate testing of offspring and reproductive monitoring for those found to have inherited deletions.

Changes in Male Reproductive Health

During the past two decades, a number of reports have raised serious concerns about the development of reproductive problems in animals and man. There have been controversial reports of changes in human semen quality (Carlsen et al 1992, Auger et al 1995, Irvine 1996), alongside reports of an increasing incidence of congenital malformations of the male genital tract, such as cryptorchidism and hypospadias (Kallen et al 1986, Ansell 1992) and of an increasing incidence of testicular cancer (Adami et al 1994, Wanderas et al 1995). However, there is controversy over whether or not these reported changes in male reproductive health are genuine, and if so, the causes and implications.

Testicular cancer

Although many of the changes seen in male reproductive health are controversial, there seems little argument that testicular cancer is increasing in frequency, with unexplained increases in the age-standardized incidence being observed in Europe (Adami et al 1994, Bergstrom et al 1996) and the USA (Devesa et al 1995). There would appear to be substantial geographical variation in both the incidence of testicular cancer and in the observed rate of increase (Adami et al 1994). Of note, this geographical variation may be linked with that seen in semen quality; testicular cancer is four times more common in Denmark, where studies have revealed rather low sperm counts (Jensen et al 1996), than in Finland, where semen quality appears to be better (Vierula et al 1996). Interestingly, the observed increases, both in Europe and the USA, would appear to be birth cohort related. Bergstrom et al (1996) evaluated data from Denmark, Norway, Sweden, East Germany, Finland and Poland, including data on over 30,000 cases of testicular cancer from 1945 to 1989 in men aged 20–84 years. They found considerable regional variation in both the incidence of testicular cancer and the observed rate of increase, ranging from a 2.3% increase annually in Sweden to a 5.2% increase annually in East Germany. In all six countries, birth cohort was a stronger determinant of testicular cancer risk than calendar time, such that men born in 1965 had a risk of testicular cancer that was 3.9 times [95% confidence interval (CI) 2.7–5.6; Sweden] to 11.4 times (95% CI 8.3–15.5; East Germany) higher than that for men born in 1905.

A recent study has looked in detail at the risk of testicular cancer in subfertile men (Moller and Skakkebaek 1999) using a population-based case–control design. This study found that paternity was associated with a reduced risk of testicular cancer (relative risk 0.63, 95% CI 0.47–0.85), and that prior to the diagnosis of testicular cancer, cases tended to have fewer children than expected for their age (relative risk 1.98, 95% CI 1.43–2.75). The study suggested that these observations are consistent with the hypothesis that testicular cancer and male subfertility share important aetiological factors.

Cryptorchidism and congenital malformations of the male genital tract

The incidence of congenital malformation of the male genital tract may also be changing, with increases observed in the prevalence of cryptorchidism and hypospadias. Cryptorchidism, for example, has increased by as much as 65–77% over recent decades in the UK (Ansell 1992). In contrast, some data from the USA have tended to suggest that rates of cryptorchidism have not changed (Berkowitz et al 1993), although one recent large study from the USA reported that rates of hypospadias doubled from the 1970s to the 1980s (Paulozzi et al 1997). Here too, though, regional differences have been observed, although the data are perhaps less robust than is the case with testicular cancer. One multicentre study of 8122 boys from seven malformation surveillance systems around the world concluded that, even when differences in ascertainment were taken into account, true geographical differences exist in the prevalence of hypospadias at birth (Kallen et al 1986).

Changing semen quality: historical data on normal men

In 1992, Carlsen et al (1992) reawakened concern over the possibility of secular trends in semen quality, publishing a meta-analysis of data on semen quality in normal men. The authors undertook a systematic review of available data on semen quality in normal men, published since 1930. Standard techniques applicable to meta-analysis were used to identify relevant papers, and care was taken to exclude data on infertile couples, men selected on the basis of their semen quality and data generated using non-classical approaches to semen analysis. Data were obtained on 14,947 men, published in 61 papers between 1938 and 1990. The authors observed a decline in sperm concentration from 113×10^6/ml in 1940 to 66×10^6/ml in 1990, along with a decline in the proportion of men with a sperm concentration above 100×10^6/ml. Predictably, the central message of this meta-analysis, that sperm counts had declined by approximately 50% over the past 50 years, attracted enormous attention and generated much controversy.

Since publication of Carlsen et al's meta-analysis, several papers have presented contemporary analyses of retrospective data. Unfortunately, the available data still fail to reach a conclusion on whether or not there is any secular trend in semen quality; at least as many studies have reported evidence of deteriorating semen quality as have reported evidence of no change. A very careful reanalysis of the historical data (Carlsen et al 1992) on semen quality in normal men (Swan et al 1997) found that there was evidence of a decline in sperm concentrations in the USA of -1.5×10^6/ml/year (95% CI -1.9 to -1.1), and in Europe of -3.13×10^6/ml/year (95% CI -4.96 to -1.30), but not in non-Western countries.

Whilst the available evidence is inconclusive and circumstantial, its weight is considerable and, at the very least, it should raise concerns that deserve to be addressed by properly designed, coordinated and funded research. Delay may compromise the fertility and reproductive health of future generations (de Kretser 1996, Irvine 1996).

References

Abdalla H, Leonard T, Pryor J, Everett D 1995 Comparison of SUZI and ICSI for severe male factor. Human Reproduction 10: 2941–2944.

Adami HO, Bergstrom R, Mohner M et al 1994 Testicular cancer in nine northern European countries. International Journal of Cancer 59: 33–38.

Aitken RJ, Clarkson JS, Hargreave TB, Irvine DS, Wu FCW 1989 Analysis of the relationship between defective sperm function and the generation of reactive oxygen species in cases of oligozoospermia. J Androl 10(3): 214–220.

Ansell PE 1992 Cryptorchidism: a prospective study of 7,500 consecutive male births. Archives of Disease in Childhood 67: 892–899.

Auger J, Kunstmann JM, Czyglik F, Jouannet P 1995 Decline in semen quality among fertile men in Paris during the past 20 years. New England Journal of Medicine 32: 281–285.

Bergstrom R, Adami HO, Mohner M et al 1996 Increase in testicular cancer incidence in six European countries: a birth cohort phenomenon. Journal of the National Cancer Institute 88: 727–733.

Berkowitz GS, Lapinski RH, Dolgin SE, Gazella JG, Bodian CA, Holzman IR 1993 Prevalence and natural history of cryptorchidism. Pediatrics 92: 44–49.

Bonde JP, Storgaard L 2002 How work-place conditions and lifestyle affect male reproductive function. International Journal of Andrology 25: 262–268.

Bonduelle M, Camus M, De Vos A et al 1999 Seven years of intracytoplasmic sperm injection and follow-up of 1987 subsequent children. Human Reproduction 14 (Suppl 1): 243–264.

Bronson RA, Cooper GW, Rosenfeld D 1984 Sperm antibodies: their role in infertility. Fertility and Sterility 42: 171–183.

Büchter D, Behre HM, Kleisch S, Nieschlag E 1998 Pulsatile GnRH or human chorionic gonadotrophin/human menopausal gonadotrophin as effective treatment for men with hypogonadotrophic hypogonadism: a review of 42 cases. European Journal of Endocrinology 139: 298–303.

Burger HG, Baker HWG 1982 Therapeutic considerations and results of gonadotrophic treatment in male hypogonadotrophic hypogonadism. Annals of the New York Academy of Sciences 438: 447–453.

Carlsen E, Giwercman A, Keiding N, Skakkebaek NE 1992 Evidence for decreasing quality of semen during past 50 years. BMJ (Clinical Research Ed.) 305: 609–613.

Chandley AC 1994 Chromosomes. In: Hargreave T (ed) Male Infertility. Springer-Verlag, London.

Comhaire FH, de Kretser D, Farley TMM 1987 Towards more objectivity in diagnosis and management of male infertility. Results of a WHO Multicentre Study. International Journal of Andrology 10 (Suppl 7): 1–53.

Cummins JM, Jequier AM 1994 Treating male infertility needs more clinical andrology, not less. Human Reproduction 9: 1214–1219.

de Kretser DM 1996 Declining sperm counts. BMJ (Clinical Research Ed.) 312: 457–458.

Devesa SS, Blot WJ, Stone BJ, Miller BA, Tarone RE, Fraumeni JF Jr 1995 Recent cancer trends in the United States. Journal of the National Cancer Institute 87: 175–182.

Dym M 1977 In: Weiss L, Greep RO (eds) Histology. McGraw Hill, New York, p 981.

Evers JH, Collins J, Clarke J 2008 Surgery or embolisation for varicoceles in subfertile men. Cochrane Database of Systematic Reviews 3: CD000479.

Fawcett DW 1975 The mammalian spermatozoon. Developmental Biology 44: 394–436.

Girardi SK 1999 Techniques for sperm recovery in assisted reproduction. Reproductive Medicine Review 7: 131–139.

Grudzinskas JG 1995 Gametes — the Spermatozoon. Cambridge University Press, Cambridge, UK.

Hackett G, Kell P, Ralph D et al 2008 British Society for Sexual Medicine guidelines on the management of erectile dysfunction. Journal of Sexual Medicine 5: 1841–1865.

Hargreave TB 1994 Varicocele. In: Hargreave TB (ed) Male Infertility. Springer Verlag, London, UK.

Hargreave TB 2000 Genetic basis of male fertility. British Medical Bulletin 56: 650–671.

Hull MGR, Glazener CMA, Kelly NJ et al 1985 Population study of causes, treatment, and outcome of infertility. BMJ (Clinical Research Ed.) 291: 1693–1697.

Irvine DS 1996 Is the human testis still an organ at risk? BMJ (Clinical Research Ed.) 312: 1557–1558.

Irvine DS 1997 Declining sperm quality: a review of facts and hypotheses. Baillières Clinical Obstetrics and Gynaecology 11: 655–671.

Ivell R, Hartung S, Anand-Ivell R 2005 Insulin-like factor 3: where are we now? Annals of the New York Academy of Sciences 1041: 486–496.

Jensen TK, Giwercman A, Carlsen E, Scheike T, Skakkebaek NE 1996 Semen quality among members of organic food associations in Zealand, Denmark. The Lancet 347: 1844.

Johnsen SG 1970 Testicular biopsy score count: a method for registration of spermatogenesis in human testes: normal values and results in 335 hypogonadal males. Hormones 1: 2–25.

Kallen B, Bertollini R, Castilla E et al 1986 A joint international study on the epidemiology of hypospadias. Acta Paediatrica Scandinavica 324 (Suppl): 1–52.

Krausz C, Degl'Innocenti S 2006 Y chromosome and male infertility: update

2006. Frontiers in Bioscience 11: 3049–3061.

Kruger TF, du Toit TC, Franken DR, Menkveld R, Lombard CJ 1995 Sperm morphology: assessing the agreement between the manual method (strict criteria) and the sperm morphology analyzer IVOS. Fertility and Sterility 63: 134–141.

Leunens L, Celestin-Westreich S, Bonduelle M, Liebaers I, Ponjaert-Kristoffersen I 2008 Follow-up of cognitive and motor development of 10-year-old singleton children born after ICSI compared with spontaneously conceived children. Human Reproduction 23: 105–111.

Liu J, Lissens W, Silber SJ, Devroey P, Liebaers I, Van Steirteghem A 1994 Birth after preimplantation diagnosis of the cystic fibrosis delta F508 mutation by polymerase chain reaction in human embryos resulting from intracytoplasmic sperm injection with epididymal sperm. Journal of the American Medical Association 272: 1858–1860.

Liu PY, Gebski VJ, Turner L, Conway AJ, Wishart SM, Handelsman DJ 2002 Predicting pregnancy and spermatogenesis by survival analysis during gonadotrophin treatment of gonadotrophin-deficient infertile men. Human Reproduction 17: 625–633.

Matsumoto AM, Paulsen CA, Bremner WJ 1984 Stimulation of sperm production by human luteinizing hormone in gonadotrophin-suppressed normal men. Journal of Clinical and Endocrinological Metabolism 59: 882–887.

Meares EM Jr, Stamey TA 1972 The diagnosis and management of bacterial prostatitis. British Journal of Urology 44: 175–179.

Moller H, Skakkebaek NE 1999 Risk of testicular cancer in subfertile men: case–control study. BMJ (Clinical Research Ed.) 318: 559–562.

Morishima A, Grumbach MM, Simpson ER, Fisher C, Qin K 1995 Aromatase deficiency in male and female siblings caused by a novel mutation and the physiological role of estrogens. Journal of Clinical Endocrinology and Metabolism 80: 3689–3698.

Mortimer D 1995 Sperm Transport in the Female Genital Tract. Cambridge University Press, Cambridge, UK.

O'Connor AE, De Kretser DM 2004 Inhibins in normal male physiology. Seminars in Reproductive Medicine 22: 177–185.

Palermo G, Joris H, Devroey P, Van Steirteghem AC 1992 Pregnancies after intracytoplasmic injection of single spermatozoon into an oocyte. The Lancet 340: 17–18.

Paradisi R, Pession A, Bellavia E, Focacci M, Flamigni C 1995 Characterization of human sperm antigens reacting with antisperm antibodies from autologous sera and seminal plasma in a fertile population. Journal of Reproductive Immunology 28: 61–73.

Paulozzi LJ, Erickson JD, Jackson RJ 1997 Hypospadias trends in two US surveillance systems. Pediatrics 100: 831–834.

Pryor JL, Kent-First M, Muallem A et al 1997 Microdeletions in the Y chromosome of infertile men. New England Journal of Medicine 336: 534–539.

Rowe PG 1993 WHO Manual for the Standardized Investigation and Diagnosis of the Infertile Couple. Cambridge University Press, Cambridge, UK.

Sandler B 1954 Recovery from sterility after mumps orchitis. BMJ (Clinical Research Ed.) 2: 795.

Schmidt L 2006 Infertility and assisted reproduction in Denmark. Epidemiology and psychosocial consequences. Danish Medical Bulletin 53: 390–417.

Schoysman RJ, Bedford JM 1986 The role of the human epididymis in sperm maturation and sperm storage as reflected in the consequences of epididymovasostomy. Fertility and Sterility 46: 293–299.

Seminara SB, Crowley WF Jr 2008 Kisspeptin and GPR54: discovery of a novel pathway in reproduction. Journal of Neuroendocrinology 20: 727–731.

Sharpe RM 1990 Intratesticular control of steroidogenesis. Clinical Endocrinology 33: 787–807.

Sharpe RM 2000 Lifestyle and environmental contribution to male infertility. British Medical Bulletin 56: 630–642.

Silber SJ 1989 Pregnancy after vasovasostomy for vasectomy reversal: a study of factors affecting long-term return of fertility in 282 patients followed for 10 years. Fertility and Sterility 31: 309–315.

Silber SJ, Nagy ZP, Liu J, Godoy H, Devroey P, Van Steirteghem AC 1994 Conventional in-vitro fertilization versus intracytoplasmic sperm injection for patients requiring microsurgical sperm aspiration. Human Reproduction 9: 1705–1709.

Smith EP, Boyd J, Frank GR et al 1994 Estrogen resistance caused by a mutation in the estrogen-receptor gene in a man. New England Journal of Medicine 331: 1056–1061.

Srinivas-Shankar U, Wu FC 2006 Drug insight: testosterone preparations. Nature Clinical Practice Urology 3: 653–665.

Swan SH, Elkin EP, Fenster L 1997 Have sperm densities declined? A reanalysis of global trend data. Environmental Health Perspectives 105: 1228–1232.

Tapanainen TS, Aittomaki K, Min J, Vasivko T, Huhtaniemi IT 1997 Men homozygous for an inactivating mutation of the follicle-stimulating hormone (FSH) receptor gene present variable suppression of spermatogenesis and fertility. Nature Genetics 15: 205–206.

Tarozzi N, Bizzaro D, Flamigni C, Borini A 2007 Clinical relevance of sperm DNA damage in assisted reproduction. Reproductive Biomedicine Online 14: 746–757.

Thonneau P, Ducot B et al 1996 Heat exposure as a hazard to male fertility. Lancet 347: 204–205.

Tulloch WS 1952 A consideration of sterility factors in the light of subsequent pregnancies: subfertility in the male. Edinburgh Obstetrical Society 52: 29–34.

van Rumste MM, Evers JL, Farquhar CM, Blake DA 2000 Intra-cytoplasmic sperm injection versus partial zona dissection, subzonal insemination and conventional techniques for oocyte insemination during in vitro fertilisation. Cochrane Database of Systematic Reviews 2: CD001301.

Van Steirteghem AC, Liu J, Joris H et al 1993 Higher success rate by intracytoplasmic sperm injection than by subzonal insemination. Report of a second series of 300 consecutive treatment cycles. Human Reproduction 8: 1055–1060.

Vermeulen A 1991 Androgens in the aging male. Journal of Clinical Endocrinology and Metabolism 73: 221–224.

Vierula M, Niemi M, Keiski A, Saaranen M, Saarikoski S, Suominen J 1996 High and unchanged sperm counts of Finnish men. International Journal of Andrology 19: 11–17.

Wanderas EH, Tretli S, Fossa SD 1995 Trends in incidence of testicular cancer in Norway 1955–1992. European Journal of Cancer 31A: 2044–2048.

World Health Organization 1992 The influence of varicocele on parameters of fertility in a large group of men presenting to infertility clinics. Fertility and Sterility 57: 1289–1293.

World Health Organization 1999 WHO Laboratory Manual for the Examination of Human Semen and Sperm–Cervical Mucus Interaction. Cambridge University Press, Cambridge.

Wu FC 2007 Guideline for male testosterone therapy: a European perspective. Journal of Clinical Endocrinology and Metabolism 92: 418–419.

Wu FC, Taylor PL, Sellar RE 1989 LHRH pulse frequency in normal and infertile men. Journal of Endocrinology 123: 149–158.

CHAPTER 22

Assisted reproduction treatments

Kannamannadiar Jayaprakasan and James Hopkisson

Chapter Contents

INTRODUCTION	312
SELECTION AND EVALUATION OF PATIENTS	312
CLINICAL MANAGEMENT OF THE TREATMENT CYCLE	316
OOCYTE RETRIEVAL	318
LABORATORY TECHNIQUES	319
EMBRYO TRANSFER	320
OUTCOME MEASURES AND FACTORS AFFECTING SUCCESS RATE	321
HEALTH RISKS ASSOCIATED WITH ASSISTED REPRODUCTION TREATMENT	325
OBSTETRIC AND PERINATAL OUTCOMES OF ASSISTED REPRODUCTION TREATMENT	328
PREIMPLANTATION GENETIC DIAGNOSIS/SCREENING	329
LOOKING INTO THE FUTURE	329
KEY POINTS	331

Introduction

Regardless of the cause of infertility, assisted reproduction treatment (ART) offers the highest pregnancy rates per cycle among all the fertility treatment options, and is therefore being used increasingly worldwide. ART involves interventions manipulating gametes to enhance fertilization and subsequent occurrence of pregnancy, and includes in-vitro fertilization (IVF), intracytoplasmic sperm injection (ICSI), gamete intrafallopian transfer (GIFT), zygote intrafallopian transfer (ZIFT), transfer of cryopreserved embryos, and treatment using donor gametes and embryos. More recently, GIFT and ZIFT have become less popular as the success rates are inferior to IVF and more invasive.

Since the first successful birth following IVF in 1978, there have been considerable advances in the field of ART and more than 3 million babies have been born across the world. ART is now widely available, and in a single year (2004), more than 360,000 treatment cycles were carried out in Europe. In the UK, a total of 44,275 IVF/micromanipulation and frozen embryo replacement (FER) cycles were reported in 2006, resulting in 12,596 livebirth events (Human Fertilisation and Embryology Authority 2008). The number of conventional IVF cycles remained reasonably steady between 1998 and 2008, while the number of ICSI treatment cycles has been increasing steadily since its introduction (Figure 22.1) Human Fertilisation and Embryology Authority 2008).

The Human Fertilisation and Embryology Authority (HFEA) was established in 1991 by the Human Fertilisation and Embryology Act 1990 to regulate and inspect all UK clinics providing ART, and was the first statutory body of its kind in the world. The introduction of guidelines into clinical practice in general and in assisted reproduction in particular has led to an ever-increasing role for an evidence-based approach to the provision of these services. Clinical guidelines for the assessment and treatment of people with fertility problems have been published by the National Institute for Clinical Excellence (2004) to streamline services and avoid unnecessary waste of resources. This chapter will review the current status of conventional IVF, ICSI and other treatments, new developments in ART and the clinical risks associated with these techniques. The obstetric and neonatal consequences of these treatments and, in particular, the impact of the number of embryos transferred on the outcome will be discussed.

Selection and Evaluation of Patients

Although IVF was initially introduced to bypass tubal blockage, the currently available techniques enable the treatment of various causes of infertility. The current indications are shown in Box 22.1.

Emphasis should be placed on the pretreatment evaluation of the individual or couple, both medically and psychologically. Assessment of the welfare of the child that may result from ART, including its need for a positive male role model, has become central to the provision of treatment in the eyes of the HFEA. With that in mind, there should be careful consideration of the duration and stability of the couple's relationship, their medical and social backgrounds, and other relevant issues. In addition, information-giving and decision-making aspects of counselling should be made available by a specially trained counsellor as a matter of

DOI: 10.1016/B978-0-7020-3120-5.00022-9

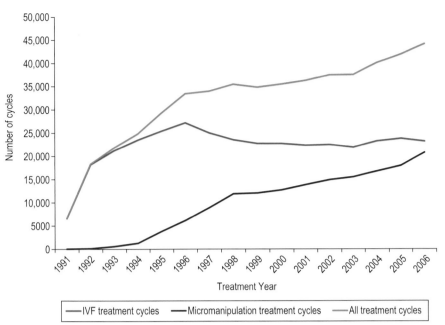

Figure 22.1 Number of treatment cycles 1991–2006.
Source: Human Fertilisation and Embryology Authority (2008).

Legend: —— IVF treatment cycles —— Micromanipulation treatment cycles —— All treatment cycles

---

Box 22.1 Indications for IVF treatment

- Tubal disease
- Unexplained infertility
- Treated endometriosis
- Male factor infertility
- Failed artificial insemination by donor
- Failed ovulation induction
- Absent or inappropriate ovaries
- IVF in association with preimplantation genetic diagnosis (PDG)
- Fertility preservation for cancer patients and social reasons
- Treatment of single women and same-sex couples

---

routine to all couples. Couples should be interviewed together, and appropriate history and clinical examination should be undertaken for both partners. For the female partner, baseline hormone profile, mid-luteal-phase progesterone assay and rubella status must be determined. Additional tests such as thyroid function, high vaginal or endocervical swabs, and cytomegalovirus status should be performed where necessary. Hepatitis B and C and human immunodeficiency virus screening are mandatory in the UK for both partners before ART.

Evaluation of pelvis

Ultrasound evaluation of the pelvis is often performed prior to ART to rule out any adnexal and uterine pathologies, such as polycystic ovary syndrome (PCOS), endometriosis, tubal disease, fibroids and endometrial polyps, which are clearly associated with aberrant and compromised outcomes during IVF.

The diagnosis of PCOS is currently based on the definition derived by the Rotterdam Consensus Workshop, which suggested the presence of 12 or more follicles measuring 2–9 mm in diameter and/or an ovarian volume of more than

$10\ cm^3$ for the ultrasound diagnosis (Balen et al 2003). Stromal vascularity and blood flow velocities are higher in women with polycystic ovaries (Agrawal et al 1998), and this may account for their tendency towards ovarian hyperstimulation in response to gonadotrophin therapy.

Endometriosis has been shown to have a negative effect on the outcome of ART, with affected women demonstrating a reduced response to ovarian stimulation (Gupta et al 2006); however, reports on its effects on embryo quality and implantation potential are conflicting. Moderate and severe degrees of endometriosis, often characterized by rectovaginal disease and the presence of ovarian endometrioma, can usually be diagnosed by transvaginal ultrasound (Moore et al 2002).

The presence of a hydrosalpinx is associated with poor implantation and pregnancy rates, and early pregnancy loss. The exact mechanism is unknown but substances toxic to the endometrium are thought to be produced that have a negative effect on endometrial receptivity (Strandell 2007). Salpingectomy, ideally performed laparoscopically, prior to IVF has been shown to be beneficial and is recommended. The diagnosis of hydrosalpinx can generally be made using transvaginal ultrasound with a high degree of confidence.

Ultrasound assessment of the uterus is generally restricted to measurement of the endometrial thickness and a description of the locality and size of any fibroids. Conventional ultrasound may also detect uterine anomalies, although these are more readily identified and correctly qualified with three-dimensional ultrasound. The diagnosis of uterine anomalies is important as they are associated with lower implantation rates and increased rates of early miscarriage, preterm labour and malpresentations (Lin 2004). The outcome appears to relate more to the length of the remaining uterine cavity than the degree of septum, and this may be measured reliably with three-dimensional ultrasound (Salim et al 2003).

The diagnosis and classification of fibroids into subserosal, intramural and submucosal is usually straightforward, and this is important as these have a progressively negative effect on pregnancy rates. Whilst intramural fibroids measuring more than 4 cm in diameter and submucous fibroids of any size are thought to have a negative effect on the outcome of fertility treatment and to be associated with lower pregnancy rates, the effect of smaller intramural fibroids on reproductive outcome is unclear (Oliveira et al 2004). There is also doubt about the exact impact of endometrial polyps, the other commonly encountered intrauterine pathology, on treatment outcome and early pregnancy. Some authors suggest conservative management, especially if the polyp is small (Isikoglu et al 2006), but this can be difficult in patients undergoing fertility treatment or with a history of miscarriage when a polyp is identified before treatment begins. Polyps are usually evident with conventional transvaginal imaging, although false-positive diagnoses are common. Saline infusion sonohysterography can reduce this and facilitate appropriate operative planning (Bartkowiak et al 2006). Delineation of the polyp with saline ensures that the size and position of the polyp can be defined accurately, allowing surgeons to modify their approach and resect the larger, more broad-based polyps rather than planning for simple polypectomy. Hysteroscopy is the gold standard technique for uterine cavity assessment, and may be necessary if diagnosis of intrauterine pathologies is in doubt.

Assessment of ovarian reserve

Evaluation of ovarian reserve has become an integral part of the pretreatment assessment of a woman about to undergo ART, and is recommended for all women planning ART (Speroff and Fritz 2005). The aim is to identify women likely to respond poorly, those who have a low chance of success and who are more likely to have their treatment cycle cancelled, and those prone to ovarian hyperstimulation which is associated with significant morbidity and even mortality. Accurate assessment of ovarian reserve and prediction of response therefore facilitates pretreatment counselling of couples of their potential risks, and allows treatment to be tailored to the individual, potentially increasing the number of oocytes retrieved without risking an exaggerated response. Ovarian reserve, defined by the size and quality of the remaining ovarian follicular pool at any given time, reflects the fertility potential of a woman (Broekmans et al 2006).

Although women's age is an important predictor of ovarian reserve and response, a great deal of interindividual variation exists, even among women of the same age (te Velde and Pearson 2002). This is indicative of a wide variation in the rate of age-related decline in the ovarian follicle population. Several endocrine and ultrasound markers have been reported, with the aim of estimating the number of gonadotrophin-responsive or 'selectable follicles' more accurately. The endocrine markers include factors produced by the developing follicles [oestradiol, inhibin B and anti-Müllerian hormone (AMH)] or hormones under the inhibitory control of these factors [follicule-stimulating hormone (FSH)]. The ultrasound markers are antral follicle count, ovarian volume and ovarian vascularity. The sensitivities, specificities and predictive values of these tests have been evaluated in many studies by correlating the test results with the number of oocytes retrieved, poor or exaggerated ovarian response, and pregnancy or livebirth rates during ART (Broekmans et al 2006).

Serum follicle-stimulating hormone

Early-follicular-phase FSH is the most widely used marker of ovarian reserve, and women with raised FSH levels (>10–15 IU/l) are more likely to have a reduced ovarian response and less successful ART outcome (Scott et al 1989, Sharif et al 1998). A meta-analysis of 21 studies looking at the value of basal FSH in the prediction of IVF outcome concluded that the performance of basal FSH as a screening test is limited in predicting poor ovarian response and non-pregnancy. Predictions with a substantial shift from pre-FSH-test probability to post-FSH-test probability are only achieved at extremely high cut-off levels (Bancsi et al 2003). Moreover, the cycle-to-cycle variability of basal FSH levels limits the reliability of a single measurement for assessment of ovarian reserve. However, it is important to note that ovarian response and pregnancy rates during IVF are low in women with high intercycle variability (Scott et al 1990) or who demonstrate abnormal FSH levels in any menstrual cycle (Abdalla and Thum 2006).

Oestradiol

Measurement of basal oestradiol in addition to FSH is recommended to improve predictive accuracy. Premature elevation of the oestradiol level due to advanced follicular development and early selection of a dominant follicle may tend to suppress the FSH level, thus masking a rise that might otherwise reflect a low ovarian reserve (Frattarelli et al 2000). An elevated level of basal oestradiol ($\geq$60 pg/ml), even in the presence of a normal FSH level, is associated with increased risk of cycle cancellation due to poor ovarian response (Evers et al 1998). However, the use of serum oestradiol estimation for ovarian reserve assessment is limited by the fact that some women with a normal ovarian reserve may have an occasional accelerated cycle with FSH levels of mid-follicular range in their true early-follicular phase (Frattarelli et al 2000). Furthermore, elevated oestrogen may simply reflect the presence of functional ovarian cysts.

Inhibin B

Inhibin B is principally produced by the granulosa cells of the developing cohort of antral follicles during the luteal–follicular transition. Its level in the early-follicular phase is considered to be indicative of the quantity or quality of developing follicles (Hall et al 1999). A low level (<45 pg/ml) of early-follicular-phase inhibin B may predict a poor ovarian response (Seifer et al 1997). However, the reliability of its measurement has been questioned because of significant intercycle variability (McIlveen et al 2007).

Anti-Müllerian hormone

Studies have shown that AMH is a promising serum marker of ovarian reserve (van Rooij et al 2002). AMH, a member of the transforming growth factor-β family of growth and differentiation factors, is primarily produced by the preantral and small antral follicles in women of reproductive age. The serum level of AMH is indicative of the growing follicle pool (de Vet et al 2002). While AMH is highly predictive of potential poor or exaggerated responders to ovarian stimulation during ART, its accuracy to predict the occurrence of pregnancy after one cycle of ART is only marginal (Broekmans et al 2008). Recent studies have suggested that AMH levels vary minimally between menstrual cycles and are cycle independent (Fanchin et al 2005, La Marca et al 2006). Therefore, AMH measurement could be undertaken during any cycle and at any time during the cycle for adequate prediction of ovarian response, and this makes it an attractive marker for routine use. However, there are potential limitations to the regular use of AMH as a marker of ovarian reserve because of different cut-off levels reported in different studies. Currently, there is no international assay standard for AMH measurement, which may contribute to the discordance between different studies and make comparison between laboratories quite difficult. Once the available assays are standardized and automated analysis systems are developed, AMH has the potential to become the test of choice for ovarian reserve.

Dynamic ovarian reserve tests

Dynamic tests have also been reported for the assessment of ovarian reserve. Dynamic testing is a provocative test of ovarian reserve that examines the endocrine dynamics of the menstrual cycle which change with the functional activity of the remaining follicles within the ovary. This involves the measurement of an endocrine marker of ovarian reserve (FSH or oestradiol) both before and after ovarian stimulation using clomiphene, gonadotrophin-releasing hormone (GnRH) agonist or FSH. The literature suggests that none of these tests offer any more predictive information than the previously described tests. Moreover, the inconvenience, expense and potential side-effects associated with the use of the additional pharmacological agents limit their use for pretreatment assessment of ovarian reserve.

Antral follicle count

Antral follicle count (AFC) is the most significant predictor of ovarian response among the ultrasound markers (Kwee et al 2007, Jayaprakasan et al 2009), although decreased ovarian volume (<3 cm^3) and stromal blood flow are also implicated for poor treatment outcome during ART. The number of gonadotrophin-responsive antral follicles measuring 2–10 mm can be measured using two- or three-dimensional ultrasound with an acceptably high level of agreement both between and within observers (Jayaprakasan et al 2008a). A total follicle count of between seven and 22 is generally considered as the optimum cut-off level for the prediction of poor and exaggerated ovarian response, respectively. AFC measurement can be performed either in the early-follicular phase of the cycle before treatment begins or after downregulation with similar predictive accuracy (Jayaprakasan et al 2008b). However, assessment prior to treatment has an additional advantage in that it provides an opportunity for pretreatment evaluation of the pelvis to screen for pathology. AFC and AMH are currently the best two predictors of ovarian reserve among all the endocrine and ultrasound markers, and are equally predictive of poor ovarian response during ART (Jayaprakasan et al 2010). AFC

is currently the test of choice for ovarian reserve assessment as it is easy to perform and due to inherent availability of ultrasound machines.

Ovarian reserve tests including AFC and AMH have limited value in the prediction of non-conception despite their adequate capacity to predict ovarian response during ART (Broekmans et al 2006). Pregnancy may occur even at extreme cut-offs for an abnormal test result; therefore, IVF treatment cannot be denied based on these tests, especially in participants who are seeking their first cycle of treatment (Broekmans et al 2007). However, the identification of participants who are likely to respond poorly during IVF treatment is clinically relevant, as a couple can be counselled accordingly. They can be made aware that they have an increased chance of cycle cancellation and a significantly lower chance of success, allowing an informed decision to be made. Such prediction also allows clinicians to formulate individualized treatment protocols to improve or at least maximize ovarian response.

Evaluation of male partner

The male partner should be evaluated carefully. Clinical examination, semen analysis including sperm function tests, genetic assessment and biochemical tests show that the aetiology of male subfertility can be divided into four main groups as follows.

- Primary spermatogenic failure, which is a testicular disorder resulting in the reduction of sperm count and abnormal sperm function. A number of different factors can induce this condition, including testicular maldescent, trauma, karyotype abnormalities, severe infection and antimitotic therapy. However, in many patients, a cause cannot be ascertained.
- Congenital or acquired obstructive lesions. Men with failed reversal of vasectomy are increasingly seen in infertility clinics and, at present, constitute up to 10% of all male problems.
- Disturbances of erection or ejaculatory disorders, including those following spinal injuries.
- Endocrine disorders, such as Cushing's disease, thyroid disorders and androgen receptor abnormalities.

Many causes of male infertility may have considerable congenital implications for the children of such patients. Sixty percent of men with congenital bilateral absence of the vas deferens were shown to have one or more of the cystic fibrosis genes. The use of ICSI in these circumstances should be considered carefully, and men must be screened with the appropriate tests before treatment.

In order to give adequate counselling to couples and their families, genetic tests should be performed before, during or after ART in cases such as women with Turner's syndrome, men with 47XXY, men or women with structural chromosomal aberrations, and men with either Yq11 deletion or congenital bilateral absence of the vas deferens (ESHRE Capri Workshop Group 2000).

The couple must be well informed about the treatment options that are suitable for them, the indications for the tests they have to undergo, details of the proposed treatment and its success rate, and risks and complications.

Clinical Management of the Treatment Cycle

The first successful birth from IVF-embryo transfer (ET) in 1978 resulted from a single oocyte obtained from the dominant follicle in a natural ovarian cycle. Success rates were found to be improved when multiple embryos were available, allowing competitive selection of the best-quality embryo/s for transfer; thus, at present, the majority of assisted reproduction programmes undertake controlled ovarian stimulation to induce multiple follicular development and subsequently to obtain many fertilizable oocytes.

The main components of typical conventional ART include:

- pituitary downregulation using GnRH analogues;
- controlled ovarian stimulation using gonadotrophins;
- monitoring follicular development using transvaginal ultrasound with or without serum oestradiol levels;
- oocyte maturation using human chorionic gonadotrophin (hCG);
- egg collection and sperm production or sperm recovery;
- fertilization (IVF/ICSI) and subsequent embryo culture;
- fresh ET into the uterus and cryopreservation of surplus good-quality embryos; and
- luteal support by progesterone administration.

Normal folliculogenesis

This involves several important and inter-related steps.

- Follicular recruitment. This occupies the first few days of the ovarian cycle and allows the follicle to continue to mature in the correct gonadotrophic environment and to progress towards ovulation.
- Selection. The mechanism whereby a single follicle is chosen and ultimately achieves ovulation.
- Dominance. The selected follicle maintains its pre-eminence over all other follicles and occupies days 8–12 of the primate ovarian cycle.

Follicular development beyond the antral stage depends on the concentration of FSH in the circulation. Once a threshold level has been attained, follicular growth beyond 4 mm occurs. The interval during which FSH remains elevated above the threshold level can be regarded as a window through which a follicle must pass to avoid atresia. The width of the window will therefore determine the number of follicles that can be selected for ovulation (Figure 22.2). The preovulatory luteinizing hormone (LH) surge is triggered by the positive feedback of oestradiol from the dominant follicle, as well as other follicular contributory factors. Ovulation occurs 24–36 h after the onset of the LH surge.

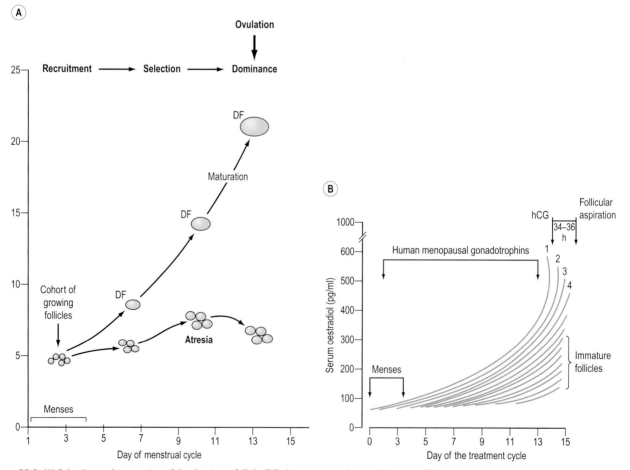

Figure 22.2 (A) Selection and maturation of the dominant follicle (DF) during a natural cycle. (B) Induced follicle maturation with gonadotrophin therapy over-riding selection of a single dominant follicle, as in the natural cycle. hCG, human chorionic gonadotrophin.

Pituitary downregulation

In the conventional ART protocol, it is standard practice to use a continuous and supraphysiological dose of GnRH agonist to obtain control over the hypothalamic–pituitary–ovarian axis. GnRH agonists cause an initial flare response, characterized by increased gonadotrophin secretion, due to upregulation of GnRH receptors. However, prolonged administration of GnRH agonists induces downregulation of GnRH receptors. This prevents a premature surge in LH and subsequent spontaneous ovulation with luteinization, which occurs in up to 23% of cycles when gonadotrophins alone are used and facilitates the timing of oocyte retrieval. The use of GnRH agonists in ART has been shown to increase the number of oocytes retrieved, improve the pregnancy rate and significantly reduce the chance of cycle cancellation (Hughes et al 1992).

Two different GnRH agonist protocols are used in most assisted conception units: long and short protocols. In the long protocol, GnRH agonists (buserelin or nafarelin) are started in the mid-luteal phase (day 21) of the previous menstrual cycle to achieve pituitary downregulation in approximately 8–21 days, after which gonadotrophins are commenced. GnRH agonists are administered for approximately 10–14 days in the short protocol. In both regimens, GnRH agonists are administered daily until the day of hCG or LH injection to trigger oocyte maturation. The short protocol takes advantage of the initial flare effect, which can be utilized to augment the ovarian response to gonadotrophin stimulation. However, a systematic review of 26 randomized-controlled trials found an increased clinical pregnancy rate per cycle and fewer cycle cancellations with the long protocol compared with the short protocol (Daya 2000). Therefore, the long GnRH agonist protocol is generally recommended in most ART cycles.

Use of the long GnRH agonist protocol often prolongs the stimulation phase, resulting in increased requirement for gonadotrophins and increased treatment cost in addition to causing undesirable side-effects of hypo-oestrogenism. It may also be associated with poor response in some patients, as well as introducing a higher risk of ovarian hyperstimulation syndrome (OHSS). Some of the disadvantages can be obviated with the use of GnRH antagonists, such as cetrorelix and ganirelix. GnRH antagonists induce immediate pituitary downregulation by competitively binding to GnRH receptors, and avoid the flare effects or the need for prolonged treatment associated with GnRH agonist protocols. Two different regimes have been described. The multiple-dose protocol involves the administration of 0.25 mg cetrorelix or ganirelix daily from day 6–7 of stimulation, or when the leading follicle is 14–15 mm, until hCG/LH administration. The single-dose protocol involves the single administration of 3 mg cetrorelix on day 7–8 of stimulation. GnRH antagonist protocols are therefore short and simple, but more importantly they reduce the incidence of severe OHSS. However, the clinical pregnancy rates following IVF treatment were significantly lower with GnRH antagonist use compared with the long GnRH agonist protocol [odds ratio (OR) 0.82, 95% confidence interval (CI) 0.68–0.97] (Al-Inany et al 2007), although data from units with experience of the GnRH antagonist protocol are encouraging. More recent trials of GnRH antagonists have reported better preg-

nancy rates than earlier trials, which used antagonist protocols that would now be recognized as suboptimal.

Controlled ovarian stimulation

The pregnancy rate with unstimulated IVF remains much lower than that in stimulated cycles, achieving a livebirth rate of 2.3% per initiated cycle and 4.7% per ET (Human Fertilisation and Embryology Authority 2000). These results have remained low over the past decade. Although an unstimulated cycle is simpler, faster, less painful, less expensive and has no risk of ovarian hyperstimulation, it requires relatively extensive monitoring which increases the cost and results in inconvenience in the timing of oocyte retrieval. Additionally, women with irregular cycles and/or hormonal imbalance or couples with male factor infertility, where fertilization may be a problem, are not suitable for natural-cycle IVF. The aims of superovulation regimens in assisted reproduction are to maximize the number of follicles that mature, to minimize the degree of asynchrony amongst developing follicles, and to minimize the deleterious effects of the abnormal follicular environment on luteal function and endometrial receptivity. Multiple follicular development and ovulation can be achieved by widening the FSH window. Several drug combinations have been used to achieve this.

Oocyte retrieval may be programmed to coincide with a working day by manipulating the onset of the menstrual cycle using norethisterone tablets, the combined oral contraceptive pill, or utilizing the hypogonadotrophic effect of GnRH agonists prior to commencing gonadotrophins on a predetermined day of the week. The downregulatory phase may be prolonged to allow a fixed number of patients to be treated each week. In the long GnRH agonist protocol, gonadotrophins are commenced following the confirmation of ovarian suppression, characterized by a thin endometrium of 5 mm less than transvaginal scan and a serum oestradiol level of less than 200 pmol/l.

The first commercially available gonadotrophin preparation used in superovulation protocols, human menopausal gonadotrophin (HMG), was extracted from the urine of menopausal women. The initial preparations were shown to be of low purity, and the major protein components were not gonadotrophins; only 5% constituted FSH and LH activity. The repeated injection of non-gonadotrophin proteins may be the cause of unwanted effects, such as pain and allergic reactions. The desirability for high-purity preparations led to the development of an immunopurified FSH product with more than 95% purity following the removal of LH activity from HMG. The introduction of highly purified urinary FSH was associated with much reduced hypersensitivity, enabling administration via the subcutaneous route. The currently available commercial preparation of HMG is also highly purified and contains both FSH and LH activity at a ratio of 1:1. The LH activity in HMG is partly due to the presence of exogenous hCG, which is added to correct imbalances in the FSH/LH ratio.

Genetic and molecular engineering has led to the production of recombinant human FSH (rFSH) with high purity (>99%), high specific bioactivity (>10,000 IU/mg protein) and absent intrinsic LH activity which is suitable for intramuscular or subcutaneous administration (Mannaerts et al

1991). Two different rFSH preparations are commercially available: follitropin alpha (Gonal F) and follitropin beta (Puregon). These two rFSH preparations differ in that follitropin alpha has a more acidic isoform profile than follitropin beta due to a slight difference in its carbohydrate component. Consequently, they differ in metabolic clearance, half-life and biological activity, but both are equally effective during ART cycles in terms of livebirth rates. A number of well-designed randomized-controlled trials have compared both preparations of rFSH against HMG in their clinical effectiveness during conventional IVF with the long GnRH agonist protocol. While none of them individually showed any statistically significant difference in livebirth rates between the two treatment arms, two recent systematic reviews have demonstrated a significant 4% increase in livebirth rate in the HMG arm (Al-Inany et al 2008, Coomarasamy et al 2008). However, the results of the meta-analysis need to be interpreted with caution because of the clinical heterogeneity of the trials; therefore, a large multicentre randomized double-blind trial is warranted. Moreover, such studies should consider reporting the more clinically relevant cumulative livebirth rates as the primary outcome.

Recombinant DNA technologies have also made it possible to produce LH (rLH). Due to the potential role of LH in follicular development according to the two-cell theory of gonadotrophin system, supplemental rLH has been suggested to improve IVF outcome if rFSH is used for ovarian stimulation. However, a recent systematic review of randomized trials failed to demonstrate any difference in livebirth rates with adding rLH to the rFSH protocol (Kolibianakis et al 2007). Although it is possible that rLH supplementation may be beneficial in a subset of the IVF population, such as poor responders (Mochtar et al 2007), its generalized use is currently limited.

The collective evidence from many studies suggests that 150–225 IU/day gonadotrophin is the appropriate starting dose for most women undergoing conventional IVF treatment. The majority of units use a daily dose according to women's age and the presence or absence of polycystic ovaries: 150 IU in women under 30 years of age or with polycystic ovaries, 225 IU for those between 30 and 39 years of age, and 300 IU for those aged 40 years or over. The lowest possible dose to achieve the optimum ovarian response should be used to reduce the risks of ovarian hyperstimulation. Although there is no consensus on what constitutes optimum ovarian stimulation, a recent study has reported that the implantation rate is maximum when 10 oocytes are retrieved following conventional IVF using the long downregulation protocol (Verberg et al 2009a).

Recently, mild ovarian stimulation protocols have gained a lot of interest in the field of ART, with the current trend of limiting the number of embryos transferred reducing the need for large numbers of oocytes. The principal aim with this approach is to reduce the number of developing follicles and thereby minimize the adverse effects of ovarian stimulation, particularly OHSS and multiple pregnancies. Three reported mild stimulation protocols include clomiphene citrate alone or in combination with gonadotrophins, delayed commencement (day 5 of the cycle) of gonadotrophins with GnRH antagonist co-medication, and late follicular replacement of FSH with administration of hCG/LH (Verberg et al 2009b). All of these protocols have been shown to reduce the gonadotrophin dosage and have the potential to reduce the cost of treatment and patient distress associated with conventional ART. As expected, the ongoing pregnancy rates/livebirth rates per cycle have been lower compared with the conventional protocol, but similar effectiveness could be achieved with more treatment cycles.

Monitoring follicular development

The purpose of monitoring ovarian response is to ensure safe practice in reducing the incidence and severity of OHSS, and also to optimize the timing of luteinization before oocyte retrieval. Ultrasound forms an integral part of monitoring. Follicular response together with endometrial thickness is monitored by ultrasound scans commencing on day 6–8 of the treatment cycle. Some units also measure serum oestradiol levels. However, current evidence does not support the adjuvant use of oestradiol for monitoring, as it does not give additional information with regard to livebirth rate or OHSS rate. The gonadotrophin dosage is adjusted according to ovarian response, although the evidence for this practice is limited. Typically, follicles are noted to grow at a rate of 2–3 mm/day, accompanied by a steady increase in serum oestradiol levels. When three or more follicles are 18 mm or greater in diameter, 5000–10,000 U hCG or 250 µg choriogonadotropin alpha (recombinant preparation) are given subcutaneously to induce oocyte maturation before oocyte retrieval.

Ovarian response is poor when no follicles or less than three follicles develop after 14 days of gonadotrophin treatment; this generally results in cancellation of the stimulation cycle. This problem is frequently encountered in women with reduced predicted ovarian reserve. Conversely, excessive ovarian response may result in OHSS, which will be discussed later. Other problems such as a premature LH surge or preoperative ovulation have been largely eliminated by the introduction of GnRH analogues in superovulation protocols.

Oocyte Retrieval

It is important to provide effective anaesthesia and analgesia for transvaginal oocyte recovery, as this is painful. No techniques for anaesthesia, analgesia or sedation are free from side-effects. Whichever technique is used, recognized standards of practice should be adhered to and all IVF professionals should follow the safe practice of administering sedative drugs published by the Academy of Medical Royal Colleges (2001). Conscious sedation should be offered to all women having the procedure as it is a safe and acceptable method of providing analgesia.

Equipment and preparation

Oocyte retrieval is performed 36 h after the trigger injection of hCG/LH. Methods of egg collection have improved considerably since the introduction of ART. At first, all egg collections were performed laparoscopically. This is now rarely used and is reserved for women whose ovaries are inaccessible through the transvaginal route. With the introduction of endovaginal transducers, the transvaginal-ultrasound-guided approach became the predominant method for egg collection. In this, the specially designed transducer is used to visualize the follicles and the aspirating needle is passed alongside it. This method is generally well tolerated when carried out under light intravenous sedation, can be learnt very quickly and is associated with minimal morbidity.

Technique

Several types of aspiration needle are available. They may have a single or double lumen to enable aspiration and flushing through different routes. The needle is usually 16-guage and must have a very sharp tip to enable easy puncture of mobile ovaries; the distal 2 cm should be roughened to enhance ultrasound visualization (Figure 22.3). The needle is connected to a test tube by tubing, and suction is applied either from a foot-operated pump (Figure 22.4) or manually. The ultrasound transducer (Figure 22.5) is enclosed in a special sterile condom and plastic sleeve prior to insertion into the vagina, and should be cleaned thoroughly with a damp cloth after each procedure.

Generally, very few technical difficulties are encountered during vaginal egg collection. The main risks of transvaginal oocyte recovery are pelvic infection (0.6%) and bleeding (>100 ml in 0.8% cases) (Bennett et al 1993), which may be serious, sometimes even fatal. Appropriate preoperative vaginal preparation and minimizing the number of repeated vaginal penetrations may serve to lower the risk of infection. While there is no evidence that routine antibiotics reduce the risk of infection, the administration of an intravenous bolus of antibiotic is generally recommended for women with a history of severe pelvic inflammatory disease or if an endometrioma is punctured. Intestinal, vascular, uterine and tubal injuries with the aspiration needle have also been reported. Bleeding and infections may be serious, sometimes even fatal, complications.

Laboratory Techniques

The oocytes obtained are fertilized by conventional IVF or ICSI treatment dependent on the quality of the sperm obtained on the day of oocyte retrieval. ICSI is indicated if there is a severe deficit in sperm quality, obstructive or non-obstructive azoospermia, and for couples in whom a

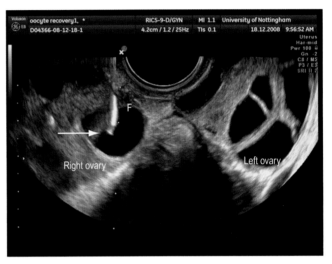

Figure 22.3 Ultrasound picture during vaginal egg recovery. The tip of the needle (arrow) is seen within the follicle (F).

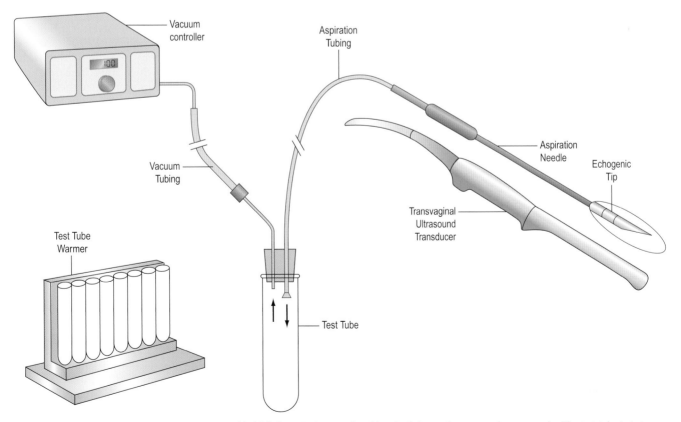

Figure 22.4 Follicle aspiration equipment. An assembled follicle aspiration needle with a single lumen is connected to a test tube. The test tube is, in turn, connected to a suction pump. The needle is attached to the transvaginal ultrasound transducer through needle guide and bracket.

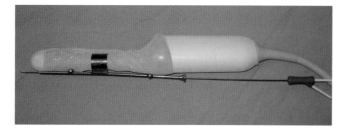

Figure 22.5 Vaginal ultrasound transducer enclosed in a sterile condom with needle guide attached. The needle tip is protruding from the proximal end of the probe.

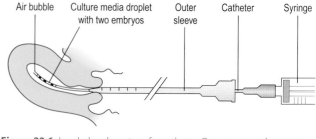

Figure 22.6 Loaded embryo transfer catheter. One or two embryos are ready to be deposited within 1 cm of the uterine fundus.

previous IVF treatment cycle has resulted in failed or very poor fertilization. Sperm utilized for conventional IVF/ICSI is obtained by masturbation. When there is azoospermia, it is aspirated from the epididymis and/or testis, or extracted from the testes.

There are numerous techniques for performing the insemination of oocytes, and these vary from laboratory to laboratory. Differences in culture systems include the quantity and volume of sperm added to oocytes, culture of oocytes either singly or in groups, and open or oil-covered culture systems. IVF in the authors' unit is performed by incubating the collected oocytes in groups of five in a media drop of 150 μl under oil; 22,500 sperm are added to this.

In cases of ICSI, meiotic maturity is assessed after denudation; only the mature oocytes are injected with sperm, following immobilization. Fertilization, as determined by the presence of two pronuclei, is assessed 18–20 h after insemination. On day 2 or 3, based on the cleavage rate, the size, shape, symmetry and cytoplasmic appearance of the blastomeres and the presence or absence of nucleus, embryo quality is graded by embryologists as grade 1, 2, 3 or 4 (Van Royen et al 1999). Grade 1 and 2 embryos are considered to be of high quality. While ET is performed with one or two of the best-available embryo/s, regardless of their grading, only top-quality (grade 1 and 2) embryos are considered eligible for freezing and this option is then offered to the couple.

Embryo Transfer

ET is a critical step in determining the final outcome of the treatment. The convention has been to replace embryos on the second or third day post insemination, when the embryos are usually at the two- to eight-cell stage of cleavage. With improvements in culture media, there is an increasing tendency for delaying ET with the aim of improving implantation rates. While there is no improvement in livebirth rates (OR 1.07, 95% CI 0.84–1.37) with delaying ET from day 2 to day 3 (Oatway et al 2004), transfer of embryos at the blastocyst stage (day 5/6) has shown a significant increase in the livebirth rate (OR 1.35, 95% CI 1.05–1.74) compared with transfers on day 2 or 3 (Blake et al 2007). It is a more physiological approach, allowing synchronization of the embryo with the endometrium, and selection of the viable embryos for transfer will be more efficient. However, the rates of embryo freezing are lower and the treatment cancellation rates are higher with blastocyst transfer. However, in certain couples, blastocyst transfer has the

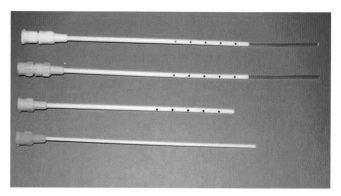

Figure 22.7 Embryo transfer catheters. From top to bottom: trial Wallace catheter (no lumen), Wallace catheter, and outer sheath and stylet of malleable catheter.

potential to favour single ET without compromising the overall success rates, but can significantly reduce the occurrence of multiple pregnancies. The most favoured couples for blastocyst transfer are those with high numbers of eight-cell embryos on day 3, in whom cycle cancellation is not increased.

Transcervical embryo replacement into the uterine cavity is a relatively simple procedure, which must be carried out meticulously to ensure appropriate placement of the embryos (Figure 22.6). Variations among clinicians in the technique of ET may influence the pregnancy rate. Avoidance of blood, mucus, bacterial contamination, excessive uterine contractions and trauma to the endometrium is associated with optimal pregnancy and implantation rates after transcervical ET. Transabdominal ultrasonographic guidance to determine the precise depth of embryo placement within the uterus appears to facilitate successful ET and is preferred (Brown et al 2007), although a recent large randomized trial from a single centre did not show any benefit over 'clinical touch' transfer (Drakeley et al 2008). The tip of the catheter is placed approximately 1 cm from the uterine fundus so that the embryo/s are expelled gently into the mid-cavity of the uterus. Soft catheters are preferable to rigid catheters as they are less likely to traumatize the cervix or endometrium, or to invoke any uterine contractions. The commonly used soft catheters (Wallace catheters) (Figure 22.7) have a softer inner cannula and a stiffer outer sheath. Occasionally, resistance to pass the soft inner cannula into the uterus, usually at the level of internal os, is encountered; in these cases, the stiffer outer sheath is advanced into the cervical canal to negotiate the resistance, and the inner cannula can be advanced into the uterine cavity. A firmer malleable catheter

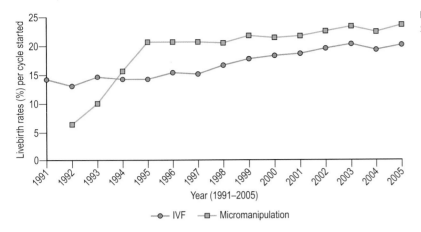

Figure 22.8 Livebirth rates per treatment cycle 1991–2005. *Source: Human Fertilisation and Embryology Authority (2008).*

with a stylet and an outer sheath is another option in diffi-cult cases, where the catheter is advanced up to the level of the internal os. The inner stylet is then removed and the softer cannula loaded with embryos is fed through the outer sheath to advance into the uterine cavity for transfer. The outer sheath or the malleable catheter should never be advanced beyond the internal os.

Following ET, women are often advised to continue their normal daily activities as prolonged bed rest has not been shown to improve IVF outcome. Luteal support is usually required as ART is associated with inadequate luteal func-tion, possibly because of suppressed LH levels secondary to supraphysiological concentrations of oestradiol, removal of the granulosa cells surrounding the oocytes while perform-ing the oocyte retrieval, and the use of GnRH agonists. hCG or progesterone is traditionally used to provide luteal support during conventional IVF cycles. However, the routine use of hCG is not recommended because of the increased likeli-hood of OHSS and no benefit over progesterone in terms of IVF success. Progesterone can be administered either 200–800 mg/day vaginally or 50–100 mg/day intramuscularly; this is continued for 14–16 days, when a pregnancy test is performed.

Outcome Measures and Factors Affecting Success Rate

Pregnancy and livebirth rates per treatment cycle for IVF and ICSI have steadily improved worldwide over the past decade. Figure 22.8 shows the improvement in the livebirth rate per treatment cycle in the UK between 1991 and 2005 (Human Fertilisation and Embryology Authority 2008). It is now widely accepted that when attempting to ascertain whether or not a treatment is required, it is essential that the time-specific or cycle-specific conception rate is used. Crude preg-nancy rate per couple is almost meaningless. Pregnancy rate per cycle can also be misleading if limited to the first cycle or two, because the rate may fall in subsequent cycles. Thus, cumulative conception or cumulative livebirth rates have been used increasingly in reporting conventional and ART outcomes. Cumulative conception rates for some of the most common causes of infertility in the untreated popula-tion were compared with those in couples following treat-ment with conventional methods (Hull 1992). The results showed that in some conditions, such as ovulatory dysfunc-tion, or in women being treated with donor insemination, the cumulative conception rate following conventional therapy is almost the same as in normal women. However, in other circumstances, such as salpingostomy for distal tubal occlusion or the use of high-dose glucocorticosteroids for seminal antisperm antibodies, the prognosis is worse and the cumulative conception rates are lower than that which can be expected in a single cycle of IVF treatment.

The effectiveness of infertility treatments (IVF, ICSI, egg and sperm donation, embryo donation) is dependent on a reasonable likelihood that embryos can be created in vitro, and then placed in the uterus with a reasonable expectation that implantation will occur. Many factors determine the outcome of treatment, such as patient selection, age, cause and duration of infertility, and the number of attempts that couples undergo. The decision to recommend ART should be based on the likelihood that a pregnancy will occur without treatment, the possibility that a less invasive form of treatment might be effective and the likely outcome of IVF treatment (National Institute for Clinical Excellence 2004). The likelihood of treatment-independent pregnancy depends on the woman's age, the cause and duration of infertility, and previous pregnancy history. In a retrospective study (Vardon et al 1995), the incidence of spontaneous treatment-independent pregnancy in couples enlisted on an IVF programme was reported to be 11% of couples with low fertility. The main difference from those in whom pregnancy did not occur was a shorter duration of infertility.

Success of ART is also dependent on where the provision of service takes place. It is clear from the HFEA annual reports that the outcome of treatment varies between small and large centres. When discussing the likelihood of birth following IVF treatment with any couple, it is essential to consider the factors that can affect the outcome significantly. These include female age, body mass index, cause and dura-tion of infertility, previous pregnancy history, number of embryos replaced, availability of surplus embryos for cryo-preservation and the number of previous treatment cycles. Such advice is particularly relevant and important in women over 40 years of age, in whom success rates are reduced considerably and the risk of miscarriage is increased.

Female age

The woman's age at the time of treatment is an important prognostic factor when the success of IVF is discussed with any couple. The number of oocytes and, consequently, the number of embryos decline with age. However, the cleavage rate does not seem to alter in the same manner. The number of embryos replaced compounds the effect of age and embryo implantation rates on pregnancy rate. The total number of embryos available for replacement influences this further. When a larger number of embryos is available for replacement, the selection of the most appropriate embryos for transfer improves the implantation and pregnancy rates.

Indeed, when women over 40 years of age had four or more embryos transferred, their pregnancy rate was not significantly different from that of younger women, whether following IVF (Widra et al 1996) or ICSI (Alrayyes et al 1997). Hence, it may be concluded that older women with a good ovarian response, producing three or more embryos suitable for transfer, have similar prospects for establishing a pregnancy as younger patients. However, other data support reduced implantation rates in older women, regardless of the number of embryos transferred (Piette et al 1990). Younger women, even if their ovarian response is poor, have a better implantation rate than women over 40 years of age experiencing a normal ovarian response (van Rooij et al 2003). This indicates that age is the major determinant of the implantation potential of oocytes and/or of endometrial receptivity. However, the reported finding of similar pregnancy rates in older women having treatment using donor eggs compared with younger women indicates that oocyte quality or implantation potential, rather than endometrial receptivity, declines with women's age (Van Voorhis 2007).

Although livebirth rates per treatment cycle following IVF and ICSI have increased consistently over the past decade, they decline with advancing age of women when using their own eggs (Figure 22.9). A number of investigators have examined different age cut-offs such as 40 years (Widra et al 1996, Sharif et al 1998) or 35 years (Preutthipan et al 1996). Mardesic et al (1994) reported that the cut-off point of effectiveness for an IVF programme was 36–37 years, with a marked decline in pregnancy rate per ET in women over 38 years of age. In an attempt to identify factors that affect the outcome of treatment, Templeton et al (1996) analysed the HFEA database between 1991 and 1994. They reported that the overall livebirth rate per treatment cycle was 13.9%. The highest livebirth rates were in women aged 25–30 years, with younger women (<25 years) having lower rates, and a sharp decline noted in older women. At all ages over 30 years, the use of donor eggs was associated with significantly higher livebirth rates compared with the use of the women's own eggs, although there was equally a downward trend in

success rates with age. After adjustment for age, increasing duration of infertility was associated with a significant decrease in livebirth rates. The indications for treatment had no significant effect on the outcome, while previous pregnancy and live birth increased treatment success significantly.

Miscarriage rates have been reported to be higher in all women following IVF, and there is a two- to three-fold increase in the rate of spontaneous abortion in women aged 40 years or more (Toner and Flood 1993). Embryo quality is more likely to be the main factor influencing the poor reproductive performance of women with advancing age than a defective response of the uterine vasculature to steroids or uterine ageing. Increasing maternal age correlates with a higher risk of fetal chromosomal aneuploidy, which results in an increased rate of miscarriage (Spandorfer et al 2004).

Obesity

Although the consequences of obesity for women's fertility are well known, there is controversy regarding the effect of obesity on the outcome of IVF treatment. Overweight [body mass index (BMI) ≥25] and obesity (BMI ≥30) have been associated with the need for higher doses of gonadotrophins, increased cycle cancellation rates and retrieval of fewer oocytes. Lower rates of ET, pregnancy and live birth have also been reported, as have higher miscarriage rates (Fedorcsak et al 2004). Other studies have not found that obesity has a negative impact on ART outcome (Dechaud et al 2006, Sneed et al 2008). However, a recent systematic review of all the reported studies confirmed that obesity has an adverse effect on the success of IVF (Maheshwari et al 2007); therefore, obese women should be advised to lose weight before commencing ART in order to improve their chance of success.

Cause of infertility

Reports have differed in their analysis of the impact of infertility factors on cumulative conception and livebirth rates. While some have found significant differences, with the lowest rates being reported in patients with male infertility or multiple infertility factors (Tan et al 1992), others found no significant effect on outcome (Templeton et al 1996). However, a history of previous pregnancy and live birth increased treatment success significantly. The IVF clinical pregnancy and livebirth rates in the HFEA report of 2000

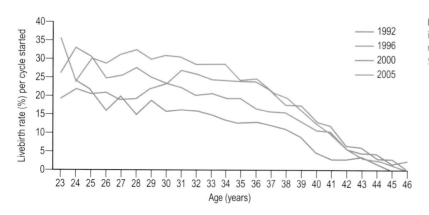

Figure 22.9 Livebirth rates by age of women who have in-vitro fertilization or intracytoplasmic injection. Success rates have improved over the years for all ages.
Source: Human Fertilisation and Embryology Authority (2008).

show similar results for tubal disease, endometriosis and unexplained infertility (Figure 22.10). Reports of higher fertilization rates after ICSI suggest that this technique may be better than the conventional method for all couples seeking IVF. A multicentre randomized-controlled trial comparing clinical outcome after ICSI or conventional IVF in couples with non-male-factor infertility showed higher implantation and pregnancy rates per cycle after IVF, hence supporting the practice of reserving ICSI for severe male factor infertility (Bhattacharya et al 2001).

All stages of endometriosis are viewed as suitable indications for ART. The timing of treatment is dependent on the severity of the disease, previous therapy and other factors, such as female age and duration of infertility. In women with severe endometriosis with mechanical tubal blockage and where surgery is inappropriate, IVF should be expedited. IVF should also be recommended 1–2 years after previous unsuccessful medical or surgical therapy, while in minimal or mild endometriosis, the balance of choice seems to be in favour of IVF after more than 2 years of expectant management. Initially, poor results were reported in women with severe disease (Matson and Yovich 1986). The introduction of ultrasound-guided techniques for oocyte collection resulted in the retrieval of more oocytes, and hence led to higher pregnancy and implantation rates in advanced-stage disease (Geber et al 1995). The use of GnRH agonists in stimulation protocols or as a pretreatment for women with endometriosis has also resulted in the retrieval and transfer of more preovulatory oocytes, lower cancellation of treatment cycles and a higher pregnancy rate, especially in women with advanced-stage disease. A recent meta-analysis indicated that the presence of ovarian endometrioma does not affect the quality of oocytes, as the pregnancy rate was similar to that of controls, although the ovarian response to gonadotrophins was reduced (Gupta et al 2006). While prospective randomized-controlled trials are lacking, evidence based on case–control studies suggests that surgery for bilateral endometrioma could impair IVF outcome significantly, possibly due to damage to the remaining healthy ovarian follicles (Somigliana et al 2008).

For male factor infertility, ICSI was successfully introduced in 1992 (Palermo et al 1992). Since then, the annual number of treatment cycles has increased steadily (see Figure 22.1). Previous techniques, such as partial zona dissection and subzonal insemination, were very disappointing (Cohen et al 1991), and comparative studies indicated that ICSI was much more efficient (Tarin 1995). It gave men who had previously been diagnosed with severe male factor infertility the chance to have their own genetic children. The sperm may be obtained either by ejaculation, percutaneous aspiration from the epididymis or testis, or testicular extraction, resulting in equally high fertilization, pregnancy and implantation rates, especially in men with borderline or very poor sperm quality. Recognized indications for ICSI include:

- very poor sperm quality;
- obstructive azoospermia;
- non-obstructive azoospermia; and
- previously failed or very poor fertilization.

Livebirth rates following ICSI are shown in Figure 22.8. A remarkable change in fertilization rate with a significant increase in the percentage of two pronuclei oocytes occurred when the technique was modified slightly by breaking the sperm's tail before injection (Fishel et al 1995). The technique requires a high-quality inverted microscope and special equipment, with holding and injection pipettes being used to stabilize and inject the oocyte, respectively. The injecting pipette is pushed almost entirely through the ooplasm before the spermatozoon is deposited inside the oocyte (Figure 22.11).

Duration of infertility

The duration of infertility remains one of the most important variables that influences the outcome of assisted reproduction, with lower pregnancy and livebirth rates associated with a longer period of infertility. Analysis of the HFEA database between 1991 and 1994 showed that, even with adjustment for age, there was a significant decrease in livebirth rate with increasing duration of infertility from 1 to 12 years (Templeton et al 1996).

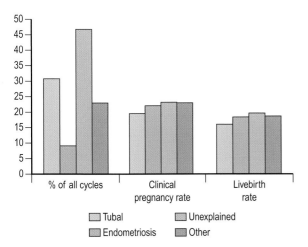

Figure 22.10 Clinical pregnancy and livebirth rates following in-vitro fertilization for female causes of infertility.
Source: Human Fertilisation and Embryology Authority (2000).

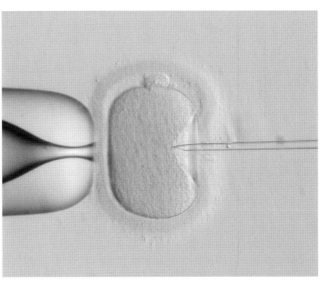

Figure 22.11 Intracytoplasmic injection of a single sperm (arrow) into the egg.

Endometrial thickness

Endometrial thickness alone is a poor predictor for pregnancy. However, no conception has been recorded for endometrial thickness below 5 mm on the day of transfer. As such, it is recommended that consideration should be given to cryopreserving all embryos and preparing the endometrium with exogenous hormones in a subsequent cycle (Friedler et al 1996).

Number of embryos transferred

Regarding the optimum number of embryos to be transferred, there is a great deal of debate and a wide variation in practice across the world. Unarguably, ART is the single most important cause for the increase in multiple pregnancies over the last two decades, which is a direct consequence of the number of embryos transferred. Retrospective studies, as early as 1985, argued that multiple pregnancies and births increased with the increase in the number of embryos replaced (Wood et al 1985). Randomized studies comparing double ET with treble ET (Staessen et al 1993) or quadruple ET (Vauthier-Brouzes et al 1994) reported similar pregnancy rates, provided that there were sufficient morphologically regular embryos available for transfer. Analysis of the HFEA database of more than 44,000 cycles (Templeton and Morris 1998) and the HFEA reports (2000) showed that when four or more fertilized eggs were available, the transfer of three embryos did not result in improved pregnancy rates compared with the elective transfer of two embryos. However, the incidence of triplets or higher order multiple births decreased considerably when two embryos were replaced (Figure 22.12).

Despite only transferring two embryos during most IVF cycles, 40% of all IVF babies are twins (Human Fertilisation and Embryology Authority 2008). In order to deal with the unacceptably high multiple birth rates following ART, there is a recent move from the IVF community, particularly in Europe, to limit the number of embryos transferred to one in carefully selected patients. In the UK, the HFEA has set a target of reducing the multiple pregnancy rate to 10% over a period of about 3 years, and has urged the fertility clinics to devise a 'multiple pregnancy minimization strategy' to achieve the agreed target. To facilitate this, the British Fertility Society in unison with the Association of Clinical Embryologists in the UK have produced guidelines for practice which focus on the effectiveness of elective single ET (eSET) and patient selection for eSET (Cutting et al 2008). The two most important criteria when choosing a couple for eSET are female age and the quality of embryos available. Twin pregnancy has increased risk for the fetuses and the mother. Given the higher risks of premature delivery (three-fold), perinatal mortality (six-fold), cerebral palsy (four- to six-fold) and pregnancy complications (hypertension, pre-eclampsia, gestational diabetes etc.), and the consequent resource implications for the health service with twin births compared with singleton deliveries, the HFEA in the UK has urged for successful IVF to be redefined as 'full-term singletons with a normal birth weight' in order to promote eSET and thereby reduce multiple births (Cutting et al 2008). A Cochrane review comparing the outcome of double ET in a single cycle compared with eSET (combined with transfer of a single frozen–thawed embryo in a subsequent cycle if necessary) identified similar pregnancy rates in both groups (OR 1.19, 95% CI 0.87–1.62) with a substantially higher multiple pregnancy rate following double ET (OR 62.83, 95% CI 8.52–463.57) (Pandian et al 2005). Several European countries have now adopted eSET coupled with effective cryopreservation programmes in patients with a good prognosis, and have reported no significant difference in pregnancy rates but a significant reduction in the rate of twin pregnancies. In carefully selected patients (e.g. women <37 years of age, undergoing their first IVF cycle and with more than one top-quality embryo), eSET plus subsequent frozen embryo replacement can be as effective as double ET.

Number of attempts

The literature appears to be somewhat divided regarding pregnancy and livebirth rates in relation to the number of ART attempts. In one study (Padilla and Garcia 1989), the pregnancy rate per ET was similar for at least seven attempts, while other studies (Tan et al 1992, Templeton et al 1996) reported a decline in pregnancy and livebirth rates with successive treatment cycles. The data from the HFEA 2000 annual report show a steady decline in pregnancy and livebirth rates per cycle after the fifth attempt, being 11.1% and 8.6%, respectively, at the 11th attempt (Figure 22.13).

When IVF cumulative pregnancy rates were estimated for a cohort of women, the rates showed a constant rise during the six initial IVF treatments and plateaued subsequently (Dor et al 1996). Similarly, the rates were reported to be as high as 80% after seven cycles, and a history of previous pregnancy improved a couple's probability of conception significantly (Croucher et al 1998).

Embryo cryopreservation

The ability to cryopreserve embryos enables any supernumerary embryos to be stored for some time before subsequent replacement when fresh ET has failed or if further children are desired. Additionally, cryopreservation has the added benefit of increasing the number of potential embryo replacement cycles without the need to undergo superovula-

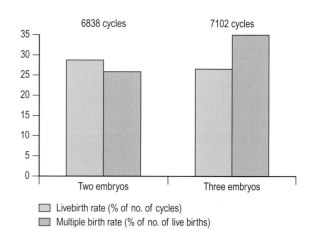

Figure 22.12 Live and multiple births following in-vitro fertilization when two or three fresh embryos were transferred after the creation of four or more embryos.
Source: Human Fertilisation and Embryology Authority (2000).

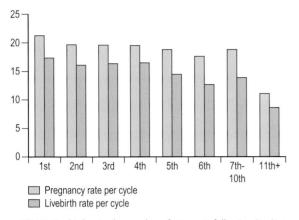

Figure 22.13 Livebirth rates by number of attempts following in-vitro fertilization.
Source: Human Fertilisation and Embryology Authority (2000).

tion and oocyte retrieval, hence reducing the risk of OHSS. Embryo quality has the most significant impact on post-thaw survival and, ultimately, pregnancy and implantation rates. As with fresh embryos, factors such as female age, number of embryos transferred and whether a pregnancy resulted from the original stimulation cycle will affect the outcome of the FER cycle.

In 2005, the HFEA annual register reported a clinical pregnancy rate of 18% and a livebirth rate of 15.6% per FER cycle in women using their own gametes (Human Fertilisation and Embryology Authority 2008). Over the past decade, considerable improvement has taken place. The French register (FIVNAT 1996) reported an increase in pregnancy rate per transfer from 11.5% to 16% between 1987 and 1995. It has been estimated that one FER cycle increases the 'take-home baby' rate by 5% (Kahn et al 1993), while treatment involving one fresh and two FER cycles achieves a cumulative viable pregnancy rate of 41% (Horne et al 1997). Frozen–thawed embryos can be replaced in natural or hormonally adjusted cycles utilizing GnRH agonist and oestrogen/progestogen preparations with comparable results. The use of GnRH agonist is useful in anovulatory or irregular cycles, and the use of different progestogens for luteal-phase support is equally effective. The cost per delivery for an FER cycle has been estimated to be between 25% and 45% of the cost of a fresh cycle. In view of these advantages, cryopreservation should be accessible and discussed with all couples where surplus good-quality embryos are available.

Oocyte donation

Oocyte donation is an effective treatment for women with premature ovarian failure, Turner's syndrome, following oophorectomy, chemo- or radiotherapy-related ovarian failure, in certain cases where there is a high risk of transmitting a genetic disorder to the child, and where repeated failure of fertilization is attributed to poor oocyte quality. High pregnancy rates have been reported following oocyte donation for patients with Turner's syndrome (Khastgir et al 1997). However, Turner's patients were reported to have significantly higher biochemical pregnancy rates and early miscarriages, and lower clinical pregnancy and delivery rates compared with other women with premature ovarian failure (Yaron et al 1996). An important factor in the establishment

of pregnancy is an endometrial thickness of greater than 6.5 mm. Other factors include the number of previous natural conceptions and live births, and the fertilization rate, while increasing female age does not affect the outcome (Burton et al 1992).

The HFEA recommends that the age limit for egg donors should be 35 years, except in exceptional circumstances. This is because there is an increased pregnancy rate and reduced risk of aneuploidy in the offspring if the treatment is performed using eggs from young donors. Oocyte donors are screened for infections (human immunodeficiency virus, hepatitis B, hepatitis C and cytomegalovirus, Venereal Disease Research Laboratory tests for syphilis), genetic diseases such as cystic fibrosis, and major chromosomal anomalies. Targeted screening based on ethnic background is also recommended: for example, Tay–Sachs disease for Jewish population, sickle cell screening in Afro-Caribbean population and thallassaemia in Asian population. If the prospective donor is found to be heterozygous for cystic fibrosis, the partner of the recipient should also be screened for cystic fibrosis.

Oocyte donation has considerable emotional and social effects on both the donor and the recipient, more so if the donor is undergoing IVF treatment herself. Both the recipient and the donor should have counselling from someone who is independent of the treatment unit regarding the physical and psychological implications of treatment for themselves and their genetic children, including any potential children resulting from donated oocytes. Apart from anonymous and known oocyte donation, an egg share scheme is an efficient use of oocytes. This aims to reduce the imbalance between the large number of potential recipients and the small number of available donors. This also allows women requiring IVF and with insufficient funds for their own treatment to access IVF treatment for free or at a significantly reduced cost. Many studies have reported a safe 'cut-off' number of oocytes to be collected from the egg share donor to share with the recipient.

Livebirth rates following treatment using oocyte donation are excellent. Pregnancy and livebirth rates per treatment cycle following oocyte donation in comparison with other treatments are depicted in Figure 22.14 where fresh embryos are replaced, and in Figure 22.15 where frozen–thawed embryos are replaced (Human Fertilisation and Embryology Authority 2008). Neither the recipient's age nor the indication of treatment affects the success of oocyte donation substantially. However, pregnancy resulting from oocyte donation should be considered as high risk, especially in those with ovarian failure, because of an increased incidence of small-for-gestational-age infants. Oocyte recipients should also be counselled regarding their increased risk for pregnancy-induced hypertension and postpartum haemorrhage.

Health Risks Associated with Assisted Reproduction Treatment

Ectopic pregnancy

The first pregnancy following IVF was an ectopic pregnancy. There is a higher rate of ectopic pregnancy after IVF/ICSI treatment, principally due to the high prevalence of tubal

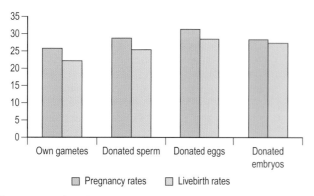

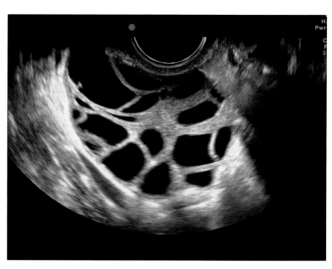

Figure 22.14 Clinical pregnancy and livebirth rates following in-vitro fertilization with fresh embryo-transfer-stimulated cycles, performed in 2005. *Source: Human Fertilisation and Embryology Authority (2008).*

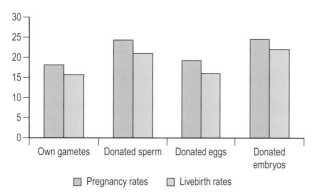

Figure 22.16 Vaginal ultrasound appearance of the hyperstimulated ovary. The enlarged ovary contains an excessive number of large, intermediate and small follicles.

Figure 22.15 Clinical pregnancy and livebirth rates following in-vitro fertilization with frozen embryo replacement, performed in 2005. *Source: Human Fertilisation and Embryology Authority (2008).*

factor infertility. The obstetric risks and outcomes of ART have always been the subject of considerable debate. Between 2% and 5% of ART pregnancies have been reported to be ectopic and 0.1–0.3% have been reported to be heterotopic (Clayton et al 2006). For comparison, the prevalence of ectopic pregnancy and heterotopic pregnancy following natural conception is approximately one in 100 and one in 30,000 respectively. The overall ectopic pregnancy rate per treatment cycle was 0.3% of over 467,778 IVF/ICSI cycles performed in the UK from 1991 to 2005 (Human Fertilisation and Embryology Authority 2008).

Ovarian hyperstimulation syndrome

OHSS remains the most serious and potentially lethal complication of ovarian hyperstimulation, correlates positively with conceptual cycles and is almost exclusively related to either exogenous or endogenous hCG stimulation. The pathophysiology of OHSS is characterized by increased capillary permeability, mediated by the vasoactive substances released from the hyperstimulated ovaries. Fluid leaks from the intravascular compartment into the third space, causing intravascular dehydration and, in severe cases, multisystem dysfunction. Young age, presence of PCOS, lean body mass and previous history of OHSS have all been reported to be risk factors for the development of OHSS. The risk increases with excessive ovarian response to gonadotrophins, characterized by the development of a large number of follicles including immature and intermediate follicles and/or high serum oestradiol levels. Mild forms are common, affecting

up to 33% of IVF cycles. The overall prevalence of moderate-to-severe OHSS varies from 3% to 8% of IVF/ICSI cycles (Mathur et al 2007). The time of onset of OHSS may determine the prognosis; late-onset OHSS is likely to be more severe and to last longer than early-onset OHSS. Early-onset OHSS is due to the effects of exogenous hCG and presents within 9 days of the ovulatory trigger hCG. Endogenous hCG from an early pregnancy triggers the development of late-onset OHSS, which develops 9 days after the ovulatory hCG.

Prevention and early recognition are the two most important components in the management of OHSS. The key to prevention is proper identification of the population at risk before treatment, and close monitoring of hormone levels as well as follicular response on ultrasound (Figure 22.16). When a high-risk situation is recognized, withholding the ovulatory dose of hCG and cancellation of the treatment cycle will almost certainly prevent OHSS. The couple should be advised to avoid intercourse as spontaneous ovulation may occur up to 11 days after discontinuing gonadotrophin treatment, resulting in conception and development of severe OHSS.

Alternative strategies have been attempted and, when effective, they usually ameliorate the severity of OHSS rather than prevent it absolutely (see Box 22.2).

A diagnosis of OHSS is usually straightforward, with typical symptoms of abdominal distension, abdominal pain, nausea and vomiting, reduced urine output and breathing difficulties. Women with OHSS should have the severity of their condition assessed (RCOG 2006). Treatment of established OHSS depends on its severity, the stage at which the diagnosis is made and whether or not the patient is pregnant. In mild cases and most moderate cases of OHSS (haematocrit <45%), bed rest, simple analgesia, increased fluid intake and close monitoring of electrolyte balance may be sufficient. Women should be encouraged to drink to thirst, rather than to excess. The patient's progress can be supervised on an outpatient basis. Hospital admission should be recommended to some women with moderate OHSS and all those with severe OHSS (haematocrit ≥45%, massive ascites). Women should be kept under review until resolution of the condition. Inpatient management is mainly aimed towards preventing or alleviating haemoconcentration, renal hypoperfusion and thromboembolic phenomena. Initiation of intravenous fluid is not always necessary unless oral intake cannot maintain renal perfusion and function. Analgesics and antiemetics should be instituted for symptomatic relief, along with subcutaneous heparin for antithrombotic prophylaxis. Diuretics should not be used in women with oliguria secondary to a reduced blood volume and decreased renal perfusion, as they may worsen intravascular dehydration. Paracentesis may be necessary for symptomatic relief or failing renal function as it results in a dramatic improvement in clinical symptoms, diuresis and improved creatinine clearance (Aboulghar et al 1992). Multidisciplinary input including critical care may be required for women who develop severe complications such as severe ascites, liver or renal dysfunction, thromboembolism or adult respiratory distress syndrome.

Risk of genital and breast cancer

The potential risk of genital cancer from follicular stimulation has initiated considerable debate (Brinton 2007). While the results of earlier studies were alarming, subsequent studies with much longer follow-up periods and better designs showed reassuring results. In a cohort study of 12,193 women, Brinton et al (2004) reported no increased risk associated with clomiphene or gonadotrophin use among subjects who had been followed-up for a median of 18.8 years. Subsequent larger studies concentrating on the effect of exposure to drugs used during IVF rather than those prescribed in earlier times also reported reassuring results (Venn et al 1999, Klip et al 2003). However, the average follow-up period in these studies was only 6–7 years. Therefore, long-term follow-up data are needed to fully evaluate the risk of exposure to gonadotrophins during IVF. Moreover, appropriate control groups should be used to determine whether the link is causal, as it is difficult to distinguish the effect of fertility treatment from that of infertility *per se* on the development of malignancies.

It is well established that endometrial cancer is sensitive to oestrogen, which is produced excessively during ovarian hyperstimulation. Most smaller cohort studies have not found any association between the fertility drugs and endometrial cancer, but the follow-up period in these studies has been less than 10 years (Brinton 2007). In a larger series with an average of over 20 years of follow-up, a significant two-fold increase in endometrial cancer was associated with

ovulation induction agents (Modan et al 1998). However, this study evaluated women who had undergone fertility treatment between 1964 and 1974, and therefore these results cannot be extrapolated to modern-day IVF treatment.

Concerns relating to the effect of high oestrogen and progesterone levels on the potential risk for the development of breast cancer have also been expressed. A large cohort study of over 90,000 subjects showed no association between exposure to ART and breast cancer (Gauthier et al 2004).

In summary, the effects of ovulation induction agents currently used in ART on genital cancer risk are unclear. Considering that the treatment protocols, preparations and dosages used during IVF are relatively new, and women exposed to IVF are only beginning to reach the cancer age range, further follow-up studies are required in this area.

Risk of congenital anomalies and malignancy in the newborn

Since IVF and ICSI became common fertility treatment modalities, concerns have been raised regarding the risk of major congenital malformations in children born following these treatments. While the majority of studies have shown an increased risk of major anomalies compared with spontaneously conceived pregnancies, some studies have been reassuring. A recent meta-analysis of 25 studies concluded that there is a statistically significant increase (30–40%) in birth defects compared with background risk (Hansen et al 2005). The authors expressed this result in terms of the number needed to harm, which in this case equates to the number of children that need to be conceived by ART for one additional child to be born with a birth defect. Therefore, for an underlying prevalence of birth defects between 1% and 4% of all births, the number needed to harm is between 250 and 62 treatments. ICSI enabled men with severe oligospermia or azoospermia to pass their genes on to their own progeny; an event that may not have been possible a few years ago. This raises certain questions about the genetic constitution of any resulting pregnancies after ICSI. A 1.2-fold increased risk of major birth defects in children born after ICSI (95% CI 0.97–1.28) compared with IVF was noted in a systematic review of the reported studies (Lie et al 2005). Sons of infertile males with Y chromosome microdeletions and born following ICSI treatment may inherit the same abnormality and are likely to be infertile.

The increased risk of congenital malformations in ART children may largely be due to the underlying parental background, rather than the treatment techniques themselves. In a recent comparative study of malformation in children born to fertile (time to pregnancy interval of ≤12 months) and subfertile parents (time to pregnancy interval of >12 months), the overall prevalence increased with increasing time to pregnancy. Compared with children in the fertile group, singletons born to infertile couples had a higher rate of congenital malformations regardless of whether they were conceived naturally (OR 1.20, 95% CI 1.07–1.35) or after infertility treatment (OR 1.39, 95% CI 1.23–1.57) (Zhu et al 2006).

There have been concerns regarding increased risk of rare imprinting disorders such as Beckwith–Wiedemann's syndrome and Angelman's syndrome in children following ART. However, the data are inconsistent, with some studies reporting increased frequency in ART children (Sutcliffe et al

2006) and other studies not finding any association (Bowdin et al 2007). Due to the rarity of these conditions, much larger studies are required for reliable detection of such associations.

Risk of malignancy in children

The issue of childhood cancer among children born after ART has been addressed in a few studies. An increased prevalence of retinoblastoma and Langerhan's histiocytosis among children born after ART in comparison with the general population has been reported in two separate studies (Moll et al 2003, Kallen et al 2005). However, the overall risk of cancer and the individual incidence of all other recorded cancers were no greater than that in the general population (Kallen et al 2005). As childhood cancers are rare, larger studies are required for reliable evaluation of any increase in risk amongst ART children.

In the context of pregnancy outcomes, the aim of ART should be a healthy singleton delivery at term. However, infertile couples may not share this target. They do not appreciate the risks associated with multiple pregnancy; indeed, between 67% and 90% of couples may desire a twin birth, while less than one-third of couples regard a single child as an ideal outcome. Increasing age or duration of infertility has been associated with greater desire for multiple births (Murdoch 1997). As discussed earlier in this chapter, an increased multiple pregnancy rate is a major reason for the increased adverse obstetric and perinatal outcomes associated with ART.

Obstetric and Perinatal Outcomes of Assisted Reproduction Treatment

Antenatal and intrapartum complications following assisted reproduction

Many studies have examined obstetric outcomes after fertility treatment. The risk of spontaneous miscarriage appears to be higher among ART pregnancies than among the general population. This comparison can be misleading as ART pregnancies are commonly under intense surveillance; losses from a very early stage of pregnancy are often carefully documented and reported, whereas miscarriage rates among natural conceptions are extremely difficult to measure and can be easily underestimated. However, a large prospective study with a meticulously chosen control group concluded that the risk of spontaneous abortion may be increased by 20–34% in ART pregnancies compared with natural pregnancies after adjusting for differences in maternal age and previous spontaneous abortion (Wang et al 2004). However, this increased risk may be as a result of infertility itself rather than due to ART, as there was no difference in miscarriage rates between patients who achieved pregnancy following any fertility treatment, including ART, and those who conceived naturally while waiting for fertility treatment (Pezeshki et al 2000).

Comparison of obstetric outcomes of IVF/ICSI pregnancies with matched normally conceived pregnancies showed a significantly increased incidence of premature delivery, intrauterine growth restriction, vaginal bleeding and hyper-

tension requiring hospitalization, pre-eclampsia and caesarean births (Halliday 2007). The increased obstetric risk can be attributed to the high rate of multiple pregnancies in most cases. However, the risk of a more complicated pregnancy was found to be increased even when the ART twin and singleton pregnancies were compared with spontaneously conceived twins and singletons, respectively, in two separate meta-analyses, even after the subjects were matched for maternal age (McDonald et al 2005a,b). A similar conclusion was drawn in another systematic review with similar objectives (Helmerhorst et al 2004).

Pregnancy following ICSI treatment has generated interest due to the additional risks involved with these pregnancies, such as the microinjection technique and the use of testicular or epidydimal sperm. However, no significant difference in obstetric outcomes between IVF and ICSI pregnancies was noted, except for prematurity which was higher in IVF singletons (Ombelet et al 2005). Couples undergoing ICSI for severe male infertility (oligoasthenoteratozoospermia) have slightly reduced fertilization rates, but have similar rates of pregnancy loss and other obstetric outcomes as other couples undergoing ICSI and IVF for non-male-factor infertility (Mercan et al 1998).

Women who conceive following oocyte donation, especially those with a history of ovarian failure, should be considered as high risk. While the majority of oocyte recipients experience a favourable outcome, an increased rate of obstetric complications in these pregnancies has been reported by many investigators (Soderstrom-Anttila 2001). Pregnancy-induced hypertension appears to occur more often than expected, even among young recipients (Wiggins and Main 2005), and the caesarean section rate is high.

Embryo cryopreservation and obstetric outcome

Cryopreservation of embryos has no apparent negative effect on obstetric outcomes. The results were comparable in pregnancies following transfer of frozen embryos derived from IVF or ICSI. However, the frozen ICSI group showed a significantly higher miscarriage rate than the frozen conventional IVF patients in one study (Aytoz et al 1999).

Perinatal outcome of assisted reproduction pregnancies

It is widely accepted that the increased incidence of multiple pregnancies following ART accounts for a disproportionately large share of adverse perinatal outcomes, including the increased incidence of very low birth weight, low birth weight, perinatal and neonatal mortality, and infant death. The increased incidence of death and morbidity in twin pregnancies compared with singleton pregnancies has been attributed mainly to prematurity and to adverse outcomes associated with premature delivery, such as hyaline membrane disease, hypocalcaemia, hypoglycaemia, hyperbilirubinaemia, small for gestational age and low Apgar scores. Slotnick and Ortega (1996) suggested that monoamniotic multiple gestations may be increased in zona-manipulated cycles (ICSI, zona drilling, assisted hatching), and although all resulting monoamniotic pregnancies ended in live births, there was a high incidence of intrauterine discordance in fetal growth. Even when compared with matched control spontaneous twin pregnancies, ART twin pregnancies had low birth weights and needed more neonatal intensive care (Helmerhorst et al 2004). However, twins conceived with IVF/ICSI have comparable perinatal mortality and morbidity rates to spontaneously conceived controls (McDonald et al 2005a).

Elimination of multiple pregnancies will not eliminate the increased risk of adverse perinatal outcomes in ART. While twins born from assisted conception are not significantly disadvantaged compared with spontaneous twin pregnancies, ART singletons have a worse perinatal outcome compared with other singletons (Helmerhorst et al 2004). Singletons born from ART are at risk for lower mean birth weight and small for gestational age. Perinatal mortality appears to be significantly higher, even after matching for maternal age, parity and infant gender. ICSI treatment does not appear to differ from conventional IVF when perinatal outcomes are compared. Retrospective comparison of births resulting from cryopreserved embryos with those after conventional IVF and fresh ET showed no difference in perinatal mortality between the two groups (Wada et al 1994).

Preimplantation Genetic Diagnosis/Screening

Preimplantation genetic diagnosis (PGD) has been developed as an alternative to prenatal diagnosis of chromosomal or sex-linked disorders in embryos formed through ART procedures. Preimplantation genetic screening (PGS) refers to the application of PGD in infertile couples undergoing conventional ART as an alternative to the traditional selection of embryos based on morphological criteria, which do not detect aneuploidy embryos that are non-viable or which could give rise to a viable but disabled child (Anderson and Pickering 2008). Aneuploid embryos most commonly result from fertilization of oocytes that are affected with meiotic non-disjunction, a common reason for age-related decline in oocyte quality. By detecting and avoiding the transfer of aneuploid embryos and only selecting euploid embryos for transfer, the success of ART cycles could potentially be improved. The application of PGD has also been extended to preimplantation human leukocyte antigen (HLA) matching to ensure the birth of HLA-identical offspring for stem cell transplantation therapy to siblings.

The procedure involves biopsy of a single cell from the human cleavage-stage embryo at around the eight-cell stage or from the blastocyst, followed by the application of a sensitive diagnostic technique to that cell. At present, biopsied polar bodies and/or blastomeres and/or trophoblast cells biopsied from blastocysts have been used, and pregnancies as well as healthy babies have resulted from biopsied and diagnosed embryos. The diagnostic technique, specific for the disorder being tested, may be the analysis of enzymes, chromosomes or a specific mutation in the DNA. If the cell shows no abnormality in the course of this analysis, the embryo is judged to be normal and is transferred to the mother to initiate pregnancy.

The enzyme approach has been disregarded, for the few genes studied, as it has been difficult to differentiate between maternal gene expression (mRNA inherited in the egg cytoplasm) and embryonic gene expression in the early embryo (Braude et al 1989). However, the analysis of chromosomes using fluorescent in-situ hybridization and the analysis of specific gene sequences using sensitive polymerase chain reaction for sexing or detection of a specific gene mutation, such as cystic fibrosis, have been used successfully.

Analysis of the first and second polar bodies is an alternative to embryonic biopsy. As the polar bodies contain the genetic information from the oocyte, it is possible to diagnose maternally derived mutations, translocations and aneuploidy. Paternally derived chromosomal abnormalities will be missed by polar body biopsies. In cases of recessive disorders, polar body biopsies are helpful as they can provide information about the maternal contribution to the embryo. It may be difficult to achieve a reliable diagnosis even with embryo biopsy, with which mosaicism and/or uniparental disomies deriving from trisomies originating from female meiotic errors will be missed. With the expanding range of PGD indications, combined testing is required when testing for the causative gene, linked markers, HLA typing and aneuploidy in the same case. Therefore, single, double or even triple biopsies may be required in order to establish an accurate PGD (Kuliev and Verlinsky 2008). Sequential or simultaneous additional biopsy procedures have been shown to have no detrimental effect on embryo development (Cieslak-Janzen et al 2006).

PGS has been proposed to improve the IVF outcome in women of advanced age, and in those with a history of recurrent miscarriage, repeated implantation failure or severe male infertility, who are at risk for having increased proportions of aneuploid embryos. Most commonly, nine chromosomes (13, 14, 15, 16, 18, 21, 22, X and Y) are screened for aneuploidy. Although PGS has no adverse effect on embryo development, the current available evidence does not support its use outside the context of research. A meta-analysis of five prospective randomized-controlled trials evaluating the effect of PGS for the indication of advanced women's age has reported a significant reduction in ongoing pregnancy rates (OR 0.56, 95% CI 0.42–0.76) compared with controls (Mastenbroek et al 2008). While the studies evaluating the use of PGS for other indications mentioned above are limited, the early evidence suggests that PGS does not improve the outcome, even in patients with a good prognosis (young age) who are undergoing single ET (Staessen et al 2008). In conclusion, the available evidence does not support the use of PGS to improve livebirth rates or reduce miscarriage rates in ART cycles, particularly for women of advanced age.

Looking into the Future

ART has improved substantially over the last three decades, and many subfertile couples are now able to have children through its application. However, clinicians and researchers continue to strive to achieve the desired outcome, i.e. a single healthy baby, with minimal side-effects and this poses new challenges. It is tempting to speculate on the areas that are most likely to witness such developments over the next few years.

Recombinant gonadotrophin preparations are now well established in superovulation protocols. While these compounds are well tolerated and as effective as the urinary products, the associated risks of OHSS and multiple pregnancies and the need for daily parenteral administration of medications do not constitute the features of a patient-friendly procedure. Active investigations are ongoing to develop a number of molecules with gonadotrophin-like activity. Longer-acting forms and orally bioactive preparations may revolutionize IVF treatment in the near future. Additionally, the use of mild ovarian stimulation protocols with a single ET policy may become the norm, leading to IVF treatment that is less drug-orientated.

Improving pregnancy and livebirth rates will remain a challenge for the future. Molecular cytogenetic procedures on polar bodies or blastomeres have indicated that more than 50% of embryos derived after ART are aneuploid. Elective transfer of euploid or top-quality embryo(s) increases the chance of a successful outcome. Currently, the embryos are scored based on morphology, but this is notoriously difficult and often subjective. Available evidence does not support the use of more invasive PGS techniques to improve livebirth rates following ART, and therefore more accurate assessment methods are needed. A number of non-invasive tests, such as embryo viability, assessment of metabolomic profile and amino acid turnover in the embryo culture media, are being evaluated in many studies and have the potential to predict which embryos have the highest implantation potential (Nagy et al 2008, Sturmey et al 2008).

The unravelling of the human genome and the increase in our knowledge of the genetic basis for many more diseases than ever imagined previously will lead to a greater understanding of the factors involved in male infertility and how to increase fecundity. This, coupled with advances in PGD, will enable accurate screening of parents for specific genes before treatment, biopsied embryos before replacement and the resulting child afterwards. Additionally, these advances will permit rapid progress in gene therapy for single or multiple gene disorders where a normal cloned gene(s) is used to replace the faulty genome.

Another challenging area for research is that of preserving fertility in children or young adults treated for cancer. As survival rates continue to improve, more young people want to know if they will be fertile, if their children will have a greater risk of developing cancer, and what alternatives exist should pelvic irradiation or chemotherapy have a permanent adverse effect on their fertility. Sperm banking is a well-recognized preservation technique for pubertal males and adults. In women, several approaches are being explored but none have been clinically established to date.

Oocyte cryopreservation is possible and requires superovulation treatment to induce multifollicular development followed by oocyte retrieval (Albani et al 2008). Oocyte cryopreservation is considered to be extremely inefficient, with approximately 100 cryopreserved oocytes needed to achieve one pregnancy. The mature oocyte is extremely fragile due to intracellular ice formation during the freezing or thawing process. There is potentially an increased risk of damage to the meiotic spindle apparatus and hardening of the zona pellucida, leading to reduced post-thaw survival, fertilization and pregnancy rates. Improvements in both advanced vitrification and slow-freezing methods have recently resulted in an increase in the efficiency of using human cryopreserved oocytes in assisted reproduction. Although the technique is currently considered experimental, this is likely to become the fastest growing area of fertility therapy in the future. It is reassuring that no increased chromosomal abnormalities, birth defects or developmental delays have been reported in children born from cryopreserved oocytes based on the limited number of pregnancies and deliveries reported to date.

Ovarian cryopreservation has been regarded as a potential method of fertility preservation for more than a decade (Anderson et al 2008). This method has the potential advantages of preservation of a large number of oocytes within primordial follicles, it does not require hormonal stimulation when time is short, and it may be appropriate for the prepubertal. Ovarian tissues can subsequently be autotransplanted, either at orthotopic (at or around the ovarian fossa) or heterotopic locations (subcutaneously at various locations including the forearm and abdominal wall), after the patient has completed treatment. Although few livebirths following either spontaneous or IVF conceptions have been reported, more research is needed in order to enhance the revascularization process, with the goal of reducing the follicular loss that takes place after tissue grafting. These technologies are still experimental, although tremendous progress has been made recently. There are many ethical concerns with these interventions, particularly their experimental nature in emotionally vulnerable patients, who often present to ART units with unrealistic expectations, the possibility of harvesting malignant cells with germ cells, and the potential for continued transmission of germ-line mutations in cancer predisposition genes. All of these highlight the need for further research and well-designed controlled clinical trials.

The technique of in-vitro maturation (IVM) of oocytes has been practised in a few IVF units worldwide (Suikkari 2008). The primary aim of IVM is to make IVF safer and simpler for women with polycystic ovaries and those at high risk of OHSS. Immature oocytes are recovered by puncture during non-stimulated cycles or after a low-dose stimulation protocol in a woman with polycystic ovaries. Priming the follicle with FSH for 2–3 days to stimulate growth to 8–12 mm diameter has been associated with improvements in implantation rates. Additional treatment with 10,000 IU hCG 36 h before oocyte retrieval has also been shown to improve the maturation rate of immature oocytes and accelerate the maturation process. Immature oocytes collected are allowed to mature in culture for approximately 30 h before insemination or ICSI. The clinical outcome has improved substantially in recent years, with pregnancy rates of over 20% in some centres. It is estimated that over 1000 children have been born following IVM worldwide. Postnatal follow-up studies of the children have been reassuring. IVM has not yet become a mainstream fertility treatment, mainly due to its lower success rate compared with conventional IVF. Knowledge regarding the molecular mechanisms of oocyte maturation and improvement in the culture system will improve the efficacy of IVM. While there is definite benefit for the use of IVM in women with polycystic ovaries and those at risk of OHSS, its role in couples with unexplained infertility or poor ovarian reserve remains to be defined.

KEY POINTS

1. IVF/ICSI is indicated not only in cases of tubal blockage, but also for various other causes of infertility. However, it should not be used as a panacea for marital or psychosexual disorders, but to fulfil the wishes of a well-adjusted couple to have a baby.

2. Pretreatment evaluation of the couple is essential as it allows the treatment to be tailored to maximize the chances of a successful outcome following ART.

3. The aims of superovulation regimens in assisted reproduction are to maximize the number of follicles, to minimize the degree of asynchrony amongst developing follicles, and to minimize the deleterious effects of the abnormal follicular environment on luteal function and endometrial receptivity.

4. The use of GnRH agonists in stimulation protocols has increased steadily since their introduction into clinical practice, and appears to result in a reduction in cancellation rates, an increase in the number of oocytes retrieved and a significantly higher clinical pregnancy rate.

5. Whilst ovarian stimulation protocols utilizing high doses of gonadotrophins are used conventionally, a milder stimulation approach has gained a lot of interest in the IVF field recently, with the aim of minimizing the adverse effects of ovarian stimulation, particularly OHSS and multiple pregnancies.

6. Transabdominal ultrasonographic guidance to determine the precise depth of embryo placement within the uterus appears to facilitate successful ET and is therefore preferred.

7. Crude pregnancy rates per couple are almost meaningless; cumulative conception or livebirth rates should be used in reporting conventional and ART outcomes.

8. The outcome of ART depends on the age of the female partner, the duration of infertility, the multiplicity of factors responsible for the couple's subfertility, the number of embryos transferred and the number of treatment cycles that a couple undergo.

9. When four or more embryos are available for transfer, the transfer of two embryos results in equally high pregnancy and livebirth rates. However, the rate of multiple pregnancy with all its pregnancy and perinatal complications is reduced dramatically.

10. In carefully selected patients (e.g. women <37 years of age, undergoing their first IVF cycle and who have more than one top-quality embryo), eSET plus subsequent FER is as effective as double ET in terms of pregnancy rates, and significantly reduces the rate of twin pregnancies.

11. In view of the potential health risks arising from ART, it is imperative that clinicians should define the risks as those associated with the medication itself, as well as the short- and long-term physical, emotional and pregnancy-related effects.

12. The effect of ovulation induction agents currently used in ART on the risk of genital cancer risk is unclear. Considering that the treatment protocols, preparations and dosages used during IVF are relatively new, and women exposed to IVF are only beginning to reach the cancer age range, further follow-up studies are required in this area before drawing any conclusions.

13. A 30–40% increase in birth defects is reported in IVF/ICSI pregnancies compared with background risk. The increased risk of congenital malformations in ART children may largely be due to the underlying parental background, rather than the treatment techniques themselves.

14. PGD is now an established technique for the diagnosis of chromosomal or sex-linked disorders in embryos formed through ART procedures. Current evidence does not support the use of PGS to improve livebirth rates or reduce miscarriage rates in ART cycles, particularly for women of advanced age.

15. Ovarian tissue cryopreservation and oocyte cryopreservation are still considered as experimental procedures, but hold promise for future female fertility preservation.

16. IVM is a safer and simpler alternative to IVF in women with polycystic ovaries and those at high risk of OHSS.

References

Abdalla H, Thum MY 2006 Repeated testing of basal FSH levels has no predictive value for IVF outcome in women with elevated basal FSH. Human Reproduction 21: 171–174.

Aboulghar MA, Mansour RT, Serour GI, Riad R, Ramzi AM 1992 Autotransfusion of the ascitic fluid in the treatment of severe ovarian hyperstimulation syndrome. Fertility and Sterility 58: 1056–1059.

Academy of Medical Royal Colleges 2001 Implementing and Ensuring Safe Sedation Practice for Healthcare Procedures in Adults. Report of an Intercollegiate Working Party Chaired by the Royal College of Anaesthetists. London: AOMRC, London.

Agrawal R, Conway G, Sladkevicius P et al 1998 Serum vascular endothelial growth factor and Doppler blood flow velocities in in vitro fertilization: relevance to ovarian hyperstimulation syndrome and polycystic ovaries. Fertility and Sterility 70: 651–658.

Al-Inany HG, Abou-Setta AM, Aboulghar M 2007 Gonadotrophin-releasing hormone antagonists for assisted conception: a Cochrane review. Reproductive Biomedicine Online 14: 640–649.

Al-Inany HG, Abou-Setta AM, Aboulghar MA, Mansour RT, Serour GI 2008 Efficacy and safety of human menopausal gonadotrophins versus recombinant FSH: a meta-analysis. Reproductive Biomedicine Online 16: 81–88.

Albani E, Barbieri J, Novara PV, Smeraldi A, Scaravelli G, Levi Setti PE 2008 Oocyte cryopreservation. Placenta 29 (Suppl B): 143–146.

Alrayyes S, Fakih H, Khan I 1997 Effect of age and cycle responsiveness in patients undergoing intracytoplasmic sperm injection. Fertility and Sterility 68: 123–127.

Anderson RA, Pickering S 2008 The current status of preimplantation genetic screening: British Fertility Society policy and practice guidelines. Human Fertility (Cambridge, England) 11: 71–75.

Anderson RA, Wallace WH, Baird DT 2008 Ovarian cryopreservation for fertility preservation: indications and outcomes. Reproduction 136: 681–689.

Aytoz A, Van den Abbeel E, Bonduelle M et al 1999 Obstetric outcome of pregnancies after the transfer of cryopreserved and fresh embryos obtained by conventional in-vitro fertilization and intracytoplasmic sperm injection. Human Reproduction 14: 2619–2624.

Balen AH, Laven JS, Tan SL, Dewailly D 2003 Ultrasound assessment of the polycystic ovary: international consensus definitions. Human Reproduction Update 9: 505–514.

Bancsi LF, Broekmans FJ, Mol BW, Habbema JD, te Velde ER 2003 Performance of basal follicle-stimulating hormone in the prediction of poor ovarian response and failure to become pregnant after in vitro fertilization: a meta-analysis. Fertility and Sterility 79: 1091–1100.

Bartkowiak R, Kaminski P, Wielgos M, Bobrowska K 2006 The evaluation of uterine cavity with saline infusion sonohysterography and hysteroscopy in infertile patients. Neuroendocrinology Letters 27: 523–528.

Bennett SJ, Waterstone JJ, Cheng WC, Parsons J 1993 Complications of transvaginal ultrasound-directed follicle aspiration: a review of 2670 consecutive procedures. Journal of Assisted Reproduction and Genetics 10: 72–77.

Bhattacharya S, Hamilton MP, Shaaban M et al 2001 Conventional in-vitro fertilisation versus intracytoplasmic sperm injection for the treatment of non-male-factor infertility: a randomised controlled trial. The Lancet 357: 2075–2079.

Blake DA, Farquhar CM, Johnson N, Proctor M 2007 Cleavage stage versus blastocyst stage embryo transfer in assisted conception. Cochrane Database of Systematic Reviews: CD002118.

Bowdin S, Allen C, Kirby G et al 2007 A survey of assisted reproductive technology births and imprinting disorders. Human Reproduction 22: 3237–3240.

Braude PR, Monk M, Pickering SJ, Cant A, Johnson MH 1989 Measurement of HPRT activity in the human unfertilised oocyte and pre-embryo. Prenatal Diagnosis 9: 839–850.

Brinton L 2007 Long-term effects of ovulation-stimulating drugs on cancer risk. Reproductive Biomedicine Online 15: 38–44.

Brinton LA, Lamb EJ, Moghissi KS, Scoccia B, Althuis MD, Mabie JE and Westhoff CL 2004 Ovarian cancer risk after the use of ovulation-stimulating drugs. Obstetrics and Gynecology 103: 1194–1203.

Broekmans FJ, Kwee J, Hendriks DJ, Mol BW, Lambalk CB 2006 A systematic review of tests predicting ovarian reserve and IVF outcome. Human Reproduction Update 12: 685–718.

Broekmans FJ, Knauff EA, te Velde ER, Macklon NS, Fauser BC 2007 Female reproductive ageing: current knowledge and future trends. Trends in Endocrinology and Metabolism 18: 58–65.

Broekmans FJ, Visser JA, Laven JS, Broer SL, Themmen AP, Fauser BC 2008 Anti-Müllerian hormone and ovarian dysfunction. Trends in Endocrinology and Metabolism 19: 340–347.

Brown JA, Buckingham K, Abou-Setta A, Buckett W 2007 Ultrasound versus 'clinical touch' for catheter guidance during embryo transfer in women. Cochrane Database of Systematic Reviews: CD006107.

Burton G, Abdalla HI, Kirkland A, Studd JW 1992 The role of oocyte donation in women who are unsuccessful with in-vitro fertilization treatment. Human Reproduction 7: 1103–1105.

Cieslak-Janzen J, Tur-Kaspa I, Ilkevitch Y, Bernal A, Morris R, Verlinsky Y 2006 Multiple micromanipulations for preimplantation genetic diagnosis do not affect embryo development to the blastocyst stage. Fertility and Sterility 85: 1826–1829.

Clayton HB, Schieve LA, Peterson HB, Jamieson DJ, Reynolds MA, Wright VC 2006 Ectopic pregnancy risk with assisted reproductive technology procedures. Obstetrics and Gynecology 107: 595–604.

Cohen J, Alikani M, Malter HE, Adler A, Talansky BE, Rosenwaks Z 1991 Partial zona dissection or subzonal sperm insertion: microsurgical fertilization alternatives based on evaluation of sperm and embryo morphology. Fertility and Sterility 56: 696–706.

Coomarasamy A, Afnan M, Cheema D, van der Veen F, Bossuyt PM, van Wely M 2008 Urinary hMG versus recombinant FSH for

controlled ovarian hyperstimulation following an agonist long down-regulation protocol in IVF or ICSI treatment: a systematic review and meta-analysis. Human Reproduction 23: 310–315.

Croucher CA, Lass A, Margara R, Winston RM 1998 Predictive value of the results of a first in-vitro fertilization cycle on the outcome of subsequent cycles. Human Reproduction 13: 403–408.

Cutting R, Morroll D, Roberts SA, Pickering S, Rutherford A 2008 Elective single embryo transfer: guidelines for practice. British Fertility Society and Association of Clinical Embryologists. Human Fertility (Cambridge, England): 1–16.

Daya S 2000 Gonadotropin releasing hormone agonist protocols for pituitary desensitization in in vitro fertilization and gamete intrafallopian transfer cycles. Cochrane Database of Systematic Reviews: CD001299.

de Vet A, Laven JS, de Jong FH, Themmen AP, Fauser BC 2002 Antimüllerian hormone serum levels: a putative marker for ovarian aging. Fertility and Sterility 77: 357–362.

Dechaud H, Anahory T, Reyftmann L, Loup V, Hamamah S, Hedon B 2006 Obesity does not adversely affect results in patients who are undergoing in vitro fertilization and embryo transfer. European Journal of Obstetrics, Gynecology and Reproductive Biology 127: 88–93.

Dor J, Seidman DS, Ben-Shlomo I, Levran D, Ben-Rafael Z, Mashiach S 1996 Cumulative pregnancy rate following in-vitro fertilization: the significance of age and infertility aetiology. Human Reproduction 11: 425–428.

Drakeley AJ, Jorgensen A, Sklavounos J et al 2008 A randomized controlled clinical trial of 2295 ultrasound-guided embryo transfers. Human Reproduction 23: 1101–1106.

ESHRE Capri Workshop Group 2000 Optimal use of infertility diagnostic tests and treatments. Human Reproduction 15: 723–732.

Evers JL, Slaats P, Land JA, Dumoulin JC, Dunselman GA 1998 Elevated levels of basal estradiol-17beta predict poor response in patients with normal basal levels of follicle-stimulating hormone undergoing in vitro fertilization. Fertility and Sterility 69: 1010–1014.

Fanchin R, Taieb J, Lozano DH, Ducot B, Frydman R, Bouyer J 2005 High reproducibility of serum anti-Müllerian hormone measurements suggests a multi-staged follicular secretion and strengthens its role in the assessment of ovarian follicular status. Human Reproduction 20: 923–927.

Fedorcsak P, Dale PO, Storeng R et al 2004 Impact of overweight and underweight on assisted reproduction treatment. Human Reproduction 19: 2523–2528.

Fishel S, Lisi F, Rinaldi L et al 1995 Systematic examination of immobilizing spermatozoa before intracytoplasmic sperm injection in

the human. Human Reproduction 10: 497–500.

FIVNAT 1996 Evaluation of frozen embryo transfers from 1987 to 1994. Contraception Fertilite Sexualite 24: 700–705.

Frattarelli JL, Bergh PA, Drews MR, Sharara FI, Scott RT 2000 Evaluation of basal estradiol levels in assisted reproductive technology cycles. Fertility and Sterility 74: 518–524.

Friedler S, Schenker JG, Herman A, Lewin A 1996 The role of ultrasonography in the evaluation of endometrial receptivity following assisted reproductive treatments: a critical review. Human Reproduction Update 2: 323–335.

Gauthier E, Paoletti X, Clavel-Chapelon F 2004 Breast cancer risk associated with being treated for infertility: results from the French E3N cohort study. Human Reproduction 19: 2216–2221.

Geber S, Paraschos T, Atkinson G, Margara R, Winston RM 1995 Results of IVF in patients with endometriosis: the severity of the disease does not affect outcome, or the incidence of miscarriage. Human Reproduction 10: 1507–1511.

Gupta S, Agarwal A, Agarwal R, Loret de Mola JR 2006 Impact of ovarian endometrioma on assisted reproduction outcomes. Reproductive Biomedicine Online 13: 349–360.

Hall JE, Welt CK, Cramer DW 1999 Inhibin A and inhibin B reflect ovarian function in assisted reproduction but are less useful at predicting outcome. Human Reproduction 14: 409–415.

Halliday J 2007 Outcomes of IVF conceptions: are they different? Best Practice and Research Clinical Obstetrics and Gynaecology 21: 67–81.

Hansen M, Bower C, Milne E, de Klerk N, Kurinczuk JJ 2005 Assisted reproductive technologies and the risk of birth defects — a systematic review. Human Reproduction 20: 328–338.

Helmerhorst FM, Perquin DA, Donker D, Keirse MJ 2004 Perinatal outcome of singletons and twins after assisted conception: a systematic review of controlled studies. BMJ (Clinical Research Ed.) 328: 261.

Horne G, Critchlow JD, Newman MC, Edozien L, Matson PL, Lieberman BA 1997 A prospective evaluation of cryopreservation strategies in a two-embryo transfer programme. Human Reproduction 12: 542–547.

Hughes EG, Fedorkow DM, Daya S, Sagle MA, Van de Koppel P, Collins JA 1992 The routine use of gonadotropin-releasing hormone agonists prior to in vitro fertilization and gamete intrafallopian transfer: a meta-analysis of randomized controlled trials. Fertility and Sterility 58: 888–896.

Hull MG 1992 Infertility treatment: relative effectiveness of conventional and assisted conception methods. Human Reproduction 7: 785–796.

Human Fertilisation and Embryology Authority 2000 Ninth annual report and accounts (http://www.hfea.gov.uk/docs/Annual-Report-9th-2000.pdf).

Human Fertilisation and Embryology Authority 2008 Facts and figures 2006 (http://www.hfea.gov.uk/docs/Facts_and_Figures_2006_fertility_probs_and_treatment_2008-10-08.pdf).

Isikoglu M, Berkkanoglu M, Senturk Z, Coetzee K, Ozgur K 2006 Endometrial polyps smaller than 1.5 cm do not affect ICSI outcome. Reproductive Biomedicine Online 12: 199–204.

Jayaprakasan K, Campbell BK, Clewes JS, Johnson IR, Raine-Fenning NJ 2008a Three-dimensional ultrasound improves the interobserver reliability of antral follicle counts and facilitates increased clinical work flow. Ultrasound in Obstetrics and Gynecology 31: 439–444.

Jayaprakasan K, Hopkisson JF, Campbell BK, Clewes J, Johnson IR, Raine-Fenning NJ 2008b Quantification of the effect of pituitary down-regulation on 3D ultrasound predictors of ovarian response. Human Reproduction 23: 1538–1544.

Jayaprakasan K, Al-Hasie H, Jayaprakasan R et al 2009 The three-dimensional ultrasonographic ovarian vascularity of women developing poor ovarian response during assisted reproduction treatment and its predictive value. Fertility and Sterility 92: 1862-1869.

Jayaprakasan K, Campbell B, Hopkisson J, Johnson I, Raine-Fenning N 2010 A prospective, comparative analysis of anti-Müllerian hormone, inhibin-B, and three-dimensional ultrasound determinants of ovarian reserve in the prediction of poor response to controlled ovarian stimulation. Fertility and Sterility 93: 855-864.

Kahn JA, von During V, Sunde A, Sordal T, Molne K 1993 The efficacy and efficiency of an in-vitro fertilization programme including embryo cryopreservation: a cohort study. Human Reproduction 8: 247–252.

Kallen B, Finnstrom O, Nygren KG, Olausson PO 2005 In vitro fertilization in Sweden: child morbidity including cancer risk. Fertility and Sterility 84: 605–610.

Khastgir G, Abdalla H, Thomas A, Korea L, Latarche L, Studd J 1997 Oocyte donation in Turner's syndrome: an analysis of the factors affecting the outcome. Human Reproduction 12: 279–285.

Klip H, van Leeuwen FE, Schats R, Burger CW 2003 Risk of benign gynaecological diseases and hormonal disorders according to responsiveness to ovarian stimulation in IVF: a follow-up study of 8714 women. Human Reproduction 18: 1951–1958.

Kolibianakis EM, Kalogeropoulou L, Griesinger G et al 2007 Among patients treated with FSH and GnRH analogues for in vitro fertilization, is the addition of recombinant LH associated with the probability of live birth? A systematic review and meta-analysis. Human Reproduction Update 13: 445–452.

Kuliev A, Verlinsky Y 2008 Preimplantation genetic diagnosis: technological advances to improve accuracy and range of applications. Reproductive Biomedicine Online 16: 532–538.

Kwee JJ, Elting MM, Schats RR, McDonnell JJ, Lambalk NC 2007 Ovarian volume and antral follicle count for the prediction of low and hyper responders with in vitro fertilization. Reproductive Biology and Endocrinology 5: 9.

La Marca A, Stabile G, Artensio AC, Volpe A 2006 Serum anti-Müllerian hormone throughout the human menstrual cycle. Human Reproduction 21: 3103–3107.

Lie RT, Lyngstadaas A, Orstavik KH, Bakketeig LS, Jacobsen G, Tanbo T 2005 Birth defects in children conceived by ICSI compared with children conceived by other IVF-methods; a meta-analysis. International Journal of Epidemiology 34: 696–701.

Lin PC 2004 Reproductive outcomes in women with uterine anomalies. Journal of Womens Health 13: 33–39.

Maheshwari A, Stofberg L, Bhattacharya S 2007 Effect of overweight and obesity on assisted reproductive technology — a systematic review. Human Reproduction Update 13: 433–444.

Mannaerts B, de Leeuw R, Geelen J et al 1991 Comparative in vitro and in vivo studies on the biological characteristics of recombinant human follicle stimulating hormone. Endocrinology 129: 2623–2630.

Mardesic T, Muller P, Zetova L, Mikova M 1994 [Factors affecting the results of in vitro fertilization — I. The effect of age]. Ceska Gynekologie 59: 259–261.

Mastenbroek S, Scriven P, Twisk M, Viville S, Van der Veen F, Repping S 2008 What next for preimplantation genetic screening? More randomized controlled trials needed? Human Reproduction 23: 2626–2628.

Mathur R, Kailasam C, Jenkins J 2007 Review of the evidence base of strategies to prevent ovarian hyperstimulation syndrome. Human Fertility (Cambridge, England) 10: 75–85.

Matson PL, Yovich JL 1986 The treatment of infertility associated with endometriosis by in vitro fertilization. Fertility and Sterility 46: 432–434.

McDonald S, Murphy K, Beyene J, Ohlsson A 2005a Perinatal outcomes of in vitro fertilization twins: a systematic review and meta-analyses. American Journal of Obstetrics and Gynecology 193: 141–152.

McDonald SD, Murphy K, Beyene J, Ohlsson A 2005b Perinatal outcomes of singleton pregnancies achieved by in vitro fertilization: a systematic review and meta-analysis. Journal of Obstetrics and Gynaecology Canada 27: 449–459.

McIlveen M, Skull JD, Ledger WL 2007 Evaluation of the utility of multiple endocrine and ultrasound measures of ovarian reserve in the prediction of cycle cancellation in a high-risk IVF population. Human Reproduction 22: 778–785.

Mercan R, Lanzendorf SE, Mayer J Jr, Nassar A, Muasher SJ, Oehninger S 1998 The outcome of clinical pregnancies following intracytoplasmic sperm injection is not affected by semen quality. Andrologia 30: 91–95.

Mochtar MH, Van der V, Ziech M, van Wely M 2007 Recombinant luteinizing hormone (rLH) for controlled ovarian hyperstimulation in assisted reproductive cycles. Cochrane Database of Systematic Reviews: CD005070.

Modan B, Ron E, Lerner-Geva L et al 1998 Cancer incidence in a cohort of infertile women. American Journal of Epidemiology 147: 1038–1042.

Moll AC, Imhof SM, Cruysberg JR, Schouten-van Meeteren AY, Boers M, van Leeuwen FE 2003 Incidence of retinoblastoma in children born after in-vitro fertilisation. The Lancet 361: 309–310.

Moore J, Copley S, Morris J, Lindsell D, Golding S, Kennedy S 2002 A systematic review of the accuracy of ultrasound in the diagnosis of endometriosis. Ultrasound in Obstetrics and Gynecology 20: 630–634.

Murdoch A 1997 Triplets and embryo transfer policy. Human Reproduction 12: 88–92.

Nagy ZP, Sakkas D, Behr B 2008 Symposium: innovative techniques in human embryo viability assessment. Non-invasive assessment of embryo viability by metabolomic profiling of culture media ('metabolomics'). Reproductive Biomedicine Online 17: 502–507.

National Institute for Clinical Excellence 2004 Fertility: Assessment and Treatment for People with Fertility Problems. National Collaborating Centre for Women's and Children's Health for the National Institute for Clinical Excellence, RCOG Press, London, p 33.

Oatway C, Gunby J, Daya S 2004 Day three versus day two embryo transfer following in vitro fertilization or intracytoplasmic sperm injection. Cochrane Database of Systematic Reviews: CD004378.

Oliveira FG, Abdelmassih VG, Diamond MP, Dozortsev D, Melo NR, Abdelmassih R 2004 Impact of subserosal and intramural uterine fibroids that do not distort the endometrial cavity on the outcome of in vitro fertilization–intracytoplasmic sperm injection. Fertility and Sterility 81: 582–587.

Ombelet W, Cadron I, Gerris J et al 2005 Obstetric and perinatal outcome of 1655 ICSI and 3974 IVF singleton and 1102 ICSI and 2901 IVF twin births: a comparative analysis. Reproductive Biomedicine Online 11: 76–85.

Padilla SL, Garcia JE 1989 Effect of maternal age and number of in vitro fertilization procedures on pregnancy outcome. Fertility and Sterility 52: 270–273.

Palermo G, Joris H, Devroey P, Van Steirteghem AC 1992 Pregnancies after intracytoplasmic injection of single spermatozoon into an oocyte. The Lancet 340: 17–18.

Pandian Z, Templeton A, Serour G, Bhattacharya S 2005 Number of embryos for transfer after IVF and ICSI: a Cochrane review. Human Reproduction 20: 2681–2687.

Pezeshki K, Feldman J, Stein DE, Lobel SM, Grazi RV 2000 Bleeding and spontaneous abortion after therapy for infertility. Fertility and Sterility 74: 504–508.

Piette C, de Mouzon J, Bachelot A, Spira A 1990 In-vitro fertilization: influence of women's age on pregnancy rates. Human Reproduction 5: 56–59.

Preutthipan S, Amso N, Curtis P, Shaw RW 1996 The influence of number of embryos transferred on pregnancy outcome in women undergoing in vitro fertilization and embryo transfer (IVF-ET). Journal of the Medical Association of Thailand 79: 613–617.

Royal College of Obstetricians and Gynaecologists 2006 The management of ovarian hyperstimulation syndrome. Greentop Guideline 5. RCOG Press, London.

Salim R, Woelfer B, Backos M, Regan L, Jurkovic D 2003 Reproducibility of three-dimensional ultrasound diagnosis of congenital uterine anomalies. Ultrasound in Obstetrics and Gynecology 21: 578–582.

Scott RT, Toner JP, Muasher SJ, Oehninger S, Robinson S, Rosenwaks Z 1989 Follicle-stimulating hormone levels on cycle day 3 are predictive of in vitro fertilization outcome. Fertility and Sterility 51: 651–654.

Scott RT, Jr, Hofmann GE, Oehninger S, Muasher SJ 1990 Intercycle variability of day 3 follicle-stimulating hormone levels and its effect on stimulation quality in in vitro fertilization. Fertility and Sterility 54: 297–302.

Seifer DB, Lambert-Messerlian G, Hogan JW, Gardiner AC, Blazar AS, Berk CA 1997 Day 3 serum inhibin-B is predictive of assisted reproductive technologies outcome. Fertility and Sterility 67: 110–114.

Sharif K, Elgendy M, Lashen H, Afnan M 1998 Age and basal follicle stimulating hormone as predictors of in vitro fertilisation outcome. British Journal of Obstetrics and Gynaecology 105: 107–112.

Slotnick RN, Ortega JE 1996 Monoamniotic twinning and zona manipulation: a survey of U.S. IVF centers correlating zona manipulation procedures and high-risk twinning frequency. Journal of Assisted Reproduction and Genetics 13: 381–385.

Sneed ML, Uhler ML, Grotjan HE, Rapisarda JJ, Lederer KJ, Beltsos AN 2008 Body mass index: impact on IVF success appears age-related. Human Reproduction 23: 1835–1839.

Soderstrom-Anttila V 2001 Pregnancy and child outcome after oocyte donation. Human Reproduction Update 7: 28–32.

Somigliana E, Arnoldi M, Benaglia L, Iemmello R, Nicolosi AE, Ragni G 2008 IVF–ICSI outcome in women operated on for bilateral endometriomas. Human Reproduction 23: 1526–1530.

Spandorfer SD, Davis OK, Barmat LI, Chung PH, Rosenwaks Z 2004 Relationship between maternal age and aneuploidy in in vitro fertilization pregnancy loss. Fertility and Sterility 81: 1265–1269.

Speroff L, Fritz MA 2005 Assisted reproductive technologies. In: Speroff L, Fritz MA (eds) Clinical Gynecologic Endocrinology and Infertility. Lippincott Williams and Wilkins, Philadelphia, pp 1215–1274.

Staessen C, Janssenswillen C, van den Abbeel E, Devroey P, van Streitegham AC 1993 Avoidance of triplet pregnancies by elective transfer of two good quality embryos. Human Reproduction 8:1650–1653.

Staessen C, Verpoest W, Donoso P et al 2008 Preimplantation genetic screening does not improve delivery rate in women under the age of 36 following single-embryo transfer. Human Reproduction 23: 2818–2825.

Strandell A 2007 Treatment of hydrosalpinx in the patient undergoing assisted reproduction. Current Opinions in Obstetrics and Gynecology 19: 360–365.

Sturmey RG, Brison DR, Leese HJ 2008 Symposium: innovative techniques in human embryo viability assessment. Assessing embryo viability by measurement of amino acid turnover. Reproductive Biomedicine Online 17: 486–496.

Suikkari AM 2008 In-vitro maturation: its role in fertility treatment. Current Opinion in Obstetrics and Gynecology 20: 242–248.

Sutcliffe AG, Peters CJ, Bowdin S et al 2006 Assisted reproductive therapies and imprinting disorders — a preliminary British survey. Human Reproduction 21: 1009–1011.

Tan SL, Royston P, Campbell S et al 1992 Cumulative conception and livebirth rates after in-vitro fertilisation. The Lancet 339: 1390–1394.

Tarin JJ 1995 Subzonal insemination, partial zona dissection or intracytoplasmic sperm injection? An easy decision? Human Reproduction 10: 165–170.

te Velde ER, Pearson PL 2002 The variability of female reproductive ageing. Human Reproduction Update 8: 141–154.

Templeton A, Morris JK, Parslow W 1996 Factors that affect outcome of in-vitro fertilisation treatment. The Lancet 348: 1402–1406.

Templeton A, Morris JK 1998 Reducing the risk of multiple births by transfer of two embryos after in vitro fertilization. New England Journal of Medicine 339: 573–577.

Toner JP, Flood JT 1993 Fertility after the age of 40. Obstetrics and Gynecology Clinics of North America 20: 261–272.

van Rooij IA, Bancsi LF, Broekmans FJ, Looman CW, Habbema JD, te Velde ER 2003 Women older than 40 years of age and those with elevated follicle-stimulating hormone levels differ in poor response rate and embryo quality in vitro fertilization. Fertility and Sterility 79: 482–488.

van Rooij IA, Broekmans FJ, te Velde ER et al 2002 Serum anti-Müllerian hormone levels: a novel measure of ovarian reserve. Human Reproduction 17: 3065–3071.

Van Royen E, Mangelschots K, De Neubourg D et al 1999 Characterization of a top quality embryo, a step towards single-embryo transfer. Human Reproduction 14: 2345–2349.

Van Voorhis BJ 2007 Clinical practice. In vitro fertilization. New England Journal of Medicine 356: 379–386.

Vardon D, Burban C, Collomb J, Stolla V, Erny R 1995 [Spontaneous pregnancies in couples after failed or successful in vitro fertilization]. Journal de Gynecologie, Obstetrique et Biologie de la Reproduction 24: 811–815.

Vauthier-Brouzes D, Lefebvre G, Lesourd S, Gonzales J, Darbois Y 1994 How many embryos should be transferred in in vitro fertilization? A prospective randomized study. Fertility and Sterility 62: 339–342.

Venn A, Watson L, Bruinsma F, Giles G, Healy D 1999 Risk of cancer after the use of fertility drugs with in-vitro fertilisation. Lancet 354: 1586–1590.

Verberg MF, Eijkemans MJ, Macklon NS et al 2009a The clinical significance of the retrieval of a low number of oocytes following mild ovarian stimulation for IVF: a meta-analysis. Human Reproduction Update 15: 5–12.

Verberg MF, Macklon NS, Nargund G et al 2009b Mild ovarian stimulation for IVF. Human Reproduction Update 15: 13–29.

Wada I, Macnamee MC, Wick K, Bradfield JM, Brinsden PR 1994 Birth characteristics and perinatal outcome of babies conceived from cryopreserved embryos. Human Reproduction 9: 543–546.

Wang JX, Norman RJ, Wilcox AJ 2004 Incidence of spontaneous abortion among pregnancies produced by assisted reproductive technology. Human Reproduction 19: 272–277.

Wennerholm WB 2000 Cryopreservation of embryos and oocytes: obstetric outcome and health in children. Hum Reprod 15 (Suppl 5): 18–25.

Widra EA, Gindoff PR, Smotrich DB, Stillman RJ 1996 Achieving multiple-order embryo transfer identifies women over 40 years of age with improved in vitro fertilization outcome. Fertility and Sterility 65: 103–108.

Wiggins DA, Main E 2005 Outcomes of pregnancies achieved by donor egg in vitro fertilization — a comparison with standard in vitro fertilization pregnancies. American Journal of Obstetrics and Gynecology 192: 2002–2006; discussion 2006–2008.

Wood C, McMaster R, Rennie G, Trounson A, Leeton J 1985 Factors influencing pregnancy rates following in vitro fertilization and embryo transfer. Fertility and Sterility 43: 245–250.

Yaron Y, Ochshorn Y, Amit A, Yovel I, Kogosowski A, Lessing JB 1996 Patients with Turner's syndrome may have an inherent endometrial abnormality affecting receptivity in oocyte donation. Fertility and Sterility 65: 1249–1252.

Zhu JL, Basso O, Obel C, Bille C, Olsen J 2006 Infertility, infertility treatment, and congenital malformations: Danish national birth cohort. BMJ (Clinical Research Ed.) 333: 679.

CHAPTER 23

Sporadic and recurrent miscarriage

William M Buckett and Lesley Regan

Chapter Contents

INTRODUCTION AND DEFINITIONS	335		CONCLUSION	347
SPORADIC MISCARRIAGE	335		KEY POINTS	347
RECURRENT MISCARRIAGE	342			

Introduction and Definitions

Miscarriage is the most common complication of pregnancy and accounts for a high proportion of gynaecological consultations and hospital admissions. It can be a traumatic and highly emotional event for a woman and her partner, and the impact may be greatly underestimated by all who are involved in their care.

Current recommendations are that the term 'abortion' should be avoided in early pregnancy loss, with more sensitive terminology substituted.

- 'Spontaneous abortion' should be replaced by 'miscarriage'.
- 'Blighted ovum', 'missed abortion' or 'anembryonic pregnancy' should be replaced by 'early embryonic or fetal demise'.
- 'Incomplete abortion' should be replaced by 'incomplete miscarriage'.
- 'Recurrent or habitual abortion' should be replaced by 'recurrent miscarriage'.

At the present time in the UK, miscarriage is defined as the loss of an intrauterine pregnancy before 24 completed weeks of gestation. The World Health Organization's definition of miscarriage is the expulsion of a fetus or embryo weighing 500 g or less and also a gestational limit of less than 22 completed weeks of pregnancy.

Threatened miscarriage is defined as uterine bleeding prior to 24 weeks of pregnancy. Inevitable miscarriage can be subdivided into complete or incomplete, depending on whether or not all fetal and placental tissues have been expelled from the uterus. Early embryonic or fetal demise is where failure of the pregnancy is identified before expulsion of the fetal and placental tissues (usually by repeated ultrasound examination). Recurrent miscarriage is defined as three or more consecutive miscarriages (Stirrat 1990). This can be further subdivided into primary recurrent miscarriage, where there have been no previous live births, and secondary recurrent miscarriage, where at least one successful pregnancy has occurred previously.

In terms of investigation and further medical and surgical management, there should be a clear distinction between sporadic and recurrent miscarriage.

Sporadic Miscarriage

Epidemiology

Problems of definition and ascertainment

Problems of definition arise very early in pregnancy, where reliable detection of pregnancy is only possible with biochemical testing using urinary or serum β-human chorionic gonadotrophin (β-hCG), and also in late pregnancy, where the distinction between a late mid-trimester miscarriage and a stillbirth can be difficult (Chard 1991). The ideal research model for determining rates of miscarriage is a prospective longitudinal study of a representative cross-section of the population which is capable of recognizing all conceptions immediately, takes account of termination of pregnancy and follows women through the first 20 weeks of pregnancy (Regan et al 1989, Alberman 1992).

Early histological work from the 1950s (Hertig et al 1959), in which fertilized ova were directly observed in 107 hysterectomy specimens from women who had intercourse around the time of expected ovulation prior to their operation, suggests a postimplantation pregnancy rate of 58% (21 of 36 possible conceptions). In a mathematical model, total pregnancy loss rates have been estimated at 78% (Roberts and Lowe 1975).

Rate of miscarriage

Following critical review of the literature, a reasonably coherent picture is emerging (Figure 23.1). Estimates of early reproductive loss rates in the peri-implantation period of approximately 50–70% still rest largely on the early work of Hertig, although data derived from in-vitro fertilization (IVF) studies support losses of this order of magnitude (Chard 1991).

Postimplantation and biochemical pregnancy loss rates appear to be of the order of 30%, whereas recognized pregnancy losses after clinical recognition of pregnancy remain consistent in most studies as 10–15% (Table 23.1).

Aetiology

Chromosomal abnormalities

Miscarriage is a heterogeneous condition, but the single largest cause of sporadic miscarriage is fetal chromosomal abnormalities, accounting for approximately 50% of all cases (Table 23.2).

It is difficult to establish the precise contribution made by fetal chromosomal abnormalities. The figures in Table 23.2 are probably an underestimate, since miscarriages occurring as a result of fetal chromosomal anomalies are maximal at the earliest and least well-documented stages of pregnancy. Evidence from preimplantation genetic diagnosis studies of embryos created as a result of IVF suggests that at least 65% of all embryos are chromosomally abnormal (Gianaroli et al 2000). However, extrapolation of these results to miscarriage in the general population must be cautious, given the high degree of selectivity of these patients and a different microenvironment at fertilization.

Trisomies are the major fetal chromosomal abnormality in sporadic cases of miscarriage, being found in 30% of all miscarriages and 60% of chromosomally abnormal miscarriages. Trisomies, together with monosomy X (15–25%) and triploidy (12–20%), account for over 90% of all chromosomal abnormalities found in sporadic cases of miscarriage.

Trisomies for all chromosomes have been described, with the exception of chromosomes 1 and Y, although the relative frequencies are vastly different. Chromosome 16 and, to a lesser extent, chromosomes 2, 13, 15, 18, 21 and 22, account for the majority of trisomic abnormalities (Figure 23.2). Most trisomies are believed to be a consequence of non-disjunction during maternal meiosis. Trisomy 16 gives rise to only the most rudimentary embryonic growth with an empty sac (Edmonds 1992), and other trisomies often result in early embryonic demise.

Monosomy X (45XO) is thought to result from paternal sex chromosome loss (which can be either X or Y). It is usually associated with the presence of a fetus, although focal abnormalities, such as encephalocoele or hygromata, may occur (Edmonds 1992).

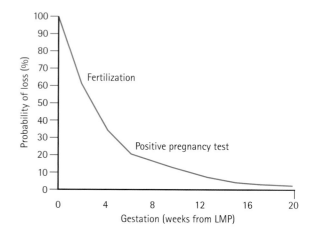

Figure 23.1 Fetal loss by gestational age.
Adapted from Kline J, Stein Z, Susser M 1989 Conception to birth — epidemiology of prenatal development. In: Kline J (ed) Monographs in Epidemiology and Biostatistics, Vol. 14. Oxford University Press, Oxford.

Table 23.1 Preclinical and clinical miscarriage rates

Authors	Preclinical loss rate (%)	Clinical loss rate (%)
French and Bierman (1962)	–	22
Miller et al (1980)	33	14
Edmonds et al (1982)	58	12
Wilcox et al (1988)	22	12
Regan et al (1989)	–	12
Brambati (1990)	–	14
Nybo Andersen et al (2000)	–	13

Table 23.2 Frequency of chromosomal abnormalities

Authors	Number of conceptions	Chromosomally abnormal	% Abnormal
Dhalial et al (1970)	547	128	23
Boué et al (1975)	1498	921	61
Creasy et al (1976)	986	290	29
Takahara et al (1977)	505	237	47
Therkelsen et al (1997)	254	139	54
Hassold et al (1980)	1000	463	46
Kajii et al (1980)	402	215	54
Warburton et al (1980)	967	312	32
Takakuwa et al (1997)	148	89	60
TOTALS	6307	3093	49

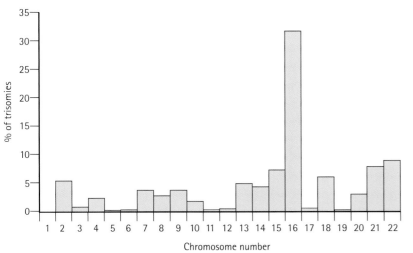

Figure 23.2 Distribution of differing trisomies in sporadic cases of miscarriage.

Polyploidy results from the addition of complete haploid sets of chromosomes. Most common are triploid micar-riages, usually 69XXY or 69XXX, which are thought to result from dispermic fertilization. These pregnancies are also characterized by multiple fetal and placental changes, such as neural tube defects, omphalocoele, hydropic villi and intrachorial haemorrhage. Tetraploid pregnancies are rare and usually do not progress beyond the third week of embryonic life.

Structural chromosome abnormalities have been reported, although minor abnormalities are no less frequent in live births compared with miscarriages. Major structural defects may arise *de novo* or be inherited. They are rarely a cause of sporadic miscarriage but are associated with recurrent miscarriage.

There appears to be a difference in the gestational age of pregnancy loss between different types of chromosomal abnormality, with trisomic and monosomic pregnancies miscarrying at a modal peak of 9 weeks and triploid pregnancy losses spanning 5–16 weeks of gestation (Alberman 1992).

Fetal malformations other than those caused by chromosomal anomaly

There is little doubt that the risk of miscarriage is increased with fetal malformation (Alberman 1992). However, since there has been no systematic search for malformations in fetal loss and since, in some cases, the malformation is secondary to a chromosomal anomaly, it is very difficult to assess the size of the increased risk. A single published study (Shephard et al 1989) has demonstrated an increased neural tube defect rate (3.6%) and an increased facial cleft rate (2.7%) amongst spontaneous miscarriages. Overall, the proportion of miscarriages as a result of fetal abnormalities without any associated chromosomal anomaly is small.

Placental abnormalities

Histological analysis of placental tissue from sporadic miscarriages has revealed several different patterns (Rushton 1995). These either point towards early fetal or embryonic demise with essentially normal placentation, or they have

shown abnormal placental villous development with marked villous hypoplasia, reduced vascularization, enlarged intra-villous spaces, often with clots and lacking significant extravillous trophoblastic infiltration, or with acute necrotic changes in the villi and associated clots which can be either patchy or global. Other reported placental changes have included inflammatory changes or a mixture of the above changes.

Amongst sporadic miscarriages, abnormalities of villous development have been reported fairly consistently at 30–40% (Hustin and Jauniaux 1997). However, the causes leading to the majority of these cases of abnormal placentation and therefore subsequent miscarriage remain unknown. Although autoimmune and infective causes can be associated with abnormal villous development, most inherently abnormal embryos probably also have abnormal placentation.

At present, although routine histological analysis of all products of conception is indicated in order to exclude molar and ectopic pregnancies, it is of little benefit in determining the cause of sporadic miscarriage.

Infection

Infection has been cited as a cause of late pregnancy loss and also early pregnancy loss for the past century. However, the precise role of infection as a cause of sporadic miscarriage is poorly and inconsistently reported (Simpson et al 1996). In many cases, whether infection has actually preceded any fetal demise or merely arose afterwards remains satisfactorily unanswered.

Several organisms have been associated with miscarriage (Box 23.1). Listeria, toxoplasmosis, herpes varicella zoster and malaria (*Plasmodium falciparum*) appear to be the most clinically important pathogens in women with early miscarriage.

Rubella infection, although a cause of first-trimester miscarriage, is now rare. The role of cytomegalovirus is unclear, although primary infection may cause miscarriage. The role of chlamydia infection, whether via an acute primary infection or a resultant chronic endometritis, also remains unclear. An association between herpes simplex virus infection and early pregnancy loss was first reported in the 1970s

Box 23.1 Infective causes associated with sporadic miscarriage

Bacteria

- *Listeria monocytogenes*
- Group B streptococcus
- Gonococcus
- *Chlamydia trachomatis*

Spirochaetes

- *Treponema pallidum*

Parasites

- *Toxoplasma gondii*
- *Trichomonas vaginalis*
- *Plasmodium falciparum*

Viruses

- Herpes simplex
- Varicella zoster
- Rubella
- Cytomegalovirus
- Parvovirus B19
- Hepatitis B
- Human immunodeficiency virus

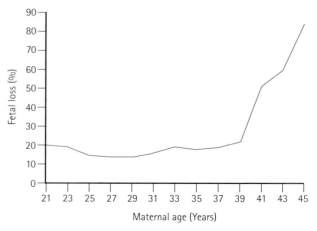

Figure 23.3 The risk of miscarriage in first pregnancies with maternal age. *Adapted from Alberman E 1992 Spontaneous abortions: epidemiology. In: Stabile I, Grudzinskas G, Chard T (eds) Spontaneous abortion — diagnosis and treatment. Springer-Verlag, London.*

(Nahmias et al 1971), although later prospective studies have failed to show any association with sporadic or recurrent miscarriage even when primary infection occurred in the first trimester (Stray-Pedersen 1993). It remains unknown whether human immunodeficiency virus (HIV) is an important cause of early pregnancy loss. Some studies have demonstrated an increased rate of early pregnancy loss with HIV (d'Ubaldo et al 1998), while others have not (Bakas et al 1996). Whether any increased risk of miscarriage is the result of the virus, the mother's general health or her immunocompromised status remains unclear.

Syphilis (*Treponema pallidum*) and parvovirus B19 are more commonly a cause of late second-trimester miscarriage and stillbirth, whilst group B streptococcus has been implicated in late miscarriage and preterm labour. Bacterial vaginosis (*Trichomonas vaginalis*) is also associated with late second-trimester miscarriage and preterm labour, but the use of metronidazole or other antibiotics in women with demonstrable bacterial vaginosis infection does not reduce late miscarriage or preterm delivery rates (Carey et al 2000).

Fetal sex, multiple pregnancy, maternal age and parity

Most studies have reported an excess of males in miscarriages and pregnancies complicated by varying degrees of placental dysfunction (Kellokumpu-Lethtinen and Pelliniemi 1984, Edwards et al 2000). However, the sex ratio of most early conceptions still remains unknown.

Multiple pregnancy is associated with an increased risk of fetal loss, either via early resorption, postimplantation loss or second-trimester miscarriage. In early pregnancy, the risk of miscarriage is twice that of singleton pregnancies (Sebire et al 1997a). The rate of late pregnancy loss is also increased, particularly in monochorionic twin pregnancies,

where late miscarriage rates can approach 12% (Sebire et al 1997b).

The risk of miscarriage rises with parity; however, the rise is a result of reproductive compensation (Alberman 1987). The risk of miscarriage in first pregnancies is low in young women (Regan et al 1989), but rises significantly after the age of 39 years (Figure 23.3). This rise is not only found in association with trisomic pregnancies (which rise with maternal age) but also in chromosomally normal pregnancies.

Maternal health

Virtually every maternal medical disorder has been associated with sporadic miscarriage. Women with severe medical disease rarely become pregnant, but if they do, their disease may deteriorate during pregnancy. Various mechanisms, including endocrinological, immunological or infective, have been suggested. Poorly controlled diabetes is associated with an increased risk of miscarriage (Mills et al 1988), whereas well-controlled and subclinical diabetes can rarely be considered a cause. Overall, only a small fraction of all early pregnancy losses can be considered to be attributable to severe maternal disease.

Cigarette smoking has been positively correlated with miscarriage, and a review of the effects of nicotine on ovarian, uterine and placental function suggests that cigarette smoking has an adverse effect on trophoblast invasion (Schiverick and Salafia 1999). Cocaine use has also been reported to increase the risk of miscarriage (Ness et al 1999). Alcohol consumption has been shown to be higher in women whose pregnancies ended in miscarriage compared with pregnancies which proceeded beyond 28 weeks of gestation (Harlap and Shapiro 1980, Kline et al 1980), although other studies have not confirmed this observation (Halmesmäki et al 1989, Parazzini et al 1990). There is some evidence to suggest that even moderate maternal alcohol consumption is associated with an increased risk of miscarriage (Windham et al 1997). Many studies have shown a relationship between coffee/caffeine intake and spontaneous miscarriage, although these have not controlled for other confounding variables. Only high levels of caffeine metabolites in maternal serum are associated with miscarriage, so it would appear that moderate consumption of caffeine is unlikely to increase the risk of miscarriage (Klebanoff et al 1999).

Some chemical agents including lead, ethylene oxide, solvents, pesticides, vinyl chloride and anaesthetic gases have been shown to have some association with fetal loss (Cohen et al 1971, Mur et al 1992, Rowland et al 1996, McDonald et al 1988). Although many environmental toxicologists accept these agents as proven, the evidence for low levels of exposure remains far from convincing.

Radiotherapy and chemotherapeutic agents are accepted causes of miscarriage (Zemlickis et al 1992), although they are only administered during pregnancy in seriously ill women. Although significant ionizing radiation for diagnostic purposes can lead to fetal malformation and miscarriage, a dose of more than 25 rads is associated with a 0.1% risk of abnormality (1 rad is the equivalent of eight to 10 abdominal/pelvic X-ray films).

There is a small increase in the risk of spontaneous miscarriage with general anaesthesia and incidental surgery during the first and second trimesters, although this is higher with gynaecological surgery (Duncan et al 1986).

It has been claimed that impaired psychological well-being predisposes to fetal loss (Stray-Pedersen and Stray-Pedersen 1984), although it has been difficult to exclude other confounding variables. Despite problems with recall bias, there are an increased number of negative life events in women with chromosomally normal as compared with chromosomally abnormal miscarriages (Neugebauer et al 1996), but no differences in hormonal markers of stress have been determined.

Pathophysiology

The exact pathophysiology resulting in the uterine expulsion of early pregnancy remains unknown. Abnormal placentation (either primary or itself secondary to early fetal demise) can either lead to reduced or shallow uterine invasion by the trophoblast, or can itself be caused by reduced invasion. In this situation, the usual reduction in maternal vascular tone cannot occur. It is presumed that this blood flow enters the intervillous space and dislodges the conceptus, thereby leading to embryonic demise if this has not already occurred (Rushton 1995). Nevertheless, even quite large intrauterine haematomata visualized by ultrasound have not prevented live births at term (Pedersen and Mantoni 1990), and the presence of haematomata *per se* does not increase the risk of miscarriage (Tower and Regan 2001).

Once the conceptus is dislodged, there is further intrauterine bleeding. Local prostaglandin release will lead to pain and ultimately expulsion of the conceptus and any associated blood.

Presentation

Threatened miscarriage

This can be defined as uterine bleeding before 24 weeks of pregnancy (the time of presumed fetal viability) with no evidence of any fetal or embryonic demise. It is usually painless. Characteristically, the bleeding is initially bright red, followed by a reducing brown loss. This can affect up to 25% of all pregnancies and is one of the most common indica-

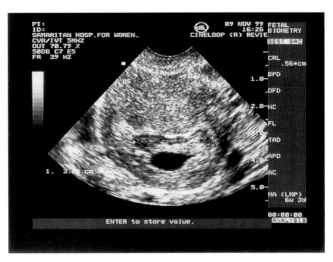

Figure 23.4 Ultrasound picture of an ongoing pregnancy with an intrauterine haematoma in a woman who presented with a threatened miscarriage.

tions for emergency early pregnancy referral. Clinical examination reveals a soft, non-tender uterus, usually of the appropriate gestational size, and a closed cervix. Transvaginal or transabdominal ultrasound scan confirms an ongoing pregnancy (Figure 23.4).

The non-specific nature of abdominal pain, vaginal bleeding and pelvic tenderness precludes their use as predictors of ultimate outcome in women with threatened miscarriage. However, continued vomiting (rather than nausea alone) in early pregnancy is associated with an increased chance of live birth (Weigel and Weigel 1989), presumably because it indicates continued placental hormone production.

Inevitable miscarriage

Miscarriage is a process rather than a single event. Of all women presenting with bleeding in early pregnancy, approximately 50% will ultimately miscarry (Stabile et al 1987). Whilst the cervix remains closed, any pain and bleeding may subside and the pregnancy may continue otherwise normally to term. However, once the cervix opens, miscarriage is inevitable.

Usually, women present with crampy abdominal pains and fresh bleeding. Symptoms alone are unreliable and the diagnosis is determined by the confirmation of cervical dilatation at vaginal examination. Examination often reveals a tender, firm uterus, which may be smaller than the expected gestational size, and the cervical os is open. Products of conception may also be felt through the os.

Occasionally, the woman may present with severe shock. This can either be secondary to massive haemorrhage, which will require appropriate emergency resuscitation, blood transfusion and uterine evacuation, or the degree of shock may be out of proportion to the blood loss and is due to the distension of the cervix by products of conception and the resultant sympathetic stimulation. This is termed 'cervical shock syndrome' and is often severe. Quick removal of the products from the os, at the bedside, results in relief of the shock. In rare cases, endotoxic shock secondary to sepsis may occur.

Complete and incomplete miscarriage

Inevitable miscarriage is either complete or incomplete depending on whether or not all fetal and placental tissues have been expelled from the uterus. The typical features of incomplete miscarriage are heavy bleeding (which may be intermittent) and abdominal cramps. The finding of a dilated cervix on examination in the presence of continued pain and bleeding is usually diagnostic. Ultrasound scan will confirm the presence of retained products of conception (Figure 23.5).

If the symptoms of incomplete miscarriage resolve spontaneously, complete miscarriage may have occurred. Nevertheless, following abdominal and pelvic examination, ultrasound may need to be perfomed to confirm that the uterus is indeed empty. Occasionally, the cervix may close despite the presence of retained products. The number of complete miscarriages is unknown. Many such early miscarriages may go unreported. Early studies of women with threatened miscarriage showed complete miscarriage rates of less than 1% (Stabile et al 1987), although more recent evidence suggests that approximately 20–30% of miscarriages are complete (Chung et al 1994, Mansur 1992). Similarly, expectant management of early fetal demise has demonstrated that, with time, up to 25% of women go on to have a complete miscarriage (Jurkovic et al 1998).

Early fetal demise (missed abortion/miscarriage)

'Early embryonic or fetal demise' is now the preferred term in both the UK and the USA, rather than 'missed abortion' or 'missed miscarriage'. Previously, this has also been termed an 'anembryonic pregnancy' (all pregnancies develop from an embryo) or 'blighted ovum' (the pregnancy cannot result from an ovum alone). These terms should also be abandoned.

Early fetal demise is where failure of pregnancy is identified before any expulsion of the products of conception occurs. The woman may report a disappearance of the symptoms and signs of early pregnancy, such as nausea and vomiting or breast tenderness. A brown vaginal loss may also be reported. The diagnosis may also be made in otherwise asymptomatic women at routine obstetric/dating ultrasound examination. The diagnosis is made by the lack of fetal heart activity in a pregnancy with a crown–rump length of over 5 mm (Pennell et al 1991), or when two ultrasound examinations 1 or 2 weeks apart have shown no growth and no fetal heart activity. In cases of doubt, a repeat ultrasound is always indicated. Occasionally, a collapsing gestational sac or a failed pregnancy surrounded by clot *in utero* may be seen (Figure 23.6). Abdominal and pelvic examination often reveals a uterus smaller than expected for the gestational age and a closed cervical os.

Sepsis

This occurs when infection complicates miscarriage or termination of pregnancy. Intrauterine sepsis rarely follows incomplete miscarriage, although the incidence is considerably higher at approximately 3.6% following termination of pregnancy (Frank 1985). The most common infecting organisms are *Escherichia coli*, Bacteroides, streptococci (both anaerobic and occasionally aerobic) and *Clostridium welchii*. Occasionally, a history of intrauterine instrumentation may be withheld. The woman usually presents with suprapubic pain, malaise, fever and, occasionally, vaginal bleeding. Findings on examination include abdominal rigidity, uterine and adnexal tenderness, and a closed cervical os. Rarely, septicaemia may ensue, leading to bacteraemic endotoxic shock and possibly maternal death.

Trophoblastic tumours

Trophoblastic tumours include complete and partial hydatidiform moles, choriocarcinoma and placental site tumours. These occasionally present as threatened miscarriage, and suggestive features are noted at ultrasound examination. Trophoblastic tumours are discussed in Chapter 43.

Investigations

Ultrasound, usually transvaginal, is essential in the diagnosis of miscarriage. It will determine the presence of an ongoing pregnancy in cases of threatened miscarriage, and distinguish between early fetal demise, incomplete miscarriage

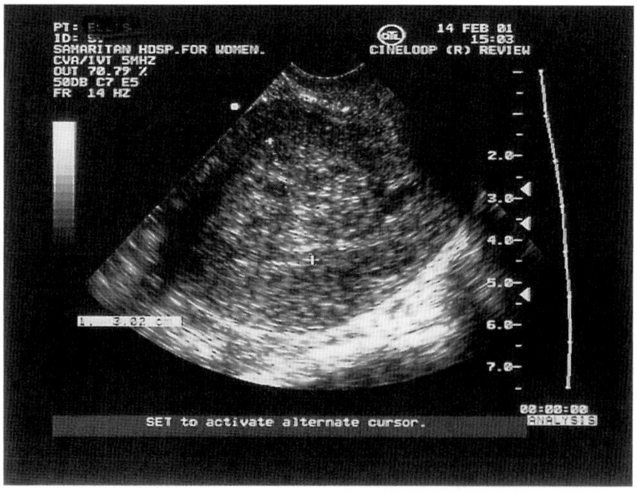

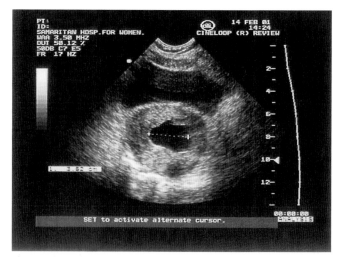

Figure 23.5 Ultrasound picture of incomplete miscarriage demonstrating retained products of conception within the endometrial cavity.

Figure 23.6 Ultrasound picture of early fetal demise, showing a collapsing gestation sac.

and complete miscarriage in failing pregnancies. Ultrasound is also important in the diagnoses of ectopic pregnancy and trophoblastic disease.

Reliable pregnancy testing, whether by urinary or serum β-hCG, is also essential in order to distinguish an early complete miscarriage or an ongoing ectopic pregnancy.

All women with uterine bleeding in early pregnancy should have their blood group determined, and all women who are Rhesus (D) negative should receive anti-D immunoglobulins regardless of the gestational age of the pregnancy.

The measurement of other fetoplacental hormones and proteins, such as α-fetoprotein, Schwangerschaft protein 1, human placental lactogen, pregnancy-associated plasma protein, oestrogen and progesterone, have all been reported as diagnostic tests in early pregnancy. In rare cases, they may improve the prediction of both early fetal demise and ectopic pregnancy (Grudzinskas and Chard 1992), but their routine use is not indicated.

Treatment

Threatened miscarriage

Early studies demonstrated that the presence of fetal heart activity at ultrasound examination in women who present with a history of bleeding in early pregnancy was associated with a high chance (97–98%) of a live birth (Stabile et al 1987). More recent evidence confirms livebirth rates of 90–95% for younger women, but for women over 40 years of age, miscarriage rates of 15–30% are reported even after the identification of fetal heart activity (Deaton et al 1997, Schmidt-Sarosi et al 1998). Nevertheless, for most women, reassurance and continued medical and emotional support are all that is required.

Bed rest and avoiding penetrative intercourse have historically been advised. If the vascular hypothesis for the pathophysiology of miscarriage is accepted (Hustin and Jauniaux 1997), bed rest may improve pressure variation and flow changes, and therefore improve the outcome. However, there is a paucity of clinical evidence to support this hypothesis. Initial presentation is usually in primary care and, currently, over 96% of general practitioners still advise bed rest and the avoidance of intercourse, although many believe that it does not improve the eventual outcome.

Progesterone supplementation in early pregnancy has been prescribed for over 30 years for women presenting with threatened (and also recurrent) miscarriage. The historical rationale was that a progesterone deficiency would lead to miscarriage. Obviously, the converse may also be true; a failed pregnancy may lead to a progesterone deficiency. There is a wealth of published data, mostly from uncontrolled treatment trials. However, several meta-analyses (Daya 1989, Goldstein et al 1989) have been unable to demonstrate a beneficial effect for progesterone treatment. The routine use of progesterone in threatened miscarriage cannot be justified.

Incomplete miscarriage

Surgical evacuation of the uterus after cervical dilatation, if necessary, has remained the cornerstone of management of incomplete miscarriage in the industrialized world since the 1940s (Hertig and Livingstone 1944). Evacuation and curettage have been regarded as essential to ensure that the uterine cavity is empty, otherwise haemorrhage, infection and later complications such as Asherman's syndrome may result. Early studies showed a maternal mortality rate of 1.6% in women who did not undergo surgical treatment (Russell 1947). In cases of haemodynamic compromise of cervical shock, appropriate resuscitation and urgent surgical evacuation are indicated. Most cases are performed under general anaesthesia, although effective outpatient curettage has been reported (Fawcus et al 1997). Suction evacuation is generally regarded as a safer technique than sharp curettage, with lower rates of perforation, blood loss and subsequent intrauterine adhesion formation (Edmonds 1992, Verkuyl and Crowther 1993).

The routine use of syntocinon or ergometrine has shown no benefit in reducing blood loss during the surgical treatment of first-trimester incomplete miscarriage (Beeby and Morgan Hughes 1984). Due to the risk of ascending infection and its sequelae, whenever uterine instrumentation is performed, screening for chlamydia infection is recommended, although the use of prophylactic doxycycline is only likely to be of benefit in areas of relatively high prevalence (Prieto et al 1995).

Although a minor procedure, surgical evacuation is associated with rare but serious morbidity. Complications include tearing or lacerations to the cervix, perforation of the uterus, which may also lead to bowel perforation, bladder perforation, damage to the broad ligament, infection, Asherman's syndrome (intrauterine adhesions) and haemorrhage (Ratnam and Prasad 1990). The incidence of serious morbidity has been estimated at 2.1% (Lawson et al 1994, Royal College of General Practitioners/Royal College of Obstetricians and Gynaecologists 1985), of which the most common problem is infection. This can lead to later sequelae including secondary infertility, ectopic pregnancy and Asherman's syndrome. The incidence of mortality associated with surgical evacuation of the uterus has been estimated at 0.5 per 100,000 (Lawson et al 1994).

Recent studies demonstrated the efficacy of expectant management or 'observation alone' in women with incomplete miscarriage (Nielsen and Hahlin 1995, Hurd et al 1997). In cases where there was no haemodynamic compromise or maternal anaemia, spontaneous resolution occurred within 3 days in up to 80% of cases with minimal retained products (15–50 ml). Therefore, in women with minimal intrauterine tissue (after ectopic pregnancy has been excluded), expectant management is safe. However, large volumes of retained products are associated with an increase in complications, primarily infection and prolonged bleeding (Hurd et al 1997). There is no evidence that future fertility is impaired following expectant management (Kaplan et al 1996).

Herbal remedies have been used in the past to encourage the uterus to expel its contents, but an effective non-surgical alternative to termination of pregnancy and miscarriage had to await the development of the antiprogesterone mifepristone and the prostaglandin analogues gemeprost and misoprostol. Their efficacy has been demonstrated in the treatment of incomplete miscarriage (Henshaw et al 1993, Ashok et al 1998), leading to complete miscarriage rates of approximately 95%.

The use of medical treatment or the adoption of an expectant approach in appropriately selected cases may have many medical and economic benefits. However, many women continue to express a preference for surgical treatment (Hamilton-Fairley and Donaghy 1997), citing fears regarding pain, bleeding and the length of time to resolution in the non-surgical group.

Early fetal demise

The treatment options for early fetal demise are essentially the same as for incomplete miscarriage. Surgical treatment should be preceded by cervical ripening agents (mifepristone or prostaglandins) in order to reduce the risks of cervical trauma or uterine perforation associated with forced cervical dilatation. Gemeprost, mifepristone, and oral or vaginal misoprostol seem to be equally effective (Gupta and Johnson 1992, Platz-Christiansen et al 1995, Ayres de Campos et al 2000). Expectant management is feasible, although less effective than in cases of incomplete miscarriage, with only 25% proceeding to complete miscarriage (Jurkovic et al 1998). The efficacy of medical treatment is also less when compared with incomplete miscarriage, although complete miscarriage rates of up to 90% have been reported with higher doses of mifepristone and misoprostol and a longer surveillance period (El-Refaey et al 1992).

Psychological aspects

Psychological consequences of early pregnancy loss differ widely among different women, different families and even different pregnancies in the same woman. Nevertheless, most women, irrespective of their attitude towards the pregnancy at the time, experience feelings of depression and anxiety following miscarriage (Seibel and Graves 1980), and up to 36% of women are 'highly symptomatic' in terms of clinical depression 4 weeks after miscarriage (Neugebauer et al 1992).

All workers caring for women with miscarriage and their families need to understand the increased psychiatric morbidity associated with pregnancy loss, and be able to offer appropriate support both at the time of diagnosis and also after treatment. Good communication with providers of primary care for the whole family and access to counselling are important, since 'miscarriages do not occur in a uterus but in a woman, and miscarriages do not occur solely in a woman but in a family' (Cain et al 1964). For some couples, the use of ritual can help them through the bereavement process (Hopper 1997).

In subsequent pregnancies, many women will need considerable reassurance and support (Hamilton 1989), and early access to ultrasound and hospital services may be required.

Recurrent Miscarriage

In contrast to sporadic miscarriage, recurrent miscarriage is relatively uncommon. A history of three or more consecutive miscarriages occurs in 0.5–2% of women (Stirrat 1990, Daya 1993, Katz and Kuller 1994). Recurrent miscarriage is obviously distressing and frustrating for both the couple concerned and those treating them. In many cases, the cause may not be apparent despite intensive and expensive clinical and laboratory testing, and there remains only a limited understanding of the causes of recurrent miscarriage.

The aetiologies are outlined below and summarized in Box 23.2. The management of recurrent miscarriage, including unexplained recurrent miscarriage, will be discussed below under specific headings. Unexplained miscarriage occurs in approximately 50% of women attending specialist recurrent miscarriage clinics (Clifford et al 1994, Stephenson 1996, Li 1998).

Genetic factors

Parental chromosomal abnormalities

Parental chromosomal abnormalities are the most important genetic anomalies currently detectable amongst couples with recurrent miscarriage. Most studies report an incidence of 3–5% (Stray-Pedersen and Stray-Pedersen 1984, Clifford et al 1994, Stephenson 1996, Li 1998), compared with an incidence of 0.5% in the general population.

Balanced or reciprocal translocations are the most frequently detected parental chromosomal anomaly in couples with recurrent miscarriage. The male:female ratio is approximately 1:2. A portion of one chromosome is exchanged with a portion of another, resulting in two abnormal chromosomes but, overall, a normal chromosomal complement. Translocations have been reported for all chromosomes in many different combinations. At gametogenesis, there is a 50% chance of a chromosomally abnormal gamete being produced. However, there appears to be a lower fertilization or implantation rate with abnormal gametes, since chorionic villus sampling and amniocentesis have demonstrated a 40% and 11% risk, respectively, of a chromosomally unbalanced fetus (Mikkelson 1985).

Robertsonian translocations are less common, occurring in approximately 1% of couples with recurrent miscarriage.

Box 23.2 Summary of the potential causes of recurrent miscarriage

Genetic
- Parental chromosomal abnormalities
- Recurrent aneuploidy
- Other genetic causes

Anatomical
- Uterine anomalies
- Cervical imcompetence

Infective
- Predisposition to infection
- Possible pathogens

Endocrine
- Luteal-phase deficiency
- Thyroid disease
- Hypersecretion of LH/polycystic ovary syndrome

Immunological
- Antiphospholipid syndrome
- Other thrombophilic defects
- Alloimmune

Here, two chromosomes adhere to each other at either the centromere or the short arms of the chromosome. This leads to a total chromosome count of 45 but a normal chromosome complement overall. The risks of recurrence and miscarriage vary in different Robertsonian translocations. The most common translocation (involving chromosomes 14 and 21) results in 10–15% of pregnancies with trisomy 21 (Boué and Gallano 1984). If homologous chromosomes are involved, the risk of a chromosomally abnormal conceptus is 100%.

Pericentric chromosomal inversions occur in approximately 1% of the general population, and are not considered to be of clinical significance for recurrent miscarriage.

Peripheral blood karyotyping should be performed in both partners of all couples with recurrent miscarriage to determine any parental chromosome abnormality. Specialized genetic counselling is essential and offers the couple a prognosis for future pregnancies; this may, in some cases, not be as bleak as anticipated. There should also be the opportunity to discuss preimplantation genetic diagnosis and antenatal fetal karyotyping, including chorionic villus sampling and amniocentesis. In cases of homologous Robertsonian translocations, gamete donation and/or effective contraception should be discussed.

It is important to note that over 35% of couples with a significant parental chromosomal abnormality have already achieved a successful pregnancy in addition to their miscarriages (Clifford et al 1994).

Recurrent aneuploidy

Some couples have an increased risk of miscarriage because they produce recurrent aneuploid fetuses. This may be the result of an increased tendency to non-disjunction, either inherited or induced environmentally. Chromosomal abnormalities are seen with a higher frequency amongst preimplantation embryos created during IVF from couples with a history of recurrent miscarriage (Vidal et al 2000). Presumably, these are the result of errors in gametogenesis, and much current research is focused on the role of sperm chromosome abnormalities in recurrent miscarriage.

Other genetic factors

The karyotype of many recurrent miscarriage conceptions may be euploid (46XX or 46XY), and in the absence of any other identifiable cause or association, these unexplained recurrent early pregnancy losses may be the result of molecular mutations or single gene defects. Chromosome analysis itself is a very crude tool to determine genetic abnormalities. So far, there has only been one report of a specific single gene locus abnormality associated with recurrent miscarriage (Pegoraro et al 1997), but much work remains to be done. The impact of other genetic factors on recurrent miscarriage is confirmed by the increased incidence amongst consanguinous couples (Hendrick 1988).

Anatomical factors

Uterine anomalies

The reported incidence of uterine anomalies in women with recurrent miscarriage varies widely from as low as 1% up to 27% (Regan 1997). Described anomalies vary from uterus

didelphis to subseptate uteri, and some studies even include submucosal fibroids. The incidence of such anomalies in the fertile population has been reported to be 1.8–3.6% (Ashton et al 1988).

The significance of such anomalies, particularly intrauterine septae, arcuate uterus and submucosal fibroids, in women with recurrent miscarriage is unclear. Historically, uterine anomalies were associated with second-trimester miscarriages, but later reports have also shown an increase in early miscarriages. The exact aetiology is unknown, although implantation over a septum or similar defect may result in decreased vascularity of the placenta.

Hysterosalpingography (HSG), laparoscopy and hysteroscopy, magnetic resonance imaging, computed tomography and three-dimensional ultrasound have all been used in the diagnosis and evaluation of uterine anomalies. Although HSG has traditionally been used as the primary screening test, three-dimensional ultrasound shows promise as a less invasive screening tool (Jurkovic et al 1995). In most cases, further evaluation at laparoscopy and hysteroscopy is indicated (Figure 23.7).

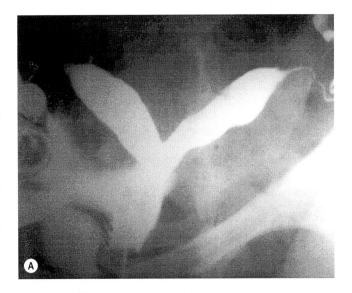

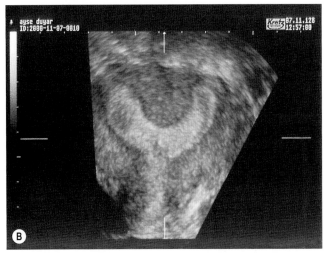

Figure 23.7 (A) Hysterosalpingogram demonstrating a septate uterus. (B) Three-dimensional ultrasound demonstrating a septate uterus.

Treatment of uterine anomalies in women with recurrent miscarriage remains controversial. Many reports demonstrate a benefit of hysteroscopic or conventional metroplasty in women with septate, subseptate or bicornuate uterus who have suffered mid-trimester miscarriage compared with matched controls (Candiani et al 1990, Ayhan et al 1992, Pabuccu et al 1995, Heinonen 1997). However, the likelihood of a live birth in untreated women is as high as 66% (Heinonen 1997), and a similar percentage of women presenting with recurrent miscarriage have already achieved a live birth (Clifford et al 1994). Open pelvic surgery, in particular, has been associated with subsequent infertility (Bennett 1987). The value of corrective uterine surgery in women with these anomalies and a history of early pregnancy loss is uncertain (Ben-Rafael et al 1991). Similarly, the value of transcervical myomectomy in women with submucous fibroids remains unknown, although there have been initial successful reports (Egwuatu 1989).

Cervical incompetence

Cervical incompetence is usually associated with miscarriage occurring after 12–14 weeks or premature labour. It usually presents as silent dilatation of the cervix without painful contractions. The membranes bulge through the cervical canal and eventually rupture spontaneously.

The diagnosis of cervical incompetence poses a difficult problem (Medical Research Council/Royal College of Obstetricians and Gynaecologists Working Party on Cervical Cerclage 1993). It is usually based on a previous history of mid-trimester miscarriage in the absence of painful uterine contractions. Vaginal ultrasound may be useful to detect early features of cervical incompetence (shortening or funnelling) (Althuisius et al 2000), but neither ultrasound nor HSG has been found to be useful in the diagnosis of cervical incompetence before pregnancy.

Treatment of cervical incompetence is cervical cerclage in pregnancy, usually after 12–14 weeks when the toll of first-trimester miscarriages has occurred and after screening for chromosomal abnormalities has been performed. It has traditionally involved the insertion of a MacDonald suture, where a tape is inserted round the exposed vaginal cervix (MacDonald 1957), or a Shirodkar suture, where the vaginal mucosa is incised and the bladder reflected, allowing insertion of the suture at a higher level of the cervical canal (Shirodkar 1960). Modifications of this procedure have included burying the suture under the vaginal mucosa at the end of the procedure. In the authors' experience, this is rarely accompanied by significant vaginal discharge. The MacDonald suture is more widely used and less traumatic to the cervix than the Shirodkar suture, although the exposed tape remains a possible focus for later infection. More recently, emergency cervical cerclage in women who present acutely in the mid-trimester with silent cervical dilatation and/or herniation of the membranes through the cervix has been reported with livebirth rates of 50–60% (Wong et al 1993, Aarts et al 1995). Nevertheless, there are high rates of premature delivery and infection, including chorioamnionitis, in over 30% of cases.

In some women, particularly where the diagnosis is unsure or in those who have other risk factors, regular ultrasound monitoring of the cervix can be performed. If there is funnelling or shortening of the cervix, emergency cerclage can be performed (Althuisius et al 2000). Ultrasound may also be useful in women who have already had cervical cerclage in order to warn of problems (Dijkstra et al 2000). Transabdominal cervical cerclage may be useful in a highly selected group of women with anatomical defects in the cervix and previous mid-trimester miscarriages or preterm labours following failed vaginal cervical cerclage (Gibb and Salaria 1995). Laparoscopic transabdominal cervical cerclage has also been reported (Scibetta et al 1998), but neither of these procedures have been assessed in appropriate trials.

Infective factors

Although any severe infection may lead to sporadic miscarriage, for infection to be a cause of repeated pregnancy failure it must persist in the genital tract and usually be asymptomatic.

Syphilis (*Treponema pallidum*) is a cause of recurrent late second-trimester miscarriage and stillbirth. Screening is performed routinely, and treatment with penicillins is effective. It is a rare cause of recurrent miscarriage in developed countries. Malaria infection in non-immune women is also associated with recurrent miscarriage in endemic areas (Royal College of Obstetricians and Gynaecologists 2001).

Bacterial vaginosis (*Trichomonas vaginalis*) is associated with recurrent late second-trimester miscarriage and preterm labour (Hay et al 1994), although there is no association with early pregnancy loss (Llahi-Camp et al 1996). Treatment with metronidazole has not been shown to be effective (Carey et al 2000).

The identification of individual organisms has proven to be disappointing in the search for causes of early or late recurrent miscarriage, which suggests that pregnancy outcome may be determined by maternal or fetal response to infection rather than the infective organism itself. Gene mutations, such as those associated with mannose-binding protein (MBP) deficiency, are an important cause of inherited immunodeficiency and increased susceptibility to infection. Early studies demonstrate a trend in association between late miscarriage and MBP genes (Baxter et al 2001). Future research regarding the role of infection in recurrent miscarriage needs to explore genetic susceptibility.

In women with a history of recurrent mid-trimester miscarriage, regular gentle sterile speculum examination to assess any cervical change, and regular high and low vaginal swabs to screen for any infection can be performed. This approach is empirical but it is difficult not to treat women with demonstrable infection. Similarly, low-dose maintenance antibiotic therapy may be used in women with repeated positive results, although this is also empirical.

Endocrine factors

Systemic endocrine disease

As discussed previously, diabetic women with good metabolic control are no more likely to miscarry than non-diabetic women. However, diabetic women with high glycosylated haemoglobin A_{1c} levels in the first trimester are at significantly higher risk of both miscarriage and fetal malformation (Hanson et al 1990). As the risk of miscarriage is only increased in women with poorly controlled diabetes mellitus, there is no value in screening for occult disease in asymptomatic women.

Although thyroid autoantibodies are associated with an increased risk of miscarriage, this is secondary to a generalized autoimmune abnormality rather than a specific thyroid dysfunction (Singh et al 1995). Screening asymptomatic women with a thyroid function test is unhelpful as they are usually normal (Clifford et al 1994, Rushworth et al 2000).

Luteal-phase deficiency

A functional corpus luteum is essential for the implantation and maintenance of early pregnancy, primarily through the production of progesterone, which is responsible for the conversion of a proliferative endometrium into a secretory endometrium available for embryo implantation. Disorders or removal of the corpus luteum can result in infertility and early pregnancy loss (Miller et al 1969, Csapo et al 1973). Although much controversy exists about luteal function, the success of oocyte donation with oestradiol and progesterone support in the absence of any ovarian activity would suggest that its effects are primarily progesterone determined.

The prevalence of a luteal-phase defect is reported to occur in 23–60% of women with recurrent miscarriage (Li and Cooke 1991), although it is difficult to determine the exact proportion of women with luteal-phase problems because of difficulties in diagnosis. The diagnosis is usually determined by low luteal-phase progesterone level and/or a non-secretory endometrium, by biopsy, in non-fertile, non-pregnant cycles (Jordan et al 1994, Serle et al 1994). Between 30% and 50% of cases of luteal-phase defect, as determined by endometrial histology, are found in the presence of normal circulating progesterone levels, suggesting that a primary endometrial defect is as common as deficient progesterone production (Li et al 1991). There is no reliable way of demonstrating a luteal-phase defect in conception cycles or early pregnancy as low levels of progesterone in early pregnancy are a reflection that the pregnancy has already failed because the trophoblast cannot produce sufficient progesterone. The use of colour-flow pulsed Doppler ultrasound may offer a non-invasive tool for diagnosis, and has been used in the diagnosis of luteal-phase defect, although only at a preliminary stage (Glock and Brumsted 1995).

There have been many reports of successful pregnancies following treatment with progesterone after the diagnosis of a luteal-phase defect. These studies have, for the most part, been uncontrolled. The only meta-analysis of controlled trials of progesterone treatment in women with recurrent miscarriage has not demonstrated any benefit (Daya 1989).

Treatment with hCG should stimulate progesterone production from the corpus luteum, and has been used in the treatment of luteal-phase defect. Although one small study demonstrated a beneficial effect of hCG treatment in women with oligomenorrhoea (Quenby and Farquharson 1994), meta-analysis has concluded that there is insufficient evidence at present concerning the effectiveness of hCG to rec-ommend its use for women with unexplained recurrent miscarriage (Prendiville 1995).

Polycystic ovary syndrome and hypersecretion of luteinizing hormone

The prevalence of polycystic ovarian morphology in women with recurrent miscarriage is 40% (Rai et al 2000), and there have been numerous reports of an increased risk of miscarriage in women with hypersecretion of luteinizing hormone (LH), hyperandrogenaemia and, more recently, hyperprolactinaemia; all the classic endocrinopathies of polycystic ovary syndrome (PCOS) (Stanger and Yovich 1985, Howles et al 1987, Homburg et al 1988, Regan et al 1990, Bussen et al 1999). Nevertheless, a degree of controversy exists.

Several reports have not confirmed the relationship between hypersecretion of LH and an increased risk of miscarriage in women with recurrent miscarriage (Tulppala et al 1993, Liddell et al 1997). Whether this is due to the radioimmunoassays or a genetic variant of LH is unclear (Tulppala et al 1998). Also, suppression of high endogenous LH secretion with gonadotrophin-releasing hormone analogues in a prospective randomized placebo-controlled trial did not improve the livebirth rate (Clifford et al 1996).

The association between raised androgens and recurrent miscarriage has similarly not been confirmed with later studies (Liddell et al 1997, Rai et al 2000), although these are not universal findings and some studies have demonstrated retarded endometrial development and increased risk of miscarriage in association with raised testosterone levels (Tulppala et al 1993, Okon et al 1998).

Hyperprolactinaemia is a common finding in women with PCOS, and has also been associated with recurrent miscarriage (Hirahara et al 1998, Bussen et al 1999). Although one study has demonstrated a beneficial effect of bromocriptine treatment, this has not been corroborated elsewhere (Hirahara et al 1998).

In summary, PCOS is over-represented in women with recurrent miscarriage but the exact mechanism or individual endocrinopathy by which miscarriage is mediated remains unclear. Until this is determined, any corrective treatment is unlikely to be effective.

Autoimmune and thrombophilic factors

Autoimmune disease

Sporadic and recurrent miscarriage are recognized complications of systemic lupus erythematosus, the most common autoimmune disorder in women of reproductive age. Since the 1980s, it has been recognized that recurrent miscarriage is associated with an increase in the detection of many autoantibodies, even in asymptomatic women. The two most common groups of autoantibodies detected have been the antiphospholipid antibodies (aPL), which in conjunction with a history of recurrent miscarriage is now known as the 'antiphospholipid syndrome' (APS) (Harris 1987), and thyroid autoantibodies (Bussen and Steck 1995). However, with the exception of APS, the mechanisms by which a generalized increase in the autoantibody pool leads to miscarriage remain unclear. Although intravenous immunoglobulin (IVIG) therapy has been used in women with recurrent miscarriage associated with non-specific autoimmunity, at present the collective evidence indicates that IVIG does not have a therapeutic effect that is clinically meaningful (Daya et al 1999).

Antiphospholipid syndrome

APS refers to the relationship between aPL, namely lupus anticoagulant (LA) and anticardiolipin antibodies (aCL), and recurrent miscarriage, thrombosis or thrombocytopenia (Harris 1987). Since this original description, it has become apparent that the three defining clinical features are too limiting, and aPL are implicated in a wide range of clinical conditions (Box 23.3).

In women with recurrent miscarriage, a previous personal or family history of thrombosis, cardiovascular disease, epilepsy and migraine is strongly predictive of a positive aPL status (Regan 1997). The overall prevalence of aPL in women with recurrent miscarriage is approximately 15% (Li 1998).

Women with APS without treatment have a miscarriage risk of 85–90%, the majority of which occur in the first trimester after establishment of a fetal heart (Rai et al 1995a,b). Pregnancy loss associated with APS is initially attributed to defective embryonic implantation and later to thrombosis of the uteroplacental vasculature and placental infarction (Rai and Regan 1998).

Diagnosis of APS and detection of aPL are subject to widespread interlaboratory variation and the fluctuating nature of the antibodies themselves. Testing for LA should follow internationally agreed guidelines (Lupus Anticoagulant Working Party on behalf of the BSCH Homeostasis and Thrombosis Task Force 1991), and the test of choice is the

dilute Russell's viper venom time which is more sensitive than the activated partial thromboplastin time and the kaolin clotting time. Testing for aCL is by standardized enzyme-linked immunosorbent assay. Testing must be repeated on at least two occasions 8 weeks apart in order to make a diagnosis of APS. Testing for aPL other than LA and aCL is of no clinical use in women with recurrent miscarriage.

Although a variety of treatments have been described for APS, including corticosteroids (Lubbe et al 1983), low-dose aspirin (Silver et al 1993), heparin alone (Rosove et al 1990) and IVIG therapy (Carreras et al 1988), treatment with subcutaneous heparin and low-dose aspirin until 34 weeks of gestation has been shown to be the most effective treatment for women with APS and recurrent miscarriage (Rai et al 1997). In cases where there are additional medical complications, such as thrombocytopenia, IVIG may be appropriate (Cowchock 1998, Piette et al 2000).

Other thrombophilic abnormalities

While APS is an acquired autoimmune thrombophilic state, recurrent miscarriage is also associated with other inherited and acquired causes of thrombophilia (Blumenfeld and Brenner 1999). Most studies are retrospective and interpretation must be cautious because of problems with acquisition and ascertainment.

Activated protein C resistance, usually but not always inherited via factor V Leiden mutation, is an important cause of acquired venous thrombosis and thrombophilia (Bertina et al 1994). It is also associated with recurrent fetal loss (Brenner et al 1997). Successful treatment with low-dose aspirin and heparin has been reported, although there are no prospective controlled studies to date.

Hyperhomocysteinaemia, as a result of congenital enzyme deficiencies or vitamin B6, B9 and B12 deficiencies, is associated with thrombosis and premature vascular disease (Boers et al 1985). It has also been reported in association with recurrent pregnancy loss (Wouters et al 1993). Thromboprophylaxis and vitamin supplementation have been reported (Aubard et al 2000), but no prospective data are yet available.

Other inherited thrombophilias, including protein S and protein C deficiency and antithrombin III deficiency, are associated with recurrent miscarriage as well as late pregnancy complications (Girling and de Swiet 1998). These need to be managed with appropriate haematological experience because of the increased risk of thromboembolism during pregnancy.

Screening women who have a history of recurrent miscarriage has shown increased incidence of thrombin generation — a global marker of a prothrombotic state — even when not pregnant (Vincent et al 1998). Further research is needed to determine whether thromboprophylaxis is appropriate for these women.

Alloimmune factors

The possibility that maternal alloimmune abnormalities lead to recurrent miscarriage has been proposed but remains contentious, and there is no reliable test. Treatments involving immunization with trophoblast or paternal leukocytes

---

> **Box 23.3** Clinical features associated with antiphospholipid antibodies
>
> ### Obstetrics and gynaecology
> - Recurrent miscarriage
> - Pre-eclampsia
> - Placental abruption
> - Intrauterine growth retardation
> - Chorea gravidarum
>
> ### Dermatological
> - Livido reticularis
> - Cutaneous necrosis
>
> ### Vascular
> - Venous thrombosis
> - Arterial thrombosis
> - Mitral valve disease
> - Thrombotic endocarditis
>
> ### Neurological
> - Transient ischaemic attacks
> - Cerebrovascular accidents
> - Migraine
> - Epilepsy
> - Multiple sclerosis

or third-party leukocytes have been successfully used in women with recurrent miscarriage. However, results of prospective randomized trials and meta-analyses have only shown minimal benefit or no benefit with treatment (Daya and Gunby 1994, Recurrent Miscarriage Immunotherapy Trialists Group 1994, Ober et al 1999). Any potential benefit must be balanced against the risk of the treatment, and at the present time, allogenic immunization should only be offered in the context of a clinical trial. Current recommendations, both in the UK and the USA, are against treatment.

Investigations

The known causes and management of recurrent miscarriage have been detailed above. Necessary investigations to identify such causes are indicated in women with recurrent miscarriage (Box 23.4). Testing thyroid function, random glucose, autoantibody screen and TORCH screen are no longer appropriate (Li 1998).

Women with recurrent miscarriage are best cared for by a careful history (ideally with a structured history sheet or questionnaire), thorough investigation, sympathetic explanation and counselling. This is best managed in the context of a dedicated recurrent miscarriage clinic. Women who conceive should then be offered early pregnancy clinic follow-up with ultrasonography and supportive care.

Treatment of unexplained recurrent miscarriage

Treatment of recurrent miscarriage where a potential cause has been identified has been discussed above. In approximately 50% of recurrent miscarriages, no cause is determined. The prognosis for this group is usually good. The value of continued reassurance and psychological support has been demonstrated (Stray-Pedersen and Stray-Pedersen 1984), with a 75% chance of a live birth in unexplained recurrent miscarriage. This support should include care in a specialist clinic, psychological support, easy access to a named contact, close monitoring including ultrasonography, appropriate reassurance, and helpful and caring staff.

Treatment of unproven value should not be offered. Any empirical treatment or treatment in clinical trials needs to have a sound scientific and statistical basis, and should

---

Box 23.4 Investigation for recurrent miscarriage

- Male and female chromosome analysis
- Anticardiolipin antibody
- Lupus anticoagulant
- Clotting studies
- Activated and modified protein C resistance
- Factor V Leiden mutation
- Early-follicular-phase LH and follicle-stimulating hormone
- Pelvic ultrasound scan
- Hysterosalpingogram
- Hysteroscopy
- Laparoscopy

---

include careful counselling and informed consent (Clifford et al 1994, Liddell et al 1997).

Counselling

Counselling should be offered to all patients attending a recurrent miscarriage clinic. It should include an explanation of the possible underlying causes and prognoses. After three consecutive early pregnancy losses, there remains a 60–70% chance that the next pregnancy will be successful (Edmonds 1992, Li 1998). This chance decreases with each subsequent miscarriage, although even after six miscarriages, the chance of a successful pregnancy is still over 45%.

Conclusion

Recurrent miscarriage needs to be differentiated from sporadic miscarriage, and investigated thoroughly. Careful evaluation and treatment of this aetiologically diverse condition are necessary. Continued research into the causes and effective treatments is appropriate and best managed through a dedicated recurrent miscarriage clinic.

Sporadic miscarriage is common and increasing in incidence because of increasing maternal age. The majority of these are unlikely to recur. Management may involve expectant and medical treatment as well as surgical evacuation.

KEY POINTS

1. Miscarriage is the most common complication of pregnancy and accounts for the majority of emergency gynaecology consultations and admissions.

2. The term 'abortion' should be avoided and more sensitive terminology substituted.

3. Miscarriage is defined as the loss of an intrauterine pregnancy before 24 completed weeks of gestation.

4. Sporadic miscarriage occurs in approximately 15% of all clinically recognized pregnancies, and this rises with maternal age.

5. Most early miscarriages are the result of chromosomal abnormalities. The most common is trisomy.

6. Treatment of miscarriage is usually with surgical uterine evacuation, although medical and expectant management should be discussed. There is a small mortality rate with miscarriage, usually due to haemorrhage or sepsis.

7. Recurrent miscarriage is defined as three consecutive miscarriages. Recurrent miscarriage should be distinguished from sporadic miscarriage.

8. Recurrent miscarriage should be investigated and managed in a specialist clinic. Empirical treatments should be avoided.

9. All treatments for recurrent miscarriage need to be evaluated in controlled randomized prospective trials because of the high likelihood of live birth in any placebo group.

References

Aarts JM, Brons JT, Bruinse HW 1995 Emergency cerclage: a review. Obstetrical and Gynecological Survey 50: 459–469.

Alberman E 1987 Maternal age and spontaneous abortion. In: Bennett MJ (ed) Spontaneous and Recurrent Abortion. Blackwell Science, Oxford.

Alberman E 1992 Spontaneous abortions: epidemiology. In: Stabile I, Grudzinskas G, Chard T (eds) Spontaneous Abortion — Diagnosis and Treatment. Springer-Verlag, London.

Althuisius SM, Dekker GA, van Geijn HP, Bekedam DJ, Hummel P 2000 Cervical incompetence prevention randomized cerclage trial (CIPRACT): study design and preliminary results. American Journal of Obstetrics and Gynecology 183: 823–829.

Ashok PW, Penney GC, Flett GM, Templeton A 1998 An effective regimen for early medical abortion: a report of 2000 consecutive cases. Human Reproduction 13: 2962–2965.

Ashton D, Amin HK, Richart RM, Neuwirth RS 1988 The incidence of asymptomatic uterine anomalies in women undergoing transcervical tubal sterilization. Obstetrics and Gynecology 72: 28–30.

Aubard Y, Darodes N, Cantaloube M, Aubard V, Diallo D, Teissier MP 2000 Hyperhomocysteinemia and pregnancy: a dangerous association. Journal of Obstetrics, Gynecology and Reproduction (Paris) 29: 363–372.

Ayhan A, Yücel I, Tuncer ZS, Kisnisçi HA 1992 Reproductive performance after conventional metroplasty: an evaluation of 102 cases. Fertility and Sterility 57: 1194–1196.

Ayres-de-Campos D, Teixeira-da-Silva J, Campos I, Patrício B 2000 Vaginal misoprostol in the management of first trimester missed abortions. International Journal of Gynecology and Obstetrics 71: 53–57.

Bakas C, Zarou DM, de Caprariis PJ 1996 First-trimester spontaneous abortions and the incidence of human immunodeficiency virus seropositivity. Journal of Reproductive Medicine 41: 15–18.

Baxter N, Sumiya M, Cheng S et al 2001 Recurrent miscarriage and variant alleles of mannose binding lectin and tumour necrosis factor genes. Clinical and Experimental Immunology 126: 529–534.

Beeby D, Morgan Hughes JO 1984 Oxytocic drugs and anaesthesia. A controlled clinical trial of ergometrine, syntocinon and normal saline during evacuation of the uterus after spontaneous abortion. Anaesthesia 39: 764–767.

Bennett MJ 1987 Congenital abnormalities of the fundus. In: Bennett MJ, Edmonds DK (eds) Spontaneous and Recurrent Abortion. Blackwell Science, Oxford.

Ben-Rafael Z, Seidman DS, Recabi K, Bider D, Mashiach S 1991 Uterine anomalies: a retrospective matched-control study. Journal of Reproductive Medicine 36: 723–727.

Bertina RM, Koeleman BP, Koster T et al 1994 Mutation in blood coagulation factor V associated with resistance to activated protein C. Nature 369: 64–67.

Blumenfeld Z, Brenner B 1999 Thrombophilic-associated pregnancy wastage. Fertility and Sterility 72: 765–774.

Boers GH, Smals AG, Trijbels FJ et al 1985 Heterozygosity for homocystinuria in premature peripheral and cerebral occlusive arterial disease. New England Journal of Medicine 313: 709–715.

Boué A, Gallano P 1984 A collaborative study of the segregation of inherited structural arrangements in 1356 prenatal diagnoses. Prenatal Diagnosis 4: 45–67.

Boué J, Boué A, Lazar P 1975 Retrospective and prospective epidemiological studies of 1500 karyotyped spontaneous human abortions. Teratology 12: 11–26.

Brambati B 1990 Fate of human pregnancies. In: Edwards RG (ed) Serono Symposia: Establishing a Successful Human Pregnancy, Vol. 66. Raven Press, New York.

Brenner B, Mandel H, Lanir N et al 1997 Activated protein C resistance can be associated with recurrent fetal loss. British Journal of Haematology 97: 551–554.

Bussen S, Steck T 1995 Thyroid autoantibodies in euthyroid non-pregnant women with recurrent spontaneous abortions. Human Reproduction 10: 2938–2940.

Bussen S, Sutterlin M, Steck T 1999 Endocrine abnormalities during the follicular phase in women with recurrent spontaneous abortion. Human Reproduction 14: 18–20.

Cain AC, Erikson ME, Fast I et al 1964 Children's disturbed reaction to their mothers' miscarriage. Psychosomatic Medicine 26: 58–66.

Candiani GB, Fedele L, Parazzini F, Zamberletti D 1990 Reproductive prognosis after abdominal metroplasty in bicornuate or septate uterus: a life-table analysis. British Journal of Obstetrics and Gynaecology 97: 613–617.

Carey JC, Klebanoff MA, Hauth JC et al 2000 Metronidazole to prevent preterm delivery in pregnant women with asymptomatic bacterial vaginosis. National Institute of Child Health and Human Development of Maternal-Fetal Medicine Units. New England Journal of Medicine 342: 534–540.

Carreras LO, Perez GN, Vega HR et al 1988 Lupus anticoagulant and recurrent fetal loss: successful treatment with gammaglobulin. Fertility and Sterility 54: 991–994.

Chard T 1991 Frequency of implantation and early pregnancy loss in natural cycles.

Baillière's Clinical Obstetrics and Gynaecology 5: 179–189.

Chung TK, Cheung LP, Lau WC, Haines CJ, Chang AM 1994 Spontaneous abortion: a medical approach to management. Australia and New Zealand Journal of Obstetrics and Gynaecology 34: 432–436.

Clifford K, Rai R, Watson H, Regan L 1994 An informative protocol for the investigation of recurrent miscarriage: preliminary experience of 500 cases. Human Reproduction 9: 1328–1332.

Clifford K, Rai R, Watson H, Franks S, Regan L 1996 Does suppressing luteinising hormone secretion reduce the miscarriage rate? Results of a randomised controlled trial. BMJ (Clinical Research Ed.) 312: 1508–1511.

Cohen EN, Belville JW, Brown BW 1971 Anesthesia, pregnancy and miscarriage: a study of operating room nurses and anesthetists. Anesthesiology 35: 343–347.

Cowchock S 1998 Treatment of antiphospholipid syndrome in pregnancy. Lupus 7 (Suppl 2): S95–S97.

Creasy MR, Crolla JA, AlbermanAlberman ED 1976 A cytogenetic study of human spontaneous abortions using banding techniques. Human Genetics 31: 177–196.

Csapo AI, Pulkinnen MO, Wiest WG 1973 Effects of lutectomy and progesterone replacement therapy in early pregnant patients. American Journal of Obstetrics and Gynecology 115: 759–765.

Daya S 1989 Efficacy of progesterone support for pregnancy in women with recurrent miscarriage. A meta-analysis of controlled trials. British Journal of Obstetrics and Gynaecology 96: 275–280.

Daya S 1993 Evaluation and management of recurrent spontaneous abortion. Current Opinion in Obstetrics and Gynecology 8: 188–192.

Daya S, Gunby J 1994 The effectiveness of allogeneic leukocyte immunization in unexplained primary recurrent spontaneous abortion. Recurrent Miscarriage Immunotherapy Trialists Group. American Journal of Reproductive Immunology 32: 294–302.

Daya S, Gunby J, Porter F, Scott J, Clark DA 1999 Critical analysis of intravenous immunoglobulins therapy for recurrent miscarriage. Human Reproduction 5: 475–482.

Deaton JL, Honoré GM, Huffman CS, Bauguess P. 1997 Early transvaginal ultrasound following an accurately dated pregnancy: the importance of finding a yolk sac or fetal heart motion. Human Reproduction 12: 2820–2823.

Dhalial RK, Machin AM, Tait SM 1970 Chromosomal anomalies in spontaneously aborted human fetuses. Lancet 2: 20–21.

Dijkstra K, Funai EF, O'Neill L, Rebarber A, Paidas MJ, Young BK 2000 Change in cervical length as a predictor of preterm delivery. Obstetrics and Gynecology 96: 346–350.

D'Ubaldo C, Pezzotti P, Rezza G, Branca M, Ippolito G 1998 Association between HIV-1 infection and miscarriage: a group retrospective study. DIANAIDS Collaborative Study Group. AIDS 12: 1087–1093.

Duncan PG, Pope WD, Cohen MM, Greer N 1986 Fetal risk of anesthesia and surgery during pregnancy. Anesthesiology 64: 790–794.

Edmonds DK 1992 Spontaneous and recurrent abortion. In: Shaw R, Soutter P, Stanton S (eds) Gynaecology, 2nd edn. Churchill Livingstone, Edinburgh.

Edmonds DK, Lindsay KS, Miller JF, Williamson E, Wood PJ 1982 Early embryonic mortality in women. Fertility and Sterility 38: 447–453.

Edwards A, Megens A, Peek M, Wallace EM 2000 Sexual origins of placental dysfunction. The Lancet 355: 203–204.

Egwuatu VE 1989 Fertility and fetal salvage among women with uterine leiomyomas in a Nigerian teaching hospital. International Journal of Fertility 34: 341–346.

el-Refaey H, Hinshaw K, Henshaw R, Smith N, Templeton A 1992 Medical management of missed abortion and anembryonic pregnancy. BMJ (Clinical Research Ed.) 305: 1399.

Fawcus S, McIntyre J, Jewkes RK et al 1997 Management of incomplete abortions at South African public hospitals. National Incomplete Abortion Study Reference Group. South African Medical Journal 87: 438–442.

Frank P 1985 Sequelae of induced abortion. In: Abortion: Medical and Social Implications. Pitman, London.

French FE, Bierman JM 1962 Probabilities of fetal mortality. Public Health Report 77: 835–847.

Gianaroli L, Magli MC, Ferraretti AP, Fortini D, Tabanelli C, Gergolet M 2000 Gonadal activity and chromosomal constitution of in vitro generated embryos. Molecular and Cellular Endocrinology 161: 111–116.

Gibb DM, Salaria DA 1995 Transabdominal cervicoisthmic cerclage in the management of recurrent second trimester miscarriage and preterm delivery. British Journal of Obstetrics and Gynaecology 102: 802–806.

Girling J, de Swiet M 1998 Inherited thrombophilia and pregnancy. Current Opinion in Obstetrics and Gynecology 10: 135–144.

Glock JL, Brumsted JR 1995 Color-flow pulsed Doppler ultrasound in diagnosing luteal phase defect. Fertility and Sterility 64: 500–504.

Goldstein P, Berrier J, Rosen S et al 1989 Hormone administration for the maintenance of pregnancy. In: Chalmers I, Enkin M, Kierse MJNC (eds) Effective Care in Pregnancy and Childbirth. Oxford University Press, Oxford.

Grudzinskas JG, Chard T 1992 Assessment of early pregnancy: measurement of fetoplacental hormones and proteins. In: Stabile I, Grudzinskas G, Chard T (eds) Spontaneous Abortion. Springer-Verlag, Berlin.

Gupta JK, Johnson N 1992 Should we use prostaglandins, tents, or progesterone antagonists for cervical ripening before first trimester abortion? Contraception 46: 489–497.

Halmesmäki E, Valimaki M, Roine R, Ylikahri R, Ylikorkala O 1989 Maternal and paternal alcohol consumption and miscarriage. British Journal of Obstetrics and Gynaecology 96: 188–191.

Hamilton SM 1989 Should follow-up be provided after miscarriage? British Journal of Obstetrics and Gynaecology 96: 743–745.

Hamilton-Fairley D, Donaghy J 1997 Surgical versus expectant management of first trimester miscarriage: a prospective observational study. In: Grudzinskas JG, O'Brien PMS (eds) Problems in early pregnancy. RCOG Press, London.

Hanson U, Persson B, Thunell S 1990 Relationship between haemoglobin A1C in early type (insulin dependent) diabetic pregnancy and the occurrence of spontaneous abortion and fetal malformation in Sweden. Diabetologia 33: 100–104.

Harlap S, Shapiro PH 1980 Alcohol, smoking and incidence of spontaneous abortions in the first and second trimester. The Lancet 2: 2.

Harris EN 1987 Syndrome of the black swan. British Journal of Rheumatology 26: 324–326.

Hassold T, Chen N, Funkhouser J et al 1980 A cytogenetic study of 1000 spontaneous abortions. Annals of Human Genetics 44: 151–178.

Hay PE, Lamont RF, Taylor-Robinson D 1994 Abnormal bacterial colonisation of the genital tract and subsequent pre-term delivery and late miscarriage. BMJ (Clinical Research Ed.) 308: 295–299.

Heinonen PK 1997 Reproductive performance of women with uterine anomalies after abdominal or hysteroscopic metroplasty or no surgical treatment. Journal of the American Association of Gynecological Laparoscopists 4: 311–317.

Hendrick PW 1988 HLA-sharing, recurrent spontaneous abortion, and the genetic hypothesis. Genetics 119: 199–204.

Henshaw RC, Cooper K, el-Refaey H, Smith NC, Templeton AA 1993 Medical management of miscarriage: non-surgical uterine evacuation of incomplete and inevitable spontaneous abortion. BMJ (Clinical Research Ed.): 894–895.

Hertig AT, Livingstone RG 1944 Spontaneous, threatened and habitual abortion: their pathogenesis and treatment. New England Journal of Medicine 230: 797–806.

Hertig AT, Rock J, Adams EC, Menkin MC 1959 Thirty-four fertilised human ova, good, bad and indifferent, recovered from 210 women of known fertility. A study of biologic wastage in early human pregnancy. Pediatrics 23: 202–211.

Hirahara F, Andoh N, Sawai K, Hirabuki T, Uemura T, Minaguchi H 1998 Hyperprolactinaemic recurrent miscarriage and results of randomised bromocriptine treatment trials. Fertility and Sterility 70: 246–252.

Homburg R, Armar NA, Eshel A, Adams J, Jacobs HS 1988 Influence of serum luteinising hormone concentrations on ovulation, conception, and early pregnancy loss in polycystic ovary syndrome. BMJ (Clinical Research Ed.) 297: 1024–1026.

Hopper E 1997 Psychological consequences of early pregnancy loss. In: Grudzinskas JG, O'Brien PMS (eds) Problems in Early Pregnancy. RCOG Press, London.

Howles CM, Macnamee MC, Edwards RG 1987 Follicular development and early luteal function of conception and non-conception cycles after in-vitro fertilization: endocrine correlates. Human Reproduction 2: 17–21.

Hurd WW, Whitfield RR, Randolph JF Jr, Kercher ML 1997 Expectant management versus elective curettage for the treatment of spontaneous abortion. Fertility and Sterility 68: 601–606.

Hustin J, Jauniaux E 1997 Mechanisms and pathology of miscarriage. In: Grudzinskas JG, O'Brien PMS (eds) Problems in Early Pregnancy. RCOG Press, London.

Jordan J, Craig K, Clifton DK, Soules MR 1994 Luteal phase defect: the sensitivity and specificity of diagnostic methods in common clinical use. Fertility and Sterility 62: 54–62.

Jurkovic D, Geipel A, Gruboeck K, Jauniaux E, Natucci M, Campbell S 1995 Three-dimensional ultrasound for the assessment of uterine anatomy and detection of congenital anomalies: a comparison with hysterosalpingography and two-dimensional ultrasound. Obstetrics and Gynecology 5: 233–237.

Jurkovic D, Ross JA, Nicolaides KH 1998 Expectant management of missed miscarriage. British Journal of Obstetrics and Gynaecology 105: 670–671.

Kajii T, Ferrier A, Niikawa N, Takahara H, Ohama K, Avirachan S 1980 Anatomic and chromosomal anomalies in 639 spontaneous abortuses. Human Genetics 55: 87–98.

Kaplan B, Pardo J, Rabinerson D, Fisch B, Neri A 1996 Future fertility following conservative management of abortion. Human Reproduction 11: 92–94.

Katz VL, Kuller JA 1994 Recurrent miscarriage. American Journal of Perinatology 11: 386–397.

Kellokumpu-Lethtinen P, Pelliniemei LJ 1984 Sex ratio of human conceptuses. Obstetrics and Gynecology 64: 220–222.

Klebanoff MA, Levine RJ, DerSimonian R, Clemens JD, Wilkins DG 1999 Maternal serum paraxanthine, a caffeine metabolite, and the risk of spontaneous abortion. New England Journal of Medicine 341: 1639–1644.

Kline J, Shrout P, Stein Z, Susser M, Warburton D 1980 Drinking during pregnancy and spontaneous abortion. The Lancet 2: 176–180.

Kline J, Stein Z, Susser M 1989 Conception to birth — epidemiology of prenatal development. In: Kline J (ed) Monographs in Epidemiology and Biostatistics, Vol. 14. Oxford University Press, Oxford.

Lawson HW, Frye A, Atrash HK, Smith JC, Shulman HB, Ramick M 1994 Abortion mortality, United States, 1972 through 1987. American Journal of Obstetrics and Gynecology 171: 1365–1372.

Li TC 1998 Recurrent miscarriage: principles of management. Human Reproduction 13: 478–482.

Li TC, Cooke ID 1991 Evaluation of the luteal phase: a review. Human Reproduction 6: 484–499.

Li TC, Dockery P, Cooke ID 1991 Endometrial development in the luteal phase of women with various types of infertility: comparison of women with normal fertility. Human Reproduction 6: 325–330.

Liddell HS, Sowden K, Farquhar CM 1997 Recurrent miscarriage: screening for polycystic ovaries and subsequent pregnancy outcome. Australia and New Zealand Journal of Obstetrics and Gynaecology 37: 402–406.

Llahi-Camp JM, Rai R, Ison C, Regan L, Taylor-Robinson D 1996 Association of bacterial vaginosis and a history of second trimester miscarriage. Human Reproduction 11: 1575–1578.

Lubbe WF, Butler WS, Palmer SJ, Liggins GC 1983 Fetal survival after prednisone suppression of maternal lupus anticoagulant. The Lancet 1: 1361–1363.

Lupus Anticoagulant Working Party on behalf of the BSCH Homeostasis and Thrombosis Task Force 1991 Guidelines on testing for the lupus anticoagulant. Journal of Clinical Pathology 44: 885–889.

MacDonald IA 1957 Suture of the cervix for inevitable miscarriage. Journal of Obstetrics and Gynecology of the British Empire 64: 731–735.

McDonald AD, McDonald JC, Armstrong B et al 1988 Fetal death and work in pregnancy. British Journal of Industrial Medicine 45: 148–157.

Mansur MM 1992 Ultrasound diagnosis of complete abortion can reduce need for curettage. European Journal of Obstetrics, Gynecology and Reproductive Biology 44: 65–69.

Medical Research Council/Royal College of Obstetricians and Gynaecologists Working Party on Cervical Cerclage 1993 Final report of the Medical Research Council/ Royal College of Obstetricians and Gynaecologists multicentre randomised

trial of cervical cerclage. British Journal of Obstetrics and Gynaecology 100: 516–523.

Mikkelson M 1985 Cytogenetic findings in first trimester chorionic villus sampling. In: Fraccaro G, Simoni G, Brambati B (eds) First Trimester Fetal Diagnosis. Springer-Verlag, Berlin.

Miller H, Durant JA, Ross DM, O'Connell FJ 1969 Corpus luteum deficiency as a cause of early recurrent abortion: a case history. Fertility and Sterility 20: 433–438.

Miller JF, Williamson E, Glue J, Gordon YB, Grudzinskas JG, Sykes A 1980 Fetal loss after implantation: a prospective study. The Lancet 2: 554–556.

Mills JL, Simpson JL, Driscoll SG et al 1988 Incidence of spontaneous abortion amongst normal women and insulin dependent diabetic women whose pregnancies were identified within 21 days of conception. New England Journal of Medicine 319: 1617–1623.

Mur JM, Mandereau L, Deplan F, Paris A, Richard A, Hemon D 1992 Spontaneous abortion and exposure to vinyl chloride. The Lancet 339: 127–128.

Nahmias AJ, Josey WE, Naib ZM, Freeman MG, Fernandez RJ, Wheeler JH 1971 Perinatal risk associated with maternal genital herpes simplex virus infection. American Journal of Obstetrics and Gynecology 110: 825–837.

Ness RB, Grisso JA, Hirschinger N et al 1999 Cocaine and tobacco use and the risk of spontaneous abortion. New England Journal of Medicine 340: 333–339.

Neugebauer R, Kline J, O'Connor P et al 1992 Depressive symptoms in women in the six months following miscarriage. American Journal of Obstetrics and Gynecology 166: 104–109.

Neugebauer R, Kline J, Stein Z et al 1996 Association of stressful life events with chromosomally normal spontaneous abortion. American Journal of Epidemiology 143: 588–596.

Nielsen S, Hahlin M 1995 Expectant management of spontaneous first trimester abortion. The Lancet 345: 84–86.

Nybo Andersen AM, Wohlfahrt J, Christens P, Olsen J, Melbye M 2000 Maternal age and fetal loss: population based register linkage. BMJ (Clinical Research Ed.) 320: 1708–1712.

Ober C, Karrison T, Odem RR et al 1999 Mononuclear-cell immunisation in prevention of recurrent miscarriages: a randomised trial. The Lancet 354: 365–369.

Okon MA, Laird SM, Tuckerman EM, Li TC 1998 Serum androgen levels in women who have recurrent miscarriages and their correlation with markers of endometrial function. Fertility and Sterility 69: 682–690.

Pabuccu R, Atay V, Urman B, Ergun A, Orhon E 1995 Hysteroscopic treatment of septate uterus. Gynaecological Endoscopy 4: 213–215.

Parazzini F, Bocciolone L, La Vecchia C, Negri E, Fedele L 1990 Maternal and paternal moderate alcohol consumption and unexplained miscarriages. British Journal of Obstetrics and Gynaecology 97: 618–622.

Pedersen JF, Mantoni M 1990 Large intrauterine haematomata in threatened miscarriage. Frequency and clinical consequences. British Journal of Obstetrics and Gynaecology 97: 75–77.

Pegoraro E, Whitaker J, Mowery-Rushton P, Surti U, Lanasa M, Hoffman EP 1997 Familial skewed X inactivation: a molecular trait associated with high spontaneous abortion rate maps to Xq28. American Journal of Human Genetics 61: 160–170.

Pennell RG, Needleman L, Pajak T et al 1991 Prospective comparison of vaginal and abdominal sonography in normal early pregnancy. Journal of Ultrasound in Medicine 10: 63–67.

Piette JC, Le Thi Huong D, Wechsler B 2000 Therapeutic use of intravenous immunoglobulins in the antiphospholipid syndrome. Annales de Médicine Interne (Paris) 151(suppl 1): S51–S54.

Platz-Christiansen JJ, Nielsen S, Hamberger L 1995 Is misoprostol the drug of choice for induced cervical ripening in early pregnancy termination? Acta Obstetrica et Gynaecologica Scandinavica 74: 809–812.

Prendiville WG 1995 HCG for recurrent miscarriage. In: Enkin MW, Keirse MJNC, Renfrew MJ et al (eds) Pregnancy and childbirth module (CD-ROM). Cochrane Database. Update Software, Oxford.

Prieto JA, Eriksen NL, Blanco JD 1995 A randomised trial of prophylactic doxycycline for curettage in incomplete abortion. Obstetrics and Gynecology 85: 692–696.

Quenby SM, Farquharson RG 1994 Human chorionic gonadotrophin supplementation in recurring pregnancy loss: a controlled trial. Fertility and Sterility 62: 708–710.

Rai RS, Clifford K, Cohen H, Regan L 1995a High prospective fetal loss rate in untreated pregnancies of women with recurrent miscarriage and antiphospholipid antibodies. Human Reproduction 10: 3301–3304.

Rai RS, Regan L, Clifford K et al 1995b Antiphospholipid antibodies and beta2-glycoprotein-I in 500 women with recurrent miscarriage: results of a comprehensive screening approach. Human Reproduction 10: 2001–2005.

Rai R, Cohen H, Dave M, Regan L 1997 Randomised controlled trial of aspirin and aspirin plus heparin in pregnant women with recurrent miscarriage associated with phospholipid antibodies (or antiphospholipid antibodies). BMJ (Clinical Research Ed.) 314: 253–257.

Rai R, Regan L 1998 Antiphospholipid syndrome and pregnancy loss. Hospital Medicine 59: 637–639.

Rai R, Backos M, Rushworth F, Regan L 2000 Polycystic ovaries and recurrent miscarriage — a reappraisal. Human Reproduction 15: 612–615.

Ratnam SS, Prasad RNV 1990 Medical management of abnormal pregnancy. Baillière's Clinical Obstetrics and Gynaecology 4: 361–374.

Recurrent Miscarriage Immunotherapy Trialists Group 1994 Worldwide collaborative observational study and meta-analysis on allogenic leukocyte immunotherapy for recurrent spontaneous abortion. American Journal of Reproductive Immunology 32: 55–72.

Regan L 1997 Sporadic and recurrent miscarriage. In: Grudizinskas JG, O'Brien PMS (eds) Problems in Early Pregnancy — Advances in Diagnosis and Management. RCOG Press, London.

Regan L, Braude P, Trembath PL 1989 Influence of past reproductive performance on risk of spontaneous abortion. BMJ (Clinical Research Ed.) 299: 541–545.

Regan L, Owen EJ, Jacobs HS 1990 Hypersecretion of luteinising hormone, infertility, and miscarriage. The Lancet 336: 1141–1144.

Roberts CJ, Lowe DB 1975 Where have all the conceptions gone? The Lancet 1: 498.

Rosove MH, Tabsh K, Wasserstrum N, Howard P, Hahn BH, Kalunian KC 1990 Heparin therapy for pregnant women with lupus anticoagulant or anticardiolipin antibodies. Obstetrics and Gynecology 75: 630–634.

Rowland AS, Baird DD, Shore DL, Darden B, Wilcox AJ 1996 Ethylene oxide exposure may increase the risk of spontaneous abortion, preterm birth and postterm birth. Epidemiology 7: 363–368.

Royal College of General Practitioners/Royal College of Obstetricians and Gynaecologists 1985 Induced abortion operations and their early sequelae. Journal of the Royal College of General Practitioners 35: 175–180.

Royal College of Obstetricians and Gynaecologists 2001 Infection and Pregnancy. RCOG Press, London.

Rushton DI 1995 Pathology of abortion. In: Fox H (ed) Haines and Taylor Obstetrical and Gynecological Pathology. Churchill Livingstone, Edinburgh.

Rushworth FH, Backos M, Rai R, Chilcott IT, Baxter N, Regan L 2000 Prospective pregnancy outcome in untreated recurrent miscarriers with thyroid autoantibodies. Human Reproduction 15: 1637–1639.

Russell PB 1947 Abortions treated conservatively: a twelve year study covering 3739 cases. Southern Medical Journal 40: 314–324.

Schiverick KT, Salafia C 1999 Cigarette smoking and pregnancy I: ovarian, uterine and placental effects. Placenta 20: 265–272.

Schmidt-Sarosi C, Schwartz LB, Lublin J, Kaplan-Grazi D, Sarosi P, Perle MA 1998 Chromosomal analysis of early fetal losses in relation to transvaginal ultrasonographic detection of fetal heart motion after infertility. Fertility and Sterility 69: 274–277.

Scibetta JJ, Sanko SR, Phipps WR 1998 Laparoscopic transabdominal cervicoisthmic cerclage. Fertility and Sterility 69: 161–163.

Sebire NJ, Thornton S, Hughes K, Snijders RJ, Nicolaides KH 1997a The prevalence and consequences of missed abortion in twin pregnancies at 10 and 14 weeks of gestation. British Journal of Obstetrics and Gynaecology 104: 847–848.

Sebire NJ, Snijders RJ, Hughes K, Sepulveda W, Nicolaides KH 1997b The hidden mortality of monochorionic twin pregnancies. British Journal of Obstetrics and Gynaecology 104: 1203–1207.

Seibel M, Graves WL 1980 The psychological implication of spontaneous abortion. Journal of Reproductive Medicine 25: 161–172.

Serle E, Aplin JD, Li TC et al 1994 Endometrial differentiation in the preimplantation phase of women with recurrent miscarriage: a morphological and immunohistochemical study. Fertility and Sterility 62: 989–996.

Shephard TH, Fantel AG, Fitzsimmons J 1989 Congenital defect rates among spontaneous abortuses: twenty years of monitoring. Teratology 39: 325–331.

Shirodkar VM 1960 Contributions to Obstetrics and Gynaecology. Churchill Livingstone, Edinburgh.

Silver RK, MacGregor SN, Sholl JS, Hobart JM, Neerhof MG, Ragin A 1993 Comparative trial of prednisone plus aspirin versus aspirin alone in the treatment of anticardiolipin antibody-positive obstetric patients. American Journal of Obstetrics and Gynecology 169: 1411–1417.

Simpson JL, Gray RH, Queenan JT et al 1996 Further evidence that infection is an infrequent cause of first trimester spontaneous abortion. Human Reproduction 11: 2058–2060.

Singh A, Dantas ZN, Stone SC, Asch RH 1995 Presence of thyroid antibodies in early reproductive failure: biochemical versus clinical pregnancies. Fertility and Sterility 63: 277–281.

Stabile I, Campbell S, Grudzinskas JG 1987 Ultrasound assessment in complications of first trimester pregnancy. The Lancet 2: 1237–1242.

Stanger JD, Yovich JL 1985 Reduced in vitro fertilisation of human oocytes from patients with raised basal luteinising hormone levels during the follicular phase. British Journal of Obstetrics and Gynaecology 92: 385–393.

Stephenson MD 1996 Frequency of factors associated with habitual abortion in 197 couples. Fertility and Sterility 66: 27–29.

Stirrat GM 1990 Recurrent miscarriage: I. Definitions and epidemiology. The Lancet 336: 673–675.

Stray-Pedersen B 1993 New aspects of perinatal infections. Annals of Medicine 25: 295.

Stray-Pedersen B, Stray-Pedersen S 1984 Etiological factors and subsequent reproductive performance in 195 couples with a prior history of habitual abortion. American Journal of Obstetrics and Gynecology 148: 140–146.

Takahara H, Ohama K, Fukiwara A 1977 Cytogenetic study in early spontaneous abortion. Hiroshima Journal of Medical Science 26: 291–296.

Takakuwa K, Asano K, Arakawa M, Yasuda M, Hasegawa I, Tanaka K 1997 Chromosome analysis of aborted conceptuses of recurrent aborters positive for anticardiolipin antibody. Fertility and Sterility 68: 54–58.

Therkelsen AJ, Grunnet N, Hjort T et al 1977 Studies in spontaneous abortion. In: Boué A, Thibault C (eds) Chromosomal Errors in Relation to Reproductive Failure. INSERM, Paris.

Tower CL, Regan L 2001 Intrauterine haematomas in a recurrent miscarriage population. Human Reproduction 16: 2005–2007.

Tulppala M, Stenman UH, Cacciatore B, Ylikorkala O 1993 Polycystic ovaries and levels of gonadotrophins and androgens in recurrent miscarriage: a prospective study of 50 women. British Journal of Obstetrics and Gynaecology 100: 438–352.

Tulppala M, Huhtaniemi I, Ylikorkala O 1998 Genetic variant of luteinizing hormone in women with a history of recurrent miscarriage. Human Reproduction 13: 2699–2702.

Verkuyl DA, Crowther CA 1993 Suction v. conventional curettage in incomplete abortion. A randomised controlled trial. South African Medical Journal 83: 13–15.

Vidal F, Rubio C, Simón C et al 2000 Is there a place for preimplantation genetic diagnosis screening in recurrent miscarriage patients? Journal of Reproduction and Fertility 55: 143–146.

Vincent T, Rai R, Regan L, Cohen H 1998 Increased thrombin generation in women with recurrent miscarriage. The Lancet 352: 116.

Warbuton D, Stein Z, Kline J et al 1980 Chromosome abnormalities in spontaneous abortions. In: Porter IH, Hook EB (eds) Human Embryonic and Fetal Deaths. Academic Press, New York.

Weigel MM, Weigel RM 1989 Nausea and vomiting of early pregnancy and pregnancy outcome. An epidemiological study. British Journal of Obstetrics and Gynaecology 96: 1304–1311.

Wilcox AJ, Weinberg CR, O'Connor JF et al 1988 Incidence of early loss in pregnancy.

New England Journal of Medicine 319: 189–194.

Windham GC, Von Behren J, Fenster L, Schaefer C, Swan SH 1997 Moderate maternal alcohol consumption and the risk of spontaneous abortion. Epidemiology 8: 509–514.

Wong GP, Farquharson DF, Dansereau J 1993 Emergency cervical cerclage: a retrospective review of 51 cases. American Journal of Perinatology 10: 341–347.

Wouters MG, Boers GH, Blom HJ et al 1993 Hyperhomocysteinemia: a risk factor in women with unexplained recurrent early pregnancy loss. Fertility and Sterility 60: 820.

Zemlickis D, Lishner M, Degendorfer P, Panzarella T, Sutcliffe SB, Koren G 1992 Fetal outcome after in utero exposure to cancer chemotherapy. Archives of Internal Medicine 152: 573–576.:

CHAPTER 24

Tubal disease

Ertan Saridogan, Essam El Mahdi and Ovrang Djahanbakhch

Chapter Contents

INTRODUCTION	353		**RESULTS**	359
AETIOLOGY OF TUBAL DISEASE	353		**CONCLUSION**	360
DIAGNOSIS	354		**KEY POINTS**	361
TREATMENT	355			

Introduction

The fallopian tube has many active roles in the process of reproduction. As the fallopian tube provides the environment in which fertilization and early development take place, these events may have a significant effect on all the subsequent events of the pregnancy. The role of the fallopian tube in the process of natural conception begins when the oocyte is released by the ruptured ovarian follicle and is picked up by the fimbrial end of the fallopian tube. It also facilitates the final maturation of sperm, which have passed through the uterus. Both the sperm and oocytes are transported within the fallopian tube to the site of fertilization and meet within well-defined, species-dependent time limits. Fertilization takes place at the ampullary–isthmic junction, and the pre-embryo is transported to the uterine cavity at the optimum time for implantation. Significantly, the sperm and pre-embryo, which differ antigenically from the mother, are not attacked by the immune system. The mechanisms by which all these complex processes are controlled are not well understood.

Ovum and embryo transport is probably the result of an interaction between the egg/embryo and the muscle contractions, ciliary activity and flow of tubal secretions. The relative importance of these factors is debatable, although there is evidence that ciliary activity plays a dominant role in gamete and embryo transport (Lyons et al 2006). Both myosalpingeal and ciliary activity are affected by a diverse range of chemical, biological and hormonal agents, including ovarian steroids, sympathomimetic agents, prostaglandins and angiotensin II (Jansen 1984, Saridogan et al 1996, Mahmood et al 1998).

Fallopian tubes probably act as sperm reservoirs, and this role may be essential for maintaining a certain number of sperm at the site of fertilization and preventing polyspermy by reducing the number of sperm available for fertilization. Sperm interaction with the tubal epithelium and secretions may also play an important role in the preparation of sperm for fertilization (Saridogan and Djahanbakhch 2009).

Tubal secretions contain proteins that derive from the plasma and also some specific substances synthesized within the oviduct itself (Maguiness et al 1992a). Both tubal proteins and the physical contact between the gametes and the tubal epithelium may play a role in gamete function (i.e. capacitation), fertilization and early embryo development (Djahanbakhch et al 1994, Kervancioglu et al 2000).

Aetiology of Tubal Disease

Tubal disease is usually defined as tubal damage caused by pelvic infection such as pelvic inflammatory disease or tuberculosis, endometriosis, surgery or salpingitis isthmica nodosa, with varying degrees of tubal damage or obstruction, sometimes involving the adjacent ovary and the pelvic peritoneum, and adhesion formation. As a result, patients with tubal damage suffer from infertility and/or pelvic pain. This definition does not cover functional defects of the fallopian tube, as our ability to describe tubal disease is currently limited to demonstrating its patency and macroscopic normality. Tubal disease is accountable for 30–40% of cases of female infertility.

Salpingitis

Most salpingitis is the result of an ascending infection from the lower genital tract, caused primarily by *Chlamydia trachomatis* and *Neisseria gonorrhoeae* (see Chapter 61, Pelvic inflammatory disease, and Chapter 62, Sexually transmitted infections, for more information). These micro-organisms cause mucopurulent endocervicitis, and break down major cervical barriers, such as the mucus plug that protects the endometrium and upper genital tract, and permits ascending infection. Other pathogens such as *Streptococcus* sp., *Escherichia coli* and anaerobes ascend through the breached barrier and reach the upper genital tract (Rice and Schachter 1991). In a significant proportion of cases, no aetiological agent is identified; this suggests that a range of other aetiological agents have a role, but the identification of novel organisms is difficult to ascertain because of the limited availability of diagnostic tests. Serological evidence has associated *Mycoplasma genitalium* with pelvic inflammatory disease (Simms and Stephenson 2009).

In the majority of patients, salpingitis is due to a sexually transmitted infection. In other cases, iatrogenic manoeuvres such as insertion of an intrauterine device, termination of pregnancy, hysterosalpingography or curettage can spread a cervical infection into the uterus and tubes. In a small proportion of women, pelvic infection may be secondary to gastrointestinal infections such as perforated appendicitis. *Mycobacterium tuberculosis* is still seen in developing countries; however, migration to developed countries has resulted in a significant increase in the number of tuberculosis notifications since the 1980s (Rose et al 2001).

Acute salpingitis causes loss of ciliated cells and distal occlusion of the fallopian tubes. Some of the deciliation may be recovered later, but subsequent immune response following the acute phase causes permanent scarring, loss of mucosal folds and flattening of the mucosa (Lyons et al 2006). Distal occlusion of the tubes together with chronic inflammatory process could result in fluid collection in the lumen of the fallopian tube, leading to hydrosalpinges. Pelvic peritonitis during the acute phase may be followed by adhesions around the fallopian tubes and ovaries, distorting the pelvic anatomy. Perihepatic inflammation may cause 'violin-string' adhesions known as 'Fitz–Hugh–Curtis syndrome' (Figures 24.1–24.3).

Other causes

Endometriosis, fibroids, previous pelvic/tubal surgery, salpingitis isthmica nodosa, endosalpingiosis and cornual polyps can be the cause of cornual obstruction or tubal damage. Endometriosis is reviewed in Chapter 33. In some patients, tubal damage is secondary to previous tubal or pelvic surgery such as salpingotomy for ectopic pregnancy, ovarian cystectomy, myomectomy, ovarian wedge resection and shortening of round ligaments. Salpingitis isthmica nodosa was described by Chiari (1887) as nodular thickening of the proximal part of the fallopian tube. The aetiology of this entity is unknown but it is probably due to a non-inflammatory process.

Diagnosis

Assessment of the fallopian tube should normally determine patency, a normal external and internal appearance, the ability to transport gametes and the embryo, and provision of an environment for the early steps of reproduction to occur. It is possible that, apart from the obvious need for tubal patency to allow passage of gametes, factors that affect the gametes and embryo, the effectors of tubal transport, the cilia, flow of tubal fluid and tubal contractions appear to constitute a higher-order system in which intact function of each may not be needed to achieve pregnancy (Verdugo 1986). However, dysfunction of this higher-order system

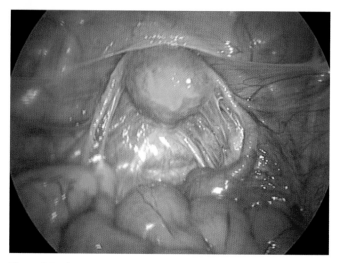

Figure 24.1 Laparoscopic view of a pelvis after pelvic inflammatory disease. There is a 'curtain' of adhesions covering the pelvic organs.

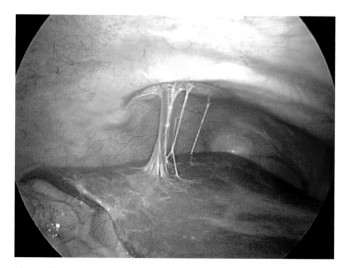

Figure 24.2 Laparoscopic photograph of perihepatic adhesions: Fitz–Hugh–Curtis syndrome.

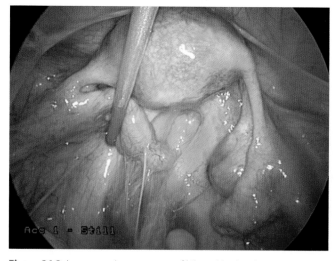

Figure 24.3 Laparoscopic appearance of bilateral hydrosalpinges as a result of previous inflammatory disease.

may be the reason for unsuccessful tubal surgery even when tubal patency has been achieved. Similarly, a functional disorder of this system may account for subfertility in some cases of unexplained infertility. Currently, tubal function is determined by demonstrating patency and normal appearance at laparoscopy.

The methods commonly used to determine tubal patency are hysterosalpingography (HSG), laparoscopy and hysterosalpingo contrast sonography (HyCoSy). The first two methods have been used for many years, whereas HyCoSy is a relatively new technique. All these methods have some degree of false-negative and false-positive results in determining tubal patency. A comparison of HSG and laparoscopy showed that complete agreement of tubal patency was found in 80.2% of cases (Maguiness et al 1992b). Laparoscopy has the ability to identify peritubal adhesions, endometriosis, polycystic ovaries, and other pelvic and intra-abdominal pathology. However, it is usually performed under general anaesthesia and does not give information about the uterine cavity. In general, these methods are considered complementary investigations, offering very important information (Figures 24.4–24.6). Laparoscopy also allows the surgeon to operate on abnormalities detected such as pelvic adhesions and endometriosis, provided that they have the relevant experience and the patient's consent has been obtained preoperatively.

The internal appearance of the fallopian tubes can be assessed by salpingoscopy. Salpingoscopy is the transabdominal examination of the tubal lumen by introducing an endoscope through the fimbrial end. Rigid endoscopes with a diameter of 2.8 mm allow excellent visualization of the infundibulum and ampulla as far as the ampullary–isthmic junction. The presence of minor intratubal lesions is not necessarily incompatible with fertility (Maguiness and Djahanbakhch 1992); however, loss of mucosal folds and intratubal fibrosis are significant. Nowadays, salpingoscopic assessment of the tubal lumen is recommended by some groups before tubal surgery for hydrosalpinges (Puttemans et al 1998). De Bruyne et al (1989) proposed a classification of ampullary findings in hydrosalpinges: grades 1 and 2 refer to normal salpingoscopic findings, grade 3 (intermediate group) refers to focal adhesions, and grades 4 and 5 refer to severe adhesions and loss of mucosal folds.

Transvaginal hydrolaparoscopy and fertiloscopy approaches utilize the advantages of laparoscopy but with a less invasive approach (Gordts et al 1998, Watrelot et al 1999). Transvaginal hydrolaparoscopy is the endoscopic examination of pelvic structures through the posterior vaginal fornix after instilling saline into the pouch of Douglas. This allows tubal patency to be checked, in addition to assessment of the pelvis for other pathology. Fertiloscopy includes salpingoscopy, microsalpingoscopy and hysteroscopy for complete examination of the female reproductive tract. These procedures can be performed under local anaesthesia or sedation.

Selective transcervical salpingography and tubal catheterization can be done in cases where it is doubtful that there is cornual obstruction (Ataya and Thomas 1991). Mucus plugs and debris can be mobilized, and a tube that was apparently obstructed can be 'opened' following such a procedure.

Treatment

The treatment of tubal disease in the infertile patient includes selective salpingography with tubal cannulation, surgery and

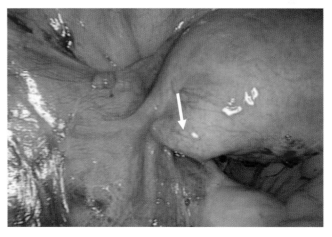

Figure 24.5 Tubal cornual block. Irregular vessels seen on the peritoneum surface as a result of previous inflammation (arrow).

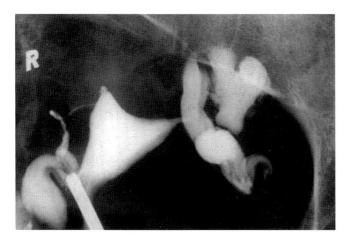

Figure 24.4 Hysterosalpingogram of a patient with bilateral hydrosalpinges.

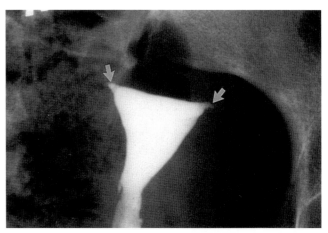

Figure 24.6 Hysterosalpingogram of a patient with bilateral tubal block (arrows).

in-vitro fertilization-embryo transfer (IVF-ET). In comparison with the other two options, IVF is now widely used for the majority of patients with tubal disease. However, it is relatively expensive, labour intensive and carries risks of multiple pregnancy and ovarian hyperstimulation syndrome (see Chapter 22, Assisted reproduction treatments, for more information).

Selective transcervical salpingography

Selective transcervical salpingography and tubal catheterization can be used for the treatment of proximal tubal obstruction in selected cases. A review of the literature on fluoroscopic tubal cannulation showed pregnancy rates of 22.7% and ectopic pregnancy rates of 3.2% (Honore et al 1999).

Reconstructive tubal surgery

With the advent of IVF-ET, the role of reconstructive tubal surgery has diminished. However, this type of surgery is still appropriate and effective for properly selected individuals (National Institute for Clinical Excellence 2004). Initial methods for tubal surgery were based on microsurgical techniques. The use of magnification and microsurgical techniques has been the traditional method. However, with advances in laparoscopic surgery, most of these methods are now possible to perform at laparoscopy.

The criteria for patient selection for treatment depend very much on the surgeon's experience and on the possibility of being able to offer alternative treatment. Other points to be considered when making the decision regarding treatment are the patient's wishes about the type of treatment that she prefers and the problem of pain. Large numbers of patients with tubal disease have pelvic pain. In some of them, the surgical freeing of the ovaries and tubes from adhesions can give symptomatic relief.

Microsurgical treatment

The microscope was first used for tubal surgery by Walz (1959). Whilst others used delicate electrosurgery and magnification (loupes) in the treatment of hydrosalpinges, Paterson and Wood (1974) in Australia and Winston and McClure-Browne (1974) in England adapted their experience from animal experiments to humans and operated on infertile women, under high magnification, using an operating microscope.

Microsurgery is not only the use of a microscope; it is based on gentle tissue handling, reperitonealization of raw areas, the use of non-resorbable suture materials, and irrigation of the tissues using Ringer's lactate solution as this tends to prevent adhesion formation.

The use of the microscope was originally much debated, but microsurgery is now well established and is a routine procedure for tubal infertility.

Coadjuvants

The use of coadjuvants can sometimes help to avoid adhesion formation, but it is important to keep in mind that no coadjuvant will replace good surgical technique. Recent reviews of methods for preventing adhesions suggest that none of the methods have been clearly shown to improve

pregnancy rates; however, some methods such as steroids, oxidized regenerated cellulose (Interceed) and polytetrafluoroethylene (Gore-Tex) reduce adhesion formation (Metwally et al 2006, Ahmad et al 2008).

Cornual occlusion

Cornual occlusion due to inflammatory causes was treated by uterotubal implantation with very poor results. Ehrler (1963) described his technique and suggested that the intramural portion of the tube could be spared in most patients. Microsurgical methods described by Winston (1977) and Gomel (1977) became the surgical technique of choice. Cornual implantation is now rarely used. Tubocornual implantation is avoided whenever possible. Destroying a possible sphincter at the uterotubal junction is associated with excessive bleeding and damage to the tubal blood supply; it shortens the tube and may increase the risk of rupture of the uterus in the event of subsequent pregnancy, which means that patients must be delivered by caesarean section.

The use of magnification allows better identification of the intramural portion of the tube by careful shaving of the cornua until healthy tissue is found, permitting a more accurate tissue apposition with a watertight anastomosis between healthy tubal tissues. Once the ends are well defined, the anastomosis is done in two layers, using 8/0 nylon as a suture. The suture material should not penetrate the mucosa, only the muscularis (Seki et al 1977). In some cases, the use of a temporary splint gives considerable help, especially in deep cornual tubal anastomosis (Figure 24.7), but this should be removed at the end of the surgical procedure; if left *in situ*, the splint should not remain for more than 48 h as longer periods of time cause mucosal damage. Tension between the anastomosed ends must be avoided. A stitch of 6/0 Prolene between both ends of the mesosalpinx should be applied as a stay suture. More details about the technique have been given elsewhere (Winston 1977, Margara 1982).

Cornual polyps

Removal of cornual polyps is still a matter of controversy. Glazener et al (1987) stated that the removal of cornual polyps does not improve fertility and they are not a cause of infertility. However, consideration should be given to removal of large polyps present in the intramural or isthmic portion of the tube. This can involve salpingotomy and resection of the polyp without tubal resection or the opening of the cornu, and removal of the affected portion of the tube followed by cornual–isthmic anastomosis in two layers. In some cases when a large polyp is implanted deep in the intramural portion of the tube, the anastomosis can be difficult due to disparity of the lumen of the tubal ends. The portion where the polyp was present is wider than the isthmic portion of the tube, and it is not always easy to achieve a watertight anastomosis. For this reason, some surgeons prefer salpingotomy whenever possible.

Tubal anastomosis

Tubal anastomosis for reversal of sterilization is the most successful technique in microsurgery for the following

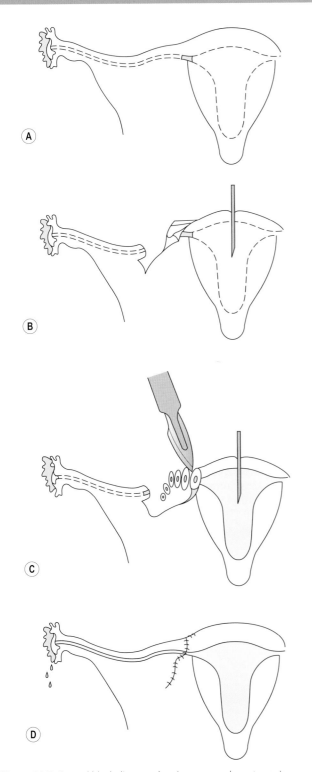

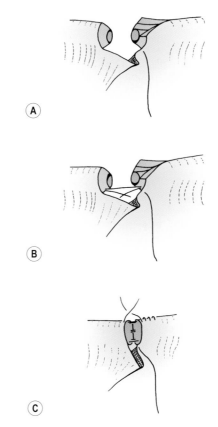

Figure 24.8 Anastomotic procedure. (A) Both tubal lumens are exposed (healthy mucosa). (B) The first stitch is at 6 o'clock and must be extramucosal. (C) The anastomosis is completed in two layers. The suture material used is 8/0 nylon.

Figure 24.7 Cornual block diagram showing a cornual anastomosis. (A) Superficial cornual block. (B) Opening of the cornua to expose the intramural part of the tube. (C) Shaving of the tube to find healthy mucosa for anastomosis. (D) Cornual anastomosis completed.

reasons: healthy tissues are anastomosed, the localized damage is removed completely (Figure 24.8) and these patients are generally fertile.

Success depends on the length of the remaining tube. The minimum length of tube necessary to maintain fertility in women is not known. In animal experiments, fertility diminished in a linear fashion depending on the length of the ampulla resected; when more than 70% was missing, none of the animals became pregnant. Resection of the ampullary–isthmic junction did not appear to alter fertility (Winston et al 1977). The rabbit is far from an ideal model for human tubal physiology, but these results emphasize the fact that the ampulla seems to be important in maintaining fertility.

The length of time between sterilization and reversal is important and has a prognostic value. Vasquez et al (1980) demonstrated that after 5 years of sterilization, the proximal portion of the tube had a severely damaged mucosa with flattening of the epithelium and polyp formation. The surgical technique of reversal of sterilization has been described by Winston (1977) and Margara (1982).

Hydrosalpinges

As well as being a cause of infertility, hydrosalpinges also have a detrimental effect on the outcome of IVF-ET treatment, with reduced pregnancy and implantation rates and increased miscarriage rates. The hydrosalpinx fluid is known to be embryotoxic and may also reduce endometrial receptivity. Removal of hydrosalpinges prior to IVF-ET seems to lead to better results (Nackley and Muasher 1998, Zeyneloglu et al 1998). However, some groups believe that salpingectomy should only be performed when there is severe tubal pathology, and other patients should be given the chance of tubal surgery (Puttemans and Brosens 1996). A Cochrane review concluded that further randomized trials are required to assess other surgical treatments for hydrosalpinx, such as salpingostomy, tubal occlusion or needle drainage of a hydrosalpinx at oocyte retrieval (Johnson et al 2004).

The value of microsurgery varies in the treatment of hydrosalpinges. In some cases, where the tube is completely free of adhesions, the use of loupes is sufficient. Where complex adhesions are present, the use of the microscope is beneficial. When performing a salpingostomy, the following points should be borne in mind. Before starting the salpingostomy, mobilization of the tube must be completed. Division of adhesions between tube and ovary or other pelvic organs is very important in order to leave the tube fully mobile, with the possibility of the new ostium being able to cover the whole ovarian surface and making egg pick-up more likely.

While dividing adhesions, special care must be taken to avoid damage to the fimbrial blood supply. These vessels are in the area of the connecting ligament between the ovary and the tube at the outer margin of the mesosalpinx. The hydrosalpinx must be opened at the most terminal part: the 'pucker point'. This is where the fimbrial end has closed; it is clearly seen under the microscope as a thin fibrous line, often with an H-shaped configuration, and is not always the thinnest part of the tube. Linear salpingostomy has a high chance of healing over. Using fine diathermy, the tube is opened and a glass probe is introduced, following the fibrous tracts parallel to the blood vessels and ensuring that the mucosal folds are not cut. Using small incisions, the new tubal ostium is completed and then the mucosa can be everted (Figure 24.9).

Two or three stitches of 8/0 nylon are used to secure the mucosal eversion. If the ovarian surface is damaged during the division of adhesions, the raw area is repaired using fine non-absorbable suture material to avoid recurrence of adhesions.

Adhesions

Omental adhesions are not infrequent and when they are more than minimal, a partial omentectomy is performed. It is best done at the beginning of the operation. Fine 2/0 linen is used to secure the pedicles. It is not used as a routine procedure, but seems to be a very effective way of avoiding recurrent adhesions in the pelvis.

The most frequent adhesions are between the ampulla, the ovary and the mesosalpinx. It is easy to work from the isthmus towards the fimbrial end. Using a glass probe, the adhesions are hooked and incised with monopolar diathermy. Care should be taken not to damage the tubal peritoneum. The use of the microscope simplifies the process because the peritoneal edges can be seen easily. If the tubal peritoneum is incised, it must be repaired using 8/0 nylon as the suture material.

Ovarian adhesions should be removed from the ovarian capsule using diathermy or scissors, leaving the ovarian capsule as free as possible. Ovulation and egg release seem to improve after careful ovariolysis and may depend on the amount of the ovarian surface left free (Figure 24.10).

Special attention must be paid to raw areas. The uterine surface and the surrounding peritoneum must be inspected carefully. Peritonealization is very important and all raw areas must be covered. If the ovarian fossa has been damaged in order to free or liberate a firmly adherent ovary, the raw area should be closed using a linear suture of 4/0 Prolene. If the raw area cannot be peritonealized using the surrounding peritoneum, a peritoneal graft can be applied. The peritoneum should be thin and without fatty tissue. It is attached to the raw area using 8/0 nylon or 6/0 Prolene. The donor

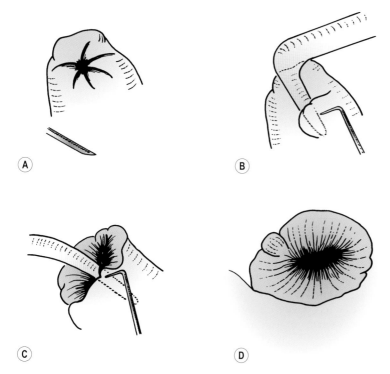

Figure 24.9 Salpingostomy. (A) Identification of the terminal part of the hydrosalpinx where the incision must be made. (B) An incision is made using diathermy, and the tip of the glass probe is inserted into the hole in the tube. (C) The salpingostomy is enlarged using the diathermy needle and glass rods. (D) The salpingostomy is completed.

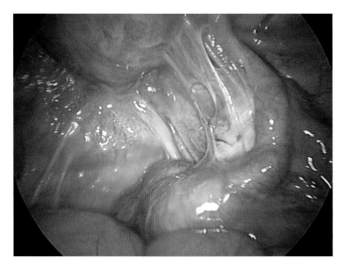

Figure 24.10 Laparoscopic appearance in a patient with severe periovarian adhesions after pelvic inflammatory disease.

1989) have been discussed. There is no evidence that one is better than the other.

After the initial experiences, procedures that can now be performed safely using operative laparoscopy include salpingo-ovariolysis, fimbrioplasty, salpingostomies, tubal reanastomosis, and management of ectopic pregnancy and endometriosis.

One of the most important attributes of this method is that it probably has a low rate of adhesion formation. There is no doubt that laparoscopic adhesiolysis is very effective for pain, and open surgery may cause more adhesion formation (Lundford et al 1991). The question still remains whether patients with severe tubal damage, not suitable for open procedures, should be operated upon using the laparoscopic approach when the prognosis is very poor and alternative methods are available to them.

Great financial advantages are offered by this method. This procedure can be done as a day case or overnight stay, and patients resume their normal activities in a very short period of time. Laparoscopic surgery, as with any other surgical procedure, has its risks and therefore intensive training is fundamental in order to diminish complications and achieve good results.

areas can be the peritoneal layer of the anterior abdominal wall, the peritoneal space between the round ligament and the bladder and, in some cases, the peritoneum of the mesentery of the small or large bowel. This technique has proved very effective in experimental animals, and the results with humans are very encouraging. Synthetic materials are available to replace peritoneum (Hunter et al 1988, Haney and Dotty 1992). They can be applied during open surgery as well as laparoscopic procedures, and can remain *in situ*, apparently without side-effects; if removal is necessary, this can be done through a laparoscope.

It must be emphasized that the treatment of tubal damage due to tuberculosis is always medical and the tubal damage cannot be repaired by surgery. In this group of patients, if the uterine cavity remains unaffected or without damage, IVF is the only option.

Laparoscopic surgery

With the development of endoscopic techniques in the last three decades, gynaecologists, using a laparoscope, have been able to perform numerous operations in the field of infertility as well as in general gynaecology.

Since the first diagnostic use of the endoscope in the 1800s, developments in optics and related technology have revolutionized the use of the laparoscope. In the 1940s, Palmer in France promoted the laparoscope as a diagnostic instrument. In the 1970s, Gomel published the first results of laparoscopic surgery. He performed salpingo-ovariolysis and fimbrioplasties using this approach, with results comparable to those he achieved using magnification in open procedures. At the same time, Semm in Germany also developed the technique and a large number of new instruments became available for laparoscopic surgery.

The development of laser beams for medical use also had an impact in laparoscopic surgery. The use of video-laparoscopy has become a standard part of laparoscopic surgery. It is less tiring, and the assistant has a more active role during surgical procedures, thus it facilitates training and teaching. Different methods of dissection using laser diathermy (Donnez and Nisolle 1989) or cold cutting (Serour et al

Results

Proximal tubal disease

Selective salpingography and tubal catheterization can achieve high patency rates and pregnancy rates of 49% (Honore et al 1999). With the exception of reversal of sterilization, laparoscopic surgery has a limited place in the treatment of proximal tubal disease. Microsurgical cornual anastomosis offers very good results in selected groups of patients. Postoperative laparoscopies show a high patency rate amongst those patients who have not conceived. The major limiting factors seem to be the recrudescence of the disease or extension of the original inflammation into the anastomotic site, rather than lack of patency. Gomel (1980) reported that 53% of patients conceived and had at least one term pregnancy.

Following tubocornual anastomosis by microsurgery, the reported term pregnancy rates in the literature vary between 22% and 57%, and ectopic pregnancy rates vary between 2% and 12%. These results are similar to cumulative delivery rates following five cycles of IVF-ET (Posaci et al 1999). In contrast, the outcome of tubouterine anastomosis is much poorer, and this procedure has mostly been replaced by tubocornual anastomosis.

The surgical treatment of salpingitis isthmica nodosa in the infertile patient is similar to that of cornual block. In nearly half of patients, the tubes are open and the diagnosis is made on the basis of the typical images of diverticulae on the hysterosalpingogram and at laparoscopy. The anastomotic procedure is generally much easier, but the length of isthmic portion that must be removed can be difficult to assess. The prognosis depends on the length of tube removed, but if insufficient tissue is removed, the surgical procedure is more likely to fail. The use of the microscope and the experience of the surgeon are very important in evaluation of the amount or length of tissue that must be resected. In general, this condition involves most of the isthmic portion of the tube, so the anastomosis is between the cornu and the ampullary–isthmic junction.

Where the intramural portion of the tube is extensively involved in the process, the patient should probably not be treated surgically. The surgical procedure itself does not vary from that of tubocornual anastomosis. When the whole of the isthmus is removed, the problem of tension at the anastomotic level can be solved using stay sutures of 6/0 Prolene between the uterus and the mesosalpinx in order to approximate the tubal ends.

Reversal of sterilization

Reversal of tubal sterilization is the most successful procedure in tubal surgery. Both open microsurgical and laparoscopic reversals offer high pregnancy rates. The pregnancy rates in the literature following reversal of sterilization with microsurgery vary between 33% and 86%, with ectopic pregnancy rates of 1–14%. Pregnancy rates of up to 87.1% have been reported following laparoscopic reversal of sterilization (Yoon et al 1999). The success rates are lower after sterilization with cautery or Pomeroy's technique compared with clip or ring sterilization (Posaci et al 1999).

Salpingostomy

In general, it is difficult to assess the results of salpingostomy because a very heterogeneous group of patients is involved. Patient selection varies widely between units and there is no agreement regarding classification, especially where salpingostomy and fimbrioplasty are concerned.

Many gynaecologists think that salpingostomy is obsolete because IVF techniques offer comparable or better results in some cases. As in any other surgical procedure, good results will be achieved in well-selected patients.

Boer-Meisel et al (1986), in a prospective study, classified hydrosalpinges as grades I, II and III, based on the nature and extent of the adhesions, the microscopic aspect of the endosalpinx, the thickness of the tubal wall and the diameter of the hydrosalpinx. In their series, 77% of patients with grade I hydrosalpinx had the possibility of conception, compared with 21% with grade II and only 3% with grade III. Thus, surgery is the obvious treatment for patients with grade I hydrosalpinges. Patients with grade III hydrosalpinges should avoid salpingostomy and should be treated using IVF techniques after salpingectomy. The difficult group is that of grade II hydrosalpinx, where treatments with IVF or tubal surgery have the same prognosis. Age, social and religious background, the possibility of alternative treatment and the patient's wishes must be considered very carefully.

The success of tubal microsurgery for distal tubal lesions depends on several factors. Patients with extensive pelvic adhesions, a thick tubal wall and abnormal tubal mucosa at salpingoscopy have poor results. Type of surgery also affects the outcome. Pregnancy rates as high as 59–60% can be achieved with fimbrioplasty, but the results after salpingostomy may not be as good (Posaci et al 1999). Patients with poor prognostic factors will have a higher chance of achieving pregnancy with IVF, whereas in the absence of poor prognostic factors, tubal microsurgery should be the first choice.

Laparoscopic surgery

Laparoscopic adhesiolysis for pelvic adhesions results in very good results, with term pregnancy rates of 47–62% and ectopic pregnancy rates of 4–8%. These results are similar to those achieved after microsurgery, so laparoscopic surgery should be the first option for suitable patients (Posaci et al 1999).

Success rates of laparoscopic surgery for distal tubal lesions also depend on several prognostic factors, including the presence of extensive pelvic adhesions, a thick tubal wall and severe endotubal damage. The reported intrauterine pregnancy rates following laparoscopic surgery for distal tubal lesions vary between 13% and 51%, with ectopic pregnancy rates of 3–23% (Posaci et al 1999). It appears that laparoscopic surgery offers similar success rates compared with microsurgery for lesser degrees of distal tubal damage. However, open microsurgery may be slightly better for more severe distal tubal disease. For the treatment of moderate to severe distal tubal disease, postoperative pregnancy rates are low, even after microsurgery, despite long periods of observation (>2 years), with remarkably high ectopic pregnancy rates. For this reason, IVF is preferable in these situations (Ozturk and Saridogan 2009).

Conclusion

Currently, in the absence of detailed information about early reproductive events which take place within the fallopian tube, the assessment of tubal function mainly depends on checking its patency and appearance at endoscopy. A better understanding of tubal physiology may enable us to test its function more effectively, and may also improve our understanding of so-called 'unexplained infertility'. There is no doubt that a large group of patients with tubal disease can be treated using IVF techniques. In a well-selected group of infertile patients with tubal damage, surgical procedures, performed using laparoscopy or open surgery (microsurgery), offer a very good prognosis and many patients can conceive more than once after a single treatment. In a highly specialized reproductive unit, these methods should be available and the choice of procedure should be adapted to each individual case.

KEY POINTS

1. Tubal disease is tubal damage caused by pelvic infection, endometriosis or iatrogenic disease with varying degrees of damage, and sometimes involving surrounding structures.

2. Tubal disease accounts for 30–40% of cases of female infertility.

3. Salpingitis most commonly results from ascending infection from the lower genital tract.

4. Salpingitis is not generally seen in women who are not sexually active.

5. *Chlamydia trachomatis* is responsible for a significant amount of salpingitis, postpartum endometritis and perihepatic adhesions.

6. Many organisms are capable of producing salpingitis. Chlamydia and gonococcal infections seem to pave the way for other micro-organisms to cross the cervical mucus and affect the uterus or tubes.

7. Although tubal damage of tuberculous origin is rare in developed countries, there has been an increase since the 1980s due to population migration.

8. A significant proportion of patients with tubal disease are best treated by IVF techniques.

9. In a well-selected group of infertile patients with tubal damage, surgical procedures, performed using laparoscopy or open surgery (microsurgery), offer a very good prognosis and many patients can conceive more than once after a single treatment.

References

Ahmad G, Duffy JMN, Farquhar C et al 2008 Barrier agents for adhesion prevention after gynaecological surgery. Cochrane Database of Systematic Reviews 2: CD000475.

Ataya K, Thomas M 1991 New techniques for selective transcervical osteal salpingography and catheterisation in the diagnosis and treatment of proximal tubal obstruction. Fertility and Sterility 56: 980–983.

Boer-Meisel ME, te Velde ER, Habbema JD, Kardaun JW 1986 Predicting the pregnancy outcome in patients treated for hydrosalpinx: a prospective study. Fertility and Sterility 45: 23–29.

Chiari H 1887 Zur pathologischen Anatomic des Eileiter-Catrrhs. Zeitschrift fur Heilkunde 8: 457–473.

De Bruyne F, Puttemans P, Boeckx W, Brosens IA 1989 The clinical value of salpingoscopy in tubal infertility. Fertility and Sterility 51: 339–340.

Djahanbakhch O, Kervancioglu E, Maguiness SD, Martin JE 1994 Fallopian tube epithelial cell culture. In: Grudzinskas JG, Chapman MG, Chard T, Djahanbakhch O (eds) The Fallopian Tube. Clinical and Surgical Aspects. Springer-Verlag, London, pp 37–51.

Donnez J, Nisolle M 1989 CO_2 laser laparoscopy surgery. Adhesiolysis, salpingostomy, laser uterine nerve ablation and tubal pregnancy. Baillière's Clinics in Obstetrics and Gynaecology 3: 525–543.

Ehrler P 1963 Die intramurale tubenanastomoze (ein Beitrag zur Uberwindung der Tubaren Steritat). Zentralblatt für Gynaekologie 85: 393–400.

Glazener CMA, Loveden LM, Richardson SJ, Jeans WD, Hull MGR 1987 Tubocornual polyps: their relevance in subfertility. Human Reproduction 2: 59–65.

Gomel V 1977 Tubal reanastomosis by microsurgery. Fertility and Sterility 28: 59.

Gomel V 1980 Clinical results of infertility microsurgery. In: Crosignani PG, Rubin BL (eds) Microsurgery in Female Infertility. Academic Press, New York, pp 77–94.

Gordts S, Campo R, Rombauts L, Brosens I 1998 Transvaginal hydrolaparoscopy as an outpatient procedure for infertility investigation. Human Reproduction 13: 99–103.

Haney AF, Dotty E 1992 Murine peritoneal injury and de novo adhesion formation caused by oxidized-regenerated cellulose (Interceed TC7) but not expanded polytetrafluoroethylene (Gore-Tex surgical membrane). Fertility and Sterility 57: 202–208.

Honore GM, Holden AE, Schenken RS 1999 Pathophysiology and management of proximal tubal blockage. Fertility and Sterility 71: 785–795.

Hunter SK, Scott JR, Hull D, Urry RL 1988 The gamete and embryo compatibility of various synthetic polymers. Fertility and Sterility 50: 110–116.

Jansen RP 1984 Endocrine response in the fallopian tube. Endocrine Reviews 5: 525–551.

Johnson N, van Voorst S, Sowter MC, Strandell A, Mol BWJ 2004 Surgical treatment for tubal disease in women due to undergo in vitro fertilisation. Cochrane Database of Systematic Reviews 3: CD002125.

Kervancioglu ME, Saridogan E, Aitken RJ, Djahanbakhch O 2000 Importance of sperm to epithelial cell contact for the capacitation of human spermatozoa in human Fallopian tube–epithelial cell coculture. Fertility and Sterility 74: 780–784.

Lundford P, Hahlin M, Kallfelt B, Thourburn J, Lindblom B 1991 Adhesion formation after laparoscopic surgery in tubal pregnancy: a randomised trial versus laparotomy. Fertility and Sterility 55: 911–915.

Lyons R, Saridogan E, Djahanbakhch O 2006 The reproductive significance of human fallopian tube cilia. Human Reproduction Update 12: 363–372.

Maguiness SD, Djahanbakhch O 1992 Salpingoscopic findings in women undergoing sterilization. Human Reproduction 7: 269–273.

Maguiness SD, Shrimanker K, Djahanbakhch O, Grudzinskas JG 1992a Oviduct proteins. Contemporary Reviews in Obstetrics and Gynaecology 4: 42–50.

Maguiness SD, Djahanbakhch O, Grudzinskas JG 1992b Assessment of the fallopian tube. Obstetrical and Gynecological Survey 47: 587–603.

Mahmood T, Saridogan E, Smutna S, Habib AM, Djahanbakhch O 1998 The effect of ovarian steroids on epithelial ciliary beat frequency in the human fallopian tube. Human Reproduction 13: 2991–2994.

Margara RA 1982 Tubal reanastomosis. In: Chamberlain G, Winston RML (eds) Tubal Infertility. Blackwell Science, Oxford, pp 106–119.

Metwally ME, Watson A, Lilford R, Vanderkerchove P 2006 Fluid and pharmacological agents for adhesion prevention after gynaecological surgery. Cochrane Database of Systematic Reviews 2: CD001298.

Nackley AC, Muasher SJ 1998 The significance of hydrosalpinx in in vitro fertilization. Fertility and Sterility 69: 373–384.

National Institute for Clinical Excellence 2004 Assessment and Treatment for People with Fertility Problems. Ref: CG011. NICE, London. Available at: http://www.nice.org.uk

Ozturk O, Saridogan E 2009 Laparoscopic surgery for tubal factor infertility. In: Allahbadia G, Saridogan E, Djahanbakhch O (eds) The Fallopian Tube. Anshan, Tunbridge Wells, pp 283–289.

Paterson P, Wood C 1974 The use of microsurgery in the reanastomosis of the rabbit fallopian tube. Fertility and Sterility 25: 757–761.

Posaci C, Camus M, Osmanagaoglu K, Devroey P 1999 Tubal surgery in the era of assisted reproductive technology: clinical options. Human Reproduction 14 (Suppl 1): 120–136.

Puttemans PJ, de Bruyne F, Heylen SM 1998 A decade of salpingoscopy. European Journal of Obstetrics, Gynecology and Reproductive Biology 81: 197–206.

Puttemans PJ, Brosens IA 1996 Preventive salpingectomy of hydrosalpinx prior to IVF. Salpingectomy improves in-vitro fertilization outcome in patients with hydrosalpinx: blind victimization of the fallopian tube. Human Reproduction 11: 2079–2084.

Rice PA, Schachter J 1991 Pathogenesis of pelvic inflammatory disease. What are the questions? JAMA: the Journal of the American Medical Association 266: 2587–2593.

Rose AM, Watson JM, Graham C et al 2001 Tuberculosis at the end of the 20th century in England and Wales: results of a national survey in 1988. Thorax 56: 173–179.

Saridogan E, Djahanbakhch O, Puddefoot JR et al 1996 Angiotensin II receptors and angiotensin II stimulation of ciliary activity in human fallopian tube. Journal of Clinical Endocrinology and Metabolism 81: 2719–2725.

Saridogan E, Djahanbakhch O 2009 Gamete and embryo transport in the human fallopian tube. In: Allahbadia G, Saridogan E, Djahanbakhch O (eds) The Fallopian Tube. Anshan, Tunbridge Wells, pp 12–19.

Seki K, Eddy CA, Smith Nk, Pauerstein CJ 1977 Comparison of two techniques of suturing in microsurgical anastomosis of the rabbit oviduct. Fertility and Sterility 28: 1215–1219.

Serour GI, Bandroui MH, Agizi HM, Hamed AF, Abdel-Aziz F 1989 Laparoscopic adhesiolysis for infertile patients with pelvic adhesive disease. International Journal of Gynaecology and Obstetrics 30: 249–252.

Simms I, Stephenson J 2009 Epidemiology of pelvic inflammatory disease. In: Allahbadia G, Saridogan E, Djahanbakhch O (eds) The Fallopian Tube. Anshan, Tunbridge Wells, pp 537–546.

Vasquez G, Winston RML, Boeckx W, Brosens I 1980 Tubal lesions subsequent to sterilisation and their relation to fertility after attempts at reversal. American Journal of Obstetrics and Gynecology 138: 86–92.

Verdugo P 1986 Functional anatomy of the fallopian tube. In: Insler V, Lunenfeld B (eds) Infertility: Male and Female. Churchill Livingstone, London, pp 26–55.

Walz W 1959 Fertilitäts Operationen mit Hilfe eines Operationemkroscopes. Geburtshilfe und Gynaekologie 153: 49–53.

Watrelot A, Dreyfus JM, Andine JP 1999 Evaluation of the performance of fertiloscopy in 160 consecutive infertile patients with no obvious pathology. Human Reproduction 14: 707–711.

Winston RML 1977 Microsurgical tubocornual anastomosis for reversal of sterilisation. Lancet i: 284–285.

Winston RML, McClure-Browne JC 1974 Pregnancy following autograft transplantation of the fallopian tube and ovary in the rabbit. Lancet i: 494–497.

Winston RML, Frantzen C, Oberti C 1977 Oviduct function following resection of the ampullary–isthmic junction. Fertility and Sterility 28: 284–289.

Yoon TK, Sung HR, Kang HG, Cha SH, Lee CN, Cha KY 1999 Laparoscopic tubal anastomosis: fertility outcome in 202 cases. Fertility and Sterility 72: 1121–1126.

Zeyneloglu H, Arici A, Olive DL 1998 Adverse effects of hydrosalpinx on pregnancy rates after in vitro fertilization-embryo transfer. Fertility and Sterility 70: 492–499.

CHAPTER 25

Ectopic pregnancy

Neelam Potdar and Justin C. Konje

Chapter Contents

INCIDENCE	363		DIFFERENTIAL DIAGNOSIS	370
AETIOLOGY AND RISK FACTORS	363		PREGNANCY OF UNKNOWN LOCATION	370
PATHOLOGY	365		MANAGEMENT OF ECTOPIC PREGNANCY	370
DIAGNOSIS	366		NON-TUBAL ECTOPIC PREGNANCY	376
FURTHER INVESTIGATIONS	368		KEY POINTS	379

Incidence

Ectopic pregnancy is defined as implantation of the fertilized ovum in a site other than the uterine endometrium. The incidence of ectopic pregnancy ranges between 0.25% and 1.5% of all pregnancies (including live births, medical termination of pregnancy and ectopic gestations). However, it varies geographically due to two reasons. Firstly, different denominators such as live births and reported pregnancies are used to express the results. Secondly, the exact incidence remains unknown as the diagnosis is often missed when the ectopic pregnancy resolves spontaneously at an early stage. Recently, the problem of ectopic pregnancies has been magnified by advancing maternal age, tubal surgery, pelvic inflammatory disease (PID) and assisted reproduction techniques.

In England and Wales between 1966 and 1996, the incidence of ectopic pregnancy increased 3.1-fold from 30.2 to 94.8 per 100,000 women aged 15–44 years, and 3.8-fold from 3.25 to 12.4 per 1000 pregnancies (Rajkhowa et al 2000). In the UK, for the 2003–2005 triennium, there were 11.1 [95% confidence interval (CI) 10.9–11.1] ectopic gestations per 1000 pregnancies reported (Lewis 2007).

In the USA, the Centers for Disease Control and Prevention have the most comprehensive data available on ectopic pregnancy. Between 1970 and 1989, there was a 5-fold increase in the incidence of ectopic pregnancies, from 3.2 to 16 per 1000 reported pregnancies (Goldner et al 1993). Women between 35 and 44 years of age have the highest risk of developing an ectopic pregnancy (27 per 1000 reported pregnancies). Data from the same centre indicate that the risk of ectopic pregnancy in African women (21 per 1000) is 1.6 times greater than the risk amongst Whites (13 per 1000); this is related to the high incidence of PID and low socioeconomic status in certain populations.

Ectopic pregnancy is still a cause of significant morbidity and mortality. In the UK, the number of deaths from ectopic pregnancies has varied in the last decade: 12 (1994–1996), 13 (1997–1999), 11 (2000–2002) and 10 (2003–2005). The death rate for the 2003–2005 triennium was 0.35 (95% CI 0.19–0.64) per 100,000 estimated ectopic pregnancies. Seven of the 10 deaths due to ectopic pregnancies during this triennium were associated with failure to diagnose or substandard care (Lewis 2007). The risk of death is higher for racial and ethnic minorities, and teenagers have the highest mortality rates.

Aetiology and Risk Factors

The aetiology of ectopic pregnancy remains enigmatic. A common denominator in most theories is the delay in ovum transport. A likely consequence of the delay is that the ovum becomes too large to pass through certain areas of the fallopian tube, particularly the isthmic segment and the uterotubal junction. In addition, the growth and proliferation of the trophoblast may be so advanced that implantation of the fertilized ovum begins prior to the departure of the ovum from the fallopian tube. Myoelectrical activity of the wall of the fallopian tube allows approximation and fertilization of gametes, as well as propulsion of the zygote and cleaving embryo from the ampulla to the uterine cavity. Oestrogens increase smooth muscle activity and progesterone decreases muscular tone. The reported increased incidence of tubal pregnancy in perimenopausal women may be related to progressive loss of myoelectrical activity along the fallopian tube, which is observed with ageing.

The cilia of the tubal epithelium are also involved in transportation of oocytes towards the uterine cavity. Salpingitis results in loss of ciliated epithelium and subsequently delayed propulsion of the embryo/blastocyst towards the uterine cavity.

Steroid hormones, oestrogens and progesterone influence cilia formation and movements. Oestrogens stimulate epithelial cell hyperplasia and ciliogenesis. High levels of

Table 25.1 Risk factors for ectopic pregnancy

Previous tubal pregnancy	Assisted conception
Previous tubal surgery	Salpingitis isthmica nodosa
Pelvic inflammatory disease	Smoking
Medical termination of pregnancy	Diethylstilbestrol
Current intrauterine contraceptive device users	

serum progesterone are associated with deciliation and atrophy of the epithelium. These changes of the ciliated epithelium of the fallopian tube may explain the increased incidence of tubal pregnancy observed in women who take the progesterone-only pill or have a progesterone-containing intrauterine contraceptive device (IUCD) *in situ*.

All sexually active women are at risk of an ectopic pregnancy. The risk factors that may be associated with an ectopic pregnancy (Table 25.1) may be present in 25–50% of women.

Independent risk factors consistently shown to increase the risk of tubal pregnancy are discussed below.

Previous tubal pregnancy

A history of prior ectopic pregnancy is a significant risk factor. A woman who has experienced one ectopic pregnancy has a 10–20% chance of presenting with an ectopic gestation in her subsequent pregnancy. Accurate assessment of the risk of recurrent ectopic pregnancy is difficult because it depends upon the size, location of previous ectopic pregnancy, status of the contralateral adenexa, treatment method and history of subfertility.

Previous tubal surgery

Sterilization

Following sterilization, the absolute risk of ectopic pregnancy is reduced. However, the ratio of ectopic to intrauterine pregnancy is higher. The greatest risk for pregnancy, including ectopic pregnancy, occurs in the first 2 years after sterilization. The cumulative probability of ectopic pregnancy for all methods of tubal sterilization is 7.3 per 1000 procedures. Fistula formation and recanalization of the proximal and distal stumps of the fallopian tube are implicated for the occurrence of ectopic gestation. Women sterilized before the age of 30 years by bipolar tubal coagulation have a 27 times higher probability of ectopic pregnancy compared with postpartum partial salpingectomy (31.9 vs 1.2 ectopic pregnancies per 1000 procedures) (Peterson et al 1997). Tubal coagulation has a lower risk of pregnancy compared with mechanical devices (spring-loaded clips or fallope rings), but the risk of ectopic pregnancy is 10 times higher when a pregnancy does occur (DeStefano et al 1982).

Reversal of sterilization

The risk depends on the method of sterilization. Following reconstruction of a cauterized tube, approximately 15% of women who conceive have an ectopic pregnancy. The risk of ectopic pregnancy is reduced to 5% when the reversal is performed following Pomeroy's method or clip sterilization.

Tubal reconstruction and repair

Reconstructive tubal surgery is a predisposing factor for ectopic pregnancy. However, it remains unclear whether the increased risk results from the surgical procedure or from the underlying pathology of the ciliated tubal epithelium and pelvic disease. In a consecutive series of 232 tubal microsurgical operations, including salpingostomies, proximal anastomoses and adhesiolyses, 12 patients (5%) presented with an ectopic pregnancy whereas 80 patients (35%) achieved an intrauterine pregnancy (Singhal et al 1991). Silva et al (1993) reported a higher risk of recurrent ectopic pregnancy following conservative surgery of salpingostomy than radical surgery of salpingectomy (18% vs 8%, relative risk 2.38, 95% CI 0.57–10.01).

Pelvic inflammatory disease

The relationship between PID, tubal obstruction and ectopic pregnancy is well documented. Infection of tubal endothelium results in damage of ciliated epithelium and formation of intraluminal adhesions and pockets. A consequence of these anatomical changes is entrapment of the zygote and ectopic implantation of the blastocyst. Westrom et al (1981) studied 450 women with laparoscopically proven PID (case–control study). The authors reported that the incidence of tubal obstruction increased with successive episodes of PID: 13% after one episode, 35% after two episodes and 79% after three episodes. Following one episode of laparoscopically verified acute salpingitis, the ratio of ectopic to intrauterine pregnancy was 1:24, a six-fold increase compared with women with laparoscopically negative results.

Tubal damage induced by *Chlamydia trachomatis* is associated with tubal pregnancy. Many cases of chlamydia infection are subclinical.

Although PID is a high risk factor for ectopic pregnancy, it is pertinent to note that only 50% of fallopian tubes removed for an ectopic pregnancy have histological evidence of salpingitis.

Current intrauterine contraceptive device users

Unmedicated, medicated and copper-coated IUCDs prevent both intrauterine and extrauterine pregnancies. However, a woman who conceives with an IUCD *in situ* is seven times more likely to have a tubal pregnancy compared with conception without contraception (Vessey et al 1974). IUCDs are more effective in preventing intrauterine than extrauterine implantation. With copper IUCDs, 4% of all accidental pregnancies are tubal, whereas with progesterone-coated IUCDs, 17% of all contraceptive failures are tubal pregnancies. The different mechanisms of action of the two devices could partially explain the difference in failure rates. Although both devices prevent implantation, copper IUCDs also interfere with fertilization by inducing cytotoxic and phagocytotic effects on the sperm and oocytes. Progesterone-containing IUCDs are probably less effective in preventing fertilization. Although the incidence of pregnancy diminishes with long-term use of the IUCD, among women who become pregnant, the likelihood of ectopic pregnancy increases. Women who have used the IUCD for more than 24 months are 2.6 times more likely to have an ectopic pregnancy compared with short-term users (<24 months).

The 'lasting effect' of the IUCD may be related to the loss of the cilia from the tubal epithelium, especially if the IUCD has been *in situ* for 3 years or more (Wollen et al 1984, Ory HW 1981).

Termination of pregnancy

Data from two French case–control studies suggest that induced abortion may be a risk factor for ectopic pregnancy for women with no history of ectopic pregnancy. There is an association between the number of previous induced abortions and ectopic pregnancy [odds ratio (OR) 1.4 for one previous induced abortion and 1.9 for two or more] (Tharaux-Deneux et al 1998). Whether this is related to the spread of asymptomatic *C. trachomatis* infection or to the procedure itself is uncertain.

Assisted conception

Induction of ovulation with either clomiphene citrate or human menopausal gonadotrophin is a predisposing factor to tubal implantation (McBain et al 1980; Marchbanks et al 1985). A number of studies indicate that 1–4% of pregnancies achieved following induction of ovulation are ectopic pregnancies. The majority of these patients had a normal pelvis and patent tubes. The incidence of tubal pregnancy following oocyte retrieval and embryo transfer is approximately 4.5%. It must be noted that some women who undergo an in-vitro fertilization (IVF) cycle have risk factors for an ectopic pregnancy (i.e. previous ectopic pregnancy, tubal pathology or surgery).

Salpingitis isthmica nodosa

Salpingitis isthmica nodosa (SIN) is diagnosed by the histological evidence of tubal isthmic diverticula, and may be suggested by characteristic changes on hysterosalpingogram. Its incidence in healthy women ranges from 0.6% to 11%, but it is significantly more common in the setting of ectopic pregnancy. Persaud (1970) reported that 49% of fallopian tubes excised for tubal pregnancy had diverticula and evidence of SIN. The reason for the high incidence of ectopic gestation in women with SIN remains largely unknown. Defective myoelectrical activity has been demonstrated over the diverticula. Entrapment of the embryo into the diverticula is a possible mechanical explanation.

Smoking

A French study found that the risk of ectopic pregnancy is significantly higher in women who smoke. The risk increases according to the number of cigarettes per day (Bouyer et al 1998). The relative risk for ectopic pregnancy is 1.3 for women who smoke one to nine cigarettes per day, 2 for women who smoke 10–12 cigarettes per day, and 2.5 for women who smoke more than 20 cigarettes per day. Inhibition of oocyte cumulus complex pick-up by the fimbrial end of the fallopian tube and a reduction of ciliary beat frequency are associated with nicotine intake (Knoll and Talbot 1998).

Diethylstilboestrol

Results of a collaborative study indicate that the risk of ectopic pregnancy in diethylstilboestrol (DES)-exposed women was 13% compared with 4% for women who had a normal uterus (Barnes et al 1980). A meta-analysis on risk factors for ectopic pregnancy confirms that exposure to DES *in utero* significantly increases the risk of ectopic pregnancy (Ankum et al 1996).

Pathology

Sites of ectopic pregnancy

A 21-year survey of 654 ectopic pregnancies (Breen 1970) revealed that the most common sites of ectopic pregnancy are as shown in Table 25.2. Similar distribution for tubal and abdominal pregnancy sites have been reported by Bouyer et al (2002) [ampullary (70.0%), isthmic (12.0%), fimbrial (11.1%), interstitial (2.4%), abdominal (1.3%)]. In this population, no cervical pregnancies were observed and slightly increased incidence was seen for ovarian pregnancies (3.2%) (Bouyer et al 2002).

Natural progression of a tubal pregnancy

Unruptured tubal pregnancy

Occasionally, in the very early stages of a tubal pregnancy, there are no obvious macroscopic features, and an ectopic pregnancy could be overlooked even after a laparoscopy. However, as pregnancy progresses, local enlargement of the tube occurs at the point of implantation. At a later stage, a large segment of the tube is distended and the tubal wall appears discoloured, dark red or purple.

Tubal rupture

One of the fundamental aspects of ectopic pregnancy is the inability of the tissues into which the blastocyst implants to offer resistance or respond to the invading trophoblast. Uncontrolled invasion of the trophoblast results in destruction of vessels, local haemorrhage and thinning of the tubal wall. Rupture of the tubal wall results in the escape of large amounts of blood, with or without the products of conception, into the peritoneal cavity. The embryo rarely survives. In rare cases, pregnancy continues if an adequate portion of the placenta is retained or if secondary implantation occurs in other organs of the pelvic or peritoneal cavity. Rupture occurs more often at the antimesenteric part of the tubal wall. Rupture of the inferior and mesenteric part of the tubal

Table 25.2 Sites of ectopic gestation

Fallopian tube	
Ampullary segment	80%
Isthmic segment	12%
Fimbrial end	5%
Interstitial and cornual	2%
Abdominal	1.4%
Ovarian	0.2%
Cervical	0.2%

wall results in haemorrhage between the two layers of the broad ligament. Intraligamentous haemorrhage could cause rupture of anterior or posterior layers of the broad ligament.

Spontaneous involution

Usually, the conceptus dies at an early stage without any notable symptoms.

Complete tubal miscarriage

At an early stage, the conceptus is extruded via the fimbriated end of the fallopian tube into the peritoneal cavity, and subsequently absorbed by the surrounding tissues.

Incomplete tubal miscarriage

The conceptus is partially extruded via the fimbrial end of the tube, and intervention is usually required.

Tubal blood mole or carneous mole

In some cases, recurrent choriodecidual haemorrhage around the dead conceptus contributes to the formation of a tubal blood mole or carneous mole. The presence and development of cellular and biochemical elements of connective tissue around the mole give rise to a semi-solid structure which could remain unresolved for years.

Time of rupture at various sites in the tube

Isthmic implantation

The isthmic segment of the fallopian tube is narrow and less distensible than the ampullary or interstitial segments. Isthmic rupture often occurs at 6–8 weeks of gestation and is usually dramatic.

Ampullary implantation

Rupture of an ampullary pregnancy usually occurs at 8–12 weeks of gestation. The ampulla is the wider segment of the fallopian tube and the site of 80% of all ectopic pregnancies.

Interstitial implantation

The interstitial segment of the fallopian tube is surrounded by myometrium which can hypertrophy to accommodate the enlarging conceptus. Rupture therefore occurs at a relatively late stage of 12–14 weeks of gestation. Rupture of an interstitial pregnancy causes damage of the highly vascularized cornual end of the uterus, resulting in severe intra-abdominal haemorrhage.

Histological changes

In the early stages of pregnancy, the myometrium responds in an identical pattern under the influence of hormones, irrespective of whether the gestation is ectopic or eutopic. The uterus becomes softened and slightly enlarged as a consequence of hypertrophy and hyperplasia of the myometrial cells. Where the gestation is ectopic, the endometrial glands

demonstrate an atypical histological pattern referred to as the 'Arias-Stella phenomenon', which is characterized histologically by: hyperplasia of glandular cells, closely packed glands with evidence of hypersecretion, large irregular hyperchromatic nuclei, cytoplasmic vacuolation and loss of cellular polarity. It is important to note that the Arias-Stella reaction is non-specific and can be found in the endometrium of patients with an intrauterine pregnancy. However, the presence of the Arias-Stella reaction and the absence of chorionic villi from endometrial curettings are both highly suspicious signs of an extrauterine pregnancy. The presence of chorionic villi is the most reliable histological feature for the definite diagnosis of pregnancy.

Simultaneous with the glandular changes, the stroma is converted into decidual tissue containing large polyhedral cells with hyperchromatic nuclei. A failing pregnancy and lower levels of associated hormones results in gradual disintegration of the decidua, giving rise to the intermittent, occasionally heavy, vaginal bleeding of uterine origin that occurs in ectopic pregnancy. In some cases, the decidua may be detached abruptly and passed as a flat, triangular, reddish-brown piece of tissue called a 'decidual cast'.

Diagnosis

Symptoms and signs

Ectopic pregnancy remains a diagnostic challenge. It should be considered as an important differential in any woman of reproductive age who presents with the triad of amenorrhoea, abdominal pain and irregular vaginal bleeding. This philosophy is particularly useful if the patient has any of the risk factor(s) identified in Table 25.1. The frequency with which various symptoms and signs were reported from a series of 300 consecutive cases are shown in Table 25.3 (Droegemueller 1982).

Abdominal pain

This is the most common symptom; however, it should be emphasized that there is no typical pain that is pathognomonic of ectopic pregnancy. Women can present with generalized abdominal or localized pain in the pelvis (unilateral or bilateral) and/or pain radiating to the shoulder.

The generalized abdominal pain is usually due to rupture of ectopic pregnancy and intraperitoneal haemorrhage. The pain is often severe. Shoulder pain is also an indirect indication of intraperitoneal haemorrhage. Accumulation of blood in the subdiaphragmatic region stimulates the phrenic nerve and creates shoulder tip pain. Localized pain may be due to distension of the fallopian tube. The pain may be sudden or progressive, and continuous or intermittent.

Amenorrhoea and abnormal uterine bleeding

Most patients present with amenorrhoea of at least 2 weeks duration. One-third of the women will either not recall the date of their last menstrual period or have irregular periods. Abnormal uterine bleeding occurs in 75% of women with an ectopic pregnancy. The bleeding is often light, recurrent and results from detachment of the uterine decidua. According to Stabile (1996a), 'If a patient who is a few weeks

Table 25.3 Symptoms and signs in 300 consecutive cases of ectopic pregnancy at admission

Symptoms and signs	Cases (%)
Abdominal pain	99
Generalized	44
Unilateral	33
Radiating to the shoulder	22
Abnormal uterine bleeding	74
Amenorrhoea ≤2 weeks	68
Syncopal symptoms	37
Adenexal tenderness	96
Unilateral adenexal mass	54
Uterus	
Normal size	71
6–8-week size	26
9–12-week size	3
Uterine cast passed away vaginally	7
Admission temperature >37°C	2

pregnant complains of a little pain and heavy vaginal bleeding, the pregnancy is probably intrauterine, whereas if there is more pain and little bleeding, it is more likely to be an ectopic pregnancy'.

Other symptoms

Although abdominal pain, amenorrhoea and abnormal vaginal bleeding are the most common and typical symptoms, patients may present with additional features such as syncopal attacks. These are related to sudden-onset haemorrhage or to hypovolaemia or anaemia. Other atypical symptoms include diarrhoea or vomiting. In the 2003–2005 Confidential Enquiry into Maternal and Child Health report (Lewis, 2007), some women who presented with these symptoms were undiagnosed and subsequently died.

Physical examination

Physical examination should include an assessment of vital signs and examination of the abdomen and pelvis. Depending on the rate and amount of blood loss, the general condition of the patient may vary from slight pallor to haemodynamic shock. Palpation of the abdomen may reveal generalized or localized mild tenderness. Occasionally, guarding and rebound tenderness are also elicited.

An unusual feature is the Cullen's sign. This is bluish discoloration of the skin around the umbilicus caused by a considerable quantity of free blood in the peritoneal cavity. However, this sign is rare and its absence does not exclude massive intraperitoneal haemorrhage.

The findings on pelvic examination vary from completely negative examination to the presence of a large, fixed, soft

and tender mass. An adnexal mass may be palpable in up to 55% of cases. In many cases, the mass is ill defined and it may consist not only of tubal pregnancy but also of adherent omentum, small and large bowel. The mass may also be an enlarged corpus luteum. The uterus may be slightly enlarged but its size does not normally correspond to the gestational age. Cervical motion tenderness may or may not be present. A tender boggy mass in the pouch of Douglas, when present, represents either a collection of blood or a dilated tube adherent to the posterior uterine wall.

Types of presentation

The presentation of symptomatic patients with a tubal ectopic pregnancy may be acute or subacute.

Acute presentation

This is usually a consequence of rupture of the ectopic gestation and the ensuing intraperitoneal haemorrhage and haemodynamic shock. These symptoms are due to the intra-abdominal haemorrhage and collection of blood into the subdiaphragmatic region and pouch of Douglas. The patient is often pale, hypotensive and tachycardic. She may complain of shoulder tip pain or urge to defaecate. Abdominal examination reveals generalized and rebound tenderness. Vaginal examination will reveal tenderness in the adnexal region and cervical motion tenderness. However, vaginal examination in patients who present with an acute abdomen due to a ruptured ectopic pregnancy is generally considered unnecessary and potentially dangerous for the following reasons: (a) generalized haemoperitoneum and pain often mean that specific information cannot be elicited, (b) the patient is very uncomfortable and the assessment is often difficult and inadequate, and (c) it could result in total rupture of the ectopic pregnancy and delay management of the patient. Although it is reported that 30% of all women with an ectopic pregnancy present after rupture (Barnhart et al 1994), acute presentation is becoming less common. This is due primarily to increased patient awareness and early referral to the hospital for evaluation of 'suspected ectopic' pregnancies. Finally, the availability of more sensitive and rapid biochemical tests for beta-human chorionic gonadotrophin (β-hCG) quantification and the wider availability of transvaginal ultrasonography and laparoscopy have significantly reduced the interval between presentation and treatment.

Subacute presentation

When the process of tubal rupture or abortion is very gradual, the presentation of ectopic pregnancy is subacute. According to Stabile (1996a,b), this is the group of women who are symptomatic but clinically stable. A history of a missed period and recurrent episodes of light vaginal bleeding may exist. The circulatory system adjusts the blood pressure, and the patient is haemodynamically stable. Progressively increasing lower abdominal pain and, occasionally, shoulder pain are typical symptoms. On bimanual examination, there may be localized tenderness in one of the fornices, and cervical motion tenderness is often present. Subacute presentation occurs in 80–90% of ectopic pregnancies. In cases with such a presentation, the establishment of an accurate diagnosis becomes more difficult, hence the need for further investigations.

Further Investigations

Biochemical tests

Quantitation of β-hCG subunit

hCG is a glycoprotein with a mass of 36,700 Da that is secreted by the syncytiotrophoblasts. It is heterodimeric, composed of two non-covalently linked α and β subunits. The α subunit is identical to that of follicle-stimulating hormone and luteinizing hormone, whereas the β subunit is specific to hCG. In response to β-hCG, the corpus luteum produces increasing concentrations of progesterone and other steroid hormones required to maintain early pregnancy, until the placenta takes over by the eighth week of gestation. β-hCG first enters the maternal circulation on the day of blastocyst implantation, i.e. 6–7 days after conception. Serum concentrations of β-hCG are approximately 1000 IU/l (third international standard) at approximately 4 weeks of pregnancy, increase exponentially during the first 6 weeks of gestation, and reach 20,000–250,000 IU/l at 10 weeks of gestation. Concentrations then decrease to 10,000–20,000 IU/l by 20 weeks of gestation and plateau thereafter.

Using highly sensitive assays (detection limit 0.1–0.3 IU/l), β-hCG can be detected in the maternal circulation around the time of implantation. This will appear in urine approximately 2 days after it appears in the blood. Most commercially available monoclonal-antibody-based urine pregnancy tests can detect β-hCG concentrations above 25 IU/l, which corresponds to day 24–25 of a regular 28-day cycle. The sensitivity of modern assays is 99–100%.

Single β-hCG measurement

A single serum β-hCG concentration has been used as a discriminatory level to detect an ectopic pregnancy as described below. A single measurement, however, has limited clinical value as there is considerable overlap of values for normal and abnormal pregnancies. When using radioimmunometric assays with a detection limit of 5 IU/l, a single measurement of β-hCG may be useful because, if negative, it can exclude the diagnosis of an ectopic pregnancy.

Serial β-hCG measurements

Serum β-hCG concentrations double every 1.4–1.6 days from the time of first detection up to the 35th day of pregnancy, and then double every 2.0–2.7 days from the 35th to the 42nd day of pregnancy (Pittaway et al 1985). Since the normal doubling time of β-hCG is 2.2 days and its half-life is 32–37 h, serial quantitative assessments of β-hCG may help to distinguish normal from abnormal pregnancies. Kadar et al (1981) first reported a method for screening for ectopic pregnancy based on β-hCG doubling time. An increase in serum β-hCG of less than 66% over 48 h was suggestive of an ectopic pregnancy (using an 85% CI for

β-hCG levels). More recently, studies have used an increase in serum β-hCG levels of 35–53% (using 99% CI) to diagnose viable intrauterine pregnancies and to reduce the potential risk of terminating an intrauterine pregnancy (Seeber et al 2006). However, another method used to help with the diagnosis of an ectopic pregnancy is the 'plateau' in serum β-hCG levels. Plateau is defined as a β-hCG doubling time of 7 days or more (Kadar and Romero 1988). If the half-life of serum β-hCG is less than 1.4 days, spontaneous miscarriage is likely, whereas a half-life of more than 7 days is more likely to be indicative of an ectopic pregnancy. Therefore, falling levels of β-hCG can distinguish between an ectopic pregnancy and a spontaneous miscarriage. As a proportion of ectopic pregnancies are tubal miscarriages (with biochemical changes similar to those of intrauterine miscarriages), and approximately 15–20% of all ectopic pregnancies can have doubling serum β-hCG levels similar to those of normal intrauterine pregnancies (Silva et al 2006), suboptimal serial β-hCG changes are not specific or sensitive enough to diagnose ectopic pregnancies.

Serum progesterone

Progesterone, a C-21 hormone, is essential in early pregnancy for decidual function, implantation, reduction in immune response and myometrial quiescence. It is produced entirely by the corpus luteum until the sixth week of gestation. The trophoblastic contribution begins from the seventh week and becomes the predominant source by the 12th week. Progesterone concentrations continue to rise until 7 weeks of gestation and then plateau until 10 weeks, after which there is a gradual increase until term. In the conception cycle, progesterone concentrations are 2–4 nmol/l on the day of the luteinizing hormone surge and rise to 20–70 nmol/l a week later. At term, concentrations vary from 200 to 600 nmol/l.

Progesterone concentrations have been widely used for the diagnosis and management of pregnancies of unknown location (PUL, i.e where ultrasound is inconclusive). In failing pregnancies, whether ectopic or miscarriage, progesterone concentrations are expected to be low compared with values in healthy ongoing pregnancies (Hahlin et al 1990). Most studies report cut-off concentrations of less than 16 nmol/l for failing pregnancies and more than 80 nmol/l for healthy ongoing pregnancies (Mathews et al 1986, Sau and Hamilton-Fairley 2003, Bishry and Ganta 2008). Progesterone levels over 25 nmol/l are 'likely to indicate' and levels over 60 nmol/l are 'strongly associated with' pregnancies subsequently shown to be normal. A progesterone concentration below 25 nmol/l in an anembryonic pregnancy has been shown to be diagnostic of non-viability (Elson et al 2003). Concentrations less than 20 nmol/l have a sensitivity of 93% and a specificity of 94% for the prediction of spontaneous resolution of PULs (Banerjee et al 2001). A meta-analysis has demonstrated that a single serum progesterone measurement is good at predicting a viable intrauterine or failed pregnancy, but is not useful for locating the site of pregnancy (Mol et al 1998). When interpreting progesterone measurements, variations in concentrations should be taken into account because of the assay methods, and a departmental protocol should state the normal range for that unit.

Other protein and steroid markers

In an effort to detect an ectopic pregnancy at an early stage, various steroid and protein markers have been studied including Schwangerschafts protein-1, human placental lactogen, pregnancy-associated plasma protein A, inhibin and insulin growth factor binding protein-1. However, none of these markers has been found to make a significant impact on clinical practice. Recently, serum CA125, creatine kinase, activin A and vascular endothelial growth factor have also been studied for the diagnosis of ectopic pregnancy; however, their sensitivity and specificity are not sufficient to allow their application in clinical practice.

Ultrasonography

Ultrasound has become an essential tool in the assessment and diagnosis of suspected ectopic pregnancies. The presence of an intrauterine pregnancy does not conclusively exclude an ectopic pregnancy; however, the occurrence of a heterotopic pregnancy is rare. The transvaginal approach is far superior to the abdominal approach, as the proximity of the vaginal probe to the pelvic structures and the use of high-frequency transducers (5–7 MHz) significantly improves resolution.

The earliest a normal intrauterine gestational sac (approximately 2 mm) can be seen is 4 weeks with a transvaginal ultrasound and 5 weeks with an abdominal ultrasound. In 20% of patients with an ectopic pregnancy, collection of fluid within the uterine cavity results in the formation of a pseudo gestational sac which mimics a true intrauterine sac. Ultrasonographic signs of a true gestational sac include an eccentrically placed gestational sac within the uterine cavity, the double ring or double decidual sac sign (DDSS) and an intact midline endometrial echo, with the pregnancy seen implanted beneath the endometrial surface. The double ring comprises chorionic villi, intervillous lakes, the extravillous trophoblast and the maternal decidua. This DDSS can also be seen in one-third of ectopic pregnancies. On the other hand, a pseudo sac is surrounded by a single layer of tissue, tends to follow the contour of the cavity, and in a longitudinal section of the uterus, the midline endometrial echo cannot be seen because of the fluid.

The most reliable sign to differentiate between a pseudo sac and a true sac is the appearance of a yolk sac within the true gestational sac. The yolk sac confirms an intrauterine pregnancy even before a live embryo is detected. A yolk sac is identified by ultrasound when the mean gestational sac diameter is greater than 8 mm.

A review of the literature by Brown and Doubilet (1994) revealed the frequency of various ultrasound features in ectopic pregnancies as detailed below:

- an empty uterus (28%);
- an empty uterus and an adnexal mass (35%);
- an intrauterine sac or pseudo gestational sac (25%);
- an empty uterus and an ectopic gestational sac (12%) with or without a yolk sac and cardiac activity; and
- varying amount of fluid in the pouch of Douglas (25%).

In ectopic pregnancies, a hyperechogenic tubal ring ('doughnut' or 'bagel' sign) is the most common finding on ultrasound scan. Others include a mixed adnexal mass representing either tubal miscarriage or tubal rupture, an ectopic sac with a yolk sac, or an embryo with or without a fetal heartbeat. The corpus luteum may be present on the ipsilateral side in 85% of cases. It has been reported that 74% of ectopic pregnancies can be visualized on initial transvaginal ultrasound scan, and more than 90% of ectopic pregnancies can be visualized prior to treatment (Kirk et al 2007).

Quantitative assessment of β-hCG levels is essential for the accurate interpretation of ultrasonographic findings. A single serum β-hCG measurement has been used as a discriminatory level to help with the diagnosis of ectopic pregnancy. Absence of an intrauterine gestational sac with serum β-hCG levels of 6500 IU/l or more has an 86% positive predictive value and a 100% negative predictive value for the presence of an ectopic pregnancy (Romero et al 1985). With transvaginal ultrasound scan, different discriminatory levels of serum β-hCG (e.g. 1000, 1500 and 2000 IU/l) have been used with no significant difference in the detection rates of ectopic pregnancies (Barnhart et al 1999, Condous et al 2005). Failure to visualize an intrauterine gestational sac by transvaginal ultrasound if β-hCG concentrations are 1000–2000 IU/l or more indicates either an abnormal intrauterine pregnancy, a recent miscarriage or an ectopic pregnancy. It must be emphasized that although the discriminatory zone for an intrauterine pregnancy is well established, there is no such discriminatory zone for ectopic pregnancies. In 15–20% of women with clinical suspicion of an early pregnancy failure, ultrasound findings are not diagnostic.

Doppler ultrasonography

Doppler ultrasound is a non-invasive biophysical method of investigating patterns of blood flow. In ectopic pregnancies, the normal high-resistance blood flow in the uterine or ovarian artery branches changes to low resistance.

Jurkovic et al (1992), in a prospective study, used colour Doppler to detect and compare changes of blood flow in the uterine and spiral arteries and the corpus luteum in ectopic and intrauterine pregnancies. In intrauterine pregnancies, the impedance to flow (resistance index) in uterine arteries decreased with gestational age, but this remained constant in ectopic pregnancies. Peak blood velocity in the uterine arteries increased with gestational age in intrauterine pregnancies, and the values were significantly higher than those seen in ectopic pregnancies. However, uterine blood flow velocity was lower in the ectopic group, indicating an overall reduction in uterine blood supply. Local vascular changes associated with a true gestational sac differentiate an intrauterine pregnancy from the pseudo sac of an ectopic pregnancy. Doppler flow imaging may thus suggest that an adnexal mass is an ectopic pregnancy from the presence of high vascularity at the periphery of the adnexal mass.

Colour and pulsed Doppler increase the sensitivity of transvaginal ultrasound and allow earlier detection of ectopic pregnancies, thereby giving the opportunity for the application of medical treatment or conservative surgery.

Three-dimensional ultrasonography

Three-dimensional (3D) ultrasound is emerging as a possible additional diagnostic tool for ectopic pregnancy. Rempen

(1998) conducted a prospective follow-up study in order to evaluate the potential of 3D ultrasound to differentiate intrauterine gestations from extrauterine gestations. Fifty-four pregnancies with a gestational age of less than 10 weeks and with an intrauterine gestational sac more than 5 mm in diameter were included in the study. The configuration of the endometrium in the frontal plane of the uterus was correlated with pregnancy outcomes. It was found that this configuration was asymmetrical in 84% of intrauterine pregnancies, whereas the endometrium showed asymmetry in 90% of extrauterine pregnancies ($P \leq 0.0001$). The conclusion was that evaluation of the endometrial shape in the frontal plane may be a useful additional means of distinguishing intrauterine from extrauterine pregnancies.

Harika et al (1995) conducted a study to assess the role of 3D imaging in the early diagnosis of ectopic pregnancy on 12 asymptomatic patients whose gestational age was less than 6 weeks. Nine of these patients had an ectopic pregnancy at laparoscopy, and of these, 3D transvaginal ultrasound showed a small ectopic gestational sac in four cases. These preliminary results suggest that 3D ultrasound may be an effective procedure for the diagnosis of ectopic pregnancy in asymptomatic patients prior to the sixth gestational week; however, its accuracy would have to be refined.

Diagnostic laparoscopy

With the availability of sensitive quantitative serum β-hCG assays and high-resolution transvaginal ultrasound, diagnostic laparoscopy is seldom used nowadays as a primary diagnostic tool. In some units, it is used to diagnose ectopic pregnancy in the presence of an empty uterus with serum β-hCG levels above the discriminatory level. A major disadvantage of laparoscopy is that a small ectopic pregnancy may not be visualized, and in 3–4% of cases the diagnosis will be missed. Therefore, careful selection of patients is crucial.

Culdocentesis

With the availability of modern equipment and biochemical tests, culdocentesis is rarely used for the diagnosis of ectopic pregnancy. However, in parts of the world where these facilities are lacking, aspirating blood from the pouch of Douglas which does not clot on standing is most likely suggestive of an ectopic pregnancy.

Differential Diagnosis

The differential diagnoses of an ectopic pregnancy should include ruptured corpus luteum cyst, threatened or incomplete miscarriage, PID and degenerating fibroids. Quantitative assessment of β-hCG, transvaginal ultrasonography and laparoscopy are powerful tools which should be used to resolve uncertain cases.

Pregnancy of Unknown Location

In recent years, PUL has been used as a diagnosis for patients with a positive pregnancy test with no signs of intrauterine or extrauterine pregnancy or retained products of conception on an initial transvaginal ultrasound scan. Studies report that PUL is identified in 8–31% of women referred for ultrasound assessment in early pregnancy (Hahlin et al 1995, Condous et al 2004).

Subsequent follow-up in woman with PUL will lead to the diagnosis of either: (a) an intrauterine pregnancy that was too early to be visualized on an initial ultrasound scan; (b) an ectopic pregnancy that was too early to be visualized or was missed on an initial ultrasound scan (7–20%); (c) a spontaneously resolving pregnancy known as a 'failing PUL' (50–70%), which would include both intrauterine and extrauterine pregnancies; or (d) persistent PUL, where biochemical findings mimic an ectopic pregnancy with suboptimal serum β-hCG levels that fail to decline, and failure to localize pregnancy on ultrasound scan or laparoscopy.

PULs present a management dilemma for health professionals in the early pregnancy unit, and inevitably increase workload and time consumption. For clinically stable women, expectant management has been demonstrated to be safe. PULs are followed up with serial hormone measurements, repeat transvaginal ultrasound scans and possibly laparoscopy with or without uterine curettage. It is important to note that in women with a history and transvaginal ultrasound findings suggestive of complete miscarriage, serial β-hCG measurements should be performed as approximately 6% of these can be ectopic pregnancies (Condous et al 2004b).

Recently, the use of β-hCG ratios (β-hCG 48 h/β-hCG 0 h) rather than absolute β-hCG values has been assessed in the diagnosis and management of PUL. A β-hCG ratio below 0.87 (or a β-hCG decrease >13%) has a 92.7% sensitivity (95% CI 85.6–96.5) and a 96.7% specificity (95% CI 90.0–99.1) for the prediction of a failing pregnancy (Condous et al 2006, Bignardi et al 2008). Various mathematical models using log regression and the Bayesian approach have been developed to predict the outcome of PULs; however (Condous et al 2004), these need to be tested prospectively in multicentre trials. Figure 25.1 shows an algorithm for the management of women with PUL.

Management of Ectopic Pregnancy

Figure 25.2 shows a summary of the algorithm for managing ectopic pregnancies. The following section should be read in tandem with this figure.

Surgical treatment

Laparoscopy or laparotomy

All the surgical procedures for the treatment of ectopic pregnancy can be accomplished via laparoscopy or laparotomy. The main factors which will determine the preferred approach are:

- haemodynamic condition of the patient;
- size and location of the ectopic pregnancy;
- laparoscopic experience of the surgeon; and
- availability of appropriate equipment for laparoscopic surgery.

Laparotomy should be considered where the patient is haemodynamically unstable, there is a suspicion of extensive abdominal and pelvic adhesions making laparoscopy

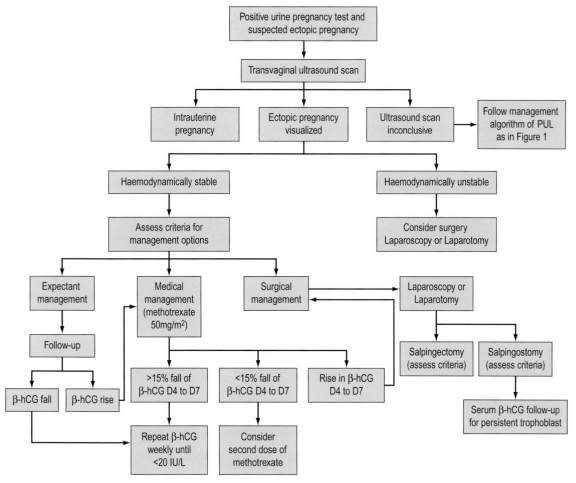

Figure 25.1 Algorithm for the management of women with pregnancy of unknown location (PUL). β-hCG, beta human chorionic gonadotrophin.

difficult, or the pregnancy is cornual or ovarian. A ruptured ectopic pregnancy does not necessarily require laparotomy, the main aim being use of the most expedient method. In the hands of an experienced laparoscopist, all the indications for laparotomy are relative rather than absolute.

A systematic review has shown that laparoscopic salpingostomy is significantly less successful than the open surgical approach in the elimination of tubal ectopic pregnancy (two randomized controlled trials, $n = 165$, OR 0.28, 95% CI 0.09–0.86) due to a significantly higher persistent trophoblast rate in laparoscopic surgery (OR 3.5, 95% CI 1.1–11). However, the laparoscopic approach is significantly less costly than open surgery. Long-term follow-up ($n = 127$) shows no evidence of a difference in intrauterine pregnancy rate, but there is a non-significant tendency to a lower repeat ectopic pregnancy rate (Hajenius et al 2007). The laparoscopic approach is associated with less intraoperative blood loss, lower analgesic requirements and a shorter duration of hospitalization and convalescence. An additional benefit of the laparoscopic approach is significantly fewer adhesions at the surgical site compared with those treated by laparotomy (Lundorff et al 1991).

Salpingectomy

Removal of the fallopian tube is still the most common method for the treatment of ectopic pregnancy. It can be performed via laparotomy or laparoscopy. When laparotomy is performed, the easiest way to remove the fallopian tube is by progressive division and ligation of the mesosalpinx. Laparoscopic salpingectomy can be performed with a pretied loop ligature, bipolar diathermy or disposable stapling devices. However, the cost associated with the use of the stapling devices has limited their popularity.

Several methods have been proposed for removal of the fallopian tube from the peritoneal cavity following laparoscopic salpingectomy:

- placement of the fallopian tube into a specially designed plastic bag introduced via a 10-mm port. The bag is then sealed at its neck and removed intact through the port;
- morcellation of the fallopian tube and removal by a 10-mm grasping forceps; or
- posterior colpotomy and removal of the tube intact via the pouch of Douglas.

When to consider salpingectomy

Salpingectomy is indicated for women with:

- ruptured tubal pregnancy;
- recurrent ectopic pregnancy in a tube already treated conservatively;
- previous sterilization and reversal of sterilization;

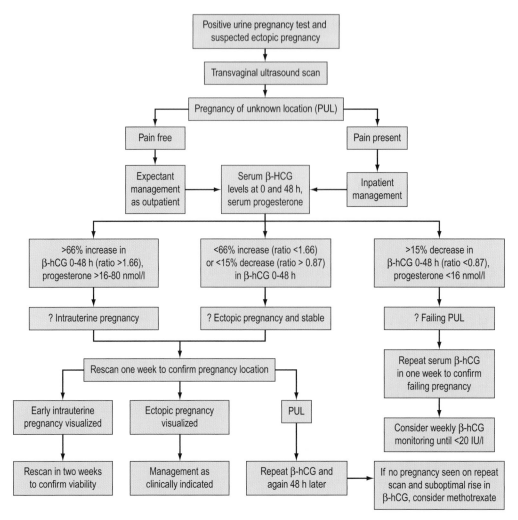

Figure 25.2 Algorithm for management of ectopic pregnancies. PUL, pregnancy of unknown location; β-hCG, beta human chorionic gonadotrophin; D4, day 4; D7, day 7.

- previous tubal surgery for infertility; or
- pre-existing tubal damage as a consequence of a frozen pelvis.

No randomized controlled trials have compared salpingectomy and salpingotomy. Results from four cohort studies suggest that there may be a higher subsequent intrauterine pregnancy rate associated with salpingotomy, but the magnitude of this benefit may be small (Royal College of Obstetricians and Gynaecologists 2004). The possibility of further ectopic pregnancies in the conserved tube should also be discussed if salpingotomy is being considered. In the presence of a healthy contralateral tube, there is no clear evidence that salpingotomy should be used in preference to salpingectomy.

Finally, the debate over salpingectomy or salpingo-oophorectomy no longer exists. Removal of a healthy ovary is now considered both unnecessary and unjustified.

Linear salpingotomy

An incision is made on the antimesenteric border of the fallopian tube with either a needle-point monopolar cutting diathermy, scalpel, scissors or laser, and the tubal lumen is exposed. The products of conception are removed with grasping forceps. Sometimes the laparoscopic suction/irrigation probe may be used for aqua dissection and removal of the products of conception by suction. Irrigation of the tubal lumen after removal of the products of conception is essential. Thereafter, haemostasis is achieved with electrocoagulation. The incision can either be closed with a fine non-absorbable suture material such as 6/0 Prolene, or left open (salpingotomy) for healing to occur by secondary intention. Either approach results in satisfactory healing of the tubal wall. A study by Tulandi and Guralnick (1991) showed that there was no significant difference in the number of subsequent intrauterine pregnancies, number of ectopic pregnancies or incidence of adhesion formation with either method.

Linear salpingotomy can be performed via an open or laparoscopic approach. However, regardless of the route used to access the ectopic pregnancy, the surgeon should remember that fallopian tubes are delicate structures. Basic microsurgical principles such as gentle handling of tissues, avoidance of peritoneal damage, thorough irrigation and suction of the peritoneal cavity to remove all the blood clots, and minimizing postoperative adhesion formation should always be applied.

Laparoscopic linear salpingotomy should be considered as the primary procedure of choice for the treatment of tubal ectopic pregnancy in the presence of contralateral tubal disease and where the patient wishes to retain her potential for future fertility.

The use of conservative surgery exposes the women to a small risk of tubal bleeding in the immediate postoperative period, persistent trophoblast and the risk of subsequent ectopic pregnancy in the conserved tube. For identification and treatment of persistent trophoblast, these women should be followed by serial β-hCG measurements post surgery. Treatment with methotrexate can be initiated if β-hCG concentrations fail to fall as expected. Sauer et al (1997) initiated treatment if serum β-hCG was more than 10% of the preoperative level by 10 days after surgery, and Pouly et al (1991) initiated treatment if serum β-hCG was more than 65% of the initial level at 48 h post surgery. Currently, there is insufficient evidence to recommend ideal cut-off concentrations of serum β-hCG for commencing treatment, but protocols for identification and treatment of persistent trophoblast should be present in every unit.

Segmental resection

When the ectopic pregnancy is located in the isthmic segment of the fallopian tube, segmental resection and end-to-end anastomosis constitute one of the conservative surgical therapeutic options. The anastomosis is usually isthmoampullary and can be performed either at the time of the resection (primary) or at a later stage (secondary). However, for isthmic tubal pregnancy, linear salpingotomy is technically less difficult and has a shorter operative time.

Fimbrial evacuation

Fimbrial evacuation is indicated when the pregnancy lies in the fimbrial segment of the fallopian tube. It involves gentle and progressive compression of the tube, starting just proximal to the side of the pregnancy and moving it systematically to the fimbrial end of the tube. When the pregnancy is located at the ampullary part, fimbrial evacuation or 'milking of the tube' is not recommended. The external pressure required to propel the ectopic pregnancy and achieve a tubal miscarriage is likely to cause severe damage to the endosalpinx and excessive bleeding from the implantation site, and the procedure is associated with a greater risk of persistent trophoblastic disease (Brosens et al 1984). When milking was compared with linear salpingotomy for ampullary ectopic pregnancy, milking was associated with a two-fold increase in the recurrent ectopic pregnancy rate (Smith et al 1987).

Reproductive outcome

The evaluation of reproductive outcome following surgical treatment for ectopic pregnancy is based on three main parameters:

- tubal patency as assessed by hysterosalpingography or second-look laparoscopy;
- subsequent intrauterine pregnancy rate; and
- recurrent ectopic pregnancy rate.

In patients who underwent radical surgery (salpingectomy), the subsequent intrauterine pregnancy rate was 49.3% (range 36.6–71.4%) and the recurrent ectopic pregnancy rate was 10% (range 5.8–12%). In patients who underwent conservative surgery, the subsequent intrauterine pregnancy rate was 53% (range 38–83%) and the recurrent ectopic pregnancy rate was 14% (range 6.4–21.2%). These results are based on a retrospective analysis of nine studies in a total of 2635 patients, and indicate that conservative surgery is associated with higher subsequent intrauterine pregnancy and higher recurrent ectopic rates compared with radical surgery (Yao and Tulandi 1997). However, the variations in the design of each study make strict comparison of the results very difficult. Similar figures of intrauterine pregnancy (83.7%) and recurrent ectopic pregnancy (8%) have been reported when expectant management is compared with salpingectomy (Helmy et al 2007).

Medical treatment with methotrexate

Early detection of an ectopic pregnancy, the desire to retain fertility, and minimizing costs and surgical morbidity are the main reasons for incorporating medical treatment as an option for managing ectopic pregnancies. The most frequently used drug is methotrexate and this will therefore be discussed in detail, although other agents have been used. Gynaecologists are familiar with methotrexate because the drug has been used very effectively for the treament of gestational trophoblastic disease since 1955 (Li et al 1956). Hreschchyshyn et al (1965) were the first to report on the use of methotrexate in the management of ectopic pregnancy. In 1982, Tanaka et al reported on the treatment of an unruptured interstitial pregnancy with a course of intramuscular methotrexate.

Mode of action and pharmacokinetics

Methotrexate, formerly known as amethopterin, is a potent folic acid antagonist. It inhibits the action of the enzyme dehydrofolate reductase and the coenzyme methyl tetrahydrofolate. These enzymes are essential for the conversion of dehydrofolic acid into tetrahydrofolic acid, and the conversion of deoxyuridylic acid into thymidylic acid which is critical for the synthesis of DNA during the S phase of the cell cycle. Prevention of incorporation of thymidylic acid into DNA results in lack of DNA synthesis and subsequent arrest of cellular division and multiplication. Methotrexate is ideal for inhibition of rapidly growing cells such as trophoblasts.

Methotrexate is almost completely absorbed if administered intramuscularly, with peak serum concentrations reached within 30–60 min. Only 10% of methotrexate undergoes hepatic and intracellular metabolism to polyglutamated products, which also act as active antimetabolites. Up to 90% of the drug is secreted unchanged in the urine within 48 h, and therefore impaired renal function can result in prolonged exposure of tissues to high levels of methotrexate or its metabolic products.

Side-effects of methotrexate

The two most significant factors that determine the intensity of methotrexate toxicity are the serum concentration of drug and the duration of exposure to methotrexate. The drug affects all rapidly proliferating cells, and therefore the main side-effects originate from suppression of bone marrow and epithelial cells of the gastrointestinal tract. The spectrum of possible side-effects include: abdominal pain in 75% of women following treatment, conjunctivitis, stomatitis, gastritis, diarrhoea, alopecia (reversible), myelosuppression, liver toxicity, photosensitivity (skin reaction), pneumonitis, renal toxicity and anaphylaxis.

The incidence of side-effects among patients treated with high-dose or multidose methotrexate is reported to be 20–30%. Single-dose regimens, however, currently used for the non-surgical treatment of ectopic pregnancy are associated with minor or no side-effects. Resolution of the adverse effects usually occurs within 72 h after termination of therapy.

Guidelines for the prescription of methotrexate

In order to achieve early identification and prevention of serious side-effects, the Committee on the Safety of Medicines has issued the following guidelines for the prescription of methotrexate.

Myelosuppression

Pretreatment full blood count needs to be documented as a baseline blood count. If an acute decrease in the white cell or platelet count occurs, treatment should be discontinued immediately.

Liver toxicity

Pre-existing abnormal liver function or concurrent abnormal liver function tests should alert medical staff to potential liver toxicity. Again, pretreatment baseline liver function tests are essential.

Renal function

Assessment of renal function is essential prior to treatment because the primary route of excretion of methotrexate is the kidney. Caution should be exercised when there is concurrent medication use with non-steroidal anti-inflammatory drugs as these may adversely affect renal function and further increase serum methotrexate concentrations.

Folinic acid rescue

Methotrexate morbidity can be minimized by the concurrent administration of the 'antidote' folinic acid in the form of calcium folinate which is then converted to 5-methyltetrahydrofolate.

Who will benefit from methotrexate?

The key for successful and safe medical treatment of ectopic pregnancy is proper selection of patients. Methotrexate should be reserved for patients who have an unruptured tubal pregnancy, are clinically asymptomatic and haemodynamically stable. The indications and contraindications for methotrexate therapy are listed below.

Indications

- Initial pretreatment plasma β-hCG concentration below 3000 IU/l.
- Tubal diameter less than 2 cm as defined by direct visualization or ultrasound.
- Absent fetal heartbeat on ultrasound scan.

Contraindications

- Symptomatic patients.
- Haemodynamically unstable patients.
- Presence of haemoperitoneum.
- Initial pretreatment β-hCG concentration greater than 3000 IU/l.
- Tubal diameter more than 2 cm.
- Presence of fetal heartbeat on ultrasound scan.
- Evidence of liver disease, renal insufficiency or myelosuppression.
- Inability of the patient to return for follow-up care.

Although medical management can be successful at serum β-hCG concentrations greater than 3000 IU/l, quality-of-life data suggest that methotrexate should only be used with serum β-hCG concentrations below 3000 IU/l. Shalev et al (1995) reported that following intratubal administration of methotrexate, the failure rate was 24% when the tubal diameter was less than 2 cm and 48% when the diameter was more than 2 cm. The authors recommend that methotrexate should only be used when the size of the ectopic pregnancy is less than 2 cm. Stovall and Ling (1993) found that the administration of methotrexate to patients who had a fetal heartbeat on ultrasound scan was associated with a 14.3% failure rate. In the group of patients without fetal cardiac activity, the failure rate was 4.7%.

Prior to commencing medical treatment, women should be given clear information about the possible need for further treatment and adverse effects following treatment, and they should be able to return easily for assessment at any time during follow-up. Patients should be advised regarding adequate compliance; no use of alcohol, aspirin, non-steroidal inflammatory drugs or folic acid supplements; avoidance of sexual intercourse and sunlight exposure; fluid intake of at least 1.5 l/day; saline mouth washes daily; and delay of pregnancy for at least 3 months after treatment because of the teratogenecity of methotrexate.

Routes of administration and dose

Methotrexate can be administered systemically (intravenously or intramuscularly) or locally using a laparoscopic or transvaginal ultrasound-guided approach. The transvaginal administration of methotrexate under sonographic guidance requires visualization of an ectopic gestational sac, and specific skills and expertise of the clinician. This mode of administration is less invasive and more effective than the laparoscopically 'blind' intratubal injection. Two randomized controlled trials (Fernandez et al 1994, Cohen et al 1996) suggested that local injection of methotrexate was equivalent in effect to systemic methotrexate. The major advantages of direct injection of methotrexate into the tube include smaller dose of the drug, higher tissue concentration and fewer systemic side-effects. In comparison, systemic methotrexate is practical, easier to administer and less dependent on clinical skills. The published literature includes a wide spectrum of protocols for the systemic administration of methotrexate, including:

- standard single dose (60–200 mg IM);
- fixed multiple dose regimen: methotrexate 1 mg/kg body weight IM on days 0, 2, 4, 6 alternated with folinic acid 0.1 mg/kg orally on days 1, 3, 5, 7 followed by 6 days without

- medication. A second course is given on day 14 if the serum hCG concentration on that day is 40% above the initial value on day 0; and
- variable single dose regimen (1 mg/kg or 50 mg/m^2 of body surface).

The success rate of all three regimens is comparable. Three trials have shown that the administration of methotrexate in a single IM dose of 50 mg/m^2 body surface area is associated with a complete reabsorption rate of 92%, a subsequent intrauterine pregnancy rate of 58% and a recurrent ectopic pregnancy rate of 9% (Hajenius et al 2007). Reabsorption rate is defined as the time interval between initiation of therapy and undetectable serum hCG concentration. The mean reabsorption time is 30 days, ranging from 5 to 100 days. Tubal patency is reported to be 50–100% (mean 71%) after systemic administration of methotrexate.

Laparoscopic surgery vs methotrexate

O'Shea et al (1994) published the results of a prospective randomized trial comparing intra-amniotic methotrexate with carbon dioxide laser laparoscopic salpingotomy. The salpingotomy group and the local methotrexate group had comparable success rates: 87.5% and 89.7%, respectively. A systematic review showed that systemic methotrexate in a fixed multiple dose IM regimen has a non-significant tendency to higher treatment success than laparoscopic salpingostomy (OR 1.8, 95% CI 0.73–4.6). No significant differences are found in long-term follow-up for intrauterine pregnancy and repeat ectopic pregnancy (Hajenius et al 2007). Methotrexate appears to be effective in a selective group of patients with ectopic pregnancy. Direct and indirect costs of medical therapy are less than half of those associated with laparoscopy. Intramuscular administration eliminates anaesthetic and surgical risks arising from laparoscopic injection of the drug. However, the long-term effect of locally injected pharmacological substances upon the endosalpinx remains largely unknown.

Serum β-hCG levels should be checked 4 and 7 days after the first dose of methotrexate, and a further dose is given if β-hCG levels have failed to fall by more than 15% between days 4 and 7. The level of serum β-hCG is likely to increase between days 1 and 4 after treatment. It has been suggested that although methotrexate is arresting mitosis in the cytotrophoblast, the syncytiotrophoblast may still be able to produce β-hCG. Also, destruction of the cells releases more β-hCG into the systemic circulation. Approximately 15% of women require more than a single dose of methotrexate, and 7% experience tubal rupture during follow-up (Yao and Tulandi 1997, Sowter et al 2001).

It is important to recognize that abdominal pain occurs in 30–50% of patients 6–7 days after the administration of methotrexate. The gynaecologist has to decide if the pain is due to imminent tubal rupture, existing tubal rupture or simply represents postmethotrexate pain. Postmethotrexate pain is localized in the lower abdomen. Its precise aetiology remains largely unknown, but it is likely to be due to a combination of factors, including destruction of the trophoblastic tissue and transtubal haemorrhage leading to peritoneal irritation. Close monitoring of patients is essential in order to avoid unnecessary surgical intervention in the form of laparoscopy or laparotomy. According to Stovall (1995), regular assessment of haemoglobin is the most useful parameter. The pain usually subsides within 24–48 h and occasionally precedes or follows an episode of vaginal bleeding.

Brown et al (1991) assessed the clinical value of serial transvaginal ultrasonography in the monitoring of ectopic pregnancies treated with methotrexate, and concluded that routine ultrasonography is not necessary after methotrexate treatment. There was no correlation between the pattern of resolution of β-hCG levels and sonographic findings.

Mifepristone and methotrexate

Mifepristone (RU486) has been used in combination with methotrexate for the medical treatment of ectopic pregnancy (Gazvani and Emery 1999). A non-randomized study from France (Perdu et al 1998) only reported one failure in the 30 patients treated with IM methotrexate and oral mifepristone, and 11 failures in 42 patients treated with methotrexate alone. The authors concluded that the combination of mifepristone and methotrexate decreased the risk of failure in medical treatment of ectopic pregnancy. However, further prospective randomized studies are needed to evaluate the role of mifepristone in the medical management of ectopic pregnancy.

Controlled expectant management

When only expectant management was available, it was associated with high morbidity and mortality because the patients who failed expectant management usually presented with significant clinical symptoms, indicating rupture of the ectopic pregnancy. Since then, due to the advancement in ultrasound and rapid access to quantitative β-hCG assays, the nature of expectant management has changed in that it is now controlled and monitored.

Ten prospective studies, with a total of 347 patients managed expectantly, demonstrated that 69% of the ectopic gestations resolved spontaneously. All patients were haemodynamically stable and had decreasing serum β-hCG levels. However, other variables such as size and location of the ectopic pregnancy or presence of fetal cardiac activity were not always specified (Yao and Tulandi 1997). Interventions are required in approximately 23–29% of cases with expectant management (Hahlin et al 1995).

The essential prerequisite for successful expectant management of ectopic gestation is appropriate selection of patients. The Royal College of Obstetricians and Gynaecologists (2004) issued guidelines for the management of tubal pregnancy. The conclusion was that expectant management is more likely to be successful in the following circumstances:

- clinically stable asymptomatic woman;
- baseline serum β-hCG concentrations below 1000–2000 IU/l;
- haemoperitoneum of less than 50–100 ml;
- a tubal mass less than 2 cm; and
- absence of recognizable fetal parts on ultrasound.

Women managed expectantly should be followed twice weekly with serial β-hCG measurements (ideally β-hCG should be <50% of the initial level within 7 days) and weekly transvaginal ultrasound examination to assess reduction in size of adnexal mass by the end of the first week. Thereafter, weekly β-hCG concentrations and transvaginal ultrasound examination should be undertaken until β-hCG concentrations are less than 20 IU/l. It must be emphasized, however, that tubal rupture has been reported in cases of very low and decreasing serum β-hCG concentration, and expectant management often involves long periods of hospitalization and follow-up. Women should be counselled about the importance of compliance and should be within easy access of medical help.

Anti-D immunoglobulin

All non-sensitized, Rhesus-negative women with suspected or confirmed ectopic pregnancy should receive 250 IU (50 μg) of anti-D immunoglobulin.

Non-Tubal Ectopic Pregnancy

Cervical pregnancy

A cervical pregnancy is one that implants entirely within the cervical canal. The reported incidence ranges from one in 2500 to one in 18,000 deliveries (0.2% of ectopic pregnancies). Predisposing factors for the development of cervical pregnancy include previous instrumentation of the endocervical canal, previous caesarean delivery, Asherman's syndrome and exposure to DES. Sporadic cases of cervical pregnancy have been reported after controlled ovarian stimulation with human menopausal gonadotrophins and intrauterine insemination, as well as IVF (Weyerman et al 1989).

Cervical pregnancy produces profuse vaginal bleeding without associated cramping pain. In some cases of advanced pregnancies, it can be associated with urinary symptoms. The clinical and ultrasound criteria for the diagnosis of cervical pregnancy are summarized below (Hofmann et al 1987).

Clinical criteria

The external os is usually dilated and the cervix feels distended or globular with a small uterus on bimanual examination. Curettage of the endometrial cavity reveals no evidence of trophoblastic tissue. The products of conception are confined within the cervix and the internal cervical os is closed.

Ultrasound criteria

No evidence of an intrauterine gestational sac, ballooned cervical canal/barrel-shaped cervix, gestational sac in the endocervix below the uterine arteries, closed internal os and Doppler blood flow around the sac.

The differential diagnoses include an intrauterine pregnancy with a low implantation site (isthmicocervical pregnancy), an ongoing spontaneous intrauterine miscarriage, a cervical carcinoma, a cervical or prolapsed submucosal myoma, placenta praevia and trophoblastic tumour.

Early forms of cervical pregnancy are managed conservatively. Conservative treatment includes the use of systemic methotrexate, intra-amniotic feticide, reduction of blood supply and tamponade. Transvaginal ultrasound-guided local injection of the ectopic pregnancy with methotrexate or potassium chloride has been shown to be successful (Benson and Doubilet 1996). This technique has been used for the treatment of heterotopic coexistent cervical and intrauterine pregnancy. Similarly, systemic methotrexate alone is 91% efficacious in the treatment of cervical ectopic pregnancy, and a combination of intra-amniotic and systemic methotrexate therapy has been used to increase the chance of successful treatment (Kung and Chang 1999). Currently, there is no recommendation for the optimal dose and route of administration of methotrexate for the treatment of cervical ectopic pregnancy, although gestational age less than 9 weeks, serum β-hCG below 10,000 IU/l, absent fetal cardiac activity and crown–rump length less than 10 mm are associated with a greater chance of success with conservative treatment (Hung et al 1998).

Removal of the products of conception from the cervical canal by suction curettage is likely to stop the haemorrhage. Conservative measures used to arrest bleeding include packing of the uterus and cervix, and insertion of an intracervical 30-ml Foley catheter to arrest bleeding, insertion of sutures to ligate the lateral cervical vessels or placement of a cervical cerclage (Kirk et al 2006). In some cases, because of the depth of trophoblastic invasion, major blood vessels are involved and more radical measures such as bilateral uterine artery or internal iliac artery ligation are necessary to control the bleeding. When all the conservative measures have failed to arrest the bleeding, hysterectomy is required. Preoperatively, the patient must be informed about the possibility of hysterectomy and sign the appropriate consent.

Caesarean scar ectopic pregnancy

This is a relatively recent description for ectopic pregnancy location. The incidence is not well known as there are only a few case reports of first trimester caesarean scar ectopic pregnancies described in the literature. Risk factors include previous caesarean section, myomectomy, adenomyosis, IVF, previous dilatation and curettage, and manual removal of the placenta. Clinical presentation can be with either hypovolaemic shock and uterine rupture or painless vaginal bleeding. Ultrasound diagnostic criteria as described by Jurkovic et al (2003) include an empty uterine cavity, a gestational sac located anteriorly at the level of the internal cervical os covering the visible or presumed site of previous lower segment caesarean scar, evidence of functional trophoblastic circulation on Doppler examination, and a negative 'sliding organs sign'. In some cases, hysteroscopy and magnetic resonance imaging have also been used to aid in the diagnosis.

Medical, expectant and surgical methods of management have all been reported. Expectant management does not seem to be an appropriate choice as there is a greater risk of scar rupture and subsequent emergency hysterectomy. As a primary treatment, transvaginal ultrasound-guided local injection of methotrexate (25 mg) in the ectopic gestation has been shown to be associated with a 70–80% success rate (Jurkovic et al 2003). In the presence of fetal cardiac activity, potassium chloride in the ectopic sac followed by local methotrexate has also been shown to be effective (Jurkovic et al 2003). Lastly, there are reports on successful outcome with the use of systemic methotrexate followed by suction evacuation (Marchiolé et al 2004, Graesslin et al 2005).

Surgical management with suction curettage under ultrasound guidance followed by balloon tamponade is successful in reducing heavy intraoperative bleeding. Uterine artery embolization can also be used as an adjunctive therapy to reduce bleeding. An alternative approach can be the use of a Shirodkar suture prior to suction evacuation, with approximately 79% of cases requiring the suture to be tied to reduce bleeding (Jurkovic et al 2007). Finally, in cases presenting with hypovolaemic shock, laparotomy followed by hysterectomy is the only option available.

Ovarian pregnancy

Ovarian pregnancy represents the most common type of non-tubal ectopic pregnancy and occurs in 0.2–1% of all ectopic pregnancies. The incidence ranges from one in 40,000 to one in 7000 deliveries. Ovarian pregnancy has been reported after IVF treatment (Marcus and Brinsden 1993) and clomifene citrate ovulation induction (De Muylder et al 1994). The only risk factor associated with the development of an ovarian pregnancy is the current use of an IUCD.

The symptoms and signs of an ovarian pregnancy are similar to those of tubal pregnancy. Usually, the diagnosis is made during a laparoscopy or laparotomy. The classic criteria of Spiegelberg (1878) for the diagnosis of an ovarian pregnancy are as follows:

- the gestational sac must occupy a portion of the ovary;
- the gestational sac must be connected to the uterus by the ovarian ligament;
- ovarian tissue must be identified in the wall of the sac; and
- the fallopian tube on the affected side of the pelvis must be intact.

Transvaginal ultrasound can help in the diagnosis of an ovarian pregnancy which usually appears on or within the ovary as a cyst with a wide outer echogenic ring. A yolk sac or an embryo is rarely seen and the appearances usually lag in comparison with the gestational age (Comstock et al 2005). These are usually mistaken for corpus luteal cysts. 3D-ultrasound imaging has been shown to be useful in differentiating a corpus luteum from an ovarian pregnancy (Ghi et al 2007), whereas Doppler ultrasound is not very helpful in differentiating between them. Differential diagnoses include tubal pregnancy or complications of an ovarian cyst.

Treatment consists of resection of the trophoblast from the ovary and preserving as much ovarian tissue as possible. Salpingo-oophorectomy is rarely necessary. Persistent trophoblast can be treated with systemic methotrexate. Systemic methotrexate as a primary treatment has also been used successfully.

Abdominal pregnancy

There are two types of abdominal pregnancy:

- primary peritoneal implantation of the blastocyst; and
- secondary peritoneal implantation of the conceptus following tubal miscarriage or rupture, or less often, after uterine rupture with subsequent implantation within the abdomen.

Secondary abdominal pregnancies are far more common. Abdominal pregnancy represents approximately 1.4% of all ectopic pregnancies, and its incidence varies from one in 3000 to one in 10,000 deliveries. Abdominal pregnancies are associated with high maternal (0.5–1.8%) and perinatal mortality (40–95%) (Atrash et al 1987). The incidence of congenital fetal abnormalities ranges from 35% to 75%. Most of the abnormalities are caused by growth restriction and external pressure on the fetus. Common fetal problems include pulmonary hypoplasia, facial asymmetry and talipes.

The classic criteria for the diagnosis of primary abdominal pregnancy are:

- no evidence of uteroplacental fistula;
- presence of normal tubes and ovaries with no evidence of a recent or past pregnancy; and
- pregnancy only attached to the peritoneal surface.

The diagnosis of an abdominal pregnancy must be made early enough to eliminate the possibility of secondary implantation after primary tubal nidation. In the first and early second trimesters, the symptoms may be the same as those of a tubal ectopic gestation. As the pregnancy advances, however, unexplained abdominal pain, occasional vomiting, diarrhoea or constipation may occur. Fetal movements are very marked or painful and felt high in the abdomen. Braxton-Hicks contractions are absent. Abdominal palpation may disclose persistently abnormal fetal lie, abdominal tenderness and easy palpation of the fetal parts. The fetus gives the impression that it lies just under the skin of the abdomen. On bimanual examination, the uterus is usually normal in size and the cervix is long, firm and displaced. Abdominal ultrasound provides an unequivocal diagnosis, although computed tomography and magnetic resonance imaging have also been used to confirm the diagnosis.

The treatment is laparotomy as soon as the diagnosis is made. This is not to be undertaken lightly. The objectives are to remove the fetus and to ligate the umbilical cord close to the placenta without disturbing it. The placenta is allowed to be absorbed; if left alone, it rarely presents problems of bleeding or infection. The placenta should only be removed when the surgeon is absolutely certain that total haemostasis can be achieved. Removal of the placenta is possible if it is attached to the ovary, the broad ligament and the posterior surface of the uterus. Attempts to remove the placenta from other intra-abdominal organs are likely to cause massive haemorrhage due to the invasive properties of the trophoblast and the lack of cleavage planes. Adjuvant treatment with methotrexate along with selective arterial embolization has been recommended to stem the haemorrhage (Oki et al 2008). Placental involution can be monitored using serial ultrasonography and β-hCG concentrations. Potential complications of leaving the placenta in place include bowel obstruction, fistula formation, haemorrhage and peritonitis. The literature reports on successful management of abdominal pregnancies laparoscopically and with systemic methotrexate (Shaw et al 2007).

Interstitial pregnancy

In interstitial pregnancy, the zygote/blastocyst implants in the portion of the uterine fallopian tube that traverses the uterine wall. It occurs in one in 2500 to one in 5000 live births and comprises 2% of all ectopic pregnancies. Predisposing factors are similar to those of other tubal pregnancies.

The implantation site may be in the utero interstitial (inner segment), the true interstitial (middle segment) or the tubo interstitial (outer segment) region. The duration of pregnancy depends on its location. Implantation in either the inner or outer segments results in early rupture. Implantation in the middle segment involves a greater mass of myometrium and permits the pregnancy to advance to a somewhat later date. Rupture of the uterine wall is the most frequent outcome and the haemorrhage is usually severe. The signs and symptoms are similar to those of tubal ectopic pregnancy. Intermittent recurrent, sharp abdominal pain occurs at 4–6 weeks. Sudden severe abdominal pain is followed by collapse. Ultrasound diagnosis is made by visualization of the interstitial line adjoining the gestational sac and the lateral aspect of the uterine cavity, and continuation of the myometrial mantle around the ectopic sac (Jurkovic and Mavrelos 2007). Interstitial pregnancy must be differentiated from cornual myoma, pregnancy in one horn of a bicornuate uterus and a large endometrioma at the utero-tubal junction.

Laparoscopy will reveal an asymmetrical enlargement of the uterus, displacement of the uterine fundus to the opposite side, elevation of the involved cornu, and rotation of the uterus on its long axis. The round ligament may be lateral to the gestational sac. Traditionally, interstitial pregnancies have been managed by laparotomy followed by wedge resection or hysterectomy. Since the 1990s, laparoscopic cornual resection and salpingotomy have become the surgical treatment of choice (Tulandi et al 1995). Laparoscopic vasopressin injection followed by excision of the pregnancy and endoloop closure or laparoscopic suturing for haemostasis has also been described.

In the presence of haemorrhagic shock, immediate laparotomy is required. In these cases, simple wedge resection, reconstruction of the uterine wall and salpingectomy will be necessary. In some cases with a severely damaged uterine wall, the only way to control haemorrhage is to perform a total abdominal hysterectomy and unilateral salpingo-oophorectomy. Cornual resection and uterine reconstruction has been associated with uterine rupture in pregnancy or during labour in subsequent gestations.

Intraligamentous pregnancy

Intraligamentous pregnancy is another rare form of non-tubal pregnancy that occurs in approximately one in 300 ectopic pregnancies. It is commonly secondary to penetration of the tubal wall by trophoblastic tissue and advancement of the trophoblast between the two layers of the broad ligament. Clinical findings are similar to those of abdominal pregnancy. The uterus is felt separately and is usually displaced to the opposite side. If the pregnancy persists, the mass may become palpable abdominally. The diagnosis is usually made at the time of surgery. The surgical principles are similar to those applied to abdominal pregnancy. Problems of extensive placental invasion of nearby structures are less likely. If possible, the placenta should be removed; when this is not possible, it can be left *in situ* and allowed to resolve.

Cornual pregnancy

The term 'cornual pregnancy' indicates that the pregnancy has occurred in one horn of a bicornuate uterus or in the rudimentary horn of a unicornuate uterus. It is very rare (one in 100,000 pregnancies) but carries a 5% maternal mortality. Asymmetrical enlargement of the early pregnant uterus should suggest a uterine anomaly. Unusual discomfort and tenderness may be described. Ultrasound criteria for diagnosis include a single interstitial part of the fallopian tube in the main uterine body, a gestational sac which is mobile and separate from the uterus, surrounded by myometrium and a vascular pedicle adjoining the gestational sac to the unicornuate uterus (Jurkovic and Mavrelos 2007).

Conservative, laparoscopic and open surgical methods of management have all been described. If the diagnosis is made earlier in pregnancy, treatment is excision of the rudimentary horn and the tube on the affected side. Congenital abnormalities of the Müllerian duct are associated with renal anomalies; therefore, renal tract imaging should be ordered postoperatively.

Heterotopic pregnancy

Heterotopic pregnancy is defined as the simultaneous occurrence of an intrauterine and an extrauterine pregnancy. In spontaneous conception, the incidence has traditionally been quoted as one in 30,000 pregnancies. However, the incidence has risen to one in 3889 pregnancies due to the increased incidence of genital infections and the use of ovulation induction agents. With assisted conception techniques, particularly IVF and embryo transfer, 1–3% of all clinical pregnancies are heterotopic; therefore, it is imperative to visualize adnexae at the time of ultrasound scan for fetal viability (Svare et al 1993).

Unusual abdominal pain in the presence of spontaneous miscarriage or profuse uterine bleeding with signs of peritoneal irritation should suggest a heterotopic pregnancy. Serial measurements of serum β-hCG concentration are not helpful. The diagnosis depends on maintaining a high index of suspicion, particularly for patients in the high-risk group, and by transvaginal ultrasound scan or laparoscopy. If the diagnosis is established at an early stage, the prognosis of the intrauterine pregnancy is more favourable. Depending upon the size and viability of the ectopic pregnancy, treatment can be conservative with local intra-amniotic injection of methotrexate in the ectopic gestation or surgery. After a surgical procedure, the intrauterine pregnancy continues in approximately 75% of patients.

KEY POINTS

1. Ectopic pregnancy is a pregnancy that is implanted outside the uterine cavity. The ampullary segment of the fallopian tube is the most common site of ectopic pregnancy.

2. Independent risk factors consistently shown to increase the risk of tubal pregnancy include previous tubal pregnancy, previous laparoscopically proven PID, previous tubal surgery and current IUCD users.

3. Ectopic pregnancy should be considered as an important differential diagnosis in any woman of reproductive age who presents with the triad of abdominal pain, irregular vaginal bleeding and amenorrhoea. The presentation of symptomatic patients with a tubal ectopic pregnancy can be acute or subacute.

4. The introduction of highly sensitive biochemical assays for the measurement of β-hCG concentration and transvaginal sonography have made early diagnosis of ectopic pregnancy possible.

5. PUL has been used as a diagnosis in women with a positive pregnancy test and no signs of intrauterine or extrauterine pregnancy or retained products of conception on an initial transvaginal ultrasound scan. PULs are primarily managed conservatively with serum β-hCG levels/ratios and serial transvaginal ultrasound scans.

6. Laparoscopic surgery is the treatment of choice for most tubal pregnancies and is superior to laparotomy. Following salpingectomy, the subsequent intrauterine pregnancy rate is 50% and the recurrent ectopic pregnancy rate is 10%. Following salpingotomy or salpingostomy, the subsequent intrauterine pregnancy rate is 53% and the recurrent ectopic pregnancy rate is 14%.

7. Administration of methotrexate allows non-invasive outpatient management of tubal pregnancy. Methotrexate should be considered when the initial pretreatment β-hCG concentration is less than 3000 IU/l, the tubal diameter is less than 2 cm, there is no evidence of fetal heartbeat on ultrasound scan, and the patient is haemodynamically stable and asymptomatic.

8. Expectant management of tubal ectopic pregnancy is more likely to be successful if the initial β-hCG concentration is less than 1000 IU/l, the diameter of the tubal mass is less than 2 cm, the fetal pole is absent on ultrasound scan, and the patient is asymptomatic.

9. Non-tubal ectopic pregnancies are rare. However, recently, the incidence of heterotopic pregnancy has increased significantly following assisted reproduction techniques.

References

Ankum WM, Mol BW, van der Veen F, Bossuyt PM 1996 Risk factors for ectopic pregnancy: a meta-analysis. Fertility and Sterility 65: 1093–1099.

Atrash HK, Frieda A, Hogue CJ 1987 Abdominal pregnancy in the United States: frequency and maternal mortality. Obstetrics and Gynecology 69: 333–337.

Banerjee S, Aslam N, Woelfer B, Lawrence A, Elson J, Jurkovic D 2001 Expectant management of early pregnancies of unknown location: a prospective evaluation of methods to predict spontaneous resolution of pregnancy. BJOG: an International Journal of Obstetrics and Gynaecology 108: 158–163.

Barnes AB, Colton T, Gundersen J et al 1980 Fertility and outcome of pregnancy in women exposed in utero to diethylstibestrol. New England Journal of Medicine 302: 609–613.

Barnhart K, Mennuti MT, Benjamin I, Jacobson S, Goodman D, Coutifaris C 1994 Prompt diagnosis of ectopic pregnancy in an emergency department setting. Obstetrics and Gynecology 84: 1010–1015.

Barnhart KT, Simhan H, Kamelle SA 1999 Diagnostic accuracy of ultrasound above and below the beta-hCG discriminatory zone. Obstetrics and Gynecology 94: 583–587.

Barnhart KT, Sammel MD, Rinaudo PF, Zhou L, Hummel AC, Guo W 2004 Symtomatic patients with early viable intrauterine pregnancy: HCG curves redefined. Obstetrics Gynecology 104: 50–55.

Benson CB, Doubilet PM 1996 Strategies for conservative treatment of cervical ectopic pregnancy. Ultrasound in Obstetrics and Gynecology 8: 371–372.

Bignardi T, Condous G, Alhamdan D et al 2008 The hCG ratio can predict the ultimate viability of the intrauterine pregnancies of uncertain viability in the pregnancy of unknown location population. Human Reproduction 23: 1964–1967.

Bishry E, Ganta S 2008 The role of single serum progesterone measurement in conjunction with beta hCG in the management of suspected ectopic pregnancy. Journal of Obstetrics and Gynaecology 28: 413–417.

Bouyer J, Coste J, Fernandez H et al 1998 Tobacco and ectopic pregnancy. Arguments in favour of a causal relation. Revue de Epidemologie et de Sante Publique 46: 93–99.

Bouyer J, Coste J, Fernandez H, Pouly JL, Job-Spira N 2002 Sites of ectopic pregnancy: a 10 year population-based study of 1800 cases. Human Reproduction 17: 3224–3230.

Breen JL 1970 A 21 year survey of 654 ectopic pregnancies. American Journal of Obstetrics and Gynecology 106: 1004–1019.

Brosens I, Gordts S, Vásquez G, Boeckx W 1984 Function-retaining surgical management of ectopic pregnancy. European Journal of Obstetrics Gynecology and Reproductive Biology 18: 395–402.

Brown DL, Felker RE, Stovall TG, Emerson DS, Ling FW 1991 Serial endovaginal sonography of ectopic pregnancies treated with methotrexate. Obstetrics and Gynecology 77: 406–409.

Brown DL, Doubilet PM 1994 Transvaginal sonography for diagnosing ectopic pregnancy: positive criteria and performance characteristics. Journal of Ultrasound in Medicine 13: 259–266.

Cohen DR, Falcone T, Khalife S 1996 Methotrexate: local versus intramuscular. Fertility and Sterility 65: 206–207.

Condous G, Okaro E, Khalid A et al 2004 The use of a new logistic regression model for predicting the outcome of pregnancies of unknown location. Human Reproduction 19: 1900–1910.

Condous G, Lu C, Van Huffel SV, Timmerman D, Bourne T 2004b Human chorionic gonadotrophin and progesterone levels in pregnancies of unknown location. International Journal of Gynaecology and Obstetrics 86: 351–357.

Condous G, Kirk E, Lu C et al 2005 Diagnostic accuracy of varying discriminatory zones for the prediction of ectopic pregnancy in women with a pregnancy of unknown location. Ultrasound in Obstetrics and Gynecology 26: 770–775.

Condous G, Kirk E, Van Calster B, Van Huffel S, Timmerman D, Bourne T 2006 Failing pregnancies of unknown location: a prospective evaluation of the human chorionic gonadotrophin ratio. BJOG: an International Journal of Obstetrics and Gynaecology 113: 521–527.

Comstock C, Huston K, Lee W 2005 The ultrasonographic appearance of ovarian ectopic pregnancies. Obstetrics and Gynecology 105: 42–45.

De Muylder X, De Loecker P, Campo R 1994 Heterotopic ovarian pregnancy after clomiphene ovulation induction. European

Journal of Obstetrics, Gynecology and Reproductive Biology 53: 65–66.

DeStefano F, Peterson HB, Layde PM 1982 Risk of ectopic pregnancy following tubal sterilization. Obstetrics and Gynecology 60: 326–330.

Droegemueller W 1982 Ectopic pregnancy. In: Danforth D (ed) Obstetrics and Gynaecology, 4th edn. Harper and Row, Philadelphia.

Elson J, Salim R, Tailor A, Banerjee S, Zosmer N, Jurkovic D 2003 Prediction of early pregnancy viability in the absence of an ultrasonically detectable embryo. Ultrasound in Obstetrics and Gynecology 21: 57–61.

Fernandez H, Bourget P, Ville Y, Lelaidier C, Frydman R 1994 Treatment of unruptured tubal pregnancy with methotrexate: pharmacokinetic analysis of local versus intramuscular administration. Fertility and Sterility 62: 943–947.

Gazvani MR, Emery SJ 1999 Mifepristone and methotrexate: the combination for medical treatment of ectopic pregnancy. American Journal of Obstetrics and Gynecology 180: 1599–1600.

Ghi T, Giunchi S, Kuleva M et al 2007 Three-dimensional transvaginal sonography in local staging of cervical carcinoma: description of a novel technique and preliminary results. Ultrasound in Obstetrics and Gynecology 30: 778–782.

Goldner TE, Lawson HW, Xia Z, Atrash HK 1993 Surveillance for ectopic pregnancy — United States 1970–1989. MMWR Morbidity and Mortality Weekly Report 42: 73–85.

Graesslin O, Dedecker F Jr, Quereux C, Gabriel R 2005 Conservative treatment of ectopic pregnancy in a cesarean scar. Obstetrics and Gynecology 105: 869–871.

Hahlin M, Wallin A, Sjöblom P, Lindblom B 1990 Single progesterone assay for early recognition of abnormal pregnancy. Human Reproduction 5: 622–626.

Hahlin M, Thorburn J, Bryman I 1995 The expectant management of early pregnancies of uncertain site. Human Reproduction 10: 1223–1227.

Hajenius PJ, Mol F, Mol BW, Bossuyt PM, Ankum WM, van der Veen F 2007 Interventions for tubal ectopic pregnancy. Cochrane Database of Systematic Reviews 1: CD000324.

Harika G, Gabriel R, Carre-Pigeon F, Alemany L, Quereux C, Wahl P 1995 Primary application of three-dimensional ultrasonography to early diagnosis of ectopic pregnancy. European Journal of Obstetrics, Gynecology and Reproduction Biology 60: 117–120.

Helmy S, Sawyer E, Ofili-Yebovi D, Yazbek J, Ben Nagi J, Jurkovic D 2007 Fertility outcomes following expectant management of tubal ectopic pregnancy. Ultrasound in Obstetrics and Gynaecology 30: 988–993.

Hofmann HM, Urdl W, Höfler H, Hönigl W, Tamussino K 1987 Cervical pregnancy: case reports and current concepts in diagnosis and treatment. Archives of Gynecology and Obstetrics 241: 63–69.

Hreschchyshyn MM, Naples JD, Randall CL 1965 Amethopterin in abdominal pregnancy. American Journal of Obstetrics and Gynecology 93: 286–287.

Hung TH, Shau WY, Hsieh TT, Hsu JJ, Soong YK, Jeng CJ 1998 Prognostic factors for an unsatisfactory primary methotrexate treatment of cervical pregnancy: a quantitative review. Human Reproduction 13: 2636–2642.

Jurkovic D, Bourne TH, Jauniaux E, Campbell S, Collins WP 1992 Transvaginal color Doppler study of blood flow in ectopic pregnancies. Fertility and Sterility 57: 68–73.

Jurkovic D, Hillaby K, Woelfer B, Lawrence A, Salim R, Elson CJ 2003 First-trimester diagnosis and management of pregnancies implanted into the lower uterine segment Cesarean section scar. Ultrasound in Obstetrics and Gynecology 21: 220–227.

Jurkovic D, Ben-Nagi J, Ofilli-Yebovi D, Sawyer E, Helmy S, Yazbek J 2007 Efficacy of Shirodkar cervical suture in securing hemostasis following surgical evacuation of Cesarean scar ectopic pregnancy. Ultrasound in Obstetrics and Gynecology 30: 95–100.

Jurkovic D, Mavrelos D 2007 Catch me if you scan: ultrasound diagnosis of ectopic pregnancy. Ultrasound in Obstetrics and Gynecology 30: 1–7.

Kadar N, Caldwell BV, Romero R 1981 A method of screening for ectopic pregnancy and its indications. Obstetrics and Gynecology 58: 162–166.

Kadar N, Romero R 1988 Serial human chorionic gonadotrophin measurements in ectopic pregnancy. American Journal of Obstetrics and Gynecology 158: 1239–1240.

Kirk E, Condous G, Haider Z, Syed A, Ojha K, Bourne T 2006 The conservative management of cervical ectopic pregnancies. Ultrasound in Obstetrics and Gynecology 27: 430–437.

Kirk E, Papageorghiou AT, Condous G, Tan L, Bora S, Bourne T 2007 The diagnostic effectiveness of an initial transvaginal scan in detecting ectopic pregnancy. Human Reproduction 22: 2824–2828.

Knoll M, Talbot P 1998 Cigarette smoke inhibits oocyte cumulus complex pick-up by the oviduct ciliary beat frequency. Reproductive Toxicology 12: 57–68.

Kung FT, Chang SY 1999 Efficacy of methotrexate treatment in viable and nonviable cervical pregnancies. American Journal of Obstetrics and Gynecology 181: 1438–1444.

Lewis G (ed) 2007 The Confidential Enquiry into Maternal and Child Health (CEMACH). Saving Mother's Lives: Reviewing Maternal Deaths to Make Motherhood Safer — 2003–2005. The Seventh Report on Confidential Enquiries into Maternal Deaths in the United Kingdom. CEMACH, London.

Li MC, Nerts R, Spence DB 1956 Effect of methotrexate therapy on choriocarcinoma and chorioadenoma. Proceedings of the Society for Experimental Biology and Medicine 93: 361–366.

Lundorff P, Thorburn J, Hahlin M, Källfelt B, Lindblom B 1991 Laparoscopic surgery in ectopic pregnancy. A randomized trial versus laparotomy. Acta Obstetricia et Gynecologica Scandinavica 70: 343–348.

Marchbanks PA, Coulman CB, Annegers JF 1985 An association between clomiphene citrate and ectopic pregnancy: a preliminary report. Fertility and Sterility 44: 268–270.

Marchiolé P, Gorlero F, de Caro G, Podestà M, Valenzano M 2004 Intramural pregnancy embedded in a previous Cesarean section scar treated conservatively. Ultrasound in Obstetrics and Gynecology 23: 307–309.

Marcus SF, Brinsden PR 1993 Primary ovarian pregnancy after in vitro fertilisation and embryo transfer: report of seven cases. Fertility and Sterility 60: 167–169.

Mathews CP, Coulson PB, Wild RA 1986 Serum progesterone levels as an aid in the diagnosis of ectopic pregnancy. Obstetrics and Gynecology 68: 390–394.

McBain JC, Evans JH, Pepperell RJ, Robinson HP, Smith MA, Brown JB 1980 An unexpectedly high rate of ectopic pregnancy following the induction of ovulation with human pituitary and chorionic gonadotrophin. BJOG: an International Journal of Obstetrics and Gynaecology 87: 5–9.

Mol BW, Lijmer JG, Ankum WM, van der Veen F, Bossuyt PM 1998 The accuracy of single serum progesterone measurement in the diagnosis of ectopic pregnancy: a meta-analysis. Human Reproduction 13: 3220–3227.

Oki T, Baba Y, Yoshinaga M, Douchi T 2008 Super-selective arterial embolization for uncontrolled bleeding in abdominal pregnancy. Obstetrics and Gynecology 112: 427–429.

Ory HW 1981 Ectopic pregnancy and intrauterine contraceptive devices: new perspectives. The Women's Health Study. Obstetrics and Gynecology 57: 137–144.

O'Shea RT, Thompson GR, Harding A 1994 Intra-amniotic methotrexate versus CO2 laser laparoscopic salpingotomy in the management of tubal ectopic pregnancy — a prospective randomized trial. Fertility and Sterility 62: 876–878.

Perdu M, Camus E, Rozenberg P et al 1998 Treating ectopic pregnancy with the combination of mifeperistone and methotrexate: a phase II nonrandomized study. American Journal of Obstetrics and Gynecology 179: 640–643.

Persaud V 1970 Etiology of tubal ectopic pregnancy. Radiologic and pathologic studies. Obstetrics and Gynecology 36: 257–263.

Peterson HB, Xia Z, Hughes JM, Wilcox LS, Tylor LR, Trussell J 1997 The risk of ectopic pregnancy after tubal sterilization. U.S. Collaborative Review of Sterilization Working Group. New England Journal of Medicine 336: 762–767.

Pittaway DE, Reish RL, Wentz AC 1985 Doubling times of human chorionic gonadotropin increase in early viable intrauterine pregnancies. American Journal of Obstetrics and Gynecology 152: 299–302.

Pouly J, Chapron C, Mage G et al 1991 The drop in the level of HCG after conservative laparoscopic treatment of ectopic pregnancy. Journal of Gynaecological Surgery 7: 211–217.

Rajkhowa M, Glass MR, Rutherford AJ, Balen AH, Sharma V, Cuckle HS 2000 Trends in the incidence of ectopic pregnancy in England and Wales from 1966 to 1996. BJOG: an International Journal of Obstetrics and Gynaecology 107: 369–374.

Rempen A 1998 The shape of the endometrium evaluated with three-dimensional ultrasound: an additional predictor of extrauterine pregnancy. Human Reproduction 13: 450–454.

Romero R, Kadar N, Jeanty P et al 1985 Diagnosis of ectopic pregnancy: value of the discriminatory human chorionic gonadotropin zone. Obstetrics and Gynecology 66: 357–360.

Royal College of Obstetricians and Gynaecologists 2004 The Management of Tubal Pregnancy. Guideline No. 21. RCOG, London.

Sau A, Hamilton-Fairley D 2003 Non surgical diagnosis and management of ectopic pregnancy. Obstetrician and Gynaecologist 5: 29–33.

Sauer M, Vidali A, James W 1997 Treating persistent ectopic pregnancy by methotrexate using a sliding scale: preliminary experience. Journal of Gynaecological Surgery 13: 13–16.

Seeber BE, Sammel MD, Guo W, Zhou L, Hummel A, Barnhart KT 2006 Application of redefined human chorionic gonadotropin curves for the diagnosis of women at risk for ectopic pregnancy. Fertility and Sterility 86: 454–459.

Shalev E, Peleg D, Bustan M, Romano S, Tsabari A 1995 Limited role for intratubal methotrexate treatment of ectopic pregnancy. Fertility and Sterility 63: 20–24.

Shaw SW, Hsu JJ, Chueh HY et al 2007 Management of primary abdominal pregnancy: twelve years of experience in a medical centre. Acta Obstetricia et Gynecologica Scandinavica 86: 1058–1062.

Silva P, Schaper A, Rooney B 1993 Reproductive outcome after 143 laparoscopic procedures for ectopic pregnancy. Fertility and Sterility 81: 710–715.

Silva C, Sammel MD, Zhou L, Gracia C, Hummel AC, Barnhart K 2006 Human chorionic gonadotrophin profile for women with ectopic pregnancy. Obstetrics and Gynecology 107: 605–610.

Singhal V, Li TC, Cooke ID 1991 An analysis of factors influencing the outcome of 232 consecutive tubal micro surgery cases. BJOG: an International Journal of Obstetrics and Gynaecology 98: 628–636.

Smith HO, Toledo AA, Thompson JD 1987 Conservative surgical management of isthmic ectopic pregnancies. American Journal of Obstetrics and Gynecology 157: 604–610.

Sowter MC, Farquhar CM, Petrie KJ, Gudex G 2001 A randomised trial comparing single dose systemic methotrexate and laparoscopic surgery for the treatment of unruptured tubal pregnancy. BJOG: an International Journal of Obstetrics and Gynaecology 108: 192–203.

Spiegelberg O 1878 Zur Casuistik der Ovarialschwangerschaft. Archives of Gynecology 13: 73–77.

Stabile I 1996a Clinical presentation of ectopic pregnancy. In: Stabile I (ed) Ectopic Pregnancy: Diagnosis and Management. Cambridge University Press, Cambridge.

Stabile I 1996b Biochemical diagnosis of ectopic pregnancy. In: Stabile I (ed) Ectopic Pregnancy: Diagnosis and Management. Cambridge University Press, Cambridge.

Stovall TG 1995 Medical management should be routinely used as primary therapy for ectopic pregnancy. Clinical Obstetrics and Gynecology 38: 346–352.

Stovall TG, Ling FW 1993 Ectopic pregnancy. Diagnostic and therapeutic algorithms minimizing surgical intervention. Journal of Reproductive Medicine 38: 807–812.

Svare J, Norup P, Grove Thomsen S et al 1993 Heterotopic pregnancies after in-vitro fertilization and embryo transfer in a Danish survey. Human Reproduction 8: 116–118.

Tanaka T, Hayashi H, Kutsuzawa T, Fujimoto S, Ichinoe K 1982 Treatment of interstitial ectopic pregnancy with methotrexate: report of a successful case. Fertility and Sterility 37: 851–852.

Tharaux-Deneux C, Bouyer J, Job-Spira N, Coste J, Spira A 1998 Risk of ectopic pregnancy and previous induced abortion. American Journal of Public Health 88: 401–405.

Tulandi T, Guralnick M 1991 Treatment of tubal ectopic pregnancy by salpingotomy with or without tubal suturing and salpingectomy. Fertility and Sterility 55: 53–55.

Tulandi T, Vilos G, Gomel V 1995 Laparoscopic treatment of interstitial pregnancy. Obstetrics and Gynecology 85: 465–467.

Vessey MP, Johnson B, Doll R, Peto R 1974 Outcome of pregnancy in women using an intrauterine device. The Lancet 1: 495–498.

Westrom L, Bengtsson LP, Mardh PA 1981 Incidence, trends and risks of ectopic pregnancy in a population of women. BMJ (Clinical Research Ed.) 282: 15–18.

Weyerman PC, Verhoeven AT, Alberda AT 1989 Cervical pregnancy after in vitro fertilisation and embryo transfer. American Journal of Obstetrics and Gynecology 161: 1145–1146.

Wollen AL, Flood PR, Sandvei R, Steier JA 1984 Morphological changes in tubal mucosa associated with the use of intrauterine contraceptive devices. BJOG: an International Journal of Obstetrics and Gynaecology 91: 1123–1128.

Yao M, Tulandi T 1997 Current status of surgical and nonsurgical management of ectopic pregnancy. Fertility and Sterility 67: 421–433.

CHAPTER 26

Hirsutism and virilization

Julian Barth

Chapter Contents

INTRODUCTION	382		SYSTEMIC ANTIANDROGEN THERAPY	387
INVESTIGATION	383		BIOCHEMICAL MONITORING OF ANDROGEN-SUPPRESSIVE THERAPY	388
HOW USEFUL ARE ENDOCRINE TESTS?	384		KEY POINTS	389
THERAPY FOR HIRSUTES	386			

Introduction

Hair follicles are stimulated by androgens to either enlarge on the face and body or to shrink on the vertex of the scalp. These changes occur in the female after puberty and probably develop to a small extent in all women. A small number of women develop excessive changes in hair, prompting advice from beauty therapists or physicians. The heaviness of facial or body hair growth that is necessary for a woman to consider herself to be hirsute is dependent on racial, cultural, social and economic factors. Although the pattern of hair growth is similar in all races, there is a variation in the heaviness of growth between ethnic groups. Furthermore, Shah (1957) in India and Lunde and Grottum (1984) in Norway have both stressed that women are more likely to consider themselves to be hirsute if they have significant growth on the upper lip, chin, chest and upper back.

The problem with defining hirsutism is that all measurements are subjective (Barth 1997). Large studies of unselected women in the USA (DeUgarte et al 2006) and Scandinavia (Lunde and Grottum 1984) have shown that it is impossible to separate hirsute from non-hirsute women on the basis of hair scoring scales, as women with similar hair scores may or may not consider that they have excessive hair growth. The problem with physician scales is that they do not consider the effect of hair localization. Is a women with facial hair but no body and limb hair more or less hirsute than a woman with a hairless face but a hairy trunk and limbs?

The standard scoring scale designed by Ferriman and Gallwey (1961) (Figure 26.1) defined 1.2% of females as hirsute, but this was based purely on mathematical grounds (i.e. 2 standard deviations from the mean). This contrasts with women's perspectives. A study of 400 unselected students, 60% of whom were Welsh, showed that 9% considered themselves to be disfigured by their facial hair growth (McKnight 1964). A study of unselected women in the USA found that approximately 20% of women had modified Ferriman and Gallwey scores greater than 3, and of these women, 70% considered themselves to have excessive facial and body hair. Furthermore, women with hirsutism give their hair growth a higher score than their physicians (Kozloviene et al 2005).

The subjectivity in the concept of hirsuties can be simplified by accepting that any woman who complains of excessive hair is hirsute. It then follows that the physician's role is to determine whether invasive investigations (see below) are required, and what sort of therapy is most appropriate for the degree of hair growth.

Hirsuties or hypertrichosis?

Hirsutism is a purely clinical diagnosis which is based on the growth and pattern of hair on the face and body of women. The pattern of hair growth in hirsute women is assumed to follow a similar pattern to that which develops on males after puberty. Hair first appears on the upper lip, followed by the chin and cheeks, and then the lower legs, thighs, forearms, abdomen, buttocks, chest, back, upper arms and shoulders. The hair shafts themselves are coarse, curly and tend to rise above the skin surface, rather than lying flush with the skin as in hypertrichosis.

Hypertrichosis needs to be differentiated as it is not androgen mediated and therefore does not respond to antiandrogen therapy. The onset of hair growth is not related to puberty; there is no hair growth pattern but there is a uniform diffuse growth of hair over the body. The individual hair shafts tend to be finer and lie flat against the skin, rather than being coarse, curly and rising above the skin surface. Hypertrichosis may be congenital or acquired due to drug therapy and some metabolic disorders (Table 26.1).

DOI: 10.1016/B978-0-7020-3120-5.00026-6

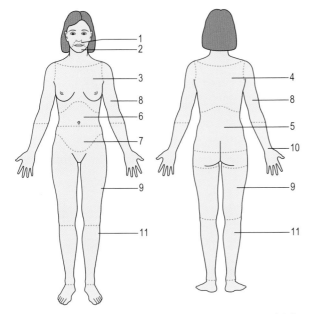

Figure 26.1 The hirsuties scoring scale designed by Ferriman and Gallwey. The body is dived into 11 zones as illustrated, and each zone is scored 0–4 giving a maximum score of 44. Ferriman and Gallwey excluded the lower arm and leg, and defined hirsuties as a score of >8. Unfortunately, there is considerable interobserver variation in scoring, so all investigators need to standardize their individual score rates.

Table 26.1 Aetiology of hirsuties and hypertrichosis

Causes of hirsutism	Causes of hypertrichosis
Ovarian, e.g. polycystic ovary syndrome, ovarian tumours	Drug therapy, e.g. cyclosporin, diazoxide, minoxidil, penicillamine etc.
Adrenal, e.g. congenital adrenal hyperplasia, adrenal tumours	Congenital disorders, e.g. hypertrichosis lanuginosa and other syndromes often associated with mental retardation
Cushing's syndrome	
Gonadal dysgenesis	
Androgen therapy	
Valproate therapy for epilepsy	Acquired hypertrichosis lanuginosa as a paramalignant condition
Obesity (due to consequent PCO)	
Prolactinoma (due to consequent PCO)	Metabolic disorders, e.g. lipodystrophy, mucopolysaccharidoses, malnutrition
Stress	
Idiopathic	

PCO, polycystic ovaries.

Investigation

A diagnosis of hirsutism is based purely on the patient's history and clinical examination. The purpose of investigation is to determine if there is any significant underlying condition which will influence further management. The majority of patients will have underlying polycystic ovary syndrome, and any investigative strategy should be designed to select those subjects who have a significant endocrinopathy that requires specific therapy.

Diagnostic approach to the hirsute woman

The history of the duration and severity of hirsutism is helpful if there is suspicion of a serious underlying cause:

- longstanding mild hirsutism with regular cycles and no features of systemic virilization; these women require no further investigation;
- longstanding moderate hirsuties with or without menstrual cycle disturbances. Most of these patients will have polycystic ovaries. Further investigation is only required if serum testosterone is elevated or if the patient seeks therapy for another symptom related to hyperandrogenism, such as infertility; and
- recent-onset hirsuties and virilization, or very severe hirsuties with a long history. Features of systemic virilism include: cliteromegaly, deepening of the voice, recent-onset temporal balding, increasing muscle bulk and decrease in breast size. These women require a comprehensive endocrine evaluation for an androgen-secreting tumour (Figure 26.2).

What is the evidence for this approach?

There have been two large studies to support this approach. Both confirmed the very low prevalence of serious endocrine disease, and it is clear that with the evidence of clinical case histories, these conditions are largely apparent on history and clinical examination.

Moran et al (1994) reported on 250 premenopausal (<38 years) women presenting with various symptoms who were noted to be hirsute. Ninety-six percent were diagnosed with polycystic ovaries, idiopathic hirsuties or obesity; 2% were diagnosed with congenital adrenal hyperplasia (CAH); and 1.6% were either iatrogenic (one case) or due to an ovarian tumour (two cases) or Cushing's syndrome (one case).

O'Driscoll et al (1994) reported a series of 350 consecutive patients who had presented with either hirsuties or androgenic alopecia. They identified eight women from this series with clear endocrine diseases; two had pituitary tumours (prolactinoma and acromegaly). The others were identified by a grossly elevated serum testosterone (>5 nmol/l). In total, 13 women had elevated testosterone; six had polycystic ovaries, two had late-onset CAH, one had virilizing CAH that had been ignored in childhood, one had an adrenal carcinoma, one had a postmenopausal Leydig cell tumour, one had corticosteroid 11-reductase deficiency, and the diagnosis in one hyperandrogenized postmenopausal woman was not elucidated. On the basis of the clinical details given in the report, only two diagnoses of late-onset CAH would have been missed by clinical evaluation alone (one had regular cycles and two children, the other had a long history of oligomenorrhoea; both had polycystic ovaries on ultrasound examination).

Arguably, the most important purpose for investigation is to identify those women with androgen-secreting tumours, since they require different therapy. Derksen et al (1994) reported a series of two adrenal adenomas and 12 carcinomas in which hirsutism was the presenting symptom. The women with adenomas were described as being severely virilized. Six of the women with carcinoma had clinical signs of Cushing's syndrome; of the remaining six cases, four were

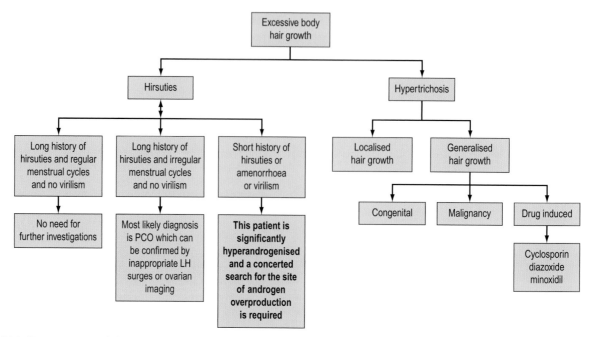

Figure 26.2 Diagnostic approach for a woman complaining of excess facial and/or body hair. PCO, polycystic ovaries; LH, luteinizing hormone.

severely virilized and the other two women presented with abdominal pain.

Functioning ovarian tumours which secrete androgens and therefore cause virilization are rare and represent only 1% of all ovarian tumours. In these cases, hirsuties is a nearly universal feature. Amenorrhoea develops rapidly in all premenopausal patients, and systemic virilization with alopecia, cliteromegaly, deepening of the voice and a male habitus develops in approximately half of patients. Meldrum and Abraham (1979) reviewed the literature of 43 women with virilizing ovarian tumours; seven had a serum testosterone level below 7.0 nmol/l but all were clinically virilized, and one 65-year-old woman was reported as not virilized but her serum testosterone level was more than 12 nmol/l.

In conclusion, the vast majority of hirsute women have polycystic ovaries, and those women with androgen-secreting tumours can be identified by clinical evaluation and a single serum testosterone estimation (Figure 26.3).

How Useful Are Endocrine Tests?

The laboratory findings in reports of hirsute women demonstrate considerable heterogeneity. This may be due to differences in diagnostic criteria for the studies; for example, hyperandrogenaemia, acne and/or hirsutism, or women with polycystic ovaries/menstrual disturbances. A further factor may be the degree of hair growth necessary to define whether a woman is considered to be hirsute (Barth et al 2007). A third point has been proposed by Toscano et al (1983) who suggested that the endocrine abnormalities are dependent on the length of the history of hirsutism. They posed the question 'is hirsutism an evolving syndrome?', and whilst their interpretation of the findings may be argued, it is clear that (i) a degree of hirsutism and/or oligomenorrhoea is necessary before hormonal abnormalities may be

present, and (ii) not all hirsute women have abnormal circulating hormones.

Investigations to diagnose polycystic ovaries

A diagnosis of polycystic ovaries was originally made on the basis of clinical signs and gross anatomical features of the ovaries; indeed, the majority of cases can be diagnosed on the basis of hirsuties and oligo-/amenorrhoea. Confirmation of the clinical diagnosis is made variably by ultrasound imaging or endocrine tests. The choice of test is largely philosophical; imaging makes a diagnosis that matches the anatomical description of the condition, whereas endocrine tests can, at best, only act as surrogates.

Ovarian imaging compares extremely favourably with anatomical appearance in those subjects who have had abdominal laparoscopy, whereas the use of gonadotrophins is less well established as a diagnostic tool. Approximately 50% of women with polycystic ovaries have an elevated concentration of luteinizing hormone (LH), and 40% of women with elevated LH have polycystic ovaries. The use of gonadotrophins is further complicated by assay methodology. In view of these factors, the latest guidelines to diagnose polycystic ovaries have abandoned their use (Rotterdam ESHRE/ASRM-sponsored PCOS Consensus Workshop Group 2004). The over-riding problem is that approximately 10% of women with ultrasound-diagnosed polycystic ovaries will have normal endocrine tests, however many are performed. This may be due to the relationship between body weight and the dynamics of testosterone production (Figure 26.4).

Most recommendations suggest a battery of androgen tests, but this is probably still based on the unreliability of testosterone assays (Rosner et al 2007). This should become less of a problem as measurement by tandem mass spectrometry becomes more routine. A single testosterone meas-

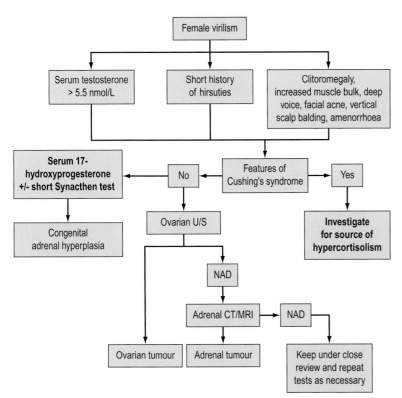

Figure 26.3 Diagnostic approach for a woman with features of systemic virilism. U/S, ultrasound; CT, computed tomography; MRI, magnetic resonance imaging; NAD, no abnormalities detected.

urement taken in the morning during the early follicular phase measured with a reliable assay is probably all that is required in the first instance (Martin et al 2008).

Short Synacthen test for late-onset congenital adrenal hyperplasia

The incidence of late-onset CAH in women with hirsutism is variously reported at 1–12% depending on the source of patient referral. Short Synacthen testing has been used extensively as a research tool, but its use in routine practice cannot be recommended. Firstly, there is no sharp cut-off value of 17-hydroxyprogesterone following Synacthen that can be used to define late-onset CAH. Secondly, treatment for hirsute women with late-onset CAH should not be influenced by the diagnosis since antiandrogen therapy with cyproterone acetate (CPA) is more effective than corticosteroids (Spritzer et al 1990). Moreover, corticosteroids aggravate insulin resistance and, theoretically, worsen the hyperandrogenism. Finally, there does not appear to be a need to identify women with late-onset CAH since they do not seem to need protection against stress-related corticosteroid deficiency.

Evaluation of metabolic factors

Polycystic ovary syndrome is now recognized to be a systemic disorder underpinned by insulin resistance. Insulin plays a key role as an amplifier of gonadotrophin-stimulated ovarian androgen production, and also as a growth factor for hair follicle. The effects of hyperinsulinaemia include android obesity, glucose intolerance, hyperlipidaemia and possibly impaired fibrinolysis. The lipid profiles show the pattern associated with patients who have ischaemic heart

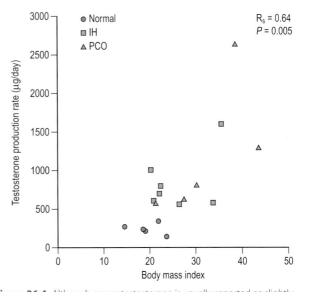

Figure 26.4 Although serum testosterone is usually reported as slightly elevated in women with polycystic ovaries (PCO) or hirsuties, it can be seen from this redrawing of the original data of Bardin and Lipsett (1967) that testosterone production rates are closely related to body mass irrespective of the patient's phenotype. IH, idiopathic hirsuties.
Data redrawn from Thomas PK, Ferriman DG. Variation in facial and pubic hair growth in white women. Am J Phys Anthropol. 1957 Jun;15(2):171–180, Wiley.

disease, namely raised triglycerides and low high-density-lipoprotein cholesterol, and hirsute women undergoing coronary angiography have more pronounced arterial disease than non-hirsute women (Wild et al 1990). Moreover, long-term studies of women with polycystic ovaries have shown an increase in diabetes and hypertension, and the central obesity phenotype in women carries an increased risk of cardiovascular disease (see Chapter 18, Polycystic ovary syndrome, for more information).

These metabolic factors are already well established during adolescence, as evidenced by the changes in bony structure. These must have been completed by the time of epiphyseal fusion at the end of the second decade. This was clearly demonstrated by Ferriman et al (1957) who noted that hirsute women had increased shoulder width and reduced bi-iliac width compared with non-hirsute women, and that these differences were greater in those women who noted that their hirsutism began during adolescence.

Recommendations for the investigation of hirsute women

Most women with hirsuties are either seeking reassurance that they are not changing sex or are seeking advice regarding therapy for their hair. Measurement of a single serum testosterone during the early follicular phase may be a useful therapy for the former, and is a useful first-line indicator of a serious endocrine disease, although, as discussed above, women with the latter will be identified by history and clinical examination. There seems to be no benefit to be gained by extensive endocrine tests in uncomplicated cases of hirsutism, since the decision to treat is not based on endocrine test results.

Since there are serious adverse metabolic factors in both lean and obese women with polycystic ovaries, it would be prudent to screen for impaired glucose tolerance by a fasting glucose and to measure a fasting plasma lipid profile.

Postmenopausal women

A different strategy is required for postmenopausal women because, unlike younger women, they cannot be stratified on the basis of menstrual pattern. However, as women age, the pattern of facial and body hair changes (Figure 26.5); hair on the face increases whilst it involutes elsewhere. Hair growth on the chest, shoulders and upper back can be considered indications for further investigation. Hormonal changes in hirsute postmenopausal women are minor with small increases in testosterone compared with appropriate controls, so an elevated testosterone more than twice the upper limit of age-related normal or approximately 3.0 nmol/l should also be considered as a trigger for further investigation. Postmenopausal women with unexplained hirsuties have normal lipids, but women with ovarian hyperthecosis should be investigated further since they appear to have a very high incidence of glucose intolerance and vascular disease (Barth et al 1997).

Therapy for Hirsuties

Most women will be satisfied with the reassurance that they are not 'turning into men' and may not require any further medical attention. Some may need advice about local destructive methods and some may need to be advised how to use those methods. The vast majority of women have experience in at least one form of depilation (Toerien and Wilkinson 2005), so many women will be seeking medical help because they have already found these methods wanting. It is important to accept that the choice of therapies

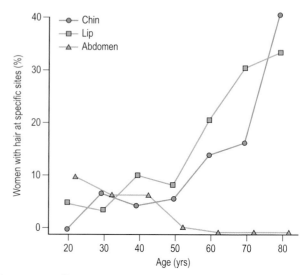

Figure 26.5 Differences in facial and abdominal hair in women aged 15–85 years. Data were collected on 584 women admitted to hospital. Hair was graded 0–4 at each site, and scores of 3 or 4 were considered to represent significant hair growth for this graph.
Redrawn from Bardin CW, Lipsett MB, Testosterone and Androstenedione Blood Production Rates in Normal Women and Women with Idiopathic Hirsutism or Polycystic Ovaries, Journal of Clinical Investigation, 1967; 46: 891–902.

will depend on the needs and desires of the patient, and not the degree of hirsutism.

Psychological factors

There is a societal expectation in Western culture for women to be hairless, and hairiness in women is overwhelmingly constructed in a negative fashion. Is it surprising, therefore, that women regard their excess hair growth with unhappiness? They spend considerable amounts of time managing their facial hair and have high levels of emotional stress, depression and anxiety. Most concerning is their poor performance in social arenas and in relationships (Lipton et al 2006), leading to an overall poor quality of life (Barnard et al 2007). Some of the symptomatology can be explained by comorbidities such as obesity and acne (Barth et al 1993), which reinforces the need to treat holistically and to provide time and sympathy rather than considering hirsuties as a purely medical condition. In the author's experience, only one-third of women want internal medical therapy after receiving a full explanation of their condition and informed advice about topical therapies.

Topical/cosmetic procedures

Hair bleaching with hydrogen peroxide and hair plucking are both useful and will have been used by most women prior to seeking medical help. Depilatory creams reduce the strength of the hair fibre by reducing the chemical sulphur–sulphur bonds which can then be sheared apart by rubbing the skin. Unfortunately, prolonged application, necessary for thick hairs, has the same effect on the stratum corneum and leads to redness and soreness. Shaving may be the only treatment that produces an acceptable cosmetic effect. This should be discouraged as no therapy can be as effective, and electrologists need a short stubble to direct their needles.

There is no evidence that shaving has any effect on hair growth despite popular belief (Peereboom-Wynia 1972).

Plucking hairs out over large areas is performed by waxing. This is a painful method and is often complicated by folliculitis since the wax oils penetrate the potential space within the outer root sheath where they establish an inflammatory reaction. This can be avoided by the use of natural sugars as a wax substitute which are not so irritant to the hair follicle; this technique is widely used in the Middle East.

Weight reduction

Holistic lifestyle changes must be considered as a primary aim in all women with polycystic ovary syndrome and hirsuties for all the reasons of cardiovascular risk outlined above and also to reduce the risk of developing diabetes. Unfortunately, weight loss is difficult to achieve in many subjects despite the beneficial effects on all the risk factors viz. lipids, insulin resistance and blood pressure. Some subjects may benefit from treatment with weight-loss medication such as orlistat and sibutramine. There is only anecdotal evidence of the benefit of weight reduction on hair growth using holistic measures. Metformin, despite its ability to improve cardiometabolic status, does not improve hirsuties unless there is weight loss and cannot be recommended (Cosma et al 2008). Weight loss following bariatric surgery does, however, result in significant reduction in hair growth (Ecobar-Morreale et al 2005).

Electrolysis

Electrolysis is a popular procedure used for permanent hair removal. It involves the insertion of a small needle or probe into the hair follicle through which an electric current is delivered. This causes tissue damage and destruction of the hair follicle, and results in a microscar surrounding the follicle which is barely perceptible at the skin surface. Focal erythema and oedema following treatment usually resolve within a few hours.

Electrolysis is more effective on anagen hairs; therefore, shaving a few days before electrolysis greatly increases its efficacy because it ensures that only growing anagen hairs are epilated. This is particularly important during the initial treatment of an area because as many as 60% of the hairs may be in telogen, which are difficult to eradicate permanently. The cosmetic outcome of electrolysis is extremely dependent on the skill of the operator, and patients should be advised to only accept therapy from appropriately trained personnel. Multiple treatment sessions are necessary due to the practice of avoiding simultaneous treatment of adjacent hair follicles (within 3–4 mm of each other) in order to reduce unnecessary thermal skin injury.

Complications are quite unusual in skilled hands but patients who are prone to hypertrophic scarring, keloids, postinflammatory hyperpigmentation or other cutaneous dyschromias should be advised that these complications may result from electrolysis treatment.

Laser depilation

Lasers cause damage to the hair follicle by irradiating the skin with high energy light. This is absorbed by melanin in the hair bulb which, in turn, suffers thermal injury as the energy is dissipated. This mechanism is fine for subjects with dark hair and light skin. Subjects with dark skin who have considerable quantities of melanin in the epidermis will suffer burns. Similarly, those subjects who burn easily in sunlight will be unable to tolerate laser therapy. However, despite these limitations, laser therapy is widely used across the globe for epilation.

Although laser therapy is routinely advertised as producing permanent hair removal, there is a lack of long-term studies. In fact, only short-term studies (≤ 6 months) have been performed. Moreover, there have been no formal comparisons against electrolysis to determine which gives the best long-term results. Adverse effects include blistering, hyperpigmentation, scabbing, hypopigmentation, scar formation and thrombophlebitis.

Systemic Antiandrogen Therapy

It is important that hirsute women are carefully selected prior to initiating therapy for the following reasons. Firstly, the effect on hair growth takes several months to become apparent and only partial improvements may be expected. Secondly, antiandrogens will potentially feminize a male fetus and it is essential that treated women do not become pregnant. Thirdly, these drugs only reduce hair scores by 25–33% and they have a suppressive effect rather than a curative effect; this wears off a few months after cessation of therapy. In view of this, therapy may need to be taken indefinitely if a favourable improvement occurs. Finally, the long-term safety of these drugs is unknown, and tumours in laboratory animals have been reported with several of the following agents.

The coexistence of obesity in many hirsute women has been discussed above. Women who are overweight should be advised to reduce their weight since a reduction as small as 5% has been shown to be associated with both a regulation in menses and a reduction in hair growth. However, once a decision has been made to treat an hirsute woman, weight does not seem to play an important role in the efficacy of treatment (Crosby and Rittmaster 1991). Weight may be an important factor in the presentation of women with hirsuties, and should be considered in the treatment possibilities since weight gain or difficulty in weight loss is experienced with oral contraceptive therapy.

Oral contraceptive agents

Cyproterone acetate

CPA is both an antiandrogen and an inhibitor of gonadotrophin secretion. It reduces androgen production, increases the metabolic clearance of testosterone and binds to androgen receptors; in addition, long-term therapy is associated with a reduction in the activity of cutaneous 5α-reductase. CPA is a potent progestogen but does not reliably inhibit ovulation and is usually administered with cyclical oestrogens in order to maintain regular menstruation and to prevent conception since there is a risk of feminization of a male fetus.

CPA is administered either as the Dianette pill alone taken for 21 days, or with supplementary CPA 50–100 mg taken for the first 10 days (the reverse sequential regimen of Hammerstein). This regimen was designed to allow for CPA stores to be cleared from adipose tissue by the end of the cycle to allow menstruation. Other regimens have been designed using intramuscular oestrogens and/or CPA.

Current dosage recommendations for CPA usually advise that 50 or 100 mg CPA should be administered for 10 days/cycle. However, three dose-ranging studies have suggested that there is no dose effect (Molinatti et al 1983, Belisle and Love 1986, Barth et al 1991).

Side-effects of CPA include weight gain, fatigue, loss of libido, mastodynia, nausea, headaches and depression. All these side-effects are more frequent with a higher dose. Contraindications to its use are the same as for the contraceptive pill and include cigarette smoking, age, obesity and hypertension. All patients should have their liver function monitored in view of the rare occurrence of liver damage.

Desogestrel (Marvelon)

Desogestrel is the progestogen used in the Marvelon contraceptive pill which contains 30 µg ethinyl oestradiol and 150 mg desogestrel. There have been few studies of its efficacy in hirsuties. All have reported subjective and/or objective reductions in hair growth of 20–25% after 6–9 months of therapy, with a high degree of patient satisfaction.

Drisperonone

Drisperonone is a novel progestogen with antiandrogenic action. It appears to help acne, and the only randomized study suggests that it is as good as Dianette (Batukan et al 2007).

Antiandrogenic compounds

Spironolactone

Spironolactone has several antiandrogenic pharmacological properties. It reduces the bioavailability of testosterone by interfering with its production and increasing its metabolic clearance. It binds to the androgen receptor and, like CPA, long-term therapy is associated with a reduction in cutaneous 5α-reductase activity.

Different dose schedules of spironolactone have been studied, varying between 50 and 200 mg taken either daily or cyclically (daily for 3 weeks in every 4). A daily dose of 200 mg produces a reduction in subjective hair growth grades of approximately 40% after 6 months of therapy, with little further effect. It is not certain that doses below 200 mg/day are effective at reducing hirsutism.

The main side-effects of spironolactone are breast soreness and menstrual irregularities, but there is considerable variation in their reported incidence. Menstrual irregularities can be eased by the concomitant use of an oral contraceptive containing either CPA or desogestrel as the gestagen.

Finasteride

Finasteride inhibits androgen action by blocking the activity of the type 2 5α-reductase enzyme. Treatment with finasteride 5 mg daily induces a reduction in hair growth within 3–6 months, as with other antiandrogens. All reported studies have noted a small, but significant, rise in plasma testosterone during therapy (approximate increase from 1.6 to 2.4 nmol/l). This rise is unexplained and does not appear to be mediated through altered gonadotrophin secretion.

Controlled trials comparing finasteride with other antiandrogens suggest that it is slightly less effective. However, no significant side-effects have been reported.

Flutamide

Flutamide acts as a pure antiandrogen and works by binding to androgen receptors. It appears to have no significant effect on gonadotrophin secretion in women, and therefore androgens do not increase during treatment, unlike the effect in men in whom androgens rise since they regulate gonadotrophin secretion.

Treatment with flutamide 250 mg twice daily, either as a sole agent or in combination with an oral contraceptive, results in reductions in hair scores after 1 year to values considered normal using the Ferriman and Gallwey scale. This therapeutic effect makes flutamide appear the most potent antiandrogen therapy, but flutamide, like all other antiandrogens, has serious hepatotoxic adverse effects (Wallace et al 1993). This adverse effect seems to develop in the first few weeks of therapy, and careful monitoring of liver function is recommended. The incidence of hepatotoxicity in males with prostate cancer is relatively low but fatal cases have occurred. At least one case of hepatic failure requiring liver transplantation has occurred as a direct result of treatment of an hirsute woman.

Other drugs

Corticosteroids

Corticosteroids are first-line therapy for CAH and were the first endocrine therapy to be employed in the treatment of hirsuties with the rationale of suppressing the production of adrenal androgens. It is uncertain how effective they are at reducing androgenic hair growth in hirsute women, and despite subjective impressions of improvement, no objective improvement has been detected (Casey et al 1966). Moreover, glucocorticoids invariably increase insulin resistance and should theoretically worsen the hyperandrogenism.

Ketoconazole

Ketoconazole is a potent inhibitor of adrenal and ovarian steroid synthesis. There have only been isolated reports of its use in hirsuties, but these have demonstrated a marked reduction in hair growth after 6 months. This treatment cannot be recommended in view of the risks of hepatic toxicity during long-term therapy.

Biochemical Monitoring of Androgen-Suppressive Therapy

Therapy for hirsute women is designed to reduce the quantity of hair and it would seem appropriate therefore to measure hair as a means of monitoring therapy. Plasma androgens fall rapidly after initiation of systemic antiandrogen therapy, whereas hair takes several months to fall to a nadir. Moreover, flutamide, which is the only systemic therapeutic agent reported to reduce hair scores into the 'normal range', does not have any effect on serum testosterone, sex-hormone-binding globulin or gonadotrophins in women.

The need for investigations during therapy should be aimed at monitoring pharmaceutical agents; for example, liver function tests for CPA, flutamide or ketoconazole, and possibly cortisol for long-term CPA as adrenal failure can rarely occur. All hirsute women should probably be periodically reassessed for glucose intolerance and hyperlipidaemia since they have such an increased risk of developing diabetes.

KEY POINTS

1. Hirsutism is the excessive growth of facial and body hair in a male-pattern distribution.
2. Hirsuties may result from increased androgen production by the ovaries and/or adrenal glands, or increased target-tissue sensitivity to androgens.
3. Virilization involves more severe features of hyperandrogenism including male body habitus, clitoromegaly, balding, voice deepening and increased libido. It is characteristically associated with androgen-producing tumours, CAH or the use of androgenic drugs.
4. The most common cause of hirsutism is polycystic ovary syndrome. Diagnosis is based on ultrasound appearance and/or raised serum testosterone.
5. All women with a serum testosterone that is greater than twice the upper limit of the local laboratory's normal value should be further investigated to exclude CAH or an androgen-secreting tumour. Investigations should include pelvic ultrasound scan, measurement of serum dehydroepiandrosterone and 17α-hydroxyprogesterone
6. and, where indicated, computed tomography or magnetic resonance imaging of the abdomen and pelvis.
7. The diagnosis of idiopathic hirsutism should be limited to those cases in which there is no identifiable pathology to account for the symptoms; the menstrual cycle is regular, the ovaries are normal on ultrasound scan and serum testosterone is less than twice the upper limit of the local laboratory's normal value.
8. A wide variety of cosmetic and medical treatments are available for removing hair. Women with excess facial and body hair should be offered the full spectrum of therapies so that they can choose the most suitable.
9. Weight reduction should be encouraged in overweight and obese women with a body mass index above 25 kg/m^2 prior to starting medical treatment.
10. CPA is the antiandrogen of choice in the management of benign hirsutism, given either in low-dose form as Dianette or at higher doses (25–100 mg) in more severe cases.

References

Bardin CW, Lipsett MB 1967 Testosterone and androstenedione blood production rates in normal women and in women with idiopathic hirsutism or polycystic ovaries. Journal of Clinical Investigation 46: 891–902.

Barnard L, Ferriday D, Guenther N, Strauss B, Balen AH, Dye L 2007 Quality of life and psychological well being in polycystic ovary syndrome. Human Reproduction 22: 2279–2286.

Barth JH 1997 How hairy are hirsute women? Clinical Endocrinology 47: 255–260.

Barth JH, Cherry CA, Wojnarowska F, Dawber RPR 1991 Cyproterone acetate for severe hirsutism: results of a double-blind dose-ranging study. Clinical Endocrinology 35: 5–10.

Barth JH, Catalan J, Cherry CA, Day AE 1993 Psychological morbidity in women referred for treatment of hirsutism. Journal of Psychosomatic Research 37: 615–619.

Barth JH, Jenkins M, Belchetz PE 1997 Ovarian hyperthecosis, diabetes and hirsuties in post menopausal women. Clinical Endocrinology 46: 123–128.

Barth JH, Yasmin E, Balen AH 2007 The diagnosis of polycystic ovary syndrome: the criteria are insufficiently robust for clinical research. Clinical Endocrinology 67: 811–815.

Batukan C, Muderris II, Ozcelik B, Ozturk A 2007 Comparison of two oral contraceptives containing either drospirenone or cyproterone acetate in the treatment of hirsutism. Gynecological Endocrinology 23: 38–44.

Belisle S, Love EJ 1986 Clinical efficacy and safety of cyprotene acetate in severe hirsutism: results of a multicentred Canadian study. Fertility and Sterility 46: 1015–1020.

Casey JH, Burger HG, Kent JR et al 1966 Treatment of hirsutism by adrenal and ovarian suppression. Journal of Clinical Endocrinology and Metabolism 26: 1370–1374.

Cosma M, Swiglo BA, Flynn DN et al 2008 Clinical review: insulin sensitizers for the treatment of hirsutism: a systematic review and metaanalyses of randomized controlled trials. Journal of Clinical Endocrinology and Metabolism 93: 1135–1142.

Crosby PDA, Rittmaster RS 1991 Predictors of clinical response in hirsute women treated with spironolactone. Fertility and Sterility 55: 1076–1081.

Derksen J, Nagesser SK, Meinders AE, Haak HR, van de Velde CJH 1994 Identification of virilising adrenal tumours in hirsute women. New England Journal of Medicine 331: 968–973.

DeUgarte CM, Woods KS, Bartolucci AA, Azziz R 2006 Degree of facial and body terminal hair growth in unselected black and white women: toward a population definition of hirsutism. Journal of Clinical Endocrinology and Metabolism 91: 1345–1350.

Escobar-Morreale HF, Botella-Carretero JI, Alvarez-Blasco F, Sancho J, San Millán JL 2005 The polycystic ovary syndrome associated with morbid obesity may resolve after weight loss induced by bariatric surgery. Journal of Clinical Endocrinology and Metabolism 90: 6364–6369.

Ferriman D, Thomas PK, Purdie AW 1957 Constitutional virilism. BMJ (Clinical Research Ed.) ii: 1410–1412.

Ferriman D, Gallwey JD 1961 Clinical assessment of body hair growth in women. Journal of Clinical Endocrinology 21: 1440–1447.

Kozloviene D, Kazanavicius G, Kruminis V 2005 The evaluation of clinical signs and hormonal changes in women who complained of excessive body hair growth. Medicina (Kaunas) 42: 487–495.

Lipton M, Sherr L, Elford J, Rustin M, Clayton W 2006 Women living with facial hair: the psychological and behavioral burden. Journal of Psychosomatic Research 61: 161–168.

Lunde O, Grottum P 1984 Body hair growth in women: normal or hirsute. American Journal of Physical Anthropology 64: 307–313.

Martin KA, Chang RJ, Ehrmann DA et al 2008 Evaluation and treatment of hirsutism in premenopausal women: an endocrine society clinical practice guideline. Journal of Clinical Endocrinology and Metabolism 93: 1105–1120.

McKnight E 1964 The prevalence of 'hirsutism' in young women. The Lancet i: 410–413.

Meldrum DR, Abraham GE 1979 Peripheral and ovarian venous concentration of various steroid hormones in virilising ovarian tumours. Obstetrics and Gynecology 53: 36–43.

Molinatti GM, Messina M, Manieri C, Massuchetti C, Biffignandi P 1983 Current approaches to the treatment of virilizing syndromes. In: Molinatti GM, Martini L, James VHT (eds) Androgenization in Women. Raven Press, New York, pp 179–193.

Moran C, Tapia MC, Hernandez E, Vazquez G, Garcia-Hernandez E, Bermudez JA 1994 Etiological review of hirsutism in 250 patients. Archives of Medical Research 25: 311–314.

O'Driscoll JB, Mamtora H, Higginson J, Pollock A, Kane J, Anderson DC 1994 A prospective study of the prevalence of clear-cut endocrine disorders and polycystic ovaries in 350 patients presenting with hirsutism or androgenic alopecia. Clinical Endocrinology 41: 231–236.

Peereboom-Wynia JDR 1972 The effect of various methods of epilation on density of hair growth in women with idiopathic hirsutism. Archiv fuer Dermatologische Forschung 243: 164–176.

Rosner W, Auchus RJ, Azziz R, Sluss PM, Raff H 2007 Utility, limitations, and pitfalls in measuring testosterone: an Endocrine Society position statement. Journal of Clinical Endocrinology and Metabolism 92: 405–413.

Rotterdam ESHRE/ASRM-sponsored PCOS Consensus Workshop Group 2004 Revised 2003 consensus on diagnostic criteria and long-term health risks related to polycystic ovary syndrome (PCOS). Human Reproduction 19: 41–47.

Shah PN 1957 Human body hair — a quantitative study. American Journal of Obstetrics and Gynecology 73: 1255–1265.

Spritzer P, Billaud L, Thalabard J-C et al 1990 Cyproterone acetate versus hydrocortisone treatment in late-onset adrenal hyperplasia. Journal of Clinical Endocrinology and Metabolism 70: 642–646.

Thomas PK, Ferriman DG 1957 Variation in facial and pubic hair growth in white women. American Journal of Physical Anthropology 15: 171–180.

Toerien M, Wilkinson S, Choi PYL 2005 Body hair removal: the 'mundane' production of normative femininity. Sex Roles 52: 399–406.

Toscano V, Adamo MV, Caiola S et al 1983 Is hirsutism an evolving syndrome? Journal of Endocrinology 97: 379–387.

Wallace C, Lalor EA, Chik CL 1993 Hepatotoxicity complicating flutamide treatment of hirsutism. Annals of Internal Medicine 118: 1150.

Wild RA, Grubb B, Hartz A, van Nort JJ, Bachman W, Bartholomew M 1990 Clinical signs of androgen excess as risk factors for coronary disease. Fertility and Sterility 54: 255–259.

CHAPTER 27

Premenstrual syndrome

Sungathi Chandru, Radha Indusekhar and P.M. Shaughn O'Brien

Chapter Contents

INTRODUCTION	391	NON-PHARMACOLOGICAL TREATMENTS	395
DEFINITION	391	PHARMACOLOGICAL TREATMENTS	397
SYMPTOMS	391	SURGERY	400
AETIOLOGY AND PATHOPHYSIOLOGY	391	CONCLUSION	400
MANAGEMENT	394	KEY POINTS	402

Introduction

Premenstrual syndrome (PMS) refers to somatic and psychological symptoms which occur in relation to the luteal phase of the menstrual cycle. Most women of reproductive age will have some symptoms related to the premenstrual phase of the cycle. These are usually very mild and are physiological. Only when the symptoms cause significant disruption to normal functioning are they considered to be PMS. The term 'premenstrual dysphoric disorder' (PMDD) is also used and this represents the severe, predominantly psychological form of PMS. It is estimated that 3–8% of women of reproductive age experience debilitating symptoms leading to functional or psychological impairment (Angst et al 2001, Wittchen et al 2002). PMS and PMDD can be debilitating conditions. The impact on society and women's lives can be very high and comparable to major depressive disorder (Pearlstein et al 2000, Halbriech et al 2003).

Definition

PMS is characterized by symptoms or clusters of symptoms that are associated with the premenstrual phase of the cycle, are recurrent, and are severe enough to cause impairment and distress (Halbriech et al 2007). Any symptom or cluster of symptoms qualify as PMS if they occur during the luteal phase of the menstrual cycle, are alleviated shortly following menses, and are not merely an exacerbation of other underlying conditions. PMDD has similar but separate criteria (Table 27.1, Figures 27.1 and 27.2)

Symptoms

A woman has PMS if she complains of psychological or somatic symptoms, or both, recurring specifically during the luteal phase of the cycle and resolving by the end of menstruation (Ismail and O'Brien 2005). This separates PMS from psychiatric disorders. The symptoms should be confirmed prospectively by daily ratings during the last two consecutive cycles. This prospective rating is best achieved using the Daily Record of Severity of Problems form (Table 27.2, Box 27.1).

Diagnostic criteria for premenstrual syndrome

An international multidisciplinary group of experts who evaluated the definitions of PMS/PMDD recommended the following diagnostic criteria (Halbriech et al 2007):

- symptom(s) occur up to 2 weeks before menses in most menstrual cycles;
- symptom(s) remit shortly following onset of menses and are absent during most of the midfollicular phase of the menstrual cycle;
- symptom(s) are associated with impairment in daily functioning and/or relationship and/or cause suffering or emotional/physical distress;
- menstrual-related cyclicity, occurrence during the luteal phase and absence during the midfollicular phase are documented by repeated observations by a clinician and/or daily monitoring by the patient (in hysterectomized women, menstrual-related cyclicity is documented by clinical determinations); and
- the symptom(s) are not just an exacerbation or worsening of another mental or physical chronic disorder. PMS may also be a concomitant condition.

Aetiology and Pathophysiology

The precise aetiology of PMS/PMDD is unknown. Various theories have been suggested. The current evidence suggests

DOI: 10.1016/B978-0-7020-3120-5.00027-8

Table 27.1 The different types of premenstrual disorders

Type	Definition
Physiological premenstrual symptoms	Symptoms occur in the luteal phase of the cycle but are so mild that they are not troublesome.
Premenstrual syndrome	PMS symptoms leading up to menstruation and completely relieved by the end of menstruation.
Mild	Does not interfere with personal/social and professional life.
Moderate	Interferes with personal/social and professional life but still able to function and interact, maybe suboptimally.
Severe	Unable to interact personally/socially/professionally, withdraws from social and professional activities (treatment resistant).
Premenstrual dysphoric disorder	Currently considered as research criteria, not yet in general use outside the USA, but increasingly addressed in Europe and other countries. This definition of the severe psychological end of the PMS spectrum has been devised by the American Psychiatric Association.
Premenstrual exaggeration	Background psychopathology, physical, medical or other condition which worsens premenstrually with incomplete relief of symptoms when menstruation ends.
Misattribution	Underlying physical, psychological or psychiatric disorder wrongly labelled as PMS by general practitioner, nurse, gynaecologist, other specialist or patient.

Adapted from Royal College Obstetricians and Gynaecologists. Management of Premenstrual Syndrome. Green-top guidelines no. 48. London : RCOG, 2007. Available at: http://www.rcog.org.uk/womens-health/clinical-guidance/management-premenstrual-syndrome-green-top-48 (Accessed: Feb 2010).

Table 27.2 Commonly reported symptoms in women with premenstrual syndrome

Psychological symptoms	Irritability, depression, crying/tearfulness, anxiety, tension, mood swings, lack of concentration, confusion, forgetfulness, unsociableness, restlessness, temper outbursts/anger, sadness/blues, loneliness.
Pain symptoms	Headache/migraine, breast tenderness/soreness/pain/swelling (collectively know as 'premenstrual mastalgia'), back pain, abdominal cramps, general pain.
Bloatedness	Weight gain, abdominal bloating, oedema of extremities (arms and legs), abdominal swelling and water retention.
Appetite symptoms	Increased appetite, food cravings, nausea.
Behavioural symptoms	Fatigue, dizziness, sleep/insomnia, decreased efficiency, accident prone, sexual interest changes, increased energy, tiredness.

Box 27.1 Diagnostic symptoms of premenstrual dysphoric disorder (DSM-IV)

- Markedly depressed mood, feelings of hopelessness or self-deprecating thoughts.
- Marked anxiety, tension or feelings of being 'keyed up or 'on edge'.
- Marked effective liability.
- Persistent and marked anger, irritability or increased interpersonal conflicts.
- Decreased interest in usual activities.
- Subjective sense of difficulty in concentrating.
- Lethargy, easy fatigability or lack of energy.
- Marked changes in appetite.
- Hypersomnia or insomnia.
- Subjective sense of being overwhelmed or out of control.
- Other physical symptoms.

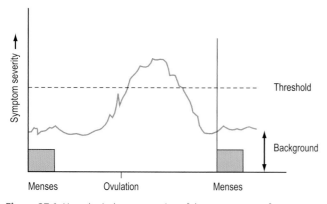

Figure 27.1 Hypothetical representation of the components of premenstrual syndrome.

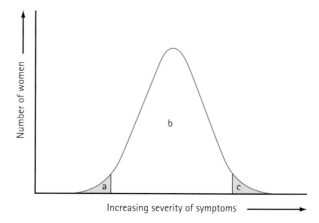

Figure 27.2 Diagrammatic representation of premenstrual syndrome (PMS) in the population of women of reproductive age. (a) Totally symptom-free women, (b) symptom severity ranges from physiological to moderate PMS, and (c) most severe PMS/premenstrual dysphoric disorder.

the possibility that both ovarian hormonal and neuroendocrine factors contribute to PMS/PMDD. The majority of women of reproductive age experience mild symptoms which are not troublesome and do not interfere with their daily activities. This should be considered as physiological rather than pathological (Figure 27.3).

Ovarian hormones

PMS only occurs in women of reproductive age during the luteal phase of the cycle; symptoms classically disappear when ovulation is absent. PMS is absent before puberty, during pregnancy and following the menopause. Suppression of ovulation with gonadotrophin-releasing hormone (GnRH) analogues (Hussain et al 1992) or following bilateral oophorectomy typically eliminates the symptoms. Conversely, postmenopausal women on sequential combined hormone replacement therapy can redevelop PMS-/PMDD-like symptoms during the progestogen phase of therapy (Hammarback et al 1985).

Previously, it was believed that hormonal or progesterone imbalances during ovulatory cycles may trigger the symptoms. However, administration of progesterone during this phase does not abolish symptoms (Wyatt et al 2001), and differences in oestrogen or progesterone levels have not been demonstrated between PMS patients and asymptomatic controls. Alternative hypotheses include the proposal that symptoms may be triggered by a preovulatory peak in oestradiol level or a postovulatory increase in progesterone level (Magos et al 1986, Schmidt et al 1998). These hypotheses do not explain why some women only develop symptoms in the late luteal phase.

It remains unclear whether oestrogen or progesterone triggers symptoms. Postmenopausal women on sequential hormone replacement therapy may report mood changes during the progesterone phase of therapy. The symptoms are likely to appear during the days when progesterone dominates over oestrogen, thus the luteal phase in ovulatory cycles.

As there is no clear evidence to implicate different levels of oestrogen or progesterone in inducing PMS, an attractive and convincing theory, partially supported by good evidence, is that an enhanced responsiveness or sensitivity exists to normal levels of these fluctuating hormones (Yonkers et al 2008) (Figures 27.4 and 27.5).

Neuroendocrine systems

Sex steroid receptors are abundant in specific regions of the brain which regulate emotions and behaviour. Serotonin is implicated in regulating mood and behaviour, and serotonin-facilitating drugs are effective as antidepressants and anxiolytic agents. In addition, certain sex steroid hormones exert their effects via serotogenic and γ-amino butyric acid (GABA) neurotransmitter systems.

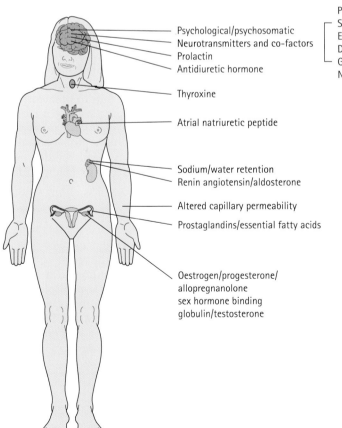

Psychological/psychosomatic
Neurotransmitters and co-factors
Prolactin
Antidiuretic hormone

Pyridoxine
Serotonin
Endorphins
Dopamine
GABA
Noradrenaline

Thyroxine

Atrial natriuretic peptide

Sodium/water retention
Renin angiotensin/aldosterone

Altered capillary permeability
Prostaglandins/essential fatty acids

Oestrogen/progesterone/
allopregnanolone
sex hormone binding
globulin/testosterone

Figure 27.3 Aetiological theories which have been proposed for premenstrual syndrome/premenstrual dysphoric disorder.

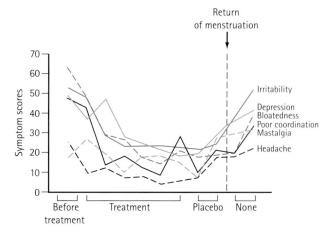

Figure 27.4 Effect of gonadotrophin-releasing hormone analogue on premenstrual symptoms, showing elimination of symptoms whilst ovarian function is suppressed, with return of symptoms prior to the return of menstruation during placebo.

Adapted from Hussain SY, Massil JH, Matta WH et al: 1992 Gynecological Endocrinology 6: 57–64.

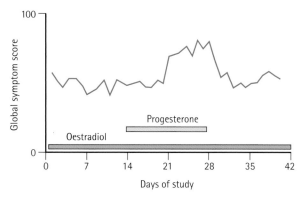

Figure 27.5 Simulation of premenstrual syndrome (PMS) symptoms on PMS patients after bilateral oopherectomy and hysterectomy. PMS symptoms recur during progesterone treatment but not during unopposed oestrogen.

Adapted from Henshaw et al (1993).

Serotonergic system

Studies undertaken on the rat model demonstrate that serotonin receptor concentrations vary with changes in oestrogen and progesterone levels (Biegen et al 1980). Serotonin depletion affects the sex-steroid-dependent behaviour; this suggests that the role of serotonin is to modulate behavioural changes by interacting with serotonin transmission, which has been demonstrated in studies performed on rodents (Carlsson and Carlsson 1988, Rubinow et al 1998) and non-human primates (Bethea et al 2002).

Selective serotonin reuptake inhibitors (SSRIs), serotonin receptor agonists (Landén et al 2001), serotonin precursors (Steinberg et al 1999) and serotonin-enhancing agents effectively dampen premenstrual symptoms. Impairment of serotonin transmission by serotonin receptor antagonists (Roca et al 2002) or a tryptophan-free diet provokes symptoms (Menkes et al 1994). Women with PMS have a low platelet concentration of serotonin and this concentration varies

during the menstrual cycle (Ashby et al 1998). This suggests that serotonin may play an important role in the pathophysiology of PMS/PMDD.

There is limited research on the genetics of serotonin in PMDD, but there does appear to be a difference in specific serotonin receptor polymorphism in PMDD sufferers (Dhingra et al 2007).

The GABAergic system

The GABA transmitter is a major inhibitory system in the central nervous system. GABA levels are low in the plasma and cerebrospinal fluid of individuals with mood disorders (Brambilla et al 2003). GABA levels have also been found to be decreased in women with PMDD during the late luteal phase compared with normal women whose plasma levels increase from the midfollicular phase (Halbriech et al 1996).

Allopregnanolone is a metabolite of progesterone, and levels vary in parallel with progesterone levels during the menstrual cycle (Genazzani et al 1998). In women with PMS, allopregnanolone levels are low in the follicular and luteal phases (Rapkin et al 1997, Bicíková et al 1998). Allopregnanolone is a positive modulator of the GABA receptor and a potent neurotransmitter with effects on mood, behaviour and cognitive function. Allopregnanolone has a bimodal effect on mood symptoms similar to benzodiazepines, barbiturates and alcohol. However, in some women with PMS, the plasma levels of allopregnanolone are low, suggesting that GABA receptor dysfunction might play a role in these women (Girdler et al 2001) (Table 27.3).

Theories related to sodium and fluid retention

Women with PMS report various somatic symptoms in the form of breast tenderness, bloating and swelling. Studies have failed to demonstrate weight gain, changes in abdominal dimensions, or any true water or sodium retention, even in women who experience bloatedness (Faratian et al 1984). There is no evidence to suggest that a shift in premenstrual water and electrolytes occurs; this is paralleled by a lack of similar changes in the hormones which influence potassium and water transport, such as components of atrial natriuretic peptide and the renin–angiotensin system. Studies have consistently shown that evidence is lacking to support this hypothesis.

Prolactin

Prolactin also promotes sodium, potassium and water retention and has direct stimulatory effects on the breast. However, prolactin levels do not undergo change during the menstrual cycle in women with PMS. Women with hyperprolactinaemia do not have symptoms of PMS, and current thinking is that prolactin or changes in prolactin levels are not involved in producing the symptoms of PMS.

Management

The diagnosis should be confirmed before commencing any form of treatment. The importance of a woman's past history is essential. This includes her contraceptive and

Table 27.3 Progesterone and allopregnanolone (progesterone metabolite) levels through the menstrual cycle

Hormone	Day	Premenstrual syndrome	Control
Allopregnanolone	19	6.32 ± 1.35	7.70 ± 1.01
	26	3.60 ± 0.75*	7.51 ± 1.25
Progesterone	19	10.66 ± 0.64	8.88 ± 0.79
	26	7.64 ± 0.91	6.39 ± 0.84
Ratio allopregnanolone: progesterone	19	0.68 ± 0.15	1.17 ± 0.25
	26	0.91 ± 0.26*	3.24 ± 1.25

Adapted from Rapkin AJ, Morgan M, Goldman L, Brann DW, Simone D, Mahesh VB: 1997 Obstetrics and Gynecology 90: 709–714.
*Statistically significant.

pregnancy wishes, previous treatment aimed at PMS/PMDD, and history of psychiatric problems, sexual abuse and illicit drug use. These latter conditions may mimic or be confused with PMS/PMDD and thus influence individualized treatment needs.

Non-Pharmacological Treatments

Lifestyle modifications

All women with PMS/PMDD should be advised regarding lifestyle changes before commencing on medications. Although there is no conclusive evidence that these changes improve symptoms of PMS/PMDD, these lifestyle habits will, at least, contribute to overall health and wellbeing. Where possible, important events can be timed to avoid the premenstrual phase. The changes should be initiated during the diagnostic process and continued throughout.

In women with mild-to-moderate symptoms, lifestyle modifications including dietary changes, exercise and cognitive behavioural therapies (CBT) may be enough to improve the symptoms. Dietary modifications in the form of reduced intake of caffeine, salt and refined sugars, a low glycaemic index diet and smaller meals may improve irritability, insomnia, fluid retention, breast tenderness, bloating and weight gain (Rapkin 2003, Kaur et al 2004). Increased intake of complex carbohydrates in the form of drink supplements decreases mood changes; this may be due to an increase in tryptophan, a precursor to serotonin (Sayegh et al 1995, Rapkin 2003). Exercise significantly improves mood and lethargy by increasing the release of endorphins (Aganoff and Boyle 1994). However, the evidence is quite limited for the effectiveness of most of these interventions.

Psychological interventions

These treatments are focused mainly on CBT and include different components. The treatment involves an analysis of triggers and stressors associated with negative emotions, problem solving and relaxation. No major randomized trials are available yet, but series of case studies with good outcomes have been reported.

In one series, women were offered eight sessions of CBT resulting in good outcomes (Slade 1989). Treatment was focused on identification of triggers and stresses associated with negative emotions, problem solving, relaxation and CBT to clarify attributions to the symptoms. Relaxation therapy was found to be superior to daily PMS symptom monitoring alone, or taking time out to read, in terms of comparative symptomatic approach (Goodale et al 1990). CBT combined with lifestyle changes is more effective in improving mood and PMS symptoms (Christensen AP et al 1995).

One randomized trial compared 10 sessions of CBT with SSRI (fluoxetine 20 mg/day) and both combined (Hunter et al 2002). There was significant improvement in all groups of symptom measures and the percentage of women fulfilling the PMDD criteria post treatment. Both treatments were equally effective at the end of 6 months; however, 1-year follow-up revealed that women who had undergone CBT maintained the improvement compared with women who had been on fluoxetine. Women with depressed mood responded poorly to both treatments, but learning active behavioural coping strategies had a good outcome at 1-year follow-up.

Vitamin or non-medical approaches

Vitamin B6 and pyridoxine

There are no well-designed randomized controlled studies to support the recommendation of any form of vitamin or herbal supplementation. A systematic review of five randomized controlled studies and one intervention study showed limited evidence for vitamin B6 (pyridoxine) supplementation in inadequate studies (Williams et al 2005). Pyridoxine 50–100 mg/day may improve premenstrual depressive symptoms provided that prescribed, daily doses do not exceed 100 mg to avoid the risk of peripheral neuropathy. Due to the poor quality of studies, pyridoxine alone cannot be recommended for treatment, although vitamin B6 and pyridoxine may have some benefit as an adjunct to treat depressive symptoms (pyridoxine is a cofactor necessary for the metabolic conversion of tryptophan to neuropeptides such as serotonin).

Calcium

In a single study, calcium supplementation 600 mg twice daily during the luteal phase of the cycle was shown to

	1	2	3	4	5	6	7	8	9	10	11	12	13	14	15	16	17	18	19	20	21	22	23	24	25	26	27	28	29	30	31	32	33	34	35	36	37	38	39	40
Bleeding	1	2	3	4	5	6	7	8	9	10	11	12	13	14	15	16	17	18	19	20	21	22	23	24	25	26	27	28	29	30	31	32	33	34	35	36	37	38	39	40
Cycle Day	1	2	3	4	5	6	7	8	9	10	11	12	13	14	15	16	17	18	19	20	21	22	23	24	25	26	27	28	29	30	31	32	33	34	35	36	37	38	39	40
Date of first day (write above)																																								
Symptoms																																								
Acne	0	0	0	0	0	0	0	0	0	0	0	0	0	0	0	0	0	0	0	0	0	0	0	0	0	0	0	0	0	0	0	0	0							
Bloatedness	3	3	2	2	0	0	0	0	0	0	0	0	0	0	0	0	2	3	3	3	3	3	3	3	3	3	3	1	1	0	0									
Breast tenderness	3	3	2	1	1	0	0	0	0	0	0	0	0	0	0	0	2	3	3	3	3	3	3	3	3	3	3	2	1	0	0									
Dizziness	3	3	3	2	0	0	0	0	0	0	0	0	0	0	0	0	2	3	3	3	3	3	3	3	3	3	3	1	1	0	0									
Fatigue	3	3	3	1	0	0	0	0	0	0	0	0	0	0	0	0	1	2	3	3	3	3	3	3	3	3	3	2	1	0	0									
Headache	3	3	1	0	0	0	0	0	0	0	0	0	0	0	0	0	0	0	0	1	2	2	1	2	3	2	3	3	3	2	2									
Hot flushes	3	3	1	0	0	0	0	0	0	0	0	0	0	0	0	0	2	3	3	3	3	3	3	3	3	3	3	0	0	0	0									
Nausea, diarrhoea, constipation	3	3	1	0	0	0	0	0	0	0	0	0	0	0	0	0	2	2	2	2	3	3	3	3	3	3	3	1	0	1	0									
Palpitations	3	3	2	1	0	0	0	0	0	0	0	0	0	0	0	0	3	3	3	3	3	3	3	3	3	3	3	3	2	0	0									
Swelling (hands, ankles, breasts)	3	3	3	1	0	0	0	0	0	0	0	0	0	0	0	0	2	3	3	3	3	3	3	3	3	3	3	3	3	1	0									
Violent tendencies	3	3	2	2	0	0	0	0	0	0	0	0	0	0	0	0	2	3	3	3	3	3	3	3	3	3	3	2	2	1	0									
Anxiety, tension, nervousness	3	2	2	2	0	0	0	0	0	0	0	0	0	0	0	0	2	3	3	3	3	3	3	3	3	3	3	2	1	0	0									
Confusion, difficulty concentrating	3	2	2	2	0	0	0	0	0	0	0	0	0	0	0	0	2	3	3	3	3	3	3	3	3	3	3	2	1	1	1									
Crying easily	3	3	3	2	0	0	0	0	0	0	0	0	0	0	0	0	2	3	3	3	3	3	3	3	3	3	3	2	2	2	1									
Depression	3	3	3	2	0	0	0	0	0	0	0	0	0	0	0	0	2	3	3	3	3	3	3	3	3	3	3	3	2	0										
Food cravings (sweets, salts)	3	2	1	1	0	0	0	0	0	0	0	0	0	0	0	0	2	3	3	3	3	3	3	3	3	3	3	2	1	1										
Forgetfulness	3	2	2	1	0	0	0	0	0	0	0	0	0	0	0	0	2	3	3	3	3	3	3	3	3	3	3	3	2	0										
Irritability	3	3	3	2	0	0	0	0	0	0	0	0	0	0	0	0	3	3	3	3	3	3	3	3	3	3	3	3	0	0										
Increase in appetite	3	2	1	0	0	0	0	0	0	0	0	0	0	0	0	0	2	3	3	3	3	3	3	3	3	3	3	2	0	0										
Mood swings	3	3	3	1	0	0	0	0	0	0	0	0	0	0	0	0	3	3	3	3	3	3	3	3	3	3	3	3	0	0										
Overly sensitive	3	3	3	1	0	0	0	0	0	0	0	0	0	0	0	0	3	3	3	3	3	3	3	3	3	3	3	2	0	0										
Wish to be alone	3	3	3	2	0	0	0	0	0	0	0	0	0	0	0	0	3	3	3	3	3	3	3	3	3	3	3	2	1	0										
Medication used	3																																							
*1																																								
*2																																								

(A)

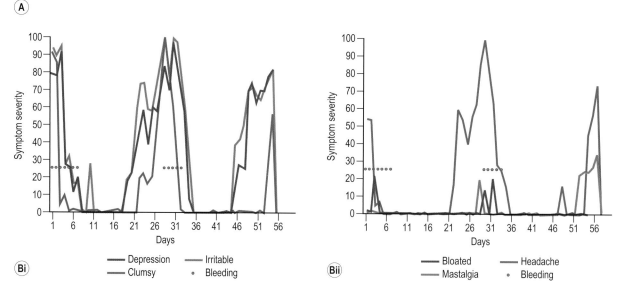

(Bi) — Depression — Irritable — Clumsy • Bleeding

(Bii) — Bloated — Headache — Mastalgia • Bleeding

Figure 27.6 Daily Record of Severity of Problems (DRSP). A typical DRSP chart of symptoms for premenstrual syndrome/premenstrual dysphoric disorder sufferer. This shows the range of symptoms, severity of symptoms, luteal phase occurrence, resolution of symptoms with menses and the impact on normal functioning.

Sources: Endicott J, Harrison W: 1990 Daily Record of Severity of Problems Form. Department of Research Assessment and Training, New York State Psychiatric Institute, New York. Endicott J, Nee J, Harrison W: 2006 Archives of Women's Mental Health 9: 41–49.

reduce emotional and physical symptoms of PMS/PMDD by the second or third treatment cycle (Thys-Jacobs et al 1998).

Agnus castus

A single randomized placebo-controlled study demonstrated that agnus castus (chaste berry) supplementation appeared to be superior to placebo in relieving irritability, anger, mood swings, headaches and breast fullness (Schellenberg 2001).

Evening primrose oil

Evening primrose oil does appear to be efficacious for cyclical mastalgia.

Box 27.2 Differential diagnoses of PMS

Psychiatric disorders

- May be confused because of the similarity in symptoms and because of the bipolar and periodic nature of some psychiatric disorders.
- Many women prefer to 'label' their psychological problem as gynaecological rather than psychiatric.
- There are no objective tests but there are many questionnaires. The general health questionnaire (Goldberg Miller 1979) may help to exclude or diagnose psychological ill health. The Daily Record of Severity of Problems form is becoming progressively more accepted as the tool to demonstrate PMS and PMDD.

Intrafamilial and psychosexual problems

- Distinguish between cause and effect.

Other causes of breast symptoms

- Cyclical breast pain may be considered as part of PMS. Can be distinguished from non-cyclical breast disease by history and symptom charts.
- Non-cyclical disease includes severe disorders requiring breast examination and possibly mammography, ultrasonography, aspiration and biopsy.
- Breast cancer must, of course, be excluded.

Other causes of abdominal bloatedness and water retention

- Only a few women exhibit significant water retention in PMS.
- More women have idiopathic oedema which is also cyclical but only occasionally coincides by chance with the menstrual cycle.

- Some women call progressive obesity 'PMS bloatedness'.
- Distinguish by twice-daily weighing.

Endometriosis, pelvic pain and dysmenorrhoea

- Primary dysmenorrhoea occurs with the period.
- Secondary dysmenorrhoea is related to pelvic pathology and may occur premenstrually.
- Laparoscopy will exclude endometriosis and pelvic infection.

Medical causes of lethargy/tiredness and anxiety/irritability

- Occasionally anaemia; haemoglobin estimation advised.
- Rarely hypothyroidism or hyperthyroidism; thyroid function tests will define.

Menopause

- May be confused with PMS in patients over 40 years of age.
- Flushes may occur in PMS; mood change can occur with the menopause.
- Usually distinguished from history.
- Raised follicle-stimulating hormone level can be helpful but not always consistent in the perimenopausal phase.

Other supplements

Supplements such as magnesium, vitamin D and St John's Wort should not be considered as effective treatment options due to a lack of evidence for or against efficacy (Douglas 2002, Kaur et al 2004).

Miscellaneous

Bromocriptine has been advocated in the past; however, in the absence of differences in prolactin levels, it does not seem to be a logical approach but may be beneficial for cyclical mastalgia.

Alternative therapy

Various treatments in the form of massage, biofeedback, acupuncture and reflexology have been proposed but none of these have been proven to be effective. Double-blind randomized and crossover studies for light therapy did not provide conclusive evidence, and there are safety issues to be taken into account before embarking on this form of treatment (Lam et al 1999) (Table 27.4).

Pharmacological Treatments

Patients with mild-to-moderate PMS/PMDD could be offered non-pharmacological treatment options, bearing in mind the limited evidence for their efficacy. In women who do not respond to such treatment and in women with severe symptoms, pharmacological treatment options should be considered at an earlier stage. The choice of treatment depends on the symptoms and their effect on lifestyle.

Progesterone

The evidence from the meta-analysis and systematic review of 10 randomized controlled trials clearly demonstrates that progesterone is not effective in treating PMS (Wyatt et al 2001). This is not surprising when one considers that progesterone deficiency has never been demonstrated in women with PMS, and when it is appreciated that the administration of sequential hormone replacement therapy to postmenopausal women commonly results in the development of mood changes similar to PMS during the progesterone phase of therapy (Hammarback et al 1985). Progesterone is not recommended in the management of PMS, although progesterone and progestogens are the only licensed products for the management of PMS in the UK (Figure 27.7).

Oestrogen

Oestrogen is effective at suppressing ovulation at doses of 100–200 µg (transdermal patches) (Smith et al 1995, Watson et al 1989). As unopposed oestrogen can cause endometrial hyperplasia and carcinoma, cyclical progestogen should also be administered (Paterson ME et al 1980). Progesterone administration can induce PMS symptoms, thereby limiting the efficacy of oestrogen. In women who are intolerant to cyclical progesterone, a shorter duration of 7 days

Table 27.4 Lifestyle modifications and alternative therapies recommended for use in the treatment of premenstrual syndrome (PMS)/premenstrual dysphoric disorder (PMDD)

Therapy	Dosage (if applicable)	Place in therapy	Level of evidence	Adverse effects/special notes
Calcium	1200 mg/day in divided doses	First-line, adjunctive	B	Nausea, dyspepsia, constipation, renal calculi
Pyridoxine (vitamin B6)	50–100 mg/day	Adjunctive	C	Peripheral neuropathy at high doses(>100 mg/day)
Evening primrose	2–4 g/day	Adjunctive	C	Benefits cyclical mastalgia
Chaste berry (Vitex agnus castus)	20–40 mg/day	Adjunctive	B	Acne, caution use with oral contraceptive pills, hormone replacement therapy, dopamine agonists/antagonist
Diet modification		First-line	C	Should be observed by all women with PMS/PMDD
Light therapy		Adjunctive	B	
Cognitive behavioural therapy (relaxation, sleep hygiene)		Adjunctive	B	
Exercise		First-line	B	
Acupuncture, massage, chiropractice, Reflexology		Adjunctive	B	
Surgery		Last-line; for severe, refractory cases of PMDD	A	Complications, permanent

Source: Jarvis et al (2008). Annals of Pharmacotherapy 42: 967–978.

Evidence level A, consistent good-quality, patient-oriented evidence; most studies found similar or coherent conclusions; high-quality systematic reviews and meta-analyses, if they exist, support the recommendation; patient-oriented outcomes that matter to patients, such as morbidity, mortality, symptom improvement , cost reduction and quality of life.

Evidence level B, inconsistent or limited-quality patient-oriented evidence; considerable variation and lack of coherence; high-quality systematic reviews and meta-analyses, if they exist, do not find consistent evidence in favour of recommendation.

Evidence level C, consensus, usual practice, opinion, disease-oriented evidence or case studies; disease-oriented evidence measures intermediate, physiological or surrogate endpoints that may or may not reflect improvements in patient outcomes.

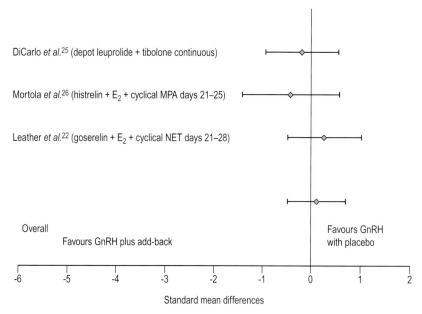

Figure 27.7 A meta-analysis of trials of progesterone in the management of premenstrual syndrome.
Adapted from Wyatt K, Dimmock P, Jones P, Obhrai M, O'Brien S: 2001 BMJ (Clinical Research Ed.) 323: 776–781.

is adequate to prevent endometrial hyperplasia (Studd 2008). A simple regimen is for progestogen to be administered on the first 7 days of each calendar month. A withdrawal bleed occurs on approximately the 10th day of the calendar month.

In women who are intolerant to oral progestogen or who have irregular or heavy bleeding, the levonorgestrel-releasing intrauterine system will usually be beneficial, providing endometrial protection and possibly amenorrhoea without producing PMS-like side-effects (Sitruk-Ware 2007). In some women, levonorgestrel can be absorbed systemically in the first months of therapy until the endometrium becomes atrophic. This is to be expected, and doctors and patients need to be forewarned, particularly of its transient nature.

Oral contraceptive pills

Oral contraceptive pills (OCPs) may be effective in improving physical symptoms such as bloating, headache, abdominal pain and breast tenderness. However, in some women, OCPs may actually worsen the symptoms. Although ovulation is effectively suppressed, exposure to the new exogenous cyclical progestogen may give rise to symptoms, as the mechanism of PMS/PMDD is thought to be the result of PMS patients being progesterone sensitive.

Newer OCPs contain the progestin drospirenone. This is a derivative of spironolactone and has similar antimineralocorticoid and antiandrogenic properties. A systematic review of all randomized controlled trials comparing the combined OCPs containing drospirenone with a placebo or other OCPs for their effect on PMS concluded that drospirenone 3 mg plus ethinyl oestradiol 20 µg may help to treat PMS in women with PMDD (Lopez et al 2008). The drospirenone group had a greater decrease in impairment of productivity, social activities and relationships. Little effect was found on less severe symptoms when comparing drospirenone plus oestrogen with another combined oral contraceptive. A 6-month study showed fewer symptoms with drosirenone, while a 2-year trial found the groups to be similar. Two OCPs, Yaz and Yasmin, containing drospirenone have been approved by the US Food and Drug Administration (FDA) for the treatment of PMDD but are not approved in Europe or the UK. FDA approval gives the manufacturer permission to make claims about the effectiveness of these OCPs for 'treating PMDD in women who require oral contraception'. It highlights the fact that the effectiveness beyond three cycles is unknown.

Danazol

Danazol has been shown to be effective when ovulation is suppressed. However, there are concerns about masculinizing side-effects. At a reduced dose (200 mg) in the luteal phase, danazol has been shown to be effective for cyclical mastalgia but not other symptoms (O'Brien and Abukhalil 1999).

Gonadotropin-releasing hormone agonists

GnRH agonist analogues are the synthetic analogues of naturally occurring GnRH. When administered, they reduce the secretion of luteinizing hormone and follicle-stimulating hormone, thereby causing anovulation with associated hypo-oestrogenization. GnRH agonists are effective in treating psychological, emotional and physical symptoms associated with ovarian steroid cycles (Brown et al 1994, Freeman et al 1997, Mezrow et al 1994).

Many women do not tolerate the adverse effects, which are in the form of menopausal symptoms including flushes, insomnia, depression, headache and muscle aches. GnRH treatment should normally be limited to no more than 6 months to reduce the risk of reduction in bone mass. There is a likelihood of return of symptoms once the treatment is discontinued. In such women, the duration of therapy may be extended in certain circumstances by the addition of 'add-back' therapy which may be achieved using continuous daily conjugated oestrogen at a dose of 0.625 mg, oestradiol valerate 2 mg or transdermal oestradiol patches 50 µg along with progestogens such as medroxyprogesterone 5–10 mg. 'Add-back' with tibolone is also very useful (Leather et al 1999, Pickersgill 1998). In the small number of women requiring such long-term therapy, bone mineral density evaluation is required and advice on adequate calcium intake should be given (Figure 27.8).

Selective serotonin reuptake inhibitors

Serotonergic neurotransmission plays an important role in the aetiology of PMS/PMDD. Serotonergic antidepressants, particularly SSRIs, have been demonstrated in several placebo-controlled studies to be significantly effective. SSRIs improve emotional and physical symptoms of PMDD, enhance psychosocial function and work performance, and improve quality of life (Pearlstein et al 2000, Wyatt et al 2002, Steiner et al 2006).

SSRIs should be commenced at the lower end of the dosing range and increased according to the response. Significant improvements in irritability, depressed mood and physical symptoms occur during the first menstrual cycle. Women with depressive disorders require at least 6–8 weeks of treatment before any improvement can be demonstrated; it is important to recognize this distinction.

SSRIs can be administered using continuous, intermittent, semi-intermittent or symptom-onset strategies. Women with an irregular menstrual cycle or those who experience intolerable symptoms on discontinuation of treatment will benefit from a continuous daily SSRI dosing regimen. The continuous regimen may also help to improve somatic symptoms associated with PMDD in the long term (Luisi and Pawasauskas 2003).

Intermittent or luteal-phase dosing can be considered in women with adverse side-effects and can be cost-effective. The luteal-phase regimen is initiated on day 14 of the menstrual cycle and is discontinued 1–2 days after the onset of menses. Semi-intermittent treatment involves continuous daily dosing of SSRIs and increasing the dose during the luteal phase. This is ideal for women who experience underlying mood symptoms throughout the cycle with worsening of symptoms during the luteal phase.

SSRIs are well tolerated in the doses used for the treatment of PMDD. Headache, fatigue, insomnia, anxiety and sexual dysfunction are common symptoms associated with the continuous dose regimen (Wyatt et al 2004).

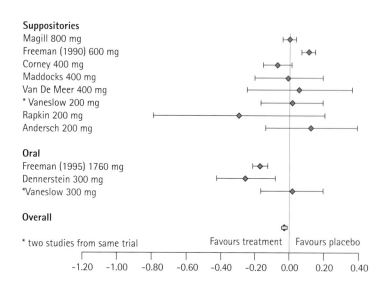

Suppositories

Magill 800 mg
Freeman (1990) 600 mg
Corney 400 mg
Maddocks 400 mg
Van De Meer 400 mg
* Vaneslow 200 mg
Rapkin 200 mg
Andersch 200 mg

Oral
Freeman (1995) 1760 mg
Dennerstein 300 mg
*Vaneslow 300 mg

Overall

* two studies from same trial

Favours treatment | Favours placebo

-1.20 -1.00 -0.80 -0.60 -0.40 -0.20 0.00 0.20 0.40

Figure 27.8 The effectiveness of gonadotrophin-releasing hormone agonist with and without 'add-back' therapy in treating premenstrual syndrome: a meta analysis.
Adapted from Wyatt et al (2007) BJOG.111: 585–593.

The US FDA has licensed various SSRIs for PMDD, but they are not licensed in the UK or Europe (Table 27.5).

Other antidepressants

Clomipramine, a tricyclic antidepressant with strong serotonergic activity, may be effective in treating severe PMDD (Sundblad et al 1993). Serotonin-norepinephrine reuptake inhibitors, venlafaxine and duloxetine have been found to be more effective than placebo for the treatment of PMDD (Mazza et al 2008).

Spironolactone

Spironolactone, a potassium-sparing diuretic and aldosterone receptor antagonist, exhibits antimineralocorticoid and antiandrogenic effects and interferes with synthesis of testosterone (Wang et al 1995, Burnet et al 1991). At doses of 25–200 mg/day during the luteal phase, spironolactone can alleviate symptoms of weight gain, bloating and breast tenderness, and may also decrease negative mood and somatic scores despite the fact that there is no evidence of water retention.

Anxiolytic agents

Anxiety is common in PMS/PMDD; anxiolytic agents during the luteal phase of the cycle can be helpful in women with persistent anxiety despite treatment with SSRIs. Alprazolam at a dose of 0.25 mg three to four times per day during the luteal phase has been shown to be effective in double-blind, placebo-controlled trials for the treatment of premenstrual depression, irritability, hostility and social withdrawal (Berger and Presser 1994, Freeman et al 1995).

Surgery

In a small group of women who have not responded or are not able to tolerate the various medical treatments or combinations of medical treatment, surgical management in the form of hysterectomy with bilateral oopherectomy or

bilateral removal of ovaries may be considered (Cronje et al 2004). Obviously, randomized trials are not possible in this form of treatment, but in open studies, 95% of carefully selected women who underwent bilateral oophorectomy and hysterectomy were shown to be very satisfied 4 years after surgery (Cronje et al 2004). These women require long-term hormone replacement therapy in the form of oestradiol; in these circumstances, it is unnecessary to give progestogen. No placebo-controlled studies have been published specifically to demonstrate the efficacy of bilateral oophorectomy alone for the management of PMS/PMDD. When bilateral oophorectomy is contemplated (with or without hysterectomy), most gynaecologists consider that a trial of a GnRH analogue for three cycles is advisable to demonstrate the potential efficacy of what is a very invasive procedure.

Conclusion

Severe PMS/PMDD continues to affect 5% of women of reproductive age. It is very important to establish the diagnosis of this condition using prospective recording Daily Record of Severity of Problems charts and to rule out other diagnoses, particularly anxiety disorders, depression and other conditions which are merely exacerbated during the premenstrual period. The treatment should be individualized according to the specific symptoms of PMS/PMDD. The dietary and lifestyle modifications should be initiated during the diagnostic phase and continued for life; however, the evidence base for these modifications is limited. The use of SSRIs or drospirenone-containing OCPs should be considered as the first line of treatment for many women, and the choice will depend on an individual woman's requirements. Achieving anovulation will effectively eliminate symptoms in the majority of women with severe PMDD, and surgery should be the last option in women who have already failed to respond to any other form of treatment. All women with PMS/PMDD should be counselled carefully, sensitively and in detail prior to treatments being commenced.

Table 27.5 Prescription medications for use in the treatment of premenstrual syndrome (PMS)/premenstrual dysphoric disorder (PMDD). None are licensed for PMS or PMDD in Europe or the UK

Drug class and agents	Dosage	Recommendation for use	Level of evidence	Adverse effects
SSRIs*				
Fluoxetine*	10–20 mg/day (max 60 mg/day)	First-line therapy for somatic and mood symptoms, continuous or intermittent therapy	A	Sexual dysfunction, sleep disturbances (insomnia, sedation, hypersomnia), GI distress, fatigue, headache, nervousness
Sertraline*	50–150 mg/day		A	
Paroxitine	10–30 mg/day		B	
Paroxetine CR	20–30 mg/day		A	
Citalopram	20–30 mg/day		B	
Escitalopram	10–20 mg/day		B	
Other serotonergic antidepressants				
Venlafaxine	50–200 mg/day		B	Sexual dysfunction, insomnia, headache, anorexia nervosa
Duloxetine	60 mg/day		B	Somnolence, dizziness, insomnia, headache, nausea, xerostomia, diarrhoea, constipation
Clomipramine	25–75 mg/day		B	Anticholinergic effects, sexual dysfunction, weight gain
Anxiolytics				
Alprazolam	0.75–1 mg/day (max 4 mg/day)	Second-line therapy for anxiety symptoms, intermittent therapy	B	Drowsiness, sedation, risk of dependence and tolerance
Buspirone	20 mg/day		B	Headache, no risk of dependence or tolerance
Danazol	**200 mg/day**	**Luteal phase for mastalgia**	**C**	**Irreversible virilizing effects**
GnRH agonists				
Leuprolide	3.75 mg IM every month or 11.25 mg every 3 months	Effective for psychoemotional and physical symptoms; adverse profile and cost limit use; 'add-back therapy' with oestrogen and/or progesterone if used >6 months	B	Hypo-oestrogenic adverse effects including atrophic vaginitis, hot flushes and osteoporosis
Goserelin	3.6 mg SC every month or 10.8 mg SC every 3 months		B	
Nafarelin	200–400 μg intranasally twice daily		B	
Histerilin	10 μg/kg SC daily		B	
Spironolactone	**25–200 mg/day during luteal phase**	**Effective in alleviating breast tenderness and bloating**	**B**	**Antioestrogenic effect and hyperkalemia**
Oral contraceptive pills				
Ethinyl oestradiol/ drospirenone	Yaz: 20 μg ethinyl oestradiol/3 mg drospirenone daily for 24 days/month. Yasmin: 30 μg ethinyl oestradiol/3 mg drospirenone daily for 21 days/month	Effective in alleviating some PMS symptoms; symptoms may worsen in some women	B	Breast tenderness, nausea, irregular bleeding, thrombosis and hyperkalemia

Source: Jarvis et al (2008). The Annals of Pharmacotherapy 42: 967–978.
CR, controlled release; GI, gastrointestinal; GnRH, gonadotrophin-releasing hormone; SSRI, selective serotonin reuptake inhibitor; SC, subcutaneous; IM, intra muscular.
*Drugs licensed in the USA for PMDD.

KEY POINTS

1. PMS refers to somatic and psychological symptoms which recur in the luteal phase of the menstrual cycle.

2. Most women of reproductive age will have some symptoms related to the premenstrual phase of the cycle. Only when the symptoms cause significant disruption to normal functioning are they considered to be PMS.

3. It is estimated that 3–8% of women of reproductive age experience debilitating symptoms, leading to functional or psychological impairment.

4. PMDD is the severe and predominantly psychological form of PMS.

5. An enormous range of symptoms have been described in PMS. The luteal-phase timing is more important than their character. The symptoms should be confirmed prospectively by daily ratings during the last two consecutive cycles. This prospective rating is best achieved by use of the Daily Record of Severity of Problems form.

6. The current evidence suggests the possibility that both ovarian hormonal and neuroendocrine factors contribute to PMS/PMDD.

7. Ideally, the diagnosis should be confirmed before commencing any form of treatment. Other factors such as contraception need and pregnancy wishes should be considered in the management decision of choice of therapy.

8. In women with mild-to-moderate symptoms, lifestyle modifications including dietary changes, exercise and CBT may be enough to improve the symptoms.

9. Suppression of ovulation using OCPs may be useful. PMS can be reintroduced by progesterone, so the choice of progesterone may be important.

10. GnRH agonists are effective in treating psychological, emotional and physical symptoms associated with ovarian steroid cycles. GnRH treatment should normally be limited to no more than 6 months to reduce the risk of a decrease in bone mass. In certain circumstances, the duration can be extended with the addition of add-back therapy.

11. SSRIs improve the emotional and physical symptoms of PMDD, enhance psychosocial function and work performance, and, in turn, improve quality of life. Their action is immediate and they can, therefore, only be used in the luteal phase.

12. Surgery needs careful consideration. Total abdominal hysterectomy and bilateral oopherectomy should normally be the last option. Women with PMS who undergo hysterectomy for gynaecological pathology reasons in addition to PMS should be offered bilateral oopherectomy at the time of surgery.

References

Aganoff JA, Boyle GJ 1994 Aerobic exercise, mood status and menstrual cycle symptoms. Journal of Psychosomatic Research 38: 183–192.

Andersch B 1983 Bromocriptine and premenstrual symptoms: a survey of double blind trials. Obstetrical and Gynaecological Survey 38: 643–646.

Angst J, Sellaro R, Merikangas KR, Endicott J 2001 The epidemiology of premenstrual psychological symptoms. Acta Psychiatrica Scandinavica 104: 110–116.

Ashby CR Jr, Carr LA, Cook CL, Steptoe MM, Franks DD 1998 Alteration of platelet serotoninergic mechanism and monoamine oxidase activity in premenstrual syndrome. Biological Psychiatry 24: 225–233.

Berger CP, Presser B 1994 Alprazolam in the treatment of two subsamples of patients with late luteal phase dysphoric disorder: a double-blind, placebo-controlled crossover study. Obstetrics and Gynecology 84: 379–385.

Bethea CL, Lu NZ, Gundlah C, Streicher JM 2002 Diverse actions of ovarian steroids in the serotonin neural systems. Frontiers in Neuroendocrinology 23: 41–100.

Bicíková M, Dibbelt L, Hill M, Hampl R, Stárka L 1998 Allopregnanolone in women with premenstrual syndrome. Hormone and Metabolic Research 30: 227–230.

Biegen A, Bercovtz H, Samuel D 1980 Serotonin receptor concentration during the oestrous cycle of the rat. Brain Research1 87: 221–225.

Brambilla P, Perez J, Barale F, Schettini G, Soares JC 2003 GABAergic dysfunction in mood disorders. Molecular Psychiatry 8: 721–731.

Brown CS, Ling FW, Andersen RN, Farmer RG, Arheart KL 1994 Efficacy of depot leuprolide in premenstrual syndrome: effect of severity and type in controlled trial. Obstetrics and Gynecology 84: 779–786.

Burnet RB, Radden HS, Easterbrook EG, McKinnon RA 1991 Premenstrual syndrome and spironolactone. Australian and New Zealand Journal of Obstetrics and Gynaecology 31: 366–368.

Carlsson M, Carlsson A 1988 A regional study of sex differences in rat brain serotonin. Progress in Neuropsychopharmacology and Biological Psychiatry 12: 53–61.

Casper RF, Hearn MT 1990 The effect of hysterectomy and bilateral oophorectomy in women with severe premenstrual syndrome. American Journal of Obstet rics and Gynecology 162: 105–109.

Christensen AP, Oei TPS 1995 The efficacy of cognitive behaviour therapy in treating premenstrual dysphoric changes. Journal of Affective Disorders 33: 57–63.

Cronje WH, Vashisht A, Studd JW 2004 Hysterectomy and bilateral oophorectomy for severe premenstrual syndrome. Human Reproduction 19 2152–2155.

Dhingra V, Magnay JL, O'Brien PM, Chapman G, Fryer AA, Ismail KM 2007 Serotonin receptor 1A C (-1019) G polymorphism associated with premenstrual dysphoric disorder. Obstetrics and Gynecology 110: 788–792.

Douglas S 2002 Premenstrual syndrome. Evidence-based treatment in family practice. Canadian Family Physician 48 1789–1797.

Endicott J, Harrison W 1990 Daily Record of Severity of Problems Form. Department of Research Assessment and Training, New York State Psychiatric Institute, New York.

Endicott J, Nee J, Harrison W 2006 Daily Record of Severity of Problems: reliability and validity. Archives of Women's Mental Health 9: 41–49.

Faratian B, Gaspar A, O'Brien PM, Johnson IR, Filshie GM, Prescott P 1984 Premenstrual syndrome: weight, abdominal size and perceived body image. American Journal of Obstetrics and Gynecology 50: 200–204.

Freeman EW, Rickels K, Sondheimer SJ et al 1995 A double-blind trial of oral progesterone, alprazolam and placebo in treatment of severe premenstrual syndrome. Journal American Medical Association 274: 51–57.

Freeman EW, Sondheimer SJ, Rickels K 1997 Gonadotropin-releasing hormone agonist in the treatment of premenstrual symptoms with and without ongoing dysphoria: a controlled study. Psychopharmacology Bulletin 33: 303–309.

Genazzani AR, Petraglia FL, Bernardi F et al 1998 Circulating levels of allopregnanolone levels in humans: gender, age and endocrine influences. Journal of Clinical Endocrinology and Metabolism 83: 2099–2103.

Girdler SS, Straneva PA, Light KC, Pedersen CA, Morrow AL 2001 Allopregnanolone levels and reactivity to mental stress in premenstrual dysphoric disorder. Biological Psychiatry 49: 788–797.

Goldberg AP, Miller B 1979 A scaled version of the general health questionnaire. Psychological Medicine 9: 139–145.

Goodale IL, Domar AD, Benson H 1990 Alleviation of premenstrual syndrome with the relaxation response. Obstetrics and Gynecology 75: 649–655.

Halbreich U, Petty F, Yonkers K, Kramer GL, Rush AJ, Bibi KW 1996 Low plasma gamma-aminobutyric levels during the late luteal phase of women with premenstrual dysphoric disorder. American Journal of Psychiatry 152: 718–720.

Halbreich U, Borenstein J, Pearlstein T, Kahn LS 2003 The prevalence, impairment, impact and burden of premenstrual dysphoric disorder (PMS/PMDD). Psychoendocrinology 28: 1–23.

Halbreich U, Backstorm T, Eriksson E et al 2007 Clinical diagnostic criteria for premenstrual syndrome and guidelines for their quantification for research studies. Gynecological Endocrinology 23: 123–130.

Hammarback S, Backstrom T, Hoist J et al 1985 Cyclical mood changes as in the premenstrual tension syndrome using sequential oestrogen — progestagen postmenopausal hormone replacement therapy. Acta Obstetrica of Gynaecologica Scandinavica 64: 393–397.

Harrison WM, Endicott J, Nee J 1990 Treatment of premenstrual dysphoria with alprazolam: a controlled study. Archives of General Psychiatry 47: 270–275.

Henshaw C, O'Brien PMS, Foreman A et al 1993 An experimental model for PMS. Neuropsychopharmacology 25: 713–719.

Hunter MS, Ussher J, Browne S et al 2002 Medical (fluoxetine) and psychological (cognitive behavioural therapy) treatments for premenstrual dysphoric disorder (PMDD): a study of treatment processes. Journal of Psychosomatic Research 53: 811–818.

Hussain SY, Massil JH, Matta WH, Shaw RW, O'Brien PM 1992 Buserelin in premenstrual syndrome. Gynecological Endocrinology 6: 57–64.

Ismail K, O'Brien S 2005 Premenstrual syndrome. Current Obstetrics and Gynaecology 15: 25–30.

Jarvis CI, Lynch AM, Morin AK 2008 Management strategies for premenstrual syndrome/premenstrual dysphoric disorder. The Annals of Pharmacotherapy 42: 967–978.

Kaur G, Gonsalves L, Thacker HL 2004 Premenstrual dysphoric disorder: a review for the treating practitioner. Cleveland Clinic Journal of Medicine 71: 303–305.

Khastgir G, Studd J, Holland N, Alaghband-Zadeh J, Sims TJ, Bailey AJ 2001 Anabolic effect of long term oestrogen replacement on bone collagen in elderly postmenopausal women with osteoporosis. Osteoporosis International 12: 456–470.

Lam RW, Carter D, Misri S, Kuan AJ, Yatham LN, Zis AP 1999 A controlled study of light therapy in women with late luteal phase dysphoric disorder. Psychiatry Research 86: 185–192.

Landén M, Eriksson O, Sundblad C, Andersch B, Naessén T, Eriksson E 2001 Compounds with affinity for serotonergic receptors in the treatment of premenstrual dysphoria: a comparison of buspirone, nefazodone and placebo. Psychopharmacology 155: 292–298.

Leather AT, Studd JW, Watson NR, Holland EF 1999 The treatment of severe premenstrual syndrome with goserelin with and without 'add-back' oestrogen therapy: a placebo controlled study. Gynecological Endocrinology 13: 48–55.

Lopez LM, Kaptein A, Helmerhorst FM 2008 Oral contraceptives containing drospirenone for premenstrual syndrome. Cochrane Database of Systematic Reviews 1: CD006586.

Luisi AF, Pawasauskas JE 2003 Treatment of premenstrual dysphoric disorder with selective serotonin reuptake inhibitors. Pharmacotherapy 23 1131–1140.

Magos AL, Brewster E, Singh R, O'Dowd T, Brincat M, Studd JW 1986 The effects of norethisterone in postmenopausal women on oestrogen replacement therapy: a model for the premenstrual syndrome. BJOG: an International Journal of Obstetrics and Gynaecology 93 1290–1296.

Mazza M, Harnic D, Catalano V, Janiri L, Bria P 2008 Duloxetine for premenstrual dysphoric disorder: a pilot study. Expert Opinion on Pharmacotherapy 9: 517–521.

Menkes DB, Coates LA, Fawcett JB 1994 Acute tryptophan depletion aggravates premenstrual syndrome. Journal of Affective Disorders 32: 37–44.

Mezrow G, Shoupe D, Spicer D, Lobo R, Leung B, Pike M 1994 Depot leuprolide acetate with oestrogen and progestin add-back for long-term treatment of premenstrual syndrome. Fertility and Sterility 62: 932–937.

O'Brien PM, Abukhalil IE 1999 Randomised controlled trial of management of premenstrual syndrome and premenstrual mastalgia using luteal phase only danazol. American Journal of Obstetrics and Gynecology 180: 18–23.

Paterson ME, Wade-Evans T, Sturdee DW, Thom MH, Studd JW 1980 Endometrial disease after treatment with oestrogens and progestogens in the climactric. BMJ (Clinical Research Ed.) 280: 822–824.

Pearlstein TB, Halbriech U, Batzed ED et al 2000 Psychosocial functioning in women with premenstrual dysphoric disorder before and after treatment with sertraline or placebo. Journal of Clinical Psychiatry 61: 101–109.

Pickersgill A 1998 GnRH agonist and add-back therapy: is there a perfect combination? BJOG: an International Journal of Obstetrics and Gynaecology 105: 475–485.

Rapkin A 2003 A review of treatment of premenstrual syndrome and premenstrual dysphoric disorder. Psychoneuroendo-crinology 28 (Suppl): 39–53.

Rapkin AJ, Morgan M, Goldman L, Brann DW, Simone D, Mahesh VB 1997 Progesterone metabolite allopregnanolone in women with premenstrual syndrome. Obstetrics and Gynecology 90: 709–714.

Roca CA, Schmidt PJ, Smith MJ, Danaceau MA, Murphy DL, Rubinow DR 2002 Effects of metergoline on symptoms in women with premenstrual dysphoric disorder. American Journal of Psychiatry 159 1876–1881.

Royal College of Obstetricians and Gynaecologists 2007 Management of Premenstrual Syndrome. Green-top Guidelines No. 48. RCOG, London. Available at: www.rcog.org.uk/resources/public/pdf/green_top48_pms.pdf.

Rubinow DR, Schmidt PJ, Roca CA 1998 Oestrogen serotonin interactions: implications for affective regulation. Biological Psychiatry 44: 839–850.

Sayegh R, Schiff I, Wurtman J, Spiers P, McDermott J, Wurtman R 1995 The effect of carbohydrate rich beverage on mood, appetite and cognitive function in women with premenstrual syndrome. Obstetrics and Gynecology 86: 520–528.

Schellenberg R 2001 Treatment for the premenstrual syndrome with agnus castus fruit extract: prospective, randomised, placebo controlled study. BMJ (Clinical Research Ed.) 322: 134–137.

Schmidt PJ, Nieman LK, Danaceau MA, Adams LF, Rubinow DR 1998 Differential behavioral effects of gonadal steroids in women with and those without premenstrual syndrome. New England Journal of Medicine 338: 209–216.

Sitruk-Ware R 2007 The levonorgestrel intrauterine system for use of in peri- and postmenopausal women. Contraception 7(Supplement): S155–S160.

Slade P 1989 Psychological therapy for premenstrual symptoms. Behavioural Psychotherapy 17: 135–150.

Smith RN, Studd JW, Zamblera D, Holland EF 1995 A randomised comparison over 8 months of 100 micrograms and 200 micrograms twice-weekly doses of transdermal oestradiol in the treatment of premenstrual syndrome. BJOG: an International Journal of Obstetrics and Gynaecology 102: 475–484.

Steinberg S, Annable L, Young S, Liyanage N 1999 A placebo controlled trial of L-tryptophan in premenstrual dysphoria. Biological Psychiatry 45: 313–320.

Steiner M, Brown E, Trzepacz P et al 2003 Fluoxetine improves functional work capacity in women with premenstrual dysphoric disorder. Archives of Women's Mental Health 6: 71–77.

Steiner M, Pearlstein T, Cohen LS et al 2006 Expert guidelines for the treatment of severe PMS, PMDD, and comorbidities: the role of SSRIs. Journal of Women's Health 15: 57–69.

Studd J 2008 Suppression of cyclical ovarian function in the treatment of severe premenstrual syndrome/premenstrual dysphoric disorder. Gynaecology Forum 13: 15–17.

Sundblad C, Hedberg MA, Eriksson E 1993 Clomipramine administered during the luteal phase reduces the symptoms of premenstrual syndrome: a placebo-controlled trial. Neuropsychopharmacology 9: 133–145.

Thys-Jacobs S, Starkey P, Bernstein D, Tian J 1998 Calcium carbonate and the premenstrual syndrome: effects on premenstrual and menstrual symptoms. Premenstrual Syndrome Study Group. American Journal of Obstetrics and Gynecology 179: 444–452.

Wang M, Hammarback S, Lindhe BA, Backstrom T 1995 Treatment of premenstrual syndrome by spironolactone: a double-blind, placebo-controlled study. Acta Obstetricia et Gynecologica Scandinavica 74: 803–808.

Watson NR, Studd JW, Savvas M, Garnett T, Baber RJ 1989 Treatment of severe premenstrual syndrome with oestradiol patches and cyclical oral norethisterone. The Lancet 2: 730–732.

Williams AL, Cotter A, Sabina A et al 2005 The role of vitamin B-6 as treatment for depression: a systematic review. Family Practitioner 22: 532–537.

Wittchen HU, Becker E, Lieb R, Krause P 2002 Prevalence, incidence and stability of premenstrual dysphoric disorder in the community. Psychological Medicine 32: 119–132.

Wyatt K, Dimmock P, Jones P, Obhrai M, O'Brien S 2001 Efficacy of progesterone and progestogens in premenstrual syndrome: systematic review. BMJ (Clinical Research Ed.) 323: 776–781.

Wyatt KM, Dimmock PW, Ismail KM, Jones PW, O'Brien PM 2004 The effectiveness of GnRHa with and without add-back therapy in treating premenstrual syndrome: a meta analysis. BJOG: an International Journal of Obstetrics and Gynaecology 111: 585–593.

Yonkers KA, O'Brien PMS, Eriksson E 2008 Premenstrual syndrome. The Lancet 371 1200–1210.

CHAPTER 28

Menopause

Margaret Rees

Chapter Contents

INTRODUCTION	405
THE MENOPAUSE: DEFINITIONS AND PHYSIOLOGY	405
CHRONIC CONDITIONS AFFECTING POSTMENOPAUSAL HEALTH	407
THERAPEUTIC OPTIONS	408
WOMEN'S HEALTH INITIATIVE AND MILLION WOMEN STUDY	409
NON-OESTROGEN-BASED TREATMENTS FOR MENOPAUSAL SYMPTOMS	412
NON-OESTROGEN-BASED THERAPY FOR OSTEOPOROSIS	413
PREMATURE OVARIAN FAILURE	417
KEY POINTS	419

Introduction

Increasing life expectancy and decreasing fertility rates mean that the number of older people is projected to grow significantly worldwide. Between 1950 and 2007, the number of people aged 65 years and older increased from 5% to 7% (Population Reference Bureau 2007). Life expectancy at birth in women in countries such as the UK is currently 81 years (World Health Organization 2006). With the menopause occurring in the early 50s, managing the postreproductive period, which extends over several decades, is an increasingly important public health issue.

The Menopause: Definitions and Physiology

The menopause is the cessation of the menstrual cycle and is caused by ovarian failure. The term is derived from the Greek *menos* (month) and *pausos* (ending). The median age at which the menopause occurs is 52 years. The age at menopause is determined by genetic and environmental factors (Gold et al 2001, Elias et al 2003, Reynolds and Obermeyer 2005, Gosden et al 2007). Japanese race and ethnicity may be associated with later age of natural menopause, while Down's syndrome is associated with an early menopause. Growth restriction in late gestation, low weight gain in infancy, starvation in early childhood and smoking may be associated with an earlier menopause. However, being breast fed, higher childhood cognitive ability and increasing parity increase the age of menopause.

Definitions

Various definitions are in use and are detailed below (Utian 1999, World Health Organization 1994).

- *Menopause*: the permanent cessation of menstruation that results from loss of ovarian follicular activity. Natural menopause is recognized to have occurred after 12 consecutive months of amenorrhoea for which no other obvious pathological or physiological cause is present. Menopause occurs with the final menstrual period, and thus is only known with certainty 1 year after the event. No adequate biological marker exists.
- *Perimenopause*: includes the period beginning with the first clinical, biological and endocrinological features of the approaching menopause, such as vasomotor symptoms and menstrual irregularity, and ends 12 months after the final menstrual period.
- *Premenopause*: often used ambiguously to refer to the 1–2 years immediately before the menopause or to the whole of the reproductive period before the menopause. Currently, this term is recommended to be used in the latter sense, encompassing the entire reproductive period from menarche to the final menstrual period.
- *Postmenopause*: from the final menstrual period, regardless of whether the menopause was induced or spontaneous. Surgical menopause is timed precisely but, as noted above, the time of natural menopause

DOI: 10.1016/B978-0-7020-3120-5.00028-X

can only be determined retrospectively after a period of 12 months of spontaneous amenorrhoea.

- *Menopausal transition*: the period of time before the final menstrual period, when variability in the menstrual cycle is usually increased.
- *Climacteric*: the phase encompassing the transition from the reproductive state to the non-reproductive state. The menopause itself is a specific event that occurs during the climacteric, just as the menarche is a specific event that occurs during puberty.
- *Climacteric syndrome*: the climacteric is sometimes, but not always, associated with symptoms. When this occurs, the term 'climacteric syndrome' may be used.
- *Induced menopause*: the cessation of menstruation that follows surgical removal of both ovaries or iatrogenic ablation of ovarian function by chemotherapy, radiotherapy or treatment with gonadotrophin-releasing hormone (GnRH) analogues. In the absence of surgery, induced menopause may be permanent or temporary.

Ovarian function and the menopause

Each ovary receives a finite endowment of oocytes, the numbers of which are maximal at 20–28 weeks of intra-uterine life. From mid-gestation onwards, a logarithmic reduction in these germ cells occurs until, approximately 50 years later, the stock of oocytes is depleted (Burger et al 2008). The main steroid hormones produced by the ovary are oestradiol, progesterone and testosterone. Premenopausally, ovarian function is controlled by the two pituitary gonadotrophins: follicle-stimulating hormone (FSH) and luteinizing hormone (LH). FSH is controlled primarily by the pulsatile secretion of hypothalamic GnRH, and is modulated by the negative feedback of oestradiol and progesterone and the ovarian peptide inhibin B. The peptide is a major regulator of FSH secretion and a product of small antral follicles. Its levels respond to the early-follicular-phase increase and decrease in FSH. The age-related decrease in ovarian primordial follicle numbers, which is reflected in a decrease in the number of small antral follicles, leads to a decrease in inhibin B, which in turn leads to an increase in FSH. LH is principally controlled by GnRH, with negative feedback control from oestradiol and progesterone for most of the cycle; positive oestradiol feedback generates the mid-cycle surge in levels of LH that triggers ovulation.

The ovary gradually becomes less responsive to gonadotrophins several years before menstruation stops, oestrogen levels fall and gondatrophin levels rise. These changes in circulating levels of hormones frequently occur with ovulatory cycles. As ovarian unresponsiveness becomes more marked, cycles tend to become anovulatory, and complete failure of follicular development eventually occurs. Production of oestradiol is no longer sufficient to stimulate the endometrium, leading to amenorrhoea, with levels of FSH and LH now persistently elevated. Levels of FSH above 30 IU/l are generally considered to be in the postmenopausal range.

The ovaries are also an important source of testosterone, which is hydroxylated to dihydrotestosterone. Testosterone can also be aromatized to oestradiol. Precursor hormones, such as androstenedione and dehydroepiandrosterone (DHEA), are produced in the ovaries and the adrenals, and both possess a less potent androgenic effect than testosterone. By the time women reach their mid-40s, mean circulating levels of testosterone, androstenedione, DHEA and DHEA sulphate are approximately half those of women in their 20s. However, menopausal status does not affect levels of androgens in women aged 45–54 years, and the postmenopausal ovary seems to be an ongoing site of testosterone production.

Stages of reproductive ageing

A staging system that uses the final menstrual period as the anchor to describe reproductive ageing was proposed by the Stages of Reproductive Aging Workshop (STRAW) (Soules et al 2001) (Figure 28.1). This incorporates both menstrual cycle and hormonal parameters. Progression through the STRAW stages is associated with elevations in serum FSH, LH and oestradiol, and decreases in luteal-phase progesterone.

Figure 28.1 The STRAW reproductive staging system. FSH, follicle-stimulating hormone.
Soules MR, Sherman S, Parrott E, et al. Executive summary: Stages of Reproductive Aging Workshop (STRAW). Fertil Steril 2001;76:874–8.

Final Menstrual Period

Stages:	-5	-4	-3	-2	-1	0	+1	+2
Terminology:	Reproductive			Menopausal transition			Postmenopause	
	Early	Peak	Late	Early	Late*		Early*	Late
				Perimenopause				
Duration of stage:	Variable			Variable		ⓐ 1yr	ⓑ 4yrs	Until demise
Menstrual cycles:	Variable to regular	Regular		Variable cycle length (>7 days different from normal)	≥2 skipped cycles and an interval of amenorrhea (≥60 days)	Amenorrhea x 12 months	None	
Endocrine:	Normal FSH		↑FSH	↑FSH			↑FSH	

*Stages most likely to be characterized by vasomotor symptoms

Menopause symptoms

Menopause symptoms include hot flushes and night sweats, depression, tiredness and sexual problems. Symptom reporting varies between cultures (Melby et al 2005). Approximately 70% of women in Western cultures will experience vasomotor symptoms, such as hot flushes and night sweats. However, Japanese women have fewer menopausal complaints than their North American counterparts. Furthermore, rural Mayan women living in the Yucatan, Mexico do not report either hot flushes or night sweats.

Vasomotor symptoms

Flushes are episodes of inappropriate heat loss mediated by cutaneous vasodilation over the upper trunk. Sympathetic nervous control of blood flow in the skin is impaired in women with menopausal flushes, in whom reflex constriction to an ice stimulus cannot be elicited. More recently, serotonin and its receptors in the central nervous system have been implicated. Hot flushes and night sweats may begin before periods stop, and their prevalence is highest in the first year after the final menstrual period. Although they are usually present for less than 5 years, some women will continue to flush beyond the age of 60 years. Although women with a higher level of education seem to have fewer symptoms, evidence about the effect of exercise is conflicting (Daley et al 2007). Current smoking and high body mass index (BMI) may also predispose a woman to more severe or frequent hot flushes (Whiteman et al 2003).

Psychological symptoms

Psychological symptoms include depressed mood, anxiety, irritability, mood swings, lethargy and lack of energy. Transition to menopause confers a higher risk for development of depression, and multiple risk factors such as previous psychological problems and current life stresses appear to increase risk (Frey et al 2008).

Sexual dysfunction

Although women may stay sexually active until their eight or ninth decades of life, sexual problems are common. It has been estimated that they affect approximately one in two women. Interest in sex declines in both sexes with increasing age, and this change is more pronounced in women. The term 'female sexual dysfunction' is now used. An international classification system was elaborated by the International Consensus Development Conference on Female Sexual Dysfunction (Table 28.1) (Basson et al 2000). The most prevalent sexual problems among women are low desire (43%), difficulty with vaginal lubrication (39%) and inability to climax (34%) (Lindau et al 2007).

Chronic Conditions Affecting Postmenopausal Health

These include cardiovascular disease (CVD), osteoporosis, dementia and urinary incontinence.

Table 28.1 Consensus classification system

Classification	Definition
I Sexual desire disorders	
A Hypoactive sexual desire disorder	The persistent or recurrent deficiency (or absence) of sexual fantasies/thoughts and/or desire for, or receptivity to, sexual activity, which causes personal distress
B Sexual aversion disorder	The persistent or recurrent phobic aversion and avoidance of sexual contact with a sexual partner, which causes personal distress
II Sexual arousal disorders	The persistent or recurrent inability to attain or maintain sufficient sexual excitement, causing personal distress, which may be expressed as a lack of subjective excitement, or genital (lubrication/swelling) or other somatic responses
III Orgasmic disorder	The persistent or recurrent difficulty, delay in or absence of attaining orgasm after sufficient sexual stimulation and arousal, which causes personal distress
IV Sexual pain disorders	
A Dyspareunia	The recurrent or persistent genital pain associated with sexual intercourse
B Vaginismus	The recurrent or persistent involuntary spasm of the musculature of the outer third of the vagina, which interferes with vaginal penetration and causes personal distress
C Non-coital sexual pain disorders	Recurrent or persistent genital pain induced by non-coital sexual stimulation

Adapted from Basson R, Berman J, Burnett A, et al. Report of the international consensus development conference on female sexual dysfunction: definitions and classifications. J Urol 2000;163:888-93.
Each of the categories above is subtyped on the basis of the medical history, physical examination and laboratory tests as: (A) lifelong vs acquired; (B) generalized vs situational; or (C) aetiology (organic, psychogenic, mixed or unknown).

Cardiovascular disease

Worldwide, CVD is the leading cause of death and disability in both sexes. It is the major cause of death in women, accounting for one-third of all deaths. As CVD increases in prevalence with age, and as women live longer than men, more women than men die from CVD each year in many countries. Coronary heart disease (CHD) and stroke are the primary clinical endpoints of CVD. In the UK, approximately half (48%) of all deaths from CVD are from CHD and more than one-quarter (28%) are from stroke. Approximately one in six women die from CHD.

Osteoporosis

Osteoporosis affects one in three women. Osteoporosis is defined in a National Institute of Health Consensus State-

Table 28.2 Definitions of osteoporosis according to the World Health Organization

Description	Definition
Normal	BMD value between −1 SD and +1 SD of the young adult mean (T-score −1 to +1)
Osteopenia	BMD reduced between −1 and −2.5 SD from the young adult mean (T-score −1 to −2.5)
Osteoporosis	BMD reduced by equal to or more than −2.5 SD from the young adult mean (T score −2.5 or lower)

BMD, bone mineral density; SD, standard deviation.

ment as 'a skeletal disorder characterized by compromised bone strength predisposing to an increased risk of fracture'. Bone strength reflects the integration of two main features: bone density and bone quality. Bone density is expressed as grams of mineral per area or volume. Bone quality refers to architecture, turnover, damage accumulation (e.g. microfractures) and mineralization. The main clinical manifestations of osteoporosis are fractures of the hip, vertebrae and wrist (Colles' fractures). They have an enormous impact on quality of life, result in significant economic burden and, particularly in the case of hip fractures, are associated with considerable excess mortality. In the year after a hip fracture, mortality is approximately 30%. Approximately 50% of patients who survive a hip fracture have permanent disability and fail to regain their previous level of independence. The number of hip fractures worldwide due to osteoporosis is expected to rise three-fold by the middle of the next century, from 1.7 million in 1990 to 6.3 million by 2050.

Definitions of osteoporosis according to the World Health Organization

The World Health Organization's definitions are based on measurement of bone mineral density (BMD) (Table 28.2). Severe osteoporosis is defined as the presence of a fragility or minimal trauma fracture and low BMD (T-score less than −2.5). The T-score is the number of standard deviations by which the bone in question differs from the young normal mean. Although BMD is a major contributor to risk, other factors, including age, BMI and falls, play a part in determining whether a person will get a fracture. The FRAX tool has been developed by the World Health Organization to evaluate fracture risk (Kanis et al 2008). It is based on individual patient models that integrate the risks associated with clinical risk factors as well as femoral neck BMD. The clinical risk factors comprise BMI (as a continuous variable), a prior history of fracture, a parental history of hip fracture, use of oral glucocorticoids, rheumatoid arthritis and other secondary causes of osteoporosis, current smoking and alcohol intake of 3 or more units/day. The FRAX algorithms give the 10-year probability of hip and other major osteoporotic fractures.

Dementia and cognitive decline

Worldwide, approximately 25 million people have dementia, with 4.6 million new cases of dementia every year (one new case every 7 seconds). It has been estimated that the number of people affected will double every 20 years to 81.1 million by 2040. Dementia is a clinical term used to describe a condition in which there is impairment of cognitive faculties, including loss of memory, language, thinking and judgement, which cause significant difficulties in functioning. A wide variety of disorders can cause dementia; the most common are Alzheimer's disease, vascular dementia and dementia with Lewy bodies.

Dementia causes significant distress to patients, their carers and families, and has an enormous impact on society. While most people with dementia live in the community, they are likely to require residential or nursing home care in the long term.

Urogenital atrophy and urinary incontinence

The lower urinary and genital tracts have a common embryological origin and are approximated closely in adult women. Oestrogen and progesterone receptors are present in the vagina, urethra, bladder and pelvic floor musculature. Urogenital atrophy is common, affecting approximately 25% of women even if they are taking systemic oestrogen replacement. A lack of oestrogen results in the vaginal epithelium becoming thinner, losing its rugae, and becoming pale or erythematous with fine petechial haemorrhages. Vaginal and cervical secretions also decrease, leading to reduced lubrication. The resulting symptoms include dyspareunia, itching, burning and dryness which can coexist with urinary symptoms.

Urinary incontinence affects millions of women throughout the world. It affects the quality of life of women of all ages and poses a large financial burden on society. The population-based prevalence of urinary incontinence in the USA has been estimated to be 45% (Melville et al 2005). Prevalence increased with age, from 28% for women aged 30–39 years to 55% for women aged 80–90 years. Eighteen percent of respondents reported severe urinary incontinence. The prevalence of severe urinary incontinence also increased notably with age, from 8% for women aged 30–39 years to 33% for women aged 80–90 years. Other surveys have reported similar findings.

Therapeutic Options

Oestrogen-based hormone replacement therapy

A wide variety of oestrogen-based preparations are available worldwide, which feature different strengths, combinations and routes of administration (Clinical Knowledge Summaries 2009). Various designations are used: hormone replacement therapy (HRT), hormone therapy, oestrogen therapy, and oestrogen and progestogen therapy for combined preparations (sequential or continuous combined).

Table 28.3 Minimum bone-sparing doses of oestrogen

Oestrogen	Dose
Oestradiol oral	1–2 mg
Oestradiol patch	25–50 µg
Oestradiol gel	1–5 g*
Oestradiol implant	50 mg every 6 months
Conjugated equine oestrogens	0.3–0.625 mg daily

*Depends on preparation.

HRT consists of an oestrogen, and a progestogen is added in non-hysterectomized women. Progestogens are given cyclically or continuously with the oestrogen.

Oestrogens

Two types of oestrogen are available: natural and synthetic. Natural oestrogens include oestradiol, oestrone and oestriol. Conjugated equine oestrogens contain approximately 50–65% oestrone sulphate, and the remainder consists of equine oestrogens, mainly equilin sulphate. These are also classified as 'natural'. The generally accepted minimum bone-sparing doses of oestrogen are listed in Table 28.3, although increasing evidence shows that even lower doses may be effective. Synthetic oestrogens, such as ethinyl oestradiol used in the combined oral contraceptive pill, are generally considered to be unsuitable for HRT because of their greater metabolic impact, apart for treating young women with premature ovarian failure (POF).

Different routes of administration are employed: oral, transdermal (patches and gels), subcutaneous (implants) and vaginal. The vaginal route is used to treat urogenital symptoms. Vaginal therapies include oestradiol by tablet or ring, or oestriol by cream or pessary. Conjugated equine oestrogen cream is also available but this is well absorbed from the vagina and can cause endometrial stimulation. Systemic absorption with oestradiol vaginal tablets or ring is low, and hormone levels remain within the postmenopausal range. Thus, if the recommended topical oestradiol and oestriol preparations are used, there is no need to add a progestogen for endometrial protection. However, if conjugated equine oestrogens are used on a long-term basis, a progestogen should also be given. Vaginal oestrogens can also be used with systemic oestrogens.

Progestogens

The progestogens used in HRT are almost all synthetic, are structurally different to progesterone and are derived from plant sources. Currently, most are given orally, although norethisterone and levonorgestrel are available in transdermal patches combined with oestradiol, and levonorgestrel can be delivered directly to the uterus. Progesterone itself is available either orally or as a vaginal gel, but availability varies worldwide.

Androgens

Testosterone may be given as patches or as subcutaneous implants to improve libido, but this is not successful in all women, as other factors, such as marital problems, may be involved. Testosterone patches have the advantage of an easily reversible delivery system, as implants cannot be removed easily.

Bioidentical hormones

In some countries, 'natural' or 'bioidentical' hormones are used as an alternative approach. In the USA, the Food and Drug Administration is concerned with the claims for safety, effectiveness and superiority of preparations that are made in compounding pharmacies.

Tibolone

Tibolone is classified as HRT in the UK British National Formulary. Tibolone is a synthetic steroid compound that is itself inert, but, on absorption, is converted *in vivo* to metabolites with oestrogenic, progestogenic and androgenic actions. Tibolone is used in postmenopausal women who wish to have amenorrhoea. It is used to treat vasomotor, psychological and libido problems, and the daily dose is 2.5 mg. Tibolone conserves bone mass and reduces the risk of vertebral and non-vertebral fracture.

Hysterectomized women

In general, hysterectomized women should be given oestrogen alone and have no need for a progestogen. However, in women who have had a subtotal hysterectomy, there may be concern about a remnant of endometrium in the cervical stump. If this is suspected to be the case, the presence or absence of bleeding induced by monthly sequential HRT may be a useful diagnostic test before giving oestrogen alone.

Non-hysterectomized women

Progestogens are added to oestrogens to reduce the increased risk of endometrial hyperplasia and carcinoma that is associated with unopposed oestrogen. Progestogen can be given 'sequentially' for 10–14 days every 4 weeks, for 14 days every 13 weeks, or every day. The first schedule leads to monthly bleeds, the second leads to bleeds every 3 months, and the last aims to achieve amenorrhoea. Progestogen must be given to women who have undergone endometrial ablative techniques or radiotherapy for gynaecological cancer, as it cannot be assumed that all of the endometrium has been destroyed.

Women's Health Initiative and Million Women Study

Publication of the results of the US Women's Health Initiative (WHI) and UK Million Women Study (MWS) since 2002 has led to considerable uncertainties regarding the use of oestrogen-based HRT (Writing Group for the Women's Health Initiative Investigators 2002, Million Women Study Collaborators 2003, Women's Health Initiative Steering Committee 2004). Several publications have questioned the design, analysis and conclusions of both these studies (Shapiro 2007). For example, in the WHI, women in their 70s were given HRT for the first time, which does not reflect usual clinical practice. In the MWS, it was not easy to control for differences between attendees and non-attendees of the National Health Service Breast Screening Programme and between attendees who agreed or declined to participate in the study. Both studies were undertaken in women aged 50 years and over, and their findings cannot be extrapolated to younger women such as those with premature menopause in their 20s and 30s.

The design of the studies will be described, together with the benefits, risks and uncertainties about oestrogen use in clinical practice.

Women's Health Initiative

The WHI is a large complex series of studies designed in the early 1990s with follow-up until 2010 of strategies for the primary prevention and control of some of the most common causes of morbidity and mortality among healthy post-menopausal women aged 50–79 years. It consisted of a randomized-controlled trial and an observational study. The randomized trial considered not only HRT but also calcium and vitamin D supplementation and a low-fat diet (Box 28.1). If eligible, women could choose to enrol in one, two or all three components of the randomized trial. The randomized trial involved 68,132 women (mean age 63 years): conjugated equine oestrogens (0.625 mg) alone (n = 10,739 hysterectomized women), conjugated equine oestrogens (0.625 mg) in combination with medroxyprogesterone acetate (2.5 mg) (n = 16,608 non-hysterectomized women), low-fat diet (n = 48,835), and calcium and vitamin D supplementation (n = 36,282). Women screened for the clinical trial who were ineligible or unwilling to participate in the controlled trial (n = 93,676) were recruited into an observational study that assessed new risk indicators and biomarkers for disease.

Million Women Study

The observational MWS examined different HRT regimens, excluding vaginal preparations, in women aged 50–64 years

---

(mean age 57 years) attending the National Health Service Breast Screening Programme in the UK. In total, 1,084,110 women were recruited between 1996 and 2001; approximately half of these women had ever used HRT. The average duration of follow-up was 2.6 years.

Benefits, risks and uncertainties of oestrogen-based hormone replacement therapy

Benefits

Vasomotor symptoms

There is good evidence from randomized placebo-controlled studies, including the WHI, that oestrogen is effective for the treatment of hot flushes, and improvement is usually noted within 4 weeks (Simon and Snabes 2007). It is more effective than non-hormonal preparations such as clonidine and selective serotonin reuptake inhibitors (see below). The most common indication for HRT prescription is relief of vasomotor symptoms, and it is often used for less than 5 years.

Urogenital symptoms and sexuality

Urogenital symptoms respond well to oestrogen administered either topically or systemically. In contrast to vasomotor symptoms, improvement may take several months. Recurrent urinary tract infections may be prevented by vaginal but not oral oestrogen replacement (Perrotta et al 2008). Topical oestrogens may have a weak effect on urinary urge incontinence, but no improvement of stress incontinence. Long-term treatment is often required as symptoms can recur when therapy is stopped. Sexuality may be improved with oestrogen alone, but testosterone may also be required, especially in young oophorectomized women.

Osteoporosis

There is evidence from randomized-controlled trials (including the WHI) that HRT reduces the risk of both spine and hip fractures, as well as other osteoporotic fractures (Writing Group on Osteoporosis for the British Menopause Society Council 2007). Most epidemiological studies suggest that continuous and lifelong use is required for fracture prevention. However, there is now some evidence that a few years of treatment with HRT around the time of the menopause may have a long-term effect on fracture reduction. While alternatives to HRT use are available for the prevention and treatment of osteoporosis in elderly women (see below), oestrogen still remains the best option, particularly in younger (<60 years) and/or symptomatic women. Few data are available on the efficacy of alternatives such as bisphosphonates in women with POF.

Colorectal cancer

Results from the combined arm, but not the oestrogen-alone arm, of the WHI concur with observational studies that HRT reduces the risk of colorectal cancer. However, little is known regarding the risk of colorectal cancer when treatment is stopped. There is no information about HRT in high-risk populations, and current data do not allow prevention as a recommendation.

> **Box 28.1** Interventions evaluated by the Women's Health Initiative
>
> - HRT (unopposed and combined): hypothesized to reduce the risk of CHD and other cardiovascular diseases and, secondarily, to reduce the risk of hip and other fractures, with increased risk of breast cancer being studied as a possible adverse outcome.
> - Low-fat eating pattern: hypothesized to prevent breast cancer and colorectal cancer and, secondarily, to prevent CHD.
> - Supplementation with calcium and vitamin D: hypothesized to prevent hip fractures and, secondarily, to prevent other fractures and colorectal cancer.

Risks

Breast cancer

HRT appears to confer a similar degree of risk as that associated with late natural menopause (2.3% compared with 2.8% per year, respectively). There is no increased risk in HRT users with a premature menopause (Ewertz et al 2005).

The WHI found that:

- combined HRT but not oestrogen-alone HRT increased the risk of breast cancer;
- the risk of breast cancer in the oestrogen-alone arm was lower than that in the placebo group. The risk of breast cancer was significantly reduced in women with no previous exposure at study entry; and
- in the combined arm, there was evidence of a duration effect with an increase in risk starting 3 years after randomization, but only in women who had used HRT before entering the study.

The MWS found:

- an increased risk with all HRT regimens (both unopposed oestrogen and combined HRT);
- the greatest degree of risk was with combined HRT and this was not influenced by route of administration; and
- different oestrogens or progestogens did not appear to alter risk, nor did the pattern of progestogen administration (i.e. cyclical or continuous).

The higher risk estimates reported in the MWS compared with the randomized WHI, especially for the oestrogen-alone arm which found a reduced risk, probably reflect the different designs of the studies.

The increased risk of breast cancer with combined HRT compared with oestrogen alone has to be balanced against the reduction in risk of endometrial cancer provided by progestogen addition. The increased risk of breast cancer with long-term use seems to be limited to lean women (BMI <25 kg/m^2) in most studies. Also, the increased risk of breast cancer with HRT is low and similar to the risk conferred by obesity, being tall, nulliparity or late age at first full-term pregnancy, and is lower than that conferred by certain inherited genetic mutations or mantle radiotherapy (American Cancer Society 2009).

Also, the risk of breast cancer decreases after stopping HRT, and after 5 years, the risk of breast cancer is no greater than that in women who have never been exposed to HRT. The incidence of breast cancer has been decreasing in the USA and this has been attributed to declining HRT use since publication of the WHI. However, the decrease started in 1998, predating the first WHI publication (Li and Daling 2007).

Endometrial cancer

Unopposed systemic oestrogen replacement therapy increases the risk of endometrial cancer (Weiderpass et al 1999). Sequential progestogen addition, especially when continued for more than 5 years, does not eliminate this risk completely. This has also been found with monthly- and long-cycle HRT. No increased risk of endometrial cancer has been found with continuous combined regimens. Very low doses of systemic oestrogen (0.014 µg/day transdermal oestradiol patch) do not seem to stimulate the endometrium, but studies are limited and require confirmation (Simon and Snabes 2007).

Furthermore, oral treatment, but not vaginal treatment, with low-potency formulations (such as oestriol) increases the relative risk of endometrial neoplasia. The increased risk of endometrial cancer with systemic oestrogen is lower than that found in obese or diabetic women.

Venous thromboembolism

HRT increases the risk of venous thromboembolism (VTE) two-fold, with the highest risk occurring in the first year of use (Canonico et al 2008). However, the absolute risk is small, being 1.7 per 1000 in women over 50 years of age not taking HRT. Advancing age, obesity and an underlying thrombophilia such as factor V Leiden increase the risk of VTE significantly. Randomized trial data strongly suggest that women who have previously suffered a VTE have an increased risk of recurrence in the first year of HRT use. However, transdermal HRT may be associated with a lower risk, even in women with a thrombophilia.

Gallbladder disease

The WHI confirmed the observation of the Heart and Estrogen/Progestin Replacement Study published in 1998 that oral HRT increases the risk of gallbladder disease. However, the MWS found that transdermal therapy confers a lower risk than oral therapy (Liu et al 2008). Gallbladder disease increases with ageing and with obesity, and HRT users may have silent pre-existing disease.

Uncertainties

CVD (CHD and stroke)

The role of HRT in both primary and secondary prevention remains uncertain.

CHD primary prevention

Until the late 1990s, oestrogen was thought to protect against CHD (Rees and Stevenson 2008). Many cohort studies showed that HRT was associated with a 40–50% reduction in the incidence of CHD. The effects were the same for both oestrogen alone and combined HRT. However, the WHI did not confirm these observational studies. It has become apparent that there are differences between regimens, and that the timing of HRT initiation may be crucial. The WHI found an early, albeit transient, increase in coronary events in the combined arm but not the oestrogen-alone arm. In the WHI oestrogen-alone arm, there was a non-significant reduction in CHD, which was most marked in younger women (50–59 years). With regard to timing, women in the WHI who started combined HRT within 10 years of the menopause had a lower risk of CHD than women who started later (Rossouw et al 2007). Combining the two HRT arms found that women who initiated hormone therapy closer to the menopause tended to have reduced CHD risk compared with the increase in CHD risk among women who initiated hormone therapy more distant from the menopause. While transdermal oestrogen has less of an effect on coagulation than oral therapy due to avoidance of the first liver pass, it is uncertain whether transdermal delivery is better than oral delivery in terms of CHD risk.

CHD secondary prevention

Although angiographic and cohort studies such as the Nurses' Health Study suggested a role of oestrogen in the secondary prevention of CHD, this has not been confirmed in randomized-controlled trials with both oral and trans-dermal therapy (Grodstein et al 2006).

Stroke

Interpretation of observational studies on HRT and stroke is difficult because of differences in design and failure to distinguish between ischaemic and haemorrhagic stroke (Billeci et al 2008). Both arms of the WHI found an increase in ischaemic stroke but not haemorrhagic stroke. However, age or time since menopause did not affect the risk of stroke. In addition, in women who have experienced a previous ischaemic stroke, oestrogen replacement does not reduce mortality or recurrence as evidenced by randomized-controlled trials.

Dementia and cognition

While oestrogen may delay or reduce the risk of Alzheimer's disease, it does not seem to improve established disease (Barber et al 2005). It is unclear if there is a critical age or duration of treatment for exposure to oestrogen to have an effect on prevention, but there may be a window of opportunity in the early postmenopause when the pathological processes that lead to Alzheimer's disease are starting and when HRT may have a preventive effect. The WHI found an increased risk of dementia and lower cognitive function in HRT users, but only in women aged over 75 and 65 years, respectively.

Ovarian cancer

Most data pertain to replacement with oestrogen alone with increasing risk in the very long term (>10 years) (Beral et al 2007). However, with continuous combined therapy, this increase does not seem apparent.

Quality of life

While some studies have shown improvement in both symptomatic and asymptomatic women, others have not. This area is difficult to evaluate because of the different questionnaires used, as well as varying levels of menopausal symptomatology.

Tibolone

Tibolone is effective in the treatment of menopausal symptoms. It conserves bone mass and reduces the risk of vertebral and non-vertebral fractures, particularly in patients who have already had a vertebral fracture. It also reduces the risk of invasive breast cancer and colon cancer. However, it does not significantly reduce the risk of hip fracture and it increases the risk of stroke (Cummings et al 2008). The LIFT study also showed that tibolone does not have a deleterious effect on CHD or VTE (Cummings et al 2008). The MWS showed an increased risk of breast cancer and endometrial cancer. However, the increased risk of endometrial cancer has not been confirmed in randomized-controlled trials (Archer et al 2007). The LIBERATE randomized trial of tibolone in breast cancer survivors was discontinued early in 2007 as there was an excess of breast cancer recurrences in the group of women randomized to receive tibolone (Kenemans et al 2009).

Non-Oestrogen-Based Treatments for Menopausal Symptoms

Non-oestrogen-based treatments are used to treat hot flushes and symptoms of urogenital atrophy. These can be either hormonal or non-hormonal (Writing Group for the British Menopause Society Council 2008).

Hormonal

Progestogens

Progestogens such as 5 mg/day norethisterone or 40 mg/day megestrol acetate can reduce hot flushes and night sweats. However, the risk of VTE may be increased with the doses of progestogen used. Also, safety with regard to the breast is uncertain. Availability of megestrol acetate 40 mg tablets varies worldwide.

Non-hormonal

Clonidine

Clonidine is a centrally acting α-adrenoceptor agonist that was originally developed for the treatment of hypertension. While it may be of limited help in women with tamoxifen-induced hot flushes, the evidence for efficacy is conflicting. Side-effects include dry mouth, sedation, dizziness, nausea and nocturnal restlessness. The dose is 50–75 μg twice daily.

Selective serotonin reuptake inhibitors and serotonin and noradrenaline reuptake inhibitors

Fluoxetine, paroxetine, citalopram and venlafaxine have been found to be effective in several studies. However, most are short lasting (only a few weeks). The most convincing data are for venlafaxine [selective serotonin and noradrenaline reuptake inhibitor (SNRI)] at a dose of 37.5 mg twice daily. A randomized trial of a new SNRI, desvenlafaxine, has shown a 64% reduction in hot flushes at 12 weeks. Side-effects include gastrointestinal symptoms (nausea) and sexual dysfunction (delayed or absent orgasm). Some early evidence suggests that selective serotonin reuptake inhibitors may cause bone loss.

Gabapentin

Gabapentin is a γ-aminobutyric acid analogue used to treat epilepsy, neurogenic pain and migraine. It reduces hot flushes at a dose of 900 mg/day by approximately 50%. Side-effects include dry mouth, dizziness and drowsiness, which may improve with continued use.

Vitamin E

Although one study showed that vitamin E reduced hot flushes, the difference between the active and placebo groups was not significant.

Vaginal lubricants and moisturizers

Lubricants usually consist of a combination of protectants and thickening agents in a water-soluble base. They are usually used to relieve vaginal dryness during intercourse. They therefore do not provide a long-term solution. Lubricants must be applied frequently for more continuous relief, and require reapplication before intercourse. Moisturizers may contain a bioadhesive polycarbophil-based polymer, which attaches to mucin and epithelial cells on the vaginal wall and retains water. Moisturizers are promoted as providing long-term relief of vaginal dryness and need to be applied less frequently. Petroleum-based products and baby oil can compromise the integrity of condoms. This is important when condoms are used for contraception and/or to prevent sexually transmitted infections.

Non-Oestrogen-Based Therapy for Osteoporosis

A wide range of pharmacological and non-pharmacological interventions are available (Table 28.4) (Writing Group on Osteoporosis for the British Menopause Society Council 2007). There are very few data regarding long-term efficacy for reducing fractures (i.e. more than 10 years of treatment) and safety of combinations of therapy. Most of these therapies have been studied in elderly women (>60 years) who have osteoporosis or who are at increased risk of the disease. Little is known about their efficacy and safety in women with premature menopause and effects on the developing fetal skeleton. This is of importance because of the long (many years) half-life of bisphosphonates and strontium ranelate.

Pharmacological interventions

All pharmacological interventions except for parathyroid hormone and strontium ranelate act mainly by inhibiting bone resorption.

Bisphosphonates

Bisphosphonates are chemical analogues of naturally occurring pyrophosphates and are classified into two groups: non-nitrogen-containing bisphosphonates, such as etidronate; and nitrogen-containing bisphosphonates, such as alendronate, risedronate, ibandronate and zoledronic acid.

All bisphosphonates are absorbed poorly from the gastrointestinal tract and must be given on an empty stomach. Food or calcium-containing drinks inhibit absorption, which at best is only 5–10% of the administered dose. The principal side-effect of all bisphosphonates is irritation of the upper gastrointestinal tract. Symptoms resolve quickly after drug withdrawal and are reduced by using weekly or monthly dosing rather than daily dosing.

Alendronate, risedronate, etidronate and ibandronate are used in the prevention and treatment of osteoporosis. The indication for zoledronic acid is the treatment of osteoporosis in postmenopausal women at increased risk of fracture. Alendronate, risedronate and etidronate are also used in corticosteroid-induced osteoporosis.

The question of how long to prescribe a bisphosphonate has not been fully clarified because of concerns about 'frozen bone', with complete turning off of bone remodelling with long-term use and also development of osteonecrosis in the jaw. Of note, most reports about ostenecrosis refer to high-dose intravenous bisphosphonates used in the oncological setting rather than oral bisphosphonates for osteoporosis. There have been concerns regarding atrial fibrillation with bisphosphonates, but mainly with intravenous regimes, and the mechanism is uncertain.

Five years of treatment with a 2-year 'holiday' have been proposed for alendronate, but differences may exist with individual bisphosphonates. This may not be applicable to glucocorticoid-induced osteoporosis.

Alendronate reduces vertebral and non-vertebral fractures by 50% in randomized-controlled trials. The dose for prevention of osteoporosis is 5 mg/day or 35 mg once weekly, and the dose for treatment of established disease is 10 mg/day or 70 mg once weekly.

Risedronate reduces vertebral and non-vertebral fractures in randomized-controlled trials. The dose for treatment of established disease is 5 mg/day or 35 mg once weekly.

Ibandronate reduces vertebral but not non-vertebral fractures by 50% in randomized-controlled trials undertaken in postmenopausal women. The dose is 2.5 mg/day or 150 mg once monthly orally or 3 mg intravenously every 3 months.

Etidronate reduces the risk of vertebral but not non-vertebral fractures. It is given intermittently (400 mg on 14

Table 28.4 Interventions for the prevention and treatment of osteoporosis

	Spine	Hip
1. Bisphosphonates		
Etidronate	A	B
Alendronate	A	A
Risedronate	A	A
Ibandronate	A	ND
Zoledronic acid	A	A
2. Calcium and vitamin D	ND	A
3. Calcium	A	B
4. Calcitriol	A	ND
5. Calcitonin	A	B
6. Oestrogen	A	A
7. Raloxifene	A	ND
8. Strontium ranelate	A	A
9. Parathyroid hormone peptides	A	ND

ND, not demonstrated.
The levels of evidence for the various agents are:
A = meta-analysis of randomized-controlled trials (RCTs) or from at least one RCT/from at least one well-designed controlled study without randomization;
B = from at least one other type of well-designed quasi-experimental study or from well-designed non-experimental descriptive studies, e.g. comparative studies, correlation studies, case–control studies.

out of every 90 days) with 1250 mg calcium carbonate (which, when dissolved in water, provides 500 mg calcium as calcium citrate) during the remaining 76 days.

Zoledronic acid significantly reduces the risk of vertebral, hip and other fractures. It is administered intravenously (5 mg annually) and has been evaluated in the treatment of postmenopausal osteoporosis.

Strontium ranelate

Strontium is an alkaline earth element like calcium and is thus incorporated into the skeleton. It reduces the risk of vertebral and hip fractures. The dose is a 2 g sachet/day. It can cause diarrhoea but this resolves on stopping treatment. There appears to be a small increased risk (<1%) of VTE and nervous system disorders (headaches, seizures, memory loss and disturbance in consciousness), but data are limited. Strontium ranelate causes a clinically significant overestimation of BMD because of the high attenuation of X-rays by strontium atoms in bone as it has a higher atomic number than calcium.

Raloxifene

Raloxifene is a selective oestrogen receptor modulator (SERM). These compounds possess oestrogenic actions in certain tissues and antioestrogenic actions in others (Palacios 2007). Other SERMs such as bazedoxifene, arzoxifene, lasofoxifene and ospemifene are currently being evaluated.

Raloxifene reduces vertebral, but not non-vertebral, fractures by 30–50%, depending on the dose. The dose is 60 mg/day. It also reduces the risk of breast cancer to the same extent as tamoxifen. Side-effects include hot flushes and calf cramps. It was thought that it could be cardioprotective from its effects on surrogate markers such as lipids; however, the Raloxifene Use for the Heart study found that it did not reduce the risk of CHD and it increased the risk of fatal stroke and VTE.

Parathyroid hormone peptides

Recombinant 1–34 parathyroid hormone, given as a subcutaneous daily injection of 20 μg, reduces vertebral and non-vertebral fractures in postmenopausal women with osteoporosis. The full 1–84 parathyroid hormone peptide is given in the same way in a daily dose of 100 μg. They both reduce the risk of vertebral fractures but not hip fractures.

Calcitonin

Calcitonin can be given by subcutaneous or intramuscular injection or by nasal spray. An oral preparation is in development. Nasal calcitonin has also been shown to reduce new vertebral fractures in women with established osteoporosis. It may help with pain in the context of an acute vertebral fracture. It may also be helpful as adjunctive treatment after surgery for hip fracture.

Calcitriol

This is the active metabolite of vitamin D and facilitates the intestinal absorption of calcium. The potential dangers of hypercalcaemia and hypercalciuria mean that levels of calcium in serum and urine should be monitored closely. Studies of the effects of calcitriol on bone loss and fractures have produced conflicting results. As such, its use is limited.

Future developments

New treatments are focusing on inhibition of bone turnover (McClung 2007). Receptor activator of nuclear factor-κB ligand (RANKL) is a pivotal regulator of osteoclast activity that provides a new therapeutic target. Denosumab, a highly specific anti-RANKL antibody, reduces bone resorption. Pharmacokinetics of the antibody allow dosing by subcutaneous injection every 3 or 6 months.

Non-pharmacological interventions

Calcium and vitamin D

Provision of adequate dietary or supplemental calcium and vitamin D is an essential part of osteoporosis management, and is the placebo component of clinical trials of agents such as bisphosphonates. Most studies show that approximately 1.5 g elemental calcium is necessary to preserve bone health in women who are not taking HRT. However, the effects of calcium and vitamin D supplements, alone or in combination, on fracture are contradictory and may depend on the study population and compliance with therapy (Tang et al 2007, Lin and Lane 2008). For example, people in sheltered accommodation or residential care may be more frail, have lower dietary intakes of calcium and vitamin D, and are at higher risk of fracture than those living in the community.

Caution has been expressed about the use of supplements in women whose diet is already adequate. Increased risk of kidney stones and CVD has been reported.

Hip protectors

Hip protectors are used to reduce the impact of falling directly on the hip, but evidence of efficacy is conflicting in both community and institutional studies. A systematic review found no evidence of the effectiveness of hip protectors from studies in which randomization was by individual patient within an institution or those living in their own homes (Parker et al 2006).

Diet and exercise

Maintaining a good diet and regular exercise are essential for healthy ageing and reducing the risk of CVD, osteoporosis, urinary incontinence and dementia (Salerno-Kennedy and Rees 2007).

Dietary components

Diet consists of macronutrients and micronutrients. Macronutrients encompass carbohydrate, protein and fat. The World Health Organization recommends that 55–75% of energy input should come from carbohydrate, with less than 10% from free sugars. Emphasis should be placed on carbohydrate-rich foods (e.g. wholegrain breakfast cereals, grains, and breads and bakery products), which also provide fibre and a number of B vitamins.

Protein is an important nutrient for older women and should comprise 10–15% of total energy intake. Total fat intake should account for 15–30% of total energy intake, with saturated fats accounting for less than 10% and polyunsaturated fats for 6–10%. Although, in the past, the main message has been to limit the total amount of fat, particular types such as omega-3 fatty acids, found mainly in oily fish, are important to health.

Micronutrients include vitamins and minerals. Those that may be associated with deficiencies in postmenopausal women include vitamin B12, vitamin A, vitamin C, vitamin D, calcium and other trace minerals. Low intakes of iron, folate and vitamin B12 can cause anaemia as well as other problems such as neuropathies and dementia.

It has been suggested that antioxidant supplements may reduce mortality. However, a systematic review found that vitamin A, beta-carotene, and vitamin E supplements may increase mortality (Bjelakovic et al 2008). No detrimental effects were found with vitamin C or selenium. Of note, most trials in the systematic review investigated the effects of supplements administered at higher doses than those commonly found in a balanced diet, and some of the trials used doses above the recommended daily allowances. These trials should not deter women from consuming fruit and vegetables which contain other substances such as fibre and flavonoids.

Functional foods

A functional food may be defined as a food with health-promoting benefits and/or disease-preventing properties over and above its usual nutritional value (Rudkovska 2008). Functional foods are also known as 'nutraceuticals' or 'designer foods'. They encompass a broad range of products, ranging from foods generated around a particular functional ingredient (e.g. stanol-enriched margarines), through to staple everyday foods fortified with a nutrient that would not normally be present to any great extent (e.g. bread or breakfast cereals fortified with folic acid). Functional foods that show promise in postmenopausal health include probiotics, prebiotics, phytosterols and stanols, omega-3 fatty acids, flavonoids and fibre.

Isoflavones can also be considered as a functional food and are discussed in the section on complementary and alternative therapies. Synbiotics are a food or supplement product containing both probiotics and prebiotics. The name derives from a proposed synergism between probiotics and prebiotics.

Probiotics are live micro-organisms that, when administered in adequate amounts, confer a health benefit on the host. Currently, the best studied probiotics are different species of *Lactobacillus* or *Bifidobacterium*, and the yeast *Saccharomyces cerevisiae (boulardii)*. These can be combined in cereals, food bars, yoghurts and drinks. Various health benefits have been proposed. These include: regulation of immune function, prolongation of inflammatory bowel conditions, shortening the duration of infectious diarrhoea in infants, enhanced gastrointestinal tolerance to antibiotic therapy, and control of symptoms associated with lactose intolerance. They may also improve therapeutic outcome for women being treated for bacterial vaginosis, and reduce the severity of symptoms or the incidence of respiratory infections.

Prebiotics are non-digestible food ingredients such as inulin that beneficially affect the host by selectively stimulating the growth and/or activity of one or a limited number of bacteria in the colon. Thus, prebiotics are food for bacterial species that are considered beneficial for health and well-being.

Phytosterols and stanols reduce low-density-lipoprotein cholesterol by 10% and thus have the potential to reduce the risk of CHD by approximately 25%. Plant sterols and stanols reduce the absorption of cholesterol from the gut, and therefore reduce serum concentrations of cholesterol. They are incorporated into a variety of foods such as spreads, yogurts and drinks. However, studies with the endpoints of cardiovascular events are awaited.

Omega-3 fatty acids include the plant-derived α-linolenic acid (18:3n-3), and the fish-oil-derived eicosapentaenoic acid (20:5n-3) and docoshexaenoic acid (22:6n-3). Consumers of oily fish have a lower risk of CVD. Consumption of a diet rich in omega-3 fatty acids may also protect against dementia and Alzheimer's disease.

Flavonoids are a large family of polyphenolic compounds synthesized by plants. They are found in a wide variety of fruit and vegetables such as grapes, berries, apples, chocolate, teas, kale and hot peppers. Isoflavones are a subclass of flavonoids with oestrogenic activity. Epidemiological evidence suggests that flavonoids reduce the risk of CVD. This would explain the inverse relationship between the consumption of red wine and CVD mortality (the 'French paradox'). Animal and in-vitro studies suggest that flavonoids may have a role in preventing cancer and neurodegenerative disease.

Dietary fibre consists of plant substances that resist hydrolysis by digestive enzymes in the small bowel, and is an extremely complex group of substances. Fibre can be classified according to its solubility and fermentability by bacteria: a soluble fibre is readily fermentable by colonic bacteria, and an insoluble fibre is only slowly fermentable. Fibres may act in several ways, including through gel-forming effects in the stomach and small intestine, fermentation by colonic bacteria, a 'mop and sponge' effect and concomitant changes in other aspects of the diet. These actions lead to potentially beneficial effects in the gastrointestinal tract and systemically, such as lowering serum cholesterol and improving glycaemic control.

The importance of diet is such that the American Heart Association recommends that 'Women should consume a diet rich in fruits and vegetables; choose wholegrain, high-fibre foods; consume fish, especially oily fish, at least twice a week; limit intake of saturated fat to <10% of energy, and if possible to <7%, cholesterol to <300 mg/day, alcohol intake to no more than 1 drink per day, and sodium intake to <2.3 g/day (approximately 1 tsp salt). Consumption of trans-fatty acids should be as low as possible (e.g. <1% of energy)' (Mosca et al 2007).

Exercise

Regular physical activity reduces the risk of CHD, osteoporotic fractures and type 2 diabetes mellitus. Hot flushes, urinary incontinence, insomnia and depression may also be helped. A systematic review found that no conclusions regarding the effectiveness of exercise as a treatment for vasomotor menopausal symptoms could be made due to a lack of trials (Daley et al 2007). With regard to CVD, the Nurses Health Study found that low intensity exercise, such as walking, conferred the same benefit as vigorous exercise, and sedentary women who became active late in life reaped similar benefits as those who remained active throughout their life (Manson et al 2002). Exercise has a key role in the prevention and treatment of osteoporosis. A Cochrane review found that fast walking improved bone density effectively in the spine and the hip, whereas weight-bearing exercises were associated with increases in bone density of the spine but not the hip (Bonaiuti et al 2003).

Exercise regimens can be very helpful in the management of established osteoporosis, and represent a component of falls prevention programmes. Pelvic floor exercises are used commonly for stress incontinence. They are also used in the treatment of women with mixed incontinence, and less commonly for urge incontinence. Systematic reviews support the view that pelvic floor muscle training and bladder training should be included in first-line conservative management programmes for women with stress, urge or mixed urinary incontinence (Shamliyan et al 2008).

Complementary and alternative medicine

Many women use complementary and alternative medicine in the belief that they are safer and 'more natural', especially with concerns regarding the safety of oestrogen-based HRT after publication of the WHI and the MWS. However, evidence from randomized trials for complementary and alternative medicine that improves menopausal symptoms or has the same benefits as HRT is poor (Nedrow et al 2006). Very little well-designed research has been undertaken. The range of approaches used includes botanicals, homeopathy, DHEA, transdermal progesterone creams and mechanical methods (e.g. acupuncture, magnetism).

Botanicals

The evidence from clinical trials on the benefit of botanicals on menopausal symptoms is limited and conflicting. Studies may use different products which are not chemically consistent, making comparison difficult. Also, the stability of individual chemicals may vary and may depend on the type of packaging. Herbs may contain many chemical compounds, the individual and combined effects of which are unknown.

A major concern is use without consulting a health professional, leading to interaction with standard pharmacopeia with potentially fatal consequences. Severe adverse reactions, including renal and liver failure and cancer, have been reported. Concern exists regarding the quality control of production. Some have been found to be contaminated or to contain unlabelled ingredients such as conventional medicines (steroids) or banned substances. While a European Union Directive on traditional herbal medicinal products was implemented in October 2005 in the UK, this will not cover preparations bought by women outside Europe.

Herbal remedies need to be used with caution in women with a contraindication to oestrogen, as some botanicals have oestrogenic properties (e.g. soy, red clover, ginseng). Thus, they should not be used by women with a hormone-dependent condition such as breast cancer or endometriosis. They may interact with selective oestrogen receptor modulators (e.g. tamoxifen, raloxifene) or aromatase inhibitors (e.g. anastrozole, letrozole). Other consequences of herb–drug interactions include bleeding when combined with warfarin or aspirin; hypertension, coma and mild serotonin syndrome when combined with serotonin reuptake inhibitors; and reduced efficacy of antiepileptics and oral contraceptives.

Phytoestrogens are plant substances that have effects similar to those of oestrogens. Preparations vary from enriched foods, such as bread or drinks (e.g. soy milk), to tablets containing plant extracts. The most important groups are the isoflavones and lignans. The major isoflavones are genistein and daidzein. The major lignans are enterolactone and enterodiol. The role of phytoestrogens has stimulated considerable interest, as people from populations that consume a diet high in isoflavones, such as the Japanese, seem to have lower rates of menopausal vasomotor symptoms; CVD; osteoporosis; and breast, colon, endometrial and ovarian cancers. PHYTOS, ISOHEART and PHYTOPREVENT are European Union studies examining the role of phytoestrogens in osteoporosis, heart disease and cancer. With regard to menopausal symptoms, the evidence from randomized placebo-controlled trials in Western populations is conflicting for soy and derivatives of red clover (Lethaby et al 2007). Similarly, debate also surrounds the effects on lipoproteins, endothelial function, blood pressure, cognition and the endometrium. Endometrial hyperplasia has been reported in soy users. Further well-designed randomized trials are needed to determine the role and safety of phytoestrogen supplements in perimenopausal and postmenopausal women and those who have survived cancer.

Actaea racemosa (black cohosh) is a herbaceous perennial plant native to North America, used widely to alleviate menopausal symptoms. The results from placebo-controlled trials are conflicting. There is no consensus regarding whether non-oestrogenic or oestrogenic actions are involved in the mechanisms by which it relieves hot flushes. Little is known regarding long-term safety, and liver toxicity has been reported.

Evening primrose oil is rich in γ-linolenic acid. One small placebo-controlled, randomized trial showed it to be ineffective for the treatment of hot flushes.

Angelica sinensis (dong quai) is a perennial plant native to south-west China. It was not found to be superior to placebo in a randomized trial, but may be effective when combined with other herbs. Interaction with warfarin and photosensitization have been reported.

Ginkgo biloba (gingko) is widely used but there is little evidence that it improves menopausal symptoms.

Panax ginseng (ginseng) is a perennial herb native to Korea and China. It does not appear to be effective for hot flushes. Case reports have associated ginseng with postmenopausal bleeding and mastalgia. Interactions have been observed with warfarin, phenelzine and alcohol.

Piper methysticum (kava kava) may be an effective symptomatic treatment for anxiety, but the data about menopausal symptoms are conflicting. Concern about liver damage has led regulatory authorities to suspend or withdraw kava kava.

Wild yam cream, dong quai, St John's wort, *Agnus castus* (Chasteberry), liquorice root and Valerian root are also popular, but no good evidence shows that they have any effect on menopausal symptoms. Claims have been made that steroids (e.g. diosgenin) in yams (*Dioscorea villosa*) can be converted to progesterone in the body, but this is biochemically impossible in humans.

Homeopathy

Samuel Hahnemann (1755–1843), a German physician and scientist, was the first to enunciate the central tenets of homeopathic philosophy. He believed in a 'vital force' that animates and regulates the human form and directs growth, healing and repair. He postulated that a homoeopathic remedy acted through the vital force. He then put forward the principle of 'similars', which claims that patients with particular signs and symptoms can be cured if given a drug that produces the same signs and symptoms in a healthy individual. He then pursued the concepts of minimum dose and succession (the curative action of certain preparations seemed to be stronger at some of the lower doses, particularly when shaken vigorously). The underlying mechanisms of homeopathy are scientifically unclear. While limited data are encouraging, further research is needed.

Dehydroepiandrosterone

DHEA is a steroid secreted by the adrenal cortex. Blood levels of DHEA decrease dramatically with age. This led to suggestions that the effects of ageing can be counteracted by DHEA 'replacement therapy'. In the USA, it is classed as a food supplement. No evidence shows that DHEA has any effect on hot flushes (Raven and Hinson 2007). Some studies have shown benefits on the skeleton, cognition, well-being, libido and vagina. The safety of long-term use is, as yet, unknown.

Progesterone transdermal creams

Progesterone is available in gels and creams. One licensed gel is available in Europe; however, it is indicated for local use on the breast but not for systemic therapy. A vaginal gel for endometrial protection has been studied. Progesterone creams have been advocated for the treatment of menopausal symptoms and skeletal protection. However, at present, insufficient published data show that transdermal progesterone has a positive effect on vasomotor symptoms or the skeleton. There is also no consistent evidence that transdermal progesterone creams can prevent mitotic activity or induce secretory change in an oestrogen-primed endometrium. Thus, it should not be used for endometrial protection in women using systemic oestrogen.

Mechanical

These approaches include acupuncture, reflexology, magnetism acupressure, Alexander technique, Ayurveda, osteopathy and Reiki. Data with regard to the menopause are scant, and well-designed adequately powered studies are required.

Premature Ovarian Failure

POF is responsible for 4–18% of cases of secondary amenorrhoea and 10–28% of cases of primary amenorrhoea. It is estimated to affect 1% of women under 40 years of age and 0.1% of those under 30 years of age. Although the terms 'POF' and 'premature menopause' are often used interchangeably, there is debate regarding which term is best. Some women with POF will have oligomenorrhoea, and have persisting sporadic ovarian activity and can become spontaneously pregnant (Nelson et al 2005). In contrast, menopause implies permanent cessation of ovarian activity and menstruation, and infertility. With regard to an age cut-off, premature menopause should ideally be defined as menopause that occurs at an age more than two standard deviations below the mean estimated for the reference population. In the absence of reliable estimates of age of natural menopause in developing countries, the age of 40 years is often used as an arbitrary limit below which the menopause is said to be premature. In the developed world, however, an age of 45 years should be taken as the cut-off point.

Aetiology

Primary premature ovarian failure

Primary POF can occur at any age, even in teenagers. It can present as primary or secondary amenorrhoea or oligomenorrhoea. In the great majority of cases, no cause is found. Traditionally, ovarian failure has been associated with one of two scenarios:

- a deficient number of primordial follicles from the onset of menarche or accelerated follicle atresia; or
- follicles resistant to stimulation by gonadotrophins.

In the absence of a non-invasive test to differentiate between follicular depletion or dysfunction, the only alternative is ovarian biopsy. The validity of single biopsies has been questioned, with pregnancies occurring despite histological lack of follicles in the biopsy material.

The causes are detailed in Box 28.2.

Box 28.2 Causes of premature ovarian failure

Primary

Chromosome abnormalities

FSH receptor gene polymorphism and inhibin B mutation

Enzyme deficiencies

Autoimmune disease

Secondary

Chemotherapy and radiotherapy

Bilateral oophorectomy or surgical menopause

Hysterectomy without oophorectomy

Infection

Chromosome abnormalities

Two intact X chromosomes are required for normal follicular development. A critical region on the X-chromosome (*POF1*), which ranges from Xq13 to Xq26, which relates to normal ovarian function has been identified, as has a second gene of paternal origin (*POF2*), which is located at Xq13.3–q21.1. Idiopathic POF can be familial or sporadic, and the familial pattern of inheritance is compatible with X-linked with incomplete penetrance or an autosomal-dominant mode of inheritance. Complete absence of one X chromosome (45XO) in Turner's syndrome results in ovarian dysgenesis and primary ovarian failure. Familial POF has been linked with fragile X permutations. Women with Down's syndrome (Trisomy 21) also have an early menopause. Blepharophimosis/ptosis/epicanthus (BEPS) syndrome is a rare autosomal-dominant condition that leads to congenital abnormalities of the eye. In BEPS I, eyelid malformation cosegregates with POF and has been mapped to chromosome 3q.17.

FSH receptor gene polymorphism and inhibin B mutation

Gonadotrophin resistance can lead to the clinical features of POF, and this has been shown in a cohort of Finnish families. This is a very rare cause. In addition, a mutation in the inhibin gene has been identified. These patients experienced ovarian failure at an early age, often before the second decade of life.

Enzyme deficiencies

A number of enzyme deficiencies have been found to be associated with an increased risk of POF. The most common is galactosaemia. Other enzyme abnormalities associated with POF include deficiencies of 17α-hydroxylase, 17–20 desmolase and cholesterol desmolase.

Autoimmune disease

POF is frequently associated with autoimmune disorders, particularly hypothyroidism (25%), Addison's disease (3%) and diabetes mellitus (2.5%). Other coexisting conditions may include Crohn's disease, vitiligo, pernicious anaemia, systemic lupus erythematosus and rheumatoid arthritis.

Secondary premature ovarian failure

Secondary POF is becoming more important as survival after the treatment of malignancy continues to improve. Techniques to conserve ovarian tissue or oocytes before cancer therapy should help with maintenance of fertility. The causes of secondary POF are detailed below.

Chemotherapy and radiotherapy

The likelihood of ovarian failure after chemotherapy or radiotherapy depends on the agent used, dosage levels, interval between treatments and, particularly, the age of the patient, which probably reflects the age-related progressive natural decline in the oocyte pool. The prepubertal ovary is relatively resistant to the effects of chemotherapeutic alkylating agents. The use of GnRH analogues to suppress ovarian activity in order to mimic prepubertal protection is, as yet, not supported by randomized-controlled trials.

Bilateral oophorectomy or surgical menopause

This results in an immediate menopause which may be intensely symptomatic. The implications of this procedure require detailed discussion with the patient in view of the increased morbidity and mortality in those who cannot, or will not, take oestrogen replacement. This area is of increasing importance in those having prophylactic oophorectomy such as BRCA1 gene carriers.

Hysterectomy without oophorectomy/uterine artery embolization

Both procedures can diminish ovarian reserve and lead to ovarian failure. Diagnosis may be difficult in women where the procedures have made them amenorrhoeic.

Infection

Tuberculosis and mumps are infections that have been implicated most commonly. Malaria, varicella and shigella infections may also cause POF.

Consequences of premature ovarian failure

Women with untreated premature menopause are at increased risk of developing osteoporosis, CVD, cognitive decline, dementia and Parkinsonism, but at lower risk of breast malignancy (Shuster et al 2008). Mean life expectancy in women with menopause before the age of 40 years is 2 years shorter than that in women with menopause after the age of 55 years.

Management

Patients must be provided with adequate information about the condition, its implications on long-term health, use of oestrogen replacement and fertility (Pitkin et al 2007). In those who have not had an oophorectomy, the return of spontaneous ovarian activity and the possibility of spontaneous pregnancy must be explained. While pregnancy may be welcomed by some, this is not true for all women. Women who do not wish to have children need to consider using an effective form of contraception.

Hormone replacement therapy

Oestrogen replacement therapy is the mainstay of treatment for women with POF and is recommended until the average age of natural menopause. This view is endorsed by regulatory bodies. This does not increase the risk of breast cancer to a level greater than that found in normally menstruating women, and women with POF do not need to start mammographic screening early (Ewertz et al 2005). HRT or the combined contraceptive pill may be used. The choice of which to use largely depends on the patient's age, with the former being more likely to be acceptable to women in their 30s and 40s and the latter being more likely to be acceptable to women in their 20s. There is no evidence to support the efficacy or safety of the use of non-oestrogen-based treatments, such as bisphosphonates, strontium ranelate or raloxifene, in these women. Some patients report reduced libido or sexual function despite apparently adequate doses of oestrogen replacement, especially oophorectomized women, and they may need testosterone addition.

Fertility and contraception

It is important to ascertain whether or not the woman wishes to have children. While women with premature menopause have traditionally been considered to be infertile, the lifetime chance of spontaneous conception in women with karyotypically normal POF has been estimated at 5–15%. A number of ovarian reserve tests (ORTs) have been designed to determine oocyte reserve and quality (Broekmans et al 2006). These include early-follicular-phase blood values of FSH, oestradiol, inhibin B and anti-Müllerian hormone, antral follicle count, ovarian volume, ovarian blood flow, the clomiphene citrate challenge test, the exogenous FSH

ORT and the gonadotrophin agonist stimulation test. A systematic review of ORTs has shown that they only have modest-to-poor predictive properties.

Donor oocyte in-vitro fertilization (IVF) is the treatment of choice for women with primary and secondary POF (Lee et al 2006). In women having chemotherapy or radiotherapy, IVF with embryo freezing prior to treatment currently offers the highest likelihood of a future pregnancy should they experience POF as a result of their treatment. Recent advances in oocyte preservation have improved livebirth rates following freezing of mature eggs. It is still less successful than embryo freezing. Ovulation induction risks delaying treatment. Cryopreservation of ovarian tissue is still largely experimental, although pregnancies have been reported. This technique would be an option for prepubertal girls in whom ovulation induction is not possible.

KEY POINTS

1. The menopause is the permanent cessation of menstruation resulting from loss of ovarian follicular activity, and occurs in the early 50s. Worldwide, the elderly population is increasing, with women forming the majority. Thus, chronic diseases affecting postreproductive health spanning over several decades are major public health issues. The major issues affecting postmenopausal women are vasomotor symptoms, psychological disorders, urogenital atrophy, sexual dysfunction, osteoporosis, CVD, dementia and urinary incontinence.

2. HRT relieves menopausal symptoms and conserves bone mass. Women with POF need HRT until their early 50s. Up to 60 years of age, the benefits of HRT outweigh the risks and mortality is reduced. There are no effective alternatives to oestrogen with long-term safety data for vasomotor symptoms. The role of oestrogen in CVD, dementia and quality of life is currently unclear.

3. With regard to the risks of HRT, the main areas of concern are breast and endometrial cancer and VTE. The increase in risk of

breast cancer is approximately equivalent to the increase in relative risk of breast cancer associated with each year the menopause is delayed after 50 years of age. In non-hysterectomized women, progestogen is added to oestrogen to reduce the risk of endometrial cancer. Oral oestrogen, but not transdermal oestrogen, increases the risk of VTE.

4. Non-hormonal treatments for osteoporosis, such as bisphosphonates and strontium ranelate, have mainly been studied in women over 60 years of age at increased risk of the disease. Data for younger women are limited, and these treatments should not be used in women contemplating pregnancy since the effects on the developing fetal skeleton and the long-term consequences are unknown.

5. The evidence that complementary and alternative therapies are effective is poor, and there are concerns about safety and interactions with standard pharmacopoeia.

References

American Cancer Society 2009. Breast Cancer Facts and Figures 2007–2008. Available at: http://www.cancer.org/downloads/STT/BCFF-Final.pdf

Archer DF, Hendrix S, Ferenczy A et al 2007 Tibolone histology of the endometrium and breast endpoints study: design of the trial and endometrial histology at baseline in postmenopausal women. Fertility and Sterility 88: 866–878.

Barber B, Daley S, O'Brien J 2005 Dementia. In: Keith L, Rees M, Mander T (eds) Menopause, Postmenopause and Ageing. RSM Press, London, pp 20–34.

Basson R, Berman J, Burnett A et al 2000 Report of the international consensus development conference on female sexual dysfunction: definitions and classifications. Journal of Urology 163: 888–893.

Beral V; Million Women Study Collaborators, Bull D, Green J, Reeves G 2007 Ovarian

cancer and hormone replacement therapy in the Million Women Study. The Lancet 369: 1703–1710.

Billeci AM, Paciaroni M, Caso V, Agnelli G 2008 Hormone replacement therapy and stroke. Current Vascular Pharmacology 6: 112–123.

Bjelakovic G, Nikolova D, Gluud L, Simonetti R, Gluud C 2008 Antioxidant supplements for prevention of mortality in healthy participants and patients with various diseases. Cochrane Database of Systematic Reviews 2: CD007176.

Bonaiuti D, Shea B, Iovine R et al 2003 Exercise for preventing and treating osteoporosis in postmenopausal women. Cochrane Database of Systematic Reviews 4: CD0000333.

Burger HG, Hale GE, Dennerstein L, Robertson DM 2008 Cycle and hormone changes during perimenopause: the key role of

ovarian function. Menopause 15: 603–612.

Canonico M, Plu-Bureau G, Lowe GD, Scarabin PY 2008 Hormone replacement therapy and risk of venous thromboembolism in postmenopausal women: systematic review and meta-analysis. BMJ (Clinical Research Ed.) 336: 1227–1231.

Clinical Knowledge Summaries. Clinical topic. Menopause. Available at: http://cks.library.nhs.uk/menopause.

Cummings SR, Ettinger B, Delmas PD et al 2008 The effects of tibolone in older postmenopausal women. New England Journal of Medicine 359: 697–708.

Daley A, MacArthur C, Mutrie N, Stokes-Lampard H 2007 Exercise for vasomotor menopausal symptoms. Cochrane Database of Systematic Reviews 4: CD006108.

Elias SG, van Noord PA, Peeters PH et al 2003 Caloric restriction reduces age at menopause: the effect of the 1944–1945 Dutch famine. Menopause 10: 399–405.

Ewertz M, Mellemkjaer L, Poulsen AH et al 2005 Hormone use for menopausal symptoms and risk of breast cancer. A Danish cohort study. Br J Cancer 92: 1293–1297.

Frey BN, Lord C, Soares CN 2008 Depression during menopausal transition: a review of treatment strategies and pathophysiological correlates. Menopause International 14: 123–128.

Gold EB, Bromberger J, Crawford S et al 2001 Factors associated with age at natural menopause in a multiethnic sample of midlife women. American Journal of Epidemiology 153: 865–874.

Gosden RG, Treloar SA, Martin NG et al 2007 Prevalence of premature ovarian failure in monozygotic and dizygotic twins. Human Reproduction 22: 610–615.

Grodstein F, Manron JE, Stampfer MJ 2006 Hormone therapy and coronary heart disease: the role of time since menopause and age at hormone initiation. Journal of Women's Health 15: 35–44.

Kanis JA, Johnell O, Oden A, Johansson H, McCloskey E 2008 FRAX and the assessment of fracture probability in men and women from the UK. Osteoporosis International 19: 385–397.

Kenemans P, Bundred NJ, Foidart JM et al 2009 Safety and efficacy of tibolone in breast-cancer patients with vasomotor symptoms: a double-blind, randomised, non-inferiority trial. Lancet Oncology 10(2): 135–146.

Lee SJ, Schover LR, Partridge AH et al 2006 American Society of Clinical Oncology recommendations on fertility preservation in cancer patients. Journal of Clinical Oncology 24: 2917–2931.

Lethaby AE, Brown J, Marjoribanks J, Kronenberg F, Roberts H, Eden J 2007 Phytoestrogens for vasomotor menopausal symptoms. Cochrane Database of Systematic Reviews 4: CD001395.

Li CI, Daling JR 2007 Changes in breast cancer incidence rates in the United States by histologic subtype and race/ethnicity, 1995 to 2004. Cancer Epidemiology, Biomarkers and Prevention 16: 2773–2780.

Lin JT, Lane JM 2008 Nonpharmacologic management of osteoporosis to minimize fracture risk. Nature Clinical Practice Rheumatology 4: 20–25.

Lindau ST, Schumm LP, Laumann EO, Levinson W, O'Muircheartaigh CA, Waite LJ 2007 A study of sexuality and health among older adults in the United States. New England Journal of Medicine 357: 762–774.

Liu B, Beral V, Balkwill A et al 2008 Gallbladder disease and use of transdermal versus oral hormone replacement therapy in postmenopausal women: prospective cohort study. BMJ (Clinical Research Ed.) 337: a386.

Manson JE, Greenland P, LaCroiz AZ et al 2002 Walking compared with vigorous exercise for the prevention of cardiovascular events in women. New England Journal of Medicine 347: 716–725.

McClung M 2007 Role of RANKL inhibition in osteoporosis. Arthritis Research and Therapy 9 (Suppl 1): S3.

Melby MK, Lock M, Kaufert P 2005 Culture and symptom reporting at menopause. Human Reproduction Update 11: 495–512.

Melville JL, Katon W, Delaney K, Newton K 2005 Urinary incontinence in US women: a population-based study. Archives of Internal Medicine 165: 537–542.

Million Women Study Collaborators 2003 Breast cancer and hormone-replacement therapy in the Million Women Study. The Lancet 362: 419–427.

Mosca L, Banka CL, Benjamin EJ et al 2007 Evidence-based guidelines for cardiovascular disease prevention in women: 2007 update. Circulation 115: 1481–1501.

Nedrow A, Miller J, Walker M, Nygren P, Huffman LH, Nelson HD 2006 Complementary and alternative therapies for the management of menopause-related symptoms: a systematic evidence review. Archives of Internal Medicine 166: 1453–1465.

Nelson LM, Covington SN, Rebar RW 2005 An update: spontaneous premature ovarian failure is not an early menopause. Fertility and Sterility 83: 1327–1332.

Palacios S 2007 The future of the new selective estrogen receptor modulators. Menopause International 13: 27–34.

Parker MJ, Gillespie WJ, Gillespie LD 2006 Effectiveness of hip protectors for preventing hip fractures in elderly people: systematic review. BMJ (Clinical Research Ed.) 332: 571–574.

Perrotta C, Aznar M, Mejia R, Albert X, Ng CW 2008 Oestrogens for preventing recurrent urinary tract infection in postmenopausal women. Cochrane Database of Systematic Reviews 2: CD005131.

Pitkin J, Rees MC, Gray S et al 2007 Management of premature menopause. Menopause International 13: 44–45.

Population Reference Bureau 2007 World Population Data Sheet. Available at: http://www.prb.org/pdf07/07WPDS_Eng.pdf.

Raven PW, Hinson JP 2007 Dehydroepiandrosterone (DHEA) and the menopause: an update. Menopause International 13: 75–78.

Rees M, Stevenson J 2008 Primary prevention of coronary heart disease in women. Menopause International 14: 40–45.

Reynolds RF, Obermeyer CM 2005 Age at natural menopause in Spain and the United States: results from the DAMES project. American Journal of Human Biology 17: 331–340.

Rossouw JE, Prentice RL, Manson JE et al 2007 Postmenopausal hormone therapy and risk of cardiovascular disease by age and years since menopause. JAMA: the Journal of the American Medical Association 297: 1465–1477.

Rudkovska I 2008 Functional foods for cardiovascular disease in women. Menopause International 14: 63–69.

Salerno-Kennedy R, Rees M 2007 Diet. In: Rees M, Keith LG (eds) Medical Problems in Women Over 70, when Normative Treatment Plans do not Apply. Informa Healthcare, Abingdon, pp 199–215.

Shamliyan TA, Kane RL, Wyman J, Wilt TJ 2008 Systematic review: randomized, controlled trials of nonsurgical treatments for urinary incontinence in women. Annals of Internal Medicine 148: 459–473.

Shapiro S 2007 Recent epidemiological evidence relevant to the clinical management of the menopause. Climacteric 10 (Suppl 2): 2–15.

Shuster L, Gostout BS, Grossardt BR, Rocca WA 2008 Prophylactic oophorectomy in pre-menopausal women and long term health — a review. Menopause International 14: 111–116.

Simon JA, Snabes MC 2007 Menopausal hormone therapy for vasomotor symptoms: balancing the risks and benefits with ultra-low doses of estrogen. Expert Opinion on Investigational Drugs 16: 2005–2020.

Soules MR, Sherman S, Parrott E et al 2001 Executive summary: Stages of Reproductive Aging Workshop (STRAW). Fertility and Sterility 76: 874–878.

Tang BM, Eslick GD, Nowson C, Smith C, Bensoussan A 2007 Use of calcium or calcium in combination with vitamin D supplementation to prevent fractures and bone loss in people aged 50 years and older: a meta-analysis. The Lancet 370: 657–666.

Utian WH 1999 The International Menopause Society menopause-related terminology definitions. Climacteric 2: 284–286.

Weiderpass E, Adami HO, Baron JA et al 1999 Risk of endometrial cancer following estrogen replacement with and without progestins. Journal of the National Cancer Institute 91: 1131–1137.

Whiteman MK, Staropoli CA, Langenberg PW, McCarter RJ, Kjerulff KH, Flaws JA 2003 Smoking, body mass, and hot flashes in midlife women. Obstetrics and Gynecology 101: 264–272.

Women's Health Initiative Steering Committee 2004 Effects of conjugated equine estrogen in postmenopausal women with hysterectomy: the Women's Health Initiative randomized controlled trial. JAMA: the Journal of the American Medical Association 291: 1701–1712.

World Health Organization 1994 Scientific Group on Research on the Menopause in the 1990s. WHO Technical Report Series 866. WHO, Geneva.

World Health Organization 2006 Life Tables for WHO Member States. Available at: http://www.who.int/whosis/database/life_tables/life_tables.cfm.

Writing Group on Osteoporosis for the British Menopause Society Council 2007 Prevention and treatment of osteoporosis in women. Menopause International 13: 178–181.

Writing Group for the Women's Health Initiative Investigators 2002 Risks and benefits of estrogen plus progestin in healthy postmenopausal women: principal results from the Women's Health Initiative randomized controlled trial. JAMA: the Journal of the American Medical Association 288: 321–333.

Writing Group for the British Menopause Society Council 2008 Non-estrogen-based treatments for menopausal symptoms. Menopause International 14: 88–90.

CHAPTER 29

Fertility control

Catherine A. Schünmann and Anna F. Glasier

Chapter Contents

INTRODUCTION	422	ABORTION	433
CONTRACEPTION	423	KEY POINTS	437
STERILIZATION	430		

Introduction

Almost everyone will use contraception at some time during their reproductive lives. While contraceptive provision in the UK is largely the role of primary care, obstetricians and gynaecologists should be familiar with all currently available methods and aware of their advantages and disadvantages. They should be able to advise women of the method most appropriate for their individual circumstances, and to deal with the side-effects which lead to referral to a gynaecologist.

Over the last 40 years, there has been a significant increase in the use of contraception worldwide. In 2008, it was estimated that up to 62% of all married women of reproductive age or their partners were using contraception. However, the prevalence of contraceptive use remains low in many less developed countries; only 13% of couples use contraception in some African countries. It has been estimated that some 120 million women in developing/restructuring countries who do not wish to become pregnant are unable, for a variety of reasons, to use contraception (Ross and Winfrey 2002).

In Great Britain, 88% of sexually active women who wish to avoid pregnancy use a method of contraception (Office for National Statistics 2007/8). Usage is lower among adolescents (56%), women over 45 years of age (69%) and less well-educated women (65%).

Worldwide, between 8 and 30 million unplanned pregnancies per year are the result of contraceptive failure. Despite the apparently high prevalence of contraceptive use in the UK, a substantial proportion of births (25.8%) occur among women who were ambivalent regarding pregnancy intention (Lakha and Glasier 2006). Moreover, large numbers of unplanned pregnancies are terminated. Scotland has an abortion rate which is one of the lowest in countries in which abortion is legal, yet for every six babies born, one pregnancy is terminated. Although abortion is a safe procedure in Western countries, it has been estimated that of the annual figure of 42 million abortions performed around the world, 20 million are unsafe and some 67,000 women die as a result (Facts on Induced Abortion Worldwide, Guttmacher Institute 2009).

The type of contraceptive method used varies around the world. The intrauterine device (IUD) is the most common method in China, while the vast majority of couples in Japan, where the combined oral contraceptive (COC) pill has only been licensed very recently, use the condom. In some of the less developed parts of the world, breast feeding is still the most important method of birth spacing. The prevalence of method use in the UK is shown in Table 29.1; condoms and the pill still prevail. In the UK in the 21st Century, the cost-effectiveness of long-acting reversible contraception (LARC) which relies little, if at all, on compliance for effectiveness has been recognized (National Institute for Health and Clinical Effectiveness 2005). In 2009, the Governments of both Scotland and England launched social marketing campaigns to increase the uptake of LARC. Increasing acceptability of LARC and, particularly, of intrauterine methods of contraception appears to be associated with a dramatic decline in female sterilization in the UK. Increased uptake of contraceptive implants and injections may reduce unintended pregnancies among sexually active teenagers.

Evidence-based recommendations on which individuals can safely use each contraceptive method were first published by the World Health Organization (WHO) in 1996, and are updated at 4-yearly intervals [WHO Medical Eligibilty Criteria (WHOMEC)]. This guidance has been further modified specifically for use in the UK by the Clinical Effectiveness Unit (CEU) of the Faculty of Sexual and Reproductive Healthcare (FSRH) of the Royal College of Obstetricians and Gynaecologists (RCOG), and is available in hard copy and online as the UK Medical Eligibility Criteria (UKMEC). Contraceptive methods are categorized according to their balance of risk and benefit in the presence of certain medical and lifestyle conditions (Table 29.2). Health professionals prescribing contraceptive methods are also directed to the National Institute for Health and Clinical Excellence guidelines on LARC published in 2005.

DOI: 10.1016/B978-0-7020-3120-5.00029-1

Table 29.1 Use of contraceptive methods in the UK

Method	%
Combined hormonal contraceptives	18
Progestogen-only pill	6
Implant/injectable	5
Intrauterine device/system	7
Barrier methods	24
Vasectomy	10
Female sterilization	7
Natural family planning	2
Withdrawal	4
No method	25[a]

Source: Office for National Statistics 2007/8 Omnibus Survey Report No. 37. Contraception and Sexual Health. Office for National Statistics, London. Available at: www.ons.gov.uk and www.statistics.gov.uk.
[a]Subcategories: 'not having sex', 14; 'pregnant or trying to conceive', 3; 'menopausal/infertile/otherwise sterile', 6; 'doesn't like/doesn't use contraception', 1.

Table 29.2 UK Medical Eligibility Criteria for Contraceptive Use (RCOG Press, London, 2009)

Classification categories

1. A condition for which there is no restriction for the use of the contraceptive method
2. A condition where the advantages of using the method generally outweigh the theoretical or proven risks
3. A condition where the theoretical or proven risks usually outweigh the advantages of using the method
4. A condition which represents an unacceptable health risk if the contraceptive method is used

Contraception

Combined hormonal contraceptives

The CHC was approved for use in Britain in 1961. In recent years, different modes of delivery have been developed, with injectable, transdermal and vaginal methods now available in some countries. Although unlikely to be substantially different from the oral preparation in terms of efficacy and safety, they do provide a wider choice of administration which may help to offset the effects of erratic pill taking.

Combined hormonal contraceptives (CHCs) contain oestrogen, usually ethinyl oestradiol, and a synthetic progesterone (progestogen). Most modern pills contain 20–35 μg ethinyl oestradiol with either a second-generation progestogen [norethisterone, levonorgestrel (LNG) or ethynodiol diacetate] or a so-called third-generation progestogen (gestodene, desogestrel or norgestimate). The newest progestogen, drospirenone, has antiandrogenic and antimineralocorticoid properties. The 20 μg pills are as effective as the 30 μg pills but, not surprisingly, are associated with poorer cycle control (Akerlund et al 1993).

The traditional CHC regimen involves taking a tablet for 21 days with a 7-day break, thus inducing a withdrawal bleed in order to mimic the body's 'natural' pattern. Variations on this theme include the everyday formulations containing dummy pills so that users do not have to remember to stop and start (common in the USA), 84-day preparations reducing the number of expected withdrawal bleeds from 13 to four per annum, and a continuous version aimed at banishing bleeding altogether. Injectable CHCs are administered intramuscularly every 28 days, with 70% of women experiencing a withdrawal bleed 18–22 days after injection. They are in common use in Latin America. Despite the plethora of transdermal hormone replacement options, there is only one contraceptive patch available. The patch is applied weekly for 3 weeks prior to a patch-free week, and may help to reduce nausea in susceptible individuals (Audet et al 2001). The latest addition to the CHC family is a vaginal ring, 54 mm in diameter and 4 mm in cross-section. It is made of a soft, ethylene–vinyl-acetate copolymer, lasts for 21 days with a 7-day break, and appears to confer more favourable cycle control than other preparations. These longer-acting CHCs may improve compliance.

Combined pills are available in monophasic, biphasic and triphasic preparations. Phasic pills were developed in order to reduce the total dose of progestogen and, by simulating the fluctuating pattern of steroid concentrations in the normal ovarian cycle, in an attempt to produce better cycle control. There is no good evidence that cycle control is superior to that achieved by monophasic pills.

Mode of action

CHCs work primarily by inhibiting ovulation. Exogenous oestrogen inhibits the secretion of follicle-stimulating hormone, while progestogens inhibit the development of the luteinizing hormone (LH) surge. The CHC also alters cervical mucus, rendering it hostile to the passage of sperm, and also causes endometrial atrophy.

CHCs are highly effective (Table 29.3). The failure rates associated with all forms of contraception depend on the inherent efficacy of the method, but also on the potential for incorrect or inconsistent use. Since ovulation is inhibited in most women who use the combined pill, failure rates of the method itself are low. However, as inhibition of ovulation depends on reliable pill taking, the overall failure rate of the COC, which includes user failure, is higher.

Contraindications

In an analysis of 25 years of follow-up of 46,000 women who took part in the Royal College of General Practitioners' (RCGP) Oral Contraceptive Study comparing 517,519 years of pill use with 335,998 years of never-use, the risk of death from all causes was similar in ever-users and never-users of oral contraception (Beral et al 1999). Among current and recent users (within 10 years), the relative risk (RR) of death from ovarian cancer was significantly decreased (RR 0.2), while the risks of dying from cervical cancer (RR 2.5) and cerebrovascular disease (RR 1.9) were increased.

Absolute contraindications to CHC use are listed in Box 29.1. They include either a past history of, or existing,

Table 29.3 Pregnancy rates for birth control methods (for 1 year of use)

Method	Typical use rate of pregnancy (%)	Lowest expected rate of pregnancy (%)
Sterilization		
Male sterilization	0.15	0.1
Female sterilization	0.5	0.5
Hormonal methods		
Implant (Implanon)	0.05	0.05
Depo-provera injection	3	0.3
Combined pill (oestrogen/progestogen)	8	0.3
Mini pill (progestogen only)	8	0.3
Evra patch	8	0.3
NuvaRing	8	0.3
IUD/IUS		
Copper T	0.8	0.6
LNG-IUS	0.1	0.1
Barrier methods		
Male condom[a]	15	23
Diaphragm[b]	16	6
Female condom	21	5
Spermicide (gel, pessary)	29	15
Sponge		
Parous women	32	20
Nulliparous women	16	9
Emergency contraception		
Levonelle	15	
Copper IUD	<5	
Natural methods		
Withdrawal	27	4
Natural family planning (calendar, temperature, mucus)	25	3
No method	85	85

Adapted from Trussel J 2007 Contraceptive efficacy. In: Hatcher RA, Trussel J, Nelson A, Kates W, Stewart F, Kowal D (eds) Contraceptive Technology, 19th edn. Ardent Media, New York.

IUD, intrauterine device; IUS, intrauterine system; LNG, levonorgestrel.

This table provides estimates of the percentage of women likely to become pregnant while using a particular contraceptive method for 1 year. These estimates are based on a variety of studies.

'Typical use' rate means that the method was not always used correctly, was not used with every act of sexual intercourse or was used correctly but failed.

'Lowest expected' rates mean that the method failed despite being used correctly with every act of sexual intercourse.

[a]Used without spermicide.

[b]Used with spermicide.

Box 29.1 Absolute contraindications to the COC pill

Arterial or venous thrombosis
Ischaemic heart disease including myopathy
Most valvular heart disease
Past cerebral haemorrhage
Hypercholesterolaemia
Conditions predisposing to thrombosis, e.g. polycythaemia
Migraine
Pulmonary hypertension
Active liver disease
Porphyria
History of a serious condition affected by sex steroids, e.g. trophoblastic disease

cardiovascular disease, migraine and most liver diseases. Women often describe headaches as migraine. CHCs are contraindicated in migraine which is or may be associated with transient cerebral ischaemia. A recent study designed to investigate the risk between migraine and stroke in young women demonstrated a significant increase in the risk of ischaemic, but not haemorrhagic, stroke in women with a personal history of migraine both with and without aura (classic and simple). Concomitant use of the CHC further increased this risk (Chang et al 1999). It is important therefore to take a clear and detailed history before refusing to prescribe a CHC because the woman has an occasional migraine.

Relative contraindications to CHC use include the following:

- factors which increase the risk of cardiovascular disease or venous thrombosis, such as obesity, smoking, hypertension and family history;
- sex-steroid-dependent conditions, including cancer;
- factors which adversely affect liver function; and
- factors which predispose to arterial wall disease.

Comprehensive discussions and lists of contraindications are available in most textbooks of contraception, and WHOMEC and UKMEC.

Side-effects of combined oral contraception

Debate continues over the increased risk of cardiovascular events in women taking CHCs. Until reliable data are available for non-oral routes of administration, it is sensible to assume that similar risks apply to all methods. Cardiovascular disease is very rare in women of reproductive age. Venous thromboembolism (VTE) is the most common cardiovascular complication of CHC use. Oestrogen and progestogen are both metabolized by the liver and alter the metabolism of most substances, including carbohydrates and lipids. Oestrogens also alter coagulation factors. A reduction in antithrombin III and alteration in platelet function increase the risk of VTE by up to seven-fold. A clear history of thromboembolism is a contraindication to CHCs. A possible history or a very strong family history are indications for investigating haemostasis, particularly circulating concentrations of antithrombin III and the factor

V Leiden thrombogenic mutation. Population screening for inherited thrombophilias is not currently considered to be cost-effective.

Studies in the mid-1990s appeared to show a differential risk of VTE between the second- and third-generation progestogens, the latter being associated with double the risk of the former (Bloemenkamp et al 1995, Jick et al 1995, WHO 1995, Spitzer et al 1996). These findings prompted the UK Committee on Safety of Medicines to advise women at risk of thrombosis to avoid third-generation progestogens. Although well designed, criticisms of these studies include prescriber bias (whereby women with cardiovascular risk factors and new users would be more likely to be prescribed a newer brand) and attrition bias (existing users susceptible to VTE would be less likely to be using older brands). Latterly, the 2005 EURAS study, funded and designed as a postmarketing cohort study to demonstrate the safety of the combined ethinylestradiol/drospirenone pill, found an increased incidence of VTE across the categories (including pregnant women and non-pregnant, non-CHC-using women) with no difference between progestogen used (Dinger et al 2007). Whilst the large numbers in the study (58,674 women and 142,475 women-years) lend strength to its findings, data from the pharmaceutical industry must always be viewed with some reservation. Of additional interest was the reported three-fold increase in risk for women with a body mass index (BMI) above 30 compared with women with a BMI of 20–25. Table 29.4 shows the comparison of risk estimates of VTE from the two sources.

Current CEU advice to prescribers acknowledges the continuing debate over progestogens, and suggests that individual risk of VTE should be a governing principle in choice of contraceptive method.

Arterial disease, including myocardial infarction (MI) and cerebrovascular accident, results from the (mainly) progestogen-related alteration to lipid profiles together with the oestrogen-associated changes in blood coagulation. A WHO expert group reviewed the data on MI, stroke and hormonal contraception; the conclusions are as follows (World Health Organization Scientific Group 1998).

Table 29.4 Absolute risk of venous thromboembolism (VTE)

Population	VTE per 100,000 women-years	
	Committee on Safety of Medicines 1995	EURAS 2005
Non-pregnant, non-user	5	44
Second-generation progestogen COC	15	80[a]
Third-generation progestogen COC	25	99
Drospirenone	–	91
Pregnant non-user	60	291

COC, combined oral contraceptive.
[a]Levonorgestrel alone.

Acute myocardial infarction

- Acute MI is uncommon in women of reproductive age.
- Women who have hypertension and who take the COC have an increased RR of MI of at least three times that of women who take the COC and are normotensive.
- Smoking increases the risk of MI by 10 times when compared with COC users who do not smoke.
- There is insufficient evidence to allow any conclusion on whether the risk of MI is influenced by the type or dose of progestogen.

There was no increased risk of mortality due to ischaemic heart disease, either during or after COC use, in the report of the RCGP study (Beral et al 1999). However, two recent meta-analyses reported odds ratios of 1.84 and 2.48 for MI with low-dose COC use compared with non-current use [Baillargeon et al (2006) and Khader et al (2003), respectively], casting some doubt on WHO's conclusion that the risk of MI is not increased in CHC users who do not smoke or have hypertension or diabetes.

Stroke

- Ischaemic and haemorrhagic stroke are both uncommon among women of reproductive age.
- The risk of ischaemic stroke is increased approximately 1.5-fold in pill users who do not smoke and are not hypertensive. In contrast, the risk of haemorrhagic stroke is not increased in these women until they reach 35 years of age, after which the increasing natural risk of haemorrhagic stroke is magnified by CHC use.
- Hypertension increases the risk of both ischaemic (by three times) and haemorrhagic (10-fold) stroke compared with never-users.
- Smoking increases the risk of ischaemic and haemorrhagic stroke ($\infty 2$–3) compared with pill users who do not smoke.
- There is insufficient evidence to determine whether the risk of either type of stroke is influenced by the type or dose of progestogen.

Thus the data are reassuring for haemorrhagic stroke, but the risk of ischaemic stroke is increased by COC use; once again, this is supported by the findings of the RCGP study (Beral et al 1999), in which the RR of death from stroke was significantly increased to 1.9 [confidence interval (CI) 1.2–3.1, $P = 0.009$]. Ten years after discontinuation of the pill, the risk of death from stroke is no longer elevated. For a useful review of hormonal contraception and cardiovascular risk, see Curtis and Marchbanks (2005).

Cancer

Overviews of the risks and benefits of the COC are dominated by breast cancer. Published data are difficult to interpret because pill formulations and patterns of reproduction (particularly age at first pregnancy) have changed with time. In 1996, the Collaborative Group on Hormonal Factors in Breast Cancer reported a meta-analysis of 54 studies involving over 53,000 women with breast cancer and 100,000 control subjects. The group concluded that use of the COC was associated with a small increase in breast cancer, and that the increased risk persisted for 10 years after discontinuation of the pill. The RCGP study (Beral et al 1999) was also reassuring in this respect, since the risk of dying from breast cancer was not significantly increased among current or recent (within 10 years) COC users. The relationship between the pill and breast cancer is difficult to explain because the risk appears to increase soon after exposure, does not increase with duration of exposure and returns to normal 10 years after discontinuation. It has been suggested that starting to use the pill may accelerate the appearance of breast cancer in susceptible women (i.e. late-stage promotion of existing dysplasia). It is also possible that women using the pill have their tumours diagnosed earlier, although it is difficult to explain why a tendency to earlier diagnosis would persist for years after discontinuation. In the large meta-analysis, the risk of breast cancer was also increased among current users of both the progestogen-only pill (RR 1.17) and Depo-provera (RR 1.07), although the number of women using progestin-only methods was small. These findings strengthen the argument for increased detection rather than late-stage promotion of breast cancer. Nonetheless, a biological effect of hormonal contraception has still not been ruled out.

Incident data from a large cohort study from the RCGP (Hannaford et al 2007) has shown significantly lower rates of cancers of the large bowel, rectum, uterine body, ovaries and tumours of unknown origin in ever-users of the COC compared with never-users. There was no material difference between groups for breast cancer, and only small, non-statistically-significant increases in cancers of the lung, cervix and central nervous system. Taken together, there was an absolute rate reduction of any cancer in ever-users of 45 per 100,000 women-years.

Conversely, women taking the COC for more than 8 years did have a significantly increased risk of cervical cancer.

An increase in the risk of squamous carcinoma of the cervix (RR 1.3–1.8) has been recognized for some time. Recent extensive analysis of existing data detected an RR of 1.9 for 5 or more years of COC use (90% CI 1.69–2.31), declining after cessation of use and, like breast cancer, no different from that of never-users at 10 years after discontinuation (International Collaboration of Epidemiological Studies on Cervical Cancer 2007). The relationship is complicated by a number of confounding factors such as patterns of sexual behaviour and the likelihood of having cervical smears. Whether the national introduction in 2008 of vaccination for girls against human papilloma virus types 16 and 18 will have an effect on these figures remains to be seen. An increase in the risk of the much less common cervical adenocarcinoma (RR 2.1, increasing to 4.4 after 12 years of use) has also been demonstrated (Ursin et al 1994).

Other side-effects

Approximately 2% of women become clinically hypertensive after starting the pill. The incidence increases with age and duration of use, obesity and family history. It does not, however, appear to be increased in women with a history of pregnancy-induced hypertension.

An increased risk of gallstones is only significant during the early years of pill use.

A few women develop chloasma on the CHC; both oestrogen and progestogen contribute to this. The chloasma may be slow to fade after the hormones are stopped.

Minor side-effects are most common during the first 3 months of use, and often lead to discontinuation of the method. More common problems include breakthrough bleeding (BTB) or spotting, nausea, breast tenderness, acne and loss of libido. Many of these resolve with time. If side-effects persist after 4 months, it is often worth changing the brand of pill, opting for a lower dose of oestrogen or a different type of progestogen, or changing the mode of delivery. Pills containing antiandrogens are particularly useful for acne.

While the CHC, in general, improves menstrual bleeding patterns, one common reason for presentation to a gynaecologist is BTB. BTB is common during the first three cycles of use. Persistence beyond 3 months may be a result of poor compliance or a coexisting gynaecological disorder such as cervical ectropion (probably more common among COC users), or cervical or uterine polyps. If pelvic examination is normal, it is worth trying a formulation containing a higher dose of oestrogen or a different type of progestogen. After 3 months' use of a pill containing 50 µg ethinyl oestradiol, the bleeding will often settle and the woman can then resume a lower-dose pill. Alternatively, the vaginal ring may confer improved bleeding patterns. If bleeding persists, try stopping hormonal contraception altogether; if it does not resolve, it should be investigated as intermenstrual bleeding, i.e. by endometrial biopsy and hysteroscopy.

Benefits of combined oral contraception

The CHC confers a number of health benefits. Withdrawal bleeds are usually more regular, lighter and less painful, and the CHC is often the treatment of choice for women with irregular heavy periods (resulting from anovulatory dysfunctional uterine bleeding), premenstrual syndrome, dysmenorrhoea and endometriosis, as ovarian suppression can be achieved without the need for additional contraception (in contrast to danazol). A Cochrane review also concluded that the CHC can improve acne (Arowojolu et al 2009). These benefits can improve compliance significantly (Courtland Robinson et al 1992).

CHC use is associated with a 70% reduction in the risk of endometrial cancer, which may be maintained for up to 15 years after discontinuation (Weiderpass et al 1999). There is a similar duration-dependent reduction in the risk of ovarian cancer (RR 0.64, 95% CI 0.57–0.73) in ever-users compared with never-users (Riman et al 2004), which probably acts through the inhibition of ovulation and lasts for at least 10 years after discontinuation.

Significant numbers of unplanned pregnancies result from women stopping the pill for a 'break'. There is no evidence that breaks in pill taking reduce the long-term risks. It is not necessary to stop the CHC before planning a pregnancy. There is no evidence of any adverse effect on the fetus of CHC use prior to conception, neither is exposure during pregnancy associated with increased risk of fetal malformation.

Fertility is restored after a delay of 1–3 months, although some women take longer to resume normal cycles. So-called 'post-pill amenorrhoea' is almost always associated with cycle irregularity before starting the pill or with coincidental factors associated with secondary amenorrhoea, such as weight loss or stress.

Progestogen-only contraceptives

Progestogen-only contraceptives (POCs) are much less commonly used than CHCs. However, POCs are available in a wider variety of systems, including pills, implants, long-acting injectables and hormone-releasing IUDs.

The mechanism of action of POCs depends on the dose of steroid administered. High doses, such as depot medroxy-progesterone acetate (DMPA), inhibit ovulation. Low doses only inhibit ovulation inconsistently, and the effect varies between individuals. All POCs affect both the quantity and physical characteristics of cervical mucus, reducing sperm penetrability and transport. All have an effect on the endometrium, probably compromising implantation. The recent addition of a 75 µg desogestrel progestogen-only pill (Cerazette®) combines inhibition of ovulation in 97% of users with the oral route of administration.

The absence of oestrogen in this group of hormonal methods is associated with an absence of cardiovascular risks including VTE. In a case–control study undertaken by WHO (World Health Organization Collaborative Study of Cardiovascular Disease and Steroid Hormone Contraception 1998), there was no significant increase in the risk of MI, stroke or VTE associated with use of oral or injectable progestogen-only methods.

The progestogen-only pill (POP or mini-pill) is a useful alternative for women who like the convenience of the COC but for whom oestrogen is contraindicated. Not only does the POP not contain oestrogen, but the dose of progestogen is significantly lower than in equivalent combined preparations. The POP is still a good alternative for women with medical contraindications to the COC, such as migraine and hypertension. It is often advocated for women with diabetes who are at increased risk of cardiovascular disease and who may find that insulin requirements fluctuate with COC cycles. However, the COC is not absolutely contraindicated for diabetic women without long-term complications, whose diabetes is well controlled and for whom pregnancy would be a disaster. The most common indication for POP use in the UK used to be for breastfeeding women, since the POP (unlike the CHC) does not interfere with either the quantity or constituents of breast milk. However, due to its mode of action and likely increased efficacy, the newest POP has wider potential. It is no longer considered necessary to advise women routinely to change from the COC to the POP when they reach the age of 35 years, since the combined pill, in the absence of risk factors for cardiovascular disease, is very safe.

Mode of action

While Cerazette inhibits ovulation in over 90% of cycles, approximately 50% of classical POP users continue to ovulate and menstruate regularly. In these women, the POP works by altering cervical mucus and probably by interfering with implantation. If follicle development is inhibited completely, amenorrhoea results (10–20% of women).

Side-effects

The mode of action of the POP explains its side-effects. Erratic bleeding is the most common cause for discontinuation of the pill; approximately 20% of women will stop using it for this reason.

Follicular growth without ovulation is associated with an increased incidence of functional ovarian cysts. Up to 20% of women using the POP will have a cyst identifiable by ultrasound. Most are symptomless and nearly all resolve spontaneously. A woman found to have a symptomless ovarian cyst should be reviewed after her next menstrual period.

POP use is associated with a slightly increased risk of ectopic pregnancy. Some 2% of pregnancies among POP failures will be ectopic, perhaps as a result of an effect of the progestogen on tubal motility. Since Cerazette inhibits ovulation in almost all cycles, the theoretical risk of ectopic pregnancy is less.

Due to its mechanism of action (50% of women continue to ovulate) and its relatively short half-life (approximately 19 h), the classical POP has a higher failure rate than the COC (see Table 29.3), with users of the established varieties having a 3-h window within which to remember to take their pill. This failure rate is dependent on age and is almost as low as the COC in women aged over 35 years. However, the ovulation-inhibiting Cerazette can be taken in much the same way as the COC with a 12-h window, making it a suitable and reliable choice for younger women as well. There is no direct evidence for advising women who weigh more than 70 kg to take two pills each day.

Injectable progestogens

Long-acting injectable progestogens are available in two forms: DMPA or Depo-provera (150 mg IM every 12 weeks) and norethisterone oenanthate (200 mg IM every 8 weeks). The latter is seldom used in the UK.

Worldwide, DMPA is a popular method of contraception used by some 9 million women in over 90 countries. DMPA appears to exert a powerful protective effect against endometrial cancer with an RR of 0.2. No association has been described between DMPA use and the risk of ovarian cancer, which is surprising if the protective effect of the COC is due to the inhibition of ovulation. The slight increase in the risk of breast cancer among users of both the POP and DMPA identified in the large meta-analysis (Collaborative Group on Hormonal Factors in Breast Cancer 1996) may be due to detection bias; however, there are some concerns that progestins alone may be associated with a real increase in risk.

Depo-provera is a highly effective (Table 29.3) long-acting method which only requires the user to attend for injection four times a year. It inhibits ovulation, and 80% of women are either amenorrhoeic (40%) or have very scanty, infrequent periods (40%) after 1 year of use. The remaining 20% of women will have prolonged regular or, more usually, irregular bleeding episodes, and approximately 2% of women will present, often to a gynaecologist, with troublesome menorrhagia. After excluding any pathology, the most effective treatment of menorrhagia is oestrogen (Fraser 1983), and it is most easily given as one packet of the COC. If bleeding problems persist, an alternative method of contraception should be considered.

Other significant long-term side-effects include:

- weight gain; up to 6 kg during the first 2 years of use;
- a delay in the resumption of fertility of up to 1 year or more after cessation of use; and
- a reduction in bone mineral density (BMD).

BMD has been shown to plateau after an initial decrease in the first year of use. Current studies (flawed by the use of surrogate measures of bone health, methodological errors, comparison of heterogeneous populations and varying sites of BMD measurements) show a 2–3% decrease in BMD in the first year of DMPA use, slowing in subsequent years. BMD is gradually regained following discontinuation of DMPA, and appears to be similar to that of never-users in adults at 30 months after the last injection (Gbolade et al 1998). Similar findings in adolescents were reported at 12 months after discontinuation of the method (Scholes et al 2005). To date, there is no good evidence for an increased risk of fractures.

The Committee on Safety of Medicines (2006) made the following recommendations in the light of the existing evidence:

- in adolescents, DMPA may be used as a first-line contraception but only after other methods have been discussed with the patient and considered to be unsuitable or unacceptable;
- in women of all ages, careful evaluation of risks and benefits of treatment should be carried out in those who wish to continue use for more than 2 years; and
- in women with significant lifestyle and/or medical risk factors for osteoporosis, other methods of contraception should be considered.

This advice is in line with the UKMEC.

Progestogen-only implants

Progestogen-only, subdermal implants are available worldwide and are used by millions of women. The original LNG-releasing Norplant® comprised six rods; modern implants with a preloaded applicator and only one or two rods are much easier to insert and remove. Jadelle® is identical to Norplant but has two rods. It is approved for 5 years. Implanon®, a single rod, is approved for 3 years of use in the UK, and consists of an ethylene–vinyl-acetate copolymer core containing 68 mg etonorgestrel. The rate-limiting membrane allows an initial release rate of approximately 60–70 μg/day, slowly decreasing to 30–40 μg/day at the end of the second year and 25–30 μg/day at the end of the third year.

Although the implants are not difficult to insert, removal can occasionally be troublesome, particularly if the rods are inserted subcutaneously rather than subdermally. Failure rates are extremely low (Table 29.3), and all failures are due to the method as implants do not depend on compliance. The dose of progestogen is sufficient to inhibit ovulation in every cycle throughout the 3 years. Cervical mucus is scanty and allows poor sperm penetration.

Approximately 20% of women experience amenorrhoea with Implanon. A further 60% may experience erratic bleeding or no effect on their usual menstrual cycle. The remaining 20% will request removal on the basis of unacceptable menstrual disturbance. Fertility resumes as soon as the implants are removed. Bleeding irregularity is the most common side-effect and reason for removal, but others include acne, hirsutism, headache, mood change, and weight gain or bloating (i.e. the metabolic side-effects of progestogens). For a useful review of contraceptive implants, see Glasier (2002).

Intrauterine devices and systems

The IUD is a cheap, effective long-acting method of contraception. It exerts a local inflammatory reaction within the cavity of the uterus which probably, acting through tubal and uterine fluid, interferes with the viability of both sperm and eggs. It also inhibits implantation. Inert devices are no longer recommended or marketed, but some older women do still have them *in utero*. Modern copper-containing devices are licensed for use over 5–10 years. After a woman reaches 40 years of age, the device need not be changed and can be removed 1 year after the last menstrual period. Copper IUDs consist of a plastic frame with copper wire round the stem and, in some cases, copper caps on the arms. The surface area of the copper determines the lifespan and efficacy of the device. IUDs with a surface area of copper of less than 200 mm² are associated with higher pregnancy rates and are no longer recommended for long-term use. A frameless IUD (Gynefix®) comprises six copper beads threaded on to a nylon line. The beads at the top and bottom are crimped to hold them on the line, and the string has a knot at the proximal end which is embedded, using a special inserter, into the myometrium, anchoring it in place.

The LNG-releasing device [known as a system (IUS) to distinguish it from copper IUDs] has been licensed in the UK since 1995 under the trade name Mirena®. It consists of a column of LNG within a rate-limiting membrane wrapped around the stem of a Nova-T frame. A total dose of 52 mg LNG is released at a rate of 20 mg/day. It is licensed for 5 years for contraception. A small amount of LNG is absorbed systemically and can give rise to androgenic side-effects such as acne. Menstrual bleeding is significantly reduced, with periods being replaced by light spotting and eventually, in many women, amenorrhoea. In the classic study of the effects of the LNG-IUS on menstrual blood loss (Andersson and Rybo 1990), women complaining of menorrhagia experienced a reduction in blood loss of 86% at 3 months and 97% at 12 months after LNG-IUS insertion. Mirena is now widely used in the UK, and is licensed for the management of menorrhagia (Royal College of Obstetricians and Gynaecologists 1999) and as the progestogen component of hormone replacement therapy. A frameless equivalent of the IUS, Fibroplant®, is the most recent modification of this technology with a silastic sleeve, suspended on a thread which is anchored into the uterine fundus with a knot.

Side-effects

Perforation is a rare event (one in 1000 insertions); if it is recognized early, it may be possible to remove the IUD via the laparoscope before adhesions form. For this reason, it is probably wise to see women for follow-up to check the tails of the device within 4–6 weeks of insertion.

Expulsion occurs in 3–10% of women in the first year of use and is related to parity, age, type of IUD and timing of insertion. The incidence of both expulsion and perforation is influenced by the skill of the person inserting the device. Both complications are increased with postpartum insertions which, according to the UKMEC, should be scheduled no earlier than 4 weeks after delivery.

The risk of pelvic infection among IUD users has been greatly exaggerated. In countries where IUDs are inserted under appropriate sterile conditions, the risk of pelvic infection is only increased for 20 days after insertion. Women infected with gonorrhoea or chlamydia have an increased risk of infection if an IUD is inserted compared with uninfected women, but the risk of salpingitis is not increased compared with infected women who are not undergoing IUD insertion. Even women who are human immunodeficiency virus (HIV) positive do not appear to have an increased risk of complications, including infection, associated with IUD insertion, and there is no evidence that IUD use increases viral shedding (Grimes 2000). In addition, there is no evidence for an increased risk of infertility among past or current IUD users. However, if an IUD user becomes pregnant, the probability of that pregnancy being ectopic is greater than that for women using no contraception or another method because the IUD does not prevent tubal implantation. In women at risk of pre-existing infection, IUD insertion can be covered with a broad-spectrum antibiotic. Routine screening for infection may be more cost-effective in services where the background rate of infection, especially with chlamydia, is high.

The most common reason for discontinuation of the copper IUD is menorrhagia. The local inflammatory response, together with increased production of prostaglandins, causes both menorrhagia and dysmenorrhoea. All IUDs are removed by steady traction on the tail of the device. Occasionally, the string snaps off during removal. It is sometimes possible to remove the device with a pair of artery forceps or a specially designed IUD remover, but some IUDs, particularly the old inert devices, appear to become deeply embedded in the endometrium and may only be removed under general anaesthetic. It is not known if an IUD without its tails can be left in the cavity of the uterus for a woman's lifetime without causing any problems. There is a small risk of actinomycosis but the inconvenience of admission to hospital for a general anaesthetic may outweigh this. It is probably best discussed with the individual concerned.

Natural family planning

Although few couples in the UK use so-called 'natural methods of family planning' (NFP), these methods are common in some parts of the world. All involve 'periodic abstinence' (i.e. avoidance of intercourse during the fertile period of the cycle). Methods differ in the way in which they recognize the fertile period. The simplest is the calendar or rhythm method, in which the woman calculates the fertile period according to the length of her normal menstrual cycle. Others use symptoms which reflect fluctuating concentrations of circulating oestrogen and progesterone, themselves reflecting follicular development, impending ovulation and completed ovulation. The mucus or Billings method relies on identifying changes in the quantity and quality of cervical and vaginal mucus as a reflection of the steroid environment. As circulating oestrogens increase with follicle growth, the mucus becomes clear and stretchy, allowing the passage of sperm. With ovulation and in the presence of progesterone, mucus becomes opaque, sticky and much less stretchy or disappears altogether. Intercourse must stop when fertile-type mucus is identified, and can start again when infertile-type mucus is recognized. Progesterone secretion is also associated with a rise in basal body temperature (BBT) of approximately 0.5 °C. The BBT method is thus able to identify the end of the fertile period. Other signs and symptoms such as ovulation pain, position of cervix and degree of dilatation of the cervical os can also be used to help define the fertile period. A personal fertility monitor called Persona, which measures urinary oestrogen and LH using a dipstick, can help to identify the fertile period but does not significantly reduce the number of days of abstinence required and is expensive. Whatever method is used, all rely on a period of abstinence and many couples find this difficult. Failure rates are high (Table 29.3) and most of the failures are due to conscious rule breaking. Perfect use of the mucus method is, in fact, associated with a failure rate of only 3.4%. There is no evidence that accidental pregnancies occurring among NFP users, which are conceived with ageing gametes, are associated with a higher risk of congenital malformations.

Lactational amenorrhoea method

Breast feeding delays the resumption of fertility, and it still has a major impact on fertility rates in developing countries. It has been calculated that breast feeding provides more than 98% protection from pregnancy during the first 6 months post partum if the mother is fully or nearly fully breast feeding and has not yet experienced vaginal bleeding after the 56th day post partum. Lactational amenorrhoea method (LAM) guidelines advise that as long as the baby is less than 6 months old, a woman can rely on breast feeding alone until she menstruates or until she starts to give her baby significant amounts of food other than breast milk. Prospective studies of the LAM confirm its effectiveness (Perez et al 1992).

Barrier methods

The male condom remains one of the most popular methods of contraception in the UK. It is cheap, widely available over the counter and, with the exception of the occasional allergic reaction, is free from side-effects. Use of the condom increased significantly with concern over the spread of HIV and acquired immunodeficiency syndrome as it is the only method of contraception which also prevents sexually transmitted infections (STIs).

In addition to protection against STIs, use of the condom, and diaphragm, is associated with a significant reduction in cervical disease (Celentano et al 1987). Female barrier methods are less popular. The diaphragm and cervical cap must be fitted by a professional and do not confer the same degree of protection against STIs/HIV. The female condom, by virtue of covering the mucus membranes of the vagina and vulva, is more effective in preventing STIs but has a high failure rate and low acceptability.

Spermicides alone are not a very effective method of contraception and are only recommended for use with a condom (most of which are already lubricated with spermicide) or diaphragm. Nonoxynol 9 (N-9) is a spermicidal product sold as a gel, cream, foam, film or pessary for use with diaphragms or caps. Many male condoms are lubricated with N-9. As frequent use of N-9 might increase the risk of HIV transmission, women who have multiple daily acts of intercourse or who are at high risk of HIV infection should not use N-9. For women at low risk of HIV infection, N-9 is probably safe (Van Damme et al 2000, www.who/int).

Emergency contraception

Hormonal preparations and the IUD can be used to prevent pregnancy after intercourse has taken place. In the UK, one hormonal preparation is available: Levonelle (LNG 1.5 g). It is licensed for use within 72 h of intercourse, but women should be encouraged to present as soon as possible for treatment. It is, in any case, very difficult to estimate the efficacy of any emergency contraceptive (EC) since the true risk of pregnancy for any one individual cannot be calculated with any degree of certainty, and many of the 'failures' are pregnancies which are, in fact, conceived with an act of intercourse which occurred earlier in the cycle or some time after the act for which EC was sought. Levonelle is now available off prescription from pharmacists.

IUD insertion is more effective (Table 29.3) and can be used up to 5 days after the estimated day of ovulation, which may be significantly longer than 5 days after the act of intercourse. The FSRH advise that intrauterine EC should be offered to all women presenting after unprotected intercourse, in the absence of contraindications, as the gold standard method. If the woman does not wish to continue with the method, it can be removed with the next period or when an alternative method has been established.

The mechanism of action of hormonal EC remains unclear. It has been shown to delay or impair ovulation in some 50% of users, but there is no good evidence that it will inhibit implantation. Neither is there any contraceptive/contragestive effect once implantation is complete. Conversely, the IUD has a toxic effect on gametes, reduces the number of sperm reaching the fallopian tubes and, if inserted after fertilization has taken place, inhibits implantation, resulting in a higher level of efficacy (Table 29.3). The LNG-IUS is not recommended as an emergency contraceptive.

Recent efforts to find a more effective, orally active emergency contraceptive with fewer side-effects have resulted in trials of the antiprogesterone mifepristone (Task Force on Postovulatory Methods of Fertility Regulation 1999). Since mifepristone is known to inhibit both ovulation and implantation, it is likely to be more effective than LNG, but its properties as an abortifacient limit its further development at present.

Sterilization

Over 42 million couples worldwide, the majority of whom live in developing countries (particularly China and India), rely on vasectomy. More than three times that number rely on female sterilization. In Britain, surgical methods of contraception are declining in popularity. Between 1998 and 2008, vasectomy fell from 12% to 10% and female sterilization fell from 12% to 7%. The more pronounced decline in female sterilization is probably due to the introduction of long-acting reversible methods.

Female sterilization

Female sterilization usually involves the blocking of both fallopian tubes either by laparotomy or minilaparotomy or, more commonly, by laparoscopy. It may also be achieved by bilateral salpingectomy (or by hysterectomy when there is coexistent gynaecological pathology such as hydrosalpinx or fibroids) or by hysteroscopic techniques.

Minilaparotomy and laparoscopic female sterilization are probably equally safe and effective; however, the latter allows sterilization to be done as a daycase procedure and is recommended by the RCOG (2004a) as the method of choice in the UK. Minilaparotomy is most commonly used when sterilization is performed immediately post partum as, at that time, the uterus is large, the pelvis is very vascular and the risks of laparoscopy are increased.

A variety of techniques exist for occluding the tube, as follows.

Ligation

Ligation is used when laparotomy or minilaparotomy are performed. The tubes can be tied with absorbable or non-absorbable sutures, and the ends can be left free or buried in the broad ligament or uterine cornu. Postpartum sterilization is associated with a higher failure rate.

Electrocautery

With electrocautery, one or more areas of the tube are cauterized by diathermy. Bipolar diathermy only allows the tissues held between the jaws of the forceps to be cauterized. The temperature of the cauterized tube may reach 300–400°C and, if allowed to touch adjacent structures, can cause local burns. Failure to cauterize all the layers of the tube results in a relatively high failure rate (2–5/1000), and cautery close to the cornual portion of the tube is thought to increase the risk of ectopic pregnancy. The RCOG (2004a) only recommends the use of diathermy if tubal occlusion proves to be difficult and mechanical methods have failed.

Falope ring

A ring of silicone rubber is placed over a loop of tube with a specially designed applicator. The ring destroys 2–3 cm of tube and may be difficult to apply if the tube is fat or rigid. As ischaemia of the loop causes significant postoperative pain, application of topical anaesthesia during sterilization is recommended.

Clips

A variety of clips are available. They destroy a much smaller length of tube, allowing easier reversal, but special care must be taken to ensure that the whole width of the tube is occluded. The Hulka–Clemens clip (stainless steel and a polycarbonate) and the smaller Filshie clip (titanium lined with silicone rubber) are probably the most commonly used in the UK.

Laser

Laser vaporization can be used to divide the tubes; however, the carbon dioxide laser divides them very cleanly and may allow a high incidence of recanalization. The neodymium:yttrium aluminium garnet laser, although probably more effective, is extremely expensive.

Efficacy

A report from the US Collaborative Review of Sterilization (Peterson et al 1996) prospectively evaluated over 10,000 women who underwent sterilization in nine US cities. The women were followed-up for between 8 and 14 years. The failure rate varied with age and the method of tubal occlusion. The 10-year lifetable cumulative probability of pregnancy for all ages combined (18–44 years) ranged from 7.5 pregnancies per 1000 procedures (for unipolar coagulation and postpartum partial salpingectomy) to 36.5 pregnancies per 1000 procedures (for clips). Failure rates were highest for women under the age of 28 years, with 52 pregnancies per 1000 procedures for spring clips. Women considering laparoscopic sterilization in the UK should be advised that the lifetime risk of failure is one in 200.

In the UK, a device called Essure® is the only licensed product available for hysteroscopic sterilization. It is a 4 cm, inert, nickel-titanium coil containing polyester fibres, designed to be inserted into each tubal ostia under direct vision and to cause fibrosis sufficient to have occluded the tubes by 3 months post procedure. A recent UK cohort study comparing Essure (developed as an 'office-based' procedure) with laparoscopic sterilization reported high levels of patient satisfaction (Duffy et al 2005). Longer-term assessment of efficacy and safety is awaited.

A number of chemical agents have been tested for their ability to occlude the fallopian tube when instilled into the tube either directly or transcervically into the uterus. The quinacrine pellet is the only one ready for large-scale use. The method involves insertion of a 252 mg quinacrine pellet into the uterine cavity through a modified IUD inserter passed through the cervical canal. Two insertions, 1 month apart, are made during the follicular phase of the cycle. Occlusion is caused by inflammation and fibrosis of the intramural segment of the tube. Efficacy can be increased by adding adjuvants such as antiprostaglandins or by increasing the number of quinacrine insertions. A failure rate of 2.6% after 1 year of follow-up has been reported (Hieu et al 1993). The method is cheaper than surgical sterilization, avoids the use of any anaesthesia and can be performed by non-medical personnel. Large numbers of women in Asia and Pakistan have been sterilized using this method. However, although quinacrine is widely used for malaria prophylaxis, the safety of quinacrine sterilization has not yet been determined and some question the ethics of using a technique which has not been approved in developed countries. Toxicology studies are presently underway.

Counselling for sterilization

Most couples seeking sterilization have been thinking about the operation for some considerable time. The initial consultation should include a discussion of:

- the procedure involved;
- the failure rate;
- the risks and side-effects;
- the possibility of wanting more children;
- which partner should be sterilized;
- the issue of reversibility. Despite careful counselling, a few couples will inevitably request reversal of sterilization. This is most likely to happen with remarriage. Immediate postpartum or postabortion sterilization is more likely to be regretted and should be avoided if possible. Although as many as 10% of couples regret being sterilized, only 1% of these will request reversal; and
- alternative long-acting methods of contraception which are reversible and equally effective, such as contraceptive implants.

The RCOG (2004a) recommends that verbal counselling advice should be backed up by accurate impartial printed information which the couple may take away.

Reversal of female sterilization is more likely to be successful after occlusion with clips which have been applied to the isthmic portion of the tube, since only a small section of tube will have been damaged. Patients should realize that reversal involves laparotomy, does not always work (microsurgical techniques are associated with approximately 70% success) and carries a significant risk of ectopic pregnancy (up to 5%). Ovulation should be confirmed and a normal semen analysis should be obtained from the partner before reversal is undertaken. Reversal is unlikely to be available on the National Health Service (NHS) in most parts of the UK.

The history should include the following:

- the reason for the request: some women seek sterilization as a cure for menstrual dysfunction, sexual problems or abdominal pain;
- gynaecological and obstetric history, and relevant medical histories of both partners;
- ages, occupations and social circumstances of both partners;
- numbers, ages and health of their children;
- previous and current contraception and any problems experienced. Some women request sterilization because they are unable to find any other acceptable method of contraception; this is not a good reason for sterilization;
- the stability of the relationship and the possibility of its breakdown; and
- the quality of the couple's sex life.

It is seldom possible to arrange sterilization for a particular time of the cycle, and women should be told to continue using their current method of contraception until their operation. It is not necessary to stop the combined pill before sterilization as the risk of thromboembolic complications is negligible.

If an IUD is *in situ*, it should be removed at the time of sterilization, unless the operation is being done at mid-cycle and intercourse has taken place within the previous few days, in which case it can be removed after the next menstrual period.

Complications

Immediate complications

- The operation carries a small operative mortality of less than eight per 100,000 operations. In a large series from the USA (Peterson et al 1983), the most common cause of death was anaesthesia. In the UK, laparoscopic sterilization is commonly performed under general anaesthesia, but local anaesthesia is an acceptable alternative.

- Vascular damage or damage to bowel or other internal organs may occur during the procedure and is usually recognized at the time of operation. Nevertheless, patients should be aware that the rare possibility of a laparotomy and longer hospital stay does exist.
- Gas embolism.
- Thromboembolic disease is rare, but is more likely if the procedure is done immediately post partum.
- Wound infection.
- Postoperative pain is common because of local tissue ischaemia and necrosis at the site of occlusion of the tube. It can be reduced by the use of local tubal anaesthesia.

Long-term complications

- Menstrual disorders: women who stop using the combined pill will almost certainly notice that their periods become heavier, perhaps more painful and less predictable, and they should be warned of this. In contrast, women whose previous method of contraception was an IUD will notice an improvement in their bleeding patterns. Although a review of the evidence concluded that female sterilization does not alter ovarian activity or menstruation (Gentile et al 1998), a number of studies have demonstrated an increased incidence of gynaecological consultation and an increased incidence of hysterectomy among women who have been sterilized (Hillis et al 1998). Bearing in mind the inevitable changes in menstrual bleeding patterns associated with advancing age and with discontinuation of the combined pill (the most commonly used method of reversible contraception), it may be that women who have been sterilized are more likely to seek hysterectomy, or more willing to accept it, if they are already incapable of further child bearing.
- The term 'post-tubal sterilization syndrome' was coined to describe a variety of symptoms that have been reported after sterilization and which women may attribute to the procedure. These symptoms include abdominal pain, dyspareunia, exacerbation of premenstrual syndrome or dysmenorrhoea, and emotional and psychosexual problems. Laparoscopy fails to demonstrate any pathology. A review of the literature (Gentile et al 1998) concluded that sterilization is not associated with an increased risk of these problems, except among young women sterilized before 30 years of age in whom the symptoms may sometimes be a manifestation of regret.
- Psychological and psychosexual problems are rare; when they do arise, they tend to do so in those who have had problems before sterilization. Many studies, in fact, report a better mental state after sterilization.
- Bowel obstruction from adhesions is a very rare complication.
- Ectopic pregnancy is a well-recognized complication of sterilization. In the US Collaborative Review (Peterson et al 1997), the risk was influenced by age and the method of occlusion. The 10-year cumulative probability of ectopic pregnancy for all ages combined ranged from 1.5 (for postpartum partial salpingectomy) to 17 (for bipolar coagulation) pregnancies per 1000 procedures, while for women aged less than 30 years, the figures were 1 and 33, respectively. Women should be advised that if they miss a period and have symptoms of pregnancy, they should seek medical advice urgently.

Vasectomy

Vasectomy involves the division or occlusion of the vas deferens to prevent the passage of sperm. The vas is exposed through a small skin incision, and ligated or occluded with small silver clips or by unipolar diathermy with a specially designed probe which can be passed into the cut end of the vas.

Excising a small portion of the vas makes reversal more difficult and probably does not increase the effectiveness unless at least 4 cm is removed. It does allow histological confirmation of a correct procedure in difficult cases, but is not routinely recommended. Interposing the fascial sheath between the cut ends or looping the cut ends of the vas back on itself may increase effectiveness. The RCOG (2004a) recommends that fascial interposition or diathermy should accompany division of the vas which, on its own, is not an acceptable technique in terms of the failure rate. This recommendation, although the opinion of experts, is not supported by scientific evidence, and the relative efficacy of any one method of occlusion and efficacy probably depends most on the skill of the surgeon.

The 'no-scalpel' vasectomy (NSV), developed in China in 1974, is now quite widely used. It makes use of specially designed instruments for isolating and delivering the vas through the scrotal skin, and substitutes a small puncture for the skin incision. Any of the standard methods of occlusion may be used. NSV is quick and associated with a lower incidence of infection and haematoma. A comparison between NSV and conventional vasectomy in Thailand reported a complication rate of 0.4% vs 3.1% (Nirapathpongporn et al 1990).

Percutaneous injection of sclerosing agents, such as polyurethane elastomers, or occlusive substances, such as silicone, is also being used in China. The technique avoids any skin incision, the silicone plug is said to be easily removed, and pregnancy rates of 100% up to 5 years after vasectomy reversal have been claimed.

The rate at which azoospermia is achieved depends on the frequency of ejaculation. In the UK, seminal fluid is examined after 12 and 16 weeks, and if sperm are still present, usually monthly thereafter. When sperm are absent from two consecutive samples, the vasectomy can be considered complete; until then, an alternative method of contraception must be used. Approximately 3% of men do not become azoospermic and the vasectomy has to be redone.

Complications of vasectomy

Local complications

Wound infection will occur in up to 5% of men and scrotal bruising is unavoidable. Postoperative bleeding will be sufficient in 1–2% of men to cause a haematoma, and perhaps 1% of these will require admission to hospital.

Sperm granulomas

Small lumps may form at the cut ends of the vas as a result of a local inflammatory response to leaked sperm. They can be painful and may need excising. Their presence may also increase the chance of failure.

Chronic intrascrotal pain and discomfort (postvasectomy syndrome)

Some men complain of a dull ache in the scrotum which may be exacerbated by sexual excitement and ejaculation. The symptoms are probably due to distension and granuloma formation in the epididymis and vas deferens. Pain may also result from scar tissue forming around small nerves. Chronic pain associated with progressive induration, tubular distension and granuloma formation in the epididymis may require excision of the epididymis and obstructed vas deferens.

Late recanalization

Failure can occur up to 10 years after vasectomy despite two negative samples of seminal fluid following the procedure. It is rare (one in 2000).

Antisperm antibodies

Most men develop detectable concentrations of autoantibodies, presumably as a result of leakage of sperm, some time after vasectomy. Their presence may compromise fertility if reversal is attempted.

Cardiovascular and autoimmune disease

Concerns about a possible link between vasectomy and cardiovascular disease were raised in the 1970s following reports that vasectomy increased atherosclerosis in monkeys, perhaps as a consequence of increased levels of autoantibodies. Several large studies, including a cohort study in the USA of over 10,000 vasectomized men, failed to substantiate increased rates of 98 diseases (McDonald 1997).

Cancer

Two studies from the USA and Scotland suggested an increased risk of testicular cancer following vasectomy. However, a large cohort study of over 73,000 men in Denmark (Moller et al 1994) demonstrated no increase in the incidence of testicular cancer among men who had a vasectomy.

A number of reports from the USA have also suggested an increased risk of prostate cancer following vasectomy. No known biological mechanism can account for any association or causal relationship between vasectomy and prostate cancer. A 1998 systematic review of 14 studies published from 1985 to 1996 (Bernal-Delgado et al 1998) reported a summary risk estimate of 1.23 (95% CI 1.01–1.49), but the authors concluded that there was evidence against a causal relationship. An editorial from the US National Cancer Institute, commenting on a large US population-based study which found no effect of vasectomy on prostate cancer (Peterson and Howards 1998), concluded that vasectomy does not appear to cause prostate cancer or there is only a relatively weak relationship.

Reversal

Reversal of vasectomy is technically feasible in many cases, with patency rates of almost 90% being reported in some series. Pregnancy rates are much less (up to 60%), perhaps as a result of the presence of antisperm antibodies.

Abortion

After the Abortion Act was passed in the UK in 1967, there was a rapid rise in the number of abortions, which reached a plateau in the late 1980s. Since then, there has been a gradual rise in the numbers each year, with 198,500 abortions being performed in England and Wales and 13,700 being performed in Scotland in 2007. The abortion rate in Britain (13 per 1000 women aged 15–45 years in Scotland and 18 per 1000 in England and Wales in 2007) is relatively low compared with many other developed countries. Nevertheless, at least one-third of British women will have had an abortion by the age of 45 years. The rate of teenage pregnancy (including both childbirth and abortion) in Britain is one of the worst in Europe. The Teenage Pregnancy Independent Advisory Group was formed in England 1998 to investigate teenage pregnancy and to make recommendations based on their findings. Their annual reports and the Government's response can be found at www.everychildmatters.gov.org.

Legal aspects

In the UK, it is illegal to induce an abortion except under specific indications, as defined by law. The conditions of the 1967 Abortion Act state that abortion can be performed if two registered medical practitioners, acting in good faith, agree that the pregnancy should be terminated on one or more of the following grounds.

- The continuance of the pregnancy would involve risk to the life of the pregnant woman greater than if the pregnancy were terminated.
- The termination is necessary to prevent grave permanent injury to the physical or mental health of the pregnant woman.
- The pregnancy has NOT exceeded its 24th week and the continuance of the pregnancy would involve risk, greater than if the pregnancy were terminated, of injury to the physical or mental health of the pregnant woman.
- The pregnancy has NOT exceeded its 24th week and the continuance of the pregnancy would involve risk, greater than if the pregnancy were terminated, of injury to the physical or mental health of the existing child(ren) of the family of the pregnant woman.
- There is a substantial risk that if the child were born it would suffer from such physical or mental abnormalities as to be seriously handicapped.

In 1990, the law was amended to reduce the upper limit from 28 to 24 weeks of gestation, reflecting the lowering of the limits of fetal viability resulting from advances in neonatal care. An exception was made in the case of a fetus with severe congenital abnormality incompatible with life (e.g. anencephaly), in which case there is no upper limit.

The 1967 Abortion Act does not apply to Northern Ireland where abortion is only legal under exceptional circumstances, such as to save the life of the mother.

The law recognizes that some doctors have ethical objections to abortion. Doctors who do have objections are obliged to refer women to a colleague who does not hold similar views.

Over 98% of induced abortions in Britain are undertaken on the grounds that the continuance of the pregnancy would involve risk to the physical or mental health of the pregnant woman.

Provision of services

In Scotland and north-east England, over 90% of abortions are performed in NHS hospitals, while in other areas of England, the majority are carried out in private clinics or by charities. In Scotland, abortion accounts for over 22% of the inpatient gynaecological workload and is thus a major issue for gynaecologists. Some hospitals have dedicated services which are quite separate from the general gynaecological service, and which are staffed by experts who are more sensitive and sympathetic. While this has obvious advantages for individual patients and is recommended as best practice by the RCOG (2004b), the approach risks separating abortion from other aspects of reproductive health care and removing it from general gynaecological training. Without exposure during their training to the issue and to women who are seeking abortion, doctors may become increasingly reluctant to be involved with the provision of services, as they are in the USA.

Counselling

Faced with the news of an unintended pregnancy, many women are emotionally devastated and the decision to have a pregnancy terminated is never an easy one. In the UK, the Committee on the Working of the Abortion Act (the Lane Committee), reporting in 1974, recommended that every woman should have the opportunity to have adequate counselling before deciding to have her pregnancy terminated. Abortion counselling should provide opportunities for discussion, information, explanation and advice in a manner which is non-judgemental and non-directional.

By the time most women see a gynaecologist, they have already seen one doctor (usually their general practitioner) and are certain of their decision. However, in order to satisfy themselves that there are grounds for termination, gynaecologists should nonetheless discuss the reasons why the pregnancy is unwanted and whether the woman is absolutely certain about her decision, since uncertainty may be more likely to lead to regret. The woman should be encouraged to think of the practical and emotional consequences of all the possible options of abortion, continuing with the pregnancy and adoption.

Not all doctors are sympathetic, and women who are seen to have conceived because of a true method failure are more likely to get a sympathetic hearing. Many women feel that they have to 'make the case' to the gynaecologist for having their pregnancy terminated, and some will claim method failure even when they have not been using contraception. One in five women who have had an abortion will present for another at some time in their lives. Women who seem to use abortion as a method of contraception and present again and again probably need psychiatric help and not a punitive approach from the gynaecologist.

In the UK, approximately 1% of women will present too late for legal abortion. These, and some of those who choose to have the baby, will need information about adoption and benefits, and sometimes referral to social services.

The gynaecologist should provide information about the procedure involved, offering, where available and appropriate, a choice of surgical or medical methods to women below 12 weeks of gestation. The possible complications and long-term side-effects of the abortion should also be discussed, together with the implications for future pregnancies. Verbal discussions should be supported by written information, and confidentiality should be emphasized.

Future contraceptive plans are usually discussed before the abortion is carried out. Although this may not be the best time, it may be one of the few opportunities to discuss contraception as many patients do not attend for follow-up.

Assessment

After it has been decided that there are grounds for abortion, it is important to make a careful medical assessment of the woman.

- The medical history should pay particular attention to conditions such as asthma which may influence the choice of method of abortion.
- The stage of gestation should be determined by menstrual history and transvaginal or transabdominal ultrasound scan. Whilst acceptable to establish gestation, pelvic examination for this purpose alone has generally been superseded by ultrasound, as the former is felt to be less accurate and seldom detects ectopic pregnancy or missed miscarriage.
- Whether the service chooses to screen for genital tract infection, particularly chlamydia, or simply to treat everyone with prophylactic antibiotics will depend on the background incidence of infection in the local population, but one or other is essential. If screening is chosen, it is emphasized that antibiotic therapy should be started before abortion is performed.
- Women considered to be at high risk of hepatitis B or HIV should be offered screening with appropriate counselling. Women who refuse screening should be treated as high risk during the abortion procedure.
- Cervical screening should be offered in accordance with national screening policies.
- Blood should be collected for measurement of haemoglobin concentration, and the blood group should be determined. All women who are Rhesus negative should be injected with anti-D immunoglobulin prior to or within 48 h of the abortion to prevent the development of Rhesus isoimmunization.

Techniques of abortion

In general, the earlier the abortion is done, the safer it is. Mortality and morbidity associated with the procedure increase with the gestation of the pregnancy at the time of termination. The risk of major complications doubles when termination is carried out at 15 weeks of gestation compared with 8 weeks.

The method of choice depends on gestation, parity, medical history and the woman's wishes. The RCOG (2004b) state that, as a minimum, all services must be able to offer abortion by one of the recommended methods for each gestation band, but that services should ideally be able to offer a choice.

Early-first-trimester abortion (≤9 weeks)

Surgical

Vacuum aspiration has been the method of choice for early surgical termination of pregnancy in industrialized countries for over 20 years. Dilatation and curettage requires more cervical dilatation and is associated with a significantly higher complication rate, including uterine injury, and a higher incidence of retained products of conception and adverse future reproductive outcome (Henshaw and Templeton 1993).

Vacuum aspiration can be performed under either local paracervical block or general anaesthesia. Some evidence suggests that the use of general anaesthesia increases the risk of the procedure. In the USA, the mortality rate is two to four times greater when general anaesthesia is used rather than local anaesthesia for first-trimester abortion. Preoperative treatment with a cervical priming agent has been shown to reduce the risk of haemorrhage and genital tract trauma associated with vacuum aspiration. Prostaglandins, bougies and mifepristone are all effective, but prostaglandins (gemeprost 1 mg vaginally or misoprostol 400 μg vaginally, both 3 h before surgery) probably achieve their effect more quickly. Pretreatment of the cervix adds to the cost of the procedure and may be difficult to organize when abortion is performed as a day case. As cervical trauma is more common in women under the age of 17 years and uterine perforation is associated with increasing parity and increasing gestation, efforts to arrange cervical ripening should be concentrated on young women (aged <18 years), highly parous women and those presenting at a gestation of greater than 10 weeks.

A curette of up to 10 mm internal diameter is passed through the cervix, and the contents of the uterus are aspirated using negative pressure created by a pump. It is advisable to use the smallest diameter curette which is adequate for the gestation; most gynaecologists use an 8 mm curette at 8 weeks, 10 mm at 10 weeks, etc.

Vacuum aspiration at this stage of pregnancy is extremely safe and effective. Failure is more likely to occur before 7 weeks of gestation when it is possible to miss the fetus with the curette. For this reason, medical methods or a rigorous protocol for early surgical abortion are recommended. The mortality from vacuum aspiration in the first trimester is less than approximately one in 100,000; considerably less than the maternal mortality from continuing pregnancy.

Medical

Medical abortion is available to women in the UK up to 63 days of amenorrhoea (9 weeks of gestation) using a combi-
nation of the antiprogesterone mifepristone 600 mg orally followed 36–48 h later by the prostaglandin gemeprost 1 mg vaginally. Mifepristone is a synthetic steroid which blocks the action of progesterone by binding to its receptor. It also binds to the glucocorticoid receptor and blocks the action of cortisol. When mifepristone is used alone, complete abortion only occurs in approximately 60% of pregnancies. The rate of complete abortion rises to over 95% if a prostaglandin is given 36–48 h after the administration of mifepristone. The antiprogesterone itself stimulates some uterine contractility, but mainly works by greatly enhancing the sensitivity of the myometrium to the tocolytic effect of prostaglandins. A 200 mg dose of mifepristone is as effective as 600 mg and, given with an oral prostaglandin misoprostol (which is not licensed for abortion) 800 μg vaginally 36–48 h later, makes for a much cheaper and now commonly used regimen.

Offered the choice of method, approximately 30% of women in Scotland prefer medical abortion. Women often choose the medical method because it avoids an anaesthetic in most cases, and because they feel more in control of the situation. It is, however, a two-stage procedure which other women find a disadvantage. The incidence of serious complications is probably similar to that associated with surgical abortion, but because 95% of women need neither anaesthesia nor instrumentation of the uterus, large randomized trials may eventually show medical abortion to be safer. Not all women are suitable for medical abortion; the contraindications are shown in Box 29.2.

There are very few side-effects following administration of mifepristone. The fetus is usually passed within 4 h of prostaglandin administration, and this is accompanied by bleeding and pain. The bleeding is usually described as being like a very heavy period, although rarely (<1%) there may be very heavy bleeding requiring resuscitation. Nulliparous women and those with a history of dysmenorrhoea are more likely to experience severe pain, and 10–20% of women may need opiate analgesia. The rest will cope with paracetamol. Prostaglandin synthetase inhibitors, such as aspirin or mefenamic acid, should be avoided for obvious reasons. A few women will abort at home in response to mifepristone with variable amounts of bleeding and discomfort.

Box 29.2 Contraindications to medical abortion

Absolute contraindications

Adrenal insufficiency

Ectopic pregnancy

Asthma

Cardiac disease

Heavy smoker

Older than 35 years

On anticoagulants or bleeding disorder

Relative contraindications

Heavy smoker

>35 years

Obesity

Hypertension (diastolic >100 mmHg)

Bleeding can continue for up to 20 days after the abortion, although most women have usually stopped after 10 days. The total amount of blood lost is similar to that occurring at the time of vacuum aspiration.

All women should be given an appointment for follow-up approximately 2 weeks after administration of the prostaglandin. This visit is absolutely essential for those (approximately 30%) who have not passed an identifiable fetus and/or placental tissue while in hospital. Although ongoing pregnancy occurs in only 1% of cases, evacuation of the uterus will be necessary in approximately 2–5% of cases because of incomplete or missed abortion. These figures are no different from those associated with surgical abortion.

The risk of fetal malformation following mifepristone alone or in combination with prostaglandins is not known. Women should be clearly advised that medical abortion is a two-stage procedure, and that it is not possible to have a change of heart after taking mifepristone and before prostaglandin administration. Women who seem even remotely uncertain about abortion should certainly not be offered the medical method. In the event of failed medical abortion and therefore ongoing pregnancy, the patient must be strongly advised to have vacuum aspiration, although babies born to the few women who have chosen to continue with the pregnancy after medical abortion has failed have been normal.

Late-first-trimester abortion (9–13 weeks)

At this stage of pregnancy, the method of choice used to be vacuum aspiration as failure rates for medical methods were thought to be higher. However, a randomized trial of women between 9 and 13 weeks of gestation to either medical or surgical abortion found completed abortion rates to be comparable (Ashok et al 2002). This is reflected in the RCOG guidelines (2004b) which detail an effective medical regimen for this purpose. Surgical evacuation is a straightforward procedure up to 12 weeks of gestation, but thereafter requires specific experience and is not undertaken in many NHS settings. Although late-first-trimester abortion remains an extremely safe procedure, blood loss and other complications increase as gestation advances. It is important, therefore, to refer the woman for abortion promptly after the decision to terminate the pregnancy has been made.

Mid-trimester abortion

Second-trimester abortion accounts for 10–15% of all legal abortions in the UK. While many are done because of fetal malformation, it is often the women who are least able to cope with an unwanted pregnancy, particularly the very young, who first present at this time.

It is possible to induce abortion at this stage of pregnancy either medically or surgically. Surgical dilatation and evacuation (D&E) is the method of choice in the USA, but in the UK, its use is confined largely to gynaecologists in private practice. It may be necessary to dilate the cervix up to a diameter of 20 mm before the fetal parts can be extracted. D&E is a safe procedure in skilled hands, but if complications such as haemorrhage and perforation of the uterus are to be avoided, surgeons should be adequately trained. D&E should be preceded by cervical preparation, as described earlier.

Medical abortion for women presenting at greater than 15 weeks of gestation can be performed with mifepristone 600 or 200 mg orally, followed 36–48 h later by either gemeprost 1 mg vaginally every 3 h, up to a maximum of five pessaries, or by misoprostol 800 µg vaginally then 400 µg orally 3-hourly to a maximum of four oral doses.

Most women find the procedure painful and distressing, and require opiate analgesia. Evacuation of the uterus is necessary in approximately 30% of women who retain all or part of the placenta.

Abortion beyond 18 weeks of gestation is rare and is usually for pregnancies complicated by severe fetal malformation. Particularly distressing for both the mother and the staff, these late abortions are often effectively managed with vaginal prostaglandins in combination with mifepristone, with intra-amniotic urea or fetal intracardiac injection of potassium to minimize the chance of a live birth.

Follow-up

Anti-D immunoglobulin should be given to all non-sensitized Rhesus-D-negative women following any therapeutic abortion. Written advice about possible post-treatment symptoms, particularly those associated with infection, together with advice about what action to take should be given to patients before discharge home. All women should receive contraceptive advice and, if appropriate, supplies before going home. Ovulation can return within 20 days following abortion, and contraception should be started at the time of abortion if possible. All should be given a follow-up appointment within 2 weeks, either with the clinic which carried out the abortion or with a suitable alternative doctor. At follow-up, a pelvic examination should confirm complete abortion and the absence of infection. Discussion should include contraceptive advice and postabortion counselling, if required.

Complications

Mortality risk

In the UK, a woman is more likely to die in childbirth than she is to die from a complication of abortion (British Medical Association 2007). Although maternal mortality is, fortunately, extremely rare following abortion, the incidence of major complications, haemorrhage, thromboembolism, operative trauma (uterine perforation and cervical trauma) and infection is approximately 2%. The main factors affecting the incidence of complications in the RCGP study (Frank 1985) undertaken in the early 1980s were the place of operation (complications were less common when the abortion was done in a private hospital), gestation, method of abortion, sterilization at the time of operation and smoking habits.

Incomplete abortion

The most common complication following abortion is the persistence of placental and/or fetal tissue. Up to 5% of women undergoing first-trimester medical abortion will require surgical evacuation of the uterus within the first month. The incidence of incomplete abortion and ongoing pregnancy after vacuum aspiration rises as the gestation increases.

The occurrence of bleeding at 2 weeks after a medical or surgical abortion is not, in itself, an indication to evacuate the uterus. Ultrasound scans often show residual trophoblastic tissue even in women who have stopped bleeding. Although an ultrasound scan of the uterus and the measurement of human chorionic gonadotrophin in plasma may be helpful in diagnosing an ongoing pregnancy, the decision to evacuate the uterus should be made on clinical grounds (i.e. continued heavy or persistent bleeding from a bulky uterus in which the cervix is still dilated). The majority of women with an incomplete or missed abortion will pass the residual tissue with time if they are prepared to be patient. The belief that all women with an incomplete abortion had a high risk of intrauterine infection until the uterus was evacuated probably stemmed from the time when illegal abortion was common.

Minor complications

Some 10% of women undergoing abortion present to their general practitioner during the 3 weeks following the procedure with a variety of complaints related to the abortion. Lower abdominal pain, vaginal bleeding and passage of clots or trophoblastic tissue are relatively common and usually only require reassurance. It is, however, important to exclude infection. Established pelvic inflammatory disease with pyrexia, abdominal pain and offensive vaginal discharge occurs in approximately 1% of women whatever method of abortion is used.

Cervical and vaginal lacerations

Lacerations to the vagina and cervix are rare, and the risk of the latter can be reduced by pretreatment of the cervix in selected cases, as discussed earlier.

Late complications

There are very few late complications from abortion if women have been counselled carefully.

Psychological sequelae

Many women feel tearful and emotional for a few days following the abortion. However, many studies have demonstrated a significant improvement in psychological well-being by 3 months post abortion compared with before abortion (Adler et al 1990, 1992). Reviewers of existing literature have concluded that adverse psychiatric outcomes are observed in a minority of women following abortion, which are most often (although not exclusively) an exacerbation of morbidity predating the procedure, and that women denied abortion often experience significant ongoing resentment (Dagg 1991, Thorp et al 2002). Lack of a supportive partner, ambivalence regarding their decision or membership of a cultural group that forbids abortion are, unsurprisingly, risk factors for adverse psychological sequelae.

Infertility

Postabortion infection is a significant cause of tubal disease and infertility following illegal abortion. However, with modern methods performed under optimal conditions, the incidence of infection is very low, particularly where preoperative screening and treatment of infection are routine.

Subsequent pregnancy

Although damage to the cervix or perforation of the uterus can predispose to cervical incompetence, preterm delivery and/or uterine rupture, there is no significant increase in adverse outcome of any subsequent pregnancy.

KEY POINTS

1. Lack of contraceptive use continues to be a major problem in many developing countries.

2. The UKMEC, available in hard copy and online, provides consensus guidance on contraceptive prescribing.

3. The risks of MI and stroke in association with the COC have been exaggerated, and are minimal in women with no other risk factors, particularly smoking and hypertension.

4. The RR of VTE is increased in women taking the COC. However, the absolute risk of VTE is very small.

5. The CHC is associated with a highly significant reduction in the risk of ovarian and endometrial cancer, but those using the method for more than 8 years have an increased risk of having breast cancer diagnosed.

6. The efficacy of long-acting progestogen-only methods (implants, injectables, IUS) rivals that of sterilization.

7. The copper IUD is a very cheap and effective method of contraception which is underused.

8. The LNG-IUS reduces menstrual blood loss significantly and has increased the popularity of the IUD as a method of contraception.

9. EC is safe and is now available without prescription.

10. Antihormones, particularly antigestogens, show great promise for the development of new contraceptives.

11. There are a variety of ways of inducing therapeutic abortion, and women should be offered a choice of method within the context of a high-quality service which meets national standards.

References

Adler NE, David HP, Major BN, Roth SH, Russo NF, Wyatt GE 1990 Psychological responses after abortion. Science 268: 41–44.

Adler NE, David HP, Major BN, Roth SH, Russo NF, Wyatt GE 1992 Psychological factors in abortion. American Psychologist 47(10): 1194–1204.

Akerlund M, Rode A, Westergaard J 1993 Comparative profiles of reliability, cycle control and side effects of two oral contraceptive formulations containing

150 μg desorgestrel and either 30 μg or 20 μg ethinyl oestradiol. British Journal of Obstetrics and Gynaecology 100: 832–838.

Andersson JK, Rybo G 1990 Levonorgestrel-releasing intrauterine device in the treatment of menorrhagia. British Journal of Obstetrics and Gynaecology 97: 690–694.

Arowojolu AO, Gallo MF, Grimes DA et al Combined oral contraceptive pills for the treatment of acne. Cochrane Database of Systematic Reviews 2009. Issue 3 Art No: CD004425. DOI: 10.1002/14651858. CD004475.pub 4.

Ashok PW, Kidd A, Flett GMM et al 2002 A randomised comparison of medical and surgical vacuum aspiration at 10–13 weeks of gestation. Human Reproduction 17: 92–98.

Audet MC, Moreau M, Koltun WD et al for the ORTHO EVRA/EVRA 004 Study Group 2001 Evaluation of contraceptive efficacy and cycle control of a transdermal contraceptive patch vs an oral contraceptive. A randomized controlled trial. JAMA: the Journal of the Americal Medical Association 285: 2347–2354.

Baillargeon JP, McClish DK, Essah PA, Nestlet JE 2006 Association between the current use of low-dose oral contraceptives and cardiovascular arterial disease: a meta-analysis. Journal of Clinical Endocrinology and Metabolism 90: 3863–3870.

Beral V, Hermon C, Kay C, Hannaford P, Darby S, Reeves G 1999 Mortality associated with oral contraceptive use: 25 year follow up of a cohort of 46,000 women from Royal College of General Practitioners' oral contraception study. BMJ (Clinical Research Ed.) 318: 96–100.

Bernal-Delgado E, Latour-Perez J, Pradas-Arnal F, Gomez-Lopez LI 1998 The association between vasectomy and prostate cancer: a systematic review of the literature. Fertility and Sterility 70: 191–200.

Bloemenkamp KWM, Rosendaal FR, Helerhorst FM, Buller HR, Vandenbroucke JP 1995 Enhancement by factor V Leiden mutation of risk of deep vein thrombosis associated with oral contraceptive containing a third generation progestagen. Lancet 364: 1593–1596.

British Medical Association 2007 Briefing Paper. First Trimester Abortion. Available at: www.bma.org.

Celentano DD, Klassen AC, Weisman CS, Rosenheim NB 1987 Role of contraceptive use in cervical cancer. American Journal of Epidemiology 126: 592–604.

Chang CL, Donaghy M, Poulter N; WHO Collaborative Study of Cardiovascular Disease and Steroid Hormone Contraception 1999 Migraine and stroke in young women: a case control study. BMJ (Clinical Research Ed.) 318: 13–18.

Clinical Effectiveness Unit Available at: www.frsh.org.

Collaborative Group on Hormonal Factors in Breast Cancer 1996 Breast cancer and hormonal contraceptives: collaborative re-analysis of individual data on 53,297 women with breast cancer and 100,239 women without breast cancer from 54 epidemiological studies. The Lancet 347: 1717–1727.

Committee on Safety of Medicines 2006 Updated Prescribing Advice on the Effect of Depo-Provera Contraception on Bone. MRHA. Available at: www.medicines.mrha. gov.uk.

Curtis KM, Marchbanks PA 2005 Hormonal contraceptive use and cardiovascular safety. In: Glasier A, Wellings K, Critchley H (eds) Contraception and Contraceptive Use. RCOG Press.

Dagg PK 1991 The psychological sequelae of therapeutic abortion denied and completed. American Journal of Psychiatry 148: 579–585.

Dinger JC, Lothar AJ, Kuhl-Habisch D 2007 The safety of a drospirenone-containing oral contraceptive: final results from the European Active Surveillance study on Oral Contraceptives (EURAS) based on 142,475 women years of observation. Contraception 75: 344–354.

Duffy S, Marsh F, Rogerson L et al 2005 Female sterilization, a cohort controlled comparative study of Essure® versus laparoscopic sterilization. BJOG: an International Journal of Obstetrics and Gynaecology 112: 1522–1528.

Fraser IS 1983 A survey of different approaches to the management of menstrual disturbances in women using injectable contraceptives. Contraception 28: 385–397.

Frank PI 1985 Sequelae of induced abortion. In: Porter R, O'Connor M (eds) Abortion: Medical Progress and Social Implications. Ciba Foundation Symposium 115. Pitman, London.

Gbolade B, Ellis S, Murby B, Randall S, Kirkman R 1998 Bone density in long term users of depot medroxyprogesterone acetate. British Journal of Obstetrics and Gynaecology 105: 790–794.

Gentile GP, Kaufman SC, Helbig DW 1998 Is there any evidence for a post-tubal sterilization syndrome? Fertility and Sterility 69: 179–186.

Glasier A 2002 Implantable contraceptives for women, effectiveness, discontinuation rates, return of fertility and outcome of pregnancies. Contraception 65: 29–37.

Grimes DA 2000 Intrauterine device and upper genital tract infection. The Lancet 356: 1013–1019.

Guttmacher Institute 1995-2003 Facts on Abortion Worldwide. Available at: www. guttmacher.org/pubs/fb_IAW.pdf.

Hannaford PC, Severaj S, Elliott AM, Angus V, Iverson L, Lee AJ 2007 Cancer risk among users of oral contraceptives: cohort data from the RCGP's oral contraception study. BMJ (Clinical Research Ed.) 335: 651.

Henshaw RC, Templeton AA 1993 Methods used in first trimester abortion. Current Obstetrics and Gynaecology 3: 11–16.

Hieu DT, Tan TT, Tan DN, Nguyet PT, Than P, Vinh DQ 1993 31 781 cases of non-surgical female sterilization with quinacrine pellets in Vietnam. The Lancet 342: 213–217.

Hillis SD, Marchbanks PA, Taylor LR, Peterson HB 1998 Higher hysterectomy risk for sterilized than nonsterilized women: findings in the U.S. Collaborative Review of Sterilization. The U.S. Collaborative Review of Sterilization Working Group. Obstetrics and Gynecology 91: 241–246.

International Collaboration of Epidemiological Studies on Cervical Cancer 2007 Cervical cancer and hormonal contraceptives: collaborative reanalysis of data from 16573 women with and 33509 women without cervical cancer from 24 epidemiological studies. The Lancet 370: 1609–1621.

Jick H, Jick SS, Gurewich V, Myers MW, Vasilakis C 1995 Risk of idiopathic cardiovascular death and nonfatal thromboembolism in women using oral contraceptives with differing progestagen components. Lancet 346: 1589–1593.

Khader YS, Rice J, John L, Abuetta O 2003 Oral contraceptive use and risk of myocardial infarction: a meta-analysis. Contraception 68: 11–17.

Lakha F, Glasier A 2006 Unintended pregnancy and the use of emergency contraception among a large cohort of women attending for antenatal care or abortion in Scotland. The Lancet 368: 1782–1787.

McDonald SW 1997 Is vasectomy harmful to health? British Journal of General Practice 47: 381–386.

Moller H, Knudsen LB, Lynge E 1994 Risk of testicular cancer after vasectomy: cohort study of over 73000 men. BMJ (Clinical Research Ed.) 309: 295–299.

National Institute for Health and Clinical Excellence 2005 CG-30 Long-acting Reversible Contraception. RCOG Press, London. Available at: www.nice.org.uk.

Nirapathpongporn A, Huber DH, Krieger JN 1990 No-scalpel vasectomy at the King's birthday vasectomy festival. The Lancet 335: 894–895.

Office for National Statistics 2007/8 Omnibus Survey Report No. 37. Contraception and Sexual Health. Office for National Statistics, London. Available at: www.ons.gov.uk and www.statistics.gov.uk.

Perez A, Labbok M, Queenan J 1992 Clinical study of the lactational amenorrhoea method for family planning. The Lancet 339: 968–969.

Peterson HB, DeStefano F, Rubin GL, Greenspan JR, Lee NC, Ory HW 1983 Deaths attributable to tubal sterilisation in the United States 1977–1981. American

Journal of Obstetrics and Gynecology 146: 131–136.

Peterson HB, Xia Z, Hughes JM, Wilkox LS, Tylor LR, Trussel J for the U.S. Collaborative Review of Sterilization Working Group 1996 The risk of pregnancy after tubal sterilization: findings from the U.S. Collaborative Review of Sterilization. American Journal of Obstetrics and Gynecology 174: 1161–1170.

Peterson HB, Xia Z, Hughes JM, Wilkox LS, Tylor LR, Trussel J for the U.S. Collaborative Review of Sterilization 1997 The risk of ectopic pregnancy after tubal sterilization. New England Journal of Medicine 336: 762–767.

Peterson HB, Howards SS 1998 Vasectomy and prostate cancer: the evidence to date. Fertility and Sterility 70: 201–203.

Riman T, Nillson S, Persson IR 2004 Review of epidemiological evidence for reproductive and hormonal factors in relation to the risk of epithelial ovarian malignancies. Acta Obstetricia et Gynecologica Scandinavica 83: 783–795.

Robinson JC, Plichta S, Weisman CS et al 1992 Dysmenorrhoea and use of oral contraceptives in adolescent women attending a family planning clinic. American Journal of Obstetrics and Gynecology 166: 578–583.

Ross JA, Winfrey WL 2002 Unmet need for contraception in the developing world and the former Soviet Union: an updated estimate. International Family Planning Perspectives 28: 138–143.

Royal College of Obstetricians and Gynecologists 1999 The Management of Menorrhagia in Secondary Care. Evidence-based Clinical Guideline No. 5. RCOG, London.

Royal College of Obstetricians and Gynaecologists 2004a Male and Female Sterilisation. Evidence-based Clinical Guideline No. 4. RCOG, London.

Royal College of Obstetricians and Gynaecologists 2004b The Care of Women Requesting Abortion. Evidence-based Guideline No. 7. RCOG, London.

Scholes D, La Croix AZ, Ichikawa LE et al 2005 Change in bone mineral density among adolescent women using and discontinuing depot medroxyprogesterone acetate contraception. Archives of Paediatric and Adolescent Medicine 159: 139–144.

Spitzer W, Lewis MA, Hainemann LAJ, Thorogood M, MacRae KD 1996 Third generation oral contraceptives and risk of venous thromboembolic disorders: an international case-control study. British Medical Journal 312: 83–88.

Task Force on Postovulatory Methods of Fertility Regulation 1999 Comparison of three single doses of mifepristone as emergency contraception: a randomised trial. The Lancet 353: 697–702.

Teenage Pregnancy Independent Advisory Group. www.dcsf.gov.uk/everychildmatters/healthandwellbeing/teenagepregnancy/tpiag.

The Lane Committee Report on the Abortion Act. Report of the Committee on the Working of the Abortion Act. Comnd 5579, 1974.

Thorp JM Jr., Hartmann KE, Shadigan E 2002 Long term physical and psychological health consequences of induced abortion: review of the evidence. Obstetrical and Gynecological Survey 58: 67–69.

Trussel J 2007 Contraceptive efficacy. In: Hatcher RA, Trussel J, Nelson A, Kates W, Stewart F, Kowal D (eds) Contraceptive Technology, 19th edn. Ardent Media, New York.

UK Medical Eligibility Criteria for Contraceptive Use 2005/2006 Faculty of Sexual and Reproductive Health, London. Available at: www.fsrh.org.

Ursin G, Peters RK, Henderson BE, d'Ablaing IIIG, Monreo KR, Pike MC 1994 Oral contraceptive use and adenocarcinoma of cervix. The Lancet 344: 1390–1394.

Van Damme L, Chandeying V, Ramjee G et al 2000 Safety of multiple daily applications of COL-1492, a nonoxynol-9 vaginal gel, among female sex workers. AIDS (London, England) 14: 85–88.

Weiderpass E, Adani H, Baron JA et al 1999 Use of oral contraceptives and endometrial cancer risk (Sweden). Cancer Causes Control 10: 277–284.

World Health Organization Collaborative Study of Cardiovascular Disease and Steroid Hormone Contraception 1995 Effect of different progestagens in low oestrogen oral contraceptives on venous thromboembolic disease. Lancet 346: 1582–1588.

World Health Organization Medical Eligibility Criteria for Contraceptive Use (WHOMEC). 2009 Department of Reproductive Health. World Health Organization, 4th ed. WHO Press. Geneva. Available at: www. whqlibdoc.who.

World Health Organization Scientific Group 1998 Cardiovascular Disease and Steroid Hormone Contraception. WHO Technical Report Series 877. WHO, Geneva.

World Health Organization Collaborative Study of Cardiovascular Disease and Steroid Hormone Contraception 1998 Cardiovascular disease and use of oral and injectable progestogen-only contraceptives and combined injectable contraceptives. Contraception 57: 315–324.

CHAPTER 30

Psychosexual medicine

Susan V. Carr

Chapter Contents

INTRODUCTION	440		SEXUAL PROBLEMS IN THE FEMALE	442
THE ROLE OF THE GYNAECOLOGIST	440		SEXUAL PROBLEMS IN THE MALE	444
HUMAN SEXUALITY	440		TREATMENTS	445
SEXUAL PROBLEMS IN GENERAL	441		CONCLUSION	446
DEFINITIONS OF SEXUAL DYSFUNCTION	441		KEY POINTS	447

Introduction

Human sexuality is important because it is inherent in everyone. It is an integral part of every human being and it is up to every individual to deal with their own sexuality in whichever way they choose. Although so fundamental to human existence, scientific documentation of sexuality is relatively recent. Historically, there was a persistent refusal to recognize that women could enjoy sex. In 1857, Acton stated that 'Happily for society the majority of women are not much troubled with sexual feelings of any kind'. At the beginning of the 20th Century, Havelock Ellis, an English doctor, gave scientific voice to the idea that sexual activity was important in its own right, not just as a means of procreation. He wrote that 'Reproduction… is not necessarily connected with sex, nor is sex necessarily concerned with reproduction'. Freud's revolutionary theories of psychoanalysis put sex and the subconscious firmly on the scientific agenda, but it was not until some decades later that Kinsey published his ground-breaking study on male and female sexual behaviour in 1948 and 1953. These reports led to uproar in their day and spearheaded the ever-increasing interest in human sexuality from the scientific viewpoint.

The Role of the Gynaecologist

The gynaecologist has a major role to play in the field of psychosexual problems, in both their prevention and detection. Gynaecology is the branch of medicine which focuses on a woman's sexual and reproductive system, which forms an essential essence of her femaleness and her perception of herself as a complete woman. Gynaecology is concerned with the area of the woman's body that is integrally involved in sexual activity. Sexual activity and emotions are closely linked, and it is therefore important to be aware of the effect that any gynaecological problem may have on the woman's sexuality and, indeed, that of her partner, if she has one.

Modern medical teaching tends to recognize the emotional needs of patients, but unfortunately, some everyday gynaecological situations may unwittingly set the scene for psychosexual problems in the future. Psychosexual therapy concentrates on individual cases, interpreting each doctor–patient interaction as unique. Nonetheless, there are patterns of aetiologies which emerge in practice, such as a history of clinical procedures. Women may often trace their problem back to what may seem a minor gynaecological procedure, such as sterilization, termination of pregnancy or even vaginal examination, which is thus of crucial importance not only from a gynaecological perspective but also from a psychosexual perspective.

Human Sexuality

For ease of understanding, human sexuality can be divided into different components: gender identity, sexual orientation and sexual response.

Gender identity

Just under 50% of the population are diagnosed at birth as being female. They are biologically and legally female, and most tend to follow female biopsychosocial pathways throughout their lifetimes. Similarly, a male gender identity is experienced by the other 50% of the population, who are diagnosed at birth to be male. However, a tiny proportion of the population are transsexual. These are individuals whose biological sex and gender identity do not match. They are, in effect, born into the wrong body and may spend many difficult years undergoing a gender reassignment process. As all transsexuals are female at some stage

DOI: 10.1016/B978-0-7020-3120-5.00030-8

in their lives, they may come into contact with gynaecology services; therefore, it is important to have an awareness of this condition. A postoperative male-to-female transsexual presents on gynaecological examination as a hysterectomized female. The Gender Recognition Act 2004 allows change of birth certificate under UK law, and transwomen can now present to a gynaecologist without disclosing their trans status.

Sexual orientation

Sexual orientation is the definition of sexual attraction: the people to whom one's sexual desire is directed. Approximately 93% of the population are heterosexual (i.e. attracted to individuals of the opposite sex). Between 5% and 10% of the population are homosexual (i.e. men who are sexually attracted to men). A further 0.5–2% of women are lesbian (i.e. women who are sexually attracted to women). Seven percent of the population are bisexual and are attracted to both men and women. In the UK National Survey of Sexual Attitudes and Lifestyles, over half of the men who had had a male sexual partner in the previous 5 years had also had a female partner; the figure was higher for females at 75.8% (Wellins et al 1994).

Sexual orientation has particular relevance in well-woman health care. Lesbians may be reluctant to discuss their sexual orientation with a clinician, but as the majority have experienced heterosexual sexual intercourse or had vaginal penetrative sexual activity with fingers or sex toys, they are at risk of cervical dysplasia and sexually transmitted infection. Lesbians should be included in national cervical screening programmes and have the same well-woman checks as the rest of the female population. Lesbians generally have positive attitudes to the new human papilloma virus vaccine programmes, but feel that any health promotion materials should recognize their sexual orientation (McNair et al 2009) in order to increase uptake (see Chapter 66, Lesbian health issues, for more information).

Bisexual women are at the highest risk of sexual morbidity, and may be reluctant to speak openly about their sexuality to clinicians.

Sexual response

The human physiological sexual response is dependent not only on intact endocrine, vascular and neurological input, but also on sensory input. This has been described as the 'psychosomatic circle of sex' (Bancroft 2008). Female sexual responsiveness is a result of sensory input through the peripheral nerves of the somatic and autonomic nervous system, as well as through the cranial nerves and psychogenic stimulation. Precisely where and how afferent information is processed within the spinal cord and brain is unknown (Yang 2000). The frontal and temporal lobes and anterior hypothalamus are all shown to have some function in mediating the sexual response, but the extent of this is still unclear. Genital motor responses include pelvic vasocongestion and vaginal lubrication. During sexual intercourse, the vagina lengthens, the labia increase in size, the uterus draws back and the clitoris retracts; at orgasm, there is also contraction of the uterine and pelvic muscles.

Clinical clarification of the human sexual response was based on the Masters and Johnson model of four phases: excitement, plateau, orgasm and resolution. This description was then modified by Kaplan to a triphasic model of desire, arousal and orgasm. These concepts provide the working models on which behavioural therapies for sexual problems are based. Recent scientific arguments have proposed that sexual desire is, in fact, the first early stage of arousal, triggered by a stimulus which has sexual meaning and is modified by situational and partner variables (Janssen et al 2000).

Most human sexuality is non-problematic and will not be within the domain of the clinician. It is only when something goes wrong with the patient's sexual response that they may seek professional help.

Sexual Problems in General

Population prevalence

The majority of the population at any one time have a trouble-free sex life. There is, however, a substantial minority for whom dealing with and expressing their sexuality is problematic. These problems may only be temporary or situational. If they persist and become increasingly distressing, the individual may seek professional help. The population prevalence of some degree of sexual dysfunction is estimated to be approximately 20%. Prevalence increases with age; overall, 40–45% of women and 20–30% of adult men report at least one sexual dysfunction at any one time (Lewis et al 2004). In the National Health and Social Life Survey (Laumann et al 1999), one-third of women reported loss of libido. Almost 25% did not experience orgasm. Approximately 20% had problems with vaginal lubrication, and a similar number did not enjoy sex. This study suggested that there was a substantial comorbidity of sexual problems. A study of US women (West et al 2008) showed that whilst 26.7% of premenopausal women had low sexual desire, 52.4% of naturally menopausal women had the same complaint. For males, the prevalence of some degree of erectile dysfunction has been reported as 30% of all males between the ages of 40 and 70 years. Premature ejaculation occurs in 10–30% of men during their lifetime. In a control group of 591 members of the general population in a Dutch study, 8.7% of men and 14.9% of women reported a sexual dysfunction unrelated to age (Diemont et al 2000), which is lower than that reported in other countries.

Definitions of Sexual Dysfunction

In the recent literature, there has been much positive debate about redefining sexual disorders, especially in the female. It is generally agreed that the definitions need clarification, especially in relation to research (Derogatis and Burnett 2008). Clinically, there is a lot of overlap in presentation, and clearer definition would help preventive and treatment strategies. Much work has concentrated on female sexual dysfunction, helping in understanding the organic basis for some problems (Meston and Bradford 2007); however, massive treatment breakthroughs have yet to follow.

Having a sexual dysfunction does not necessarily mean that the individual has a sexual problem. This will depend on the effect, if any, that the dysfunction has on the life of the individual in terms of their feelings, relationships and lifestyle. Conversely, restoration of sexual function may not solve the sexual problem; in fact, it may serve to highlight an underlying emotional or relationship discord. Individuals with psychosexual problems usually have no organic sexual dysfunction whatsoever.

Problems of function or desire

Sexual disorders can be divided into problems of function or desire. They are often interlinked. For example, impaired sexual function, such as some degree of erectile problem, can result in the man protecting himself from the distress of failure by emotionally shutting himself off from coitus altogether. This results in loss of libido. If a woman is experiencing loss of function such as dyspareunia, she may subconsciously employ the same defensive mechanisms, and loss of desire develops.

The most common female sexual problems are vaginismus, loss of libido, dyspareunia and inorgasmia. There will be differences in the frequency of presenting sexual complaints in different clinical settings. An American gynaecology clinic sample showed loss of libido (87.2%) with inorgasmia (83%) and dyspareunia (72%) (Nusbaum et al 2000). In a community-based setting such as a family planning clinic, however, loss of libido, dyspareunia and vaginismus are the most common presenting complaints, with a low incidence of inorgasmia.

In males, erectile dysfunction, ejaculatory disorders and loss of libido are the most frequent presenting complaints, all of which will affect the partner to some degree.

Problems relevant to gynaecology

There are many gynaecological conditions which may predispose to sexual problems. Any disease or its treatment which results in alteration of the genitalia may cause functional sexual difficulties. These conditions may range from having colposcopy, where spontaneous interest in sex was found to be lower 6 months post procedure, irrespective of whether or not treatment was needed (Hellsten 2008), to traumatic obstetric delivery or gynaecological malignancy. Trauma or disease, however, may cause an alteration in the woman's perception of herself, such as distorted body image causing sexual problems. This may or may not be directly related to physical reality. An exceptionally high rate of sexual dissatisfaction was found in a gynaecology clinic sample in the USA. Over 98.8% of the sample reported one or more sexual worries, and body image concerns were reported by 68.5% of the 1480 women who attended (Nusbaum et al 2000). A study of Dutch gynaecologists found that one in 14 of their patients presenting in the previous week had problems of a sexual nature, mainly dyspareunia or lack of sexual desire (Frenken and van Tol 1987). A significant degree of deterioration of sexual function was described in a study of 41 women who had undergone vulvectomy, attributed to disturbed body image rather than physical impairment (Green et al 2000). The rate of sexual problems in women with gynaecological cancers is approximately 50%. The main complaint of this client group is lack of opportunity to discuss these problems.

Once any gynaecological treatment is completed, the treatment approach for the sexual problem is the same as for any other patient.

Sexual Problems in the Female

Vaginismus

Vaginismus is a condition in which nothing is able to enter the vagina. This means that penetrative sexual intercourse does not take place. It is caused by psychogenically mediated involuntary spasm of the vaginal muscles. Vaginismus can be primary or secondary. In primary vaginismus, nothing has ever entered the woman's vagina. A useful diagnostic question is 'Have you ever used a tampon'. In a case of primary vaginismus, the answer will always be 'no'. Secondary vaginismus can appear at any time in a woman's life, sometimes after childbirth or any other life-changing event.

The vagina is physiologically intact in a case of vaginismus. There is no stenosis or organic disorder. This is a psychogenic condition for which the treatment is psychosexual, never surgical.

Presentation

Vaginismus is a condition which usually has a masked presentation. One of the most common presentations is the avoidance of cervical smears. No woman likes having a vaginal examination or smear. The alert clinician, however, will observe a patient's persistent avoidance of examination or a fear of being examined which is in excess of that usually observed by the clinician. If vaginismus is suspected, a forced vaginal examination should not be done. This is the equivalent of medical rape, which can have a long-lasting traumatic effect on the woman.

Vaginismus can present initially as dyspareunia or painful sexual intercourse. In this case, the couple are not really having sex; as the erect penis attempts vaginal entry, the vaginal muscles contract and the interaction becomes painful. Vaginismus can also be a cofactor in loss of libido, although more commonly the woman has a strong desire to have sex, 'just like everybody else'.

Vaginismus may present as infertility. It is essential to ask the infertile couple whether or not they are having vaginal intercourse. Patients still reach tertiary referral centres for assisted conception where it is discovered that sexual intercourse has never taken place and vaginismus is the primary diagnosis.

Unconsummated relationships are usually due to vaginismus, but can occasionally be due to male sexual dysfunction.

Treatment

There are various different approaches to the treatment of vaginismus. There are no data to suggest which method is best, and to date there has been no randomized controlled trial comparing methods of treatment. Treated by a skilled clinician, the reported cure rate is 90%.

Psychodynamic methods

The trained clinician helps the patient to understand the basis for her problem and to recognize the barriers to sex. This method can take up to 2 years to cure the vaginismus, but deals with the root causes of the problem as well as offering practical solutions.

Behavioural methods

Evidence shows that cognitive behavioural therapy is effective (van Lankveld 2006), and can also be used with couples (Kabakci and Batur 2003). A useful adjunct to therapy is the use of vaginal trainers, which are plastic 'pseudopenises' made in graduated sizes, which the woman is taught to insert into her own vagina. The same effect can be gained by using fingers. This teaches her that she can be in control of what enters her body. This can be a good adjunct to psychodynamic therapy.

Supplying vaginal trainers without supportive therapy is unlikely to show sustained benefit.

Classic couple therapy, based on the Masters and Johnson model, is also shown to be effective, with success rates of 93% reported (Jeng 2006). Recent reports of the intravaginal use of botulinum toxin are promising (Ghazizadeh and Nikzad 2004). The use of surrogate male partners was shown to be effective in women without a cooperative partner (Ben-Zion 2007), but clearly raises many social and ethical issues in treatment.

Surgery has no place in the treatment of vaginismus.

Inorgasmia

Inorgasmia is the lack of ability to experience orgasm. There are two main areas of innervation in the female genital region that can produce orgasmic symptoms if stimulated. The main area is the clitoris and there is another inside the vagina, about two-thirds of the way up, close to the urethra. This is known as the 'G-spot'.

Presentation

The woman will either complain of inability to experience orgasm or may say that she does not know whether or not the feelings she is having constitute orgasm. Presentation at a clinic with this complaint will usually have been prompted by the acquisition of a new partner, the inability to find a partner or by popular media interest in the topic.

Treatment

There are some women who have no feelings at all in the clitoral area. Women with selective serotonin reuptake inhibitor (SSRI)-induced loss of sensation and sexual dysfunction showed improvement on taking sildenafil (Nurnberg et al 2008). Combined oestrogen and androgen therapy may improve sexual sensation in menopausally triggered inorgasmia. Sildenafil may also improve clitoral blood flow in menopausal women with orgasmic dysfunction and women with type 1 diabetes.

With women who have never experienced orgasm, however, drug treatment alone is unlikely to work. Encouraging body self-awareness, by discussion of female genital anatomy and physiology, will help. Encouraging masturba-

tion is very rewarding. If this is combined with psychodynamic input, the patient usually responds.

Loss of libido

Loss of libido is loss of sexual desire. It is generally associated with loss of self-esteem due to a multitude of underlying causes. There may be a traumatic event in the past which has not been dealt with emotionally and which may cause problems, such as loss of libido, at a later stage in the woman's lifetime. Examples of this are rape, sexual or emotional abuse, or a loss such as bereavement or redundancy leading to loss of status and loss of self-esteem.

There are associations between loss of desire and hormonal status in postmenopausal women. Hypoactive sexual desire disorder is much more common in menopausal women, especially young women with surgical menopause. There is, however, no physiological marker for loss of libido, and there is rarely a 'quick fix' solution to the problem.

Presentation

Loss of libido may present as depression or as a relationship problem. The woman may be uncomfortable broaching the subject but, if prompted by an empathetic clinician, may disclose the problem. In areas of gynaecological health care where body image becomes problematic, such as oncology, menopause and continence, loss of libido may be an overlooked complaint.

Treatment

The core treatment for loss of libido is psychosexual therapy, which deals with the underlying psychogenic origin of the problem. Counselling before procedures can allow women to explore their feelings in relation to these procedures. A past history of abortion is not uncommon in women with loss of libido. Pretermination of pregnancy counselling is, of necessity, information based and time limited. After termination of pregnancy, however, there is an opportunity for the woman to come to terms with what has happened, thus preventing the development of sexual problems later in life and hopefully preventing repeat unwanted pregnancy. After sterilization, there will be some women who suffer loss of libido. Even if they have no regrets over the procedure, they may not have realized the emotional impact of losing their fertility as they have not understood the difference between choosing not to have a child and not being able to conceive.

In cases where the loss of libido can be clearly linked to a hormonal trigger, such as starting a different combined oral contraceptive, changing contraception can improve the problem.

There is some evidence for the addition of androgens to oestrogen replacement therapy for menopausal loss of libido (Kingsberg 2007). Hormonal therapy alone, however, can only return a woman to her premenopausal status and cannot change any underlying emotional blocks to sexual desire. The menopause is a time of major social and emotional upheaval for many women, which can be as overwhelming as adolescence, so psychosexual therapy combined with appropriate hormone replacement therapy would seem to be best practice.

Dyspareunia

Dyspareunia is painful sexual intercourse. It may be described as deep or superficial. There are organic causes for this, such as post delivery, after gynaecological operations, genital infections and in any condition which causes vaginal dryness, such as menopause. Vulval pain syndrome, or vulvodynia, is a complex condition which causes severe dyspareunia.

Vaginal dryness can be physiological, caused by lack of sufficient sexual stimulation during intercourse.

Presentation

Dyspareunia is a common presenting complaint to the gynaecologist. Some women (and doctors!) find it easier to discuss than some other sexual problems, as it seems more likely than other sexual complaints to have an organic origin. Postdelivery dyspareunia is reported frequently but, on average, women resume sexual intercourse at 7 weeks post partum (Byrd et al 1998). Approximately 15% of women have chronic dyspareunia of unclear origin (Weijmar Schultz et al 2005), and as well as causing distress to the patient, this presents an enormous challenge to the gynaecologist.

Treatment

If dyspareunia persists despite clinical evidence of cure of the underlying condition, or no clinical findings despite full appropriate genitourinary and gynaecological investigation, psychosexual therapy should be considered. Recommended therapy for vulval pain syndromes is multidisciplinary with psychosexual input in coordination with gynaecological treatment (Nunns 2000). There is now a recognition that more research and clarification of definitions of sexual pain, particularly in relation to vulvar vestibulitis and vaginismus, is required in order to focus treatment (Weijmar Schultz et al 2005).

Various treatments now have evidence to recommend their use. Pelvic floor physiotherapy is an important tool of modern assessment and treatment (Rosenbaum 2005). The use of vibrators (Zolnoun et al 2008) is helpful and can be easily accessed and used by the women without clinical intervention. Hypnosis (Pukall et al 2007) and vaginal botulinum toxin type A have been reported as having positive therapeutic effects, and can increase the ability to have relatively pain-free and pleasurable sexual intercourse.

The emotional aspects of vulvar pain should never be ignored. Sometimes the memory of a previous painful condition may lead to expectation of pain on intercourse. This can produce involuntary vaginal muscle spasm, causing secondary vaginismus and thereby perpetuating the dyspareunia despite treatment of the original cause.

Physiological dyspareunia is caused by vaginal dryness due to lack of sufficient and appropriate sexual stimulation. It is treated by helping the woman to understand the cause of the problem. Discussion of sexual technique may help, emphasizing foreplay. Enabling the woman to gain insight into the nature of her relationship with her partner is an essential part of this process.

Sexual problems of lesbians

Gynaecologists should remember that not all women are heterosexual. Lesbians have similar sexual problems to other women but, as they find it difficult to disclose their sexual orientation to doctors, it may be even harder for them to discuss sexual problems than it is for heterosexuals. Women complaining of loss of libido, inorgasmia or dyspareunia may be in same-sex relationships. Vaginal penetration, as with all women, may occur with fingers and sex toys. Once organic causes have been excluded, psychosexual therapy should be offered. Synchronicity of menstruation in women living together, possibly due to pheromonal influence, has been documented (McClintock 1998). This is not universal but, where it exists, the coincidence of severe premenstrual symptoms can trigger domestic violence in lesbian couples, which can be an underlying cause of sexual problems (see Chapter 66, Lesbian health issues, for more information).

Sexual Problems in the Male

Gynaecologists are unlikely to be in the front line when dealing with male sexual problems, but as many of their female patients have male partners, it is important to have an overview of this area. If her partner has sexual problems, the woman can feel hurt and rejected, and will frequently blame herself, presenting at a clinic for help in solving the problem.

Erectile dysfunction

Erectile dysfunction is the inability to sustain a penile erection sufficient to achieve satisfactory penetrative sexual intercourse. According to the oft-quoted Massachusetts Male Aging Study, the incidence of erectile dysfunction in men aged 40–69 years is 25.9 cases per 1000 man-years; 60% of cases are organic in origin, 15% are psychogenic and 25% are of mixed origin (Aytac et al 2000).

Aetiology

Erectile dysfunction can be caused by any disruption of the neurological, endocrine or vascular supply to the genitalia. It can also occur for entirely psychogenic reasons. Associated factors are age, diabetes, alcohol intake, hypertension and the side-effects of many medications. Erectile dysfunction reduces quality of life and may lead to other associated sexual problems, such as loss of libido.

Presentation

The man with erectile dysfunction may present to a doctor himself, although it is not unusual for the female partner of a male with a sexual problem to present herself as the patient. She may say that she is experiencing either loss of sexual interest or painful sex. The couple themselves may not recognize where the problem lies.

Treatment

The treatment depends on the cause and falls into four basic categories: chemical, mechanical, surgical and psychosexual.

Oral therapy is now available which has revolutionized treatment of this distressing condition. The phosphodiesterase type 5, cyclic GMP inhibitors are now widely used worldwide. The drugs are facilitators, not initiators, of erections. These oral medications have reported efficacy rates of approximately 70% for sexual intercourse. They produce a vasodilatory effect and must not be used routinely for patients with coronary insufficiency on nitrates. The recreational use of amyl nitrate 'poppers', employed to facilitate anal intercourse, is strongly contraindicated with these drugs.

Locally acting chemical treatments can also be used. Alprostadil, which is prostaglandin E, can be injected into the base of the penis, causing smooth muscle relaxation and resulting in an erection. It can also be introduced by a tiny pellet into the urethra, causing an erection. Both methods have success rates of approximately 70%. Success rates with this urethral medication have been improved by the use of a penile constriction band which augments local retention. A newer combination of alprostadil and an α-adrenergic antagonist enhances erection rates, and other medications are being researched. This causes smooth muscle relaxation, leading to engorgement of the corpora cavernosa and erection of the penis. Although there can be some local discomfort, there are few contraindications to this therapy. It does, however, require manual dexterity and a willingness to inject or to insert medication into the penis. Unsurprisingly, there are fairly high discontinuation rates for this type of invasive therapy.

The simplest, non-invasive treatments are vacuum devices. A constriction ring is first applied to the base of the flaccid penis, then a vacuum is created, causing engorgement of the corpora cavernosa which is maintained by the constriction ring. This method creates a slightly blue, cold erection which may be sufficient for intercourse, and which is suitable for some men who prefer non-chemical treatment methods. Surgery is required if a venous shunt has been demonstrated or to insert a prosthesis, if there are no other options for treatment.

Psychosexual therapy is an important therapy to consider in cases of erectile dysfunction, either on its own or as an adjunct to physical therapy, as 40% of cases of erectile dysfunction have a psychogenic element. This form of treatment allows the man to explore all the issues surrounding his problem, and also allows him to include his partner in treatment if he wishes. It also takes a whole-person approach, rather than merely focusing on the genitalia.

Premature ejaculation

Premature ejaculation is the most common male sexual problem worldwide. It is a condition where the male reaches the point of orgasm and ejaculates very rapidly, before satisfactory sexual intercourse has taken place. It is frequently a complaint of young men but may present in all age groups.

Presentation

The man suffering from premature ejaculation will ask for clinical help if it is affecting his sexual satisfaction or relationships.

Treatment

A psychodynamic approach will help the man to understand and cope with his anxieties related to the problem.

The 'squeeze' technique can be used. If the thumb and forefinger are used to squeeze firmly at the base of the glans penis at the point of ejaculation, ejaculation will be delayed. This technique, however, requires a good degree of coordination.

The mainstay of treatment, however, is the use of antidepressant medication, such as clomipramine or SSRIs, which have been shown to increase ejaculation latency. Daily use of SSRIs is more effective than on-demand treatment (Waldinger 2007).

Delayed ejaculation

Delayed ejaculation is a condition which is usually psychogenic in origin. Infrequently, it can be a side-effect of some medications. It can be extremely distressing to the female partner, and if penetrative, thrusting sexual intercourse becomes prolonged due to a failure of the man to become orgasmic, it can lead to dyspareunia. The male may be able to ejaculate when masturbating but is unable to do so intravaginally. This could be for various subconscious reasons, some of which are fear of losing control, fear of causing pregnancy or unwillingness to make a commitment to his partner (Thexton 1992).

Treatment

Psychosexual therapy is the treatment of choice. This problem may take a prolonged course of therapy before positive outcomes are achieved.

Loss of libido

This can affect men as well as women. Rarely, lack of testosterone may be implicated but the cause is usually emotional and will frequently be linked to some cause of loss of self-esteem in the man.

Treatments

Most problems of a sexual nature have a psychogenic origin. Even sexual problems with clear organic origins tend to have some degree of psychogenic overlay, as sexual activity, or the lack of it, has emotional impacts.

There are three main treatment modalities for sexual problems: psychodynamic methods, behavioural methods and drug treatments.

Psychodynamic methods

Psychodynamic medicine is concerned with understanding how emotional factors interfere with sexual activity and enjoyment. These emotional factors may not be at the conscious level. The aim of treatment is to enable the patient to resolve the problem by removing the psychological blocks to satisfactory sexual activity and relationships (Skrine 1989). This is achieved by taking a 'mind–body' approach to the patient and their sexual problem. The psychosexually trained clinician will explore the problem with the patient by interpreting the doctor–patient interaction, and feeding these observations back to the patient in order to elicit their response.

An important part of this treatment is the psychogenic genital examination. Many of the patient's underlying attitudes, fears and fantasies related to their sexual problem may be revealed in relation to this part of the consultation.

The philosophy of treatment is that the patient is 'whoever presents' at the consultation. This mode of treatment is suitable for individuals, regardless of whether or not they are in a relationship. It is also appropriate for couples, regardless of gender identity or sexual orientation.

Not all psychosexual problems require prolonged specialist treatment. A single consultation with a suitably trained doctor is sufficient help for some patients.

Behavioural methods

Behavioural methods involve a more didactic, 'hands-on' approach to treatment. This philosophy of treatment was developed through the early work of Masters and Johnson, and Helen Singer Kaplan. Patients are given practical tasks in order to learn or relearn how to experience and enjoy sexual activity. This approach maintains that the many causes of sexual dysfunction can be treated effectively by a programme combining education, homework assignments and counselling. A staged approach to re-establishing healthy sexual contact can be a useful therapeutic tool when dealing with couples, and has been modified to treat single individuals although it is felt to be of most use for people with partners.

Cognitive behavioural therapy is increasingly used as a practical and effective method of treatment of sexual problems.

Drug treatments

Drug treatment of male erectile dysfunction has been shown to have a high success rate, and there is some evidence for improvements in premature ejaculation with antidepressants (e.g. SSRIs) or anticholinergics (e.g. clomipramine). Medication may restore genital function, but associated emotional and relationship issues should also be addressed appropriately.

For women, there has been increased interest in the possibility of drug treatment for sexual dysfunction. Despite much research, the only evidence-based conclusion is that appropriate hormone replacement therapy with the addition of androgen will improve sexual functioning in some postmenopausal women. Research has shown an influence of adrenergic compounds on physiological sexual arousal, but not on the woman's subjective sexual experience (Everaerd and Laan 2000), which is, in fact, what matters most in sexual functioning. Compounds used to increase male penile blood flow have been shown to have limited success in women in clearly defined circumstances. If the woman's medication is thought to be causally associated with loss of libido, such as some hormonal contraceptives, antiepileptics and psychotropic drugs, a change of drug may help.

The mainstay of treatment for sexual problems, however, particularly for women, is therapy which deals with the emotional and interpersonal blocks to satisfactory sexual activity. Sensitivity to the emotional aspects of the consultation, and possible sexual sequelae of the gynaecological condition or its treatment, may prevent the onset of sexual problems in the future.

Service provision

Over the last few years, the amount of research into all aspects of women's sexual problems has proliferated. Sadly, service provision and professional training do not seem to have kept up the same pace. Many localities have some provision of service for the treatment of psychosexual problems; however, rural and outlying areas often have none. Sexual and reproductive healthcare services may have an attached sexual problems clinic, which provides treatment in a non-threatening and non-judgemental, community-based environment. In areas of gynaecological care, such as cancer services, where the prevalence of sexual problems can be as high as 50%, the provision of sexual problems services is not uniformly available, despite women's wishes for the provision of these services.

Many people find it very embarrassing to disclose a sexual problem to anyone, and a self-referral facility for making appointments can encourage patients to come forward for treatment.

Conclusion

With such a large minority of women experiencing some form of sexual difficulty in their lifetime, from adolescence to menopause and beyond, it is vital for the gynaecologist to be aware of these conditions and to allow the woman to voice her concerns in a confidential, empathetic and non-threatening environment. Just being listened to and having her concerns acknowledged in an empathetic and non-judgemental manner can be enough to initiate the therapeutic process. If she wishes, referral can be made to the appropriate local sexual problems service. With suitable training, however, it is possible to employ brief focused analytical techniques within the context of a routine gynaecological appointment. This allows the gynaecologist to assess the psychosexual element of the situation, and enhances the quality of care for the patient.

KEY POINTS

1. Sexual problems are prevalent in society and have either an organic, emotional or mixed origin. The mode of treatment depends on the cause.

2. Sexual problems can present unexpectedly in any clinical setting, and commonly in community or hospital gynaecology clinics.

3. Patients find it difficult to disclose problems of a sexual nature. Increased awareness by the gynaecologist and a willingness to introduce the topic is helpful.

4. A gynaecologist trained in basic psychosexual techniques can provide help to the patient within the context of the gynaecology clinic setting.

5. Dyspareunia presenting to the gynaecologist with negative clinical findings may have a psychogenic origin.

6. Primary vaginismus is of psychogenic origin and surgery has no place in its treatment.

7. Loss of libido is mostly of emotional origin, but the addition of testosterone to hormone replacement therapy is beneficial in some menopausal women.

References

Acton W 1857 The functions and disorders of the reproductive organs. In youth, adult age and advanced life. John Churchill, Condon.

Aytaç IA, Araujo AB, Johannes CB, Kleinman KP, McKinlay JB 2000 Sep Socioeconomic factors and incidence of erectile dysfunction: findings of the longitudinal Male Aging Study. Soc Sci Med 51(5): 771–778.

Bancroft J 2008 Human Sexuality and its Problems. Churchill Livingstone, Edinburgh.

Ben-Zion I, Rothschild S, Chudakov B, Aloni R 2007 Surrogate versus couple therapy in vaginismus. Journal of Sexual Medicine 4: 728–733.

Byrd JE, Hyde JS, de Lamater JD, Plant E, Ashby MS 1998 Sexuality during pregnancy and the year postpartum. Journal of Family Practice 47: 305–308.

Derogatis LR, Burnett AL 2008 The epidemiology of sexual dysfunctions. Journal of Sexual Medicine 5: 289–300.

Diemont WL, Wruggink P, Meuleman E, Doesburg W, Lemmens W, Berden J 2000 Sexual dysfunction after renal replacement therapy. American Journal of Kidney Diseases 35: 845–851.

Everaerd W, Laan E 2000 Drug treatments for women's sexual disorders. Journal of Sex Research 37: 195–204.

Frenken J, van Tol P 1987 Sexual problems in gynaecological practice. Journal of Psychosomatic Obstetrics and Gynaecology 6: 143–155.

Freud Sigmund 1987 Fall-Winter The origin and development of psychoanalysis. 1910. Am J Psychol 100 (3–4): 472–488. Freud S. PMID: 3322053.

Ghazizadeh S, Nikzad M 2004 Botulinum toxin in the treatment of refractory vaginismus. Obstetrics and Gynecology 104: 922–925.

Green MS, Naumann R, Elliott M, Hall J, Higgins R, Grigsby J 2000 Sexual dysfunction following vulvectomy. Gynaecologic Oncology 77: 73–77.

Helen Singer Kaplan 1974 The New Sex Therapy. Brunner/Mazel, New York.

Havelock Ellis Studies in the psychology of sex (reprint General Books LCC 2009).

Hellsten C, Lindqvist PG, Sjöström K 2008 A longitudinal study of sexual functioning in women referred for colposcopy: a 2-year follow up. BJOG 115: 205–211.

Janssen E, Everaerd W, Spiering M, Janssen J 2000 Automatic processes and the appraisal of sexual stimuli. Journal of Sex Research 37: 8.

Jeng CJ, Wang LR, Chou CS, Shen J, Tzeng CR 2006 Oct-Dec Management and outcome of primary vaginismus. J Sex Marital Ther 32 (5): 379–387.

Kabakci E, Batur S 2003 Who benefits from cognitive behavioural therapy for vaginismus? Journal of Sex and Marital Therapy 29: 277–288.

Kingsberg S 2007 Testosterone treatment for hypoactive sexual desire disorder in postmenopausal women. Journal of Sexual Medicine 4 (Suppl 3): 227–234.

Kinsey AC, Wardell B, Pomoroy C, Martin E 1947 Sexual behaviour In Human male. Saunders, New York.

Laumann EO, Paik A, Rosen RC 1999 Sexual dysfunction in the United States: prevalence and predictors. JAMA: the Journal of the American Medical Association 281: 537–544.

Lewis RW, Fugl-Meyer KS, Bosch R et al 2004 Epidemiology/risk factors of sexual dysfunction. Journal of Sexual Medicine 1: 35–39.

Masters and Johnson's 2008 Sex Research and Sex. Routledge, New York. Hollie J. Fuhrmann; Eric R. Buhi.

Meston CM, Bradford A 2007 Sexual dysfunctions in women. Annual Review of Clinical Psychology 3: 233–256.

McClintock M 1998 Whither menstrual synchronicity? Annual Review of Sex Research 9: 77–95.

McNair R, Power J, Carr S 2009 Comparing knowledge and perceived risk related to the human papilloma virus amongst Australian women of diverse sexual identities. Australian and New Zealand Journal of Public Health 33: 87–93.

Nunns D 2000 Vulval pain syndromes. British Journal of Obstetrics and Gynaecology 107: 1185–1193.

Nurnberg HC, Hensley PL, Heiman JR, Croft HA, Debattista C, Paine S 2008 Sildenafil treatment of women with anti-depressant associated sexual dysfunction: a randomized controlled trial. JAMA: the Journal of the American Medical Association 300: 395–404.

Nusbaum M, Gamle G, Skinner B, Heiman J 2000 The high prevalence of sexual concerns among women seeking routine gynaecology care. Journal of Family Practice 49: 229–232.

Pukall C, Kandyba K, Amsel R, Khalife S, Binik Y 2007 Effectiveness of hypnosis for the treatment of vulvar vestibulitis syndrome: a preliminary investigation. Journal of Sexual Medicine 4: 417–425.

Rosenbaum TV 2005 Physiotherapy treatment of sexual pain disorders. Journal of Sex and Marital Therapy 31: 329–340.

Skrine R (ed) 1989 Introduction to Psychosexual Medicine. Chapman and Hall, London.

Thexton R 1992 Ejaculatory disturbances. In: Lincoln R (ed) Psychosocial Medicine: a Study of Underlying Themes. Chapman and Hall, Boston.

Van Lankveld JJ, ter Kuile MM, de Groot HE, Melles R, Nefs J, Zandbergen M 2006 Cognitive-behavioural therapy for women with lifelong vaginismus; a randomised waiting-list controlled trial of efficacy. Journal of Consulting and Clinical Psychology 74: 168–178.

Waldinger MD 2007 Premature ejaculation: state of the art. Urologic Clinics of North America 34: 591–599.

Weijmar Schultz W, Bason R, Binik Y, Eschenbach D, Wesselmann U, Van Lankveld J 2005 Womens sexual pain and its management. Journal of Sexual Medicine 2: 301–306.

West SL, D'Aloisio AA, Agans RP, Kalsboek WD, Borisov NN, Thorp JM 2008 Prevalence of low sexual desire and hypoactive sexual desire disorder in a nationally representative sample of US women. Archives of Internal Medicine 168: 1441–1449.

Wellins K, Field J, Johnson A, Wadsworth J 1994 Sexual Behaviour in Britain. Penguin, London.

Yang C 2000 Female sexual function in neurologic disease. Journal of Sex Research 37: 205–212.

Zolnoun D, Lamvu G, Steege J 2008 Patient perceptions of vulvar vibration therapy for refractory vulvar pain. Journal of Sexual and Relationship Therapy 23: 345–353.

Psychosexual Training Information

Institute of Pyschosexual Medicine www.ipm.org.uk.

British Association of Sexual and Relationship Therapy www.basrt.org.uk.

Faculty of Sexual and Reproductive Healthcare of the Royal College of Obstetrics and Gynaecology www.ffprhc.org.uk.

CHAPTER 31

Menstruation and menstrual disorders

Sujan Sen and Mary Ann Lumsden

Chapter Contents

INTRODUCTION	448
MENSTRUATION	448
MECHANISMS OF NORMAL MENSTRUATION AND CONTROL OF BLOOD LOSS	450
NORMAL MENSTRUAL CYCLE	453
ABNORMAL MENSTRUATION	453
EPIDEMIOLOGY OF MENSTRUAL ABNORMALITY	456
PRESENTATION	457
INVESTIGATION	457
TREATMENT	459
DYSMENORRHOEA	467
CONCLUSIONS	467
KEY POINTS	468

Introduction

Menstrual abnormality is a common reason why women present at gynaecological outpatient clinics, and heavy menstrual bleeding (HMB) is one of the most common causes of iron-deficiency anaemia in Western women (Cohen and Gibor 1980). The average woman now experiences approximately 400 cycles, in contrast to the 40 or so she would have experienced 50 years ago. This is mainly due to smaller family size, availability of effective contraception, occurrence of an earlier menarche and later onset of menopause (Higham 1994). In addition to having an increased number of cycles, a significant number of women now work outside home, where disruption of work due to episodes of flooding is even less tolerable. Consequently, disorders of menstruation have become a significant public health issue.

Menstruation

At the end of the ovarian cycle, a major portion of the endometrium in primates undergoes periodic necrosis and sloughing associated with blood loss. Hence, the endometrium is a site of recurrent physiological injury and repair (Critchley et al 2001). During menstruation, the gonadal steroids reach their lowest levels. The nature of the supportive effect on the endometrium is unknown, although possible mechanisms will be discussed later.

Anatomy of the uterus

The uterus is a muscular, pear-shaped organ consisting of a fundus, body and cervix. The uterus receives the fallopian tubes at the cornua, whilst the cervix protrudes and opens into the vaginal vault.

The wall of the uterus consists of three layers: the serous coat, the myometrium and the endometrium. The serous coat is firmly adherent to the myometrium, which consists of smooth muscle fibres, the main branches of the blood vessels, and the nerves of the uterus and connective tissue. The endometrium consists principally of glandular and stromal cells, although its structure does vary spatially within the uterus and temporally with the stage of the menstrual cycle. The human endometrium is a dynamic tissue that, in response to the prevailing steroid environment of sequential oestrogen and progesterone exposure, undergoes well-characterized cycles of proliferation, differentiation and tissue breakdown on a monthly basis (Jabbour et al 2006).

Blood supply of the uterus

The blood supply of the uterus (Figure 31.1) is via the uterine artery, a branch of the anterior division of the internal iliac artery. It passes medially across the pelvic floor above the ureter, reaching the uterus at the supravaginal part of the cervix. Giving a branch to the cervix and vagina, the vessel turns upwards between the leaves of the broad ligament to run alongside the uterus as far as the entrance of the fallopian tube, where it anastomoses with the tubal branch of the ovarian artery. In its course, it gives off branches that penetrate the walls of the uterus. Within the myometrium, the uterine and ovarian arteries form the arcuate arteries. These, in turn, give rise to the radial arteries which, after passing through the endometrial–myometrial junction, branch into the basal arterioles, supplying the basal endometrium, and

DOI: 10.1016/B978-0-7020-3120-5.00031-X

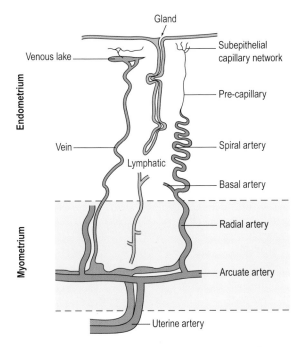

Gland

Venous lake

Subepithelial capillary network

Pre-capillary

Vein

Spiral artery

Lymphatic

Basal artery

Radial artery

Arcuate artery

Uterine artery

Endometrium

Myometrium

Figure 31.1 Schematic representation of the blood supply of the uterus.

the spiral arterioles, supplying the superficial layer of the endometrium. Spiral arterioles are end arterioles and are only present in species that menstruate. Each supplies an area of 4–9 mm^2. Branching of the spiral arterioles occurs throughout the superficial layer of the endometrium. Just below the surface epithelium, they break up into a prominent subepithelial plexus that drains into venous sinuses.

The endometrial vasculature is unlike any other vascular bed owing to its cyclic remodelling and regression during the menstrual cycle. These vessels are sensitive to changes in gonadal steroid levels, and at menstruation, the capillaries are shed with the glands and stroma (Rogers et al 1998). A recent study confirmed that crucial structural components in the endometrium during the menstrual process are the component blood vessels and the dynamic population of leukocytes that influx at this time (Jabbour et al 2006).

Histology of the uterus

The endometrium

The endometrium is composed of heterogeneous cell types that undergo cyclic synchronized waves of proliferation and differentiation in response to the rise and fall of oestrogen and progesterone. Histologically, it is divided into a superficial or functional layer, which lies adjacent to the uterine cavity, and a basalis, or deeper layer.

In the uterus, the superficial endometrial layer is characterized by rapid proliferation during the follicular phase of the cycle, followed by secretory transformation of the glandular epithelium, predecidualization of the stromal compartment and influx of uterine natural killer cells in the luteal phase of the cycle (King et al 1998).

During the proliferative phase, the short, straight epithelial glands elongate and become tortuous (Figure 31.2A). Changes occur in the position of the nuclei and the number

of mitoses. During the secretory phase, the glands increase in diameter and tortuosity, and vacuoles appear in the cellular cytoplasm (Figure 31.2B). The tissue also becomes markedly oedematous.

These morphological events are controlled by highly coordinated activation of certain gene sets essential for the regulation of uterine function. For instance, after ovulation, the sequential expression of progesterone-dependent genes defines a limited period of uterine receptivity or, in the absence of pregnancy, maintains vascular integrity prior to menstruation (Tabibzadeh and Babaknia 1995, Lockwood et al 1998). In addition, recent application of knowledge from the human genome, utilizing microarray technologies, has allowed several groups to contribute to a rapidly expanding literature on gene profiles during the 'putative window' of implantation (Carson et al 2002, Kao et al 2002, Riesewijk et al 2003).

In contrast, the basal endometrium shows no 'classic' sex steroid hormone response and is characterized by low proliferative activity, absence of glandular secretory transformation and lack of a predecidualization reaction in the late luteal phase. This absence of the 'classic' sex steroid hormone response does not, however, imply refractoriness to ovarian hormones. The basal layer is an important source of uterotonins and the site of active metaplasia of basal endometrial stromal cells into myofibroblasts and vice versa. It is further characterized by the presence of resident CD-3-positive T-lymphocyte aggregates.

The microvascular blood supply of the endometrium undergoes the unique process of benign angiogenesis, and is under the control of ovarian steroids during reproductive life. Following cessation of menstruation, they are simple in form, extending just into the endometrium. The secretory phase is characterized by the growth of arterioles. In the late secretory phase, coiling occurs due to proliferation and extension of the arterioles (Figure 31.2C). With the fall in steroid concentrations, menstrual shedding of the functional layer of the endometrium occurs (Figure 31.2D). Dramatic changes occur in the spiral arterioles at menstruation. These changes were described by Markee (1948) after experiments involving the transplantation of endometrium into the anterior chamber of the eye of the Rhesus monkey. This work was the cornerstone of current concepts of menstruation. On observing the bleeding process, Markee suggested that the arteriolar coiling caused constriction of the vessel lumen with vascular stasis and leukocytic infiltration. Approximately 24 h premenstrually, intense vasoconstriction led to ischaemic damage, followed by vasodilatation with haemorrhage from both arterial and venous vessels: 75% of the loss was arteriolar, 15% was venous and 10% was diapedesis of erythrocytes (Markee 1940).

The myometrium

The human myometrium is structurally and functionally polarized during the reproductive years. Compared with the outer myometrium, the subendometrial layer or junctional zone (JZ) is characterized by higher cell density, lower cellular nuclear:cytoplasmic ratios and the expression of different extracellular matrix (ECM) components (Brosens et al 1998, Campbell et al 1998). Additionally, evidence from ^{31}P nuclear magnetic resonance spectroscopic studies has dem-

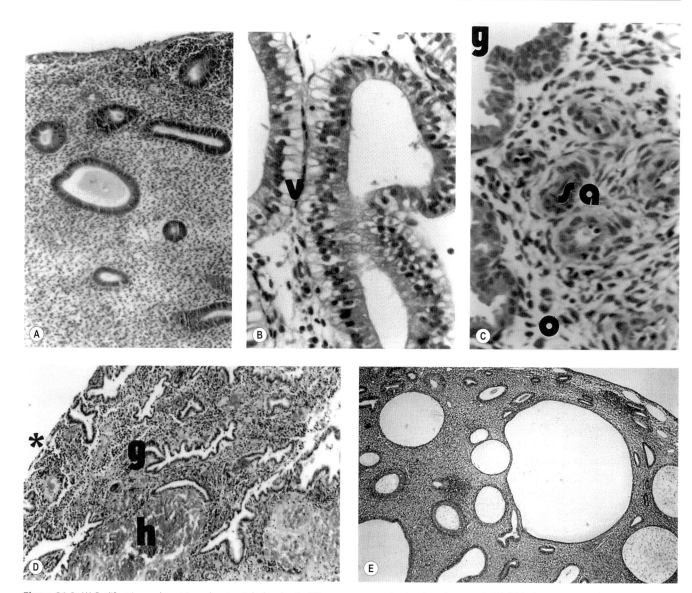

Figure 31.2 (A) Proliferative endometrium showing tubular glands. Mitoses are present in glands and stroma (×10). (B) Early secretory endometrium showing subnuclear vacuolation (v) and the presence of secretions. There are now few mitoses (×40). (C) Midsecretory endometrium (day 23) characterized by 'saw-toothed' glands (g), convoluted spiral arterioles (sa) and stromal oedema (o) (×40). (D) Menstruating endometrium. The glands (g) are now thin and show little secretory activity. There are lakes of haemorrhage (h) and the endometrium is beginning to break up (*). There is infiltration with white blood cells (×10). (E) Cystic glandular hyperplasia (×4).

onstrated biochemical heterogeneity between both myometrial layers (Xu et al 1997).

The differentiation of the myometrium into two distinct layers is strictly under ovarian hormonal control. In premenarchal girls and postmenopausal women, the zonal anatomy is often indistinct. Ovarian suppression with gonadotrophin-releasing hormone (GnRH) analogues leads to a magnetic resonance imaging (MRI) appearance of the uterus mimicking that of postmenopausal women, whilst hormone replacement therapy in postmenopausal women results in the reappearance of myometrial zonal anatomy (Demas et al 1985).

Further evidence for hormone responsiveness of the JZ is provided by the work of Wiczyk et al (1988), who demonstrated changes in JZ thickness throughout the menstrual cycle in conjunction with endometrial thickness.

Mechanisms of Normal Menstruation and Control of Blood Loss

The tissue components of the endometrium are a surface epithelium and associated glands, with a connective tissue stroma in which an elaborate vascular tree is embedded. The endometrial surface area is large (10–45 cm²), indicating that haemostasis during menstruation is usually very efficient.

Withdrawal of progesterone from an oestrogen-primed endometrium results in menstrual shedding. Shedding arises because of the induction of matrix metalloproteinases (MMPs) from the endometrium, in particular MMPs 1, 2 and 9 (Jeziorska et al 1996, Marbaix et al 1996). This arises through a mechanism of upregulation of transforming growth factor-beta (TGF-β) (Bruner et al 1995). The blood vessels are thus denuded of their support. Spiral arterioles and venules are cleaved at the level of the JZ between the endometrial functionalis and basalis, with subsequent bleeding.

Factors involved in the control of menstrual blood loss are:

- haemostasis;
- vasoconstriction; and
- endometrial repair.

Derangement of any of these mechanisms is likely to lead to excessive menstrual loss.

Haemostasis

Coagulation occurs in the distal endometrium, and platelets found within the endometrial cavity are deactivated and do not respond to collagen, as they would elsewhere. Once clinical bleeding and tissue shedding have started, haemostatic plug formation occurs, but less rapidly and less completely than is observed in human skin wounds (Christiaens et al 1982). Certain haemorrhagic conditions (e.g. thrombocytopenic purpura) are associated with increased incidence of HMB, suggesting that abnormalities of platelet structure may be important.

The coagulation cascade operates in the uterus and endometrium as in other tissues. Platelet accumulation, platelet degranulation and fibrin deposition occur within hours of the onset of menstruation, sealing endometrial vessels. The platelet count in menstrual discharge is only one-tenth of that seen in peripheral blood. This is probably due to the consumption of platelet aggregates in endometrial blood vessels early in the haemostatic processes of menstruation (de Merre et al 1967). Additionally, these platelets have been found to be devoid of granules, and they fail to aggregate when challenged with aggregating stimuli such as adenosine diphosphate and collagen. Compared with peripheral blood platelets, those in menstrual fluid do not produce appreciable cyclo-oxygenase products from arachidonic acid (Christiaens et al 1981, Sheppard et al 1983, Rees et al 1984).

Since prevention of clot formation is necessary to deter scarring and obliteration of the endometrial cavity, there appears to be an active fibrinolytic system in the endometrium mediated by plasmin through proteolytic cleavage of plasminogen by the activators urokinase-type plasminogen activator (uPA) and tissue-type plasminogen activator (tPA). These activators are regulated by plasminogen activator inhibitor 1 (PAI-1) and PAI-2, both of which are expressed in the endometrium. The presence of these fibrinolytic agents suggests that coagulation occurs but is rapidly reversed. Oestradiol stimulates uPA, whilst progesterone inhibits uPA (Casslen et al 1986). Furthermore, progesterone inhibits production of tPA, and this effect is amplified by production of PAI. Blood coagulation products have also been found to be severely depleted in menstrual fluid, suggesting consumption during menstruation (Hahn 1980).

Fibrin formation occurs during the process of menstruation (Beller 1971, Sheppard et al 1983). The high levels of fibrin degradation products in menstrual fluid are not solely due to direct digestion. Although menstrual blood contains high levels of fibrin and fibrin degradation products, it contains no fibrinogen. Similar levels of protein C_1 inactivator, α_2-macroglobulin and α_2-antitrypsin have been found in peripheral and menstrual blood (Daly et al 1990). However, compared with peripheral plasma, lower levels of activated prothrombin, antithrombin, antiplasmin, plasminogen, protein C and factors V, VII, VIII and X have been reported in menstrual fluid (Rees et al 1985, Daly et al 1990).

Compared with peripheral plasma, menstrual blood has a marked increase in the level of tPA antigen with reduced levels of PAI. Levels of fibrinolytic enzymes in menstrual fluid vary according to cycle stage. Throughout the cycle, higher levels of tPA are found in the myometrium compared with the endometrium in the normal menstrual cycle (Sheppard 1992), whilst during the late secretory phase, several studies have demonstrated a significant increase in endometrial tPA levels.

The above mechanisms ensure that progesterone falls and oestradiol rises during menstruation. There is increased fibrinolytic activity in the endometrium of women with increased menstrual blood loss. The endometrium also generates factors that inhibit platelet aggregation and platelet adhesion. Such factors include prostacyclin, nitric oxide and platelet-activating factor (PAF) (Kelly et al 1984, Alecozay et al 1991).

Vasoconstriction

In the menstruating uterus, haemostatic events are strikingly different from the rest of the body (Christiaens et al 1980). At the onset of menstruation, damaged blood vessels are sealed by intravascular thrombi of platelets and fibrin. However, as menstruation progresses, the functional endometrium is shed and so these haemostatic thrombi are lost. Subsequently, during the first 20 h of menstruation, intense vasoconstriction of the spiral arterioles occurs; this assures haemostasis until regeneration of the endometrial surface is complete.

The role of prostaglandin $F_{2\alpha}$ ($PGF_{2\alpha}$) in vasoconstriction is well established. The effects of the vasoconstricting $PGF_{2\alpha}$ are balanced by those of the vasodilating prostaglandin E_2 (PGE_2). Concentrations of both these prostaglandins are increased in the luteal phase. Overproduction of the vasodilatory prostaglandins or reduced production of the vasoconstrictors is likely to lead to excessive blood loss at the time of menstruation. This is confirmed by work showing an elevated $PGE_2/PGF_{2\alpha}$ ratio, increased endometrial PGE_2 or increased PGE_2 receptor concentrations in women with HMB (Smith et al 1981, Adalantado et al 1988). Steroid hormones influence endometrial prostaglandin synthesis, and the highest levels of the latter are found during menstruation. This is particularly true for $PGF_{2\alpha}$, the synthesis of which rises significantly during the secretory phase of the menstrual cycle under the influence of progesterone. It is also likely that the upregulation of the cyclo-oxygenase pathway impacts on angiogenesis in the endometrium.

Other vasoconstrictors, such as endothelins and PAF, may also contribute. Endothelins are powerful vasoconstrictors, and are found in human endometrium (Cameron et al 1992). They are thought to be involved in paracrine regulation of a number of endometrial functions, such as the induction of vascular and myometrial smooth muscle contractions, fibroblast mitogenesis and the release of other paracrine agents (Ohbuchi et al 1995). Endothelins can also induce $PGF_{2\alpha}$. It has been proposed that as endometrial glandular epithelium breaks down during menstruation, stored endothelin gains access to the spiral arterioles, causing long-lasting vasoconstriction (Cameron and Davenport 1992).

PAF is present in the endometrium in the luteal phase and has an ambiguous effect on spiral arteriolar tone. PAF itself is a vasoconstrictor but it stimulates production of the vasodilator PGE_2 (Björk and Smedegård 1983, Smith and Kelly 1988).

Endometrial repair

Vasculature

Seventy percent of menstrual loss arises from the spiral arterioles, and most of this bleeding occurs within the first 3 days of menses (Haynes et al 1977). Concordantly, vessel repair begins within the first 2–3 days of the onset of bleeding. As might be expected, the endometrium is a rich source of angiogenic growth factors (Smith 1998). The fibroblast growth factor (FGF) and the vascular endothelial growth factor (VEGF) families are the best known.

Vascular endothelial growth factor

VEGF is a heterodimeric angiogenic growth factor which is expressed and secreted by a variety of endometrial cells, including macrophages and large decidualized cells. They cluster around the spiral arterioles during the late luteal phase (Gospodarowicz et al 1989, Charnock-Jones et al 1993). The variants of VEGF differ in their cellular localization.

Steroids and hypoxia regulate VEGF, with steroid regulation being around two orders of magnitude lower than that of hypoxia. VEGF mRNA is abundant in the endometrium at the time of menstruation (Charnock-Jones et al 1993). This upregulation probably follows the hypoxia induced by spiral arteriole vasoconstriction (Sharkey et al 2000). Its expression is followed by rapid angiogenesis when the functional endometrium is lost.

Vascular smooth muscle cells (VSMCs) in endometrium also express certain VEGF receptors. This provides a direct link between the development of spiral arterioles and VEGF-A expression. The finding of reduced proliferation of VSMCs in patients with HMB could be explained by altered VEGF-A expression. A novel angiogenic factor, endocrine gland VFGF, and its receptors have recently been reported to be expressed in the uterus (Battersby et al 2004).

Fibroblast growth factor

The FGF family consists of at least eight members, some of which are expressed in the endometrium and are hormone dependent with expression during the proliferative phase and reduction during the secretory phase (Basilico and Moscatelli 1992, Ferriani et al 1993). FGF synergizes with VEGFs in inducing angiogenesis (Pepper et al 1992). Inhibition of FGF action does not fully inhibit angiogenesis, but this is possible when anti-VEGF agents are used. VEGFs promote the release of FGF from the ECM. FGF and platelet-derived growth factor are also known to stimulate angiogenesis, and have been demonstrated in the endometrium of a number of a species (Weston and Rogers 2000).

Angiopoietins

The angiopoietins are another family of molecules which influence vascular development and maintenance by stabilizing the endothelial cell and vascular smooth muscle structure (Suri et al 1998). Recently, expression patterns of the angiopoetin family in the human endometrium have been examined, although results have been conflicting, perhaps reflecting relatively low expression of these factors (Rogers and Abberton 2003). It is possible that this will alter the function of the VSMCs that are essential for controlling the blood loss at menstruation, and that HMB is due to aberrant build-up of VSMCs. Angiopoietin expression and signalling are regulated by the cyclo-oxygenase enzymes.

Epithelium

Once the functional layer of the endometrium is shed, the regeneration of all cell types (epithelial, endothelial and stromal) occurs rapidly. This regeneration occurs from the cells of the remaining basal layer, which acts as the germinal compartment of the functional endometrium (Chan et al 2004).

Given its dynamic nature, growth factors and cytokines are especially important in the development of the endometrium. In addition, tissue remodelling is dependent on the integrity of the ECM. Profound hormone-dependent tissue remodelling is seen in the endometrium, although currently there is no direct evidence linking disorders of tissue regeneration with HMB. Proliferation of the endometrium is most active during menstruation. The proliferation starts on day 2 in the basal glands and is complete by day 5, leaving a completely re-epithelialized endometrial surface. Various agents regulate this process, the best-known being epidermal growth factor (EGF). EGF is expressed in human epithelial cells throughout the cycle and stimulates endometrial epithelial proliferation (Haining et al 1991, Zhang et al 1995). Oestradiol induces the expression of EGF and its receptor. However, during menstruation, when the concentration of oestradiol is at its lowest, there are sufficient amounts of residual EGF remaining in the epithelial cells as growth continues before oestradiol levels increase during the proliferative phase. Additionally, EGF has been shown to mimic the proliferative effect of oestradiol in the endometrium of transgenic mice lacking the oestradiol receptor (Ignar Trowbridge et al 1993). Numerous other growth factors (insulin-like growth factor, FGF) and their binding proteins are expressed in the endometrium, and all promote cell proliferation. The complexities of tissue remodelling suggest that altered wound healing may be a factor in the aetiology of HMB, and its role warrants further investigation.

Matrix

The ECM is a dynamic structure composed of collagens, fibronectin, laminin, gelatins, entactins, hyaluronic acid and proteoglycans, all of which provide the tissue with structural integrity.

Integrins are the agents which link the ECM with epithelial cells of the endometrium (Hynes 1987, Lessey et al 1992). The MMPs are a highly regulated family of calcium and zinc endopeptidases, which are able to degrade most components of the ECM in the activated state. These enzymes are active in normal and pathological processes involving tissue remodelling. MMP activity is greatest during days 1–4 of the cycle. Progesterone withdrawal and migratory leukocytes activate some MMPs, and this may be a significant step in the initiation of menstruation. Local release of agents such as MMP-1 and MMP-3 from stromal cells may activate other proteases released from the invading neutrophils (Schatz et al 1999). This is supported by the presence of substantially more latent MMP-9 than active MMP-9 before menstruation (Rigot et al 2001). Abnormalities in the dynamic turnover of collagen production are likely to be important in menstrual upset given their importance in other vascular and fibrotic processes.

Normal Menstrual Cycle

The majority of cycles lie between 24 and 32 days, and a normal cycle is considered to last for 28 days. Menstrual cycle length varies during reproductive life, being most regular between the ages of 20 and 40 years. It tends to be longer after the menarche and shorter as the menopause approaches. The mean menstrual blood loss per menstruation in a healthy Western European population ranges between 37 and 43 ml; 70% of the loss occurs in the first 48 h. Despite large interpatient variability, loss between consecutive menses in the same woman does not vary largely (Figure 31.3). Only 9–14% of women lose more than 80 ml per menses, and 60% of these women are actually anaemic. The upper limit of normal menstruation is thus taken as 80 ml per menses (Rybo 1966). However, total fluid loss (mucus, tissue, etc.) may be considerably more than the blood loss alone and amounts vary. These parameters have been reviewed recently (Fraser and Inceboz 2000).

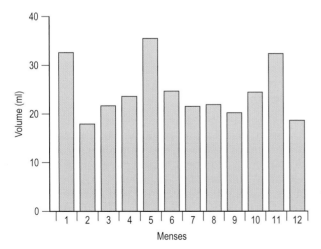

Figure 31.3 The variability in menstrual blood loss in a single individual: values for 12 consecutive periods.
From Hallberg L, Nilsson L 1964 Consistency of individual menstrual blood loss. Acta Obstetrica et Gynecologica Scandinavica 43:352–359, Blackwell Science.

During the first day or two of the menses, uterine contractility is at its greatest. This may aid expulsion of the degenerating endometrium from the uterus. Activity is extremely variable between women, although it is remarkably constant between menses in the same woman. There is no objective method of separating normal and abnormal contractility; normal contractility does not cause debility to a woman, although mild discomfort may occur.

The pattern of spontaneous myometrial contractions varies during the menstrual cycle (Lumsden et al 1983). Time-lapse ultrasound studies have shown that propagated myometrial contractions in the non-pregnant uterus emanate from the JZ. The frequency and direction of these contractions depend on the phase of the cycle. In the follicular and periovulatory phases, cervicofundal subendometrial contractions can be seen, the amplitude and frequency of which increase notably towards ovulation. Short, asymmetrical myometrial waves are present during the luteal phase, but propagated fundocervical subendometrial contraction waves are noted during menstruation (de Vries et al 1990, Chalubinski et al 1993).

Kunz et al (1996) demonstrated the role of preovulatory cervicofundal contractions in assisting the rapid transport of sperm through the female reproductive tract. Others have postulated that the asymmetrical myometrial peristalsis during the luteal phase serves to maintain the developing blastocyst within the uterine fundus. The role of fundocervical contractions during menstruation is likely to be important in controlling menstrual flow and limiting retrograde menstruation (Chalubinski et al 1993).

Abnormal Menstruation

This part of the chapter will consider abnormalities of menstrual bleeding including HMB, with particular reference to dysfunctional uterine bleeding (DUB) and dysmenorrhoea. The defects most usually associated with infertility, e.g. oligo- and amenorrhoea, will not be discussed further.

Heavy menstrual bleeding (HMB)

In the past, this was known as 'menorrhagia' but this term means different things to different people and should be avoided.

The causes of HMB fall into four categories:

- DUB;
- pelvic pathology;
- medical disorders; and
- coagulation disorders.

Dysfunctional uterine bleeding

Disturbances in the pattern of menstruation are a common clinical presentation for abnormalities of the hypophyseal–pituitary–ovarian axis. DUB is defined as HMB, in the absence of recognizable pelvic pathology, pregnancy or general bleeding disorder, which interferes with a woman's physical, social, emotional and/or material quality of life. It commonly occurs at the extremes of reproductive life (adolescence and perimenopausally). The abnormalities of ovarian activity may be classified as anovulatory [i.e. inadequate signal, such as in polycystic ovary syndrome (PCOS) or premenopausally, and impaired positive feedback, such as in adolescence] and ovulatory.

Anovulatory dysfunctional uterine bleeding

Occasionally, anovulatory cycles occur in all women. Chronic anovulation, however, is associated with an irregular and unpredictable pattern of bleeding ranging from short cycles with scanty bleeding to prolonged periods of irregular heavy loss. Normal bleeding occurs in response to withdrawal of both progesterone and oestradiol. If ovulation does not occur, the absence of progesterone results in an absence of secretory changes in the endometrium, accompanied by abnormalities in the production of steroid receptors, prostaglandins and other locally active endometrial products. Unopposed oestrogen gives rise to persistent proliferative or hyperplastic endometrium, and oestrogen withdrawal bleeding is characteristically painless and irregular. It tends to occur at the extremes of reproductive life but is rare at other times. Only 20% of those cycles with excessive menstrual blood loss are anovulatory (Haynes et al 1979); this same study failed to demonstrate any abnormalities in gonadotrophin or circulating steroid concentrations. In anovulatory cycles, the endometrium is unable to produce factors whose synthesis is controlled by progesterone, such as $PGF_{2\alpha}$ (Smith et al 1982). This may account for the painless nature of the bleeds. Ovulation occurs in response to the mid-cycle surge of luteinizing hormone (LH). If this fails to occur due to insufficient oestradiol secretion or impaired positive feedback, ovulation will not occur.

Failure of follicular development

Follicular development which is insufficient to produce an oestrogen signal strong enough to induce an LH surge is one of the common reasons for the irregularities in menstrual cycle pattern in premenopausal women. This occurs perimenopausally and in PCOS (see Chapter 18 for information regarding the aetiology and treatment of PCOS).

Anovulatory bleeding may be associated with cystic glandular hyperplasia of the endometrium (see Figure 31.2E). This occurs in some older women and also in peripubertal girls where unopposed oestrogen secretion occurs. The first few cycles after the menarche are commonly anovulatory. However, if anovulation persists, a long period of amenorrhoea is accompanied by endometrial hyperplasia. This is probably a result of multiple follicular development (multicystic ovaries) with failure of antral follicle formation. Endometrial hyperplasia may cause excessive bleeding, anaemia, infertility and even cancer of the endometrium.

In the younger patient (<40 years of age) with anovulatory HMB, assessment of the hypothalamic–pituitary–ovarian axis is indicated. The diagnosis of PCOS has increased over recent years, with the finding of altered LH/follicle-stimulating hormone ratios in the follicular phase of the cycle and the identification of micro- and macrocystic disease by vaginal ultrasound. Obesity alone can produce a similar picture in the absence of any other sign of PCOS.

Ovulatory dysfunctional uterine bleeding: idiopathic bleeding

As described above, an important factor in the control of menstrual blood loss is vasoconstriction. It appears that there are a number of endometrial products which alter the degree of vasoconstriction, and thus may affect the volume of menstrual blood lost. In the mid-1970s, a relationship between prostaglandin production and HMB was suggested by work showing that total endometrial prostaglandin content was proportional to menstrual loss. It appears that a shift in endometrial conversion of endoperoxide from the vasoconstrictor prostaglandins ($PGF_{2\alpha}$) to the vasodilator prostaglandins (PGE_2 or prostacyclin) occurs. However, it is likely that it is not only prostaglandins that are of importance, and work is now being performed on the role of endothelin in heavy menstrual loss. Endothelins are very potent vasoconstrictors that are produced within the endometrial vessels; their receptors are also present, although it is not yet clear whether either of these two factors differ in women with heavy menstrual loss. Although studies to date are limited, Marsh (1996) showed reduced immunostaining for endothelin in the endometrium of women with HMB, implicating this peptide in the pathophysiology of increased menstrual blood loss. This is a rapidly changing area of knowledge, and it is likely that other elements will come to light which will be significant. According to Jabour et al (2006): 'Further challenge in the future will be the development of experimental strategies that will allow us to assess the exact role of the various factors deduced from gene mining studies in menstrual function/dysfunction and which of these gene pathways constitute a sensible target for novel therapeutic application in the clinic.'

It is still uncertain why there is a difference in production of local factors in those with heavy menstrual loss compared with those with normal loss. Interest has centered on the role of steroid hormones, but it has been impossible to demonstrate either a difference in the circulating levels of oestradiol and progesterone or in the receptor concentration within the endometrium (Critchley et al 1994). It is possible that there is a genetic difference altering the production of local hormones and growth factors, or that there is a multifactorial aetiology. Reference has been made above, in discussion of the control of menstrual blood loss, to areas of research which may throw new light on the mechanism of HMB.

Heavy menstrual bleeding in the presence of pelvic pathology

HMB is thought to be associated with uterine fibroids, adenomyosis, pelvic infection, endometrial polyps and the presence of a foreign body such as an intrauterine contraceptive device (IUD). In addition, the rare conditions of myometrial hypertrophy and vascular abnormality may be associated with severe, even life-threatening HMB. However, objective evidence of HMB in most of these situations is limited. In women with menstrual blood loss greater than 200 ml, over half will have fibroids, although only 40% of those with adenomyosis actually have menstrual blood loss in excess of 80 ml per menses. It is not clear if chronic pelvic inflammatory disease or endometrial polyps are associated with above-average blood loss.

Although vasoactive peptides may contribute to HMB associated with pathology, non-steroidal anti-inflammatory drugs (NSAIDs) are less effective in HMB associated with IUD presence than in DUB, making it likely that other factors are also important.

Medical problems

HMB is associated with various endocrine disorders such as hypothyroidism (thyrotoxicosis is more commonly associated with cycle disturbance) and Cushing's disease, although the mechanism is unknown. Thyroid disease is often considered to be a common cause for HMB, but it is rare for thyroid disease to present in this way without other associated symptoms, e.g. weight gain, hair loss, constipation, etc. Thyroid function tests do not need to be performed in all women presenting with HMB.

Coagulation disorders

Although certain haemorrhagic conditions, e.g. thrombocytopenic purpura and von Willebrand's disease, are associated with an increased incidence of HMB, coagulation disorders have a variable effect overall. There is no impairment of systemic coagulation in those with excess menstrual loss, nor are fibrin degradation products elevated in the menstrual fluid of those with heavy menstrual loss (Bonnar et al 1983). In women with thrombocytopenia, menstrual blood loss correlates broadly with platelet count at the time of the menses. Splenectomy has been known to reduce menstrual blood loss dramatically in these patients.

Women with factor VII deficiency exhibit a spectrum of bleeding symptoms, with HMB being one of the most common (Kulkarni et al 2006). There is no need to test for these routinely unless HMB has been present from adolescence or the woman encountered bleeding problems with dental extraction.

Dysmenorrhoea

Dysmenorrhoea comes from Greek and means 'difficult monthly flow', but is now taken to mean painful menstruation. It is a symptom complex, with cramping lower abdominal pain radiating to the back and legs, often accompanied by gastrointestinal and neurological symptoms as well as general malaise. As with HMB, it may be associated with pathology or may be idiopathic in origin.

Idiopathic (primary) dysmenorrhoea

There are many different theories regarding why women suffer from dysmenorrhoea. The following factors may be of importance.

Uterine hyperactivity

The significance of uterine hyperactivity in women with dysmenorrhoea was first proposed in 1932. Since then, there has been much research which suggests that women with dysmenorrhoea have increased uterine activity during menstruation (Novak and Reynolds 1932, Filler and Hall 1970). Patients often describe the pain as 'labour-like', and an increase in uterine contractility can be demonstrated by measuring intrauterine pressure in those with dysmenorrhoea compared with women without dysmenorrhoea (Lumsden and Baird 1985). The increased uterine contractility also appears to be related to uterine blood flow and the presence of pain (Åkerlund and Anderssen 1976).

During the reproductive years, the myometrium is structurally and functionally polarized (see above). Using transvaginal ultrasound scanning or MRI, it is possible to delineate between the myometrial zones (Brosens et al 1998, Lesny et al 1999).

Patients with endometriosis and adenomyosis have been found to have structural and functional abnormalities of the JZ (Brosens et al 2000). Leyendecker et al (1996) demonstrated marked hyperperistalsis of the JZ during the early- and mid-follicular phase in women with endometriosis, associated with a marked increase in the transport of inert particles from the vaginal depot to the peritoneal cavity.

Dysmenorrhoeic patients have been found to exhibit profound structural changes in the JZ, including irregular thickening, and smooth muscle hyperplasia characterized by closely packed smooth muscle fibres which are poorly oriented and less vascular than the smooth muscle of normal inner myometrium (Togashi et al 1989, Brosens et al 1998). Consequently, the term 'junctional zone hyperplasia' was coined for this disorder (Brosens et al 1998).

Dysperistalsis and hyperactivity of the uterine JZ are important mechanisms of primary dysmenorrhoea, and possibly menstrual pain associated with adenomyosis and endometriosis (Brosens et al 2000).

Endothelins

Endothelins are potent uterotonins in the non-pregnant uterus. They are thought to be involved in the induction of myometrial smooth muscle contraction in a juxtacrine fashion. The greatest density of endothelin-binding sites is found on glandular epithelium in the endomyometrial junction, and recent evidence suggests that endothelins in the endometrium can induce $PGF_{2\alpha}$ and further endothelin release in a paracrine and autocrine fashion (Bacon et al 1995). Local ischaemia could further increase the expression of endothelins and prostaglandins, which could further aggravate uterine dysperistalsis.

Prostaglandins

It has been shown that dysmenorrhoeic women have increased endometrial synthesis of $PGF_{2\alpha}$ and enhanced concentrations of $PGF_{2\alpha}$ and PGE_2 in menstrual blood compared with asymptomatic women (Lundstrom and Green 1978, Lumsden et al 1983). $PGF_{2\alpha}$ is a potent oxytocic and vasoconstrictor. When administered into the uterus, it will give rise to dysmenorrhoea-like pain and occasionally menstrual bleeding. Menstrual fluid $PGF_{2\alpha}$ concentrations also correlate with uterine work during the menses in women with dysmenorrhoea (Lumsden et al 1983). These properties of $PGF_{2\alpha}$ could thus lead to 'angina' of the myometrium. The role of PGE_2 is less clear, although its administration may increase the sensitivity of nerve endings.

The reason for the abnormal prostaglandin levels is unknown. Primary dysmenorrhoea occurs almost exclusively in ovulatory cycles, and steroid hormones affect both uterine prostaglandin concentration and myometrial contractility. However, no consistent abnormality of hormone levels has been demonstrated in those with dysmenorrhoea. Treatment with prostaglandin synthetase inhibitors reduces uterine $PGF_{2\alpha}$ production, uterine activity and dysmenorrhoea.

Vasopressin

The treatment of HMB with desmopressin is efficacious and safe if patients are instructed to self-administer the agent only during the first 2 or 3 days of heavy menstrual blood loss, for a maximum of three to four doses and with no more than two consecutive administrations during a 12-h interval (Rodeghiero 2008).

There are other stimulants of the non-pregnant uterus, such as vasopressin, a vasoconstrictor that also stimulates uterine contractility. On the first day of menstruation, circulating vasopressin levels are higher in those with dysmenorrhea than in those without dysmenorrhea (Åkerlund et al 1979). Infusion of hypertonic saline results in increased uterine contractility and pain in women with dysmenorrhoea as a result of stimulation of endogenous vasopressin release, as well as a reduction in concentrations of $PGF_{2\alpha}$ metabolites. Preliminary studies also indicate that vasopressin analogues may have a place in the treatment of dysmenorrhoea.

Other factors

PAF is present in a higher concentration in women with dysmenorrhoea (Migram et al 1991). This is somewhat surprising as PAF inhibits $PGF_{2\alpha}$ production, although it does stimulate overall phospholipid metabolism, and other factors, which have not been measured, may be elevated.

Another factor of potential importance is the destruction of nerve endings in the myometrium and cervix by pregnancy. This may explain the observation that primary dysmenorrhoea is relieved by the birth of a baby. The literature suggests that psychological and physical causes for dysmenorrhoea are mutually exclusive. The evidence for physical factors is strong, treatment is very effective and it is unlikely that psychological problems would be removed simply by taking tablets. However, recurring, debilitating pain may cause depression and anxiety in women of any age.

Secondary dysmenorrhoea

As with HMB, this may be associated with uterine and pelvic pathology such as fibroids, the presence of an inert copper-containing IUD, pelvic inflammatory disease, adenomyosis, endometriosis or cervical stenosis. The cause of the pain is not always clear. Abnormal uterine contractility has been observed in those with fibroids, and prostaglandins may be involved when dysmenorrhoea is associated with an IUD, pelvic inflammatory disease, adenomyosis and possibly endometriosis. However, the use of prostaglandin synthetase inhibitors is less effective in the presence of pathology, making it likely that other factors also exist.

Those women presenting with dysmenorrhoea who have no other complaints or abnormalities on examination can be safely treated without further investigation. Pierzynski et al (2006) have shown that tamoxifen, a selective oestrogen-receptor modulator, directly inhibits uterine contractions, causing improvement in uterine blood flow and a decrease in menstrual pain and cramps. This could be considered for application in selected groups of dysmenorrheic women; for instance, carriers of breast-cancer-associated

antigen genes, breast cancer survivors or women with advanced endometriosis (Pierzynski et al 2006).

Letzel et al (2006) reported that aceclofenac (100 mg) and naproxen (500 mg) effectively reduced the pain associated with primary dysmenorrhoea, and both were more effective than placebo at easing menstrual pain assessed by various pain relief criteria. Laparoscopy is indicated for those with a provisional diagnosis of endometriosis or pelvic inflammatory disease. Hysteroscopy, endometrial sampling and examination under anaesthetic are only required if uterine abnormality is suspected. The standard treatment for dysmenorrhoea (prostaglandin synthetase inhibitors and the oral contraceptive pill) is so effective that laparoscopy in treatment failures will often demonstrate previously unsuspected abnormalities such as mild endometriosis, even in teenage girls.

Epidemiology of Menstrual Abnormality

The distribution of blood loss for a normal population shows a positively skewed distribution, as mentioned above (Figure 31.4) (Cole et al 1971). Age *per se* does not influence menstrual blood loss until the sixth decade (Figure 31.5, Table 31.1). This may be due to an increased incidence of pathology (e.g. fibroids or perimenopausal endocrine abnormalities). An hereditary influence has been demonstrated following twin studies, and parity is thought to be an important factor; parous women have greater menstrual blood loss than nulliparous women. Uterine pathology, particularly fibroids, is a well-documented cause for HMB, although endometrial pathology is rather uncommon in these women; it is found as a reasonable cause for HMB in approximately 6% of cases.

The variation between menses for an individual (intra-menses) is between 20% and 40%. Approximately 90% of blood is lost during the first 3 days of the menses in women with normal blood loss and women with HMB. These studies are based on objective measurement of menstrual blood loss, which is rarely done except for research purposes

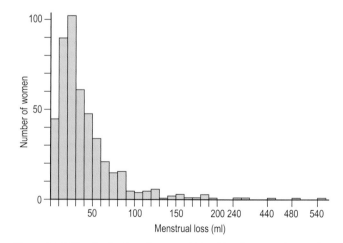

Figure 31.4 The distribution of menstrual blood loss for a population of women who did not consider they had any menstrual abnormality.
Source: From Hallberg L, Nilsson L. 1964 Consistency of individual menstrual blood loss. Acta Obstetricia et Gynecologica Scandinavica 43:352–359, Blackwell Science.

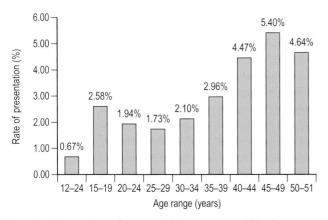

Figure 31.5 Annual rate of women with heavy menstrual bleeding presenting to services.

Table 31.1 Costs and savings

Recommendations with significant resource impact	Annual cost (£millions)
Full blood count investigations	0.9
Transvaginal ultrasound investigations	10.4
Endometrial biopsy for suspected endometrial cancer	−0.9
Pharmaceutical treatments levonorgestrel-releasing intrauterine system	−0.6
Substitution of hysterectomy with endometrial ablation	−1.2
Total net cost of implementing the HMB guideline	8.7

Source: National Institute for Health and Clinical Excellence 2007 NICE Clinical Guideline No. 44. HMB, heavy menstrual bleeding.

(Hallberg and Nilsson 1964). New methods of measuring menstrual symptoms are being designed in order to allow for better objective assessment, with consideration given to the variety of symptoms that contribute to the overall complaint such as irregularity, HMB, pain and premenstrual syndrome.

The results of epidemiological studies performed over the last 50 years give a variable incidence for dysmenorrhoea. This is because pain is a subjective symptom and cannot be assessed accurately by an outsider. Different women will react to the same pain in different ways. How each woman perceives the pain will vary according to her individual circumstances. In addition, the definition and diagnosis allow different interpretations by different workers. Severe dysmenorrhoea, which causes disruption of daily routine with time off work or study, occurs in 3–10% of 19-year-olds (Andersch and Milsom 1982), while mild discomfort occurs in the majority of women. The relative risk of dysmenorrhoea in those who have smoked for 10–20 years is up to six-fold higher than the risk in non-smokers (Parazzini et al 1994). The incidence of dysmenorrhoea is inversely correlated with age, and parous women are less likely to report the condition. There is no correlation between the incidence of emotional stress factors and dysmenorrhoea.

Presentation

Clinical history

Menstrual problems are a common reason for presentation to both general practitioners and gynaecologists. A history of heavy, regular, cyclical menstrual blood loss over several consecutive cycles without additional irregular bleeding suggests DUB. A detailed history may suggest other underlying pathology; for example, heavy painful menses and dyspareunia might suggest endometriosis, whilst heavy bleeding with a vaginal discharge and abdominal pain points to pelvic inflammatory disease.

Risk factors for endometrial carcinoma should be noted carefully in the history (Box 31.1, Figure 31.6).

Examination

General examination may reveal signs of hypothyroidism, anaemia or blood clotting disorders. Abdominal and pelvic examination is only mandatory in women complaining of HMB if structural abnormality is expected (National Institute for Health and Clinical Excellence 2007). Clues to diagnosis may be revealed on pelvic examination. A tender fixed uterus may suggest endometriosis or pelvic inflammatory disease, whilst fibroids can often be palpated. A symmetrically enlarged uterus is more typical of adenomyosis or endometrial carcinoma. Atrophic and inflammatory vulvar and vaginal lesions can be visualized, and cervical polyps and invasive lesions of cervical carcinoma that may present with irregular bleeding can be seen. Anaemia may also be present since HMB is the most common cause of iron-deficiency anaemia in the Western world. HMB may arise because of disorders of the haemopoietic system, as described above.

Investigation

Haemoglobin concentration should be determined in all women with HMB, and iron supplementation should be given if required. Although thyroid disease is a cause of

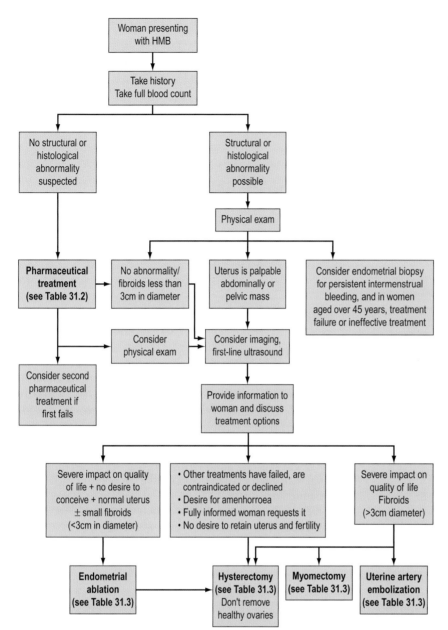

Figure 31.6 National Institute for Health and Clinical Excellence care pathway for heavy menstrual bleeding (HMB).
Source: National Institute for Health and Clinical Excellence 2007 Clinical Guideline No. 44. Heavy Menstrual Bleeding at www.nice.org

menstrual derangement in some women, screening thyroid-stimulating hormone and thyroxine measurements are not justified unless there are other features in the history suggestive of thyroid disease (Fraser et al 1986, National Institute for Health and Clinical Excellence 2007). Similarly, routine screening for bleeding diatheses is not appropriate.

Assessment of the uterine cavity

The main indication for assessment of the uterine cavity is to exclude sinister pathology, the likelihood of which increases with age in the presence of risk factors. A history of irregular bleeding or the presence of risk factors for endometrial cancer will determine the need for endometrial assessment.

A wide array of methods are available for endometrial assessment including:

- ultrasonography for evaluation of uterine architecture and endometrial thickness;
- endometrial sampling;
- hysteroscopy and endometrial biopsy;
- sonohysterography;
- cytological examination; and
- dilatation and curettage (D&C) alone should not be used as a diagnostic tool (National Institute for Health and Clinical Excellence 2007).

Ultrasonography

Ultrasonography allows evaluation of the uterine architecture and endometrial thickness, and is an important adjunct to endometrial sampling. Transvaginal ultrasound scanning is a useful tool allowing better resolution than abdominal scanning because of the close proximity of the ultrasound probe with the pelvic organs. It has a specificity of 96% and a sensitivity of 89%. Endometrial thickness is only of value after the menopause. Ultrasound assessment should be combined with endometrial biopsy when endometrial thickness exceeds 5 mm.

Abnormalities on pelvic examination should be investigated by ultrasound, and laparoscopy if required.

Endometrial sampling

In 1882, Moriche obtained the first endometrial sample using a catheter. Endometrial biopsy has been performed in an outpatient setting since 1935. The 1970s saw the introduction of the Vabra curette, followed by the Pipelle sampler in the 1980s. The Pipelle is easier to use and more comfortable for the patient but it only samples 4% of the endometrium, whereas the Vabra aspirator samples approximately 40%. The main disadvantage of blind sampling of the uterine cavity is that pathology such as polyps or submucous fibroids may be missed.

The risk of endometrial carcinoma in women with perimenopausal HMB is approximately 1%; hence, all women with irregular bleeding that is unresponsive to treatment need endometrial assessment. Although women under 40 years of age have a very low risk of developing endometrial carcinoma, further investigation may be needed in high-risk symptomatic women (Royal College of Obstetricians and Gynaecologists 1994).

Hysteroscopy

Hysteroscopy facilitates intrauterine surgical procedures such as endometrial ablation. Hence, it has long been accepted into UK gynaecological practice for diagnostic and therapeutic purposes. Hysteroscopy and directed biopsy appear to be superior in identifying benign endometrial pathology (Gimpleson and Rappold 1988, Loffer 1989). More pertinently, in a significant minority of women with endometrial carcinoma, the diagnosis is missed when conventional curettage is used (Stovall et al 1989), and it appears that hysteroscopy and directed biopsy is more sensitive in the diagnosis of this condition. Ultrasound is better at identifying fibroids unless it is intracavity, and hysteroscopy should only be used when ultrasound is unsatisfactory.

The development of a narrow diameter (4 mm) scope allows this investigation to be performed in the outpatient setting in a carefully selected patient group following counselling (Taylor and Hamou 1983). Patient selection is important to maximize the success of the procedure; for example, women with a previous cervical cone biopsy or Manchester repair may have cervical stenosis, making passage of the hysteroscope through the internal os difficult.

Hysteroscopy should always be combined with an endometrial biopsy. It should be avoided during menstruation as blood in the cavity obscures the view. The cavity is distended with either gas or fluid. In addition, hysteroscopy enables detection of polyps, submucous fibroids and uterine synechiae in women who have previously had multiple previous 'negative' curettages.

These studies provide increasing evidence that hysteroscopy and endometrial sampling in combination is a superior diagnostic tool. This has therefore replaced D&C as the investigation of choice in menstrual disorders (Lewis 1990, 1994).

Sonohysterography

In sonohysterography, ultrasound is performed following injection of saline by a narrow catheter into the uterus. This may increase the sensitivity of transvaginal ultrasonography. Hence, sonohysterography has been used to evaluate the endometrial cavity for polyps, submucous fibroids and uterine abnormality, especially septate and subseptate uterus.

Cytologic examination

Cytological examination is normally used to diagnose asymptomatic intraepithelial lesions of the cervix. This is not reliable for the diagnosis of endometrial pathology. The presence of endometrial cells in the smear of a postmenopausal woman is abnormal, unless she has been exposed to exogenous oestrogen. Similarly, women in the secretory phase of the menstrual cycle should not shed endometrial cells. However, a smear that is positive or suspicious for endometrial cancer needs evaluation.

The investigation of women presenting with heavy menstrual loss is summarized in Figure 31.6.

Quantification of Menstrual Blood Loss

The objective assessment of menstrual blood loss is rarely made, except for research purposes. However, menstrual blood loss can be assessed either in a semiquantitative manner, relying on the patient's assessment of the bleeding, or by the use of pictorial aids (Higham et al 1990). The pictorial method has been shown to correlate well with the gold standard alkaline haematin method (Higham et al 1990, Wyatt et al 2001). However, this correlation has also been challenged (Reid et al 2000). Attention is being given to the development of aids, including the use of hand-held computers, to assess the menstrual complaint as a whole, which consists of more than heavy bleeding. Many women also complain of pain and premenstrual syndrome. Again, these are not yet available for general use.

Treatment

General principles of management

A detailed history should be taken and examination performed as required. The importance of desiring a pregnancy when using the oral contraceptive pill, Depo-Provera, Implanon and IUDs must be considered. The most likely cause of the abnormal bleeding, the work-up strategy and the treatment will depend upon the woman's age, medical condition and desire for future fertility. Women should be given information prior to an outpatient appointment. Treatment options should be discussed, and rapid, safe and effective treatment should be instituted to improve menstrual problems and quality of life.

Medical treatment

Current medical therapy falls into two broad groups: non-hormonal (prostaglandin synthetase inhibitors, antifibrinolytics and ethamsylate) and hormonal (progestogens, oral contraceptives, hormone replacement therapy, danazol, gestrinone, GnRH analogues) (see Table 31.2). Non-hormonal treatment may be taken during menstruation, which avoids teratogenicity and is therefore suitable for women who wish to conceive. Some women, once reassured that there is no major pathology, will require no further treatment.

Non-hormonal treatment

Prostaglandin synthetase inhibitors

NSAIDs remain a popular choice for the treatment of HMB (Coulter et al 1995). Their principal mechanism of action is to decrease endometrial prostaglandin concentrations. The endometrium is a rich source of PGE_2 and $PGF_{2\alpha}$, and a number of studies have shown that prostaglandin concentrations are greater in the endometrium of women with HMB than they are in the endometrium of women with normal blood loss (Cameron and Norman 1995).

There are four groups of prostaglandin synthetase inhibitors, of which the fenamates are the most widely used. These are unique amongst the prostaglandin synthetase inhibitors in that, in addition to inhibition of prostaglandin synthesis, they bind and block the prostaglandin receptor (Rees et al 1988). Menstrual blood loss is reduced by a median of 25–40% in three-quarters of women with HMB (Figure 31.7). The beneficial effect of mefenamic acid on menstrual blood loss (and other symptoms including dysmenorrhoea, headache, nausea, diarrhoea and depression) can be long term, but if it is not effective within 3 months, treatment should be stopped. Side-effects, mainly gastrointestinal (dyspepsia, nausea and diarrhoea), are mild and not frequently reported.

In summary, mefenamic acid and related compounds are effective first-line medical treatments for women with HMB. The mean reduction of menstrual blood loss is not as great as that for antifibrinolytic agents, but the NSAIDs have a lower side-effect profile in otherwise healthy women and are more effective for the treatment of pain.

Antifibrinolytics

As discussed above, the endometrium possesses an active fibrinolytic system which is more active in the endometrium of women with HMB than in those without HMB. Antifibrinolytic agents such as tranexamic acid reduce menstrual loss by approximately 50%. This is greater than the reduction following administration of prostaglandin synthetase inhibitors (Ylikorkala and Viinikka 1983, Milsom et al 1991).

The incidence of adverse effects is dose dependent. One-third of women experience gastrointestinal side-effects following treatment with tranexamic acid 3–6 g/day. As 90% of menstrual blood is lost in the first 3 days of full flow, dose-related side-effects can be reduced by limiting the number of days on which the drug is taken to the first 3 or 4 days of the menses. Serious side-effects are uncommon. No increase in the incidence of thromboembolic disease has been seen in women of reproductive age in Scandinavia, where tranexamic acid has been used since the early 1970s as a first-line treatment for HMB (Rybo 1991). Antifibrinolytic agents therefore represent a relatively effective first-line treatment to reduce the degree of menstrual bleeding.

Ethamsylate

Systematic evaluation clinical trials suggest that ethamsylate is ineffective and its use in HMB is no longer recommended.

Hormonal treatment

Hormonal treatments for HMB are summarized in Box 31.2.

Progestogens

Synthetic progestogens are widely used to treat HMB. They have an endometrial suppressive effect, resulting in small depleted glands lined with a thin epithelium and decidualized transformation of the stroma.

Cyclical progestogens

It has been shown that low-dose, short-duration therapy of oral progestogens during the luteal phase is ineffective for the reduction of menstrual loss (Figure 31.8) (Cameron et al 1990). However, they may be successful if given at a dose of 5 mg three times daily from days 5 to 26 of the cycle. On this regime, menstrual loss can be reduced by up to 30% (Irvine et al 1998). Cyclical progestogens can be used to regulate the onset of bleeding and are useful for those with an irregular, unpredictable cycle.

Continuous progestogens

Various continuous preparations are available including oral tablets, long-acting intramuscular injections and subdermal

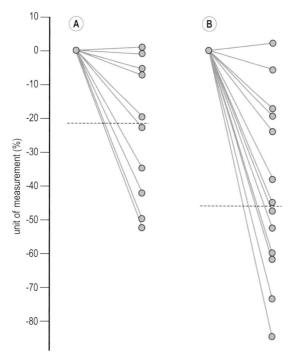

Figure 31.7 Percentage change in menstrual blood loss (mean of two cycles) of women receiving (A) norethisterone (5 mg bd, days 19–25) and (B) mefenamic acid (250 mg tds, days 1–5).

Table 31.2 Pharmaceutical treatments proven to reduce menstrual bleeding*

Discuss hormonal and non-hormonal options, and provide time and support to help the woman to decide which option is best for her.

	Pharmaceutical treatment	How it works	Is it a contraceptive?	Will it impact on future fertility?	Potential unwanted outcome experienced by some women§
First line	Levonorgestrel-releasing intrauterine system†‡	A device which slowly releases progestogen and prevents proliferation of the endometrium. A physical examination is needed before fitting	Yes	No	Common: irregular bleeding that may last for over 6 months; hormone-related problems such as breast tenderness, acne or headaches, if present, are generally minor and transient. Rare: uterine perforation at the time of insertion
Second line	Tranexamic acid (non-hormonal). Can be used in parallel with investigations. If no improvement, stop treatment after three cycles	Oral antifibrinolytic tablets	No	No	Less common: indigestion, diarrhoea and headache
	Non-steroidal anti-inflammatory drugs (non-hormonal). If no improvement, stop treatment after three cycles. Can be used in parallel investigations. Preferred over tranexamic acid dysmenorrhoea	Oral tablets that reduce production of prostaglandin	No	No	Common: indigestion and diarrhoea. Rare: worsening of asthma in sensitive individuals, and peptic ulcer with possible bleeding and peritonitis
	Combined oral contraceptives‡	Oral tablets that prevent proliferation of the endometrium	Yes	No	Common: mood change, headache, nausea, fluid retention and breast tenderness
Third line	Oral progestogen (norethisterone)‡	Oral tablets that prevent proliferation of the endometrium	Yes¶	No	Common: weight gain, bloating, breast tenderness, headaches and acne (but usually minor and transient). Rare: depression
	Injected progestogen†‡	Intramuscular injection that prevents proliferation of the endometrium	Yes	No	Common: weight gain, irregular bleeding, amenorrhoea and premenstrual-like syndrome (including bloating, fluid retention and breast tenderness). Less common: bone density loss
Other	Gonadotrophin-releasing hormone analogue. If used for more than 6 months, add-back hormone replacement therapy is recommended	Injection that stops production of oestrogen and progesterone	No	No	Common: menopausal-like symptoms (e.g. hot flushes, increased sweating and vaginal dryness). Less common: osteoporosis, particularly trabecular bone with use for more than 6 months

Source: National Institute for Health and Clinical Excellence (2007) CG 44 Heavy menstrual bleeding. London: NICE. Available from www.nice.org.uk/CG44 Reproduced with permission.

* The evidence for effectiveness can be found in the full guidelines.
† Check the Summary of Product Characteristics for current licensed indications. Informed consent is needed when using outside the licensed indications.
‡ See World Health Organization Pharmaceutical Eligibility Criteria for Contraceptive Use: www.ffprhc.org.uk/admin/uploads/298_UKMEC_200506.pdf.
§ Common: one in 100 chance; less common: one in 1000 chance; rare: one in 10,000 chance; very rare: one in 100,000 chance.
¶ The recommended dosing regimen for norethisterone is not licensed for use as a contraceptive, but may affect a woman's ability to become pregnant while it is being taken.

Box 31.2 Hormonal treatment for heavy menstrual bleeding

Progestogens

Norethisterone

Medroxyprogesterone acetate

Dydrogesterone

Intrauterine progestogens

LNG-IUS

Progestasert intrauterine system

Combined oestrogen/progestogens

Oral contraceptives

Hormone replacement therapy

Others

Danazol

GnRH analogues

Gestrinone

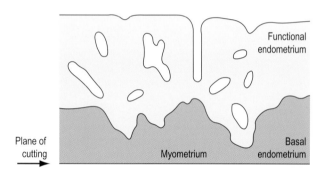

Figure 31.8 The uterine wall.

implants. Irregular bleeding and oligomenorrhoea (in many cases, amenorrhoea) are common consequences. Progestogen-only contraceptive pill users may also report a decrease in their menstrual loss.

Intrauterine progestogens

The most recently described medicated device is the levonorgestrel intrauterine system (LNG-IUS; Mirena). This delivers LNG 20 µg to the endometrium every 24 h in a sustained-release formulation that can last for up to 5 years (Luukkainen et al 1986). Direct administration of the progestogen to the uterus results in minimal systemic absorption (Andersson and Rybo 1990), giving a better side-effect profile (Cheng Chi 1991).

The efficacy of the LNG-IUS for the treatment of HMB compares well with transcervical resection of the endometrium (TCRE) at 12 months post treatment (Crosignani et al 1997, Rauramo et al 2004). It has also been suggested that it might be an acceptable alternative to hysterectomy (Lahteenmaki et al 1998). Moreover, it also appears to be cost-effective when compared with thermal balloon ablation for treatment of HMB (Brown et al 2006).

The LNG-IUS has a local effect on the endometrium causing endometrial glandular atrophy, stromal decidualization and epithelial cell inactivation. This is seen within 1 month of insertion and occurs independently of ovarian

activity (Silverberg et al 1986). When removed, the endometrium recovers quickly and biopsies taken at 1–3 months show no sign of progesterone administration, regardless of duration of treatment. The LNG-IUS has a weak effect on ovarian function, with ovulation continuing in approximately 75% of women. The most significant side-effect is irregular bleeding that may present for more than 6 months; women require careful counselling prior to insertion if this is not to lead to removal of the device.

Oestrogen/progestogen regimes

The combined oral contraceptive pill is widely used to treat HMB. It causes endometrial atrophy and, in this way, reduces endometrial prostaglandin synthesis and fibrinolysis. Menstrual loss can be reduced by as much as 50% (Fraser and McCarron 1991). Although the use of the low-dose oestrogen pill in the management of HMB has been affected by adverse publicity associated with its use in older women, it is now felt to be quite safe in women of any age who are not obese, do not smoke and are not hypertensive. It has the added advantage of providing a regular menstrual cycle and being effective in the treatment of dysmenorrhoea (Ekstrom et al 1989, Davis 2005). The limiting factor is that many of the women will have been sterilized and are therefore reluctant to continue with something they see as a contraceptive agent. Hormone replacement therapy can be used in perimenopausal women with excessive menstrual bleeding (Rees and Barlow 1991).

Danazol

Danazol, a derivative of testosterone, causes endometrial atrophy by inhibiting release of the pituitary gonadotrophins and can reduce menstrual loss by as much as 50% (Chimbira et al 1980, Dockeray et al 1989). The use of danazol is limited by its androgenic side-effects, which include weight gain, acne, depression and other long-term metabolic sequelae, all of which reduce compliance. This drug is no longer recommended.

Gonadotropin-releasing hormone analogues

GnRH analogues act by causing pituitary downregulation and subsequent inhibition of cyclical ovarian activity, resulting in amenorrhoea. Their use is limited to less than 6 months because of problems related to the hypo-oestrogenic state, including hot flushes, dry vagina and decreased bone mineral density unless 'add-back' oestrogen/progestogen therapy is used concurrently. They are useful in a minority of women (Shaw and Fraser 1984) and also in those with fibroids before surgery.

Surgical treatment

Surgical treatments range from minor conservative procedures to hysterectomy (see Table 31.3). First- and second-generation ablation methods are a less invasive alternative to hysterectomy and are associated with high levels of satisfaction, but in a proportion, surgery may be required repeatedly, and there is some risk of perioperative morbidity. Hysterectomy is the definitive treatment to stop HMB, with satisfaction rates consistently greater than 90%. However, hysterectomy is a major operation with the potential for serious morbidity and, rarely, mortality. The inconvenience to the patient and the cost to both the patient and the health services need to be balanced against the high levels of satisfaction that are reported after hysterectomy (Lethaby and Farquhar 2003).

Endometrial ablation techniques

Attempts at endometrial destruction in cases of heavy menstruation have been made by a variety of techniques. Early trials involved the intrauterine application of cytotoxic chemicals, intracavity radium, steam and cryosurgery. However, these were either ineffective or had unacceptable side-effects. They were also carried out blindly and, since the endometrium has remarkable powers of regeneration, any missed areas resulted in failure.

Endometrial ablation can be considered in a woman with HMB whose quality of life is affected to such an extent that she does not wish to preserve menstrual or reproductive function. This is suitable in woman with a normal uterus, and in those with small uterine fibroids (less than 3 cm) and a uterus no bigger than 10-week pregnancy size. Women wishing to have endometrial ablation should be provided with evidence-based information about its risks and benefits, and other available treatment options. Women must avoid pregnancy after endometrial ablation.

Hysteroscopic techniques (first generation) allow visualization of the uterine cavity, and enable the endometrium to be ablated under direct vision. Since regeneration of the endometrium occurs from the basal layer, it is essential to destroy all the endometrium. As the endometrial–myometrial border is irregular, the superficial layer of myometrium must also be included (Figure 31.8). There are a number of methods of achieving this, including removal of the tissue using a cutting loop, or coagulation or vaporization of the tissue using laser.

First-generation (hysteroscopic) ablation techniques (TCRE and rollerball endometrial ablation) are only appropriate if hysteroscopic myomectomy is to be included in the procedure.

Endometrial resection

The technique for TCRE is essentially similar to that of transurethral prostatectomy in men, and is performed through a continuous flow resectoscope. In this technique, a loop diathermy electrode is used to scrape out and remove the tissues through the cervix, and rollerball ablation uses an electrode with a movable ball or cylinder to coagulate and stop the bleeding tissues. It is important to destroy all the endometrium, otherwise regeneration will occur and the operation will fail. TCRE requires considerable skill if it is to be effective and safe. It is currently only used when hysteroscopic myomectomy is performed at the same time.

Laser ablation

Neodymium:yttrium-aluminium-garnet laser is optimal for intrauterine surgery, since it can be delivered along a flexible fibre through a liquid medium and the depth of tissue penetration can be controlled. The beam produces warming, coagulation, evaporation and carbonization. Tissue destruction typically occurs to a depth of 4–5 mm. Heat transmission through the myometrium is minimized by the continuous flow of cold irrigation fluid.

More recently, second-generation (non-hysteroscopic) ablation techniques are widely used because of a better safety profile compared with first-generation techniques. The second-generation techniques include: fluid-filled thermal balloon endometrial ablation, microwave endometrial ablation (MEA) and impedance-controlled bipolar radiofrequency ablation

Thermal balloon ablation (Figure 31.9)

This involves the blind insertion of a balloon through the cervix, which is then filled with fluid until a pressure of 160–180 mmHg is reached. The fluid is then heated to 75–90°C (average 87°C). Endometrial destruction occurs over the next 8 min. The diameter of the insertion tube is very small and no cervical dilatation is required. This means that the procedure is particularly appropriate for women who are not suitable for or who do not wish to have a general anaesthetic. It is uncomfortable but pain relief can be improved by prior administration of a preparation such as diclofenac. Some sedation may be useful in certain instances. The success rate of this procedure appears to be similar to that for TCRE. One of the main advantages appears to be that pretreatment with a GnRH agonist is not required. Since the procedure is done in the outpatient setting in a number of units and has even been performed in general practice, it is likely to be a cheap and popular modality in the future. Outpatient thermal balloon ablation (Thermachoice III) can be performed in the majority of women, and is associated with similar overall pain scores but significantly less nausea, vomiting, need for antiemetics and less time spent in hospital compared with day-case Thermachoice III (Marsh et al 2007)

The procedure is effective and patient satisfaction is rated between good and excellent in more than 90% of cases. Complications of thermal balloon ablation include endometritis, urinary tract infection and haemorrhage, but all are uncommon (National Institute for Health and Clinical Excellence 2003).

Microwave endometrial ablation

MEA requires the insertion of a probe that emits microwaves into the uterus. The probe is then slowly moved across the fundus and down through the uterine cavity, destroying the

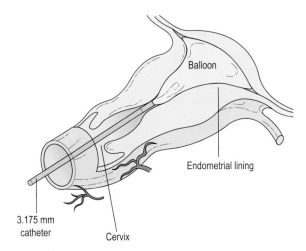

Figure 31.9 A thermal balloon inside the uterus (Thermachoice®, Gynecare, Edinburgh).

Table 31.3 Surgical and radiological treatment options for women whose quality of life is severely impacted

Provide information to the woman before her outpatient appointment.

Indication	Type of surgery	How it works	Will it impact on future fertility?	Other considerations	Potential unwanted outcomes experienced by some women*
Severe impact on quality of life + no desire to conceive + normal uterus +/− small fibroids (<3 cm diameter). Consider as first line only after full discussion of risks and benefits. Preferable to hysterectomy if uterus no bigger than 10-week pregnancy.	Endometrial ablation. Second-generation • Impedance-controlled bipolar radiofrequency • Balloon thermal • Microwave • Free fluid thermal First generation • Rollerball • Transcervical resection of the endometrium	It destroys the womb lining.	Yes	Discuss impact on fertility. Use second-generation technique in women with no structural or histological abnormality. Advise use of effective contraception following this procedure.	Common: vaginal discharge, increased period pain or cramping (even if no further bleeding), and need for additional surgery. Less common: infection. Rare: perforation (but very rare with second-generation techniques).
Fibroids (>3 cm diameter) + severe impact on quality of life. Consider as first line if there are other significant symptoms, pain or pressure. Recommended for women who want to retain uterus +/− avoid surgery.	Uterine artery embolization	Small particles are injected into the blood vessels that take blood to the uterus. The blood supply to the fibroids is blocked and this causes them to shrink.	Fertility is potentially retained	Discuss impact on fertility	Common: persistent vaginal discharge, postembolization syndrome – pain, nausea, vomiting and fever (not involving hospitalization). Less common: need for additional surgery, premature ovarian failure, particularly in women over 45 years of age, and haematoma. Rare: haemorrhage, non-target embolization causing tissue necrosis, infection causing septicaemia.
Fibroids (>3 cm diameter) + severe impact on quality of life. Recommended for women who want to retain uterus.	Hysteroscopic myomectomy	Surgical removal of the fibroids using hysteroscope.	Fertility is potentially retained	Discuss impact on fertility. Consider pretreatment with GnRH analogue. Following with a first-generation ablation technique is appropriate.	Less common: adhesions (which may lead to pain and/or impaired fertility), need for additional surgery, perforation, recurrence of fibroids and infection. Rare: haemorrhage
Fibroids (>3 cm diameter) + severe impact on quality of life.	Myomectomy	Surgical removal of the fibroids.	Fertility is potentially retained	Discuss impact on fertility. Consider pretreatment with GnRH analogue.	Less common: adhesions (which may lead to pain and/or impaired fertility), need for additional surgery, recurrence of fibroids and infection. Rare: haemorrhage

Continued

Fibroids (>3 cm diameter) + severe impact on quality of life	Hysterectomy. Decide route based on individual assessment. First line: vaginal; second line: abdominal. Do not remove any healthy ovaries	Surgical removal of the uterus. Ovaries may also be removed (oophorectomy)	Yes	Discuss impact on sexual feelings, fertility, bladder function and psychology. Discuss complications, expectations and alternatives. Consider pretreatment with GnRH analogue. Discuss increased risk in women with fibroids. Discuss total and subtotal methods in abdominal surgery. If considering oophorectomy, discuss impact on well-being. If concerned, discuss risks and benefits with women. Offer genetic grief counselling	Common: infection. Less common: intraoperative haemorrhage, damage to other abdominal organs (e.g. urinary tract or bowel) and urinary dysfunction (frequent passing of urine and incontinence). Rare: thrombosis (DVT and clot on the lung). Very rare: death. *With oophorectomy at time of hysterectomy:* Common: menopausal-like symptoms
Not first line solely for heavy menstrual bleeding. Consider when: • other treatments have failed, are contraindicated or declined • desire for amenorrhoea • fully informed woman requests it • no desire to retain uterus and fertility	Hysterectomy. Decide route based on individual assessment. First line: vaginal; second line: abdominal. Consider laparoscopic vaginal hysterectomy in morbidly obese/oophorectomy. Do not remove healthy ovaries	Surgical removal of the uterus. Ovaries may also be removed (oophorectomy)	Yes	Discuss impact on sexual feelings, fertility, bladder function and psychology. Discuss complications, expectations and alternatives. Consider pretreatment with GnRH analogue. Discuss total and subtotal methods in abdominal surgery. If considering oophorectomy, discuss impact on well-being. If concerned about health of ovaries, discuss risks and benefits. Other genetic counselling	Common: infection. Less common: intraoperative haemorrhage, damage to other abdominal organs (e.g. urinary tract or bowel) and urinary dysfunction (frequent passing of urine and incontinence). Rare: thrombosis (DVT and clot on lung). Very rare: death. *With oophorectomy at time of hysterectomy:* Common: menopausal-like symptoms

Source: National Institute for Health and Clinical Excellence (2007) CG 44 Heavy menstrual bleeding. London: NICE. Available from www.nice.org.uk/CG44 Reproduced with permission.

GnRH, gonadotrophin-releasing hormone; DVT, deep vein thrombosis.

*Common: one in 100 chance; less common: one in 1000 chance; rare: one in 10,000 chance; very rare: one in 100,000 chance.

endometrium. Provided that the probe is in the cavity of the uterus, this is a very safe procedure as the temperature rises as the endometrium is treated and the probe moved to another area. Randomized comparisons of this technique with TCRE suggest that it is equally effective; like TCRE, MEA also requires pretreatment with a GnRH agonist. In addition, since it requires dilatation of the cervix to 9 mm, it is unusual to perform this procedure under local anaesthetic. However, it is likely that smaller probes will be developed in order to achieve this result. The curative effect of MEA is similar to that of total hysterectomy, especially when preservation of the uterus and postoperative recovery is considered (Lin 2006).

These procedures are attractive alternatives to endometrial resection, although they are less valuable in the presence of uterine fibroids, particularly if the cavity is enlarged.

Success rates

There is little variation in success rates between the different methods. Overall, approximately 30% of women will be amenorrhoeic and a further 45–50% will have significantly decreased loss, giving a satisfaction rate of approximately 75% (Magos et al 1991, Scottish Hysteroscopy Audit Group 1995, Cooper et al 1999). Careful counselling is essential in that if a woman is keen to have amenorrhoea, this will not be the treatment of choice for her. Some women also experience relief from symptoms of dysmenorrhoea and premenstrual tension.

Complications

The most significant complications are those of uterine perforation and fluid absorption. Uterine perforation occurs in less than 1% of cases and is not usually associated with major problems, unless the device is activated within the abdominal cavity, when bowel or blood vessels may be damaged. Fluid absorption is rare since surgeons have become aware of the risk and stop the operation if absorption becomes excessive. Infection may also occur and most surgeons give prophylactic antibiotics routinely. MEA should be used with caution if there is a thin lower segment caesarean section scar.

Comparison of endometrial resection with hysterectomy

Endometrial resection was developed as an alternative to hysterectomy. However, it appears that the number of hysterectomies being performed is continuing to rise, suggesting that it is not serving this purpose. There have been a number of randomized comparisons between endometrial ablation and hysterectomy which show that satisfaction with both procedures is high (Pinion et al 1994). In addition, the operation can be performed on a day-case basis and recovery time is short, making it a cheap alternative to hysterectomy. However, it does appear that 20% of patients will require further surgical treatment, and there is still uncertainty regarding whether or not the number of failures will increase with time.

Endometrial resection is most likely to be successful in women over 40 years of age who have a normal-sized uterus and no intrauterine pathology. Its use in dysmenorrhoea is equivocal since it appears to make women worse in approximately 12% of cases, which may be due to the formation of haematometra. However, approximately 40% will improve so the presence of dysmenorrhoea is not an absolute con-traindication. The menstrual cycle length will not be changed by the procedure, and hysterectomy may be an appropriate alternative in women with very irregular bleeding (Lewis 1994).

Hydrothermal ablation (fluid-filled thermal endometrial ablation)

Hydrothermal ablation is a procedure in which high-temperature water is used to destroy the lining of the uterus. It is used to treat abnormal uterine bleeding even when there are small submucous fibroids. The procedure is safe, effective and can be performed as a day-case procedure.

Novasure

The NovaSure system is safe and effective for the treatment of women with abnormal uterine bleeding. Endometrial pre-treatment is not necessary, and the presence of blood in the uterine cavity during treatment is not a limiting factor. The procedure is quick, safe and simple. This minimally invasive procedure controls heavy bleeding by using energy to remove the lining of the uterus. The average treatment time is approximately 90 s, and the procedure only needs to be performed once to lighten or stop menses. NovaSure can be performed in the hospital or outpatient setting.

Without the side-effects of hormones or the risks of hysterectomy, NovaSure has a quick recovery time. Most women experience no pain after the procedure and can return to work the next day. With more than 500,000 patients treated to date, NovaSure is proven to be safe and successful. A clinical trial has shown that more than nine out of 10 women return to normal or lower than normal bleeding levels following treatment with NovaSure (Cooper et al 2002). For some women, their menses stopped completely. In a small percentage of patients, side-effects include cramping, nausea/vomiting, discharge and spotting.

Uterine artery embolization

This procedure is usually performed to treat fibroids associated with HMB, under local anaesthesia by an interventional radiologist. Particles are injected to block both uterine arteries. This shrinks the fibroids. This procedure is safe and there is symptomatic improvement in bleeding. There is no proven permanent effect on the uterus (National Institute for Health and Clinical Excellence 2007).

Uterine artery embolization (UAE), myomectomy or hysterectomy should be considered in HMB where large uterine fibroids (>3 cm diameter) are affecting the woman's quality of life. Women should be informed that UAE or myomectomy may potentially allow them to retain their fertility. MRI can be used, if required, prior to UAE or myomectomy to assess the position, size, number and vascularity of the fibroids. Three to four months of treatment with a GnRH analogue should be considered before myomectomy or hysterectomy where fibroids have enlarged or distorted the uterus. However, GnRH analogues should be stopped prior to UAE as they decrease the calibre of the vessels and make cannulation more difficult.

Hysterectomy

Hysterectomy is no longer recommended as a first-line treatment for HMB. Conservative surgery should be considered prior to hysterectomy. Woman's expectations and the possible impact of hysterectomy on personal, psychological, sexual, family and social life should also be discussed in full and documented in the notes. Women should also be informed about the possible loss of ovarian function and its consequences (such as the need for hormone replacement therapy and its benefits and risks) even if the ovaries are preserved.

However, hysterectomy can be considered when other management options are contraindicated or have failed, or if the woman (being fully informed) requests it because she no longer wishes to retain her menstrual and reproductive function.

Hysterectomy, although an effective treatment for menstrual problems, is a major operation and is not without risk in terms of both mortality and morbidity. The major risks include intraoperative bleeding and damage to other abdominal organs, such as bladder, ureter or bowel. Complications are greater in the presence of fibroids.

The incidence of hysterectomy is gradually increasing in the Western world as a whole, but it varies considerably from one country to another, reflecting differences in the attitudes of both patients and gynaecologists rather than a variation in pathology. Women in Scotland have a 20% chance of losing their uterus before 60 years of age, whereas the figure is 50% in California.

In deciding the route of hysterectomy (vaginal, laparoscopic-assisted vaginal or abdominal), individual assessment is essential. Factors that influence this decision include: uterine size, mobility and descent; number, size and site of uterine fibroids; size, shape and prolapse of vaginal wall; history of previous surgery; and presence of comorbidities such as obesity, diabetes, hypertension or heart disease. The possibility of total and subtotal hysterectomy should also be discussed when abdominal hysterectomy is considered.

Healthy ovaries should not be removed at the time of hysterectomy. This should be discussed prior to the operation, and bilateral oophorectomy should only be performed with the express wish and consent of the woman. In the presence of a significant family history of breast or ovarian cancer, the woman needs appropriate genetic counselling. This is likely to help her make an informed decision about oophorectomy. In premenopausal women, especially those under 45 years of age, considering hysterectomy for HMB with other symptoms that may be related to ovarian dysfunction (e.g. premenstrual syndrome), a trial of ovarian suppression for 3–6 months should be used as a guide to the necessity for hysterectomy. Once oophorectomy is decided, the impact of this on the woman's well-being and the possible need for hormone replacement therapy should also be discussed.

Abdominal hysterectomy involves a laparotomy incision that is transverse or longitudinal. A vaginal hysterectomy involves an incision through the vaginal wall. For many surgeons, vaginal hysterectomy is the preferred method for women with some degree of uterine descent and where the uterus is not excessively large. Abdominal hysterectomy allows better visualization of the pelvic cavity should there be pathology or where difficulty is anticipated. Non-randomized studies indicate that the complication rate for abdominal hysterectomy is greater than that for vaginal hysterectomy, and women who have vaginal procedures are able to go home sooner than women who have abdominal operations (Dicker et al 1982, Clinch 1994).

Recently, it has become possible to convert an abdominal hysterectomy to a vaginal hysterectomy using endoscopic techniques. The laparoscope allows visualization of the pelvic cavity, and all or part of the hysterectomy may be performed using specially designed laparoscopic instruments. A laparoscopic-assisted vaginal hysterectomy allows tissues accessible through the vagina to be ligated and the uterus to be removed by the vaginal route. This method facilitates the removal of ovaries and aids the operation when there is no uterine descent. It allows for dissection of adhesions and the treatment of pelvic pathology, such as endometriosis, prior to the hysterectomy. Published complication rates are low but recovery does not appear to be quicker than that following abdominal hysterectomy (Lumsden et al 2000), although the length of hospital stay is reduced (Boike et al 1993). Compared with abdominal hysterectomy, laparoscopic hysterectomy is associated with a higher rate of major complications, less postoperative pain and shorter hospital stay, but takes longer to perform (Boike et al 1993). The ovarian pedicles were only secured with laparoscopic sutures in 7% of cases, but this was associated with 25% of the complications. Abdominal laparoscopic hysterectomy is associated with a significantly higher risk of major complications and takes longer to perform than abdominal hysterectomy. Abdominal laparoscopic hysterectomy is, however, associated with less pain, quicker recovery and better short-term quality of life after surgery than abdominal hysterectomy. The cost-effectiveness of laparoscopic hysterectomy is finely balanced and is also influenced by the choice of reusable vs disposable equipment (Garry et al 2004).

Dysmenorrhoea

In young women, dysmenorrhoea is frequently the only menstrual abnormality. Prostaglandin synthetase inhibitors and the oral contraceptive pill are very effective (Anderson 1981), but in a minority of women, even in the absence of disease, these measures are insufficient. Calcium channel blockers (e.g. nifedipine) have been used in Scandinavia and are effective, although their use is limited by cardiovascular side-effects. Oxytocin/vasopressin receptor antagonists may become available when effective oral agents are developed.

In the past, presacral neurectomy was performed but this involved major abdominal surgery and was only effective in approximately 50% of cases. Recently, presacral neurectomy has been performed using intra-abdominal lasers. The long-term effect of this treatment has not been reported and it is only available in a few UK centres.

In older women where child bearing is completed, hysterectomy is often the solution since dysmenorrhoea in this group is frequently associated with other menstrual problems.

Conclusions

Menstrual dysfunction remains one of the most common reasons why women seek medical advice, yet the process of menstruation is poorly understood. Strategies to improve the investigation and management of this problem are likely to arise from two directions. First, a thorough investigation of the medicosociological factors is required. Second, the role of vasoactive substances in the endometrium needs to be further investigated, as well as determination of the factors that control endometrial proliferation. HMB affects work, family and social life. Investigations and management should be evidence based. When management options are discussed, there should be the flexibility to provide an acceptable solution for each individual woman.

KEY POINTS

1. HMB is the most common cause of iron-deficiency anaemia in Western women.
2. The menstrual cycle consists of proliferative, secretory and menstrual phases.
3. Menstruation is initiated by a withdrawal of progesterone and oestrogen support to the endometrium.
4. Menstrual loss is dependent upon the degree of platelet plug formation, vasoconstriction and endometrial repair. Abnormality in these mechanisms can result in menstrual dysfunction. Paracrine factors are also thought to play a role in the control of menstruation.
5. The mean menstrual blood loss is 37–43 ml per menses. Loss in excess of 80 ml per menses is considered to be HMB.
6. Abnormal menstrual loss may arise from pelvic pathology, clotting disorders, medical disorders or DUB.
7. DUB is defined as heavy or irregular bleeding in the absence of pelvic pathology, pregnancy or clotting disorder.
8. Anovulatory cycles may be associated with cystic glandular hyperplasia. This can occur in both older women and peripubertal girls, and may result in excessive menstrual loss.
9. Primary dysmenorrhoea occurs almost exclusively in ovulatory cycles, and prostaglandin secretion is strongly implicated in its aetiology.
10. Subjective and objective assessments of menstrual loss are poorly correlated. Medical treatment of HMB is less effective if the blood loss is within normal limits, unless there are other associated symptoms which are relieved.
11. Hysteroscopy and endometrial biopsy is more sensitive than endometrial curettage in the diagnosis of endometrial abnormality.
12. Hysterectomy is a very effective remedy for menstrual dysfunction but is associated with postoperative morbidity and mortality. It is the only treatment that is guaranteed to lead to amenorrhoea.
13. Laparoscopic-assisted vaginal hysterectomy allows conversion of an abdominal hysterectomy to a vaginal hysterectomy. It is associated with a shorter hospital stay, but the recovery time is similar to that following abdominal hysterectomy.
14. Endometrial ablation is a useful alternative to medical treatment or hysterectomy in cases of DUB and can be performed under local anaesthesia.
15. Medical treatment of HMB may result in good symptomatic relief and is safe but does not result in long-term cure.

References

Adalantado JM, Rees MCP, Bernal AL, Turnbull AC 1988 Increased intrauterine prostaglandin E receptors in menorrhagic women. British Journal of Obstetrics and Gynaecology 95: 162.

Åkerlund M, Anderssen KE 1976 Vasopressin response and turbutaline inhibition of the uterus. Obstetrics and Gynecology 48: 528–536.

Åkerlund M, Stromberg P, Forsling ML 1979 Primary dysmenorrhoea and vasopressin. British Journal of Obstetrics and Gynaecology 86: 484–487.

Alecozay AA, Harper MJK, Schenken RS, Hanahan DJ 1991 Paracrine interactions between platelet-activating factor and prostaglandins in hormonally-treated human luteal phase endometrium in vitro. Journal of Reproduction and Fertility 91: 301–312.

Andersch B, Milsom I 1982 An epidemiologic study of young women with dysmenorrhoea. American Journal of Obstetrics and Gynecology 144: 655–660.

Anderson A 1981 The role of prostaglandin synthetase inhibitors in gynaecology. Practitioner 225: 1460–1470.

Andersson K, Rybo G 1990 Levonorgestrel-releasing intrauterine device in the treatment of menorrhagia. British Journal of Obstetrics and Gynaecology 97: 690–694.

Bacon CR, Morrison JJ, O'Reilly G, Cameron IT, Davenport AP 1995 ETA and ETB endothelin receptors in human myometrium characterised by the subtype selective ligands BQ123, BQ3020, FR139317 and PD15142. Journal of Endocrinology 144: 127–134.

Basilico C, Moscatelli D 1992 The FGF family of growth factors and oncogenes. Advances in Cancer Research 59: 115–165.

Battersby S, Critchley HOD, Morgan K, Millar RP, Jabbour HN 2004 Expression and regulation of prokineticins (endocrine-gland-derived vascular endothelial growth factor and Bv8) and their receptors in the human endometrium across the menstrual cycle. Journal of Clinical Endocrinology and Metabolism 89: 2463–2469.

Beller FK 1971 Observations on the clotting of menstrual blood and clot formation. American Journal of Obstetrics and Gynecology 11: 535–546.

Björk J, Smedegård G 1983 Acute microvascular effects of PAF-acether, as studied by intravital microscopy. European Journal of Pharmacology 96: 87.

Boike GM, Elfstrand EP, Del Priore G et al 1993 Laparoscopically assisted vaginal hysterectomy in a university hospital: report of 82 cases and comparison with abdominal and vaginal hysterectomy. American Journal of Obstetrics and Gynecology 168: 1690–1701.

Bonnar J, Sheppard BL, Dockeray CJ 1983 The haemostatic system and dysfunctional uterine bleeding. Research and Clinical Forums 5: 27–36.

Brosens JJ, Barker FG, deSouza NM 1998 Myometrial zonal differentiation and uterine junctional zone hyperplasia in the non-pregnant uterus. Human Reproduction Update 4: 496–502.

Brosens JJ, Mak I, Brosens I 2000 Mechanisms of dysmenorrhoea. In: O'Brien S, Cameron IT, MacLean A (eds) Disorders of the Menstrual Cycle. RCOG Press, London, pp 113–132.

Brown PM, Farquhar CM, Lethaby A, Sadler LC, Johnson NP 2006 Cost-effectiveness analysis of levonorgestral intrauterine system and thermal balloon ablation for heavy menstrual bleeding. BJOG: an International Journal of Obstetrics and Gynaecology 113: 797–803.

Bruner KL, Rodgers WH, Old LI et al 1995 Transforming growth factor beta mediates progesterone suppression of an epithelial metalloproteinase by adjacent stroma in the human endometrium. Proceedings of the National Academy of Sciences USA 92: 7362–7366.

Cameron IT, Haining R, Lumsden MA, Reid-Thomas V, Smith SK 1990 The effects of mefenamic acid and norethisterone on measured menstrual blood loss. Obstetrics and Gynecology 76: 85–88.

Cameron IT, Davenport AP 1992 Endothelins in reproduction. Reproductive Medicine Review 1: 99–113.

Cameron IT, Davenport AP, van Papendorp CL et al 1992 Endothelin-like immunoreactivity in human endometrium. Journal of Reproduction and Fertility 95: 623–628.

Cameron IT, Norman JE 1995 Endometrial biochemistry in menorrhagia. In: Studd J, Asch R (eds) Progress in Reproductive Medicine, Volume II. Parthenon Publishing Group, London, pp 267–279.

Campbell S, Young A, Stewart CJR et al 1998 Laminin beta 2 distinguishes inner and outer myometrial layers of the human myometrium. Journal of Reproduction and Fertility 22: 12.

Carson DD, Lagow E, Thathiah A et al 2002 Changes in gene expression during the early to mid-luteal (receptive phase) transition in human endometrium detected by high density microarray screening. Molecular Human Reproduction 8: 871–879.

Casslen B, Andersson A, Nilsson IM, Astedt B 1986 Hormonal regulation of the release of plasminogen activators and of a specific activator inhibitor from endometrial tissue in culture (42360). Proceedings of the Society for Experimental Biology and Medicine 182: 419–424.

Chalubinski K, Deutinger J, Bernaschek G 1993 Vaginosonography for recording of cycle-related myometrial contractions. Fertility and Sterility 59: 225–228.

Chamberlain G, Freeman R, Price F, Kennedy A, Green D, Eve L 1991 A comparative study of ethamsylate and mefenamic acid in dysfunctional uterine bleeding. British Journal of Obstetrics and Gynaecology; 98: 707–711.

Chan RW, Schwab KE, Gargett CE 2004 Clonogenicity of human endometrial epithelial and stromal cells. Biology of Reproduction 70: 1738–1750.

Charnock-Jones DS, Sharkey AM, Rajput-Williams J et al 1993 Identification and localization of alternately spliced mRNAs for vascular endothelial growth factor in human uterus and estrogen regulation in endometrial carcinoma cell lines. Biology of Reproduction 48: 1120–1128.

Cheng Chi I 1991 An evaluation of the levonorgestrel-releasing IUD: its advantages and disadvantages when compared to the copper-releasing IUDs. Contraception 44: 573–587.

Chimbira TH, Anderson ABM, Turnbull AC 1980 Relation between measured menstrual blood loss and patients' subjective assessment of loss, duration of bleeding, number of sanitary towels used, uterine weight and endometrial surface area. British Journal of Obstetrics and Gynaecology 87: 603–609.

Christiaens G, Sixma JJ, Haspels AA 1980 Morphology of haemostasis in menstrual endometrium. British Journal of Obstetrics and Gynaecology 87: 425–439.

Christiaens G, Sixma JJ, Haspels AA 1981 Fibrin and platelets in menstrual discharge before and after the insertion of an intrauterine contraceptive device. American Journal of Obstetrics and Gynecology 140: 793–798.

Christiaens G, Sixma JJ, Haspels AA 1982 Haemostasis in menstrual endometrium: a review. Obstetrical and Gynecological Survey 37: 281–303.

Clinch J 1994 Length of hospital stay after vaginal hysterectomy. British Journal of Obstetrics and Gynaecology 101: 253–254.

Cohen BJB, Gibor Y 1980 Anaemia and menstrual blood loss. Obstetrical and Gynecological Survey 35: 597–618.

Cole SK, Billewicz WZ, Thomson AM 1971 Sources of variation in menstrual blood loss. Journal of Obstetrics and Gynaecology of the British Commonwealth 78: 933–939.

Cooper KG, Parkin DE, Garrett AM, Grant AM 1999 Two year follow-up of women randomised to medical management or transcervical resection of the endometrium for heavy menstrual loss; clinical and quality of life outcomes. British Journal of Obstetrics and Gynaecology 106: 258–265.

Cooper J, Gimpleson R, Laberge P et al 2002 A randomized, multicenter trial of safety and efficacy of the NovaSure® system in the treatment of menorrhagia. Journal of the American Association of Gynecologic Laparoscopists 9: 418–428.

Coulter A, Kelland J, Peto V, Rees M 1995 Treating menorrhagia in primary care: an overview of drug trials and a survey of prescribing practice. International Journal of Health Technology Assessment in Health Care 11: 456–471.

Critchley H, Abberton KM, Taylor NH, Healy DL, Rogers AW 1994 Endometrial sex steroid receptor expression in women with menorrhagia. British Journal of Obstetrics and Gynaecology 101: 428–434.

Critchley HO, Kelly RW, Brenner RM, Baird DT 2001 The endocrinology of menstruation — a role for the immune system. Clinical Endocrinology 55: 701–710.

Crosignani PG, Vercellini P, Mosconi P, Oldani S, Cortesi I, de Giorgi O 1997 Levonorgestrel-releasing intrauterine device versus hysteroscopic endometrial resection in the treatment of dysfunctional uterine bleeding. Obstetrics and Gynecology 90: 257–263.

Daly L, Sheppard BL, Carroll E, Hennelly B, Bonnar J 1990 Coagulation and fibrinolysis in menstrual and peripheral blood in dysfunctional uterine bleeding. Irish Journal of Medical Science 159: 24–25.

de Merre LJ, Moss JD, Pattison OS 1967 The haematological study of menstrual discharge. Obstetrics and Gynecology 30: 830–833.

de Vries K, Lyons EA, Ballard G, Levi CS, Lindsay DJ 1990 Contractions of the inner third of the myometrium. American Journal of Obstetrics and Gynecology 162: 679–682.

Demas BE, Hricak H, Jaffe RB 1985 Uterine MR imaging: effects of hormonal stimulation. Radiology 159: 123–126.

Davis AR 2005 Oral contraceptives for dysmenorrhoea in adolescent girls: a randomized trial. Obstetrics and Gynecology 106: 97–104.

Dicker RC, Greenspan JR, Strauss LT et al 1982 Complications of abdominal and vaginal hysterectomy among women of reproductive age in the United States. American Journal of Obstetrics and Gynecology 144: 841–848.

Dockeray CJ, Sheppard BL, Bonnar J 1989 Comparison between mefenamic acid and danazol in the treatment of established menorrhagia. British Journal of Obstetrics and Gynaecology 96: 840–844.

Ekstrom P, Juchnicka E, Laudanski T, Åkerlund M 1989 Effect of an oral contraceptive in primary dysmenorrhoea — changes in uterine activity and reactivity to agonists. Contraception 40: 39–47.

Ferriani RA, Charnock-Jones DS, Prentice A, Thomas EJ, Smith SK 1993 Immunohistochemical localization of acidic and basic fibroblast growth factors in normal human endometrium and endometriosis and the detection of their mRNA by polymerase chain reaction. Human Reproduction 8: 11–16.

Filler WW, Hall WC 1970 Dysmenorrhoea and its therapy: a uterine contractility study. American Journal of Obstetrics and Gynecology 106: 104–109.

Fraser IS, McCarron G, Markham R, Resta T, Watts A 1986 Measured menstrual blood loss in women with menorrhagia associated with pelvic disease or coagulation disorder. Obstetrics and Gynecology 68: 630–633.

Fraser IS, McCarron G 1991 Randomised trial of two hormonal and two prostaglandin-inhibiting agents in women with a complaint of menorrhagia. Australian and New Zealand Journal of Obstetrics and Gynaecology; 31: 66–70.

Fraser IS, Inceboz US 2000 Defining disturbances of the menstrual cycle. In: O, Brien PMS, Cameron I, Maclean A (eds) Disorders of the Menstrual Cycle. RCOG Press, London, pp 141–152.

Garry R, Fountain J, Brown J et al 2004 EVALUATE hysterectomy trial: a multicentre randomized trial comparing abdominal, vaginal and laparoscopic methods of hysterectomy. Health Technology Assessment 8: 1–154.

Gimpleson RJ, Rappold HO 1988 A comparative study between panoramic hysteroscopy with directed biopsies and dilatation and curettage. American Journal of Obstetrics and Gynecology 158: 489–492.

Gospodarowicz D, Abraham JA, Schilling J 1989 Isolation and characterization of a vascular endothelial cell mitogen produced by pituitary-derived follicular stellate cells. Proceedings of the National Academy of Sciences USA 86: 7311–7315.

Hahn L 1980 Composition of menstrual blood. In: Diczfalusy E, Fraser IS, Webb FTG (eds) Endometrial Bleeding and Steroidal Contraception. Pitman Press, Bath, pp 107–137.

Haining REB, Cameron IT, van Papendorp CL et al 1991 Epidermal growth factor in human endometrium: proliferative effects in culture and immunocytochemical localisation in normal and endometriotic tissues. Human Reproduction 6: 1200.

Hallberg L, Nilsson L 1964 Consistency of individual menstrual blood loss. Acta Obstetrica et Gynecologica Scandinavica 43: 352–359.

Haynes P, Hodgson H, Anderson A, Turnbull A 1977 Measurement of menstrual blood loss in patients complaining of menorrhagia. British Journal of Obstetrics and Gynaecology 84: 763–768.

Haynes P, Anderson ABM, Turnbull AC 1979 Patterns of menstrual blood loss in menorrhagia. Research and Clinical Forums 1: 73–78.

Higham JM 1994 Medical treatment of menorrhagia. Progress in Obstetrics and Gynaecology 68: 335–337.

Higham JM, O'Brien PMS, Shaw RW 1990 Assessment of menstrual blood loss using a pictorial chart. British Journal of Obstetrics and Gynaecology 97: 734–739.

Hynes RO 1987 Integrins: a family of cell surface receptors. Cell 48: 549–554.

Ignar Trowbridge DM, Teng CT, Ross KA, Parker MG, Korach KS, McLachlan JA 1993 Peptide growth factors elicit estrogen receptor-dependent transcriptional activation of an estrogen-responsive element. Molecular Endocrinology 7: 992–998.

Irvine GA, Campbell-Brown MB, Lumsden MA, Heikkila A, Walker JJ, Cameron IT 1998 Randomised comparative trial of the levonorgestrel intrauterine system and norethisterone for treatment of idiopathic menorrhagia. British Journal of Obstetrics and Gynaecology 105: 592–598.

Jabbour HN, Kelly RW, Fraser HM, Critchley HO 2006 Endocrine regulation of menstruation. Endocrine Reviews 27: 17–46.

Jeziorska M, Nagase H, Salamonsen LA, Woolley DE 1996 Immunolocalisation of the matrix metalloproteinase gelatinase B and stromelysin 1 in human endometrium throughout the menstrual cycle. Journal of Reproductive Fertility 107: 43–51.

Kao LC, Tulac S, Lobo S et al 2002 Global gene profiling in human endometrium during the window of implantation. Endocrinology 143: 2119–2138.

Kelly RW, Lumdsen MA, Abel MH, Baird DT 1984 The relationship between menstrual blood loss and prostaglandin production in the human: evidence for increased availability of arachidonic acid in women suffering from menorrhagia. Prostaglandins, Leukotrienes and Medicine 16: 69–78.

King A, Burrows T, Vernas S, Hiby S, Loke YW 1998 Human uterine lymphocytes. Human Reproduction Update 5: 480–485.

Kulkarni A, Lee CA, Griffeon A, Kadir RA 2006 Disorders of menstruation and their effect on the quality of life in women with congenital factor VII deficiency. Haemophilia 12: 248–252.

Kunz G, Beil D, Deininger H, Wildt L, Leyendecker G 1996 The dynamics of rapid sperm transport through the female genital tract: evidence from vaginal sonography of uterine peristalsis and hysterosalpingoscintigraphy. Human Reproduction 11: 627–632.

Lahteenmaki P, Haukkamaa M, Puolakka J et al 1998 Open randomised study of use of levonorgestrel releasing intrauterine system as an alternative to hysterectomy. BMJ (Clinical Research Ed.) 316: 1122–1126.

Lesny P, Killick SR, Tetlow RL et al 1999 Ultrasound evaluation of the uterine zonal anatomy during in-vitro fertilization and embryo transfer. Human Reproduction 14: 1593–1598.

Lessey BA, Castelbaum AJ, Buck CA, Lei Y, Yowell CW, Sun J 1992 Integrin adhesion molecules in the human endometrium. Correlation with the normal and abnormal menstrual cycle. Journal of Clinical Investigation 90: 188–195.

Lethaby S, Farquhar C 2003 Treatments for heavy menstrual bleeding. BMJ (Clinical Research Ed.) 327: 1243–1244.

Letzel H, Megard Y, Lamarca R, Raber A, Fortea J 2006 The efficacy and safety of aceclofenac versus placebo and naproxen in women with primary dysmenorrhoea. European Journal of Obstetrics, Gynaecology and Reproductive Biology 129: 162–168.

Lewis BV 1990 Hysteroscopy for the investigation of abnormal uterine bleeding. British Journal of Obstetrics and Gynaecology 97: 283–284.

Lewis BV 1994 Guidelines for endometrial ablation. British Journal of Obstetrics and Gynaecology 101: 470.

Leyendecker G, Kunz G, Wildt L, Beil D, Deiniger H 1996 Uterine hyperperistalsis and dysperistalsis as dysfunctions of the mechanism of rapid sperm transport in patients with endometriosis and infertility. Human Reproduction 11: 1542–1551.

Lin H 2006 Comparison between microwave endometrial ablation and total hysterectomy. Chinese Medical Journal 119: 1195–1197.

Lockwood CJ, Krikun G, Hausknecht VA, Papp C, Schatz F 1998 Matrix metalloproteinase and matrix metalloproteinase inhibitor expression in endometrial stromal cells during progestin-initiated decidualisation and menstruation. Endocrinology 139: 4607–4613.

Loffer FD 1989 Hysteroscopy with selective endometrial sampling compared with D&C for abnormal uterine bleeding: the value of a negative hysteroscopic view. Obstetrics and Gynecology 73: 16–20.

Lumsden MA, Kelly RW, Baird DT 1983 Is prostaglandin F_2 involved in the increased myometrial contractility of primary dysmenorrhoea? Prostaglandins 25: 683–692.

Lumsden MA, Baird DT 1985 Intrauterine pressure in dysmenorrhoea. Acta Obstetrica et Gynecologica Scandinavica 64: 183–186.

Lumsden MA, Twaddle S, Hawthorn R et al 2000 A randomised comparison and economic evaluation of laparoscopic-assisted hysterectomy and abdominal hysterectomy. British Journal of Obstetrics and Gynaecology 107: 1386–1391.

Lundstrom V, Green K 1978 Endogenous levels of prostaglandin $F_{2\alpha}$ and its main metabolites in plasma and the endometrium of normal and dysmenorrhoeic women. American Journal of Obstetrics and Gynecology 130: 640–646.

Luukkainen T, Allonen H, Haukkamaa M, Lahteenmaki P, Nilsson CG, Toivonen J 1986 Five years experience with levonorgestrel-releasing IUCDs. Contraception 33: 139–148.

Magos AL, Baumann R, Lockwood GM, Turnbull AC 1991 Experience with the first 250 endometrial resections for menorrhagia. The Lancet 337: 1074–1078.

Marbaix E, Kokorine I, Moulin P, Donnez J, Eeckhout Y, Courtoy PJ 1996 Menstrual breakdown of human endometrium can be mimicked in vitro and is selectively and reversibly blocked by inhibitors of matrix metalloproteinases. Proceedings of the National Academy of Sciences USA 93: 9120–9125.

Markee JE 1940 Menstruation in intraocular endometrial transplants in the rhesus monkey. Contributions to Embryology, Carnegie Institute 28: 219–308.

Markee JE 1948 Morphological basis for menstrual bleeding. Relation of regression to the initiation of bleeding. Bulletin of the New York Academy of Medicine 24: 253–270.

Marsh M 1996 Endothelin and menstruation. Human Reproduction 11: 83–89.

Marsh F, Thewlis J, Duffy S 2007 Randomised controlled trial comparing Thermachoice III in the outpatient versus day-case setting. Fertility and Sterility 87: 642–650.

Migram S, Benedetto C, Zonka M, Leo Rosscerg I, Lubbert H, Hammerstein J 1991 Increased concentrations of eicosanoids and platelet-activating factor in menstrual fluid in women with primary dysmenorrhoea. Eicosanoids 4: 137–141.

Milsom I, Andersson K, Andersch B, Rybo G 1991 A comparison of flurbiprofen, tranexamic acid, and a levonorgestrel-releasing intrauterine contraceptive device in the treatment of idiopathic menorrhagia. American Journal of Obstetrics and Gynecology 164: 879–883.

National Institute for Health and Clinical Excellence 2003 Balloon thermal endometrial ablation. Interventional Procedure Guidance 6. NICE. Available at: www.nice.org.

National Institute for Health and Clinical Excellence 2007 Heavy Menstrual Bleeding. Clinical Guideline 44. NICE. Available at: www.nice.org.

Novak E, Reynolds SRM 1932 The cause of primary dysmenorrhoea with special reference to hormonal factors. JAMA: the Journal of the American Medical Association 99: 1466–1472.

Ohbuchi H, Nagai K, Yamaguchi M et al 1995 Endothelin-1 and big endothelin-1 increase in human endometrium during menstruation. American Journal of Obstetrics and Gynecology 173: 1483–1490.

Parazzini F, Tozzi L, Mezzopane R, Luchini L, Marchini M, Fedele L 1994 Cigarette smoking, alcohol consumption, and risk of primary dysmenorrhoea. Epidemiology 5: 469–472.

Pepper MS, Ferrara N, Orci L, Monteano R 1992 Potent synergism between vascular endothelial growth factor and basic fibroblast growth factor in the induction of angiogenesis in vitro. Biochemical and Biophysical Research Communications 189: 824–831.

Pierzynski P, Swiatecka J, Oczeretko E, Laudanski P, Batra S, Laudanski T 2006 Effect of short-term, low-dose treatment with tamoxifen in patients with primary dysmenorrhoea. Gynecological Endocrinology 22: 698–703.

Pinion SB, Parkin DE, Abramovich DR et al 1994 Randomised trial of hysterectomy, endometrial laser ablation and transcervical endometrial resection for dysfunctional uterine bleeding. BMJ (Clinical Research Ed.) 309: 979–983.

Rauramo I, Elo I, Isre O 2004 Long-term treatment of menorrhagia with levonorgestral intrauterine system versus endometrial resection. Obstetrics and Gynecology 104: 1314.

Rees MCP, Demers LM, Anderson ABM, Turnbull AC 1984 A functional study of platelets in menstrual fluid. British Journal of Obstetrics and Gynaecology 91: 667–693.

Rees MCP, Cederholm-Williams SA, Turnbull AC 1985 Coagulation factors and fibrinolytic proteins in menstrual fluid collected from normal and menorrhagic women. British Journal of Obstetrics and Gynaecology 92: 1164–1168.

Rees MCP, Canete-Soler R, Lopez-Bernal A, Turnbull A 1988 Effect of fenamates on prostaglandin E receptor binding. The Lancet ii 541–542.

Rees MCP, Barlow DH 1991 Quantitation of hormone replacement induced withdrawal bleeds. British Journal of Obstetrics and Gynaecology 98: 106–107.

Reid PC, Coker A, Coltart R 2000 Assessment of menstrual blood loss using pictorial chart: a validation study. British Journal of Obstetrics and Gynaecology 107: 320–322.

Riesewijk A, Martin J, van Os R et al 2003 Gene expression profiling of human endometrial receptivity on days LH+2 versus LH+7 by microarray technology. Molecular Human Reproduction 9: 253–264.

Rigot V, Marbaix E, Lemoine P, Courtoy PJ, Eechout Y 2001 In vivo perimenstrual activation of progelatinase B (ProMMP-9) in the human endometrium and its dependence on stromelysin 1(MMP-3) ex vivo. Biochemical Journal 358: 275–280.

Rodeghiero F 2008 Management of menorrhagia in women with inherited bleeding disorders: general principles and use of desmopressin. Haemophilia 14 (Suppl 1): 21–30.

Rogers PAW, Lederman F, Taylor N 1998 Endometrial microvascular growth in normal and dysfunctional states. Human Reproduction Update 4: 503–508.

Rogers PA, Abberton KM 2003 Endometrial arteriogenesis: vascular smooth muscle cell proliferation and differentiation during the menstrual cycle and changes associated with endometrial bleeding disorders. Microscopy Research and Technique 60: 412–419.

Royal College of Obstetricians and Gynaecologists 1994 Inpatient Treatment 1-1 D&C in Women Aged 40 or Less. Guideline No. 3. RCOG, London.

Rybo G 1966 Plasminogen activator in the endometrium. II. Clinical aspects. Acta Obstetrica et Gynecologica Scandinavica 45: 97–118.

Rybo G 1991 Tranexamic acid therapy: effective treatment in heavy menstrual bleeding. Clinical update on safety. Therapeutic Advances 4: 1–8.

Schatz F, Krikun G, Runic R, Wang EY, Hausknecht V, Lockwood CJ 1999 Implications of decidualization-associated protease expression in implantation and menstruation. Seminars in Reproductive Endocrinology 17: 3–12.

Scottish Hysteroscopy Audit Group 1995 A Scottish audit of hysteroscopic surgery for menorrhagia — complications and follow up. British Journal of Obstetrics and Gynaecology 102: 249–254.

Sharkey AM, Day K, McPherson A et al 2000 Vascular endothelial growth factor expression in human endometrium is regulated by hypoxia. Journal of Clinical Endocrinology and Metabolism 85: 402–409.

Shaw RW, Fraser HM 1984 Use of a superative luteinizing hormone-releasing hormone (LHRH) agonist in the treatment of menorrhagia. British Journal of Obstetrics and Gynaecology 91: 913–916.

Sheppard BL 1992 Physiology of dysfunctional uterine bleeding. In: Lowe D, Fox H (eds) Advances in Gynaecological Pathology. Churchill Livingstone, Edinburgh, pp 191–204.

Sheppard BL, Dockeray CJ, Bonnar J 1983 An ultrastructural study of menstrual blood in normal menstruation and dysfunctional uterine bleeding. British Journal of Obstetrics and Gynaecology 90: 259–265.

Silverberg SG, Haukkamaa M, Arko H, Nilsson CG, Luukkainen T 1986 Endometrial morphology during long-term use of levonorgestrel-releasing intrauterine devices. International Journal of Gynecological Pathology 5: 235–241.

Smith SK 1998 Angiogenesis, vascular endothelial growth factor and the endometrium. Human Reproduction 4: 519.

Smith SK, Abel MH, Kelly RW, Baird DT 1981 Prostaglandin synthesis in the endometrium of women with ovular dysfunctional uterine bleeding. British Journal of Obstetrics and Gynaecology 88: 434–442.

Smith SK, Abel MH, Kelly RW, Baird DT 1982 The synthesis of prostaglandins from persistent proliferative endometrium. Journal of Clinical Endocrinology and Metabolism 55: 284–289.

Smith SK, Kelly RW 1988 Effect of platelet-activating factor on the release of $PGF_{2\alpha}$ and PGE_2 by separated cells of human endometrium. Journal of Reproduction and Fertility 82: 271–276.

Stovall TG, Solomon SK, Ling FW 1989 Endometrial sampling prior to hysterectomy. Obstetrics and Gynecology 73: 405–408.

Suri C, McClain J, Thurston DM et al 1998 Increased vascularization in mice overexpressing angiopoietin-1. Science 282: 468–471.

Tabibzadeh S, Babaknia A 1995 The signals and molecular pathways involved in implantation, a symbiotic interaction between blastocyst and endometrium involving adhesion and tissue invasion. Molecular Human Reproduction 1: 1579–1602.

Taylor PJ, Hamou J 1983 Hysteroscopy. Journal of Reproductive Medicine 28: 359–389.

Togashi K, Ozasa H, Konishi I et al 1989 Enlarged uterus: differentiation between adenomyosis and leiomyoma with MR imaging. Radiology 171: 531–534.

Weston G, Rogers PA 2000 Endometrial angiogenesis. Baillières Best Practice and Research Clinical Obstetrics and Gynaecology 14: 919–936.

Wiczyk HP, Janus CL, Richards CJ et al 1988 Comparison of magnetic resonance imaging and ultrasound in evaluating follicular and endometrial development throughout the normal cycle. Fertility and Sterility 49: 969–972.

Wyatt KM, Dimmok PW, Walker TJ, O'Brien PMS 2001 Determination of total menstrual blood loss. Fertility and Sterility 76: 125–131.

Xu S, Yang Y, Gregory CD et al 1997 Biochemical heterogeneity in hysterectomised uterus measured by 31P NMR using SLIM localisation. Magnetic Resonance in Medicine 37: 736–743.

Ylikorkala O, Viinikka L 1983 Comparison between anti-fibrinolytic and anti-prostaglandin treatment in the reduction of increased menstrual blood loss in women with intrauterine contraceptive devices. British Journal of Obstetrics and Gynaecology 90: 78–83.

Zhang L, Rees MCP, Bicknell R 1995 The isolation and long term culture of normal human endometrial epithelium and stroma. Journal of Cell Science 108: 323–331.

Further Reading

Cameron IT 1993 Medical treatment of menorrhagia. In: Yearbook of the RCOG. RCOG Press, London, pp 55–64.

Cameron IT, Fraser IS, Smith SK (eds) 1998 Clinical Disorders of the Endometrium and Menstrual Cycle. Oxford University Press, Oxford.

Fraser IS, Jansen RPS, Lobo RA, Whitehead M (eds) 1998 Estrogens and Progestogens in Clinical Practice. Churchill Livingstone, London.

O'Brien S, Cameron I, Maclhean A (eds) 2000 Disorders of the Menstrual Cycle. RCOG Press, London.

Sheth S, Sutton C 1999 Menorrhagia. Isis Medical Media, Oxford.

Swiet MD, Chamberlein G, Bennet P 2002 Basic Science in Obstetrics and Gynaecology, 3rd edn. Churchill Livingstone, London.

Vollenhoven B (ed) 1998 Uterine fibroids. Baillière's Clinical Obstetrics and Gynaecology 12: 177–195.

CHAPTER 32

Uterine fibroids

Gareth Weston and David L. Healy

Chapter Contents

INTRODUCTION	473	INVESTIGATIONS FOR UTERINE FIBROIDS	479
INCIDENCE	473	TREATMENT METHODS	480
CLASSIFICATION AND PATHOPHYSIOLOGY	474	FUTURE DIRECTIONS	486
CLINICAL PRESENTATION	477	KEY POINTS	486

Introduction

Uterine fibroids are the most common type of tumour in women. Benign tumours, they arise from the uterine myometrium or, less commonly, from the cervix. The term 'fibroid' is inaccurate, as these tumours comprise smooth muscle cells contained within varying proportions of elastin, collagen and extracellular matrix proteins. They are more accurately termed 'leiomyomata' or 'myomas'.

There continues to be an appalling paucity of research on this tumour and its treatment. This is of particular concern given that it occurs in more than two-thirds of women at some stage of their lives, and is the leading indication for the most common major gynaecological operation in women — hysterectomy. The annual cost of inpatient surgery for fibroids is estimated to be $US2.1 billion in the USA (Parker 2007), with additional indirect costs from outpatient treatment and lost time at work.

Incidence

The true incidence of uterine fibroids in the general female population is unknown. This is because most studies on fibroids have only included women with symptoms or women having treatments such as hysterectomy. Given that up to 50% of fibroids are asymptomatic (Buttram and Reiter 1981), the former approach can be expected to underestimate the true population incidence. However, studies of incidence based on histological examination of hysterectomy specimens may similarly overestimate the incidence of fibroids, as they concentrate the worst cases of menorrhagia where medical treatments have failed. Cramer and Patel (1990) found that 77% of hysterectomy specimens had fibroids on histology, although fibroids were only detected in 33% of patients clinically and 50% of patients by ultrasound examination.

The lifetime risk of a woman over 45 years of age developing fibroids is greater than 60%, with reported incidences in different studies varying from 30% to 70% for premenopausal women (Okolo 2008).

Aetiology

The precise aetiology of fibroids remains unknown. It is known that each fibroid is monoclonal, developing from a single cell. Electrophoresis patterns of glucose-6-phosphate dehydrogenase isoenzyme (A or B) demonstrated this in early studies (Townsend et al 1970). Later, polymerase chain reaction experiments confirmed monoclonality by the pattern of inactivation of the X-chromosome-linked phosphoglycerokinase gene (Hashimoto et al 1995). In the development of fibroid tumours, some form of initiation event must transform a normal myometrial cell into an abnormal 'founding' cell. Possible factors initiating this change include intrinsic myometrial abnormalities, elevated oestrogen receptors in the myometrium, hormonal changes and ischaemic injury (Parker 2007).

The initial transformation of the myometrial cell is likely to be accompanied in many cases by some form of cytogenetic or molecular alteration. Non-random chromosomal changes, such as translocations, duplications and deletions, can be identified in almost 50% of fibroids. The most frequent cytogenetic changes are translocations involving chromosomes 7, 12 and 14, and deletions in chromosome 7. The critical region affected in chromosome 7 appears to be on the long arm (7Q21–22). Several known genes are coded in this apparently critical region. These include genes for collagen type 1a 2, the MET proto-oncogene and the cytochrome P450 gene. There are rare instances of fibroids being due to mutations in a single gene, such as the mitochondrial enzyme, fumarate hydratase, involved in Krebs cycle and responsible for Reed's syndrome (multiple cutaneous and uterine leiomyoma syndrome). However, in the

DOI: 10.1016/B978-0-7020-3120-5.00032-1

vast majority of cases, uterine fibroids are not a single gene disorder. Once the fibroid tumour has been initiated, growth of the tumour occurs under the influence of sex steroid hormones (oestrogen and progesterone), peptide growth factors and the alteration of processes such as angiogenesis, apoptosis and extracellular matrix production.

It has long been known that fibroid growth is dependent on both oestrogen and progesterone. Fibroids only occur after the menarche, and they normally show a reduction in size after the menopause. They display reversible shrinkage after treatment with gonadotrophin-releasing hormone (GnRH) agonists. Although circulating serum oestradiol and progesterone levels are not altered in women with fibroids, fibroids have increased local oestrogen levels relative to the surrounding normal myometrium, partly due to increased fibroid expression of the aromatase enzyme (Parker 2007). They also have increased oestrogen receptor levels and increased responsiveness to oestrogen compared with normal myometrial cells. As for progesterone, the receptor levels have been shown to be increased in fibroids relative to the myometrium (Brandon et al 1993), and to upregulate the levels of some proteins which influence cell proliferation, such as the antiapoptotic protein Bcl-2 (Matsuo et al 1999). During the secretory phase of the menstrual cycle, when serum progesterone levels are at their peak, the highest mitotic activity is seen in fibroids. Similarly, high mitotic activity is seen during pregnancy. Treatment with the antiprogestin, mifepristone, has been shown to cause a marked decrease in fibroid tumour volume.

A large number of growth factors are produced locally in uterine fibroids and the myometrium. Some of them are overexpressed in fibroids, partially due to an exaggerated response to oestrogen. Some of the growth factors that have been found to have a potential role in the promotion of fibroid growth include: transforming growth factor-β, epidermal growth factor, basic fibroblast factor, insulin-like growth factor, platelet-derived growth factor and vascular endothelial growth factor (VEGF). The differential effects of these growth factors on cell proliferation, angiogenesis, extracellular matrix production and apoptosis are due to a variety of mechanisms including altered receptor levels and signalling pathways. For a detailed review, see Fleischer et al (2008).

Epidemiology

Age is the most common risk factor for uterine fibroids (Marshall et al 1997), although many of the studies examining incidence are cross-sectional or retrospective, rather than prospective and longitudinal. Race has been identified as an epidemiological factor in fibroid development. Black women are three to five times more likely to have uterine fibroids than White, Asian or Hispanic women (Marshall et al 1997). In addition, the fibroids in Black women are larger, more numerous, more symptomatic and diagnosed at an earlier age.

There is evidence of hereditary factors influencing fibroid development, despite no specific gene being identified. The development of fibroids clusters in families, and 'familial' fibroids appear to be more likely to cause symptoms than 'non-familial' fibroids (Okolo 2008). Twin studies show an increased incidence of fibroids in monozygotic twin pairs compared with dizygotic twin pairs.

Uterine fibroids are more common in nulliparous women, presumably due to the increased number of cycles over their premenopausal lifespan compared with parous women. Increasing parity decreases the incidence and number of fibroids. It is a myth that fibroids increase in size during pregnancy. In pregnancy, fibroids initially increase in size in the first trimester, but then decrease in size for the remaining two trimesters, with an overall volume that is either reduced or unchanged throughout the pregnancy (Hammoud et al 2006). Obesity, diabetes mellitus, polycystic ovary syndrome and hypertension all appear to be associated with an increased risk of uterine fibroids. In these conditions, a combination of insulin resistance, increased androgen levels and increased peripheral conversion of circulating androgens to oestrogen may alter the ovarian steroid hormonal stimulus to the fibroids. Smoking decreases the risk of uterine fibroids, presumably through a reduction in oestrogen levels.

The effects of exogenous sex steroid hormones on fibroid growth are particularly important as they comprise some of the most common treatments for menorrhagia, itself the most common symptom of uterine fibroids. Use of the combined oral contraceptive pill (COCP) has been associated with fibroid growth in some earlier studies (particularly older pill formulations with a higher oestrogen dosage), although the majority show no association or even a reduced risk of developing fibroids with COCP use. Therefore, fibroids are not a contraindication to the use of the COCP to treat menorrhagia. Both systemic and local administration of progestins to the uterus have been shown to be safe with fibroids. Depot medroxyprogesterone acetate injections reduce the risk of fibroids, and the levonorgestrel-containing intrauterine system (LNG-IUS; Mirena) reduces the overall volume of fibroid uteri. The LNG-IUS is also an effective treatment for menorrhagia associated with fibroids, although it is less effective than for dysfunctional uterine bleeding. In some patients, it may be difficult to insert the LNG-IUS due to cavity distortion by the fibroids. The effect of hormone therapy in postmenopausal women on fibroids has been reviewed by Ang et al (2001). They found that use of hormone therapy in women with fibroids caused continued fibroid growth, especially in the first 6 months of therapy, or at least a failure in normal postmenopausal regression. However, this did not correspond to an increase in symptoms.

Classification and Pathophysiology

Macroscopic appearance

Fibroids have a characteristically firm fibrous texture, from which the clinical term 'fibroid' is presumably derived. They frequently become calcified; rarely, they become ossified so that they are rock hard. Fibroids are round or oval-shaped tumours with a characteristic white whorled appearance on cross-section. They may be single but are more commonly multiple, present in varying sizes and in different sites (Figure 32.1). Tiny 'seedling' fibroids are commonly seen in association with larger tumours, possibly accounting for the high recurrence rate after surgical removal at myomectomy.

Surgical removal of over 120 individual fibroids from a single patient has been recorded in the literature!

Clinical classification

Subserosal fibroids

Subserosal fibroids project outwards from the uterine surface, covered with peritoneum, and may reach a very large size. Greater than 50% of the fibroid mass must project beyond the myometrium for the fibroid to be classified as subserosal. Many subserosal fibroids are pedunculated (Figure 32.2), making torsion a potential, although rare, complication. Sessile subserosal fibroids projecting from the fundal region may adhere to omentum or bowel, particularly if there has been coincidental inflammatory disease. Fibroids rarely become attached to the omentum; if they develop an alternative blood supply, they may become separated from the uterus, forming a so-called 'parasitic' fibroid. Subserosal fibroids arising from the lateral uterine wall may lie between the layers of the broad ligament where large tumours may displace the ureters, or bulge between the layers of the sigmoid mesocolon. Broad ligament fibroids arising from the lateral uterine wall differ from true broad ligament fibroids, which have no attachment to the uterus but have their origin in smooth muscle fibres within the broad ligament; for example, from the round ligament, ovarian ligament or perivascular connective tissue.

Intramural fibroids

Intramural fibroids lie within the wall of the uterus. A strict definition requires more than 50% of the fibroid mass to lie within the myometrial layer of the uterus, although smaller percentages of the tumour mass may project either into the uterine cavity or out from the serosal layer. They are separated from the adjacent normal myometrium by a thin layer of connective tissue which forms the so-called 'pseudocapsule' or 'false capsule'. This pseudocapsule is of great help when performing a myomectomy, as it provides a plane of easy cleavage to enucleate the fibroid tumour but leave the remainder of the uterus.

Submucosal fibroids

Submucosal fibroids are less common, comprising approximately 5% of all leiomyomata. By definition, more than 50% of the fibroid mass projects into the uterine cavity and is covered by endometrium. Submucosal fibroids may cause abnormal uterine bleeding and infertility. Uterine enlargement is not usually evident unless other fibroids are also present. Submucous fibroids are regarded as suitable for hysteroscopic resection. Pedunculated submucous fibroids on a long stalk may prolapse through the cervix (Figure 32.3), where they may cause intermenstrual bleeding or become ulcerated and infected.

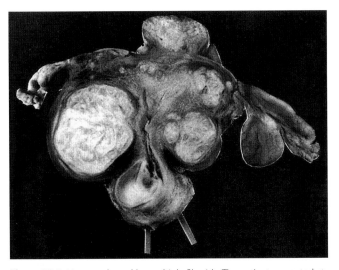

Figure 32.1 Uterus enlarged by multiple fibroids. The patient presented at 43 years with menorrhagia; she had a 13-year history of primary infertility. Septate vagina and double cervix (marked with rods).

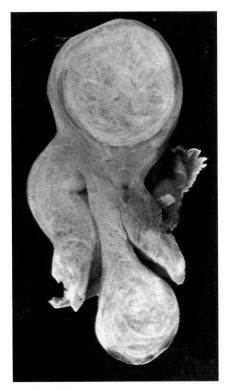

Figure 32.3 Submucous fibroid protruding through cervix. The patient, aged 44 years, presented with a 3-week history of continuous bleeding; haemoglobin level was 6.9 g/dl.

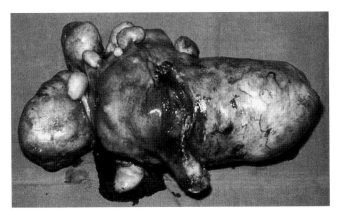

Figure 32.2 Multiple subserous fibroids, some pedunculated. Specimen width 350 mm.

475

Cervical fibroids

Cervical fibroids are relatively uncommon but give rise to the greatest surgical difficulty by virtue of their relative inaccessibility and close proximity to the bladder and ureters. Enlargement causes upward displacement of the uterus, and the fibroid may become impacted in the pelvis, causing urinary retention and ureteric obstruction. During labour, a cervical fibroid may prevent descent of the fetal head, resulting in obstructed labour; if on the anterior surface of the uterus, a cervical fibroid may complicate caesarean section surgery.

Vascular supply

Perfusion studies with injections of ^{133}Xe radiocontrast and gadolinium-enhancement contrast material during magnetic resonance imaging (MRI) show reduced blood flow through fibroids compared with myometrium, but increased blood flow in a compressed rim around the fibroid. Immunohistochemical studies of the microvascular density of fibroids demonstrate reduced vessel area staining in fibroids compared with the myometrium (Casey et al 2000), and with the difference increasing after the menopause (Weston et al 2005); this is probably due to relatively faster collapse of the myometrial cellular and extracellular matrix volume relative to that of the fibroid. Electron microscopy of corrosion vessel casts of fibroids performed by Walocha et al (2003) shed even greater insight into the vasculature of fibroids. A single larger artery usually provides the major blood supply to the fibroid, sending small nutrient arteries to penetrate the capsule. The vasculature of fibroids is reduced compared with the surrounding myometrium, but is most markedly reduced in smaller fibroids, with the only area of greater vascularity than the myometrium being the compressed rim of perifibroid tissue around the periphery of larger fibroids. Walocha et al (2003) proposed an initial regression of the vasculature within smaller fibroids, followed by an intense proangiogenic response, whereby the vascular rim around the fibroid acts as the source for neovascularization of the growing fibroid.

The relative avascularity of the fibroid core appears to be at odds with the finding of increased VEGF in fibroids compared with the myometrium. However, the VEGF within the interior of the fibroid may be trapped in a biologically inactive fashion within the expanded extracellular matrix of the fibroid. A gene expression microarray experiment performed by Weston et al (2003) specifically targeting angiogenesis-related genes found a reduced level of two angiogenesis promoters (CTGF and CYR61) and increased expression of collagen IVa 2; a precursor for the angiogenesis inhibitor, canstatin. This triad of gene expression differences may, in part, explain the relatively avascular fibroid tissue.

Microscopic appearance

Microscopically, fibroids are composed of smooth muscle cell bundles, also arranged in whorl-like patterns (Figure 32.4A), admixed with a variable amount of connective tissue, although the latter rarely predominates. The relatively poor blood supply to individual fibroids may result in degenerative changes, particularly within large tumours. Hyaline degeneration (Figure 32.4B) is the most common, resulting in a smoother and more homogeneous consistency, which may become cystic if liquefaction occurs. Much more rarely, fatty change may develop. This is distinct from the true lipoma of the uterus, which is extremely uncommon. Calcification (Figure 32.5) is a later consequence of degeneration secondary to circulatory impairment. It characteristically occurs after the menopause, although it may occur earlier in subserosal fibroids with narrow pedicles.

There are a number of recognized histological variants of the usual microscopic appearance of uterine leiomyomata. The term 'cellular leiomyoma' is used when the density of the smooth muscle cells is significantly greater than usual, but there are no other atypical features such as increased mitotic activity or abnormal mitoses. Some pathologists use the term 'neurilemmoma-like leiomyoma' when there is striking lining-up or palisading of the tumour nuclei. This resembles nerve sheath tumours. Sometimes, fibroids are composed of polygonal cells rather than spindle cells. This type of nuclear pleomorphism is associated with giant cell formation; such tumours are called 'symplasmic', 'bizarre' or 'atypical' leiomyomas.

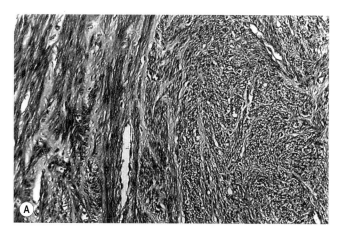 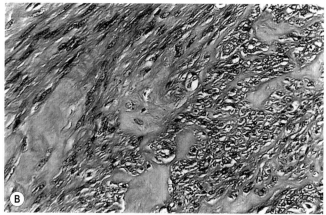

Figure 32.4 Leiomyoma of uterus. (A) Bundles of elongated smooth muscle cells in both longitudinal (left) and transverse planes (×160). (B) Focal hyalinization. Smooth muscle bundles are separated by dense hyalinized connective tissue (×320). *Images courtesy of Dr K. Maclaren.*

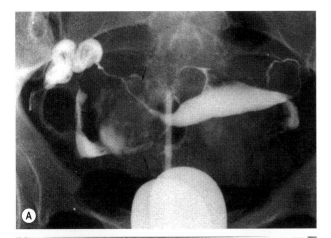

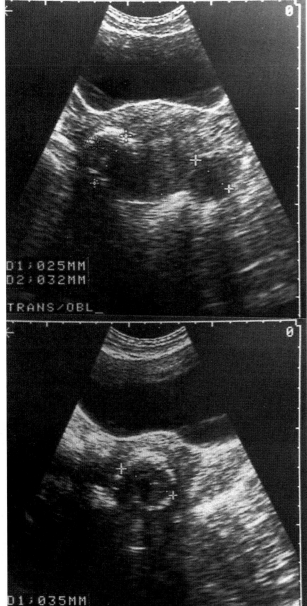

Figure 32.5 (A) Calcified fibroid seen on hysterosalpingogram. (B) Ultrasound appearance of the uterus: two fibroids seen in transverse plane with calcified fibroid to left (top); calcified fibroid shown in longitudinal plane (bottom).

Image (A) courtesy of Dr B. Muir.

One differential diagnosis of uterine fibroids is that of adenomyosis, which may have a similar macroscopic appearance to uterine fibroids. However, in adenomyosis, there is no clear demarcation from the adjacent normal tissue. Leiomyosarcoma is a malignant tumour of the smooth muscle of the uterus. The macroscopic appearance of leiomyosarcoma shows an irregular invasive margin and a variegated cut surface. The microscopic appearance of leiomyosarcoma shows high cellularity, nuclear pleomorphism, a high mitotic rate with abnormal mitoses and areas of necrosis with infiltrating margins. Typically, the number of mitoses per 10 high-power fields in leiomyosarcoma is greater than 10, in contrast to standard leiomyoma where the number of mitoses per 10 high-power fields is less than five.

Finally, there are rare groups of uterine tumours with histological features intermediate between fibroids and leiomyosarcomas. These are termed 'smooth muscle tumours of uncertain malignant potential'. Other rare tumours include endometrial stromal nodule, diffuse leiomyomatosis and endometrial stromal sarcoma.

Crow et al (1995) examined the microscopic appearance of uterine fibroids after treatment with GnRH agonists. They found considerable variation between fibroids after a course of treatment and subsequent myomectomy or hysterectomy. Decreases in the extracellular matrix, in particular, cause extreme crowding of tumour nuclei, resulting in a densely cellular appearance of such fibroids on microscopic examination. For the inexperienced pathologist, this will be worrying in terms of possible malignancy. There should not, however, be mitotic activity, cytological atypia or coagulative necrosis.

Clinical Presentation

Abnormal bleeding/menorrhagia

The proportion of uterine fibroids causing abnormal uterine bleeding — menorrhagia being the most common abnormal pattern observed — is uncertain but is usually quoted as 30–50%. The exact mechanism by which fibroids cause menorrhagia is unknown. The many theories include: increase in endometrial surface area (Figure 32.6), increased vascularity of the uterus, vascular congestion due to fibroid compression of the myometrial venous drainage, abnormal uterine contractility, dysregulation of growth factors causing disordered angiogenesis of the uterine vasculature, and ulceration of the endometrial layer overlying submucous fibroids.

As fibroids are so common, and so often asymptomatic, menorrhagia in a woman with uterine fibroids should not automatically be ascribed to the fibroids themselves. Other possible aetiologies for menorrhagia should always be considered and excluded, including coagulopathies such as von Willebrand's disease (Munro and Lukes 2005). In a study of self-reported bleeding patterns by 878 women (aged 35–49 years) screened for the presence and size of myomas, Wegienka et al (2003) reported findings on the association between fibroids and bleeding pattern. Of women with fibroids, 46% reported 'gushing' episodes during their periods, compared with 28% without fibroids. Gushing episodes and length of periods were related to the size of the

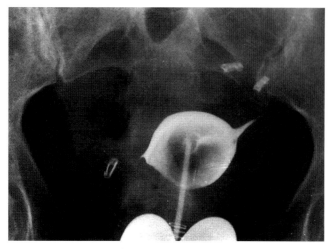

Figure 32.6 Hysterosalpingogram showing enlargement of uterine cavity and filling defect from intramural fibroid. Extensive endometriosis had complicated laparoscopic sterilization (hence the two clips on the left tube). *Image courtesy of Dr B. Muir.*

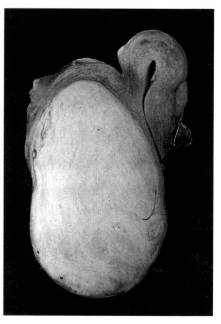

Figure 32.7 Cervical fibroid growing anteriorly in the supravaginal cervix. Presentation was with frequency of micturition followed by acute urinary retention.

myomas, but not to their number or location. The worst bleeding was found with fibroids over 5 cm in diameter, with women using three more pads or tampons on heavy bleeding days than women with smaller fibroids.

Pelvic pain and pressure symptoms

Fibroids do not usually give rise to pain. In a cohort study of 635 non-care-seeking women, symptoms of dyspareunia, dysmenorrhoea and non-cyclic pelvic pain were examined for their association with the presence and size of uterine fibroids (Lippman et al 2003). The 96 women with fibroids had only a slight increase in non-cyclic pain or dyspareunia, but no increase in dysmenorrhoea, and no relationship was found between the size or total volume of fibroids and pain symptoms. Where fibroids are associated with pain or abdominal discomfort, it is usually described as 'pressure' or a 'dragging' sensation. It is surprising that even in the presence of multiple fibroids, menstruation may be painless.

Exceptionally, the presentation of fibroids may be acute on account of torsion of a fibroid on a narrow pedicle, or degeneration. Attempted expulsion of a large submucous fibroid through the cervix causes uterine cramp associated with bleeding, and may be mistaken for spontaneous abortion, particularly with the finding of a dilated cervix and a protruding mass. This situation has been described as a complication of treatment with GnRH analogues. Rarely, it can result in uterine inversion. Torsion or painful degeneration presents with an acute abdomen, and is commonly confused with complications of ovarian neoplasia. Distinction between these conditions is particularly important in pregnancy complicated by red degeneration of a fibroid, in order to avoid subjecting the woman to unnecessary laparotomy.

The location and size of fibroids determines symptoms from pressure on adjacent organs. A posterior wall fibroid can cause lower back pain, or constipation and tenesmus if the rectosigmoid is compressed. Anterior wall fibroids compressing the bladder may cause urinary frequency, nocturia

and urgency in some women. It has been shown that reduction in size of such fibroids after either GnRH agonists or uterine artery embolization (UAE) causes a decrease in associated urinary symptoms (Parker 2007). Cervical fibroids causing compression of the bladder outlet may present with acute retention of urine (Figure 32.7), although this is rare.

Reproductive outcomes

Infertility/miscarriage

Fibroids are associated with infertility, although it has been estimated that fibroids are only responsible for 2–3% of cases (Buttram and Reiter 1981). Increasing maternal age increases the likelihood of both fibroids and infertility, making it a possible confounding factor. It is not known why fibroids increase infertility. Hypothetical mechanisms include interference with embryo implantation or sperm/embryo transport due to distortion of the cavity or tubal ostium, and an altered uterine environment due to increased local oestrogen levels or a local inflammatory effect. Embryo implantation may be reduced due to endometrial oedema, atrophy or ulceration, which in turn could be due to either the pressure effects of the uterine fibroid or its effects on the local blood supply. There have been series indicating postoperative pregnancy rates of 50–60% in women after myomectomy, but these studies have usually been uncontrolled or poorly controlled.

The effect of fibroids on assisted reproductive technology (ART) has been the subject of many studies, often with conflicting results. In an excellent systematic literature review, Klatsky et al (2008) summarized the evidence for the effects of fibroids on the results of in-vitro fertilization (IVF). It is generally accepted that subserosal fibroids, with more than 50% of their mass outside the myometrial border, are unlikely to have an adverse effect on IVF outcomes or to increase the risk of miscarriage. This was confirmed by Eldar-Geva et al (1998), with subserosal fibroids not influencing treatment outcome after ART. However, in a series of 88 patients, treatment outcome after ART was impaired with either submucosal fibroids or intramural fibroids, even without uterine cavity distortion. Established wisdom is that submucosal fibroids should undergo hysteroscopic resection prior to ART. Submucosal fibroids, if not removed, are associated with an overall 70% reduction in pregnancy rate and 72% reduction in implantation rate compared with controls (Klatsky et al 2008), as well as an approximate doubling of the risk of miscarriage. Intramural fibroids are where controversy begins. Surgery to remove them is more risky and involved than that for submucosal fibroids, while the evidence is for a smaller and less consistent effect. Some authors (Khaund and Lumsden 2008) believe that intramural fibroids have an adverse effect on fertility where they cause distortion of the uterine cavity, and should be removed if they do so. Others (Klatsky et al 2008), citing disparity of study results, possible biases including publication bias and the small effect, feel that more prospective studies of intramural fibroids are required before a strong recommendation on desired treatment can be given. Their cumulative results from 18 controlled studies showed a slight decrease in implantation rate (18% vs 22%) and clinical pregnancy rate (37% vs 41%), and an increase in miscarriage rate (8% vs 15%) associated with intramural fibroids.

Pregnancy complications

The best-available evidence points to an increased risk of caesarean section delivery with fibroids, mainly due to malpresentation of the fetus. Incoordinate uterine action and labour dystocia were increased in at least one study on pregnant women with fibroids, but fibroids are not a contraindication to a trial of labour. The results for placenta praevia and placental abruption are conflicting, with some studies showing an increased risk and other studies showing no increased risk. Preterm labour and delivery are more common with uterine fibroids (odds ratio 1.5–1.9). At least four studies showed an increased risk of postpartum haemorrhage with uterine fibroids (Klatsky et al 2008). Despite the considerable evidence of adverse pregnancy outcomes with uterine fibroids, it should be noted that the data are often conflicting in different studies. Also, confounding factors such as advanced maternal age, and ascertainment bias from increased use of ultrasound in complicated pregnancies, need to be considered.

In approximately 5% of pregnant women with fibroids, the fibroids undergo red degeneration. This is a form of coagulative necrosis resulting in a haemorrhagic, meaty, cut surface and areas of cystic degeneration or mucinous change. One hypothesis is that changes in orientation of the myoma to its vascular supply during uterine growth cause obstruction of the vascular supply and ischaemic necrosis of the fibroid tissue (Parker 2007). Red degeneration causes severe abdominal pain and mild fever, and often requires a short hospital stay and treatment with non-steroidal anti-inflammatory drugs, such as ibuprofen. A similar clinical presentation can occur after GnRH agonist treatment or uterine artery embolisation UAE.

Malignant transformation in fibroids: where is the evidence?

For the 'worried well', the diagnosis of a uterine fibroid naturally raises the issue 'Can it become cancer, doctor?'. Some women continue to have a hysterectomy or a myomectomy 'just in case' the uterine fibroid grows into a uterine sarcoma. Gard et al (1999) reviewed uterine leiomyosarcomas in Australia, conducting a retrospective survey of major teaching hospitals in Sydney and Melbourne. They identified 49 patients treated over a 28-year period, equating to approximately one leiomyosarcoma of the uterus per million Australian women per year. There is considerable doubt regarding whether or not a myomectomy would be protective in any case, as most leiomyosarcomas are believed to arise *de novo*, unrelated to existing benign fibroids. Malignant transformation of fibroids is believed to be exceedingly rare; genetic differences between uterine fibroids and leiomyosarcomas point to distinct origins. Given that leiomyosarcomas can also arise outside the uterus, even a hysterectomy may not be completely protective of this rare tumour. Removing asymptomatic fibroids from women on this basis cannot be justified. Until proven otherwise, sarcomatous 'change' in a fibroid is a myth. Even rapid myoma growth almost never indicates a uterine sarcoma. No cases of sarcoma were found in a study of 198 fibroid uteri with an increase in size greater than 6 weeks over a 1-year period (Parker et al 1994).

There are many types of uterine sarcoma, all differing in their biological behaviour. The clinical benefits of oophorectomy, lymphadenectomy and cytotoxic chemotherapy remain controversial for these various types of leiomyosarcoma, not least because they are rare, even in the clinical experience of gynaecological oncologists.

Investigations for Uterine Fibroids

The investigations outlined below are those intended to diagnose the condition. However, required investigations will vary depending on the presenting problem. With menorrhagia, for example, a full blood examination should be performed to look for anaemia. Also, if surgery is anticipated, investigations to establish fitness for surgery should be performed.

Ultrasound

Ultrasound should always be used to confirm or clarify the nature of a pelvic mass. Both the transabdominal and transvaginal route should be taken in examining possible fibroids. Larger fibroid uteri may only be fully visible via the abdominal route, but smaller lesions and submucosal fibroids may be better visualized via the vagina. Ultrasound is rapid, inexpensive and uses no ionizing radiation, making it the undisputed first-line imaging investigation for fibroids. Even in relatively unskilled hands, it will diagnose pregnancy and differentiate between cystic and solid lesions (Figure 32.8). With appropriate training and experience, the site and nature of a pelvic mass may be predicted with accuracy in over 80% of cases. Fibroids appear as an enlarged uterus with patchy echogenicity. Serial ultrasound examination is of value in

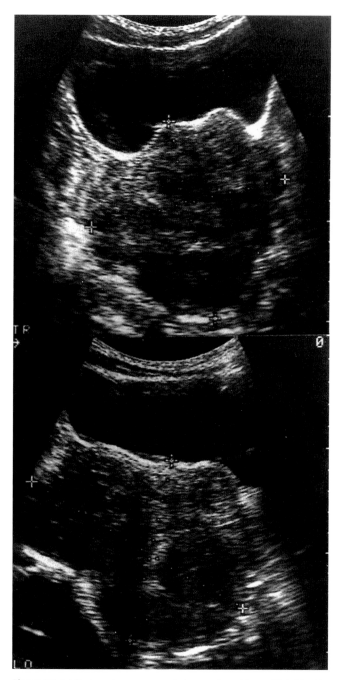

Figure 32.8 Ultrasound appearance of uterus enlarged by multiple fibroids, showing patchy echogenicity.
Image courtesy of Dr B. Muir.

monitoring fibroid size during medical or conservative treatment. The volume of individual fibroids or of the whole uterus can be calculated by measuring the diameter in three planes at right angles and using the formula $4/3\pi r^3$, where r is the radius.

Sonohysteroscopy, where the use of ultrasound is accompanied by the instillation of sterile saline into the uterine cavity via a balloon catheter, enables improved delineation of intrauterine pathology, such as submucosal fibroids. It also allows the diagnosis of endometrial polyps and intrauterine adhesions. Even large submucosal fibroids, up to 4–5 cm in diameter, can then be considered for hystero-scopic resection, especially if more than 50% of the volume of the tumour is projecting into the uterine cavity.

Magnetic resonance imaging

While it is an excellent imaging modality for mapping the precise location and size of uterine fibroids, the use of MRI is limited by its expense and availability. While the accuracy of ultrasound is operator dependent, MRI has an overall low interobserver variability. It allows the diagnosis of adenomyosis, a common differential diagnosis of uterine fibroids. Nonetheless, until the cost and access to this imaging modality improve, it will not be a routine investigation for the diagnosis of myomas.

Hysteroscopy

Hysteroscopy as an investigational procedure is very effective for the diagnosis of submucosal fibroids. Diagnosis and treatment can occur at the same time if the appropriate equipment (a resecting hysteroscope) is available. The use of hysteroscopy allows endometrial sampling to be performed at the same time to diagnose coexisting endometrial pathology (endometrial hyperplasia, cancer or polyps). However, it is an invasive procedure, with both surgical and anaesthetic risks that are not incurred by the use of ultrasound alone.

Laparoscopy

Diagnostic laparoscopy can be of clinical value if the uterus is not larger than a 12-week gestation size and there is associated infertility or pelvic pain. It may reveal the presence of coincidental endometriosis, pelvic adhesions or other tubal pathology. Laparoscopy will also differentiate between a pedunculated fibroid and an ovarian neoplasm if there is an individual patient where this diagnosis is unclear on the basis of clinical and ultrasound findings.

Treatment Methods

Expectant management

At least 50% of fibroids are asymptomatic, and provided that their nature can be determined with reasonable certainty, active treatment is unnecessary. While traditionally, surgical removal has been advocated when the uterine size exceeds that of a 12-week pregnancy, this policy has been challenged (Reiter et al 1992). The mere presence of a fibroid uterus carries no long-term detrimental effects; spontaneous regression of the fibroid(s) after the menopause may be anticipated. Sarcomatous change in fibroids if they are left *in situ* is a myth.

Medical management

There are two main objectives in the medical treatment of uterine fibroids: relief of symptoms associated with fibroids, and reduction in fibroid size. No medical treatment has been show to cause complete regression of fibroids. Where medical treatments cause fibroid shrinkage, there is a high rate of regrowth following cessation of treatment, as well as a recurrence of symptoms. This has severely limited the use of medical treatment for fibroids.

Medical treatment of menorrhagia associated with fibroids

Since fibroids are often associated with menorrhagia, the effect of medical treatments for menorrhagia, with respect to both symptoms and fibroid growth, is important. As mentioned above, oral contraceptive pills with a high dose of oestrogen have been reported to cause fibroid growth. Later studies with current lower oestrogen-containing pills have shown either no change or a reduction in size. Similarly, the de-novo incidence of fibroids in users of the oral contraceptive pill appears to be decreased or no different compared with controls. Thus, the use of the oral contraceptive pill to treat menorrhagia in the setting of a fibroid uterus is not contraindicated (Benagiano and Primiero 2006).

There have been very few studies examining the effect of non-hormonal treatments for menorrhagia in women with fibroids. There have been no published randomized-controlled trials examining the effect of tranexamic acid on menstrual blood flow in women with fibroids. Non-steroidal anti-inflammatory drugs, such as ibuprofen and naproxen, have been shown to be ineffective in treating fibroid-related menorrhagia, despite their effectiveness for idiopathic menorrhagia and dysfunctional uterine bleeding. While not addressing the cause of the anaemia, iron tablets, often in combination with vitamin C tablets to aid absorption, are an effective treatment for mild-to-moderate iron-deficiency anaemia associated with menorrhagia.

The LNG-IUS is highly effective for the treatment of menorrhagia. It is also effective for the treatment of menorrhagia associated with fibroids, although less effective than for dysfunctional uterine bleeding. There is an increased risk of expulsion or failed insertion with fibroids, particularly where they cause cavity distortion. Regarding the effect of the LNG-IUS on fibroid growth, the data are conflicting (Benagiano and Primiero 2006). Despite initial reports of regression in the size of fibroids, subsequent studies have shown no decrease in size.

Gonadotrophin-releasing hormone analogues

GnRH analogues reduce the size of uterine fibroids significantly, thus relieving pressure symptoms as well as menorrhagia. However, their use as a primary treatment for fibroids is hampered by the rapid and high rate of recurrence after cessation of therapy, as well as menopausal symptoms and bone demineralization with long-term use. Due to these problems, as well as their high cost, their use is now largely restricted to an adjunct or pretreatment to surgery.

GnRH agonists should be commenced in the mid-luteal phase of the ovarian cycle for the most rapid pituitary down-regulation. Bleeding in response to oestrogen withdrawal occurs during the initial treatment cycle, but amenorrhoea is usual thereafter. Gonadal suppression results in vasomotor symptoms and vaginal dryness. Uterine volume assessed by MRI reduces by 35% after 3 months, and 50% after 6 months, with little change thereafter. The effects of treatment only persist for the duration of administration. The optimal duration of presurgical treatment with GnRH agonists is 3

months, which will also correct associated anaemia. Appropriate doses of currently available GnRH agonists include goserelin 3.6 mg (Zoladex) or leuprolin 3.75 mg (Lupron) by monthly subcutaneous depot insertion, and buserelin 900–1200 µg or nafarelin 800 µg (Synarel) intranasal sprays in divided doses. Therapy should be initiated in the mid-luteal phase of the cycle with no sexual intercourse that month in order to avoid accidental initiation during early pregnancy. Compliance may be a problem with the nasal spray; as erratic usage may result in stimulation rather than suppression of pituitary–ovarian function, hence administration by subcutaneous depot is preferable.

For women nearing the menopause who are particularly keen to avoid surgery, the use of GnRH analogues as a stand-alone therapy, with 'add-back' therapy to reduce menopausal symptoms, has been proposed as a viable alternative to surgical treatment. Low-dose oestrogen/progesterone combinations, oral progesterone alone and tibolone have been used to ameliorate the vasomotor symptoms associated with GnRH agonist gonadal suppression, but without compromising fibroid shrinkage (Sankaran and Manyonda 2008).

Other medical treatments

Danzol cannot be recommended for long-term treatment for fibroids because of marked androgenic activity. After short-term treatment, there is rapid return of size and symptoms, as with GnRH analogues. Selective oestrogen receptor modulators have no proven role in the medical treatment of fibroids in humans, despite their success in animal models. Aromatase inhibitors such as anastrozole are only effective for the treatment of fibroids in postmenopausal women. Given that their fibroids are regressing due to the naturally hypo-oestrogenic state of menopause, the number of patients for whom aromatase inhibitors would be a useful treatment is extremely small. GnRH antagonists have been shown to have a similar effect as GnRH agonists in the treatment of fibroids, although with faster effects. However, GnRH antagonists are more costly than agonists at present, limiting their feasibility as a treatment for most patients.

Antiprogesterone treatment

The use of antiprogesterone RU486, mifepristone, has been reported to reduce fibroid size and fibroid-related symptoms, making it a potentially promising new medical treatment. However, there have been varying reports of increased incidence of endometrial hyperplasia following prolonged use of mifepristone, due to its antiprogestin effects on the endometrium (Tropeano et al 2008). Recurrence rates after cessation of therapy are likely to be high, and risk to any potential pregnancies makes its use for women with infertility particularly troublesome. Further studies are required with larger numbers of patients over longer periods to reliably determine the long-term efficacy and safety of treatment.

Asoprisnil, a selective progesterone receptor modulator (SPRM) with mixed agonist/antagonist effects, has also been used to treat fibroids. It inhibits the proliferation of endometrial cells, unlike mifepristone, theoretically reducing the risk of endometrial hyperplasia with treatment. Only one randomized, double-blind, placebo-controlled trial of aso-prisnil for the treatment of fibroids has been reported (Chwalisz et al 2007). It found that asoprisnil treatment for 3 months reduced fibroid-related symptoms and size in a dose-dependent manner, without hypo-oestrogenic symptoms or endometrial hyperplasia. Clearly, longer-term and larger trials are needed, but the initial results are promising. Other SPRMs are likely to be trialled for the treatment of fibroids over the next few years.

Hysterectomy

Management of symptomatic uterine fibroids has tradition-ally been surgical. Despite the existence of newer, less inva-sive techniques, their lack of availability in most centres means that, for most women, the decision for treatment continues to be between hysterectomy or myomectomy. The decision to perform a hysterectomy should not be under-taken without due consideration of the alternatives. For women who wish to preserve their reproductive function, myomectomy or medical treatment must be considered. Hysterectomy is clearly an effective treatment for fibroids, but it carries considerable risk of major complications (up to 10% with a large fibroid uterus).

The route selected for hysterectomy will depend on the size of the uterus, the situation of the fibroids and the history of any previous surgical procedures. Abdominal hysterec-tomy with ovarian conservation (Figure 32.9) will be the procedure of choice where fibroids are very large. For gynae-cologists who favour vaginal hysterectomy, consideration should be given to preoperative shrinkage with a GnRH agonist, as described below. Similarly, a reduction in volume and vascularity may facilitate removal of a very large uterus by the abdominal route. Abdominal hysterectomy is ren-dered difficult in the presence of large fibroids arising from the cervix or situated in the broad ligament. It is also more complicated if there are adhesions from previous myomec-tomies, or from associated endometriosis or pelvic inflam-

matory disease. Difficult access to the pelvis during hysterectomy for large fibroids will be rendered easier by prior enucleation of the fibroids. The ureters may be vulner-able during an operation to remove a broad ligament fibroid, and their pathway must always be identified. Regardless of the direction of displacement, they are always extracapsular. In the case of a large cervical fibroid, an alternative approach is hemisection of the uterus, followed by enucleation of the fibroid in order to gain access to the uterine arteries and cervix. These techniques are described in detail elsewhere (Monaghan 1986).

The increasing popularity of minimal access surgery has led to the use of laparoscopic-assisted methods of vaginal hysterectomy in women with large fibroids, sometimes fol-lowing prior shrinkage with a GnRH agonist. Even a large fibroid uterus can be removed via the laparoscopic method, using a morcellator to remove the fibroid and/or uterus piecemeal. However, the place of laparoscopic-assisted or total laparoscopic hysterectomy in the treatment of uterine fibroids remains unclear due to the lack of comparative studies with more traditional surgical methods.

Abdominal myomectomy

Removal of individual fibroids was first reported in the middle of the 19th Century, although current surgical tech-niques are largely attributable to Victor Bonney who described a personal series of 403 cases. The main indication for myomectomy is a woman with symptomatic fibroids who wishes to retain her uterus.

Unless the fibroid uterus is exceptionally large (greater than a 20-week gestation uterus), a Pfannenstiel or lower transverse incision should provide adequate access, as the uterus can usually be mobilized through the wound with the assistance of a myoma screw. If it is a repeat myomectomy, however, bowel adhesions are common and may necessitate a vertical midline incision. The uterus with the fibroid(s) is exteriorized after careful inspection of the pelvis for coexist-ent pathology. The uterine incision is made with either cold knife or cutting diathermy, the fibroid(s) grasped with either a myoma screw or tenaculum, and the fibroid enucleated either with finger or scissors around the usually clear tissue plane of the pseudocapsule. Every effort should be made to remove all palpable fibroids. After removal, the cavities left behind should be closed meticulously with figure-8 sutures (the authors usually use absorbable Vicryl sutures) to prevent haematoma collection, and the serosal layer should be closed with a continuous subserosal suture.

Complications

The two major problems associated with abdominal myo-mectomy are intraoperative blood loss (which can be severe and may necessitate a hysterectomy to control bleeding in 1–2% of patients) and postoperative adhesion formation. The risk of adhesions is increased with posterior and multi-ple uterine incisions. They are usually a consequence of difficulties with haemostasis and oozing from incision lines. Adhesions after incisions on the posterior wall are poten-tially more serious because of involvement of the uterine tubes and ovaries. To minimize adhesion formation, as many fibroids as possible should be removed through a

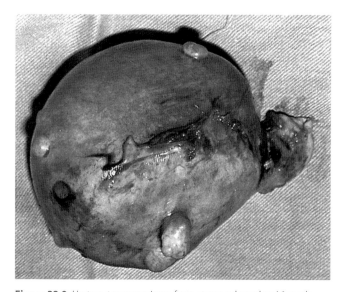

Figure 32.9 Hysterectomy specimen from uterus enlarged to 16-week gestation size by single intramural fibroid and several small seedling fibroids. Uterine volume was 575 ml.

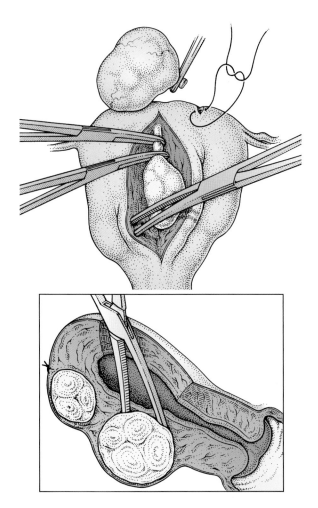

Figure 32.10 Removal of subserous, intramural, submucous and posteriorly located intramural fibroids through a single anterior incision. *Reproduced with permission of the American Society for Reproductive Medicine, formerly the American Fertility Society.*

increase both preoperative and postoperative haemoglobin and haematocrit (Lethaby et al 2000). This also reduced the size of the fibroids by approximately 50%, and reduced pelvic symptoms, operating time, duration of hospital stay, blood loss and rate of requiring a vertical incision. Disadvantages of the use of GnRH analogues include the cost, menopausal symptoms during treatment and bone demineralization with prolonged use. While an increased risk of fibroid recurrence has been reported, due to shrinkage of smaller fibroids making them undetectable at surgery, this was not confirmed in a systematic review. While the use of GnRH analogues has been criticized for making the pseudo-capsule plane of cleavage between the fibroid and the surrounding myometrium less well defined, this has not been the authors' experience. Intraoperative interventions to reduce blood loss during myomectomy have undergone a Cochrane review by Kongnyuy and Wiysonge (2007). One such method is the use of Bonney's myomectomy clamp (Figure 32.11A), which is placed across the lower uterus to occlude the uterine arteries. It can be used in conjunction with ring forceps to occlude the ovarian blood supply. An alternative is the use of a rubber tourniquet or catheter, placed around the uterus through an incision in the broad ligament at the level of the lower segment. During a long operation, intermittent release of the clamps or tourniquet is recommended every 10–20 min to prevent ischaemic damage to the tissues. Many intraoperative techniques have been advocated to reduce blood loss. Those that have been found to be effective (with weighted mean difference in blood loss with their use given in parentheses) include intramyometrial vasopressin (−299 ml), intramyometrial bupivacaine plus epinephrine (−69 ml), pericervical tourniquet (−1870 ml) and vaginal misoprostol (−149 ml).

The issue of mode of delivery in subsequent pregnancies following myomectomy where the uterine cavity has been breached is controversial. While common advice given to patients is that all myomectomies involving breach of the uterine cavity mandate caesarean sections in subsequent pregnancies, the evidence for this advice is limited (Parker 2007). During pregnancy and labour, rupture of the uterus after fibroid surgery is an extremely rare event. However, rupture after laparoscopic myomectomy may be higher than after abdominal myomectomy.

Hysteroscopic resection

Submucosal fibroids (such as those illustrated in Figure 32.12) are best removed hysteroscopically. Resection of the fibroid via the hysteroscope may be combined with endometrial ablation for the relief of menorrhagia if the woman has completed childbearing. Hysteroscopic surgery has been used for the removal of lesions measuring up to 7 cm in diameter, although many authorities would set a maximum of 3–4 cm (Agdi and Tulandi 2008). With larger fibroids, GnRH analogues can be used to shrink the tumour prior to surgery. Preoperatively, some surgeons use intravaginal misoprostol to soften and dilate the cervix, and allow easier insertion of the instruments. The uterine cavity is distended with a non-conductive glycine solution, and continuous irrigation with an infusion pump is employed to maintain visibility. A loop electrode is placed distal to the myoma, and sliced towards the cervix under vision. At all times, the

single incision (Figure 32.10), preferably at the fundus or anterior uterine wall. Some authorities recommend removal of posterior wall fibroids via the uterine cavity through an incision on the anterior abdominal wall, although this causes a deliberate breach of the uterine cavity and entails a risk of intrauterine adhesions. Bonney (Monaghan 1986) described a 'hood' method of closure of the cavity left after enucleation of a large single posterior tumour (Figure 32.11), suturing the redundant flap of serosal-covered myometrium over the fundus and low down on to the anterior abdominal wall to avoid adhesion formation. Keeping tissues moist, using wet packs to displace the bowel and minimal tissue handling is thought to reduce adhesions. The use of barrier agents, such as Interceed, Seprafilm and Gore-Tex, to reduce adhesions has been the subject of a recent Cochrane review (Ahmad et al 2008). While the use of Interceed does reduce postoperative adhesion formation after surgery, there is insufficient evidence to show that the reduced adhesion rates correspond with increased fertility and pregnancy rates.

Both mechanical and medical methods have been described to reduce intraoperative blood loss. Preoperative treatment with GnRH analogues for at least 3 months prior to either hysterectomy or myomectomy has been shown to

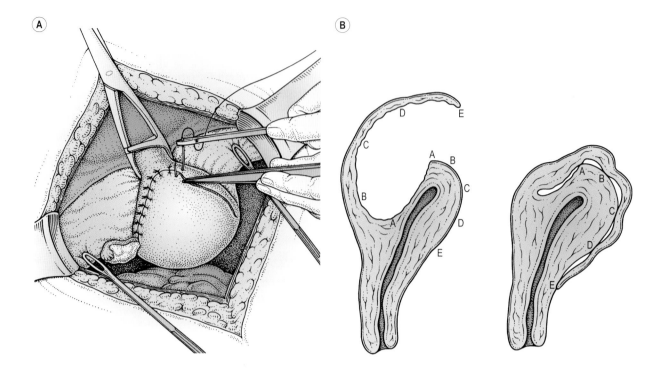

Figure 32.11 (A) Closure of myomectomy through transverse posterior incision using Bonney's 'hood', showing final anterior suture line and Bonney's clamp in place. (B) Construction of Bonney's hood showing the capsule after enucleation (left) and the hood in place (right).
EFFECTIVE GYNECOLOGICAL DAY SURGERY, DAVID HEALY & OSWALD PETRUCCO, 1998 LIPPINCOTT—RAVEN PUBLISHERS.

loop should remain under vision to reduce the risk of perforation of the uterus and damage to bowel or other internal organs. Any uterine perforation necessitates abandoning the procedure. Lengthy procedures carry the risk of 'water intoxication' and electrolyte disturbances, and a strict check should be made on the amount of glycine absorbed. The major advantage of hysteroscopic resection is the avoidance of major surgery, as well as easier access to submucosal fibroids compared with the abdominal route.

Some authors (Donnez et al 1990) advocate the use of the neodynium:YAG laser for larger fibroids, after prior shrinkage with a GnRH analogue. Laser ablation can also be used for smaller fibroids.

Laparoscopic myomectomy

Despite laparoscopic myomectomy being performed for almost two decades, there is little evidence and considerable debate about its place in the treatment of uterine fibroids. It is still not clear how the complications of the procedure compare with open myomectomy, and reported results from studies and case series are highly operator dependent. The purported advantages of the technique include shorter hospital stay, less postoperative pain, faster recovery and better visualization of adjacent organs (Agdi and Tulandi 2008). However, there have been reports of a higher risk of recurrence of fibroids, due to the inability to palpate the uterus and remove smaller coexisting fibroids laparoscopically. There is also a possible increased risk of uterine rupture in pregnancy and labour. Larger fibroid uteri may be impossible to remove laparoscopically, although preoperative

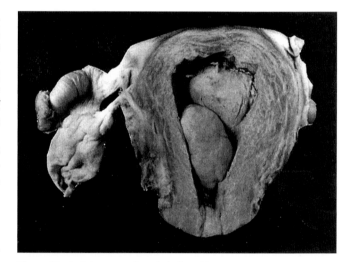

Figure 32.12 Submucous fibroids (subtotal hysterectomy specimen).

shrinkage with GnRH analogues may help in these cases. The procedure is challenging, with skills only available at a few centres, and is time consuming compared with an open myomectomy, subjecting the patient to a longer period of anaesthesia.

Generally, the procedure involves intramyometrial injection of epinephrine, followed by enucleation of the fibroid via diathermy incision, laparoscopic suturing in multiple layers of the remaining cavity, and morcellation and removal of the fibroid through one of the laparoscopic ports.

Recurrent fibroids after surgery

Reported cumulative recurrence rates after myomectomy are up to 50% at 5 years, with approximately 20% of women undergoing hysterectomy. It is not clear whether 'recurrent' fibroids after conservative treatment represent regrowth of existing tumours or de-novo development of additional fibroids. The literature is of poor quality with inconsistent reports regarding the definition of 'recurrence', the length of follow-up, the percentage of women lost to follow-up and why, and the use of other treatments which might affect recurrence. From the available literature, a larger preoperative fibroid size, an increased number of fibroid tumours, increasing fibroid penetration into the myometrium and any residual tissue at the completion of the procedure were all associated with increased risk of recurrence. These factors, leading to the development of further symptomatic fibroids after treatment, seem to occur with medical therapies, UAE or myomectomy.

Uterine artery embolization

Transarterial embolization for the successful treatment of obstetric and gynaecological haemorrhage has been practised for 30 years. It has also been used subsequently to treat uterine arteriovenous malformations. The initial report of the use of UAE to treat symptomatic fibroids was by Ravina et al in 1995. Its use has increased in popularity since then, and has been the subject of thorough recent reviews (Hickey and Hammond 2008, Tropeano et al 2008).

Technique

UAE is a percutaneous, image-guided procedure performed by an interventional radiologist. With regional anaesthesia or sedation, an angiographic catheter is placed under X-ray guidance into the uterine arteries via the common femoral artery. Embolic agents (usually polyvinyl alcohol particles or tris-acryl gelatin microspheres) are then injected into both uterine arteries to occlude them. Occlusion is confirmed angiographically and the catheters are removed (Figure 32.13). While the normal myometrium rapidly re-establishes its blood supply due to an extensive collateral circulation, the fibroids are supplied by end-arteries and undergo necrosis. The procedure takes approximately 1 h, and exposes the woman's ovaries to 20 rads, the equivalent of most routine diagnostic imaging procedures. The date of the last menses should be assessed, and a urine pregnancy test should be performed prior to the procedure to exclude pregnancy. Pretreatment with GnRH agonists may hamper UAE treatment for fibroids and is contraindicated, unlike for surgery.

Clinical outcomes

Treatment efficacy for menorrhagia associated with fibroids is high, with an 85% reduction in heavy menstrual bleeding immediately post procedure, and approximately 80% patient satisfaction at 5 years. While treatment is associated with a 50% reduction in fibroid volume, the reduction in fibroid volume does not appear to correlate with the reduction in symptoms. In comparison with surgical treatment, UAE is associated with a shorter hospital stay (usually 24 h) and faster return to work (7–10 days). It has less risk of major

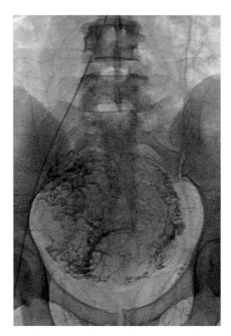

Figure 32.13 Catheter inserted via right femoral artery. The contrast medium clearly shows marked vasculature around a fibroid prior to embolization.

intraprocedural morbidity, such as bladder and bowel damage. However, long-term patient satisfaction appears to be greater with hysterectomy, with approximately 8–9% of women treated with UAE each year requiring either further UAE or surgery for recurrent symptoms.

Complications

Short-term complications include failure to cannulate either or both uterine arteries (8–11%), local haematoma formation or thrombosis, and femoral artery damage. 'Post-embolization syndrome' occurs in 40% of patients, lasting 3–7 days, and consists of general malaise, mild fever and flu-like symptoms. Severe pain following the procedure is common, requiring hospitalization and narcotic analgesia. Medium-term complications include vaginal expulsion of an infarcted fibroid (10%), which may become obstructed at the cervix. This is more common with submucosal fibroids. The most serious complication in the medium term is intrauterine sepsis associated with necrosis of the fibroid (1–2%). Two deaths from overwhelming sepsis after UAE have been reported.

Long-term complications include treatment failure (up to 25% of women will require a second procedure within 5 years), permanent ovarian failure and effects on fertility. After UAE, up to 8% of women have permanent ovarian failure, with higher rates for older women. Effects on future fertility and pregnancies are unknown at this time, but could include uterine rupture and intrauterine growth retardation. Although successful pregnancies have been reported following UAE, it should not be recommended at this time for women planning on having children.

MRI-guided focused ultrasound

MRI-guided focused ultrasound uses high-intensity ultrasound waves directed to a precise area of tissue via MRI (performed concurrently), causing a temperature rise sufficient to induce coagulative necrosis in the tissue (Tropeano et al 2008). The aim is controlled localized thermal ablation of the fibroid tissue, while leaving the surrounding normal tissues undamaged. The ultrasound waves are delivered to the fibroids via the anterior abdominal wall while the patient is sedated and lying prone on the MRI table. The procedure takes approximately 3 h, but patients go home 1 h post procedure and return to work in 48 h.

Preliminary reports suggest that the procedure is associated with less pain and postoperative complications than UAE, but is less effective as the maximum volume of fibroid tissue that can be treated is limited. While there is theoretically less risk of collateral damage to the ovaries, larger scale studies need to be performed before the safety of this new procedure can be compared with UAE.

Future Directions

There continues to be a lack of quality research into the pathophysiology and treatment of uterine fibroids. This is, in part, due to a lack of desire on the part of government bodies to fund research into a condition that does not cause an increase in mortality. With a lack of quality data from clinical trials, the treatment provided for uterine fibroids continues to be largely driven by individual clinician and patient preference. More comparative trials of alternative treatments for fibroids and related symptoms are required.

Development of non-surgical treatments for uterine fibroids, as well as improvement in understanding of pathogenesis, is hampered by a lack of suitable in-vitro or in-vivo models. Most studies in the literature consist of observational comparisons between fibroid and adjacent normal myometrial tissue. The best available animal model is the Eker rat model, in which 65% of the female $Tsc^{EK/+}$ carriers develop fibroids (Walker and Stewart 2005), but their applicability to fibroids in humans is still unclear and they are expensive to maintain. In-vitro models using smooth muscle cells isolated from the fibroids and adjacent myometrium have also been used. However, recent gene expression microarray work has shown that the differences in gene expression patterns of the two cell types diminish over time in culture (Zaitseva et al 2006), including the oestrogen and progesterone receptors that are critical to fibroid growth *in vivo*. This makes work from in-vitro cultures more difficult to translate into clinically relevant data.

KEY POINTS

1. Uterine fibroids occur in 60% of women by 45 years of age, are the most common cause of hysterectomy, and cost the US health system $US2.1 billion each year in direct surgical costs.

2. The growth of fibroids is sex steroid dependent. They do not occur until the menarche, and regress after the menopause. Progesterone appears to be as important in fibroid growth as oestrogen.

3. Increasing age, Black race, nulliparity, diabetes mellitus, obesity and hypertension have been associated with an increased risk of uterine fibroids.

4. Uterine fibroids are asymptomatic in at least 50% of cases. If asymptomatic, they require no treatment.

5. Sarcoma (leiomyosarcoma) occurs in one in one million women each year, and typically presents as postmenopausal bleeding. Fear of sarcoma is not an indication for surgical treatment of a fibroid.

6. Menorrhagia is the most common symptom attributed to fibroids, occurring in 30–50% of women with fibroids.

7. Adverse reproductive function (reduced implantation and increased miscarriage) is attributable to submucosal fibroids, and possibly intramural fibroids with uterine cavity distortion, but not to subserosal fibroids.

8. Pelvic ultrasound is the best diagnostic test for uterine fibroids at present.

9. Medical management of fibroids may control patient symptoms, but does not result in complete fibroid regression.

10. GnRH analogues may be used to shrink fibroids for 3 months prior to surgery with reduced intraoperative blood loss, reduced length of stay in hospital and less risk of requiring a vertical incision.

11. More comparative data of laparoscopic vs open surgery is required before firm recommendations can be made regarding the relative benefits and disadvantages of each technique.

12. UAE and MRI-guided focused ultrasound are two relatively non-invasive interventional radiological techniques for treating uterine fibroids which show great promise. However, their use is limited by availability and expertise.

References

Agdi M, Tulandi T 2008 Endoscopic management of uterine fibroids. Best Practice and Research Clinical Obstetrics and Gynaecology 22: 707–716.

Ahmad G, Duffy JM, Farquhar C et al 2008 Barrier agents for adhesion prevention after gynaecological surgery. Cochrane Database of Systematic Reviews 2: CD000475.

Ang WC, Farrell E, Vollenhoven B 2001 Effect of hormone replacement therapies and selective estrogen receptor modulators in postmenopausal women with uterine leiomyomas: a literature review. Climacteric 4: 284–292.

Benagiano G, Primiero FM 2006 Uterine leiomyomata: medical treatment. In: Brosens I (ed) Uterine Leiomyomata: Pathogenesis and Management. Taylor and Francis, London.

Brandon DD, Bethea CL, Strawn EY et al 1993 Progesterone receptor messenger ribonucleic acid and protein are overexpressed in human uterine leiomyomas. American Journal of Obstetrics and Gynecology 169: 78–85.

Buttram VC, Reiter RC 1981 Uterine leiomyomata: etiology, symptomatology and management. Fertility and Sterility 36: 433–445.

Casey R, Rogers PAW, Vollenhoven BJ 2000 An immunohistochemical analysis of fibroid vasculature. Human Reproduction 15: 1469–1475.

Chwalisz K, Larsen L, Mattia-Goldberg C et al 2007 A randomized, controlled trial of asoprisnil, a novel selective progesterone receptor modulator, in women with uterine leiomyomata. Fertility and Sterility 87: 1399–1412.

Cramer SF, Patel A 1990 The frequency of uterine leiomyomas. Americal Journal of Clinical Pathology 94: 435–438.

Crow J, Gardner RL, McSweeney G et al 1995 Morphological changes in uterine leiomyomas treated by GnRH agonist goserilin. International Journal of Gynaecological Pathology 14: 235–248.

Donnez J, Gillerot S, Bougonjon D et al 1990 Neodynium:YAG laser hysteroscopy in large submucous fibroids. Fertility and Sterility 54: 999–1003.

Eldar-Geva T, Meagher S, Healy DL et al 1998 Effect of intramural, subserosal and submucosal uterine fibroids on the outcome of assisted reproductive technology treatment. Fertility and Sterility 70: 687–691.

Fleischer R, Weston GC, Vollenhoven BJ et al 2008 Pathophysiology of fibroid disease: angiogenesis and regulation of smooth muscle proliferation. Best Practice and Research Clinical Obstetrics and Gynaecology 22: 603–614.

Gard GB, Mulvany NJ, Quinn MA 1999 Management of uterine leiomyosarcoma in Australia. Australia and New Zealand Journal of Obstetrics and Gynaecology 39: 93–98.

Hammoud AO, Asaad R, Berman J et al 2006 Volume change of uterine myomas during pregnancy: do myomas really grow? Journal of Minimally Invasive Gynecology 13: 386–390.

Hashimoto K, Azuma C, Kamiura S et al 1995 Clonal determination of uterine leiomyomas by analysing differential inactivation of the X-chromosome-linked phosphoglycerokinase gene. Gynecologic and Obstetric Investigation 40: 204–208.

Hickey M, Hammond I 2008 What is the place of uterine artery embolisation in the management of symptomatic uterine fibroids? Australian and New Zealand Journal of Obstetrics and Gynaecology 48: 360–368.

Khaund A, Lumsden MA 2008 Impact of fibroids on reproductive function. Best Practice and Research Clinical Obstetrics and Gynaecology 22: 749–760.

Klatsky PC, Tran ND, Caughey AB et al 2008 Fibroids and reproductive outcomes: a systematic literature review from conception to delivery. American Journal of Obstetrics and Gynecology 198: 357–366.

Kongnyuy EJ, Wiysonge CS 2007 Interventions to reduce haemorrhage during myomectomy for fibroids. Cochrane Database of Systematic Reviews 1: CD005355.

Lethaby A, Vollenhoven B, Sowter M 2000 Pre-operative GnRH analogue therapy before hysterectomy or myomectomy for uterine fibroids. Cochrane Database of Systematic Reviews 2: CD000547.

Lippman SA, Warner M, Samuels S et al 2003 Uterine fibroids and gynaecologic pain symptoms in a population-based study. Fertility and Sterility 80: 1488–1494.

Marshall LM, Spiegelman D, Barbieri R et al 1997 Variation in the incidence of uterine leiomyoma among premenopausal women by age and race. Obstetrics and Gynecology 90: 967–973.

Matsuo H, Kurachi O, Shimomura Y et al 1999 Molecular bases for the actions of ovarian sex steroids in the regulation of proliferation and apoptosis of human uterine leiomyoma. Oncology 57 (Suppl 2): 49–58.

Monaghan JM 1986 Bonney's Gynaecological Surgery, 9th edn. Baillière Tindall, London.

Munro MG, Lukes AS 2005 Abnormal uterine bleeding and underlying haemostatic disorders: report of a consensus process. Fertility and Sterility 84: 1335–1337.

Okolo S 2008 Incidence, aetiology and epidemiology of uterine fibroids. Best Practice and Research Clinical Obstetrics and Gynaecology 22: 571–588.

Parker WH, Fu YS, Berek JS 1994 Uterine sarcoma in patients operated on for presumed leiomyoma and rapidly growing leiomyoma. Obstetrics and Gynecology 83: 414–418.

Parker WH 2007 Etiology, symptomatology, and diagnosis of uterine myomas. Fertility and Sterility 87: 725–736.

Ravina JH, Herbreteau D, Cirau-Vigneron N et al 1995 Arterial embolisation to treat uterine myomata. The Lancet 346: 671–672.

Reiter RC, Wagner PL, Gambone JC 1992 Routine hysterectomy for large asymptomatic uterine leiomyomata: a reappraisal. Obstetrics and Gynecology 79(4): 481–484.

Sankaran S, Manyonda IT 2008 Medical management of fibroids. Best Practice and Research Clinical Obstetrics and Gynaecology 22: 655–676.

Townsend DE, Sparkes RS, Baluda MC et al 1970 Unicellular histogenesis of uterine leiomyomas as determined by electrophoresis by glucose-6-phosphate dehydrogenase. American Journal of Obstetrics and Gynecology 107: 1168–1173.

Tropeano G, Amoroso S, Scambia G 2008 Non-surgical management of uterine fibroids. Human Reproduction Update 14: 259–274.

Walker CL, Stewart EA 2005 Uterine fibroids: the elephant in the room. Science 308: 1589–1592.

Walocha JA, Litwin JA, Miodonski AJ 2003 Vascular system of intramural leiomyomata revealed by corrosion casting and scanning electron microscopy. Human Reproduction 18: 1088–1093.

Wegienka G, Baird DD, Hertz-Picciotto I et al 2003 Self-reported heavy bleeding associated with uterine leiomyomata. Obstetrics and Gynecology 101: 431–437.

Weston G, Trajstman AC, Gargett CE et al 2003 Fibroids display an anti-angiogenic gene expression profile when compared with adjacent myometrium. Molecular Human Reproduction 9: 541–549.

Weston GC, Cattrall F, Lederman F et al 2005 Differences between the pre-menopausal and post-menopausal uterine fibroid vasculature. Maturitas 51: 343–348.

Zaitseva M, Vollenhoven BJ, Rogers PA 2006 In vitro cuture significantly alters gene expression profiles and reduces differences between myometrial and fibroid smooth muscle cells. Molecular Human Reproduction 12: 187–207.

CHAPTER **33**

Endometriosis

Robert W. Shaw

Chapter Contents

INTRODUCTION	488	DIAGNOSIS	494
DEFINITION	488	CLASSIFICATION SYSTEMS	500
PREVALENCE	488	TREATMENT: GENERAL PRINCIPLES	500
PATHOGENESIS	489	MEDICAL TREATMENTS	501
PERITONEAL FLUID ENVIRONMENT IN ENDOMETRIOSIS	490	SURGICAL TREATMENT	504
		RECURRENT ENDOMETRIOSIS	505
PRESENTATION	491	KEY POINTS	506
ENDOMETRIOSIS AND INFERTILITY	493		

Introduction

Endometriosis is one of the most common benign gynaecological conditions. It is second only to uterine fibroids as the most common reason for major surgical procedures in women under 45 years of age. It has been estimated that it is present in between 10% and 25% of women presenting with gynaecological symptoms in the UK and USA (Tyson 1974). These figures are based on the findings of patients who have undergone laparoscopy for diagnostic indications, such as pelvic pain or infertility, or in patients undergoing laparotomy. Although it is such a widespread condition, it is true to say that there is limited understanding regarding its aetiology and pathogenesis, and the condition still arouses much controversy with regard to its diagnosis, treatment and management. Endometriosis varies in severity from minimal disease with a few peritoneal implants to severe disease producing adhesions, deep infiltrating lesions and involvement with ovarian cyst formation.

Definition

Endometriosis is defined as a disease characterized by the presence of tissue that is morphologically and biologically similar to normal endometrium, and contains functional endometrial glands and stroma, in ectopic locations outside the uterine cavity. This ectopic endometrial tissue initially responds to hormones and drugs in a generally similar manner to eutopic endometrium undergoing cyclical changes. Cyclical bleeding from the endometriotic deposit appears to contribute to the induction of a local inflammatory reaction, fibrous adhesion and formation, and, in the

case of deep ovarian implants in the ovary, leads to the formation of an endometrioma or chocolate cyst. Endometrial tissue deep within the myometrium of the uterine wall is termed 'adenomyosis'. This condition is increasingly viewed as a separate pathological entity to that of endometriosis, since it affects a different population of women, probably has a different aetiology and is most often found in the absence of other evidence of pelvic endometriosis.

Prevalence

Continued growth of endometriotic tissue, as with that of the endometrium, is dependent on ovarian steroid hormones, particularly oestrogen. Thus, endometriosis is prevalent in the reproductive years with a peak incidence between 30 and 45 years of age, although it is increasingly being diagnosed in much younger women as the threshold for investigation of gynaecological symptoms utilizing diagnostic laparoscopy has altered. Endometriosis is thus primarily a disease of the reproductive years and is only rarely described in adolescence, when it is associated with obstructing genital tract abnormalities, or in postmenopausal women, where it has been reactivated because of hormone replacement therapy.

No racial differences in the incidence of the disease have been found, except for Japanese women who have been reported to have twice the incidence of Caucasian women (Miyazawa 1976).

The exact prevalence of endometriosis is unknown since precise diagnosis depends on observation of implants, predominantly at the time of laparoscopy or laparotomy. Until simple non-invasive screening tests are developed, the true

DOI: 10.1016/B978-0-7020-3120-5.00033-3

prevalence will remain unknown. Current prevalence therefore depends upon identification in women who are either symptomatic or undergoing various operative procedures. The incidence is markedly variable as the data in Table 33.1 show, but the prevalence of endometriosis in the reproductive years is estimated to be approximately 10% (Eskenazi and Warner 1997). Endometriosis commonly affects women during their childbearing years. In the main, this is reflected in deleterious sexual, reproductive and social consequences as a result of its associated painful symptoms and often associated infertility. Symptomatology may extend over several decades of a patient's life because of its often late diagnosis and the recurrent nature of the disease. For individual patients and healthcare systems, it represents a major call upon resource use.

Pathogenesis

The precise aetiology of endometriosis still remains unknown. Indeed, it is often called the 'disease of theories' because of the many mechanisms postulated to explain its pathogenesis. It is likely that no single theory can explain all forms of endometriosis. Different types of endometriosis may have different origins (i.e. they are multifactorial in origin). Peritoneal endometriosis could arise as a result of retrograde menstruation, ovarian endometriosis via coelomic metaplasia, and rectovaginal endometriosis from development within Müllerian duct remnants. The major theories of causation of endometriosis are metaplasia (transformation) of coelomic epithelium, and implantation of endometrial fragments through retrograde menstruation.

Transformation of coelomic epithelium

This theory, first described by Meyer (1919), postulated the possibility of differentiation by metaplasia towards an endometrial-like tissue of the original coelomic membrane following prolonged irritation and oestrogen stimulation. It is proposed that these adult cells undergo dedifferentiation back to their primitive origin and then transform to endometrial cells. If this theory is correct, metaplasia should occur wherever coelomic membranes are present. This theory has many attractions which could explain the occurrence of endometriosis in nearly all the ectopic sites in the presence of aberrant Müllerian cells. What induces this transformation — whether it is hormonal stimuli, inflammatory irritation or other processes — is uncertain. If coelomic metaplasia is similar to metaplasia elsewhere, the frequency of the disorder should increase with advancing age. The clinical pattern of endometriosis is distinctly different from this, with an abrupt halt in the disease with the cessation of menses at the menopause and reduced oestrogen production, thus raising some questions over this theory.

Menstrual regurgitation and implantation (metastatic theory)

As early as 1927, Sampson proposed the metastatic theory, postulating that retrograde menstrual flow transported desquamated endometrial fragments through the fallopian tubes

Table 33.1 Prevalence of endometriosis through various presentations

Presentation	Prevalence (%)
Unexplained infertility	70–80*
Infertile women (all causes)	15–20*
At diagnostic laparoscopy	0–53†
At treatment laparoscopy	0.1–50†
Women undergoing sterilization	2‡
In women with diagnosed first-degree relatives	7§

* Source: Kistner RW 1977 In: Sciarra J (ed) Gynaecology and Obstetrics, Vol. 1. Harper and Row, London.
† Source: Houston DE 1984 Epidemiology Reviews 6: 167–191.
‡ Source: Strathy JH, Molgaard GA, Coulam CB, Molton LJ III 1982 Fertility and Sterility 38: 667–672.
§ Source: Simpson JL, Elias S, Malinak LR, Buttram VC Jr 1980 American Journal of Obstetrics and Gynecology 137: 327–331.

into the peritoneal cavity (Sampson 1927). Once there, the still viable cells subsequently implanted and began growth and invasion. In support of this theory, experimental endometriosis has been induced in animals with replacement of menstrual fluid or endometrial tissue in the peritoneal cavity. Supporting this theory in humans is the finding that endometriosis is commonly found in young girls with associated abnormalities in the genital tract causing obstruction to the outflow of menstrual fluid (Schifrin et al 1973). Halme et al (1984) observed bloody fluid at the time of menstruation in the pelvis during laparoscopic assessment, but as this finding occurs in up to 90% of all women, it is regarded as a physiological phenomenon. The high incidence of retrograde menstruation suggests that this phenomenon alone does not give rise to endometriosis, but that some other factor(s) must be involved in development of the disease. These factors could include some alteration in the (uterine) endometrium, altered immune response to retrograde menstruation (hence failure to clear the peritoneal cavity of debris efficiently), or a more favourable peritoneal environment which may stimulate the growth and implantation of ectopic endometrium within the peritoneal cavity itself.

Genetic and immunological factors

Many studies have indicated that there may be a genetic factor related to endometriosis since the disease is more prevalent in certain families. It has been shown that women with an affected first-degree relative have a seven times higher risk of developing endometriosis, which may be severe (Simpson et al 1980, Halme et al 1986). Endometriosis is also more common in monozygotic twin sisters than dizygotic twins, but no association was found with specifically identified tissue types (Simpson et al 1984). Whilst Dmowski et al (1981) demonstrated a decreased cellular immunity to endometriotic tissue in women with endometriosis, no clinically significant immune system abnormality has been observed in women with the disease; hence, the precise genetic or immune components increasing an individual's potential to develop this disorder are yet to be defined.

Vascular and lymphatic metastasis (Halban's theory)

Halban's theory suggests that distant endometriosis (outwith the abdominal cavity) occurs via vascular or lymphatic spread of viable endometrial cells or fragments. The theory would explain the rare occurrence of endometriosis in lung, limbs and brain, but not in more common sites within the peritoneal cavity and pelvis.

Endometrial disease theory

Many view the superficial implants as 'physiological' lesions which may regress spontaneously. Deep infiltrating lesions and ovarian endometriotic cysts are pathological and arise from cells that have undergone somatic mutations. Such mutations may have been produced by environmental factors (e.g. pollutants, dioxins). These abnormal cells then develop into a 'benign tumour' consisting of endometriotic glands and stroma. For a review on environmental factors in the aetiology of endometriosis, the reader is directed to Missmer and Mohllagee (2008).

Further support of the above theory stems from biochemical differences demonstrated in the endometrium in patients with and without endometriosis (Guidice and Kao 2004). These include differences in the expression of metalloproteinases, tumour susceptibility genes and angiogenic factors. Such changes may allow certain types of retrograde endometrial fragments to implant more readily than others, and this may be due to an underlying inherited genetic tendency.

Iatrogenic dissemination

Transplantation of endometrial cells can occur during gynaecological surgical procedures. This would explain the development of endometriotic nodules in abdominal wall scars following caesarean section, myomectomy and hysterectomy, and in laparoscopic port scars. In addition, implantation at perineal repair can cause endometriosis to develop in episiotomy scars.

Conclusion

The conclusion reached from the above theories is that pelvic endometriosis is probably a consequence of transplantation of viable endometrial cells regurgitated at the time of menstruation from the fallopian tubes into the peritoneal cavity. In addition, transport of endometrial cells may occur by other routes (some iatrogenic). It is unclear whether endometriotic implants are derived from in-situ pluripotential cells generated by metastatic seeding, but it is known that endocrine and immunological factors allow growth and spread within the pelvis and neighbouring organs. Delayed childbearing, either by choice or infertility, has been implicated as a risk factor for the development of endometriosis. The risk of developing endometriosis also corresponds with cumulative menstruation, menstrual frequency and volume.

Women with shorter menstrual cycles of less than 27 days and longer flows (more than 7 days) are twice as likely to develop the disease compared with women with longer cycles and shorter flows. Thus, many components are necessary to allow endometriotic deposits to implant and subsequently grow (Figure 33.1).

The cell-mediated efferent arm of the immune system controls implantation or rejection of such fragments. In most women, these fragments are not in a favourable state or in a favourable environment for implantation, and are engulfed by macrophages and thus disposed. In women with deficient or altered cell-mediated immunity, implantation of the ectopic fragments allows implantation to occur with subsequent development of endometriotic implants. Such immune changes could be transmitted genetically and could be both qualitative and quantitative, resulting in variable ages of onset, extent and duration of expression. Autoantibody production would be a secondary phenomenon, developing as the number and extent of endometriotic deposits increase.

Peritoneal Fluid Environment in Endometriosis

It has been suggested that peritoneal fluid volume and its contents may be adversely affected by the presence of endometriotic tissue in the pelvis, with possible consequent interference with tubo-ovarian function and/or fertilization and early implantation. Peritoneal fluid is an ultrafiltrate of plasma, and the volumes are very low in normal women. Endometriosis may alter the peritoneal fluid volume by increasing fluid production in the ovary, altering mesothelial permeability or increasing the hydrostatic pressure as a result of altered protein content.

Peritoneal macrophages

Normal peritoneal fluid contains approximately 10^6 cells per ml; 90% are macrophages, and the remainder are lymphocytes and desquamated mesothelial cells. The role of peritoneal macrophages in women with endometriosis has been the source of much interest, and women with endome-

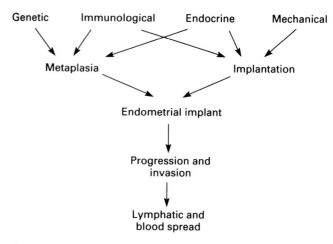

Figure 33.1 Suggested aetiological factors in the pathogenesis of endometriotic implants.

triosis associated with infertility have been reported to have significantly higher concentrations of macrophages in peritoneal fluid than either fertile women or infertile women without endometriosis. Macrophages in patients with endometriosis appeared to be highly phagocytic against spermatozoa *in vitro* compared with those from fertile women or infertile women without endometriosis (Muscato et al 1982). In addition, they are also able to survive better *in vitro* than those from fertile controls (Halme et al 1986). Peritoneal fluid from patients with endometriosis has also been shown to have a cytotoxic effect on in-vivo cleavage of mouse embryos. These findings on the quantitative and qualitative properties of macrophages in peritoneal fluid may partially explain the mechanisms of infertility in patients with endometriosis.

Prostaglandins and prostanoids

The role of prostaglandins and their metabolites in peritoneal fluid in the pathogenesis and symptomatology of endometriosis is controversial. It has been reported that increased levels of prostaglandin $F_{2\alpha}$ ($PGF_{2\alpha}$) are found in the peritoneal fluid of patients with the disease (Meldrum et al 1977). In addition, increased peritoneal fluid volume and increased concentrations of the prostaglandin metabolites thromboxane B_2 and 6-keto $PGF_{2\alpha}$ have been noted. Other investigators have found no increase in either the volume of peritoneal fluid or its concentrations of prostaglandins or metabolites (Rock et al 1982). These conflicting reports may reflect the timing of peritoneal fluid sampling and difficulties in assay measurement of the small quantities of substrates, all of which have very short half-lives.

In recent years, it has been appreciated that more subtle forms of endometriosis may be present with only minimal evidence of visual changes in the peritoneum. However, if there are changes in the prostaglandin content of the peritoneal fluid, the mechanisms by which these changes influence endometriosis or its association with infertility remain unclear.

Cytokines and growth factors

A large number of cells, including macrophages, lymphocytes, fibroblasts and epithelial cells, synthesize a wide range of polypeptides of high biological activity within the cytokine/growth factor group. They have multiple effects including the regulation of differentiation, growth and function of a wide variety of cell types. It was generally believed that cytokines were produced in increased amounts as part of the inflammatory process or as part of a response to infection or immune challenge. Cytokines are very potent and active at picogram to nanogram levels, and are difficult to detect and identify. Research activity has been concentrated on the measurement of various cytokines including various interleukins, colony stimulating factors, human necrosis factor and transforming growth factors. To date, no consistent changes between normal, infertile women with and without endometriosis and patients with endometriosis who are not infertile have been reported to satisfactorily explain the aetiology or pathogenesis of the disease.

Peritoneal environment: conclusions

Peritoneal macrophages play an important role in the peritoneal cavity where endometrial tissue fragments often arrive and are likely to adhere to the mesothelial lining. The adherence may be mediated by cell adhesion molecules and other factors produced by activated macrophages. Endometrial tissue will potentially adhere if the regurgitated amount of the tissue is too great, or if the capacity of the intra-abdominal cells to clear the cellular debris is in any way impaired. Once an endometrial fragment has gained adherence, further tissue growth may be promoted by steroids, cytokines, growth factors and angiogenic factors present in peritoneal fluid in a paracrine and autocrine fashion.

Presentation

Endometriosis commonly presents between the ages of 25 and 35 years, although it can present in early adolescence and in postmenopausal women on hormone replacement therapy. The symptoms of endometriosis are variable and often unrelated to the extent of the disease process as currently quantified. The three most common complaints amongst women with endometriosis are dysmenorrhoea, dyspareunia and pelvic pain. The pain symptoms are often cycle related and increase premenstrually. However, it must be stated that the finding of endometriosis may not conclusively link it with painful symptoms in an individual, since the severity of symptoms is rarely correlated with the extent of the disease, and endometriosis is often found coincidentally (during surgery or investigation for other gynaecological conditions, such as infertility) at similar levels in patients not complaining of pain.

Atypical bleeding patterns are a leading symptom in a variety of gynaecological diseases, but may also characterize patients with endometriosis. Premenstrual spotting and menometrorrhagia are frequently noted. On the other hand, cyclical rectal bleeding or haematuria is pathognomonic of the disease and, although rarely observed (1–2% of cases), these symptoms give strong evidence for bowel or bladder involvement. Painful micturition or defaecation at the time of menstruation may be the first signs of progressing disease. The various symptoms of endometriosis as found in various sites of implantation are shown in Table 33.2.

Dysmenorrhoea

Dysmenorrhoea is the most common presenting symptom, affecting 70–80% of women with proven endometriosis. Dysmenorrhoea often occurs with pelvic pain, but patients commonly describe a background of constant dragging, aching pain which may be exacerbated by the menses but is often a different type of pain from the typical cramping nature of spasmodic dysmenorrhoea and often in a different site. Typically, pain starts some days before menstruation as an ache or discomfort, similar to congestive pelvic pain. It worsens and becomes spasmodic with the start of the menses and continues throughout days of bleeding, lessening as menstrual flow ebbs. Unlike 'primary dysmenorrhoea' which starts soon after the establishment of ovulatory cycles, endometriosis-related dysmenorrhoea often starts in the

Table 33.2 Symptoms of endometriosis related to sites of implants

Symptoms	Site
Dysmenorrhoea	Reproductive organs
Lower abdominal pain	
Pelvic pain	
Low back pain	
Menstrual irregularity	
Rupture/torsion endometrioma	
Infertility	
Cyclical rectal bleeding	Gastrointestinal tract
Tenesmus	
Diarrhoea/cyclic constipation	
Cyclical haematuria	Urinary tract
Dysuria (cyclical)	
Ureteric obstruction	
Cyclical haemoptysis	Lungs
Cyclical pain and bleeding	Surgical scars/umbilicus
Cyclical pain and swelling	Limbs

early 20s, and is usually very severe, incapacitating and unresponsive to simple/mild analgesics or antiprostaglandins. If endometriosis is untreated, dysmenorrhoea progressively increases in duration, but severity tends to remain constant.

Dyspareunia

Another common symptom of endometriosis is deep dyspareunia resulting from stretching at intercourse of the involved pelvic tissues such as a fixed retroverted uterus, the uterosacral ligaments or rectovaginal septum; or pressure on an involved enlarged, often adherent, ovary. The presence of endometriotic tissue within these areas, however, is not always associated with dyspareunia; perhaps less than half of patients who are coitally active admit to this symptom when deposits are found in these areas. The pain continues for a variable time after intercourse, often as a dull ache. Typically, dyspareunia is exaggerated in the phase before menstruation commences. This pain is more severe in women with deep rectovaginal septum involvement and may result in complete apareunia.

Origin of pain

The basis of the pelvic pain and dysmenorrhoea is uncertain but could reflect stretching of tissues by the menstrual process and an effect of the local production of prostaglandins within the endometriotic implants. The pain also relates to tissue damage and fixity of organs from scar and adhesion formation. What is immediately clear when reviewing patients with endometriosis is the huge variation in extent of symptomatic disease, which does not correlate

with the extent of the observed disease process. In addition, many patients who are asymptomatic are found to have endometriosis, and in some of these patients, severe disease is discovered following laparoscopy during infertility investigations. One possible explanation for this is that in these individuals, the disease may have disrupted the pelvic sensation altogether. Pain may arise from mediator release from the endometriotic deposits (prostaglandins, inflammatory products from macrophages or interleukins) in the early stages of the disease at menstruation. Pain associated with more advanced disease is likely caused by extensive adhesions, ovarian endometriotic cysts or deep infiltration of disease. The pain may result from mechanical compression or disruption of nociceptors, particularly around the uterosacral ligaments.

Non-cyclic chronic pelvic pain

In approximately 30–50% of women with pelvic endometriosis, chronic pelvic pain (CPP) of varying severity, pattern and location is reported. Pelvic pain is arguably the symptom causing the most misery amongst endometriosis sufferers, and is more distressing than infertility. CPP, as with other forms of pain, often produces a serious long-term detrimental effect on the personality, and affects working ability and social and marital life. Possible causes include adhesions, ovarian cysts, peritoneal inflammatory reaction around implants, or involvement of bladder or bowel. Pain may be triggered by ovulation, bowel evacuation or micturition. Pain resulting from adhesions may be provoked or worsened by certain body positions or movements. A common feature of CPP is worsening before and during menstruation.

Menstrual irregularities

In 16% of women, the disease is associated with heavy and/or irregular periods or premenstrual spotting, the causes of which are undetermined.

Other symptoms associated with the menstrual cycle

Direct involvement of the bladder wall can result in haematuria and dysuria occurring at the time of menstruation. Invasion into the muscular coat of the descending colon and rectum (most commonly) can cause cyclical rectal bleeding and painful defaecation (dyschezia), whilst involvement of the small bowel or colon elsewhere may not present until a narrowing of the bowel lumen has occurred with complete or partial obstruction. Rarely, dysmenorrhoea may be associated with symptoms due to extrapelvic endometriosis (e.g. sciatica, groin pain), or cyclical haemoptysis or pneumoperitoneum with lung/pleural involvement. Other rare associations include bleeding, swelling and/or pain in surgical scars, umbilicus or episiotomy site affected by endometriosis.

Correlation of symptoms and severity of endometriosis

The frequencies of the more common symptoms in endometriosis patients are summarized in Table 33.3. Whilst the

Table 33.3 Frequency of the more common symptoms in endometriosis patients

Symptom	Likely frequency (%)
Dysmenorrhoea	60–80
Pelvic pain	30–50
Infertility	30–40
Dyspareunia	25–40
Menstrual irregularities	10–20
Cyclical dysuria/haematuria	1–2
Dyschezia	1–2
Rectal bleeding (cyclic)	<1

Table 33.4 Possible mechanisms of causation of infertility with mild endometriosis

Problem area	Mechanism
Ovarian function	Endocrinopathies • Anovulation • Luteinized unruptured follicle syndrome • Altered prolactin release • Altered gonadotrophin midcycle surge
	Luteolysis caused by prostaglandin $F_{2\alpha}$
	Oocyte maturation defects
Coital function	Dyspareunia causing reduced penetration and coital frequency
Tubal function	Alterations in tubal and cilial motility by prostaglandins
	Impaired fimbrial oocyte pick-up
Sperm function	Phagocytosis by macrophages
	Inactivation by antibodies
Endometrium	Interference by endometrial antibodies
	Luteal-phase deficiency
Early pregnancy failure	Increased early abortion
	Prostaglandin induced or immune reaction

symptoms of dysmenorrhoea, dyspareunia and pelvic pain can occur with other gynaecological disorders, it is the combination, cyclical and menstrually related component of several symptoms which should alert the clinician to the potential underlying presence of endometriosis. Many women have delayed diagnosis of their condition, which may mean that it has progressed to a more extensive and potentially less reversible or curable stage at the time of diagnosis.

There appears to be little correlation between sites involved in endometriosis and symptoms. Various 'types' of symptoms can, however, be related to some degree to the system involved (see Table 33.2). However, these do not always correlate with the anatomy and type of pain innervation of the pelvis (for review, see MacLaverty and Shaw 1995).

One reason for the apparent lack of correlation between disease severity and symptom severity is that the classification systems for endometriosis thus developed have primarily been directed towards infertility prediction rather than pain symptom severity.

Deeply infiltrating endometriosis is very strongly associated with the presence and severity of pelvic pain. In addition, superficial non-pigmented endometriosis has the capacity to produce more prostaglandin F (PGF) than pigmented classic powder burn lesions. PGF is implicated in pain causation (Vernon et al 1986). Thus, in the early, less florid stages before it has become destructive and more easily recognized, endometriosis may be producing large quantities of PGF and hence possesses greater potential to increase the severity of pain. The type of pain may alter with disease progression, with constant pain and exacerbation at the menses initially in the disease, and pain later becoming continuous due to scar formation and organ fixity.

Endometriosis and Infertility

It is accepted that endometriosis resulting in structural damage to the tubes and ovaries causes infertility. However, what is less clear is whether the milder forms of endometriosis are also the cause of infertility in otherwise asymptomatic patients.

Endometriosis was one of the most frequently made diagnoses in couples undergoing infertility investigation, when routine use of laparoscopy for investigation of such couples was employed, in past years. The assumption was made that endometriotic implants are responsible for the patient's inability to conceive. Estimates of the incidence of endometriosis in the general population of reproductive age vary between 2% and 10%. From retrospective studies in infertile patients, the incidence has been reported as being between 20% and 40% (Mahmood and Templeton 1990). This increased incidence in infertile patients has led many clinicians to consider the endometriotic implants to be responsible, in some way, for the associated infertility. The question is how, and a number of suggested mechanisms have been reported. These are summarized in Table 33.4. For the majority of these potential causes, there are few or no consistent data to provide a sustainable explanation. Thus, the nature of the relationship between mild endometriosis and infertility remains unresolved.

Although there may be some debate about the role of filmy peritubal or periovarian adhesions in infertility, it is accepted that with increasing severity of endometriosis, adhesions become more common and the chances of a natural conception decrease. The majority of specialists would divide such adhesions if found at laparoscopy and if appropriate consent had been obtained, although laparoscopy is no longer routinely undertaken in asymptomatic infertile women. Evidence that the treatment of endometriosis benefits fertility would provide proof that endometriosis is linked with infertility. Historically, many studies have utilized ovarian-suppression treatments with progestogens, danazol and/or gonadotrophin-releasing hormone (GnRH) analogues in the hope of treating endometriosis and enhancing fertility. The majority of these patients had minimal or mild endometriosis (see later for classification). These studies show that 3–6 months of medication prevents fertility during treatment, but does not increase pregnancy rates following treatment cessation. Meta-analysis showed no difference in pregnancy rate between ovarian suppression and no treatment (relative risk 0.98; confidence interval 0.81–1.15) (Hughes et al 1993, Adamson and Pasta 1994). There was no difference among different ovarian-suppression agents, and the current recommendation is that ovarian suppression in the infertile patient is not justified because of lack of effectiveness on improving conception rates over a conservative approach alone.

Laparoscopic surgical destruction, excision or laser ablation of endometriotic deposits has become popular in recent years and is helpful in pain management of selective endometriosis patients (see later). However, its role in patients with endometriosis and infertility without tubo-ovarian adhesion, endometriomas or other pathology is in question. The ENDOCAN randomized trial from Canada showed a higher pregnancy rate at 9 months in patients who had undergone surgical destruction of endometriotic deposits (and any adhesions present) compared with the control (no treatment) arm (37.5% vs 22.5%). The number needed to treat to create a pregnancy was 7.7 (Marcoux et al 1997). However, a smaller, prospective randomized controlled trial from Italy did not show any difference in pregnancy rates between the treatment and control groups (19.6% vs 22.2%) (Parazzinni 1999). There is a need for more large randomized controlled trials to investigate the role of surgery in such patients.

Conclusions

To date, it is not known how mild endometriosis (without tubo-ovarian disease or adhesions) causes infertility, but it is recognized that such patients have a reduced fecundity rate. Until the underlying cause (if any) is found and appropriate corrective therapies are available, such asymptomatic patients are best treated along the lines of unexplained infertile couples (see Chapters 20 and 22) with treatment options based on age and duration of infertility.

Diagnosis

The diagnosis of endometriosis still presents several problems resulting from the similarities in clinical symptoms produced by endometriosis to other benign gynaecological disorders, and to several non-gynaecological disorders, particularly related to the gastrointestinal system.

Symptomatic pointers

No single symptom is pathognomic of endometriosis, but severe dysmenorrhoea (pain sufficient to require time off work and/or to interfere with normal everyday activity) is highly predictive. Dyspareunia and pelvic pain are less predictive in the absence of severe dysmenorrhoea (Overton and Kennedy 1993). These gynaecological symptoms may, however, be of diagnostic help in the suspicion of endometriosis, which should be a differential diagnosis in any patient presenting with worsening dysmenorrhoea, pelvic pain and/or dyspareunia or with other cycle-associated symptoms relating specifically to the bowel, bladder or localized skin lesions (see Table 33.2 and Box 33.1). In endometriosis, the associated dysmenorrhoea extends to the pre- and postmenstrual phase, and is typically of secondary onset and progressive rather than being present from the onset of the menarche. In women presenting with pelvic pain, a history of whether or not this relates to the menstrual cycle is helpful in differentiating other aetiological causes of pain. In those with associated marked bowel symptoms, a trial of treatment for irritable bowel syndrome may be worthwhile before considering referral for diagnostic laparoscopy, although other pathologies may be present concurrently (see Box 33.2).

Clinical examination

Clinical abdominal examination may demonstrate local tender nodular lesions in a caesarean section or laparotomy scar, or at the umbilicus or other site of a laparoscopy port. Gynaecological speculum examination may visualize endometriotic lesions as clear red or bluish cysts or nodules in the vagina, most commonly in the posterior fornix, or on the cervix. This visual diagnosis cannot substitute for histological confirmation even if bleeding occurs from the lesions at the time of menstruation.

Box 33.1 Symptoms suggestive of the presence of endometriosis

Primary symptoms

- Dysmenorrhoea: secondary onset
- Pain not normally controlled by simple analgesics or oral contraceptive pill
- Pain severe enough to cause significant incapacitation

Plus two or more in addition

- Dyspareunia: deep
- Pelvic pain: worse in premenstrual phase
- Dysmenorrhoea/pain continues with postmenstrual days

Less common associated symptoms

- Infertility
- Bleeding from rectum coinciding with menstruation
- Pain at micturition or defaecation: worse or only at time of menses

---

Box 33.2 Differential diagnosis of endometriosis

- Pelvic infection: chronic pelvic inflammatory disease
- Adhesions: postoperative or following pelvic inflammation
- Ovarian cyst: torsion or haemorrhage into a cyst
- Haemoperitoneum: ruptured corpus luteum or ectopic
- Large bowel: irritable bowel syndrome, diverticulitis, ulcerative colitis, obstruction
- Small bowel: Crohn's disease, obstruction
- Musculoskeletal

Pelvic examination often reveals induration of the uterosacral ligaments or nodules in the pouch of Douglas or rectovaginal septum. Involvement of the ovaries can lead to the development of endometriotic cysts which eventually become large enough to be palpable. There may be fixation of the uterus in retroversion, with the immobilization of the ovaries by adhesion formation, and tenderness, particularly when the patient is examined in the immediate premenstrual phase of the cycle. These clinical findings, whilst not specific to endometriosis, may add to the suspicion of the presence of the disease from the pointers obtained in the history.

Pelvic endometriosis

Pelvic endometriosis has been defined as endometriotic implants involving the peritoneum, anterior and posterior cul-de-sac and pelvic side walls, and the surfaces of the uterus, tubes and ovaries.

Diagnosis of pelvic endometriosis cannot be made with absolute certainty from symptoms or examination alone, and laparoscopic examination may be required to confirm the initial clinical diagnosis. The role of laparoscopy is to:

- provide direct visualization of the endometriotic lesions;
- present an opportunity to biopsy suspected areas, if desired;
- stage the disease by extent, type and site of lesions;
- evaluate the extent and type of adhesions present; and
- provide an opportunity for concomitant laparoscopic surgical treatment, if felt appropriate.

The laparoscopic features of pelvic endometriosis are many and varied, and it is clear that a carefully undertaken laparoscopy by an experienced surgeon is essential if cases are not to be missed at this diagnostic opportunity. Whenever there is any doubt, the need for biopsy confirmation is paramount. Careful recording of the laparoscopic findings is essential and photographic records are most helpful if patients are to be referred on for further management.

Morphology of the typical black lesions

The typical peritoneal endometriotic lesion is described as a 'powder burn' which results from tissue bleeding and retention of blood pigments, producing a brown–black discoloration of the tissue. In the early stages, these lesions may appear more pink, red and haemorrhagic, and develop into brown–black lesions with increasing time. Eventually, discoloration disappears altogether and a white plaque of old collagen is all that remains of the endometriotic implant (Figure 33.2).

Scarring in the peritoneum surrounding implants is also a typical finding. Apart from encapsulating an isolated implant, the scar tissue may deform the surrounding peritoneum, resulting in development of adhesions between adjacent pelvic structures. These adhesions are commonly found between the mobile pelvic structures, particularly the posterior leaf of the broad ligament and the ovary, and the dependent sigmoid colon and posterior aspect of the vagina and/or cervix.

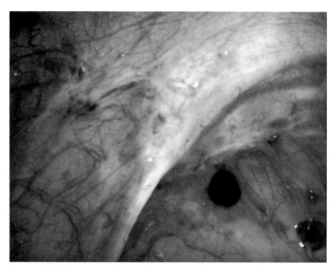

Figure 33.2 Black deposits on the uterosacral ligament with the uterus in anteversion.
Source: Overton C, Davis C, McMillan L, Shaw RW 2007 An Atlas of Endometriosis, 3rd edn. Informa Healthcare, London.

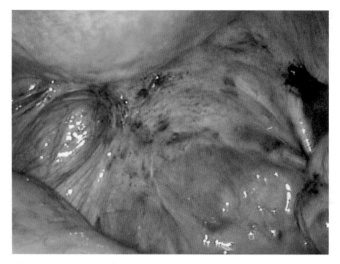

Figure 33.3 Active endometriosis on the uterosacral ligament.
Source: Overton C, Davis C, McMillan L, Shaw RW 2007 An Atlas of Endometriosis, 3rd edn. Informa Healthcare, London.

Classification and morphology of subtle appearances

More recently, more subtle laparoscopic appearances have been reported which were confirmed on biopsy as being due to endometriosis (Donnez and Nisolle 1991). The subtle forms are more common and may be more active and more important than the puckered black lesions that represent the later stages of the disease. These other peritoneal lesions include red lesions and white lesions.

Red lesions

- Red flame-like lesions on the peritoneum, with the appearance of red vascular excrescences in the broad ligament and uterosacral ligaments, largely due to the presence of active endometriosis surrounded by stroma (Figure 33.3).

- Glandular excrescences which closely resemble the mucosa of the endometrium as seen at hysteroscopy; biopsy reveals the presence of numerous glandular elements (Figures 33.4 and 33.5).

White lesions

- White opacification of the peritoneum. These lesions contain an occasional retroperitoneal glandular structure, scanty stroma surrounded by fibrotic tissue and connective tissue (Figure 33.6).
- Yellow–brown peritoneal patches called 'café-au-lait spots', found in the cul-de-sac, broad ligament or over the bladder. Histologically, they are similar to findings of white opacification; the yellow–brown patches indicate the presence of haemosiderin.
- Circular peritoneal defects of the pelvic peritoneum, uterosacral ligaments or broad ligament. Serial section has demonstrated the presence of endometrial glands in approximately 50% of these structures (Figure 33.7).

Ovarian endometriosis

The ovary represents a unique site for implantation of endometrial fragments, as levels of gonadal steroids are several times higher than those in the general circulation or peritoneal cavity.

Superficial endometriosis

Superficial implants on the ovary resemble implants in other peritoneal sites. Comparable features are typical black, red or white lesions (Figure 33.8).

Subovarian adhesions

Subovarian adhesions may be confined to the peritoneum of the ovarian fossa, and are distinct from adhesions characteristic of previous salpingitis or peritonitis; this connective tissue often contains sparse endometrial glands.

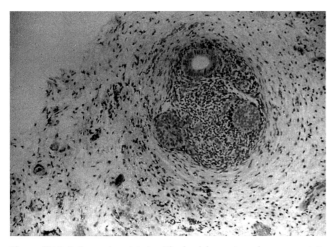

Figure 33.4 Active endometriosis with glandular or stromal components in a biopsy specimen from a red lesion.

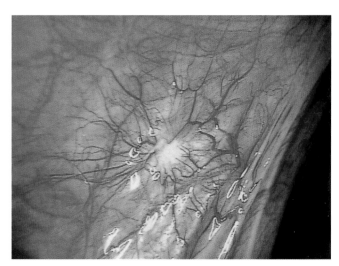

Figure 33.6 Scarring neovascularization of the left uterosacral ligament.
Source: Overton C, Davis C, McMillan L, Shaw RW 2007 An Atlas of Endometriosis, 3rd edn. Informa Healthcare, London.

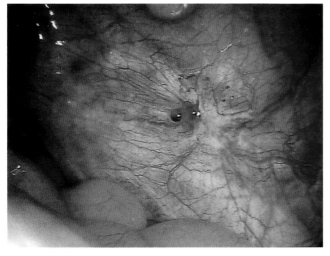

Figure 33.5 Vesicular implant of the ovarian fossa.
Source: Overton C, Davis C, McMillan L, Shaw RW 2007 An Atlas of Endometriosis, 3rd edn. Informa Healthcare, London.

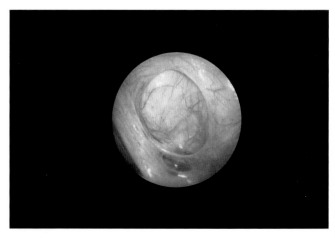

Figure 33.7 Peritoneal pouches near right uterosacral ligament associated with endometriosis.

Endometrioma

The pathogenesis of the typical ovarian endometriotic cyst or endometrioma has now been clarified. It is a process originating from a free superficial implant which is in contact with the ovarian surface and is sealed off by adhesions (Figure 33.9). A pseudocyst is thus formed by accumulation of menstrual debris from shedding and bleeding of the small implant, resulting in fluid collection. Progressive invagination of the ovarian cortex occurs and the associated inflammatory reactive tissue progressively thickens the inverted cortex. Outgrowths through the endometrial epithelium, with or without stroma, extend over the surface or become embedded in the fibroreactive tissue covering the wall. This pathogenesis explains the typical features of an endometrium such as frequent location of the cyst, adhesions on the anterior side of the ovary opposing the posterior side of the parametrium or, when on the posterior aspect of the ovary, adhesions to the ovarian fossa. The contents of the cyst are, to a large extent, fluid which represents the debris from cyclical menstruation (Figures 33.10 and 33.11).

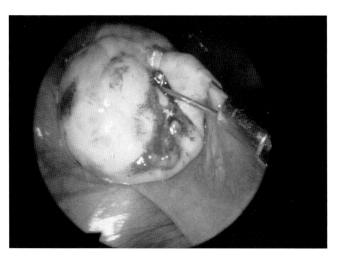

Figure 33.8 Superficial lesions on posterior aspect of ovary.

There is usually a well-defined separation between the normal adjacent ovarian stroma and the cyst wall, but whilst the epithelial lining of the cyst may initially resemble the endometrium, with increasing time and size, pressure atrophy compresses the epithelium to a flat cuboidal pattern.

Ovarian endometriomas rarely occur in the adolescent, but incidence increases with age. Laparoscopic features of a typical endometrioma include ovarian cysts not greater than 12 cm in diameter, adhesions to the pelvic side wall and/or the posterior broad ligament, powder burns, minute red or blue spots with adjacent puckering on the surface, and the presence of the characteristic tarry, thick, chocolate-coloured fluid content (see Figure 33.10).

Extrapelvic endometriosis

Extrapelvic endometriosis is defined as endometriotic-like implants elsewhere in the peritoneal cavity or other body cavities. Extrapelvic endometriosis has been reported in virtually every organ, system and tissue, but far less frequently than pelvic endometriosis. Overall, the incidence of extrapelvic disease represents less than 12% of reported cases of endometriosis, and it appears that the frequency of occurrence decreases with the distance from the pelvis.

Urinary tract endometriosis

Endometriotic implants can be found over the pelvic ureter and bladder, with unilateral involvement of the ureter and potential obstruction to drainage of the kidney more common than bilateral involvement. The highest incidence of involvement of endometriosis of the urinary tract involves the bladder, followed by the lower ureter and the upper ureter, with the kidney itself being the least common site.

Common symptoms associated with bladder endometriosis are cyclical haematuria, dysuria, urgency and frequency. Ureteral endometriosis eventually induces partial or complete obstruction of the ureter which will always require surgical management; either segmental resection

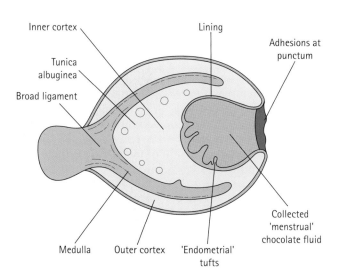

Figure 33.9 Diagrammatic representation of endometriosis formation, beginning on serosal surface and invaginating into cortex.

Inner cortex
Lining
Adhesions at punctum
Tunica albuginea
Broad ligament
Medulla
Outer cortex
'Endometrial' tufts
Collected 'menstrual' chocolate fluid

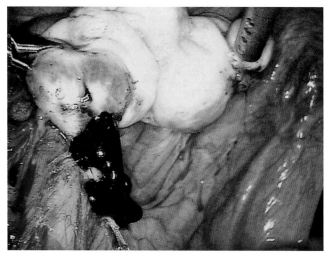

Figure 33.10 Left ovarian endometrioma.
Source: Overton C, Davis C, McMillan L, Shaw RW 2007 An Atlas of Endometriosis, 3rd edn. Informa Healthcare, London.

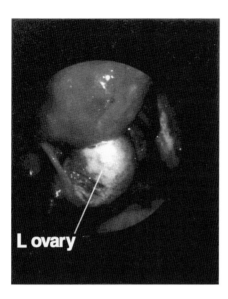

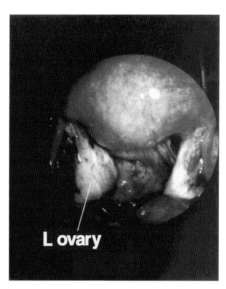

Figure 33.11 Enlarged left ovary containing a deep-seated endometrioma (left) and another ovary with superficial deposits on the ovarian capsule, in addition to others on the peritoneal surface in the pouch of Douglas (right).

and reanastomosis, or reimplantation of the ureter. For temporary resolution of hydronephrosis, the insertion of a ureteric stent may be necessary until definitive surgery is undertaken.

Gastrointestinal tract endometriosis

Extrapelvic endometriosis is most commonly found with involvement of the gastrointestinal tract. The most common site for involvement is the sigmoid colon, followed by the rectum, the ileocaecal area and the appendix. The transverse colon and small bowel are infrequently involved.

When there is involvement of the gastrointestinal tract, endometriosis is not the first diagnosis in the majority of patients. Symptoms are non-specific and include abdominal pain, distension, disturbed bowel function and rectal bleeding. The occurrence of cyclical rectal bleeding at the time of menstruation is the key pointer to endometriosis. Discomfort and pain at defaecation (dyschezia) is a hallmark of involvement of the rectosigmoid area. Besides rectal bleeding, there is often little to observe in the mucosal lining at endoscopy since involvement is deep within the smooth muscle wall. In advanced stages, a typical irregular stricture formation can be demonstrated on barium enema, and the use of magnetic resonance imaging (MRI) demonstrates the extent of involvement in the rectovaginal septum. Superficial implants on the serosal surface of the bowel are not uncommon and can be treated by laser destruction or medical suppressive therapy. However, involvement of the smooth muscle of the bowel wall and evidence of stricture formation will require surgical excision by open or laparosopic approaches, depending upon the localized site of involvement.

Involvement in surgical scars

Endometriosis in surgical scars has been reported in the umbilicus or other port sites following laparoscopy, in abdominal incisions following gynaecological surgery and caesarean section, and in the perineum within episiotomy scars following childbirth (Figure 33.12). Such patients

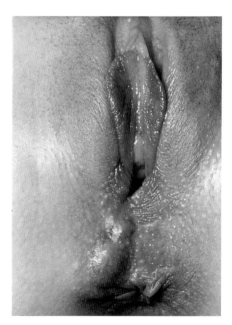

Figure 33.12 Endometriosis in episiotomy scar. The patient presented with cyclic, tender swelling in the perineum.

present with a painful, palpable swelling, usually more symptomatic at the time of menstruation. Occasionally, some women report discharge or cyclical bleeding occurring perimenstrually from the lesions. While medical treatment will control the symptoms with effective suppression of menstruation, surgical excision of the nodule will normally be necessary in the long term.

Vaginal endometriosis

Endometriosis of the vagina may occur following hysterectomy, most commonly in patients with a past history of endometriosis and in whom an ovary has been conserved. It has also been reported in women who have undergone bilateral oophorectomy, but who have been commenced on hormone replacement therapy soon after surgery.

However, endometriosis involving the posterior vaginal fornix is found in most instances as a continuance of deep infiltrating disease from the cul-de-sac and rectovaginal septum. Bimanual examination of these patients is essential as the small vaginal lesions do not represent the full extent of involvement, and assessment at or near the time of menstruation may be the most informative.

Pulmonary and thoracic endometriosis

Cyclical haemoptysis and cyclical haemo-/pneumothorax have been reported in patients in whom endometriosis has been found involving the lungs and thorax. Pulmonary thoracic endometriosis is uncommon. Hormone therapy is of value as an interim measure, but as with other deep-seated extrapelvic endometriosis, recurrence is inevitable on cessation of medical treatment, and surgical excision would be the eventual treatment of choice.

Non-invasive methods of diagnosis

It is an unsatisfactory situation that in order to diagnose endometriosis with certainty, an invasive, albeit minor, surgical procedure in the form of laparoscopy needs to be performed. This can readily be justified for making the initial diagnosis, but if the nature of the disease is of recurrence for the majority of patients throughout their reproductive life, this may involve repeat laparoscopies on many occasions if one is to be certain that the disease process has returned. Attempts have therefore been made to provide a non-invasive test which is highly sensitive and specific for endometriosis. Currently, such a test eludes investigators, although a number of adjunctive non-invasive tests may be contributory in the management of patients.

Serum markers: CA125

The most widely used serum marker for endometriosis has been the monoclonal antibody OC125, raised against a human ovarian cancer cell line containing the antigen designated 'CA125'. CA125 is a high-molecular-weight glycoprotein found in over 80% of cases of epithelial ovarian carcinoma. Investigation leads to the conclusion that CA125 is possessed by many tissues present in the pelvis, as well as more distant sites including the pericardium and the pleura. Moderate elevation of serum CA125 has been observed in endometriosis, particularly in patients with severe disease (Barbieri et al 1986, Pittaway and Douglas 1989). In these studies, serum levels in excess of 35 u/ml were used as a cut-off point, but sensitivity and specificity have proved inadequate for the use of CA125 as a screening test for endometriosis. However, in individuals in whom the disease has been confirmed and treated, an increase in serum levels above 35 u/ml may be a useful marker of disease recurrence.

Monocyte chemotactic protein-1

Monocyte chemotactic protein-1 (MCP-1) is a member of the small inducible gene family which plays a role in the recruitment of monocytes to sites of injury and inflammation. Levels of MCP-1 have been shown to be increased in the peritoneal fluid of women with endometriosis (Arici et al 1997) and in the serum of such patients compared with controls (Pizzo et al 2002), particularly in patients with early disease. Further investigation needs to be undertaken to evaluate the potential value of measuring MCP-1 in the non-invasive diagnosis of endometriosis.

Other potential markers

Since endometriosis is an inflammatory process, a number of possible inflammation markers are being investigated (e.g. RANTES, interleukins), and proteomic analysis may subsequently provide a serum non-invasive marker. However, to date, these remain research tools and have lacked enough specificity to be adopted clinically.

Imaging techniques

Ultrasound

Ultrasound examination of the pelvis may be useful in delineating the presence and aetiology of ovarian cystic structures. The characteristic pictures on ultrasound are different when there is a large proportion of blood, such as haemorrhagic corpus luteum cysts or endometriomas, which in a minority of cases may be echo free. However, the walls of an endometrioma are irregular as opposed to the smooth wall of the simple ovarian cyst. The most common pattern is for the chocolate cyst to contain low-level echoes or lumps of dense high-level echoes representing blood clots. The picture may sometimes be confused if there are several cysts in different phases of evolution (see Figure 33.13).

Transrectal ultrasound may be of value before surgery in patients in whom rectal/rectovaginal septum involvement is suspected. This method permits measurement of the distance between the lesion and anal verge, as well as assessment of extrinsic compression and lesions in the rectal submucosal layer (Abrão et al 2004). This method is limited to evaluating the rectosigmoid and retrocervical region. It is

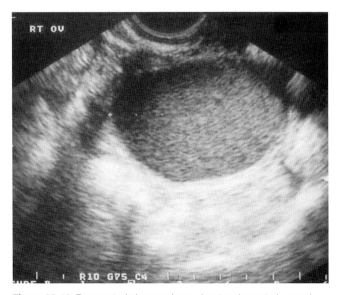

Figure 33.13 Transvaginal ultrasound scan showing the typical ground-glass appearance of endometrioma.
Source: Overton C, Davis C, McMillan L, Shaw RW 2007 An Atlas of Endometriosis, 3rd edn. Informa Healthcare, London.

advisable to undertake such examinations 1 h after a simple rectal enema.

Ultrasound may also be useful to identify hypoechogenic nodules in the bladder wall when bladder involvement is suspected, most often in the vesico-uterine fold.

Computed tomography scans and magnetic resonance imaging

Computed tomography (CT) provides better definition than ultrasound in many situations, but it has not established a role in the assessment of pelvic endometriosis. MRI, which is more expensive and has currently been used in a limited number of patients with ovarian endometriomas, has not proved to be diagnostic since, again, there has been a significant overlap between the MRI scanning appearances of endometriomas and cystic adenomas.

Ultrasound, CT and MRI scanning do not appear to be of any help in the diagnosis of peritoneal endometriosis, the deposits of which are too small to be detected by current technology, although various strategies utilizing enhancement agents are being investigated. However, MRI of the pelvis is an additional tool for the diagnosis of pelvic deep infiltrating endometriosis (Bazot and Darai 2005). MRI is unable to precisely define the intestinal layer affected by the lesion, and rectosigmoidoscopy or colonoscopy may be necessary. Even when cyclical rectal bleeding occurs at menstruation, no overt mucosal lesion may be visualized in such patients since the lesions are submucosal. However, external compression or stricture formation may be seen and may also be demonstrated by barium enema studies.

Cystoscopy

The bladder lesions of endometriosis are extrinsic, invading the muscular layer and then finally the mucosa. Hence in the earlier stages of development, cystoscopy may show no mucosal lesions, but is useful to exclude other causes of haematuria and dysuria (interstitial cystitis, vescular neoplasias) and in the follow-up of excised/treated lesions involving the bladder.

Classification Systems

Over the last three decades, various classification systems have been proposed which attempt to standardize criteria on which the severity of endometriosis could be based. Such a system, if available, would help in the critical assessment of performance of various forms of treatment, and hopefully provide meaningful prognostic indicators. No classification system so far devised has received uniform acceptance; all have suffered from various pitfalls which make it difficult to compare treatment results. The most recent attempt to provide a standardized classification for uniform use has been the Revised American Society for Reproductive Medicine Classification of Endometriosis (American Society for Reproductive Medicine 1996), shown in Figure 20.4. This serves to record the sites of deposits accurately and makes some effort to differentiate between superficial and deep-seated disease, as well as the presence or absence of adhesions. Whilst it offers a differential weighting to the score given to different types of endometriosis,

it must be appreciated that these scores are arbitrary. Classification of the extent of the disease as minimal, mild, moderate or severe is certainly helpful in explaining the problem to the patient, and perhaps in determining whether a medical, surgical or combined medical and surgical approach is the most logical treatment step, at least in relation to fertility outcome.

In addition to the Revised American Fertility score, it may be helpful to chart the exact sites of all implants and their sizes; a method used in the scheme of Additive Diameter of Implants (ADI score) described by Doberl et al (1984), gives a simple quantitative valuation of alteration of the volume of endometriotic disease, although not the activity. For each square millimetre of disease, a score of 1 is given. The ADI score helps to quantify the volume of disease and may be useful in evaluating the response to treatment options.

The major pitfall of any scoring system has been the lack of correlation between the score, or severity of the disease, and the degree of symptoms experienced. What is most important for patient management is an accurate record of the extent and site of each deposit.

These days, most laparoscopic camera systems have the facility to record pictures, and representative pictures before and following treatment are useful records to record the stage of disease and for referral on to other colleagues.

With increasing understanding of the morphological changes of deposits and their relationship to ovarian steroid hormones, and the precise colour and type of each lesion, more accurate selection of treatment options may become possible. Accurate records are vitally important to prevent needless repeat laparoscopies for patients referred to secondary and tertiary referral centres when laparoscopies have been performed previously.

Treatment: General Principles

Endometriosis is a particularly difficult disease to treat. Often, response to therapy relies on recognition of the disease in its earliest possible stages. With most treatment modalities, there is eventual recurrence in up to 60% of cases. Thus, there is no known permanent cure and eventually clinicians have to proceed to surgical oophorectomy in selected cases; this offers the most effective available treatment to date. In addition, in minimal and mild disease (according to the Revised American Fertility Society Classification), particularly in asymptomatic cases presenting with infertility alone, controversy exists as to whether treatment should be given, since no control studies have shown a significant increase in fertility rates following such ovarian-suppression therapies. However, placebo-controlled studies in such cases have shown that endometriosis tends to be a progressive disease for many patients (Thomas and Cooke 1987), and hence treatment may at least arrest progression or eradicate disease for significant intervals.

When endometriosis is associated with symptoms, particularly pain, there can be no doubt that treatment is of benefit, at least in relieving those symptoms for a period of time.

The treatment should be individualized, taking into account the patient's age, wish for fertility, severity of symptoms and extent of disease (see Box 33.3). An important aspect of therapy is a sympathetic approach, with adequate counselling and explanation to the patient that will also ensure her compliance whilst on therapy.

Medical Treatments

Ectopic endometrial tissue responds to endogenous and exogenous ovarian steroid hormones in a fashion similar to that of normal endometrium. Thus, a hormonal approach which suppresses oestrogen–progesterone levels and which prevents cyclical changes and menstruation should be beneficial in its treatment. In the hypo-oestrogenic state following the menopause, atrophy of the normal endometrium and atrophy and regression of endometriotic deposits occur. Administration of progestogens opposes the effect of oestrogen on endometrial tissue by inhibiting the replenishment of cytosolic oestrogen receptors. Progestogens also induce secretory activity in endometrial glands and decidual reaction in the endometrial stroma.

The success of various hormonal therapies depends to a large extent on the localization and type of the endometriotic lesions. Superficial peritoneal and ovarian serosal implants may respond better to hormone therapy than deep ovarian or peritoneal lesions or lesions within organs (e.g. bladder and rectum), where symptoms rapidly recur after medical therapy and most require ultimate surgical excision.

Box 33.3 Planning endometriosis treatment: factors to consider

- Patient's age
- Wish for future conception
- Contraception need
- Severity of pain and impact on life style
- Type, extent and location of deposits
- Involvement bowel, bladder or renal tract
- Availability of resources
- Surgical expertise of gynaecologist
- Patient's preference

The treatment of endometriosis has undergone a remarkable evolution in the last 40 years. In the past, testosterone, diethylstilboestrol and high-dose combination oestrogen–progestogen pill preparations were used with some success. However, therapies which induce decidualization (pseudopregnancy regimes) or suppress ovarian function (pseudomenopausal regimes) appear to offer the best chance of inducing clinical remission of endometriosis (Table 33.5).

Analgesics

Simple analgesics (e.g. paracetamol, aspirin) can be used but have often been tried and failed prior to referral to a specialist gynaecologist. They are helpful to a degree for the mild-to-moderate pain of endometriosis. A clinical feature in many women with the disease, as it progresses, is the failure of simple analgesics to work, and more potent agents (Tramadol, Dicolfenac etc.) may be required.

Prostaglandin synthetase inhibitors

An association with prostaglandin release and dysmenorrhoea has long been established. One might therefore expect that prostaglandin synthetase inhibitors (PGSIs) might have a beneficial effect in treating the symptoms of endometriosis. PGSIs are a heterogeneous group of non-steroidal inflammatory agents which act mainly by inhibiting the production of prostaglandins, although some (fenamates) also antagonize prostaglandins at the target level. These agents are perhaps beneficial in the early stages of initial or recurrent disease, but when symptoms become more severe, they are usually inadequate by themselves to control symptomatology.

There are surprisingly few data on the evaluation of the effectiveness of analgesics or PGSIs in treating endometriosis-associated pain.

Gestagen and antigestagen treatment

A state of pseudopregnancy can be induced effectively by the continuous administration of progestogenic preparations. The progestogens used are derivatives of progesterone (dydogesterone or medroxyprogesterone acetate) or

---

Table 33.5 Various hormonal states and their effects upon normal endometrium and ectopic endometrial deposits

Hormonal state	Effects on endometrium	Effects on endometriotic implants
Oestrogenic e.g. exogenous oestrogens	Proliferative activity and hyperplasia	Proliferative activity and hyperplasia
Hypo-oestrogenic e.g. postmenopause, pseudomenopause regimens, posto-ophorectomy, GnRH analogues, aromatase inhibitors	Atrophic changes	Atrophy, regression and resorption
Progestational e.g. pregnancy, exogenous progestogens, pseudopregnancy treatment, LNG-IUS	Secretory activity and decidualization	Secretory activity, necrobiosis and resorption
Androgenic e.g. danazol and its metabolites, gestrinone	Atrophy	Atrophy and regression

GnRH, gonadotrophin-releasing hormone; LNG-IUS, levonorgestrel intrauterine system.

19-nor-testosterone (norethisterone, norethisterone acetate, norgestrel, ethynodrel and lynoestrenol).

The use of progestogens induces a hyperprogestogenic/hypo-oestrogenic state. Treatments are available orally or injected as a depot formulation, and are administered for 6–9 months. The results achieved appear to be comparable to those achieved with combined oral oestrogen–progestogen preparations in the past. The side-effects most commonly seen with progestogen usage include breakthrough bleeding, weight gain, abdominal bloating, oedema, acne and mood changes.

The adverse effects of some progestogens on circulating levels of low- and high-density lipoproteins may determine the choice of progestogen if long-term administration is planned.

The oral progestogens used most commonly to attempt to induce amenorrhoea are:

- medroxyprogesterone acetate (30–40 mg/day);
- dydrogesterone (20–30 mg/day); and
- norethisterone (10–25 mg/day).

Long-acting depot preparations of progestogens (Depo-Provera 150 mg, 3 monthly) can be used. However, the author's personal experience has been that in order to avoid the initial problems (e.g. erratic/irregular vaginal bleeding), this may be best commenced once amenorrhoea has been achieved with other agents (e.g. GnRH analogues) for a few months. Depo-Provera has been shown to be as effective as the combined oral contraceptive pill (COCP) or danazol in reducing endometriosis-associated pain (Vercellini et al 1996).

Levonorgestrel intrauterine system

The levonorgestrel intrauterine system (LNG-IUS) was introduced as a long-acting contraceptive coil method, but its utility as a treatment option in gynaecology has been expanded into the treatment of menorrhagia due to dysfunction (unexplained) causes (see Chapter 31) and more recently in the treatment of endometriosis.

The steady low level of LNG achieved in the peripheral circulation appears to have a direct effect on the growth of endometriotic deposits through peritoneal fluid. The suppression of menstruation, or marked reduction of flow, may also be beneficial in reducing the amount of retrograde menstrual regurgitation, which may help to prevent new disease induction.

Effectiveness data come from two randomized controlled trials. In a study comparing LNG-IUS with expectant management, significantly lower pain scores were achieved in the LNG-IUS women at 12 months (Vercellini et al 2003). In the second trial, LNG-IUS was compared with GnRH analogue; after 6 months of treatment, both treatments were equally effective in reducing pain scores (Petta et al 2005).

Larger trials are required, along with long-term data, to enable clinicians to determine the types of disease and subjects with endometriosis in which the LNG-IUS may be of benefit.

Combined oral contraceptive pill

The COCP reduces pain associated with endometriosis, is well tolerated and can be continued long term for the control of symptoms in healthy women without risk factors. One of a number of 'high-dose' COCPs may be administered, and regimes often utilize COCPs prescribed continuously for three cycles to reduce the frequency of menstruation. If breakthrough bleeding occurs before planned interval bleeding, changing to another preparation with a higher progestogenic content is advocated.

Side-effects such as weight gain, headaches, breast enlargement and/or tenderness, nausea and depression may occur. The risk of thromboembolism is increased, and a personal previous history or family history of venous thromboembolism may involve screening for risk factors, including factor V Leiden polymorphism, prior to administration.

Gonadotrophin-releasing hormone agonists

Surgical castration is known to be an effective therapy for severe endometriosis. Thus, the possibility of inducing a reversible medical castration with the continued administration of GnRH agonists has been investigated as an alternative therapy in endometriosis. Modification of the native GnRH molecule with substitution, particularly in positions 6 and 10, with alternative amino acids produces agonistic analogues with a reduced susceptibility to degradation and hence a prolonged therapeutic half-life (Figure 33.14). Continued administration of these analogues induces pituitary gonadotrophin desensitization via downregulation of GnRH

	1	2	3	4	5	(6)	7	8	9	(10)	
	Pyro –	GLU –	HIS –	TRP –	SER –	TYR –	GLY –	LEU –	ARG –	PRO	GLY – NH$_2$	LHRH
Nonapeptides						D-SER (Bu^t)			PRO – NET		Buserelin
						D-LEU			PRO – NET		Leuprolide
Decapeptides						D-TRP					Tryptorelin
						(D-NAL)$_2$					Nafarelin
						D-SER (Bu^t)			AZA – GLY		Goserelin

Figure 33.14 Amino acid sequence of native luteinizing-hormone-releasing hormone (LHRH) and some of the agonistic gonadotrophin-releasing hormone (GnRH) analogues used in the treatment of endometriosis.

receptors and an eventual state of hypogonadotrophic hypogonadism. Reduced gonadotrophic stimulation of the ovaries leads to cessation of follicular growth and reduction in ovarian steroidogenesis, with circulating 17β-oestradiol levels falling to those observed in the postmenopausal range (typically less than 100 pmol/l).

A large amount of data has now appeared in the literature from both controlled and randomized comparative trials of GnRH analogues and danazol (for review, see Shaw 1995). These trials have all confirmed the value of GnRH analogues for the treatment of endometriosis. Rapid and effective symptomatic relief is achieved with these agents, as well as a marked degree of resolution of the endometrial deposits in the majority of patients. However, for both symptomatic relief and the resolution of endometrial deposits, there is essentially no significant difference in comparative trials between GnRH analogues and danazol. However, patient acceptability and the profile of side-effects may be slightly in favour of GnRH analogues (Matta and Shaw 1987, Henzl et al 1988).

Side-effects of GnRH analogues include those which are predictable from induction of a pseudomenopause. These include hot flushes (in virtually all patients), headaches and, less commonly, atrophic vaginitis, vaginal dryness and reduced libido.

Dosage varies depending on the analogue used and its formulation, but regimens include: nafarelin 200 µg twice daily intranasally, buserelin 300–400 µg three times daily intranasally, goserelin 3.6 mg subcutaneous depot monthly, triptorelin 3.0 mg monthly, and leuprorelin 3.75 mg intramuscular depot monthly.

Metabolic side-effects include (as in the menopause) increased excretion of urinary calcium. Over a 6-month period, there is a 3–5% loss in the vertebral trabecular bone density of the lumbar spine as assessed by dual energy X-ray absorptiometry. In most patients, the bone density changes induced following a 6-month course of therapy with GnRH analogues are reversed 6 months after return of ovarian function (Matta et al 1987, Henzl et al 1988). However, the implications of such changes in calcium homeostasis with prolonged and repetitive treatment with GnRH analogues are being further investigated. This has led to the development of protective 'add-back' regimens which reduce the symptomatic effects of the GnRH-agonist-induced hypo-oestrogenism, particularly the frequency of hot flushes and bone loss, but do not result in reduced therapeutic effectiveness on symptom relief or implant resolution. A recent meta-analysis of 15 studies assessing GnRH agonists with add-back with oestrogen and progestogen showed protection to the lumbar spine for up to 12 months following cessation of treatment (Sagsveen et al 2003).

A new series of GnRH antagonists are currently being developed, and these peptides contain multiple and complex substitutions of the GnRH molecule. There is little evidence on long-term use of GnRH antagonists in the treatment of endometriosis to date, and their structural complexity and costs may make substitution of GnRH antagonists for the current widely used GnRH agonists unlikely. However, orally administered non-peptide GnRH receptor antagonists are being developed and may present alternative therapies in the future.

Danazol

Danazol is an isoxazol derivate of 17-α-ethinyl testosterone. Due to its base structure, it has both androgenic and anabolic properties. Danazol was one of the first approved medical treatments for endometriosis. Its mechanism of action is complex and includes suppression of the hypothalamic–pituitary axis with interference in pulsatile gonadotrophin secretion and inhibition of the midcycle gonadotrophin surge, but with no change in basal gonadotrophin levels. It achieves direct inhibition of ovarian steroidogenesis by inhibiting several enzymatic processes and by competitive blockage of androgen, oestrogen and progesterone receptors in the endometrium. An increase in free testosterone occurs because of a reduction in sex-hormone-binding globulin, and this explains many of danazol's androgenic side-effects. The increase in free testosterone may also contribute to its direct action in inducing endometrial atrophy. The degree of endocrine changes described above is dose related.

In the treatment of endometriosis, danazol is administered in a dose range of between 400 and 800 mg daily, titrated to endeavour to induce amenorrhoea. In the case of mild-to-moderate endometriosis, there is highly effective symptomatic improvement in over 85% of cases.

Objective resolution of endometriotic lesions has been observed at post-treatment laparoscopic evaluation in between 70% and 95% of patients, depending upon the stage of the disease (Barbieri et al 1982). However, recurrence rates of up to 40% have been reported in the 36 months after completion of a course of danazol.

Danazol therapy should be commenced in the early follicular phase of the menstrual cycle. It is recommended that the patient should use additional barrier methods of contraception in order to avoid the drug being administered during early pregnancy, where continued use could lead to androgenization of a developing female fetus. The drug dosage should be related to the patient's clinical staging, response and severity of side-effects, starting with a dose of 400 mg/day in mild disease and 600–800 mg/day in moderate-to-severe cases for a recommended treatment course of at least 6 months.

Danazol is associated with side-effects related to its androgenic and anabolic properties. These include weight gain, acne, oily skin, fluid retention, muscle cramps, hot flushes, depression and mood changes. Less commonly, hirsutism, skin rash and voice deepening are noted. It is recommended that patients should discontinue treatment immediately if they develop hirsutism, a skin rash or deepening of the voice.

Metabolic side-effects include elevation of low-density lipoproteins, and reduction of high-density lipoproteins and cholesterol concentrations. In addition, changes in liver enzymes are noted, and danazol is contraindicated in patients with liver disease.

Gestrinone

Gestrinone is a synthetic trienic 19-norsteroid (13-ethyl-17-α-ethinyl-17-hydroxy-gona-4,o,ll-triene-3-one). It has been shown in clinical trials to be another effective clinical treatment for endometriosis (Thomas and Cooke 1987). The drug exhibits mild androgenic and antigonadotrophic properties. The combined effect is to induce progressive endometrial atrophy. Gestrinone has a high binding affinity for progesterone receptors; it also binds to androgen receptors but not to oestrogen receptors. The combined endocrine effect of gestrinone therapy is similar to that of danazol in that the midcycle gonadotrophin surge is abolished, although basal gonadotrophin levels are not significantly reduced, together with inhibition of ovarian steroidogenesis and reduction of sex-hormone-binding globulin levels. Gestrinone has a prolonged half-life and may be administered orally at a dosage of 2.5–5.0 mg twice weekly for a period of 6–9 months in patients with endometriosis. This dosage schedule effectively induces endometrial atrophy, with 85–90% of patients becoming amenorrhoeic within 2 months.

Gestrinone compares favourably with danazol in terms of both symptomatic relief and resolution of endometrial deposits (Mettler and Semm 1984).

The side-effects, occurring in up to 50% of patients, include weight gain, breakthrough bleeding, reduced breast size, muscle cramps and, uncommonly, hirsutism, voice change and hoarseness.

Aromatase inhibitors

Aromatase P-450 is the key enzyme for oestrogen biosynthesis, and catalyses the conversion of andostenedione and testosterone to oestrone and oestradiol. Aromatase activity is expressed inappropriately in endometriotic deposits and their eutopic endometrium, but not in the endometrium of normal women. Prostaglandin E_2 is a potent inducer of aromatase activity in endometriotic cells, and hence there is a link between repeated proliferation and inflammation within endometriosis deposits.

Limited data have been published on the use of aromatase inhibitors in endometriosis. A meta-analysis of 40 women from seven published case studies utilizing aromatase inhibitors in combination with progestogens, COCP or GnRH-A reported reduced mean pain scores and lesion size, and improved quality-of-life scores (Nawathe et al 2008). More data are needed to establish the efficacy and safety of aromatase inhibitors, and which combination of drugs produces the best results.

Other drug therapies tried or in development

A number of potential new drug therapies to treat endometriosis have been postulated, investigated in animals or are under development. These include progesterone antagonists, selective oestrogen receptor modulators and statins. However, scant, often only research data exist, and further data or modification of regimens to reduce side-effects would be necessary before they become clinically viable therapies.

In addition, research is underway to evaluate selective progesterone receptor modulators, selective oestrogen receptor β-agonists, angiogenesis inhibitors and immunomodulators/inflammatory modulators. It will be some considerable time before it is known if any of these approaches prove to be effective and tolerable as therapeutic options in the treatment of endometriosis.

Surgical Treatment

Many forms of severe endometriosis do not respond to drug treatment, including deep-seated invasive disease, endometriomas, extrapelvic endometriosis of the bladder and bowel, or within surgical scars. In these instances, surgery may be required to relieve the symptomatology and effect a longer term cure.

Conservative surgery

Endometriotic deposits may be excised, destroyed by electrocautery, or evaporated utilizing carbon dioxide or KTP/YAG lasers or argon beam.

With the increasingly widespread availability of laparoscopic expertise, improved instrumentation and experience of laser technology, minimal access surgery is becoming a more popular treatment option. There have been few appropriately conducted randomized trials, but one small double-blind placebo-controlled study measured pain relief following laser ablation and/or laparoscopic uterosacral nerve ablation or placebo (no treatment). At 6 month follow-up, 53% of those treated with laser compared with only 23% from the placebo diagnostic laparoscopy group had improvements in symptoms (Sutton et al 1994). It was of interest that in minimal disease, only 38% of women had a reduction in pain. Therefore, this approach appeared to be more effective in reducing pain symptoms in women with more severe disease.

Sutton et al (1997) published the results of a longer term follow-up of this cohort of patients. Sadly, 1 year after the initial treatment, 44% had recurrence of pain requiring additional treatment. The reasons for failure of the surgical approach may result from missing lesions, incomplete destruction and, of course, recurrence of the disease.

An alternative approach to ablation of lesions is excision. Advocates of this approach argue that excision is the only way to ensure complete treatment because it may be difficult to determine the depth of the implant. Local excision can achieve good results in terms of pain reduction — 67% improvement up to 12 months (Wykes et al 2006) — but another study reported a high reoperation rate with longer term follow-up of 46% at 5 years and 55% at 7 years (Shakiba et al 2008) (see Figures 33.15 and 33.16).

Laparoscopic uterosacral nerve ablation

The uterosacral ligaments are a commonly affected site in patients suffering with endometriosis, and infiltration of endometriotic deposits results in invasion, inflammation and fibrosis of the anterior extension of the inferior hypogastric nerve, the uterovaginal plexus (or Lee-Frankenhauser plexus). Ablation of the uterosacral ligaments, forming two small craters, can be performed at the time of laparoscopy. The risks of the procedure are haemorrhage from a vessel within the uterosacral ligaments and damage to the ureter, which needs to be identified before laser treatment commences.

In a double-blind randomized controlled study, the addition of laparoscopic uterosacral nerve ablation to laparoscopic laser vaporization of endometriotic lesions alone was

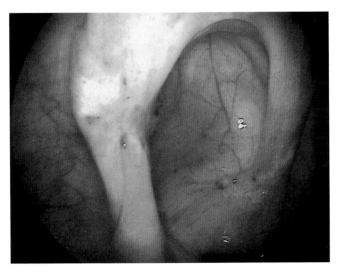

Figure 33.15 Left uterosacral nodule.
Source: Overton C, Davis C, McMillan L, Shaw RW 2007 An Atlas of Endometriosis, 3rd edn. Informa Healthcare, London.

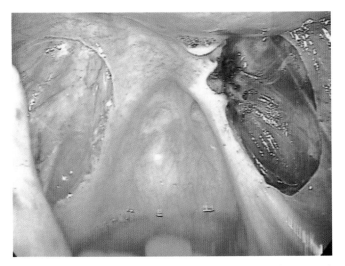

Figure 33.16 Excision of the uterosacral ligaments and bilateral uterosacral nodules.
Source: Overton C, Davis C, McMillan L, Shaw RW 2007 An Atlas of Endometriosis, 3rd edn. Informa Healthcare, London.

not found to improve pelvic pain responses (Sutton et al 2001). This procedure should not be performed if the uterosacral ligaments have a normal appearance, whilst excision of deep infiltrating lesions on the uterosacral ligament seems to be beneficial.

Radical surgery: hysterectomy and oophorectomy

Radical surgery is reserved for those patients with severe symptoms, where there is no desired fertility potential and especially when other forms of treatment have failed. Total abdominal hysterectomy and bilateral salpingo-oophorectomy are performed along with resection of any endometriotic lesions as completely as possible. As the majority of these patients are relatively young, hormone replacement

therapy should be commenced but kept to a minimum to control oestrogen-deficiency symptoms, as a small percentage of those patients may develop a recurrence of endometriosis when on such oestrogen replacement.

Combined oestrogen–testosterone implants may minimize the risk of recurrence as well as offering the beneficial effects of the androgens in maintaining libido in young women who are sexually active. However, no data exist from randomized trials to define if one particular hormone replacement therapy regimen is superior to others.

Surgical treatment of endometriomas

The definitive treatment of the typical endometrioma is the surgical release of the adhesions and fibrosis at the site of invagination, and the eversion of the invaginated cortex. Simply puncturing and draining the endometrioma, whether this is followed by GnRH agonist therapy or not, has no beneficial effects in the long term (Vercellini et al 1992). Medical treatment is highly effective for the destruction of active implants located on the surface of the normal ovarian cortex. However, when a definite endometrioma is present, surgery is necessary. This can be performed laparoscopically for smaller endometriomas using laser destruction. With endometriomas larger than 3 cm in diameter, treatment may be facilitated to enable laparoscopic surgery if, following initial drainage, patients are pretreated for 3 months with a GnRH agonist prior to laser ablation (Donnez et al 1990).

On the other hand, fibrotic larger endometriomas have a thickened capsule which is more likely to be removed effectively by excisional techniques.

In many instances, however, because of other associated extensive adhesions and fixity of ovaries on to other structures, a laparotomy rather than a laparoscopy may be necessary.

Whatever the surgical approach, be it minimal access or open laparotomy, if dense and extensive adhesions are present at the time of original surgery, it is likely that such patients will have recurrence of adhesions with attendant problems of fixity of the ovary following such approaches (Shaw et al 2001).

Recurrent Endometriosis

The natural course of the disease remains a mystery. It has been suggested that the disease is only progressive in one-third of cases, whilst in the remainder, the endometriosis remains in a steady state or eventually even resolves spontaneously.

After medical suppression of the disease or surgical destruction of all visible deposits, residual viable (microscopic) implants can regenerate once ovarian function is re-established. In other cases, new disease develops at new sites, perhaps indicating the potential for an entire 'field change' within the pelvic peritoneum. The degree of differentiation of a lesion may also correlate with persistence of disease following medical therapy. Two-thirds of lesions that were most highly differentiated disappeared following 6 months of medical therapy, whilst three-quarters of poorly differentiated lesions persisted (Schweppe 1984).

However, as far as therapeutic options are concerned, there is no essential difference between primary and recurrent endometriosis. The choice of treatment in a patient with recurrent disease is not determined by the manifestations of the disease as such, but more by the extent of distortion of the pelvic anatomy and the severity of symptomatology. In many instances, repeat medical therapy or repeat conservative surgery is appropriate, but when there are severe symptoms and repeated recurrence, a radical surgical approach may be the patient's best option to achieve longstanding relief of pain and other symptoms.

KEY POINTS

1. Endometriosis is one of the most common gynaecological conditions and is present in 10–25% of women presenting with gynaecological symptoms.

2. Endometriosis is most commonly found inside the pelvis, but rarely it has been described in sites such as the urinary tract, bowel, lungs and umbilicus.

3. The growth of endometriotic tissue depends on oestrogen; thus, endometriosis occurs almost exclusively in the reproductive years, with a peak incidence between 30 and 45 years of age.

4. The theories of aetiology of endometriosis include Sampson's theory of retrograde menstruation and implantation, and Meyer's theory of transformation of coelomic epithelium. Genetic predisposition and immunological factors are also thought to be important in rendering individuals susceptible to the disease.

5. The peritoneal fluid in women with endometriosis contains higher concentrations of more active macrophages and prostaglandins than in normal women. These factors may be important in explaining the link between infertility, pain and endometriosis.

6. Endometriosis that is associated with tubal and ovarian damage and the formation of adhesions can compromise fertility. The link between mild endometriosis and infertility is more controversial.

7. Suppression of ovarian function is not effective at improving fertility in women with endometriosis.

8. The best means to diagnose endometriosis is by direct visualization at laparoscopy or laparotomy, with histological confirmation where uncertainty persists.

9. Non-invasive tests are being developed, and additional investigations are of value in diagnosing extrapelvic disease.

10. The typical blue–black peritoneal endometriotic lesion is described as a 'powder burn'. Recently, non-pigmented lesions and red lesions have been described together with many other visual appearances now recognized as hallmarks of the disease process.

11. The medical treatment of endometriosis involves suppressing oestrogen–progesterone levels to prevent cyclical changes and menstruation. Treatments include progestogens, gestrinone, danazol and gonadotrophin-releasing hormone analogues.

12. Induction of complete amenorrhoea is the key to successful control of pain symptoms.

13. The surgical treatment of endometriosis is either minimally invasive (e.g. laparoscopic diathermy or laser vaporization) or radical (e.g. total abdominal hysterectomy or bilateral salpingo-oophorectomy). Extrapelvic and deep-seated endometriosis invariably requires a surgical approach.

14. The performance of laparoscopic uterosacral nerve ablation where the uterosacral ligaments appear normal provides no added benefit in reducing pain levels.

15. The natural course of the disease is not clearly defined. However, in perhaps one-third of cases, the disease is progressive, whilst in the remainder, the disease remains in a steady stage or may even resolve spontaneously. For many patients, the disease is one of recurrent episodes of treatment cycles and recurrence throughout reproductive life.

16. There seems to be no justification to treat minimal-to-mild endometriosis where infertility and not pain is the predominant symptom. Such cases are best assessed for infertility treatment options based on the woman's age, duration of infertility and the presence/absence of other infertility factors.

17. Classification systems are subjective and correlate poorly with the severity of pain symptoms. They may help to determine the prognosis of infertility outcomes.

References

Abrão MS, Neme RM, Averbach M, Petta CA, Aldrighi JM 2004 Rectal endoscopic ultrasound with a radial probe in the assessment of rectovaginal endometriosis. Journal of the American Association of Gynecologic Laparoscopists 11: 50–54.

Adamson GD, Pasta DJ 1994 Surgical treatment of endometriosis-associated infertility: meta-analysis compared with survival analysis. American Journal of Obstetrics and Gynecology 171: 1488–1504.

American Society for Reproductive Medicine 1996 Revised ASRM classification of endometriosis. Fertility and Sterility 67: 817–821.

Arici A, Oral E, Attar E, Tazuke SI, Olive DL 1997 Monocyte chemotactic protein-1 concentration in peritoneal fluid in patients with endometriosis and its modulation in human mesothelial cells. Fertility and Sterility 67: 1065–1072.

Barbieri RL, Evans S, Kistner RW 1982 Danazol in the treatment of endometriosis: analysis of 100 cases with a 4-year follow-up. Fertility and Sterility 37: 737–749.

Barbieri RL, Niloff JM, Bast RC, Shaetzl E, Kistner RW, Knapp RC 1986 Elevated serum concentrations of CA-125 in patients with advanced endometriosis. Fertility and Sterility 45: 630–634.

Bazot M, Darai E 2005 Sonography and MR imaging for the assessment of deep pelvic endometriosis. Journal of Minimally Invasive Gynecology 12: 178–185.

Dmowski WP, Steele RW, Baker GF 1981 Deficient cellular immunity in endometriosis. American Journal of Obstetrics and Gynecology 141: 377–383.

Doberl A, Bergquist A, Jeppson S, Koskimies AI, Ronnberg L, Segerbrand E 1984 Repression of endometriosis following shorter treatment with or lower dose of danazol. Acta Obstetricia et Gynecologica Scandinavica 123 (Suppl): 51–58.

Donnez J, Nisolle M, Clerckx F et al 1990 The ovarian endometrial cyst: combined (hormonal and surgical) therapy. In: Brosens I, Jacobs HS, Runnebaum B (eds) LHRH Analogues in Gynaecology. Parthenon, Carnforth, pp 165–175.

Donnez J, Nisolle M 1991 Appearance of peritoneal endometriosis. Third Laser Surgery Symposium, March 1991, Brussels.

Drake TS, O'Brien WF, Ramwell P, Metz SA 1981 Peritoneal fluid thromboxane B2 and 6-keto-prostaglandin F1 alpha in endometriosis. American Journal of Obstetrics and Gynecology 140: 401–404.

Eskanazi B, Warner ML 1997 Epidemiology of endometriosis. Obstetrics and Gynecological Clinics of North America 24: 235–258.

Giudice LC, Kao LC 2004 Endometriosis. The Lancet 364: 1789–1799.

Halme J, Beecher S, Wing R 1984 Accentuated cyclic activation of peritoneal macrophages in patients with endometriosis. American Journal of Obstetrics and Gynecology 148: 85–90.

Halme J, Becher S, Haskill S 1986 Altered life span and function of peritoneal macrophages: a new hypothesis for pathogenesis of endometriosis. Society of Gynecologic Investigation, Toronto, Abstract 48.

Henzl MR, Corson SL, Moghissi K, Buttram VC, Bergquist C, Jacobson C 1988 Administration of nasal nafarelin as compared with oral danazol for endometriosis. New England Journal of Medicine 318: 485–489.

Houston DE 1984 Evidence for the risk of pelvic endometriosis by age, race and socioeconomic status. Epidemiology Reviews 6: 167–191.

Hughes EG, Fedorkow DM, Collins JA 1993 A quantitative overview of controlled trials in endometriosis-associated infertility. Fertility and Sterility 59: 963–970.

Ingamells S, Thomas EJ 1995 Infertility and endometriosis. In: Shaw RW (ed) Endometriosis — Current Understanding and Management. Blackwell Science, Oxford, pp 147–167.

Kennedy SH, Soper NDW, Mojiminiyi OA, Shepstone BJ, Barlow DH 1988 Immunoscintigraphy of ovarian endometriosis. A preliminary study. BJOG: an International Journal of Obstetrics and Gynaecology 95: 693–697.

Kistner RW 1977 In: Sciarra J (ed) Gynaecology and Obstetrics, Vol. 1. Harper and Row, London.

Koninckx PR, de Moor P, Brosens IA 1980 Diagnosis of the luteinizing unruptured follicle syndrome by steroid hormone assays in peritoneal fluid. BJOG: an International Journal of Obstetrics and Gynaecology 87: 929–934.

Landazabal A, Diaz I, Valbuena D 1999 Endometriosis and in vitro fertilisation: a meta-analysis. Human Reproduction 14: 181–182.

MacLaverty CM, Shaw RW 1995 Pelvic pain and endometriosis. In: Shaw RW (ed) Endometriosis — Current Understanding and Management. Blackwell Science, Oxford, pp 112–146.

Mahmood TA, Templeton A 1990 The impact of treatment on the natural history of endometriosis. Human Reproduction 5: 965–970.

Marcoux S, Maheux R, Berube S 1997 The Canadian collaborative group on endometriosis laparoscopic surgery in infertile women with minimal–mild endometriosis. New England Journal of Medicine 337: 217–222.

Matta WH, Shaw RW 1987 A comparative study between buserelin and danazol in the treatment of endometriosis. British Journal of Clinical Practice 41 (Suppl 48): 69–73.

Matta WM, Shaw RW, Hesp R, Katz D 1987 Hypogonadism induced by luteinizing hormone releasing hormone agonist analogues: effects on bone density in premenopausal women. BMJ (Clinical Research Ed.) 294: 1523–1524.

Meldrum DR, Shamonki IM, Clarke KE 1977 Prostaglandin content of ascitic fluid in endometriosis: a preliminary report. 25th Annual Meeting of the Pacific Coast Fertility Society, Palm Springs, CA.

Mettler L, Semm K 1984 Three-step therapy of genital endometriosis in cases of human infertility with lynestrenol, danazol or gestrinone administration. In: Raynaud JP, Ojasoo T, Martini L (eds) Medical Management of Endometriosis. Raven Press, New York, pp 233–247.

Meyer R 1919 Uber den Staude der Frage der Adenomyosites Adenomyoma in allegemeinen und Adenomyometitis Sarcomastosa. Zentralblatt für Gynäkologie 36: 745–759.

Missmer SA, Mohllagee AP 2008 The etiology of endometriosis: environment. In: Rombauts L, Tsaltas J, Maher P, Healy D (eds) Blackwell Publishing, Sydney, Australia, pp 49–67.

Miyazawa K 1976 Incidence of endometriosis among Japanese women. Obstetrics and Gynecology 48: 407–409.

Nawathe A, Patwardhan S, Yates D, Harrison GR, Khan KS 2008 Systematic review of the effects of aromatase inhibitors on pain associated with endometriosis. BJOG: an International Journal of Obstetrics and Gynaecology 115: 818–822.

Overton C, Kennedy S 1993 Endometriosis and pelvic pain. Contemporary Reviews of Obstetrics and Gynaecology 5: 94–97.

Overton C, Davis C, McMillan L, Shaw RW 2007 An Atlas of Endometriosis, 3rd edn. Informa Healthcare, London.

Parazzinni F 1999 Ablation of lesions or no treatment in minimal–mild endometriosis in infertile women: a randomized trial. Human Reproduction 14: 1332–1334.

Petta CA, Ferriani RA, Abra MS et al 2005 Randomized clinical trial for a levonorgestrel-releasing intrauterine system and a depot GnRH analogue for the treatment of chronic pelvic pain in women with endometriosis. Human Reproduction 20: 1993–1998.

Pittaway DE, Douglas JW 1989 Serum CA-125 in women with endometriosis and chronic pelvic pain. Fertility and Sterility 51: 68–70.

Pizzo A, Salmeri FM, Ardita FV, Sofo V, Tripepi M, Marsico S 2002 Behaviour of cytokine levels in serum and peritoneal fluid of women with endometriosis. Gynecologic and Obstetric Investigation 54: 82–87.

Rock JA, Dubin NM, Ghodgaonkar RB, Bergquist CA, Erozan YS, Kimball AW Jr 1982 Cul-de-sac fluid in women with endometriosis: fluid volume and prostanoid concentration during the proliferative phase of the cycle — days 8–12. Fertility and Sterility 37: 747–752.

Sagsveen M, Farmer JE, Prentice A, Breeze A 2003 Gonadotrophin-releasing hormone analogues for endometriosis: bone mineral density. Cochrane Database of Systematic Reviews 4: CD001019.

Sampson JA 1927 Perforating haemorrhagic (chocolate) cysts of the ovary, their importance and especially their relation to pelvic adenomas of endometrial type. Archives of Surgery 3: 245–323.

Schifrin BS, Erez S, Moore JG 1973 Teenage endometriosis. American Journal of Obstetrics and Gynecology 116: 973–980.

Schweppe KW 1984 Morphologie und Klinik der Endometriose. F.K. Schattauer Verlag, Stuttgart, pp 198–207.

Shakiba K, Bena JF, McGill KM, Minger J, Falcone T 2008 Surgical treatment of endometriosis: a 7 year follow-up on the requirement for further surgery. Obstetrics and Gynecology 111: 1285–1292.

Shaw RW 1995 Evaluation of treatment with gonadotrophin-releasing hormone analogues. In: Shaw RW (ed) Endometriosis — Current Understanding and Management. Blackwell Science, Oxford, pp 206–234.

Shaw RW, Garry R, McMillan L et al 2001 A prospective randomized open study comparing goserelin (Zoladex) plus surgery and surgery alone in the management of ovarian endometriomas. Gynaecological Endoscopy 10: 151–157.

Simpson JL, Elias S, Malinak LR, Buttram VC Jr 1980 Heritable aspects of endometriosis. I. Genetic studies. American Journal of Obstetrics and Gynecology 137: 327–331.

Simpson JL, Malinak LR, Elias S, Carson SA, Redvary RA 1984 HLA associations in endometriosis. American Journal of Obstetrics and Gynecology 148: 395–397.

Strathy JH, Molgaard GA, Coulam CB, Molton LJ III 1982 Endometriosis and infertility: a laparoscopic study of endometriosis among fertile and infertile women. Fertility and Sterility 38: 667–672.

Sutton CJ, Ewen SP, Whitelaw N, Haines P 1994 Prospective, randomized double blind, controlled trial of laser laparoscopy in the treatment of pelvic pain associated with minimal mild, and moderate endometriosis. Fertility and Sterility 62: 696–700.

Sutton CJ, Polley AS, Ewen SP, Haines P 1997 Follow-up report on a randomized controlled trial of laser laparoscopy in the treatment of pelvic pain associated with minimal to moderate endometriosis. Fertility and Sterility 68: 1070–1074.

Sutton C, Pooley AS, Jones KD et al 2001 A prospective, randomized, double-blind controlled trial of laparoscopic uterine nerve ablation in the treatment of pelvic pain associated with endometriosis. Gynecological Endoscopy 10: 217–222.

Templeton A, Morris DJK, Parslow W 1996 Factors that affect the outcome of in vitro fertilisation treatment. The Lancet 348: 1402–1406.

Thomas EJ, Cooke ID 1987 Impact of gestrinone on the course of asymptomatic endometriosis. BMJ (Clinical Research Ed.) 294: 272–274.

Tyson JEA 1974 Surgical consideration in gynecologic endocrine disorders. Surgical Clinics of North America 54: 425–442.

Vercellini P, Vendola N, Bocciolone L, Colombo A, Rognoni MT, Bolis G 1992 Laparoscopic aspiration of ovarian endometriomas: effect with postoperative gonadotropin releasing hormone agonist treatment. Journal of Reproductive Medicine 37: 577–580.

Vercellini P, De Giorgi O, Oldani S, Cortesi I, Panazza S, Crosignani PG 1996 Depot medroxyprogesterone acetate versus an oral contraceptive combined with low-dose danazol for long-term treatment of pelvic pain associated with endometriosis. American Journal of Obstetrics and Gynecology 175: 396–401.

Vercellini P, Frontino G, De Giorgi O et al 2003 Comparison of levonorgestrel-releasing intrauterine device versus expectant management after conservative surgery for symptomatic endometriosis: a pilot study. Fertility and Sterility 80: 305–309.

Vernon M, Beard J, Graves K, Wilson EA 1986 Classification of endometriotic implants in morphologic appearance and capacity to synthesize prostaglandin F. Fertility and Sterility 46: 801–805.

Wykes CB, Clark TJ, Chakravati S, Mann CH, Gupta JK 2006 Efficacy of laparoscopic excision of visually diagnosed peritoneal endometriosis in the treatment of chronic pelvic pain. European Journal of Obstetrics, Gynecology and Reproductive Biology 125: 129–133.

Epidemiology of gynaecological cancer

Peter Sasieni, Alejandra Castañón and Jack Cuzick

Chapter Contents

INTRODUCTION	509		OVARIAN CANCER	516
GENERAL OVERVIEW	509		CANCERS OF THE VULVA AND THE VAGINA	517
CERVICAL CANCER	509		KEY POINTS	519
ENDOMETRIAL CANCER	514			

Introduction

Epidemiology is the study of disease in populations as opposed to individuals. Its scope ranges from description of the incidence and mortality from disease at a national level, through analytical studies of disease causation, to interventions leading to disease prevention and mortality reduction. Epidemiology has made significant contributions to our understanding of the causes and control of gynaecological cancers. Human papilloma virus (HPV) is the primary cause of cervical cancer, but requires cofactors to cause malignancy. Obesity, nulliparity and use of unopposed oestrogens are major risk factors for endometrial cancer. Oral contraceptives are highly protective for ovarian cancer. Screening programmes have resulted in a substantial reduction in cervical cancer. Introduction of vaccination against HPV 16 and 18 in conjunction with established screening programmes is expected to reduce the incidence of cervical cancer by an additional 60% (allowing for incomplete coverage), and to have a substantial impact on vaginal (80%) and vulval (40%) cancers.

General Overview

Globally, breast cancer and cancer of the cervix are the two most common female malignancies. However, both ovarian and endometrial cancer rank in the top 10 female malignancies. Cervical cancer is most common in developing countries, while cancer of the uterine corpus and ovarian cancer have higher incidence in industrialized countries. Indeed, in the presence of cervical screening, these cancers are more common than cervical cancer in most Western countries. Table 34.1 provides an overview of age-standardized incidence and mortality rates of these three gynaecological cancers around the world. Other gynaecological cancers (i.e. cancers of the vulva and vagina) are relatively rare in all parts of the world. The age-standardized rates are less than one per 100,000 in most countries (Curado et al 2007).

The variation in the rates of gynaecological cancers around the world is enormous (Table 34.1). Cervical cancer rates in East Africa are 12 times greater than in West Asia (the Middle East). The rates for cancer of the uterine corpus are nearly 10 times higher in North America than in West Africa, and ovarian cancer is two and a half times more common in Northern Europe than in Middle Africa. Some, but certainly not all, of these variations can be explained in terms of differences in lifestyle and public health interventions.

Cervical Cancer

The cervical epithelium is composed of two distinct cell types. The ectocervix is covered by non-keratinized squamous cells similar to those of the lining of the vagina. The endocervical canal is covered by columnar cells of the same origin as those of the endometrium. Cervical cancers initiate in the region where these two cell types meet — the squamo-columnar junction. There are three main types of cervical cancer (squamous, adenocarcinoma and adenosquamous carcinoma), with squamous cell carcinoma being the most common. It used to be said that this accounted for approximately 90% of all cases of cervical cancer. However, more recent data show that the proportion of cervical cancer that is adenocarcinoma or adenosquamous carcinoma has doubled, particularly in younger women. Squamous cell carcinoma now only accounts for approximately 75% of all cases of cervical cancer. The reason for the increasing proportion of adenocarcinoma seems to be three-fold: adenocarcinoma really is becoming more common, having been very rare; due to the introduction of mucin staining and greater awareness of adenocarcinoma, it is being reported more often on pathology reports; and cytological screening is more able to detect precancerous squamous lesions than

Table 34.1 Age-standardized rates (per 100,000 women-years) for cancer of the cervix, corpus uterus and ovary (world standard population)

Region	Cervix		Corpus uterus		Ovary	
	Cases	Deaths	Cases	Deaths	Cases	Deaths
E. Africa	42.7	34.6	3.2	1.2	5.8	4.1
M. Africa	28.0	23.0	2.5	0.9	3.3	2.3
N. Africa	12.1	9.8	2.4	1.0	2.6	1.8
S. Africa	38.2	22.6	3.5	1.5	5.2	3.2
W. Africa	29.3	23.8	2.2	0.9	4.6	3.2
Caribbean	32.6	16.0	8.8	4.3	4.3	2.6
C. America	30.6	15.0	4.5	2.0	7.2	3.6
S. America	28.6	12.9	6.7	2.0	7.7	3.7
N. America	7.7	2.3	22.0	2.6	10.7	6.1
E. Asia	7.4	3.7	2.5	0.5	3.7	1.8
S.E. Asia	18.7	10.2	4.2	1.6	7.2	4.1
S.C. Asia	26.2	15.0	2.3	1.0	5.3	3.8
W. Asia	5.8	2.9	5.8	2.7	5.3	3.4
E. Europe	14.5	7.1	11.8	3.6	10.2	6.0
N. Europe	9.0	3.6	12.2	2.1	13.3	7.9
S. Europe	10.7	3.3	11.8	2.2	9.7	4.5
W. Europe	10.0	3.4	12.5	2.1	11.3	6.3
Aust/NZ	7.4	2.0	10.6	1.7	9.4	5.1
Melanesia	38.1	21.7	6.7	2.7	6.6	3.9
World	16.2	9.0	6.5	1.6	6.6	4.0

Source: Ferlay J, Bray F, Pisani P, Parkin DM 2004 Globocan 2002: Cancer Incidence, Mortality and Prevalence Worldwide. IARC CancerBase No. 5. IARC Press, Lyon.

precancerous glandular (adeno) lesions, and thus the relative incidence of the two types of cancer has changed (Sasieni et al 2009).

Invasive cervical cancer is preceded by precancerous neoplasia variously referred to as high-grade squamous intraepithelial lesion, cervical intraepithelial neoplasia (CIN) or carcinoma *in situ* (CIS). Epidemiological studies have focused not only on invasive cancer, but also on the more common preinvasive disease. A similar preinvasive phase has also been identified for adenocarcinoma (or adenocarcinoma *in situ*).

Descriptive epidemiology

Cervical cancer is the second most commonly diagnosed cancer in women. Worldwide, it is estimated that there are approximately half a million new cases of cervical cancer each year, accounting for approximately 12% of all female cancers (Garcia et al 2007). The cumulative incidence rate up to 74 years of age (assuming no prior death) ranges from 5% in parts of Latin America to approximately 0.5% in parts of the Middle East and Finland. In most European countries, it is under 2% (Curado et al 2007). Cervical cancer is also extremely common in sub-Saharan Africa, but African incidence data are unreliable, particularly for older women.

The incidence of cervical cancer in most countries has decreased significantly since the 1960s. In the UK, mortality from cervical cancer has been declining since 1950. The difference between mortality rates in 1950–1952 compared with 2005–2007 varies with age, from an extraordinary 85% reduction in women aged 55–64 years to a more moderate 15% reduction in women aged 25–34 years. Figure 34.1 shows the age-specific mortality rates for cervical cancer in the UK since 1971. It is seen that the greatest decreases have been in older women (aged ≥65 years), and that the increasing rates in younger women between 1970 and 1985 reversed in the 1990s.

The differing cervical cancer mortality and incidence trends by age can be examined by birth cohort analysis in addition to analysis by year of death. Plotting the rate of disease against age for women born in different 5-year periods yields a series of curves, approximately parallel, but with some higher than others. In other words, women born at one time might be at relatively high risk of cervical cancer in their 20s and 30s, and remain at relatively high risk through their 40s, 50s, 60s and 70s. The authors' understanding of this effect is that there is an underlying characteristic of increasing rate of disease with age, but the level is determined by environmental exposure (to a sexually transmitted agent) in the late teens and 20s. So, for example, for women born at the end

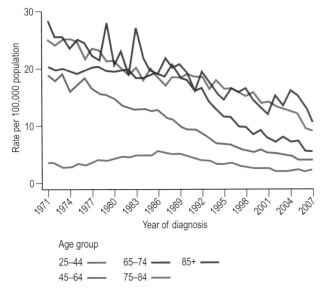

Figure 34.1 Age-specific mortality rates for cervical cancer, UK 1971–2007.

Age group
25–44 —— 65–74 —— 85+ ——
45–64 —— 75–84 ——

of the 19th century or around 1920, cervical cancer mortality was higher throughout their lives than for previous and subsequent birth cohorts. These two cohorts of women with increased risk would have become sexually active around the times of World War I and World War II.

The level of environmental exposure will be determined by social norms and will vary between ethnic groups and over time. Modelling shows that the idea that incidence and mortality rates can be modelled by age and cohort effects works well until the 1980s. However, more recent data require the addition of age-specific time trends corresponding to a beneficial effect of screening, particularly in younger women, to provide a satisfactory model (Sasieni and Adams 2000). From a public health perspective, it is important to note that women born in the 1960s are at three- to four-fold higher risk of cervical cancer compared with women born in the 1930s.

Risk factors

Evidence for an association between cervical cancer and sexual activity dates back to 1842, when Rigorni-Stern published data showing that whereas married women were more likely to die of cancer of the uterus (predominantly cervix) than breast cancer, nuns very rarely died of cancer of the uterus. Since then, the epidemiological evidence suggestive of a sexually transmitted agent causing cervical cancer has grown steadily. Traditional risk factors include the number of sexual partners and age at first sexual intercourse. The behaviour of men is also important, as shown by increasing risk in women with just one partner according to the number of partners of their husband (Buckley et al 1981). More recently, the sexually transmitted agent has been identified as certain types of HPV. The evidence that the relationship between HPV infection and cervical cancer is causal is overwhelming (Bosch et al 2002). Several large studies have been carried out to determine the prevalence of HPV in cervical cancer and precancerous lesions. Over 90% of cervical cancers have been found to include HPV DNA (Smith et al 2007), and when full adjustment for tissue adequacy and a range of polymerase chain reaction primers are used, the

estimates rise to almost 100% (Walboomers et al 1999). Several studies have shown that HPV-negative women have an extremely low risk of CIN 3 or cancer (Bulkmans et al 2007, Cuzick et al 2008a, Dillner et al 2008). Furthermore, a recent study (Sankaranarayanan et al 2009) found no cancer deaths among 30,000 HPV-negative women in the subsequent 8-year period.

There are over 100 types of HPV, and only some of these infect the anogenital region. These can be split into low-risk types, which cause genital warts, and high-risk types, which can lead to cervical cancer. Types 16 and 18 are strongly associated with cervical cancer; other types including 31, 33, 35, 39, 45, 51, 52, 56, 58 and 66 are associated with a more moderate elevated risk. Table 34.2 details the prevalence of the most common high-risk types of HPV in women with normal cytology, precancerous cervical lesions and invasive cervical cancer in the UK and worldwide.

It has been estimated that HPV is a very common sexually transmitted infection worldwide, with the majority of people being exposed to the virus by 30 years of age. Most infections with high-risk types are transitory and harmless. In a minority of women, the infection may become persistent and lead to high-grade cervical lesions with a potential for progression to cancer. Immune factors are certainly associated with persistence, but are poorly understood. Similarly, it is largely unknown why some women with persistent infection develop cervical cancer whereas others do not.

Other risk factors are less clear cut. Smoking is generally found to be associated with cervical cancer, but it is difficult to disentangle the confounding caused by the sociological link between smoking and increased number of sexual partners. Nevertheless, the body of evidence available suggests that smoking increases the risk of cervical cancer two- to three-fold by reducing the local immune response to HPV (Kapeu et al 2009). The association between oral contraceptive use and cervical cancer is also confounded by sexual behaviour; however, a large pooled analysis including 24 studies found that women who had used oral contraceptives for 5 years or more were at almost double the risk of cervical cancer compared with women who had never used oral contraceptives. This risk declines after the use of oral contraceptives is stopped; within 10 years, the risk is similar to non-users (Appleby et al 2007). High parity and young age at first full-term pregnancy have, independently, been found to increase the risk of invasive cervical carcinoma, and this association remains after adjusting for other reproductive factors. Women with seven or more pregnancies are at approximately 78% greater risk than women with one or two pregnancies. It is estimated that cervical cancer could be reduced by 30% in developing countries if parity and age at first intercourse were the same as in developed countries (International Collaboration of Epidemiological Studies of Cervical Cancer 2006). Previous exposure to sexually transmitted diseases, in particular *Chlamydia trachomatis* and herpes simplex virus type 2, also increases the risk of cervical cancer, even after adjusting for HPV infection (Bosch and de Sanjose 2007).

Immunosuppression certainly conveys an increased risk of cervical cancer, as shown in studies on renal transplant patients receiving immunosuppressive drugs (Birkeland et al 1995) and on women who are human immunodeficiency virus (HIV) positive (Grulich et al 2007). It seems likely that diet plays a role in the immune response to HPV, but studies

Table 34.2 High-risk human papilloma virus (HPV) prevalence in women with normal cytology, precancerous cervical lesions and invasive cervical cancer

Population	High-risk HPV prevalence[a]					
	16	18	33	45	31	Negative
Normal cytology (overall)[b]	2.5%	0.9%	0.6%	0.4%	0.7%	90.0%
Normal cytology (UK)[b]	2.3%	0.8%	0.3%	0.7%	0.5%	92.5%
Low-grade cytology (overall)[b]	20.3%	6.1%	4.7%	3.7%	8.3%	28.9%[c]
Low-grade cytology (UK)[b]	20.4%	8.9%	4.6%	3.9%	8.3%	
High-grade cytology[d]	45.4%	6.9%	7.3%	2.3%	8.6%	15.1%[d]
High-grade cytology (UK)[b]	58.7%	10.5%	9.6%	4.2%	18.3%	
Cancer[d]	54.4%	15.9%	4.3%	3.7%	3.6%	0.3%[e]
Cancer (UK)[b]	66.7%	15.4%	4.3%	2.3%	7.0%	

[a]Women with multiple infections contribute to more than one column.
[b]WHO/ICO Information Centre on Human Papilloma Virus (HPV) and Cervical Cancer (2007).
[c]Clifford et al (2005).
[d]Smith et al (2007).
[e]Walboomers et al (1999).

on diet and cervical cancer have found little evidence for a strong effect of intake of fruit and vegetables on the risk of cervical cancer (IARC Handbooks of Cancer Prevention 2003). It has been shown recently that cervical neoplasia (including CIS) exhibits familial clustering and that the strength of association increases with increasing genetic relatedness (Magnusson et al 1999). Independently, several groups have found an association between certain human leukocyte antigen class II antigens and cervical neoplasia. However, much more remains to be done in understanding the factors that determine why some women infected with oncogenic HPVs develop cervical cancer but the vast majority do not.

Natural history

There are few data from studies that directly observe the natural history of cervical cancer development because it is generally felt to be unethical not to treat precancerous cervical disease. The situation is further complicated by the possibility that the process of taking a biopsy, required for definitive diagnosis of disease, may affect the natural history by stimulating regression. Therefore, most of what is known of the natural history of cervical precancer is derived from the follow-up of women with cytological abnormalities and the study of the incidence and prevalence of cervical lesions. There is one exception — cervical CIS in Auckland, New Zealand between 1965 and 1974. Women with CIS were not treated. A judicial inquiry in 1988 concluded that this practice was unethical, but allowed the histological and other material to be used for further research. Two studies have been published using this data (McIndoe et al 1984, McCredie et al 2008), with the most recent paper including over 25 years of follow-up (McCredie et al 2008). This study provides the most direct estimates available of the rate of progression from CIS to invasive cancer; the results show that approximately 30% of CIS progress to cancer within 30 years.

For the vast majority (estimated as well over 95%) (Walboomers et al 1999) of cervical cancers, the first step is exposure to one of the oncogenic HPVs. The time from infection to the development of invasive cancer is thought to be many years; typically between 10 and 40. Longitudinal studies on young women show that the majority of HPV infections are transient (Moscicki et al 2004) and that the virus is indeed sexually transmitted (Burk et al 1996). Persistence of infection has been shown to be associated with the development of cervical lesions (Ho et al 1995). It is generally believed that one of the key steps in the development of cancer is integration of the viral DNA in the host genome (Das et al 1992), although some carcinomas only have episomal viral DNA (Cullen et al 1991).

Cervical neoplasia appears to constitute a disease continuum ranging from CIN grades I to III, to microinvasive cancer and, finally, fully invasive cancer. More recent evidence shows that CIN I is frequently not associated with HPV infection and may not be part of the continuum. However, histology is not currently able to distinguish CIN I associated with oncogenic HPV infection from CIN I without HPV DNA. The histological report of HPV infection is based on morphological features, and is not particularly tightly correlated with the presence of oncogenic HPV DNA.

Follow-up studies of women with CIN have found that approximately 60% of CIN I regresses compared with approximately 33% of CIN III; 11% and 22% of CIN I and II, respectively, progressed to CIN III (Östör 1993). Modellers find that regression is more common in younger women, and that three-quarters of CIN in women under 35 years of age will regress (van Ballegooijen et al 1997). They estimate the mean duration of CIN to be 12 years, and that the time from HPV infection to CIN is between 1 and 10 years. Although the details of progression and regression are largely speculative, it is clear that, at most, approximately one-third of high-grade CIN will progress to cancer over approximately 15 years and that the majority of CIN I will regress.

CIN III rates rise rapidly before 30 years of age. Rates then decrease, rather more slowly, being at approximately half their peak by 40 years of age and just 10–20% of their peak by 50 years of age (Office for National Statistics 2006). The extent to which published CIN III rates reflect the prevalence of an untreated condition and the extent to which they mirror incidence is not completely clear.

Prevention and screening

Prevention of cervical cancer could be approached in several ways. Strategies aimed at promoting safe sex (use of condoms, particularly with an occasional partner), delaying the age of first sexual intercourse and reducing the number of women who smoke are only likely to have modest effects on cervical cancer rates. However, if successful, they would also have additional health benefits in terms of control of sexually transmitted diseases (including chlamydia with the resultant pelvic inflammatory disease), reduction in teenage pregnancies and reduction in heart disease and lung cancer, respectively.

The impact of vaccination on rates of cytological abnormalities, CIN III and invasive cancer will not be seen for at least 12–16 years after vaccination is rolled out. It is possible that, in 30 years time, prevention of cervical cancer may be achievable by vaccination of teenage girls (within a well-organized high-coverage programme) against a large subset of HPV oncogenic types. Until that time, the most likely route to reducing the morbidity associated with cervical cancer is through the detection and treatment of precancerous cervical lesions. Screening by cytological analysis of cervical smears has proven to be an effective means of reducing the incidence of cervical cancer in many industrialized countries. It satisfies most of the criteria that should be considered before introducing a public screening programme. Cervical screening programmes were set up with the intention of preventing cervical cancer. They also have the additional benefit of reducing mortality from cervical cancer by diagnosing occult invasive tumours at an early stage when they are more treatable. Cervical screening was offered to women well before its effectiveness had been demonstrated. By the time that people considered the possibility of evaluating cervical screening in a randomized controlled clinical trial, the indirect evidence of the benefits of such screening made a trial in which some women were deprived of screening unethical in a setting where screening is already routine. In the absence of randomized trials, researchers sought evidence from population trend studies and studies that looked at screening at the individual level rather than in populations. The individual-level studies have mainly been carried out as case–control studies, comparing the screening experience of women diagnosed with or dying from cervical cancer with that of healthy women. Ideally, case–control and population trend studies should be interpreted together. The fact that women with cervical cancer are less likely to have been screened than healthy women could be confounded, to some extent, by socioeconomic status and attitudes to healthy lifestyles. Women who do not attend for screening may be at greater risk than those who attend even if screening is useless, simply because they are more likely to smoke, to have a poor diet and to be exposed to oncogenic HPVs. Taken together, however, one sees a picture in which overall cancer rates are falling and women who have been screened are less likely to develop cancer than those who have not.

Estimates of the sensitivity of cytology are available from studies in which a large number of women with negative cytology have colposcopy. Ideally, colposcopy should be offered to all women, but this would be expensive and taking a biopsy from all women would be unethical. Many studies comparing two or more screening tests (such as cytology, HPV testing, direct visual inspection) offer colposcopy to all women who are positive on one or more of the screening tests. From such studies, the sensitivity of cytology for high-grade CIN is found to be between 50% and 75% (Nanda et al 2000, Cuzick et al 2006). However, most cases of missed CIN 3 would not become cancerous within 5 years. It is for this reason that screening is recommended, in most countries, to start around the age of 20 years and continue at regular intervals (of between 3 and 5 years) up to the age of 65 years.

There is now sufficient evidence that testing for HPV infections with a primary screening tool can reduce cervical cancer incidence and mortality rates (IARC Monographs 2007). Although HPV testing has high sensitivity (>90%), it is, on average, 6% less specific than cytology (Cuzick et al 2008b). This leads to a higher number of women being referred to colposcopy with no visible lesions. This is especially important in women under 30 years of age, in whom transient HPV infection and cervical lesions are most common. In many high-resource settings, HPV testing is being used in the triage of women over 30 years of age with borderline or mild smears. However, in low-resource settings where organized cytology is not feasible, introduction of HPV testing with subsequent ablative treatment for those women that are positive is an attractive alternative (Sankaranarayanan et al 2009). The introduction of HPV testing to the screening programme would allow the screening interval to be extended (Bulkmans et al 2007, Cuzick et al 2008b, Dillner et al 2008).

Human papilloma virus vaccines

Prophylactic HPV vaccines are L1 virus-like particles (VLPs) in which the surface L1 protein is made to aggregate into particles, mimicking the virus in antigenic respects but not containing the viral DNA. VLPs have been shown to induce a high titre of in-vitro neutralizing antibodies and to protect against experimental challenge with homologous virus in animal models. As VLPs do not contain any viral genes, they are non-infectious and non-oncogenic. To date, two vaccines are commercially available (Cervarix™ and Gardasil™); both are licensed to be applied in three doses within 6 months. Both preparations immunize against HPV 16 and 18, and Gardasil also immunizes against HPV 6 and 11. Results from a number of randomized controlled trials have been published to date. The phase III trials are designed to evaluate the endpoint of CIN 2/3 associated with the HPV types included in the vaccine (Harper et al 2006, Garland et al 2007, Paavonen et al 2007). The smaller phase II trials were powered primarily to evaluate protection from infection by the vaccine types (Villa et al 2005, Mao et al 2006).

There is no evidence that vaccination is effective against an HPV infection that is already present at the time of vaccination (i.e. vaccines do not induce HPV clearance or reduce progression) (Hildesheim et al 2007). This is important when interpreting the results from clinical trials. There are three main types of analysis for efficacy studies. The according-to-protocol analysis (ATP) only included those women who were HPV negative at enrolment, received all three vaccine doses and remained HPV negative up to the final dose. The modified intention-to-treat (MITT) analysis included study participants who received at least one dose of vaccine, and who were negative for relevant HPV types at enrolment (Cervarix studies) or were randomly assigned to study group irrespective of their baseline HPV status (Gardasil studies). Finally, the intention-to-treat analysis included all randomized subjects.

The vaccine trial subjects differed in age (mostly aged 15–26 years) from the recommended age at vaccination (10–14 years). As younger women are less likely to be infected with HPV at the time of vaccination, the ATP or MITT analysis will more closely reflect the efficacy that one would expect to observe in individuals vaccinated at 10–14 years of age. Vaccine efficacy results by analysis type are detailed in Table 34.3. Overall, HPV vaccines are over 95% effective against vaccine HPV types in HPV-naïve women. Recent results from the PATRICIA trial suggest that this vaccine also confers a high degree of cross-protection against other HPV types (specifically HPV 31, 45 and 33), and that the overall efficacy against CIN 2 or worse associated with any HPV type in the ATP analysis is 70% (Paavonen et al 2009).

HPV vaccination has been approved and is being rolled out in over 90 countries worldwide. In England, vaccination was introduced in 2008–2009 to girls aged 12–13 years, with a catch-up campaign for girls up to 17–18 years of age.

Endometrial Cancer

Most cancers of the uterine corpus are adenocarcinomas of the endometrium. Sarcomas of the myometrium (muscle) are rare and are not considered in this chapter. Endometrial cancer comprises approximately 4% of all female cancers worldwide (Bray et al 2005). Incidence rates of endometrial cancer in Western countries are three to eight times as great as mortality rates, reflecting the high cure rate for these cancers (Table 34.1). In fact, 5-year survival for endometrial cancer patients relative to the general population is approximately 70% (Garcia et al 2007). Endometrial cancer is rare in premenopausal women, but becomes relatively common in postmenopausal women; in 2006, the incidence of endometrial cancer in England was 14 per 100,000 in women aged 45–49 years, compared with 29 per 100,000 in women aged 50–54 years. In recent years, endometrial cancer rates have been substantially greater in women over 60 years of age compared with women aged 50–59 years, whereas the rates were similar in the past (Figure 34.2A). Incidence rates are highest in North America; up to 10 times higher than in parts of Africa and almost double those in Northern Europe (Table 34.1). Data from the US Cancer Statistics 2001–2005 show that incidence rates are higher among US Whites (23.5 per 100,000) than Blacks (19.1 per 100,000) (US Cancer Statistics Working Group 2009).

When studying trends in endometrial cancer, it is important to look at 'cancer of the uterus, site not specified' since, in many countries, the majority of those cancers will have originated in the endometrium. In both England (Sasieni et al 1997) and the USA (Ries et al 2001), mortality rates fell steadily and substantially (approximately 60%) between 1950 and 1990. More recent UK trends are shown in Figure 34.2B. Incidence rates in women over 55 years of age have been increasing in the UK and across Northern Europe. In contrast, rates in premenopausal women have been declining (Bray et al 2005). The observed trends in younger women have been attributed to the widespread use of the combined oral contraceptive pill (COCP), while the increasing incidence observed in older women is believed to be linked to the increased prevalence of obesity. Interpretation of trends is complicated by the prevalence of women who have had a hysterectomy, since women without a uterus are obviously not susceptible to uterine cancer.

Risk factors

The main aetiological factors for endometrial cancer are obesity, hormonal levels and reproductive history.

Table 34.3 Efficacy of two prophylactic vaccines against human papilloma virus type 16/18-related cervical intraepithelial neoplasia (CIN)

| Vaccine | Study | No. of subjects | | | Efficacy against 16/18-related lesions* | | |
		Vaccine	Placebo	Endpoints	ATP	MITT	ITT
Gardasil Quadrivalent (16/18/6/11)	Merck 007 (Villa et al 2005)	235	233	CIN 1–3, AIS	100% (<0–100)	100% (31–100)	NR
	FUTURE I (Garland et al 2007)	2241	2258	CIN 1–3, AIS	100% (94–100)	98% (92–100)	55% (40–66)
	FUTURE II (2007)	6087	6080	CIN 2/3, AIS	98% (86–100)	95% (85–99)	44% (26–58)
Cervarix Bivalent (16/18)	GSK 001/07 (Harper et al 2006)	481	470	CIN 2/3	100% (8–100)	NR	NR
	PATRICIA (Paavonen et al 2007, 2009)	7788	7838	CIN 2/3	98%* (90–100)	90%[†] (53–99)	30.4%* (16–42)

ATP, according to protocol; MITT, modified intention to treat; ITT, intention to treat; NR, not reported.
95% confidence intervals, except 97.9%[†] and 96.1% confidence intervals for PATRICIA.

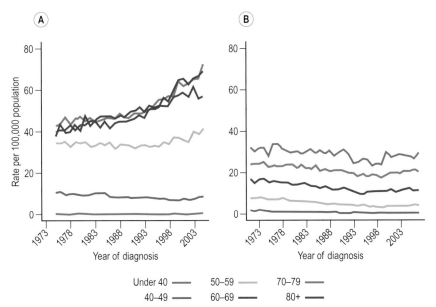

Figure 34.2 Age-specific (A) incidence and (B) mortality rates for corpus uterine cancer (including uterine unspecified), UK 1971–2007.

Obesity is consistently found to be associated with endometrial cancer in both case–control and cohort studies. Due to the high prevalence of obesity in many populations, is likely to be responsible for a significant proportion of cases of endometrial cancer. Typically, studies report a two- to three-fold risk of endometrial cancers associated with obesity (Schouten et al 2004), but some studies have found much stronger effects (Weiderpass et al 2000). Obesity is likely to affect cancer rates by increasing the level of circulating oestrogens, particularly in postmenopausal women. This occurs due to increased conversion of androstenedione to oestrogen, and decreased levels of sex-hormone-binding globulin (Cook et al 2006). There is some evidence that greater upper body fat, as opposed to overall obesity, might be a better indicator of the risk of endometrial cancer, and that waist circumference and waist:hip ratio could be a better predictor of risk than body mass index (BMI; Xu et al 2005). Diabetes has been associated with a two-fold increased risk of endometrial cancer (Friberg et al 2007). Although it is difficult to distinguish between the risks associated with increased body weight and the risks of diabetes *per se,* there is evidence that hyperinsulinaemia increases the risk of endometrial cancer (Lukanova et al 2004).

Oestrogens are the primary stimulation for endometrial proliferation. In premenopausal women, oestrogens are counteracted by progestagens; however, in postmenopausal women, they go unopposed. Any state that reduces the exposure of uterine tissue to oestrogen or oestrogen-like substances reduces the risk of endometrial cancer, and inversely, any medical condition that results in high levels of endogenous oestrogens increases the risk (i.e. polycystic ovaries, oestrogen-secreting ovarian tumours). Pregnancy and parity reduce the risk of this cancer by 30% for the first birth and by 25% for each successive birth. The use of the COCP reduces the risk by 10% for each year of use, so that there is approximately a 65% reduction with 10 years of use. The protective effect of the COCP lasts for at least 15 years after last use (Pike et al 2004). Oestrogen replacement therapy has been consistently found to be associated with an increase in endometrial cancer. A meta-analysis estimated a relative risk of 2.3 in ever-users compared with never-users, and found that the risk remains elevated for several years after cessation of use (Grady et al 1995). The risk appears to increase both with increasing duration of use and increased dose of oestrogen, with a relative risk of 10 associated with 10 years of use (Grady et al 1995). Newer hormone replacement therapy preparations including a progestogen either as a continuous combined replacement or used sequentially for the last 10 days per month cause minimal, if any, increased risk of endometrial cancer (Beresford et al 1997). The oestrogen receptor modulator hormone used in the treatment and prevention of breast cancer, tamoxifen, has been shown to increase the risk of endometrial cancer two- to three-fold (Cuzick et al 2003). Physical activity and smoking have been shown to decrease the risk of endometrial cancer. Physical activity independent of body weight has been shown to reduce the risk of endometrial cancer by 23% (Voskuil et al 2007). Smoking has consistently been associated with a decreased risk of endometrial cancer; this effect might be linked to the fact that smokers metabolize oestrogens into less harmful metabolites than non-smokers. A recent study (Viswanathan et al 2005) found that smoking reduced the risk of endometrial cancer by 30–40% among current and past smokers, and that the effect was greater in those who had been smoking for longer.

Women with Lynch syndrome (hereditary non-polyposis colorectal cancer) are at very high risk of endometrial cancer from 40 years of age. The risks differ depending on the affected gene, but lifetime risk is thought to be between 40% and 60% (Meyer et al 2009). For this reason, most women with Lynch syndrome will have a prophylactic hysterectomy between 40 and 50 years of age.

Prevention and screening

Primary prevention of endometrial cancer should be aimed at weight loss and careful monitoring of women taking oestrogen-only hormone replacement therapy, both of which would have net benefits on woman's health. Screening is unlikely to have a role in the foreseeable future. The COCP reduces the risk of endometrial cancer and the protection lasts for at least 15 years after use. Since the COCP increases the risk of breast cancer, the overall risk benefit is not likely to be favourable in women over 40 years of age.

Ovarian Cancer

Ovarian cancer is the sixth most common type of cancer and the sixth most common cause of cancer mortality in women in the developed world (Garcia et al 2007). Survival is very poor, except when the tumour is detected early, which is rare in most countries. Overall 5-year survival statistics estimate survival to be 46% in the USA (Horner et al 2008) and 39% in England (Office for National Statistics 2008). However, when the cancer is detected at an early stage, 5-year survival increases to over 70%. Approximately 90% of ovarian cancers are adenocarcinomas of the epithelium, but germ cell tumours are the most common histological type in women under 30 years of age.

Descriptive epidemiology

Variation in the rates of ovarian cancer around the world is less marked for ovarian cancer than for other gynaecological cancers (Table 34.1). The highest rates are found in Northern Europe and in White women in North America and Western Europe. Similarly, rates tend to be lower in most Asian countries, but women of Japanese and Chinese descent in the USA have rates that are higher than in their countries of origin.

Trends in ovarian cancer in England and Wales differ by age. Mortality rates in premenopausal women have fallen considerably since the 1970s (Figure 34.3). By 1999, the rates in women aged 30–44 years were just half of what they had been in 1970. The picture for older women is dramatically different. Rates in women over 65 years of age have increased, and by 2006, the rates in women over 65 years of age were over 30% greater than they were in 1971. The incidence of ovarian cancer is only slightly greater than the mortality rates, reflecting the poor cure rate for this disease. Consequently, trends in incidence are similar to the trends in mortality. Recently, however, survival has improved substantially due to a combination of earlier detection and the use of platinum-based chemotherapies (Kitchener 2008).

Risk factors

The main factors affecting the risk of epithelial cancers of the ovary are reproductive history and contraceptive use, although a small proportion of women are at greatly increased risk due to inherited genetic susceptibility. Overall, the main risk factor appears to be the lifetime number of ovulatory cycles.

One of the first observations linking reproductive history to ovarian cancer risk was that never-married women were at approximately one and a half times the risk of ever-married women. Subsequently, decreasing risk with increasing numbers of full-term pregnancies has been shown in over a dozen case–control studies (Whittemore et al 1992). Typically, having had one or two children is associated with a decrease in risk of approximately 30%, and having had three or more children is associated with a decrease in risk of approximately 60%. In a recent US study of 563 cases and

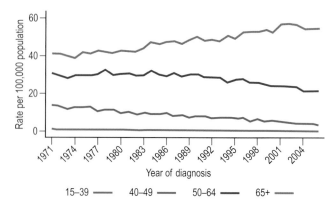

Figure 34.3 Age-specific mortality rates for ovarian cancer, UK 1971–2007.

523 controls, one child was associated with a 40% reduction in risk, two children with a 60% reduction in risk and five or more children with a 80% reduction in risk (Titus-Ernstoff et al 2001). A large cohort study in Sweden including 4128 ovarian cancer cases found that having had one child was associated with a 25% reduction in risk and having had two children was associated with a 43% reduction in risk (Granstrom et al 2008). The effect of parity does not appear to be attributable to confounding by age at first birth, age at last birth, age at menarche or age at menopause, none of which seem to be associated with ovarian cancer risk to any significant extent.

Infertility, however, does have an independent effect on ovarian cancer risk. In a pooled analysis of eight case–control studies (Ness et al 2002), nulliparous women who tried to conceive for more than 5 years had a 2.7-fold risk of ovarian cancer compared with women who had not tried to conceive for more than 1 year. There have been claims that women who received fertility treatment had an increased risk compared with those who had never been treated with fertility drugs, but there is no evidence to support this claim (Kashyap et al 2004).

Although not established conclusively, breast feeding seems to reduce the risk of ovarian cancer, even after adjusting for parity. A recent prospective study found that women who had breast fed for 18 months or more were at significantly lower risk of ovarian cancer compared with women who had not breast fed (Danforth et al 2007).

Exogenous hormones

The protective effect of the COCP on ovarian cancer risk has been demonstrated beyond any reasonable doubt (Collaborative Group on Epidemiological Studies of Ovarian Cancer 2008). Pooled estimates of the protection indicate that the risk is reduced by approximately 50% with 5 years of use, and that protection increases with the duration of use (Whittemore et al 1992). The protective effect of oral contraceptives persists for up to 30 years after cessation of use, and is not confined to any particular formulation of the pill. The benefit in absolute terms can be expected to increase over the next few decades as the cohort of women with extensive use of oral contraceptives reaches the peak age of ovarian cancer incidence. Hormone replacement therapy has been associated with a 19–24% increased risk of ovarian cancer; however, the risk is not increased in women using hormone replacement therapy for less than 5 years, and decreases once a woman stops taking it (Zhou et al 2008).

Family history

It is a well-known clinical observation that ovarian cancer tends to aggregate in families. Rarely, such clustering can be extreme with increased risk of breast cancer (in *BRCA1* and *BRCA2* gene mutation carriers) and colon and endometrial cancer in cancer family syndromes. The risk of ovarian cancer associated with *BRCA1* and *BRCA2* mutation carriers is 40% and 18%, respectively (Chen and Parmigiani 2007). Case–control studies generally find a relative risk of approximately 3 associated with one affected family member, and a relative risk of approximately 7 with two affected relatives. More recently, the Swedish Cancer Family Database reported relative risks of 2.54 in women with an affected mother and 2.76 in women with an affected sister (Granstrom et al 2008). Relative risks of such magnitude are typical of most cancers, but the high absolute risk in women with a family history of both early breast cancer and ovarian cancer is such that many such women consider having a prophylactic oophorectomy once they have completed their families, particularly since having an oophorectomy before the natural menopause also reduces the risk of breast cancer.

Other factors

Inconsistent results have been found from epidemiological studies regarding BMI (Vaino and Bianchini 2002). A recent meta-analysis (Schouten et al 2008) concluded that a BMI of 30 or more in premenopausal women increases the risk of ovarian cancer by 30% compared with women with a BMI below 24. No effect was observed in postmenopausal women.

There has been great interest in whether talcum powder applied to the perineal area increases the risk of ovarian cancer. In an attempt to clarify the evidence, a systematic review was carried out in 2003. This found a significantly increased risk associated with talc use (relative risk 1.33, 95% confidence interval 1.16–1.45). However, there was no clear association with dose, and the authors concluded that the association could be confounded or biased (Huncharek et al 2003). A further two case–control studies (Gates et al 2008, Merritt et al 2008) have been published, both of which seem to suggest a significant trend of increasing risk with more frequent use. Despite this finding, the authors advise caution because the majority of studies failed to observe a dose–response relationship and there is the possibility of recall bias differentially affecting cases and controls.

The relationship between smoking and ovarian cancer is unclear. A meta-analysis including 10 studies found that the risk of mucinous ovarian cancer was doubled in current smokers compared with never-smokers; however, a risk reduction for clear cell cancers was also observed (Jordan et al 2006). In 2008, the Norwegian–Swedish Women's Lifestyle and Health cohort including 103,081 women found a doubling of risk for borderline tumours for former and current smokers compared with non-smokers. They also found a dose–response relationship according to smoking intensity and duration for borderline and serous tumours (Gram et al 2008).

Prevention and screening

No effective screening methods are available for the detection of early ovarian cancer. Recent hopes are centred on multimodal screening involving serum tumour marker CA125 for primary screening followed by ultrasound (Menon et al 2009). Transvaginal ultrasound examination on its own is not justified as a screening technique at population level due to its lack of specificity and predictive value, because it is unable to differentiate benign cysts from malignant disease. The serum tumour marker CA125 is present in approximately 80% of epithelial cancers, but is also raised in the presence of other cancers (i.e. pancreatic, breast, bladder) as well as in some benign diseases (e.g. diverticulitis, endometriosis) and some physiological conditions (e.g. pregnancy, menstruation) (Menon 2004). The best evidence to date regarding multimodal screening comes from a large randomized-controlled trial in the UK; although this trial did not find a difference in deaths from ovarian cancer, it did find a significant difference in the median rate of survival in the screened group compared with the control group (Jacobs et al 1999). Currently, the UK Collaborative Trial of Ovarian Cancer Screening has randomized over 200,000 women to multimodal screening or no screening. The main endpoint is death from ovarian cancer, and the results are expected in 2015. In the multimodal arm, triage is offered based on a substantial increase in CA125 and not simply on the absolute level. There is much interest in other proteomic markers detectable in serum, but it is too early to evaluate these fully (Rifai et al 2006, Gagnon and Ye 2008).

Cancers of the Vulva and the Vagina

Cancers of the vulva and vagina account for 7% and less than 2% of all gynaecological cancers in the UK, respectively. Over 80% are squamous in origin, with 10% of vulva cancers being melanomas. Incidence and mortality of both cancers is highest in women over 60 years of age (Figure 34.4). The incidence of vaginal cancer in women over 60 years of age is three per 100,000 in England (compared with less than one per 100,000 in women under 60 years of age). The risk in women over 60 years of age is much more pronounced for vulval cancer; incidence increases from approximately three per 100,000 in women aged 40–59 years to 11 per 100,000 in women aged over 60 years. The incidence of vaginal cancer in the UK has remained at approximately 0.6 per 100,000 for the past 15 years. The incidence of vulval cancer fell during the 1970s and 1980s; however, it has increased in recent years and the incidence rate is now comparable to that observed in 1975 (Figure 34.5). This increase reflects the sharp rise of vulval cases in women under 50 years of age, which in turn is thought to be caused by the high prevalence of HPV infection in younger women (Joura et al 2000). The increase in HPV infection of the vulva has been attributed to changing attitudes towards oral sex. Mortality rates from both cancers have fallen considerably since the 1970s. For vaginal cancer, the rates have fallen by 38% since the 1970s (from 0.4 per 100,000 to 0.2 per 100,000), and for vulva cancer, the corresponding figure is 53% (from 1.3 per 100,000 in 1971 to 0.6 per 100,000 in 2006).

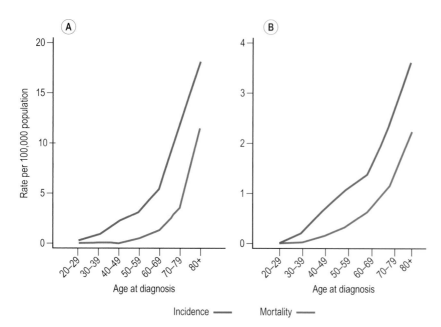

Figure 34.4 Incidence and mortality rates for (A) vulval and (B) vaginal cancer, England 2006.

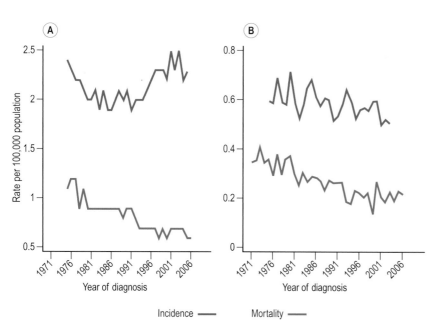

Figure 34.5 Age-standardized (European) incidence and mortality rates for (A) vulval and (B) vaginal cancers, Great Britain 1971–2006.

Rates of vaginal cancer vary around the world, with the lowest rates observed in Eastern and Western Asia (approximately 0.2 per 100,000) and the highest rates seen in the Caribbean and Southern Asia (0.7 per 100,000). Vulval cancer is much more common in North America and Europe (1.6 per 100,000), and relatively rare in Eastern Asia and Northern Africa (0.3 per 100,000). The geographical distribution for vaginal cancer most probably reflects not only HPV prevalence but the extent of cervical screening available in different populations, as many vaginal lesions are identified at the time of screening for cervical cancer.

Risk factors for these cancers appear to be similar to those for cervical cancer. A well-defined precancerous stage has been identified for both these cancers: vaginal intraepithelial neoplasia and vulval intraepithelial neoplasia. It is estimated that 65–90% of vaginal cancers and 30–35% of vulval cancers can be attributed to HPV infection [WHO/ICO Infor-

mation Centre on Human Papilloma Virus (HPV) and Cervical Cancer 2007]. HPV 16 has been found to be the most prevalent HPV type in both these cancers; it compromised approximately 60% of the HPV found in vaginal cancer (Hampl et al 2006) and 20–60% of the HPV found in vulval cancer. HPV-positive vulvar cancer is much more common in women under 50 years of age, where high-risk HPV types can be detected in up to 60% of cancers (Hampl et al 2008). It has been hypothesized that vulval cancer arises from two distinct diseases (Trimble et al 1996, Basta et al 1999). The first type develops from in-situ vulval neoplasia, in which a much higher proportion of high-risk HPV types are found (70–90%) (Madeleine et al 1997) and which is more prevalent in young women. The second type, which more often afflicts older women, develops from non-cancerous vulvar epithelial disorders as a result of chronic inflammation (the itch–scratch–lichen sclerosus hypothesis) (Canavan and Cohen 2002). Antibodies to herpes simplex virus type 2 have been associated with increased risk of both vaginal and vulval cancer, even after controlling for HPV infection (Hildesheim et al 1997, Madeleine et al 1997). Smoking increases the risk of vulval cancer six-fold, and this increases to 25-fold when heavy smoking (>20 cigarettes a day) and HPV infection interact (Hildesheim et al 1997, Madeleine et al 1997). The association between smoking and vaginal cancer still remains uncertain.

The one risk factor that is very strongly associated with cancer of the vulva is immunosuppression; the risk of invasive vulval cancer is increased 100-fold in women with renal transplants (Penn 1986). It has also been documented that the incidence of vulval intraepithelial neoplasia is increased in women who are HIV positive (Frisch et al 2000).

Vaginal cancer in adolescents has been attributed to in-utero exposure to diethylstilbestrol (DES), a synthetic oestrogen used to prevent spontaneous abortions between 1940 and 1970 (Greenwald et al 1971). Vaginal cancer is almost never diagnosed in cohorts who could not have been exposed to DES *in utero* (either because they were born prior to 1945 or because DES was never prescribed in the country). The current estimates suggest a 40-fold increase in the risk of vaginal cancer in the daughters of exposed women (Hatch et al 1998).

KEY POINTS

1. Breast cancer and cervical cancer are the two most common female malignancies in the world.
2. Cervical cancer is most common in developing countries while uterine corpus and ovarian cancer have a higher incidence in industrialized countries.
3. The variation in the rates of gynaecological cancers around the world is enormous.
4. Well-organized cytological screening has had a dramatic effect on the incidence and mortality rates of cervical cancer.
5. HPV infection is very common, but only a tiny minority of women infected with HPV develop cervical cancer. The development of cancer depends on the persistence of HPV infection.
6. HPV testing offers the potential for improving the effectiveness and feasibility of cervical screening, particularly in the developing world.
7. In the long term, vaccination against HPV may eliminate cervical cancer completely.
8. The incidence of endometrial cancer in women over 55 years of age has been increasing in the UK, while rates in premenopausal women have been decreasing.
9. Obesity and oestrogens are the main factors associated with endometrial cancer.
10. The oral contraceptive pill has reduced the incidence of ovarian cancer in women aged 30–44 years. The rise in incidence in older women has been attributed to increased prevalence of obesity.
11. Incidence of ovarian cancer is only slightly greater than the mortality rates, reflecting the poor cure rate.
12. Reproductive history and contraceptive use are the main risk factors for ovarian cancer.
13. Detecting ovarian cancer at an early stage is key to increasing survival. A large randomized controlled trial is ongoing assessing the effectiveness of serum tumour marker CA125 followed by ultrasound examination as a screening tool.
14. A large proportion of vaginal and vulval cancers are attributed to HPV infection.

References

Appleby P, Beral V, Berrington de Gonzalez A et al 2007 Cervical cancer and hormonal contraceptives: collaborative reanalysis of individual data for 16,573 women with cervical cancer and 35,509 women without cervical cancer from 24 epidemiological studies. The Lancet 370: 1609–1621.

Basta A, Adamek K, Pitynski K 1999 Intraepithelial neoplasia and early stage vulvar cancer. Epidemiological, clinical and virological observations. European Journal of Gynaecological Oncology 20: 111–114.

Beresford SA, Weiss NS, Voigt LF, McKnight B 1997 Risk of endometrial cancer in relation to use of oestrogen combined with cyclic progestagen therapy in postmenopausal women. The Lancet 349: 458–461.

Birkeland SA, Storm HH, Lamm LU et al 1995 Cancer risk after renal transplantation in the Nordic countries 1964–1986. International Journal of Cancer 60: 183–189.

Bosch FX, Lorincz A, Munoz N, Meijer CJ, Shah KV 2002 The causal relation between human papillomavirus and cervical cancer. Journal of Clinical Pathology 55: 244–265.

Bosch FX, de Sanjose S 2007 The epidemiology of human papillomavirus infection and cervical cancer. Disease Markers 23: 213–227.

Bray F, dos Santos Silva I, Moller H, Weiderpass E 2005 Endometrial cancer incidence trends in Europe: underlying determinants and prospects for prevention. Cancer Epidemiology, Biomarkers and Prevention 14: 1132–1142.

Buckley JD, Harris RW, Doll R, Vessey MP, Williams PT 1981 Case–control study of the husbands of women with dysplasia or carcinoma of the cervix uteri. The Lancet 2: 1010–1015.

Bulkmans NW, Berkhof J, Rozendaal L et al 2007 Human papillomavirus DNA testing for the detection of cervical intraepithelial neoplasia grade 3 and cancer: 5-year follow-up of a randomised controlled implementation trial. The Lancet 370: 1764–1772.

Burk RD, Ho GY, Beardsley L, Lempa M, Peters M, Bierman R 1996 Sexual behavior and partner characteristics are the predominant risk factors for genital human papillomavirus infection in young women. Journal of Infectious Diseases 174: 679–689.

Canavan TP, Cohen D 2002 Vulvar cancer. American Family Physician 66: 1269–1274.

Chen S, Parmigiani G 2007 Meta-analysis of BRCA1 and BRCA2 penetrance. Journal of Clinical Oncology 25: 1329–1333.

Clifford GM, Rana RK, Franceschi S et al 2005 Human papillomavirus genotype distribution in low-grade cervical lesions: comparison by geographic region and with cervical cancer. Cancer Epidemiology, Biomarkers & Prevention 14: 1157–1164.

Collaborative Group on Epidemiological Studies of Ovarian Cancer, Beral V, Doll R, Hermon C, Peto R, Reeves G 2008 Ovarian cancer and oral contraceptives: collaborative reanalysis of data from 45 epidemiological studies including 23,257 women with ovarian cancer and 87,303 controls. The Lancet 371: 303–314.

Cook LS, Weiss NS, Doherty JA, Chen C 2006 Endometrial Cancer. Oxford University Press, Oxford.

Cullen AP, Reid R, Campion M, Lorincz AT 1991 Analysis of the physical state of different human papillomavirus DNAs in intraepithelial and invasive cervical neoplasm. Journal of Virology 65: 606–612.

Curado MP, Edwards B, Shin HR et al (eds) 2007 Cancer Incidence in Five Continents, Vol. IX. IARC Scientific Publications No. 160. Lyon, IARC.

Cuzick J, Powles T, Veronesi U et al 2003 Overview of the main outcomes in breast-cancer prevention trials. The Lancet 361: 296–300.

Cuzick J, Clavel C, Petry KU et al 2006 Overview of the European and North American studies on HPV testing in primary cervical cancer screening. International Journal of Cancer 119: 1095–1101.

Cuzick J, Szarewski A, Mesher D et al 2008a Long-term follow-up of cervical abnormalities among women screened by HPV testing and cytology — results from the Hammersmith study. International Journal of Cancer 122: 2294–2300.

Cuzick J, Arbyn M, Sankaranarayanan R et al 2008b Overview of human papillomavirus-based and other novel options for cervical cancer screening in developed and developing countries. Vaccine 26 (Suppl 10): K29–K41.

Danforth KN, Tworoger SS, Hecht JL, Rosner BA, Colditz GA, Hankinson SE 2007 Breastfeeding and risk of ovarian cancer in two prospective cohorts. Cancer Causes and Control 18: 517–523.

Das BC, Sharma JK, Gopalakrishna V, Luthra UK 1992 Analysis by polymerase chain reaction of the physical state of human papillomavirus type 16 DNA in cervical preneoplastic and neoplastic lesions. Journal of General Virology 73: 2327–2336.

Dillner J, Rebolj M, Birembaut P et al 2008 Long term predictive values of cytology and human papillomavirus testing in cervical cancer screening: joint European cohort study. BMJ (Clinical Research Ed.) 337: a1754.

Ferlay J, Bray F, Pisani P, Parkin DM 2004 Globocan 2002: Cancer Incidence, Mortality and Prevalence Worldwide. IARC CancerBase No. 5. IARC Press, Lyon.

Friberg E, Orsini N, Mantzoros CS, Wolk A 2007 Diabetes mellitus and risk of endometrial cancer: a meta-analysis. Diabetologia 50: 1365–1374.

Frisch M, Biggar RJ, Goedert JJ 2000 Human papillomavirus-associated cancers in patients with human immunodeficiency virus infection and acquired immunodeficiency syndrome. Journal of the National Cancer Institute 92: 1500–1510.

FUTURE II Study Group 2007 Quadrivalent vaccine against human papillomavirus to prevent high-grade cervical lesions. New England Journal of Medicine 356(19):1915–1927.

Gagnon A, Ye B 2008 Discovery and application of protein biomarkers for ovarian cancer. Current Opinions in Obstetrics and Gynecology 20: 9–13.

Garcia M, Jemal A, Ward EM et al 2007 Global Cancer Facts & Figures 2007. American Cancer Society, Atlanta, GA.

Garland SM, Hernandez-Avila M, Wheeler CM et al 2007 Quadrivalent vaccine against human papillomavirus to prevent anogenital diseases. New England Journal of Medicine 356: 1928–1943.

Gates MA, Tworoger SS, Terry KL et al 2008 Talc use, variants of the GSTM1, GSTT1, and NAT2 genes, and risk of epithelial ovarian cancer. Cancer Epidemiology, Biomarkers and Prevention 17: 2436–2444.

Grady D, Gebretsadik T, Kerlikowske K, Ernster V, Petitti D 1995 Hormone replacement therapy and endometrial cancer risk: a meta-analysis. Obstetrics and Gynecology 85: 304–313.

Gram IT, Braaten T, Adami HO, Lund E, Weiderpass E 2008 Cigarette smoking and risk of borderline and invasive epithelial ovarian cancer. International Journal of Cancer 122: 647–652.

Granstrom C, Sundquist J, Hemminki K 2008 Population attributable fractions for ovarian cancer in Swedish women by morphological type. British Journal of Cancer 98: 199–205.

Greenwald P, Barlow JJ, Nasca PC, Burnett WS 1971 Vaginal cancer after maternal treatment with synthetic estrogens. New England Journal of Medicine 285: 390–392.

Grulich AE, van Leeuwen MT, Falster MO, Vajdic CM 2007 Incidence of cancers in people with HIV/AIDS compared with immunosuppressed transplant recipients: a meta-analysis. The Lancet 370: 59–67.

Hampl M, Sarajuuri H, Wentzensen N, Bender HG, Kueppers V 2006 Effect of human papillomavirus vaccines on vulvar, vaginal, and anal intraepithelial lesions and vulvar cancer. Obstetrics and Gynecology 108: 1361–1368.

Hampl M, Deckers-Figiel S, Hampl JA, Rein D, Bender HG 2008 New aspects of vulvar cancer: changes in localization and age of onset. Gynecological Oncology 109: 340–345.

Harper DM, Franco EL, Wheeler CM et al 2006 Sustained efficacy up to 4.5 years of a bivalent L1 virus-like particle vaccine against human papillomavirus types 16 and 18: follow-up from a randomised control trial. Lancet 367: 1247–1255.

Hatch EE, Palmer JR, Titus-Ernstoff L et al 1998 Cancer risk in women exposed to diethylstilbestrol in utero. JAMA: the Journal of the American Medical Association 280: 630–634.

Hildesheim A, Han CL, Brinton LA, Kurman RJ, Schiller JT 1997 Human papillomavirus type 16 and risk of preinvasive and invasive vulvar cancer: results from a seroepidemiological case–control study. Obstetrics and Gynecology 90: 748–754.

Hildesheim A, Herrero R, Wacholder S et al 2007 Effect of human papillomavirus 16/18 L1 viruslike particle vaccine among young women with preexisting infection: a randomized trial. JAMA: the Journal of the American Medical Association 298: 743–753.

Ho GY, Burk RD, Klein S et al 1995 Persistent genital human papillomavirus infection as a risk factor for persistent cervical dysplasia. Journal of the National Cancer Institute 87: 1365–1371.

Horner MJ, Ries LAG, Krapcho M et al (eds) 2008 SEER Cancer Statistics Review 1975–2006. National Cancer Institute, Bethesda, MD.

Huncharek M, Geschwind JF, Kupelnick B 2003 Perineal application of cosmetic talc and risk of invasive epithelial ovarian cancer: a meta-analysis of 11,933 subjects from sixteen observational studies. Anticancer Research 23: 1955–1960.

IARC Handbooks of Cancer Prevention 2003 Fruit and Vegetables. IARC Press, Lyon.

IARC Monographs 2007 Human Papillomaviruses. IARC Monographs on the Evaluation of Carcinogenic Risks to Humans. IARC Press, Lyon.

International Collaboration of Epidemiological Studies of Cervical Cancer 2006 Cervical carcinoma and reproductive factors: collaborative reanalysis of individual data on 16,563 women with cervical carcinoma and 33,542 women without cervical carcinoma from 25 epidemiological studies. International Journal of Cancer 119: 1108–1124.

Jacobs IJ, Skates SJ, MacDonald N et al 1999 Screening for ovarian cancer: a pilot randomised controlled trial. The Lancet 353: 1207–1210.

Jordan SJ, Whiteman DC, Purdie DM, Green AC, Webb PM 2006 Does smoking increase risk of ovarian cancer? A systematic review. Gynecological Oncology 103: 1122–1129.

Joura EA, Losch A, Haider-Angeler MG, Breitenecker G, Leodolter S 2000 Trends in vulvar neoplasia. Increasing incidence of vulvar intraepithelial neoplasia and squamous cell carcinoma of the vulva in young women. Journal of Reproductive Medicine 45: 613–615.

Kapeu AS, Luostarinen T, Jellum E et al 2009 Is smoking an independent risk factor for invasive cervical cancer? A nested case–control study within Nordic biobanks. American Journal of Epidemiology 169: 480–488.

Kashyap S, Moher D, Fung MF, Rosenwaks Z 2004 Assisted reproductive technology and the incidence of ovarian cancer: a meta-analysis. Obstetrics and Gynecology 103: 785–794.

Kitchener HC 2008 Survival from cancer of the ovary in England and Wales up to 2001. British Journal of Cancer 99 (Suppl 1): S73–S74.

Lukanova A, Zeleniuch-Jacquotte A, Lundin E et al 2004 Prediagnostic levels of C-peptide, IGF-I, IGFBP -1, -2 and -3 and risk of endometrial cancer. International Journal of Cancer 108: 262–268.

Madeleine MM, Daling JR, Carter JJ et al 1997 Cofactors with human papillomavirus in a population-based study of vulvar cancer. Journal of the National Cancer Institute 89: 1516–1523.

Magnusson PK, Sparen P, Gyllensten UB 1999 Genetic link to cervical tumours. Nature 400: 29–30.

Mao C, Koutsky LA, Ault KA et al 2006 Efficacy of human papillomavirus-16 vaccine to prevent cervical intraepithelial neoplasia: a randomized controlled trial. Obstetrics and Gynecology 107: 18–27.

McCredie MR, Sharples KJ, Paul C et al 2008 Natural history of cervical neoplasia and risk of invasive cancer in women with cervical intraepithelial neoplasia 3: a retrospective cohort study. The Lancet Oncology 9: 425–434.

McIndoe WA, McLean MR, Jones RW, Mullins PR 1984 The invasive potential of carcinoma in situ of the cervix. Obstetrics and Gynecology 64: 451–458.

Menon U 2004 Ovarian cancer screening. CMAJ: Canadian Medical Association Journal 171: 323–324.

Menon U, Gentry-Maharaj A, Hallett R et al 2009 Sensitivity and specificity of multimodal and ultrasound screening for ovarian cancer, and stage distribution of detected cancers: results of the prevalence screen of the UK Collaborative Trial of Ovarian Cancer Screening (UKCTOCS). The Lancet Oncology 10: 327–340.

Merritt MA, Green AC, Nagle CM, Webb PM 2008 Talcum powder, chronic pelvic inflammation and NSAIDs in relation to risk of epithelial ovarian cancer. International Journal of Cancer 122: 170–176.

Meyer LA, Broaddus RR, Lu KH 2009 Endometrial cancer and Lynch syndrome: clinical and pathologic considerations. Cancer Control 16: 14–22.

Moscicki AB, Shiboski S, Hills NK et al 2004 Regression of low-grade squamous intra-epithelial lesions in young women. The Lancet 364: 1678–1683.

Nanda K, Mccrory DC, Myers ER et al 2000 Accuracy of the Papanicolaou test in screening for and follow-up of cervical cytologic abnormalities: a systematic review. Annals of Internal Medicine 132: 810–819.

Ness RB, Cramer DW, Goodman MT et al 2002 Infertility, fertility drugs, and ovarian cancer: a pooled analysis of case–control studies. American Journal of Epidemiology 155: 217–224.

Office for National Statistics 2006 Cancer Statistics Registrations. Series MB1 No. 34. Office for National Statistics, London.

Office for National Statistics 2008 Cancer survival, England, patients diagnosed 2001–2006 and followed up to 2007: one year and five-year survival for 21 common cancers, by sex and age. Cancer Survival Trends. SMPS No. 61. Office for National Statistics, London.

Östör AG 1993 Natural history of cervical intraepithelial neoplasia: a critical review. International Journal of Gynecological Pathology 12: 186–192.

Paavonen J, Jenkins D, Bosch FX et al 2007 Efficacy of a prophylactic adjuvanted bivalent L1 virus-like-particle vaccine against infection with human papillomavirus types 16 and 18 in young women: an interim analysis of a phase III double-blind, randomised controlled trial. Lancet 369: 2161–2170.

Paavonen J, Naud P, Salmeron J et al 2009 Final phase III efficacy analysis of cervarix in young women. Abstract O-29.06. 25th International Papilloma Virus Conference, Malmo.

Penn I 1986 Cancers of the anogenital region in renal transplant recipients. Analysis of 65 cases. Cancer 58: 611–616.

Pike MC, Pearce CL, Wu AH 2004 Prevention of cancers of the breast, endometrium and ovary. Oncogene 23: 6379–6391.

Ries LAG, Eisner MP, Kosary CL et al (eds) 2001 SEER Cancer Statistics Review, 1973–1998. National Cancer Intitute, Bethesda, MD.

Rifai N, Gillette MA, Carr SA 2006 Protein biomarker discovery and validation: the long and uncertain path to clinical utility. Nature Biotechnology 24: 971–983.

Sankaranarayanan R, Nene BM, Shastri SS et al 2009 HPV screening for cervical cancer in rural India. New England Journal of Medicine 360: 1385–1394.

Sasieni PD, Adams J, Cuzick J 1997 Trends in gynaecological cancers in England and Wales. Journal of Epidemiology and Biostatistics 2: 187–195.

Sasieni PD, Adams J 2000 Analysis of cervical cancer mortality and incidence data from England and Wales: evidence of a beneficial effect of screening. Journal of the Royal Statistics Society Series A, Issue 163: 191–209.

Sasieni P, Castanon A, Cuzick J 2009 Screening and adenocarcinoma of the cervix. International Journal of Cancer 125: 525–529.

Schouten LJ, Goldbohm RA, van den Brandt PA 2004 Anthropometry, physical activity, and endometrial cancer risk: results from the Netherlands Cohort Study. Journal of the National Cancer Institute 96: 1635–1638.

Schouten LJ, Rivera C, Hunter DJ et al 2008 Height, body mass index, and ovarian cancer: a pooled analysis of 12 cohort studies. Cancer Epidemiology, Biomarkers and Prevention 17: 902–912.

Smith JS, Lindsay L, Hoots B et al 2007 Human papillomavirus type distribution in invasive cervical cancer and high-grade cervical lesions: a meta-analysis update. International Journal of Cancer 121: 621–632.

Titus-Ernstoff L, Perez K, Cramer DW, Harlow BL, Baron JA, Greenberg ER 2001 Menstrual and reproductive factors in relation to ovarian cancer risk. British Journal of Cancer 84: 714–721.

Trimble CL, Hildesheim A, Brinton LA, Shah KV, Kurman RJ 1996 Heterogeneous etiology of squamous carcinoma of the vulva. Obstetrics and Gynecology 87: 59–64.

US Cancer Statistics Working Group 2009 United States Cancer Statistics: 1999–2005 Incidence and Mortality Web-based Report. US Department of Health and Human Services, Centers for Disease Control and Prevention, and National Cancer Institute, Atlanta, GA.

Vaino F, Bianchini F (eds) 2002 IARC Handbooks of Cancer Prevention: Weight Control and Physical Activity. IARC Press, Lyon.

van Ballegooijen M, van den Akker-van Marle ME, Warmerdam PG, Meijer CJ, Walboomers JM, Habbema JD 1997 Present evidence on the value of HPV testing for cervical cancer screening: a model-based exploration of the (cost-) effectiveness. British Journal of Cancer 76: 651–657.

Villa LL, Costa RL, Petta CA et al 2005 Prophylactic quadrivalent human papillomavirus (types 6, 11, 16, and 18 L1 virus-like particle vaccine in young women: a randomised double-blind placebo-controlled multicentre phase II efficacy trial. The Lancet Oncology 6: 271–278.

Viswanathan AN, Feskanich D, de Vivo I et al 2005 Smoking and the risk of endometrial cancer: results from the Nurses' Health Study. International Journal of Cancer 114: 996–1001.

Voskuil DW, Monninkhof EM, Elias SG, Vlems FA, van Leeuwen FE 2007 Physical activity and endometrial cancer risk, a systematic review of current evidence. Cancer Epidemiology, Biomarkers and Prevention 16: 639–648.

Walboomers JM, Jacobs MV, Manos MM et al 1999 Human papillomavirus is a necessary cause of invasive cervical cancer worldwide. Journal of Pathology 189: 12–19.

Weiderpass E, Persson I, Adami HO, Magnusson C, Lindgren A, Baron JA 2000 Body size in different periods of life, diabetes mellitus, hypertension, and risk of postmenopausal endometrial cancer (Sweden). Cancer Causes and Control 11: 185–192.

Whittemore AS, Harris R, Itnyre J 1992 Characteristics relating to ovarian cancer risk: collaborative analysis of 12 US case–control studies. IV. The pathogenesis of epithelial ovarian cancer. Collaborative Ovarian Cancer Group. American Journal of Epidemiology 136: 1212–1220.

WHO/ICO Information Centre on Human Papilloma Virus (HPV) and Cervical Cancer 2007 Human Papillomavirus and Cervical Cancer [cited 17 April 2009]; available from: http://www.who.int/hpvcentre/en.

Xu WH, Matthews CE, Xiang YB et al 2005 Effect of adiposity and fat distribution on endometrial cancer risk in Shanghai women. American Journal of Epidemiology 161: 939–947.

Zhou B, Sun Q, Cong R et al 2008 Hormone replacement therapy and ovarian cancer risk: a meta-analysis. Gynecologic Oncology 108: 641–651.

CHAPTER 35

The genetics and molecular biology of gynaecological cancer

Martin Widschwendter, Simon Gayther and Ian J. Jacobs

Chapter Contents

INTRODUCTION	522
MOLECULAR BASIS OF CARCINOGENESIS	523
GENETICS OF FAMILIAL GYNAECOLOGICAL CANCER	526
MANAGEMENT OF FAMILIAL GYNAECOLOGICAL CANCER	528
MOLECULAR GENETICS OF SPORADIC GYNAECOLOGICAL CANCER	529
CLINICAL ASPECTS OF THE GENETICS OF GYNAECOLOGICAL CANCER	535
KEY POINTS	536

Introduction

Enormous progress has been made in understanding the molecular basis of disease during the last decade, and this has transformed our understanding of the process of carcinogenesis. In recent years, these developments have started to have an impact in gynaecological cancer. Although the details of molecular research and technology are frequently complex and often of limited relevance to clinicians, the underlying principles provide a coherent and comprehensible framework of the process of carcinogenesis. The fundamental understanding of the process of carcinogenesis achieved using molecular technology provides exciting opportunities for the prevention, early detection and treatment of cancer. Molecular knowledge has not yet had a major impact in clinical oncology, but the potential impact is clear and is likely to emerge during the next decade.

During the past century, human cancers have been categorized by their microscopic appearance (histology), and each category has been linked to a certain clinical behaviour and prognostic significance. However, cancer patients with similar histological tumour types and stage of disease may have a different clinical outcome. It has become clear that biological diversity of tumours cannot be explained by microscopic appearance alone. The current focus of profiling tumours is the large-scale analysis of gene expression using new DNA microarray technology. By surveying thousands of genes at once, it is now possible to read the molecular signature of an individual patient's tumour. Analysing these complex data sets might introduce new tumour classes. The ultimate goal is to move beyond standard tumour classification to achieve more detailed insight into the biological aggressiveness of tumours, and to develop more specific potential therapeutic targets (e.g. gene therapy). It will,

therefore, become increasingly important for clinicians involved in the management of gynaecological malignancies to have a working knowledge of the molecular basis of carcinogenesis.

Gynaecological cancers provide examples of a number of contrasting mechanisms of carcinogenesis (Figure 35.1). For example, ovarian and endometrial cancer can occur as components of familial cancer syndromes (familial breast/ovarian cancer and Lynch II syndrome) due to germline inheritance of predisposing genetic abnormalities. However, most ovarian cancers are not thought to be due to inherited genetic alterations, but result from somatic mutations occurring in ovarian cells with an initially normal genome. These somatic mutations are thought to be secondary to environmental factors that act to increase the opportunity for spontaneous mutation in a number of critical genes. One of the genetic alterations that lead to cervical cancer is caused by an environmental factor, human papilloma virus (HPV), and in at least some endometrial cancers, unopposed oestrogen exposure or hyperinsulinism leads to carcinogenesis. High-risk subtypes of HPV are much less common in vulval cancer. This suggests that vulval and cervical carcinomas are not identical aetiologically, and that factors other than HPV are more important in vulval carcinogenesis. There is recent evidence that different genetic events occur between HPV-positive and -negative vulval cancers, with a greater number of molecular alterations in HPV-negative vulval cancers compared with HPV-positive tumours (Flowers et al 1999). HPV-positive vulval cancers are more frequently found in younger patients. Vulval cancers in older patients are more often HPV negative, and more frequently show allelic loss of the *TP53* gene.

The histological features, and biological and clinical behaviour of fallopian tube cancers are similar to those of

DOI: 10.1016/B978-0-7020-3120-5.00035-7

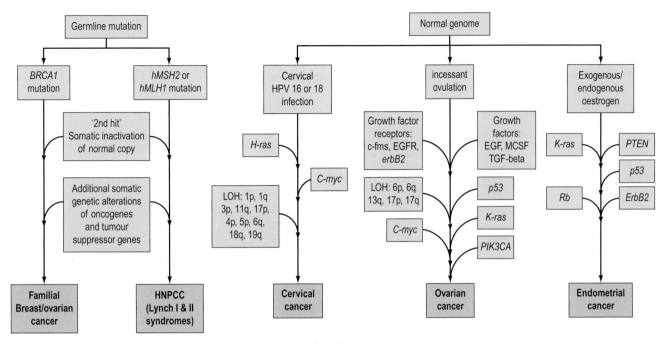

Figure 35.1 Pathways of carcinogenesis in familial and sporadic gynaecological cancer.

ovarian cancer. In addition, there is evidence that similar genetic alterations occur with the same frequency in fallopian tube and ovarian cancers of the same histological subtype. This suggests a common molecular pathogenesis between these cancer types (Levanon et al 2008).

To date, little is known about the molecular genetics of vaginal cancer.

Molecular Basis of Carcinogenesis

A fundamental characteristic of cancer cells is loss of the normal restraints controlling cell division, cell-to-cell interaction and cellular mobility. The fact that this characteristic is passed on to cells arising from the division of cancer cells has long been regarded as evidence for a genetic basis for carcinogenesis, and is supported by a number of other observations. First, agents which cause damage to DNA (chemical mutagens, ionizing radiation and some viruses) also increase susceptibility to cancer. Second, studies of the clonal origin of tumours indicate that the vast majority of cancers arise from a single cell which passes on its abnormality to daughter cells. An initial genetic alteration provides a selective advantage for proliferation of a clone of cells, and further genetic alterations within this expanded population of cells increase the selective proliferative advantage and eventually lead to the formation of a clinically recognizable tumour.

During the last decade, it has become clear that the genetic changes in cancer involve genes which control normal cell growth and proliferation. Cells communicate via a complex interacting set of signalling pathways, the principles of which, unlike the details, are well established (Figure 35.2). The best understood mechanism of communication between cells is via the release of molecules which interact as agonists with receptors either within the cell or, more frequently, in

the cell membrane. This interaction results in a further signal within the cell which, via transducer proteins and secondary mechanisms, results in modified cell behaviour either by activating already synthesized target enzymes directly or by initiating transcription of genes and synthesis of their protein product. The genetic abnormalities observed in cancer are known to affect genes coding for all of the groups of molecules in Figure 35.2.

Oncogenes

The identification of oncogenes resulted from in-vitro and animal work with virus-induced cancers. As the viral genome is relatively small, it was possible to identify the specific genes (viral oncogenes) involved in the transforming activity of retroviruses, such as the Rous sarcoma virus. It was possible to identify homologous genes in normal cells, and a number of viral oncogenes were found to have normal cellular homologues known as 'proto-oncogenes'. Other workers identified oncogenes by transfecting cell lines with DNA from human cancer cell lines, and found that some of the transforming oncogenes identified were mutated versions of the proto-oncogene identified by the retroviral approach. Subsequently, it was demonstrated that chromosome translocations such as the Philadelphia chromosome in chronic myeloid leukaemia involved known oncogenes (de Klein et al 1982).

Approximately 100 proto-oncogenes have been identified, and many can be assigned to the groups of functions summarized in Figure 35.2. The mutation resulting in conversion of a proto-oncogene into an oncogene may occur in several different ways (Figure 35.3), and may result in an abnormal protein produced in a normal quantity, a normal protein produced in an excessive amount, or a normal protein produced inappropriately due to loss or alteration of control regions of the gene.

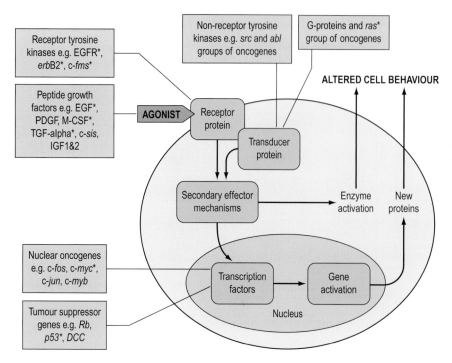

Figure 35.2 An overview of the role of oncogenes and tumour suppressor genes in the control of cell growth and proliferation. The purpose of this figure is to emphasize that the genetic abnormalities in cancer are a result of alterations to or abnormal expression of genes which are normally involved in cell regulation. Genes which are implicated in ovarian carcinogenesis are marked with an asterisk. Note that many aspects of the figure are oversimplified for clarity; for example, although a function of *p53* and *Rb* is transcriptional regulation, this is not true of all tumour suppressor genes.

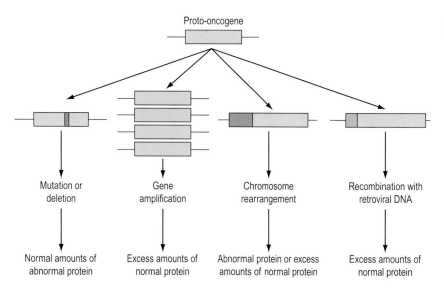

Figure 35.3 A summary of the mechanisms of activation of oncogenes.

Tumour suppressor genes

The existence of tumour suppressor genes was suggested by cell fusion studies of transformed cells and non-transformed cells which resulted in a non-transformed hybrid cell. The subsequent identification of the first tumour suppressor gene followed from the study of retinoblastoma, a rare childhood cancer which may occur in a hereditary and sporadic form. On the basis of epidemiological and statistical analysis, Knudson suggested that development of the cancer required two events. He postulated that in the hereditary form, the first event was a germline mutation present in every cell of the individual, and that a second event in any of the many million retinoblasts could result in tumour formation. The rarity, later onset and unilateral nature of the sporadic form could be attributed to the need for two events in a single retinal cell in the absence of a germline mutation. When the retinoblastoma (*Rb*) gene was mapped to chromosome 13q and cloned, it was confirmed that in both familial and sporadic retinoblastoma, the two copies of the gene were inactivated in tumour cells, consistent with Knudson's 'two-hit' hypothesis (Cavenee et al 1983).

Knudson's hypothesis that two hits are required for the full inactivation of a tumour suppressor gene has been shown to be fundamentally correct in almost all cases of human cancer. However, the fact that methylation of CpG islands located in the promoters of genes can cause transcriptional silencing, coupled with the observation that DNA methylation patterns are perturbed in cancer cells, has led to the suggestion that abnormal methylation of the promoters of tumour suppressor genes might be implicated in carcinogenesis, and can serve as a third pathway to inactivation of

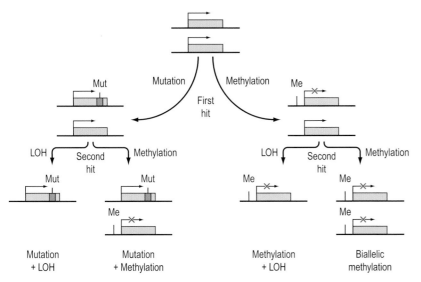

Figure 35.4 Besides loss of heterozygosity (LOH) and mutations (mut), DNA methylation (Me) is the third possibility to inactivate a tumour suppressor gene. *Source: From Nature Genetics, Laird and Jones; Cancer-epigenetics comes of age; 21: 163–7; 1999.*

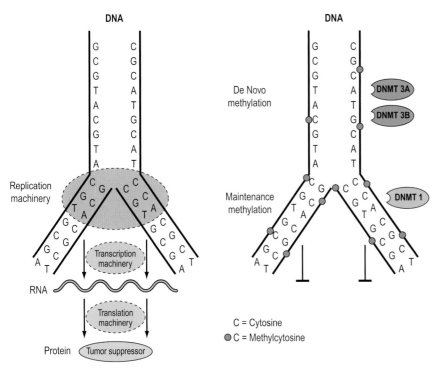

Figure 35.5 DNA methylation and regulation of gene activity. Genes without methylation at their 5′ region can be transcribed into RNA and translated into protein (e.g. tumour suppressing proteins). De-novo DNA methyltransferases (DNMT3A and 3B) inititate methylation of cytosines which are located in front of a guanosine (CpGs), and the maintenance DNA methyltransferase (DNMT1) ensures that once a cytosine is methylated, it will become methylated immediately after cell division. Methylated genes attract proteins which modify the chromatin and therefore suppress the expression of these genes.

a tumour suppressor gene (Figure 35.4) (Jones and Laird 1999).

Epigenetics and DNA methylation in cancer

As outlined above, aberrant gene function and altered patterns of gene expression are key features of cancer. Growing evidence shows that acquired epigenetic abnormalities participate with genetic alterations to cause this dysregulation. The modern definition of epigenetics is modifications of the DNA or associated proteins, other than DNA sequence variation, that carry information content during cell division. The best understood example of epigenetic modification is DNA methylation, a covalent addition of a methyl group derived from S-adenosyl-L-methionine to the fifth carbon of the cytosine ring to form the fifth base, 5-methylcytosine (5meC) (Laird 2003, Jones and Baylin 2007). The reaction is catalysed by DNA methyltransferases together with accessory proteins. Among all eukaryotic species, methylation occurs predominantly in cytosines located 5′ of guanines, and known as 'CpG dinucleotides' (CpGs). In the mammalian genome, the distribution of CpGs is far from random. CpGs are greatly under-represented in the genome through evolutionary loss of 5meC through deamination to thymine. However, clusters of CpGs known as 'CpG islands' (CGIs) are present in 1–2% of the genome. Typically, they range in length from 200 to 5000 base pairs (bp). Most are unmethylated under normal circumstances, with the exception of those associated with imprinted genes, genes subjected to X-chromosome inactivation and transposable elements. In this last respect, DNA methylation is thought to repress faulty expression of endogenous transposons that may disrupt the genome. It is also involved in the parental-specific silencing of one allele of imprinted genes. In addition, approximately 70% of CGIs are associated with DNA sequences 200–2000 bp long found in the promoter, the first and second exons, and the first intron regions of all genes (5′ CGIs). This suggests that CGIs are critical in gene regulation. There is, for instance, usually an inverse relationship between the degree of methylation of a regulatory CGI and the extent of gene transcription (Figure 35.5) (Laird 2003, Jones and Baylin 2007).

DNA methylation patterns are established during defined phases in embryonic development. With the exception of imprinted genes, gamete methylation patterns are erased by a genome-wide demethylation at around the eight-cell stage of blastocyst formation. During the implantation stage, methylation patterns are re-established via de-novo methylation. During adulthood, the degree and patterns of methylation are both tissue- and cell-type specific. Disruption of these preset patterns of DNA methylation in adult life has been linked to ageing and to disease. Furthermore, dysregulation of developmental programming by maternal factors or environmental mimics is thought to induce abnormal DNA methylation of specific genes and hence their faulty expression, leading to disease (Laird 2003, Jones and Baylin 2007).

Over the last decade, the importance of epigenetic gene regulation has become increasingly evident as studies have shown that each epithelial tumour only contains approximately 10–15 tumour suppressor genes silenced through mutations, but several hundred silenced through DNA methylation (Jones and Baylin 2007, Thomas et al 2007). Numerous genes involved in central pathways can be silenced by means of DNA methylation (Figure 35.3).

Germline and somatic genetic alterations

A common feature of tumours is that they accumulate somatic genetic changes during the development of the cancer. A proportion of cancers may also develop as a result of germline mutations in cancer predisposing genes. An important distinction must be made between germline and somatic mutations. Somatic mutations are found in the tumour cells but not the normal cells of an individual with cancer, and cannot therefore be passed on to descendants through the germline. Germline mutations, however, are present in all the cells of the individual and can initiate tumour development. They can be passed on to descendants of the individual, and can be identified in DNA obtained from all diploid cell populations (e.g. peripheral blood samples) and not just the tissues that are susceptible to disease. It is worth pointing out that the same genes mutated in the germline are also frequently mutated in the somatic cells of a cancer, which suggests a functional significance for specific genes in cancer development. For example, mutations of the *p53* gene are one of the most common genetic changes found in human cancer. In most cancers, *p53* mutations occur as somatic events, but germline *p53* mutations are often found in patients from families with the rare Li-Fraumeni syndrome, which is characterized by sarcomas, breast cancer and other malignancies occurring at a young

age. Another example is the colorectal cancer predisposition syndrome, familial adenomatous polyposis (FAP), caused by germline mutations in the *APC* gene (Kinzler et al 1991). The FAP syndrome is responsible for approximately 1% of all colorectal cancers, but somatic mutations of *APC* have been detected in over 80% of sporadic colorectal cancers and appear to be one of the earliest events in colorectal carcinogenesis.

Most of the familial cancer syndromes identified to date are rare, single gene disorders and have an autosomal-dominant pattern of inheritance. Individuals inheriting the germline abnormality are generally at high risk of developing malignancy because the penetrance of most of these genes is of the order of 80%. Another class of cancer predisposition genes that confer more modest penetrance has been identified recently. Although these genes are associated with much lower penetrance, they are also much more common in the population than the rare high-risk genes, and so are probably responsible for a greater proportion of cancer overall (reviewed in Easton and Eeles 2008). However, the identification of individuals in the population that are likely to carry these low penetrance genes is not easy because they are not often associated with a significant family history of disease.

Genetics of Familial Gynaecological Cancer

Although there are anecdotal reports of more than one case of vulval cancer occurring in close relatives, there is no good evidence of inherited predisposition to this disease. For cervical cancer, the absence of any obvious clustering of multiple cases within families suggests that no highly penetrant susceptibility loci for the disease await identification. However, population-based epidemiological studies suggest that shared genetic factors do play a role in the development of cervical cancer, and possibly account for approximately 27% of cases. This perhaps suggests the presence of several common genetic variants that confer low penetrance disease risk. Ovarian and endometrial cancers occur as part of well-defined cancer family syndromes with an autosomal-dominant inheritance pattern. Pedigree studies of cancer within families have revealed three main syndromes associated with ovarian cancer. The most common hereditary form of ovarian cancer occurs in association with breast cancer. A large number of hereditary breast/ovarian cancer families have been described in which there is a high frequency of both cancers and an association with an early age of onset. Hereditary ovarian cancer may also occur as a site-specific disease, although genetic studies suggest that a large proportion of site-specific ovarian and breast/ovarian cancer families are part of the same disease spectrum. Nevertheless, there remains evidence that there is a rare genetic component that confers high penetrance susceptibility specifically to ovarian cancer (reviewed in Ramus and Gayther 2009). Less frequently, ovarian cancer occurs in hereditary non-polyposis colorectal cancer (HNPCC) families, and germline genetic mutations in highly penetrant genes that cause HNPCC have been found in ovarian cancer cases from these families. Women from HNPCC families most frequently develop colorectal or endometrial cancer, and this is the syndrome most commonly associated with genetic predisposition to endometrial cancer. Some families have recently been described with an apparently high risk of site-specific endometrial cancer. It is important to recognize that when all of these familial syndromes are combined, they are probably responsible for less than 5% of ovarian cancer cases and a smaller proportion of endometrial cancer cases.

The *BRCA1* and *BRCA2* genes

The identification and detailed pedigree-based descriptions of families at high risk of breast and ovarian cancer, together with the development of polymorphic DNA markers, made it possible to perform detailed linkage analysis with the aim of locating genes involved in familial cancer. A major step forward was the report of linkage of early-onset breast cancer to the polymorphic marker CMM86 located on chromosome 17q (Hall et al 1990). Subsequently, linkage to 17q in 214 families was confirmed by a consortium of 13 research groups from Europe and the USA (Easton et al 1993). Almost all breast/ovarian cancer families and 40% of families with breast cancer alone were found to have a linkage with the *BRCA1* (Breast Cancer 1) locus on chromosome 17q. Subsequently, the consortium localized the gene to a 2cM region on 17q, and in 1994, a group in Utah described a large gene on 17q within which they had identified mutations in five affected families (Miki et al 1994). Subsequent work by other research groups has confirmed that this gene is the *BRCA1* gene, and over 12,000 carriers of a *BRCA1* mutation have now been described in breast/ovarian cancer families and cancer cases unselected for a family history [described on the Breast Cancer Information Core (BIC) database: http://research.nhgri.nih.gov/bic/].

BRCA1 is a large gene with 22 exons encoding a protein of 1863 amino acids. There are no specific hotspots for mutation in the gene, and only a small proportion of mutations are recurrent. Overall, the penetrance of a *BRCA1* mutation for ovarian cancer and breast cancer appears to be 40–50% and 80%, respectively Ford et al 1994, 1998). However, there is evidence that penetrance may be modified by both environmental factors and other genetic influences. Furthermore, the location of a mutation within the *BRCA1* gene may influence both the overall risk of cancer and the type of cancer. Gayther et al (1995') reported a correlation between mutations toward the 3' end of the gene and a greater risk of ovarian cancer than breast cancer. Well-defined founder mutations have been described in *BRCA1*. Mutations at 185delAG and 5382insC have been documented in approximately 1% of Ashkenazi Jewish cancers, and up to 40% of Ashkenazi Jewish women with ovarian cancer or early-onset breast cancer. Identification of *BRCA2* closely followed the cloning of *BRCA1*. Wooster et al (1995) identified the gene following studies involving high-risk families in which the disease pattern was not linked to *BRCA1*.

BRCA2, located on chromosome 13q, is also a large gene with 26 coding exons encoding a protein with 3418 amino acids. More than 11,000 mutation carriers have been described to date (the BIC database). As for *BRCA1*, there are no hotspots for mutation, although there are founder mutations in some ethnic groups such as Ashkenazi Jews (Levy-Lahad et al 1997, Thorlacius et al 1997). Although the penetrance for breast cancer is approximately 80%, the penetrance for ovarian cancer seems to be lower than that for *BRCA1* mutations at approximately 25% (Ford et al 1998).

There is a suggestion that mutations in exon 11 confer a higher risk of ovarian cancer than mutations in other areas (Gayther et al 1997). This has been confirmed in a more recent meta-analysis (reviewed in Ramus and Gayther 2009). Overall, *BRCA1* and *BRCA2* are believed to account for over 95% of hereditary cases of ovarian cancer and over 80% of hereditary cases of breast cancers.

The functions of *BRCA1* and *BRCA2* are still unclear. Most of the mutations of *BRCA1* are small insertions or deletions, which result in loss of protein synthesis or production of a truncated protein. This observation supports the concept that *BRCA1* functions as a tumour suppressor gene. In this 'two-hit' model, although one copy of the gene is inherited as an inactive mutant form, the development of cancer requires somatic mutation of the other wild-type ('normal') gene copy. Analysis of tumours from familial breast/ovarian cancer families has demonstrated that loss of heterozygosity (LOH) in these tumours involves the wild-type gene, thus providing further evidence that the *BRCA1* gene is a tumour suppressor (Smith et al 1992). Both *BRCA1* and *BRCA2* are expressed in the largest amounts in the testis and thymus, and at lower levels in the breast and ovary. Although the genes have limited sequence homology, they do have similarities including being A-T rich, having a large exon 11 with the start of translation at codon 2. The presence of a zinc finger motif in *BRCA1* has suggested a role as a transcription factor, whilst *BRCA2* has homology with known transcription factors. However, the most compelling functional evidence indicates that *BRCA1* and *BRCA2* both play a major role in homologous and non-homologous DNA double-strand break (DSB) repair through their interaction with the RAD51 DSB protein. It is still not known why abrogation of such a ubiquitous cellular function should predispose individuals specifically to breast and ovarian cancer.

HNPCC-associated gynaecological cancer and DNA repair genes

HNPCC is associated with autosomal-dominant inheritance of colorectal cancer in those who do not have the multiple adenomas which occur in FAP. The identification of the genetic basis of Lynch II syndrome is a notable example of the power of molecular technology. HNPCC was classified by Henry Lynch into site-specific hereditary colon cancer (Lynch I syndrome), and families with a predisposition to non-polyposis colorectal cancer in association with other cancers including stomach, small bowel, ureter, renal pelvis and brain, as well as ovarian and endometrial cancer (Lynch II syndrome) (Lynch 1985). The identification of the genes responsible for HNPCC was a result of several developments which showed that HNPCC is associated with hereditary defects in one of five DNA mismatch repair genes [mutS homolog 2 (*MSH2*), mutL homolog 1 (*MLH1*), postmeiotic segregation increased 1 (*PMS1*), postmeiotic segregation increased 2 (*PMS2*) and mutS homolog 6/G/T mismatch-binding protein (*MSH6/GTBP*)]. Hundreds of mutations have been identified in these five genes in HNPCC families, making mutation testing a difficult challenge in these families (Lynch and de la Chapelle 1999). Available evidence suggests that these genes function as tumour suppressor genes in a manner consistent with Knudson's 'two-hit' model. The inherited germline mutation inactivates one copy of the mismatch repair gene, but inactivation of the remaining wild-type copy by a second somatic mutation is required prior to tumour formation. The secondary, acquired mutations which result from loss of DNA repair gene function include defects of *APC*, *K-ras*, *DPC4* and *p53* (Huang et al 1996, Kinzler and Vogelstein 1996). The penetrance for colorectal cancer in mutation carriers is in excess of 80% in men and 30% in women, and HNPCC accounts for approximately 5% of colorectal cancers (Dunlop et al 1997, Aarnio et al 1999, Salovaara et al 2000). Endometrial cancer is the second most common cancer in HNPCC families, with female carriers having a 42% risk by 70 years of age (Dunlop et al 1997). The penetrance for ovarian cancer is less, with a reported lifetime risk of 9% (Marra and Roland 1995).

Management of Familial Gynaecological Cancer

Risk assessment

At present, risk assessment is based largely upon information derived from a detailed family tree. Important information includes the number of cases of cancer relative to the number of people at risk, the pattern of cancers of different types, and the age at diagnosis of cancer. For a number of reasons, risk assessment should ideally be undertaken in the setting of a multidisciplinary specialist familial cancer clinic run by a geneticist working with a team of genetic counsellors and with close links to specialists in areas such as gynaecological, colorectal and breast cancer. Obtaining a detailed family history and confirming the history with clinical and histopathological information is time consuming and requires an organization and resources specifically established for this purpose. The interpretation of family histories is not always straightforward, particularly when there are a variety of different primary sites in the family. Specialist training is required to counsel patients about the implications and consequences of genetic testing. Particular expertise is also required to provide the patient with sound advice about methods of prevention and screening.

Although it is difficult to precisely define the minimum family history necessary to satisfy the description of a familial cancer syndrome involving a gynaecological cancer, some broad guidelines can be outlined:

- families in which two first-degree relatives have ovarian cancer;
- families in which first-degree relatives have breast cancer at less than 50 years of age and ovarian cancer; and
- families in which two first-degree relatives have breast cancer at less than 60 years of age and a third relative has ovarian cancer.

The likelihood that the high frequency of cancer in such families is due to an inherited predisposition rather than a chance event is in excess of 60%. Families in which one relative has ovarian or endometrial cancer and two or more first-degree relatives have cancer of the colon/rectum, at least one at less than 50 years of age, can be classified as HNPCC families. Although the *BRCA1* gene and DNA repair genes have now been identified, there are still limitations in the

analysis of these genes for mutations in the clinical setting. The genes are large and the mutations are not localized to specific regions of the gene. Nevertheless, the availability and speed of techniques for the detection of mutations is improving rapidly. Mutation testing is now widely available for high-risk families via clinical genetics centres in the UK after thorough counselling about the implications of testing.

Prevention of familial cancer

Use of the oral contraceptive pill may be suggested for HNPCC and breast/ovarian cancer family members on the basis of case–control studies in the general population which indicate a protective effect against ovarian and endometrial cancer. While one study has suggested a protective effect of the oral contraceptive pill in *BRCA1* and *BRCA2* carriers, this was not confirmed in a second study and the situation remains unclear (Modan et al 2001). Furthermore, there is concern in breast/ovarian cancer families that a reduction in risk of ovarian cancer may be offset by an increased risk of breast cancer.

Prophylactic salpingo-oophorectomy and hysterectomy as a primary procedure is justifiable in women from breast/ovarian cancer and HNPCC families after completion of their family and after thorough counselling. There is convincing evidence that salpingo-oophorectomy is an effective method of prevention of cancer of the ovary, fallopian tube and breast. A recent meta-analysis (Rebbeck et al 2009) of all reports of preventative surgery in *BRCA1* and *BRCA2* mutation carriers from 1999 to 2007 revealed a reduction in risk of breast cancer (hazard ratio 0.49) and ovarian/fallopian tube cancer (hazard ratio 0.21). Women undergoing prophylactic surgery should be counselled that the procedure will prevent ovarian and tubal cancer, but that they may still be at risk of primary peritoneal cancer.

It should also be noted that cases of intra-abdominal carcinomatosis following oophorectomy have been reported in which subsequent review of the oophorectomy specimen revealed a small focus of ovarian cancer (Chen et al 1985). Surgery should therefore include a careful inspection of the abdomen and pelvis, and thorough histological examination of the ovary. Fallopian tube cancer does seem to be more common in *BRCA1* and *BRCA2* families, so prophylactic surgery should include salpingectomy. Hysterectomy should be advised for women from HNPCC families, but women from breast/ovarian cancer families do not appear to be at increased risk of endometrial cancer and the decision regarding hysterectomy will depend on other factors.

Screening for familial cancer

The efficacy of ovarian cancer screening is unproven to date, although a survival benefit was noted in a pilot randomized trial in the general population (Jacobs et al 1999). The preliminary results of the UK Collaborative Trial of Ovarian Cancer Screening (UKCTOCS), a larger randomized trial involving 202,000 postmenopausal women from the general population, are encouraging (Menon et al 2009) but there will not be definitive data on mortality impact until 2015. Although the value of ovarian cancer screening is therefore unclear, there is a consensus that it is reasonable to screen women from breast/ovarian cancer families with transvaginal ultrasonography and serum CA125 measurement in view of their level of risk. Screening is usually performed on an annual basis from the mid 30s or 5 years prior to the earliest age of onset of ovarian cancer in the family.

It should be noted that both CA125 and ultrasound are associated with a substantial risk of false-positive results, leading to unnecessary surgery (Campbell et al 1993, Jacobs et al 1993). It is essential to warn women clearly about this risk. The false-positive rate for both CA125 and ultrasonography is approximately 1–2% in postmenopausal women and higher in premenopausal women. It is therefore likely that a 30-year-old woman undergoing annual screening for up to 50 years will have a false-positive result at some stage, with consequent anxiety and the risk of unnecessary surgery.

Women from breast/ovarian cancer families may be advised to commence screening with mammography from the mid 30s or 5 years prior to the earliest age of onset of breast cancer in their family, although the value of mammography in premenopausal women is controversial. Women from HNPCC families should be advised to undergo regular colonoscopy and mammography in addition to ovarian cancer screening. Ultrasound screening for endometrial cancer has a significant false-positive rate and lack of evidence for a mortality benefit, but is often offered to this group of women because of the particularly high risk. Ultrasound measurement of endometrial thickness can be performed at the time of screening for ovarian size and morphology. It is reasonable to add an outpatient form of endometrial sampling, such as pipelle aspiration. These screening strategies are currently recommended on a pragmatic basis in view of the high risk of cancer, rather than on the basis of clear evidence concerning their efficacy.

Women with a family history not consistent with a familial syndrome

Most women who seek advice about a family history of gynaecological cancer have one affected first-degree relative and do not fall into a familial syndrome. Requests for advice from this group of women have increased dramatically following recent media publicity about screening for ovarian cancer and identification of the BRCA1 and BRCA2 genes. Although women with a first-degree relative with ovarian cancer are at increased risk compared with the general population, the absolute risk remains small. They should be reassured that although their risk of ovarian cancer may be increased several fold, it remains low (lifetime risk of 4–5% vs 1% in the general population). Screening with either CA125 or ultrasound should not be offered routinely on a population basis to these women for two reasons. First, an improvement in prognosis for ovarian cancer through detection by screening has not been demonstrated. Second, because the incidence of ovarian cancer in this population is relatively low, the risk of a false-positive result resulting in surgical investigation is likely to be more than 10 times that of a true positive result (i.e. the positive predictive value of screening is <10%). The value of screening for women in this group and for those without a family history awaits evaluation in the UKCTOCS trial. Oophorectomy should not be recommended as a primary procedure, but may be considered as a secondary procedure at the time of surgery for benign disease (e.g. hysterectomy).

Molecular Genetics of Sporadic Gynaecological Cancer

Cervical cancer

The histopathological progression of cervical neoplasia from mild to increasingly severe dysplasia and ultimately invasive cervical cancer is well described, as is the evidence for an association with HPV infection. HPV infection is a necessary but insufficient cause for cervical cancer. Infection with oncogenic types of HPV is very common, but most of these infections go unnoticed. Carcinogenesis is a very rare outcome of HPV infection and it clearly involves interactions of the host, the environment and the virus. During recent years, important progress has been made in understanding the mechanism of HPV-induced carcinogenesis and incorporating these findings with the principles of multistep carcinogenesis. HPVs form a group of more than 80 viruses, most of which give rise to benign tumours such as wart infections. The risk of cervical neoplasia is associated with particular HPV types (HPV 16 and 18) (zur Hausen 1987). The genomes of all HPVs have a similar organization which encodes eight major open reading frames encoding early (E1–7) and late (L1–2) viral proteins. It is the early proteins E6 and E7 which are responsible for the transforming activity of the virus (Whiteside et al 2008). The E6 and E7 proteins of high-risk HPV types (HPV 16 and 18), but not those of low-risk types, cause in-vitro changes which parallel the changes in cervical intraepithelial neoplasia (Whiteside et al 2008).

During a normal viral infection resulting in production and release of new virus, the viral genome exists episomally (closed circular DNA) without integration in the nucleus of the infected cell. In tumour cells, the viral DNA is integrated with the DNA of the host cell. Although the sites of integration of viral DNA are random in cancer cell lines and many of the viral genes are lost, the E6 and E7 viral open reading frames are always conserved and are the most abundant viral transcripts in such cell lines (Whiteside et al 2008). Furthermore, integration of E6 and E7 usually occurs in a manner which disrupts the normal viral regulation of expression of these proteins. These observations suggest that E6 and E7 have an important role in cervical carcinogenesis, and are supported by evidence that these proteins can interact with and inactivate several important cellular proteins. E7 binds to the product of the Rb tumour suppressor gene, interfering with normal protein complex formation and disrupting the normal function of Rb protein. E6 interacts with the protein product of the p53 tumour suppressor gene, causing rapid breakdown of the protein and loss of normal p53 function. The overall effect of E6 and E7 expression in the cell is therefore equivalent to loss of the Rb and p53 tumour suppressor genes. This is consistent with the observation that p53 mutation is uncommon in cervical cancer but is found in HPV-16- and HPV-18-negative cervical cancer cell lines. E6 and E7 also interact with several other important cellular proteins (involved in adhesion, apoptosis, cell cycle, DNA repair, signal transduction and transcription) affecting the integrity of key pathways, as demonstrated in several in-vitro studies (Whiteside et al 2008).

Clinical and experimental evidence suggests that in common with other mechanisms of carcinogenesis, HPV infection alone is not sufficient to cause cervical cancer, but requires other factors which may influence local immune responses or result in other genetic alterations. First, high-risk genital HPV infection is very common, and the majority of individuals clear their infection with time. However, a proportion of women, approximately 15%, cannot clear the virus effectively, and the persistence of a high-risk HPV is the major risk factor for the development of anogenital malignancies. Immunosuppressed women (e.g. human immunodeficiency virus infection, transplant recipients) have a substantially increased risk of developing cervical cancer. Second, epidemiological studies suggest that other factors such as smoking and herpes simplex infection may play a role. Third, a number of genetic abnormalities have been identified in cervical cancers. These include amplification or overexpression of *c-myc*, mutation of *c-H-ras* and LOH at a number of chromosomal loci. Recurrent LOH is identified in chromosome regions 3p14–22, 4p16, 5p15, 6q21–22, 11q23, 17p, 18q12–22 and 19q13. All these regions may harbour potential tumour suppressor genes. Several studies reported amplification of chromosome 3q24–28 in up to 90% of cervical cancers. Comparative genomic hybridization (CGH) is a powerful molecular tool which allows screening of the entire genome of a tumour for genetic alterations by highlighting regions of altered DNA sequence copy numbers. CGH from preinvasive (dysplastic) cervical cells reveals several chromosomal imbalances. Most frequent gains were found on chromosomes 1p, 2q, 4 and 5, whereas losses could be found on chromosome 13q (Aubele et al 1998). As outlined above, epigenetic alterations regulate gene expression without changing the DNA sequence. As well as methylation of cytosine in DNA, these alterations include acetylation of histone proteins. Epigenetic alterations are increasingly recognized as important oncogenic mechanisms, and HPV-associated oncogenesis is no exception (reviewed in Whiteside et al 2008). DNA methylation is also presumed to be a cellular defence to silence foreign DNA transcription. Methylation of HPV is known to occur. Recent studies of HPV 16 and 18 have shown that the extent of methylation varies by region of the genome, and changes in the methylation patterns may be associated with the grade of neoplasia. Epigenetic changes could also occur through direct interaction between HPV and the cellular proteins involved in DNA methylation and chromatin remodelling, including histone deacetylase, DNA methyltransferase and p300 (reviewed in Whiteside et al 2008). Numerous genes [e.g. cadherin 1 (*CDH1*), fragile histidine triad gene (*FHIT*), telomerase reverse transcriptase (*TERT*), cadherin 13 (*CDH13*), O-6-methylguanine–DNA methyltransferase (*MGMT*), tissue inhibitor of metallopeptidase 3 (*TIMP3*) and hypermethylated in cancer 1 (*HIC1*)] have been demonstrated to be methylated in preneoplastic and neoplastic cervical tissue (reviewed in Wentzensen et al 2009). Currently, studies are underway to determine whether aberrant epigenetic changes are a prerequisite for HPV-mediated carcinogenesis.

Ovarian cancer

The majority of cases of ovarian cancer are not associated with familial predisposition. Although it is widely believed that ovarian epithelial tumours arise in the coelomic epithelium that covers the ovarian surface, there is now accumulating evidence suggesting that they could arise from tissues that are embryologically derived from the Müllerian ducts. The observation that women with a greater number of ovulatory cycles have an increased risk of ovarian cancer led to the incessant ovulation hypothesis by Fathalla in 1971. According to this hypothesis, as ovulation occurs, ovarian surface epithelial cells are internalized and damaged, and the subsequent repair mechanisms place the cells at an increased risk of developing mutations and subsequent malignancies. Consistent with this hypothesis, women with a history of multiple pregnancies, increased time of lactation and oral contraceptive use are at decreased risk. However, this theory is weakened by other observations. For example, endometriosis, the presence of endometrium outside the uterus, is associated with increased risk of ovarian cancer (Melin et al 2006). Likewise, hysterectomy (particularly at an early age) and tubal ligation, both of which result in either removal or alteration of Müllerian tissue, are associated with decreased risk of epithelial ovarian cancer (Irwin et al 1991, Hankinson et al 1993, Parazzini et al 1993, Narod et al 2001). The fact that a substantial residual risk for peritoneal cancer in *BRCA1* and *BRCA2* mutation carriers remains for a long time following prophylactic salpingo-oophorectomy (Finch et al 2006) supports the view that the cell of origin for ovarian cancer may originate from outside the ovary. Dubeau was the first to challenge the coelomic hypothesis (Dubeau 1999), as it is surprising that tumours currently regarded as being of primary ovarian origin would resemble tumours derived from various segments of the Müllerian tract (cervix, endometrium and fallopian tube), despite the fact that the ovary is not embryologically related to this tract. Proponents of the coelomic metaplasia hypothesis account for the Müllerian appearance of ovarian tumours by stipulating that the coelomic epithelium is not the direct precursor of ovarian tumours, but must first change into Müllerian-like epithelium by metaplasia. This implies that ovarian carcinomas are better differentiated than the cells from which they originate. This notion is at odds with our current understanding of cancer development (Dubeau 2008a).

Early events in ovarian carcinogenesis

Like most cancers, epithelial ovarian cancers are thought to arise from a single cell in 90% of cases. Evidence for the clonality of ovarian cancer lies in the similarity between primary and metastatic lesions during the examination of LOH, X-chromosome inactivation and specific gene mutations (reviewed in Landen et al 2008). In contrast to cervical cancer, where early changes can be studied due to the fact that the cervix is easily accessible, it is very difficult to identify early changes in ovarian carcinogenesis, even more so because the cell of origin is still under debate.

Studying genetic disorders can provide great insight into the aetiology and early events in carcinogenesis. As outlined above, hereditary genetic disorders account for approximately 10% of ovarian cancers, and 90% of these are either *BRCA1* or *BRCA2* mutations. In recent years, a major effort to prevent serous cancer in genetically susceptible women with mutations in *BRCA1* or *BRCA2* has spawned the practice of prophylactic salpingo-oophorectomy. Histological surveillance of prophylactic salpingo-oophorectomy specimens revealed that many early cancers in these women arise in the fallopian tube, and further studies have pinpointed the distal (fimbrial) portion as the most common site of origin. In addition, a high proportion of histologically normal fimbriae from *BRCA* mutation carriers stain positive for *p53* (Crum et al 2007). Another convincing piece of molecular evidence favouring the idea that the cell of origin for ovarian cancer comes from the Müllerian duct is provided by recent expression profiling studies. Gene expression profiles of laser capture microdissected non-malignant distal fallopian tube epithelium from *BRCA1* and *BRCA2* mutation carriers and control women, as well as high-grade tubal and ovarian serous carcinoma, have been analysed (Tone et al 2008). Interestingly, fallopian tube samples from mutation carriers clustered closely with serous carcinomas rather than normal control fallopian tube epithelium. These findings support a common molecular pathway for adnexal serous cancers, and provide further evidence that cells from the Müllerian duct serve as the cells of origin for ovarian cancer. All this leaves us with the question of why *BRCA* mutation carriers do not carry an exaggerated high risk for endometrial cancer. The endometrium contains by far the highest number of epithelial cells originating from the Müllerian duct, and hence the statistical chances would be higher for a cancer in this organ rather than in the ovary, where cancers develop extremely frequently in *BRCA* mutation carriers. This paradox can be resolved by looking at the contribution of the stroma and the microenvironment to tumorigenesis. Dubeau's group inactivated the *BRCA1* gene in mouse granulosa cells (Chodankar et al 2005, Dubeau 2008b). Two-thirds of the mice developed epithelial cysts in their reproductive organs by the time they reached 12–18 months of age. Some of those cysts involved the ovary and were very similar to human ovarian cystadenomas. Although the tumours were benign, preliminary results suggested that crossing the mutant mice with mice carrying a homozygous knock-out of *p53* increases the rate of malignant transformation. The fact that the cystic tumours showed no evidence of rearrangement of *BRCA1*, implying that they expressed a functional BRCA1 protein, strongly supports the view that the ovarian stroma — in particular, granulosa cells — influences the development of ovarian epithelial tumours (Chodankar et al 2005, Dubeau 2008b).

Most of the evidence on genetic and epigenetic alterations in ovarian cancer is based on studies of late-stage cancers. However, current understanding of these processes allows speculation that many alterations must occur early to achieve a clinically recognized tumour. The genetic and epigenetic abnormalities in ovarian cancer involve genes at each step in the complex pathway of cell regulation, which are summarized in Figure 35.1. These include involving growth factors [macrophage colony-stimulating factor, transforming growth factor (TGF)-β], growth factor receptors [fms, epidermal growth factor receptor (EGFR), Her-2/neu], genes involved in signal transduction (*ras*), genes involved in transcriptional regulation (*myc*, *p53*) and LOH at various loci, which occur in a proportion of epithelial ovarian cancers.

Oncogenes in sporadic ovarian cancer

Over 60 different oncogenes have been identified and they are categorized according to their cellular location and func-

tion. The subject is reviewed in detail by Landen et al (2008) and Barton et al (2008).

Growth signals

There is good evidence that the response of ovarian cancer cells to growth factors is altered. The proliferative response of ovarian cancer cells in culture to epidermal growth factor (EGF) and TGF-α is variable but usually less than normal ovarian epithelium (Berchuck et al 1990), whilst the inhibitory effect of TGF-β is less marked in ovarian cancer cell lines than in normal ovarian epithelium. TGF-β appears to function as an autocrine inhibitory factor in normal ovarian epithelial growth, and the loss of this regulatory loop may represent a step in the process of ovarian carcinogenesis. During early phases of carcinogenesis, antigrowth signals must be overcome. The restriction point after which a cell is committed to divide is controlled by cyclin D and E's regulation of E2F release by *Rb*. Cyclin E is overexpressed in malignant tumours and is associated with poor prognosis in early-stage ovarian cancer (Marchini et al 2008).

The initiation of DNA replication represents a final and critical step in growth regulation, and lies downstream at the convergence point of growth regulatory pathways (Williams et al 1998). Minichromosome maintenance proteins (Mcm2–7) participate in the assembly of prereplicative complexes to establish competence for initiation of DNA synthesis (DNA replication licensing). All six Mcm proteins are essential for replication, are present in all phases of the proliferative cell cycle, but are tightly downregulated in the quiescent, terminally differentiated and senescent 'out-of-cycle' states. The presence of one protein reflects the presence of the other five, as all six are loaded together on to DNA as a heterohexamer on exit from metaphase. Mcm proteins have not been shown to be good prognostic markers in ovarian cancer (Gakiopoulou et al 2007, Marchini et al 2008).

Telomeres are tandem repeats of a short DNA sequence at the end of each chromosome. The length of telomeres decreases in somatic cells each time they divide. Most mammalian cells are therefore limited in terms of the number of times they can undergo cell division, because chromosomes cannot replicate unless their telomeres are longer than a minimal critical length. This mitotic clock does not operate in cancer cells because almost all cancers express telomerase, ensuring maintenance of the telomeres above the critical length necessary to support cell division, activating p53 and other policing proteins that propel a cell into an apoptotic pathway. Most ovarian cancer cells maintain telomere length by production of telomerase, a reverse transcriptase composed of an RNA component (hTR) and a catalytic subunit (hTERT). The hTR subunit is expressed by all cells, but hTERT expression increases with increasing tumorigenicity, which suggests that it is the rate-limiting step in telomerase activity (reviewed in Landen et al 2008).

Growth factor receptors

The growth factor receptors are a family of cell membrane tyrosine kinases which act as receptors for growth factors and are involved in signal transduction via autophosphorylation and phosphorylation of intracellular proteins. EGFR (also referred to as erbB) and Her-2/neu (also referred to as erbB2) are structurally similar, and both have been shown to be overexpressed in human cancers. EGFR is expressed by most advanced-stage ovarian cancers and there is some evidence that EGFR-positive tumours have a worse prognosis than tumours that do not express the receptor. Her-2/neu is overexpressed in approximately one-third of ovarian cancers (Slamon et al 1989), and overexpression is associated with gene amplification. Many proliferation pathways mediate signals through the RAS (rat sarcoma viral oncogene homolog) oncoprotein, a G-protein attached to the cell membrane and activated by many tyrosine kinase receptors, and BRAF (v-raf murine sarcoma viral oncogene homolog B1), which is downstream of RAS. RAS activates a cascade of serine/threonine and tyrosine non-receptor kinases, which leads to phosphorylation and activation of Erk1 and Erk2 transcription factors that make their way to the nucleus to initiate signals of growth and progression through the cell cycle. *RASSF1A* (Ras association domain family 1 isoform A) is a recently discovered tumour suppressor whose inactivation — mainly by DNA methylation (Barton et al 2008) — is implicated in the development of many human cancers. *RASSF1A* lacks apparent enzymatic activity but contains a Ras association domain and is potentially an effector of the Ras oncoprotein. *RASSF1A* modulates multiple apoptotic and cell cycle checkpoint pathways. Current evidence supports the hypothesis that it serves as a scaffold for the assembly of multiple tumour suppressor complexes, and may relay proapoptotic signalling by *K-ras*.

Oncogenes

Chromosome 3q26 is found to be increased in copy number in approximately 40% of ovarian cancers. This region contains a recently identified oncogene, *PIK3CA*, which encodes the p110-α subunit of phosphatidylinositol 3-kinase (PI 3-kinase). PI 3-kinase-mediated signalling is involved in a broad range of cancer-related functions, including glucose transport, catabolism, apoptosis, cell adhesion, RAS signalling and oncogenic transcription. Little is known about the role of most nuclear oncogenes in ovarian cancer. Amplification of *c-myc* and increased expression of the protein product has been described in approximately one-third of ovarian cancers. Overexpression of *c-myc* is found in 38% of ovarian tumours (Tashiro et al 1992).

Tumour suppressor genes in sporadic ovarian cancer

Mutations of the *p53* gene are the most frequent genetic alterations in cancer, and occur most frequently in regions of the gene which show the greatest degree of conservation between p53 proteins of different species. Immunohistochemical studies have revealed overexpression of the p53 protein in 50% of advanced-stage ovarian cancers (Marks et al 1991). Sequencing of *p53* from ovarian cancers overexpressing the p53 protein has, in most cases, confirmed point mutations in conserved regions of the gene (Marks et al 1991). In most of these tumours, LOH studies have revealed that the second copy of the gene is inactivated through deletion of the gene. *p53* mutations are less common in stage I disease than advanced-stage disease, and clonal analysis suggests that the occurrence of *p53* mutations precedes but is

temporally associated with metastases (Jacobs et al 1992). No clear relationship between *p53* mutation and histological grade or prognosis has been established. The location and nature of *p53* mutations in ovarian cancer have now been reported in 149 tumours. Over 100 different mutations involving approximately 60 different codons have been identified, and most occur in the highly conserved exons 5–8 of the gene. The codons most frequently involved in *p53* mutations are the same as those described in other cancers. The pattern of mutations suggests that most *p53* alterations in ovarian cancer arise due to endogenous mutagenic processes rather than exposure to a carcinogen.

Several novel potential candidate tumour suppressor genes have recently been reported for ovarian cancer, and their role in ovarian carcinogenesis has yet to be elucidated. Analysis of LOH at 11q25 identified *OPCML* (opioid binding protein/cell adhesion molecule-like), a member of the IgLON family of immunoglobulin domain-containing glycosylphosphatidylinositol-anchored cell adhesion molecules, as a candidate tumour suppressor gene in ovarian cancer (Sellar et al 2003). *OPCML* is frequently somatically inactivated by allele loss, and up to 83% of ovarian cancers demonstrate CGI methylation of this gene.

Defects in programmed cell death can promote oncogenesis and resistance to chemotherapy. Apoptosis (type I programmed cell death) has been well studied as a caspase-regulated cellular response to environmental stress and to the activation of oncogenes. Numerous genes involved in apoptosis are methylated and silenced in ovarian cancer (Barton et al 2008, Figure 35.3). Autophagy (type II programmed cell death) is characterized by the accumulation of multilamellar vesicles that engulf cytoplasm and organelles, forming autophagosomes marked by microtubule-associated protein light chain 3. The maternally imprinted Ras-related tumour suppressor gene, aplasia Ras homolog member I (*ARHI*), is downregulated in more than 60% of ovarian cancers, and re-expression of *ARHI* in multiple human ovarian cancer cell lines induces autophagy (Lu et al 2008). In addition, death-associated protein kinase (DAPK) also contributes to the autophagic pathways, and loss of their function — a feature frequently observed in ovarian cancer — could inhibit the induction of autophagy and increase the incidence of cancer.

Loss of heterozygosity

Studies of LOH in ovarian cancer have revealed a number of regions with high frequencies of loss. The reported frequency of LOH for each chromosome arm is summarized in Figure 35.6. Losses have been observed on almost all chromosome arms, and the background 'random' rate of loss in ovarian cancer is high (range 15–25%). A high frequency of allelic deletion (>33%) based upon more than 50 tumours in at least three separate studies has been documented for seven chromosome arms: 6p, 6q, 13q, 17p (possibly associated with *p53*), 17q, 18q and Xp. A number of other chromosome arms have frequencies of loss in the range 25–33% which may be above background rates: 4p, 8p, 9p, 9q, 11p, 14q, 16q, 19p and 21q and 22q (McCluskey and Dubeau 1997). Some of these allelic deletions have been correlated with clinicopathological parameters. Recent studies have shown a distinct relationship between allelic

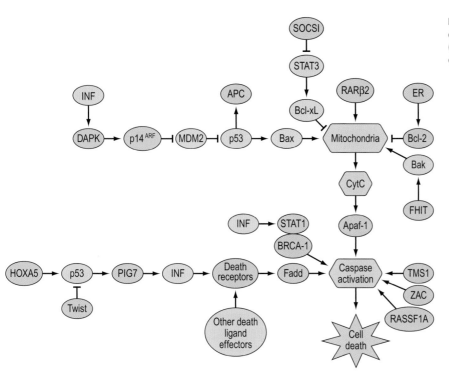

Figure 35.6 Genes which are involved in the cascade which leads to programmed cell death (apoptosis). Genes in red have a CpG island and can be silenced by means of DNA methylation.

imbalance at 8p12-p21 and 8p22-pter in ovarian cancer and tumour grade, stage and histological subtype. Poorly differentiated tumours, advanced-stage cancers and serous tumours were more prone to allelic imbalance at these regions (Pribill et al 2001).

Further localization of putative tumour suppressor genes in regions with a high rate of LOH requires detailed analysis with a panel of polymorphic markers for the relevant chromosome arm. Available data suggest that a number of as yet unidentified tumour suppressor genes are involved in ovarian carcinogenesis, and recent reports have defined deletion units on chromosome arms with the highest rates of LOH including 6p, 6q, 11p, 13q, 17q and Xp. The nature of specific chromosomes affected by LOH can influence tumour biological aggressiveness, as losses on certain chromosomes such as 13q and Xq are strongly associated with poorly differentiated tumours (Cheng et al 1996). LOH in chromosomes 6q or 17 is more frequently found in well-differentiated tumours.

Comparative genomic hybridization

The application of this technique has shown that 53–69% of human ovarian cancers demonstrate amplifications on chromosomes 1q, 3q, 8q, 13q, 19p and 20q (Kiechle et al 2001). Under-representations were found for chromosomes 4q, 13q and 18q in approximately 50% of ovarian cancers. Undifferentiated tumours were found to correlate significantly with under-representation of 11p and 13q, as well as with amplification of 7p and 8q.

cDNA microarrays

The development of cancer is the result of a series of molecular changes at DNA level, and these events lead to changes in gene expression (mRNA) levels of numerous genes resulting in different phenotypic characteristics of tumours. cDNA microarray analysis enables the identification of differences in gene expressions between normal and malignant tissues by analysing thousands of genes at the same time. A recent study comparing 5766 different gene expressions between normal and malignant ovarian tissue revealed that several genes were under- or overexpressed (Wang et al 1999). Several genes were highly overexpressed in ovarian cancer, such as epithelial glycoprotein (*GA733*, gene antigen 733), *PUMP1* (Pump-1 protease) (*MMP7*, matrix metallopeptidase 7) and *cytokeratin 8*, and some of these have also been shown to be overexpressed in other cancers such as colorectal cancer. This illustrates that phenotypical similarity between different tumour types is also reflected at molecular level.

Another study, using a DNA microarray of 9121 genes, identified 55 genes commonly upregulated and 48 genes downregulated in ovarian cancer specimens compared with the corresponding normal ovarian tissues (Ono et al 2000). The 55 genes that were often upregulated in the nine adenocarcinomas analysed represent candidates for stimulating cell growth and preventing apoptosis. Serial analysis of gene expression has recently been introduced to generate global gene expression profiles from various ovarian cell lines and tissues including primary ovarian cancers, ovarian surface epithelial cells and cystadenoma cells. More than 56,000 gene expressions (10 different libraries) were generated (Hough et al 2000). Interestingly, ovarian cancer cell lines showed high levels of similarity to libraries from other cancer cell lines such as colorectal cancer, indicating that these cell lines had lost many of their tissue-specific expression patterns. Many of the genes upregulated in ovarian cancer represent surface or secreted proteins such as mucin-1, HE4 (human epididymal protein 4), epithelial cellular adhesion molecule, mesothelin and several keratins (e.g. keratins 18 and 19).

MicroRNAs

MicroRNAs (miRNAs) are endogenous non-coding small RNAs which negatively regulate gene expression. In human cancer, miRNAs might function as either oncogenes or tumour suppressor genes. Increasing evidence shows that expression of miRNAs is deregulated in human cancer. High-throughput miRNA quantification technologies have provided powerful tools to study global miRNA profiles. It has become progressively obvious that although the number of miRNAs (~600) is much smaller than that of the protein-coding genes (~22,000), miRNA expression signatures reflect the developmental lineage or tissue origin of human cancers more accurately. Recently, it has been demonstrated that genomic copy number loss and epigenetic silencing, respectively, may account for the downregulation of ~15% and at least ~36% of miRNAs in advanced ovarian tumours, and miRNA downregulation contributes to a genome-wide transcriptional deregulation. Eight miRNAs located in the chromosome 14 miRNA cluster (Dlk1–Gtl2 domain) were identified as potential tumour suppressor genes. Tumours with lower expression of these eight miRNAs were associated with a higher proliferation index and significantly shorter survival. Although the function of this miRNA cluster is largely unknown, it may play a critical role in embryonic development (Zhang et al 2008).

DNA methylation

As outlined above, genome-wide demethylation of normally methylated and silenced chromosomal regions, and hypermethylation and silencing of genes including tumour suppressors are among the most common features of cancer cells (reviewed in Barton et al 2008). Epigenetic alterations, including CGI DNA methylation, frequently occur in ovarian cancer, and the identification of specific genes that are altered by epigenetic events is currently an area of intense research. Aberrant DNA methylation in ovarian cancer is observed in early cancer development, can be detected in serum/plasma DNA and hence provides the promise of a non-invasive cancer detection test. In addition, identification of ovarian-cancer-specific epigenetic changes has promise in molecular classification and disease stratification.

Endometrial cancer

Endometrial cancers have long been classified into two major divisions (types I and II) based on light microscopic appearance, clinical behaviour and epidemiology. Type I (endometrioid histology) comprise 70–80% of newly diagnosed cases of endometrial cancer. They are associated with unopposed oestrogen exposure and are often preceded by premalignant disease (atypical complex hyperplasia). In contrast, type II endometrial cancers (usually papillary serous or clear cell histology) have not been identified in association with hormonal factors, and do not have a readily observed premalignant phase. In addition, they demonstrate an aggressive clinical course compared with the type I tumours. The morphologic and clinical differences are paralleled by genetic distinctions, in that type I and II cancers carry mutations of independent sets of genes (Hecht and Mutter 2006). While most type II cancers contain mutations of *p53*, type I adenocarcinomas demonstrate larger numbers

of genetic changes in which the temporal sequence of mutation and the final combination of defects differ substantially between individual examples. Common genetic changes in endometrioid endometrial cancers (type I) include, but are not limited to, microsatellite instability or specific mutation of *PTEN* (phosphatase and tensin homolog), *K-ras* and *β-catenin* genes (Hecht et al 2006). With regard to epigenetics, promoter hypermethylation is common in type I but not type II tumours. Many of the tumour suppressor pathways that are mutated in type I endometrial cancer such as *PTEN*, *hMLH1*, *MGMT* and *APC* can also be inactivated by hypermethylation. In addition, *PR-B* (progesterone receptor B) promoter hypermethylation is established as the dominant mechanism of *PR-B* silencing (Zhou et al 2007).

Vulval cancer

Neoplasias of the vulva are rare malignancies accounting for less than 5% of all female genital tract cancers. However, in recent years, the incidence of vulval intraepithelial neoplasia (VIN), a precursor of vulval cancer, has increased in young women, generating considerable interest in its molecular pathogenesis.

CGH has recently been used to study alterations (losses or gains) on all chromosomes in vulval cancer (Jee et al 2001). Frequent chromosomal losses were found on 3p, 4p13-pter and 5q, and less frequent losses were found on 6q, 11q and 13q. Most frequent chromosomal gains were observed on 3q and 8p, and less frequent gains were found on 9p, 14, 17 and 20q. The pattern of chromosomal imbalance in vulval cancer detected by CGH was revealed to be very similar to that in cervical cancer. These results suggest that the molecular pathways in vulval and cervical carcinomas may be similar. However, it is not clear whether HPV-positive and -negative vulval cancers have similar or different molecular pathways.

Vulval squamous cell carcinomas (VSCCs) exhibit a broad range of allelic losses irrespective of HPV status, with high frequencies of LOH on certain chromosomal arms. High frequencies of LOH are found on 1q, 2q, 3p, 5q, 8p, 8q, 10p, 10q, 11p, 11q, 15q, 17p, 18q, 21q and 22q (Pinto et al 1999). This suggests that despite their differences in pathogenesis, both HPV-positive and -negative VSCCs share similarities in type and range of genetic losses during their evolution. Another study observed a greater number of molecular alterations in HPV-negative vulval cancers compared with HPV-positive tumours (Flowers et al 1999). Allelic losses at 3p are common early events in vulval carcinogenesis in HPV-negative cancers, and are detected at a high rate in the corresponding high-grade precursor lesions (VIN II/III). *TP53* gene mutations with associated 17p13.1 LOH are also more common in HPV-negative cancers. Fractional regional loss index, an index of total allelic loss at chromosomal regions 3p, 13q14 and 17p13.1, is greater in HPV-negative vulval cancers than in HPV-positive tumours (Flowers et al 1999). Similar observations have been found in HPV-negative high-grade VINs compared with HPV-positive lesions. Overall, LOH at any 3p region is common (80%) in both groups of cancers and in their associated VIN lesions. Although *TP53* gene mutations are present in a minority of vulval cancers (20%), allelic losses at the *TP53* locus are frequently present, especially in HPV-negative vulval cancers, compared with HPV-positive tumours.

Fallopian tube cancer

The histological features, and biological and clinical behaviour of fallopian tube cancer are similar to those of ovarian cancer. In addition, there is recent evidence that similar genetic alterations occur with the same frequency between fallopian tube and ovarian cancer when considering the same histological subtype. This suggests a common molecular pathogenesis between these cancer types (Crum et al 2007). Recent molecular genetic analyses using CGH reveal that different histological subtypes differ in respect to their genomic alterations, but similar subtypes of different cancers have similar patterns of genomic abnormalities. For example, the frequency and pattern of chromosomal changes detected in serous tubal carcinomas (95% of all fallopian tube carcinomas) are strikingly similar to those observed in serous ovarian carcinomas, suggesting a common molecular pathogenesis. In fallopian tube carcinoma, frequent gains are found on chromosomes 3q and 8q and frequent losses are found on chromosomes 4q, 5q, 8q and 18q (Pere et al 1998). There is also evidence that fallopian tube cancer is similar to ovarian cancer with respect to the proportion of tumours with abnormal expression of *Her-2/neu* and *p53*. The prognostic significance and predictive drug response of these two genes needs to be explored in fallopian tube cancer.

Clinical Aspects of the Genetics of Gynaecological Cancer

Cancer prevention

Vaccines against HPV have become available over the last few years. Two HPV vaccines — a quadrivalent vaccine against HPV types 6, 11, 16 and 18 (Gardasil) and a bivalent vaccine against HPV types 16 and 18 (Cervarix) — are now licensed in the European Union for the prevention of premalignant cervical lesions and cervical cancer. The quadrivalent vaccine is also licensed for prevention of premalignant vulval and vaginal lesions, and external genital warts. Both vaccines show high efficacy in preventing high-grade premalignant cervical lesions. Studies to date have been too brief to confirm the effectiveness of the vaccines for the prevention of cervical cancer. There are also uncertainties about the duration of protection, whether booster doses are needed and whether the vaccines protect against infection with non-vaccine HPV types. A national programme to vaccinate girls aged 12–13 years began in the UK in September 2008.

Early detection of cancer

Knowledge of specific genetic and epigenetic alterations associated with cancer, along with the high sensitivity of molecular techniques such as the polymerase chain reaction, may provide new methods for detection of cancer. As direct sampling of the ovary requires an invasive procedure, any screening test for ovarian cancer based upon genetic markers will be directed towards identification of a gene product in peripheral blood. Tumour-specific hypermethylation of at least one of a panel of six tumour suppressor gene promoters, including *RASSF1A* (Ras association domain family member 1A), *BRCA1* (breast cancer 1 early onset), *APC* (adenomatous polyposis coli), *CDKN2A* (cyclin-dependent kinase inibitor 2A) and *DAPK* (death-associated protein kinase 1), could be detected in the serum or plasma of ovarian cancer patients with 100% specificity and 82% sensitivity, including 13/17 cases of stage I (confined to the ovary) disease. Methylation was only observed in one peritoneal fluid sample from 15 stage IA or B patients, but 11/15 paired sera were positive for methylation (Ibanez de Caceres et al 2004). In addition to proof of principle, these data indicate that circulating ovarian tumour DNA is more readily accessible in the bloodstream than in the peritoneum. In addition, serum DNA methylation of *SFRP1* (secreted frizzled-related protein 1), *SOX1* (SRY(sex determining region Y)-box 1) and *LMX1A* (LIM homeobox transcription factor 1 alpha) revealed sensitivity and specificity of 73% and 75%, respectively (Su et al 2009).

DNA is a very stable molecule compared with RNA or protein. It can easily be analysed in any body fluid, including vaginal secretions. In a proof of principle study, the authors aimed to define a new and simple strategy for detection of endometrial cancer using epigenetic markers. They investigated DNA isolated from vaginal secretions collected from tampons for aberrant methylation of five genes [(*CDH13*, *HSPA2* (heat shock 70kDa protein 2), *MLH1*, *RASSF1A*, and *SOCS2* (suppressor of cytokine signalling 2)] using MethyLight in 15 patients with endometrial cancer and 109 patients without endometrial cancer. All endometrial cancer patients revealed three or more methylated genes, whereas 91% (99 of 109) of the patients without endometrial cancer had fewer than three genes methylated in their vaginal secretion. The methods developed in this study provided the basis for a prospective clinical trial to screen asymptomatic women who are at high risk for endometrial cancer (Fiegl et al 2004).

Prognostic and predictive indicators

Numerous genetic and epigenetic prognostic and predictive markers have been discovered over the past few years (reviewed in Crijns et al 2006, Barton et al 2008), but none of these markers have yet been integrated into clinical practice. Silencing of *hMLH1*, a DNA mismatch repair gene, by hypermethylation of its promoter CGI has been linked with acquired resistance to platinum-based drugs in ovarian cell line models. Moreover, methylation of *MLH1* is increased at relapse in epithelial ovarian cancer patients, with 25% (34/138) of plasma samples from relapsed patients showing methylation of *MLHI* which is not evident in matched prechemotherapy plasma samples (Barton et al 2008). The acquisition of *MLH1* methylation at relapse predicts poor overall patient survival, and is associated with drug resistance (Gifford et al 2004, Barton et al 2008). The concept of predicting and monitoring response to systemic therapies by means of serum/plasma DNA analysis is currently under investigation.

Strategies for gene therapy

Promising preclinical and clinical data led to the initiation of an international randomized phase II/III trial of *p53* gene therapy for first-line treatment of patients with ovarian cancer. In that trial, replication-deficient adenoviral vectors carrying wild-type *p53* were given intraperitoneally in combination with standard chemotherapy to patients with ovarian cancers harbouring *p53* mutations. The study was closed after the first interim analysis because an adequate therapeutic benefit was not shown (Zeimet and Marth 2003). There may be various reasons for the failure of this strategy; for example, the repair of single genes might not be a suitable strategy for the treatment of cancer, heterogeneity or

lack of expression of coxsackie-adenovirus receptors and integrin coreceptors in ovarian tumours, and the presence of adenovirus-neutralizing antibodies in ovarian cancer-related ascites. Although the safety of many other treatment strategies has been demonstrated in early-phase clinical trials, efficacy has been mostly limited. Major challenges include improving the vectors used, with the aim of more effective and selective delivery. In addition, effective penetration into and spreading within advanced and complex tumour masses and metastases remains challenging (Kanerva et al 2007).

KEY POINTS

1. Oncogenes result in a gain in function which will take effect even in the presence of the remaining normal copy of the gene; tumour suppressor genes involve a loss of function that requires inactivation or deletion of both copies of the gene before cellular regulation is affected.

2. Epigenetic events, particularly silencing of tumour suppressor genes by DNA methylation, are early key events in carcinogenesis.

3. The genetic changes required for cancer usually occur in the somatic cells and are random events. However, some individuals develop oncogenic mutations in their germ cells which can then be passed on to their progeny.

4. Among gynaecological cancers, inherited malignancies only occur in the ovary, endometrium and breast. These are rare, accounting for less than 5% of ovarian or endometrial cancers.

5. Two genes, termed *BRCA1* and *BRCA2*, have been identified. *BRCA1* is found in almost all families with both breast and ovarian cancer, and in 40% of families with breast cancer alone.

6. These genes have high penetrance, with 80% of affected individuals developing a malignancy between 30 and 70 years of age.

7. Genetic advice to women who may have inherited a cancer gene should only be given by clinical geneticists or gynaecological oncologists with a special knowledge of these conditions.

8. The efficacy of screening such women is unproven. There is a substantial risk of false-positive results.

9. Oophorectomy and hysterectomy should be considered if the risk of inheritance seems high.

10. Identifying the genetic basis for cancer allows for the investigation and development of therapy targeted at the underlying abnormality.

References

Aarnio M, Sankila R, Pukkala E et al 1999 Cancer risk in mutation carriers of DNA-mismatch-repair genes. International Journal of Cancer 12: 214–218.

Aubele M, Zitzelsberger H, Schenck U, Walch A, Hofler H, Werner M 1998 Distinct cytogenetic alterations in squamous intraepithelial lesions of the cervix revealed by laser-assisted microdissection and comparative genomic hybridization. Cancer 84: 375–379.

Barton CA, Hacker NF, Clark SJ, O'Brien PM 2008 DNA methylation changes in ovarian cancer: implications for early diagnosis, prognosis and treatment. Gynecological Oncology 109: 129–139.

Berchuck A, Rodriguez G, Kamel A, Soper JT, Clarke-Pearson DL, Bast RC Jr 1990 Expression of epidermal growth factor receptor and HER-2/neu in normal and neoplastic cervix, vulva, and vagina. Obstetrics and Gynecology 76: 381–387.

Campbell S, Bourne T, Bradley E 1993 Screening for ovarian cancer by transvaginal sonography and colour Doppler. European Journal of Obstetrics, Gynecology and Reproductive Biology 49: 33.

Cavenee WK, Dryja TP, Phillips RA et al 1983 Expression of recessive alleles by

chromosomal mechanisms in retinoblastoma. Nature 305: 779–784.

Chen KT, Schooley JL, Flam MS 1985 Peritoneal carcinomatosis after prophylactic oophorectomy in familial ovarian cancer syndrome. Obstetrics and Gynecology 66: 93.

Cheng PC, Gosewehr JA, Kim TM et al 1996 Potential role of the inactivated X chromosome in ovarian epithelial tumor development. Journal of the National Cancer Institute 88: 510–518.

Chodankar R, Kwang S, Sangiorgi F et al 2005 Cell-nonautonomous induction of ovarian and uterine serous cystadenomas in mice lacking a functional Brca1 in ovarian granulosa cells. Current Biology 15: 561–565.

Crijns AP, Duiker EW, de Jong S, Willemse PH, van der Zee AG, de Vries EG 2006 Molecular prognostic markers in ovarian cancer: toward patient-tailored therapy. International Journal of Gynecological Cancer 16 (Suppl 1): 152–165.

Crum CP, Drapkin R, Kindelberger D, Medeiros F, Miron A, Lee Y 2007 Lessons from BRCA: the tubal fimbria emerges as an origin for pelvic serous cancer. Clinical Medicine and Research 5: 35–44.

de Klein A, van Kessel AG, Grosveld G et al 1982 A cellular oncogene is translocated to the Philadelphia chromosome in chronic myelocytic leukaemia. Nature 300: 765–767.

Dubeau L 1999 The cell of origin of ovarian epithelial tumors and the ovarian surface epithelium dogma: does the emperor have no clothes? Gynecological Oncology 72: 437–442.

Dubeau L 2008a The cell of origin of ovarian epithelial tumours. The Lancet Oncology 9: 1191–1197.

Dubeau L 2008b BRCA1-induced ovarian oncogenesis. Advances in Experimental Medicine and Biology 622: 89–97.

Dunlop MG, Farrington SM, Carothers AD et al 1997 Cancer risk associated with germline DNA mismatch repair gene mutations. Human Molecular Genetics 6: 105–110.

Easton DF, Eeles RA 2008. Genome-wide association studies in cancer. Human Molecular Genetics 17(R2): R109–R115.

Easton DF, Bishop DT, Ford D, Crockford GP 1993 Genetic linkage analysis in familial breast and ovarian cancer: results from 214 families. The Breast Cancer Linkage

Consortium. American Journal of Human Genetics 52: 678.

Fathalla MF 1971 Incessant ovulation: a factor in ovarian neoplasia? Lancet 2(7716): 163.

Fiegl H, Gattringer C, Widschwendter A et al 2004 Methylated DNA collected by tampons — a new tool to detect endometrial cancer. Cancer Epidemiology, Biomarkers and Prevention 13: 882–888.

Finch A, Beiner M, Lubinski J et al 2006 Salpingo-oophorectomy and the risk of ovarian, fallopian tube, and peritoneal cancers in women with a BRCA1 or BRCA2 mutation. JAMA: the Journal of the American Medical Association 296: 185–192.

Flowers LC, Wistuba II, Scurry J et al 1999 Genetic changes during the multistage pathogenesis of human papillomavirus positive and negative vulvar carcinomas. Journal of the Society for Gynecologic Investigation 6: 213–221.

Ford D, Easton DF, Bishop DT et al 1994 Risks of cancer in BRCA1-mutation carriers. Breast Cancer Linkage Consortium. Lancet 343: 692–695.

Ford D, Easton DF, Stratton M et al 1998 Genetic heterogeneity and penetrance analysis of the BRCA1 and BRCA2 genes in breast cancer families. The Breast Cancer Linkage Consortium. American Journal of Human Genetics 62: 676–689.

Gakiopoulou H, Korkolopoulou P, Levidou G et al 2007 Minichromosome maintenance proteins 2 and 5 in non-benign epithelial ovarian tumours: relationship with cell cycle regulators and prognostic implications. British Journal of Cancer 97: 1124–1134.

Gayther SA, Warren W, Mazoyer S et al 1995 Germline mutations of the BRCAI gene in breast and ovarian cancer families provide evidence for a genotype-phenotype correlation. Nature Genetics 11: 428–433.

Gayther SA, Mangion J, Russell P et al 1997 Variation of risks of breast and ovarian cancer associated with different germline mutations of the BRCA2 gene. Nature Genetics 15: 103–105.

Gifford G, Paul J, Vasey PA, Kaye SB, Brown R 2004 The acquisition of hMLH1 methylation in plasma DNA after chemotherapy predicts poor survival for ovarian cancer patients. Clinical Cancer Research 10: 4420–4426.

Hall JM, Lee MK, Newman B et al 1990 Linkage of early-onset familial breast cancer to chromosome 17q21. Science 250: 1684–1689.

Hankinson SE, Hunter DJ, Colditz GA et al 1993 Tubal ligation, hysterectomy, and risk of ovarian cancer. A prospective study. JAMA: the Journal of the American Medical Association 270: 2813–2818.

Hecht JL, Mutter GL 2006 Molecular and pathologic aspects of endometrial carcinogenesis. Journal of Clinical Oncology 24: 4783–4791.

Hough CD, Sherman-Baust CA, Pizer ES et al 2000 Large-scale serial analysis of gene expression reveals genes differentially expressed in ovarian cancer. Cancer Research 60: 6281–6287.

Huang J, Papadopoulus N, McKinley AJ et al 1996 APC mutations in colorectal tumours with mismatch repair deficiency. Proceeding of the National Academy of Sciences USA 93: 9049–9054.

Ibanez de Caceres I, Battagli C, Esteller M et al 2004 Tumor cell-specific BRCA1 and RASSF1A hypermethylation in serum, plasma, and peritoneal fluid from ovarian cancer patients. Cancer Research 64: 6476–6481.

Irwin KL, Weiss NS, Lee NC, Peterson HB 1991 Tubal sterilization, hysterectomy, and the subsequent occurrence of epithelial ovarian cancer. American Journal of Epidemiology 134: 362–369.

Jacobs I, Davies AP, Bridges J et al 1993 Prevalence screening for ovarian cancer in postmenopausal women by CA 125 measurement and ultrasonography [see comments]. British Medical Journal 306: 1030.

Jacobs IJ, Kohler MF, Wiseman RW et al 1992 Clonal origin of epithelial ovarian carcinoma: analysis by loss of heterozygosity, p53 mutation, and X-chromosome inactivation. Journal of the National Cancer Institute 84: 1793–1798.

Jacobs IJ, Skates SJ, MacDonald N et al 1999 Screening for ovarian cancer: a pilot randomized controlled trial. Lancet 353(9160): 1207–1210.

Jee KJ, Kim YT, Kim KR, Kim HS, Yan A, Knuutila S 2001 Loss in 3p and 4p and gain of 3q are concomitant aberrations in squamous cell carcinoma of the vulva. Modern Pathology 14: 377–381.

Jones PA, Baylin SB 2007 The epigenomics of cancer. Cell 128: 683–692.

Jones PA, Laird PW 1999 Cancer epigenetics comes of age. Nature Genetics 21: 163–167.

Kanerva A, Raki M, Hemminki A 2007 Gene therapy of gynaecological diseases. Expert Opinion on Biological Therapy 7: 1347–1361.

Kiechle M, Jacobsen A, Schwarz-Boeger U, Hedderich J, Pfisterer J, Arnold N 2001 Comparative genomic hybridization detects genetic imbalances in primary ovarian carcinomas as correlated with grade of differentiation. Cancer 91: 534–540.

Kinzler KW, Vogelstein B 1996 Lessons from hereditary colorectal cancer. Cell 87: 159–170.

Kinzler KW, Nilbert MC, Su L-K et al 1991 Identification of FAP locus genes from chromosome 5q21. Science 253: 661–665.

Laird PW 2003 The power and the promise of DNA methylation markers. Nature Reviews. Cancer 3: 253–266.

Landen CN Jr, Birrer MJ, Sood AK 2008 Early events in the pathogenesis of epithelial ovarian cancer. Journal of Clinical Oncology 26: 995–1005.

Levanon K, Crum C, Drapkin R 2008 New insights into the pathogenesis of serous ovarian cancer and its clinical impact. Journal of Clinical Oncology 26: 5284–5293.

Levy-Lahad E, Catane R, Eisenberg S et al 1997 Founder BRCA1 and BRCA2 mutations in Ashkenazi Jews in Israel: frequency and differential penetrance in ovarian cancer and in breast-ovarian cancer families. American Journal of Human Genetics 60: 1059–1067.

Lu Z, Luo RZ, Lu Y et al 2008 The tumor suppressor gene ARHI regulates autophagy and tumor dormancy in human ovarian cancer cells. Journal of Clinical Investigation 118: 3917–3929.

Lynch HT, de la Chapelle H 1999 Genetic susceptibility to non-polyposis colorectal cancer. Journal of Medical Genetics 36: 801–808.

Lynch HT, Kimberling W, Albano WA et al 1985 Hereditary nonpolyposis colorectal cancer (Lynch syndromes I and II). Cancer 15: 938–938.

Marchini S, Mariani P, Chiorino G et al 2008 Analysis of gene expression in early-stage ovarian cancer. Clinical Cancer Research 14: 7850–7860.

Marks JR, Davidoff AM, Kerns BJ et al 1991 Overexpression and mutation of p53 in epithelial ovarian cancer. Cancer Research 51: 2979–2984.

Marra G, Boland CR 1995 Hereditary nonpolyposis colorectal cancer. Journal of the National Cancer Institute 87: 1114–1125.

McCluskey LL, Dubeau L 1997 Biology of ovarian cancer. Current Opinion in Oncology 9: 465–470.

Melin A, Sparen P, Persson I, Bergqvist A 2006 Endometriosis and the risk of cancer with special emphasis on ovarian cancer. Human Reproduction 21: 1237–1242.

Menon U, Gentry-Maharaj A, Hallett R et al 2009 Sensitivity and specificity of multimodal and ultrasound screening for ovarian cancer, and stage distribution of detected cancers: results of the prevalence screen of the UK Collaborative Trial of Ovarian Cancer Screening (UKCTOCS). The Lancet Oncology 10: 327–340.

Miki Y, Swensen J, Schattuck-Eidens D et al 1994 Isolation of BRCA1, the 17q linked breast and ovarian cancer susceptibility gene. Science 266: 66–71.

Modan B, Hartge P, Hirsh-Yechezkel G et al for the National Israel Ovarian Cancer Study Group 2001 Parity, oral contraceptives, and the risk of ovarian cancer among carriers and noncarriers of a BRCA1 or BRCA2 mutation. New England Journal of Medicine 345(4): 235–240.

Narod SA, Sun P, Ghadirian P et al 2001 Tubal ligation and risk of ovarian cancer in carriers of BRCA1 or BRCA2 mutations: a case–control study. The Lancet 357: 1467–1470.

Ono K, Tanaka T, Tsunoda T et al 2000 Identification by cDNA microarray of genes involved in ovarian carcinogenesis. Cancer Research 60: 5007–5011.

Parazzini F, Negri E, La Vecchia C, Luchini L, Mezzopane R 1993 Hysterectomy, oophorectomy, and subsequent ovarian cancer risk. Obstetrics and Gynecology 81: 363–366.

Pere H, Tapper J, Seppala M, Knuutila S, Butzow R 1998 Genomic alterations in fallopian tube carcinoma: comparison to serous uterine and ovarian carcinomas reveals similarity suggesting likeness in molecular pathogenesis. Cancer Research 58: 4274–4276.

Pinto AP, Lin MC, Mutter GL, Sun D, Villa LL, Crum CP 1999 Allelic loss in human papillomavirus-positive and -negative vulvar squamous cell carcinomas. American Journal of Pathology 154: 1009–1015.

Pribill I, Speiser P, Leary J et al 2001 High frequency of allelic imbalance at regions of chromosome arm 8p in ovarian carcinoma. Cancer Genetics and Cytogenetics 129: 23–29.

Ramus SJ, Gayther SA 2009 The contribution of BRCA1 and BRCA2 to ovarian cancer. Molecular Oncology 3(2): 138–150.

Rebbeck TR, Kauff ND, Domchek SM 2009 Meta-analysis of risk reduction estimates associated with risk-reducing salpingo-oophorectomy in BRCA1 or BRCA2 mutation carriers. Journal of the National Cancer Institute 101: 80–87.

Salovaara R, Loukola A, Kristo P et al 2000 Population-based detection of hereditary nonpolyosis colorectal cancer. Journal of Clinical Oncology 18: 2193–2200.

Sellar GC, Watt KP, Rabiasz GJ et al 2003 OPCML at 11q25 is epigenetically inactivated and has tumor-suppressor function in epithelial ovarian cancer. Nature Genetics 34: 337–343.

Slamon DJ, Godolphin W, Jones LA et al 1989 Studies of the HER-2/neu proto-oncogene in human breast and ovarian cancer. Science 244: 707–712.

Smith SA, Easton DF, Evans DG, Ponder BA 1992 Allele losses in the region 17q12-21 in familial breast and ovarian cancer involve the wild-type chromosome. Nature Genetics 2: 128.

Su HY, Lai HC, Lin YW, Chou YC, Liu CY, Yu MH 2009 An epigenetic marker panel for screening and prognostic prediction of ovarian cancer. International Journal of Cancer 124: 387–393.

Tashiro H, Miyazaki K, Okamura H, Iwai A, Fukumoto M 1992 c-myc over-expression in human primary ovarian tumours: its relevance to tumour progression. International Journal of Cancer 50: 828–833.

Thomas RK, Baker AC, Debiasi RM et al 2007 High-throughput oncogene mutation profiling in human cancer. Nature Genetics 39: 347–351.

Thorlacius S, Sigurdsson S, Bjarnadottir H et al 1997 Study of a single BRCA2 mutation with high carrier frequency in a small population. American Journal of Human Genetics 60: 1079–1084.

Tone AA, Begley H, Sharma M et al 2008 Gene expression profiles of luteal phase fallopian tube epithelium from BRCA mutation carriers resemble high-grade serous carcinoma. Clinical Cancer Research 14: 4067–4078.

Wang K, Gan L, Jeffery E et al 1999 Monitoring gene expression profile changes in ovarian carcinomas using cDNA microarray. Gene 229: 101–108.

Wentzensen N, Sherman ME, Schiffman M, Wang SS 2009 Utility of methylation markers in cervical cancer early detection: appraisal of the state-of-the-science. Gynecological Oncology 112: 293–299.

Whiteside MA, Siegel EM, Unger ER 2008 Human papillomavirus and molecular considerations for cancer risk. Cancer 113 (Suppl): 2981–2994.

Williams GH, Romanowski P, Morris L et al 1998 Improved cervical smear assessment using antibodies against proteins that regulate DNA replication. Proceedings of the National Academy of Science USA 95: 14932–14937.

Wooster R, Bignell G, Lancaster J et al 1995 Identification of the breast cancer susceptibility gene BRCA2. Nature 378: 789–792.

Zeimet AG, Marth C 2003 Why did p53 gene therapy fail in ovarian cancer? The Lancet Oncology 4: 415–422.

Zhang L, Volinia S, Bonome T et al 2008 Genomic and epigenetic alterations deregulate microRNA expression in human epithelial ovarian cancer. Proceedings of the National Academy of Science USA 105: 7004–7009.

Zhou XC, Dowdy SC, Podratz KC, Jiang SW 2007 Epigenetic considerations for endometrial cancer prevention, diagnosis and treatment. Gynecological Oncology 107: 143–153.

zur Hausen H 1987 Papillomaviruses in human cancer. Applied Pathology 5: 19–24.

CHAPTER 36

Principles of radiotherapy and chemotherapy

Nawaz Walji and Indrajit Fernando

Chapter Contents

RADIOTHERAPY	539	**KEY POINTS**	553
CHEMOTHERAPY	547		

Radiotherapy

Radiotherapy is the utilization of ionizing radiation, primarily for the treatment of malignant cancers and infrequently for some preinvasive and benign conditions. It is central to the curative treatment of women with cervical carcinoma, and is used in the adjuvant and palliative treatment of other gynaecological malignancies.

Radiation physics

Therapeutic ionizing radiation can be electromagnetic or particulate. Particulate radiation causes ionization directly and electromagnetic radiation indirectly by ejecting fast-moving electrons from atoms, resulting in potentially significant biochemical, cellular and tissue changes within biological systems. Radiation energy absorbed in tissue is measured in grays (Gy), with 1 Gy being equivalent to 1 joule per kilogram.

Electromagnetic radiation

X-rays and gamma-rays (γ-rays) are part of the electromagnetic spectrum; the former are produced artificially and the latter from naturally occurring or artificially produced radio-isotopes. Megavoltage X-rays for therapeutic purposes are produced by a linear accelerator (Figure 36.1) by accelerating electrons to high kinetic energies on to a target composed of tungsten or gold. Kinetic energy given up by the electrons is converted to high-energy X-rays. γ-rays are emitted as byproducts of radioactive isotopes (e.g. iridium-192) undergoing decay to reach a stable nuclide.

X-rays and γ-rays are characterized by very short wavelengths and high frequencies, and consist of packets of energies (photons) capable of tissue ionization. Higher energy photons have greater tissue penetration. Photon energies in the range of 6–15 million electron volts (megavolts, MV) are typically used for pelvic irradiation, although higher energies may be required for obese patients to achieve adequate dose to the centre of the pelvis. Use of photon energies less than 4 MV can result in greater dose variation within the patient.

Particulate radiation

This consists of atomic subparticles: electrons (negatively charged), protons (positively charged), neutrons (no charge) and negative π-mesons. Only electrons are commonly used in clinical practice. High-energy electrons are produced in a linear accelerator from which the target has been removed. Electrons react more rapidly with tissue compared with photons, and have a depth–dose profile which follows a plateau for a distance depending on the electron energy, followed by a rapid dose fall-off. Electrons are useful for the treatment of superficial tumours, allowing sparing of deeper structures which reduces treatment-related morbidity.

Proton beam radiotherapy has generated increasing interest in recent years. The dose distribution of a monoenergetic proton beam increases slowly with depth but reaches a sharp maximum near the end of the particle's range (Bragg peak) with subsequent rapid dose fall-off. This has the attraction of precisely confining the high-dose region to the deep-seated tumour volume whilst minimizing the dose to the surrounding normal tissues. The availability of proton beam therapy remains restricted by the limited number of cyclotron machines available globally for the production of protons.

Radiobiology

Radiobiology is the study of the effects of ionizing radiation on biological systems. Ionizing radiation acts on both normal and cancer cells. The primary ionization event in living cells usually occurs within intracellular water molecules, with subsequent ionization occurring in surrounding macromolecules. Deoxyribose nucleic acid (DNA) is the critical intracellular target for radiation therapy. Following DNA damage, some cells undergo immediate apoptosis. More frequently, death occurs at subsequent mitosis and the main effect of radiation is to delay or prevent mitosis. The onset of the latter depends on the cellular turnover time, hence more rapidly dividing systems (e.g. intestinal epithelium) show the effects of radiation earlier compared with slowly dividing systems (e.g. central nervous system).

DOI: 10.1016/B978-0-7020-3120-5.00036-9

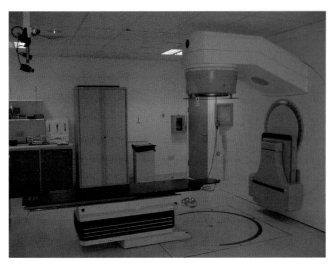

Figure 36.1 A linear accelerator and radiotherapy treatment room. The linear accelerator can rotate 360° around the treatment couch, which is also able to rotate about its axis, allowing the patient to be treated using beams from multiple directions. The patient is monitored during treatment using cameras, and communication is possible using a microphone.

Eradication of a cancer is only possible if irreversible DNA damage in all tumour clonogens is achieved. The success or otherwise of ionizing radiation in achieving this is governed by the five 'Rs' of radiobiology: reoxygenation, redistribution, repair, repopulation and (intrinsic) radiosensitivity. *Intracellular oxygen* is important for the ionizing effects of radiation, and total hypoxia results in a dose reduction of a factor of 2–3 in most biological systems. *Reoxygenation* of hypoxic cells occurs as a consequence of tumour regression during fractionated radiotherapy, resulting in increased radiation efficacy. Anaemia is a poor prognostic factor in the treatment of cervical carcinoma, and is thought to relate to reduced oxygen partial pressures secondary to a low haemoglobin concentration. Patients having radiotherapy for cervical carcinoma should have their haemoglobin concentration maintained above 12 g/dl. *Redistribution* of cells into the cell cycle from the resting phase during a course of fractionated radiotherapy increases the number of cells undergoing mitotic division, increasing the probability of tumour cell kill. Despite radiation, some tumour clonogens may undergo successful *repair* of DNA damage, and subsequent *repopulation* of these cells results in treatment failure. Finally, *intrinsic radiosensitivity* is an inherent property of tumours; some tumours (e.g. lymphomas) are successfully eradicated with relatively low doses of radiotherapy, whilst others (e.g. gliomas) frequently recur despite high radiation doses. Indirect effects of radiation on tumours include loss of small blood vessels leading to tumour necrosis and subsequent activation of the reticuloendothelial system.

A major challenge for radiotherapists is to eradicate tumours without causing significant permanent damage to normal tissue. Three important factors need consideration when planning a radical course of radiation: the total dose of radiation required to achieve tumour eradication, the number of fractions required to deliver the total dose, and the length of time over which the treatment is delivered. Normal tissues have a greater capacity for repair of sublethal DNA damage compared with cancer cells, provided that the overall dose is not too large and is given over a period of time. However, significant prolongation of treatment increases the risk of treatment failure for some cancers, including squamous cell carcinoma of the cervix. Advantages of fractionated radiotherapy include:

- repair of DNA damage and repopulation of cells in normal tissues between treatment fractions;
- recruitment of cancer cells from the resting phase into the more radiosensitive phases of the cell cycle; and
- reoxygenation of hypoxic tumour cells following tumour regression.

Normal tissue tolerance is an important concept in radiotherapy. Accepted tolerance ranges of total radiation dose which result in a clinically acceptable low incidence of treatment-related morbidity have been established. A number of factors adversely influence the radiation tolerance of normal tissues, including: volume of tissue irradiated, previous surgery, exposure to previous or concomitant cytotoxic treatment, vascular insufficiency, diabetes mellitus and connective tissue disorders.

Concomitant chemoradiation

Cisplatin-based chemoradiation became the standard of care in cervical cancer following an alert issued by the National Cancer Institute in 1999. The benefit of chemoradiation in cervical cancer over radiotherapy alone has been confirmed by recent meta-analyses. Concomitant chemotherapy may have an additive or synergistic effect when combined with radiotherapy. Perceived benefits include increased tumour sensitization to radiotherapy and eradication of systemic micrometastatic disease.

Radiation dose and scheduling

Radiotherapy fractionation

Conventional practice involves once-daily treatment giving five fractions per week using 1.8–2 Gy/fraction. Modified dose-fractionation schedules have been investigated in an attempt to improve cure rates. Hyperfractionated radiotherapy is the delivery of two or more fractions per day using smaller doses per fraction to deliver a higher total dose over the same time period compared with standard fractionated radiotherapy. An interfraction gap of a minimum of 6 h is recommended for recovery of normal cells. Advantages of this approach include delivery of a higher total dose to improve tumour eradication whilst allowing sufficient time for normal tissue repair between fractions. Accelerated radiotherapy refers to the delivery of radiotherapy over a significantly shorter period of time by delivering six or more fractions per week, with an interfraction gap of a minimum of 6 h. The total dose and dose per fraction remain the same as for standard treatment. Delivering radiotherapy over a shorter period of time reduces the negative effects of accelerated repopulation seen in some cancers. Hypofractionated radiotherapy delivers radiation treatment over a shorter period of time by using fraction sizes larger than 2 Gy/fraction. However, such an approach increases the risk of late normal tissue toxicity, as normal tissues are more sensitive to larger doses per fraction compared with tumour cells. In order to reduce this risk, the total dose of radiotherapy is reduced to deliver the same biologically effective dose. Hypofractionated radiotherapy is commonly used in palliative radiotherapy to minimize patient inconvenience and to optimize resource utilization.

Dose prescription

A radiotherapy prescription specifies the total dose to be given, the total number of fractions to be used, the dose per fraction, and the overall treatment duration. The total dose required to eradicate a tumour is dependent on the tumour volume to be treated. Whereas a dose of 50 Gy in 25 fractions treating five times per week over 5 weeks is sufficient to eradicate microscopic disease in 90% of cases, doses above 66 Gy using 2 Gy/fraction over 6.5 weeks are required to eradicate macroscopic disease. Where delivery of radical radiotherapy with curative intent is not possible because of tumour-related (e.g. tumour volume, metastatic disease) or patient-related (e.g. poor performance status) factors, palliative radiotherapy may be considered to alleviate distressing symptoms. Doses typically used include 8 Gy in a single fraction, 20 Gy in five fractions over 1 week or 30 Gy in 10 fractions over 2 weeks.

Radiotherapy techniques

Teletherapy, also referred to as 'external beam radiotherapy', and brachytherapy are commonly utilized in the treatment of gynaecological malignancies and are discussed below. Instillation of radioactive fluids into the peritoneal or pleural cavity for treating small volume disease is rarely used and will not be discussed in detail.

External beam radiotherapy

This is irradiation of tumours at a 'long' distance away from the source of ionizing radiation. Pelvic external beam radiotherapy remains integral to the treatment of gynaecological malignancies as it permits irradiation of the primary tumour and regional lymph nodes. The dose that can be delivered to the tumour is limited by the tolerance of the normal tissues, also referred to as the 'organs at risk', which include the small bowel, rectum and bladder. Technological advances in the methods of radiation delivery are increasingly permitting the use of techniques which minimize the dose received by normal tissues whilst allowing a higher dose to be delivered to the tumour. Radiotherapy treatment planning remains a vital component of radiation treatment.

Radiotherapy planning

The aim of radiotherapy planning is to deliver a homogenous dose to the primary tumour and potential areas of micrometastatic disease whilst minimizing the dose to the organs at risk. Accurate tumour localization is central to radiotherapy planning, and it is important to have the following information to hand: findings of clinical examination including examination under anaesthesia, operation notes and intraoperative findings, histopathology report and the results of any radiological investigations including computed tomography (CT), magnetic resonance imaging (MRI) and [18]FDG-positron emission tomography (PET) scans.

Simulator-based radiotherapy planning has been superseded by CT-based planning which allows more accurate visualization of the tumour and organs at risk. Where appropriate, coregistration of MRI and CT images provides greater certainty and clarification of anatomy. Coregistration of functional imaging scans (e.g. PET scan) with planning CT scans may provide yet more sophisticated radiotherapy planning. The simulator — a diagnostic X-ray machine connected to a television screen which emulates a treatment machine — continues to have a useful role for palliative radiotherapy planning. It is also useful in the minority of cases where CT scanning is not possible due to patient obesity or other patient-related factors.

Planning procedure

A vaginal examination is performed prior to the CT scan to determine the extent of vaginal involvement and the most inferior aspect of the tumour. The patient is scanned in the supine position unless a belly board is used to displace the small bowel anteriorly to minimize small bowel irradiation, in which case she is placed in the prone position. A vaginal probe can aid in defining the extent of vaginal involvement, although this is not universally utilized. Rectal contrast may be used to delineate the rectum and sigmoid. Intravenous contrast may be administered to enhance identification of blood vessels which are anatomical landmarks for the regional lymph nodes. A CT scan is performed using 2.5–5-mm slices from the third lumbar vertebra to 5 cm below the ischial tuberosities. The superior border is extended to include the lower thoracic vertebrae if para-aortic lymph node irradiation is required. The patient is asked to have a comfortably full bladder to reduce the volume of small bowel within the pelvis. Following acquisition of CT images, permanent tattoos are marked on the patient's skin as reference points for aligning her in the correct position for each fraction of treatment.

Conformal radiotherapy

The CT scan images are subsequently transferred to a computer terminal (Figure 36.2) with software allowing delineation of target volumes and organs at risk according to recommendations from the International Commission on Radiation Units and Measurements. The gross tumour volume includes the palpable and/or radiologically visible tumour; it is absent if it has been surgically resected. The clinical target volume (CTV) involves the gross tumour volume and potential areas of microscopic disease (e.g. pelvic lymph nodes and parametria in cervical cancer). The CTV is grown by a margin to allow for internal organ motion and geometric uncertainties in treatment delivery; this is called the 'planning target volume' (PTV). The organs at risk for pelvic radiation include the rectum, bladder, small bowel and both hip joints. The kidneys and spinal cord are the dose-limiting organs at risk when radiating the para-aortic lymph nodes. The clinician specifies the dose fractionation to be used in the radiation treatment of the patient.

Following the process described above, a radiotherapy treatment plan is produced by medical physicists using complex computer algorithms which simulate the effects of a radiation beam passing through the designated area and the radiation dose deposited at any one site. Three or more

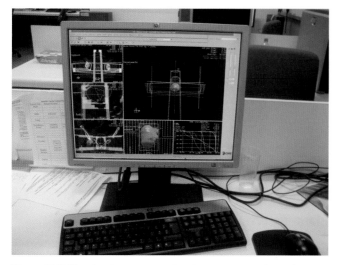

Figure 36.2 The planning computer showing a treatment plan and dose–volume histogram.

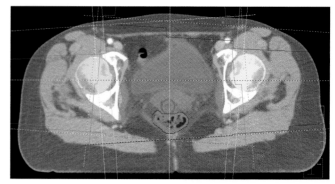

Figure 36.3 A computed tomography (CT) slice from a four-field conformal radiotherapy plan to treat a patient with carcinoma of the cervix. The green area represents the clinical target volume (CTV) consisting of the primary tumour plus a margin for microscopic disease and the pelvic nodes. The organs at risk are also drawn on the CT slice: rectum (blue), urinary bladder (purple) and femoral heads (yellow).
Image courtesy of Professor Peter Hoskin, Mount Vernon Hospital, Northwood.

beams are typically required to produce a homogenous dose for the radiation of pelvic cancers; the use of two beams increases the volume of bowel receiving radiotherapy and risk of radiation enteropathy. However, the use of two opposing anterior–posterior beams is necessary for irradiation of carcinoma of the vulva due to irradiation of inguinal lymph nodes. Modern linear accelerators contain computer-driven multi-leaf collimators which shape the radiation beams to improve conformity to the PTV and to shield the organs at risk. These have replaced the lead blocks previously manually placed in the beam to provide shielding of the organs at risk, thus speeding up the treatment process and reducing the heavy manual work required of therapy radiographers.

The final radiotherapy plan comprises the following information: the number of beams used to optimize conformity to the PTV, beam energies, beam direction, use of wedge angles and multi-leaf collimators to improve PTV conformity, and the dose distribution and percentage dose received by the PTV. A dose–volume histogram is provided to determine the dose being received by the PTV and organs at risk. The final plan is checked and approved by the clinician prior to implementation of the radiotherapy plan (Figure 36.3). Verification checks are performed to validate the treatment plan and to detect for any unforeseen errors prior to starting radiation treatment. A standard dose prescription for carcinoma of the cervix is 45–50 Gy in 25–28 fractions using 1.8 Gy/fraction over 5–5.5 weeks.

The patient is treated in a specially designed room to prevent radiation of personnel outside the room. The patient is positioned on the treatment couch with reference to the tattoo marks (Figure 36.4). Computerized transfer of planning data from the planning computer to the linear accelerator minimizes the risk of human error in transferring data. The radiographers control the linear accelerator from outside the room using a console which is used to start and stop the radiation beam, and to set the duration of treatment and the dose to be delivered. The patient is monitored using cameras in the treatment room, and communication with the patient is possible via a microphone. These safety features are designed to optimize radiation treatment and are subject to frequent quality assurance checks.

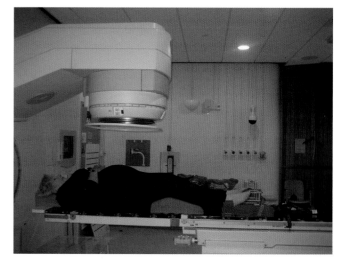

Figure 36.4 Patient lying on the couch of a linear accelerator.

Virtual simulation

The planning CT scan images can be reconstructed using computer software to provide a digitally reconstructed radiograph (DRR). Bony landmarks are used for radiotherapy planning with the clinician using the computer software to place the radiation beams on to the DRR. This is akin to conventional radiotherapy. The advantages of virtually simulated radiotherapy planning include: the clinician is able to visualize the pelvic soft tissues by using the CT scan images, thus ensuring the tumour is encompassed within the radiation field; radiotherapy planning is less time-consuming compared with conformal radiotherapy; the clinician can apply multi-leaf collimators at the time of planning to optimize shielding of the organs at risk; and a dose distribution can be provided by the medical physicists to ensure that the PTV is receiving the prescribed dose. The disadvantages of virtually simulated radiotherapy planning are that it is not suitable for producing complex radiotherapy plans, and a dose–volume histogram cannot be provided to determine the dose being received by the organs at risk. Virtually simulated radiotherapy (Figure 36.5) is frequently utilized for pelvic radiotherapy for the reasons outlined above.

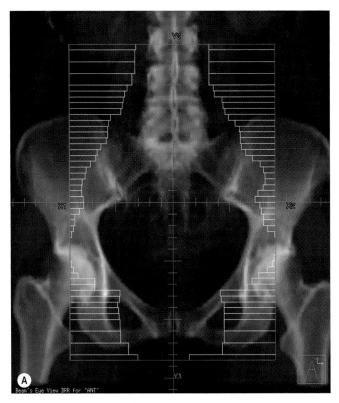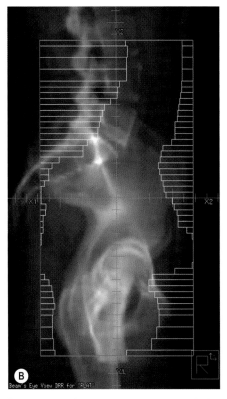

Figure 36.5 Anterior (A) and right lateral (B) views of a virtually simulated radiotherapy plan for carcinoma of the cervix. The superior border has been extended superiorly to include the common iliac lymph nodes. The red (A) and green (B) delineated areas denote the planning target volume; the white rectangles represent the multi-leaf collimators used to shield organs at risk which do not need to be irradiated.
Images courtesy of Professor Peter Hoskin, Mount Vernon Hospital, Northwood.

Conventional radiotherapy

Conventional external beam radiotherapy uses bony landmarks to define the target volume for pelvic radiotherapy. A simulator film is obtained after the patient is aligned on the simulator couch using orthogonal lasers. Cross wires mounted in the light beam from the simulator define the size of the area to be treated, and anterior–posterior and lateral pelvic X-rays are obtained as permanent records. The clinician is able to identify areas where shielding can be applied to reduce dose to the organs at risk (Figure 36.6). As diagnostic X-rays have poor soft tissue resolution, the clinician must rely on information gathered from clinical examination and radiological investigations to determine the target volume. Studies have reported underdosing of the regional lymph nodes in up to 40% of patients using conventional radiotherapy. However, conventional radiotherapy planning still has a role in centres where access to CT planning software is restricted due to resource implications, in patients unable to fit into a CT scan machine due to gross obesity, and in palliative radiotherapy.

Intensity-modulated radiotherapy

Intensity-modulated radiotherapy (IMRT) is generally regarded as a significant advancement in the development of conformal radiotherapy. A major advantage of IMRT is the ability to generate PTVs which conform to targets which are concave in the plane of the incident beams, which is not possible with standard conformal radiation. This is achieved by using numerous non-coplanar beams of varying intensity to improve conformity to treatment targets whilst further reducing the dose to selected organs at risk. However, IMRT results in a larger volume of normal tissue receiving low doses of radiation; one of the concerns of IMRT is that, over a period of time, this may result in a higher incidence of secondary malignancies and other unwanted late toxicities.

IMRT may be inverse- or forward-planned. In inverse-planned IMRT, the clinician specifies the dose constraints within the patient and an inverse-planning algorithm computes the beam modulations required to produce the specified dose distribution. A number of planning cycles may be required to produce an 'optimized' dose distribution. Forward-planned IMRT utilizes a limited number of non-coplanar beams of different weighting to deliver a more conformal plan. An additional advantage of IMRT is that it is possible to allocate different dose targets within a single treatment volume by a process called 'simultaneous integrated boost IMRT'.

A number of studies investigating the role of IMRT in cervical and endometrial cancer have been published in the literature. The majority are single-centre retrospective analyses involving fewer than 100 patients.

Whilst the use of IMRT may be promising, there are insufficient long-term data regarding its efficacy and safety in the treatment of gynaecological malignancies. Concerns have been raised regarding the use of IMRT because of the poor visualization of the cervix on CT scans. The use of MRI/CT fusion is currently being explored. IMRT should be regarded as an experimental treatment in gynaecological cancers, and its use should be confined to clinical trials until there are convincing data for its role in these cancers.

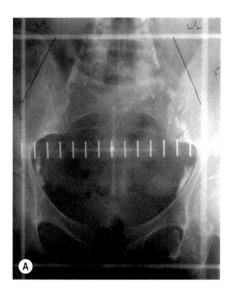

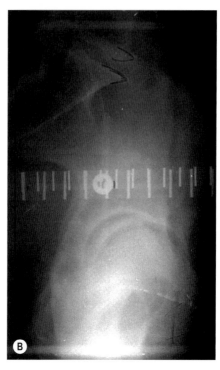

Figure 36.6 Anteroposterior (A) and lateral (B) X-rays of the pelvis showing the superior, inferior and lateral margins. The triangular areas are protected from the beam. The patient has had a lymphangiogram.

Brachytherapy

This entails the delivery of ionizing radiation using sealed sources placed as close to the tumour as possible. The principal advantage of brachytherapy lies in the delivery of a very high dose of radiation to the tumour whilst relatively sparing normal tissues due to a rapid fall-off of dose away from the source according to the principle of the inverse square law. Other advantages over external beam radiation include: the accurate localization of tumour and immobilization of the area being treated reduces set-up errors; and delivery of treatment over a significantly shorter period, thus eliminating the risk of accelerated tumour repopulation associated with protracted courses of radiotherapy. A major disadvantage includes the need to access the tumour, which frequently requires an operative procedure subject to the competency of the brachytherapist. In gynaecological cancers, brachytherapy is commonly used to boost the tumour following external beam radiotherapy, as in cervical cancer. It may be used as the primary treatment for early cancers where surgery is contraindicated (e.g. early cervical and vaginal cancers). Vaginal vault brachytherapy is increasingly used as the sole adjuvant treatment following surgery for endometrial cancer with a good prognosis.

Radionuclides used in gynaecological malignancies

Radium-226 was the first radionuclide used in gynaecological brachytherapy. It has a half-life of 1620 years and decays by alpha emission to its gaseous daughter product, radon-222. There were several disadvantages associated with the use of radium-226, including emission of high-energy photons which required thick shielding and storage of the daughter nuclides for prolonged time periods. Radium-226 has been replaced with more convenient radionuclides such as caesium-137, cobalt-60 and iridium-192. Other artificially produced radionuclides are likely to become available for brachytherapy use in the future.

Dose rates in brachytherapy

Moderate-dose-rate (MDR) and high-dose-rate (HDR) brachytherapy are commonly used in gynaecological malignancies. Whilst there is no universally accepted definition of dose rate, it is generally accepted that MDR uses dose rates of 1–12 Gy/h whereas HDR refers to dose rates greater than 12 Gy/h. Sufficient data are available to suggest that both are equally effective in achieving tumour control when used in the treatment of gynaecological malignancies. MDR brachytherapy is typically delivered over a period of 12–14 h, and thus requires inpatient treatment in an appropriately designed room. The patient is required to remain flat and immobile during this period to prevent displacement of the applicators. MDR brachytherapy has the radiobiological attraction of allowing treatment to be completed in a short period of time, thus reducing the negative effects of tumour repair and repopulation. Advantages of HDR brachytherapy include shorter treatment times, allowing outpatient-based treatment and the reduced risk of applicator displacement during treatment. However, HDR brachytherapy requires fractionation of treatment to reduce the risk of late tissue toxicity, with three to six fractions being delivered on a weekly basis. This leads to prolongation of the overall treatment time, associated with a theoretical disadvantage of allowing tumour repair and repopulation between treatment fractions. Pulsed-dose-rate (PDR) brachytherapy utilizes HDR treatment to simulate LDR brachytherapy to minimize the radiobiological disadvantages of prolonging overall treatment time. In PDR brachytherapy, pulses of HDR treatment are repeated at short intervals to simulate LDR brachytherapy.

Delivery systems in gynaecological brachytherapy

The manual insertion of radioactive sources into tumours has almost become obsolete and has been superseded by afterloading systems. Afterloading involves the initial placement of non-radioactive applicators within the patient with subsequent insertion of the radioactive material. This has the advantage of significantly reducing the risk of exposing personnel to the radioactive sources. The use of machine (remote) afterloading techniques virtually eliminates the risk of radiation exposure for all personnel, and has become the standard of care in gynaecological brachytherapy.

Intracavitary brachytherapy

This technique is routinely used for the radical treatment of cervical cancer where hysterectomy has not been performed, and occasionally in patients with inoperable endometrial cancer. The procedure is carried out under general anaesthesia unless contraindicated, in which case spinal anaesthesia provides a suitable alternative. The patient is examined to assess tumour size and parametrial involvement, and a urinary catheter is inserted. Following cervical dilatation, a sound is used to assess the uterine length. The width of the vaginal vault is estimated to guide the applicator sizes required. The intrauterine tube is inserted first, followed by the vaginal applicators. A rectal retractor may also be inserted to push the anterior rectal wall further away from the applicators; alternatively, a gauze pack may be used to achieve this purpose and also to secure the applicators in place. A simulator film is taken with the applicators in place once the patient is awake, which is then transferred on to a planning computer to allow dosimetry calculations to be performed. The patient is treated in an appropriately shielded room using a remote afterloading system (Figure 36.7). The patient is monitored via a camera inside the treatment room, and a microphone can be used to communicate with the patient. Once treatment is completed, the applicator and gauze packing are removed and the patient is discharged home.

A number of applicator systems are available for intracavitary brachytherapy, all of which are based around the principle of delivering a high radiation dose to the cervix, parametrium and upper vagina. Two main types of applicator are available (Figure 36.8a,b,c).

- A central intrauterine tube and lateral vaginal sources (ovoid). Several variations on this theme are available for use.
- A central tube and ring applicator. This technique is considered to allow greater individualization of dose distribution. It is a variation of the intrauterine and ovoids mentioned above.
- A single line source, which is advocated by some brachytherapists. It is useful for treatment where the cervical carcinoma is extending down into the vagina.

The Manchester system was developed to calculate and describe the dose distribution for intracavitary brachytherapy. The system specified activity loadings for the intrauterine tube and each ovoid to give a dose defined to a defined reference point, called 'Point A'. This is defined as being 2 cm lateral to the centre of the uterine canal and 2 cm superior to the mucous membrane of the lateral fornix along the line of the uterine canal. An additional point (Point B)

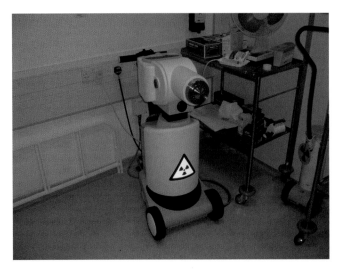

Figure 36.7 A remote afterloading high-dose brachytherapy machine. Once the applicators are inserted and a radiotherapy plan is produced, the applicators are attached to the machine using cathethers. The patient is treated in the room in isolation to allow protection of staff from the ionizing radiation.

placed 3 cm lateral to Point A is used to calculate the dose received by the pelvic side wall.

Conventionally, a total dose of 75–85 Gy is delivered to Point A. Following external beam radiotherapy with a dose of 45–50 Gy in 25–28 fractions, a dose of 25–27 Gy is delivered to Point A using MDR brachytherapy. A number of recommendations exist for the total dose and number of fractions used for HDR brachytherapy. The most commonly used dose fractionation is 21 Gy in three fractions using 7 Gy per fraction.

Vaginal vault brachytherapy

Following hysterectomy, women with cervical or endometrial cancer with pathological features suggestive of a high risk of relapse are often recommended to have adjuvant radiotherapy, including vaginal vault brachytherapy where appropriate. Vaginal vault brachytherapy is increasingly being used as the sole adjuvant treatment for endometrial cancer in women with intermediate–high risk of pelvic relapse. A number of vaginal applicators are available for use, including vaginal cylinders (Figure 36.8D) of varying sizes, vaginal ovoids or individualized vaginal moulds. Applicator insertion may be carried out on the ward or in the brachytherapy suite, although some brachytherapists prefer the procedure to be carried out in theatre under general anaesthesia.

Following insertion of the applicators, patients undergo the same planning process as for intracavitary brachytherapy. Following external beam radiotherapy (45 Gy in 25 fractions), a dose of 15 Gy is prescribed to 5 mm if using MDR brachytherapy. If using HDR brachytherapy, 12 Gy in two or three fractions may be prescribed.

Interstitial brachytherapy

Interstitial brachytherapy is used for the treatment of tumours of the vagina and vulva, either as primary treatment for small tumours or to boost the primary tumour following external

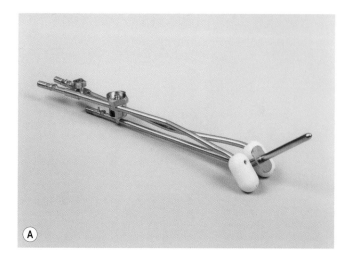

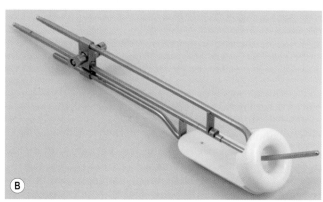

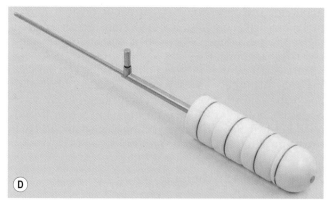

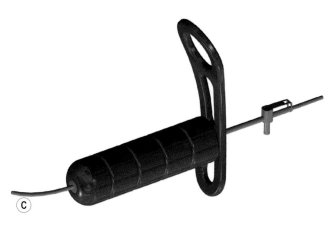

Figure 36.8 Different types of applicators available for intracavitary brachytherapy. (A) Intrauterine tube and two ovoids, which is used as the standard applicator system for delivering intrauterine brachytherapy, although some centres use the intrauterine tube and ring applicator shown in (B). Other brachytherapists advocate the use of a single line source as shown in (c). An example of a vaginal cylinder applicator used for vaginal vault brachytherapy is also shown (D).
Image B–D courtesy of Nucletron.

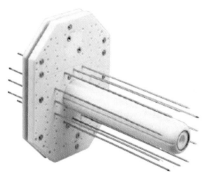

Figure 36.9 A Martinez universal perineal interstitial template for interstitial treatment of carcinoma of the vagina.
Image courtesy of Nucletron.

beam radiotherapy. It can also be used for palliating symptoms for locally recurrent or metastatic cancers of the vagina and vulva. Either LDR iridium wire interstitial implants or HDR afterloading implant techniques can be used for perineal implants using some form of perineal template (Figure 36.9). Perineal implants are performed under general or spinal anaesthesia. Computer-based planning allows for more accurate visualization of the tumour in relation to the implant (Figure 36.10).

Image-guided adaptive brachytherapy

Simulator-based dosimetry for intracavitary brachytherapy relies on doses to points (e.g. Point A) rather than to volumes. For advanced cervical tumours, prescribing to Point A may lead to tumour underdosage as a proportion of the tumour may lie outside the high-dose envelope. Image-guided adaptive brachytherapy uses CT and/or MRI imaging to allow visualization of the tumour in relation to the applicator and the organs at risk at the time of brachytherapy to enable dose adaptation to the target whilst improving the sparing of normal tissues (Figure 36.11). The possibility of fusing FDG-PET images with planning CT software provides another potential avenue for the use of adaptive brachytherapy to improve tumour control.

Image-guided adaptive brachytherapy is a relatively new concept for the treatment of cervical cancer, and is only available in a few centres. Some of the challenges to the widespread adaptation of this technique include: the availability of CT- and MRI-compatible applicators, the availability of software to define applicator geometry for CT and MRI, coregistration of pelvic CT and MRI images, and a limited number of published clinical results. Image-based adaptive brachytherapy continues to generate significant interest, with the potential of improving tumour control and significantly reducing treatment-related morbidity.

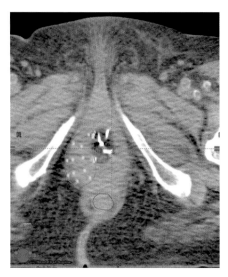

Figure 36.10 Computed tomography slice showing perineal brachytherapy to treat carcinoma of the right vaginal wall. Packing is applied within the vagina to keep the left vaginal wall away from the radioactive sources, thus minimizing radiation toxicity.
Image courtesy of Professor Peter Hoskin, Mount Vernon Hospital, Northwood.

Radiation morbidity

Treatment-related morbidity is the dose-limiting factor when utilizing radiotherapy for the curative treatment of any cancer, and has potentially important physical and psycho-social consequences for the patient. The risk of unwanted radiation effects is determined by the interaction of tumour- and patient-related factors. Unwanted radiation effects are divided into early effects, arbitrarily defined as those occurring within 90 days of starting treatment, and late effects, defined as those occurring more than 90 days after starting treatment. In pelvic radiotherapy, the small bowel, rectum and bladder are the main organs at risk. The kidneys and spinal cord are the vital organs at risk when para-aortic lymph node irradiation is required. Table 36.1 summarizes the early and potential late effects associated with pelvic radiation.

Conclusion

Radiotherapy continues to play a central role in the treatment of gynaecological malignancies. Technological advances are allowing increasingly sophisticated ways of planning and delivering radiation treatment in this group of patients. This is accompanied by ongoing research in ways to improve tumour control whilst minimizing the unwanted effects of radiotherapy.

Chemotherapy

Cytotoxic chemotherapy as a primary treatment modality cures less than 5% of all malignancies. It is the definitive mode of treatment in gestational trophoblastic tumours and germ cell tumours of the ovary. Chemotherapy is often used in conjunction with other treatment modalities such as surgery and radiotherapy in the treatment of gynaecological malignancies, either in an attempt to effect cure (radical), or to palliate symptoms and prolong survival in patients with

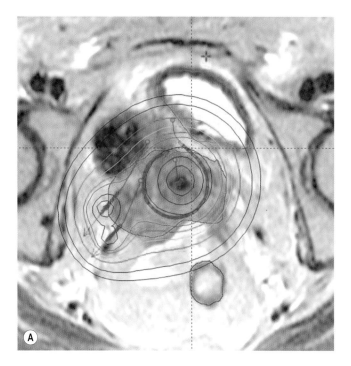

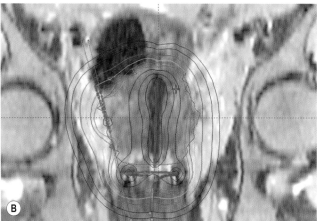

Figure 36.11 (A, B) Image-guided brachytherapy showing the treatment of a patient with cervical carcinoma with right parametrial involvement using interstitial brachytherapy. Treatment is performed using standard intracavitary treatment and interstitial brachytherapy to boost the right parametrium, thus allowing greater conformity of treatment using image-guided brachytherapy.
Images courtesy of Professor Peter Hoskin, Mount Vernon Hospital., Northwood.

advanced or metastatic disease (palliative chemotherapy). Adjuvant chemotherapy is utilized where disease is known or suspected to be present after surgery, with the intent of prolonging disease-free and overall survival (e.g. in ovarian or endometrial carcinoma). There is increasing interest in the role for neoadjuvant chemotherapy to reduce the burden of tumour prior to definitive surgery in advanced ovarian carcinoma. The use of concurrent chemoradiation is well established in the radical treatment of cervical carcinoma. It is also used for the radical treatment of selected cases of vulval cancer. The use of chemotherapy in patients with metastatic incurable cancers poses unique challenges; whilst chemotherapy may extend survival, treatment is often associated with unwanted side-effects which can negatively impact on the patient's quality of life. On the other hand,

Table 36.1 Early and late unwanted radiation effects

Organ	Early effect	Late effect
Skin	Erythema, desquamation	Telangiectasia, fibrosis
Small bowel, sigmoid and rectum	Radiation colitis or proctitis	Radiation proctitis, diarrhoea, bowel stenosis, fistulae
Bladder	Radiation cystitis	Radiation cystitis, fistulae
Hip joints and pelvic bones		Osteoradionecrosis, insufficiency fractures
Ovaries		Infertility, menopause
Vagina	Mucositis	Vaginal stenosis, fistulae
Lymph nodes		Lymphoedema
Spinal cord		Radiation myelopathy
Kidneys		Renal failure, hydronephrosis
General		Secondary cancers

response to palliative chemotherapy can lead to improvement in the patient's symptoms with subsequent improvement in quality of life. Prior to embarking on a course of palliative chemotherapy, several factors must be taken into account, including performance status, previous treatments, response rates to chemotherapy, utility of other treatments to alleviate symptoms and, ultimately, the patient's wishes and expectations.

Drug discovery and clinical trials

Historically, the process of drug discovery relied on highly empirical approaches based on testing randomly selected compounds against rapidly proliferating murine leukaemic cells. This has been replaced by rational drug design based on the expanding knowledge of the molecular mechanisms of cancer, and the use of automated in-vitro screens using panels of human tumour cell lines, some chosen for their resistance to existing agents.

Of the hundreds of thousands of chemical and biological agents tested in laboratories, only a small number find their way into routine clinical use. Before any new agent can be tested on humans, it undergoes preclinical studies to assess both its efficacy and toxicity in animal models. A promising agent is then studied in phase I studies to determine the appropriate dose of the drug to be used in its subsequent development. Phase I trials are designed to define a drug's dose-limiting toxicities and the maximum tolerated dose. Pharmacokinetic studies form an integral part of phase I studies. Phase II studies are designed to assess the activity of a particular drug in different tumour types, measured as response rates. A drug demonstrating 'activity' in a particular tumour type is subsequently tested in phase III trials to further define its effectiveness and clinical utility.

Pharmacology

For a given chemotherapeutic agent to be effective, several features must be present, including: the drug must reach the cancer cells, sufficiently toxic amounts of the drug or its metabolites must enter the cell and remain there for an adequate period of time, and the cancer cells must be sensitive to the drug or its metabolites and must not overcome its effects by developing resistance to treatment. Pharmacology involves the study of drug pharmacokinetics and pharmacodynamics.

Pharmacokinetics is the study of processes that determine the concentration of the drug and its metabolites within the body (i.e. absorption, distribution, metabolism and excretion). Pharmacodynamics is the study of the relationship between drug concentration and effect. In oncological treatment, this therapeutic index may be quite narrow in that the dose required for therapeutic effect may be close to that which could cause severe side-effects. In most studies, drug plasma concentration is taken as the conventional measure for drug concentration at the site of action. The shape of the concentration–time curve is a predictor of effect and is defined by the pharmacokinetics.

Drugs can only be taken orally if they are well absorbed from the alimentary tract. Parenteral administration — intravenous, intramuscular or intra-arterial — is the optimal route for most chemotherapy agents as oral administration can result in poor absorption and uncertain bioavailability, particularly because of first-pass metabolism through the liver. However, after a bolus injection, redistribution will account for the initial fall in plasma concentration and is controlled by both redistribution and elimination. The latter is the sum of metabolism and excretion, although some drugs are excreted unchanged and others are metabolized and excreted. Excretion of drugs is a complicated process but usually involves both the liver and kidneys.

Another factor which determines drug concentration is protein binding. A number of cytotoxic drugs (e.g. etoposide) are heavily protein bound, and small reductions in binding could lead to a significant increase in drug concentration. Changes in protein binding may be caused by other drugs competing for binding sites. Redistribution of a drug increases clearance and factors such as cachexia may reduce this, as can hepatic and renal dysfunction. It can therefore be seen that knowledge of a drug's pharmacokinetics and pharmacodynamics is essential in order to predict and avoid either potential under- or overdosing.

In a clinical setting, factors such as serum albumin, liver function tests, creatinine, patient's age and performance status, and previous exposure to chemotherapy can guide the clinician in estimating the dose of chemotherapy to be used.

Routes of administration

Systemic chemotherapy

With intravenous administration, drugs are normally given at intervals of 1–4 weeks which permits recovery of bone marrow function between pulses of treatment. Although some cancer cells will also recover, there is a net loss of cancer cells in every cycle.

Intraperitoneal chemotherapy

The use of the intraperitoneal route to deliver chemotherapy in ovarian cancer has a long history. The attraction of such an approach is that high concentrations of drugs can be delivered into the peritoneal cavity which acts as a reservoir, releasing the drugs slowly into the systemic circulation. This results in very high and prolonged local concentration of the drug. However, absorption of cytotoxic drugs directly into tumour nodules is limited as penetration will only be three to six cells deep. Some agents are unsuitable because they cause a severe local chemical peritonitis. Cisplatin can be given by this route, but if the dose is too high, systemic complications ensue. Three randomized phase III trials have now shown that intraperitoneal delivery of a cisplatin-based regimen results in a 20–25% relative reduction in mortality for patients with small-volume residual advanced ovarian cancer. A variety of strategies are being investigated to improve the toxicity profile of platinum-based intraperitoneal chemotherapy.

Dose calculation

To give equivalent dosages to patients, the dose of chemotherapy drugs is based on an estimate of the patient's surface area (m^2), calculated from height and weight. Use of granulocyte-stimulating colony factors or dose modification may be required where bone marrow toxicity is encountered in order to prevent severe neutropenia and risk of infection. With renal or hepatic impairment, doses of drugs excreted by the kidneys or metabolized by the liver are reduced. Carboplatin dosage is often based upon a measurement of renal function, rather than surface area. This is called the 'Calvert formula' and allows the clinician to calculate a dose which will provide a specified area under the concentration–time curve.

Duration of therapy

The optimum duration of chemotherapy remains unknown. The duration of chemotherapy is determined by a number of factors including the indication for treatment, tumour response to chemotherapy, and patient tolerance to side-effects of chemotherapy. In practice, chemotherapy is usually given for 12–24 weeks, with prolongation of treatment being associated with a greater risk of toxicity.

Rarely, where tumours release a specific tumour marker such as β-human chorionic gonadotrophin in trophoblastic disease, marker measurements allow the treatment period to be defined more accurately for individual patients. Sufficiently sensitive and specific tumour markers are not yet developed for the common gynaecological tumours.

Drug resistance

The development of resistance to chemotherapeutic drugs by neoplastic cells remains one of the major obstacles in attempts to cure cancers with chemotherapy alone. Whilst some cells are inherently resistant, others adapt by using various detoxification pathways to acquire resistance. One common process that may cause resistance to virtually all chemotherapy agents is referred to as suppression or inactivation of cell-damage-induced apoptosis or loss of the apoptotic pathway, which results from inactivation of the *p53* tumour suppressor gene.

Other mechanisms of drug resistance include: overexpression of the Bcl-2 protein; overexpression of the multidrug resistance (*MDR-1*) gene enhancing production of the transmembrane protein P-170 which functions as a pump capable of ejecting cytotoxic agents from the cell; alteration of topoisomerase enzyme activity; and increased levels of intracellular concentrations of gluthathione and glutathione S-transferase isoenzymes.

Principles of combination therapy

Single-agent chemotherapy rarely cures human cancers, and combination chemotherapy was developed to provide maximal remission in most tumour types. The guiding principles of combination chemotherapy include:

- each agent must have single-agent activity against the tumour under study;
- drugs acting at different intracellular targets can be combined to give a synergistic effect;
- drugs with different toxicities can be combined to avoid the cumulative toxic effects of each individual drug;
- drugs must be administered as close as possible to their optimal dose and at a minimal interval, taking into account the toxicity of therapy; and
- the ability of tumour cells to develop resistance to cytotoxic therapy is reduced.

The case for combination chemotherapy in gynaecological cancers has not been proven completely in first-line treatment of ovarian cancer. Similar controversies also exist in advanced or metastatic cervical cancer, where potentially higher response rates have been associated with increased toxicity, possibly negating any therapeutic gain.

An alternative method of preventing the development of drug resistance is to give different drugs in turn. This also allows for a shorter treatment time, as severely myelotoxic drugs can be alternated with those which have no effect on the bone marrow. This approach has been effective in treating germ cell tumours and trophoblastic disease, but not epithelial tumours.

Classification

The most common classification of cytotoxic drugs is based on their mechanisms of action. Drugs are divided into alkylating agents, antimetabolites, vinca alkaloids, antibiotics, topoisomerase inhibitors, tubulin-binding agents and others. Table 36.2 summarizes the mechanism of action and toxicity of some of the chemotherapy agents mentioned below.

Alkylating agents

These drugs cross-link DNA strands and intracellular proteins by forming covalent bonds between highly reactive alkylating groups and nitrogen groups on the DNA helix. This either prevents division of the helix at mitosis or transcription of RNA, and results in imperfect division and cell death.

The most frequently used alkylating agents in gynaecological cancers are carboplatin and cisplatin. Previously used agents include cyclophosphamide, ifosfamide, chlorambucil, melphalan and treosulfan. Some alkylating agents may be taken orally.

Both cisplatin and carboplatin contain platinum. They act in a similar way to alkylating agents, forming DNA adducts. Both are given intravenously but, because of its potential nephrotoxicity and associated hypomagnesaemia and hypokalaemia, cisplatin requires a forced diuresis and elec-

Table 36.2 Chemotherapeutic agents used in gynaecological cancers, mechanisms of action and toxicities

Drug	Mechanism of action	Toxicity	Clearance
5-Fluorouracil	Antimetabolite, inhibits thymidine synthesis	Bone marrow suppression, mucositis, nausea, vomiting, diarrhoea, PPE	Hepatic, renal
Bleomycin	Antitumour antibiotic, DNA strand breakage	Anorexia, skin pigmentation and peeling, fever, rigors, interstitial pneumonitis, pulmonary fibrosis	Renal
Carboplatin	DNA cross-link, covalent adduct	Thrombocytopenia, neutropenia, nausea, vomiting	Renal
Cisplatin	DNA cross-link, covalent adduct	Neutropenia, thrombocytopenia, nausea, vomiting, peripheral neuropathy, ototoxicity, autonomic neuropathy, renal impairment, hypokalaemia, hypomagnesaemia	Renal
Docetaxel	Promotes tubulin synthesis and inhibits microtubule depolymerization, interferes with cell division	Bone marrow suppression, alopecia, nausea, vomiting, mucositis, peripheral neuropathy, fluid retention, arthralgia, myalgia, capillary leak syndrome, allergic reactions	Hepatic
Epirubicin	Topoisomerase II inhibitor	Bone marrow suppression, alopecia, vesicant, nausea, vomiting, cardiomyopathy	Hepatic
Etoposide	Topoisomerase II inhibitor	Bone marrow suppression, alopecia	Renal
Ifosfamide	Alkylating agent	Bone marrow suppression, alopecia, nausea, vomiting, haemorrhagic cystitis, encephalopathy	Renal
Liposomal doxorubicin	Topoisomerase II inhibitor	Bone marrow suppression, alopecia, PPE, cardiomyopathy	Hepatic
Methotrexate	Antifolate antimetabolite	Bone marrow toxicity, mucositis, exfoliative dermatitis, renal impairment	Renal
Paclitaxel	Tubulin synthesis deregulation	Bone marrow toxicity, nausea, vomiting, alopecia, allergic reactions, peripheral neuropathy, autonomic neuropathy	Hepatic
Topotecan	Topoisomerase I inhibitor	Bone marrow toxicity, alopecia, nausea, vomiting	Renal

PPE, palmar–plantar erythrodysesthesia.

trolyte replacement. It is also associated with severe nausea and vomiting which require potent antiemetic therapy. Peripheral neuropathy and ototoxicity are recognized side-effects which can be disabling and are usually dose related. Cisplatin has little myelotoxicity except for anaemia.

Carboplatin is less frequently associated with nephrotoxicity or neurotoxicity, and is also less emetogenic. It may be given as a short outpatient infusion. The most common side-effect of carboplatin is bone marrow suppression, with thrombocytopenia being a particular problem, especially in the context of impaired renal function. There is increasing recognition that platinum-associated hypersensitivity reactions are seen when carboplatin is used in the second-line setting. Data suggest that more than 10% of patients treated with carboplatin will experience this reaction, which can vary from a mild rash to hypotensive shock. A variety of desensitization schedules have been devised; however, patients can be challenged with cisplatin if it is felt to be too dangerous to continue with carboplatin.

Ifosfamide is an alkylating agent which is activated by hepatic microsomal enzymes. Bone marrow suppression is the dose-limiting toxicity and it also causes marked alopecia. It is excreted in the urine in the form of active metabolites, which can cause severe chemical cystitis when given in high doses unless mesna (sodium 2-mercaptoethanesulphonate) is administered at the same time to protect the bladder mucosa. In addition, ifosfamide may cause a fatal encephalopathy and must only be given after reference to a treatment nomogram.

Antimetabolites

These compounds closely resemble metabolites essential for the synthesis of nucleic acids and proteins. They are incorporated into natural metabolic pathways and enzyme systems, and disrupt the cellular mechanism. Each antimetabolite acts at different sites in the pathway of nucleic acid synthesis. These drugs include 5-fluorouracil (5-FU), methotrexate, capecitabine and gemcitabine.

Methotrexate

Methotrexate is a folic acid antagonist. It inhibits the enzyme dihydrofolate reductase, which reduces dihydrofolate to tetrahydrofolate; the precursor of coenzymes essential for the formation of purines and pyrimidines (nitrogen bases of DNA). These effects are bypassed by giving folinic acid. Folinic acid rescue is given from approximately 12 h after the methotrexate dose to all patients receiving 100 mg or more. The most common complication with methotrexate is oral ulceration. As it is excreted in urine, the dose must be reduced in women with renal impairment or with large fluid collections such as ascites which delays excretion.

5-fluorouracil

5-FU is a pyrimidine analogue which blocks thymidine synthesis and inhibits the incorporation of uracil into DNA. Myelosuppression and mucositis are the most common toxic effects. Patients with a rare inherited deficiency of the enzyme dihydropyrimidine dehydrogenase (DPD) can develop unexpectedly severe toxicity, including 5-FU-induced colitis. Capecitabine is an oral prodrug of 5-FU which is metabolized by intracellular enzymes into the active metabolite. Palmar–plantar erythrodysesthesia (PPE) is a commonly recognized side-effect.

Gemcitabine

Gemcitabine is converted to gemcitabine diphosphate, which inhibits the activity of ribonucleotide reductase and production of intracellular nucleotides. It competes with cytaribine, thus inhibiting DNA synthesis. Common toxicities include bone marrow suppression, nausea and vomiting.

Vinca alkaloids

Vinka alkaloids act during the metaphase of mitosis, probably through toxicity to the microtubules of the mitotic spindle. Peripheral and autonomic neuropathy are particular problems with vinca alkaloids, particularly vincristine. In addition, they are very irritant and are best injected into a fast-flowing drip. Vincristine is one of the very few chemotherapeutic drugs that is not myelotoxic.

Topoisomerase inhibitors

There are two different types of topoisomerase inhibitors. Both interfere with the transformation of DNA which is required for mitosis. Topoisomerase-1 inhibitors include topotecan and irinotecan, and topoisomerase-2 inhibitors include the epipodophyllotoxins (e.g. etoposide) and the anthracyclines [e.g. doxorubicin (including liposomal doxorubicin) and epirubicin].

Topotecan

Topotecan inhibits DNA replication by inhibiting the enzyme topoisomerase-1. Bone marrow suppression, particularly neutropenia, is the dose-limiting toxicity. Other side-effects include nausea, vomiting, stomatitis and asthenia. It is not recommended in women with renal or significant hepatic impairment.

Etoposide

Etoposide is a semisynthetic derivative of podophyllotoxin that blocks the cell cycle in G1 as well as DNA replication in the S phase. It prevents topoisomerase-2 from completing relegation repair. Cell cycle progression ceases and DNA strands break up, leading to cell death. Etoposide can cause telomeric shortening which accounts for the associated increased risk of leukaemia.

Anthracyclines

Doxorubicin is an antibiotic with antitumour activity that forms a stable irreversible complex by binding to DNA and topoisomerase enzymes, resulting in DNA damage that interferes with replication and transcription. It also interacts with cell membranes altering their function and generating hydroxy radicals which are highly destructive to cells. It causes marked alopecia, is myelosuppressive and should always be given as a fast-running infusion as it is very irritant and will cause a necrotic ulcer if it extravasates. Cardiomyopathy results from high cumulative doses unless the total dose is limited to 450 mg/m^2. The dose should be modified in the presence of hyperbilirubinaemia.

Pegylated liposomal doxorubicin (PLDH) consists of doxorubicin encapsulated in liposomes that have been pegylated (i.e. have surface-bound methoxy-poly-ethylene-glycol). This pegylation protects the liposomes from destruction in the circulation, and enhances the drug concentration and localization in tumour cells with a consequent increase in therapeutic efficacy and reduction in toxicity. Patients may exhibit infusion reactions which can be prevented with antihistamine and steroid premedication, and can develop PPE, stomatitis and haematological toxicity. PPE usually results in a painful macular rash affecting the hands, feet and skin folds (e.g. groin and axillae). These cutaneous side-effects are often self-limiting but occasionally result in significant toxicity, including crusting, ulceration and necrosis, which may require dose modification or even cessation of treatment. Patients receiving PLDH may need monitoring for cardiac toxicity.

Bleomycin

Bleomycin is another antitumour antibiotic which causes DNA strand breakage, thus interfering with DNA replication. It is not myelotoxic; however, the most important side-effect is pulmonary fibrosis, which is dose related and not often seen at a cumulative dose below 300 mg/m^2.

Taxanes

The taxanes include paclitaxel (Taxol) and docetaxel. They work by promoting microtubule assembly and stabilizing tubulin polymers, which results in the formation of nonfunctional microtubules, thus inhibiting mitosis. Taxol is active in ovarian and breast cancers as well as in many other tumours. Hypersensitivity reactions are less commonly experienced with a premedication cocktail of antihistamines, H$_2$ antagonists and steroids. The vast majority of patients develop total alopecia. Other side-effects include nausea, vomiting, peripheral neuropathy and myalgia. It is now usually given as a 3-h infusion in a non-PVC system by the manufacturers. When combined with a platinum agent, Taxol should be administered first to reduce toxicity and increase synergism. The reverse is the case for combination with doxorubicin.

Docetaxel has a slightly different side-effect profile compared with Taxol, with a reduced incidence and severity of peripheral neuropathy but a higher incidence of bone marrow suppression.

Chemotherapy-related toxicity

Tissues affected by toxic effects include the bone marrow, injection site, skin, hair, mucosa, gastrointestinal tract, reproductive system, heart, lungs, liver, renal system and nervous system. Knowledge of these toxic effects is essential for the safe management of chemotherapy. The most common toxicities for each of the commonly used drugs are shown in Table 36.2. Patients with poor performance, multiple comorbidities and heavily pretreated patients are less likely to tolerate chemotherapy.

Bone marrow suppression

This is a side-effect of almost all of the chemotherapy agents because of their action on bone marrow stem cells, the exceptions being vincristine and bleomycin. The blood count must be checked regularly and before each course of treatment. Neutropenia can result in infections not only from infective organisms such as *Staphylococcus aureus*, but also from opportunistic organisms which normally cause no problems in healthy individuals. Fungal infections also occur. Infections need to be treated aggressively as they can be life-threatening. Granulocyte colony-stimulating factors increase the tolerance of bone marrow to chemotherapy, reducing the incidence of secondary infections. Thrombocytopenia and anaemia may also occur and may need correction.

Alimentary tract toxicity

Nausea and vomiting are common side-effects of chemotherapy but can be well controlled with the armamentarium of antiemetics currently available to oncologists. Mucositis can result in patient discomfort, but is usually manageable with appropriate advice and appropriate treatment. Diarrhoea is a commonly encountered side-effect of 5-FU and its prodrug capecitabine, but it is usually self-limiting and can be easily managed with loperamide or codeine phosphate. Patients with DPD deficiency can develop fulminant diarrhoea due to 5-FU-induced colitis.

Alopecia

Alopecia is a common problem encountered with some agents but is seldom permanent.

Reproductive system

Chemotherapy may cause permanent infertility, but many young women successfully treated for germ cell tumours have had normal pregnancies. Cytotoxic drugs during pregnancy, particularly in the first trimester, can result in spontaneous abortion or congenital abnormalities. Young women undergoing treatment for gynaecological cancers are often rendered postmenopausal and may require hormone replacement therapy to reduce the long-term effects of early menopause. Other associated effects, such as loss of libido and vaginal dryness, can have a significant impact on the patient's quality of life.

Heart

Doxorubicin can cause cardiomyopathy which can result in heart failure. The risk is dose related. If the total dose is kept below 450 mg/m^2 and it is not used in patients with impaired cardiac function, cardiotoxicity is rarely seen.

Lungs

Bleomycin can cause pulmonary fibrosis and severe respiratory distress. Therefore, chest X-rays and respiratory function tests are essential before treatment. Anaesthesia after bleomycin also carries an increased risk, and anaesthetists need to be aware that the drug has been given in the past.

Kidneys

Nephrotoxicity is a serious complication of cisplatin and resulted in fatalities until forced diuresis was found to reduce renal damage. The toxicity is dose related. To avoid serious renal damage, serum creatinine should be measured before every course. If it increases by more than 25% over the pre-treatment value, a creatinine or ethylenediaminetetra-acetic acid clearance should be performed. If the clearance is less than 50 ml/min, the dose should be reduced by 50%. If the clearance is less than 40 ml/min, cisplatin should be discontinued.

Carboplatin has largely replaced cisplatin in the treatment of ovarian cancer as it is less nephrotoxic.

Nervous system

Cisplatin causes a dose-dependent peripheral neuropathy and high-tone deafness. The taxanes, paclitaxel in particular, are associated with peripheral neuropathy which can lead to loss of sensation and muscle weakness. Autonomic neuropathy is also a recognized side-effect of the taxanes. Vincristine can also result in peripheral and autonomic neuropathy. Treatment with ifosfamide can result in encephalopathy, especially in patients with a low serum albumin concentration.

Skin toxicity

Extravasation of some intravenously administered chemotherapeutic agents (e.g. vincristine and doxorubicin) can give rise to phlebitis or thrombosis which can be avoided by giving bolus injections into a free-running infusion. If such drugs leak out into the subcutaneous tissues, they can result in marked morbidity, including large painful ulcers and loss of function. 5-FU, capecitabine and liposomal doxorubicin are associated with PPE, which is usually self-limiting and resolves on cessation of treatment. The taxanes are associated with nail toxicity manifesting as hyperpigmentation, cracking and loss of nails.

Allergic reactions

This can be encountered with any chemotherapeutic agent, usually in the context of rechallenging patients with the same agent, but is also infrequently seen with the first cycle of treatment. Reactions can vary from mild symptoms to anaphylactic reactions requiring inpatient treatment including cardiopulmonary resuscitation.

Hormones

Tamoxifen is a selective oestrogen receptor modulator which has shown activity in the treatment of platinum-resistant ovarian cancer. Histological confirmation of overexpression of the oestrogen- or progesterone-receptor status must be obtained prior to commencing patients on tamoxifen. Common side-effects include hot flushes, night sweats and an increased risk of thromboembolic disease. It also increases the risk of endometrial cancer; however, most women with ovarian carcinoma undergo hysterectomy as part of routine surgical management.

Progestins such as medroxyprogesterone acetate are used in the palliative treatment of hormone-positive endometrial cancer. There is little evidence that doses higher than 200 mg twice daily are more effective. Although widely regarded as free of side-effects and toxicity, many patients do complain of fluid retention and there is some concern that prolonged use may increase the risk of cardiovascular disease. Glucocorticoids are often useful as antiemetics and in terminal care.

Conclusion

Chemotherapy plays an important part in the management of ovarian cancer, and its use can largely explain the improved prognosis for this disease which has been seen over the last decade in the West. The rare trophoblastic and germ cell tumours are now cured by these drugs in the vast majority of patients. In the treatment of solid tumours, it may be used in combinations with surgery and radiotherapy, and in cervical cancer, there is evidence that concurrent chemoradiation improves outcome compared with radiotherapy alone.

The dramatic increase in the number of potential drugs available as well as those in the developmental pipeline means that toxicity has been improved, and quality of life is an important goal. Indeed, no new agent is likely to be developed without an assessment of quality of life.

The most important contribution from chemotherapy is likely to be improved quality and duration of survival. This has already been achieved in ovarian cancer and there are reasons for optimism over the forthcoming years.

KEY POINTS

1. Most radiotherapy is delivered in the form of electromagnetic radiation using either high-energy X-rays generated by linear accelerators or radioactive isotopes.

2. Radiotherapy is usually given over many fractions to exploit the radiobiological differences between tumour clonogens and normal tissues.

3. Cisplatin-based chemoradiation is the generally accepted standard of care for the radical treatment of cervical carcinoma.

4. Technological advances are improving the accuracy with which radiotherapy is delivered, and also lead to reduced exposure of staff to ionizing radiation.

5. A major advantage of brachytherapy is the principle of the inverse square law which permits the delivery of high doses of radiation with relative sparing of normal tissues.

6. Late effects of radiotherapy including the effects on the gastrointestinal tract, bladder and bone marrow can have a significant impact on patients' quality of life.

7. Chemotherapy as a primary treatment modality cures approximately 5% of all cancers, and is the definitive mode of treatment for gestational trophoblastic tumours and ovarian germ cell tumours.

8. Chemotherapy is often used with other treatment modalities such as surgery and radiotherapy for the radical treatment of gynaecological malignancies.

9. All chemotherapeutic agents are associated with toxicity and can sometimes have an adverse effect on patients' quality of life, which is particularly important in the palliative setting.

10. All chemotherapeutic agents undergo stringent clinical trials prior to being approved for general clinical use.

11. Knowledge of pharmacokinetics and pharmacodynamics is vital to ensure that patients are treated effectively and safely.

12. Resistance to chemotherapeutic agents is one of the major unsurpassed hurdles which continues to pose significant challenges for the role of chemotherapy in curing cancers.

Acknowledgements

The authors would like to convey their gratitude to Professor Peter Hoskin, Mount Vernon Hospital, Northwood, for providing Figures 36.3, 36.5(A,B), 36.10 and 36.11(A,B); and to Ruth Wyatt, Queen Elizabeth Hospital, Birmingham, and Nucletron, for providing Figures 36.8(B,C) and 36.9.

References

Green J, Kirwan J, Tierney J et al 2005 Concomitant chemotherapy and radiotherapy for cancer of the uterine cervix. Cochrane Database of Systematic Reviews 3: CD002225.

King M, McConkey C, Latief TN, Hartley A, Fernando IN 2006 Improved survival after concurrent weekly cisplatin and radiotherapy for cervical carcinoma with assessment of acute and late side effects. Clinical Oncology (Royal College of Radiologists) 18: 38–45.

Tanguay JS, Ansari J, Buckley L, Fernando I 2009 Epithelial ovarian cancer: role of pegylated liposomal doxorubicin in prolonging the platinum-free interval and cancer antigen 125 trends during treatment. International Journal of Gynecological Cancer 19: 361–366.

Further Reading

Dale RG, Jones B 1998 The clinical radiobiology of brachytherapy. British Journal of Radiobiology 71: 465–483.

Fischer DS, Knobf MT, Durivage HJ, Beaulieu NJ 2003 The Cancer Chemotherapy Handbook, 6th edn. Mosby Inc., Philadelphia.

Hoskin P (ed) 2006 Radiotherapy in Practice: External Beam Radiotherapy. Oxford University Press, Oxford.

Hoskin P, Coyle C (eds) 2005 Radiotherapy in Practice: Brachytherapy. Oxford University Press, Oxford.

Poole CJ, Palmer D 2001 Chemotherapy for gynaecological malignancies. In: Shafi MI, Leusley DM, Jordan JA (eds) Handbook of Gynaecological Oncology. Harcourt Publishers Limited, London.

CHAPTER 37

Novel therapies in gynaecological cancer

Debra Josephs, Susannah Stanway and Martin Gore

Chapter Contents

INTRODUCTION	554		Src	559
VASCULAR ENDOTHELIAL GROWTH FACTOR AND ANGIOGENESIS INHIBITION	554		ALPHA FOLATE RECEPTOR	560
			NOVEL TAXANES	560
THE EPIDERMAL GROWTH FACTOR RECEPTOR FAMILY	556		EPOTHILONES	560
POLY(ADP-RIBOSE) POLYMERASE INHIBITORS	557		MISCELLANEOUS	560
mTOR	558		CONCLUSION	561
PROTEIN KINASE C	559		KEY POINTS	562
CA125	559			

Introduction

Ovarian cancer is the fourth most common cause of cancer death in women, with a worldwide incidence of 200,000 cases causing 115,000 deaths per year. As described elsewhere, the current standard of care for women with stage IC (and stage IB with adverse histological features) to stage III disease is surgery followed by adjuvant chemotherapy. Further lines of treatment can be given when patients relapse but cure is not possible. Ovarian cancer is considered to be a chemosensitive disease, with nearly 75% of patients initially responding to platinum-based treatment. The choice of agent upon relapse depends on the timing of relapse; if this is over 6 months from previous platinum administration, this can be repeated either as a single agent or as part of a combination regimen, as patients are still considered to be platinum sensitive. If relapse occurs within 6 months of previous platinum administration, non-platinum drugs such as pegylated liposomal doxorubicin are used. There is an increased understanding of the complicated biological pathways involved in the development of gynaecological cancers, their subsequent metastagenesis and the mechanisms involved in chemoresistance. Many clinical studies are underway investigating the use of novel agents in patients with gynaecological malignancies, either alone, concurrently with chemotherapy or sequentially, in an attempt to improve response rates/durations and thereby survival. This chapter will outline several of the new classes of novel agents which are at various stages of development, detail their putative mechanisms of action and their potential indications, and

include brief summaries of their toxicity profiles from studies to date. Many of the phase II studies of new agents include patients in the platinum-refractory group, whose tumours are intrinsically resistant to chemotherapy and radiotherapy, and who therefore have low rates of response to conventional treatment.

Vascular Endothelial Growth Factor and Angiogenesis Inhibition

Angiogenesis or neovascularization is a normal physiological process involving the remodelling of vasculature and formation of new blood vessels. Angiogenesis plays a vital role in tumour formation and metastasis because both primary lesions and metastatic tumours must develop a new vascular supply in order to survive (Folkman 1971, 1990). Early initiation of angiogenesis is essential for cancer survival, and occurs when stimulatory factors overcome inhibitory factors, promoting the formation of new blood vessels (Bergers and Benjamin 2003).

Research investigating the molecular basis of angiogenesis has identified multiple pathways that contribute to tumour angiogenesis. These include vascular endothelial growth factor (VEGF), fibroblast growth factor and platelet-derived growth factor (PDGF). Based on the central role of VEGF in tumour angiogenesis and growth, this has emerged as the most promising therapeutic target for angiogenesis inhibition. The VEGF molecule interacts with cell surface VEGF receptors (VEGFRs) that initiate signalling through

DOI: 10.1016/B978-0-7020-3120-5.00037-0

downstream pathways to promote growth and differentiation of vascular endothelial cells and formation of new blood vessels.

The biological roles of VEGF predict that its expression should be related to clinical outcome in cancer patients. Indeed, VEGF expression has been correlated with both disease-free survival and overall survival (OS) in a variety of gynaecological cancers. VEGF expression has been evaluated in women with ovarian carcinoma in several studies, which collectively provide consistent evidence that higher VEGF levels are associated with aggressive clinical behaviour in ovarian carcinoma. Kassim et al (2004) found some degree of VEGF expression in all ovarian cancer specimens examined, and the level of VEGF expression was significantly higher in tumour specimens compared with benign ovarian tissue. In addition, rising titres of VEGF from tumour specimens correlated with increasing stage and decreased survival. This relationship seems to be independent of important clinical and pathological prognostic factors. Furthermore, in women with ovarian cancer, high serum levels of VEGF are an independent risk factor for ascites, advanced-stage disease, undifferentiated histology, more metastases and decreased survival (Cooper et al 2002, Li et al 2004).

There are limited data regarding VEGF expression in endometrial cancer specimens. Holland et al (2003) documented VEGF expression in 100% of the endometrial cancer specimens examined. In addition, they found no expression of VEGF in benign endometrial tissue. The functional significance of the VEGF/VEGFR axis in endometrial cancer remains to be demonstrated.

In tissue specimens from patients with cervical cancer, VEGF expression has been noted immunohistochemically in 94% of samples (Loncaster et al 2000). Intratumour levels of VEGF are increased in patients with cervical cancer compared with levels in normal cervical tissue. For these women with cervical cancer, increasing intratumoral levels of VEGF also correlated with higher stage, increased risk of lymphovascular space invasion, greater likelihood of parametrial spread, and lymph node metastasis (Cheng et al 1999).

The biological and clinical significance of the VEGF pathway in tumour angiogenesis suggests its value as a therapeutic target in gynaecological malignancies. There are three main strategies for inhibition of the VEGF pathway for therapeutic applications. The first is to target VEGF itself, the second is to target VEGFR so as to prevent binding of VEGF, and the third is to inhibit tyrosine kinase activation and downstream signalling with small molecules that work at the intracellular level.

Bevacizumab (Avastin) is the first targeted agent to show significant single-agent activity in ovarian carcinoma. It is a recombinant humanized monoclonal antibody directed against VEGF. Bevacizumab has been tested in a number of phase II trials as monotherapy in epithelial ovarian cancer (EOC). Two such trials using single-agent bevacizumab in relapsed high-grade carcinoma of the ovary were presented at the American Society of Clinical Oncology (ASCO) meetings in 2005 and 2006 (Burger et al 2007, Cannistra et al 2007). They convincingly demonstrate bevacizumab's significant single-agent activity in patients with relapsed EOC, with objective response rates (ORR) of 21% and 16%, respectively. Additionally, 52% and 64% of cases, respectively, achieved disease stabilization with median progression-free survival (PFS) of 4.4 and 4.5 months. These results are as good or better than typical rates from traditional second-line chemotherapeutic agents in this group of patients.

Cytotoxic and antiangiogenic agents can be used in combination for enhanced activity. It has been hypothesized that combining VEGF-targeted agents with frequently administered low-dose so-called 'metronomic chemotherapy' may have additive or synergistic antiangiogenic or antitumour effects. In 2005, Garcia et al presented preliminary data from a phase II trial of patients with recurrent ovarian cancer who were given bevacizumab biweekly with metronomic oral cyclophosphamide. The ORR was 28% and a further substantial proportion (57%) achieved disease stabilization for at least 6 months. The median PFS was 7.5 months and OS was 13 months. This protocol is now closed and the data are undergoing final analysis, but if consistent with preliminary results, these findings would provide the rationale for a phase II randomized trial of combination versus single-agent therapy. Additional reports of outcomes for patients with EOC and primary peritoneal cancer treated with bevacizumab include three historical case series of patients treated outside clinical trials with single-agent therapy or in combination with cytotoxic drugs, suggesting activity in more heavily pretreated patients with recurrent disease, and preliminary data in 2006 demonstrating the feasibility of the combination of traditional carboplatin/paclitaxel chemotherapy combined with bevacizumab in front-line therapy (Cohn et al 2006, Monk et al 2006, Penson et al 2006, Wright et al 2006a).

Based on the encouraging phase II trial data, bevacizumab has been rapidly incorporated into phase III trials, the major focus of which is on first-line treatment. Two similar randomized trials are now underway. The Gynaecologic Oncology Group 218 trial is designed to explore the role of bevacizumab in first-line treatment and in the maintenance setting, with a three-way randomization whereby all patients receive carboplatin/paclitaxel plus bevacizumab or placebo for six cycles, with those receiving bevacizumab further randomized to drug or placebo maintenance for 15 months, with the primary endpoint being OS. It is limited to patients with stage III or IV disease. In contrast, the Gynaecological Cancer Intergroup trial (ICON 7) is a non-placebo-controlled, smaller, two-arm trial in which patients receive either carboplatin/paclitaxel for six cycles or the same treatment plus bevacizumab every 3 weeks during chemotherapy and continuing for an additional 9 months, with the primary endpoint being PFS. The patient population for this trial includes all patients with at least high-risk, early-stage disease. Bevacizumab has also been tested in the phase II setting in combination with topotecan in women with platinum-refractory ovarian cancer (McGonigle et al 2008). To date, 22 patients have been enrolled, 18 of whom were evaluable; 22.2% had a partial response (PR) and 27.8% achieved disease stabilization. Toxicity was described as being acceptable.

Bevacizumab has also been given to women with cervical carcinoma. Wright et al (2006b) gave combination bevacizumab and 5-fluorouracil or capecitabine to women with recurrent cervical cancer. In this small retrospective group of six women, one patient achieved a complete response (CR), one achieved a PR and two achieved disease stabilization.

Unfortunately, all four women eventually had disease progression at a median time of 4.3 months, and none had a progression-free interval of more than 6 months.

Unique toxicities have been ascribed to the administration of bevacizumab and other anti-VEGF molecules. Most of these toxicities (such as proteinurea, hypertension and bleeding) are generally mild and are either self-limiting or easily manageable. Other adverse effects, although uncommon, may be serious; these include arterial thromboembolism, wound-healing complications, and gastrointestinal perforation or fistulae.

Targeting the VEGF/VEGFR axis may affect the survival of both proliferating and quiescent endothelial cells, leading to the disruption of normal vasculature. The increase in arterial thromboembolic events, including cerebral infarction, transient ischaemic attacks, myocardial infarction and angina, may be related to this phenomenon. Hypertension is one of the most common side-effects of bevacizumab therapy, with an overall incidence of 22–32% (Gordon and Cunningham 2005). The mechanism responsible for bevacizumab-related hypertension is not fully understood, but it is thought to be related to decreased production of nitric oxide as a result of VEGF inhibition. Most patients with hypertension can be managed with oral antihypertensive agents.

VEGF is known to play a critical role in the physiological angiogenesis required for wound healing. This could be of particular importance when considering antiangiogenic therapy as front-line adjuvant treatment of ovarian cancer after cytoreductive surgery. Concerns about wound healing in postoperative patients have resulted in the decision to start bevacizumab/placebo therapy at cycle 2 within the Gynaecologic Oncology Group 218 trial. This would be more than 28 days after surgery.

The complication of bowel perforation is now well documented with bevacizumab and, although uncommon, is of concern. It has been suggested that the number of prior cytotoxic regimens and the presence of bowel obstruction might predispose to this complication, although our ability to identify high-risk patients requires further investigation.

Other agents targeting the VEGF pathway are also being developed rapidly. VEGF-Trap inactivates VEGF by acting as a decoy receptor for VEGF, preventing binding of the ligand to its natural receptors. Promising data have been reported regarding VEGF-Trap in preclinical and phase I studies in patients with advanced solid malignancies (Dupont et al 2004, Hu et al 2005). One patient in the phase I study had carboplatin-, taxane- and gemcitabine-resistant advanced ovarian cancer and achieved a response evaluation criteria in solid tumours (RECIST)-defined PR, a 67% reduction in CA125 levels, radiographic resolution of abdominal ascites and subjective improvement of performance status after four cycles of VEGF-Trap. It is currently being evaluated in the phase II setting in patients with recurrent ovarian carcinoma.

Cediranib (AZD2171) is a potent oral tyrosine kinase inhibitor (TKI) of VEGF1, 2, 3 and c-Kit. It has been tested in a phase II study reported at the ASCO meeting in 2008 as a single agent in recurrent ovarian, peritoneal or tubal cancer (Matulonis et al 2008). Preliminary results from 28 patients, 16 of whom had platinum-resistant disease, revealed an ORR of 18.5%. Common toxicities included hypertension ($n = 13$), fatigue ($n = 5$) and diarrhoea ($n = 3$). A further

phase II study of this agent, reported in 2008, has shown similar promising efficacy data and toxicity profiles (Hirte et al 2008).

Sunitinib, an oral multitargeted TKI known to be effective against, amongst others, VEGFR and PDGF receptors, has recently been tested in the phase II setting as a single agent in patients with EOC, primary peritoneal and fallopian tube cancers (Biagi et al 2008). Preliminary results reported at the ASCO meeting in 2008 revealed that 12 out of 17 patients had a PR or disease stabilization. The tolerability profile of this drug is well known from its extensive use in other tumour types, and includes fatigue, mucositis, dysgeusia, hypertension, nausea and hand–foot reaction. Further studies involving larger patient groups are warranted in order to further assess the efficacy of sunitinib in gynaecological cancers.

Sorafenib, another multitargeted TKI (predominantly affecting VEGFR, PDGF receptors, Flt3 and c-Kit) has also been tested in the phase II setting in patients with recurrent EOC and primary peritoneal cancer, the results of which were presented at the recent ASCO meeting (Matel et al 2008). Seventy-three patients who had persistent or recurrent EOC who had been treated previously with one or two cytotoxic regimens, and who had progressed within 12 months of platinum-based therapy, were treated until disease progression or toxicity requiring cessation. The primary endpoint was PFS at 6 months. Response, OS and toxicity were also documented. Toxicities (grade three to four) included rash ($n = 12$), metabolic ($n = 10$), gastrointestinal ($n = 3$), cardiovascular ($n = 2$) and pulmonary ($n = 2$). Twelve out of 59 evaluable patients were progression free for at least 6 months. Two PRs were reported and 20 patients achieved disease stabilization. Mature data are awaited to further define the utility of this agent.

Sorafenib has also been studied in patients with uterine cancer in the phase II settting, and preliminary results have been reported (Nimeiri et al 2008). Patients with advanced or recurrent disease who had experienced one or fewer prior regimens were treated with sorafenib 400 mg bd. Fifty-five patients were enrolled. Grade three to four toxicities included hypertension (13%), hand–foot syndrome (13%) and anaemia (6%). The response rate in patients with advanced/recurrent disease was 5% (PR), and 50% of patients achieved disease stabilization. The median OS was 10.1 months. In patients with carcinosarcoma, 27% achieved disease stabilization. The completion of the trial is awaited.

The Epidermal Growth Factor Receptor Family

The human epidermal growth factor receptor (EGFR) family of transmembrane receptor tyrosine kinases has four identified members: EGFR or HER1, HER2, HER3 and HER4. This subgroup of receptors mediate cell growth, differentiation and survival, and are dysregulated in many types of cancer. Ligand binding to the extracellular domain of the receptors enables receptor homo- or heterodimerization, which initiates phosphorylation of the intracellular tyrosine kinase domain and activation of cell signalling to reduce apoptosis and increase tumour cell proliferation.

The HER pathway is involved in ovarian cancer pathogenesis (Berchuck et al 1990, Bartlett et al 1996, Campiglio et al

1999). The majority of ovarian cancer cell lines and tumours express high levels of a number of HER receptor ligands, as well as exhibiting amplification of EGFR and HER2, and expressing all HER receptors (Campiglio et al 1999). In EOC, attention has focused on EGFR (HER1) which is expressed in 19–92% of tumours, and expression of which is associated with a poor prognosis (Ford et al 1994, Lin et al 1994, Goff et al 1996, Ilekis et al 1997, Fischer-Colbrie et al 1997).

The goal of EGFR-targeted therapies is to disrupt phosphorylation, thereby increasing apoptosis and reducing cell proliferation signals. This disruption can be achieved in several ways: inhibition of dimerization, blocking of EGFR receptor ligand binding with humanized monoclonal antibodies, and inhibition of tyrosine kinase activity with small-molecule TKIs. In the majority of trials of anti-EGFR agents in patients with EOC, the agents are investigated as monotherapy in heavily pretreated women. Objective responses are relatively low but prolonged disease stabilization has been seen in a subset of women.

The small-molecule TKIs erlotinib (Tarceva) and gefitinib (Iressa) have been tested in phase II trials of patients with relapsed and pretreated EOC. A trial of erlotinib as monotherapy in women with advanced EGFR-positive cancers treated with a mean of three prior regimens was presented at the ASCO meeting in 2001 (Finkler et al 2001). The ORR was 8.8%, with a further 7% of patients achieving disease stabilization for more than 6 months. A similar trial of gefitinib in patients with recurrent or persistent ovarian carcinoma or primary peritoneal cancer, but in which EGFR expression was not required for inclusion, led to a response rate of only 3.7% and long-term disease stabilization for more than 6 months in a further 14.8% of patients (Schilder et al 2003). The median time to progression was approximately 2 months, but 10% of patients remained progression free at 8–12 months. Interestingly, all of these patients had EGFR-positive tumours. Unlike in lung cancer, where EGFR expression and the presence of a mutation in the tyrosine kinase domain of EGFR confer sensitivity to EGFR TKIs, the relationship between EGFR positivity, EGFR mutation and response to EGFR TKIs is not clearly defined in EOC. Better definition of this relationship may help to identify the subset of women with EOC that are likely to achieve clinically meaningful responses to TKIs, and therefore define the appropriate treatment population.

Monoclonal antibodies against EGFR have also been investigated. The most established anti-EGFR antibody is cetuximab (Erbitux). This has been evaluated in previously untreated women with EOC in combination with standard first-line carboplatin/paclitaxel chemotherapy and as maintenance therapy. An ORR of 87% was seen and toxicity was acceptable (Aghajanian et al 2005). Its use as monotherapy is currently under investigation. Another anti-EGFR monoclonal antibody, matuzumab, has been investigated in women with recurrent EGFR-positive EOC (Seiden et al 2005); although no objective responses were seen, 21% of women achieved disease stabilization for more than 6 months.

Monoclonal antibodies directed against HER2 have also been investigated in advanced EOC. Laboratory studies have suggested that 10–15% of women have tumours that over-express HER2 graded as 2+ or 3+ positivity by immunohis-tochemistry (IHC). It is unclear whether this is predictive of clinical outcome in EOC. In breast cancer, where the role of HER2 receptor overexpression is well defined, it is only a predictive factor in those with IHC 3+ positivity and it is only this subset who derive clinical benefit from anti-HER2 therapies (Slamon et al 2001). In a phase II study of the anti-HER2 monoclonal antibody trastuzumab (Herceptin) in EOC, of the 837 patients who were registered and screened, only 95 (11%) had tumours with grade 2+ or 3+ positivity. Of these patients, only 41 were treated, with an ORR of only 7.3% (Bookman et al 2003). The study concluded that the clinical value of single-agent trastuzumab in recurrent ovarian cancer is limited by the low frequency of HER2 overexpression and low rate of objective response among patients with HER2 overexpression.

The monoclonal antibody pertuzumab was the first in a new class of targeted anticancer agents termed 'HER dimerization inhibitors'. It binds to the dimerization site of HER2, inhibiting its interaction with other HER family members. Unlike HER1, -3 and -4, HER2 has no known ligand and assumes an open conformation, with its dimerization domain permanently exposed for interaction with other ligand-activated HER receptors. HER2 is the preferred partner for dimer formation, and subsequent pathway activation via receptor phosphorylation has been shown to drive ovarian tumour cell proliferation, even in the absence of HER2 over-expression. Pertuzumab was investigated as monotherapy in a phase II trial in patients with advanced, refractory or recurrent ovarian cancer (Gordon et al 2006). A PR was achieved in 4.3% of subjects, with 41% achieving disease stabilization. However, median PFS was 20.9 weeks for HER2-positive patients compared with 5.8 weeks for HER2-negative patients and 9.1 weeks for those of unknown HER2 status. It should be noted that these patients were heavily pretreated and the median number of prior therapies was five. The study concluded that given that pertuzumab blocks all HER2-mediated signalling, in contrast to targeted blockade of EGFR or HER2 overexpression, pertuzumab may result in higher rates of clinical activity in an appropriately selected population. A randomized phase II study evaluating the combination of carboplatin-based chemotherapy with pertuzumab in comparison with carboplatin-based therapy alone in patients with relapsed, platinum-sensitive ovarian cancer is currently underway. Preliminary data presented at the ASCO meeting in 2008 reveal that the addition of pertuzumab to carboplatin-based chemotherapy is well tolerated, but efficacy data are awaited.

The small-molecule TKI lapatinib is similar to gefitinib and erlotinib, except that it has similar specificity for EGFR and HER2. Data from initial clinical experience with lapatinib have only shown mild adverse events (rash, diarrhoea, nausea, vomiting) and no grade four events. In the original phase I trial, three subjects showed a PR and 12 patients achieved disease stabilization, including two with ovarian cancer (Spector et al 2005).

Poly(ADP-Ribose) Polymerase Inhibitors

BRCA1 and *BRCA2* belong to a class of genes known as tumour suppressor genes. Their protein products are important for DNA double-strand break repair (Tutt and Ashworth

2002). Mutations in *BRCA1* and *BRCA2* predispose to a number of hereditary cancers, including breast and ovarian. Poly(ADP-ribose) polymerase (PARP) is a DNA-binding enzyme involved in base excision repair, a key pathway in the repair of DNA single-strand breaks. Tumours in carriers of *BRCA1* or *BRCA2* mutations lack wild-type *BRCA1* or *BRCA2*, but normal tissues retain a single wild-type copy of the relevant gene. This biochemical difference provides the rationale for an approach involving PARP inhibition to generate specific DNA lesions that require functional *BRCA1* and *BRCA2* for their repair. In a study by Farmer et al in 2005, *BRCA1* and *BRCA2* dysfunction was shown to profoundly sensitize cells to the inhibition of PARP enzymatic activity, resulting in chromosomal instability, cell cycle arrest and subsequent apoptosis. In other words, PARP inhibitors were found to be selectively cytotoxic to tumours lacking *BRCA1* and *BRCA2*, where the specific mechanism that repairs damaged DNA is absent. In addition, PARP inhibitors have been shown to significantly enhance the effect of a number of widely used cytotoxics that damage DNA. Results from a phase I study of AZD2281, a novel, potent, orally active PARP inhibitor in patients with *BRCA*-deficient ovarian cancer, were presented at the ASCO meeting in 2008 (Fong et al 2008). The study demonstrated compelling activity in patients with *BRCA*-deficient ovarian cancer, with efficacy data revealing a PR rate of 44% and a further 25% of patients achieving disease stabilization. AZD2281 was well tolerated, toxicities being mainly gastrointestinal and mild, and little myelosuppression was seen. A randomized study of AZD2281 in *BRCA*-deficient ovarian cancer is planned.

mTOR

It is known that intracellular signal transduction pathways interact to regulate the cell cycle, apoptosis, cytoskeletal organization and senescence. An example of this is the mammalian target of rapamycin (mTOR), a serine/threonine protein kinase that is a central regulator of cell growth, proliferation and survival (Beevers et al 2006). mTOR, in turn, is regulated by the phosphatidylinositol3-kinase (PI3K)/ AKT pathway, a signalling cascade that is aberrant in over 70% of tumours (Meric-Bernstam and Mills 2004). Dysregulation of this pathway has been demonstrated in ovarian cancer.

The inhibition of mTOR results in a profound decrease in the transmission of proliferative signals through the PI3K/ AKT pathway, leading to antiproliferative effects and angiogenesis inhibition. IHC analysis of ovarian cancer specimens has shown that both AKT and mTOR are frequently activated (phosphorylated) in these tumours (Altomare et al 2004). In the same study, the effects of AKT/mTOR activation on the therapeutic sensitivity of ovarian cancer cells to cytotoxic agents was tested. Augmentation of cisplatin-induced apoptosis was seen in cells exhibiting constitutive AKT activity when pretreated with the PI3K inhibitor LY294002. In contrast, ovarian cancer cell lines with low basal levels of AKT activity did not show increased cisplatin-induced apoptosis. In addition, inhibition of mTOR activity with rapamycin resulted in cell cycle arrest in those cells exhibiting constitutive AKT activity, but not in those cells with low levels of AKT activity. Collectively, these findings indicate that active AKT and downstream mTOR represent potentially important therapeutic targets in ovarian cancer.

Preclinical studies have demonstrated that rapamycin (a highly specific inhibitor of mTOR kinase) and its analogues inhibit proliferation not only in ovarian cancer cell lines but also in cervical and endometrial cancer cell lines, and in a broad range of murine syngeneic tumour models and human xenografts. Three rapamycin analogues are currently in clinical development as anticancer agents: AP23573, CCI-779 (temsirolimus) and RAD001 (everolimus).

AP23573 has been tested in a phase I trial in patients with advanced solid malignancies (Mita et al 2004). The dose-limiting toxicity was mucositis, and common treatment-related adverse events included mouth sores and rash. Four out of 32 (12.5%) patients experienced a confirmed PR and three (9%) additional patients had minor tumour regression. AP23573 has also been tested in a phase Ib combination trial with paclitaxel in patients with progressive solid tumours (Cresta et al 2007). The dose-limiting toxicities were mucositis, fatigue, myelotoxicity with prolonged moderate neutropenia, and skin rash. Pharmacodynamic analysis in peripheral blood mononuclear cells demonstrated no interference by paclitaxel on mTOR inhibition by AP23573. The trial concluded that combined therapy with AP23573 and paclitaxel is feasible and well tolerated, and recommended evaluation of the combination in phase II trials examining efficacy in specific tumours.

Preliminary results of a phase II trial of single-agent AP23573 in patients with advanced metastatic endometrial cancer were presented at the ASCO meeting in 2007 (Colombo et al 2007). The trial involved 45 patients, all of whom had progressive disease. The primary endpoint was a clinical benefit response, defined as a CR or PR or prolonged disease stabilization for at least four cycles. This was achieved, with 29% of patients having a clinical benefit response, including 10% with a PR. The most common toxicities were mucositis, fatigue, anaemia, diarrhoea and nausea/vomiting. This study reveals promising results of single-agent AP23573 in progressing endometrial cancer, and warrants further evaluation of the drug as monotherapy and in combination with other agents.

In preclinical models, CCI-779 or temsirolimus, an ester derivative of rapamycin, has shown antitumour effects across a wide variety of tumour types. An initial dose-escalation phase I trial administered temsirolimus weekly (Raymond et al 2004). Although thrombocytopenia was dose limiting and a reversible maculopapular rash and stomatitis were observed, the formal definition of a maximum tolerated dose was not met. In addition, objective partial and minor responses were observed at lower dose levels. Encouraging data from a phase II study of single-agent temsirolimus in chemotherapy-naïve patients with metastatic or recurrent endometrial cancer were presented at the ASCO meeting in 2006 (Oza et al 2006). The ORR was 21%, with 48% of patients achieving prolonged disease stabilization. These results are equivalent to those of currently used cytotoxic chemotherapy. A subsequent phase II study assessed the level of activity of temsirolimus in patients with metastatic and/or locally advanced recurrent endometrial cancer who had previously received chemotherapy (Oza et al 2008). The results of this study indicated that temsirolimus had modest activity, with only 7.4% of patients achieving a PR; however, 44% achieved disease stabilization with a mean duration of 3.5 months. A phase II trial of temsirolimus in the treatment of persistent or recurrent EOC or primary peritoneal cancer is currently underway.

RAD001 (everolimus) is an oral rapamycin analogue that selectively inhibits mTOR. It has shown encouraging single-agent clinical benefit in pretreated patients with recurrent endometrial carcinoma in a phase II study presented at the ASCO meeting in 2008 (Slomovitz et al 2008). Although none of the patients achieved a PR, 44% of patients achieved disease stabilization of more than 8 weeks. Interestingly, loss of *PTEN* expression, a tumour suppressor gene found in 40–60% of endometrial cancers, the loss of which leads to constitutive AKT activation and upregulation of mTOR activity, was found to be predictive of prolonged disease stabilization.

Protein kinase C

Protein kinase C (PKC) is a family of serine/threonine protein kinases which are centrally involved with the regulation of angiogenesis, cell growth and survival. Activated PKC-β promotes VEGF-mediated angiogenesis and has been implicated in the progression of malignancy, cell proliferation and inhibition of apoptosis. The activated form of PKC-β has been identified in a number of human tumours, including ovarian cancer.

Enzastaurin, an oral selective inhibitor of the PKC-β isozyme, has been shown to have antiangiogenic effects and to promote apoptosis by downregulating signalling through the PI3K pathway in several cancers (Graff et al 2005, Lee et al 2008). Preclinical studies have shown enzastaurin to have anticancer effects as a single agent and in combination with carboplatin and paclitaxel in breast and ovarian carcinomas (Teicher et al 2002, Keyes et al 2004). In a study of the effect of enzastaurin on ovarian cancer cell lines with selective resistance against various cytostatic drugs, taxane-resistant cells showed the most prominent response to low concentrations of enzastaurin (Meinhold-Heerlein et al 2006). In phase I trials, prolonged stabilization of disease was seen in several patients treated with enzastaurin, with acceptable toxicities (Carducci et al 2006). Synergistic activity with standard-of-care chemotherapies was seen, with no significant alterations in the pharmacokinetic variables of the cytotoxic drugs with which it was combined (Beerepoot et al 2006, Rademaker-Lakhai et al 2007). Enzastaurin is now being tested in ovarian cancer in the phase II setting by the Gynaecologic Oncology Group.

CA125

CA125 is a surface antigen that is expressed on the majority of EOCs and occurs at elevated levels in the serum of patients with ovarian cancer. Serum levels of CA125 are used to monitor responses to chemotherapy, relapse and disease progression in ovarian cancer patients. In 2001, the gene for the peptide moiety of CA125 was cloned and termed 'MUC16' because of its similarities to the mucin family of proteins (Yin and Lloyd 2001). The biological

functions of CA125 are complex but, based on current knowledge, CA125 seems to enhance the malignant potential of ovarian cancer cells.

Monoclonal antibodies that target CA125 are now in development as a therapeutic strategy. One such drug, ovregovomab (Mab-813.13, Ovarex), behaves as an immunotherapeutic agent. Infusion of low-dose antibody results in the formation of circulating immune complexes which can trigger a cellular immune response targeting CA125 and the ovarian cancer. Reported data have shown an association between intratumoral T cells and improved clinical outcome, lending support for immune-mediated disease control (Zhang et al 2003). Ovregovomab has been compared with placebo in a randomized trial of women with ovarian cancer who had achieved complete remission after first-line chemotherapy. There was no OS advantage but subset analysis showed that half of the treated women generated an immune response to ovregovomab, and these women had superior survival to those without an immune response (Ehlen 2002, Berek et al 2004).

A phase III randomized trial was reported at the ASCO meeting in 2008 of maintenance oregovomab monoimmunotherapy versus placebo in patients with stage III/IV ovarian cancer (Berek et al 2008). Patients were treated until recurrence or for up to 5 years, and the primary endpoint was time to recurrence. Three hundred and seventy-one patients were randomized, but unfortunately there were no significant differences in the clinical outcomes between the two groups. Conclusions drawn were that although it was not effective as a single agent, its use in combination with other cytotoxic agents should be investigated further. Ovregovomab has been evaluated in combination with carboplatin/paclitaxel as front-line chemoimmunotherapy in patients with advanced ovarian cancer (Braly et al 2007). Chemotherapy-induced bone marrow suppression has been assumed to inhibit the generation of augmented immune responses; however, contrary to expectations, concurrent carboplatin/paclitaxel resulted in enhanced immune stimulation with ovregovomab.

A second drug, abagovomab (formerly ACA125), is an antibody which functionally mimics the CA125 antigen and induces humoral and cellular CA125-specific immunity. Abagovomab has been shown to generate immune responses in women with EOC (Wagner et al 2001). Indeed, those women who generated an immune response had a mean survival of 19.9 ± 3.1 months, compared with 5.3 ± 4.3 months in those women who did not develop a response. Efficacy testing is underway, although it is not yet clear whether this strategy will have clinical impact in EOC.

Src

Src, a non-receptor tyrosine kinase, is an attractive therapeutic target in ovarian cancer because it is expressed and activated in the majority of ovarian cancers and regulates a myriad of intracellular signal cascades responsible for critical tumour cell functions, including cell proliferation and differentiation, through extracellular stimulation by growth factors, growth hormones and integrins (Ishizawar and Parsons 2004). Moreover, the emerging role of Src in angiogenesis has recently been noted because of its upregulation of proangiogenic cytokines such as VEGF and interleukin-8 (Summy et al 2005). The ability of VEGF to disrupt endothelial barrier function, which has been correlated with tumour cell extravasation and metastasis, is mediated through Src.

Src has been found to be overexpressed in the majority of late-stage ovarian tumours, as well as a panel of ovarian cancer cell lines (Wiener et al 2003). A study by Han et al in 2006 showed that Src inhibition, through a novel small-molecule inhibitor AP23994, alone and in combination with cytotoxic chemotherapy, significantly reduced tumour growth *in vivo* in both chemotherapy-sensitive and chemotherapy-resistant preclinical ovarian cancer models. They concluded that Src inhibition might be an attractive therapeutic approach for patients with ovarian carcinoma.

Alpha Folate Receptor

Alpha folate receptor is a membrane-bound protein with high affinity for binding and transporting physiological levels of folate into cells. Folate is a basic component of cell metabolism and DNA synthesis and repair. Rapidly dividing cancer cells have an increased requirement for folate to maintain DNA synthesis; an observation supported by the widespread use of antifolates in cancer chemotherapy. Alpha folate receptor is overexpressed in the majority of EOCs but is largely absent from normal tissue. Overexpression is associated with increased tumour aggressiveness (Toffoli et al 1997). MORAb-003 is a humanized monoclonal antibody against alpha folate receptor. Binding of MORAb-003 to alpha folate receptor blocks phosphorylation, mediates the killing of alpha-folate-receptor-expressing tumour cells, and suppresses tumour growth in xenograft models. A phase I study of single-agent MORAb-003 showed no dose-limiting toxicities and no significant adverse events, and suggested efficacy in platinum-resistant EOC (Bell-McGuinn et al 2008).

A phase II trial of MORAb-003 as monotherapy or in combination with platinum and taxane in women with recurrent, platinum-sensitive EOC was presented at the ASCO meeting in 2008 (Armstrong et al 2008). In subjects receiving MORAb-003 with platinum and taxane, CA125 normalized in 58% of women after two cycles, 88% of women after four cycles and 100% of subjects after six cycles; RECIST scores of measurable disease improved in parallel. This is a significant increase in ORR compared with historical data for platinum/taxane alone. Based on these data, additional studies of MORAb-003 with chemotherapy in platinum-sensitive and platinum-resistant EOC are planned.

Novel Taxanes

Paclitaxel conjugates have an extended half-life compared with paclitaxel, leading to increased exposure of a tumour to the agent. One such agent that has shown activity in both platinum-sensitive and platinum-resistant ovarian cancer is CT2103. A phase II study of CT2103 in 99 heavily pretreated patients with recurrent ovarian, fallopian tube or peritoneal cancer has been carried out. Platinum-sensitive

($n = 42$) and platinum-refractory/-resistant ($n = 57$) patients were recruited, 61% of whom had received between three and 12 prior regimens (Sabbatini et al 2004). The response rate was 14% and 7% in platinum-sensitive patients and platinum-resistant patients, respectively, with a median time to progression of 2 months. Common toxicities reported were neuropathy (30% grade two or three) and hypersensitivity (8%).

Epothilones

Like the taxanes, epothilones are microtubule stabilizers and have activity against cancer cell lines which are resistant to paclitaxel and other cytotoxic drugs (Rowinsky 1997). They show activity in taxane-resistant tumours *in vivo* (Kolman 2005). This is partially due to the fact that they are not substrates for multidrug transporter proteins. Epothilone B (patupilone) has led to disease stabilization and responses in the phase I/II setting in various malignancies including cancer of the ovary, prostate, breast, colon, stomach and kidney (Mani et al 2004). Six epothilones are in early clinical trials for cancer treatment. Dilawari et al (2008) reported an expanded phase I study of ixabepilone 40 mg/m^2 in patients previously treated with taxanes ($n = 44$) who had ovarian, endometrial, fallopian tube, cervical, breast or another cancer. A range of one to 14 cycles was given, primarily to examine activity and neurotoxicity. Tumour marker response was seen in one-quarter of patients. Three patients had a PR and two had a minimal response. One-quarter of the patients had grade two to three neuropathy, which was preceded by vibration perception threshold changes. Other toxicities included hypersensitivity ($n = 1$) and neutropenia (grade three or more in 18 patients). There are also phase I data on the epothilone patupilone (EPO 906), both as a single agent and in combination with other chemotherapeutics, such as carboplatin (Gore et al 2005, Smit et al 2005, Baggstrom et al 2008, Fracasso et al 2008, Reid et al 2008).

Miscellaneous

Trabectedin (Yondelis, ecteinascidin-743) is a tetrahydroisoquinoline alkaloid derived from a Mediterranean marine organism which is able to bind to the minor groove in DNA. It thereby affects transcription factors involved in cell proliferation, blocks cell division in the G(2) phase and inhibits overexpression of the multidrug resistance-1 gene that leads to development of resistance to many anticancer drugs. It also interferes with nucleotide excision repair. Two phase II trials have reported single-agent activity in patients with platinum-sensitive and platinum-refractory recurrent ovarian cancer (Sessa et al 2005, Krasner et al 2007). In the platinum-sensitive group, 62 evaluable patients had an ORR of 29% [95% confidence interval (CI) 18.2–41.9] and median PFS was 5.1 months (95% CI 2.8–6.2). In the platinum-resistant group, out of 79 evaluable patients, the ORR was 6.3% (95% CI 2.1–14.2) and median PFS was 2 months (95% CI 1.7–3.5). The toxicity profile was manageable with 10% of patients having alanine aminotransferase elevation and 8% of patients having neutropenia (Krasner et al 2007).

A second phase II study including patients with ovarian cancer resistant to platinum and taxanes ($n = 30$) or not ($n = 29$) has been reported (Sessa et al 2005). After two, three-weekly cycles, two PRs were seen and other responses were evident for up to 12.9 months (median 5 months). In the platinum-sensitive group, response rates were 43% (95% CI 23–65). The treatment was well tolerated.

The drug TLK-286 is thought to work by inhibiting glutathione-S-transferaseⅡ, a detoxifying mechanism. A phase II study recruited 36 patients with platinum- and paclitaxel-refractory or -resistant ovarian carcinoma (Kavanagh et al 2005). Of the 94% of patients that were evaluable for response, 15% had objective tumour responses, one had a CR and four had a PR. Twelve patients achieved disease stabilization and this was associated with a decrease in CA125 and improvement in performance status. Median survival was 423 days. The compound was well tolerated and phase III studies are now underway.

A study investigating the additive benefit of proteosome inhibition in combination with liposomal doxorubicin in platinum-sensitive ($n = 15$) and platinum-resistant ($n = 15$) patients was reported at the ASCO meeting in 2008 (Scambia et al 2008). Preliminary results in the platinum-resistant cohort of patients showed prolonged disease stabilization, and four PRs were seen in the platinum-sensitive cohort. The main adverse events were gastrointestinal (77% grade two or less), neurotoxicity (25% grade two or less) and haematological toxicity (21% grade three or less). The study is still open and complete results are awaited with interest to further define the possible synergy with this combination.

Brostacillin is a drug that forms a covalent interaction with DNA when glutathione is present. Twenty-one platinum-resistant and platinum-refractory patients with EOC were treated with brostacillin in a phase II study (Lorusso et al 2008). Two patients had a PR which lasted over 6 months, one patient achieved disease stabilization for 24 weeks and the rest of the patients progressed. Reported toxicity included haematological toxicity (neutropenia in 71% of patients and thrombocytopenia in 43%) and weight decrease (9.5%). Further studies were felt to be warranted to further investigate the use of brostacillin in this patient group.

Integrins are molecules which are vital in forming cell-to-cell adhesions. Volociximab is an $\alpha5\beta1$ integrin antibody that has been tested in patients with relapsed advanced EOC and primary peritoneal carcinoma in the phase I/II setting (Delmonte and Sessa 2008). Three patients were treated with 7 mg/kg qwk and six patients were treated with 15 mg/kg qwk in combination with liposomal doxorubicin until disease progression. Preliminary data suggest that this is a well-tolerated combination, with the main toxicities reported as asthenia ($n = 6$), nausea ($n = 3$), abdominal pain ($n = 2$), flu-like sumptoms ($n = 2$) and vomiting ($n = 1$). A phase II study is planned comparing liposomal doxorubicin alone with the combination of liposomal doxorubicin and volociximab.

Farnesyl transferase inhibitors block the activity of the RAS oncoprotein in tumours. BMS-214662 is a farnesyl transferase inhibitor that has been tested in the phase I setting in patients with advanced solid tumours in combination with paclitaxel and carboplatin (Dy et al 2005). Paclitaxel and carboplatin were given three weekly, and escalating doses of BMS-214662 were given on the first day of each cycle. Thirty patients were treated, and no pharmacokinetic interactions were seen between the three drugs. One patient with endometrial cancer and one patient with ovarian cancer had a PR. Disease stabilization was achieved in eight other patients. The combination was well tolerated with dose-limiting toxicities including neutropenia, thrombocytopenia, nausea and vomiting. A further phase I study tested BMS-214662 in combination with paclitaxel alone in patients with advanced solid tumours. Patients were treated ($n = 26$) with weekly paclitaxel and escalating doses of BMS-214662, and up to 94 courses of treatment (Bailey et al 2007). All the pretreated ovarian cancer patients had a PR, and pharmacokinetic studies showed no interaction with paclitaxel. Peripheral blood lymphocytes (PBLs) were taken to test for significant farnesyl transferase inhibition (>80%), which was seen at the end of the BMS-214662 infusion. Dose-limiting toxicities included grade four neutropenia, rises in serum transaminases and grade three diarrhoea.

Histone deacetylase (HDAC) inhibitors block the deacetylation of histones, a mechanism by which the regulation of gene expression is mediated. Two phase II studies were reported at the ASCO meeting in 2008 detailing results of HDAC inhibition in platinum-resistant epithelial ovarian tumours. The first study used belinostat (PXD101) in platinum-resistant patients ($n = 18$, group 1) or patients with micropapillary/borderline ovarian tumours ($n = 12$, group 2) (Mackay et al 2008). Tumour biopsies and PBLs were taken prior to treatment, and on the fourth day (out of 5 days) of treatment. Of the patients in group 1, nine patients achieved disease stabilization and six progressed. Of the patients in group 2, one patient had a PR, nine achieved disease stabilization and one patient had a CA125 response. Grade three adverse events included thrombosis ($n = 3$), dyspnoea ($n = 2$), fatigue ($n = 2$), elevated alkaline phosphatase ($n = 2$) and nausea ($n = 2$). The second study also tested belinostat but in combination with carboplatin and paclitaxel in platinum-resistant and platinum-sensitive patients. Eleven patients relapsed within 6 months of first platinum therapy. The ORR was 31%, which included one CR and 10 PRs. Sixteen patients achieved disease stabilization. Common grade three to four adverse events were neutropenia ($n = 4$), transaminitis ($n = 4$) and fatigue ($n = 3$). Recruitment to both studies is still ongoing.

Conclusion

The treatment of gynaecological malignancies in the future will no doubt make use of our increased understanding of the biology of these diseases. Whether the novel agents discussed above are used alone, in combination with each other or with other chemotherapeutics remains to be defined. The exact benefit of many of these agents in terms of response rates and disease-free survival is also largely unknown. In addition, it is uncertain whether they will simply be unaffordable in most health economies. However, this is certainly an exciting time in the field of gynaecological oncology, and it is hoped that the use of targeted agents will have a significant impact on disease progression and outcome in the near future.

KEY POINTS

1. Advances in the molecular biology of gynaecological malignancies has led to a number of potential therapeutic targets being identified: VEGF, EGFR, PARP, PI3K/AKT, PKC pathways and the alpha folate receptor.

2. Early initiation of angiogenesis is essential for cancer survival, and VEGF expression has been correlated with outcome for gynaecological cancers.

3. A number of antiangiogenic agents are showing activity in gynaecological cancers, including monoclonal antibodies, TKIs and decoy receptor molecules.

4. Mutations in *BRCA1* or *BRCA2* result in specific DNA repair mechanism defects. PARP inhibitors have been shown to be active against such tumours, and also enhance the effect of cytotoxics.

5. Inhibition of mTOR results in a profound decrease in signalling via the PI3K/AKT pathway. mTOR inhibitors have activity in gynaecological malignancies, particularly endometrial cancer.

6. Inhibitors of PKC and Src have potential as targeted therapy against ovarian cancer, and are currently the subject of clinical studies.

7. The alpha folate receptor is overexpressed in the majority of ovarian cancers but is largely absent from normal tissue, and is a promising target.

8. It remains to be defined whether the novel targeted agents will be best utilized as single agents or in combination with each other or cytotoxics.

9. Target agents have the potential to be used as maintenance therapy following remission induction.

References

Aghajanian C, Sabbatini P, Derosa F 2005 A phase II study of cetuximab/paclitaxel/carboplatin for the initial treatment of advanced stage ovarian, primary peritoneal and fallopian tube cancer. Journal of Clinical Oncology 23 (Suppl): a5047.

Altomare DA, Wang HQ, Skele KL 2004 AKT and mTOR phosphorylation is frequently detected in ovarian cancer and can be targeted to disrupt ovarian tumor cell growth. Oncogene 23: 5853–5857.

Armstrong DK, Bicher A, Coleman RL et al 2008 Exploratory phase II efficacy study of MORAb-003, a monoclonal antibody against folate receptor alpha, in platinum-sensitive ovarian cancer in first relapse. Journal of Clinical Oncology 26 (Suppl): a5500.

Bailey HH, Alberti DB, Thomas JP et al 2007 Phase I trial of weekly paclitaxel and BMS-214662 in patients with advanced solid tumours. Clinical Cancer Research 13: 3623–3629.

Bartlett JM, Langdon SP, Simpson BJ et al 1996 The prognostic value of epidermal growth factor receptor mRNA expression in primary ovarian cancer. British Journal of Cancer 73: 301–306.

Baggstrom MQ, Ravaud A, Fracasso PM 2008 Patupilone combined with carboplatin in patients (pts) with advanced solid tumours: preliminary safety and activity results. Journal of Clinical Oncology 26 (Suppl): a13538.

Beerepoot L, Rademaker-Lakhai J, Witteveen E et al 2006 Phase I and pharmacokinetic evaluation of enzastaurin combined with gemcitabine and cisplatin in advanced cancer. Journal of Clinical Oncology 24 (Suppl): 2046.

Beevers C, Li F, Liu L, Huang S 2006 Curcumin inhibits the mammalian target of rapamycin-mediated signaling pathways in cancer cells. International Journal of Cancer 119: 757–764.

Bell-McGuinn KM, Konner JA, Pandit-Taskar N et al 2008 A phase I study of MORAb-003, a humanized monoclonal antibody against folate receptor alpha, in advanced epithelial ovarian cancer. Journal of Clinical Oncology 26 (Suppl): a5517.

Berchuck A, Kamel A, Whitaker R 1990 Overexpression of HER-2/neu is associated with poor survival in advanced epithelial ovarian cancer. Cancer Research 50: 4087–4091.

Berek J, Taylor PT, Gordon A 2004 Randomized, placebo-controlled study of ovregovomab for consolidation of clinical remission in patients with advanced ovarian cancer. Journal of Clinical Oncology 22: 3507–3516.

Berek J, Taylor PT, McGuire WP, Smith LM, Suhulte B, Nicodemus CF 2008 Evaluation of maintenance mono-immunotherapy to improve outcomes in advanced ovarian cancer (OV CA). Journal of Clinical Oncology 26 (Suppl): a5507.

Bergers G, Benjamin LE 2003 Tumorigenesis and the angiogenic switch. Nature Reviews Cancer 3: 401–410.

Biagi JJ, Oza AM, Grimshaw R et al 2008 A phase II study of sunitinib (SU11248) in patients (pts) with recurrent epithelial ovarian, fallopian, tube or primary peritoneal carcinoma — NCIC CTG IND 185. Journal of Clinical Oncology 26 (Suppl): a5522.

Bookman MA, Darcy KM, Clarke-Pearson D, Boothby RA, Horowitz IR 2003 Evaluation of monoclonal humanized anti-HER2 antibody, trastuzumab, in patients with recurrent or refractory ovarian or primary peritoneal carcinoma with overexpression of HER2: a phase II trial of the Gynecologic Oncology Group. Journal of Clinical Oncology 21: 283–290.

Braly P, Chu C, Collins Y et al 2007 Prospective evaluation of front-line chemo-immunotherapy with oregovomab (2 alternative dosing schedules) carboplatin–paclitaxel in advanced ovarian cancer. Proceedings of the American Society of Clinical Oncology 25: 3024.

Burger RA, Sill MW, Monk BJ et al 2007 Phase II trial of bevacizumab in persistent or recurrent epithelial ovarian cancer or primary peritoneal cancer: a Gynecologic Oncology Group study. Journal of Clinical Oncology 25: 5165–5171.

Campiglio M, Ali S, Knyazev PG 1999 Characteristics of EGFR family-mediated HRG signals in human ovarian cancer. Journal of Cell Biochemistry 73: 522–532.

Cannistra SA, Matulonis UA, Penson RT et al 2007 Phase II study of bevacizumab in patients with platinum resistant ovarian cancer or peritoneal serous cancer. Journal of Clinical Oncology 25 (Suppl): 5180–5186.

Carducci MA, Musib L, Kies MS et al 2006 Phase I dose escalation and pharmacokinetic study of enzastaurin, an oral protein kinase C beta inhibitor, in patients with advanced cancer. Journal of Clinical Oncology 24: 4092–4099.

Cheng WF, Chen CA, Lee CN et al 1999 Vascular endothelial growth factor in cervical carcinoma. Obstetrics and Gynecology 93: 761–765.

Cohn DE, Valmadre S, Resnick KE et al 2006 Bevacizumab and weekly taxane chemotherapy demonstrates activity in refractory ovarian cancer. Gynecological Oncology 102: 134–139.

Colombo N, McMeekin S, Schwartz P et al 2007 A phase II trial of the mTOR inhibitor AP23573 as a single agent in advanced endometrial cancer. Journal of Clinical Oncology 25 (Suppl): 5516.

Cooper BC, Ritchie JM, Broghammer CL et al 2002 Preoperative serum vascular endothelial growth factor levels: significance in ovarian cancer. Clinical Cancer Research 8: 3193–3197.

Cresta S, Tosi D, Sessa C et al 2007 Phase Ib study defining the optimal dosing combinations of the mTOR inhibitor AP23573 and paclitaxel (PTX). Journal of Clinical Oncology 25 (Suppl) 3509.

Delmonte A, Sessa C 2008 Molecule-targeted agents in endometrial cancer. Current Opinion in Oncology 20(5): 554–559.

Desai AA, Mita M, Fetterly GJ et al 2005 Development of pharmacokinetic (PK) model and assessment of patient covariate effects on dose-dependent PK following different dosing schedules in two phase I trials of AP23573, a mTOR inhibitor. Journal of Clinical Oncology 23 (Suppl): a3043.

Dilawari A, Goel S, Assai A, Moore S, Muggia FM, Mani S 2008 Ixabepilone (Ixa) in taxane-pretreated women with breast and gynaecologic cancers: overall tolerance neurotoxicity (NT) assessment and evidence of activity. Journal of Clinical Oncology 26 (Suppl): a16529.

Dupont J, Bienvenu B, Aghajanian C et al 2004 Phase I and pharmokinetic study of the novel oral cell-cycle inhibitor Ro 31-7453 in patients with advanced solid tumors. Journal of Clinical Oncology 22: 3366–3374.

Dy GK, Bruzek L, Croghan GA et al 2005. A phase I trial of thenovel farnesyl protein transferase inhibitor, BMS-214662, in combination with paclitaxel and carboplatin in patients with advanced cancer. Clinical Cancer Research 11: 1877–1883.

Ehlen T 2002 Adjuvant treatment with monoclonal antibody, Ovarex Mab-843.13 targeting CA125 induces robust immune responses associated with prolonged time to relapse in a randomized, placebo controlled study in patients with advanced epithelial ovarian cancer. Proceedings of the American Society of Clinical Oncology 21: a31.

Farmer H, McCabe N, Lord CJ et al 2005 Targeting the DNA repair defect in BRCA mutant cells as a therapeutic strategy. Nature 434: 917–921.

Finkler N, Gordon A, Crozier M 2001 Phase II evaluation of OSI-774, a potential oral antagonist of the EGFR-TK in patients with advanced ovarian cancer. Proceedings of the American Society of Clinical Oncology 20: a831.

Fischer-Colbrie J, Witt A, Heinzl H et al 1997 EGFR and steroid receptors in ovarian carcinoma: comparison with prognostic parameters and outcome of patients. Anticancer Research 17: 613–619.

Folkman J 1971 Tumor angiogenesis: therapeutic implications. New England Journal of Medicine 285: 1182–1186.

Folkman J 1990 What is the evidence that tumors are angiogenesis dependent? Journal of the National Cancer Institute 82: 4–6

Fong PC, Boss DS, Carden CP et al 2008 AZD2281 (KU-0059436), a PARP (poly ADP-ribose polymerase) inhibitor with single agent anticancer activity in patients with BRCA deficient ovarian cancer: results from a phase I study. Journal of Clinical Oncology 26 (Suppl): a5510.

Ford M, Richter A, Thomas EJ et al 1994 Expression of EGF receptor ligands and their receptor status in ovarian tumors. British Journal of Cancer 71 (Suppl. 24): 16.

Fracasso PM, Ravaud A, Baggstrom MQ et al 2008 Patupilone combined with carboplatin in patients (pts) with advanced solid tumours: preliminary safety and activity results. Journal of Clinical Oncology 26 (Suppl): a13544.

Garcia AA, Oza AM, Hirte H et al 2005 Interim report of a phase II clinical trial of bevacizumab and low dose metronomic oral cyclophosphamide in recurrent ovarian and primary peritoneal cancer; a California Cancer Consortium Trial. Journal of Clinical Oncology 23 (Suppl): a5000.

Goff BA, Shy K, Greer BE, Muntz HG, Skelly M, Gown AM 1996 Overexpression and relationships of HER2/neu, epidermal growth factor receptor, p53, Ki-67, and tumor necrosis factor α in epithelial ovarian cancer. European Journal of Gynaecological Oncology 17: 487–492.

Gordon MS, Cunningham D 2005 Managing patients treated with bevacizumab combination therapy. Oncology 69 (Suppl 3): 25–33.

Gordon MS, Matei D, Aghajanian C et al 2006 Clinical activity of pertuzumab (rhuMab2C4), a HER dimerization inhibitor, in advanced ovarian cancer: potential predictive relationship with HER2 activation status. Journal of Clinical Oncology 24: 4324–4332.

Gore M, Kaye S, Oza A et al 2005 Phase I trial of patupilone plus carboplatin in patients with advanced cancer. Journal of Clinical Oncology 23 (Suppl): 5087.

Graff JR, McNulty AM, Hanna KR 2005 The protein kinase Cβ-selective inhibitor, enzastaurin (LY317615.HCl), suppresses signalling through the AKT pathway, induces apoptosis, and suppresses growth of human colon cancer and glioblastoma xenografts. Cancer Research 65: 7462–7469.

Han LY, Landen CN, Trevino JG et al 2006 Antiangiogenic and antitumor effects of Src inhibition in ovarian carcinoma. Cancer Research 66: 8633–8639.

Hirte HW, Vidal L, Fleming GF et al 2008 A phase II study of cediranib (AZD2171) in recurrent or persistent ovarian, peritoneal or fallopian tube cancer. Final results of a PMH, Chicago and California Consorts Trial. Journal of Clinical Oncology 26 (Suppl): a5521.

Holland CM, Day K, Evans A et al 2003 Expression of the VEGF and angiopoietin genes in endometrial atypical hyperplasia and endometrial cancer. British Journal of Cancer 89: 891–898.

Hu L, Hofmann J, Holash J et al 2005 Vascular endothelial growth factor trap combined with paclitaxel strikingly inhibits tumor and ascites, prolonging survival in a human ovarian cancer model. Clinical Cancer Research 11: 6966–6971.

Ilekis JV, Connor JP, Prins GS, Ferrer K, Niederberger C, Scoccia B 1997 Expression of epidermal growth factor and androgen receptors in ovarian cancer. Gynecological Oncology 66: 250–254.

Ishizawar R, Parsons SJ 2004 C-Src and cooperating partners in human cancer. Cancer Cell 6(3): 209–214.

Kassim SK, El-Salahy EM, Fayed ST et al 2004 Vascular endothelial growth factor and interleukin-8 are associated with poor prognosis in epithelial ovarian cancer patients. Clinical Biochemistry 37: 363–369.

Kavanagh JJ, Gershenson Dm, Choi H et al 2005 Multi-institutional phase II study of TLK286 (TELCYTA, a glutathione S-transferase P1-1 activated glutathione analog prodrug) in platinum and paclitaxel refractory or resistant ovarian cancer. International Journal of Gynecological Cancer 15: 593–600.

Keyes KA, Mann L, Sherman M 2004 LY317615 decreases plasma VEGF levels in human tumor xenograft-bearing mice. Cancer Chemotherapy and Pharmacology 53: 133–140.

Kolman A 2005 Activity of epothilones. Current Opinion in Investigative Drugs 6: 616–622.

Krasner CN, McMeekin DS, Chan S et al 2007 A phase II study of trabectedin single agent in patients with recurrent ovarian cancer previously treated with platinum based regimens. British Journal of Cancer 97: 1618–1624.

Lee KW, Kim SG, Kim H-P et al 2008 Enzastaurin, a protein kinase C{beta} inhibitor, suppresses signaling through the ribosomal S6 kinase and bad pathways and induces apoptosis in human gastric cancer cells. Cancer Research 68: 1916–1926.

Lin J, Chew K, Sauter G, Waldman F, Benz C 1994 Prevalence and prognostic significance of HER2/neu and epidermal growth factor receptor (EGFR) overexpression in ovarian cancer. Proceedings of the American Society of Clinical Oncology 13: 258.

Li L, Wang L, Zhang W et al 2004 Correlation of serum VEGF levels with clinical stage, therapy efficacy, tumour metastasis and patient survival in ovarian cancer. Anticancer Research 24: 1973–1979.

Loncaster JA, Cooper RA, Logue JP et al 2000 Vascular endothelial growth factor (VEGF) expression is a prognostic factor for radiotherapy outcome in advanced carcinoma of the cervix. British Journal of Cancer 83: 620–625.

Lorusso D, Zanaboni F, Scalone S et al 2008 Phase II exploratory study of brostacillin in patients with ovarian cancer resistant/refractory to platinum based chemotherapy. Journal of Clinical Oncology 26 (Suppl): a16520.

Mackay H, Hirte HW, Covens A et al 2008 A phase II trial of the histone deacetylase inhibitor belinostat (PXD101) in patients with platinum resistant epithelial ovarian tumours and micropapillary/boarderline (LMP) ovarian tumours. A PMH phase II consortium trial. Journal of Clinical Oncology 26 (Suppl): a5518.

Mani S, McDaid H, Hamilton A et al 2004 Phase I clinical and pharmacokinetic study of BMS-247550, a novel derivative of epothilone B, in solid tumours. Clinical Cancer Research 10: 1289–1298.

Matel D, Sill MW, DeGeest K, Bristow RE 2008 Phase II trial of sorafenib in persistent or recurrent epithelial ovarian cancer (EOC) or primary peritoneal cancer (PPC): a Gynaecologic Oncology Group (GOG) study. Journal of Clinical Oncology 26 (Suppl): a5537.

Matulonis UA, Berlin ST, Krasner CN et al 2008 Cediranib (AZD2171) is an active agent in recurrent epithelial ovarian cancer. Journal of Clinical Oncology 26 (Suppl): a5501.

McGonigle KF, Muntz HG, Vuky JL et al 2008 Phase II prospective study of weekly topotecan and bevacizumab in platinum refractory ovarian cancer or peritoneal cancer (OC). Journal of Clinical Oncology 26 (Suppl): a5551.

Meinhold-Heerlein I, Bauerschlag DO, Bräutigam K et al 2006 Effects of PKC beta inhibitor enzastaurin on parental and chemoresistant ovarian cancer cell lines. Journal of Clinical Oncology 24 (Suppl): 20037.

Meric-Bernstam F, Mills GB 2004 Mammalian target of rapamycin. Seminars in Oncology 31 (Suppl 16): 10–17.

Mita M, Rowinsky E, Mita A et al 2004 Phase I, pharmacokinetic (PK) and pharmacodynamic (PD) study of AP23573, an mTOR inhibitor administered IV daily × 5 every other week in patients with refractory or advanced malignancies. Journal of Clinical Oncology 22 (Suppl): 3076.

Monk BJ, Han E, Josephs-Cowan CA et al 2006 Salvage bevacizumab (rhuMAB VEGF)-based therapy after multiple prior cytotoxic regimens in advanced refractory epithelial ovarian cancer. Gynecological Oncology 102: 140–144.

Nimeiri HS, Oza AM, Morgan RJ et al 2008 Sorafenib (SOR) in patients (pts) with advanced/recurrent uterine carcinoma (UCA) or carinosarcoma (CS): a phase II trial of the University of Chicago, PMH and California Phase II Consortia. Journal of Clinical Oncology 26 (Suppl): a5585.

Oza AM, Elit L, Biagi J et al 2006 Molecular correlates associated with a phase II study of temsirolimus (CCI-779) in patients with metastatic or recurrent endometrial cancer. Journal of Clinical Oncology 24 (Suppl): 3003.

Oza AM, Elit L, Provencher D et al 2008 A phase II study of temsirolimus (CCI-779) in patients with metastatic and/or locally advanced recurrent endometrial cancer previously treated with chemotherapy: NCIC CTG IND 160b. Journal of Clinical Oncology 26 (Suppl): a5516.

Penson RT, Cannistra SA, Seiden MV et al 2006 Phase II study of carboplatin, paclitaxel and bevacizumab as first line chemotherapy and consolidation for advanced mullerian tumors. Journal of Clinical Oncology 24 (Suppl): a5020.

Rademaker-Lakhai JM, Beerepoot LV, Mehra N et al 2007 Phase I pharmacokinetic and pharmacodynamic study of the oral protein kinase C {beta}-inhibitor enzastaurin in combination with gemcitabine and cisplatin in patients with advanced cancer. Clinical Cancer Research 13: 4474–4481.

Raymond E, Alexandre J, Faivre S et al 2004 Safety and pharmacokinetics of escalated doses of weekly intravenous infusion of CCI-779, a novel mTOR inhibitor, in patients with cancer. Journal of Clinical Oncology 2: 2336–2347.

Reid TR, Takimoto CH, Vershraegen CF et al 2008 Evaluation of safety, tolerability and pharmacokinetics (PK) of patupilone in patients (pts) with advanced solid tumours and varying degrees of hepatic function: an open label phase I study. Journal of Clinical Oncology (Suppl): a2557.

Rivkin SE, Muller C, Iriarte D, Arthur J, Canoy A, Reid TR 2008 Phase I/II lapatinib plus carboplatin and paclitaxel in stage III or IV relapsed ovarian cancer patients. Journal of Clinical Oncology 26 (Suppl): a5556.

Rowinsky EK 1997 The development and clinical utility of the taxane class of antimicrotubule chemotherapy agents. Annual Review of Medicine 48: 353–374.

Sabbatini P, Aghajanian C, Dizon D et al 2004 Phase II study of CT-2103 in patients with recurrent epithelial ovarian, fallopian tube or primary peritoneal carcinoma. Journal of Clinical Oncology 22: 4523–4531.

Scambia G, Parma G, Del Conte G et al 2008 A phase II study of bortezomib with pegylated-liposomal doxorubicin in patients with ovarian cancer failing platinum containing regimens. Journal of Clinical Oncology 26 (Suppl): a5581.

Schilder RJ, Kohn E, Sill MW 2003 Phase II trial of gefitinib in patients with recurrent ovarian or primary peritoneal cancer. Gynecologic Oncology Group 170C. Proceedings of American Society of Clinical Oncology 22: a1814.

Seiden M, Burris HA, Matulonis U 2005 A phase II trial of EMD72000 (matuzumab) a humanized anti-EGFR monoclonal antibody in subjects with heavily pretreated and platinum resistant advanced Mullerian malignancies. Journal of Clinical Oncology 23 (Suppl): a3151.

Sessa C, De Braud F, Perotti A et al 2005 Trabectedin for women with ovarian carcinoma after treatment with platinum and taxanes fails. Journal of Clinical Oncology 23: 1867–1874.

Slamon DJ, Leyland-Jones B, Shak S et al 2001 Use of chemotherapy plus a monoclonal antibody against HER2 for metastatic breast cancer that overexpresses HER2. New England Journal of Medicine 344: 783–792.

Slomovitz BM, Lu KH, Johnston T et al 2008 A phase II study of oral mammalian target or rapamycin (mTOR) inhibitor, RAD001 (everolimus), in patients with recurrent endometrial carcinoma. Journal of Clinical Oncology 26 (Suppl): a5502.

Smit WM, Sufilarsky J, Spanik S et al 2005 Phase I/II dose escalation trial of patupilone every 3 weeks in patients with relapsed/refractory ovarian cancer. Journal of Clinical Oncology 23 (Suppl): 5056.

Spector NL, Xia W, Burris H III et al 2005 Study of the biologic effects of lapatinib, a reversible inhibitor of ErbB1 and ErbB2 tyrosine kinases, on tumor growth and survival pathways in patients with advanced malignancies. Journal of Clinical Oncology 23: 2502–2512.

Summy JM, Trevino JG, Lesslie DP et al 2005 AP23846, a novel and highly potent Src family kinase inhibitor, reduces vascular endothelial growth factor and interleukin-8 expression in human solid tumour cell lines and abrogates downstream angiogenic processes. Molecular Cancer Therapies 4: 1900–1911.

Teicher BA, Menon K, Alvarez E 2002 Antiangiogenic and antitumor effects of a protein kinase Cβ inhibitor in human breast and ovarian cancer xenografts. Investigational New Drugs 20: 241–251.

Toffoli G, Cernigoi C, Russo A et al 1997 Overexpression of folate binding protein in ovarian cancers. International Journal of Cancer 74: 193–198.

Tutt A, Ashworth A 2002 The relationship between the roles of BRCA genes in DNA repair and cancer predisposition. Trends in Molecular Medicine 8: 571–576.

Wagner U, Kohler S, Reinartz S 2001 Immunological consolidation of ovarian carcinoma with monoclonal anti-idiotype antibody ACA125: immune responses and survival in palliative treatment. Clinical Cancer Research 7: 1112–1115.

Wiener JR, Windham TC, Estrella VC et al 2003 Activated SRC protein tyrosine kinase is overexpressed in late-stage human ovarian cancers. Gynecoloogical Oncology 88: 73–79.

Wright JD, Hagemann A, Rader JS et al 2006a Bevacizumab combination therapy in recurrent, platinum-refractory, epithelial ovarian carcinoma: a retrospective analysis. Cancer 107: 83–89.

Wright JD, Viviano D, Powell MA et al 2006b Bevacizumab combination therapy in heavily pretreated, recurrent cervical cancer. Gynecological Oncology 103: 489–493.

Yin BW, Lloyd KO 2001 Molecular cloning of the CA125 ovarian cancer antigen: identification as a new mucin, MUC16.

Journal of Biological Chemistry 276: 27371–27375.

Zhang L, Conejo-Garcia JR, Katsaros D et al 2003 Intratumoral T cells, recurrence, and survival in epithelial ovarian cancer. New England Journal of Medicine 348: 203–213.

CHAPTER 38

Premalignant disease of the genital tract

Esther Moss, Charles W. Redman and Raji Ganesan

Chapter Contents

INTRODUCTION	566	THE UTERINE CORPUS	577
THE CERVIX	566	THE OVARY	579
THE VAGINA	575	KEY POINTS	580
THE VULVA	576		

Introduction

The key to the effective management of premalignancy is to understand its aetiology, pathogenesis and natural history. Our knowledge and understanding of premalignant disease of the genital tract has progressed from descriptive morphology to a molecular biological level; a shift that is reflected by the evolution of clinical management from the detection and surgical removal of premalignant lesions to their prevention.

The tissues of the female genital tract differ in terms of embryological origin, responsiveness to intrinsic factors such as hormones, and exposure to external mutagens. Cellular transformation, leading to the development of cancer, is brought about by a variety of events, in part responding to various agents, acting alone or in combination, termed 'carcinogens'. In the female genital tract, these may be viruses, chemicals, hormones or ionizing radiation. It follows that a single chapter under the heading of 'Premalignant disease of the female genital tract' will necessarily cover a variety of issues that are best considered by anatomical site.

The Cervix

In 1886, Sir John Williams described eight cases of cervical cancer, one of which was equivalent to carcinoma *in situ*:

> *'this is the earliest condition of undoubted cancer of the portio vaginalis that I have met with, and it is the earliest condition that is recognisable as cancer. It presented no distinct symptoms and was discovered accidentally.'*

This described the cardinal features of cervical premalignancy; it is asymptomatic, clinically undetectable and has malignant potential. Its recognition had profound therapeutic significance as detection and treatment offered the potential to prevent cancer. The challenge has been to realize this

therapeutic goal effectively with as little collateral damage as possible.

The terminology of cervical premalignancy

Most cervical cancers are squamous in origin, but a significant, and increasing, proportion arise from cervical glandular epithelium (estimates ranging from 5% to 30% of the precancerous lesions found on the cervix). Both cancer types have premalignant lesions.

The premise that cervical squamous premalignancy was a continuum underpinned the concept of cervical intraepithelial neoplasia (CIN), which was suggested by Richart (1967). The usefulness of this system was limited by significant interobserver variability in the diagnosis and grading of CIN, particularly in differentiating CIN1 from human papilloma virus (HPV) lesions, and separating CIN1 from CIN2 lesions. Furthermore, there is no clear evidence that CIN3 arises from earlier lesions.

These considerations were addressed by the Bethesda classification which was initially introduced as a cervical cytological grading system. Cervical lesions are classified into high- and low-grade squamous intraepithelial lesions; the latter group includes HPV lesions. This has the potential advantage of simplicity and tends to reflect the way in which clinicians practise, in that high-grade lesions are thought to be genuinely premalignant and should be treated.

Currently, whilst CIN terminology is used in the UK, clinical practice reflects the Bethesda classification in that CIN1 is regarded as a low-grade lesion, which tends to be managed conservatively, and CIN2 and CIN3 are regarded as high-grade lesions which are treated.

Attempts to classify premalignant glandular lesions have been bedevilled by a number of problems. In the UK, they are termed 'cervical glandular intraepithelial neoplasia' (CGIN) and are classified as high- or low-grade lesions. Low-grade CGIN lesions are difficult to distinguish from a number

DOI: 10.1016/B978-0-7020-3120-5.00038-2

of benign and reactive changes. The biological behaviour of low-grade CGIN is not understood.

Pathology of cervical premalignancy

Cervical intraepithelial neoplasia

CIN relates to lesions that are confined to the squamous epithelium. The diagnosis of CIN is based upon the architectural and cytological appearances of the squamous epithelium. It is characterized by abnormal cellular proliferation, abnormal epithelial maturation and cytological atypia. Grading depends on the level in the epithelium to which abnormal changes extend.

The proportion of the thickness of the epithelium showing differentiation is a useful feature to be taken into account when deciding the severity of a CIN; roughly lower-, middle- and upper-third involvement equate to CIN1, CIN2 and 3, respectively. It is not the most important criterion despite the fact that it is one of the easiest to assess. In CIN1, at least the upper half of the epithelium usually shows good differentiation and stratification, whereas in CIN3, differentiation may be very slight or even absent.

CIN may affect the gland crypts as well as the surface epithelium (Figure 38.1). It is recognized that the degree and depth of crypt involvement increases with the grade of CIN. Histological assessment of crypt involvement in women with CIN3 has shown a mean depth of 1–2 mm, with a maximum of 5.22 mm and a mean ±3 standard deviations (99.7%) of 3.8 mm (Anderson and Hartley 1980). These figures suggested that treatment of ectocervical lesions to a depth of 7 mm should be sufficient to eradicate most CIN.

Cervical glandular intraepithelial neoplasia

CGIN is characterized by columnar cells with hyperchromatic nuclei and stippled chromatin (Figure 38.2). The nuclei show increased stratification and abnormal mitotic figures with loss of normal mucin. In some cases, the whole of a gland may be involved, but the lesion often occurs as a sharply demarcated area. It may be multifocal. CGIN is often associated with goblet cells or intestinal metaplasia of the endocervical cells. In two-thirds of cases, there are associated squamous abnormalities, and CGIN is often serendipitously discovered in the management of these abnormalities.

Histological problems

The histological diagnosis of these lesions is based largely upon subjective criteria and is dependent on the adequacy of sampling. It is not surprising to find substantial inter- and intraobserver variation in the grading of CIN and the identification of CGIN. Variation is greatest at the lower end of the spectrum.

These considerations have important implications. Firstly, understanding of the risk of progression of CIN and its subgroups, on which treatment strategies are based, is inevitably flawed by bias of one form or another. Furthermore, in any given patient, there will be a spectrum of disease so that the reliability of the histological diagnosis is dependent on the quality and extent of sampling.

Pathogenesis of cervical premalignancy

The development of squamous precancerous abnormalities is intimately associated with the region of the cervical squamocolumnar junction (SCJ) and the changes that occur at puberty and adolescence.

The position of the SCJ is influenced by the hormonal changes that occur during a woman's life (Figure 38.3). With the onset of puberty, the uterus enlarges and the cervix swells with a resultant eversion, exposing columnar epithelium to the acid environment of the vagina. This induces metaplasia

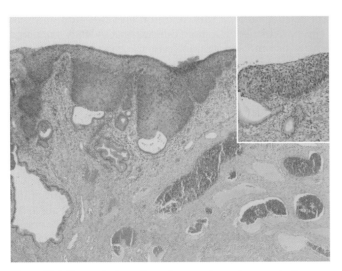

Figure 38.1 The cervical transformation zone shows the metaplastic squamous epithelium replaced by full-thickness lack of maturation amounting to cervical intraepithelial neoplasia 3 (long arrow). This is seen extending down the gland cleft (block arrow). The inset shows brisk epithelial mitotic activity. Original magnification ×100, inset ×200.

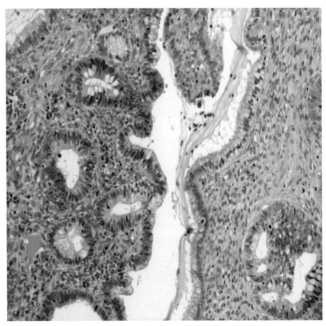

Figure 38.2 High-grade cervical glandular intraepithelial neoplasia, characterized by hyperchromatic glandular cells with pseudostratification, relative paucity of mucin, brisk mitotic activity and abrupt junction with normal epithelium (long arrow). Intestinal metaplasia (short arrow) is noted. Original magnification ×40.

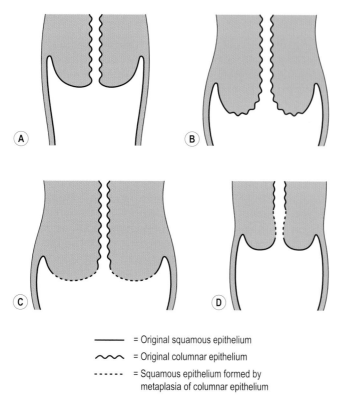

——— = Original squamous epithelium

∿∿∿ = Original columnar epithelium

- - - - - = Squamous epithelium formed by metaplasia of columnar epithelium

Figure 38.3 The different stages in the development and involution of the cervix. (A) Before puberty, the ectocervix is covered with squamous epithelium, and columnar epithelium is usually confined to the endocervical canal. (B) The cervix enlarges and everts when oestrogen levels rise. This exposes columnar epithelium on the ectocervix. (C) The columnar epithelium on the ectocervix is replaced with squamous epithelium by a process of metaplasia. (D) Following the climacteric when oestrogen levels fall, the cervix shrinks, drawing the squamocolumnar junction up the canal.

Table 38.1 Risk factors for cervical intraepithelial neoplasia

- Early age at first intercourse (16 years or younger)
- History of multiple sexual partners
- Human papilloma virus infection, chlamydia or other sexually transmitted diseases
- Presence of other genital tract neoplasia
- History of previous cervical intraepithelial neoplasia
- Multiparity
- Cigarette smoking
- Combined oral contraception
- Dietary factors

in the exposed columnar epithelium, resulting in the development of metaplastic squamous epithelium. This area of transformation is termed the 'cervical transformation zone' (cervical TZ), and it is within this area that preneoplastic changes can occur with the development of CIN. It is thought that these dysplastic changes occur at the time of metaplasia, indicating that this is the time when the cervix is most vulnerable to potential carcinogenic factors, such as HPV and other cofactors.

These considerations have important clinical significance with regards to detecting and treating CIN, as these changes occur within the cervical TZ and it is accessible. Furthermore, the recognition that the development of precancerous changes can occur early in a woman's sexual and reproductive life provided some indication that these events were potentially associated with some form of environmental exposure related to sexual activity. In other words, most of the identified risk factors for CIN are thought to be largely surrogate markers of HPV infection (Table 38.1).

Malignant potential of cervical premalignant lesions

Cervical intraepithelial neoplasia

The malignant potential of CIN3 was shown by McIndoe et al (1984) in a crucial paper. This indicated that approxi-

mately 30% of women with CIN3 would develop invasive cancer over a 20-year period.

The authors' rationale for treating CIN3 is based upon this paper, which implies that when CIN3 is discovered, it should be treated. However, there are caveats. Firstly, the patients in this study had large carcinoma in situ lesions, and can we be sure that the undoubted premalignant potential for the lesions managed in this paper are shared by patients with smaller lesions that have small foci of CIN3? For example, it has been estimated that perhaps one-third of cases with CIN3 regress (Östör 1993).

Overall, it is thought that 1% of all CIN progresses to invasive cancer. Studies indicate that approximately 45–60% of CIN1 regress, 22–45% persist without progression and 10–16% progress to CIN3; whereas 28–40% of CIN2 regress, 20–40% persist and up to 50% progress to CIN3. However, all these studies are blighted by the difficulty in accurately determining the grade of the initial lesion and methodological variations.

These data indicate that treatment should always be considered for CIN3, but not necessarily for lesser grades of CIN. However, given the shortcomings in accurate assessment and the risk of progression of these cases, careful follow-up of untreated cases is mandatory.

Cervical glandular intraepithelial neoplasia

The relative rarity of this condition and classification problems have made this a more difficult area to study compared with squamous lesions. However, there is good evidence to support the concept that high-grade CGIN is a premalignant condition.

Aetiology of cervical premalignancy

The epidemiological risk factors for both squamous and glandular cervical premalignant lesions are similar and include young age at first intercourse and multiple sexual partners. It is now well established that infection with oncogenic high-risk HPV types is the central causal factor in the development of cervical neoplasia (Walboomers et al 1999).

The fact that virtually all cervical malignancies contain HPV DNA illustrates the central role of HPV in cervical carcinogenesis. It has now been proven beyond reasonable doubt that HPV infection is a necessary prerequisite for cervical carcinogenesis.

HPVs are small double-stranded DNA viruses which have an icosahedral protein capsid (Figure 38.4). They are typed according to the DNA sequence homology in particular

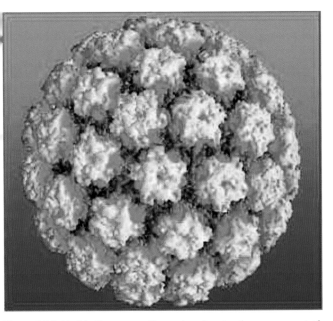

Figure 38.4 Model of human papilloma virus showing the arrangement of capsid proteins.

genes, specifically *L1* (which codes for the viral capsid) and *E6* and *E7* (which have important carcinogenic functions). Nearly 30 HPV types can infect the genital tract and can be classified into high-, intermediate- and low-risk oncogenic types. HPV types 16 and 18 are by far the most common high-risk types, accounting for 60% of HPV-positive invasive cervical cancers.

HPV infection can lead to integration of viral DNA into the host's genome, with expression of the viral oncogenes *E6* and *E7* which produce proteins that interfere with tumour-suppression genes controlling the cell cycle. As a result, the cell loses the ability to repair DNA damage and to undergo apoptosis, becoming susceptible to additional mutations and genomic instability. It is therefore postulated that HPV integration can lead to carcinogenesis.

HPV infection is very common. It can be detected in up to 20% of sexually active women in the reproductive age group, and approximately 80% of women will, at some point, be infected. In most cases, genital HPV infections are transient with only a small proportion developing persistent infection, but the risk of subsequent development of CIN increases substantially in this group. HPV alone is not thought to lead to neoplastic change, and other cofactors are thought to be involved, such as smoking-related carcinogens, and dietary and hormonal factors.

Prevention of cervical premalignancy

The recognition that risk factors for cervical neoplasia were sexually related suggested the potential for a number of primary preventive strategies.

Primary prevention using behavioural changes

An obvious strategy was modification of sexual behaviour. Options included the use of sexual heath education, particu-

larly advocating the use of barrier methods of contraception which are associated with a reduced incidence of CIN. Smoking is another consideration. Reducing or quitting smoking is associated with improvements in CIN. Nonetheless, the potential of these approaches is limited by the reality of only limited success in persistently changing human behaviour.

Primary prevention using immunization

Recognition of the central role of HPV in the pathogenesis of cervical neoplasia suggested that primary prevention was possible through the development of prophylactic HPV vaccines. These have been shown to be highly immunogenic, to generate high levels of neutralizing immunoglobulin G antibodies, and to persist for at least 5 years. Antibody responses are higher around the time of puberty (9–15 years), indicating that this should be the target population. What is not known is how long the duration of protection lasts, and whether or not booster immunization is needed.

Several phase III trials (Ault 2007) have shown that more than 90% of persistent HPV 16/18 infections can be prevented for up to 5 years after vaccination, and that more than 90% of precancerous lesions can be prevented in subjects who were HPV negative prior to vaccination. The long-term effects on cervical cancer incidence will require another 10–20 years of follow-up.

The optimal target age for prophylactic vaccination is just before the start of sexual activity (i.e. 9–14 years), as HPV infection may occur soon afterwards. The UK HPV vaccination programme began in 2007. Girls in Year 8 at school (aged 12–13 years) are offered a bivalent HPV vaccine (Cervarix) which protects against infection with HPV 16/18 types. The programme involves three injections over 6 months.

Women will still develop cervical cancer despite HPV vaccination. It is estimated that 70% of cervical cancers might be prevented by HPV vaccination, so primary cervical screening will still be needed, albeit in a modified version.

Detection of cervical premalignancy

Population-based screening should be conducted using well-organized and high-quality programmes with high coverage, as well as providing adequate treatment for detected lesions.

In the developed world, cervical cytology has formed the basis of screening programmes, but the resources and infrastructure required have precluded its use in poorer countries. Current debate concerns the use of the HPV detection assay as a screening tool, whereas in poorer countries, attention has focused on cheaper screening techniques that involve visually assessing the cervix, such as cervicography and visual inspection with acetic acid.

Cervical cytology

The recognition that cervical cytology could be used to detect precancerous change led to the introduction of cervical cytology as a screening test (Figure 38.5). Early detection and treatment can prevent the development of 75% of cancers. Whilst cytology is used to detect women at risk of having cervical premalignancy, most abnormalities are not precancerous. Only a small proportion of women with abnormal

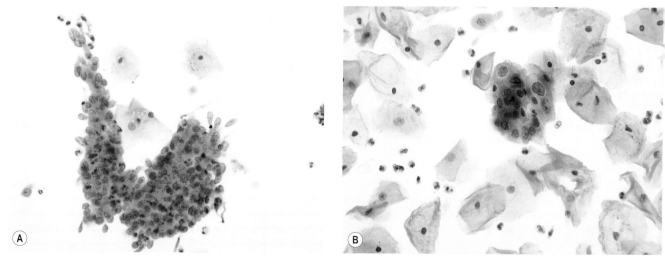

Figure 38.5 (A) Dyskaryotic squamous cells showing mild and moderate dyskaryosis. There is cytoplasmic clearing resulting in a clear area around the nucleus indicative of koilocytosis, which is a papilloma-virus-related cytopathic change (Sure Path, original magnification ×60). (B) Glandular cells show disturbance in the normal honeycomb architecture. There is nuclear hyperchromasia, crowding of cells and 'feathering' of outline. These are features of glandular dyskaryosis (Thin Prep, original magnification ×60).
Images courtesy of Dr C.A. Waddell, Birmingham Cytology Training Centre.

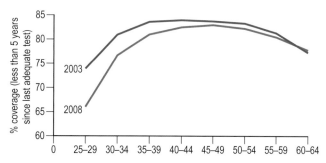

Figure 38.6 Cervical screening: coverage by age, England, 2003 and 2008, showing the fall in screening uptake in younger women.
Source: Health and Social Care Information Centre, 2009. Cervical Screening Programme 2007/2008. The Health and Social Care Information Centre, Sheffield.

smears would develop cancer, although these women are high risk compared with the normal population. There is therefore huge potential for overtreatment unless one can accurately select which lesions require treatment.

In the UK, the incidence of cervical cancers has halved since the National Health Service's (NHS) cervical screening programme was introduced in 1988. The NHS cervical screening programme is highly organized. In the UK, women aged 25–65 years are invited for screening every 3 or 5 years. It is thought that screening under the age of 25 years may do more harm than good as cervical cancer is rare in this age group (Sasieni and Adams 1999). There are clear service guidelines, effective data collection systems using a number of mandatory returns from cytological laboratories, and internal and external quality assurance systems. Target population coverage is the key to success. The programme aims for coverage of over 80% of the target population, but there has been a worrying fall in levels in recent years, falling as low as 66% in women aged 25–30 years (Figure 38.6).

In spite of the success achieved by cervical cytology, it is not without its shortcomings. The assessment and definition of cytological abnormality are subjective with considerable interobserver variation. The process is laborious and tiring with considerable scope for operator error, especially when the workload is high. Furthermore, cytology screening has little effect on the incidence of adenocarcinoma of the cervix.

False-negative results have been variously estimated as being between 2.4% and 26% in various types of study. False-negative results can occur because of inadequate sampling, incorrect laboratory processing, or detection and interpretative errors of the cell samples. This type of error is potentially serious, as a falsely reassuring result may result in no further investigation for 3–5 years, but it is relatively uncommon. There is a need for less labour-intensive and more reliable screening methods.

HPV detection assay

Up to 20% of women, depending on their age, will have evidence of HPV infection using sensitive techniques, such as hybrid capture 2. These assays have high sensitivity but poor specificity, making this a poor test for identifying women with CIN, although specificity rises with age. However, the negative predictive value of these assays is high, making them useful as a means of identifying women who do not have CIN.

It is likely that the combination of prophylactic HPV vaccination and the use of HPV testing as a primary test will be the most cost-effective strategy. Assuming a protective effect of prophylactic HPV vaccination of 15–20 years, nationwide prepubertal vaccination may allow delaying the onset of the cervical screening programme to 30 years instead of 25 years as is the current guidance (Bulkmans et al 2007).

Colposcopy

Colposcopy should not be regarded as an effective primary screening tool, but is essential for diagnosing and treating premalignant lesions detected by either cytology or HPV testing.

Colposcopy involves the visual examination of the cervix under magnification and with enhancement from dilute acetic acid. It is usually performed in women with abnormal smears or an abnormal-looking cervix. It aims to detect macroscopic changes in tissue features such as colour and morphology which are used to classify the lesion.

Colposcopy aims primarily to examine the whole of the cervical TZ, extending from its innermost margin at the SCJ to the outer margin where the metaplastic squamous epithelium adjoins native squamous epithelium.

Colposcopic examination

Women are examined in a modified lithotomy position, often using a colposcopy couch which facilitates easy adjustment of height and position. A bivalve speculum is then introduced and the cervix visualized.

At the initial examination, obvious macroscopic abnormality is sought, including leukoplakia, viral condylomata and invasion. Invasion is associated with the surface of the cervix appearing raised or ulcerated (Figure 38.7). Atypical vessels seen on invasive lesions run a bizarre course and are often corkscrew- or comma-shaped (Figure 38.8). Condylomata are usually obvious from their regular frond-like surface (Figure 38.9).

Having completed the initial inspection of the cervix, 5% acetic acid is applied liberally and gently. This turns abnormal epithelium white, producing the so-called 'acetowhite' changes of CIN. The position of the SCJ must then be ascertained to define the upper limits of the abnormality. On the basis of these findings, the cervical TZ can be classified into one of three types (Figure 38.10). In a type III TZ, the SCJ is not visible and the examination cannot be regarded as satisfactory. This has important management implications.

Colposcopic abnormalities

The key colposcopic features of suspected abnormalities are acetowhitening, abnormal vasculature and topography.

Acetowhite change is the most important of all colposcopic features. Its actual mechanism is uncertain, but it is a reversible reaction which has an association with the activity of the epithelium and results in a temporarily increased reflection of light (Figure 38.11). These changes are non-specific. There is a spectrum of change from low- to high-density acetowhitening which corresponds with an increasing likelihood of high-grade CIN.

Abnormal vascular patterns comprise punctuation, mosaicism (Figure 38.12) and abnormal vessels. In general terms, the coarser the vascular pattern, the greater the likelihood of high-grade change. Abnormal vessels are typically irregular in size, shape and arrangement, and can suggest the presence of invasion.

CIN is usually a distinct acetowhite lesion with sharp margins. It often shows a mosaic vascular pattern with

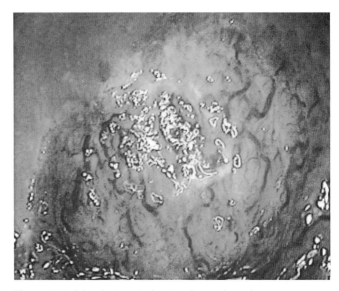

Figure 38.8 Colpophotograph showing abnormal vessels.
Image courtesy of Dr Lázló Szalay, Györ, Hungary.

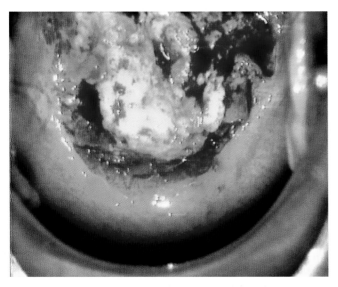

Figure 38.7 Colpophotograph of a stage Ib cervical cancer showing the irregular surface.
Image courtesy of Dr Lázló Szalay, Györ, Hungary.

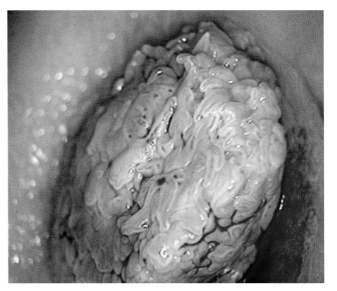

Figure 38.9 Colpophotograph of a cervical condylomata.
Image courtesy of Dr Lázló Szalay, Györ, Hungary.

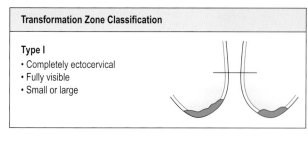

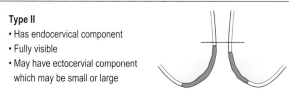

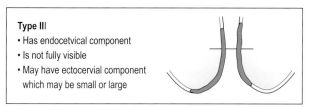

Figure 38.10 Types of cervical transformation zone. (A) Type I, (B) type II, (C) type III.

Images courtesy of Professor Walter Prenderville, Coombe Women's Hospital, Dublin.

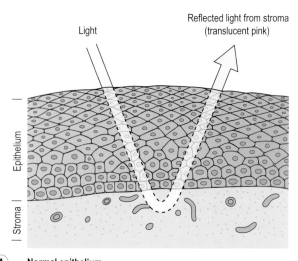

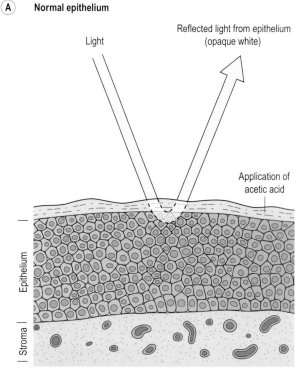

Figure 38.11 Tissue basis for colposcopy. (A) Normal epithelium, (B) abnormal (atypical) epithelium.

Source: Singer A, Monaghan J 2000. Lower Genital Tract Precancer. Blackwell Science, Oxford, p 10.

patches of acetowhite separated by vessels like red weeds between white flagstones. Where the vessels run perpendicular to the surface, punctation is seen as the vessels are viewed end-on. This appears as red spots on a white background. In general, the more quickly and strongly the acetowhite changes develop, the clearer and more regular the margins of the lesion, and the more pronounced the mosaic or punctation, the more severe the lesion is likely to be.

Colposcopic diagnosis

Colposcopic diagnosis is multifaceted. In part, it involves comparing the visual findings with the established patterns of disease as described above. These skills and abilities require training and experience. In addition, there are other important factors that a colposcopist uses to make a diagnostic decision, and these include the referring cytology, patient's age and parity, and smoking history. These other factors are, on occasions, at least as important as the colposcopic image in making a diagnosis, especially when the colposcopic features are low grade or normal. This observation has led to the use of a number of scoring systems to facilitate diagnosis (Table 38.2), although these are not recommended for routine clinical use.

Colposcopy is not reliable when the SCJ cannot be seen, when glandular lesions are suspected, and when there has been previous treatment. In these circumstances, if a high-grade lesion is suspected, an excisional biopsy of the cervix should be performed.

As with any subjective test, a high variation in colposcopic performance has been reported in terms of specificity, sensitivity, and inter- and intraobserver variability. The sensitiv-

ity of colposcopy to distinguish normal from abnormal tissue is relatively high, but it is less good at differentiating low-grade lesions from high-grade lesions. The sensitivity of colposcopy for detecting high-grade disease is approximately 50%. Women undergoing colposcopy are therefore at risk from both overtreatment and underdiagnosis.

Colposcopic diagnostic performance might be improved using some technological innovations such as digital image enhancement (Figure 38.13), and reflective and impedance spectroscopy (Louwers et al 2008). Despite a number of promising initial reports, these newer techniques have not been adopted, principally because of expense, inconvenience and insufficient high-quality evidence.

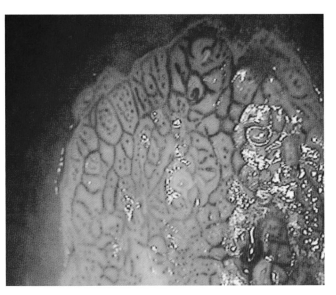

Figure 38.12 Colpophotograph showing coarse mosaicism.
Image courtesy of Dr Lázló Szalay, Györ, Hungary.

Table 38.2 Clinicocolposcopic index

Variable	Score		
	Zero points	One point	Two points
Index cytology	Low grade	—	High grade
Smoking	No	—	Yes
Age (years)	≤30	>30	—
Acetowhitening	Slight	Marked	—
Surface area (cm²)	≤1	>1	—
Intercapillary distance (µm)	≤350 (fine or no mosaic/ punctation)	>350 (coarse mosaic/punctation)	—
Focality of lesion	Unifocal or multifocal	Annular	—
Surface pattern	Smooth	Irregular	—

Source: Shafi MI, Nazeer S: 2006 Colposcopy — A Practical Guide. Fivepin Publishers, Salisbury.
For each individual patient, a maximum score of 10 can be achieved. The higher the score, the more significant the lesion: score of 0–2, insignificant lesions; score of 3–5, low-grade lesions; score 6–10, high-grade lesions.

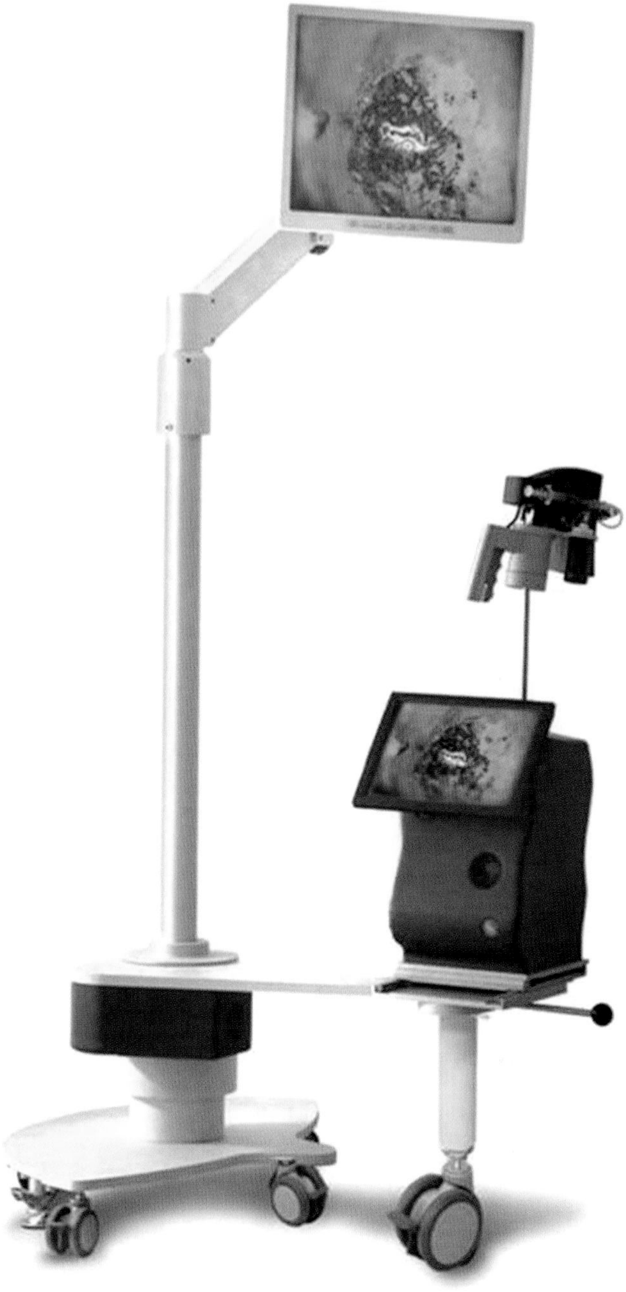

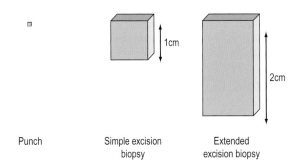

Figure 38.13 Dynamic Spectral Imaging System (DySIS; Forth Phototonics, Athens, Greece) is a colposcope that measures the acetowhitening of every image pixel of the cervix after the application of acetic acid.

Colposcopic biopsy

Colposcopy is often viewed as a means of deciding whether or not to take a biopsy and where to take it from. Colposcopic biopsies can be classified as in Figure 38.14. An extended excisional biopsy aims to sample most of the endocervical canal and can be performed when the SCJ is not visible or a glandular lesion is suspected. It is accepted that excisional biopsy is the gold standard for histological diagnosis, but this is best avoided when low-grade lesions are suspected.

The colposcopically-directed punch biopsy (CDB) is often used, but the reliability and validity of this test is question-

Punch   Simple excision biopsy   Extended excision biopsy

Figure 38.14 Classification of cervical biopsies.

able for a variety of reasons. Few studies have been performed that have assessed the reliability of CDB, and these have been of poor quality. CDB should be avoided when the TZ cannot be fully seen, or when glandular lesions or high-grade lesions are suspected. If CDB is to be used, multiple biopsies must be taken.

Treatment of cervical premalignancy

Effective treatment involves striking a balance between the risks of persistent and recurrent disease from undertreatment and excessive damage due to overtreatment. This is particularly pertinent in the management of cervical precancerous change, as many women undergoing treatment will not have started or completed their child bearing.

A failure to appreciate the nature and behaviour of cervical premalignancy has bedevilled its treatment. In the past, CIN was treated by radical hysterectomy but it soon became evident that this was unnecessary, and simple hysterectomy became the method of choice. In time, it was realized that cone biopsy was just as effective, and hysterectomy is now reserved for women with difficult-to-treat recurrent disease or who have additional indications for hysterectomy. The introduction of colposcopy and a better appreciation of the limited location of CIN led to the introduction of more conservative methods of treatment (Soutter and Fletcher 1994).

There is no doubt that high-grade CIN (CIN2/3) and high-grade CGIN should be treated, but there is uncertainty about the therapeutic value of treating CIN1. Whilst conservative treatment is increasingly adopted, follow-up should be performed until spontaneous regression or treatment is performed.

The treatment morbidity is a function of the amount of tissue removed or destroyed. The potential complications are:

- intraoperative haemorrhage;
- secondary haemorrhage;
- pelvic infection;
- cervical stenosis; and
- cervical incompetence.

With the exception of radical diathermy, ablative treatments were not associated with a significantly increased risk of serious adverse pregnancy outcomes. However, all excisional procedures used to treat CIN seem to be associated with adverse obstetric morbidity, but among these, only cold knife conization is associated with a significantly increased rate of severe outcomes (Kyrgiou et al 2006). The risk of serious obstetric morbidity has not been confirmed with the use of loop excision, but excisions that remove large amounts of cervical tissue probably have the same effect as knife cone biopsies. Most loop excisions in young women with fully visible transformation zones only need to be 1 cm deep, and this should protect against serious obstetric outcomes.

Types of treatment

Ablation

A number of ablative methods are available (Table 38.3). The potential advantages of ablative treatments are that general anaesthesia is not usually required (with the exception of radical electrodiathermy) and the associated damage

Table 38.3 Treatment for cervical intraepithelial neoplasia

	Method	Anaesthesia	Obstetric morbidity*
Ablation	Radical electrodiathermy	GA	++
	Laser vaporization	LA	+/−
	'Cold' coagulation	LA	+/−
Excision	LLETZ	LA	+/−
	NETZ	LA	+/−
	Laser conization	LA	+
	Knife conization	GA	++
	Hysterectomy	GA	+++

*Based on Arbyn M, et al 2008 Perinatal mortality and other severe adverse pregnancy outcomes associated with treatment of cervical intraepithelial neoplasia: meta-analysis. BMJ 337: a1284.
GA, general anaesthesia; LA, local anaesthesia; LLETZ, large loop excision of the transformation zone; NETZ, needle excision of the transformation zone.

Table 38.4 Contraindications for ablative treatment

- Suspected invasive disease
- Suspected glandular disease
- Squamocolumnar junction not clearly visible
- Previous cervical surgery, including cryocautery
- Unexplained cytological abnormality, i.e. significant smear/colposcopy discrepancy

might be less. This might mean less obstetric morbidity. However, there are caveats. Firstly, the treatment method has to be fit for purpose; cryotherapy, for example, is easy to use but it destroys insufficient tissue to treat CIN adequately.

Secondly, ablative therapy can only be undertaken when the whole of the cervical TZ can be examined reliably, so the SCJ must be visible. When ablative treatment is contraindicated (Table 38.4), excisional therapy must be performed.

Finally, a disadvantage common to all these techniques is that they depend upon the exclusion of invasion by colposcopy and directed biopsy, which is not necessarily sufficiently reliable. Furthermore, as the treated tissue is destroyed, it is not possible to know for certain what has been treated and whether it has been treated adequately.

Excision

Excisional treatments range from local treatments to hysterectomy (Table 38.3). The extent of local excision depends on the context. When treating ectocervical lesions, the aim is to excise to a depth of approximately 10 mm. However, the depth of excision may need to be extended if the SCJ is not visible or if a glandular lesion is suspected.

When high-grade CGIN is suspected and conservative treatment is preferred, local excision is appropriate provided that the lesion is excised completely. When the margins are not free of disease, a simple hysterectomy is probably the safest treatment, provided that invasive disease has been excluded. A further cone biopsy as definitive treatment would be acceptable management for young women who want more children. If the margins are clear, close observation with 6-monthly cervical smears is reasonable management provided that both patient and physician are aware of the relatively high likelihood of the need for further treatment for suspected recurrence.

The principle advantage of excisional treatments is that there is histological confirmation of what has been treated and whether or not excision is complete. Compared with ablative treatments, there might be greater scope for damage but that is a function of the amount of tissue removed.

Large loop excision of the transformation zone (LLETZ) is the most common method. It is simple and easy to use on an outpatient basis, usually only requiring local analgesia. The amount of tissue removed and the shape of the sample is largely predetermined by the shape and size of the loop. Wherever possible, the specimen should be removed as a single specimen. Unfortunately, larger lesions (i.e. those at greatest risk of being high grade and incompletely excised) are often removed in multiple fragments, making orientation of the specimen and assessment of the completeness of excision impossible.

Knife cone biopsy still has utility when larger specimens are needed or when greater histological certainty of excision status is required. However, this requires general anaesthesia.

Choice of treatment

None of the methods of treating CIN are more effective than any of the others when used appropriately by a well-trained and experienced operator. Each has particular advantages with regards to cost, ease of use, speed or precision. The particular method chosen will depend upon local circumstances. It seems sensible to choose a method which will allow abnormalities to be treated under local anaesthesia. In spite of its greater capital cost, the laser does have the advantage that it can be used to excise and vaporize lesions when it is appropriate to do so. However, needle excision of the TZ and LLETZ have largely replaced the laser because of the reduced capital cost, greater simplicity in maintenance of the instrument, and more rapid treatment with less blood loss.

Results of treatment

Treated adequately, some 5% of patients treated for CIN will have recurrent disease within 2 years. Thereafter, the number of recurrences is small. However, long-term follow-up is necessary as these women remain at higher risk of CIN or invasive cervical cancer than the general population. Currently, it is recommended that patients treated for high-grade CIN should have increased cytological surveillance for 10 years.

The Vagina

Terminology and pathology of vaginal intraepithelial neoplasia

The terminology and pathology of vaginal intraepithelial neoplasia (VAIN) is analogous to that of CIN (VAIN1–3).

The main difference is that vaginal epithelium does not normally have crypts so the epithelial abnormality remains superficial until invasion occurs. The common exception to this is found following surgery (usually hysterectomy) when abnormal epithelium can be buried below the suture line or in suture tracks.

Natural history of vaginal intraepithelial neoplasia

VAIN is seldom seen as an isolated vaginal lesion. It is more usual for it to be coexistent with CIN. In most cases, it is diagnosed colposcopically prior to any treatment during the investigation of an abnormal smear. However, it may not be recognized until after a hysterectomy has been performed. When this happens, abnormal epithelium is likely to be buried behind the sutures used to close the vault and cannot be assessed (Figure 38.15). Untreated or inadequately treated VAIN may progress to frank invasive cancer. Very rarely, VAIN may be seen many years after radiotherapy for cervical carcinoma, when it is probably a new lesion. Care must be taken in these women to ensure that postradiotherapy changes are not being misinterpreted as VAIN.

Assessment of vaginal intraepithelial neoplasia

VAIN is often detected by abnormal cytology following hysterectomy. Colposcopy of the vagina is more difficult than that of the cervix, particularly if the patient has had a hysterectomy, as it is very difficult to see into the angles of the vagina, and impossible to visualize epithelium that lies above the suture line or vaginal adhesions. The colposcopic features of VAIN are very similar to those of CIN, except that mosaic is seen less often. Punch biopsy can indicate whether or not there is an abnormality, but assessment short of complete excision must be regarded as suboptimal.

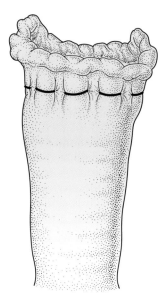

Figure 38.15 Sutures in the vaginal vault isolate a cuff of the vagina above the suture line.

Treatment of vaginal intraepithelial neoplasia

As with the cervix, excision avoids suboptimal assessment and inadvertent inadequate management of invasive lesions. Ablative treatments appeal because of their apparent simplicity, but they can be associated with morbidity as well as compounding the dangers of undertreatment with future difficulties in assessment.

In the past, a number of ablative techniques such as carbon dioxide laser, topical 5-fluorouracil and radiotherapy have been used, but surgical excision gives better results and is the only effective option available to patients previously treated with radiotherapy. Following hysterectomy, an abdominal or combined abdominal and vaginal approach is preferable to vaginal excision (Ireland and Monaghan 1988).

The Vulva

Vulvar intraepithelial neoplasia (VIN) is seen more commonly than was the case 10–20 years ago. It is not certain whether this represents a real increase or is simply the result of a greater awareness of the problem.

Pathology of premalignant disease of the vulva

Premalignant squamous lesions of the vulva are labelled 'vulvar intraepithelial neoplasia' (VIN). This term has been adopted by the International Society for the Study of Vulvar Disease and the International Society for Gynecologic Pathologists. This replaces previous terminology such as 'hyperplastic dystrophy', 'Bowen's disease', 'squamous dysplasia' and 'carcinoma in situ'.

VIN is classified into two distinct clinicopathological subtypes: classic (Bowenoid, usual type) and simplex (differentiated). Classic VIN is seen in younger women and is associated with HPV. Multifocal involvement of the vulva occurs in more than 40% of cases, and multicentric involvement affecting the vagina, cervix and perianal region occurs in 18–52% of patients. Approximately 50% of women with VIN present with symptoms of pruritus, irritation or a mass lesion, and in the remainder it is an incidental finding. Local recurrence or persistence has been noted in 7–32% of patients following therapy. Occult areas of invasive carcinoma are seen in approximately 6–18% of patients treated surgically for VIN. Histologically, classic VIN may have a warty pattern with an undulating surface, and frequent koilocytosis or multinucleation or a basaloid pattern with a relatively flat lesion where the normal epithelium is replaced by a fairly homogeneous proliferation of abnormal cells. Both types can coexist. Classic VIN is graded depending on the level of involvement of the affected epithelium by abnormal cells. This grading scheme is similar to that used in CIN: VIN1, when the lowest third is involved; VIN2, when the lower two-thirds are involved; and VIN3, when the abnormality extends to the upper third of epithelium. VIN1 is uncommon.

Simplex (differentiated) VIN is much less common and accounts for less than 10% of VIN cases. It occurs in postmenopausal women and is associated with lichen sclerosis. HPV is uncommon with differentiated VIN; however, it has a strong association with vulvar squamous cell carcinoma. Histologically, simplex VIN is a subtle lesion with a generally well-preserved architecture, thickened epidermis, abnormal basal keratinocytes and deeply situated abnormal individual cell keratinization.

Vulvar Paget's disease is said to represent adenocarcinoma in situ and is very rare. The histological appearance of Paget's disease is similar to the lesion seen in the breast. In one-third of cases of Paget's disease, there is an associated invasive cancer, often an adenocarcinoma, in underlying apocrine glands and these carry an especially poor prognosis

Natural history of vulvar intraepithelial neoplasia

Forty per cent of women with VIN are under 41 years of age. Although histologically very similar to CIN and often occurring in association with it, VIN does not seem to have the same malignant potential. However, this opinion is based largely on studies of women who have been treated by excision biopsy or vulvectomy.

Diagnosis and assessment of vulvar intraepithelial neoplasia

VIN often presents with itching, but 20–45% are asymptomatic and are frequently found after treatment of preinvasive or invasive disease at other sites in the lower genital tract, particularly the cervix.

These lesions are often raised above the surrounding skin and have a rough surface. The colour is variable: white, due to hyperkeratinization; red, due to thinness of the epithelium; or dark brown, due to increased melanin deposition in the epithelial cells. They are very often multifocal.

Adequate biopsies must be taken from abnormal areas to rule out invasive disease. This can usually be done under local anaesthesia in the outpatient clinic using a disposable 4-mm Stiefel biopsy punch or a Keyes punch.

Treatment of vulvar intraepithelial neoplasia

Treatment of VIN is difficult. Uncertainty about the malignant potential, the multifocal nature of the disorder, and the discomfort and mutilation resulting from therapy suggest that recommendations should be cautious and conservative in order to avoid making the treatment worse than the disease. The youth of many of these patients is a further important consideration. In view of the mutilating nature of treatment, the high recurrence rate and the uncertainty about the risk of invasion, there is a place for careful observation, especially of young women without severe symptoms.

The documented progression of untreated cases of VIN3 to invasive cancer underlines the potential importance of these lesions. If the patient has presented with symptoms, therapy is required. Asymptomatic patients, particularly those under 50 years of age, may be observed closely with biopsies repeated if there are any suspicious changes.

Medical therapy

The main role for medical treatment is in relieving symptoms in women for whom surgery may be avoided.

Provided invasion has been excluded as far as possible, topical steroids provide symptomatic relief for many women. A strong, fluorinated steroid is usually required. This may be applied twice daily for not more than 6 months because of the thinning of the skin which can result. Frequent review is necessary initially.

Surgery

If the lesion is small, an excision biopsy may be both diagnostic and therapeutic. If the disease is multifocal or covers a wide area, wider excision may require plastic surgery using split skin grafting or transpositional skin flaps.

Assessment of the results of treatment should include consideration of the length of follow-up. Surgical excision is associated with crude recurrence rates of 15–43%.

Carbon dioxide laser

An alternative approach is to vaporize the abnormal epithelium with a carbon dioxide laser. Careful control of the depth of destruction is essential for good cosmetic results. Given the very irregular surface of the vulva, it is very difficult to achieve a uniform depth of destruction. Moreover, the depth of treatment required for VIN is still unclear. In some cases, hair follicles may be involved for several millimetres below the surface, but it may not always be necessary to destroy the whole depth of involved appendages. In any case, treatment of the whole vulva to such a depth would result in a third-degree burn which would need skin grafting. In practice, laser vaporization has proved to be disappointing in UK practice and is seldom used (Shafi et al 1989).

Paget's disease

This is an uncommon condition and is similar to that found in the breast. It is characterized by large malignant cells arranged singly and in clusters. The typical Paget's cell has a vesicular nucleus and abundant cytoplasm which contains demonstrable mucin (Figure 38.16). The cells of primary Paget's disease are characteristically positive with cytokeratin 7, carcinoembryonic antigen, CAM 5.2, androgen receptor, gross cystic disease fluid protein 15 and human epidermal growth factor receptor 2 (HER 2) (Goldblum and Hart 1997).

The disease is often extensive or multifocal, so clinically unsuspected positive resection margins are not uncommon. No underlying regional malignancy is identified in the majority of cases, but up to 30% of cases have invasion of the dermis, microscopically noted but often clinically unsuspected. The main differential diagnosis of Paget's disease is superficial spreading malignant melanoma which will, in contrast to Paget's disease, show positivity for S100, HMB45 and Melan A. Concomitant genital malignancies are found in 15–25% of women with Paget's disease of the vulva; these are most commonly vulval or cervical, but transitional cell carcinoma of the bladder (or kidney), and ovarian, endometrial, vaginal and urethral carcinomas have all been reported.

Pruritis is the presenting complaint and it often presents as a red, crusted plaque with sharp edges (Figure 38.17), sometimes with multiple erosions. The diagnosis is made histologically on biopsy.

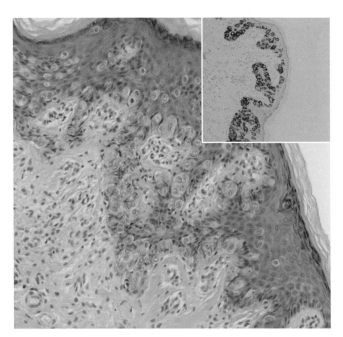

Figure 38.16 Single and nested Paget cells showing characteristic abundant cytoplasm and vesicular nuclei (block arrow). The inset shows the cells highlighted by cytoplasmic and membranous staining with cytokeratin 7 (arrowed). Original magnification x100.

The treatment of Paget's disease is very wide local excision, usually involving total vulvectomy because of the propensity of this condition to involve apparently normal skin. The specimen must be examined histologically with great care to exclude an apocrine adenocarcinoma.

The Uterine Corpus

Introduction

The concept of premalignancy in the uterine corpus is confined to the endometrium. Myometrial neoplasms, such as leiomyomas, leiomyosarcomas and endometrial stromal sarcomas, do not have a recognized preneoplastic phase.

Terminology of endometrial premalignancy

Endometrial carcinoma is the most common malignancy of the female genital tract in the Western world. Simplistically and conceptually, there are two types of endometrial carcinomas: type 1, oestrogen-related, endometrioid carcinoma; and type 2, non-oestrogen-related, prototypically serous carcinomas. Type 1 carcinoma is more common and has a precursor termed 'endometrial hyperplasia'. Endometrial hyperplasia is best described as a non-physiological, non-invasive proliferation of glands visibly resulting in an increase in the volume of endometrial glands relative to the stroma. The precursor of type 2 carcinoma is termed 'endometrial intraepithelial carcinoma' (EIC).

The World Health Organization (WHO) classification of endometrial hyperplasia is into simple and complex hyperplasia. Both simple and complex hyperplasia can be associated with cellular atypia. Simple atypical hyperplasia is exceedingly rare. Complex atypical hyperplasia is

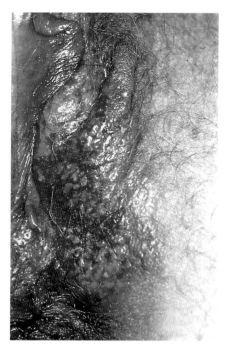

Figure 38.17 Paget's disease of the vulva. Note the crusted surface and clear margins.

commonly termed 'atypical hyperplasia', and is closely related to progression or coexistence of endometrial carcinoma. In women who undergo hysterectomy soon after a biopsy that shows atypical hyperplasia, the uterus shows an established endometrioid adenocarcinoma in 17–45% of cases in various series reported in the literature. When such a cancer is discovered, it is almost always a low-grade, low-stage carcinoma.

Histopathology of endometrial premalignancy

On histopathological examination, all forms of hyperplasia show an increase in the number of glands in comparison with the stroma. Simple and complex forms of hyperplasia are distinguished by the gland morphology. Simple hyperplasia is characterized by variably sized cystically dilated glands. The stroma is abundant relative to the lesser volumes of stroma seen in complex hyperplasia. The latter shows more densely crowded glands with irregular outlines, and outpouching and infoldings of the lumen. The glands are closely packed, although stroma is consistently identified between the glands. In any sample of endometrium, a combination of simple and complex hyperplasia may be seen. Cellular atypia is identified by nuclear enlargement, rounded outlines and irregularity of nuclear chromatin.

The diagnosis of endometrial hyperplasia has been shown in several studies to be an area of gynaecological pathology with low diagnostic reproducibility. Even after accounting for extrinsic factors such as scanty sample or low volume changes, there is disagreement amongst general and specialist pathologists in the diagnosis of complex hyperplasia and cytological atypia. These difficulties in reproducibility of diagnosis are likely to be secondary to lack of strict definition and objective criteria in the present WHO clas-

sification. There is a proposal from Mutter and colleagues from Boston to use more specific diagnostic criteria for precancerous changes in the endometrium termed 'endometrial intraepithelial neoplasia'. This classification is currently under discussion and has not replaced the current WHO classification.

EIC represents the precursor lesion of type 2 endometrial carcinoma. This lesion occurs in a background of atrophic endometrium, and has cells with pleomorphic nuclei that are immunoreactive for *p53*. By definition, EIC does not show myometrial invasion. Biologically, however, EIC can be aggressive with extrauterine spread noted at the time of diagnosis. This diagnosis of EIC can trigger management as carcinoma.

Aetiology and molecular pathology of endometrial premalignancy

Type 1 endometrial carcinoma is associated with hyperoestrinism. The development of endometrial hyperplasia is strongly influenced by steroid hormones; oestrogen induces glandular proliferation leading to thickening of the uterine lining, whereas growth is suppressed by progesterone. This is reflected by the risk factors for endometrial hyperplasia, including obesity, nulliparity and oestrogen-only hormone replacement therapy, which are associated with states of prolonged unopposed oestrogen. Hyperoestrogenic states such as polycystic ovary syndrome have a greater incidence of endometrial hyperplasia, as do patients taking the partial oestrogen agonist tamoxifen for breast cancer. Although there is no association with hyperoestrinism, hereditary non-polyposis colonic cancer is known to have an increased incidence of hyperplasia.

The most frequently altered gene in type 1 carcinoma is *PTEN*, located on chromosome 10. Up to 55% of preneoplastic lesions reveal loss of *PTEN* expression. This loss of *PTEN* is an early event in endometrial tumorigenesis. Mutations of *p53* are found in approximately 80% of precursors of type 2 carcinoma.

Screening for endometrial premalignancy

Endometrial hyperplasia is typically diagnosed in perimenopausal women. There are few data in the literature regarding screening of asymptomatic women for endometrial hyperplasia. Both ultrasonography for endometrial thickness and outpatient endometrial biopsy have yields too low to justify investigation of asymptomatic women.

Clinical presentation of endometrial hyperplasia

Endometrial hyperplasia usually presents with abnormal uterine bleeding. This includes menorrhagia, intermenstrual bleeding, postcoital bleeding and postmenopausal bleeding. Occasionally, endometrial hyperplasia might be detected in asymptomatic women being investigated for smears containing atypical endometrial cells. Endometrial hyperplasia can occur in both pre- and postmenopausal women, accounting for approximately 15% of women presenting with postmenopausal bleeding.

Investigation of endometrial hyperplasia

In the UK, the cancer waiting time and 18-week waiting time initiatives have increasingly focused attention on one-stop assessment and diagnosis. Women over the age of 45 years with irregular bleeding or postmenopausal women are referred on the cancer pathway and seen within 14 days. Transvaginal ultrasound (TVS) is the primary investigation of choice in postmenopausal women as it can assess the endometrium and detect other relevant pelvic pathologies. The endometrial thickness is measured and, using a cut-off of more than 5 mm, has a high sensitivity and specificity for detecting endometrial pathology, as well as a true negative predictive value approaching 100% (Smith-Bindman et al 1998). If the endometrial thickness exceeds 5 mm, endometrial assessment is required. Whilst the diagnostic gold standard is hysteroscopy, blind endometrial sampling using tests such as Pipelle (Punimar, Wilton, Connecticut, USA) are frequently used and are cost-effective. When outpatient sampling is not feasible or is unsatisfactory, or in the context of the patient being on tamoxifen or in whom symptoms have persisted despite negative findings on initial assessment, hysteroscopy should be undertaken. Hysteroscopy allows the whole surface of the uterine cavity to be inspected and facilitates targeted biopsy or curettage. Hysteroscopy with biopsy has an excellent sensitivity and specificity for detecting endometrial pathology in women aged less than 45 years who have symptoms of irregular and/or heavy bleeding that is non-responsive to first-line management. In this clinical scenario, an endometrial sample should be the primary test, as TVS is less specific. Notwithstanding the above, TVS should always be considered when clinical findings are abnormal or examination is suboptimal.

Management of endometrial hyperplasia

The management will depend upon the nature of the abnormality and upon the patient's wishes for further children. As most types of endometrial hyperplasia do not progress to endometrial cancer, treatment regimens should be individualized; hysterectomy is unnecessary in the majority of cases. On the other hand, the presence of cytological atypia with its risk of concomitant cancer or risk of progressing to endometrial cancer should be managed as if cancer was there, unless there are powerful considerations to do otherwise, such as fertility issues or significant medical comorbidity.

Non-atypical endometrial hyperplasia (simple or complex hyperplasia)

Given the low risk of progression to carcinoma, there is no indication for hysterectomy or for progestin therapy in asymptomatic women, and subsequent management can probably be decided on the basis of further symptoms. Available data suggest that persistent or progressive disease will occur in one-third of conservatively managed cases (Clark et al 2006). Progestin therapy may result in its complete disappearance. Progestogens can be delivered systemically, either alone or in combination with oestrogen (as in the oral contraceptive pill or hormone replacement therapy), or locally in the form of the levonorgestrol intrauterine device (Mirena, Schering Health). Both systemic and local administration of progestogens show a 75–100% conversion rate to normal endometrium.

Atypical hyperplasia

Most women with atypical hyperplasia should have a hysterectomy and bilateral salpingo-oophorectomy because of the high risk of coexistent carcinoma. However, younger women who wish to preserve their fertility may be managed with medical therapy and repeated endometrial sampling. One study reported a 94% success rate with 3–18 months of therapy, allowing five women to become pregnant, delivering at full term (Randall and Kurman 1997). However, these encouraging results have to be weighed against those where a 25% risk of progression to carcinoma was described (Ferenczy and Gelfand 1989). Most data relate to the use of various progestins given for short-term courses or as continuous therapy for many years. Most of the studies only include carefully selected cases, and the results of the different studies are not really comparable because of the selection criteria applied. It is clear that these results should be regarded with considerable caution, and that long-term follow-up is essential because recurrences may not appear for many years (Ferenczy and Gelfand 1989).

The Ovary

Introduction

Ovarian cancer is a heterogeneous disease including epithelial neoplasms, germ cell and stromal tumours, and metastatic malignancies. The concept of ovarian premalignant disease is currently confined to epithelial neoplasms; however, its clinical usefulness has been limited by the diverse histological subtypes and the lack of an obvious precursor.

As a result, attention has focused on the detection of small early-stage cancers in certain situations, such as the need for careful examination of ovaries and fallopian tubes removed at prophylactic surgery in patients with *BRCA1* or *BRCA2* mutations since small areas of malignant change can easily be missed. Similarly, it is recognized that endometriosis can be coexistent in up to 25–40% of cases of endometrioid and clear cell ovarian cancers (Fukunaga et al 1997), and consequentially all endometriotic cysts must be sampled optimally, especially to include any solid or suspicious areas. Only a small percentage of women with endometriosis will develop an ovarian cancer, and the mechanisms responsible for the malignant transformation have still to be elucidated. However, evidence is emerging of genetic mutations common to both ovarian endometriosis and endometriosis-associated ovarian cancer (Prowse et al 2006).

Ovarian carcinogenesis

Based on morphological and molecular genetic studies, a dualistic model has been suggested (Shih and Kurman 2004) in which ovarian cancers can be divided into two broad categories: type I and II tumours (Figure 38.18). The type I pathway resembles the adenoma–carcinoma pathway in

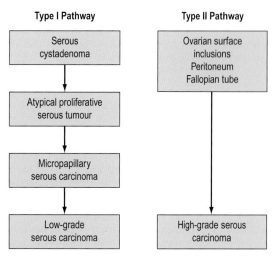

Type I Pathway	Type II Pathway
Serous cystadenoma	Ovarian surface inclusions Peritoneum Fallopian tube
↓	↓
Atypical proliferative serous tumour	
↓	
Micropapillary serous carcinoma	
↓	
Low-grade serous carcinoma	High-grade serous carcinoma

Figure 38.18 The dualistic model of ovarian cancer pathogenesis. *Adapted from Kurman RJ, Shih IM 2008 International Journal of Gynecological Pathology 27: 151–160.*

colorectal cancer and is characterized by clearly recognized precursor lesions, namely cystadenoma and borderline lesions. Type I tumours evolve slowly in a stepwise fashion and are associated with distinct molecular changes that are not shared by the more common type II tumours. Type II tumours comprise high-grade tumours, such as poorly differentiated serous lesions and mixed mesodermal tumours, which arise and metastasize early.

The pathological evidence for the progression of type I tumours arises from studies which have shown the frequent occurrence of a transition or coexistence between malignant and benign areas in mucinous ovarian cancers, and between low-grade serous cancers and areas of borderline change (Malpica et al 2004). Also, borderline serous tumours typically recur as low-grade serous cancers (Crispens et al 2002).

The significance of this dualistic theory is that it provides a basis for further morphological and molecular genetic studies that might help to explain ovarian carcinogenesis.

Prevention of premalignancy of the ovary

Due to the lack of a clearly identifiable premalignant phase, prevention strategies have concentrated on either trying to identify early-stage lesions or removing the ovaries before disease develops, thereby aiming to impact on disease-associated morbidity and mortality. Various approaches have been tried in order to achieve this aim, including clinical, chemoprevention and prophylactic surgery.

The clinical approach has been predominantly aimed at screening with the serum tumour marker CA125, pelvic ultrasound or a combination of both modalities. Large clinical trials are currently underway, investigating the potential of such screening programmes in both low- and high-risk populations (i.e. UK Collaborative Trial of Ovarian Cancer Screening, UK Familial Ovarian Cancer Screening Study).

Chemoprevention has particularly focused on the use of the oral contraceptive pill, which has been shown to reduce the risk of ovarian cancer in both low- and high-risk populations (Hankinson et al 1992, McLaughlin et al 2007). The use of oral contraceptives in *BRCA* mutation carriers is currently not advised due to an apparent increase in the rate of breast cancer, although the data on this are limited.

Bilateral salpingo-oophorectomy has also been shown to reduce the risk of ovarian and fallopian tube cancer in *BRCA1* or *BRCA2* mutation carriers (Rebbeck et al 2009). The timing of surgery is dependent on the individual, their fertility requirements, the potential surgical morbidity and long-term hormonal sequelae. The current advice is that surgery should be considered once a woman reaches 35 years of age. Prophylactic surgery, however, does not completely remove the risk of malignancy since women in some high-risk populations are still at risk of developing primary peritoneal carcinoma (Finch et al 2006).

KEY POINTS

1. Infection with oncogenic high-risk HPV types is the central causal factor in the development of cervical neoplasia.
2. High-grade CIN has the potential to develop into invasive cancer in up to 30% of cases over a 20-year period.
3. 70% of cervical cancers might be prevented by HPV vaccination alone.
4. Cervical cytology can prevent 75% of cervical cancers by enabling early detection and treatment.
5. Colposcopy is subjective, has significant inter- and intraobserver error, and a sensitivity for high-grade disease of only 50%.
6. The diagnostic precision of cervical punch biopsies is not good. Invasive disease is not always detected and CIN2/3 may be substantially undercalled.
7. All excisional procedures used to treat CIN are associated with adverse obstetric morbidity, but only cold knife conization is associated with an increased rate of perinatal mortality.
8. The malignant potential of VAIN and VIN is uncertain.
9. Atypical endometrial hyperplasia should be managed as if cancer, as up to 45% of cases will be found to have endometrial cancer at hysterectomy.

References

Anderson MC, Hartley RB 1980 Cervical crypt involvement by intraepithelial neoplasia. Obstetrics and Gynecology 55: 546–550.

Arbyn M, Kyrgiou M, Simoens C, et al 2008 Perinatal mortality and other severe adverse pregnancy outcomes associated with treatment of cervical intraepithelial neoplasia: meta-analysis. BMJ 337: a1284.

Ault KA; The Future II Study Group 2007 Effect of prophylactic human papillomavirus L1 virus-like-particle vaccine on risk of cervical intraepithelial neoplasia grade 2, grade 3, and adenocarcinoma in situ: a comparison of four randomised clinical trials. The Lancet 369 1861–1868.

Bulkmans NW, Berkhof J, Rozendaal L, van Kemendade FJ, Snijders PJ, Meijer CJ 2007

Human papillomavirus DNA testing for the detection of cervical intraepithelial neoplasia grade 3 and cancer: 5 year follow-up of a randomised controlled implementation trial. The Lancet 370 1764–1772.

Clark TJ, Neelakantan D, Guptal JK 2006 The management of endometrial hyperplasia. An evaluation of current practice. European Journal of Obstetrics, Gynecology and Reproductive Biology 125: 259–264.

Crispens MA, Bodurka D, Deavers M, Lu K, Silva EG, Gershenson DM 2002 Response and survival in patients with progressive or recurrent serous ovarian tumors of low malignant potential. Obstetrics and Gynecology 99: 3–10.

Ferenczy A, Gelfand M 1989 The biologic significance of cytologic atypia in progestogen-treated endometrial hyperplasia. American Journal of Obstetrics and Gynecology 160: 126–131.

Finch A, Beiner M, Lubinski J et al; Hereditary Ovarian Cancer Clinical Study Group 2006 Salpingo-oophorectomy and the risk of ovarian, fallopian tube, and peritoneal cancers in women with a BRCA1 or BRCA2 mutation. Journal of the American Medical Association 296: 185–192.

Fukunaga M, Nomura K, Ishikawa E, Ushigome S 1997 Ovarian atypical endometriosis: its close association with malignant epithelial tumours. Histopathology 30(3):249–255.

Goldblum JR, Hart WR 1997 Vulvar Paget's disease: a clinicopathologic and immunohistochemical study of 19 cases. American Journal of Surgical Pathology 21 1178–1187.

Hankinson SE, Colditz GA, Hunter DJ, Spencer TL, Rosner B, Stampfer MJ 1992 A quantitative assessment of oral contraceptive use and risk of ovarian cancer. Obstetrics and Gynecology 80: 708–714.

Health and Social Care Information Centre, 2009. Cervical Screening Programme 2007/2008. Health and Social Care Information Centre, Sheffield.

Ireland D, Monaghan JM 1988 The management of the patient with abnormal vaginal cytology following hysterectomy.

BJOG: an International Journal of Obstetrics and Gynaecology 95: 973–975.

Jimbo H, Yoshikawa H, Onda T, Yasugi T, Sakamoto A, Taketani Y 1997 Prevalence of ovarian endometriosis in epithelial ovarian cancer. International Journal of Gynaecology and Obstetrics 59: 245–250.

Kyrgiou M, Koliopoulos G, Martin-Hirsch P, Arbyn M, Prendiville W, Paraskevaidis E 2006 Obstetric outcomes after conservative treatment for intraepithelial or early invasive cervical lesions: systematic review and meta-analysis. The Lancet 367: 489–498.

Louwers JA, Kocken M, ter Harmsel WA, Verheijen RHM 2008 Digital colposcopy: ready for use? An overview of the literature. BJOG: an International Journal of Obstetrics and Gynaecology 116: 220–229.

Malpica A, Deavers MT, Lu K et al 2004 Grading ovarian serous carcinoma using a two-tier system. American Journal of Surgical Pathology 28: 496–504.

McIndoe WA, McLean MR, Jones RW, Mullins PR 1984 The invasive potential of carcinoma in situ of the cervix. Obstetrics and Gynecology 64: 451–458.

McLaughlin JR, Risch HA, Lubinski J et al; Hereditary Ovarian Cancer Clinical Study Group 2007 Reproductive risk factors for ovarian cancer in carriers of BRCA1 or BRCA2 mutations: a case–control study. The Lancet Oncology 8: 26–34.

Mutter GL, Baak JPA, Crum CP, Richart RM, Ferenczy A, Faquin WC 2000 Endometrial precancer diagnosis by histopathology, clonal analysis and computerized morphometry. Journal of Pathology 190: 462–469.

Östör AG 1993 Natural history of cervical intraepithelial neoplasia: a critical review. International Journal of Gynecologic Pathology 12: 186–192.

Prowse AH, Manek S, Varma R et al 2006 Molecular genetic evidence that endometriosis is a precursor of ovarian cancer. International Journal of Cancer 119: 556–562.

Randall TC, Kurman RJ 1997 Progestin treatment of atypical endometrial hyperplasia and well-differentiated carcinoma of the endometrium in women

under the age of 40. Obstetrics and Gynecology 40: 434–440.

Rebbeck TR, Kauf ND, Domchek SM 2009 Meta-analysis of risk reduction estimates associated with risk-reducing salpingo-oophorectomy in BRCA1 or BRCA2 mutation carriers. Journal of the National Cancer Institute 101: 80–87.

Richart RM 1967 Natural history of cervical intraepithelial neoplasia. Clinics in Obstetrics and Gynecology 10: 748–784.

Sasieni P, Adams J 1999 Effect of screening on cervical cancer mortality in England and Wales: analysis of trends with an age cohort model. BMJ (Clinical Research Ed.) 318: 1244–1245.

Shafi MI, Luesley DM, Byrne P et al 1989 Vulval intraepithelial neoplasia — management and outcome. BJOG: an International Journal of Obstetrics and Gynaecology 96: 1339–1344.

Shafi MI, Nazeer S 2006 Colposcopy — A Practical Guide. Fivepin Publishers, Salisbury.

Shih IEM, Kurman RJ 2004 A proposed model based on morphological and molecular genetic analysis. American Journal of Pathology 164: 1511–1518.

Singer A, Monaghan J 2000. Lower Genital Tract Precancer. Blackwell Science, Oxford, p 10.

Smith-Bindman R, Kerlickoske K, Feldstein V et al 1998 Endovaginal ultrasound to exclude endometrial cancer and other endometrial pathologies. Journal of the American Medical Association 280: 1510–1517.

Soutter WP, Fletcher A 1994 Invasive cancer of the cervix in women with mild dyskaryosis followed cytologically. BMJ (Clinical Research Ed.) 308: 1421–1423.

Shih IM, Kurman RJ 2009 Pathogenesis of ovarian cancer: lessons from morphology and molecular biology and their clinical implications. International Journal of Gynecological Pathology 27: 151–160.

Walboomers JM, Jacobs MV, Manos MM et al 1999 Human papillomavirus is a necessary cause of invasive cervical cancer. Journal of Pathology 189: 12–19.

Williams J 1886 Cancer of the Uterus. Harverian Lectures for 1886. HK Lewis, London.

CHAPTER 39

Cancer of the uterine cervix

Kavita Singh and Janos Balega

Chapter Contents

EPIDEMIOLOGY	582		RECURRENT CERVICAL CANCER	594
AETIOLOGY	582		FOLLOW-UP AFTER TREATMENT FOR CERVICAL CANCER	595
NATURAL HISTORY AND SPREADING PATTERN OF CERVICAL CANCER	583		MANAGEMENT OF COMPLICATIONS IN ADVANCED DISEASE	595
CLINICAL PRESENTATION	584		CERVICAL CANCER IN PREGNANCY	596
DIAGNOSIS AND STAGING	584		CONCLUSIONS	596
HISTOLOGY	587		KEY POINTS	596
TREATMENT OF CERVICAL CANCER	587			

Epidemiology

Cervical cancer is the most common gynaecological malignancy in the world with an estimated 493,000 new cases diagnosed each year (Ferlay et al 2004). It accounts for nearly 10% of all cancers in women. Although the incidence of cervical cancer has decreased in industrialized countries in the past 20 years, it still remains a major problem in the developing world. In most parts of Africa, South-Central Asia and Central America, cervical cancer accounts for 7–13% of all newly diagnosed cancers, with an incidence of 30–40 new cases per 100,000 population (Cancer Research UK, 2005).

In the UK, 2800 patients are diagnosed with cervical cancer per year, which accounts for approximately 2% of all female cancer cases, and 950 patients die from the disease (Cancer Research UK, 2005). With the introduction of the cervical screening programme in the UK, the incidence of cervical cancer has decreased from 16/100,000 in 1985 to 8/100,000 in 2005, while the incidence of carcinoma *in situ* has risen because of early detection with screening (Cancer Research UK, 2005). Carcinoma *in situ* is most common in women aged 35–39 years, while the incidence of cervical cancer is highest in women aged 30–34 years (17/100,000). The distribution of cervical cancer is bimodal, with a second peak reached in women aged over 85 years (14/100,000) (Cancer Research UK, 2005). Only 30% of cervical cancers are detected by screening, and the majority of cases occur in women who have never had a smear test or who have not been regular participants in the screening programme.

Aetiology

Epidemiological studies have long indicated a positive correlation between sexual activity and cervical cancer (Schiffman and Brinton 1995). Promiscuity, a sexual partner with promiscuous sexual behaviour and early age at first sexual intercourse have all been associated with a high risk of cervical cancer. It has been well demonstrated that human papilloma virus (HPV) infection is the major and probably a necessary causal factor, enhanced by several cofactors for both squamous cell carcinoma and adenocarcinoma of the cervix (Muñoz et al 1992, Schiffman et al 1993, Bosch et al 2002). HPV viral particles have been detected in almost all cases of cervical cancer (99.7%) (Walboomers and Meijer 1997, Franco et al 1999, Walboomers et al 1999).

Human papilloma virus

HPV is a double-stranded DNA virus that contains eight genes: six early (*E1, E2, E4, E5, E6, E7*) and two late (*L1, L2*). The early genes are expressed when the virus enters the host cell and encodes those proteins that regulate viral replication and the interaction with the host cell. The late genes code for capsid proteins.

E6 and *E7* encode oncoproteins. After the virus enters the host cell, *E6* and *E7* integrate into the host DNA and encode for oncoproteins. The E6 oncoprotein binds to and destabilizes the host's *p53* tumour suppressor gene, resulting in a shorter half-life and inactivation. The E7 oncoprotein binds to tumour suppressor genes *pRB, p21* and *p27*, resulting in increased cell proliferation.

DOI: 10.1016/B978-0-7020-3120-5.00039-4

Table 39.1 Risk groups of human papilloma virus (HPV)

| High-risk HPV | 16, 18, 31, 33, 35, 45, 51, 52, 58, 59, 68, 73, 82 |
| Low-risk HPV | 6, 11, 40, 42, 43, 44, 54, 61, 70, 72, 81 |

To date, more than 200 subtypes of HPV have been identified. According to oncogenic potential, HPVs can be classified as low-risk or high-risk types (Table 39.1) (Duenas-Gonzalez et al 2005, Smith et al 2007). Approximately 75% of cervical cancers are related to HPV 16 and 18 in Europe, and 90% of genital warts are caused by HPV 6 and 11 (Smith 2003). However, the distribution of HPV subtypes varies in other parts of the world (Smith et al 2007).

It is estimated that nearly 80% of sexually active women will acquire an HPV infection during their lifetime, while oncogenic subtypes are identified in 15% of the population (Brown et al 2005, Dunne et al 2007). Ninety percent of HPV infections will be eradicated by the host immune system, and only a minority of women will develop preinvasive disease or cancer (Pagliusi and Teresa Aguado 2004). The prevalence of HPV infection decreases with age, from approximately 20% in women aged 20–25 years to approximately 5% in women aged 50 years (Woodman et al 2001).

Cofactors

Cigarette smoking

Cigarette smoking has been linked with a higher risk of cervical cancer and has been demonstrated to be an independent risk factor (Winkelstein 1990, Kapeu et al 2009). High concentrations of nicotine metabolites have been detected in cervical mucus, and their molecular interaction with fragile histidine triad (*FHIT*) tumour suppressor gene has been investigated (Schiffman et al 1987, Holschneider et al 2005). The loss of function of *FHIT* plays an important role in early carcinogenesis (Pichiorri et al 2008). In comparison with non-smokers, smokers have impaired immune responses in the cervical epithelium and produce reduced levels of HPV 16/18 antibodies (Simen-Kapeu et al 2008).

A recent meta-analysis confirmed that smoking is an independent risk factor for squamous cell cervical cancer, but failed to demonstrate the same for adenocarcinoma (Berrington de González et al 2004).

Oral contraceptives

The association between long-term oral contraceptive (OC) use and cervical cancer is unclear. Recent analyses have shown an increased risk (relative risk 1.3–1.9) of cervical cancer amongst OC users (Smith 2003, Appleby et al 2007, Hannaford et al 2007). In contrast, others have reported that sexual behaviour differs between OC users and non-users, and that OC use is not an independent risk factor (Miller et al 2004, Syrjänen et al 2006).

Immunodeficiency

It has been observed that patients with immunodeficiency disorders, those on immunosuppressive therapy and those with human immunodeficiency virus (HIV) infection are at higher risk of developing anogenital HPV-related premalignant changes and cancers. Cervical cancer is an acquired-immunodeficiency-syndrome-defining disease. One meta-analysis estimated a six-fold increased risk of developing cervical cancer for patients with HIV infection, and a two-fold increased risk for those with previous transplant surgery (Grulich et al 2007).

HPV vaccination

Cervical cytology

Cervical cytology is an effective secondary preventive measure. Since the identification of HPV as a causative factor for cervical cancer, laboratory research has focused on developing a primary preventive method, i.e. a vaccine against HPV.

HPV-virus-like particles have been developed that have similar antigenic properties to the virus itself, and therefore provoke a host immune response.

Two types of HPV vaccine have been developed: the bivalent Cervarix targeting HPV 16 and 18, and the quadrivalent Gardasil for HPV 6, 11, 16 and 18. The efficacy of Gardasil and Cervarix has been demonstrated in large, prospective, randomized trials (FUTURE II and PATRICIA) (FUTURE II Study Group 2007, Paavonen et al 2007). The vaccines are prophylactic and are not effective in patients with existing HPV infection. There is some cross-protection against other high-risk types of HPV.

Vaccination programme in the UK

The routine vaccination of 12–13-year-old girls with Cervarix has been introduced in the UK, and catch-up vaccination is available until 18 years of age. Three 0.5 ml injections are given at 0, 2 and 6 months. Immunity has been demonstrated for at least 5 years and long-term follow-up studies are ongoing.

Natural History and Spreading Pattern of Cervical Cancer

Cervical cancers can arise from the ectocervix or endocervix. Most ectocervical cancers are squamous in histology, and endocervical cancers arise from squamous and columnar epithelium. All cervical cancers are preceded by a preneoplastic stage (cervical intraepithelial neoplasia and cervical glandular intraepithelial neoplasia). Cervical cancers may present as an exophytic growth or an endophytic expansion without any visible tumour on the surface of the cervix.

The pattern of spread may be direct, lymphatic or haematogenous. The cancer can spread directly to the parametria, vagina, corpus, bladder and rectum. Primary sites of lymphatic spread are the external and internal iliac and obturator lymph nodes, while secondary sites are the presacral, common iliac and para-aortic lymph nodes. The most common sites of haematogenous metastases are lungs and liver.

Clinical Presentation

Patients with cervical cancer may be symptomatic or asymptomatic. Symptoms associated with cervical cancer are often non-specific, such as postcoital bleeding, intermenstrual bleeding, postmenopausal bleeding, excessive foul-smelling vaginal discharge and pelvic pain. Patients with locally advanced cancer can present with loin pain secondary to obstructive uropathy; sciatic pain due to compression of pelvic nerves; and fistula formation between the rectum, vagina and bladder. Renal failure is regarded as the most common cause of death by cervical cancer.

The positive predictive value of postcoital and intermenstrual bleeding for the diagnosis of cervical cancer in younger women is very low (Shapley et al 2006). Only 2% of patients with postcoital bleeding will be diagnosed with cervical cancer (Shapley et al 2006).

Asymptomatic patients are usually referred with either abnormal appearance of the cervix, a suspicious smear or an incidental discovery of cervical cancer on loop biopsy performed for treatment of intraepithelial neoplasia.

Diagnosis and Staging

Clinical examination

Apart from the routine medical history, special emphasis must be placed on the patient's desire for future fertility. Detailed examination is essential, including physical examination to exclude any obvious peripheral lymphadenopathy, speculum examination to assess the size of tumour and vaginal extension, and a rectovaginal examination to assess the size of cervical tumour and its extension to the parametria, vaginal vault and rectal mucosa. In cases of suspected bladder and bowel involvement, an examination under anaesthesia with cystoscopy and rectosigmoidoscopy is required, and biopsies are obtained for histological confirmation.

Pathology review

All patients referred with cervical cancer need to have their histology reviewed by a gynaecological oncopathologist. Information is obtained regarding the tumour histological type, differentiation, size (breadth × horizontal width × depth of invasion), pattern of invasion (uni- or multifocal, pushing or spreading), and presence or absence of lymphovascular space invasion.

Imaging in cervical cancer

Although cancer of the uterine cervix is staged clinically worldwide, a more precise assessment of the extent of cancer by cross-sectional imaging results in more tailored management. Magnetic resonance imaging (MRI) of the abdomen and pelvis is performed to assess the size and volume of tumour, the presence of parametrial invasion by analysing the integrity of the high-intensity stromal ring around the tumour, and to exclude bladder or rectum involvement. MRI is more accurate than computed tomography (CT) for assessment of local spread, and both modalities are superior to clinical examination.

Positron emission tomography (PET) is a functional scan that assesses the increased uptake of fluorodeoxyglucose (FDG). Organs with high metabolic activity (liver, brain, neoplastic tissue) have high FDG uptake. Addition of CT to PET (PET–CT) provides improved assessment of tumour localization. PET–CT has been used to assess para-aortic nodal status to facilitate planning of radiotherapy fields (Figure 39.1F) (Grigsby et al 2001). A further role of PET–CT is to assess the response to primary chemoradiotherapy, as well as early detection of cancer recurrences (Figure 39.2D).

Laparoscopic para-aortic lymph node sampling

Laparoscopic para-aortic lymph node sampling has been performed to assess the para-aortic lymph nodes; however, the only prospective randomized study failed to confirm therapeutic benefit (Lai et al 2003). The detection of micrometastasis in the para-aortic nodes has been used to modify radiation treatment fields (Leblanc et al 2007). Superiority of lymphadenectomy over PET–CT in assessment of the para-aortic nodes has not been established.

Multidisciplinary discussion

All patients must be discussed by a multidisciplinary team of gynaecological oncologists, clinical oncologists, medical oncologists, radiologists, pathologists and clinical nurse practitioners. Factors which influence management include:

- clinical staging;
- histological type;
- tumour size;
- volume of occult cancer;
- presence of adverse pathological risk factors;
- performance status and associated comorbidities;
- fertility status and plans; and
- patient's choice.

Staging

The International Federation of Obstetricians and Gynecologists (FIGO) staging of cervical cancer is based on clinical findings and, in the early stages, on the microscopic extent of the disease, and is not changed by intraoperative findings or the postoperative histological result (Table 39.2). When doubt exists regarding the stage of a particular cancer, the earlier stage should be chosen.

Surgical staging in cervical cancer is an issue that continues to generate discussion. Should lymph node status influence the staging? Should further substages be included? Should the histological findings and cross-sectional imaging influence the process of staging? A consensus statement from the International Gynecological Cancer Society meeting in 2006 reported as follows (Odicino et al 2007).

- Surgical staging is not practical, feasible or beneficial in the majority of cervical cancer patients, hence it is not recommended for staging. Nearly 80% of cervical cancer patients are diagnosed in the developing world, and the majority are diagnosed in late stages and are not suitable for surgical staging. Therefore, cervical cancer should remain a clinically staged disease.
- Pathological extent and other pathological findings such as lymphovascular space invasion (LVSI) should

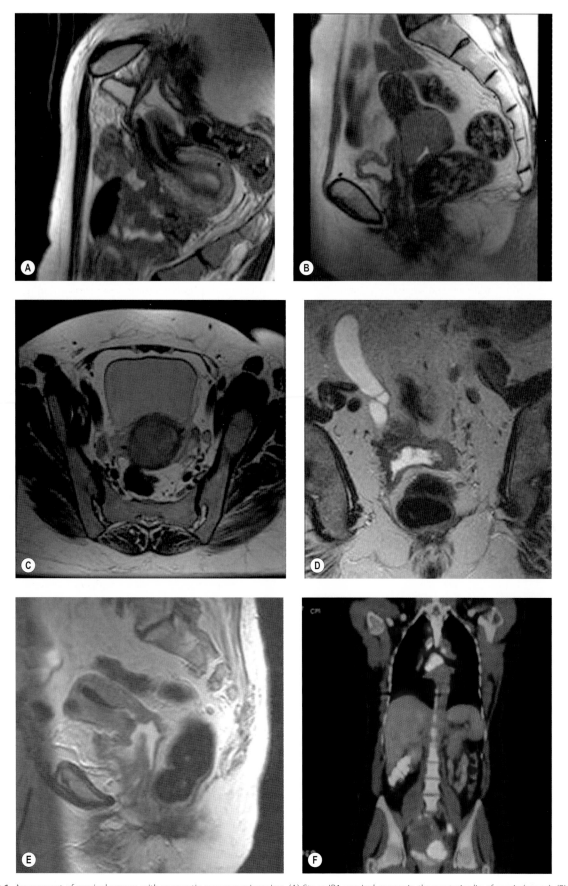

Figure 39.1 Assessment of cervical cancer with magnetic resonance imaging. (A) Stage IB1 cervical cancer in the posterior lip of cervix (arrow). (B) Stage IB2 cervical cancer with bulky tumour replacing the cervix (arrow). (C) Stage IIB cervical cancer with right parametrial invasion. Note the interruption of the high-signal-intensity ring around the cervix on the right side (arrow). (D) Stage IIIB cervical cancer causing right hydronephrosis (arrow). (E) Stage IVA cervical cancer with fistula formation between the bladder and vagina (arrow). (F) Stage IVB cervical cancer with mediastinal lymphadenopathy (star). Note the increased uptake of left common iliac lymph nodes (arrow).

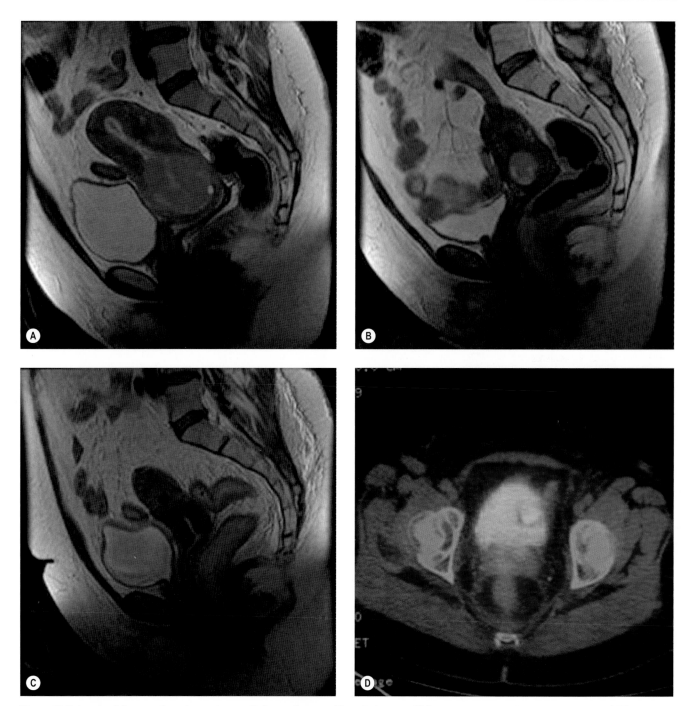

Figure 39.2 Imaging follow-up after primary chemoradiotherapy for stage IIB cervical cancer. (A) Pretreatment magnetic resonance imaging (MRI) scan. (B) Three months post chemoradiation. (C) Six months post treatment MRI scan. (D) Six months post treatment positron emission tomography–computed tomography scan with no uptake of fluorodeoxyglucose in the cervix. Note the increased uptake in the bladder.

be reported but not included in the staging of cervical cancer.

- Use of imaging techniques such as MRI, if available, is encouraged but not mandatory.
- Clinical investigations, including examination under anaesthesia, cystoscopy or sigmoidoscopy, which were previously mandatory for staging purposes are now optional and adopted for selected cases.
- The following modifications in cervical cancer staging would be adopted at the next FIGO meeting in 2009:
  - Stage 0 will be erased, as it is not an invasive disease.

- Stage IIA: should be subgrouped similar to stage IB based on tumour size as stage IIA1 with tumour size less than 4 cm with involvement of up to two-thirds of the upper vagina, and stage IIA2 with tumour size greater than 4 cm with involvement of up to two-thirds of the upper vagina.
- Stage IIB and IIIB: inclusion of unilateral or bilateral parametrial involvement. Stage IIB1 and IIIB1 indicate unilateral parametrial involvement, and stage IIB2 and IIIB2 indicate bilateral parametrial involvement.

Table 39.2 Revised FIGO staging of cervical cancer (2009)

Stage I	The carcinoma is strictly confined to the cervix (extension to the corpus would be disregarded)
IA	Invasive carcinoma which can be diagnosed only by microscopy, with deepest invasion ≤5.0 mm and largest extension ≤7.0 mm
IA1	Measured stromal invasion of ≤3.0 mm in depth and horizontal extension of ≤7.0 mm
IA2	Measured stromal invasion of >3.0 mm and not >5.0 mm with an extension of not >7.0 mm
IB	Clinically visible lesions limited to the cervix uteri or preclinical cancers greater than stage IA*
IB1	Clinically visible lesion ≤4.0 cm in greatest dimension
IB2	Clinically visible lesion >4.0 cm in greatest dimension
Stage II	Cervical carcinoma invades beyond the uterus, but not to the pelvic wall or to the lower third of the vagina
IIA	Without parametrial invasion
IIAI	Clinically visible lesion ≤4.0 cm in greatest dimension
IIA2	Clinically visible lesion >4.0 cm in greatest dimension
IIB	With obvious parametrial invasion
Stage III	The tumour extends to the pelvic wall and/or involves lower third of the vagina and/or causes hydronephrosis or non-functioning kidney§
IIIA	Tumour involves lower third of the vagina, with no extension to the pelvic wall
IIIB	Extension to the pelvic wall and/or hydronephrosis or non-functioning kidney
Stage IV	The carcinoma has extended beyond the true pelvis or has involved (biopsy proven) the mucosa of the bladder or rectum. A bullous oedema, as such, does not permit a case to be allotted to stage IV
IVA	Spread of the growth to adjacent organs
IVB	Spread to distant organs

* All macroscopically visible lesions, even with superficial invasion, are allotted to stage IB carcinomas. Invasion is limited to a measured stromal invasion with a maximal depth of 5.0 mm and a horizontal extension of not >7.0 mm. Depth of invasion should not be >5.0 mm taken from the base of the epithelium of the original tissue — superficial or glandular. The depth of invasion should always be reported in mm, even in those cases with 'early (minimal) stromal invasion' (~1.0 mm). The involvement of vascular/lymphatic spaces should not change the stage allotment.
§ On rectal examination, there is no cancer-free space between the tumour and the pelvic wall. All cases with hydronephrosis or non-functioning kidney are included, unless they are known to be due to another cause.

Histology

The vast majority of cervical cancers (75%) are squamous cell carcinomas. The clinical appearance is usually exophytic, but it is not uncommon to have an endophytic tumour with a normal ectocervix. Histologically, three types of squamous cell carcinoma can be distinguished: large cell keratinizing, large cell non-keratinizing and small cell squamous carcinoma.

Adenocarcinoma is the second most common histological type and represents 20% of cervical cancers. The proportion of adenocarcinomas compared with squamous cell carcinomas has increased significantly over the past three decades. The cause of this change is two-fold: relative, due to the gradual decrease in incidence of squamous cell carcinoma following the introduction of the cervical screening programme; and absolute, probably due to factors such as increased use of OCs (Ursin et al 1994, Smith et al 2000, Sasieni and Adams 2001). The gross appearance of adenocarcinomas is similar to squamous lesions; however, nearly 15% of patients present with clinically non-apparent lesions due to the endophytic expansion of the cancer (barrel-shaped cervix).

Microscopically, several subtypes are distinguished. The most common types are the endocervical (mucinous), intestinal and endometrioid variants.

It is a common clinical dilemma to distinguish between endocervical cancer with extension to the uterus and endometrial cancer of isthmic origin involving the cervical stroma. Clinical impression, cross-sectional imaging (MRI scan) and immunohistochemistry studies using p16 antibody can be of help to determine the origin of the cancer. The p16 protein is mainly expressed by HPV-related cancer cells.

Adenosquamous carcinomas consist of both squamous and glandular elements. A dedifferentiated form of adenosquamous carcinoma is the glassy cell carcinoma, which tends to occur in young patients and has a particularly aggressive clinical behaviour with poor outcome. Microscopically, it is characterized by large cells with glassy cytoplasm.

Neuroendocrine cervical carcinomas are rare histological subtypes, accounting for less than 5% of cervical cancers. They are characterized by highly aggressive clinical behaviour, manifesting as early nodal and distant diseases in more than half of patients. This results in poor survival despite multimodal treatment. Neuroendocrine cervical carcinomas are similar to the neuroendocrine cancers of the lung, both clinically and histologically. There are four subgroups: classical carcinoid, atypical carcinoid tumour, neuroendocrine large cell carcinoma and neuroendocrine small cell (oat cell) carcinoma (Albores-Saavedra et al 1997).

Clear cell carcinomas of the cervix are rare and have been linked with diethylstilboestrol exposure *in utero*. They usually present with large, exophytic tumours and are chemoradioresistant. Surgery is therefore the cornerstone of management, followed by chemoradiotherapy.

Treatment of Cervical Cancer

Surgical management

The method of surgical treatment of cervical cancer depends on the stage of disease, tumour volume, histological features, patient's desire for future fertility and performance status. Treatment options for different stages of cervical cancer are shown in Table 39.3. The Wertheim-Meigs radical hysterectomy with pelvic lymphadenectomy has been the standard treatment for over a century in patients with stage IA2–IIA cervical cancer. Critical analysis of the data on the role of parametrectomy and pelvic lymphadenectomy has changed the practice significantly, and narrowed the indication for the radical operation. In stage IA2 and low-volume stage IB1 (<500 m³) cervical cancer, the risk of parametrial

Table 39.3 Management of cervical cancer

Stage	Treatment	LND
IA1	Cone biopsy/simple trachelectomy/simple hysterectomy	No
IA2	Cone biopsy/simple trachelectomy/simple hysterectomy	+/− (variable practice)
IA1/IA2 + LVSI	Cone biopsy/simple trachelectomy/simple hysterectomy	+
IB1: low volume (<500 mm³)	Simple trachelectomy/simple hysterectomy	+
IB1: <2 cm diameter	Radical trachelectomy/radical hysterectomy	+
IB1: 2–4 cm diameter	Radical hysterectomy	+
IB2/IIA	Chemoradiation/radical hysterectomy	+
IIB–IVA	Chemoradiation/palliative surgery	
IVB	Chemotherapy +/− palliative radiotherapy	

LND, lymph node dissection.

involvement is low (<2%); therefore, simple hysterectomy is recommended (Stegeman et al 2007). Novel developments in surgical technique, such as fertility-sparing surgery (trachelectomy), laparoscopic radical hysterectomy, pelvic lymphadenectomy and para-aortic lymphadenectomy, have been developed and are practised increasingly. Sentinel node biopsy in cervical cancer is also being explored (Levenback et al 2002).

Stage IA1

The rate of metastasis to lymph nodes is less than 1%. Treatment options in the absence of lymphovascular space invasion are as follows.

- Conization for women who wish to preserve their fertility. Cold-knife cone biopsy is the preferred technique to prevent cauterized margins, which may affect histological assessment.
- Simple hysterectomy for women who do not wish to retain their fertility. This can be performed with ovarian conservation if desired.
- Simple trachelectomy for women with a short infravaginal cervix, where conization may be difficult to perform. Unlike radical vaginal trachelectomy (RVT), dissection of the ureter and removal of a vaginal cuff and parametrial tissue is not necessary. The technique is simple and involves a circular incision at the cervicovaginal junction, dissection of the vesicocervical space anteriorly and the pouch of Douglas posteriorly. The cervix is transsected 1 cm below the level of the internal os. Insertion of a

cervical cerclage is necessary to retain the function of the cervical canal. This procedure is less morbid than a hysterectomy.

If therapeutic conization or trachelectomy is performed, the minimum desired surgical margin of clearance is 10 mm. Intraoperative frozen section analysis can exclude the presence of cancer at the surgical margin. If cervical intraepithelial neoplasia (CIN) extends to the resection margins, a repeat excision should be performed to remove the residual CIN and to exclude further invasive disease.

The presence of LVSI is generally considered to be a poor prognostic factor in cervical cancer (relative risk of recurrence 2.0) (Marchiole et al 2005). Therefore, for stage IA1 cervical cancer with extensive LVSI, pelvic lymphadenectomy might be considered in addition to simple hysterectomy or simple trachelectomy. However, this approach does not have a robust evidence base.

Stage IA2

The reported incidence of nodal involvement in stage IA2 cervical cancer varies from 0.5% to 10% due to the lack of uniformity in measurement of tumour dimensions (Hasumi et al 1980, van Nagell et al 1983, Simon et al 1986, Maiman et al 1988, Creasman et al 1998). The accepted surgical treatment for stage IA2 cervical cancer is pelvic lymphadenectomy with simple hysterectomy. However, in the presence of extensive LVSI, modified radical hysterectomy or RVT with pelvic node dissection has been recommended. It is debatable whether lymphadenectomy should be performed routinely in this substage as, by strict histological subgrouping of stage IA2 cervical cancer (i.e. depth of invasion 3–5 mm and horizontal dimension up to 7 mm), the true incidence of positive lymph node metastasis is 0.5% (1/205 histologically confirmed stage IA2) (Rogers and Luesley 2009).

Stage IB1 and IIA cervical cancer

Both surgery and chemoradiotherapy are thought to be equally effective for the management of stage IB1 and IIA cervical cancer. Surgical treatment which involves radical hysterectomy with pelvic lymphadenectomy has potential advantages in younger women by preserving ovarian function and avoiding radiotherapy-related late complications (e.g. vaginal stenosis, radiation cystitis and radiation-induced bowel damage). Complications related to radical surgery are usually temporary and short term (e.g. autonomic dysfunction of the bladder and rectum, shortening of the vagina, lymphoedema and lymphocysts). Careful preoperative selection of patients for radical surgery avoids subjecting them to double treatment (surgery followed by adjuvant treatment). If adverse histological factors are found in the surgical specimen, postoperative chemoradiotherapy is required (Table 39.4). Approximately 20% of patients with stage IB1 and IIA cervical cancer will require adjuvant chemoradiotherapy, which results in increased treatment-related morbidity.

The reported incidence of parametrial involvement in stage IB1 cervical cancer with tumour size less than 2 cm, depth of invasion less than 10 mm, negative pelvic lymph nodes and absent LVSI is low (0.4–0.6%) (Stegeman et al 2007, Wright et al 2007). This suggests that it may be advisable to avoid parametrectomy in this subgroup.

Table 39.4 Adverse histological prognostic factors in cervical cancer

Major risk factors	Minor risk factors
Positive pelvic nodes	Presence of lymphovascular space invasion
Parametrial invasion	Deep cervical stromal invasion (>1/3)
Positive or close (<5 mm) surgical margins	Large tumour size (≥4 cm)

Table 39.5 Modified Piver/European Organization for Research and Treatment of Cancer classification of radical hysterectomy

Class	Description
Type I	Simple hysterectomy.
Type II	Modified radical hysterectomy: the uterus, paracervical tissues and upper vagina (1–2 cm) are removed after dissection of the ureters to the point of their entry to the bladder. The uterine arteries are ligated at the site of crossing the ureters, and the medial half of the parametria and proximal uterosacral ligaments are resected.
Type III	Radical hysterectomy: en-bloc removal of the uterus with the upper third of the vagina along with the paravaginal and paracervical tissues. The uterine vessels are ligated at their origin, and the entire width of the parametria is resected bilaterally. Removal of as much of the uterosacral ligaments as possible.
Type IV	Extended radical hysterectomy: the difference from the type III procedure is that three-quarters of the vagina and paravaginal tissue are excised.
Type V	Partial exenteration: the terminal ureter or a segment of the bladder or rectum is removed, along with the uterus and parametria (supralevator exenteration).

Stage IB2 cervical cancer

The rate of pelvic lymph node metastasis in patients with bulky cervical cancer (>4 cm) is approximately 44% (Finan et al 1996). Although primary surgery is feasible and has some advantages (e.g. removal of tumour bulk, removal of bulky lymph nodes, proper assessment of tumour extension), due to the high likelihood of requiring double treatment, the logical option is primary chemoradiotherapy (NIH Consensus Development Conference Statement on Cervical Cancer 1997). The rate of pelvic relapse is significantly higher in patients with stage IB2 disease who had radiation alone compared with patients who had surgery followed by adjuvant radiotherapy (30% vs 20%) (Landoni et al 1997).

Neoadjuvant chemotherapy has been used with a rationale of reducing tumour bulk prior to surgery or radiotherapy, but no survival benefit has been demonstrated over conventional radiotherapy (Sananes et al 1998, Benedetti-Panici et al 2002).

Stage IIB–IVA cervical cancer

Surgical procedures (defunctioning colostomy, percutaneous nephrostomy) are performed in advanced cervical cancer, mainly for symptom control.

Surgical techniques

Radical hysterectomy

Radical hysterectomy was classified into five types by Piver et al in 1974 based upon the site of ligation of the uterine vessels and the radicality of parametrial resection. The Surgery Committee of the Gynecological Cancer Group of the European Organization for Research and Treatment of Cancer have produced, approved and adopted a revised version of the original Piver classification (Table 39.5) (Trimbos et al 2004). The salient steps of radical hysterectomy are (Figure 39.3):

- division of the round ligaments and dissecting the paravesical spaces;
- dissecting the uterovesical space;
- isolating and dissecting the ureters and dissecting the pararectal spaces;
- ligating the uterine vessels at their origin;
- dissecting the ureteric tunnels and displacing the ureters laterally;
- dissecting the rectovaginal space;
- excising the cardinouterosacral complex;

- excising the vaginal cuff; and
- completing the pelvic lymphadenectomy.

Landoni et al (2001) conducted a prospective randomized study comparing survival, relapse and morbidity between type II and type III radical hysterectomy for patients with stage IB and IIA cervical cancer. They found similar outcomes but a higher rate of late morbidity in the group with type III radical hysterectomy.

Okabayashi's nerve-sparing radical hysterectomy preserves both the hypogastric nerves and the splanchnic nerves in order to reduce bladder and bowel dysfunction (Fujii et al 2007). Laparoscopic radical hysterectomy is a novel approach with similar efficacy and recurrence rates to open radical hysterectomy, but with reduced blood loss and wound-related complications, and a shorter recovery period (Abu-Rustum et al 2003, Ghezzi et al 2007).

Removal of the tubes and ovaries is not routinely part of a radical hysterectomy. The risk of ovarian metastasis is 0.5% in early squamous cell carcinomas and 1.7% in adenocarcinomas (Sutton et al 1992). Therefore, for women under 45 years of age with cervical cancer, the ovaries can usually be preserved and can be transposed into the paracolic gutters out of the pelvis (outwith the potential radiation field). Conventionally, patients with adenocarcinoma are offered salpingo-oophorectomy; however, isolated ovarian metastasis in the absence of adverse pathological features is rare. The ovarian failure rate after transposition is 50% (Anderson et al 1993, Feeney et al 1995).

Type II–V radical hysterectomies are completed with systematic bilateral pelvic lymphadenectomy. The anatomical borders of the lymphadenectomy are the bifurcation of the common iliac vessels cranially, the deep circumflex iliac vein and the bladder caudally, the obturatour internus muscle and the genitofemoral nerve laterally, the internal iliac artery medially, and the obturator nerve inferiorly (Figure 39.4).

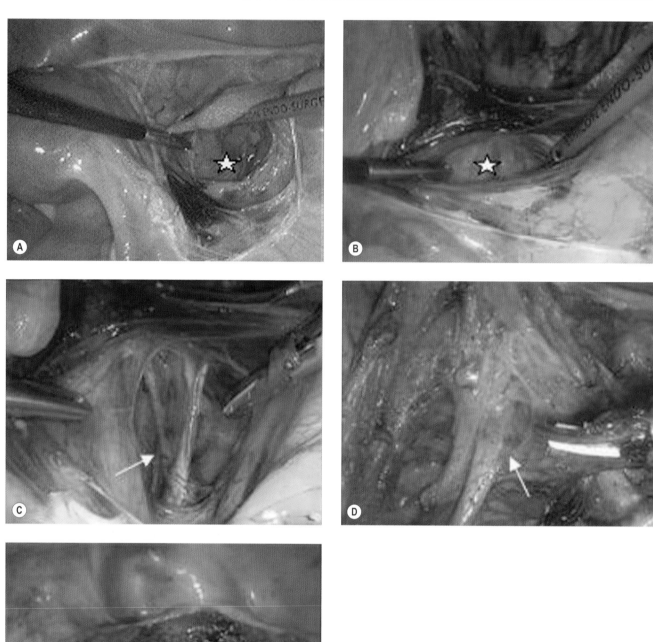

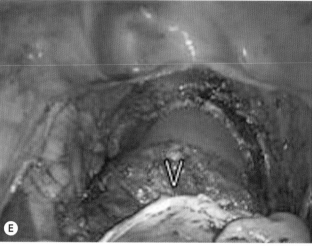

Figure 39.3 Surgical steps of laparoscopic radical hysterectomy. (A) Division of round ligament and dissecting paravesical space (☆paravesical space). (B) Dissecting pararectal space (☆pararectal space). (C) Isolation of uterine artery at origin (arrow points to origin of uterine artery from internal iliac artery). (D) Dissection of the ureteric tunnel (arrow points to entry of ureter within the ureteric tunnel). (E) Excision of the vagina (V, vaginal cuff being excised).

Any bulky para-aortic nodes should also be resected, given that radiation therapy cannot sterilize metastatic nodes larger than 2 cm in diameter (Hacker et al 1995).

Complications of radical hysterectomy

The complications of radical hysterectomy can be related directly or indirectly to the surgical procedure. Direct com-

plications can arise from injury to bladder, ureters, rectum, pelvic vessels and nerves, and these have to be managed intraoperatively. Indirect complications can result from devascularization of the ureters and can manifest as urogenital fistulae, usually 2–3 weeks postoperatively. Extensive parametrial dissection can damage the autonomic nerve supply of the bladder and rectum, resulting in voiding and

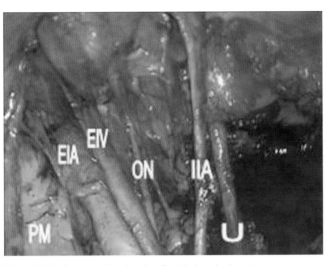

Figure 39.4 Anatomical landmarks of pelvic lymphadenectomy. EIA, external iliac artery; EIV, external iliac vein; IIA, internal iliac artery; U, ureter; ON, obturator nerve; PM, psoas muscle.

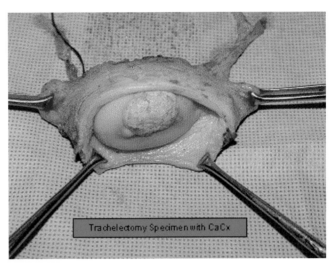

Figure 39.5 Trachelectomy specimen. PM, parametrium.

evacuating difficulties. Removal of the upper part of the vagina may cause sexual dysfunction. Pelvic lymphadenectomy can result in formation of lymphocysts and development of leg lymphoedema. Damage to the obturator nerve during lymphadenectomy impairs the function of the adductor muscles.

Trachelectomy

In the UK, the peak incidence of cervical cancer is in women aged 35–39 years. As maternal age at first childbirth has increased progressively, it is not uncommon to find women with cervical cancer who have not yet started or completed their families (Cancerstats 2003). RVT is a fertility-preserving operation for the treatment of invasive cervical cancer, and was first reported by Dargent et al in 1994.

Selection criteria for trachelectomy

- Women wanting a further pregnancy.
- Size of cervical cancer less than 2 cm (up to 3 cm in selected cases with an exophytic tumour).
- Stage I1 and IA2 cervical cancer with LVSI.
- Stage IB1 cervical cancer.
- No evidence of pelvic lymph node metastasis.
- Presence of cervical cancer at least 1 cm away from internal cervical os on MRI.
- Non-neuroendocrine cervical cancers.

Procedure and technique

RVT is performed in two steps. Firstly, the pelvic lymph nodes are assessed laparoscopically to exclude metastasis. The second step is radical resection of the cervix along with a vaginal cuff and the paracervical tissue (Figure 39.5). Both procedures can be performed on the same day if a reliable frozen section facility is available. If not, laparoscopic lymphadenectomy can precede the radical trachelectomy by a few days. A circumferential incision is made on the upper vagina creating a 1–2 cm vaginal cuff. The vesicovaginal and paravesical spaces are dissected anteriorly and the pouch of Douglas is opened posteriorly. The knee of the ureter is palpated in the bladder pillar, which is reflected upwards and medially. The bladder pillars are divided inferiorly, further releasing the bladder and ureters superiorly. The cardinal–uterosacral complex is clamped and divided just below the ureters. The cervix is then amputated leaving 0.5–1.0 cm of normal cervical tissue below the internal os. Cervical cerclage suture is inserted, the vagina is sutured in a circular fashion around the cervix and a new, vagino–isthmic junction is created.

Radical trachelectomy can also be performed abdominally and laparoscopically (Cibula et al 2005). The abdominal approach is suitable in women with poor vaginal access, when the cervix is flush with the vault or in the presence of a large, exophytic cervical growth (Cibula et al 2008). Pelvic lymphadenectomy is usually performed laparoscopically, but can also be performed by an extraperitoneal approach.

Outcome after radical vaginal trachelectomy

Potential morbidities after RVT are bladder and ureteral injury, bladder dysfunction, haematoma, lymphoedema and cervical stenosis with haematometra (Plante et al 2005). The reported recurrence rate after RVT is 4% (Milliken and Shepherd 2008). Common sites of recurrence are the vagina, parametrium, pelvic sidewall and para-aortic lymph nodes. Central recurrences may be attributable to either persistent disease in the isthmus or persistent high-risk HPV infection (Morice et al 2004). In the presence of poor histological prognostic factors, additional treatment may be recommended, including completion radical hysterectomy if the margins of clearance are less than 1 cm, or chemoradiation if more than one poor prognostic factor is present (Table 39.4).

Obstetric outcome after radical trachelectomy

Out of 780 RVT procedures reported to date, there have been 302 pregnancies with 190 live births (Shepherd and Milliken 2008). Following RVT, a significant proportion (57%) of patients did not attempt any further pregnancy. In those who did, there was a 70% conception rate with a 30% pregnancy loss during the first and second trimesters, and a preterm delivery rate of 20%. Pregnancies after RVT should be accorded high-risk status because of the increased risk of miscarriage, ascending infection, premature membrane rupture and preterm labour. Regular screening for bacterial vaginosis, prophylactic antibiotics, antenatal steroid therapy and elective caesarean section are recommended.

Follow-up after radical vaginal trachelectomy

Follow-up practices are varied in terms of intervals, duration and modalities used. Shepherd and Milliken (2008) recommend 4-monthly visits for 3 years, and 6-monthly visits until 5 years. Endocervical and vaginal vault cytology and colposcopy are performed during follow-up. HPV testing may be recommended in the presence of persistent dyskariotic cytology on follow-up smears (Singh et al 2004).

Sentinel lymph node biopsy in cervical cancer

The sentinel node is defined as the first lymph node or group of nodes that drains the anatomical site of the tumour. The status of the sentinel node should represent the whole lymphatic area, meaning that if the sentinel node is negative, the non-sentinel lymph nodes should also be negative. The application of sentinel node dissection in breast and vulval cancer has resulted in a decrease in treatment-related morbidity.

Sentinel lymph node biopsy in cervical cancer has not become a routine practice outside clinical trials. Potential advantages of sentinel node biopsy in cervical cancer are to facilitate treatment planning; for example, if the sentinel node is positive, the radical surgery can be abandoned in favour of chemoradiotherapy. Similarly, if the sentinel node is negative, extensive lymphadenectomy can be avoided and the surgical morbidity of complete pelvic lymphadenectomy can be minimized. Sentinel lymph node biopsy is feasible in cervical cancer as the tumour is visible and it is easy to inject radionucleotide colloid (99m technetium) and blue dye. All potential sites of lymphatic drainage of the uterine cervix are accessible through the laparoscope.

Limitations of sentinel node dissection in cervical cancer are:

- multiple sentinel nodes may be identified and there is a risk of skip metastases to para-aortic, common iliac and presacral lymph nodes in 4%, 5% and 8% of cases, respectively; and
- a sentinel node may be identified in more than one site.

Technique of sentinel node biopsy in cervical cancer

Radionucleotide tracer 99m technetium sulphur colloid (1 ml) is injected around the cervical tumour in four quadrants, followed by lymphoscintigraphy performed a few hours prior to surgery. Immediately prior to surgery, 2 ml of blue dye diluted with 2 ml of normal saline is injected in four quadrants around the cervical tumour. Laparoscopic identification and retrieval of the sentinel node using a gamma probe is performed (Figure 39.6). Using a combination of radioactive colloid and blue dye increases the identification of sentinel nodes to 98%. Histological ultrastaging and immunostaining with pancytokeratin further increase the detection of micrometastases.

Radiotherapy

Radiation therapy can be used as primary treatment for all stages of cervical cancer, and as an adjuvant treatment after surgery in the presence of adverse histological features. In cases of disseminated cancer, it can be administered with palliative intent to achieve symptom control in the pelvis. Radiotherapy can be used as curative or palliative therapy for recurrent cervical cancer.

Recently, three randomized trials administering concurrent chemotherapy (cisplatin) and radiotherapy to patients with locally advanced cervical cancer demonstrated a significant benefit in progression-free and overall survival compared with radiotherapy alone (Keys et al 1999, Morris et al 1999, Rose et al 1999, Bekkers et al 2002). Since these seminal trials, chemoradiation therapy has become the standard treatment for medically fit patients with locally advanced cervical cancer. Concurrent chemotherapy enhances the effect of radiotherapy in two ways: certain chemotherapeutics (e.g. cisplatin, hydroxyurea) behave as radiation sensitizers, and the chemotherapy itself is cytotoxic.

Primary radiotherapy

Although all stages of cervical cancer can be treated with radiotherapy, surgical management is preferred in the early stages (stage IA1, IA2 and IB1) to avoid complications of radiotherapy. Primary radiation therapy with chemotherapy, however, is the cornerstone of management for stage IB2, IIA–B, IIIA–B and IVA cervical cancers. There are two main types of radiotherapy: external beam radiation and vaginal brachytherapy. They are usually used in combination.

External beam radiotherapy (teletherapy)

The objectives are to control the primary tumour as well as the parametria and the pelvic sidewalls containing lymphatic tissue. The borders of the radiation field are:

- inferior: the mid-pubic line;
- superior: the superior aspect of the L5 vertebra; and
- lateral: 1 cm lateral to the bony pelvis.

In cases of positive para-aortic lymph nodes, the field can be extended up to the level of the renal vessels. The maximum dose of radiation to the tumour can be delivered using two opposed fields (anterior and posterior) or the four-field technique (anterior, posterior, left and right lateral). The latter usually produces a more favourable dose distribution, delivering less radiation to the bladder and rectum.

Radiation dose

The treatment consists of 25 fractions of external beam radiation therapy (50 Gy) with weekly cisplatin (40 mg/m^2), which reduces the central tumour mass and facilitates subsequent brachytherapy to optimally control the rest of the disease.

Brachytherapy

Placement of radioactive material into a body cavity is called 'brachytherapy'. Various delivery techniques are used. The Manchester applicator consists of a uterine probe and a pair of intravaginal receptacles (Figure 39.7). The patient is

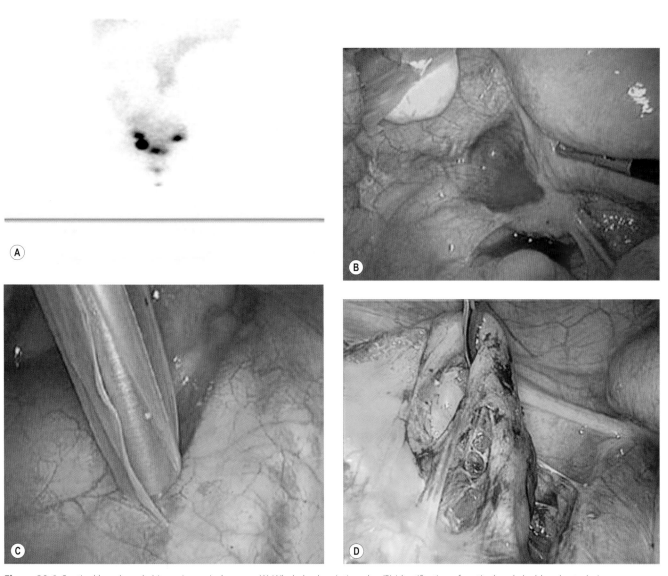

Figure 39.6 Sentinel lymph node biopsy in cervical cancer. (A) Whole-body scintigraphy. (B) Identification of sentinel node by blue dye technique. (C) Identification of sentinel node using gamma probe. (D) Laparoscopic retrieval of sentinel node.

isolated in a shielded room and remote control is used to deliver the radioactive particles into the applicators. There are two main forms of brachytherapy:

- low-dose-rate brachytherapy, which delivers a single dose of 25–27 Gy over 10–15 h; and
- high-dose-rate brachytherapy, with shorter (20 min) but multiple (two to three) applications of a total dose of 15–20 Gy.

Brachytherapy delivers a high dose of radiation to a small volume of target tissue surrounding the applicator. The radiation dose falls off rapidly over a short distance, minimizing the radiation effects to normal surrounding tissues. Retraction of the rectum and bladder with vaginal packing can further reduce radiation-related complications.

Vaginal brachytherapy is critically important to control the central tumour mass adequately. The omission of brachytherapy will result in a higher locoregional relapse rate (Lanciano et al 1991, Logsdon and Eifel 1999).

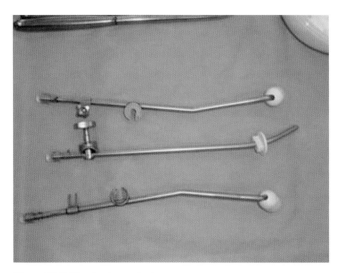

Figure 39.7 Manchester applicator.

Two primary reference points are identified to deliver the optimal dose of radiation to the cervical tumour:

- point A: 2 cm lateral and 2 cm superior to the external cervical os; and
- point B: 3 cm lateral to point A.

Adjuvant radiotherapy

Adjuvant radiation therapy is administered in combination with chemotherapy. Adjuvant therapy in the presence of one major risk factor or at least two of the three minor adverse factors (Table 39.4) reduces the risk of recurrence, and increases recurrence-free survival (Sedlis et al 1999).

Emergency and palliative radiotherapy

Patients with advanced cervical cancer presenting with profuse haemorrhage can be managed effectively with a total dose of 5–30 Gy external beam pelvic radiation in multiple fractions. Patients with unresectable para-aortic lymph node mass, symptomatic supraclavicular or mediastinal lymph node enlargement, or bony metastasis may also benefit from palliative radiotherapy and chemotherapy.

Complications of radiation therapy

Complications of radiotherapy depend on radiation-related factors and patient-related characteristics. The total dose of radiation, the dose per fraction and the total volume irradiated are proportionately related to radiation-related complications. Factors related to the patient, such as previous pelvic inflammatory disease, history of smoking, diabetes, hypertension or previous pelvic surgery, will increase the risk of complications. Acute complications (e.g. skin reactions, diarrhoea and anaemia) are usually mild.

Late complications can occur many months or years after treatment and are usually chronic.

- Bladder complications: radiation cystitis manifesting as haematuria, frequency and dysuria.
- Bowel complications: radiation enteritis presents with severe diarrhoea, malabsorption, cachexia or bowel obstruction.
- Fibrosis of the pelvic structures resulting in reduced bladder capacity and pelvic pain.
- Fusion of the vaginal walls and shortening of the vaginal resulting in dyspareunia and altered sexual function.
- Fistulae: rectovaginal or vesicovaginal fistula formation is a major complication with a significant adverse impact on quality of life.

Recurrent Cervical Cancer

The risk of recurrence depends on the extent of the primary cancer at presentation. Approximately 10–20% of patients with stage IB–IIA cervical cancer with negative lymph nodes will recur, compared with up to 70% of patients with nodal metastasis or locally advanced disease (Table 39.6).

Recurrences can be locoregional or distant (Table 39.7). Patients with pelvic recurrence usually present with vaginal bleeding, discharge, pelvic pain and sciatic pain. Patients with disseminated recurrence will develop systemic symptoms associated with cachexia.

When such symptoms are present, the following investigations should be considered:

- clinical examination (rectovaginal and speculum examination, assessment of peripheral lymph nodes);
- cross-sectional imaging (MRI of pelvis and abdomen, CT of chest);
- examination under anaesthesia, biopsies, cystoscopy and rectosigmoidoscopy; and
- PET–CT scan in cases of central pelvic recurrence to exclude extrapelvic disease.

Treatment of recurrent cervical cancer depends upon the site and extent of recurrence, type(s) of previous treatment, time elapsed since primary treatment and the patient's performance status. The aim of treatment may be curative or palliative depending upon the distribution of disease.

Pelvic recurrence after surgery

Patients not initially treated with radiation therapy can be considered for external beam radiotherapy for their recurrence.

Pelvic recurrence after radiotherapy

Patients with local pelvic relapse who have previously been treated with primary or adjuvant radiotherapy may be considered for curative surgical treatment provided that the

Table 39.6 Rate of pelvic and distant recurrences in cervical cancer

Stage	Pelvic recurrence (%)	Distant metastasis (%)
IB	10–14	16
IIA	17–20	31
IIB	23	26
III	42	39
IVA	74	75

Source: Chan YM, Ng TY, Ngan HY, Wong LC 2002 Monitoring of squamous cell carcinoma antigen levels in invasive cervical cancer: is it cost effective? Gynecological Oncology 84: 7–11.

Table 39.7 Distribution of distant metastases

Site	Rate (%)
Lung	21
Para-aortic lymph nodes	11
Abdominal cavity	8
Supraclavicular lymph nodes	7
Bone (lumbar/thoracic)	16

Source: Chan YM, Ng TY, Ngan HY, Wong LC 2002 Monitoring of squamous cell carcinoma antigen levels in invasive cervical cancer: is it cost effective? Gynecological Oncology 84: 7–11.

esion is confined to the pelvis and does not extend to the pelvic sidewall. All patients should undergo PET–CT to exclude extrapelvic disease. The classic triad of leg oedema (suggestive of nodal infiltration), leg pain (suggestive of nerve infiltration) and hydronephrosis (suggestive of pelvic side wall infiltration) are contraindications to therapeutic exenteration. Depending on the site and extent of recurrence, pelvic exenteration, originally described by Brunschwig, can be either total, anterior or posterior. Total exenteration involves removal of the anterior (bladder and urethra), middle (vulva, vagina and perineum) and posterior (anal canal, rectum and sigmoid) compartments; anterior exenteration involves removal of the anterior and middle compartments; and posterior exenteration involves removal of the middle and posterior compartments. Depending upon the cranio-caudal extent of tumour involvement, the exenteration is termed 'supralevator' when the levator ani muscle is preserved, and 'translevator' when both the supra- and infralevator compartments are resected.

Exenterations are significantly morbid surgical procedures with a major degree of psychosexual impact. Patients require extensive preoperative counselling and postoperative support. With careful selection, the 5-year survival rate after anterior and posterior exenteration is 30–60% and 20–40%, respectively (Friedlander and Grogan 2002).

Patients with sidewall recurrences of less than 5 cm in diameter can be considered for laterally extended endopelvic resection, and can achieve a 5-year survival rate of up to 60% (Hockel 2003).

Disseminated recurrence

For multiple site or distant recurrence, chemotherapy can be administered with a palliative intent. Cisplatin is usually administered in doses of 50–100 mg/m^2 every 3 weeks, either alone or in combination with paclitaxel or gemcitabine.

Follow-up after Treatment of Cervical Cancer

Follow-up is aimed to detect recurrent disease, assess treatment-related morbidity, and analyse psychosocial and psychosexual morbidity. There is no standardized effective protocol for follow-up in cervical cancer. Vault cytology is not effective in detecting recurrences of cervical cancer and is not recommended (Bodurka-Bevers et al 2000). Symptom status at the time of recurrence is a significant predictor of survival; the median survival is 11 months for symptomatic recurrence and 42 months for asymptomatic recurrence. Routine clinical examination in asymptomatic patients appears to lack sensitivity, as a high proportion of recurrences are not detected until symptoms are apparent.

In an observational study of 993 cases of stage IB cervical cancer treated with surgery or radiotherapy, 63% of recurrences occurred before 24 months and 77% occurred before 36 months. The median time to relapse was 16 months (Bodurka-Bevers et al 2000). Patients should be followed-up every 4 months for at least 2 years. MRI and CT are performed whenever recurrence is suspected, but have limitations in differentiating postradiotherapy fibrosis from recurrent tumour. PET–CT scan has been demonstrated as a more sensitive modality for post-therapy surveillance for the detection of recurrent and persistent cervical cancer in both symptomatic and aymptomatic patients. There is limited evidence regarding the optimal timing and frequency of post-therapy scans (Figure 39.2). PET–CT scans should not be used within 3 months of the primary treatment to reduce false-positive results, as the therapeutic effect of radiation continues even after completion of treatment. PET–CT scan is able to identify persistent disease in patients following completion of chemoradiotherapy to select patients for salvage hysterectomy or exenteration.

The tumour marker squamous cell carcinoma antigen is neither sensitive nor cost-effective in the follow-up of cervical cancer and is not recommended (Chan et al 2002).

Management of Complications in Advanced Disease

Patients with advanced cervical cancer may develop the following distressing symptoms.

- Pain: due to direct nerve infiltration or nodal enlargement impinging on pelvic nerves. This can be managed with oral analgesics such as acetaminophen, non-steroidal anti-inflammatory drugs (NSAIDs), opiates given as oral or intramuscular morphine, fentanyl patches, nerve blocks and gabapentin for neuropathic pain.
- Renal failure: due to bilateral ureteric obstruction caused by bilateral parametrial infiltration extending to the pelvic sidewalls, or extrinsic compression from an enlarged nodal mass. Prerenal and renal causes of failure should always be excluded. The management of obstructive uropathy is dependent upon the general condition of the patient, quality of life, and the wishes of the patient and her relatives. Management of ureteric obstruction is controversial as the medical intervention to relieve ureteric obstruction may convert a peaceful death from uraemia to a more painful and distressing terminal phase. If further useful palliative intervention is available, the treatment options include either percutaneous nephrostomy, retrograde stenting or urinary diversions.
- Thrombosis: patients with advanced cervical cancer are at high risk of thrombosis. Thrombosis can result from the compression of pelvic vessels by tumour masses, impaired mobility, the effects of treatment or cancer-related vascular factors. Treatment with low-molecular-weight heparin is recommended if thrombosis is confirmed.
- Haemorrhage: this can result from erosion of blood vessels on the surface of an exophytic or ulcerating growth. Invasion of the bladder or bowel can result in haematuria or rectal bleeding. Treatment is dependent upon the extent of bleeding. Minor bleeding is improved with oral tranexamic acid, withholding any NSAID therapy, vaginal packing or a single fraction of radiotherapy. Heavier arterial bleeding is usually fatal.

It is essential to forewarn the relatives or carers of the patient with advanced cervical cancer so that they will be prepared for any of the above events. If the patient is in a preterminal stage, treatment is aimed at keeping the patient comfortable with sedation and anxiolytics such as midazolam.

- Malodorous discharge: results from tumour necrosis or fistulae. Oral or topical metronidazole reduces the odour.
- Fistulae: cervical cancer can erode into both the bladder and the bowel. If the patient is not suitable for any exenterative procedure, urinary diversion surgery such as an ileal conduit can be performed when both ureters are implanted into a segment of ileum and drained via a stoma. Ileostomy or colostomy can be performed to relieve symptoms from bowel fistulae.

Cervical Cancer in Pregnancy

Pregnancy has no adverse effects on the natural history or the prognosis of cervical cancer. If cervical cancer is detected prior to 16 weeks of gestation, immediate treatment is recommended irrespective of its stage. If cervical cancer is detected after 16 weeks of gestation and is at an early stage (1A1–IB1), treatment can be delayed until fetal maturity. Antenatal steroid administration will promote fetal lung maturity. Elective caesarean section with simple hysterectomy is performed for stage IA2 cervical cancer, and Wertheim's radical hysterectomy is performed for stage IB1 cervical cancer. Patients with stage IA1 cervical cancer require laser loop excision of the transformation zone or cold-knife conization 6 weeks postnatally. For pregnant patients with advanced cervical cancer (stage IB2 or greater) diagnosed after 16 weeks of gestation, consideration for delay up to 4 weeks must be based on the gestational age at the time of diagnosis. Classical caesarean section is the recommended mode of delivery if the fetus has reached the stage of viability, in order to avoid damage to the cervix.

Conclusions

The management of cervical cancer continues to develop and become more individualized to meet each patient's needs. This has occurred against a background of decreasing incidence in the developed world. Efforts have been focused to reduce treatment-related morbidity and prolong survival with improved quality of life. Recent developments in the management of cervical cancer include wider use of laparoscopic techniques (laparoscopic Wertheim's radical hysterectomy, and pelvic and para-aortic lymphadenectomy), use of the sentinel node technique, use of PET–CT scan for pretreatment assessment and post-treatment follow-up, neoadjuvant chemotherapy prior to chemoradiation and radical primary surgery. The techniques of extensive pelvic sidewall resection for primary (total mesometrial resection) or recurrent cancer (laterally extended endopelvic resection) have been developed recently to enhance patient survival with acceptable morbidity.

The more difficult challenge will be to impact on cervical cancer cases occurring outwith the developed world.

KEY POINTS

1. In England and Wales, the incidence and mortality of cervical cancer have been decreasing as a result of the introduction of organized screening. Cervical cancer remains the second most common cancer in women worldwide.

2. The cause remains unknown, but HPV infection is widely believed to be a key step. HPV infection is very common in young people, implying that some other factors are necessary before cancer will develop.

3. Conservative treatment of microinvasive lesions should only be considered where invasion is less than 3 mm from the nearest basement membrane and lymphatic channel involvement is not seen.

4. Squamous cell carcinoma is the most common type of cervical cancer and has a similar prognosis to adenocarcinoma. Undifferentiated tumours have a poor prognosis.

5. Metastatic spread is mainly lymphatic, and involvement of the parametria is initially focal rather than confluent.

6. The volume of the primary tumour is one of the most important indications of prognosis after the status of the lymph nodes.

7. MRI with an endovaginal coil gives the best estimate of the volume of the tumour, but MRI is not reliable in identifying nodal disease.

8. Overall, 42% of women with cervical cancer die within 5 years.

9. Surgery is most often performed on the younger patient with lower-volume stage IB disease.

10. Radiotherapy is used for older and less fit patients, regardless of the size of the tumour, and for women with bulky stage IB and IIA tumours or with more advanced disease.

11. Chemoradiation offers a small increase in cure rate but at the cost of increased immediate toxicity.

References

Abu-Rustum NR, Gemignani ML, Moore K et al 2003 Total laparoscopic radical hysterectomy with pelvic lymphadenectomy using the argon-beam coagulator: pilot data and comparison to laparotomy. Gynecological Oncology 91: 402–409.

Albores-Saavedra J, Gersell D, Gilks CB et al 1997 Terminology of endocrine tumors of the uterine cervix: results of a workshop sponsored by the College of American Pathologists and the National Cancer Institute. Archives of Pathology and Laboratory Medicine 121: 34–39.

Anderson B, LaPolla J, Turner D, Chapman G, Buller R 1993 Ovarian transposition in cervical cancer. Gynecological Oncology 49: 206–214.

Appleby P, Beral V, Berrington de González A et al 2007 Cervical cancer and hormonal contraceptives: collaborative reanalysis of individual data for 16,573 women with cervical cancer and 35,509 women without cervical cancer from 24 epidemiological studies. The Lancet 370: 1609–1621.

Bekkers RL, Keyser KG, Bulten J et al 2002 The value of loop electrosurgical conization in the treatment of stage IA1 microinvasive carcinoma of the uterine cervix. International Journal of Gynecological Cancer 12: 485–489.

Benedetti-Panici P, Greggi S, Colombo A et al 2002 Neoadjuvant chemotherapy and radical surgery versus exclusive radiotherapy in locally advanced squamous cell cervical cancer: results from the Italian multicenter randomized study. Journal of Clinical Oncology 20: 179–188.

Berrington de González A, Sweetland S, Green J 2004 Comparison of risk factors for squamous cell and adenocarcinomas of the cervix: a meta-analysis. British Journal of Cancer 90: 1787–1791.

Bodurka-Bevers D, Morris M, Eifel PJ et al 2000 Posttherapy surveillance of women with cervical cancer: an outcome analysis. Gynecological Oncology 78: 187–193.

Bosch FX, Lorincz A, Muñoz N, Meijer CJ, Shah KV 2002 The causal relation between human papillomavirus and cervical cancer. Journal of Clinical Pathology 55: 244–265.

Brown DR, Shew ML, Qadadri B et al 2005 A longitudinal study of genital human papillomavirus infection in a cohort of closely followed adolescent women. Journal of Infectious Diseases 191: 182–192.

Cancer Research UK 2005 www.cancerresearchuk.org.

Cancerstats 2003 Cervical Cancer UK. Cancer Research UK.

Chan YM, Ng TY, Ngan HY, Wong LC 2002 Monitoring of squamous cell carcinoma antigen levels in invasive cervical cancer: is it cost effective? Gynecological Oncology 84: 7–11.

Cibula D, Ungar L, Palfalvi L, Bino B, Kuzel D 2005 Laparoscopic abdominal radical trachelectomy. Gynecological Oncology 97: 707–709.

Cibula D, Slama J, Fischerova D 2008 Update on abdominal radical trachelectomy. Gynecological Oncology 111 (Suppl): S111–S115.

Creasman WT, Zaino RJ, Major FJ, DiSaia PJ, Hatch KD, Homesley HD 1998 Early invasive carcinoma of the cervix (3 to 5 mm invasion): risk factors and prognosis. A Gynecologic Oncology Group study. American Journal of Obstetrics and Gynecology 178: 62–65.

Dargent D, Burn JL, Roy M, Remi I 1994 Pregnancies following radical trachelectomy for invasive cevical cancer. Gynecological Oncology 52: a14.

Duenas-Gonzalez A, Cetina-Perez L, Lopez-Graniel C et al 2005 Pathologic response and toxicity assessment of chemoradiotherapy with cisplatin versus cisplatin plus gemcitabine in cervical cancer: a randomized phase II study. International Journal of Radiation Oncology, Biology and Physics 61: 817–823.

Dunne EF, Unger ER, Sternberg M et al 2007 Prevalence of HPV infection among females in the United States. JAMA: the Journal of the American Medical Association 297: 813–819.

Feeney DD, Moore DH, Look KY, Stehman FB, Sutton GP 1995 The fate of the ovaries after radical hysterectomy and ovarian transposition. Gynecological Oncology 56: 3–7.

Ferlay J et al 2004 Cancer Incidence, Mortality and Prevalence Worldwide. IARC CancerBase No. 5, Version 20. IARC Press, Lyon.

Finan MA, DeCesare S, Fiorica JV et al 1996 Radical hysterectomy for stage IB1 vs IB2 carcinoma of the cervix: does the new staging system predict morbidity and survival? Gynecological Oncology 62: 139–147.

Franco EL, Rohan TE, Villa LL 1999 Epidemiologic evidence and human papillomavirus infection as a necessary cause of cervical cancer. Journal of the National Cancer Institute 91: 506–511.

Friedlander M, Grogan M 2002 Guidelines for the treatment of recurrent and metastatic cervical cancer. The Oncologist 7: 342.

Fujii S, Takakura K, Matsumura N et al 2007 Anatomic identification and functional outcomes of the nerve sparing Okabayashi radical hysterectomy. Gynecological Oncology 107: 4–13.

FUTURE II Study Group 2007 Quadrivalent vaccine against human papillomavirus to prevent high-grade cervical lesions. New England Journal of Medicine 356: 1915–1927.

Ghezzi F, Cromi A, Ciravolo G et al 2007 Surgicopathologic outcome of laparoscopic versus open radical hysterectomy. Gynecological Oncology 106: 502–506.

Grigsby PW, Siegel BA, Dehdashti F 2001 Lymph node staging by positron emission tomography in patients with carcinoma of the cervix. Journal of Clinical Oncology 19: 3745–3749.

Grulich AE, van Leeuwen MT, Falster MO, Vajdic CM 2007 Incidence of cancers in people with HIV/AIDS compared with immunosuppressed transplant recipients: a meta-analysis. The Lancet 370: 59–67.

Hacker NF, Wain GV, Nicklin JL 1995 Resection of bulky positive lymph nodes in patients with cervical carcinoma. International Journal of Gynecological Cancer 5: 250–256.

Hannaford PC, Selvaraj S, Elliott AM, Angus V, Iversen L, Lee AJ 2007 Cancer risk among users of oral contraceptives: cohort data from the Royal College of General Practitioner's oral contraception study. BMJ (Clinical Research Ed.) 335: 651.

Hasumi K, Sakamoto A, Sugano H 1980 Microinvasive carcinoma of the uterine cervix. Cancer 45: 928–931.

Hockel M 2003 Surgical treatment of locally advanced and recurrent cervical carcinoma: overview on current standard and new developments. Onkologie 26: 452–455.

Holschneider CH, Baldwin RL, Tumber K, Aoyama C, Karlan BY 2005 The fragile histidine triad gene: a molecular link between cigarette smoking and cervical cancer. Clinical Cancer Research 11: 5756–5763.

Kapeu AS, Luostarinen T, Jellum E et al 2009 Is smoking an independent risk factor for invasive cervical cancer? A nested case–control study within Nordic biobanks. American Journal of Epidemiology 169: 480–488.

Keys HM, Bundy BN, Stehman FB et al 1999 Cisplatin, radiation, and adjuvant hysterectomy compared with radiation and adjuvant hysterectomy for bulky stage IB cervical carcinoma. New England Journal of Medicine 340: 1154–1161.

Lai CH, Huang KG, Hong JH et al 2003 Randomized trial of surgical staging (extraperitoneal or laparoscopic) versus clinical staging in locally advanced cervical cancer. Gynecological Oncology 89: 160–167.

Lanciano RM, Won M, Coia LR, Hanks GE 1991 Pretreatment and treatment factors associated with improved outcome in squamous cell carcinoma of the uterine cervix: a final report of the 1973 and 1978 patterns of care studies. International Journal of Radiation Oncology, Biology and Physics 20: 667–676.

Landoni F, Maneo A, Colombo A et al 1997 Randomised study of radical surgery versus radiotherapy for stage Ib–IIa cervical cancer. The Lancet 350: 535–540.

Landoni F, Maneo A, Cormio G et al 2001 Class II versus class III radical hysterectomy in stage IB–IIA cervical cancer: a prospective randomized study. Gynecological Oncology 80: 3–12.

Leblanc E, Narducci F, Frumovitz M et al 2007 Therapeutic value of pretherapeutic extraperitoneal laparoscopic staging of locally advanced cervical carcinoma. Gynecological Oncology 105: 304–311.

Levenback C, Coleman RL, Burke TW et al 2002 Lymphatic mapping and sentinel node identification in patients with cervix cancer undergoing radical hysterectomy and pelvic lymphadenectomy. Journal of Clinical Oncology 20: 688–693.

Logsdon MD, Eifel PJ 1999 Figo IIIB squamous cell carcinoma of the cervix: an analysis of prognostic factors emphasizing the balance between external beam and intracavitary radiation therapy. International Journal of Radiation Oncology, Biology and Physics 43: 763–775.

Maiman MA, Fruchter RG, Dimaio TM, Boyce JG 1988 Superficially invasive squamous cell carcinoma of the cervix. Obstetrics and Gynecology 72: 399–403.

Marchiole P, Buenerd A, Benchaib M, Nezhat K, Dargent D, Mathevet P 2005 Clinical significance of lymphovascular space involvement and lymph node micrometastases in early-stage cervical cancer: a retrospective case–control surgico-pathological study. Gynecological Oncology 97: 727–732.

Miller K, Blumenthal P, Blanchard K 2004 Oral contraceptives and cervical cancer: critique of a recent review. Contraception 69: 347–351.

Milliken DA, Shepherd JH 2008 Fertility preserving surgery for carcinoma of the cervix. Current Opinion in Oncology 20: 575–580.

Morice P, Dargent D, Haie-Meder C, Duvillard P, Castaigne D 2004 First case of a centropelvic recurrence after radical trachelectomy: literature review and implications for the preoperative selection of patients. Gynecological Oncology 92: 1002–1005.

Morris M, Eifel PJ, Lu J et al 1999 Pelvic radiation with concurrent chemotherapy compared with pelvic and para-aortic radiation for high-risk cervical cancer. New England Journal of Medicine 340: 1137–1143.

Muñoz N, Bosch FX, de Sanjosé S et al 1992 The causal link between human papillomavirus and invasive cervical cancer: a population-based case–control study in Colombia and Spain. International Journal of Cancer 52: 743–749.

NIH Consensus Development Conference Statement on Cervical Cancer 1997. Gynecological Oncology 66: 351–361.

Odicino F, Tisi G, Rampinelli F, Miscioscia R, Sartori E, Pecorelli S 2007 New development of the FIGO staging system. Gynecological Oncology 107 (Suppl): S8–S9.

Paavonen J, Jenkins D, Bosch FX et al 2007 Efficacy of a prophylactic adjuvanted bivalent L1 virus-like-particle vaccine against infection with human papillomavirus types 16 and 18 in young women: an interim analysis of a phase III double-blind, randomised controlled trial. The Lancet 369: 2161–2170.

Pagliusi SR, Teresa Aguado M 2004 Efficacy and other milestones for human papillomavirus vaccine introduction. Vaccine 23: 569–578.

Pichiorri F, Palumbo T, Suh SS et al 2008 Fhit tumor suppressor: guardian of the preneoplastic genome. Future Oncology 4: 815–824.

Piver MS, Rutledge F, Smith JP 1974 Five classes of extended hysterectomy for women with cervical cancer. Obstetrics and Gynecology 70: 172–175.

Plante M, Renaud MC, Roy M 2005 Radical vaginal trachelectomy: a fertility-preserving option for young women with early stage cervical cancer. Gynecological Oncology 99 (Suppl 1): S143–S146.

Rogers LJ, Luesley DM 2009 Stage 1A2 cervical cancer: how much treatment is enough? International Journal of Gynecological Cancer 19: 1620–1624.

Rose PG, Bundy BN, Watkins EB et al 1999 Concurrent cisplatin-based radiotherapy and chemotherapy for locally advanced cervical cancer. New England Journal of Medicine 340: 1144–1153.

Sananes C, Giaroli A, Soderini A et al 1998 Neoadjuvant chemotherapy followed by radical hysterectomy and postoperative adjuvant chemotherapy in the treatment of carcinoma of the cervix uteri: long-term follow-up of a pilot study. European Journal of Gynaecological Oncology 19: 368–373.

Sasieni P, Adams J 2001 Changing rates of adenocarcinoma and adenosquamous carcinoma of the cervix in England. The Lancet 357: 1490–1493.

Schiffman MH, Haley NJ, Felton JS et al 1987 Biochemical epidemiology of cervical neoplasia: measuring cigarette smoke constituents in the cervix. Cancer Research 47: 3886–3888.

Schiffman MH, Bauer HM, Hoover RN et al 1993 Epidemiologic evidence showing that human papillomavirus infection causes most cervical intraepithelial neoplasia. Journal of the National Cancer Institute 85: 958–964.

Schiffman MH, Brinton LA 1995 The epidemiology of cervical carcinogenesis. Cancer 76: 1888–1901.

Sedlis A, Bundy BN, Rotman MZ, Lentz SS, Muderspach LI, Zaino RJ 1999 A randomized trial of pelvic radiation therapy versus no further therapy in selected patients with stage IB carcinoma of the cervix after radical hysterectomy and pelvic lymphadenectomy: a Gynecologic Oncology Group study. Gynecological Oncology 73: 177–183.

Shapley M, Jordan J, Croft PR 2006 A systematic review of postcoital bleeding and risk of cervical cancer. British Journal of General Practice 56: 453–460.

Shepherd JH, Milliken DA 2008 Conservative surgery for carcinoma of the cervix. Clinical Oncology (Royal College of Radiologists) 20: 395–400.

Simen-Kapeu A, Kataja V, Yliskoski M et al 2008 Smoking impairs human papillomavirus (HPV) type 16 and 18 capsids antibody response following natural HPV infection. Scandinavian Journal of Infectious Diseases 40: 745–751.

Simon NL, Gore H, Shingleton HM, Soong SJ, Orr JW Jr, Hatch KD 1986 Study of superficially invasive carcinoma of the cervix. Obstetrics and Gynecology 68: 19–24.

Singh N, Titmuss E, Chin AJ et al 2004 A review of post-trachelectomy isthmic and vaginal smear cytology. Cytopathology 15: 97–103.

Smith JS 2003 Cervical cancer and use of hormonal contraceptives: a systematic review. The Lancet 361: 1159–1167.

Smith JS, Lindsay L, Hoots B et al 2007 Human papillomavirus type distribution in invasive cervical cancer and high-grade cervical lesions: a meta-analysis update. International Journal of Cancer 121: 621–632.

Smith HO, Tiffany MF, Qualls CR, Key CR 2000 The rising incidence of adenocarcinoma relative to squamous cell carcinoma of the uterine cervix in the United States — a 24-year population-based study. Gynecological Oncology 78: 97–105.

Stegeman M, Louwen M, van der Velden J et al 2007 The incidence of parametrial tumor involvement in select patients with early cervix cancer is too low to justify parametrectomy. Gynecological Oncology 105: 475–480.

Sutton GP, Bundy BN, Delgado G et al 1992 Ovarian metastases in stage IB carcinoma of the cervix: a Gynecologic Oncology Group study. American Journal of Obstetrics and Gynecology 166: 50–53.

Syrjänen K, Shabalova I, Petrovichev N et al 2006 Oral contraceptives are not an independent risk factor for cervical intraepithelial neoplasia or high-risk human papillomavirus infections. Anticancer Research 26: 4729–4740.

Trimbos JB, Franchi M, Zanaboni F, Velden J, Vergote I 2004 'State of the art' of radical hysterectomy; current practice in European oncology centres. European Journal of Cancer 40: 375–378.

Ursin G, Peters RK, Henderson BE, d'Ablaing G 3rd, Monroe KR, Pike MC 1994 Oral contraceptive use and adenocarcinoma of cervix. The Lancet 344: 1390–1394.

van Nagell JR Jr, Greenwell N, Powell DF, Donaldson ES, Hanson MB, Gay EC 1983 Microinvasive carcinoma of the cervix. American Journal of Obstetrics and Gynecology 145: 981–991.

Walboomers JM, Meijer CJ 1997 Do HPV-negative cervical carcinomas exist? Journal of Pathology 181: 253–254.

Walboomers JM, Jacobs MV, Manos MM et al 1999 Human papillomavirus is a necessary cause of invasive cervical cancer worldwide. Journal of Pathology 189: 12–19.

Winkelstein W 1990 Smoking and cervical cancer: current status — a review. American Journal of Epidemiology 131: 945–957.

Woodman CB, Collins S, Winter H et al 2001 Natural history of cervical human papillomavirus infection in young women: a longitudinal cohort study. The Lancet 357: 1831–1836.

Wright JD, Grigsby PW, Brooks R et al 2007 Utility of parametrectomy for early stage cervical cancer treated with radical hysterectomy. Cancer 110: 1281–1286.

CHAPTER 40

Benign disease of the vulva and the vagina

Allan Maclean and Wendy Reid

Chapter Contents

DEVELOPMENT AND ANATOMY	599	VULVAL ULCERATION	606
CLASSIFICATION OF VULVAL DISEASE	600	VULVAL INFECTION	606
PRESENTATION OF VULVAL DISEASE	600	BENIGN TUMOURS OF THE VULVA	608
EXAMINATION OF THE PATIENT	600	VAGINAL INFECTION	608
PREVALENCE OF VULVAL LESIONS	601	OTHER VAGINAL PATHOLOGY	609
USE OF TOPICAL CORTICOSTEROIDS	601	BENIGN TUMOURS OF THE VAGINA	610
DERMATOSES	602	FEMALE CIRCUMCISION/GENITAL MUTILATION	610
VULVAL PAIN/VULVODYNIA	605	KEY POINTS	610

Patients with vulval symptoms are not uncommon in gynaecological practice. The complaint is often longstanding, distressing and frequently induces a feeling of despair in both patient and doctor. A careful, sympathetic approach and a readiness to consult colleagues in other disciplines are essential. Even when it seems that no specific therapy can be offered, many patients are helped by the knowledge that there is no serious underlying pathology and by a supportive attitude.

Development and Anatomy

The vulva and vagina develop in association with the urogenital sinus, the caudal end of the paramesonephric or Müllerian ducts, and the development of the anus posteriorly and bladder and urethra anteriorly. Debate continues regarding how much of the lower vagina, hymen and vestibule originate from the ectoderm, the endoderm of the hindgut forming the urogenital sinus and the mesoderm of the paramesonephric ducts. Developmental abnormalities are not unusual and range from a single cloaca to variations in vaginal development, including agenesis or the presence of a transverse or midline septum.

The vulva consists of the labia majora, labia minora, mons pubis, clitoris, perineum and the vestibule. The labia join anteriorly at the anterior commissure and merge posteriorly into the perineum, the anterior margin of which is the posterior commissure. From puberty, the mons and lateral parts of the labia majora are covered in strong coarse hair and are distended with subcutaneous fat. In addition to hair follicles, they contain sebaceous and sweat (eccrine and apocrine) glands. The labia minora are two smaller, longitudinal, cutaneous, non-hair-bearing folds medial to the labia majora and extending from the clitoris for a variable distance beside the vestibule to end before reaching the perineum. The labia majora and minora are separated from each other by the interlabial fold, and may contain prominent or tortuous veins during pregnancy and later life. The labia minora contain numerous blood vessels, nerve endings and sebaceous glands. There is considerable variation in size and shape from woman to woman, and gross enlargement or asymmetry can occur. Anteriorly, they fuse above the clitoris to form the prepuce and below the clitoris to form the frenulum. The labia minora have an important role during sexual arousal when they become engorged and extend or are pushed outwards to allow coital entry; when flaccid, they serve to protect the vestibule and access to the urethra and vagina (O'Connell et al 2008).

The clitoris consists of a body formed of the two corpora cavernosa composed of erectile tissue enclosed in a fibrous membrane and attached to the puboischial ramus on each side by the crus. The body of the clitoris ends in the glans which also contains spongy tissue and nerve endings. The clitoris has a rich blood supply which comes from the terminal branches of the pudendal arteries.

The vagina consists of a non-keratinized squamous epithelial lining supported by connective tissue and surrounded by circular and longitudinal muscle coats. Vaginal epithelium

DOI: 10.1016/B978-0-7020-3120-5.00040-0

has a longitudinal column on the anterior and posterior walls, and from each column, numerous transverse ridges or rugae extend laterally on each side. The squamous epithelium is thick and rich in glycogen during the reproductive years. It does not change significantly during the menstrual cycle. The prepubertal and postmenopausal vaginal epithelium is thin or atrophic. Engorgement and transudation of the distal vagina are important components of normal sexual response.

The vulvovaginal vestibule is the cleft between the labia minora. It is covered by non-keratinized squamous epithelium and extends cranially from the hymen to reach the keratinized skin at Hart's line. The vestibule contains the entrance to the vagina, the urethral meatus, and the ducts of the greater (Bartholin's) and lesser vestibular and periurethral glands. Further features are included below in the section on vulvodynia.

Classification of Vulval Disease

Terminology of lesions and conditions of the vulva has caused confusion because of the many and complex names used, sometimes for similar changes. The International Society for the Study of Vulvovaginal Disease (ISSVD) has published a classification of vulvar dermatoses (Lynch et al 2007) (Box 40.1). Its use is not universal but it serves as a starting point to group some of the diseases described in this chapter.

Presentation of Vulval Disease

The majority of women present with vulval pruritus (itch) and associated scratching. Others will present with pain, burning, soreness, rawness, stinging or irritation but without scratching. However, the symptoms do not necessarily imply a particular condition. Sometimes a lesion will be noted as white, red or pigmented, or as raised or ulcerated. Some lesions will be asymptomatic.

The onset of symptoms will sometimes be associated with other life events such as following a course of antibiotics, a diagnosis of certain medical disorders, the introduction of certain therapeutic drugs or withdrawal of systemic corticosteroids. A full medical history will sometimes identify other conditions with vulval manifestations, and dental details should not be overlooked. Some patients with vulvovaginal lichen planus will already have a diagnosis of oral lichen planus; Belfiore et al (2006) found that 57% of women with oral lichen planus also had vulval lichen planus. Many patients will present with a list or bag full of topical treatments that they have used previously. A comprehensive list is useful because those drugs that have helped or caused deterioration can be identified, and this will also allow confident prescription of a preparation not yet tried.

Examination of the Patient

General examination of the patient should include inspection of the buccal, lingual and gingival mucosa and the skin of the face, hands, finger nails, wrists, elbows, scalp, trunk and knees. Evidence of systemic disease such as diabetes, and hepatic, renal or haematological disease should be sought. Where appropriate, urinalysis or blood testing should also be performed.

A combined clinic conducted by gynaecologists, dermatologists and genitourinary physicians has considerable merit (McCullough et al 1987). Facilities should include adequate lighting, a tilting examination chair to obtain access to the posterior part of the pudendum, a colposcope, and a camera for colpophotography and clinical photography.

Examination should consist of inspection of the vulva including the vestibule, urethral meatus, perineum and perianal area. Patients with neoplastic disorders must also have the cervix and vagina examined, but many older patients and those with lichen sclerosus will not tolerate a speculum examination and, unless there is any specific symptom, it is unnecessary to include this as part of the examination.

Colposcopic assessment of the vulva is not essential if there is an obvious, readily diagnosed lesion and there are

---

Box 40.1 ISSVD 2006 classification of vulvar dermatoses: pathological subsets and their clinical correlates

Spongiotic pattern
Atopic dermatitis
Allergic contact dermatitis
Irritant contact dermatitis

Acanthotic pattern (formerly squamous cell hyperplasia)
Psoriasis
Lichen simplex chronicus
Primary (idiopathic)
Secondary (superimposed on lichen sclerosus, lichen planus or other vulvar disease)

Lichenoid pattern
Lichen sclerosus
Lichen planus

Dermal homogenization/sclerosis pattern
Lichen sclerosus

Vesiculobullous pattern
Pemphigoid, cicatricial type
Linear immunoglobulin A disease

Acantholytic pattern
Hailey–Hailey disease
Darier's disease
Papular genitocrural acantholysis

Granulomatous pattern
Crohn's disease
Melkersson–Rosenthal syndrome

Vasculopathic pattern
Aphthous ulcers
Behçet's disease
Plasma cell vulvitis

no suggestions of neoplastic change. However, colposcopy is valuable if the patient is symptomatic but no lesion can be seen, if there is difficulty in interpreting or defining the limits of the visible lesions, and to select an appropriate site for biopsy. The techniques are described elsewhere (MacLean and Reid 1995). The vascular patterns can be complex and may be associated with neoplasia. Sometimes, sites of previous biopsies will develop unusual vascular patterns associated with healing. Excessive applications of potent topical corticosteroids will exaggerate vascularity with prominent telangiectasia and thinned epidermis.

Once the vulva has been scanned with the colposcope, aqueous acetic acid solution should be applied. It is important to realize that the aceto-white changes will not be as dramatic as those seen on the cervix, and may not be apparent in areas of abnormal keratinization. Aceto-white epithelium may represent vulvar intraepithelial neoplasia (VIN) or viral changes with human papilloma virus (HPV) and Epstein-Barr virus, as well as tissue repair with ulcers and erosions, scratch damage or coital trauma. It is incorrect to interpret the papillae seen in the vestibule as 'microwarts'; Jonsson et al (1997) showed that aceto-white changes in the vulva were a poor predictor of viral presence.

In the past, histological diagnosis of the vulval lesions depended on inpatient biopsy performed under general anaesthesia. Very appropriate biopsy material can be obtained using a 4 mm diameter Stiefel disposable sterile biopsy punch, and this can be performed as an outpatient procedure under local anaesthesia (McCullough et al 1987). A silver nitrate stick with a small plug of cotton wool or, alternatively, ferric subsulphate (Monsel's solution) is applied for haemostasis.

Prevalence of Vulval Lesions

Box 40.2 shows the range of lesions seen in a combined vulva clinic (MacLean et al 1998). There may be some bias

Box 40.2 Prevalence of vulval lesions seen in 1000 women	
Lichen sclerosus	243
Dermatitis/lichen simplex	56
Lichen planus	23
Localized provoked vulvodynia	98
Generalized vulvodynia	32
Psoriasis	25
Diabetic vulvitis	9
Vulval Crohn's disease	5
Acute contact vulvitis	2
Cicatricial pemphigoid	2
Plasma cell vulvitis	2
Neoplastic	
Cancer	23
VIN, usual type	82
Paget's disease	4
Melanoma	2

Source: MacLean AB, Roberts DT, Reid WMN 1998 Review of 1000 women seen at two specially designated vulval clinics. Current Opinion in Obstetrics and Gynaecology 8: 159–162.

in these figures because the clinic received referrals from gynaecologists, and because the authors' research interests included vulval precancer and pain.

Infections included recurrent candidiasis, bacterial vaginosis, trichomoniasis, herpes simplex virus, condyomata acuminata, ulcers associated with human immunodeficiency virus, hidradenitis suppurativa, *Enterobius vermicularis* (threadworms) and vulva lymphoedema secondary to filariasis, and were not enumerated because they sometimes coexisted with other conditions.

Use of Topical Corticosteroids

As many gynaecologists are apprehensive about the use of topical corticosteroids in the vulval area, some basic information is desirable.

Topical steroids are effective in the management of inflammatory changes but are contraindicated in the presence of untreated infection. In some situations, corticosteroids can be combined with an antifungal or antibacterial agent, but care must be taken with the latter because an allergic contact dermatitis can develop.

Topical preparations are suspended in a vehicle, usually as a cream or ointment. Creams are miscible with skin secretions, easy to apply smoothly (and sparingly) but may contain additive to which the patient will become sensitized. Ointments are usually insoluble in water, greasy in texture and therefore more difficult to apply and more occlusive than creams. As they encourage hydration, they are better suited for dry lesions. Pastes are stiffer but useful for localized lesions. They are less occlusive than ointments and can be used to protect excoriated or ulcerated lesions.

Topical corticosteroids are graded according to their potency, which reflects the degree of absorption or penetration through a lesion to be effective. A very potent steroid is necessary if there is lichenification or hyperkeratosis, or if the inflammatory changes are predominantly within the dermis. These include clobetasol propionate 0.05% (Dermovate) and diflucortolone valerate 0.3% (Nerisone Forte). Potent preparations include betamethasone 0.1% (Betnovate) and triamcinolone acetonide 0.1% (Adcortyl), moderately potent preparations include clobetasone butyrate 0.05% (Eumovate) and mild preparations include hydrocortisone 1%.

Patients will have anxieties about applying potent topical corticosteroids, particularly because some of the patient information with the packaging advises against their use in the genital area. This can be reduced by giving the patient written instructions on their use, either as an information sheet or in a letter with specific instructions for the patient.

Long-term use of potent corticosteroids does have side-effects which include the development of telangiectasia, striae, thinning of the skin, increased hair growth and mild depigmentation. However, clinical experience finds that this is rare for vulval applications, and is more likely when large amounts are spread over the buttocks or inner thighs. There is a risk of worsening infection if steroids are applied where yeast or fungal organisms are present. Systemic absorption is rarely seen. Side-effects can be reduced by using less potent preparations where possible. However, it is better to use more potent steroids to gain relief and then reduce either the potency or the frequency of application to maintain control. Sudden cessation will often produce a rebound of symptoms. A 30 g tube of Dermovate, if used appropriately [i.e. one application using a fingertip length (approximately 0.5 g) as squeezed from the tube] should last between 3 and 6 months.

On nights when topical steroids are not being applied or during the day, emollients can be applied to soothe and smooth the surface and to act as a moisturizer. Some emollients must be used with care in certain patients, such as those who have a history of irritation with wool, as components [e.g. wool fat (lanolin) or preservatives] can cause sensitization. Examples of emollients include aqueous cream BP, E45, Sudocrem, Ultrabase and Unguentum Merck (creams); Diprobase (cream or ointment); and emulsifying ointment BP, zinc and castor oil ointment BP (ointments). Some of these are suitable as soap substitutes (emulsifying ointment, aqueous cream), or preparations such as Alphakeri, Balneum or Oilatum can be added to the bath or shower (but can make the bath or shower dangerously slippery for the unsuspecting).

Dermatoses

While dermatologists will have little difficulty in reaching a diagnosis with these lesions, most gynaecologists are likely to be less certain. One of the confusing issues is the interchangeable use of the terms 'eczema' and 'dermatitis'; essentially they mean the same thing. Dermatitis is found in 64% of patients with chronic vulval symptoms (Fischer et al 1995). Many of these patients will have skin manifestations elsewhere and will be identified by history and examination. The term 'atopic dermatitis' is used when there is clinical evidence of atopy (e.g. asthma, hayfever or allergic rhinitis in the patient or immediate family). In some cases, biopsy and histology will be diagnostic. Many lesions will respond to topical corticosteroids, although the required potency will depend on the diagnosis.

Contact and irritant dermatitis

Contact dermatitis occurs as an allergic response to various allergens including topical antibiotics, anaesthetic and antihistamine creams, deodorants and perfumes (e.g. Balsam of Peru as used in various haemorrhoid creams), lanolin, azo-dyes in nylons, biological washing powders, spermicidals, latex of sheaths or diaphragms, etc. An increasing number of referrals to vulval clinics are being seen because of the current trend to remove vulval hair. Some women have applied depilatory creams or waxes with subsequent irritant reaction, while others have inflicted skin damage by shaving.

Clinically, there is a diffuse erythema and oedema with superimposed infection or lichenification. Patch testing may identify the allergen to allow removal or avoidance of the factor, and moisturizing cream or mild steroids should provide local control. Haverhoek et al (2008) reported that 81% of the patients that they saw with vulval pruritus had at least one contact allergen detected on patch testing.

Some topical preparations will cause irritation over time (i.e. in a chronic fashion). The vulval appearances will be less obvious, with minimal erythema but with pallor or

pigmentation, and with dryness, thickening and cracking — lichenification, or lichen simplex chronicus. Lichen simplex chronicus (previously known as 'neurodermatitis') occurs in normal skin which becomes thick and fissured in response to the trauma of constant scratching. Lichenification is a similar change which is superimposed on another pathology such as dermatitis. These lesions are not usually symmetrical and occur in vulval areas accessible to scratching.

Treatment consists of the use of emollients or topical corticosteroids of low-to-moderate potency. Sometimes, sedation at night is useful to stop nocturnal scratching. Once control is gained, assessment for an underlying cause or lesion is often necessary.

Psoriasis

Psoriasis may occur exclusively on the vulva, but often there are lesions elsewhere and a family history. It affects approximately 2% of the population. Unlike psoriatic lesions elsewhere on elbows, knees and scalp, they are unlikely to show the hyperkeratotic silvery scales but are often salmon-pink in appearance with a sharp but irregular outline and with satellite lesions. Vulval psoriasis is treated with mild or moderately potent topical corticosteroids.

Lichenoid lesions and vulval intraepithelial neoplasia

Terms such as 'ichthyosis', 'leucoplakia', 'kraurosis', 'lichen planus sclereux' and 'dystrophy' have created confusion in describing vulval lesions (Ridley 1988). The current terminology has evolved from the ISSVD's 1976 classification of hyperplastic dystrophy, lichen sclerosus (no longer with 'et atrophicus') and mixed dystrophy; the abandonment of the term 'dystrophy' (MacLean 1991); and the use of the term 'non-neoplastic epithelial disorder of vulval skin and mucosa' (Ridley et al 1989) which included lichen sclerosus, squamous cell hyperplasia (formerly hyperplastic dystrophy) and other dermatoses. This did not cover those lesions with neoplastic potential or association, and the latest terminology incorporates 'differentiated vulvar intraepithelial neoplasia' for those lichenoid lesions with basal atypia and a significant association with vulval cancer (Sideri et al 2005, Scurry and Wilkinson 2006). This new terminology has met opposition, firstly because it removes the VIN 1, 2 and 3 classification which sat comfortably with CIN 1, 2 and 3 of the cervix, and replaces it with a single-grade system VIN (which groups together VIN 2 and 3 plus differentiated VIN). VIN 1 is uncommon compared with CIN 1. There is no evidence that it is a cancer precursor, and it is best considered as a warty lesion with no need for treatment and follow-up as one would do for the former VIN 2 and 3 lesions. The VIN frequently associated with HPV is now known as 'usual or classic type' (sometimes divided into basaloid and Bowenoid or warty subtypes, but this is not always meaningful because both subtypes are linked with HPV 16, and both appearances can occur in the same vulva). On the other hand, atypia or abnormality confined to the basal layer of lichen sclerosus (previously designated 'hyperplastic/ hypertrophic or mixed dystrophy with atypia' may appear consistent with VIN 1 but has a significant association with vulval carcinoma, and thus differentiated VIN is regarded as high grade (Jeffcoate and Woodcock 1961, Leibowitch et al 1990, Scurry et al 1997). There are opinions that differentiated VIN is only found in the immediate vicinity when vulval cancer develops within an area of lichen sclerosus, but also a growing awareness of the basal cell changes (e.g. overexpression of *p53*, *Ki-67* and *CD1a*) (Mulveny and Allen 2008) to provide the diagnosis in biopsies taken when cancer is not coexistent. Such cases are believed to have a greater risk of progressing to invasive cancer than cases with lichen sclerosus alone. Eva et al (2008) reported that there is an almost four-fold higher risk of recurrence when vulval cancer occurs in association with differentiated VIN.

Lichen sclerosus

The importance of lichen sclerosus is that it is common, occurring in at least one in 800 girls (Powell 2006) and increasing to one in 30 elderly women (Leibovitz et al 2000). It accounts for up to one-quarter of women seen in vulval clinics (MacLean et al 1998), 1.7% of patients seen in general gynaecological practice (Goldstein et al 2005) and 0.3–1 per 1000 of all new patients seen in a general hospital (Wallace 1971). It occurs in men, where it is known as balanitis xerotica obliterans, but at approximately one-sixth to one-tenth of the incidence in women. It is an inflammatory dermatosis and is frequently symptomatic, causing pruritus, sleeplessness, dyspareunia and constipation. It may produce major architectural changes and alteration in vulval appearance and function, and has a small but important risk of cancer; 60–70% of vulval squamous cell cancers occur against a background of or in association with lichen sclerosus. Lichen sclerosus involves the pudendum, either partially or completely as a figure-of-eight lesion encircling the vestibule and involving the clitoris, labia minora, inner aspects of the labia majora and the skin surrounding the anus. It is usually bilateral and symmetrical. It does not involve the vestibule or extend into the vagina or anal canal.

The lesions consist of thin, pearly, ivory or porcelain white crinkly plaques. Sometimes, there is marked shrinkage and absorption of the labia minora, coaptation of the labia across the clitoris to form a phimosis, and narrowing of the introitus to obscure the urethra and make intercourse impossible. Scratching will produce lichenification or may produce epidermal erosion and ulceration. Areas of ecchymoses and subsequent pigmentation are common. Lichen sclerosus may also involve the trunk or limbs in 18% of patients (Meyrick-Thomas et al 1988).

The histological features of lichen sclerosus typically show epidermal atrophy, dermal oedema, hyalinization of the collagen and subdermal chronic inflammatory cell infiltrate. There is a correlation between clinical appearance and histology, with the clinically thin area showing marked epidermal thinning with loss of rete ridges and vacuolation of the basal cells, while thick white fissured areas will histologically show hyperkeratosis, parakeratosis (abnormal keratinization) acanthosis and elongation, widening and blunting of the rete ridges (lichen sclerosus with lichenification; Ridley 1988). The inflammatory infiltrate may extend into the superficial dermis. These histological features are often modified secondary to trauma, with the presence of red blood cells or haemosiderin. However, histological changes may be minimal, and the histology may appear normal in some clinically obvious cases.

Cause of lichen sclerosus

The aetiology of lichen sclerosus remains unknown. Its uneven distribution between countries raises the possibility of an infectious cause (e.g. *Borrelia burgdorferi* spread by tick bites), but while there has been demonstration of these spirochaetes (Aberer and Stanek 1987), subsequent studies have not supported this theory.

The possibility of a hormonal (androgen-associated) cause has been examined without conclusive results (Friedrich and Kalra 1984, Kohlberger et al 1998). There is recognition that the incidence is higher among postmenopausal women, but no evidence that it is due to oestrogen deficiency. Young girls with lichen sclerosus seem to gain symptom improvement at puberty, but one study has documented that 75% of these teenagers have persistent features of lichen sclerosus (Powell and Wojnarowska 2002).

The suggestion that lichen sclerosus might be related to an autoimmune process is supported by finding associations with other autoimmune manifestations, a family history of autoimmune-related disease in first-degree relatives or the presence of circulating autoantibodies in patients with lichen sclerosus (Goolamali et al 1974, Meyrick-Thomas et al 1988). Recently, circulating basement membrane zone antibodies have been found in the serum of patients with lichen sclerosus (Howard et al 2004), and a specific circulating autoantibody to extracellular matrix protein 1 (ECM1) has been described (Oyama et al 2003). The nature of ECM1 epitopes in the serum of patients with lichen sclerosus has been examined, and an enzyme-linked immunosorbent assay has been developed which is highly sensitive and specific for lichen sclerosus, and discriminates between lichen sclerosus and other disease/control sera (Oyama et al 2004). Higher anti-ECM1 titres correlated with more longstanding and refractory disease and cases complicated by carcinoma. The factors that initiated this antibody are unknown, or its appearance may predate the development of lesions or symptoms. Investigation of the inflammatory process has demonstrated oxidative damage to lipids, proteins and DNA in biopsies taken from untreated patients with lichen sclerosus (Sander et al 2004). Interferon-γ has been demonstrated within lesional epidermis, underlying dermis and the zone of inflammation, along with other cytokines including tumour necrosis factor-α, interleukin-1α, IL-2 receptor CD25, intercellular adhesion molecule _1 CD11a and ICAM-1 ligand ICAM-1 (Farrell et al 2006).

Some supportive evidence for a genetic cause has been described (Marren et al 1995), and a link with human leukocye antigen (HLA) DQ7 has been demonstrated (Tasker and Wojnarowska 2003). Gao et al (2005) reported an increased frequency of DRB1*12 (DR12) and the haplotype DRB1*12/DQB1*0308/04/08/010, and a lower frequency of DRB1*0301/04 (DR17) among 187 women with lichen sclerosus, suggesting that HLA DR and DQ antigens or their haplotypes are involved in susceptibility and protection from lichen sclerosus.

Treatment of lichen sclerosus

Most dermatologists and gynaecologists now use topical steroids, such as clobetasol, and bland emollients to treat lichen sclerosus (Tidy et al 1996). However, it is only relatively recently that the effectiveness of topical steroids has been confirmed (Dalziel et al 1989, 1991, Lorenz et al 1998, Sinha et al 1999). Most patients will respond to nightly applications within a few weeks, but treatment can be continued for 1 month followed by alternate nights for the second month and twice weekly in the third month. A fingertip amount (approximately 0.5 g) is applied each time, and a 30 g tube of clobetasol should last for 3 months (Neill et al 2002). If patients do not improve, coexisting fungal infection, sensitization to the cream or coexisting carcinoma must be considered.

Renaud-Vilmer et al (2004) used a similar protocol for 83 women with lichen sclerosus, and calculated that the estimated incidence of remission at 3 years was 72% in women under 50 years of age, 23% in women aged 50–70 years and 0% in women over 70 years of age. The incidence of relapse was estimated to be 50% at 16 months and 84% at 4 years, and age was not a factor in relapse rate. Thus, discontinuation of treatment is likely to lead to a return of symptoms. Cooper et al (2004) reported on 327 patients managed in Oxford; 96% had symptom improvement with treatment (66% complete responses and 30% partial responses). Among the 253 patients who had clinical appearances recorded, 23% showed a total response with return to normal colour and texture, 68% showed a partial response, 7% showed a minor response and 2% showed a poor response.

Patients with squamous hyperplasia are less likely to respond (Clark et al 1999), but longer use or very potent steroids might be more successful. There is no advantage in applying oestrogen cream or testosterone ointment to the vulva.

Physical destruction by cryotherapy or laser ablation of areas of lichen sclerosus no longer seems justified, and nor is vulvectomy. Very occasionally, it may be necessary to divide labial or preputial adhesions.

Relationship between lichen sclerosus and vulval squamous cell carcinoma

This relationship continues to be an area of debate, and the positive side of the argument has been presented elsewhere (MacLean 1993, 2000a). Several authors have reported a prevalence of carcinoma of 2.5–5% in women who present with lichen sclerosus (Friedrich 1985, Meyrick-Thomas et al 1988). It is unlikely that the development of malignancy led to the appearance of lichen sclerosus, although many of these women denied having had symptoms for any duration. Nevertheless, there are individual cases or series of cases that document carcinoma occurring some time after a clinical diagnosis of lichen sclerosus, in spite of the use of appropriate clobetasol therapy. Jones et al (2004) reported that women who develop cancer with lichen sclerosus are more likely to show clinical evidence of squamous hyperplasia, and are more likely to have been symptomatic for 5 years or more (Jones and Joura 1999). Cooper et al (2004) reported that six women developed carcinoma in spite of treatment in their series. Renaud-Vilmer et al (2004) reported that among eight women who developed cancer, one had discontinued treatment 3 years earlier, and a second patient had used treatment irregularly.

There are concerns that certain treatments may increase the risk of cancer. There have been publications advocating the application of tacrolimus or pimecrolimus as alternatives to steroids, but following reports of apparently rapid progression to cancer, the US Food and Drug Administration released a warning advising caution with their use (Edwards 2008).

Many vulval cancers have lichen sclerosus in the adjacent skin, and the changes have been studied for various molecular alterations including changes in tumour suppressor gene activity and increased expression of mutant *p53* (Kagie et al 1997, Kohlberger et al 1995), and allelic imbalance with loss of heterozygosity or allelic gain (Pinto et al 2000). The authors' group have identified a mutation in codon 136 of exon 5 for *p53* found in the areas of invasion and also in the adjacent lichen sclerosus (Rolfe et al 2003). Several patients with lichen sclerosus plus hyperplasia have progressed to carcinoma, and it is suggested that immunohistochemical staining of increased expression of *p53* and *Ki-67* may be a useful predictor of progression before invasion occurs (Rolfe et al 2001).

Until we have a better way of anticipating which patients with lichen sclerosus are at greatest risk of developing cancer, it is recommended that any patient who has difficulty with symptom control should be referred to a specialist/specialist clinic. This includes women who require topical potent corticosteroid application three or more times a week, or who use more than 30 g clobetasol in 6 months for symptom control. Women with clinical evidence of localized skin thickening/hyperkeratosis require biopsies. If the skin contains differentiated VIN or other features of concern, a short intensive course of topical treatment should be followed by review biopsies. Persistent areas of differentiated VIN require excision. Particular care is needed in the follow-up of patients who have already been managed for cancer, because their chance of recurrence is higher than for other patients with lichen sclerosus (Jones et al 2008).

The following mnemonic may be helpful when assessing lichen sclerosus:

Labial changes (e.g. reduction or fusion)
Introital changes (e.g. narrowing)
Clitoral changes including phimosis
Hyperkeratosis
Elevated or eroded areas
Neoplastic or suspicious area with hyperkeratosis or contour changes
Symptom control
Colour, usually with pallor but also ecchymoses
Localization, usually central
Extension posteriorly, causing anal symptoms and constipation
Rest of body; involvement elsewhere
Other autoimmune conditions or associated symptoms
Sexual difficulties
Urinary difficulties
Steroid use and misuse

Lichen planus

The lesions of lichen planus may be seen on mucous membranes or on cutaneous surfaces such as the inner surfaces of the wrists and lower legs. These cutaneous lesions are usually red or purple flat-topped nodules, or papules with an overlying white lacy-patterned appearance.

Involvement of the vulva is usually with white patterned areas that are sometimes elevated and thickened (hypertrophic lichen planus), or may appear red and raw with features of erosion. Changes in the mouth are often seen. The vulval lesions may extend into the vagina where scarring, stenosis and adhesions make intercourse painful or impossible. In a small number of cases, 'crossover' from lichen sclerosus (involving the vulval skin) to lichen planus (involving the vestibule and vaginal mucosa) occurs.

Histology will show liquefactive degeneration of the basal epidermal layer, long and pointed rete ridges, with parakeratosis, acanthosis and a dense dermal infiltrate of lymphocytes close to the dermal epidermal margin. Immunohistochemistry shows differences in the expression of interleukin-4 and interferon-α between lichen planus and lichen sclerosus (Carli et al 1997).

When the condition is severe, treatment can be difficult, requiring systemic steroids, azathioprine or other immune-modifying agents. Lesser symptoms, particularly those externally on the vulva, can be managed with the application of topical corticosteroids; vaginal lesions can be managed with Colifoam (hydrocortisone) or Predfoam (prednisolone). Rarely, vulval cancer will arise in association with lichen planus (Dwyer et al 1995, Zaki et al 1996).

Paget's disease of the vulva

This is an uncommon lesion with uncertain malignant potential. Its appearance is of an eczematoid lesion with a scaly surface but vague margins, or it may be sharply bordered with a red and velvety texture, with areas or islands of hyperkeratosis. Histology classically shows large round atypical cells with oval nuclei and pale cytoplasm, singly or within clusters among the basal cells of the epidermis. These cells stain positively with cytokeratin 7, PAS para-aminosalcylic and CEA carcinomaembryonic antigen, and are regarded by many as carcinoma *in situ*. Their origin is uncertain. Their similarity to Paget's cells seen in the nipple, usually with underlying breast carcinoma, questions their association with cancers. Studies of large numbers of vulval Paget's cases report that less than 10% of cases will have an underlying adenocarcinoma of the vulva arising from an adnexal structure, and another 20% or more will have a carcinoma arising from adjacent viscera including rectocolon, endocervix or endometrium, ovary, urinary tract or breast. Wilkinson and Brown (2002) have proposed a classification that separates the lesions into those where the Paget's lesion is *in situ* without any associated cancer, those with an underlying adenocarcinoma of a skin appendage or a subcutaneous gland, and those that are secondary to an underlying anorectal adenocarcinoma, a urothelial cancer or an adenocarcinoma arising from elsewhere (this latter group may be suspected by finding cytokeratin 20 expression in the Paget's lesion). A small number of cases appear to progress from *in situ* to invasive adenocarcinoma if left untreated or undertreated.

Treatment by surgery is complicated with difficulty with primary closure, and plastic and reconstructive surgical techniques will be required. Achieving clear excision margins is difficult, and even when frozen section or definitive histology suggest clearance, recurrence will occur in 50% of cases or more. Currently, there is some enthusiasm for using topical imiquimod, although series are small and follow-up is short (MacLean 2000b, MacLean et al 2004).

Vulval Pain/Vulvodynia

Vulval pain is a common complaint in specialist vulval clinics, with many woman complaining that other doctors have either dismissed their symptoms or been unable to make a diagnosis or treat the condition effectively. However, the lack of clarity in the diagnostic categories reflects the complexity of the problem and the relative paucity of pathophysiological research in this area of medicine. Women with vulval pain are referred to genitourinary medicine, gynaecology, dermatology, urology, psychosexual medicine, physiotherapy and many other services. There are relatively few dedicated vulval clinics in the UK, and the majority exist to manage dermatoses and premalignant conditions, such as lichen sclerosus and VIN, rather than vulval pain.

Classification

The classification of vulval pain syndromes has been as difficult and confusing as vulval disorders in general; however, the most recent ISSVD classification logically uses a descriptive, anatomical and historical method. Vulval pain is not a single entity, and a detailed history and careful examination must be made before diagnosis is attempted. Vulval pain has been described in the medical literature for over 100 years (Skene, 1880). Previous definitions of these symptoms have referred to vulvar vestibulitis syndrome or burning vulvar syndrome, and to dysaesthetic vulvodynia. However, the lack of clarity in the diagnostic categories reflects the complexity of the problem, and the relative paucity of pathophysiological research in this area of medicine. Pain is described as either primary or secondary, provoked or unprovoked, and located anatomically, i.e. vestibulodynia, clitorodynia or the more generalized vulvodynia (Moyal-Barracco and Lynch 2004).

Pain characteristics

The predominant characteristic of vulval pain is a burning sensation. This can be accompanied by a description of 'rawness' or 'soreness'. Provoked pain with entry dyspareunia as the primary complaint is usually described as a burning pain, and may be accompanied by superficial splitting or fissuring at the fourchette. The burning sensation may last several hours or even days after attempted intercourse. Similar pain may be associated with tampon insertion or withdrawal.

Unprovoked vulval pain is described as a constant unremitting sensation of pain, characteristically a burning or raw sensation that is not exacerbated by contact.

In clinical practice, there is inevitably a crossover of provoked and unprovoked pain, with women either having an element of 'background' pain or developing a complex pain syndrome with both provoked and unprovoked elements. Using the anatomical site of pain as a descriptor allows careful clinical examination, and will improve understanding of other urogenital pain syndromes such as interstitial cystitis.

Management

In younger women, the predominant symptom of dyspareunia is more commonly a secondary provoked vestibulodynia. Attempted coitus is accompanied by severe pain at entry that has a burning character and splitting of the skin at the fourchette. The pain may last for several hours or even days after contact. The appearance of the external vulval skin is normal, but there is a band of erythema in the vestibule; pressure from a cotton bud over the vestibular gland openings causes severe pain (Q-tip tenderness). This pressure can be quantified using an algesiometer, but is most often judged clinically (Eva et al 1999). It is helpful to define any triggers for this syndrome, particularly candida or bacterial vaginosis infections, or urinary tract problems. Local anaesthetic gel can be used on a cotton ball to 'desensitize' as well as to allow coitus to continue. Some patients respond to topical steroids, possibly because their symptoms are due to an underlying dermatosis. Pain-modifying drugs such as pregabalin, gabapentin or amitriptyline may be beneficial, particularly in longstanding pain or when there is a mixed picture of provoked and unprovoked pain. Increasingly, biofeedback techniques are utilized, ranging from pelvic floor physiotherapy (Glazer et al 1995) to cognitive behavioural therapy. Rarely, surgical removal of the vestibular skin is the treatment of choice. Reports of this procedure in the 1990s suggested a high level of success, but long-term follow-up data are less convincing. It should, however, not be dismissed as an option.

Unprovoked vulvodynia is rarely a primary complaint and is more common in older women. The characteristic burning is unremitting and is not influenced or exacerbated by contact. It is equated to other pain syndromes such as trigeminal neuralgia, and these patients may themselves have more than one pain syndrome. Treatment is with one or a combination of the pain-modifying agents amitriptyline, gabapentin or pregabalin.

The treatment of vulval pain requires a sympathetic, professional approach. The consultation needs to be long enough for the complex history to be explored fully and for patients' anxieties to be discussed. Providing a diagnosis, no matter how limited, is reassuring. Simple measures such as advising the use of soap substitutes, managing precipitating factors and prescribing local anaesthetic gel are helpful. It may be worth considering physical therapies as described, but some women find using a transcutaneous electrical nerve stimulation machine beneficial. The use of pain-modifying agents means that patients must have clear advice about side-effects. It can be very helpful to work with colleagues in pain clinics, particularly in cases where there is clear evidence of pudendal neuropathy or in those cases where a combination of techniques is deemed necessary.

For a proportion of women, there is no resolution of pain despite all attempts at treatment. These women and many others require psychological support, and those that benefit from treatment may benefit from psychosexual counselling. Very little is known about how vulval pain affects partners, but anecdotally, couples report gaining benefit from counselling service. Women should be told about the patient support groups available in order to have the opportunity to talk to others similarly afflicted.

Vulval Ulceration

Vulval ulceration may be infective, aphthous or associated with Behçet's syndrome, Stevens-Johnson syndrome, dermatitis artefacta, benign mucous membrane pemphigoid, familial benign chronic pemphigus (Hailey–Hailey disease), pyoderma gangrenosum, Crohn's disease, histiocytosis X or toxic epidermal necrolysis (Lyell's syndrome). These conditions are uncommon, but may be serious or even fatal. Sometimes, the diagnosis can be made clinically or with a good history. However, occasionally, biopsy will be necessary and may require immunofluorescent techniques.

Vulval Infection

Some lesions will be due to primary infection, while in other cases, a lesion has become secondarily infected. The commensal flora of the vulva consists of staphylococci, aerobic and anaerobic streptococci, Gram-negative bacilli and yeasts. Increased temperature, humidity and lower pH of vulval skin make it more susceptible to infection compared with skin elsewhere.

Fungal infections

Genital candida infection is caused by the yeast *Candida albicans* in the majority of cases. Occasionally, non-albicans species or yeasts such as *Saccharomyces cerevisiae* are identified, and these should be considered if there is limited response to the usual antifungal therapies. Candida are frequently found within the vagina, but incidence is increased with pregnancy, the use of oral contraceptives, the concurrent use of broad-spectrum antibiotics, the presence of glucosuria or diabetes mellitus, and in association with the wearing of nylon underwear and tights. Fungal infections are less likely to be seen in postmenopausal women unless they are diabetic or immunocompromised, and other causes of pruritus should be sought. Infection produces acute vulval pruritus associated with a crusting discharge, and white plaques will be seen within the vagina and on the vulva. With more extensive infection, the vulva will become acutely erythematous with oedema and superficial maceration. Culture on appropriate medium or direct microscopy will demonstrate the presence of fungus or hyphae.

Treatment of simple infection may be with a topical imidazole preparation (topical nystatin seems to have been discontinued). More extensive or recurrent infections can be treated with fluconazole 150 mg capsule as a single dose and repeated 1–2 weeks later, or itraconazole 200 mg morning and evening for 1–3 days.

Tinea cruris is relatively uncommon in females but may be transmitted from a partner; appropriate enquiry may be rewarding.

Genital warts

These are known as condylomata acuminata and are caused by HPV types 6 and 11 in the majority of cases. Descriptions of the role of oncogenic or high-risk HPV can be found in Chapter 38. Such lesions may involve not only vulval skin but also the vagina and the cervix, and may extend around the perianal area or out on to non-genital skin. Typical lesions are elevated with epithelial proliferation, usually discrete but sometimes confluent and covering large areas. The typical lesion shows koilocytosis in the upper third of the epithelium, acanthosis, parakeratosis, dyskeratosis and basal hyperplasia. The majority of condylomata acuminata are diploid, and only 10% may show nuclear atypia of various degrees, requiring differentiation from VIN with associated viral changes. The transmission of this virus is usually by sexual contact. The diagnosis is usually made on clinical appearance.

The treatment of single or small numbers of condylomata consists of the application of 25% trichloracetic acid followed by 25% podophyllin at weekly intervals. This combination should be applied to the lesion and the patient asked to bathe some 6–8 h later to remove any excess. Prolonged application can lead to excessive skin excoriation. Podophyllin should not be used during pregnancy. Those condylomata that are resistant to such treatment can be treated with imiquimod or some form of physical therapy. Atypical or resistant condylomata should be biopsied in order to exclude verrucous carcinoma.

Due to the widespread distribution of HPV and the difficulty in eradicating this virus from genital skin of immunosuppressed women, it may not always be appropriate to apply repeated, painful treatments that damage the vulval skin. For some, the repeated use of imiquimod may be useful. It is hoped that, in the future, the use of the quadrivalent vaccine, which will provide immunity against HPV 6 and 11, will reduce the clinical load from condylomata. Unfortunately, the recently introduced bivalent vaccine for British teenage girls is unlikely to prevent HPV 6 and 11 infection.

Herpes simplex

Vulval herpes lesions are usually associated with type 2 herpes simplex virus rather than type 1. The primary episode is associated with an incubation period of some 2–20 days, with an average of 1 week. There is often an associated prodromal illness before a localized area of vulval skin becomes erythematous, followed by the appearance of blisters and subsequent ulceration. These lesions are usually acutely painful and may be associated with inguinal lymphadenitis. Vulval discomfort associated with micturition may cause urinary retention. Secondary bacterial infection can occur. Resolution of discomfort and healing occurs some 7–14 days after the onset of symptoms. Frequently, the primary infection is much less dramatic. Following the primary episode, the virus enters the dorsal ganglia where it becomes dormant or latent. Reactivation may occur and a secondary episode results. Recurrences are less painful than primary lesions and rarely last more than 48 h.

The diagnosis and management of vulval herpes can be found in Chapter 63.

Bacterial infections

Bartholinitis

This is the most common bacterial infection of the vulva. It is usually found between menarche and menopause, but is not necessarily associated with sexual activity. It results from infection of the duct leading from the gland. Obstruction of the duct will produce an abscess in the acute situation, or a cyst if infection is low grade or recurrent. Causative organisms may be from the vulval flora or may be sexually transmitted.

The management of bartholinitis requires appropriate swabs for bacteriology, analgesia, antibiotics and surgical drainage of a cyst or abscess by marsupialization. In women over 40 years of age, the edges of the cyst should be sent for histological examination to exclude carcinoma.

Staphylococcal infection

This may take the form of perifolliculitis, involving the hair follicles and adjacent glandular structures within the dermis, or furunculosis which are larger, deeper lesions involving subcutaneous tissue that eventually discharge through multiple sinuses. Occasionally, staphylococcal impetigo is seen. Management consists of the application of povidone iodine washes or mupirocin ointment, or use of an antistaphylococcal antibiotic such as flucloxacillin. Occasionally, surgical drainage of the pus is required.

Hidradenitis

Similar features of recurrent staphylococcal infection are seen with hidradenitis suppurativa, a chronic inflammatory disease involving the apocrine glands (Thomas et al 1985). This condition is more likely to involve the axilla but will occasionally involve the vulva, perianal areas or the genitofemoral fold. These abscesses are deep and may often involve anaerobic organisms. Acute cases will require intravenous antibiotics such as flucloxacillin and metronidazole, and may require surgical deroofing of the abscess. Long-term antibiotic treatment may be combined with hormone control of apocrine gland activity. This appears to be best achieved using a combination of oestrogen and cyproterone. There is a small risk of carcinoma developing in areas of chronic scarring.

Other bacterial infections

Streptococcal infection of the vulva may be relatively superficial or localized, as in erysipelas. This will be associated with sharply defined erythema, oedema and pain. Streptococci may cause deeper infection involving tissue down to the fascia or periostium. Gangrene of the skin (necrotizing fasciitis) may complicate any form of vulval surgery, especially in diabetic women. High doses of penicillin are required. In cases with deep infection, other aerobic and anaerobic organisms are often involved, and a combination of antibiotics and very wide surgical excision is required. Infection of the vulva with *Neisseria gonorrhoeae* is rare in adults. The urethra, however, will be infected in approximately 75% of cases of gonorrhoea, and this may lead to infection of periurethral glands. Involvement of the duct of Bartholin's gland is described above. Gonococcal vulvitis can occur in children.

Other bacterial infections involving the vulva include erythrasma, trichomycosis, tuberculosis (lupus vulgaris), syphilis, chancroid, granuloma inguinale and lymphogranuloma venereum, and is described in Chapter 63.

Protozoal and parasitic infections

Trichomonas vaginalis

This involves the vagina initially, although the patient may present with vulval symptoms. This infection is due to *Trichomonas vaginalis*, a flagellated protozoan, and is associated with vaginal discharge (which is often frothy and brown or green), vaginal irritation and dyspareunia. The organisms may be identified in a wet film by their motility or may be recognized in cervical smears. Colposcopic assessment of the vagina shows characteristic double-looped coarse punctation of the vagina and cervix, which may be diffuse and extensive or patchy and localized (strawberry vagina). Treatment of this infection is with metronidazole 200 mg three times a day for 7 days or a single 2 g dose. The partner should be treated concurrently and both should be warned not to take alcohol with this antibacterial agent.

Threadworms

Enterobius vermicularis live in the large bowel, lay eggs on the anal margins and cause pruritus ani; vulval irritation may also occur. The ova can be recognized on microscopy of a strip of Sellotape left in position overnight. Treatment is with piperazine or mebendazole.

Other infections that may involve the vulva include pediculosis (crabs), scabies, amoebiasis, schistosomiasis, filariasis and leishmaniasis. Vulval lesions due to entamoeba, schistosoma, filarial worms and leishmania are uncommon in Western countries. They should be considered in anyone returning from overseas, and may cause diagnostic difficulties if considering a 'tropical' venereal infection or even syphilis.

Benign Tumours of the Vulva

Lipomas and fibromas are the most common benign tumours of the vulva which arise from other than the epithelial tissues. Haemangiomas are benign tumours composed of blood vessels, with the capillary type (strawberry haemangioma) being most commonly encountered in infants and young children. A variety of site-specific stromal tumours can occur in the vulvovaginal area, including aggressive angiomyxoma, angiomyofibroblastoma and cellular angiofibroma (McCluggage 2009). In young to middle-aged women, fibroepithelial stromal polyps occur more frequently in the vagina, but also in the vulva or cervix. They are benign and are lined by normal squamous epithelium, which may be keratinized depending on the location; the stroma varies from bland to cellular and pleomorphic, especially in pregnancy-associated cases. There is potential for local recurrence, particularly if incompletely excised.

Angiomyofibroblastoma is a well-circumscribed lesion which occurs almost exclusively in the vulvovaginal region, and is often clinically thought to be a cyst of Bartholin's gland. The stromal cells may have an epithelioid appearance and tend to cluster around vessels; they show reactivity for vimentin and desmin, and are actin negative.

Cellular angiofibroma occurs exclusively in the vulva of middle-aged women, and behaves in a benign fashion. It is composed of spindle cells arranged in short fascicles in a meshwork of thick-walled vessels. The cells express vimentin but not desmin or actin.

Aggressive angiomyxoma is a locally infiltrative tumour that recurs in 30–40% of cases if incompletely excised. It occurs most commonly in the reproductive years and usually has a gelatinous appearance. Histologically, it is a myxoid, poorly cellular neoplasm composed of bland spindle cells which merge imperceptibly into the surrounding stroma. There is no specific immunohistochemical marker, although high mobility group AT-hook2 HMGA2 expression may be useful.

Superficial angiomyxoma arises in the dermis and subcutaneous tissue, and therefore often appears polypoid. If multiple lesions involving other sites are present, Carney's complex may be suspected and further investigations are warranted to exclude a cardiac myxoma.

Prepubertal vulval fibromas have been described which may be a childhood variant of aggressive angiomyxomas or may be enlargement secondary to hormonal changes approaching puberty. Superficial myofibroblastoma of the female lower genital tract may involve the vulva, vagina or cervix, are usually polypoidal or nodular, and are benign in behaviour (McCluggage 2009). Other smooth muscle tumours of the vulva are much rarer than the uterine counterpart; the presence of mitotic activity, nuclear pleomorphism or an infiltrative margin is associated with locally recurrent potential (atypical smooth muscle tumours), while tumours with any three of the following features are considered sarcomas: more than 50 mm in size, infiltrative margins, more than five mitoses/10 High-Power Fields, and moderate to severe atypia.

Granular cell tumours are of peripheral nerve sheath origin and arise in the vulva of children or adults as painless subcutaneous nodules of the mons pubis, labia majora or clitoris. They are often associated with pseudoepitheliomatous hyperplasia of the overlying epithelium, and are composed of epithelioid, granular cells infiltrating the stroma and typically exhibiting S-100 protein. Wide local excision is the treatment of choice. Neurofibromas may affect the vulva as part of von Recklinghausen disease. Benign angiokeratoma may be difficult to distinguish from a melanoma, especially if the initial red colour has given way to the later brown or black hue, and the lesion has started to bleed due to trauma.

Squamous papillomata and 'skin tags' are common, benign and similar in appearance. They may be solitary or multiple (vestibular or squamous papillomatosis, microwarts). They lack significant correlation with HPV DNA and histology may overestimate viral changes.

Seborrhoeic keratosis may also occur on the hair-bearing skin of the vulva of elderly women. The rare keratoacanthoma might well be mistaken for invasive squamous cancer because of its rapid growth over a matter of weeks. Spontaneous involution usually begins after approximately 6 months. The centre of this well-demarcated, regular dome contains a plug of keratin, which may suggest the diagnosis, but complete excision of the lesion is required for histological confirmation.

Vaginal Infection

Between puberty and the menopause, the presence of lactobacilli maintains a vaginal pH of between 3.8 and 4.2; this protects against infection. Before puberty and after the menopause, the higher pH and urinary and faecal contamination increase the risk of infection. Normal physiological vaginal discharge consists of transudate from the vaginal wall, squames containing glycogen, polymorphs, lactobacilli, cervical mucus, residual menstrual fluid and a contribution from the greater and lesser vestibular glands.

Vaginal discharge varies with hormonal levels and does not automatically mean infection. Non-specific vaginitis may be associated with sexual trauma, allergies to deodorants or contraceptives, or the chemical irritation of topical antimicrobial therapy. Infection may be aggravated by the presence of foreign bodies, continuing use of tampons and the presence of an intrauterine contraceptive device.

Vaginal infection may produce vulval symptoms, and the above descriptions of genital candidiasis, trichomoniasis, herpes simplex virus, HPV and syphilis are relevant to vaginal lesions. *Neisseria gonorrhoeae* will not infect the vaginal epithelium, except in prepubertal girls or postmenopausal women. If there is suspicion of sexual abuse in a young girl, an appropriate vaginal swab should be taken.

Bacterial vaginosis

Bacterial vaginosis is now believed to be due to a vibrio or comma-shaped organism named *Mobiluncus*. Other organisms, including anaerobes, may have a contributory role. These organisms are believed to be sexually transmitted, although the condition may be due to imbalance in the vaginal ecosystem. Usually, the vagina is not inflamed and therefore the term 'vaginosis' is used rather than 'vaginitis'. Nearly half of 'infected' patients will not have symptoms (Thomason et al 1990), while others will complain of increased or unpleasant discharge, soreness and irritation.

Examination will reveal a thin, grey-white discharge and a vaginal pH greater than 5. A Gram stain of the discharge will show 'clue cells' which consist of vaginal epithelial cells covered with micro-organisms. The absence of lactobacilli will be confirmed if a characteristic fishy amine smell is released when a drop of vaginal discharge is added to saline on a glass slide, along with one drop of 10% potassium hydroxide. The diagnosis is made if three of these four criteria are met.

There are claims that bacterial vaginosis is associated with increased risk of preterm labour (Hay et al 1994), pelvic inflammatory disease and postoperative pelvic infection (Paavonen et al 1987, Eschenbach et al 1988). The treatment of bacterial vaginosis is metronidazole, either as 400 mg two or three times a day for 7 days or as a single 2 g dose. Alternatively, clindamycin 2% can be used as a vaginal cream but, unlike metronidazole, this is active against lactobacilli and will delay the restoration of normal vaginal flora.

Toxic shock syndrome

This topic has been included here because it is associated with the use of vaginal tampons during menstruation or less frequently in the puerperium (Shands et al 1980). Although there is a link between this syndrome and certain organisms (e.g. group A streptococci and *Staphylococcus aureus*) found within the vagina of affected women, it is not a vaginal infection. The manifestations are usually systemic with occasionally life-threatening consequences. Removal of superabsorbent brands of tampons from the market in the USA, and greater care in tampon use and insertion reduced the frequency of the syndrome. Early effective treatment of hypovolaemia in severe cases is essential. Treatment is the same as for septicaemia, and includes intravenous fluids and inotropic support where necessary. The cause should be eliminated where possible, and a β-lactamase-resistant penicillin should be given parenterally. Further attacks can occur and it is recommended that tampons should not be used until *Staphylococcus aureus* has been eradicated from the vagina.

Other Vaginal Pathology

Atrophy

This is seen following the menopause, but can also occur prior to puberty and during prolonged lactation. Examination shows loss of rugal folds and prominent subepithelial vessels, sometimes with adjacent ecchymoses. The patient may present with vaginal bleeding, vaginal discharge, or vaginal dryness and dyspareunia. Superficial infection, with Gram-positive cocci or Gram-negative bacilli, may be associated.

Treatment requires oestrogen to restore the vaginal epithelium and pH. This is usually by topical oestrogen cream or pessary. Systemic absorption will increase blood levels of oestrogen. Alternatively, hormone replacement therapy can be used.

Trauma

A torn hymen following a first attempt at intercourse may result in profuse, frightening haemorrhage. Suture of the bleeding vessel under general anaesthesia should be accompanied by one or more radial incisions in the hymen to prevent recurrence.

Trauma in young girls or women may be the result of falling astride an object like a bicycle or fence. It may result from sexual abuse, sometimes self-inflicted, but may represent sexual assault or rape. It may also occur following normal sexual intercourse, particularly in a postmenopausal woman who has not had intercourse for some time. In these cases, the laceration is usually at the vault of the vagina in the posterior fornix.

An indwelling catheter may be necessary and ice packs will give some comfort. Damage to the vagina, rectum, urethra, bladder or ureter may also occur. Pain relief with opiates and replacement of blood loss may be needed urgently. Examination under anaesthesia is often required to determine the extent of the damage. A closed haematoma is best managed conservatively, but bleeding lacerations will require suture. Devitalized tissues will need to be excised, and tears in bowel or bladder must be repaired in layers.

Seminal fluid allergy

Patients may present with a history of dyspareunia with itching, burning or swelling, or occasionally more widespread symptoms such as urticaria, bronchospasm or even angioneurotic oedema, after intercourse. The allergic reaction appears to be due to sensitization to seminal fluid

(Poskitt et al 1995). Symptoms may arise following first coitus or after exposure to several sexual partners.

Treatment has included long-term immunotherapy following skin testing (Friedman et al 1984). Treatment with desensitization may be helpful, and antihistamines and intravaginal cromoglycate are described (Poskitt et al 1995).

Sjogren's syndrome

Patients with vaginal dryness and pain may have Sjogren's syndrome if there is ocular or oral dryness. They may have arthralgia, myalgia or Raynaud's phenomenon. The diagnostic criteria include ocular and oral symptoms, ocular signs, salivary gland histology, other evidence of salivary gland involvement and the presence of autoantibodies. Vaginal symptoms may predate the oral or ocular symptoms.

Benign Tumours of the Vagina

Tumours in the vagina are uncommon. Condylomata acuminata are by far the most common type seen. The frond-like surface is usually characteristic, but it is wise to await the result of a biopsy before instituting treatment.

Endometriotic deposits may be seen in the vagina. They are most common in an episiotomy wound and may lie deep to the epithelium.

Simple mesonephric (Gartner's) or paramesonephric cysts may be seen, especially high up near the fornices. If asymptomatic, they are best left untreated. If treatment is required, marsupialization is effective and safer than excision. Similarly, management of anterior wall cysts must include the exclusion of a bladder or urethral diverticulum.

Adenosis (multiple mucus-containing vaginal cysts) is a rare condition which, even more rarely, gives rise to symptoms. A variety of abnormalities are reported in the daughters of women who took diethylstilboestrol during their pregnancy. Most of these are of no significance (see Chapters 38 and 39).

Female Circumcision/Genital Mutilation

It is inevitable that obstetricians and gynaecologists will encounter patients with female genital mutilation (FGM), and management will sometimes cause more harm than good. Gordon et al (2007) emphasized that reversal procedures are better performed in non-pregnant or antenatal patients, rather than when the patient presents in labour and is dealt with by junior or inexperienced staff.

The World Health Organization (http://www.who.int/topics/female_genital_mutilation/en/) has defined FGM as all procedures involving partial or total removal of the external female genitalia, or other injury to the female genital organs for non-medical reasons. FGM is classified into four types, as follows.

- Type I: partial or total removal of the clitoris and/or prepuce (clitoridectomy).
- Type II: partial or total removal of the clitoris and labia minora, with or without excision of the labia majora (excision).
- Type III: narrowing of the vaginal orifice with creation of a covering seal by cutting and appositioning the labia minora and/or the labia majora, with or without excision of the clitoris (infibulation).
- Type IV: all other harmful procedures to the female genitalia for non-medical purposes; for example, pricking, piercing, incising, scraping and cauterization.

Most of the cases described by Gordon et al (2007) and managed in North London were of type III and the clitoris was found intact after reversal.

It is estimated that more than 2 million women and children undergo some form of FGM each year, mainly in Africa, but also in the Middle East and Asia. It is a cultural rather than a religious requirement or duty. Performing FGM in the UK became illegal in 1985, and in 2003, it became an offence for UK citizens to perform FGM in other countries. Nevertheless, many young girls appear to leave the UK to have the procedure performed between their birth and reaching puberty. Acute complications include pain, infection, bleeding, injury to the urethra/vagina/rectum, urinary retention, faecal incontinence and death. More chronic complications include urinary and menstrual difficulty, haematocolpos, sexual difficulty if not impossibility from fibrous scarring, and epidermoid cysts. Incompetent attempts at defibulation have caused urethral and rectal injuries, further scarring and persistent dyspareunia.

As mentioned above, Gordon et al (2007) advocated reversal as an elective procedure rather than during labour. If it is performed during labour, the fused labia minora should be incised in the midline anteriorly as far as the urethral meatus, and further anterior dissection of clitoral structures should be deferred because of risk of urethral damage and difficult haemostasis. It is illegal to close the infibulations following delivery, even if the husband insists. When performed electively, the CO_2 laser provides a bloodless incision, but care must be taken of underlying structures. Examples have been seen where careless use of electrodiathermy has left damage to underlying clitoral glans when dissecting a paraclitoral epidermoid cyst.

Gordon et al (2007) emphasized the requirement of providing an interpreter and nurse/midwife who will meet the psychosexual and social aspects of FGM. Certainly, the scenario of a patient presenting in advanced labour with undisclosed infibulated labia and the threat of imminent tearing should be avoided.

KEY POINTS

1. A multidisciplinary team approach to vulval disease is helpful.
2. The presenting symptoms will not indicate the nature of the pathology.
3. Topical steroids are effective and safe in the treatment of many vulval disorders.
4. Topical oestrogens have little to offer the woman with a vulval disorder.
5. There is no place for vulvectomy in the management of lichen sclerosus.

References

Aberer E, Stanek G 1987 Histological evidence for spirochetal origin of morphoea and lichen sclerosis et atrophicus. American Journal of Dermatopathology 9: 374–379.

Belfiore P, Di Fede O, Cabibi D et al 2006 Prevalence of vulval lichen planus in a cohort of women with oral lichen planus: an interdisciplinary study. British Journal of Dermatology 155: 994–998.

Carli P, Moretti S, Spallanzani A et al 1997 Fibrogenic cytokines in vulvar lichen sclerosus. Journal of Reproductive Medicine 42: 161–165.

Clark TJ, Etherington IJ, Luesley DM 1999 Response of the vulvar lichen sclerosus and squamous cell hyperplasia to graduated topical steroids. Journal of Reproductive Medicine 44: 958–962.

Cooper SM, Gao XH, Powell JJ, Wojnarowska F 2004 Does treatment of vulvar lichen sclerosus influence its prognosis? Archives of Dermatology 140: 702–706.

Dalziel K, Millard P, Wojnarowska F 1989 Lichen sclerosus et atrophicus treated with a potent topical steroid (clobetasol dipropionate 0.05%). British Journal of Dermatology 121 (Suppl 34): 34–35.

Dalziel KL, Millard PR, Wojnarowska F 1991 The treatment of vulval lichen sclerosus with a very potent topical steroid (clobetasol propionate 0.05%) cream. British Journal of Dermatology 124: 461–464.

Dwyer CM, Kerr RE, Millan DW 1995 Squamous cell carcinoma following lichen planus of the vulva. Clinical and Experimental Dermatology 20: 171–172.

Edwards L 2008 Lichen sclerosus. In: Black MM, Ambros-Rudolph C, Edwards L, Lynch P (eds) Obstetric and Gynecologic Dermatology. Mosby-Elsevier, pp 133–145.

Eschenbach DA, Hillier S, Critchlow C 1988 Diagnosis and clinical manifestations of bacterial vaginosis. American Journal of Obstetrics and Gynecology 158: 819–828.

Eva LJ, Reid WMN, MacLean AB, Morrison GD 1999 Assessment of response to treatment in vulvar vestibulitis syndrome by means of the vulvar algesiometer. American Journal of Obstetrics and Gynecology 181: 99–102.

Eva LJ, Ganesan R, Chan KK, Honest H, Malik S, Luesley DM 2008 Vulval squamous cell carcinoma occurring on a background of differentiated vulval intraepithelial neoplasia is more likely to recur: a review of 154 cases. Journal of Reproductive Medicine 53: 397–401.

Farrell A, Dean D, Millard PR, Charnock FM, Wojnarowska F 2006 Cytokine alterations in lichen sclerosus: an immunohistochemical study. British Journal of Dermatology 155: 931–940.

Fischer G, Spurett B, Fischer A 1995 The chronically symptomatic vulva: aetiology and management. British Journal of Obstetrics and Gynaecology 102: 773–779.

Friedman SA, Bernstein IL, Enrione M et al 1984 Successful long-term immunotherapy for human seminal plasma anaphylaxis. JAMA: the Journal of the American Medical Association 251: 2684–2687.

Friedrich EG 1985 Vulvar dystrophy. Clinical Obstetrics and Gynecology 28: 178–187.

Friedrich EG, Kalra PS 1984 Serum levels of sex hormones in vulvar lichen sclerosus and the effect of topical testosterone. New England Journal of Medicine 310: 488–491.

Gao XH, Barnardo MC, Winsey S et al 2005 The association between HLA DR, DQ antigens and vulval lichen sclerosus in the UK: HLA DRB 112 and its associated DRB112/DQB 10301/04/09/010 haplotype confers susceptibility to vulval lichen sclerosus, and HLA DRB10301/04 and its associated DRB10301/04/DQB10201/02/03 haplotype protects from vulval lichen sclerosus. Journal of Investigative Dermatology 125: 895–899.

Glazer HI, Rodke G, Swencionis C et al 1995 Treatment of vulvar vestibulitis syndrome with electromyographic biofeedback of pelvic floor musculature. Journal of Reproductive Medicine 40: 283–290.

Goldstein AT, Marinoff SC, Christopher K, Srodon M 2005 Prevalence of vulvar lichen sclerosus in a general gynecology practice. Journal of Reproductive Medicine 50: 477–480.

Goolamali SK, Barnes EW, Irvine WJ et al 1974 Organ-specific antibodies in patients with lichen sclerosus. BMJ (Clinical Research Ed.) ii: 78–79.

Gordon H, Comerasamy H, Morris NH 2007 Female genital mutilation: experience in a west London clinic. Journal of Obstetrics and Gynaecology 27: 416–419.

Haverhoek E, Reid C, Gordon L, Marshman G, Wood J, Selva-Nayagam P 2008 Prospective study of patch testing in patients with vulval pruritus. Australasian Journal of Dermatology 49: 80–85.

Hay PE, Lamont RF, Taylor-Robinson D et al 1994 Abnormal bacterial colonisation of the genital tract and subsequent preterm delivery and late miscarriage. BMJ (Clinical Research Ed.) 308: 295–298.

Howard A, Dean D, Cooper S, Kirtshig G, Wojnarowska F 2004 Circulating basement membrane zone antibodies are found in lichen sclerosus of the vulva. Australasian Journal of Dermatology 45: 12–15.

Jeffcoate TNA, Woodcock AS 1961 Premalignant conditions of the vulva, with particular reference to chronic epithelial dystrophies. BMJ (Clinical Research Ed.) 2: 127–134.

Jones RW, Joura EA 1999 Analyzing prior clinical events at presentation in 102 women with vulvar carcinoma: evidence of diagnostic delays. Journal of Reproductive Medicine 44: 766–768.

Jones RW, Sadler L, Grant S, Whineray J, Exeter M, Rowan D 2004 Clinically identifying women with vulvar lichen sclerosus at increased risk of squamous cell carcinoma: a case control study. Journal of Reproductive Medicine 49: 808–811.

Jones RW, Scurry J, Neill S, MacLean AB 2008 Guidelines for the follow-up of women with vulvar lichen sclerosus in specialist clinics. American Journal of Obsterics and Gynecology 198: 496.e1–496.e3.

Jonsson M, Karlsson R, Evander M 1997 Acetowhitening of the cervix and vulva as a predictor of subclinical human papillomavirus infection: sensitivity and specificity in a population based study. Obstetrics and Gynecology 90: 744–747.

Kagie MJ, Kenter GG, Tollenaar RAE et al 1997 p53 protein overexpression, a frequent observation in squamous cell carcinoma of the vulva and in various synchronous vulva epithelia, has no value as a prognostic parameter. International Journal of Gynecological Pathology 16: 124–130.

Kohlberger PD, Joura EA, Bancher D et al 1998 Evidence of androgen receptor expression in lichen sclerosus: an immunohistological study. Journal of the Society for Gynecological Investigation 5: 331.

Kohlberger PD, Kainz CH, Breitenecker G et al 1995 Prognostic value of immunohistochemically detected p53 expression in vulvar carcinoma. Cancer 76: 1786–1789.

Leibovitz A, Kaplun V, Saposhnicov N, Habot B 2000 Vulvovaginal examinations in elderly nursing home women residents. Archives of Gerontology and Geriatrics 31: 1–4.

Leibowitch M, Neill S, Pelisse M, Moyal-Baracco M 1990 The epithelial changes associated with squamous cell carcinoma of the vulva: a review of the clinical, histological and viral findings in 78 women. British Journal of Obstetrics and Gynaecology 97: 1135–1139.

Lorenz B, Kaufman RF, Kutzner SK 1998 Lichen sclerosus. Therapy with clobetasol propionate. Journal of Reproductive Medicine 43: 790–794.

Lynch PJ 2007 2006 International Society for the Study of Vulvovaginal Disease classification of vulvar dermatoses: a synopsis. Journal of Lower Genital Tract Disease 11(1): 1–2.

MacLean AB 1991 Vulval dystrophy — the passing of a term. Current Opinion in Obstetrics and Gynaecology 1: 97–102.

MacLean AB 1993 Precursors of vulval cancers. Current Opinion in Obstetrics and Gynaecology 3: 149–156.

MacLean AB 2000a Are 'non-neoplastic' disorders of the vulva premalignant? In:

Luesley D (ed) Cancer and Precancers of the Vulva. Arnold, London.

MacLean AB 2000b Paget's disease of the vulva. Journal of Obstetrics and Gynaecology 20: 7–9.

MacLean AB, Reid WMN 1995 Benign and premalignant disease of the vulva. BJOG: an International Journal of Obstetics and Gynaecology 102: 359–363.

MacLean AB, Roberts DT, Reid WMN 1998 Review of 1000 women seen at two specially designated vulval clinics. Current Opinion in Obstetrics and Gynaecology 8: 159–116.

MacLean AB, Makwana M, Ellis PE, Cunnington F 2004 The management of Paget's disease of the vulva. Journal of Obstetrics and Gynaecology 24: 124–128.

Marren P, Yell J, Charnock FM et al 1995 The association between lichen sclerosus and antigens of the HLA system. British Journal of Dermatology 132: 197–203.

McCullough AM, Seywright M, Roberts DT, MacLean AB 1987 Outpatient biopsy of the vulva. Journal of Obstetrics and Gynaecology 5: 166–169.

McCluggage WG 2009 Recent developments in vulvovaginal pathology. Histopathology 54: 156–173.

Meyrick-Thomas RH, Ridley CM, MacGibbon DH, Black MM 1988 Lichen sclerosus and autoimmunity — study of 350 women. British Journal of Dermatology 118: 41–46.

Moyal-Barracco M, Lynch PJ 2004 2003 ISSVD terminology and classification of vulvodynia: a historical perspective. Journal of Reproductive Medicine 49: 772–777.

Mulveny NJ, Allen DG 2008 Differentiated intraepithelial neoplasia of the vulva. International Journal of Gynecologic Pathology 27: 125–135.

Neill SM, Tatnall FM, Cox NH 2002 Guidelines for the management of lichen sclerosus. British Journal of Dermatology 147: 640–649.

O'Connell HE, Eizenberg N, Rahman M, Cleeve J 2008 The anatomy of the distal vagina: towards unity. Journal of Sexual Medicine 5: 1883–1891.

Oyama N, Chan I, Neill SM et al 2003 Autoantibodies to extracellular matrix protein 1 in lichen sclerosus. The Lancet 362: 118–123.

Oyama N, Chan I, Neill SM et al 2004 Development of antigen-specific ELISA for circulating autoantibodies to extracellular matrix protein 1 in lichen sclerosus. Journal of Clinical Investigation 113: 1550–1559.

Paavonen J, Teisala K, Heinonen PK et al 1987 Microbiological and histopathological findings in acute pelvic inflammatory disease. British Journal of Obstetrics and Gynaecology 94: 454–460.

Pinto AP, Lin MC, Sheers EE et al 2000 Allelic imbalance in lichen sclerosus, hyperplasia and intraepithelial neoplasia of the vulva. Gynecologic Oncology 77: 171–176.

Poskitt BL, Wojnarowska FT, Shaw S 1995 Semen contact urticaria. Journal of the Royal Society of Medicine 88: 108–109.

Powell J, Wojnarowska F 2002 Childhood vulvar lichen sclerosus: the course after puberty. Journal of Reproductive Medicine 47: 706–709.

Powell J 2006 Paediatric vulval disorders. Journal of Obstetrics and Gynaecology 26: 596–602.

Renaud-Vilmer C, Cavelier-Balloy B, Porcher R, Dubertret L 2004 Vulvar lichen sclerosus — effect of long-term application of a potent steroid on the course of the disease. Archives of Dermatology 140: 709–712.

Ridley CM 1988 The Vulva. Churchill Livingstone, London.

Ridley CM, Frankman O, Jones ISC et al 1989 New nomenclature for vulvar disease. Human Pathology 20: 495–496.

Rolfe KJ, Eva LJ, MacLean AB et al 2001 Cell cycle proteins as molecular markers of malignant change in lichen sclerosus. International Journal of Gynecological Cancer 11: 113–118.

Rolfe KJ, MacLean AB, Crow JC, Benjamin E, Reid WM, Perrett CW 2003 TP53 mutations in vulval lichen sclerosus adjacent to squamous cell carcinoma of the vulva. British Journal of Cancer 89(12): 2249–2253.

Sander CS, Ali I, Dean D, Thiele JJ, Wojnarowska F 2004 Oxidative stress is implicated in the pathogenesis of lichen sclerosus. British Journal of Dermatology 151: 627–635.

Scurry J, Vanin K, Osters A 1997 Comparison of histological features of vulvar lichen sclerosis with and without adjacent squamous cell carcinoma. International Journal of Gynecological Cancer 7: 392–399.

Scurry J, Wilkinson EJ 2006 Review of terminology of precursors of vulvar squamous cell carcinoma. Journal of Lower Genital Tract Disease 10: 161–169.

Shands KN, Schmid GP, Dan BB 1980 Toxic shock syndrome in menstruating women. Association with tampon use and Staphylococcus aureus, and clinical features in 52 cases. New England Journal of Medicine 303: 1436–1442.

Sideri M, Jones RW, Wilkinson EJ et al 2005 Squamous vulvar intraepithelial neoplasia: 2004 modified terminology, ISSVD Vulvar Oncology Subcommittee. Journal of Reproductive Medicine 50: 807–810.

Sinha P, Sorinola O, Luesley DM 1999 Lichen sclerosus of the vulva. Long-term steroid maintenance therapy. Journal of Reproductive Medicine 44(7): 621–624.

Skene AJC 1880 The anatomy and pathology of two important glands of the female urethra. American Journal of Obstetrics and Diseases of Women 13: 265–270.

Tasker G, Wojnarowska F 2003 Lichen sclerosus. Clinical and Experimental Dermatology 28: 128–133.

Thomas R, Barnhill D, Bibro M 1985 Hidradenitis suppurativa: a case presentation and review of the literature. Obstetrics and Gynecology 66: 592–595.

Thomason JL, Gelbart SM, Anderson B et al 1990 Statistical evaluation of diagnostic criteria for bacterial vaginosis. American Journal of Obstetrics and Gynecology 162: 155–160.

Tidy JA, Soutter WP, Luesley DM et al 1996 Management of lichen sclerosus and intraepithelial neoplasia of the vulva in the U.K. Journal of the Royal Society of Medicine 89: 699–701.

Wallace HJ 1971 Lichen sclerosus et atrophicus. Transactions of St John's Dermatology Society 57: 9–30.

Wilkinson EJ, Brown H 2002 Vulvar Paget disease of urothelial origin: a report of three cases and a proposed classification of vulvar Paget disease. Human Pathology 33: 549–554.

Zaki l, Dalziel KL, Solomonsz FA et al 1996 The under reporting of skin disease in association with squamous cell carcinoma of the vulva. Clinical and Experimental Dermatology 21: 334–337.

CHAPTER 41

Malignant disease of the vulva and vagina

Shing Shun N. Siu and David Luesley

Chapter Contents

INTRODUCTION	613	TREATMENT	617
AETIOLOGY	613	ADVANCED DISEASE	621
HISTOLOGY	614	RECURRENCES	621
LYMPHATIC DRAINAGE	614	MALIGNANT MELANOMA	621
NATURAL HISTORY OF SQUAMOUS CANCERS	614	BARTHOLIN'S GLAND CARCINOMA	622
PRESENTATION	614	INVASIVE PAGET'S DISEASE	622
ASSESSMENT	615	VERRUCOUS CARCINOMA	622
EXAMINATION	615	BASAL CELL CARCINOMA	623
DIAGNOSIS	615	SARCOMA	623
STAGING	615	CANCER OF THE VAGINA	623
PROGNOSTIC FACTORS	616	KEY POINTS	625

Introduction

Vulval cancer is an uncommon condition that largely affects elderly women (Figure 41.1). The Office of National Statistics recorded 842 cases in 2005 (Office of National Statistics 2008). This incidence of 3.3 per 100,000 ranks vulvar cancer as the 20th most common cancer in women. The most recent mortality figures recorded 270 deaths for all age groups, giving a death rate of 1.05 per 100,000 women (0.53/105 persons), ranking it the 19th most common cause of cancer death in women.

The changing population demographics will result in an increase in the incidence of the disease as a result of an ageing population, and an increase in the associated comorbidity, providing additional medical challenges to effective multimodality care.

The disease is potentially curable in most cases, even in the elderly and unfit. However, if the diagnosis is delayed or if managed inappropriately, the outcome is variable with the potential for a miserable, degrading death. Effective surgical treatment seems deceptively simple, but few gynaecologists and their nursing colleagues acquire sufficient experience of this disease to offer the highest quality of care for these women. This is a disease where there is a compelling case for centralized care, and where one might expect the reorganization of gynaecological cancer services to benefit women significantly.

Aetiology

There seem to be two distinct types of vulval carcinoma: the first type occurs predominantly in older women, is typically a well-differentiated keratinizing tumour that is not associated with usual-type vulvar intraepithelial neoplasia (VIN) or human papilloma virus (HPV) infection, but which often shows adjacent epithelial disorders such as lichen sclerosus and/or differentiated VIN; and a second type which mainly occurs in younger women, is associated with usual-type VIN, shows evidence of oncogenic HPV infection, and may be associated with synchronous or metachronous squamous preneoplastic or neoplastic lesions of the cervix, vagina and anal canal (Crum et al 1997, van der Avoort et al 2006). Smoking may be an important cofactor involved in the aetiology of HPV-related vulvar tumours (Hussain et al 2008).

Case-controlled studies have failed to confirm an association with diabetes mellitus, obesity, vascular disease and syphilis.

The following are recognized risk factors for all types of vulval cancer:

- immunosuppression;
- advanced age;
- history of cervical neoplasia (Ansink and Heintz 1993);
- lichen sclerosus (4–7% risk of developing cancer) (MacLean and Reid 1995, Meffert et al 1995);

DOI: 10.1016/B978-0-7020-3120-5.00041-2

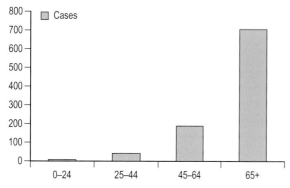

Figure 41.1 Age distribution of vulval cancer.

Source: Office of National Statistics 2008 Cancer Statistics Registration, Registration of Cancer Diagnosed in 2005, England. Series MB1 No. 36. Her Majesty's Stationery Office, London.

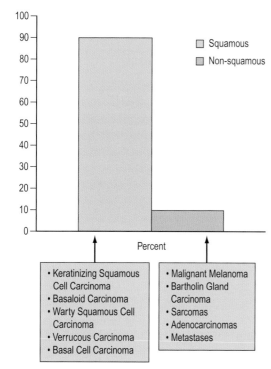

Figure 41.2 The histological subtypes of vulval cancer.

- VIN and multifocal disease (5–90%) (Herod et al 1996, Jones et al 1997);
- Paget's disease (Fishman et al 1995);
- melanoma in situ (Bradgate et al 1990, Ragnarsson-Olding et al 1993); and
- smoking (Hussain et al 2008).

Histology

The majority of vulvar cancers (90%) are squamous in origin (Figure 41.2). Verrucous and basal cell cancers are squamous cell variants.

Non-squamous cancers include Bartholin's gland cancer and other adenocarcinomas, malignant melanoma, Paget's disease and sarcomas. The vulva may also be a site for lym-

phoma and metastases from elsewhere (Finan 2003). Rarely, primary breast cancers have been reported (Piura et al 2002).

The histology has a bearing on management, largely because of the different risks of nodal metastases and the predilection for distant spread.

Lymphatic Drainage

An understanding of the lymphatic drainage is important as the regional nodes are a potential site of metastases.

Lymph drains from the vulva to the superficial inguinal glands and then to the deep femoral glands in the groin. Drainage continues to the external iliac glands. Drainage to both groins occurs from midline structures — the perineum and the clitoris — but some contralateral spread may take place from other parts of the vulva (Iversen and Aas 1983). Direct spread to the pelvic nodes along the internal pudendal vessels occurs very rarely, and no direct pathway from the clitoris to the pelvic nodes has been demonstrated consistently. An important aspect of the lymphatic drainage is the concept of sentinel nodes in each groin. This is the first node that draining lymph encounters as it drains bilaterally from the vulvar basin (Cabanas 1977). This anatomical concept has been exploited recently to develop selective lymphadenectomy in this disease.

Natural History of Squamous Cancers

Malignant transformation may occur in more than one site, and this appears to apply in both HPV-negative and -positive scenarios, although more commonly in the latter. The earliest recognizable phase of vulval cancer is termed 'superficially invasive disease' (stage Ia). The tumour is less than 2 cm in lateral dimension, and there is less than 1 mm invasion when measured from the base of an adjacent dermal papilla. Accurate identification and classification of this stage requires expert pathological interpretation, and is exceptionally important as the current consensus would suggest a virtually negligible risk of lymph node metastases. As the cancer gradually increases in size and progressively invades the deeper layers of the dermis, it spreads locally. The tumour will eventually involve the local lymphatics, hence the propensity for groin lymph node involvement (Table 41.1).

Local progression will eventually lead to involvement of adjacent structures. The urethra, anus and vagina can all become involved. In advanced stages, there can be extensive local destruction and involvement (often with superadded infection), groin node metastases and potentially lymph node involvement in the pelvis, para-aortic and neck nodes. Metastases in adjacent skin may also be noted, and haematogenous spread can also occur in late disease.

If widespread disease is seen with small vulvar tumours, a more aggressive histotype may be present, such as a melanoma or sarcoma.

Presentation

The medial aspects of the labia majora are the most common sites for disease to develop (70%). The labia minora, clitoris,

Table 41.1 Groin recurrences in women who did not undergo any form of groin node surgery. None had clinically suspicious lesions in the groin, and all were regarded as 'low-risk cases'. In many, groin node surgery was omitted because of associated medical problems

Reference	Lesion		n	Groin recurrences	Deaths due to groin disease
	Depth (mm)	Diameter (cm)			
Magrina (1979)	5	2	35	4	3
Hacker et al (1984a)	>1	2	23	2	2
Thomas GM (1991)	NK	2	27	6	NK
Sutton (1991)	1	2	10	0	0
Kelly (1972)	1	2	13	0	0
Lingard (1992)	NK	NK	20	7	7
			128	19 (14%)	

NK, not known.

periurethral areas, posterior fourchette and perineum account for the remainder (30%). Small lesions may be asymptomatic and go unnoticed by the patient. However, both Hacker et al (1981) and Monaghan (1990) have commented that, in a significant minority of patients, there appears to be considerable delay in presentation. The intimate nature of the disease, fear and/or ignorance and the advanced age of many patients might partly explain this observation. The fact that the disease is uncommon may also be contributory, as primary carers may not recognize the significance of symptoms or fail to recognize the clinical signs. Whatever the cause, a significant number of cases continue to present in advanced stages.

The reasons for presenting have been analysed by Podratz et al (1983a). Pruritus is the most common presenting symptom (71%), and an ulcer or mass will have been noted in nearly 80% of cases. Surprisingly, pain is only a feature in 23% of cases. Bleeding (26%), discharge (13%) and urinary tract dysfunction (14%) are other common reasons for presentation.

Assessment

The assessment of these women should include confirmation of the diagnosis, an assessment of disease extent, and an holistic approach to the patient to assess relevant comorbidity and/or other factors that may impact on the management plan.

Examination

The character, size and location(s) of all lesions should be documented. Particular attention should be paid to assess any involvement of the vagina, urethra, bladder base or anus. Palpation is important to determine possible involvement of the surrounding bony structures. Discomfort and tenderness may necessitate an examination (and biopsies) under general anaesthesia. The groin should be examined, although a negative assessment cannot reliably exclude cancer. Hard, enlarged, fixed or ulcerated nodes (Figure

41.3) need to be documented as this will almost certainly influence management.

Due to the potential for other genital tract malignancies, the vagina and cervix should also be assessed thoroughly and biopsied as necessary.

Diagnosis

Diagnosis is based upon a representative biopsy of the tumour. The biopsy should include an area where there is a transition from normal to malignant tissue (Figure 41.4). Biopsies should be of a sufficient size to allow differentiation between superficially invasive tumours and frankly invasive tumours, and orientated to allow quality pathological interpretation. Radical excision should not be undertaken without prior biopsy confirmation of malignancy unless there are extenuating circumstances.

The histopathological report should include:

- site;
- size (in three dimensions);
- associated features (such as the presence of VIN or condylomata);
- tumour type;
- depth of invasion;
- maximum horizontal measurement;
- whether the tumour is completely excised and tumour-free margin measurement;
- presence or absence of lymphovascular invasion; and
- nature of the adjacent non-malignant squamous epithelium.

The grading of the tumour is based on the percentage of undifferentiated cells, with grade 1 having no undifferentiated cells, grade 2 having less than half undifferentiated cells and grade 3 having more than half poorly differentiated cells.

Staging

There are two staging systems: the Tumour, Node, Metastasis system and the International Federation of Gynaecology and

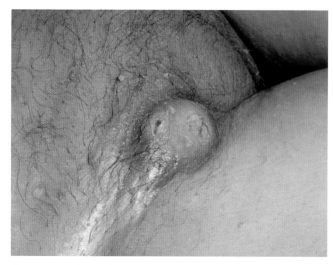

Figure 41.3 Enlarged fungating lymph node.

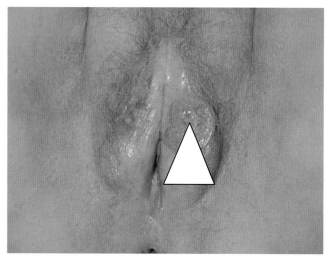

Figure 41.4 Diagnostic 'wedge biopsy' to include tumour and adjacent 'normal' epithelium.

Obstetrics (FIGO) system. Most gynaecologists use the latter which, since its last update in 2000, is based upon clinical and surgical findings. Table 41.2 details both staging systems.

Prognostic Factors

The size of the primary tumour and the status of the regional lymph nodes are the only two factors that have been consistently associated with outcome (Homesley et al 1991). The 5-year survival rate in cases without lymph node involvement is in excess of 80%, falling to less than 50% if the inguinal nodes are involved and 10–15% if the iliac or other pelvic nodes are involved.

Tumour size

Tumours larger than 2 cm in diameter have a greater chance of being frankly invasive and metastasizing to lymph nodes.

Table 41.2 FIGO staging of vulval cancer

FIGO stage	Description
I	Tumour confined to the vulva
Ia	Lesions ≤2 cm in size, confined to the vulva or perineum and with stromal invasion ≤1 mm. No nodal metastasis
Ib	Lesions >2 cm in size or with stromal invasion >1 mm confined to the vulva or perineum. No nodal metastasis
II	Tumour of any size with extension to adjacent perineal structures (lower 1/3 urethra; lower 1/3 vagina; anus) with negative nodes
III	Tumour of any size with or without extension to adjacent perineal structures (lower 1/3 urethra; lower 1/3 vagina; anus) with positive inguinofemoral nodes
IIIa	(i) With 1 lymph node metastasis (≥5 mm), or (ii) 1–2 lymph node metastasis(es) (<5 mm)
IIIb	(i) With 2 or more lymph node metastase (≥5 mm), or (ii) 3 or more lymph node metastases (<5 mm)
IIIc	With positive nodes with extracapsular spread
IV	Tumour invades other regional (upper 2/3 urethra; 2/3 vagina) or distant structures
IVa	Tumour invades any of the following (i) Upper urethral and or vaginal mucosa; bladder mucosa; rectal mucosa or fixed to pelvic bone, or (ii) Fixed or ulcerated inguinofemoral lymph nodes
IVb	Any distant metastasis including pelvic lymph nodes

FIGO, International Federation of Gynaecology and Obstetrics.

Depth of invasion

Invasion less than 1 mm (superficially invasive or stage Ia) has a negligible risk of lymph node involvement, and groin node dissection may be omitted (Hacker et al 1984b). The risk of nodal metastasis rises to 8% for a depth of 1–2 mm, 11% for 2–3 mm, and over 25% for lesions with a depth greater than 3 mm (Morrow et al 1993) (Figure 41.5).

Lymphovascular space permeation

This factor along with tumour border pattern (infiltrating vs pushing) and perineural invasion are not included in the surgicopathological staging of vulvar cancer, although they are associated with an increased risk of metastasis (Heaps et al 1990, Hopkins et al 1991).

Lymph node status

This is the most important prognostic variable. The number of lymph nodes involved and the nature of involvement influence the prognosis. Microscopic involvement of a single groin node, without extracapsular involvement, represents a low risk of recurrence, and adjuvant therapy is not necessary (Hacker et al 1983). Conversely, multiple nodal diseases and macroscopic and/or capsular involvement are indications for adjuvant radiotherapy in order to reduce the risk

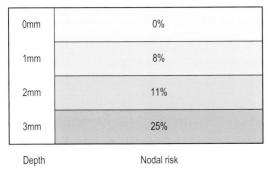

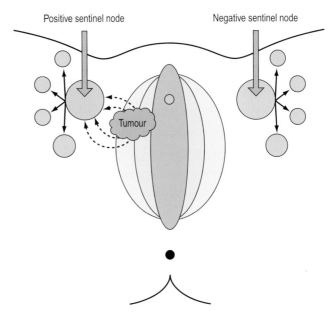

Figure 41.5 The relationship between depth of invasion and groin node metastases (squamous lesions).

Figure 41.6 Diagramatic illustration of the sentinel node concept.

of groin recurrence, which is usually fatal (van der Velden et al 1995). It is well recognized that groin node dissection is associated with significant morbidity. Almost 50% of patients undergoing groin node dissection will suffer post-operative complications, most commonly wound infection, wound breakdown and lymphoedema (Gaarenstroom et al 2003). For these reasons, a presurgical investigation that could identify those at risk could have a significant thera-peutic benefit. Assessment by clinical palpation of the groins is inadequate; of patients with clinically normal lymph nodes, 16–24% have metastases, while 24–41% of those with clinically involved nodes are negative when examined histologically (Sedlis et al 1987, Homesley et al 1993). Even though the majority of vulval cancers are still assessed clini-cally, there is increasing interest in utilizing additional imaging, particularly of the regional node groups. Ultra-sonography, computed tomography (CT), magnetic reso-nance imaging (MRI) and positron emission tomography have all been assessed but lack the sensitivity to exclude microscopic disease reliably (Selman et al 2005). Sentinel node sampling (vide infra) has shown promise, and the col-lective experience of this technique now suggests that it is reliable, at least in early-stage disease.

Sentinel lymph node detection

The concept of the 'sentinel lymph node' (SLN) was intro-duced in 1977 by Cabanas (1977). He defined the SLN as the first node in the lymphatic basin that receives primary lymphatic flow. Subsequent studies have confirmed that a tumour-free SLN implies absence of lymph node metastases in the entire draining lymphatic basin (Balega and van Trappen 2006). The last two decades have seen the tech-nique become established in the management of cutaneous melanoma and breast cancer. The concept (Figure 41.6) has now been introduced for the management of early vulval cancers, and the published performance data to date are promising (Table 41.3).

There are two ways to detect the SLN: blue dyes and radio-active tracer. Both are injected around the edge of the tumour prior to surgery; they are complementary and combining these techniques achieves a higher sensitivity compared with a single tracer. Excised SLNs are subjected to frozen section analysis and ultrastaging. Full inguinofemoral lymphadenec-tomy is avoided if SLNs are negative. Since unrecognized groin disease is nearly always fatal, the negative predictive value of this method is of particular concern. Early studies

included full inguinofemoral lymphadenectomy following the SLN procedure to provide a 'gold standard' for com-parison. The results confirmed a negative predictive value approaching 100%.

A large-scale international trial, the Groningen Interna-tional Study on Sentinel Nodes in Vulvar Cancer (GROINSS-V), was established to test the safety and clinical utility of SLN dissection in early-stage vulvar cancer. This was an observational study. Patients with stage I and II disease with tumour size less than 4 cm were recruited. Only patients found to have disease in either SLN underwent full inguinofemoral lymphadenectomy. Among 259 patients with unifocal vulvar cancer and a negative sentinel node, groin recurrences occurred in six (2.3%) women, and the 3-year survival rate was 97%. This result was comparable with similar historical groups of patients that had full inguinofemoral lymphadenectomy. However, both short- and long-term morbidity were significantly reduced, includ-ing shorter hospital stay and less wound breakdown and lymphoedema (van der Zee et al 2008). The authors thus proposed that sentinel node dissection should be the stand-ard treatment for patients with unifocal early-stage vulvar cancer. In the second phase of the GROINSS-V study, inves-tigators are evaluating radiotherapy, rather than complete inguinofemoral lymphadenectomy, in patients with meta-static SLNs. The objective is to further reduce morbidity by avoiding double-modality treatment.

Treatment

Factors influencing the management plan

Site of the tumour

Centrally located tumours lie close to midline structures such as the clitoris, urethra, vagina and anus, and are associ-ated with a higher risk of bilateral inguinal nodal spread compared with more lateral tumours. If the medial margin

Table 41.3 Performance of the sentinel lymph node technique in early vulval cancer

Author	Detection method	Groins dissected	Detection rate	Positive SLN	False-negative SLN	NPV
Ansink et al 1999	BD	93	56	9	2	95
de Hullu et al 2000	BD + RA	107	100	31	0	100
De Cicco et al 2000	RA	55	100	8	0	100
Levenback et al 2001	BD	76	75	10	0	100
Sliutz et al 2002	RA	46	100	9	0	100
Moore et al 2003	BD + RA	31	100	9	0	100

BD, blue dye; RA, radioactive tracer; SLN, sentinel lymph node; NPV, negative predictive value.

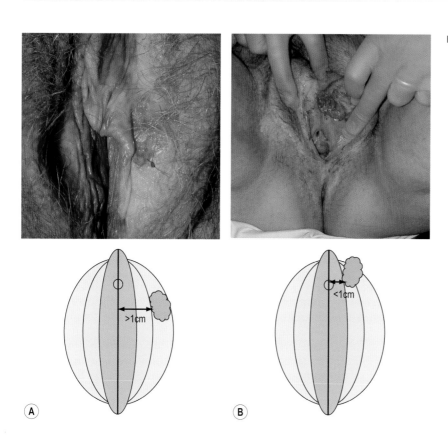

Figure 41.7 Laterality.

lies within 1 cm of the midline, they should be defined as central (de Hullu and van der Zee 2006). Bilateral groin node dissection is recommended for central tumours, and ipsilateral groin node dissection is recommended for lateralized tumours (Figure 41.7). Furthermore, if central tumours approximate to the urethra or anal canal such that these structures would be sacrificed to achieve satisfactory clearance, urinary or bowel diversion may be necessary.

Surgery

Surgery is the mainstay of treatment. The traditional 'butterfly' incision en-bloc radical (Figure 41.8) vulvectomy introduced by Taussig (1940) and Way (1960) clearly improved survival. The excised tissues included the vulvar lesion, the inguinofemoral lymph nodes and the lymphat-

ics in between. Large areas of normal tissue were frequently included, and primary wound closure was rarely achieved. Protracted postoperative recovery and severe wound complications and disfigurement were associated with this procedure. This postoperative morbidity has been the main driver for progress over the last two decades. Surgical treatment has become more individualized and conservative, aimed at reducing morbidity without compromising survival.

Separate incisions

The use of three separate incisions for groin dissections and vulvectomy instead of the traditional 'butterfly incision' has improved wound healing and reduced the frequency of wound breakdown (Hacker et al 1981). The suggestion that

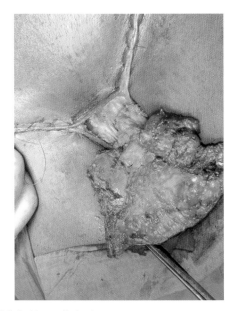

Figure 41.8 En-bloc radical vulvectomy.

this lesser approach might result in an increase in skin bridge recurrence was not born out in a Cochrane review, which showed a skin bridge recurrence rate of less than 1% (Ansink and van der Velden 2000). The hypothesis underpinning this strategy is based upon the belief that in early tumours, cells disseminate by embolization rather than in continuity (Willis 1973); therefore, there should be no residual tumour in the lymphatic channels between the tumour and the groin nodes. Reported cases of skin bridge recurrences were mainly seen in women with large groin node metastasis (Rose 1999). No prospective randomized controlled studies have been performed comparing the traditional radical vulvectomy with en-bloc inguinofemoral lymphadenectomy with the separate incision technique. However, de Hullu et al (2002) did undertake a retrospective comparison and noted a significant increase in groin and skin bridge recurrence with the less radical procedure (6.3% vs 1.3%, P=0.029). This, however, did not result in a difference in overall survival. They concluded that in view of the morbidity of the 'butterfly incision' and relatively low skin bridge recurrence rate, separate incisions were the preferable technique for stage I and II disease.

Modified radical vulvectomy or wide local excision

The main factor causing severe morbidity and disfigurement following radical vulvectomy is the extensive dissection and removal of normal tissue from the vulvar region. In the last two decades, less radical surgery, such as modified radical vulvectomy, hemivulvectomy and wide local excision, has been introduced to reduce morbidity without compromising survival. Tumour-free margins are the most important predictive factor for local recurrences. Both Heaps et al (1990) and de Hullu et al (2002) showed that a tumour-free margin of more than 8 mm was associated with significantly lower local recurrence rate. These studies found that suboptimal tumour-free margins (<8 mm) were more likely when the

intentional macroscopic margin was 1 cm or less. A lesion might extend further than judged by macroscopic inspection, and tissues usually shrink during preparation for histological examination (Balega et al 2008). A macroscopic surgical margin of 2 cm is thus recommended. This may be difficult to achieve in some cases where the tumour is adjacent to the urethra and anus, but every effort should be made to maximize the margins. The tumour-free margins should be the same regardless of whether a radical vulvectomy or a wide local excision is performed.

Unilateral inguinofemoral lymphadenectomy

Lateralized vulvar tumours rarely metastasize to the contralateral inguinofemoral lymph nodes without the ipsilateral nodes being involved. van der Velden (1996) pooled 489 patients with unilateral vulvar cancers and found only 0.9% with isolated contralateral lymph node metastases in lateralized stage I disease. Similarly, Gonzalez Bosquet et al (2007) reviewed 320 patients who underwent bilateral groin lymph node dissection. Among 163 patients with unilateral vulvar lesions, only three (1.8%) had an isolated contralateral nodal metastasis. No patients with a tumour diameter equal to or less than 2 cm and depth of invasion less than 5 mm had bilateral groin lymph node involvement. Given the recognized higher morbidity and low numbers of patients with contralateral metastases, it is now a generally accepted practice to perform a unilateral inguinofemoral lymphadenectomy in patients with stage I and II lateralized tumours, without suspicious lymph nodes on palpitation. If nodal disease is found in one groin, the opposite groin should also be explored. Normal lymph flow may be disturbed in cases of ipsilateral groin node metastases with alternate channels developing, thus allowing contralateral spread.

Superficial inguinal lymphadenectomy

In order to reduce lymphoedema and wound breakdown associated with groin dissection, DiSaia et al (1979) proposed removing only the superficial inguinal lymph nodes lying anterior to the cribriform fascia, without exploration of the deeper femoral nodes. The rationale for this was that lymphatic drainage from the vulva passes first to the superficial inguinal nodes before subsequently draining to the femoral nodes. The superficial inguinal nodes were assessed by frozen section, and a deep dissection was performed if the superficial nodes were found to be positive. However, the results of subsequent studies have not been encouraging. Unexpected groin recurrences occurred in patients with early-stage disease and presumed negative inguinal nodes (Hacker et al 1984b, Kelley et al 1992, Stehman et al 1992a). The current practice is that a full inguinofemoral lymphadenectomy including all superficial inguinal lymph nodes and femoral lymph nodes medial to the femoral veins should be performed whenever there is an indication for node dissection.

Pelvic lymphadenectomy

Routine pelvic lymphadenectomy is no longer considered in the surgical management of vulvar carcinoma. The incidence of pelvic node metastases is approximately 5% and is very rare in the absence of inguinofemoral lymph node metastases (Gadducci et al 2006). One randomized trial (Homesley et al 1986) compared pelvic lymphadenectomy with pelvic radiotherapy in patients with inguinofemoral lymph node metastases after radical vulvectomy and bilateral inguinofemoral lymphadenectomy. The 2-year survival rate for the radiation group was significantly better than that for the pelvic lymphadenectomy group (68% vs 54%, $P<0.03$). The incidence of groin recurrence was less in the radiation group (5.1% vs 23.6%, $P<0.02$). However, the rate of pelvic recurrence was increased in patients who received pelvic irradiation. It was postulated that radiation may not be able to sterilize bulky pelvic metastatic nodes. Therefore, removal of enlarged pelvic nodes seen on CT scan via an extraperitoneal approach was suggested before starting radiotherapy.

Surgical morbidity

Incremental reduction in the radicality of treatment has resulted in less morbidity. Wound breakdown, wound infections, lymphocysts, lymphoedema, vulvar disfigurement and psychosexual disturbance remain problematic.

Vulvar morbidity

Primary wound closure was often difficult if not impossible when the traditional 'butterfly incision' was used. This is still the case when large excisions are required, but even in these instances, more frequent use of plastic reconstructive techniques results in improved healing and better cosmetic outcomes. In smaller vulvar tumours, wide local excision with separate groin wounds has decreased the wound breakdown rate significantly.

Problems with micturition (spraying, angulation of urine, urethral stenosis) are not uncommon if the distal third of the urethra is excised. Surgery for perineal and perianal lesions may give rise to problems with defaecation (constipation, tenesmus and faecal incontinence), localized pain when sitting and coital difficulties (Barton 2003). Occasionally, repeat surgery is needed to excise fibrotic tissue or to widen the stenotic introitus in order to facilitate coitus.

Groin morbidity

Lymphocysts and infection are the two most common short-term groin complications. Despite the routine use of drains and antibiotics, complications are still as high as 66% (Gaarenstroom et al 2003). More troublesome is the long-term complication of lower limb lymphoedema, which is often difficult to treat and can cause significant distress to patients. The incidence of lymphoedema is further increased if adjuvant radiotherapy is given after surgery (Barton 2003). The simplest approach to reduce groin morbidity is less radical surgery and avoidance of double treatment. SLN dissection goes some way to addressing this need without compromising disease control, at least in early vulval cancer. The incidence of wound breakdown, infection and lymphoedema decreased to 11.7%, 4.5% and 1.9%, respectively (van der Zee et al 2008).

Psychological morbidity

Vulvar disfigurement, coital difficulties and lower limb oedema are all chronic problems that continually remind patients of their past disease and treatment. This can impact adversely on relationships and self-esteem. Leg oedema is distressing as it is a visible disfigurement, can reduce mobility and impact on independent living. Such complications may eventually result in depression, low self-esteem and loss of confidence. Consideration should be given to provide psychological and psychosexual support for these patients.

Radiotherapy

Radiotherapy was traditionally considered to have a limited role in the management of vulvar cancer. Vulvar skin does not tolerate irradiation well, especially so when orthovoltage equipment was in use. Vulvar skin is thin, delicate, very sensitive and highly vascularized. Radiotherapy to this area frequently causes both acute and chronic reactions, making treatment difficult to tolerate, particularly in the elderly. Acute inflammation with both dry and moist desquamation is very painful, and may be exacerbated by associated urinary incontinence. Tolerance of radiotherapy has improved with megavoltage therapy. Late reactions include scarring, fibrosis and telangiectasia causing functional compromise and cosmetic impairment.

Postoperative adjuvant therapy

Patients with risk factors for local recurrence, such as a close surgical margin, lymphovascular space permeation, poorly differentiated tumour grade or diffuse infiltrative growth pattern, should be considered for adjuvant external beam radiation therapy to reduce the risk of recurrence (Perez et al 1998, Blake 2003).

With regard to the nodal status, no additional treatment is recommended if there is only one microscopically positive lymph node (Hacker et al 1983). However, if two or more metastatic nodes are present, or there is capsular involvement in a single metastatic node, postoperative adjuvant radiotherapy is usually recommended (van der Velden et al 1995). In a subgroup analysis of Homesley et al's study, the survival advantage of radiotherapy was limited to those patients with clinically evident groin nodes or more than one positive groin node (Homesley et al 1986).

Neoadjuvant therapy

In order to achieve an adequate surgical margin with large tumours close to the urethra and/or anal canal, it may be necessary to compromise urethral and/or anal function with an associated diversion. In 1973, Boronow suggested a combined radiosurgical approach to shrink the tumour preoperatively, aiming to spare this group of patients from exenterative surgery. Subsequent reports (Hacker et al 1984a, Boronow et al 1987) confirmed the feasibility of this function-sparing approach. More recently, concurrent chemoradiation has been used with the same intent. Moore et al (1998) gave concurrent cisplatin/5-fluorouracil (5FU) and radiation therapy to 71 patients with stage III–IV disease. Thirty-three patients (46.5%) had no visible tumour after chemoradiation, and only three patients were not able to preserve urinary and/or gastrointestinal continence after surgery. van Doorn et al (2006) reviewed the available literature and concluded that preoperative chemoradiotherapy reduces tumour size and improves operability. However, complications are considerable, especially in delayed wound healing, and overall increased treatment-related morbidity.

Primary treatment

Radiotherapy alone as a treatment for vulvar cancer is not recommended in operable tumours, mainly because of the perceived intolerance of vulvar tissue. However, it is an option in patients who cannot undergo surgery because of advanced disease or comorbidity issues. In selected cases, primary radiotherapy can cure vulvar cancer with acceptable morbidity (Busch et al 1999). Chemotherapy can be added to the regimen, either as a neoadjuvant to reduce tumour bulk or as concomitant chemoradiotherapy to improve cure rates (Moore et al 1998).

Although the groin tolerates radiotherapy better than the vulva, primary radiotherapy to treat groin disease is not recommended. One study has reported a higher recurrence rate when comparing radiation therapy with inguinofemoral lymphadenectomy (Stehman et al 1992b). However, this study has been criticized on the basis of suboptimal radiotherapy technique, particularly that the maximum dose did not reach the deep inguinofemoral nodes. More recently, Katz et al (2003) re-evaluated the value of primary radiotherapy for groin disease. Comparable recurrence rates were observed when radiotherapy alone was compared with inguinofemoral lymphadenectomy (15% vs 16.6%). The authors concluded that radiotherapy alone was as effective as surgery in preventing groin recurrence. This study was criticized largely because of difficulties in interpreting the individualized treatment. There were also doubts about the radicality of lymphadenectomy.

Although the available data are somewhat confused, radiotherapy appears to be an effective treatment for microscopic (residual) disease in the groin, but less effective when gross disease is present.

Palliation

Patients with advanced disease and distant metastasis might not derive much overall benefit from radical surgery. Radiotherapy may offer a palliative option in some of these cases.

Chemotherapy

The role of chemotherapy in vulvar cancer is either as concomitant therapy with radiation or as a palliative manoeuvre in recurrent or metastatic disease. Several cytotoxic drugs (cisplatin, methotrexate, bleomycin, mitomycin C and 5FU) have been shown to have activity when used alone or in combination (Shimizu et al 1990, Benedetti Panici et al 1993). 5FU appears to be the most effective agent. In a series of 12 patients with advanced vulvar cancer involving either or both the anus and urethra, a combination of cisplatin and 5FU gave a 100% response rate. The anal sphincter and urethra were conserved in these patients during subsequent

radical surgery. However, three patients receiving cisplatin alone showed no response or even progression (Geisler et al 2006). However, all of the studies were small and uncontrolled, and should be interpreted with caution.

Advanced Disease

Advanced vulvar cancer (T3/T4) is characterized by local extension to neighbouring structures (urethra, vagina, bladder and anus). Regional lymph node metastases are present in over 50% of these patients (Hacker et al 1983). Ultraradical surgery with urinary tract and/or bowel diversion is required for complete excision. Unfortunately, most of these patients are elderly and frail, having significant comorbidities rendering them unsuitable for such extensive surgery. Radiation therapy with or without chemotherapy can shrink some tumours before surgery, sparing them from stoma formation and reducing surgical morbidity (Hacker et al 1984a, Boronow et al 1987). Furthermore, preoperative chemoradiation can result in fixed groin nodes becoming resectable (Montana et al 2000). Radiation therapy with or without concurrent chemotherapy should be considered as an alternative option for patients with advanced vulvar cancer who would otherwise require exenterative surgery.

Recurrences

Rouzier et al (2002) identified three patterns of local recurrence:

- primary site recurrence, defined as within 2 cm of the vulvectomy scar (39%);
- recurrence remote from the primary tumour site, regarded as reoccurrence of cancer (39%); and
- skin bridge recurrence (22%).

Tumour size, surgical margins and depth of invasion (Rouzier et al 2002) are risk factors for primary site relapse. It is usually salvageable with repeat surgical excision or radiotherapy (Thomas et al 1989, Hopkins et al 1990). Local recurrence remote from the primary tumour site should be considered as a new primary lesion and is seen more frequently in patients with a background of lichen sclerosus or differentiated VIN. Again, surgical excision is the first choice of treatment. The prognosis is generally good, with more than 60% of patients surviving for more than 3 years. Patients with skin bridge recurrence seldom live for more than 1 year (Rouzier et al 2002).

Almost one-third of all recurrences occur in the groin. Groin recurrence is seen more often when previous node dissection was omitted, or when positive nodes were present at primary surgery. The prognosis is poor, with more than 90% of patients dying within 1 year (Hacker et al 1984b).

Malignant Melanoma

Malignant melanoma is the second most common vulvar malignancy, accounting for 5–10% of cases of vulvar cancer. The incidence is less than 0.2 per 100,000 women per year (Piura 2008). It is a disease of the elderly, occurring in the fifth to seventh decades, and is more common in

Caucasians. They usually present with a vulvar mass, bleeding and pruritus. The labia minora, clitoris or inner aspects of the labia majora are the most common sites. A variety of pigmented lesions mimic vulvar melanoma, including vulvar melanosis, different types of nevi and acanthosis nigricans. Biopsy is essential for diagnosis. Three histological subtypes have been described (Ragnarsson-Olding et al 1999a):

- lentiginous melanoma;
- superficial spreading melanoma; and
- nodular melanoma.

Up to 25% of tumours are amelanotic.

Various staging systems have been proposed for vulvar melanoma. The most commonly used are the Clark et al (1969), Breslow (1970) and Chung et al (1975) systems. However, in 1994, a Gynecologic Oncology Group study showed that the American Joint Committee on Cancer melanoma staging system is more accurate in predicting outcome (Phillips et al 1994).

Radical vulvectomy has been recommended for vulvar melanoma in the past. However, the available literature suggests no survival difference in patients having a radical vulvectomy, simple vulvectomy or wide local excision (Rose et al 1988, Tasseron et al 1992). The current consensus is to aim for a tumour-free margin of at least 1 cm for tumour less than 1 mm thick, a tumour-free margin of 2 cm for tumours 1–4 mm thick, and a tumour-free margin of at least 1 cm at the subcutaneous layer for all cases. The role of elective regional node dissection is controversial for both cutaneous and vulvar melanoma. A prospective study by the Gynecologic Oncology Group in 1994 failed to find a definite survival benefit for elective lymph node dissection in patients with vulvar melanoma (Phillips et al 1994). The role of adjuvant therapy for treatment of vulvar melanoma is also unclear. Radiotherapy has been suggested for incomplete tumour resection or positive groin/pelvic lymph nodes (Piura 2008). Interferon α-2b seems to be a promising adjuvant therapy for cutaneous melanoma (Kirkwood et al 2001), but data in vulvar melanoma are lacking.

Vulvar melanoma is usually highly aggressive, with a tendency to recur locally and spread haematogenously to distant organs such as the liver, lung and brain. Reported 5-year survival rates range from 21% to 54% (Podratz et al 1983b, Blessing et al 1991, Ragnarsson-Olding et al 1999b, Verschraegen et al 2001). As with cutaneous melanoma, the survival rate correlates with depth of invasion.

Bartholin's Gland Carcinoma

Primary carcinoma of Bartholin's gland is rare, accounting for 0.1–7% of all vulvar carcinomas (Nasu et al 2005). Bartholin's gland carcinomas may initially be confused with Bartholin's cyst or an abscess. The tumour may arise from either the gland or the duct, thus various histological types may occur, including adenocarcinomas, squamous carcinomas, transitional cell carcinomas, adenosquamous carcinomas and adenoid cystic carcinomas. Since most of these lesions are located deep in the vulva, radical excision usually involves removing part of the vagina, levator muscles and the ischiorectal fat in order to achieve an adequate tumour-free margin. If regional groin or pelvic lymph nodes are

positive, adjuvant radiotherapy is indicated to reduce the risk of recurrence (Copeland et al 1986). Adenoid cystic carcinoma is a rare variant, characterized by slow growth, with a marked tendency for perineural and local invasion. The tumour seldom metastasizes and carries a better prognosis (Nasu et al 2005).

Invasive Paget's Disease

Paget's disease of the vulva is a rare intraepithelial neoplasia, probably originating from the vulvar apocrine glands. Approximately 10% of cases are invasive and 4–8% are associated with adenocarcinoma (Fanning et al 1999). The disease predominantly affects postmenopausal Caucasian women, usually presenting with vulvar pruritus and soreness. The lesion is usually multifocal, well demarcated and characterized by red eczematous patches (Figure 41.9). These originate on the hair-bearing regions of the vulva. Notoriously, vulvar Paget's disease extends beyond the macroscopic lesions, and recurrence frequently occurs despite a clear surgical margin obtained at wide local excision (MacLean et al 2004). Thus, it is not uncommon for patients to undergo multiple recurrences and re-excisions over years of surveillance. In the event of finding invasive carcinoma, the patient should be treated with radical vulvectomy and groin node dissection, as for squamous cell carcinoma.

An additional concern with extramammary Paget's disease is its association with other malignancies, including breast, uterine, vagina, bladder, pancreas, lung and stomach. Appropriate management includes investigations to try and exclude other cancers.

Verrucous Carcinoma

Verrucous carcinoma is a rare variant of squamous cell carcinoma, characterized by local invasion without nodal or distant metastases. The gross appearance resembles a giant condyloma. Histologically, there is an exophytic papillary component of well-differentiated squamous epithelium with hyperparakeratosis and well-demarcated

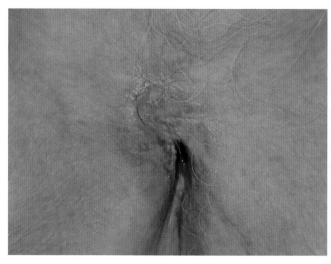

Figure 41.9 Recurrent Paget's disease after vulval excision.

pushing borders. The treatment is modified radical vulvectomy. Lymphadenectomy is not indicated (Finan 2003).

Basal Cell Carcinoma

Basal cell carcinoma accounts for approximately 2–4% of all cases of vulvar cancer. It usually appears as a small (1–2 cm), raised, nodular lesion with well-defined edges. Wide local excision with a 1 cm margin is usually curative, and recurrence and metastases are rare (Mulayim et al 2002).

Sarcoma

Vulvar sarcoma is extremely rare and treatment options are derived from anecdotal case reports. Leiomyosarcoma, rhabdomyosarcoma, malignant fibrous histiocytoma, dermatofibrosacroma protuberans and epithelioid sarcoma are all reported in the literature. The usual treatment is radical vulvectomy and groin node dissection (Aartsen and Albus-Lutter 1994, Hensley 2000).

Cancer of The Vagina

Introduction

Vaginal carcinoma accounts for less than 2% of gynaecological cancers (Kirkbride et al 1995). In 2005, 216 cases were registered in the UK, equivalent to 0.8/100,000 women (Office of National Statistics 2008). Seventy percent of these patients were 60 years of age or older. Squamous cell carcinoma was the most common variant (Grigsby 2002). The evidence base is drawn from case reports and retrospective reviews.

Aetiology

The exact aetiology for primary vaginal cancer is unknown. Up to one-third of patients have a history of a cervical lesion, either benign or malignant (Peters et al 1985). Stock et al (1995) reviewed 100 cases of vaginal cancer and found that patients who had a previous hysterectomy were more likely to develop a lesion in the upper third of the vagina compared with women who had not had an hysterectomy (62% vs 34%, $P<0.005$). Possible explanations for this are: occult residual disease from a cervical lesion, HPV as a persisting carcinogenic agent (Daling et al 2002), an effect of radiation therapy given for previous genital tract cancer may induce vaginal cancer, and the disease interval is usually more than 10 years (Chaturvedi et al 2007).

Similar to cervical cancer, there is a premalignant condition in the vagina, vaginal intraepithelial neoplasia (VAIN). However, the true malignant potential of VAIN is unclear. Vaginal cancer caused by chronic irritation, such as procidentia and vaginal pessaries, has been reported (Ghosh et al 2009) but the incidence is extremely low. Intrauterine exposure to diethylstilboestrol was thought to be a causative agent for clear cell adenocarcinoma of the vagina in the past (Herbst et al 1971). However, with the cessation of its use in the 1970s, it is rarely seen nowadays.

Pathology

More than 80% of primary vaginal tumours are squamous cell carcinomas; adenocarcinomas are the second most common, accounting for approximately 15% (Grigsby 2002). The remainder are sarcomas, malignant melanomas, small cell carcinomas, lymphomas and carcinoid tumours. Metastatic lesions from non-gynaecological sites have also been reported, including bladder, kidney, colon and rectum (Tarraza et al 1998, Parikh et al 2008).

Clinical assessment

The most common presenting symptoms are painless vaginal bleeding (81%) and abnormal discharge (33%) (Pingley et al 2000). Large, posteriorly sited tumours may cause tenesmus. When disease has spread beyond the vagina, patients may present with pelvic pain. Occasionally, vaginal cancer may be recognized after an abnormal Pap smear (Pride et al 1979).

The majority of lesions are located in the upper posterior vagina, usually in the form of an exophytic mass with contact bleeding (Pingley et al 2000). It is not uncommon to miss a small lower vaginal lesion at the initial examination, when it may be hidden by the blades of the speculum. If vaginal cancer is to be excluded, a full and thorough inspection of the entire vagina is required.

In order to make a diagnosis of vaginal cancer, apart from histological confirmation, certain criteria are to be met (Benedet et al 2000):

- the primary site has to be in the vagina;
- the lesion should not involve the uterine cervix, vulva or urethra, otherwise they should be considered as the likely primary cancer; and
- this is not a recurrence of genital tract cancer.

The diagnosis of vaginal cancer should only be made with a biopsy, which may be taken either in the office or under anaesthesia. The latter is preferable because it provides an opportunity to examine the patient in total relaxation, and a generous full-thickness excisional biopsy may be obtained. Cystoscopy and proctosigmoidoscopy are indicated when local spread is suspected. Chest radiography and an intravenous pyelogram are necessary to exclude lung metastasis and ureteric involvement. Cross-sectional imaging (CT scan or MRI) is useful in evaluate the extent of disease and intraabdominal metastasis.

Staging

The FIGO staging system for vaginal cancer is shown in Table 41.4. It is a clinical staging system based on findings from physical examination, cystoscopy, proctoscopy and chest X-ray.

Pattern of spread

Vaginal cancer initially spreads by local invasion; it may infiltrate adjacent pelvic organs and the side walls by direct extension. Tumour in the upper vagina embolizes to the pelvic and para-aortic lymph nodes, while those in the lower vagina metastasize to the groin lymph nodes and

Table 41.4 International Federation of Gynaecology and Obstetrics (FIGO) staging for carcinoma of the vagina

FIGO stage	Description
Stage 0	Carcinoma in situ, intraepithelial carcinoma, high-grade vaginal intraepithelial neoplasia
Stage I	The carcinoma is limited to the vaginal wall
Stage II	The carcinoma has invaded the subvaginal tissues but has not extended on to the pelvic sidewall
Stage IIa	The carcinoma has invaded the subvaginal tissues but has not extended to the parametrium
Stage IIb	The carcinoma involves the parametrium but has not extended to the pelvic sidewall
Stage III	The carcinoma has extended to the pelvic sidewall
Stage IV	The carcinoma extends beyond the true pelvis or has clinically involved the mucosa of the bladder or rectum. Bullous oedema as such does not permit a case to be allocated to stage IV
Stage IVa	The carcinoma has spread to adjacent organs and/or direct extension beyond the true pelvis
Stage IVb	The carcinoma has spread to distant organs

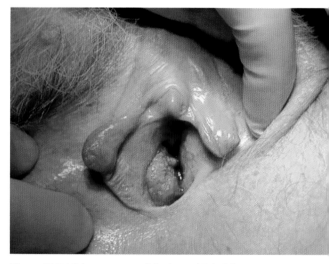

Figure 41.10 Primary tumour of the lower third of the vagina.

secondarily to pelvic nodes. Haematogenous dissemination to distant organs is a late event.

Treatment

Due to the rarity of this disease, there is no consensus on the treatment, be it radiation or surgery. Patients should be managed in tertiary centres, and all treatment should be individualized according to stage and site of disease.

Radiotherapy is the most commonly used treatment modality for vaginal cancer. The close proximity of the bladder and rectum limit the ability of surgery to radically excise tumour without significant functional compromise. Exenterative surgery is often needed in order to achieve adequate margins, especially with lower vaginal tumours (Figure 41.10).

Both teletherapy and brachytherapy are used in managing these cancers. A number of reports have shown that sequential use of teletherapy followed by brachytherapy results in a better outcome (Perez et al 1999, Pingley et al 2000). External radiation is used to treat disease with lateral infiltration; the irradiation field is similar to that for cervical cancer. The pelvis receives 50 Gy, covering the side walls, pelvic nodes and the whole vagina (Grigsby 2002). The irradiation field should be extended to the groin if the tumour is located in the lower third of the vagina. External beam irradiation also results in shrinkage of large tumours, facilitating subsequent brachytherapy. Interstitial implants using premade templates may be indicated for deeply invasive tumours. Early-stage disease (stage I–II) may be treated by brachytherapy alone.

Although surgery has a limited role in the treatment of vaginal cancer, it is indicated in certain situations. Stage I–II upper vaginal lesions can be treated surgically. Upper vaginectomy in combination with radical hysterectomy and bilateral pelvic lymphadenectomy can be performed for patients with an intact uterus. If the patient has had a hysterectomy, radical upper vaginectomy and pelvic lymphadenectomy may be considered. In a retrospective study of 89 stage I and II patients, Davis et al (1991) reported no survival differences when comparing surgery and radiotherapy.

Pelvic exenteration can be considered for localized recurrent disease after radiotherapy. It should also be considered in medically fit patients with stage IVa disease, especially in those with symptomatic fistulae.

There is limited information in the literature regarding concurrent chemoradiation therapy for vaginal cancer. The use of this modality of treatment for vaginal cancer is a logical extension of its use in cervical cancer.

Prognosis

Staging is the only consistent prognostic factor in predicting outcome. The 5-year survival rates for stage I, II, III and IV disease are 73%, 51%, 33% and 20%, respectively (Beller et al 2001).

Uncommon vaginal tumours

Rhadbomyosarcoma (sarcoma botryoides)

This rare tumour mainly affects children below 5 years of age. The polypoid tumour protrudes from the vagina, resembling a bunch of grapes. Treatment is based upon primary chemotherapy using vincristine, actinomycin D and cyclophosphamide plus doxorubicin, followed by conservative organ-sparing surgery or radiotherapy. Survival rates of over 80% are now achievable (Andrassy et al 1999, Harting et al 2004).

Clear cell adenocarcinoma

Approximately 15% of primary vaginal cancers are adenocarcinomas, predominantly affecting young women. In the main, they arise from vaginal adenosis, which is a consequence of disrupted Müllerian development. This malformation may or may not be related to in-utero diethylstilboestrol exposure (Herbst and Anderson 1990). The treatment is similar to that of squamous cell carcinoma of the vagina. However, every effort should be made to retain vaginal and ovarian function as most of these patients are still in their reproductive years.

Malignant melanoma

Primary malignant melanoma of the vagina constitutes less than 0.3% of all melanomas and less than 3% of malignant vaginal tumours (Siu et al 2004). It is highly malignant and is notoriously more aggressive than non-genital and vulvar melanoma. Most patients are diagnosed at an advanced stage with a deeply invasive tumour. The 5-year survival rate is 17%. Radical surgery does not appear any better than conservative surgery (wide local excision) in terms of survival (Reid et al 1989). Radiotherapy is mainly used as an adjuvant therapy to decrease recurrence.

KEY POINTS

1. Vulval cancer probably arises through two oncogenic pathways: one related to oncogenic HPVs and the other related to lichen sclerosus.
2. It is predominantly a disease of the elderly and comorbidity is common.
3. Surgery is the mainstay of treatment and has become progressively less radical over time.
4. Management must always address the possibility of regional disease in the groin lymph nodes.
5. Sentinel node detection is likely to further reduce treatment-related morbidity for early vulval cancer.
6. Multimodality treatment with reconstructive surgery should improve outcomes in more locally advanced disease.
7. Groin node dissection is not routinely required for vulval melanoma as the depth of invasion is the most potent prognostic indicator.
8. The squamous variants, basal cell and verrucous carcinoma, have a very low risk of regional spread, and therefore do not require groin lymphadenectomy.

REFERENCES

Aartsen EJ, Albus-Lutter CE 1994 Vulvar sarcoma: clinical implications. European Journal of Obstetrics and Gynecology and Reproductive Biology 56: 181–189.

Andrassy RJ, Wiener ES, Raney RB et al 1999 Progress in the surgical management of vaginal rhabdomyosarcoma: a 25-year review from the Intergroup Rhabdomyosarcoma Study Group. Journal of Pediatric Surgery 34: 731–735.

Ansink AC, Heintz AP 1993 Epidemiology and etiology of squamous cell carcinoma of the vulva. European Journal of Obstetrics and Gynecology and Reproductive Biology 48: 111–115.

Ansink AC, Sie-Go DM, van der Velden J et al 1999 Identification of sentinel lymph nodes in vulvar carcinoma patients with the aid of a patent blue V injection: a multicenter study. Cancer 86: 652–656.

Ansink A, van der Velden J 2000 Surgical interventions for early squamous cell carcinoma of the vulva. Cochrane Database of Systematic Reviews 2: CD002036.

Balega J, van Trappen PO 2006 The sentinel node in gynaecological malignancies. Cancer Imaging 6: 7–15.

Balega J, Butler J, Jeyarajah A et al 2008 Vulval cancer: what is an adequate surgical margin? European Journal of Gynaecological Oncology 29: 455–458.

Barton DPJ 2003 The prevention and management of treatment related morbidity in vulval cancer. Best Practice and Research Clinical Obstetrics and Gynaecology 17: 683–701.

Beller U, Sideri M, Maisonneuve P et al 2001 Carcinoma of the vagina. Journal of Epidemiology and Biostatistics 6: 141–152.

Benedet JL, Bender H, Jones H 3rd, Ngan HY, Pecorelli S 2000 FIGO staging classifications and clinical practice guidelines in the management of gynecologic cancers. FIGO Committee on Gynecologic Oncology. International Journal of Gynecology and Obstetrics 70: 209–262.

Benedetti-Panici P, Greggi S, Scambia G, Salerno G, Mancuso S 1993 Cisplatin (P), bleomycin (B), and methotrexate (M) preoperative chemotherapy in locally advanced vulvar carcinoma. Gynecologic Oncology 50: 49–53.

Blake P 2003 Radiotherapy and chemoradiotherapy for carcinoma of the vulva. Best Practice and Research Clinical Obstetrics and Gynaecology 17: 649–661.

Blessing K, Kernohan NM, Miller ID, Al Nafussi AI 1991 Malignant melanoma of the vulva: clinicopathological features. International Journal of Gynecological Cancer 1: 81–87.

Boronow RC 1973 Therapeutic alternative to primary exenteration for advanced vulvovaginal cancer. Gynecologic Oncology 1: 233–255.

Boronow RC, Hickman BT, Reagan MT, Smith RA, Steadham RE 1987 Combined therapy as an alternative to exenteration for locally advanced vulvovaginal cancer. II. Results, complications, and dosimetric and surgical considerations. American Journal of Clinical Oncology 10: 171–181.

Bradgate MG, Rollason TP, McConkey CC, Powell J 1990 Malignant melanoma of the vulva: a clinicopathological study of 50 women. British Journal of Obstetrics and Gynaecology 97: 124–133.

Breslow A 1970 Thickness, cross-sectional areas and depth of invasion in the prognosis of cutaneous melanoma. Annals of Surgery 172: 902–908.

Busch M, Wagener B, Dühmke E 1999 Long-term results of radiotherapy alone for carcinoma of the vulva. Advances in Therapy 16: 89–100.

Cabanas RM 1977 An approach for the treatment of penile carcinoma. Cancer 39: 456–466.

Chaturvedi AK, Engels EA, Gilbert ES et al 2007 Second cancers among 104,760 survivors of cervical cancer: evaluation of long-term risk. Journal of the National Cancer Institute 99: 1634–1643.

Chung AF, Woodruff JM, Lewis JL Jr 1975 Malignant melanoma of the vulva: a report of 44 cases. Obstetrics and Gynecology 45: 638–646.

Clark WH Jr, From L, Bernardino EA, Mihm MC 1969 The histogenesis and biologic behavior of primary human malignant melanomas of the skin. Cancer Research 29: 705–727.

Copeland LJ, Sneige N, Gershenson DM, McGuffee VB, Abdul-Karim F, Rutledge FN 1986 Bartholin gland carcinoma. Obstetrics and Gynecology 67: 794–801.

Crum CP, McLachlin CM, Tate JE, Mutter GL 1997 Pathobiology of vulvar squamous neoplasia. Current Opinion in Obstetrics and Gynecology 9: 63–69.

Daling JR, Madeleine MM, Schwartz SM et al 2002 A population-based study of squamous cell vaginal cancer: HPV and cofactors. Gynecologic Oncology 84: 263–270.

Davis KP, Stanhope CR, Garton GR, Atkinson EJ, O'Brien PC 1991 Invasive vaginal carcinoma: analysis of early-stage disease. Gynecologic Oncology 42: 131–136.

De Cicco C, Sideri M, Bartolomei M et al 2000 Sentinel node biopsy in early vulvar cancer. British Journal of Cancer 82: 295–299.

de Hullu JA, Hollema H, Piers DA et al 2000 Sentinel lymph node procedure is highly accurate in squamous cell carcinoma of the vulva. Journal of Clinical Oncology 18: 2811–2816.

de Hullu JA, Hollema H, Lolkema S et al 2002 Vulvar carcinoma. The price of less radical surgery. Cancer 95: 2331–2338.

de Hullu JA, van der Zee AGJ 2006 Surgery and radiotherapy in vulvar cancer. Critical Reviews in Oncology/Hematology 60: 38–58.

DiSaia PJ, Creasman WT, Rich WM 1979 An alternate approach to early cancer of the vulva. American Journal of Obstetrics Gynecology 133: 825–832.

Fanning J, Lambert HC, Hale TM, Morris PC, Schuerch C 1999 Paget's disease of the vulva: prevalence of associated vulvar adenocarcinoma, invasive Paget's disease, and recurrence after surgical excision. American Journal of Obstetrics and Gynecology 180: 24–27.

Finan MA 2003 Bartholin's gland carcinoma, malignant melanoma and other rare tumours of the vulva. Best Practice and Research Clinical Obstetrics and Gynaecology 17: 609–633.

Fishman DA, Chambers SK, Schwartz PE, Kohorn EI, Chambers JT 1995 Extramammary Paget's disease of the vulva. Gynecologic Oncology 56: 266–267.

Gaarenstroom KN, Kenter GG, Trimbos JB et al 2003 Postoperative complications after vulvectomy and inguinofemoral lymphadenectomy using separate groin incisions. International Journal of Gynecological Cancer 13: 552–557.

Gadducci A, Cionini L, Romanini A, Fanucchi A, Genazzani AR 2006 Old and new perspectives in the management of high-risk, locally advanced or recurrent, and metastatic vulvar cancer. Critical Reviews in Oncology/Hematology 60: 227–241.

Geisler JP, Manahan KJ, Buller RE 2006 Neoadjuvant chemotherapy in vulvar cancer: avoiding primary exenteration. Gynecologic Oncology 100: 53–57.

Ghosh SB, Tripathi R, Mala YM, Khurana N 2009 Primary invasive carcinoma of vagina with third degree uterovaginal prolapse: a case report and review of literature.

Archives of Gynecology and Obstetrics 279: 91–93.

Gonzalez Bosquet J, Magrina JF, Magtibay PM et al 2007 Patterns of inguinal groin metastases in squamous cell carcinoma of the vulva. Gynecologic Oncology 105: 742–746.

Grigsby PW 2002 Vaginal cancer. Current Treatment Options in Oncology 3: 125–130.

Hacker NF, Leuchter RS, Berek JS, Castaldo TW, Lagasse LD 1981 Radical vulvectomy and bilateral inguinal lymphadenectomy through separate groin incisions. Obstetrics and Gynecology 58: 574–579.

Hacker NF, Berek JS, Lagasse LD, Leuchter RS, Moore JG 1983 Management of regional lymph nodes and their prognostic influence in vulvar cancer. Obstetrics and Gynecology 61: 408–412.

Hacker NF, Berek JS, Juillard GJ, Lagasse LD 1984a Preoperative radiation therapy for locally advanced vulvar cancer. Cancer 54: 2056–2061.

Hacker NF, Berek JS, Lagasse LD, Nieberg RK, Leuchter RS 1984b Individualization of treatment for stage I squamous cell vulvar carcinoma. Obstetrics and Gynecology 63: 155–162.

Harting MT, Blakely ML, Andrassy RJ 2004 Surgical management of gynecologic rhabdomyosarcoma. Current Treatment Options in Oncology 5: 109–118.

Heaps JM, Fu YS, Montz FJ, Hacker NF, Berek JS 1990 Surgical-pathologic variables predictive of local recurrence in squamous cell carcinoma of the vulva. Gynecologic Oncology 38: 309–314.

Hensley ML 2000 Uterine/female genital sarcomas. Current Treatment Options in Oncology 1: 161–168.

Herbst AL, Ulfelder H, Poskanzer DC 1971 Adenocarcinoma of the vagina. Association of maternal stilbestrol therapy with tumor appearance in young women. New England Journal of Medicine 284: 878–881.

Herbst AL, Anderson D 1990 Clear cell adenocarcinoma of the vagina and cervix secondary to intrauterine exposure to diethylstilbestrol. Seminars in Surgical Oncology 6: 343–346.

Herod JJ, Shafi MI, Rollason TP, Jordan JA, Luesley DM 1996 Vulvar intraepithelial neoplasia: long term follow up of treated and untreated women. British Journal of Obstetrics and Gynaecology 103: 446–452.

Homesley HD, Bundy BN, Sedlis A, Adcock L 1986 Radiation therapy versus pelvic node resection for carcinoma of the vulva with positive groin nodes. Obstetrics and Gynecology 68: 733–740.

Homesley HD, Bundy BN, Sedlis A et al 1991 Assessment of current International Federation of Gynecology and Obstetrics staging of vulvar carcinoma relative to prognostic factors for survival (a Gynecologic Oncology Group study). American Journal of Obstetrics and Gynecology 164: 997–1003, discussion 1003–1004.

Homesley HD, Bundy BN, Sedlis A et al 1993 Prognostic factors for groin node metastasis in squamous cell carcinoma of the vulva (a Gynecologic Oncology Group study). Gynecologic Oncology 49: 279–283.

Hopkins MP, Reid GC, Morley GW 1990 The surgical management of recurrent squamous cell carcinoma of the vulva. Obstetrics and Gynecology 75: 1001–1005.

Hopkins MP, Reid GC, Vettrano I, Morley GW 1991 Squamous cell carcinoma of the vulva: prognostic factors influencing survival. Gyncologic Oncology 43: 113–117.

Hussain SK, Madeleine MM, Johnson LG et al 2008 Cervical and vulvar cancer risk in relation to the joint effects of cigarette smoking and genetic variation in interleukin 2. Cancer Epidemiology, Biomarkers and Prevention 17: 1790–1799.

Iversen T, Aas M 1983 Lymph drainage from the vulva. Gynecologic Oncology 16: 179–189.

Jones RW, Baranyai J, Stables S 1997 Trends in squamous cell carcinoma of the vulva: the influence of vulvar intraepithelial neoplasia. Obstetrics and Gynecology 90: 448–452.

Katz A, Eifel PJ, Jhingran A, Levenback CF 2003 The role of radiation therapy in preventing regional recurrences of invasive squamous cell carcinoma of the vulva. International Journal of Radiation Oncology, Biology, Physics 57: 409–418.

Kelley JL 3rd, Burke TW, Tornos C et al 1992 Minimally invasive vulvar carcinoma: an indication for conservative surgical therapy. Gynecologic Oncology 44: 240–244.

Kelly J 1972 Malignant disease of the vulva. Journal of Obstetrics and Gynaecology of the British Commonwealth 79: 265–272.

Kirkbride P, Fyles A, Rawlings GA, Manchul L, Levin W, Murphy KJ, Simm J 1995 Carcinoma of the vagina — experience at the Princess Margaret Hospital (1974–1989). Gynecologic Oncology 56: 435–443.

Kirkwood JM, Ibrahim JG, Sosman JA et al 2001 High-dose interferon alfa-2b significantly prolongs relapse-free and overall survival compared with the GM2-KLH/QS-21 vaccine in patients with resected stage IIB–III melanoma: results of intergroup trial E1694/S9512/C509801. Journal of Clinical Oncology 19: 2370–2380.

Levenback C, Coleman RL, Burke TW, Bodurka-Bevers D, Wolf JK, Gershenson DM 2001 Intraoperative lymphatic mapping and sentinel node identification with blue dye in patients with vulvar cancer. Gynecologic Oncology 83: 276–281.

Lingard D, Free K, Wright, Battistutta D 1992 Invasive squamous cell carcinoma of the vulva: behaviour and results in the light of changing management regimens. A review of clinicohistological features predictive of regional lymph node involvement and local recurrence. Australian & New Zealand Journal of Obstetrics and Gynaecology 32: 137–145.

MacLean AB, Reid WM 1995 Benign and premalignant disease of the vulva. British Journal of Obstetrics and Gynaecology 102: 359–363.

MacLean AB, Makwana M, Ellis PE, Cunnington F 2004 The management of Paget's disease of the vulva. Journal of Obstetrics and Gynaecology 24: 124–128.

Magrina JF, Webb MJ, Gaffey TA, Symmonds RE 1979 Stage I squamous cell cancer of the vulva. American Journal of Obstetrics and Gynecology 15: 453–459.

Meffert JJ, Davis BM, Grimwood RE 1995 Lichen sclerosus. Journal of the American Academy of Dermatology 32: 393–416.

Monaghan JM 1990 Management of Vulval Carcinoma in Clinical Gynaecological Oncology. Blackwell Scientific Publications, Oxford, p 145.

Montana GS, Thomas GM, Moore DH et al 2000 Preoperative chemo-radiation for carcinoma of the vulva with N2/N3 nodes: a gynecologic oncology group study. International Journal of Radiation Oncology, Biology, Physics 48: 1007–1013.

Moore DH, Thomas GM, Montana GS, Saxer A, Gallup DG, Olt G 1998 Preoperative chemoradiation for advanced vulver cancer: a phase II study of the Gynecologic Oncology Group. International Journal of Radiation Oncology, Biology, Physics 42: 79–85.

Moore RG, DePasquale SE, Steinhoff MM et al 2003 Sentinel node identification and the ability to detect metastatic tumor to inguinal lymph nodes in squamous cell cancer of the vulva. Gynecologic Oncology 89: 475–479.

Morrow CP, Curtin JP, Townsend DE 1993 Tumour of the vulva. In: Synopsis of Gynaecologic Oncology, 4th edn. Wiley, New York. pp 65–92.

Mulayim N, Foster Silver D, Tolgay Ocal I, Babalola E 2002 Vulvar basal cell carcinoma: two unusual presentations and review of the literature. Gynecologic Oncology 85: 532–537.

Nasu K, Kawano Y, Takai N, Kashima K, Miyakawa I 2005 Adenoid cystic carcinoma of Bartholin's gland. Case report with review of the literature. Gynecologic and Obstetric Investigation 59: 54–58.

Office of National Statistics 2008 Cancer Statistics Registration, Registration of Cancer Diagnosed in 2005, England. Series MB1 No. 36. Her Majesty's Stationery Office, London.

Parikh JH, Barton DP, Ind TE, Sohaib SA 2008 MR imaging features of vaginal malignancies. Radiographics 28: 49–63.

Perez CA, Grigsby PW, Chao C et al 1998 Irradiation in carcinoma of the vulva: factors affecting outcome. International Journal of Radiation Oncology, Biology, Physics 42: 335–344.

Perez CA, Grigsby PW, Garipagaoglu M, Mutch DG, Lockett MA 1999 Factors affecting long-term outcome of irradiation in carcinoma of the vagina. International Journal of Radiation Oncology, Biology, Physics 44: 37–45.

Peters WA 3rd, Kumar NB, Morley GW 1985 Carcinoma of the vagina. Factors influencing treatment outcome. Cancer 55: 892–897.

Phillips GL, Bundy BN, Okagaki T, Kucera PR, Stehman FB 1994 Malignant melanoma of the vulva treated by radical hemivulvectomy. A prospective study of the Gynecologic Oncology Group. Cancer 73: 2626–2632.

Pingley S, Shrivastava SK, Sarin R et al 2000 Primary carcinoma of the vagina: Tata Memorial Hospital experience. International Journal of Radiation Oncology, Biology, Physics 46: 101–108.

Piura B, Gemer O, Rabinovich A, Yanai-Inbar I 2002 Primary breast carcinoma of the vulva: case report and review of literature. European Journal of Gynaecological Oncology 23: 21–24.

Piura B 2008 Management of primary melanoma of the female urogenital tract. The Lancet Oncology 9: 973–981.

Podratz KC, Symmonds RE, Taylor WF, Williams TJ 1983a Carcinoma of the vulva: analysis of treatment and survival. Obstetrics and Gynaecology 61: 63–74.

Podratz KC, Gaffey TA, Symmonds RE, Johansen KL, O'Brien PC 1983b Melanoma of the vulva: an update. Gynecologic Oncology 16: 153–168.

Pride GL, Schultz AE, Chuprevich TW, Buchler DA 1979 Primary invasive squamous carcinoma of the vagina. Obstetrics and Gynecology 53; 218–225.

Ragnarsson-Olding B, Johansson H, Rutqvist LE, Ringborg U 1993 Malignant melanoma of the vulva and vagina. Trends in incidence, age distribution, and long-term survival among 245 consecutive cases in Sweden 1960–1984. Cancer 71: 1893–1897.

Ragnarsson-Olding BK, Kanter-Lewensohn LR, Lagerlöf B, Nilsson BR, Ringborg UK 1999a Malignant melanoma of the vulva in a nationwide, 25-year study of 219 Swedish females: clinical observations and histopathologic features. Cancer 86: 1273–1284.

Ragnarsson-Olding BK, Nilsson BR, Kanter-Lewensohn LR, Lagerlöf B, Ringborg UK 1999b Malignant melanoma of the vulva in a nationwide, 25-year study of 219 Swedish females: predictors of survival. Cancer 86: 1285–1293.

Reid GC, Schmidt RW, Roberts JA, Hopkins MP, Barrett RJ, Morley GW 1989 Primary melanoma of the vagina: a clinicopathologic analysis. Obstetrics and Gynecology 74: 190–199.

Rose PG, Piver MS, Tsukada Y, Lau T 1988 Conservative therapy for melanoma of the vulva. American Journal of Obstetrics and Gynecology 159: 52–55.

Rose PG 1999 Skin bridge recurrences in vulvar cancer: frequency and management. International Journal of Gynecological Cancer 9: 508–511.

Rouzier R, Haddad B, Plantier F, Dubois P, Pelisse M, Paniel BJ 2002 Local relapse in patients treated for squamous cell vulvar carcinoma: incidence and prognostic value. Obstetrics and Gynecology 100: 1159–1167.

Sedlis A, Homesley H, Bundy BN et al 1987 Positive groin lymph nodes in superficial squamous cell vulvar cancer. A Gynecologic Oncology Group Study. American Journal of Obstetrics and Gynecology 156: 1159–1164.

Selman TJ, Luesley DM, Acheson N, Khan KS, Mann CH 2005 A systematic review of the accuracy of diagnostic tests for inguinal lymph node status in vulvar cancer. Gynecologic Oncology 99: 206–214.

Shimizu Y, Hasumi K, Masubuchi K 1990 Effective chemotherapy consisting of bleomycin, vincristine, mitomycin C, and cisplatin (BOMP) for a patient with inoperable vulvar cancer. Gynecologic Oncology 36: 423–427.

Siu SSN, Lo KWK, Chan ABW, Yu MY, Cheung TH 2004 Nodal detection in malignant melanoma of vagina using laparoscopic ultrasonography. Gynecologic Oncology 92: 985–988.

Sliutz G, Reinthaller A, Lantzsch T et al 2002 Lymphatic mapping of sentinel nodes in early vulvar cancer. Gynecologic Oncology 84: 449–452.

Stehman FB, Bundy BN, Dvoretsky PM, Creasman WT 1992a Early stage I carcinoma of the vulva treated with ipsilateral superficial inguinal lymphadenectomy and modified radical hemivulvectomy: a prospective study of the Gynecologic Oncology Group. Obstetrics and Gynecology 79: 490–497.

Stehman FB, Bundy BN, Thomas G et al 1992b Groin dissection versus groin radiation in carcinoma of the vulva: a Gynecologic Oncology Group study. International Journal of Radiation Oncology, Biology, Physics 24: 389–396.

Stock RG, Chen AS, Seski J 1995 A 30-year experience in the management of primary carcinoma of the vagina: analysis of prognostic factors and treatment modalities. Gynecologic Oncology 56: 45–52.

Sutton GP, Miser MR, Stehman FB, Look KY, Ehrilich CE 1991 Trends in the operative management of invasive squamous carcinoma of the vulva at Indiana University, 1974 to 1988. American Journal of Obstetrics and Gynecology 164: 1472–1478.

Tarraza HM Jr, Meltzer SE, DeCain M, Jones MA 1998 Vaginal metastases from renal cell carcinoma: report of four cases and review of the literature. European Journal of Gynaecological Oncology 19: 14–18.

Tasseron EW, van der Esch EP, Hart AA, Brutel de la Rivière G, Aartsen EJ 1992 A clinicopathological study of 30 melanomas of the vulva. Gynecologic Oncology 46: 170–175.

Taussig FJ 1940 Cancer of the vulva — an analysis of 155 cases (1911–1940). American Journal of Obstetrics and Gynecology 40: 764–779.

Thomas G, Dembo A, DePetrillo A et al 1989 Concurrent radiation and chemotherapy in vulvar carcinoma. Gynecologic Oncology 34: 263–267.

Thomas GM, Dembo AJ, Bryson SC, Osborne R, DePetrillo AD 1991 Changing concepts in the management of vulvar cancer. Gynecological Oncology 42: 9–21.

van der Avoort IA, Shirango H, Hoevenaars BM et al 2006 Vulvar squamous cell carcinoma is a multifactorial disease following two separate and independent pathways. International Journal of Gynecological Pathology 25: 22–29.

van der Velden J, van Lindert AC, Lammes FB et al 1995 Extracapsular growth of lymph node metastases in squamous cell carcinoma of the vulva. The impact on recurrence and survival. Cancer 75: 2885–2890.

van der Velden J 1996 Some Aspects of the Management of Squamous Cell Carcinoma of the Vulva. Thesis. Amsterdam.

van Doorn HC, Ansink A, Verhaar-Langereis M, Stalpers L 2006 Neoadjuvant chemoradiation for advanced primary vulvar cancer. Cochrane Database of Systematic Reviews 3: CD003752.

van der Zee AG, Oonk MH, de Hullu JA et al 2008 Sentinel node dissection is safe in the treatment of early-stage vulvar cancer. Journal of Clinical Oncology 26: 884–889.

Verschraegen CF, Benjapibal M, Supakarapongkul W et al 2001 Vulvar melanoma at the M. D. Anderson Cancer Center: 25 years later. International Journal of Gynecological Cancer 11: 359–364.

Way S 1960 Carcinoma of the vulva. American Journal of Obstetrics and Gynecology 79: 692–697.

Willis RA 1973 The Spread of Tumours in the Human Body, 3rd edn. Butterworth, London.

CHAPTER 42

Malignant disease of the uterus

Sudha S. Sundar and Suhail Anwar

Chapter Contents

INTRODUCTION	629	PREOPERATIVE EVALUATION	638
EPIDEMIOLOGY	629	TREATMENT	638
PATHOLOGY	630	UTERINE SARCOMAS	645
SPREAD OF DISEASE	635	PROGNOSIS	646
FIGO STAGING	635	TARGETED THERAPIES	646
DIAGNOSIS OF ENDOMETRIAL CANCER	636	FOLLOW-UP IN ENDOMETRIAL CANCER	647
INVESTIGATIONS AND DIAGNOSIS OF ENDOMETRIAL CANCER	637	CHALLENGES AND FUTURE DIRECTIONS	647
SCREENING FOR ENDOMETRIAL CANCER	638	KEY POINTS	647

Introduction

Worldwide, approximately 200,000 women are diagnosed with endometrial cancer each year (Ferlay et al 2004). Of these, more than two-thirds arise in developed countries where age-standardized incidence is four times higher than in developing countries (Ferlay et al 2007). Endometrial cancer is now the most common gynaecological malignancy in Western Europe and North America, with an annual incidence of 81,500 women in the European Union and 40,100 women in North America. In the UK, the incidence of endometrial cancer increased by 29.3% between 1993 and 2005, with an incidence of 6891 women in 2005 (Office for National Statistics 2008). This increase is attributable to an increase in obesity, tamoxifen use for breast cancer and increased life expectancy (Reich 1992, Kitchener 2008). Given the anticipated increase in obesity, it is likely that this trend will continue.

Endometrial cancer has traditionally been believed to have a relatively good outcome. Whilst commonly believed to be a curable cancer in contrast to other gynaecological malignancies, the overall 5-year survival rate is disappointing considering that 75% of patients present with early (stage I) disease. Relative survival at both 1 and 5 years after diagnosis has risen steadily from 85% and 72%, respectively, in the late 1980s to 88% and 76% in the late 1990s (Cooper et al 2008). However, there is a significant gap in survival between the most affluent and the most deprived groups of approximately 4% based on data from England and Wales, with survival lagging 2–6% behind Europe (Sant et al 2003, Cooper et al 2008). This deprivation gap may be best explained by comorbidities such as obesity, hypertension and cardiovascular disease, which are more common in deprived communities (Kitchener 2008). In addition, survival in advanced-stage endometrial cancer and poor prognostic types of endometrial cancer continues to be poor.

With the implementation of improving outcomes guidance in endometrial cancer, women with higher grade and poor prognostic types of endometrial cancer should be managed in gynaecological oncology centres, thus centralizing resources and experience, and facilitating trials that investigate new therapies for these patients (Department of Health 1999).

Epidemiology

Most studies focus on the epidemiology of endometrioid cancers, as the epidemiology for non-endometrioid histotypes is less clear (Box 42.1).

Obesity

Body mass index (BMI) plays an important role with a strong linear increase in risk with increasing BMI. There is a six-fold increase in women with a BMI greater than 40 kg/m^2 compared with those with a normal BMI (20–24 kg/m^2), whereas women with a BMI under 20 kg/m^2 have half the risk (Lindemann et al 2008). The fact that obesity increases risk

DOI: 10.1016/B978-0-7020-3120-5.00042-4

Box 42.1 Factors known to alter the risk of developing endometrial cancer

Increase	Decrease
Obesity	Late age at last birth
Diabetes mellitus	Combined oral
High-fat/low complex carbohydrate diet	contraceptive
Sedentary lifestyle	Smoking
Early menarche	Diet with high intake of
Late menopause	fruit and vegetables
Prolonged/irregular bleeding	Physical exercise
Nulliparity	
Polycystic ovary syndrome	
Functioning ovarian tumours	
Unopposed oestrogen therapy	
Personal history of breast or colon cancer	
Family history of breast, colon or endometrial cancer	
Tamoxifen use	

Box 42.2 Lifetime risk of malignancy in women with HNPCC

Colorectal	30–50%
Endometrial	40–60%
Ovarian	9–12%
Gastric	2–7%
Biliary	13–15%
Urinary	4–5%

has been attributed to changes in concentrations of endogenous hormones in obese women. Oestrogens produced in adipose tissue have a direct mitogenic effect on endometrial cells. In postmenopausal women, oestrogens derived from peripheral adipose tissue are the primary source of endogenous oestrogen, and the rate of production is related to the size of the adipose depots. In younger premenopausal women, obesity can also be associated with anovulatory cycles, resulting in the absence of counterbalancing progesterone. Oligo- and amenorrhoeic women with polycystic ovary syndrome can develop endometrial hyperplasia and later carcinoma. There is a weight-related increase in insulin and insulin-like growth factor-I, both of which are endometrial growth factors. Cytokines produced in fat tissue (leptin and adiponectin) may play a direct role in endometrial carcinogenesis, as well as transcription factors that can modulate both cellular lipid metabolism and tumorigenesis. There is also a strongly increased risk of endometrial cancer in diabetics, possibly because of shared underlying mechanisms.

Tamoxifen

Tamoxifen improves the survival of postmenopausal women with hormone-receptor-positive breast cancer. Breast and endometrial cancer share several risk factors including age of menopause, unopposed oestrogen use and obesity, and breast cancer patients have an increased rate of endometrial cancer regardless of endocrine therapy. The risk of endometrial cancer rises with both the use of higher doses and increasing duration of tamoxifen use. Treatment beyond 5 years increases the risk at least four fold. However, the absolute risk of endometrial cancer is still very small in tamoxifen-treated women (Early Breast Cancer Trialists' Collaborative Group 1998). The use of aromatase inhibitors for postoperative adjuvant therapy instead of tamoxifen significantly reduces the risk of adverse gynaecological events (Duffy et al 2009). Switching from tamoxifen to an aromatase inhibitor may reduce the risk of endometrial cancer, but needs to be balanced against the side-effects and costs of therapy.

Hereditary non-polyposis colorectal cancer

Hereditary non-polyposis colorectal cancer (HNPCC) is one of the most common cancer family syndromes. The estimated lifetime risk of developing endometrial cancer in women carrying these mutations is approximately 42–60%. HNPCC results from germline mutations in DNA mismatch repair genes and is autosomal dominant in inheritance (Froggatt et al 1996). As well as an increased risk of malignancies in the colon, cancers of the endometrium, ovary, biliary tract, stomach, small intestine and renal tract occur more commonly in these women (Box 42.2). Endometrial cancer is the most common and usually occurs in the premenopausal period. The majority of mismatch repair gene defects involve the genes *MSH2* and *MLH1*, with defects in *PMS1* and *PMS2* being less common (Papadopoulos and Lindblom 1997). A good family history will help to identify women who may carry these mutations. If such a mutation is found or if the woman is thought to be at high risk, there may be a role for prophylactic hysterectomy and bilateral salpingo-oophorectomy. Screening may be offered to those who do not wish to have surgery but with the caveat that there is no evidence that it is effective. There may also be a role for prophylactic progesterone in these women, and studies are currently investigating the role of the Mirena™ intrauterine system for prophylaxis.

Hormones

The combined oral contraceptive pill has a large protective effect that lasts for at least 20 years after cessation. Older hormone replacement therapy (HRT) regimens that utilized unopposed oestrogen in women with an intact uterus increase the relative risk of endometrial carcinoma approximately six fold after 5 years of use (Weiderpass et al 1999). It is strongly recommended that women with intact uteri should not be started on regimes containing oestrogen alone, and should be offered endometrial protection by regimes with either 10–12 days of cyclical progestogens or continuous combined regimens (Lethaby et al 2004).

Pathology

There is a growing consensus that endometrial cancers can be classified into two types based on clinical and molecular characteristics. Type I endometrial cancers (80%) are oestrogen dependent, usually arise in a background of endometrial hyperplasia, have well to moderately differentiated endometrioid histology, tend to be biologically indolent and have a good prognosis (Bokhman 1983). Type II cancers are not oestrogen driven, have a higher grade, occur in a background of atrophic endometrium and have a poorer prognosis (Bokhman 1983). Uterine papillary serous carcinomas and clear cell carcinomas are considered to be type II endometrial cancers. These cancers, and uterine serous papillary cancer in particular, are characterized by early metastasis, resistance to therapy and a high mortality rate. Within the type II cancer histological subtypes, Creasman et al (2004) found 5-year survival of 81% for surgically staged stage I clear cell cancer and 72% for uterine papillary serous cancer. This is in comparison with over 95% for well to moderately differentiated stage IA endometrioid cancers. Although unusual cancers only account for 10% of endometrial cancers, they account for more than 50% of recurrences and deaths (Acharya et al 2005).

The morphological and clinical differences are paralleled by genetic distinctions (Hecht and Mutter 2006). Type I cancers are associated with mutations in the *K-ras2* oncogene, loss of the *PTEN* tumour suppressor gene, defects in DNA mismatch repair and near-diploid karyotype, whereas type II cancers are associated with mutations in *TP 53* and *ERBB-2* expression, and most are non-diploid. A dualistic model of endometrial tumorigenesis has been proposed which could explain the very different clinical outcomes in these groups of patients (Table 42.1, Figure 42.1). An understanding of the molecular heterogeneity of various histological types of endometrial cancer has the potential to lead to better individualization of treatment in the future (Maxwell et al 2005).

Malignancy may develop in either the glands or the stroma of the endometrium. Endometrial adenocarcinoma, derived from the endometrial glandular cells, is overwhelmingly the most common malignant tumour arising in the body of the uterus; the stroma is the origin of the much less common endometrial stromal sarcoma. Carcinosarcoma or malignant mixed Müllerian tumour comprises both glandular and stromal elements; however, carcinosarcomas are monoclonal and epithelial in origin, contrary to popular belief.

Histopathology

Endometrial carcinoma is usually seen as a raised, rough, perhaps papillary area occupying at least half of the endometrium. It often arises in the fundal region of the uterus; the internal os is rarely involved early in the disease (Figure 42.2). Myometrial invasion may be obvious to the naked eye. There seems to be no correlation between the degree of exophytic growth of the tumour within the uterine cavity and the presence of myometrial invasion.

There are several different histological subtypes of endometrial carcinoma (Table 42.2).

Microscopically, approximately 80% of malignant endometrial epithelial tumours are conventional adenocarcinomas which can be graded into well (grade 1, 50%), moderately (grade 2, 35%) and poorly differentiated (grade

Table 42.1 Clinicopathological characteristics and genetic abnormalities in type I and type II endometrial carcinomas

Characteristic	Type I	Type II
Unopposed oestrogen	Yes	No
Background endometrium	Hyperplastic	Atrophic
Morphology	Endometrioid	Serous, clear cell
Microsatellite instability	20–40%	0–5%
p53 mutations	10–20%	90%
β-Catenin mutations	31–47%	0–3%
K-ras mutations	15–30%	0–5%
PTEN inactivation	35–50%	10%
HER-2/neu	No information	18–80%

Source: From Doll A, Abal M, Rigau M, Monge M, Gonzalez M, Demajo S, et al. Novel molecular profiles of endometrial cancer-new light through old windows. J Steroid Biochem Mol Biol 2008;108(3–5):221–9.

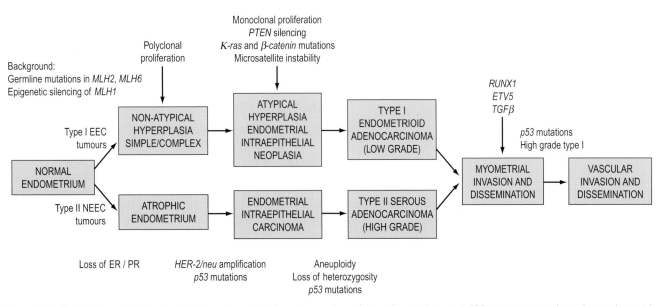

Figure 42.1 A dualistic model of endometrial tumorigenesis. EEC, oestrogen-dependent endometrial cancer; NEEC, non-oestrogen-dependent endometrial cancer; ER, oestrogen receptor; PR, progesterone receptor.

Source: Doll A, Abal M, Rigau M et al 2008 Journal of Steroid Biochemistry and Molecular Biology 108: 221–229.

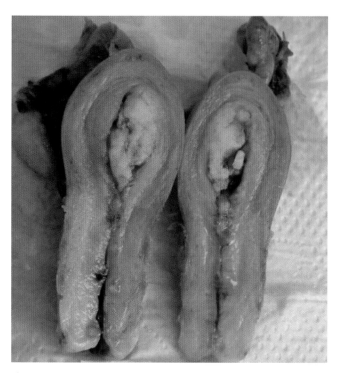

Figure 42.2 Macroscopic pathology of endometrial cancer.

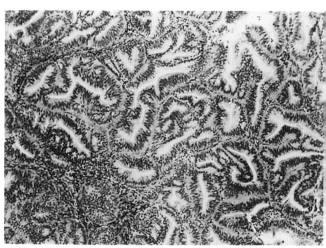

Figure 42.3 A well-differentiated (grade 1) endometrial carcinoma of endometrioid pattern. Haematoxylin and eosin ×170.

Table 42.2 Classification of endometrial carcinomas

Endometrioid (usual) carcinoma (includes glandular and villoglandular patterns)
Secretory
Ciliated cell
With squamous differentiation (includes adenoacanthoma and adenosquamous carcinoma)
Special variant carcinomas
Papillary serous adenocarcinoma
Clear cell carcinoma
Mucinous carcinoma
Pure squamous cell carcinoma
Mixed
Undifferentiated
Carcinosarcoma

3, 15%). The International Confederation of Gynecology and Obstetrics (FIGO) grading takes into account the relative proportion of glandular and solid areas, as well as nuclear atypia. Approximately one-quarter of well-differentiated tumours have a papillary or villoglandular component. Such tumours need to be distinguished from serous papillary adenocarcinomas, which also show a papillary pattern but belong to the non-endometrioid, poorly differentiated type. Numerous morphological forms of endometrial adenocarcinomas exist, but while adenoacanthoma, adenosquamous carcinoma, secretory carcinoma and ciliated carcinoma are variants of ordinary endometrioid adenocarcinoma, papillary serous carcinoma, clear cell carcinoma and mucinous carcinoma are considered to be non-endometrioid.

Endometrioid adenocarcinoma

The most common endometrial carcinoma is referred to as endometrioid adenocarcinoma, the glandular pattern of which generally resembles that of normal proliferative-phase endometrium, although sometimes showing extreme complexity of the glands and cribriform pattern (Figure 42.3). Multilayering of the epithelial cells is nearly always seen. The secretory and ciliated cell variants are rare and well differentiated by definition. Secretory adenocarcinoma is a well-differentiated adenocarcinoma characterized by neoplastic glands with a subnuclear vacuolization resembling normal 17-day secretory endometrium. Mucinous adenocarcinoma is a low-grade neoplasm in which most of the cells contain prominent intracytoplasmic mucin, and should be distinguished from otherwise typical endometrioid carcinomas with abundant extracellular mucin but no intracellular mucin.

Endometrial adenocarcinoma with squamous metaplasia (adenoacanthoma)

Up to 25% of endometrioid-pattern endometrial adenocarcinomas contain areas of squamous metaplasia. Those tumours in which the squamous component is morphologically benign are commonly termed 'adenoacanthomas'. The squamous change is seen as islands of typical squamous epithelium, very often situated within the gland lumina or as surface or diffuse squamous metaplasia (Figure 42.4).

Adenosquamous carcinoma

Adenosquamous carcinoma is composed of malignant glands with a morphologically malignant squamous element. Histologically, the glandular element always predominates, making up at least 70% of the tumour. When matched by stage and grade, there are no prognostic differences between

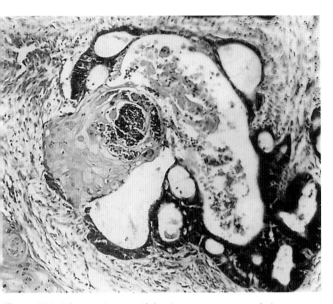

Figure 42.4 Adenocarcinoma with benign squamous metaplasia (adenoacanthoma). Haematoxylin and eosin ×195.

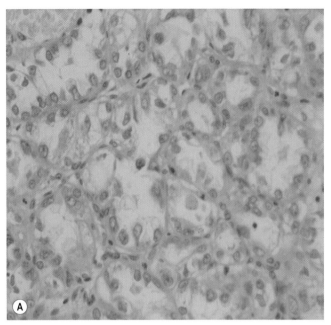

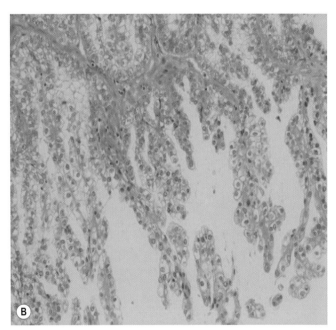

Figure 42.5 Clear cell endometrial carcinoma with (A) acinar pattern and (B) papillary pattern.

these variants. It is recommended that such tumours should be graded according to the grade of the glandular component. Squamous cell carcinoma is a rare primary tumour of the endometrium and can only be diagnosed as such in the absence of cervical involvement.

Papillary serous and clear cell adenocarcinomas

These are less common histological subtypes, both associated with a poor prognosis. Clear cell carcinoma is composed of large, clear cells containing glycogen, often forming papillary structures lined by 'hobnail' cells (Figure 42.5). Papillary serous carcinoma closely resembles ovarian papillary serous carcinoma, featuring severe atypia, a complex papillary pattern, high mitotic index, prominent myometrial invasion and psammoma bodies (Figure 42.6). Most patients are postmenopausal.

Mixed cancers

The conventional approach is to use a minimum 10% tumour volume of a specific histological type to warrant a specific diagnostic heading. Management should be guided by the worst component in histology.

Histopathological reporting

It is essential not only to recognize specific subtypes and to grade carcinomas accurately, but also to record the extent of myometrial invasion. The maximum depth of myometrial invasion, overall thickness of the myometrium, and minimum distance of the tumour from the serosal surface should be recorded. The presence of lymphovascular invasion should be noted. The cervical stroma, fallopian tubes and ovaries should all be examined carefully for tumour. Histopathological examination of the omentum would be valuable in uterine papillary serous carcinoma and clear cell carcinoma. The number of lymph nodes removed, the number of lymph nodes positive for malignancy, extracapsular spread and the extent of lymphatic spread (e.g. node replaced with malignancy or not) should also be reported. There is no convincing evidence for routine ultrastaging or special immunohistochemical analysis of surgically removed lymph nodes (Figure 42.7).

The national minimum dataset published by the Royal College of Pathologists provides a useful tool for both gynaecologists and histopathologists. Serous carcinoma, clear cell carcinoma, and squamous and undifferentiated carcinoma are not graded, these tumours being highly malignant neoplasia. Sarcomas are also highly malignant neoplasms (Figures 42.8–42.11). The architectural grade, nuclear grade and FIGO grade of tumours can be used to separate patients

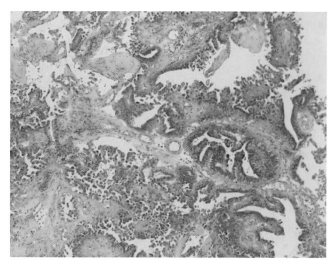

Figure 42.6 Uterine papillary serous carcinoma.

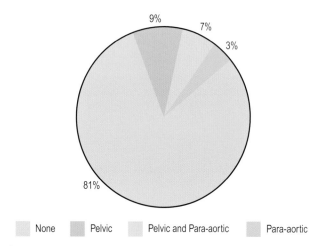

9%

7%

3%

81%

| None | Pelvic | Pelvic and Para-aortic | Para-aortic |

Figure 42.7 Lymph node involvement in clinical stage I endometrial carcinoma
Source: Ayhan et al 1994 Surgical pathological spread patterns of endometrial cancer: A Gynecologic Oncology Group Study. Cancer 60: 2035–2041.

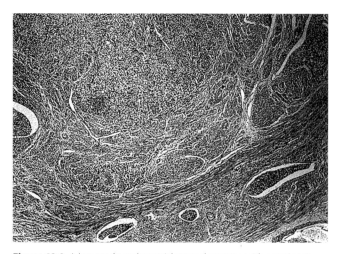

Figure 42.8 A low-grade endometrial stromal sarcoma with prominent lymphatic channel involvement. Haematoxylin and eosin ×64.

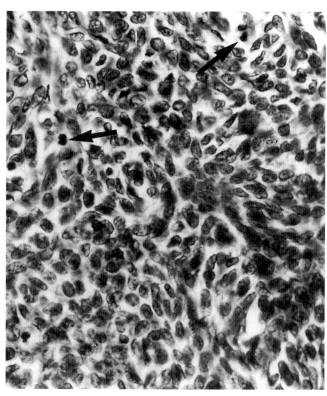

Figure 42.9 A high-grade endometrial stromal sarcoma. Nuclear crowding and pleomorphism are apparent and although mitotic figures (arrowed) are not conspicuous, this tumour contains more than 10 mitotic figures per 10 high-power fields. Haematoxylin and eosin ×650.

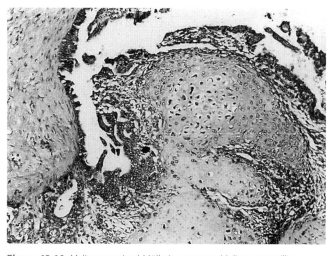

Figure 42.10 Malignant mixed Müllerian tumour. Malignant papillary epithelium and malignant cartilage are both present in this illustration. Haematoxylin and eosin ×195.

into groups with significantly different rates of progression of disease and relative survival.

Useful immunohistochemical markers

With improvements in immunohistochemistry, a panel of markers is frequently used by pathologists to improve the accuracy of histology and inform patient management.

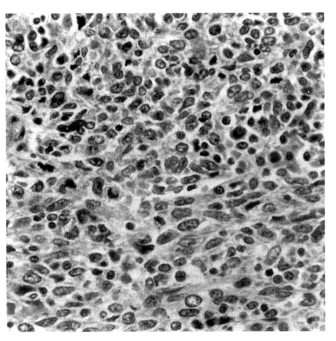

Figure 42.11 Leiomyosarcoma. Although a few cells are spindled, most are poorly differentiated and show marked nuclear pleomorphism. Haematoxylin and eosin ×720.

Immunohistochemistry for oestrogen receptors (ER) and progesterone receptors (PR) is performed to assess the sensitivity of tumours for hormonal therapy and to guide oncologists in the management of later relapse. Type I tumours tend to be ER and PR positive, *p53* negative and express low levels of the proliferation antigen Ki-67. Type II cancers tend to be ER and PR negative, *p53* positive with high Ki-67 labelling. Other markers can be performed to help in diagnosis. Wilms' tumour-1 (WT1) antibody staining is usually positive in uterine papillary serous cancers and can help distinguish from endometrioid adenocarcinomas with a papillary pattern of proliferation. In contrast to endometrial adenocarcinoma, endocervical adenocarcinoma is usually carcinoembryonic antigen positive, ER and PR negative and vimentin negative. *p16* is a marker for human papilloma virus and may be useful in distinguishing a cervical adenocarcinoma from endometrial adenocarcinoma with cervical extension.

Endometrial hyperplasia

Endometrioid endometrial cancers may be preceded by a preinvasive phase of background endometrial hyperplasia. However, the natural history and progression from endometrial hyperplasia to endometrial cancer is poorly understood, unlike preneoplasia of the cervix. Endometrial hyperplasia may be divided into simple, complex and atypical hyperplasia. In simple glandular hyperplasia, the endometrium is increased in volume and the glands show marked variations in shape, with many cystically dilated forms and pseudostratified lining epithelium that may show mitoses but lacks cytological atypia. In complex hyperplasia, there is more epithelial and glandular proliferation, with glandular budding and reduction in the stroma between glands. In atypical hyperplasia, epithelial cytological atypia is seen which is defined as loss of nuclear polarization, enlarged rounded nuclei with hyperchromatism, chromatin clumping and enlarged nucleoli, and may be associated with a simple or a complex glandular pattern. Atypia is more often associated with complex than simple hyperplasia. Unfortunately, the diagnosis of atypical hyperplasia depends upon subjective criteria so there is substantial interobserver variability in the diagnosis. To date, no special techniques, such as ploidy, histochemistry or molecular biology, have demonstrated reproducible differences between atypical hyperplasia and well-differentiated adenocarcinoma.

Simple glandular hyperplasia is no longer considered to be a premalignant condition, but atypical hyperplasia is an ominous finding. Approximately 10–20% of all cases with atypia will have an underlying carcinoma present, and invasive cancer will develop later in up to 50% of cases. These figures are higher in the case of complex atypical hyperplasia than simple atypical hyperplasia (Silverberg 2000). Women with hyperplasia without cytological atypia may be treated with cyclical or continuous progestogens for 6 months and then undergo rebiopsy. Women with lesions showing cytological atypia who have finished childbearing should be offered a hysterectomy. The management of younger women with atypical hyperplasia is more difficult. Hyperplasia is discussed further in Chapter 38.

Spread of Disease

Endometrial carcinoma spreads by invading the myometrium. In some cases, it extends over the endometrial surface before penetrating the muscle layer. The more deeply it invades, the greater the likelihood of lymphatic or, less commonly, vascular involvement. Usually, initial lymphatic spread occurs to the external iliac, internal iliac and obturator group of lymph nodes. Further involvement of common iliac lymph nodes and para-aortic nodes can also occur. In approximately 5% of cases, para-aortic lymph nodes are involved without obvious histological involvement of the pelvic lymph nodes. Lymphatic spread may rarely include the supraclavicular or the inguinal nodes. Spread to the cervix may occur by extension along the surface (implants). This does not affect the prognosis, unlike infiltration of the cervical stroma. This is difficult to assess clinically (see below). Direct infiltration into the parametria is uncommon except when the cervix is involved.

In women with metastatic disease, spread to the ovaries is common. In 5% of cases (Gynecologic Oncology Group 2001), a synchronous primary ovarian cancer is noted. Transperitoneal spread occurs either when myometrial invasion reaches the serosal surface or via the fallopian tubes. This will involve the peritoneal surfaces and omentum in the same way as ovarian carcinoma. Clear cell and papillary serous carcinomas have a propensity to spread in this way, often without deep myometrial invasion.

The current FIGO staging criteria are shown in Box 42.3.

FIGO Staging

The FIGO surgical staging system is based on histopathological findings including myometrial invasion, and is important in determining prognosis and treatment post hysterectomy. This staging system is based on findings in the uterus. As deep myometrial invasion or serosal involvement cannot always be visualized grossly, it is imperative that the pathologist samples the uterine corpus and cervix adequately for microscopic examination. Indicators of poor prognosis include high histological grade, deep myometrial invasion, unfavourable histological subtypes, lower uterine segment involvement by tumour, and myometrial vascular space invasion. The presence or absence of endometrial hyperplasia should be included in the report as aggressive carcinoma types are not associated with hyperplasia.

Depth of myometrial penetration is a more important guide to the likelihood of nodal metastases than tumour grade (Table 42.3; Creasman et al 1987). Serous papillary and clear cell cancers have the highest risk of spread to para-aortic nodes. Only 10% of cases subsequently proven to have nodal spread had clinically enlarged nodes but, on the other hand, enlarged lymph nodes are not necessarily involved with metastatic disease. Serous papillary carcinoma of the endometrium, histologically similar to serous papillary cancer of the ovary, has a very poor prognosis and a pattern of spread akin to ovarian malignancy.

Positive peritoneal washings are present in approximately 12–15% of all cases of endometrial cancer, with half of these having no histological evidence of extrauterine spread. The Gynaecological Cancer Intergroup have proposed changes to the FIGO staging which have been incorporated into the revised FIGO staging for endometrial cancer (Box 42.3). They recommend that the grading of tumours is added to stage I tumours as this carries a direct clinical relevance. They also recommend removing the upgrading to stage IIIC on the basis of positive peritoneal washings, as these are very likely due to handling at the time of surgery and do not have independent prognostic significance; and that metastasis to positive inguinal lymph nodes is considered stage IIIC rather than stage IV. Although not part of FIGO staging, some centres perform a serum CA125 in women with endometrial cancer as reports suggest that an elevated serum CA125 at diagnosis indicates a high risk of subsequent recurrence but is less effective at predicting myometrial invasion than ultrasound.

Box 42.3 FIGO surgical staging of endometrial carcinoma

Stage I[a]	Tumor confined to the corpus uteri
IA[a]	No or less than half myometrial invasion
IB[a]	Invasion equal to or more than half of the myometrium
Stage II[a]	Tumor invades cervical stroma, but does not extend beyond the uterus[b]
Stage III[a]	Local and/or regional spread of the tumor
IIIA[a]	Tumor invades the serosa of the corpus uteri and/or adnexae[c]
IIIB[a]	Vaginal and/or parametrial involvement[c]
IIIC[a]	Metastases to pelvic and/or para-aortic lymph nodes[c]
IIIC1[a]	Positive pelvic nodes
IIIC2[a]	Positive para-aortic lymph nodes with or without positive pelvic lymph nodes
Stage IV[a]	Tumor invades bladder and/or bowel mucosa, and/or distant metastases
IVA[a]	Tumor invasion of bladder and/or bowel mucosa
IVB[a]	Distant metastases, including intra-abdominal metastases and/or inguinal lymph nodes

[a]Either G1, G2, or G3.
[b]Endocervical glandular involvement only should be considered as Stage I and no longer as Stage II.
[c]Positive cytology has to be reported separately without changing the stage.
Source: FIGO Committee on Gynecologic Oncology 2009 Revised FIGO staging for carcinoma of the vulva, cervix, and endometrium. International Journal of Gynecology and Obstetrics 105: 103–104.

Diagnosis of Endometrial Cancer

Presenting symptoms

The vast majority of women diagnosed with endometrial cancer present with abnormal bleeding. This is usually postmenopausal or irregular perimenopausal bleeding. The remainder have discharge or pain. Only a tiny minority are diagnosed by abnormal cervical cytology or the fortuitous finding of thickened endometrium observed on an ultra-

---

Table 42.3 Incidence of nodal involvement when disease is clinically confined to corpus

Grade	No. of cases	None (*n* = 86)	Inner (*n* = 281)	Mid (*n* = 115)	Outer (*n* = 139)	All cases (*n* = 621)
Positive pelvic nodes (%)						
1	180	0	3	0	11	2.8
2	288	3	5	9	19	8.7
3	153	0	9	4	34	18.3
All cases	621	1.2	5.3	6.1	25.2	9.3
Positive para-aortic nodes (%)						
1	180	0	1	5	6	1.7
2	288	3	4	0	14	4.9
3	153	0	4	0	24	11.1
All cases	621	1.2	2.8	0.9	17.3	5.5

Modified from: Creasman W, Morrow C, Bundy B et al 1987 Surgical pathological spread patterns of endometrial cancer: a Gynecologic Oncology Group study. Cancer 60: 2035–2041.

sound scan performed for some other purpose. Endometrial cancer usually presents at an early stage as patients present with postmenopausal bleeding.

Postmenopausal bleeding

Postmenopausal bleeding is defined as an episode of bleeding 12 months or more after the last period. Postmenopausal bleeding is the most common presenting symptom, as 75–80% of women with the disease are in this age group. The most common mistake made that delays the diagnosis is to assume that vaginal spotting is due to atrophic vaginitis. Postmenopausal bleeding represents one of the most common reasons for referral to gynaecological services, largely due to suspicion of an underlying endometrial malignancy. Endometrial cancer is present in approximately 10% of patients referred with postmenopausal bleeding. No evidence has been identified to determine whether different patterns of postmenopausal bleeding, such as one-off or more frequent bleeds, are more or less likely to be associated with endometrial cancer.

Postmenopausal discharge

Diagnostic curettage in the patient with foul-smelling postmenopausal discharge due to a pyometra will reveal a carcinoma in approximately 50% of cases. It is usually in these women that the rare, pure squamous carcinoma is found.

Pelvic pain

The presence of pain usually indicates metastatic disease. It is often due to nerve compression on the pelvic side wall. Pyometra may present with a constant dull pain or cramping pain.

Symptoms in premenopausal women

Premenopausal women with endometrial carcinoma usually present with irregular bleeding, but over one-third complain of heavy but regular periods. All women over the age of 40 years who present with irregular menstrual bleeding persisting over 6 months should be investigated with an endometrial sample. Women at particular risk in the premenopausal age group include obese women with anovulatory cycles and women with polycystic ovary syndrome, and most gynaecological oncologists will remember anecdotal cases of endometrial cancer in the under 40s diagnosed during investigations for infertility. Consideration should be given to performing a pipelle sample in women under 40 years of age with irregular menstrual bleeding who are in high-risk groups (e.g. obese women with infertility, women with polycystic ovary syndrome).

Clinical examination

Physical examination will seldom suggest the diagnosis of endometrial carcinoma, but several signs should be sought in women with postmenopausal or perimenopausal bleeding.

- Enlarged lymph nodes in the groin or supraclavicular fossa.

- A metastatic focus in the vagina may lie behind the blades of the speculum, commonly on the anterior wall.
- The uterus may be enlarged, an unusual finding in a postmenopausal woman, or spread to the adnexae or parametrium may be felt.
- The breasts should be palpated because breast cancer can sometimes present with the symptoms caused by uterine or ovarian spread (Scottish Intercollegiate Guidelines Network 2002).

Investigations and Diagnosis of Endometrial Cancer

Patients with suspicious symptoms should initially be investigated with a transvaginal ultrasound to investigate the endometrial cavity. Transvaginal ultrasound is useful in the investigation of women with postmenopausal bleeding because it helps to identify those at higher risk of endometrial cancer who require further investigation, and is also an effective means of excluding endometrial cancer. Transvaginal ultrasound measurement of endometrial thickness of less than 5 mm can be a good diagnostic index (Scottish Intercollegiate Guidelines Network 2002). The pooled sensitivity and specificity of endovaginal ultrasound in the detection of endometrial cancer if a cut-off of 5 mm was used were 96% [95% confidence interval (CI) 94–98%] and 61% (95% CI 59–63%), respectively. Sensitivity decreased and specificity increased with increasing thresholds. Thin (<5 mm) endometrial measurement on endovaginal ultrasound can exclude endometrial disease in the majority of postmenopausal women with vaginal bleeding, regardless of hormone replacement use (Smith-Bindman et al 1998).

The mean endometrial thickness in women on sequential HRT with postmenopausal bleeding is greater than that in women with postmenopausal bleeding who are not on sequential HRT. Thus, an abnormal endometrial thickness in women with postmenopausal bleeding who are not using sequential HRT represents a greater probability of endometrial disease than in women taking HRT (Gupta et al 2002). Women presenting with postmenopausal bleeding and taking tamoxifen have a higher probability of malignancy (substantially >10%). In these cases, the ultrasound image is more difficult to interpret. Therefore, it is advisable to sample the endometrium initially and examine the cavity hysteroscopically.

Endometrial biopsy

A definitive diagnosis in postmenopausal bleeding is made by histology. The diagnosis of endometrial cancer is made by an endometrial sample obtained either in the outpatient setting by a pipelle endometrial sample, or through outpatient hysteroscopy which allows the operator the advantage of targeted biopsy and removing small polyps if necessary. Hysteroscopy under anaesthetic should be reserved for selected cases where the os does not admit an endometrial sampling device despite lithotomy, gentle volsellum traction on the cervix and adequate illumination.

Historically, endometrial samples have been obtained by dilatation and curettage (D&C). This involves curetting the walls of the uterine cavity in a systematic fashion. The significant drawback of D&C is that it is a 'blind' procedure and the uterine cavity is not likely to be sampled adequately. Hysteroscopy offers the advantage of a visually targeted biopsy, particularly in focal lesions on a background of atrophic endometrium. Endometrial samplers work on the principle that cancer cells are more likely to detach from the endometrium and be aspirated by suction exerted by the device. These plastic-tube-like devices are inserted into the uterine cavity and a plunger is withdrawn, resulting in 'negative' pressure which permits aspiration of tissue into the device. In a small proportion of patients, outpatient endometrial sampling is not technically possible. Outpatient endometrial sampling has a procedure failure rate as well as a tissue-yield failure rate, each of approximately 10%. It should be noted that yield failures are not unexpected in women with atrophic endometrium, whereas failure to obtain tissue would be less likely if cancer was present.

Hysteroscopy

Hysteroscopy allows the operator to visualize the endometrial cavity. The procedure can be performed either in an outpatient setting with the patient awake or under general anaesthesia. A biopsy of the endometrium is usually taken following hysteroscopy, either with a sampler or by curettage. Hysteroscopy in the outpatient setting appears to have an accuracy and patient acceptability equivalent to inpatient hysteroscopy under general anaesthetic. Facilities to perform hysteroscopy and curettage under general anaesthetic should be available for occasions when the outpatient procedure is not possible or the patient has a strong preference for a general anaesthetic.

One-stop postmenopausal bleeding clinic

The current standard of care in the UK is to establish a one-stop rapid access clinic with facilities for transvaginal ultrasound and endometrial biopsy with or without hysteroscopic evaluation of the uterus to investigate these women. Following such assessment, reassurance can be given or further investigations undertaken.

Investigation of women using tamoxifen

Women with breast cancer who take tamoxifen on a long-term basis are at increased risk of endometrial cancer. In view of the increased risk of endometrial cancer associated with tamoxifen therapy, there is a case for heightened vigilance for postmenopausal bleeding by both the women and the clinician(s) responsible for their care. Current evidence does not justify the use of any investigation (ultrasonography, hysteroscopy, endometrial biopsy or D&C) in postmenopausal women receiving treatment with tamoxifen in the absence of vaginal bleeding. Ultrasonography is poor at differentiating potential cancers from other tamoxifen-induced thickening because of the distorted endometrial architecture associated with long-term use of tamoxifen. Furthermore, endometrial thickness is not a useful discriminator in this group. Hysteroscopy with biopsy is preferable as the first line of investigation in women taking tamoxifen who experience postmenopausal bleeding.

Recurrent postmenopausal bleeding

There is no evidence to recommend when reinvestigation should take place following recurrent or persistent postmenopausal bleeding. Clinical judgement is required, but consideration of reinvestigation must be given if postmenopausal bleeding persists after 6 months in view of the false-negative rate associated with all methods of diagnosis. 'Beware the weeping womb' is an old but useful aphorism.

Screening for Endometrial Cancer

As most patients with endometrial carcinomas present early, it is unlikely, based on current technology, that a population screening programme would be of any value. Routine screening in asymptomatic women for endometrial carcinomas is currently not justified. Women at risk, including those on tamoxifen and families with hereditary non-polyposis colon cancer, have a higher risk of endometrial cancer and should report any bleeding or spotting. Ultrasound screening is not recommended for women on tamoxifen. Whilst a Pap smear is not a screening test for endometrial cancer, the incidental finding of endometrial cells on a Pap smear in a postmenopausal woman requires investigation.

Preoperative Evaluation

A transvaginal ultrasound report should also include an assessment of ovarian morphology as synchronous primary ovarian cancers, oestrogen-producing tumours or endometrial cancer metastasis can be identified in this way. Some centres also perform magnetic resonance imaging (MRI) in order to plan management such as reserving pelvic lymphadenectomy for deeply invasive lesions. Computed tomography (CT) scan of the abdomen and pelvis in uterine papillary serous cancer is advisable to detect upper abdominal disease. A CT of the chest is advisable in women with carcinosarcoma to exclude pulmonary metastasis. If the diagnosis of endometrial carcinoma is confirmed, a chest X-ray is essential. A full blood count, urea, creatinine and electrolyte estimations are required, as is urinalysis for sugar and protein.

If preoperative radiological assessment is undertaken, it seems that MRI is the most accurate for assessing local spread to the cervix and through the myometrium. Neither CT nor MRI is sufficiently sensitive to detect small, involved lymph nodes. Many patients also require medical optimization as these patients are frequently elderly with multiple comorbidities. Assessment by an anaesthetist may be helpful in determining fitness for surgery.

Treatment

Surgery for early-stage endometrial cancer

The mainstay of treatment in stage I endometrial cancer is a total abdominal hysterectomy and bilateral salpingo-oophorectomy, with pelvic and para-aortic lymphadenectomy in selected cases. Both transverse incisions and midline incisions can be utilized; however, a midline umbilical incision allows the best access to the abdominal cavity since it can be extended easily to above the umbilicus if para-aortic nodes are thought to be involved or if unsuspected upper abdominal metastases are detected. In the very obese patient with an 'apron', it is best not to straighten out the abdominal wall by pulling up the panniculus of fat over the pubic symphysis. Retraction of this fat is often tiresome, exposure can be suboptimal and the incidence of wound infection in the skinfold is high. 'Panniculectomy' with removal of skin and fat to the fascia using a wide transverse elliptical incision does give good access to the pelvic side walls, although it adds to the duration of the procedure. The other option, favoured at the authors' centre, is to perform a midline incision extended above the umbilicus if necessary to avoid the infraumblical apron of fat.

Once the abdominal cavity is entered, washings should be taken from around the uterus, bladder and pouch of Douglas, and a full laparotomy performed with particular attention being paid to the liver, omentum, uterine adnexal and retroperitoneal node-bearing areas. A simple extrafascial total abdominal hysterectomy and bilateral salpingo-oophorectomy is undertaken. There is no need to remove a vaginal cuff. A complete pelvic lymphadenectomy involving common iliac nodes, external iliac nodes, internal iliac nodes and obturator nodes down to the level of the obturator nerve may then be performed in selected patients with a higher risk of lymph node metastasis (see below).

In patients with high-risk histology features on preoperative biopsy, particularly uterine papillary serous cancer, the upper abdomen, omentum and liver should be assessed as these cancers metastasize to the upper abdomen like ovarian cancer. Surgery for carcinosarcoma can be challenging as the uterus is frequently fixed and pelvic spread is common. Removal of a large piece of infracolic omentum is recommended in women with uterine papillary serous cancer and clear cell cancer, since microscopic disease in the omentum may be present. In approximately 5% of cases, positive para-aortic nodes can be identified in the absence of involved pelvic lymph nodes. The incidence of nodal positivity is summarized in Table 42.3.

Role of lymphadenectomy

Two large independent surgical randomized controlled trials found that routine pelvic and/or para-aortic lymphadenectomy confer no therapeutic benefit. The Italian randomized controlled trial and the Medical Research Council's ASTEC (A Study in the Treatment of Endometrial Cancer) trial differed in the extent of lymphadenectomy and use of postoperative radiotherapy (Benedetti Panici et al 2008, Kitchener et al 2009). However, lymphadenectomy may still play a role in accurate surgical staging and tailoring of adjuvant therapy. In the authors' institution, regional lymphadenectomy is performed for patients estimated to have a risk of nodal metastasis greater than 10%; this includes stage IC, grade 3, unusual histology subtypes of patients. A pelvic lymphadenectomy is performed in patients with a preoperative biopsy showing grade 2–3 endometrial cancer and myometrial invasion greater than 50% on MRI (presumed stage IC, grade 2–3). Para-aortic lymphadenectomy is reserved for clinically enlarged lymph nodes at MRI or laparotomy. However, practice differs among centres in the UK and elsewhere regarding the extent of lymphadenectomy.

This protocol is based on balancing the risks of adjuvant radiotherapy and the knowledge of lymph node involvement conferred by surgical staging. Omitting pelvic radiotherapy in adequately staged patients with a stage IC, grade 3 tumour spares the not-inconsiderable risks of external beam radiotherapy to the pelvis in approximately two-thirds of patients. Pelvic lymphadenectomy should only be performed in the context of a trial unless it is used to guide adjuvant management. Sentinel nodes to identify the draining lymph node in endometrial cancer have been investigated, but at present this is solely a research technique. The role of positron emission tomography (PET) scanning to estimate nodal status in this group of patients has not been established in prospective trials.

Laparoscopic surgery for endometrial cancer

Laparoscopic surgery for primary management of endometrial cancer has been successfully reported, with several case series reporting satisfactory outcomes for both survival and morbidity (O'Hanlan et al 2004, 2005, Ghezzi et al 2006, Barakat et al 2007, Istre et al 2007). A meta-analysis of laparoscopic surgery for endometrial cancer establishing its feasibility and efficacy has been published (Lin et al 2008). Three techniques exist: laparoscopically assisted vaginal hysterectomy and laparoscopic hysterectomy where the uterine arteries are divided laparoscopically; and total laparoscopic hysterectomy (TLH) where the entire procedure is completed laparoscopically. In TLH for endometrial cancer, the entire hysterectomy procedure is performed laparoscopically, including division of the uterine vessels, the uterus is removed through the open vault of the vagina and the vagina is sutured laparoscopically. TLH may have technical advantages in the obese nulliparous population where vaginal access may be difficult and there is no vaginal descent (O'Hanlan et al 2004, Ramirez et al 2006).

A large randomized trial of laparoscopy vs laparotomy for surgical staging of endometrial cancer has been published in abstract form by the Gynecologic Oncology Group (GOG) (Walker et al 2006). The trial established the efficacy of laparoscopic surgical staging, with 74.2% of patients randomized to receive laparoscopy undergoing successful staging. Other benefits favouring the laparoscopic arm were improvement in quality of life, decreased hospital stay and fewer complications greater than grade 2. Survival results are pending at this time. However, the survival and morbidity associated with TLH compared with conventional open surgery have not been established in a randomized clinical trial, and this is being addressed in LACE (Janda et al 2006).

The majority of endometrial cancers in the UK have been managed through laparotomy; in a recent randomized controlled trial of lymphadenectomy and external beam radiotherapy in endometrial cancer (ASTEC), less than 10% of hysterectomies in the UK were performed using minimal access techniques. However, laparoscopic expertise amongst gynaecological oncologists is increasing, and more surgeons are now offering laparoscopic surgery for women with endometrial cancer. In the authors' centre, all patients with endometrial cancer are considered for laparoscopic surgery. Exclusion criteria are uterine size greater than 10–12 weeks, multiple previous laparotomies and anaesthetic factors preventing steep Trendelenberg position.

Surgery for advanced-stage endometrial cancer

In patients with clinically suspected stage II endometrial cancer with cervical involvement, a radical hysterectomy to achieve tumour clearance may be performed. Occasionally, at laparotomy for stage I disease, particularly for poor prognostic histotypes, macroscopic spread to the omentum and pelvic/para-aortic lymph nodes is identified. It is reasonable to attempt a macroscopic clearance of all deposits in an attempt to 'debulk', akin to ovarian cancer prior to adjuvant chemotherapy, as this may improve outcome. Most patients with advanced-stage endometrial cancer may be best managed by total abdominal hysterectomy and bilateral salpingo-oophorectomy with primary palliative intent to prevent troublesome vaginal bleeding. Carcinosarcomas in particular deeply infiltrate the pelvis and may prove inoperable. A hysterectomy may also be performed in stage IV disease with distant metastasis as effective palliation to reduce bleeding.

Non-surgical management of endometrial carcinoma

Non-surgical management of endometrial carcinoma involves radiotherapy, chemotherapy and hormonal therapy.

Radiotherapy

After surgery, radiotherapy is the most common modality of treatment used in endometrial cancer. It has a role in most stages of this disease. The use of radiotherapy began empirically, but, more recently, randomized trials have confirmed its benefits. The most important role is as adjuvant therapy following surgery in early-stage disease, but it also provides good palliation in advanced-stage disease. In circumstances where surgery may be very high risk, definitive treatment

with radiotherapy alone can be considered. The following discussions will present evidence for adjuvant radiotherapy as per the old FIGO staging for endometrial cancer.

Stages IA and IB, grades 1 and 2

For the usual histological type of endometrioid adenocarcinoma which is well differentiated (grade 1) or moderately differentiated (grade 2), there is usually no indication for any adjuvant treatments. This is because the risk of local recurrence is very low (0–9%) (GOG 33) and radiotherapy is unlikely to be of significant benefit, especially when the majority of recurrences are salvageable by further treatment.

Stages IA and IB, grade 3 or high-risk histology

Poorly differentiated endometrioid adenocarcinoma, clear cell carcinoma and papillary serous carcinoma pose a higher risk of not only locoregional but also systemic recurrence. This is evident from their poorer relapse-free survival (RFS) and overall survival (OS) compared with grades 2 and 3 endometrioid adenocarcinomas (Creasman et al 2004). Five-year survival rates for papillary serous carcinoma, grade 3 endometrioid carcinoma and clear cell carcinoma are 72%, 76% and 80%, respectively. Almost half of those perceived to have early-stage uterine papillary serous carcinoma are found to have advanced-stage disease at surgery or in the definitive pathology. OS and progression-free survival (PFS) slip down to 80% and 68%, respectively, for stage I uterine papillary serous carcinoma. Recurrence rates were as high as 29% for stage IB–IC uterine papillary serous carcinoma (Havrilesky et al 2007a). While systemic management of this particular category is still evolving, radiotherapy has been in use for decades to at least reduce the risk of locoregional recurrence. Historically, this has been achieved mainly by external beam radiotherapy as this would encompass most pelvic lymph nodes including obturator, internal iliac, external iliac and common iliac, which are the main lymph node

Table 42.4 Trials of adjuvant radiotherapy in endometrial cancer

Publication year	Trial	No. of patients	Inclusion criteria	Outcome
2000	PORTEC 1*	715	Stage IA, grade 3; stage IB, any grade; or stage IC, grade 1–2	Local recurrence 13.7% vs 4.2%
2004	Gynecologic Oncology Group 99[†]	392	Stages IB–C or IIA–B	Local recurrence 26% vs 6%
2001[§]	Fanning[‡]	66/265	Stage IC, grade 3; or stage IIA–B	5-year overall survival 84%, disease-free survival 97%
2008[∥]	PORTEC 2	427	Age >60 years: stage IC, grade 2–3; or stage IB, grade 3. Any age: stage IIA, grade 1–2	3-year pelvic nodal recurrence rate 3.5% vs 0.6%
2009[¶]	ASTEC	789	Stage IA–B, grade 3; stage IC, any grade; stage IIA; or serous papillary	NA

*Creutzberg CL, van Putten WL, Koper PC et al 2000 The Lancet 355: 1404–1411.
[†]Keys HM, Roberts JA, Brunetto VL et al 2004 Gynecologic Oncology 92: 744–751.
[‡]Fanning J 2001 Long-term survival of intermediate risk endometrial cancer (stage IG3, IC, II) treated with full lymphadenectomy and brachytherapy without teletherapy. Gynecologic Oncology 82: 371–374.
[§]Non-randomized, [∥]posting date, [¶]publication expected.

groups to which endometrial cancer would metastasize (Table 42.4).

In the largest postoperative radiotherapy trial in endometrial cancer (PORTEC 1), 715 patients with FIGO stage IC, grades 2 and 3, stage IB, any grade and stage IA, grade 3 endometrioid carcinoma, serous papillary carcinoma and clear cell carcinoma were randomized to receive either external beam radiotherapy or no adjuvant radiotherapy following total abdominal hysterectomy, bilateral salpingo-oophorectomy and washings (Creutzberg et al 2000). Adjuvant radiotherapy reduced the risk of locoregional recurrence from 13.7% to 4.2%, which was statistically significant. The distant metastasis rate (7.9% vs 7%, respectively) and death due to distant metastases (6.4% vs 4.5%, respectively) at 5 years were similar in the radiotherapy and observation arms. There was no significant difference in survival between the treated and non-treated groups. Higher age of the patient ($\geq$60 vs <60, hazard ratio 3.1, P = 0.02) and poor differentiation of the tumour (grade 3 vs grade 2, hazard ratio 4.9, P = 0.0008) were significant risk factors for cancer-related deaths. The risk of gastrointestinal toxicity was increased from 1% to 17% (P = 0.0001) in the treated group. PORTEC 1 registered 99 patients with FIGO stage IC, grade 3 endometrial carcinoma for analysis purposes only as they all received radiotherapy (Creutzberg et al 2004). Five-year distant metastasis rate was higher for FIGO stage IC, grade 3 compared with FIGO stage IC, grade 2 endometrial carcinoma (31% vs 20%, respectively) in patients treated with adjuvant radiotherapy. Five-year survival was 74% vs 58% for stages IB and IC, respectively.

Another study by the GOG looked at the value of adjuvant radiotherapy following definitive surgery that involved selective pelvic lymph node dissection (Keys et al 2004). Three hundred and ninety-two patients with intermediate risk of recurrence (FIGO stages IB, IC, IIA and IIB) who underwent total abdominal hysterectomy, bilateral salpingo-oophorectomy, selective pelvic lymphadenectomy and selective para-aortic lymph node dissection were randomized to either adjuvant radiotherapy to the pelvis or no further adjuvant treatment. Based on GOG 33 trial, three factors were considered as risk factors: grade 2–3, involvement of outer third of myometrium and lymphovascular space invasion. Patients were considered to be at high–intermediate risk of recurrence if they were aged 70 years or more with one risk factor, 50 years or more with two risk factors, or any age with all three risk factors. It is interesting to note that one-third of stage I patients meet this criteria and that two-thirds of recurrences occur in this group. Risk of recurrence in patients at high–intermediate risk was reduced to 6% with radiotherapy compared with 26% when no adjuvant radiotherapy was given. At 4 years, there was a trend towards better survival with radiotherapy (92% vs 86%), although this was not statistically significant. The trial, however, was not powered to detect a survival advantage.

Two trials have evaluated the usefulness of brachytherapy without external beam radiotherapy, also labelled as 'teletherapy'. The first of these studies was a prospective non-randomized study (Fanning 2001). Two hundred and sixty-five patients underwent complete surgical staging with full lymphadenectomy up to the duodenum, undertaken by one surgeon. Sixty-six patients were identified to have intermediate-risk disease on the basis of grade 3, involvement of outer myometrium (FIGO stage IC) or involvement of cervix (FIGO stage IIA–B), and all received adjuvant brachytherapy but no external beam radiotherapy. Five-year survival was reported to be 84% and PFS was 97%. Although one should avoid comparing the results of two different trials, it was noted with interest that this PFS was comparable with the PFS observed in GOG 99 trial for a similar group of patients who received teletherapy. The second pivotal randomized trial of adjuvant brachytherapy compared with external beam radiotherapy was planned on the basis of similar observations in phase II trials (PORTEC 2). Patients at high–intermediate risk (on the basis of PORTEC 1 results) were randomized to receive either external beam radiotherapy or brachytherapy. The primary endpoint was vaginal recurrence rate, and secondary endpoints were quality of life, OS and locoregional recurrence. The analysis was by intention to treat. A total of 427 patients were randomized into the two treatment groups. Three-year vaginal recurrence rate was 1.9% (P = 0.97 in both groups). Three-year pelvic nodal recurrence rate was 0.6% in the external beam radiotherapy group compared with 3.5% in the brachytherapy alone arm (P = 0.03). Three-year OS and RFS rates were 90.4% and 90.8% (P = 0.55) and 89.5 and 89.1 (P = 0.38), respectively. The distant recurrence rates were similar in both groups.

ASTEC is a large phase III, randomized trial which addressed two issues, namely the role of lymphadenectomy and adjuvant radiotherapy in early-stage endometrial cancer (Kitchener et al 2009). Although the results of the lymphadenectomy part of the trial have recently been published, the results of the radiotherapy part are not yet in the public domain.

Usually, a dose between 40 and 50 grays (Gy) is given in 20–28 fractions over 4–5.5 weeks using megavoltage (MV) photons of higher energy (typically between 8 and 15 MV). The side-effects of radiotherapy are described as early (usually temporary and appearing during treatment and up to 3 months after) or late (usually permanent and typically occurring more than 3 months after radiation therapy). Early side-effects include tiredness, diarrhoea, local soreness of skin/vagina, local hair loss and radiation cystitis. Delayed toxicity includes the risk of chronic proctitis or a weak bladder leading to poor control, urinary urgency and occasionally incontinence, but most importantly the risk of a fistula (involving bowel, vagina or urinary bladder) or narrowing of the bowel which may require colostomy. Obviously, this risk is directly proportional to the dose of radiotherapy and the amount of bowel in the radiation field. The risk is less than 5% over 5 years at the doses mentioned above (Milano et al 2007). Comorbidity, especially previous pelvic operations and inflammatory bowel disease, increase this risk significantly and therefore are relative contraindications to radiotherapy to the pelvis. Similarly, hereditary conditions including ataxia telangiectasia and xeroderma pigmentosum markedly increase radiation sensitivity, and are absolute contraindications to adjuvant radiotherapy.

Stages IC, IIA and IIB

Involvement of the outer half of the myometrium and cervical stroma are well known to increase the risk of local recurrence as well as regional lymph node spread. As many as one-third of patients with apparent stage IC, grade 2 tumours may have pelvic nodes involved, and one-quarter may have para-aortic nodes involved. There has been a definite role for radiotherapy in these stages following surgery to reduce that risk. The modality of radiotherapy, the dose and the extent of the area radiated have not been without controversy. While preliminary results of the largest phase III randomized trial of adjuvant radiotherapy in the UK do not show any advantage for external beam radiotherapy for stage IC disease, the fact that some centres were allowed to use brachytherapy in accordance with their local guidelines has made interpretation difficult. In fact, most radiation/clinical oncologists continue to offer radiotherapy to this group of patients, and were reluctant to recruit these patients into any trials of adjuvant radiotherapy or not. For these reasons, the PORTEC 1 trial excluded stage IC, grade 3 patients from randomization although they were registered in the trial to follow their progress (Creutzberg et al 2004).

With the adoption of pelvic lymphadenectomy, the use of external beam radiotherapy in early-stage cancer is being replaced by localized brachytherapy, eliminating the need for radiating a large pelvic volume including pelvic nodes. While the issue of pelvic node surgery in early endometrial cancer has been controversial and open to debate, patients who do undergo this type of surgery and who are node negative may be eligible for brachytherapy alone. The PORTEC 2 trial has shown no differences in vaginal vault recurrence rates between patients who had external beam radiotherapy or brachytherapy. However, the recent ASTEC publication discouraged the routine use of pelvic lymphadenectomy outside of a clinical trial (Kitchener et al 2009). This is unfortunate as it would lead to inadequate staging of endometrial cancer patients and hence deny adjuvant treatments to those with higher stage disease. Obviously, there are also significant implications of this in terms of acute and long-term toxicity of radiotherapy. There is a definite need for more evidence to finally resolve this issue. Detailed discussion on this subject is outwith the scope of this chapter.

If the cervix is involved, external beam radiotherapy is usually followed by brachytherapy. Brachytherapy is administered by a remote afterloading system. The intention is to boost the vaginal vault with a higher dose of radiotherapy without giving an excessive dose to the small bowel. In brachytherapy, sources of radiation are placed near the area of interest so that the area nearest to the source receives a higher dose, and the normal tissues (organs at risk) away from the source receive a much smaller dose, thereby reducing the risk of serious morbidity.

Stages IIIA, IIIB and IIIC

Locally advanced endometrial cancer has a lower OS rate but there is also a significant risk of local recurrence. While the prognosis is usually determined by distant recurrence, local relapse can be distressing and uncomfortable, with intractable symptoms such as pain, bleeding, discharge, and fistulation into the vagina, bladder and rectum. Involvement of ureters or bladder usually leads to renal impairment, compromising further cytotoxic therapy. If patients are suitable for chemotherapy, they usually receive this first, followed by radiotherapy.

Stage IVA

An attempt should be made to deliver a radical dose of radiotherapy in otherwise fit patients. This may include external beam radiotherapy as well as brachytherapy. The aim in the first place is to control the local disease, and hence the local symptoms, but a small number of patients may be salvaged. They may go on to live for many years (Churn and Jones 1999). For the majority, a palliative dose of radiation is given to help local symptoms.

Stage IVB

The aim of radiotherapy is almost always palliation in this situation. Virtually any part of the body can receive a palliative dose, but, for obvious reasons, the most common site to be treated is the pelvis. Either external beam radiotherapy or brachytherapy can be used. This aims to help symptoms such as pain, bleeding and spinal cord compression, but also those that arise from the mass effect of raised intracranial pressure from brain metastases. The total dose and number of fractions depend on the site, extent, tempo of the disease and fitness of the patient. Most commonly used doses are 8 Gy in a single fraction, 20 Gy in five fractions over 1 week, and 30 Gy in 10 fractions over 2 weeks.

Radiotherapy technique

The quality of planning and delivery of radiotherapy has improved remarkably over the last few years in line with the improvements in computer and technological advances (Figure 42.12). The latest state-of-the-art multi-leaf-collimator-equipped linear accelerators with ability to deliver gated, conformal MV radiotherapy are in stark contrast with the old orthovoltage (KV) machines with limited planning techniques. For external beam radiotherapy, the patient first undergoes a planning scan which is usually a CT scan, although MR scans are likely to replace CT for this purpose. Work is also ongoing to explore the usefulness of PET-CT and PET-MRI in radiotherapy planning (Figure 42.13). After the planning CT, patients are marked with tattoos (usually pin head size) to ensure reproducibility of the treatment position during each fraction of radiotherapy. Clinical or radiation oncologists then draw the target volume, i.e. the area to be treated (Figures 42.14 and 42.15). Most patients are treated using a four-field plan (brick technique) to reduce the dose of radiation to normal tissues around the target volume (Figures 42.16 and 42.17). Once the physicist

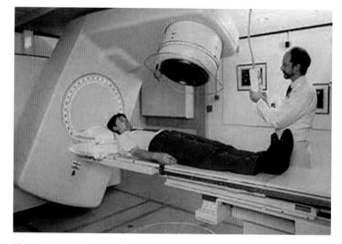

Figure 42.12 Linear accelerator; delivery of megavoltage external beam radiotherapy.

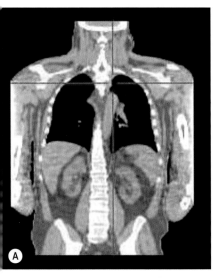
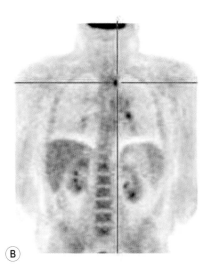
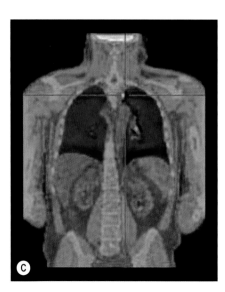

Figure 42.13 Computed tomography/positron emission tomography image fusion.

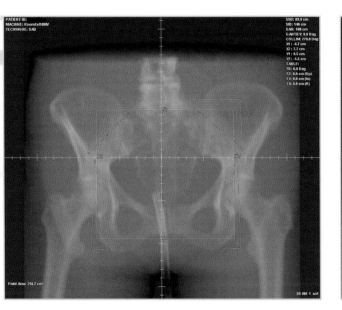

Figure 42.14 Superior, inferior and lateral limits of anterior and posterior beams of external beam radiotherapy for endometrial cancer. Note lead shielding at all four corners.

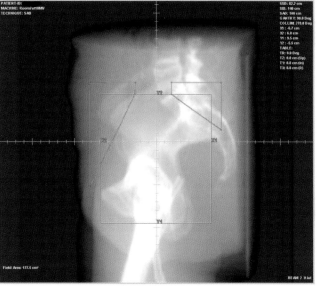

Figure 42.15 Superior, inferior, anterior and posterior borders of right and left lateral fields of four-field external beam radiotherapy plan for endometrial cancer. Top anterior and posterior corners are shielded.

has planned the treatment and it is approved by the oncologist, treatment can be started. There are many quality assurance and safety nets at different stages to ensure safe radiation exposure in line with the local radiation protection laws. One treatment is given per day, Monday to Friday, with no treatment over the weekend. Patients can be treated over the weekend or even twice a day depending upon the availability of resources and staff. If treated twice a day, there has to be a minimum gap of 6 h between treatments to allow the normal tissue repair to take place. Patients are reviewed weekly to assess for any side-effects.

Where needed, brachytherapy is delivered using afterloading devices. In recent years, there has been a gradual move from low- (LDR) to medium-dose-rate (MDR) brachytherapy (dose rates <1200 cGy/min) and now to high-dose-rate (HDR) brachytherapy (dose rates >1200 cGy/min), meaning

that the treatment can now be given in a few minutes rather than many hours. The results of HDR brachytherapy in cervical cancer confirm its efficacy at no significant additional toxicity (Lertsanguansinchai et al 2004). LDR and MDR brachytherapy require a single insertion, while HDR brachytherapy requires two to four treatments depending on the dose needed. Also, the total dose required is less for HDR systems.

Depending upon the dose required and the aim of treatment, one to three applicators are placed vaginally to treat the uterus, vaginal vault or both. This is usually done under general or spinal anaesthetic, but can be carried out under local or even no anaesthetic, especially in postoperative cases where only vault radiation is required. Patients are treated in isolation rooms for radiation protection. The applicators are connected to the tubes from the radiation delivery

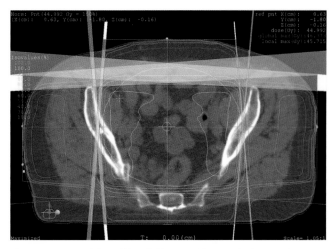

Figure 42.16 Axial slice of four-field external beam radiotherapy plan showing isodose distribution including planning target volume (red line) and shielding anteriorly (grey bands)

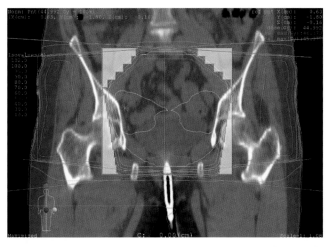

Figure 42.17 Isodose distribution on coronal section. Lead shielding at all four corners of anterior and posterior radiation fields. Red line represents 90% isodose (planning target volume).

machine holding radiation sources. Once all planning is complete and rechecked and all staff have left the room, the machine can be switched on. Patients should be able to lie on their backs and keep their legs straight for many hours for LDR and MDR brachytherapy, although they can be treated while under anaesthetic for HDR brachytherapy.

Radiotherapy for recurrent disease

Proponents of radiotherapy claim that many of the recurrences are not localized, while advocates of no adjuvant radiotherapy for early disease stress that the majority of recurrences (although not all) are localized and therefore are salvageable, the so-called 'Alabama approach' (Barnes and Kilgore 2000). This approach, although not widely popular, is being adopted by some in view of no survival advantage of adjuvant radiotherapy and a definite, although small, risk of late serious toxicity of radiotherapy. Recurrent, localized disease at the vault can be treated with radiotherapy or surgery, and success rates are high (Creutzberg et al 2003).

If radiotherapy is used, the doses required are high and the risk of toxicity is proportionally high. Nevertheless, any patient with localized recurrence should be viewed as potentially curable.

Chemotherapy

The role of chemotherapy is less well established. There are many reasons for this, but mainly the comorbidities of typical endometrial cancer patients such as hypertension, diabetes mellitus, obesity and related problems, combined with the myth that early endometrial cancer has excellent survival, have discouraged oncologists from exploring this avenue in the past. However, improvements in general health care, refinements of cytotoxic agents, the use of granulocyte colony-stimulating factor and 24-h medical/nursing support for such patients has resulted in a refreshed interest in assessing the role of chemotherapy.

Early-stage localized disease has excellent survival after surgery and it would be difficult to demonstrate any benefit from adjuvant chemotherapy. In high-risk early-stage disease, the risk of systemic relapse is high and so is the 5-year disease-specific mortality rate. Papillary serous carcinoma, clear cell carcinoma and poorly differentiated endometrioid carcinoma infiltrating the outer half of the myometrium are particularly associated with poor OS (5-year OS 70–80%) (Murphy et al 2003). These high-risk scenarios may benefit from adjuvant chemotherapy. Until recently, there were no convincing phase III data to show a survival benefit for the use of chemotherapy; based on retrospective data, many oncologists were considering fitter patients for adjuvant chemotherapy, especially if they had serous carcinoma or even elements of clear cell carcinoma. Evidence is now gradually accumulating to support this approach. Most oncologists now agree that serous papillary carcinoma should be treated as ovarian carcinoma with adjuvant chemotherapy. A recently published systematic review (Table 42.5) evaluated data collected from 2288 patients recruited into 11 trials of chemotherapy for advanced disease.

A GOG study showed better OS of 15.3 vs 12.3 months, PFS of 8.3 vs 5.3 months and overall response rate of 57 vs 34% in favour of the addition of paclitaxel to the combination of doxorubicin and cisplatin, but at the cost of much higher toxicity (Fleming et al 2004). Combinations of an anthracycline and platinum are still probably the most commonly used regimes in endometrial carcinoma.

The Japanese GOG study showed that early-stage high-risk patients, including stages IC, grade 3, II and IIIA, had higher PFS (83.8% vs 66.2%, $P = 0.024$) and OS (89.7% vs 73.6%, $P = 0.006$) when treated with combination chemotherapy comprising cyclophosphamide, adriamycin and cisplatin compared with treatment with pelvic radiotherapy alone (Susumu et al 2008). A phase II feasibility study by the Radiation Therapy Oncology Group used concurrent chemotherapy (cisplatin 50 mg/m² on days 1 and 28) during external beam radiotherapy of 45 Gy in 25 fractions followed by four cycles of adjuvant combination chemotherapy with cisplatin 50 mg/m² and paclitaxel 175 mg/m² four weekly (Greven et al 2006). Forty-six patients with grade 2 or 3 endometrial adenocarcinoma with FIGO stages between IC, IIB and IIIB were treated and followed-up to a median of 4.3

Table 42.5 Systematic reviews of chemotherapy in advanced endometrial carcinoma

Year	Author	Size	Study arm	Control arm	Median PFS (months)	ORR (%)	Overall survival (months)
1978	Horton	40	Dox	Cyclo	NA	19 vs 0	NA
1984	Cohen	155	Dox, 5-FU, cyclo, mega	Mel, 5-FU, mega	6.1 vs 5.2	37.7 vs 35.9	10.6 vs 10.1
1987	Edmondson	30	Cis, dox, cyclo	Cis	2.9 vs 1.9	31 vs 21	6.7 vs 7.5
1994	Thigpen	222	Dox, cyclo	Dox	3.9 vs 3.2	30 vs 22	7.3 vs 6.9
1995	Long	28	Dox, cyclo, meth, vin	Dox, cyclo	6.9 vs 6.2	69 vs 26	15 vs 15
1999	Pawinski	59	Ifosf	Cyclo	2 vs 1.75	12 vs 7	NA
2003	Gallion	342	Circadian timed dox	Standard timed dox	5.9 vs 6.5	49 vs 46	13.2 vs 11.2
2003	Aapro	177	Dox, cis	Dox	8 vs 7	43 vs 17	9 vs 7
2004A	Fleming	263	Dox, cis, paclitaxel	Dox, cis	8.3 vs 5.3	57 vs 34	15.3 vs 12.3
2004B	Fleming	317	Dox, cis, filgrastim	Dox, cis	6 vs 7.2	43 vs 40	13.6 vs 12.6
2004	Thigpen	284	Dox, cis	Dox	3.8 vs 5.7	43 vs 25	9.2 vs 9

Source: Humber CE, Tierney JF, Symonds RP et al 2007 Chemotherapy for advanced, recurrent or metastatic endometrial cancer: a systematic review of Cochrane collaboration. Annals of Oncology 18: 409–420.

PFS, progression-free survival; ORR, overall response rate; NA, not available; dox, doxorubicin; cyclo, cyclophosphamide; 5-FU, 5-fluorouracil; mel, melphalan; cis, cisplatin; meth, methotrexate; vin, vinblastin; ifosf, ifosfamide.

years. At 4 years, pelvic, regional and distant recurrence rates were observed to be 2%, 2% and 19%, respectively. Four-year DFS and OS were 81% and 85%, respectively. Grade 2 and 4 late toxicity was seen in 21% of cases and grade 1 and 2 in 57% of cases. The inferences drawn were that this was a feasible regime with acceptable toxicity showing excellent locoregional control, and should be tested in a randomized controlled trial. It has become the basis of the PORTEC 3 trial.

There seems to be a stronger view in favour of adjuvant chemotherapy in locally advanced disease as the risk of distant spread and resultant mortality is high. The response rates to different chemotherapeutic agents used alone range between 4% and 77%. A systematic review of chemotherapy in advanced endometrial carcinoma by Humber et al reported an improvement in OS to 15 months from 6.9 months for best supportive care (Humber et al 2007). Median PFS improved from 3.2 months to 8.3 months. Overall response rates ranged between 17% and 34% for single agents, but between 30% and 69% for combination chemotherapy. Unfortunately, randomized evidence is lacking but retrospective data have shown some improvement in RFS but not OS. A randomized trial of adjuvant chemotherapy with cisplatin and adriamycin has been completed by the European Organization for Research and Treatment of Cancer, and the results are encouraging (Aapro et al 2003). Many oncologists feel uncomfortable not giving adjuvant chemotherapy to this group of patients (FIGO stage IIIA onwards), and treat them with platinum +/− anthracycline/taxane.

Metastatic endometrial cancer carries a very poor prognosis. Palliative treatments range from radiotherapy to hormonal therapy to chemotherapy depending on the symptoms of the patients, comorbidities and their wishes. Cytotoxic options include platinum +/− anthracycline/taxane.

Hormonal therapy

A proportion (11–25%) of endometrial carcinomas express ER and/or PR. Published data do not support the routine use of adjuvant hormones in early-stage disease. This is because of a high rate of recurrence following endocrine treatment in spite of very significant initial complete response rates (Ushijima et al 2007). However, in exceptional circumstances where, due to extreme comorbidities or patient choice, surgery or radiotherapy cannot be used, consideration may be given to the use of hormone treatment. For advanced endometrial carcinomas, especially those that are well differentiated, showing strong progesterone positivity and metastatic to the lungs, hormone therapy is a reasonable choice and should always be considered (Bouros et al 1996, Thigpen et al 1999). Long-term responses have been documented. The most commonly used agent is medroxyprogesterone in high doses such as 200 mg two to three times a day. Fluid retention and heart failure are recognized complications. Other hormonal agents such as aromatase inhibitors have been used with some efficacy (Rose et al 2000).

Uterine Sarcomas

The uterus is not an uncommon site for the development of sarcomas. The principles of management are very similar to those for endometrial carcinomas and soft tissue sarcomas at other sites. The mainstay of treatment is surgery for early and localized disease. Radical radiotherapy can be considered for surgically unfit patients. The common perception of these tumours being radioresistant is only true for leiomyosarcomas.

The indications for adjuvant treatment are somewhat variable but mainly depend on the type of sarcoma, size and degree of surgical clearance. For small (≤5 cm) low-grade sarcomas with complete microscopic clearance, radiotherapy is unnecessary as the risk of local recurrence is low. Similarly, there is insufficient evidence to suggest that radiotherapy is beneficial in cases of endometrial stromal sarcomas. Tumours larger than 5 cm, of higher grade and malignant mixed Müllerian tumours, also known as 'carcinosarcomas', should be considered for adjuvant radiotherapy. Incomplete surgical clearance usually requires higher doses of radiotherapy. Previous history of radiotherapy to the pelvis is very important as this may be a causative factor in some pelvic sarcomas (Nakanishi et al 2001).

Retrospective data suggest no definite survival benefit with adjuvant radiotherapy for early disease, but a significant reduction in the risk of local recurrence. The Royal Marsden experience shows local recurrence rates as high as 70% without radiotherapy. With external beam radiotherapy, the rate of local recurrence fell to 40%, and, with the addition of brachytherapy, fell as low as 23%. Local DFS improved to 70% from 55% with the use of radiotherapy in stage I disease. In stage II and III disease, the best results are achieved with external beam radiotherapy and brachytherapy combined.

Since publication of the meta-analysis of adjuvant chemotherapy in soft tissue sarcoma and the small associated benefit, many oncologists have extrapolated the data to include uterine sarcomas of high grade, especially leiomyosarcomas (Sarcoma Meta-analysis Collaboration 2000). More recent updates have only shown a marginal benefit against significant toxicity (Pervaiz et al 2008). Doxorubicin and ifosfamide are given as a three-weekly cycle to a total of six. Common side-effects include nausea and vomiting, hair loss, cardiotoxicity, confusion and neutropenic sepsis. Another challenge is the management of malignant mixed Müllerian tumours. The prognosis of this aggressive subtype remains very poor, with 3-year OS of approximately 22%. The only randomized trial of cisplatin and ifosfamide that showed some benefit also revealed that the toxicity was quite significant (Sutton et al 2000, 2005). Although the use of adjuvant chemotherapy is gradually increasing, there is, as yet, no set standard. The relatively low incidence of these tumour types and frailty of many patients makes it difficult to plan randomized trials.

Recurrent disease might be localized in a small proportion of cases. The history of previous treatments, relapse-free interval, distribution of the disease and comorbidities determine further management which may include localized surgery to exenterative surgery to radical radiotherapy or only palliative measures. For metastatic disease, the goal is palliation at the outset. Radiotherapy for localized symptoms, chemotherapy for more widespread disease, occasionally surgery for intractable local symptoms, and even hormonal treatment with progestogens for low-grade endometrial stromal sarcomas have a place.

Prognosis

The aura of good prognosis surrounding endometrial cancer may just be a reflection of diagnosis and prompt treatment at an early stage. The prognosis for advanced-stage disease is quite poor, with the exception of metastatic disease responsive to progestogens. In this situation, years of control can sometimes be achieved with very significant improvement of symptoms. Although hormone-resistant disease may respond to chemotherapy, the responses are short-lived. Aggressive/high-risk histologies also carry a poorer prognosis (Table 42.6).

Stage IC poorly differentiated endometrioid, papillary serous and clear cell tumours have 5-year survival rates of 50–70% (Murphy et al 2003, Havrilesky et al 2007b). Uterine sarcomas are also aggressive histiotypes, but the prognosis ranges from approximately 30% OS for malignant mixed Müllerian tumours (Callister et al 2004) to 50–90% for endometrial stromal sarcomas (Chan et al 2008). Leiomyosarcomas probably fall in the middle, with a 5-year survival rate of 40% (Kahanpaa et al 1986) (Box 42.4).

Targeted Therapies

Currently, approximately 250 clinical trials involving endometrial cancer are registered internationally. Fifty-nine of these include some form of targeted therapy. These studies focus almost exclusively on recurrent or persistent disease. Agents are used as monotherapy or in combination with chemo- or radiotherapy, and also with other targeting agents.

Forty-six trials cover three groups of agents: tyrosine kinase receptor inhibitors or antibodies ($n = 23$), mTOR (mammalian target of rapamycin) inhibitors ($n = 14$) and oestrogen inhibitors (selective ER modulators, aromatase inhibitors) ($n = 9$). The remaining 13 trials include agents such as cell cycle inhibitors, mitogen-activated protein

Table 42.6 Five-year overall survival by International Federation of Gynecologists and Obstetricians (FIGO) stage

FIGO stage	Substage	5-year overall survival (%)
I	A	91
	B	90
	C	81
II	A	79
	B	71
III	A	60
	B	55
	C	50
IV	A	15
	B	5

Source: Creasman WT, Carcinoma of the corpus uteri; Int J Gynecol Obstet 2003;83:79, with permission of Elsevier.

Box 42.4 Staging system for uterine sarcomas

Stage I	Sarcomas confined to the uterus
Stage II	Sarcomas involving the corpus and cervix
Stage III	Sarcomas spreading beyond the uterus but not outside the pelvis
Stage IV	Sarcomas spreading outside the pelvis or into the bladder or rectum

kinase inhibition, gonadotrophin-releasing hormone agonism, folic acid analogism, histone deacetylase inhibition, the monoclonal antibody RAV12, CALAA-01 (RNA interference), UCN-01 (protein kinase C inhibition) and cyclo-oxygenase II inhibition.

Amongst these, the most widely researched molecules are the epidermal growth factor receptor and the vascular endothelial growth factor (VEGF) receptor families. The growth and progression of tumours is unequivocally angiogenesis dependent. The main proangiogenic factor, namely VEGF, also known as 'vascular permeability factor', is a potent angiogenic cytokine that induces mitosis and also regulates the permeability of endothelial cells. VEGF is an endothelial-cell-specific growth factor and the principal regulator of angiogenesis under normal and pathological conditions in most organs. Increased levels of VEGF and angiogenic markers are associated with poor outcome in endometrioid endometrial cancer patients (Kamat et al 2007).

The human epidermal growth factor receptor-2 (HER-2 protein), which is also known as c-erbB-2 or neu, is a member of subclass 1 of the superfamily of receptor tyrosine kinases. HER-2 is an independent prognostic factor in endometrial cancer and an important oncogene in high grade and stage endometrial cancer (Morrison et al 2006). Overexpression of HER-2/neu was associated with an overall worse prognosis in uterine papillary serous cancer (Slomovitz et al 2004). Inhibition of the epidermal growth factor receptor in poor prognostic types of endometrial cancer may be of benefit. There is limited research into new therapies for endometrial cancer, despite the increasing incidence. Identification of new drugs and targeted therapies for poor prognostic types of endometrial cancer will benefit treatment at initial presentation and relapse.

Follow-Up in Endometrial Cancer

Recurrence from endometrioid endometrial cancer tends to be pelvic and frequently occurs at the vaginal vault, usually within the first 2 years after diagnosis. In patients who have received adjuvant radiotherapy, recurrences can be sited outside the radiotherapy field. Recurrence in sarcomas can be distant and occur in the chest. Vaginal bleeding and discharge is the most common presentation at relapse. During follow-up, symptoms such as vaginal bleeding and/or discharge, and any urinary or gastrointestinal disturbance should raise the suspicion of relapse and prompt appropriate investigation. The history should also aim to identify morbidity associated with radiotherapy, such as troublesome diarrhoea which can be managed with the use of codeine or over-the-counter medication. Vaginal dilators are also beneficial to preserve vaginal capacity after radiotherapy in patients keen to preserve vaginal capacity, and also to aid clinical examination at follow-up. An abdominal examination and vaginal examination to detect vaginal/pelvic masses is of value. Patients with early-stage endometrial cancer stage IA with grade 1 endometrioid cancer can be discharged safely. All patients with poor prognostic types of histology and patients who have received adjuvant radio-/chemotherapy should be seen at regular intervals for the first 2 years and then less frequently in the subsequent 3 years after diagnosis. The value of clinician-led follow-up compared with patient-initiated follow-up in the presence of symptoms for early-stage endometrial cancer has never been proven. However, it remains conventional practice to institute a regime of follow-up for patients at greatest risk of recurrence. HRT can be safely instituted in symptomatic young women with adequately staged and treated stage I endometrial cancer.

Challenges and Future Directions

The rising incidence in endometrial cancer is likely to continue and this will impact on current resources. Laparoscopic surgery will become more established in the management of this disease, as will tailoring adjuvant therapy for those at greatest risk of recurrence. Results of trials of targeted therapies in poor prognostic types of endometrial cancer are eagerly awaited, and may pave the way for individualization of treatment in the future.

KEY POINTS

1. The incidence of endometrial cancer is increasing, attributable to an increase in obesity, adjuvant tamoxifen therapy in breast cancer and life expectancy.

2. Endometrial cancer can be characterized on molecular pathology into an oestrogen-dependent type I, comprising well to moderately differentiated endometrioid histologies, and non-oestrogen-dependent type II, comprising grade 3 endometrioid, uterine serous papillary cancer, clear cell carcinoma and carcinosarcoma.

3. The diagnosis of endometrial cancer is made by a pipelle sample or hysteroscopically obtained endometrial biopsy.

4. Surgical treatment of early-stage endometrial cancer is the mainstay of treatment, followed by adjuvant radiotherapy in selected cases based on the risk of recurrence.

5. Laparoscopic surgery is feasible and safe in women with endometrial cancer, and may reduce the morbidity associated with surgery in obese women.

6. Early-stage endometrial cancer can be classified into low risk, intermediate risk and high risk based on the risk of recurrence.

7. For low-risk endometrial cancers, adjuvant radiotherapy can be safely omitted. External beam radiotherapy for intermediate-risk patients can be confined to patients over 60 years of age with lymphovascular invasion on histology.

8. External beam radiotherapy to the pelvis in intermediate-risk patients reduces the risk of recurrence but does not improve survival.

9. The optimum adjuvant therapy for patients with high-risk endometrial cancer is currently not known and is being investigated.

10. Pelvic lymphadenectomy in intermediate–high-risk endometrial cancer does not confer survival benefit, but knowledge of lymph node status enables accurate staging. This may have an impact on selecting patients for adjuvant therapy, and thereby reducing morbidity from external beam radiotherapy.

References

Aapro MS, van Wijk FH, Bolis G et al 2003 Doxorubicin versus doxorubicin and cisplatin in endometrial carcinoma: definitive results of a randomised study (55872) by the EORTC Gynaecological Cancer Group. Annals of Oncology 14: 441–448.

Acharya S, Hensley ML, Montag AC, Fleming GF 2005 Rare uterine cancers. The Lancet Oncology 6: 961–971.

Barakat RR, Lev G, Hummer AJ et al 2007 Twelve-year experience in the management of endometrial cancer: a change in surgical and postoperative radiation approaches. Gynecologic Oncology 105: 150–156.

Barnes MN, Kilgore LC 2000 Complete surgical staging of early endometrial adenocarcinoma: optimizing patient outcomes. Seminars in Radiation Oncology 10: 3–7.

Benedetti Panici P, Basile S, Maneschi F et al 2008 Systematic pelvic lymphadenectomy vs. no lymphadenectomy in early-stage endometrial carcinoma: randomized clinical trial. Journal of the National Cancer Institute 100: 1707–1716.

Bokhman JV 1983 Two pathogenetic types of endometrial carcinoma. Gynecologic Oncology 15: 10–17.

Bouros D, Papadakis K, Siafakas N, Fuller AF Jr 1996 Natural history of patients with pulmonary metastases from uterine cancer. Cancer 78: 441–447.

Callister M, Ramondetta LM, Jhingran A, Burke TW, Eifel PJ 2004 Malignant mixed Müllerian tumors of the uterus: analysis of patterns of failure, prognostic factors, and treatment outcome. International Journal of Radiation Oncology, Biology, Physics 58: 786–796.

Chan JK, Kawar NM, Shin JY et al 2008 Endometrial stromal sarcoma: a population-based analysis. British Journal of Cancer 99: 1210–1215.

Churn M, Jones B 1999 Primary radiotherapy for carcinoma of the endometrium using external beam radiotherapy and single line source brachytherapy. Clinical Oncology 11: 255–262.

Cooper N, Quinn MJ, Rachet B, Mitry E, Coleman MP 2008 Survival from cancer of the uterus in England and Wales up to 2001. British Journal of Cancer 99: S68–S69.

Creasman W, Morrow C, Bundy B et al 1987 Surgical pathological spread patterns of endometrial cancer: a Gynecologic Oncology Group study. Cancer 60: 2035–2041.

Creasman WT, Kohler MF, Odicino F, Maisonneuve P, Boyle P 2004 Prognosis of papillary serous, clear cell, and grade 3 stage I carcinoma of the endometrium. Gynecologic Oncology 95: 593–596.

Creutzberg CL, van Putten WL, Koper PC et al 2000 Surgery and postoperative radiotherapy versus surgery alone for patients with stage-1 endometrial carcinoma: multicentre randomised trial. PORTEC Study Group. Post Operative Radiation Therapy in Endometrial Carcinoma. The Lancet 355: 1404–1411.

Creutzberg CL, van Putten WL, Koper PC et al 2003 Survival after relapse in patients with endometrial cancer: results from a randomized trial. Gynecologic Oncology 89: 201–209.

Creutzberg CL, van Putten WL, Warlam-Rodenhuis CC et al 2004 Outcome of high-risk stage IC, grade 3, compared with stage I endometrial carcinoma patients: the Postoperative Radiation Therapy in Endometrial Carcinoma Trial. Journal of Clinical Oncology 22: 1234–1241.

Department of Health 1999 Guidance on Commissioning Cancer Services: Improving Outcomes in Gynaecological Cancers — the Manual. Department of Health, London. http://www.dh.gov.uk/en/Publicationsandstatistics/Publications/PublicationsPolicyAndGuidance/DH_4005385

Doll A, Abal M, Rigau M et al 2008 Novel molecular profiles of endometrial cancer — new light through old windows. Journal of Steroid Biochemistry and Molecular Biology 108: 221–229.

Duffy SR, Distler W, Howell A, Cuzick J, Baum M 2009 A lower incidence of gynecologic adverse events and interventions with anastrozole than with tamoxifen in the ATAC trial. American Journal of Obstetrics and Gynecology 200: 80 e1–7.

Early Breast Cancer Trialists' Collaborative Group 1998 Tamoxifen for early breast cancer: an overview of the randomised trials. The Lancet 351(9114): 1451–1467.

Fanning J 2001 Long-term survival of intermediate risk endometrial cancer (stage IG3, IC, II) treated with full lymphadenectomy and brachytherapy without teletherapy. Gynecologic Oncology 82: 371–374.

Ferlay J, Bray F, Pisani P, Parkin DM 2004 GLOBOCAN 2002.Cancer Incidence, Mortality and Prevalence Worldwide. IARC CancerBase No.5, Version 2.0. IARC Press, Lyon.

Ferlay J, Autier P, Boniol M, Heanue M, Colombet M, Boyle P 2007 Estimates of the cancer incidence and mortality in Europe in 2006. Annals of Oncology 18: 581–592.

Fleming GF, Brunetto VL, Cella D et al 2004 Phase III trial of doxorubicin plus cisplatin with or without paclitaxel plus filgrastim in advanced endometrial carcinoma: a Gynecologic Oncology Group Study. Journal of Clinical Oncology 22: 2159–2166.

Froggatt NJ, Brassett C, Koch DJ et al 1996 Mutation screening of MSH2 and MLH1 mRNA in hereditary non-polyposis colon cancer syndrome. Journal of Medical Genetics 33: 726–730.

Ghezzi F, Cromi A, Bergamini V et al 2006 Laparoscopic management of endometrial cancer in nonobese and obese women: a consecutive series. Journal of Minimally Invasive Gynecology 13: 269–275.

Greven K, Winter K, Underhill K, Fontenesci J, Cooper J, Burke T 2006 Final analysis of RTOG 9708: adjuvant postoperative irradiation combined with cisplatin/paclitaxel chemotherapy following surgery for patients with high-risk endometrial cancer. Gynecologic Oncology 103: 155–159.

Gupta JK, Chien PF, Voit D, Clark TJ, Khan KS 2002 Ultrasonographic endometrial thickness for diagnosing endometrial pathology in women with postmenopausal bleeding: a meta-analysis. Acta Obstetrica et Gynecologica Scandinavica 81: 799–816.

Havrilesky LJ, Secord AA, Bae-Jump V et al 2007a Outcomes in surgical stage I uterine papillary serous carcinoma. Gynecologic Oncology 105: 677–682.

Havrilesky LJ, Cragun JM, Calingaert B et al 2007b The prognostic significance of positive peritoneal cytology and adnexal/serosal metastasis in stage IIIA endometrial cancer. Gynecologic Oncology 104: 401–405.

Hecht JL, Mutter GL 2006 Molecular and pathologic aspects of endometrial carcinogenesis. Journal of Clinical Oncology 24: 4783–4791.

Humber CE, Tierney JF, Symonds RP et al 2007 Chemotherapy for advanced, recurrent or metastatic endometrial cancer: a systematic review of Cochrane collaboration. Annals of Oncology 18: 409–420.

Istre O, Langebrekke A, Qvigstad E 2007 Changing hysterectomy technique from open abdominal to laparoscopic: new trend in Oslo, Norway. Journal of Minimally Invasive Gynecology 14: 74–77.

Janda M, Gebski V, Forder P, Jackson D, Williams G, Obermair A 2006 Total laparoscopic versus open surgery for stage I endometrial cancer: the LACE randomized controlled trial. Contemporary Clinical Trials 27: 353–363.

Kahanpaa KV, Wahlstrom T, Grohn P, Heinonen E, Nieminen U, Widholm O 1986 Sarcomas of the uterus: a clinicopathologic study of 119 patients. Obstetrics and Gynecology 67: 417–424.

Kamat AA, Merritt WM, Coffey D et al 2007 Clinical and biological significance of vascular endothelial growth factor in endometrial cancer. Clinical Cancer Research 13: 7487–7495.

Keys HM, Roberts JA, Brunetto VL et al 2004 A phase III trial of surgery with or without adjunctive external pelvic radiation therapy in intermediate risk endometrial adenocarcinoma: a Gynecologic Oncology Group study. Gynecologic Oncology 92: 744–751.

Kitchener HC 2008 Survival from endometrial cancer in England and Wales up to 2001. British Journal of Cancer 99 (Suppl 1): S68–S69.

Kitchener H, Swart AM, Qian Q, Amos C, Parmar MK 2009 Efficacy of systematic pelvic lymphadenectomy in endometrial cancer (MRC ASTEC trial): a randomised study. The Lancet 373: 125–136.

Lertsanguansinchai P, Lertbutsayanukul C, Shotelersuk K et al 2004 Phase III randomized trial comparing LDR and HDR brachytherapy in treatment of cervical carcinoma. International Journal of Radiation Oncology, Biology, Physics 59: 1424–1431.

Lethaby A, Suckling J, Barlow D, Farquhar CM, Jepson RG, Roberts H 2004 Hormone replacement therapy in postmenopausal women: endometrial hyperplasia and irregular bleeding. Cochrane Database of Systematic Reviews 3: CD000402.

Lin F, Zhang QJ, Zheng FY et al 2008 Laparoscopically assisted versus open surgery for endometrial cancer — a meta-analysis of randomized controlled trials. International Journal of Gynecological Cancer 18: 1315–1325.

Lindemann K, Vatten LJ, Ellstrom-Engh M, Eskild A 2008 Body mass, diabetes and smoking, and endometrial cancer risk: a follow-up study. British Journal of Cancer 98: 1582–1585.

Maxwell GL, Chandramouli GV, Dainty L et al 2005 Microarray analysis of endometrial carcinomas and mixed Müllerian tumors reveals distinct gene expression profiles associated with different histologic types of uterine cancer. Clinical Cancer Research 11: 4056–4066.

Milano MT, Constine LS, Okunieff P 2007 Normal tissue tolerance dose metrics for radiation therapy of major organs. Seminars in Radiation Oncology 17: 131–140.

Morrison C, Zanagnolo V, Ramirez N et al 2006 HER-2 is an independent prognostic factor in endometrial cancer: association with outcome in a large cohort of surgically staged patients. Journal of Clinical Oncology 24: 2376–2385.

Murphy KT, Rotmensch J, Yamada SD, Mundt AJ 2003 Outcome and patterns of failure in pathologic stages I–IV clear-cell carcinoma of the endometrium: implications for adjuvant radiation therapy. International Journal of Radiation Oncology, Biology, Physics 55: 1272–1276.

Nakanishi K, Yoshikawa H, Ueda T et al 2001 Postradiation sarcomas of the pelvis after treatment for uterine cervical cancer: review of the CT and MR findings of five cases. Skeletal Radiology 30: 132–137.

Office for National Statistics 2008 Cancer Statistics Registrations: Registrations of Cancer Diagnosed in 2005, England. Series MB1 no. 36. Office for National Statistics, London.

O'Hanlan KA, Huang GS, Lopez L, Garnier AC 2004 Total laparoscopic hysterectomy for oncological indications with outcomes stratified by age. Gynecologic Oncology 95: 196–203.

O'Hanlan KA, Huang GS, Garnier AC et al 2005 Total laparoscopic hysterectomy versus total abdominal hysterectomy: cohort review of patients with uterine neoplasia. Journal of the Society of Laparoendoscopic Surgeons 9: 277–286.

Papadopoulos N, Lindblom A 1997 Molecular basis of HNPCC: mutations of MMR genes. Human Mutatation 10: 89–99.

Pervaiz N, Colterjohn N, Farrokhyar F, Tozer R, Figueredo A, Ghert M 2008 A systematic meta-analysis of randomized controlled trials of adjuvant chemotherapy for localized resectable soft-tissue sarcoma. Cancer 113: 573–581.

Ramirez PT, Slomovitz BM, Soliman PT, Coleman RL, Levenback C 2006 Total laparoscopic radical hysterectomy and lymphadenectomy: the M.D. Anderson Cancer Center experience. Gynecologic Oncology 102: 252–255.

Reich H 1992 Laparoscopic hysterectomy. Surgical Laparoscopy and Endoscopy 2: 85–88.

Rose PG, Brunetto VL, VanLe L, Bell J, Walker JL, Lee RB 2000 A phase II trial of anastrozole in advanced recurrent or persistent endometrial carcinoma: a Gynecologic Oncology Group study. Gynecologic Oncology 78: 212–216.

Sant M, Aareleid T, Berrino F et al 2003 EUROCARE-3: survival of cancer patients diagnosed 1990–94 — results and commentary. Annals of Oncology 14 (Suppl 5): 61–118.

Sarcoma Meta-analysis Collaboration 2000 Adjuvant chemotherapy for localised resectable soft tissue sarcoma in adults. Cochrane Database of Systematic Reviews 2: CD001419.

Scottish Intercollegiate Guidelines Network 2002 Investigation of Post-menopausal Bleeding. SIGN Publication No. 61. SIGN, Edinburgh.

Silverberg SG 2000 Problems in the differential diagnosis of endometrial hyperplasia and carcinoma. Modern Pathology 13: 309–327.

Slomovitz BM, Broaddus RR, Burke TW et al 2004 Her-2/neu overexpression and amplification in uterine papillary serous carcinoma. Journal of Clinical Oncology 22: 3126–3132.

Smith-Bindman R, Kerlikowske K, Feldstein VA et al 1998 Endovaginal ultrasound to exclude endometrial cancer and other endometrial abnormalities. Journal of the American Medical Association 280: 1510–1517.

Susumu N, Sagae S, Udagawa Y et al 2008 Randomized phase III trial of pelvic radiotherapy versus cisplatin-based combined chemotherapy in patients with intermediate- and high-risk endometrial cancer: a Japanese Gynecologic Oncology Group study. Gynecologic Oncology 108: 226–233.

Sutton G, Brunetto VL, Kilgore L et al 2000 A phase III trial of ifosfamide with or without cisplatin in carcinosarcoma of the uterus: a Gynecologic Oncology Group Study. Gynecologic Oncology 79: 147–153.

Sutton G, Kauderer J, Carson LF, Lentz SS, Whitney CW, Gallion H 2005 Adjuvant ifosfamide and cisplatin in patients with completely resected stage I or II carcinosarcomas (mixed mesodermal tumors) of the uterus: a Gynecologic Oncology Group study. Gynecologic Oncology 96: 630–634.

Thigpen JT, Brady MF, Alvarez RD et al 1999 Oral medroxyprogesterone acetate in the treatment of advanced or recurrent endometrial carcinoma: a dose–response study by the Gynecologic Oncology Group. Journal of Clinical Oncology 17: 1736–1744.

Ushijima K, Yahata H, Yoshikawa H et al 2007 Multicenter phase II study of fertility-sparing treatment with medroxyprogesterone acetate for endometrial carcinoma and atypical hyperplasia in young women. Journal of Clinical Oncology 25: 2798–2803.

Walker JL, Piedmote M, Spirtos N et al 2006 Surgical staging of uterine cancer: randomized phase III trial of laparoscopy vs laparotomy — a Gynecologic Oncology Group Study (GOG): preliminary results. Journal of Clinical Oncology 2006 ASCO Annual Meeting Proceedings Part I 24 (Suppl 18): 5010.

Weiderpass E, Adami HO, Baron JA et al 1999 Risk of endometrial cancer following estrogen replacement with and without progestins. Journal of the National Cancer Institute 91: 1131–1137.

CHAPTER 43

Gestational trophoblastic tumours

Thomas Newsom-Davis and Michael J. Seckl

Chapter Contents

INTRODUCTION	650		MANAGEMENT	657
GENETICS AND PATHOLOGY	650		PATIENT FOLLOW-UP AFTER CHEMOTHERAPY	663
EPIDEMIOLOGY AND AETIOLOGICAL FACTORS	652		TIMING OF PREGNANCY AFTER TREATMENT	663
GENETIC FACTORS: THE ROLE OF IMPRINTING	653		CONTRACEPTIVE ADVICE	663
RISK OF GESTATIONAL TROPHOBLASTIC TUMOURS FOLLOWING COMPLETE OR PARTIAL HYDATIDIFORM MOLE	654		LONG-TERM COMPLICATIONS OF THERAPY	664
			PROGNOSIS	664
HUMAN CHORIONIC GONADOTROPHIN	654		CONCLUSION	664
CLINICAL FEATURES	655		KEY POINTS	664
INVESTIGATIONS	656			

Introduction

The World Health Organization (WHO) has classified gestational trophoblastic disease (GTD) into two premalignant diseases, termed 'complete hydatidiform mole' (CM) and 'partial hydatidiform mole' (PM), and three malignant disorders, termed 'invasive mole', 'gestational choriocarcinoma' and 'placental-site trophoblastic tumour' (PSTT) (World Health Organization 1983). These malignant disorders are also frequently referred to as 'gestational trophoblastic tumours' (GTTs) or 'neoplasia' (GTN). GTTs are important to recognize because they are nearly always curable and fertility can be preserved in most cases. This is mainly because:

- GTTs are exquisitely chemosensitive;
- all GTTs produce human chorionic gonadotrophin (hCG), a serum tumour marker with a sensitivity and accuracy in screening, monitoring, management and follow-up of patients which is unparalleled in cancer medicine; and
- detailed prognostic scoring has permitted fine-tuning of treatment intensity so that each patient only receives the minimum therapy required to eliminate her disease.

Genetics and Pathology

Complete hydatidiform mole

CMs nearly always contain paternal DNA alone and are therefore androgenetic. This occurs in most cases because a single sperm bearing a 23X set of chromosomes fertilizes an ovum lacking maternal genes, and then duplicates to form the homozygote, 46XX (Figure 43.1A). However, in up to 25% of CMs, fertilization can take place with two spermatozoa, resulting in the heterozygous 46XY or 46XX configuration (Figure 43.1B). A 46YY conceptus has not yet been described and is presumably non-viable. Very rarely, a CM can arise from a fertilized ovum which has retained its maternal nuclear DNA and is therefore biparental in origin (Fisher and Newlands 1998). Macroscopically, the classic CM resembles a bunch of grapes due to generalized (complete) swelling of chorionic villi. However, this appearance is only seen in the second trimester and the diagnosis is usually made earlier when the villi are much less hydropic. Indeed, in the first trimester, the villi microscopically contain little fluid, are branching and consist of hyperplastic syncytio- and cytotrophoblast with many vessels. Although it was previously thought that CM produced no fetal tissue, histology from 6–8-week abortions reveals evidence of embryonic

DOI: 10.1016/B978-0-7020-3120-5.00043-6

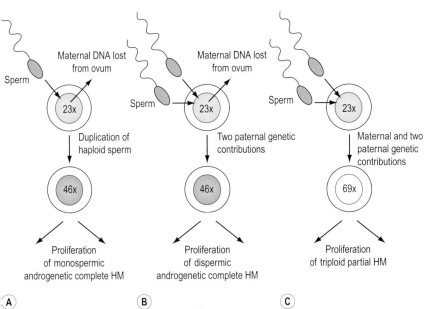

Figure 43.1 Schematic diagram showing that the androgenetic diploid complete hydatidiform mole is formed either (A) by duplication of the chromosomes from a single sperm, or (B) by two sperm fertilizing the ovum which, in both cases, has lost its own genetic component. The triploid genetic origin of a partial hydatidiform mole (HM) is demonstrated in (C).

elements, including fetal red cells (Paradinas 1998). This has resulted in pathologists incorrectly labelling CMs as PMs. The presence of embryonic tissue from a twin pregnancy comprising a fetus and a CM is another source of error which can lead to the incorrect diagnosis of PM.

Partial hydatidiform mole

Genetically, PMs are nearly all triploid with two paternal and one maternal sets of chromosomes (Figure 43.1C). Rarely, tetraploid PMs are found. Triploidy occurs in 1–3% of all recognized conceptions and in approximately 20% of spontaneous abortions with an abnormal karyotype, but at least two paternal sets of chromosomes are needed for PM development. Triploids due to two sets of maternal chromosome do not become PMs (Lawler et al 1982). Although a variety of reports have suggested that diploid PMs exist, genetic analysis of such lesions has not supported this. In general, a diploid molar gestation is believed to be a CM (Genest et al 2002). Flow cytometry, which can be done in formalin-fixed, paraffin-embedded tissues (Seckl et al 2000), can help in differentiating CM from PM, and PM from diploid non-molar hydropic abortions.

In PMs, villous swelling is less intense and only affects some villi. Both swollen and non-swollen villi can have trophoblastic hyperplasia which is mild and focal. The villi have characteristic indented outlines and round inclusions. An embryo is usually present and can be recognized macroscopically or inferred from the presence of nucleated red cells in villous vasculature. It may survive into the second trimester, but usually dies at approximately 8–9 weeks of gestation and this is followed by loss of vessels and stromal fibrosis. In PMs evacuated early, villous swelling and trophoblastic excess can be so mild and focal that the diagnosis of PM may be missed (Paradinas 1998). Indeed, at uterine evacuation for a 'miscarriage', it is likely that many PMs are misclassified as products of conception. Fortunately, the authors only see about one patient per year with persistent GTD related to a previously unrecognized PM. Of the increas-

ing number of PMs which are correctly diagnosed, very few go on to develop persistent GTD. Indeed, in approximately 3000 PMs reviewed and followed at Charing Cross Hospital between 1973 and 1997, only 15 (0.5%) have required chemotherapy (Seckl et al 2000).

Other pregnancies mistaken for hydatidiform mole

Over half of first-trimester non-molar abortions are due to trisomy, monosomy, maternally derived triploidy and translocations. These often develop hydrops but are small (<3 mm), and PM can be excluded if they are diploid on flow cytometry. A significant recent development in the pathological analysis of hydatidiform mole (HM) is the use of $p57^{kip2}$ immunostaining to make a definitive diagnosis of androgenetic CM as opposed to a hydropic abortion or a PM. $p57^{kip2}$, a cyclin-dependent kinase inhibitor, is a paternally imprinted gene which is maternally expressed. The absence of maternal genes in androgenetic CM means that the gene cannot be expressed in CM cytotrophoblast. Consequently, $p57^{kip2}$ staining is negative with CMs, in contrast to PMs, hydropic abortion and normal placenta. This technique is well validated, easy and inexpensive to perform (Sebire et al 2004, Popiolek et al 2006).

Syndromes such as Turner's, Edward's and Beckwith-Wiedemann's can also cause histological confusion with PMs (Paradinas 1998).

Invasive hydatidiform mole

Invasive hydatidiform mole is common and is clinically identified by the combination of an abnormal uterine ultrasound (US) and a persistent or rising hCG level following uterine evacuation of a CM or PM. Pathological confirmation of this condition is rarely required. Moreover, repeat dilatation and curettage (D & C) is often contraindicated because of the risks of uterine perforation, infection, life-threatening haemorrhage and subsequent hysterectomy. In occasional cases where histology is available, invasive mole can be distinguished from choriocarcinoma by the presence of chorionic villi. Identification of cases of CM and PM that will subsequently undergo malignant transformation would be an important development. There is accumulating evidence that such HMs are more likely to show telomerase activity (i.e. have limitless replicative potential) and increased expression of the anti-apoptotic gene *Mcl-1* (Wells 2007). These findings need further prospective evaluation.

Choriocarcinoma

Most choriocarcinomas have been shown to have grossly abnormal karyotypes with diverse ploidies and several chromosome rearrangements, none of which are specific for the disease (Arima et al 1994). Studies of the origin of GTTs have confirmed that choriocarcinoma may arise from any type of pregnancy including a normal term pregnancy, or homozygous or heterozygous CM. Until recently, it was thought that PMs could not give rise to choriocarcinoma. However, there is now incontrovertible genetic evidence that PMs can indeed transform into choriocarcinomas (Seckl et al 2000). This is important as some centres wrongly believe that it is safe to discontinue hCG follow-up following the diagnosis of a PM.

Interestingly, choriocarcinoma may not always be due to the antecedent pregnancy. A patient with a history of CM 4 years previously developed choriocarcinoma following the delivery of a twin pregnancy. Using polymerase chain reaction to amplify short tandem repeat polymorphisms in DNA, this tumour was shown to be genetically identical to the previous CM (Fisher et al 1995). As for invasive moles, obtaining tissue to make a formal histological diagnosis of choriocarcinoma is often not appropriate, so doubt frequently exists regarding whether patients have one or the other form of GTT.

Choriocarcinoma is highly malignant in behaviour, appearing as a soft, purple, largely haemorrhagic mass. Microscopically, it mimics an early implanting blastocyst with central cores of mononuclear cytotrophoblast surrounded by a rim of multinucleated syncytiotrophoblast and a distinct absence of chorionic villi. There are extensive areas of necrosis and haemorrhage, and frequent evidence of tumour within venous sinuses. Interestingly, the disease fails to stimulate the connective tissue support normally associated with tumours, and induces hypervascularity of the surrounding maternal tissues. This probably accounts for its highly metastatic and haemorrhagic behaviour.

Placental-site trophoblastic tumour

PSTTs have been shown to follow term delivery, non-molar abortion or CM. Furthermore, a recent case has shown that PSTTs can develop after a PM (Palmieri et al 2005). Like choriocarcinoma, the causative pregnancy may not be the immediate antecedent pregnancy (Fisher et al 1995). Genetic analysis of some PSTTs has demonstrated that they are mostly diploid, originating from either a normal conceptus and therefore biparental, or androgenetic and arising from a CM (Newlands et al 1998a).

In the normal placenta, placental-site trophoblast is distinct from villous trophoblast and infiltrates the decidua, myometrium and spiral arteries of the uterine wall. PSTTs are rare, slow-growing malignant tumours composed mainly of intermediate trophoblast derived from cytotrophoblast, and so produce little hCG. However, they often stain strongly for human placental lactogen (hPL) and β1-glycoprotein. Elevated Ki-67 levels may help in distinguishing PSTTs from regressing placental nodules (Shih and Kurman 1998). In contrast to other forms of GTT, spread tends to occur late by local infiltration and via the lymphatics, although distant metastases can occur. More than five mitoses per 10 high-power fields may predict tumours with metastasizing potential (Newlands et al 1998a).

Epithelioid trophoblastic tumour

Epithelioid trophoblastic tumours (ETTs) are a recently described neoplastic proliferation of intermediate trophoblast that are thought, by some investigators, to be distinct from PSTTs and choriocarcinoma. It has been proposed that ETTs arise from the intermediate trophoblasts of the chorionic laeve (Shih and Kurman 2001). Histologically, ETTs display a relatively uniform, nodular proliferation of intermediate-sized epithelioid trophoblasts, forming nests and cords. Islands of trophoblast are typically surrounded by areas of hyalinization or eosinophilic debris simulating tumour cell necrosis and resembling keratinous material in a squamous cell carcinoma. ETTs can be associated with focal replacement of the cervical glandular epithelium with stratified neoplastic cells, simulating squamous cervical intraepithelial neoplasia. ETT cells are positive for cytokeratin, epithelial membrane antigen and inhibin-A, whereas trophoblastic markers hPL, hCG and melanoma cell adhesion molecular are only expressed focally (Hui et al 2005).

Whether ETT is really a distinct disease entity in the GTD spectrum remains a contentious issue. Indeed, the authors have only seen this appearance in patients who have previously had chemotherapy for an invasive mole or choriocarcinoma, so this may simply represent the differentiating effects of treatment (as seen with germ cell tumours) rather than a separate type of GTT.

Epidemiology and Aetiological Factors

Hydatidiform mole

Incidence and ethnic origin

The incidence of HM in the UK is one in 714 pregnancies (Tham et al 2003). Recent results indicate that the previously documented higher rates in the Far East have fallen towards the stable levels found in Europe and North America (Hando et al 1998), possibly because of dietary changes. The incidence of PM has been underestimated in the past and is currently three per 1000 pregnancies (Newlands et al 1998b).

Age

CMs are more common at the extremes of reproductive age. In one study, compared with the lowest rate between 25–29 years, the relative increased risk was six-fold in girls under

15 years, three-fold between 40 and 45 years, 26-fold between 45 and 49 years and more than 400-fold over 50 years of age (Bagshawe and Begent 1983, Newlands et al 1998b). PMs are also more common at the extremes of reproductive age, although the effect is less pronounced (Sebire et al 2002a).

Previous pregnancies

Increasing gravidity does not increase the risk of CM. However, following one CM, the risk of a subsequent pregnancy being a CM rises from one in 1000 to one in 76, and to one in 6.5 with two previous CMs (Bagshawe and Begent 1983). Therefore, patients with a previous CM must be followed-up after each subsequent pregnancy to confirm that their hCG levels return to normal. Similar results have been reported for PMs, with the risk for subsequent molar pregnancies rising to one in 59 for women with one previous PM (Sebire et al 2003).

Choriocarcinoma

The incidence of choriocarcinoma following term delivery without a history of CM is approximately one in 50,000. However, CM is probably the most common antecedent to choriocarcinoma, comprising 29–83% in various studies across the world (World Health Organization 1983). Consequently, the overall incidence of choriocarcinoma after a CM is much higher. Proof of this is frequently difficult to obtain, but when histology was available, these tumours were identified as choriocarcinoma in 3% and invasive mole in 16% of previous CMs (seldom as PSTT). Rarely, PMs can give rise to choriocarcinoma (Seckl et al 2000). Unlike HM, choriocarcinoma does not exhibit any clear geographical trends in incidence, but the effect of age remains important.

Placental-site trophoblastic tumours

First described as a separate disease entity in 1976 (Kurman et al 1976), there are currently approximately 150 recorded cases of this tumour in the literature; therefore, estimates of its true incidence may be quite inaccurate (Newlands et al 1998a, Papadopoulos et al 2002, Hassadia et al 2005, Baergen et al 2006). In the largest series described — 62 patients between 1976 and 2006 — PSTTs represented 0.2% of all trophoblastic tumours (Schmid et al 2008) The relative incidence in the UK has been stable over the past 15 years following an increase in the first years after the introduction of this new disease classification.

Genetic Factors: The Role of Imprinting

Hydatidiform mole

The theory of an underlying genetic cause of HM is based on two observations: women who have had one mole have an excess risk of having another mole; and the discovery of an inherited syndrome of recurrent CM pregnancies, which has been identified in a handful of families globally. Familial CM is diagnosed by the presence of more than one woman in a single family with two CMs or more, and is inherited in an autosomal-recessive pattern. These families are being studied with the aim of identifying specific genetic abnormalities and their role in the pathogenesis of HM.

All autosomal genes consist of two alleles (paternal and maternal). However, some alleles are only expressed from one parent and not the other; a phenomenon called 'genomic imprinting'. Underexpression of an imprinted gene has been demonstrated in cases of both familial and sporadic CM, and abnormal methylation patterns have been described in another family (Fisher et al 2002, Judson et al 2002).

Extensive mapping studies have been performed on the families with CM. These have demonstrated a defective locus at 19q13.4 in five families which has been localized to a single gene — NALP7 (Murdoch et al 2006). This is the first causative single gene defect identified in CM. NALP7 is a member of the CATERPILLER family which is involved in inflammation and apoptosis. It is expressed in oocytes and the endometrium, and is a negative regulator of the proinflammatory cytokine interleukin-1β, which is involved in regulating trophoblast invasion during implantation. It is unclear how defects in NALP7 result in CM formation, but abnormal inflammation during embryogenesis may be involved.

NALP7 does not appear to be involved in the establishment of imprinting; therefore, defects in NALP7 may be a consequence of abnormal imprinting rather than its cause. Further families have been identified that do not map to 19q13.4, proving that familial CM is a genetically heterogeneous condition (Zhao et al 2006). Moreover, to date, abnormal NALP7 has not been demonstrated in sporadic CM or PM cases.

Three other, closely related, genes are imprinted and may be involved in GTT development. These are H19, a putative tumour suppressor gene (Hao et al 1993), and $p57^{kip2}$ (discussed previously) (Matsuoka et al 1996), both of which are normally expressed by the maternal allele; and the paternally expressed IGF-2, a growth factor commonly implicated in tumour proliferation (Ogawa et al 1993). While $p57^{kip2}$ showed the expected pattern of expression in CM and choriocarcinoma (Chilosi et al 1998), CM and postmole tumours were unexpectedly found to express H19 (Walsh et al 1995), and some post-term tumours showed biallelic expression of both H19 and IGF-2 (Hashimoto et al 1995). This suggests that loss of the normal imprinting patterns of these genes may be an important factor in the development of GTT.

Choriocarcinoma

Historically, cytogenetic studies of choriocarcinoma have demonstrated a diverse range of abnormalities. Microsatellite studies have shown loss of heterozygosity at specific regions: deletions of 7p12-q11.2, amplification of 7q21-q31 and loss of 8p12-p21 (Matsuda et al 1997) Abnormalities in the latter two are also found in some cases of ovarian and breast cancer, and are postulated to encode novel tumour suppressor genes. Several groups have reproduced these findings in non-molar choriocarcinoma, but results in postmolar choriocarcinoma have been inconsistent (Burke et al 2006). Only a minority of tumours showed loss of heterozygosity for all three regions, suggesting that these defects are acquired late in the development of choriocarcinoma and are not essential for malignant transformation.

Risk of Gestational Trophoblastic Tumours Following Complete or Partial Hydatidiform Mole

Following evacuation of a CM or PM, the risk of developing a GTT is less than 16% and 0.5%, respectively (Bagshawe et al 1990, Seckl et al 2000). Since it is not yet possible to predict which patients with a CM or PM will develop persistent GTD, all patients must be registered for hCG monitoring. Following this strict protocol enables the identification of individuals with persistent trophoblastic growth who could benefit from life-saving chemotherapy.

Human Chorionic Gonadotrophin

Beta-human chorionic gonadotrophin assays

The family of pituitary/placental glycoprotein hormones includes hCG, follicle-stimulating hormone, luteinizing hormone (LH) and thyroid-stimulating hormone (TSH). Each hormone comprises an α-subunit which is common between the family members and a distinct β-subunit. Consequently, assays to measure hCG are directed against the β-subunit. Many different β-hCG assays are available. Some detect intact β-hCG, and others are either selective for individual fragments or detect various combinations of fragments (Cole 1998). In pregnancy, hCG is usually intact and fragments of β-hCG are not produced, although the β chain is hyperglycosylated during the first trimester. However, in cancer, β-hCG may circulate in many different forms which can vary in their glycosylation status. Therefore, assays used in patients with GTD and cancer need to be able to detect all forms of β-hCG. The ideal assay should be able to recognize all forms equally well and be sufficiently sensitive to limit the risk of false-negative results (Mitchell and Seckl 2007). Moreover, the assay should not produce false-positive results as this is well recognized to be associated with unnecessary medical interventions and potentially life-threatening complications (Cole et al 2001). So how good are the existing β-hCG assays?

Commercially available β-hCG tests are based on the sandwich assay principle and rely on two antibodies which generally target different regions of the molecule. These assays are primarily licensed for use in pregnancy detection. However, they are frequently employed for monitoring patients with cancer. The assays can produce both false-positive and false-negative results (Cole et al 2001, Mitchell and Seckl 2007). The false-positive results occur because there is another molecule (often a heterophile antibody) which sticks the capture and detection antibodies together. This can usually be avoided by measuring the hCG in urine, as cross-reacting antibodies are large and cannot pass through the renal glomerulus into the urine. Alternatively, if a false-positive result is suspected, remeasuring the hCG on an alternative assay or serially diluting the serum sample usually resolves the issue. Real hCG will be seen in another assay and will dilute appropriately, whilst a cross-reacting molecule will be negative in another assay and does not serially dilute away. Recent work from the authors' laboratory shows that commercial assays may be particularly prone to false-negative results, either because they completely fail to detect or as a

consequence of poor sensitivity for a particular β-hCG isoform (Mitchell and Seckl 2007). False-negative results can potentially result in failure to diagnose disease or early termination of treatment, and therefore higher relapse rates.

In addition to the commercial assays, there are also several in-house assays in various centres around the world which are usually based on a single antibody to capture the hormone on a competitive basis with labelled (often radioactively) β-hCG. These assays may also produce false-positive and false-negative results. Indeed, all types of assay are only as good as the antibodies used. At Charing Cross Hospital, a rabbit polyclonal antibody is used in a radio-immunoassay (RIA); this recognizes all forms of β-hCG equally well and with sufficient sensitivity that false-negative results appear to be rare (Mitchell and Seckl 2007). Moreover, since this RIA is performed on both serum and urine samples which are serially diluted, the risk of false-positive results is very low (Mitchell and Seckl 2007).

Currently, the authors believe that the Charing Cross RIA for β-hCG remains the gold standard assay for use in the management of GTD and other cancers. The assay is sensitive to 1 IU/l in serum and 20 IU/l in urine.

New assays designed to detect specific hCG variants are in development and are leading to further increases in the specificity and sensitivity of hCG monitoring. Elevation of hyperglycosylated hCG (hCG-H) levels may be specific to cases of HM that subsequently require chemotherapy. This rise occurs earlier than in conventional hCG and before clinically apparent GTTs develop (Cole et al 2006a). However, further work is required, and since no commercial hCG-H assays are available, progress in this area is likely to be slow.

Recent data have also shown that proportionately higher levels of free β-hCG fragments are produced in PSTTs, and that this is a highly sensitive test for discriminating PSTTs from choriocarcinoma (Cole et al 2006b, Harvey et al 2008), although β-hCG may also be elevated in some non-trophoblastic malignancies.

Beta-human chorionic gonadotrophin as a tumour marker

hCG has a half-life of 24–36 h and is the most sensitive and specific marker for trophoblastic tissue. However, hCG production is not confined to pregnancy and GTD. Indeed, hCG is produced by any trophoblastic tissue found, for example, in germ cell tumours and in up to 15% of epithelial malignancies (Vaitukaitis 1979). The hCG levels in such cases can be just as high as those seen in GTD or in pregnancy. Therefore, measurements of hCG do not reliably discriminate between pregnancy, GTD or non-gestational trophoblastic tumours.

However, serial measurements of hCG have revolutionized the management of GTD for several reasons. The amount of hCG produced correlates with tumour volume, such that a serum hCG level of 5 IU/l corresponds to approximately 10^4–10^5 viable tumour cells. Consequently, these assays are several orders of magnitude more sensitive than the best imaging modalities available today. In addition, hCG levels can be used to determine prognosis (Bagshawe 1976). Serial measurements allow monitoring of disease progression or response to therapy (Figure 43.2). Develop-

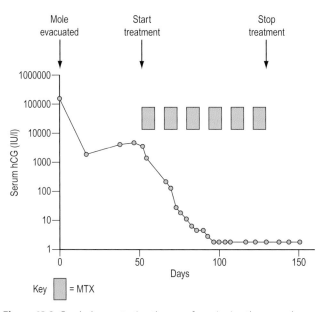

Figure 43.2 Graph demonstrating the use of monitoring the serum human chorionic gonadotrophin (hCG) concentration following evacuation of a hydatidiform mole (HM). In this case, after an initial fall, the hCG level started to rise, indicating the development of invasive HM or choriocarcinoma, so the patient was called up for staging. The prognostic score was low risk (see Table 43.4) and the patient was successfully treated with methotrexate (MTX) and folinic acid (see Table 43.5).

ment of drug resistance can be detected at an early stage, which facilitates appropriate changes in management. Estimates may be made of the time for which chemotherapy should be continued after hCG levels are undetectable in serum in order to reduce the tumour volume to zero. For these reasons, hCG is the best tumour marker known.

Clinical Features

Complete and partial moles

These most commonly present in the first trimester as a threatened abortion with vaginal bleeding. If the diagnosis is delayed, patients may notice the passing of grape-like structures (vesicles), and occasionally the entire mole may be evacuated spontaneously. The uterus may be any size but is commonly large for gestational age. Patients with marked trophoblastic growth and high hCG levels are particularly prone to hyperemesis, toxaemia and the development of theca lutein cysts which may sometimes be palpable above the pelvis. Toxaemia was diagnosed in 27% of patients with CM (Berkowitz et al 1981), but is seen less frequently today because of early US diagnosis. Convulsions are rare. The high hCG levels may also produce hyperthyroidism because of cross-reactivity between hCG and TSH at the TSH receptor. Although pulmonary, vaginal and cervical metastases can occur, they may disappear spontaneously following removal of the mole. Thus the presence of metastases does not necessarily imply that an invasive mole or choriocarcinoma has developed. Patients may rarely present with acute respiratory distress, not only because of pulmonary metastases or anaemia but occasionally as a result of tumour embolization (Savage et al 1998). The risk of embolization is reduced by avoiding agents which induce uterine contrac-

tion before the cervix has been dilated to enable evacuation of the CM.

Patients with PMs do not usually exhibit the dramatic clinical features characteristic of CM (Goldstein and Berkowitz 1994). The uterus is often not enlarged for gestational age, and vaginal bleeding tends to occur later so that patients most often present in the late first or early second trimester with a missed or incomplete abortion. In fact, the diagnosis is often only suspected when the histology of curettings is available. The pre-evacuation hCG level is less than 100,000 IU/l at diagnosis in over 90% of cases.

At present, a proportion of CMs and PMs still go undiagnosed because of miscarriage at home or because termination centres do not carry out histopathological examination of all abortions (Seckl et al 2004a). This can result in late presentation of disease, sometimes with life-threatening complications. Clearly, there is little that can be done about miscarriages at home. However, for women attending termination centres, it may be possible to establish a screening procedure to help prevent subsequent problems from missed diagnosis.

Twin pregnancies

Twin pregnancies comprising a normal fetus and an HM occur in between one in 20,000 and one in 100,000 pregnancies. Some probably abort in the first trimester and so go undiagnosed. However, some are discovered on US examination either routinely or because of complications such as bleeding, excessive uterine size or problems related to a high hCG level. With specialist obstetric care, 40% of such cases have continued into the third trimester and delivered live babies (Sebire et al 2002b).

Invasive moles

Invasive moles are usually diagnosed because serial urine or serum hCG measurements reveal a stable or rising hCG level in the weeks after molar evacuation. Patients may complain of persistent vaginal bleeding and lower abdominal pains and/or swelling. This may occur as a result of haemorrhage from leaking tumour-induced vasculature as the trophoblast invades through the myometrium, or because of vulval, vaginal or intra-abdominal metastases. The tumour may also involve other pelvic structures, including the bladder or rectum, producing haematuria or rectal bleeding, respectively. Enlarging pulmonary metastases or tumour emboli growing in the pulmonary arteries can contribute to life-threatening respiratory complications (Seckl et al 1991). The risk of these complications is clearly higher in patients where the initial diagnosis of a molar pregnancy was missed and who are not, therefore, on hCG follow-up.

Choriocarcinoma

Choriocarcinoma can present after any form of pregnancy, but most commonly occurs after a CM. Histological proof of choriocarcinoma is not usually obtained after a CM because of the risk of fatal haemorrhage caused by biopsy, and so it is impossible to distinguish from an invasive mole. Choriocarcinoma following a normal pregnancy or non-molar abortion usually presents within 1 year of delivery but can occur 17 years later (Tidy et al 1995). The presenting features may be similar to HM with vaginal bleeding, abdominal pain and a pelvic mass.

However, one-third of all choriocarcinomas present without pelvic symptoms but have symptoms from distant metastases. In these cases, lives can be saved by remembering to include choriocarcinoma in the differential diagnosis of metastatic malignancy (particularly in lungs, brain or liver) presenting in a woman of childbearing age. Any site may be involved, including skin (producing a purple lesion), cauda equina and the heart. Pulmonary disease may be parenchymal, pleural or may result from tumour embolism and subsequent growth in the pulmonary arteries (Savage et al 1998). Thus, respiratory symptoms and signs can include dyspnoea, haemoptysis and pulmonary artery hypertension. Cerebral metastases may produce focal neurological signs, convulsions, evidence of raised intracranial pressure, and intracerebral or subarachnoid haemorrhage. Hepatic metastases may cause local pain or referred pain in the right shoulder. Although none of these presentations are specific to choriocarcinoma, performing a simple pregnancy test or quantitative hCG assay can provide a vital clue to the diagnosis.

Infantile choriocarcinoma

Choriocarcinoma in the fetus or newborn is exceptionally rare, with approximately 30 reported cases (Blohm and Gobel 2004, Sebire et al 2005). While a primary choriocarcinoma within the infant is possible, the mother also had the tumour in 17 cases. Interestingly, the diagnosis was often made in the neonate before the mother. In all cases, the infant was anaemic and had a raised hCG level, but the site of metastasis was variable, including brain, liver, lung and skin. Only a few cases have been treated successfully with platinum chemotherapy (Johnson et al 2003), with the rest dying within weeks of the initial diagnosis, which may have been delayed. Consequently, serum or urine hCG levels should be measured in all babies of mothers with choriocarcinoma. As the disease can present up to 6 months after delivery, an argument could be made for serial monitoring of hCG in these infants.

Placental-site trophoblastic tumour

PSTTs grow slowly and can present years after term delivery, non-molar abortion, CM or PM. Unlike choriocarcinoma, PSTTs tend to metastasize late in their natural history, so patients frequently present with gynaecological symptoms alone. In addition to vaginal bleeding, the production of hPL by the cytotrophoblastic cells may cause hyperprolactinaemia which can result in amenorrhoea and galactorrhoea. Rarely, patients can develop nephrotic syndrome, haematuria and disseminated intravascular coagulopathy. Metastases may occur in the vagina, extrauterine pelvic tissues, retroperitoneum, lymph nodes, lungs and brain (Newlands et al 1998a).

Epithelioid trophoblastic tumours

There are currently only a few recorded cases of this recently described tumour in the literature. Although most ETT

patients are women of childbearing age, a significant percentage of women are peri- or postmenopausal with a remote history of pregnancy (Coulson et al 2000). Similar to PSTTs, patients present with vaginal bleeding and low levels of serum β-hCG (<2500 IU/l). In half of the reported cases, tumours arise in the lower uterine segment or cervix, and the distinction from a keratinizing squamous cell carcinoma can sometimes be difficult. Extrauterine locations such as broad ligament as the primary site have also been observed (Kuo et al 2004). Similar to PSTTs, ETTs appear to respond less well to conventional chemotherapy compared with choriocarcinoma. Consequently, management of ETT cases is currently identical to that for PSTT cases, with hysterectomy for localized disease and careful follow-up until more experience of this rare lesion becomes available.

Investigations

Human chorionic gonadotrophin, chest X-ray and pelvic Doppler ultrasound

All patients who are suspected of having GTTs should have an hCG, a chest X-ray and pelvic Doppler ultrasound. The most common metastatic appearance on chest X-ray is of multiple, discrete, rounded lesions, but large solitary lesions, a miliary pattern or pleural effusions can occur (Bagshawe and Noble 1965). Furthermore, tumour emboli to the pulmonary arteries can produce an identical picture to venous thromboembolism, with wedge-shaped infarcts and areas of decreased vascular markings. Pulmonary artery hypertension can cause dilatation of the pulmonary arteries. Routine computed tomography (CT) scanning of the chest does not add anything to the management of these cases.

US and colour Doppler imaging are not diagnostic but highly suggestive of persistent GTD when there is a combination of a raised hCG level, no pregnancy and a vascular mass within the uterus (Figure 43.3). The last is seen in more than 75% of patients at the authors' centre. Detection rates are higher for CM compared with PM, and improve after 14 weeks of gestation (Fowler et al 2006). The uterine volume and uterine artery blood flow correlate with the amount of disease and the degree of abnormal tumour vasculature, respectively. Doppler frequently demonstrates a change in the waveform of the uterine arteries (Figure 43.3). This is attributed to large vascular channels forming in the myometrium, resulting in arteriovenous shunting (Long et al 1992). The uterine artery pulsatility index, an indirect measure of the functional tumour vascularity, has been shown to independently predict the response to chemotherapy in GTTs (Agarwal et al 2002). Furthermore, the increased sensitivity of modern colour Doppler US now reveals abnormal blood vessel encroachment through the myometrium into the endometrium. Although this has not been shown to have prognostic significance, the degree of vascular endometrial encroachment may aid in assessing the risk of major haemorrhage in patients with GTT (Boultebee and Newlands 1995). Interestingly, the vascular abnormalities within the pelvis and uterus can persist long after the disease has been eradicated with chemotherapy. Indeed, patients with repeated vaginal haemorrhage from these vas-

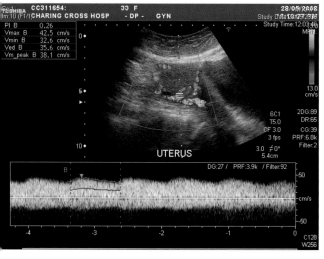

Figure 43.3 Ultrasonography with colour Doppler showing persistent gestational trophoblastic disease following a complete hydatidiform mole within the body and wall of the uterus. Typical vesicular or 'snow storm' appearance of residual molar tissue can be seen within the uterus, together with a rich blood supply through the endometrium and myometrium. There is no evidence of a fetus. Uterine artery pulsatility index showing low values indicative of arteriovenous shunting associated with an abnormal tumour vasculature.

cular malformations may require selective arterial emboliza-tion. This is usually successful and does not appear to affect fertility.

Pelvic US can also demonstrate ovarian theca lutein cysts and other ovarian masses. Metastatic spread outside the pelvis, such as to the liver or kidneys, can also be identified and shown to have an abnormal Doppler signal.

Investigation of drug-resistant disease

When patients develop drug-resistant disease, further inves-tigation is required to more accurately define where the residual tumour is located, as resection can be curative. CT of the chest and abdomen together with magnetic resonance imaging (MRI) of the brain and pelvis are often helpful and can detect deposits not previously seen. If the CT and MRI are normal, a lumbar puncture to measure the hCG level in cerebrospinal fluid can be useful to detect disease in the central nervous system (CNS). An hCG level greater than 1:60 of that found in the serum is highly indicative of the presence of trophoblastic disease.

Experimental imaging techniques

Radiolabelled anti-hCG antibodies given intravenously can localize tumours producing hCG when the serum hCG level is more than 100 IU/l (Begent et al 1987). However, both false-positive and false-negative results occur, so anti-hCG scanning should be regarded as complementary to other imaging investigations. More recently, positron emission tomography (PET) has provided a novel approach to image many tumour types using a variety of labels. Whole-body PET has already been reported to distinguish GTT emboli from blood clots in two patients with choriocarcinoma (Hebart et al 1996).

Other case reports demonstrate the potential value of PET in the differential diagnosis of undefined pulmonary nodules or in the localization of disease (Numnum et al 2005, Shaw et al 2005). [18]Fluorodeoxyglucose (FDG)-PET may be used to locate sites of disease in cases showing serological relapse without visible abnormality on conventional imaging (Dhillon et al 2006). However, the role of PET has yet to be confirmed in larger series of patients with GTTs.

Genetic analysis

On some occasions, it can be helpful to perform a compara-tive genetic analysis of the patient's trophoblastic tumour with their normal tissue and, if available, that of their partner. Thus, if the tumour is suspected of being of non-gestational origin, this can be confirmed by the presence of maternal DNA alone and the complete absence of paternal DNA. Genetic studies can also determine which of several antecedent pregnancies is the causal pregnancy of the current GTT. This can have an impact on determining appropriate therapy and prognosis (Fisher and Newlands 1998, Fisher et al 2007). In addition, genetic studies can help to identify whether a woman with repeated CM pregnancies has the rare biparental variant of CM. The latter condition is rarely com-patible with a normal pregnancy, and preimplantation diag-nosis is not yet possible. In contrast, a woman with repeated androgenetic CM can be offered in-vitro fertilization and preimplantation selection of unaffected concepti.

Management

Molar evacuation

Evacuation of the uterine cavity using suction gives the lowest incidence of sequelae. When the molar trophoblast invades the myometrium, it is relatively easy to perforate the uterus if a metal curette is used. Medical induction involving repeated contraction of the uterus induced by oxytocin or prostaglandin, or other surgical approaches including hysterectomy or hysterotomy increase the risk of requiring chemotherapy two- to three-fold compared with suction evacuation. This is thought to be because tumour is more likely to be disseminated by uterine contraction and manipulation. For similar reasons, the use of prostanoids to ripen a nulliparous cervix is not recommended, even in nulliparous women (Royal College of Obstetricians and Gynaecologists 2004). If bleeding is severe immediately after suction evacuation, a single dose of ergometrine to produce one uterine contraction may stem the haemorrhage, and does not appear to increase the chance of requiring chemotherapy.

In the past, it has been common practice for gynaecolo-gists to perform a second and sometimes a third evacuation of the uterine cavity in patients with a molar pregnancy. However, the chance of requiring chemotherapy after one evacuation is only 2.4%, but rises markedly to 18% after two evacuations and 81% after four evacuations (Table 43.1). Patients with an hCG plateau or with rising hCG levels are at particularly high risk of this, and 74% require chemo-therapy despite undergoing a second evacuation. In addi-tion, high hCG values have been shown to be an indicator

Table 43.1 Correlation between the number of evacuations performed following an hydatidiform mole and the subsequent requirement for chemotherapy at Charing Cross Hospital (1973–1986)

Number of evacuations	Patients not treated	Patients treated	% Patients treated
1	4481	109	2.4
2	1495	267	18
3	106	106	50
4	5	22	81

for low rates of benefit of a second evacuation, with 80% of patients with a preintervention hCG level of more than 5000 IU/l subsequently requiring chemotherapy (Savage and Seckl 2005). However, second evacuations may be useful for symptom control in selected patients with heavy vaginal bleeding in the presence of persisting molar tissue, or curative if the recurrent molar tissue is confined to the uterine cavity, particularly in those with hCG levels below 1500 IU/l (Pezeshki et al 2004). Such cases should be discussed first with the local GTD centre. The use of US control during this procedure may help to reduce the risk of uterine perforation.

Twin pregnancies

At Charing Cross Hospital, there have been 77 confirmed cases of CM with a separate normal conceptus; 25% of these resulted in a live birth, while the remainder had non-viable pregnancies which mostly ended in spontaneous abortions or suction D & Cs. Interestingly, in both the viable and non-viable pregnancies, only 20% of women subsequently needed chemotherapy to eliminate persistent GTD and none of these women died of resistant disease. Furthermore, although the incidence of pre-eclampsia was 5–10% in those continuing their pregnancies, there were no maternal deaths. Thus, it appears reasonably safe to allow patients with twin pregnancies in which one of the conceptions is a CM to continue to term provided that there are no other complications. This is in line with observations on singleton CMs which suggest that later gestational age at termination does not increase the risk of subsequently requiring chemotherapy (Seckl et al 2004b).

Registration and follow-up after uterine evacuation

The majority of patients require no further treatment after evacuation, but 16% of patients with a CM and less than 0.5% with a PM develop persistent GTD. It is vital that patients with persistent GTD are identified as virtually all of them can be cured with appropriate therapy.

In 1973, under the auspices of the Royal College of Obstetricians and Gynaecologists, a national follow-up service was instituted in the UK whereby patients with GTD are registered with one of three laboratories located in Dundee, Sheffield and London. Approximately 1400 women are registered per annum and 110–120 require subsequent chemotherapy. After registration, the patient's details and pathology, together with two weekly blood and urine samples, are sent through the post to one of the reference laboratories for confirmation of diagnosis and serial hCG estimations. Following the success of this scheme, other countries have now established or are attempting to establish a similar registration programme to reduce GTT mortality rates.

In the majority of cases, the molar tissue dies out spontaneously, the hCG concentration returns to normal (= 4 IU/l) and the patient can start a new pregnancy after a further 6 months. If the hCG level has fallen to normal within 8 weeks of evacuation, marker follow-up can be safely reduced to 6 months as 98% of patients requiring chemotherapy presented within this timeframe (Sebire et al 2007). Since patients who have had a previous mole or GTT are at greater risk of having another, all patients should have a further estimation of hCG at 6 and 10 weeks following the completion of each subsequent pregnancy.

Indications for chemotherapy

Factors associated with an increased risk of requiring chemotherapy are summarized in Table 43.2. The hormones in the oral contraceptive pill are probably growth factors for trophoblastic tumours; for this reason, patients are advised not to use the pill until hCG levels have returned to normal.

The indications for intervention with chemotherapy in patients who have had a CM or PM are shown in Box 43.1. An hCG value = 20,000 IU/l 4 weeks after evacuation of a mole or rising values in this range at an earlier stage indicate that the patient is at increased risk of severe haemorrhage or uterine perforation with intraperitoneal bleeding. These complications can be life-threatening and their risk can be reduced by starting chemotherapy. Withholding chemotherapy from women with metastases in the lung, vulva and vagina is only safe if the hCG levels are falling. However, chemotherapy is required if the hCG levels are not dropping or if the patient has metastases at another site, which can indicate the development of choriocarcinoma.

Prognostic factors: scoring vs International Federation of Gynaecology and Obstetrics staging

The principal prognostic variables for GTTs, which were originally identified by Bagshawe in 1976 and since modified by WHO and the authors' own experience, are summarized in Table 43.3. Anatomical staging systems, such as that of the International Federation of Gynaecology and Obstetrics (FIGO), have been used by several centres managing GTTs. However, surgery is virtually never indicated in the initial management of this disease, so the FIGO system does not appear to add anything in treatment planning to the existing scoring system. Furthermore, the original FIGO staging system did not always predict prognosis correctly, so some patients were under- or overtreated (Smith et al 1992). This problem was overcome by modifying the FIGO system to include some of the WHO variables (Goldstein et al 1998). An international committee was then established, and recommended a new combined WHO/FIGO scoring system in 2000. This was internationally accepted in 2002, so that all centres managing this rare group of diseases can compare their results more easily (Kohorn 2002).

The authors currently use both the Charing Cross system and the new combined system as outlined in Tables 43.3 and 43.4. In both systems, each variable carries a score which, when added together for an individual patient, correlates with the risk of the tumour becoming resistant to single-agent therapy. It is this score, rather than the stage, that determines treatment; thus far, there appears to be excellent concordance for assigning patients to either low- or high-risk groups (see section on chemotherapy below). The most important prognostic variables carry the highest score and include:

- duration of the disease because drug resistance of GTTs varies inversely with time from the original antecedent pregnancy;
- serum hCG concentration which correlates with the volume of viable tumour in the body; and
- presence of liver or brain metastases.

Liver metastases correlate with a worse prognosis than brain metastases (Bower et al 1997), so patients with liver involvement score six points rather than four. Since the ABO blood groups contribute little to the scoring system and it is difficult to have complete data on both patients and relevant partners, this has been dropped from the system.

Chemotherapy

At Charing Cross Hospital, the prognostic scoring system in Table 43.3 has been used to subdivide the patients into three groups (low, medium and high risk) depending on their overall score. Formerly, each risk group corresponded with a separate treatment regimen and so there were three types of therapy (low, medium and high risk). Ten years ago, the medium-risk treatment was discontinued for three reasons:

Box 43.1 Indications for chemotherapy following the diagnosis of GTD

- Evidence of metastases in brain, liver or gastrointestinal tract, or radiological opacities more than 2 cm on chest X-ray
- Histological evidence of choriocarcinoma
- Heavy vaginal bleeding or evidence of gastrointestinal or intraperitoneal haemorrhage
- Pulmonary, vulval or vaginal metastases unless hCG falling
- Rising hCG after evacuation
- Serum hCG = 20,000 IU/l more than 4 weeks after evacuation, because of the risk of uterine perforation
- Raised hCG 6 months after evacuation, even if still falling

---

Table 43.2 Factors increasing the risk of requiring chemotherapy following evacuation of an hydatidiform mole

Factor
• Uterine size greater than gestational age (Curry et al 1975)
• Pre-evacuation serum hCG above 100,000 IU/l (Berkowitz and Goldstein 1981)
• Oral contraceptives given before hCG falls to normal (Stone et al 1976)
• Bilateral cystic ovarian enlargement (Berkowitz and Goldstein 1981)

Sources: Berkowitz RS, Goldstein DP, Marean AR, Bernstein M 1981 Obstetrics and Gynecology 58: 474–477.
Curry SL, Hammond CB, Tyrey L, Creasman WT, Parker RT 1975 Obstetrics and Gynecology 45: 1–8.
Stone M, Dent J, Kardana A, Bagshawe KD 1976 BJOG: an International Journal of Obstetrics and Gynaecology 86: 913–916.
hCG, human chorionic gonadotrophin.

Table 43.3 Scoring system for gestational trophoblastic tumours (Charing Cross Hospital)

Prognostic factor	Score			
	0	1	2	6
Age (years)	<39	>39	–	–
Antecedent pregnancy	Mole	Abortion or unknown	Term	–
Interval (end of antecedent pregnancy to chemotherapy in months)	<4	4–7	7–12	>12
hCG (IU/l)	$10^3–10^4$	$<10^3$	$10^4–10^5$	$>10^5$
Number of metastases	0	1–3	4–8	>8
Site of metastases	None, lung, vagina	Spleen, kidney	Gastrointestinal tract	Brain, liver
Largest tumour mass	–	3–5 cm	>5 cm	–
Prior chemotherapy	–	–	Single drug	Two drugs or more

hCG, human chorionic gonadotrophin.
The total score for a patient is obtained by adding the individual scores for each prognostic factor. Low risk, 0–8; high risk, ≥9. Patients scoring 0–8 currently receive single-agent therapy with methotrexate and folinic acid, while patients scoring ≥9 receive combination drug therapy with EMA/CO (see Table 43.6).

Table 43.4 Scoring system for gestational trophoblastic tumours (World Health Organization/ International Federation of Gynaecology and Obstetrics)

Prognostic factor	Score			
	0	1	2	4
Age (years)	<40	≥40	–	–
Antecedent pregnancy	Mole	Abortion	Term	–
Interval (end of antecedent pregnancy to chemotherapy in months)	<4	4–6	7–13	>13
hCG (IU/l)	$<10^3$	$10^3–10^4$	$10^4–10^5$	$>10^5$
Number of metastases	0	1–4	5–8	>8
Site of metastases	Lung	Spleen, kidney	Gastrointestinal tract	Brain, liver
Largest tumour mass	–	3–5 cm	>5 cm	
Prior chemotherapy	–	–	Single drug	Two drugs or more

hCG, human chorionic gonadotrophin.
The total score for a patient is obtained by adding the individual scores for each prognostic factor. Low risk, 0–6; high risk, ≥7.

- the short- and long-term toxicity of this treatment is probably not significantly different from that of high-risk therapy;
- some patients that receive medium-risk treatment have developed drug resistance and subsequently require high-risk treatment; and
- approximately 30% of medium-risk patients can be cured on low-risk chemotherapy, which is less toxic than either medium- or high-risk chemotherapy (Rustin et al 1996). Moreover, there is no evidence that prior treatment failure with methotrexate is an adverse prognostic variable (Bower et al 1997, McNeish et al 2002).

Accordingly, patients who score between five and eight now receive low-risk chemotherapy, which was previously only given to those with a score = five. Patients scoring nine are given high-risk treatment. The details of both low- and high-risk treatment are discussed below. Patients are admitted for the first 3 weeks of either therapy, principally because the tumours are often highly vascular and may bleed vigorously in this early period of treatment.

Low-risk patients

Patients with low-risk disease have a 5-year survival rate of nearly 100% (Bower et al 1997). The regimen used since 1964 at Charing Cross Hospital and widely followed in other centres is shown in Table 43.5. This schedule is well tolerated with no alopecia, and since the folinic acid dose has been increased from 7.5 mg to 15 mg, the incidence of mucosal ulceration has reduced from 20% to just 2%. Methotrexate can induce serositis, resulting in pleuritic chest pain or abdominal pain. Myelosuppression is rare, but a full blood count should be obtained before each course of treatment. Liver and renal function should also be monitored regularly. All patients are advised to avoid sun exposure or use complete sun block for 1 year after chemotherapy because the drugs can induce photosensitivity.

Table 43.5 Chemotherapy regimen for low-risk patients

Methotrexate/folinic acid	
Methotrexate	50 mg by intramuscular injection repeated every 48 h for a total of four doses
Calcium folinate	15 mg orally 30 h after each injection of methotrexate (folinic acid)

Courses repeated every 2 weeks, i.e. days 1, 15, 29, etc.

Approximately 33% of low-risk patients will need to change therapy: 31% because of drug resistance and 2% due to treatment toxicity (usually mucositis, occasionally severe pleuritic pain or drug-induced hepatitis) (McNeish et al 2002). However, in the authors' experience, all such patients are cured and the only deaths in this group of patients over the last 30 years were one from concurrent but not therapy-induced non-Hodgkin's lymphoma and one from hepatitis (Bagshawe et al 1989). Moreover, there is no evidence that methotrexate alone increases the risk of developing a second cancer (Rustin et al 1996).

High-risk patients

These patients are at high risk of developing drug resistance, and since 1979 have been treated with an intensive regimen consisting of etoposide, methotrexate and actinomycin D (EMA) alternating weekly with cyclophosphamide and vincristine, otherwise known as 'Oncovin' (CO; see Table 43.6). A recent meta-analysis has failed to demonstrate superiority of any other chemotherapy combination (Xue et al 2006). The EMA/CO regimen requires one overnight stay every 2 weeks and causes reversible alopecia. It is also myelosuppressive, but prolonged gaps in therapy, which may permit tumour regrowth, can usually be avoided by the following measures: continuing to treat unless the white cell count is less than 1.5×10^9/l and/or platelets fall below 60×10^9/l

Table 43.6 Chemotherapy regimen for high-risk patients

EMA		
Day 1	Etoposide	100 mg/m² by IV infusion over 30 min
	Actinomycin D	0.5 mg IV bolus
	Methotrexate	300 mg/m² by IV infusion over 12 h
Day 2	Etoposide	100 mg/m² by IV infusion over 30 min
	Actinomycin D	0.5 mg IV bolus
	Folinic acid rescue (starting 24 h after commencing the methotrexate infusion)	15 mg IM or orally every 12 h for four doses
CO		
Day 8	Vincristine	1 mg/m² IV bolus (max. 2 mg)
	Cyclophosphamide	600 mg/m² IV infusion over 30 min

EMA, etoposide, methotrexate and actinomycin D; CO, cyclophosphamide and vincristine.
EMA alternates with CO every week. To avoid extended intervals between courses caused by myelosuppression, it may occasionally be necessary to reduce the EMA by omitting the day 2 doses of etoposide and actinomycin D.

and/or mucosal ulceration develops. The introduction of granulocyte colony-stimulating factor in patients who have a low neutrophil count also helps to maintain treatment intensity and has reduced the number of neutropenic febrile episodes.

The cumulative 5-year survival of patients treated with this schedule is 86%, with no deaths from GTTs beyond 2 years after the initiation of chemotherapy (Bower et al 1997). While these results were good, the presence of liver or brain metastases correlated with only 30% or 70% long-term survival, respectively. Indeed, long-term survival in patients with both liver and brain metastases is only 10% (Newlands et al 2002). Interestingly, for patients with brain metastasis, if one excludes patients who were too sick to receive chemotherapy and died within a few days of admission, the survival rates appear to be the same as those for patients without brain involvement (Newlands et al 2002). The authors are currently undertaking a new analysis on patients with liver metastasis; of 38 patients treated more recently, the overall survival rate appears to be higher at just under 50% (Seckl et al, unpublished observations). This improvement in outcome may be because of changes in treatment. Other adverse prognostic variables include a longer interval from the antecedent pregnancy, and term delivery in the antecedent pregnancy (Powles et al 2007).

Early deaths accounted for a significant proportion of the overall mortality, with the causes being respiratory failure, cerebral metastases, hepatic failure and pulmonary embolism (Bower et al 1997). Importantly, these women did not have an HM, were not registered for follow-up and consequently presented with extensive disease. Clearly, it will be difficult to improve the survival of this particular subgroup. However, any woman of childbearing age presenting with widespread malignancy should have an hCG measurement as very high levels of this hormone are highly suggestive of choriocarcinoma.

The long-term risk of chemotherapy-induced second tumours in patients treated for GTTs in the authors' centre has been reviewed previously (Rustin et al 1996), and is discussed below in the section on long-term complications of therapy.

Management of drug-resistant disease

GTN is one of a very small minority of malignant conditions where patients who progress on or after primary chemotherapy still have a good chance of cure [>90% overall 5-year survival in a recent case series (Powles et al 2007)].

Low-risk disease

Frequent (twice-weekly) measurement of serum hCG is a simple way to detect drug resistance at an early stage as the hormone levels will stop falling and may start to rise long before there are other clinical changes. Decisions to alter treatment are not made on the basis of a single hCG result but on a progressive trend over two to three values. For patients receiving methotrexate for low-risk disease, if the hCG is below 100 IU/l when drug resistance occurs, the disease can often be cured simply by substituting actinomycin D (0.5 mg IV total dose daily for 5 days every 2 weeks) (McNeish et al 2002). This drug is more toxic than methotrexate, inducing some hair thinning (occasional complete alopecia), myelosuppression and more oral ulceration. However, it is preferable to EMA/CO. Indeed, more recently, in order to reduce the number of patients proceeding directly to this more toxic regimen, the authors have raised the hCG level for switching from methotrexate to actinomycin D therapy to less than 300 IU/l. The cure rate, even in those rare cases that need three or more lines of treatment, remains nearly 100% (Powles et al 2007).

Low-risk patients failing methotrexate whose serum hCG level is above 300 IU/l are treated with EMA/CO.

High-risk disease

Seventy per cent of patients who have failed EMA/CO for high-risk disease can still be salvaged by further chemotherapy and/or surgery (Bower et al 1997). Indeed, the combination of surgical removal of the main site of drug resistance (usually uterus, lung or brain) together with chemotherapy is particularly effective. Preoperative investigations include those outlined above. If all of these investigations are negative, hysterectomy should be considered. Following surgery or when surgery is not appropriate, the authors use the cisplatin-containing regimen, EP (etoposide 150 mg/m² and cisplatin 75 mg/m² with hydration) alternating weekly with EMA (omitting day 2 except the folinic acid). Although this regimen is very toxic, the outcome has been impressive with survival rates in excess of 80% (Newlands et al 2000).

Other options that can be considered include use of some of the newer anticancer agents such as the taxanes, topotecan, gemcitabine and temozolomide. Several cases of drug-resistant GTTs that have responded to paclitaxel-based single-agent or combination therapy have been reported (Jones et al 1996, Termrungruanglert et al 1996, Osborne et al 2004, Shorbagi et al 2005). An alternating doublet of paclitaxel/cisplatin and paclitaxel/etoposide (TP/TE) has been found to be well tolerated and effective in patients with relapsed and/or refractory GTN (Wang et al 2008). Overall survival ranged from 44% for patients who failed previous cisplatin-based chemotherapy to 75% for those receiving TP/TE as a result of discontinuing prior chemotherapies due to toxicities.

Another approach in patients with refractory disease involves high-dose chemotherapy with autologous bone marrow or peripheral stem cell transplantation. Patient selection here is important in determining outcome as it has been shown for refractory germ cell tumours that patients with drug-sensitive disease stay in remission (Beyer et al 1996, Lyttelton et al 1998). In the largest series of high-dose chemotherapy for refractory GTT, five out of 11 patients showed a temporary partial or complete response, although all but one patient progressed eventually (El-Helw et al 2005). Since the time of writing, the authors have treated several more cases and now appear to have two long-term survivors. Therefore, high-dose chemotherapy with autologous stem cell support for GTN remains investigational. Further studies are needed to better define the role of high-dose chemotherapy, in particular in patients with high-risk GTN who fail their first salvage treatment for recurrent disease.

Management of acute disease-induced complications

Haemorrhage

Heavy vaginal or intraperitoneal bleeding is the most frequent immediate threat to life in patients with GTTs. The bleeding mostly settles with bed rest and appropriate chemotherapy. However, occasionally, the bleeding can be torrential, requiring massive transfusion. In this situation, if the bleeding is coming from the uterus, it may be necessary to consider a uterine pack or emergency embolization of the tumour vasculature. Fortunately, hysterectomy is rarely required. If the bleeding is intraperitoneal and does not settle with transfusion and chemotherapy, laparotomy may be required. Indeed, patients occasionally present this way.

Respiratory failure

Occasionally patients present with respiratory failure due to multiple pulmonary metastases or, more rarely, as a result of massive tumour embolism to the pulmonary circulation (Savage et al 1998). However, in the authors' experience, these patients can be cured with appropriate management. Oxygen support may be required, including masked continuous positive airway pressure ventilation, but mechanical ventilation is usually contraindicated as it results in trauma to the tumour vasculature, leading to massive intrapulmonary haemorrhage and death.

Management of cerebral metastases

The presence of neurological symptoms and signs may alert the clinician to the presence of brain metastases. However, some high-risk patients do not have either overt pulmonary or CNS disease at presentation, but subsequently develop cerebral metastases which are then drug resistant. Consequently, careful investigation of patients at risk of developing brain metastases is warranted so that appropriate CNS-penetrating chemotherapy is given rather than the standard low- or high-risk treatments.

Prophylaxis against possible CNS disease, i.e. in the presence of a normal MRI brain, is given to patients from all risk categories with lung metastases and all high-risk patients regardless of the absence or presence of lung deposits. The prophylaxis consists of 12.5 mg methotrexate administered intrathecally, followed 24 h later by 15 mg folinic acid orally. This is given with every course of low-risk therapy, or with each CO in the high-risk therapy for three doses. Since the introduction of this policy, the development of brain metastases without evidence of drug resistance elsewhere has been much less frequent (Athanassiou et al 1983).

Overt CNS disease requires careful management as therapy can induce haemorrhage into the tumour, leading to a rise in intracranial pressure and subsequent loss of life (Athanassiou et al 1983). Early resection of solitary brain deposits in patients with serious neurological signs can sometimes be life-saving (Ishizuka 1983, Song and Wu 1988, Rustin et al 1989). Cerebral oedema can be reduced with high-dose corticosteroids, so patients are given 24 mg dexamethasone in divided doses before starting chemotherapy. The EMA/CO regimen is modified by increasing the dose of methotrexate to 1 g/m^2, given as a 24-h infusion on day 1. The folinic acid rescue is increased to 30 mg given 8-hourly intravenously for 3 days, commencing 32 h after the start of methotrexate infusion. Provided that there is no evidence of raised intracranial pressure, 12.5 mg methotrexate is given intrathecally with each CO until the serum hCG level is normal. Modified EMA/CO is then continued for a further 6–8 weeks. Overall, long-term remission can be achieved in approximately 80% of patients with cerebral metastases (Newlands et al 2002). Patients who survive the first 3 weeks of such treatment have a good prognosis, with an 86–89% chance of cure (Athanassiou et al 1983, Rustin et al 1989, Newlands et al 2002).

Patients who develop cerebral tumours during chemotherapy have a poor prognosis because their disease is almost certainly drug resistant. Nevertheless, a combination of immediate surgery to remove the deposit(s) and modified chemotherapy designed to provide better CNS penetration can be curative in this situation (Athanassiou et al 1983, Rustin et al 1989). Radiotherapy has been advocated as an alternative therapeutic approach. However, it has not been shown to eradicate tumour in its own right, and in combination with chemotherapy has produced less effective results than chemotherapy alone. Nevertheless, stereotactic radiotherapy probably has a role in the treatment of isolated deep lesions that cannot be removed surgically, especially if still present at the end of chemotherapy.

Management of placental-site trophoblastic tumours

PSTTs differ from the other forms of GTD in that they grow slowly, metastasize late and produce little hCG. This is because hCG is produced in high levels by syncytiotrophoblasts, which are not present in PSTTs, and only in low levels by intermediate trophoblasts. However, in the authors' experience of over 60 cases, it is still an accurate biomarker.

PSTTs are relatively resistant to combination chemotherapy regimens, and therefore hysterectomy with pelvic lymph node clearance and ovarian preservation remains the treatment of choice provided that the disease is localized to the uterus (stage I). In these patients, 10-year survival is 90% and there is no clear benefit from pre- and/or postoperative chemotherapy (Schmid et al 2008). However, for patients with disease in the resection margin or lymphovascular invasion, the authors routinely offer adjuvant EP/EMA and, more recently, TE/TP chemotherapy for 8 weeks until more data are available.

When disease has spread beyond the uterus, patients can respond to and be cured by chemotherapy (EP/EMA) either alone or in combination with surgery (Newlands et al 1998b). Ten-year survival rates are 52% for locoregional (stage II) disease and 49% for metastatic (stage III/IV) disease. In the largest series of 62 patients, 9% had refractory disease and died of PSTTs (Schmid et al 2008).

Nineteen per cent of patients treated for PSTTs experience disease recurrence, all within the first 5 years (Schmid et al 2008). In this group, the outlook is poor with a minority achieving long-term survival. Radiotherapy does not appear to add much to the management, and it is unlikely that a high dose will be curative, although the latter should be considered in chemoresponsive patients who have failed first-line therapies. The most important prognostic variable is the interval from the antecedent pregnancy (Newlands et al 2000). A cut-off of 4 years discriminates patients with a positive predictive value of 100% and a negative predictive value of 98% (Schmid et al 2008). PSTTs are so rare that it is unlikely that their treatment will ever be fully optimized.

The major question in the management of PSTTs, which frequently affect women of childbearing age, is whether fertility-sparing surgery is safe in a minority of cases with good prognostic factors and disease localized to a single uterine site. There have been five reported cases of attempted fertility-sparing surgery using a variety of surgical techniques with and without postoperative chemotherapy, with mixed results. One case had a successful pregnancy, two cases achieved long-term remission but no term pregnancy, and two cases went on to need a hysterectomy for relapsed disease (Leiserowitz and Webb 1996, Tsuji et al 2002, Machtinger et al 2005, Pfeffer et al 2007). In one case at relapse, it was found post hysterectomy that disease that appeared localized to a single uterine site on imaging, including [18]FDG-PET, was in fact multifocal throughout the uterus. Any attempts at fertility-sparing surgery should be undertaken cautiously with preoperative counselling of the patient and close postoperative follow-up.

Patient Follow-Up after Chemotherapy

On completion of their chemotherapy, patients are followed-up regularly with hCG estimations (Table 43.7) to confirm that their disease is in remission. The risk of relapse is approximately 3% and is most likely in the first year of follow-up. However, the authors currently continue follow-up for life, until a full set of data are available to more accurately indicate when it may be safe to stop.

Table 43.7 Follow-up of patients with gestational trophoblastic tumours who have been treated with chemotherapy

		Low-/high-risk postchemotherapy patients, hCG concentration sampling	
		Urine	Blood
Year 1	Weeks 1–6 after chemotherapy	Weekly	Weekly
	Months 2–6	2-weekly	2-weekly
	Months 7–12	2-weekly	–
Year 2		4-weekly	–
Year 3		8-weekly	–
Year 4		3-monthly	–
Year 5		4-monthly	–
After Year 5		6-monthly	–

hCG, human chorionic gonadotrophin.

Timing of Pregnancy after Treatment

Patients are advised not to become pregnant until 12 months after completing their chemotherapy. This minimizes the potential teratogenicity of treatment and avoids confusion between a new pregnancy and relapsed disease as the cause of rising hCG. Despite this advice, 230 women on follow-up at the authors' centre between 1973 and 1997 have become pregnant during the first year. Fortunately, this does not appear to be associated with an increased risk of relapse or fetal morbidity, and there were no maternal deaths. Indeed, 72% of women continued their pregnancy to term (Blagden et al 2002). Consequently, although the authors continue to advise women to avoid pregnancy for 1 year after completing chemotherapy, those that become pregnant can be reassured of a likely favourable outcome. When a patient becomes pregnant, it is important to confirm by US and other appropriate means that the pregnancy is normal. Follow-up is then discontinued until 3 weeks after the end of pregnancy, when the hCG due to the pregnancy should have returned to normal.

Patients who do not require chemotherapy following evacuation of their first mole, although not on life-long follow-up, should have their hCG levels measured 6 and 10 weeks after any subsequent pregnancy. This is because they are at increased risk compared with the general population of a further molar pregnancy (Sebire et al 2003). In addition, with a subsequent pregnancy, there is a small risk of reactivation of 'dormant' residual molar tissue, even if the pregnancy itself is normal.

Contraceptive Advice

Patients using oral contraceptives before the hCG level is normal following evacuation of an HM have an increased risk of developing persistent GTD (Stone et al 1976). Other centres have not been able to reproduce this finding, so this area is controversial. Nevertheless, the authors' data set is very large; for this reason, patients in the UK are advised to avoid the oral contraceptive pill until the hCG level has returned to normal after removal of an HM. Patients who have had chemotherapy for their GTT are advised not to use the oral contraceptive pill until their hCG level is normal and chemotherapy is completed.

Long-Term Complications of Therapy

Most patients, including those who have received intensive chemotherapy, return to normal activity within a few months, and the majority of the side-effects are reversible, including alopecia. Late sequelae from chemotherapy have been remarkably rare. In 15,279 patient-years of follow-up, there was no significant increase in the incidence of second tumours (Rustin et al 1996) following methotrexate therapy. In contrast, 26 patients receiving combination chemotherapy for GTTs developed another cancer when the expected rate was only 16.45; a significant difference (Rustin et al 1996).

Fertility is an important issue in the management of patients with GTTs. Although combination chemotherapy induces the menopause 3 years earlier than expected (Bower et al 1998), fertility does not otherwise appear to be affected. In 392 patients receiving single-agent methotrexate, 327 (83.4%) had successful live births, whilst in the 336 patients receiving multi-agent chemotherapy, including EMA/CO, 280 (83.3%) also succeeded in having normal

pregnancies (Woolas et al 1998). There is no increase in the incidence of congenital malformations compared with the general population (Rustin et al 1984, Woolas et al 1998).

Prognosis

All patients in the low-risk groups can be expected to be cured of their GTTs (Bagshawe and Begent 1983, Newlands et al 1986). For high-risk patients, survival has improved progressively and is currently 86% (Bower et al 1997). The diagnosis of choriocarcinoma is often not suspected until the disease is advanced. As a result, some deaths occur before chemotherapy has a chance to be effective. The number of such patients can be diminished by a greater awareness of the possibility that multiple metastases in a woman of child-bearing age may be due to choriocarcinoma. The simple measurement of the hCG level in such individuals is a very strong indicator of choriocarcinoma, and could help to hasten referrals for life-saving chemotherapy.

Conclusion

In the past, many women have died from GTD. However, during the last 50 years, much has been learnt about the biology, pathology and natural history of this group of disorders. Furthermore, accurate diagnostic and monitoring methods have been developed, together with effective treatment regimens. As a result, the management of GTD today represents one of the modern success stories in oncology, with few women dying from trophoblastic tumours.

KEY POINTS

1. CM and PM are the most common forms of GTD.
2. First-trimester bleeding is the most common presentation.
3. Prostanoids are contraindicated prior to evacuation, even in nulliparous women.
4. Second evacuation should be discussed with a GTD centre, and more than two evacuations is contraindicated.
5. All confirmed cases should be registered for hCG follow-up.
6. If in doubt, get histology reviewed by GTD centre.
7. RIA remains the gold standard for hCG testing in GTD.
8. Sixteen per cent of CM and 0.5% of PM will require chemotherapy and all can expect to be cured.
9. Deaths from GTTs are usually due to late recognition of a post-term choriocarcinoma or from metastatic PSTTs which are less chemosensitive.
10. Chemotherapy does not affect fertility significantly, but EMA/CO increases the risk of second tumours.
11. Further information can be found at http://www.hmole-chorio.org.uk

---

References

Agarwal R, Strickland S, McNeish IA et al 2002 Doppler ultrasonography of the uterine artery and the response to chemotherapy in patients with gestational trophoblastic tumors. Clinical Cancer Reseach 8: 1142–1147.

Arima T, Imamura T, Amada S, Tsuneyoshi M, Wake N 1994 Genetic origin of malignant trophoblastic neoplasms. Cancer Genetics and Cytogenetics 73: 95–102.

Athanassiou A, Begent RH, Newlands ES, Parker D, Rustin GJ, Bagshawe KD 1983 Central nervous system metastases of

choriocarcinoma: 23 years' experience at Charing Cross Hospital. Cancer 52: 1728–1735.

Baergen RN, Rutgers JL, Young RH, Osann K, Scully RE 2006 Placental site trophoblastic tumor: a study of 55 cases and review of the literature emphasizing factors of prognostic significance. Gynecologic Oncology 100: 511–520.

Bagshawe KD 1976 Risk and prognostic factors in trophoblastic neoplasia. Cancer 38: 1373–1385.

Bagshawe, KD, Noble MI 1965 Cardiorespiratory effects of trophoblastic tumours. Quarterly Journal of Medicine 137: 39–54.

Bagshawe KD, Begent RH 1983 Staging markers and prognostic factors in germ cell tumours. In: Bagshawe KD, Newlands EH, Begent RH (eds) Clinics in Oncology 2, Germ Cell Tumours. pp 159–181.

Bagshawe KD, Dent J, Newlands ES, Begent RH, Rustin GJ 1989 The role of low dose methotrexate and folinic acid in gestational trophoblastic tumours (GTT). BJOG: an

International Journal of Obstetrics and Gynaecology 96: 795–802.

Bagshawe KD, Lawler SD, Paradinas FJ, Dent J, Brown P, Boxer GM 1990 Gestational trophoblastic tumours following initial diagnosis of partial hydatidiform mole. The Lancet 334: 1074–1076.

Begent RH, Bagshawe KD, Green AJ, Searle F 1987 The clinical value of imaging with antibody to human chorionic gonadotrophin in the detection of residual choriocarcinoma. British Journal of Cancer 55: 657–660.

Berkowitz RS, Goldstein DP 1981 Pathogenesis of gestational trophoblastic neoplasms. Pathology Annual 11: 391.

Berkowitz RS, Goldstein DP, Marean AR, Bernstein M 1981 Oral contraceptives and postmolar trophoblastic disease. Obstetrics and Gynecology 58: 474–477.

Beyer J, Kramar A, Mandanas R et al 1996 High-dose chemotherapy as salvage treatment in germ cell tumors: a multivariate analysis of prognostic variables. Journal of Clinical Oncology 14: 2638–2645.

Blagden SP, Foskett MA, Fisher RA et al 2002 The effect of early pregnancy following chemotherapy on disease relapse and foetal outcome in women treated for gestational trophoblastic tumours. British Journal of Cancer 86: 26–30.

Blohm ME, Gobel U 2004 Unexplained anaemia and failure to thrive as initial symptoms of infantile choriocarcinoma: a review. European Journal of Pediatrics 163: 1–6.

Boultebee JE, Newlands ES 1995 New diagnostic and therapeutic approaches to gestational trophoblastic tumours. In: Bourne TH, Jauniaux E, Jurkovic D (eds) Transvaginal Colour Doppler. The Scientific Basis and Practical Application of Colour Doppler in Gynaecology. Springer, pp 57–65.

Bower M, Newlands ES, Holden L et al 1997 EMA/CO for high-risk gestational trophoblastic tumours: results from a cohort of 272 patients. Journal of Clinical Oncology 15: 2636–2643.

Bower M, Rustin GJ, Newlands ES et al 1998 Chemotherapy for gestational trophoblastic tumours hastens menapause by 3 years. European Journal of Cancer 34: 1204–1207.

Burke B, Sebire NJ, Moss J et al 2006 Evaluation of deletions in 7q11.2 and 8p12-p21 as prognostic indicators of tumour development following molar pregnancy. Gynecologic Oncology 103: 642–648.

Chilosi M, Piazzola E, Lestani M et al 1998 Differential expression of p57kip2, a maternally imprinted cdk inhibitor, in normal human placenta and gestational trophoblastic disease. Laboratory Investigation 78: 269–276.

Cole LA 1998 hCG, its free subunits and its metabolites. Roles in pregnancy and trophoblastic disease. Journal of Reproductive Medicine 43: 3–10.

Cole LA, Shahabi S, Butler SA et al 2001 Utility of commonly used commercial human chorionic gonadotropin immunoassays in the diagnosis and management of trophoblastic diseases. Clinical Chemistry 47: 308–315.

Cole LA, Butler SA, Khanlian SA et al 2006a Gestational trophoblastic diseases: 2. Hyperglycosylated hCG as a reliable marker of active neoplasia. Gynecologic Oncology 102: 151–159.

Cole LA, Khanlian SA, Muller CY, Giddings A, Kohorn E, Berkowitz R 2006b Gestational trophoblastic diseases: 3. Human chorionic gonadotropin-free beta-subunit, a reliable marker of placental site trophoblastic tumors. Gynecologic Oncology 102: 160–164.

Coulson LE, Kong CS, Zaloudek C 2000 Epithelioid trophoblastic tumor of the uterus in a postmenopausal woman: a case report and review of the literature. American Journal of Surgical Pathology 24: 1558–1562.

Curry SL, Hammond CB, Tyrey L, Creasman WT, Parker RT 1975 Hydatidiform moles; diagnosis, management and long term follow-up of 347 patients. Obstetrics and Gynecology 45: 1–8.

Dhillon T, Palmieri C, Sebire NJ et al 2006 Value of whole body 18FDG-PET to identify the active site of gestational trophoblastic neoplasia. Journal of Reproductive Medicine 51: 879–887.

El-Helw LM, Seckl MJ, Haynes R et al 2005 High-dose chemotherapy and peripheral blood stem cell support in refractory gestational trophoblastic neoplasia. British Journal of Cancer 93: 620–621.

Fisher RA, Soteriou BA, Meredith L, Paradinas FJ, Newlands ES 1995 Previous hydatidiform mole identified as the causative pregnancy of choriocarcinoma following birth of normal twins. International Journal of Cancer 5: 64–70.

Fisher RA, Newlands ES 1998 Gestational trophoblastic disease: molecular and genetic studies. Journal of Reproductive Medicine 43: 81–97.

Fisher RA, Hodges MD, Rees HC et al 2002 The maternally transcribed gene p57(KIP2) (CDNK1C) is abnormally expressed in both androgenetic and biparental complete hydatidiform moles. Human Molecular Genetics 11: 3267–3272.

Fisher RA, Savage PM, MacDermott C et al 2007 The impact of molecular genetic diagnosis on the management of women with hCG-producing malignancies. Gynecologic Oncology 107: 413–419.

Fowler DJ, Lindsay I, Seckl MJ, Sebire NJ 2006 Routine pre-evacuation ultrasound diagnosis of hydatidiform mole: experience of more than 1000 cases from a regional referral center. Ultrasound in Obstetrics and Gynecology 27: 56–60.

Genest DR, Ruiz RE, Weremowicz S, Berkowitz RS, Goldstein DP, Dorfman DM 2002 Do nontriploid partial hydatidiform moles exist? A histologic and flow cytometric reevaluation of nontriploid specimens. Journal of Reproductive Medicine 47: 363–368.

Goldstein DP, Berkowitz RS 1994 Current management of complete and partial molar pregnancy. Journal of Reproductive Medicine 39: 139–146.

Goldstein DP, Zanten-Przybysz IV, Bernstein MR, Berkowitz RS 1998 Revised FIGO staging system for gestational trophoblastic tumors. Journal of Reproductive Medicine 43: 37–43.

Hando T, Ohno M, Kurose T 1998 Recent aspects of gestational trophoblastic disease in Japan. International Journal of Gynaecology and Obstetrics 60 (Suppl 1): S71–S76.

Hao Y, Crenshaw T, Moulton T, Newcomb E, Tycko B 1993 Tumor suppressor activity of H19 RNA. Nature 365: 764–767.

Harvey RA, Pursglove HD, Schmid P, Savage PM, Mitchell HD, Seckl MJ 2008 Human chorionic gonadotrophin free beta-subunit measurement as a marker of placental site trophoblastic tumours. Journal of Reproductive Medicine 53: 643–648.

Hashimoto K, Azuma C, Koyama M et al 1995 Loss of imprinting in choriocarcinoma. Nature Genetics 9: 109–110.

Hassadia A, Gillespie A, Tidy J et al 2005 Placental site trophoblastic tumour: clinical features and management. Gynecologic Oncology 99: 603–607.

Hebart H, Erley C, Kaskas B et al 1996 Positron emission tomography helps to diagnose tumor emboli and residual disease in choriocarcinoma. Annals of Oncology 7: 416–418.

Hui P, Martel M, Parkash V 2005 Gestational trophoblastic diseases: recent advances in histopathologic diagnosis and related genetic aspects. Advances in Anatomic Pathology 12: 116–125.

Ishizuka T 1983 Intracranial metastases of choriocarcinoma: a clinicopathologic study. Cancer 52: 1896–1903.

Johnson EJ, Crofton PM, O'Neill JM et al 2003 Infantile choriocarcinoma treated with chemotherapy alone. Medical and Pediatric Oncology 41: 550–557.

Jones WB, Schneider J, Shapiro F, Lewis JL Jr 1996 Treatment of resistant gestational choriocarcinoma with taxol: a report of two cases. Gynecologic Oncology 61: 126–130.

Judson H, Hayward BE, Sheridan E, Bonthron DT 2002 A global disorder of imprinting in the human female germ line. Nature 416: 539–542.

Kohorn EI 2002 Negotiating a staging and risk factor scoring system for gestational trophoblastic neoplasia. A progress report. Journal of Reproductive Medicine 47: 445–450.

Kuo KT, Chen MJ, Lin MC 2004 Epithelioid trophoblastic tumor of the broad ligament: a case report and review of the literature. American Journal of Surgical Pathology 28: 405–409.

Kurman RJ, Scully RE, Norris HJ 1976 Trophoblastic pseudotumor of the uterus: an exaggerated form of syncytial endometritis simulating a malignant tumor. Cancer 38: 1214–1226.

Lawler SD, Fisher RA, Pickthall VJ, Povey S, Evans MW 1982 Genetic studies on hydatidiform moles I: the origin of partial moles. Cancer Genetics and Cytogenetics 4: 309–320.

Leiserowitz GS, Webb MJ 1996 Treatment of placental site trophoblastic tumor with hysterotomy and uterine reconstruction. Obstetrics and Gynecology 88: 696–699.

Long MG, Boultbee JE, Langley R, Newlands ES, Begent RH, Bagshawe KD 1992 Doppler assessment of the uterine circulation and the clinical behaviour of gestational trophoblastic tumours requiring chemotherapy. British Journal of Cancer 66: 883–887.

Lyttelton MP, Newlands ES, Giles C et al 1998 High-dose therapy including carboplatin adjusted for renal function in patients with relapsed germ cell tumor: outcome and prognostic factors. British Journal of Cancer 77: 1672–1676.

Machtinger R, Gotlieb WH, Korach J et al 2005 Placental site trophoblastic tumor: outcome of five cases including fertility preserving management. Gynecologic Oncology 96: 56–61.

Matsuda T, Sasaki M, Kato H et al 1997 Human chromosome 7 carries a putative tumor suppressor gene(s) involved in choriocarcinoma. Oncogene 15: 2773–2781.

Matsuoka S, Thompson JS, Edwards MC et al 1996 Imprinting of the gene encoding a human cyclin-dependent kinase inhibitor, p57kip2, on chromosome 11p15. Proceedings of the National Academy of Sciences USA 93: 3026–3030.

McNeish IA, Strickland S, Holden L et al 2002 Low risk persistent gestational trophoblastic disease: outcome following initial treatment with low-dose methotrexate and folinic acid, 1992–2000. Journal of Clinical Oncology 20: 1838–1844.

Mitchell H, Seckl MJ 2007 Discrepancies between commercially available immunoassays in the detection of tumour-derived hCG. Molecular and Cellular Endocrinology 260–262: 310–313.

Murdoch S, Djuric U, Mazhar B et al 2006 Mutations in NALP7 cause recurrent hydatidiform moles and reproductive wastage in humans. Nature Genetics 38: 300–302.

Newlands ES, Bagshawe KD, Begent RH, Rustin GJ, Holden L, Dent J 1986 Development of chemotherapy for medium- and high-risk patients with gestational trophoblastic tumours 1979–1984. BJOG: an International Journal of Obstetrics and Gynaecology 93: 63–69.

Newlands ES, Bower M, Fisher RA, Paradinas FJ 1998a Management of placental site trophoblastic tumours. Journal of Reproductive Medicine 43: 53–59.

Newlands ES, Paradinas FJ, Fisher RA 1998b Recent advances in gestational trophoblastic disease. Hematology/ Oncology Clinics of North America 13: 225–244.

Newlands ES, Mulholland PJ, Holden L, Seckl MJ, Rustin GJ 2000 Etoposide and cisplatin/etoposide, methotrexate, and actinomycin D (EMA) chemotherapy for patients with high-risk gestational trophoblastic tumors refractory to EMA/ cyclophosphamide and vincristine chemotherapy and patients presenting with metastatic placental site trophoblastic tumors. Journal of Clinical Oncology 18: 854–859.

Newlands ES, Holden L, Seckl MJ, McNeish I, Strickland S, Rustin GJ 2002 Management of brain metastases in patients with high-risk gestational trophoblastic tumors. Journal of Reproductive Medicine 47: 465–471.

Numnum TM, Leath CA 3rd, Straughn JM Jr, Conner MG, Barnes MN 3rd 2005 Occult choriocarcinoma discovered by positron emission tomography/computed tomography imaging following a successful pregnancy. Gynecologic Oncology 97: 713–715.

Ogawa O, Eccles MR, Szeto J et al 1993 Relaxation in insulin-like growth factor II gene imprinting implicated in Wilm's tumour. Nature 362: 749–751.

Osborne R, Covens A, Mirchandani D, Gerulath A 2004 Successful salvage of relapsed high-risk gestational trophoblastic neoplasia patients using a novel paclitaxel-containing doublet. Journal of Reproductive Medicine 49: 655–661.

Palmieri C, Fisher RA, Sebire NJ et al 2005 Placental site trophoblastic tumour arising from a partial hydatidiform mole. The Lancet 366: 688.

Papadopoulos AJ, Foskett M, Seckl MJ et al 2002 Twenty-five years' clinical experience of placental site trophoblastic tumors. Journal of Reproductive Medicine 47: 460–464.

Paradinas FJ 1998 The diagnosis and prognosis of molar pregnancy. The experience of the National Referral Centre in London. International Journal of Gynaecology and Obstetrics 60 (Suppl 1): S57–S64.

Pezeshki M, Hancock BW, Silcocks P et al 2004 The role of repeat uterine evacuation in the management of persistent gestational trophoblastic disease. Gynecologic Oncology 95: 423–429.

Pfeffer PE, Sebire N, Lindsay I, McIndoe A, Lim A, Seckl MJ 2007 Fertility-sparing partial hysterectomy for placental-site trophoblastic tumour. Lancet Oncology 8: 744–746.

Popiolek DA, Yee H, Mittal K et al 2006 Multiplex short tandem repeat DNA analysis confirms the accuracy of p57(KIP2) immunostaining in the diagnosis of complete hydatidiform mole. Human Pathology 37: 1426–1434.

Powles T, Savage PM, Stebbing J et al 2007 A comparison of patients with relapsed and chemo-refractory gestational trophoblastic neoplasia. British Journal of Cancer 96: 732–737.

Royal College of Obstetricians and Gynaecologists 2004 The Management of Gestational Trophoblastic Neoplasia. Guideline No. 38. RCOG, London.

Rustin GJ, Booth M, Dent J, Salt S, Rustin F, Bagshawe KD 1984 Pregnancy after cytotoxic chemotherapy for gestational trophoblastic tumours. BMJ (Clinical Research Ed.) 288: 103–106.

Rustin GJ, Newlands ES, Begent RH, Dent J, Bagshawe KD 1989 Weekly alternating chemotherapy (EMA/CO) for treatment of central nervous systems of choriocarcinoma. Journal of Clinical Oncology 7: 900–903.

Rustin GJ, Newlands ES, Lutz JM et al 1996 Combination but not single agent methotrexate chemotherapy for gestational trophoblastic tumours (GTT) increases the incidence of second tumours. Journal of Clinical Oncology 14: 2769–2773.

Savage P, Roddie M, Seckl MJ 1998 A 28-year-old woman with a pulmonary embolus. The Lancet 352: 30.

Savage P, Seckl MJ 2005 The role of repeat uterine evacuation in trophoblast disease. Gynecologic Oncology 99: 251–252; author reply 252–253.

Schmid P, Nagai Y et al 2008 Prognostic markers and long-term outcome of placental-site trophoblastic tumours: 30 years of UK experience. Submitted to The Lancet.

Sebire NJ, Foskett M, Fisher RA, Rees H, Seckl M, Newlands ES 2002a Risk of partial and complete hydatidiform molar pregnancy in relation to maternal age. BJOG: an International Journal of Obstetrics and Gynaecology 109: 99–102.

Sebire NJ, Foskett M, Paradinas FJ et al 2002b Outcome of twin pregnancies with complete hydatidiform mpole and healthy co-twin. The Lancet 359: 2165–2166.

Sebire NJ, Fisher RA, Foskett M, Rees H, Seckl MJ, Newlands ES 2003 Risk of recurrent hydatidiform mole and subsequent pregnancy outcome following complete or partial hydatidiform molar pregnancy. BJOG: an International Journal of Obstetrics and Gynaecology 110: 22–26.

Sebire NJ, Rees HC, Peston D, Seckl MJ, Newlands ES, Fisher RA 2004 p57(KIP2) immunohistochemical staining of gestational trophoblastic tumours does not identify the type of the causative pregnancy. Histopathology 45: 135–141.

Sebire NJ, Lindsay I, Fisher RA, Seckl MJ 2005 Intraplacental choriocarcinoma: experience from a tertiary referral center and relationship with infantile choriocarcinoma. Fetal and Pediatric Pathology 24: 21–29.

Sebire NJ, Foskett M, Short D et al 2007 Shortened duration of human chorionic gonadotrophin surveillance following complete or partial hydatidiform mole: evidence for revised protocol of a UK regional trophoblastic disease unit. BJOG: an International Journal of Obstetrics and Gynaecology 114: 760–762.

Seckl MJ, Rustin GJ, Newlands ES, Gwyther SJ, Bomanji J 1991 Pulmonary embolism, pulmonary hypertension, and choriocarcinoma. The Lancet 338: 1313–1315.

Seckl MJ, Fisher RA, Salerno G et al 2000 Choriocarcinoma and partial hydatidiform moles. The Lancet 356: 36–39.

Seckl MJ, Gillmore R, Foskett M, Sebire NJ, Rees H, Newlands ES 2004a Routine terminations of pregnancy — should we screen for gestational trophoblastic neoplasia. The Lancet 364: 705–707.

Seckl MJ, Dhillon T, Dancey G et al: 2004b Increased gestational age at evacuation of a complete hydatidiform mole: does it correlate with increased risk of requiring chemotherapy? Journal of Reproductive Medicine 49: 527–530.

Shaw SW, Wang CW, Ma SY, Ng KK, Chang TC 2005 Exclusion of lung metastases in placental site trophoblastic tumor using [18F]fluorodeoxyglucose positron emission tomography: a case report. Gynecologic Oncology 99: 239–242.

Shih IM, Kurman RJ 1998 Ki-67 labeling index in the differential diagnosis of exaggerated placental site, placental site trophoblastic tumour, and choriocarcinoma: a double staining technique using Ki-67 and Mel-CAM antibodies. Human Pathology 29: 27–33.

Shih IM, Kurman RJ 2001 The pathology of intermediate trophoblastic tumors and tumor-like lesions. International Journal of Gynecological Pathology 20: 31–47.

Shorbagi A, Aksoy S, Kilickap S, Güler N 2005 Successful salvage therapy of resistant gestational trophoblastic disease with ifosfamide and paclitaxel. Gynecologic Oncology 97: 722–723.

Smith DB, Holden L, Newlands ES, Bagshawe KD 1992 Correlation between clinical staging (FIGO) and prognostic groups in gestational trophoblastic disease. BJOG: an International Journal of Obstetrics and Gynaecology 100: 157–160.

Song HZ, Wu PC 1988 Treatment of brain metastases in choriocarcinoma and invasive mole. In: Song HZ, Wu PC (eds) Studies in Trophoblastic Disease in China. Pergamon, Oxford, pp 231–237.

Stone M, Dent J, Kardana A, Bagshawe KD 1976 Relationship of oral contraceptive to development of trophoblastic tumour after evacuation of hydatidiform mole. BJOG: an International Journal of Obstetrics and Gynaecology 86: 913–916.

Termrungruanglert W, Kudelka AP, Piamsomboon S et al 1996 Remission of refractory gestational trophoblastic disease with high-dose paclitaxel. Anti-Cancer Drugs 7: 503–506.

Tham BW, Everard JE, Tidy JA, Drew D, Hancock BW 2003 Gestational trophoblastic disease in the Asian population of Northern England and North Wales. BJOG: an International Journal of Obstetrics and Gynaecology 110: 555–559.

Tidy JA, Rustin GJ, Newlands ES et al 1995 Presentation and management of choriocarcinoma after nonmolar pregnancy. BJOG: an International Journal of Obstetrics and Gynaecology 102: 715–719.

Tsuji Y, Tsubamoto H, Hori M, Ogasawara T, Koyama K 2002 Case of PSTT treated with chemotherapy followed by open uterine tumor resection to preserve fertility. Gynecologic Oncology 87: 303–307.

Vaitukaitis JL 1979 Human chorionic gonadotrophin — a hormone secreted for many reasons. New England Journal of Medicine 301: 324–326.

Walsh C, Miller SJ, Flam F, Fisher RA, Ohlsson R 1995 Paternally derived H19 is differentially expressed in malignant and non-malignant trophoblast. Cancer Research 55: 1111–1116.

Wang J, Short D, Sebire NJ et al 2008 Salvage chemotherapy of relapsed or high-risk gestational trophoblastic neoplasia (GTN) with paclitaxel/cisplatin alternating with paclitaxel/etoposide (TP/TE). Annals of Oncology 19: 1578–1583.

Wells M 2007 The pathology of gestational trophoblastic disease: recent advances. Pathology 39: 88–96.

World Health Organization 1983 Gestational Trophoblastic Diseases. Technical Report Series 692. WHO, Geneva, pp 7–81.

Woolas RP, Bower M, Newlands ES, Seckl M, Short D, Holden L 1998 Influence of chemotherapy for gestational trophoblastic disease on subsequent pregnancy outcome. BJOG: an International Journal of Obstetrics and Gynaecology 105: 1032–1035.

Xue Y, Zhang J, Wu TX, An RF 2006 Combination chemotherapy for high-risk gestational trophoblastic tumour. Cochrane Database Systematic Reviews 3: CD005196.

Zhao J, Moss J, Sebire NJ et al 2006 Analysis of the chromosomal region 19q13.4 in two Chinese families with recurrent hydatidiform mole. Human Reproduction 21: 536–541.

CHAPTER **44**

Benign tumours of the ovary

Ulises Zanetto and Gabrielle Downey

Chapter Contents

INTRODUCTION	668		INVESTIGATION	669
PHYSIOLOGICAL OVARIAN CYSTS	668		MANAGEMENT	671
CLINICAL PRESENTATION OF SYMPTOMATIC OVARIAN CYSTS	668		PATHOLOGY	672
			KEY POINTS	677
DIFFERENTIAL DIAGNOSIS	669			

Introduction

Ovarian cysts are common, frequently asymptomatic and often resolve spontaneously. They are the fourth most prevalent gynaecological cause of hospital admission. By 65 years of age, 4% of all women in England and Wales will have been admitted to hospital for this reason. Ovarian cysts are found either during the course of investigation of abdominal pain or as a result of imaging for other reasons. It is important to distinguish between ovarian cysts that will require assessment and management and those that will resolve spontaneously. In addition, reliable prediction of their benign or malignant nature would be beneficial in order to arrange appropriate referral and management, as per Improving Outcome Guidance (NHS Executive 1999).

In order to fully understand the nature of an ovarian cyst, one must understand the natural changes that occur in the ovary during the normal menstrual cycle. In the normal menstrual cycle, the ovary responds to an increased level of follicle-stimulating hormone by recruitment of eight to 10 follicles. By day 8, under the influence of an increased level of luteinizing hormone (LH), one follicle becomes the lead follicle and the rest regress. This lead follicle grows to approximately 16–20 mm and ovulation occurs 36 h after the LH surge. Thereafter, the cyst persists as a lipid-filled corpus luteum, producing the progesterone required to mature and maintain the endometrium for possible implantation of a fertilized ovum.

Physiological Ovarian Cysts

As pelvic ultrasound, particularly transvaginal scanning, is now used more frequently, physiological cysts are detected more often. The corpus luteum may persist and continue to secrete progesterone beyond its natural lifespan, and thus cause some menstrual irregularity, or haemorrhage may occur into the cyst at or just after ovulation. Most good radiologists will recognize the features of a follicle, corpus luteum or haemorrhagic cyst and will report these as such. Most simple cysts will resolve spontaneously over a period of 6 months (Zanetta et al 1996, Saasaki et al 1999). Occasionally, they can persist for longer or grow in size to become a clinical problem. Physiological cysts should simply be regarded as large versions of the cysts which form in the ovary during the normal cycle.

Failure of development of the lead follicle results in anovulation and is a classical finding in polycystic ovary syndrome (PCOS). PCOS is predominantly an endocrine abnormality, and polycystic ovaries do not cause abdominal pain (see Chapter 18, Polycystic ovary syndrome, for more information).

Clinical Presentation of Symptomatic Ovarian Cysts

Benign ovarian cysts present as follows:

- acute and chronic pain;
- abdominal swelling, bloating and pressure effects; and
- menstrual disturbances and hormonal effects.

Pain

Acute-onset pain

For a woman to present with acute-onset abdominal pain in the presence of an ovarian cyst suggests a cyst accident such as torsion, rupture or haemorrhage. Torsion usually gives rise to an acute-onset sharp, constant pain caused by ischaemia of the cyst. Areas may subsequently become infarcted if there is delay in treatment, and pyrexia may develop. Haemorrhage may occur into the cyst and cause pain as the capsule is stretched. Intraperitoneal bleeding mimicking ectopic pregnancy may result from rupture of the cyst, which is most often a ruptured, bleeding corpus luteum.

If the patient is haemodynamically unstable at the time of presentation, resuscitation and stabilization are priorities. At a minimum, a full blood count, cross-match and urinary human chorionic gonadotrophin (hCG) should be performed. If the urinary hCG is positive, a serum quantitative hCG would help in the diagnostic process. If it is possible to obtain emergency ultrasound imaging, this may be beneficial but surgery should not be delayed whilst waiting for investigations which would not necessarily affect the management.

Chronic pain

Pelvic inflammatory disease may give rise to a mass of adherent bowel, hydrosalpinx or pyosalpinx. In such circumstances, the pain will be gradual in onset rather than acute. It is often difficult to distinguish between a hydrosalpinx and an ovarian mass on ultrasound; if there is a diagnostic dilemma, laparoscopy should be considered.

Abdominal swelling, bloating and pressure effects

Patients seldom note abdominal swelling until the tumour is very large. A benign mucinous cyst may occasionally fill the entire abdominal cavity. Bloating is a common symptom which can be associated with ovarian tumours but most often is not. Gastrointestinal or urinary symptoms may result from pressure effects. In extreme cases, oedema of the legs, varicose veins and haemorrhoids may result. Sometimes, uterine prolapse is the presenting complaint in a woman with an ovarian cyst.

An attempt to assess symptoms qualitatively and quantitatively in order to distinguish women who may have an ovarian cyst from those unlikely to have a cyst suggests that recent-onset, severe and persistent symptoms should warrant further investigation (Bankhead et al 2008).

Hormonal effects

Occasionally, the patient will complain of menstrual disturbances but this may be coincidence rather than due to the tumour. Rarely, ovarian tumours present with oestrogen effects such as precocious puberty, menorrhagia, glandular hyperplasia, breast enlargement and postmenopausal bleeding. Secretion of androgens may cause hirsutism and acne initially, progressing to frank virilism with deepening of the voice and clitoral hypertrophy. Very rarely indeed, thyrotoxicosis may occur. Some of these tumours are malignant, but are mentioned here because of their ability to produce hormones in some cases. The hormonal effects and histology are discussed later.

Predominantly oestrogen-secreting tumours

- Granulosa cell tumours
- Thecoma
- Sertoli cell tumours (sex cord tumour with annular tubules)

Predominantly androgen-secreting tumours

- Sertoli-Leydig tumours (androblastomas)
- Adrenal-like tumours
- Gonadoblastoma

Differential Diagnosis

The differential diagnosis of benign ovarian tumours is broad, reflecting the wide range of presenting symptoms.

Pain

- Ectopic pregnancy
- Spontaneous abortion
- Pelvic inflammatory disease
- Appendicitis
- Meckel's diverticulum
- Diverticulitis

Abdominal swelling

- Pregnant uterus
- Fibroid uterus
- Full bladder
- Distended bowel
- Ovarian malignancy
- Colorectal carcinoma

Pressure effects

- Urinary tract infection
- Constipation

Hormonal effects

- All other causes of menstrual irregularities, precocious puberty and postmenopausal bleeding

A full bladder should be considered in the differential diagnosis of any pelvic mass. In premenopausal women, a gravid uterus must always be considered. Fibroids can be impossible to distinguish from ovarian tumours. Rarely, a fimbrial cyst may grow sufficiently to cause anxiety.

Investigation

The investigations required will depend upon the circumstances of the presentation. The patient presenting with acute symptoms will usually require emergency surgery, whereas the asymptomatic patient or the woman with chronic problems may benefit from more detailed preliminary assessment.

Gynaecological history

Details of the presenting symptoms and a full gynaecological history should be obtained, with particular reference to the date of the last menstrual period, the regularity of the menstrual cycle, any previous pregnancies, contraception, medication and family history (particularly of ovarian or breast cancer).

General history and examination

Indigestion or dysphagia combined with profound weight loss might indicate a primary gastric cancer metastasizing to the pelvis. Similarly, a history of altered bowel habit or rectal bleeding should be sought as evidence of diverticulitis or large bowel carcinoma. Ovarian carcinoma may also present with these features.

If the patient has presented as an emergency, evidence of hypovolaemia should be sought. Hypotension is a relatively late sign of blood loss, as the blood pressure will be maintained for some time by peripheral and central venous vasoconstriction. When decompensation of this mechanism occurs, it often does so very rapidly. It is vital to recognize the early signs (i.e. tachycardia and cold peripheries). In these circumstances, it is not appropriate to delay surgery pending further investigations, and laparotomy is the correct course of action.

If a cyst is found, the chest should be examined for signs of a pleural effusion. Peripheral oedema can indicate both pressure symptoms and hypoproteinaemia. It is also important to rule out other sites of tumours that are known to metastasize to the ovary, such as the breasts; thus, a full clinical examination is indicated.

Abdominal examination

The abdomen should be inspected for signs of distension by fluid or by the tumour itself. Dilated veins may be seen on the lower abdomen. Gentle palpation will reveal areas of tenderness and peritonism. The best way of detecting a mass that arises from the pelvis is to palpate gently with the left hand, starting in the upper abdomen and working caudally. This is the reverse of the process taught to every medical student for feeling the liver edge. Use of the right hand alone is the most common reason for failing to detect pelvic–abdominal masses.

Shifting dullness is probably the easiest way of demonstrating ascites, but it remains a very insensitive technique. If present, examination of the chest is required to determine if a pleural effusion is also present. It is always worth listening for bowel sounds in any patient with an acute abdomen. Their complete absence in the presence of peritonism is an ominous sign.

Bimanual examination

This is an essential component of the assessment because, even in expert hands, ultrasound examination is not infallible. By palpating the mass between both the vaginal and abdominal hands, its mobility, texture and consistency, the presence of nodules in the pouch of Douglas and the degree of tenderness can be determined. While it is impossible to make a firm diagnosis with bimanual examination, a hard, irregular, fixed mass is likely to be invasive.

Investigations

As a minimum, urine should be tested for the presence of infection and pregnancy. Blood should be obtained for a full blood count, blood grouping and cross-match if the patient is haemodynamically unstable. If the clinical signs suggest the possibility of upper gastrointestinal pathology, liver function tests and serum amylase should be performed.

Serum tumour markers

CA125 is well established in the investigation of ovarian cysts. It is a tumour marker for peritoneal disease/irritation, and whilst not specific for ovarian cancer, a level above 30 u/ml is abnormal. Benign conditions that increase the level of CA125 are endometriosis and pelvic inflammatory disease. In an acute cyst accident, it may also be raised, however, levels above 250 u/ml are almost always associated with malignant disease. The level of CA125 is increased in 80% of ovarian cancers. Other tumour markers may be useful in certain circumstances. If the tumour has features suggestive of a teratoma (dermoid), alpha-fetoprotein and hCG help to determine its malignant potential. Carcinoembryonic antigen, C15.3 and C19.9 are indicated when there is a possibility of pathology other than primary ovarian. Occasionally, the ovary may contain a rare tumour called a 'granulosa cell tumour'; in this case, serum inhibin levels are useful in tracking the course of disease.

Ultrasound

The techniques of transabdominal and transvaginal ultrasound are discussed in detail in Chapter 6. Ultrasound is the single most important investigation and can demonstrate the presence of an ovarian mass with 81% sensitivity and 75% specificity. Most ovarian masses are cystic, whilst the presence of solid areas makes a malignancy more likely. Reporting of an ultrasound finding of an ovarian cyst has been standardized in order to allow for the allocation of a scoring system to assist in the preoperative assessment of the risk of any ovarian cyst being malignant. The ultrasound is awarded a U score of 0 if no cyst is present, 1 if only one characteristic is found, and 3 if two or more characteristics are found:

- Multilocular
- Evidence of solid areas
- Evidence of metastases
- Presence of ascites
- Bilateral lesions

Computed tomography (CT) scanning has no significant advantages over ultrasound in cyst assessment, but can be useful in the presence of obvious extrapelvic disease to assess tumour bulk prior to chemotherapy. Magnetic resonance imaging (MRI) has a marginal advantage over CT in determining if a cyst is more likely to be benign or malignant, but both have no benefit over good transvaginal ultrasound and should not be used routinely. Initial studies using colour flow Doppler were promising but, once again, its use has not been proven to improve cyst assessment.

Risk of malignancy index

There is good evidence that primary surgery undertaken by a gynaecological oncologist improves survival in ovarian cancer by allowing for adequate staging and optimal debulking. It is not practical for all cysts to be managed by gynaeological oncologists; thus, in order to triage cysts for the appropriate surgeon, the Royal College of Obstetricians and Gynaecologists (RCOG) recommend use of the risk of malignancy index (RMI). In order to calculate the RMI, the menopausal status is also taken into account, with premenopausal being awarded a score of 1 and postmenopausal being awarded a score of 3. This simple formula is used:

$$RMI = CA125 \times U \text{ score} \times \text{Menopausal status}$$

A score below 25 can be managed by any gynaecologist, a score of 25–250 should be managed by a cancer unit lead, and a score above 250 should be referred to a cancer centre. This assessment allows for 70% of ovarian cancers to be managed in a cancer centre. The specificity is 90%. The cysts most likely to result in confusion regarding their benign or malignant nature are endometriomas. The clinical history and examination may better inform the clinician but, as a general principle, a significantly raised CA125 (>300 u/ml) is almost always associated with malignant disease.

The Scottish Collegiate also uses an RMI scoring system but gives different weightings to the ultrasound findings and menopausal status. If there are two or more abnormal ultrasound features, they award a U score of 4, whilst a postmenopausal status also has a score of 4. In addition, referral to a cancer centre is recommended when the RMI score is above 200. These adaptations increase the sensitivity of the RMI for prediction of malignant disease from 70% to 80%, and increase the specificity from 89% to 92%. Many centres in the UK also apply this RMI.

Ultrasound-guided diagnostic ovarian cyst aspiration

This investigation has been introduced gradually into gynaecological practice without the benefit of appropriate trials to indicate its potential efficacy. Unfortunately, this technique has a false-negative rate of up to 71% and a false-positive rate of 2% for the cytological diagnosis of malignancy (Diernaes et al 1987). The degree of risk of dissemination of malignant cells along the needle track or into the peritoneal cavity is not established. Most simple cysts will resolve, and most complex cysts require definitive management. Thus, due to its poor prognostic value and the potential for upstaging an early malignancy, cyst aspiration is not recommended for the assessment or management of ovarian cysts.

Management

The management will depend upon the severity of the symptoms, the size and ultrasound characteristics of the cyst, the CA125 results and the age of the patient, and therefore the risk of malignancy and her desire for further children.

The asymptomatic patient

This includes women whose cysts were diagnosed incidentally during investigation of another problem or during investigation of lower abdominal symptoms that may or may not be related to the cyst.

Simple cysts less than 8 cm in diameter with normal CA125 levels

A normal follicular cyst up to 3 cm in diameter requires no further investigation. A simple cyst which is unilocular, echo-free without solid parts or papillary formations less than 8 cm in diamater with a normal CA125 level should have a repeat ultrasound in 3–6 months. If the cyst persists or grows, laparoscopic removal is advised. Premenopausal women under 40 years of age are more likely to want the option of further children and less likely to have a malignant epithelial tumour. In a study by Ekerhovd et al (2001), only three (0.73%) of 413 premenopausal women who underwent surgery for simple echo-free cysts without solid parts or papillary formations had borderline ($n = 2$) or malignant ($n = 1$) tumours.

The use of a combined oral contraceptive is unlikely to accelerate the resolution of a functional cyst (Steinkampf and Hammond 1990). Hormonal treatment of endometriosis does not usually benefit an endometrioma, the mainstay management of which is surgical.

The older woman

Women over 50 years of age are far more likely to have a malignancy and have less to gain from the conservative management of a pelvic mass. However, the capacity of the postmenopausal ovary to generate benign cysts is greater than previously thought, occurring in up to 17% of asymptomatic women (Levine et al 1992). Over 50% of simple cysts will resolve spontaneously and almost 30% will remain static (Levine et al 1992, Bailey et al 1998, Saasaki et al 1999).

Considerable efforts have been made to safely avoid unnecessary surgery in this older age group. However, one group found malignant tumours in 8.9% of 112 postmenopausal women with monolocular simple cysts studied between 1987 and 1993 with transvaginal ultrasound (Osmers et al 1998). They did not find internal echoes helpful in identifying malignancies. They found malignancies in 4.6% of cysts less than 40 mm in diameter, 10.8% of cysts 40–69 mm in diameter, and 18.2% of cysts more than 69 mm in diameter. Their view was that only cysts less than 3 cm in diameter could be managed conservatively. The results of other studies are more reassuring. In particular, a more recent study running from 1992 to 1997 found that only 1.6% of 247 echo-free cysts in postmenopausal women were malignant and that all of these were more than 7.9 cm in diameter (Ekerhovd et al 2001). It was only cysts with small solid areas or papillary formations on the internal side of the cyst wall or echogenic cyst content that carried a 10% risk of malignancy in the 130 cysts studied. Of the nine invasive cancers detected in this group, five were in cysts less than 8 cm in diameter.

This suggests that simple, echo-free, unilateral cysts without solid parts or papillary formations and less than 8 cm in diameter are very likely to be benign, and may safely be managed conservatively with 3–6-monthly ultrasound and CA125 estimation (Goldstein 1993, Ekerhovd et al 2001).

All other cysts

Echo-free ovarian cysts more than 7.9 cm in diameter are unlikely to be physiological or to resolve spontaneously, and will be malignant in approximately 5% of premenopausal women and approximately 15% of postmenopausal women (Ekerhovd et al 2001). These are probably better removed or, at the very least, rescanned 3 months later if the woman is unwilling to undergo surgery.

If the cyst is not echo-free, unilocular or unilateral, or if the CA125 level is raised, surgical removal must be advised to all postmenopausal women regardless of the size of the lesion. In premenopausal women, a corpus luteum or an endometrioma will have a complex appearance on ultrasound and the CA125 level is often slightly raised. When these are suspected, a repeat scan in 3 months is reasonable, with surgery advised if the tumour persists. Otherwise, surgical removal should be advised.

The patient with symptoms

If the patient presents with severe, acute pain or signs of intraperitoneal bleeding, an emergency laparoscopy or laparotomy will be required. More chronic symptoms of pain or pressure may justify pelvic ultrasound if no mass can be felt.

The pregnant patient

An ovarian cyst in a pregnant woman may undergo torsion or may bleed. There is said to be increased incidence of these complications in pregnancy, although the evidence for this is poor. Very occasionally, it can prevent the presenting fetal part from engaging. An ovarian cyst is usually discovered incidentally at the antenatal clinic or on ultrasound. These are usually physiological and resolve by the time of the midtrimester scan.

A recent RCOG publication in The Obstetrician and Gynaecologist (2006) has clarified the position somewhat:

- If the cyst is symptomatic, remove it.
- If the cyst is less than 5 cm in diameter and simple, leave it alone.
- If the cyst is simple and more than 5 cm in diameter, or complex of any size, repeat scan in 4 weeks.
- If the cyst is more than 5 cm in diameter and complex in nature, arrange an MRI and MDT discussion:
  - If thought to be benign, remove post natally.
  - If thought to be malignant (7–11%), remove in the midtrimester.

The pregnant woman with an ovarian cyst is a special case because of the dangers of surgery to the fetus. These have probably been exaggerated in the past and no urgent operation should be postponed solely because of a pregnancy. Thus, if the patient presents with acute pain due to torsion or haemorrhage into an ovarian tumour, or if appendicitis is a possibility, the correct course is to undertake a laparotomy regardless of the stage of the pregnancy. The likelihood of labour ensuing is small; however, the operation should be covered by tocolytic drugs and performed in a centre with intensive neonatal care when possible.

The tumour marker CA125 is not useful in pregnant women, since elevated levels occur frequently as an apparent physiological change.

Cysts found by chance at caesarean section can also have a variety of management options. In summary:

- If the cyst is simple and less than 5 cm in diameter, leave it alone.
- If the cyst is complex or more than 5 cm in diameter, consider the following options:
  - Perform an ovarian cystectomy and open cyst. If any atypical feature (inclusions), remove ovary. Counsel patient of a 10% chance of a second operation if cystectomy only performed.
  - Perform oophorectomy and staging.

If there is a high clinical suspicion of malignancy, advice from an appropriately trained consultant colleague should be sought.

Pathology (Box 44.1)

Physiological ovarian cysts

These are included here because they can present as tumours when increased in size. However, most are asymptomatic, being found incidentally as a result of pelvic examination or ultrasound scanning. Although they may occur in any premenopausal woman, they are most common in young women. They are an occasional complication of ovulation induction, when they are commonly multiple. They may

---

Box 44.1 Pathology of benign ovarian tumours

Physiological cysts

Simple follicular cysts
Cysts of corpus luteum
Massive oedema of the ovary

Benign germ cell tumours

Dermoid cyst (mature cystic teratoma)
Mature solid teratoma

Benign epithelial tumours

Serous cystadenoma
Mucinous cystadenoma
Endometrioid cystadenoma
Transitional cell tumours
Clear cell (mesonephroid tumours)

Benign sex cord stromal tumours

Thecoma–fibroma group of tumours

Fibroma
Stromal cell tumour with minor sex cord elements
Theca cell tumour
Thecafibroma
Sclerosing stromal tumour
Signet ring stromal tumour
Androblastomas (Sertoli-Leydig cell tumours)

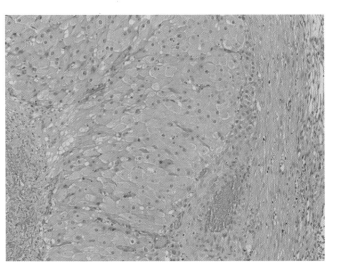

Figure 44.1 Cyst of corpus luteum. Note luteinized theca cells. Haematoxylin & eosin, original magnification ×20.

also occur in premature female infants and in women with trophoblastic disease.

Simple follicular cyst

Lined by granulosa cells, a simple follicular cyst is the most common type of benign ovarian tumour and is most often found incidentally in women of reproductive age, particularly during the early years after the menarche. It results from the non-rupture of a dominant follicle, or the failure of normal atresia in a non-dominant follicle which is thought to result from continuous hormone stimulation of a developing cycle without the midcycle surge of LH that normally triggers ovulation. Follicular cysts may be associated with menstrual irregularities. They may rupture with the consequent clinical syndrome of acute abdominal presentation. Occasionally, oestrogen production may persist, leading to menstrual disturbances and endometrial hyperplasia.

Histologically, follicular cysts show a lining of variably luteinized granulosa cells.

Corpus luteum cyst

Sometimes, corpora lutea undergo central cystification, often associated with haemorrhage into their lumen. Not uncommonly, these will present as an acute haemorrhagic abdominal episode. The degree of cystic dilatation exceeding 2 or 3 cm (according to different authors) justifies the designation of 'corpus luteum cyst'.

Macroscopic identification is straightforward due to the intense yellowish colour resulting from mature luteinized theca cells (Figure 44.1).

Massive oedema

Massive oedema is not a physiological cyst but presents as a tumour. It occurs in young patients (average 21 years of age) presenting with abdominal pain and swelling. Presentation is largely unilateral, and torsion of the involved ovary is seen in half of cases.

Macroscopically, the size varies greatly from 5 to 35 cm in diameter. The external surface is smooth and the cut section surface typically exudes watery fluid. Microscopically, the stromal oedema is more intense towards the central parenchyma, sparing the fibrous cortex.

Ninety per cent of all ovarian tumours are benign, although this varies with age, and they can arise from any tissue in the ovary. Approximately one in eight ovarian tumours in patients under 45 years of age is malignant; by contrast, the proportion is one in three in older women (Scully et al 2004). Most benign ovarian tumours are cystic, and the finding of solid elements makes malignancy more likely. However, fibromata, thecomata, dermoids and some transitional cell tumours are totally benign despite being partly or predominantly solid.

Pathological ovarian cysts

The diagnosis of ovarian tumours ultimately depends upon histological examination.

Benign germ cell tumours

Germ cell tumours account for approximately 30% of all ovarian tumours (Young et al 2004). Ninety five per cent of germ cell tumours are dermoid cysts (mature cystic teratomas) and most of the remainder are malignant. Malignant tumours are usually solid, although benign forms also commonly have a solid element. As the name suggests, they arise from totipotential germ cells, and may therefore contain elements of all three germ layers. Most malignant germ cell tumours are composed of primitive or immature elements.

Dermoid cyst (mature cystic teratoma)

Mature cystic teratoma accounts for 27–44% of all ovarian tumours and up to 58% of benign tumours (Koonings et al 1989).

Although most mature cystic teratomas occur in women of reproductive age, they have a wide age distribution (2–80 years) and 5% occur in postmenopausal women.

Most mature cystic teratomas present with a mass, but up to 60% are discovered incidentally. Complications that have been described include torsion of the pedicle and rupture. Rupture is rare (1% of cases) and can elicit chemical peritonitis with granulomatous nodules. The differential diagnosis here has to be made with tuberculosis and carcinomatosis.

Macroscopically, dermoid cysts appear as ovoid tumours, commonly multilocular, with diameters ranging from 0.5 to 40 cm (average 15 cm) with a smooth external surface and filled with sebaceous and hairy material. Not uncommonly, a nodule composed of teeth or bone (Rokitansky protuberance) is found. This area is known to harbour the greatest variety of tissue types, and therefore histological examination is recommended, even when decalcification is required (Rosai 2004).

Histologically, most tumours show derivatives of the three embryonal layers, with ectodermal structures usually predominating and reported in 100% of cases.

The cystic cavities are lined by mature epidermis, with skin adnexae found frequently. Neural (particularly glial), cartilage, respiratory and gastrointestinal tract tissues are also common.

By definition, all these tissues should be histologically mature; very occasionally, one may see foci of immature tissues. The behaviour of tumours with histological foci of up to 21 mm^2 of immature neuroepithelial tissue is excellent. They have to be distinguished from immature (malignant) teratomas.

'Somatic-type' tumours developing in mature cystic teratoma

Approximately 2% of mature cystic teratomas are known to contain a malignant somatic-type component. The most common is squamous carcinoma, followed by carcinoid tumour and adenocarcinoma. The list includes malignant melanoma, Paget's disease, sarcoma, carcinosarcoma, glioblastoma multiforme and neuroblastoma/primitive neuroectodermal tumour. Even when these behave comparably to their somatic counterparts, they are believed to arise from the germ cell elements.

Not surprisingly, benign somatic-type tumours have also been described, such as blue nevus, sebaceous adenoma, sweat gland adenoma, glomus tumour and prolactinoma.

Mature solid teratoma

These are rare and occur mainly in the first two decades of life. They are usually large and solid with multiple cysts, although multiple small cystic areas are common. By definition, they should be composed entirely of adult tissues. They must be differentiated from immature teratomas which are malignant.

Benign epithelial tumours

Most ovarian tumours (approximately two-thirds of all benign tumours and up to 90% of all malignant tumours) are classified as surface epithelial tumours. Most of these are derived from the ovarian surface epithelium, which in turn develops from the mesothelium–coelomic epithelium that covers the embryonic gonad. It is important to note that in the embryo, this epithelium is continuous with the coelomic epithelium that penetrates the underlying mesenchyme to form the Müllerian duct. This proximity is, in turn, reflected in the various directions of differentiation: towards fallopian tube epithelium in serous neoplasms, endometrial epithelium in endometrioid and clear cell tumours, and endocervical epithelium in some of the mucinous and transitional tumours.

The majority of these tumours are thought to derive from precursor lesions such as serosal inclusions, surface proliferations, metaplasias and endometriosis in the ovary. Although benign epithelial tumours tend to occur at a slightly younger age than their malignant counterparts, they are most common in women over 40 years of age.

Benign serous tumours

Serous tumours are most commonly endophytic (serous cystadenoma), but they may grow to the surface in the form of papillomas.

Serous cystadenomas are the most common type of benign epithelial tumour. Approximately 10% are bilateral. They can occasionally attain huge dimensions (Figure 44.2) and can be uni- or multilocular. Characteristically, the cysts are

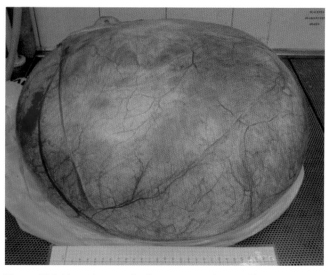

Figure 44.2 Macrophotograph of a serous cystadenoma. This specimen measured 40 cm in diameter and weighed over 5 kg.

thin walled and feature watery contents. The cysts may have a smooth lining, but not uncommonly polypoid excrescences can be seen.

Serous surface papillomas appear as polypoid excrescences on the outer surface of the ovaries. Serous adenofibromas are hard and white due to a predominance of the fibromatous component.

Histologically, all three variants are typically lined by epithelium similar to that of the fallopian tube, with variable degrees of ciliation. Psammoma bodies are usually absent.

When papillae are found, these are made almost entirely of stroma. In cystadenofibromas, the fibromatous stroma is prominent. By definition, none of these tumours show cellular atypia.

Benign mucinous tumours (mucinous cystadenoma)

These are the second most common type of ovarian epithelial tumour and tend to be the largest, some of them exceeding 30 cm in diameter and weighing more than 4 kg. The lining epithelium consists of columnar mucus-secreting cells. The most common type is referred to as of intestinal-type lining, in which goblet cells are almost always found. Less frequently, the epithelial lining is of endocervical type. The cyst fluid is generally thick and gelatinous.

A rare complication is pseudomyxoma peritonei which is more often present before the cyst is removed rather than following intraoperative rupture. Pseudomyxoma peritonei is most commonly associated with mucinous tumours of the ovary or appendix. Synchronous tumours of the ovary and appendix are common. There is, however, strong evidence that ovarian mucinous tumours associated with pseudomyxoma peritonei are almost all metastatic rather than primary.

Benign endometrioid tumours

These are ovarian tumours with histological features of benign glands or cysts lined by well-differentiated cells of endometrial type. They are very rare, usually unilateral and have no specific clinical symptoms. The histological diagnosis of an endometrioid adenoma or cystadenoma is based on the presence of well-differentiated glands lined by endometrial-type cells with scanty or absent surrounding endometrial stroma. When the latter is prominent, the lesion is classified as endometriosis.

Transitional cell (Brenner) tumours

These are neoplasms composed of epithelial elements histologically resembling urothelium (transitional epithelium). They account for only 1–2% of all ovarian tumours, and are bilateral in 10–15% of cases.

The tumour consists of nests and islands of transitional-type epithelial cells with characteristically grooved nuclei and abundant amphophilic cytoplasm set in a dense fibrotic stroma, giving a largely solid appearance. The nests show central lumina containing mucin and may be lined by columnar cells with a mucinous or ciliated appearance (Figure 44.3).

Despite the transitional appearance of the epithelium, immunohistochemical studies have demonstrated that it lacks a urothelial phenotype, and it closely resembles that of ovarian surface epithelium. As with the other ovarian tumours of epithelial derivation, the whole spectrum from benign to malignant is possible.

Clear cell (mesonephroid) tumours

These arise from serosal cells showing little differentiation, and are only rarely benign. The typical histological appearance is of clear or 'hobnail' cells with varying proportions of fibromatous component. Other cells that may be present include cuboidal, flat, oxyphilic and, rarely, signet ring.

Benign sex cord stromal tumours

Oestrogen-secreting tumours

Granulosa cell tumours

These slowly growing malignant tumours are the most common sex cord stromal tumours occurring in the ovary.

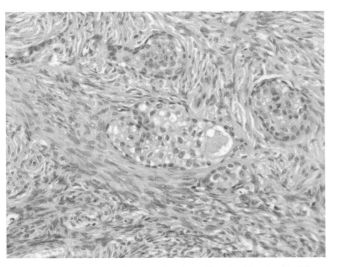

Figure 44.3 Transitional cell (Brenner) tumour showing bland epithelial cells with well-formed lumina. Haematoxylin & eosin, original magnification ×20.

While the great majority occur in postmenopausal women, 5% present in prepubertal or pubertal girls.

Approximately 70% of these tumours secrete oestrogens or, very rarely, androgens. Among postmenopausal women, 60% will present with vaginal bleeding due to oestrogen secretion from the tumour. Endometrial hyperplasia will develop in 25–50% of these women, and 5–10% will develop adenocarcinoma of the endometrium. Approximately 50% of women of reproductive age will complain of menstrual abnormalities, and 16% will have secondary amenorrhoea. In the rare cases when the tumour is secreting androgens, hirsutism may be the presenting feature. Precocious puberty is the usual presentation in young girls. The typical signs of abdominal swelling and pain seen in advanced epithelial ovarian cancer only appear when the granulosa cell tumour is more than 10 cm in diameter.

Thecoma

Thecomas account for less than 1% of all ovarian tumours. They occur in women of postmenopausal age and only a few cases have been reported in women under 30 years of age.

Approximately 70% of thecomas secrete oestrogens but they are less often associated with postmenopausal bleeding than granulosa cell tumours. On the other hand, they are more often associated with endometrial cancer (7% vs 2%). Endometrial hyperplasia is found in a further 19.8% of cases. Postmenopausal bleeding and abdominal pain are the main presenting features. In the presence of luteinized cells, these tumours can secrete androgens and result in hirsutism.

Pure Sertoli cell tumours (sex cord tumour with annular tubules)

These resemble well-differentiated Sertoli-Leydig tumours but contain no Leydig cells. They are benign. The sex cord tumour with annular tubules is a specific variety which resembles gonadoblastomas histologically. Although first described in association with Peutz-Jeghers syndrome, they have also been described in women without this syndrome.

Approximately half of these tumours produce oestrogen and very few secrete androgens. Those secreting oestrogen may cause endometrial hyperplasia, amenorrhoea, menorrhagia or sexual pseudoprecosity. Those associated with Peutz-Jeghers syndrome are usually small, benign, bilateral and partly calcified. In women unaffected by this syndrome, the tumours tend to be larger, unilateral and may be associated with granulosa or Sertoli-Leydig cell tumours. Some are malignant.

Predominantly androgen-secreting tumours

Sertoli-Leydig tumours (androblastoma)

Sertoli-Leydig cell tumour, also called 'androblastoma', is another rare, malignant, sex cord stromal tumour. Like the normal Leydig cell in males, these tumour cells in female ovaries may produce androgens, resulting in virilization. These tumours should be suspected in women in their second or third decades with an adnexal mass and virilization. However, some Sertoli-Leydig tumours can secrete oestrogen and approximately 80% are inactive. These usually present as unilateral stage I disease when the prognosis is good, even after fertility-conserving surgery, unless the tumour is poorly differentiated.

Adrenal-like tumours of the ovary

The nomenclature of these tumours is a source of great confusion. The current term, 'adrenal-like tumours', is now preferred but many others remain in wide use. The alternative names include 'hilar cell tumours', 'lipoid cell tumours', 'luteomas' and 'adrenal rest tumours'. These are often very small tumours less than 5 mm in diameter. Most are unilateral and benign. Surgical removal will result in reversal of the symptoms of virilization.

Gonadoblastoma

Gonadoblastoma is the most common neoplasm arising in dysgenetic gonads and arises almost exclusively in them. Although gonadoblastomas are benign, more than half are accompanied by malignant germ cell tumours, usually dysgerminomas, which have probably arisen from premalignant cells within the gonadoblastoma. Metastasis of the dysgerminoma component is uncommon but the other combinations can be highly malignant.

They vary in size from a few millimetres to large masses when other germ cell tumours are present. Most are only a few centimetres in diameter. They are often calcified and can be recognized on plain X-ray. More than half are bilateral.

The great majority occur in phenotypic females who are usually virilized. The age range of reported cases is 1–40 years. The clinical presentation may be abnormal genitalia in phenotypic male infants, or primary amenorrhoea with or without hirsutism in phenotypic females. Most have high levels of gonadotrophins due to ovarian virilization failure.

Bilateral gonadectomy is indicated in all these patients because of the risk of malignancy in the non-functioning gonads. This is usually curative for those associated with dysgerminoma, even when large, but chemotherapy will be required for those with other germ cell tumours. The prognosis for such individuals is good, with modern chemotherapy regimens offering 90% survival.

Thecoma–fibroma group of tumours

These arise from the stroma of the ovary and display a spectrum of morphology, from simple fibromas to thecomas. They are classified as fibromas unless an appreciable component of luteinized cells is present.

Fibroma

These are the most common type of sex cord stromal tumour (>66%), with more than 90% occurring in women aged 30 years or older.

Ascites is present in approximately 10% of cases and this occurs in tumours larger than 10 cm in diameter. Approximately 1% of cases are associated with Meigs syndrome (ascites and pleural effusion).

Fibromas are typically uniformly solid, white and rarely show yellowish foci, haemorrhage or necrosis. The classic appearance is that of a spindle cell tumour with variable collagen production and frequent storiform pattern. They are usually cellular but lack atypia or mitotic activity. A subgroup exists in which cellularity is dense but still not atypical (i.e. cellular fibromas). When luteinized cells are present, they should be classified as luteinized thecoma (see below).

Stromal cell tumour with minor sex cord elements

These are rare fibrothecomatous tumours containing scattered sex cord elements (<10%). The latter vary in appearance from granulosa cells to tubules resembling immature Sertoli cells.

Theca cell tumours

Thecomas are benign tumours composed of plump lipid-containing cells resembling the cells of the theca interna of the follicle. The mean age at presentation is 55 years and they typically manifest with symptoms secondary to oestrogen production. They are almost always unilateral, and macroscopically characterized by a solid and bright yellowish cut surface.

Histologically, there is a typical form featuring a varied arrangement of masses of plump eosinophilic or vacuolated cells with intervening fibrous connective tissue. Occasional small nests of granulosa cells can be present.

There is another well-defined histological pattern known as luteinized thecoma commonly seen in a younger age group, with bilateral presentation in which the fibrotic tissue predominates. Ten per cent of these tumours are androgenic.

Theca fibromas

These resemble the largely hormonally inactive fibromas and sclerosing stromal tumours (see below) in that most of them are clinically inactive. Their macroscopy is also indistinguishable from that of the fibromas, as is the histology with the addition of small clusters of theca cells.

Sclerosing stromal tumours

These occur in a younger group than typical thecoma or fibroma (>80% in women under 30 years of age) presenting with symptoms secondary to an ovarian mass, and very rarely give rise to oestrogen-related manifestations. They are unilateral, solid white and clearly demarcated from the adjacent ovarian tissue. The low-power histology is that of pseudolobules separated by bands of sclerotic or oedematous tissue. Within the pseudolobules are two characteristic groups of cells: (i) rounded and vacuolated luthela cells; and (ii) spindle cell fibroblasts. The differential diagnoses here include luteinized thecoma and Krukenberg tumour.

Signet ring stromal tumour

These are rare and are composed of signet ring cells with no mucin content. The numbers of signet ring cells are variable and the main differential diagnosis is Krukenberg tumour.

KEY POINTS

1. Asymptomatic, benign ovarian cysts in young women often resolve spontaneously.
2. Ovarian cysts with a simple appearance on ultrasound and less than 10 cm in diameter are very rarely malignant.
3. Solid ovarian tumours are often malignant; in young women, these are usually germ cell or sex cord stromal tumours.
4. There is no place for ultrasound-directed aspiration of cysts.
5. Laparoscopic removal of ovarian cysts should be confined to those with no features of malignancy.
6. Women over 44 years of age with a unilocular ovarian cyst with a diameter greater than 10 cm or with any other type of ovarian tumour should usually be advised to have a total abdominal hysterectomy and bilateral salpingo-oophorectomy.
7. A bimanual examination under anaesthesia should be performed prior to any surgery for ovarian tumours to confirm that a mass is still palpable.

References

Bailey CL, Ueland FR, Land GL et al 1998 The malignant potential of small cystic ovarian tumors in women over 50 years of age. Gynecological Oncology 69: 3–7.

Bankhead CR, Collins C, Stokes-Lampard H et al 2008 Identifying symptoms of ovarian cancer: a qualitative study. British Journal of Obstetrics and Gynaecology 115: 1008–1014.

Diernaes E, Rasmussen J, Soersen T, Hasche E 1987 Ovarian cysts: management by puncture? Lancet i: 1084.

Ekerhovd E, Wienerroith H, Staudach A, Granberg S 2001 Preoperative assessment of unilocular adnexal cysts by transvaginal ultrasonography: a comparison between ultrasonographic morphological imaging and histopathologic diagnosis. American Journal of Obstetrics and Gynecology 184: 48–54.

Goldstein SR 1993 Conservative management of small postmenopausal cystic masses. Clinical Obstetrics and Gynecology 36: 395–401.

Koonings PP, Campbell K, Mishell DR Jr, Grimes DA 1989 Relative frequency of primary ovarian neoplasms: a 10 year review. Obstetrics and Gynecology 74: 921–926.

Levine D, Gosink B, Wolf SI, Feldesman MR, Pretorius DH 1992 Simple adnexal cysts: the natural history in postmenopausal women. Radiology 184: 653–659.

NHS Executive 1999 Guidance on Commissioning Cancer Services: Improving Outcomes in Gynaecological Cancers. No. 16149. Department of Health.

Osmers RGW, Osmers M, von Maydell B, Wagner B, Kuhn W 1998 Evaluation of ovarian tumors in postmenopausal women by transvaginal sonography. European Journal of Obstetrics, Gynecology and Reproductive Biology 77: 81–88.

Rosai J 2004 Ackerman's Surgical Pathology, 9th edn. Mosby, Edinburgh, Chapter 19.

Russell P, Robboy S, Anderson MC 2002 Sex cord-stromal and steroid cell tumours of the ovaries. In: Pathology of the Female Genital Tract. Harcourt Publishers Ltd, London, Chapter 21.

Saasaki H, Oda M, Ohmura M et al 1999 Follow up of women with simple ovarian cysts detected by transvaginal sonography in the Tokyo metropolitan area. British Journal of Obstetrics and Gynaecology 106: 415–420.

Scully RE, Clement PB, Young RH 2004 Ovarian surface epithelial-stromal tumours. In: Sternberg's Diagnostic Surgical Pathology, 4th edn. Lippincott Williams & Wilkins, Philadelphia, Chapter 44.

Spencer CP, Robarts PJ 2006 Management of adnexal masses in pregnancy. The Obstetrician and Gynaecologist 8: 14–19.

Steinkampf MP, Hammond KR 1990 Hormonal treatment of functional ovarian cysts: a randomised, prospective study. Fertility and Sterility 54: 775–777.

Tavassoli FA, Devilee P 2003 WHO Classification of Tumours of the Breast and Female Genital Organs. IARC Press, Lyon, Chapter 2.

Young RH, Scully RE 1987 Non neoplastic disorders of the ovary. In: Haines and Taylor's Gynaecological Pathology. Churchill Livingstone, London, Chapter 17.

Young RH, Clement PB, Scully RE 2004 Sex cord stromal, steroid cell and germ cell tumours of the ovary. In: Sternberg's Diagnostic Surgical Pathology, 4th edn. Lippincott Williams & Wilkins, Philadelphia, Chapter 55.

Zanetta G, Lissoni A, Torri V et al 1996 Role of puncture and aspiration in expectant management of simple ovarian cysts: a randomised study. British Medical Journal 313: 1110–1113.

CHAPTER 45

Carcinoma of the ovary and fallopian tube

Sean Kehoe

Chapter Contents

CARCINOMA OF THE OVARY	678	CONCLUSIONS	686
CARCINOMA OF THE FALLOPIAN TUBE	684	KEY POINTS	686

Carcinoma of the Ovary

Epidemiology

The incidence of ovarian carcinoma varies around the world, with lower rates recorded in Japan (3/100,000 women) and some of the highest rates recorded in the Nordic countries (20/100,000 women). Variations are also noted within Europe, with lower rates occurring in Mediterranean countries (Figure 45.1). In the UK, approximately 7000 cases are reported each year, with a mortality rate of 4500. As such, ovarian cancer remains the most lethal of the gynaecological cancers, and the fourth most common malignant cause of death in women. The majority of women present with disease spread outside the ovaries, normally stage III–IV disease (Table 45.1), and this has a 5-year survival rate of approximately 40%. Ovarian cancer is mainly a disease of postmenopausal women, with the bulk of cases occurring in women aged 50–75 years. The main histological tumours are epithelial in origin, accounting for 90% of cases. Serous tumours are the most common, and as tubal tumours are also serous, accurate identification of the true primary site of disease can be difficult.

Aetiology

The main theory recounted for many years, called the 'incessant ovulation theory', is derived from the association between a woman's number of lifetime ovulations and the risk of ovarian cancer. The greater the number of ovulations, the greater the risk of ovarian cancer. Prevention of ovulation by either pregnancy or use of the combined contraceptive pill should reduce the risk of ovarian cancer, and this has indeed been noted. Some of the proposed explanations for this theory are that the milieu of rapid cellular turnover (in the development of the ovum), the injury caused with release of the ovum and stromal invagination (which occurs at ovulation) contribute to the risk of malignancy. However, more complex factors are likely to be involved. For example, the progesterone in the contraceptive pill is known to cause apoptosis of ovarian cells, and this is being investigated in a phase II trial by the Gynecologic Oncology Group in high-risk patients to determine the apoptotic effect on ovarian tissues. This may potentially become a preventative therapy in the future.

Infertility

For many years, it has been recognized that there may be an association between infertility and risk of ovarian cancer. The relationship has never been absolutely clarified, and there are many conflicting reports in the literature (Mahdavi et al 2006, Jensen et al 2009). The difficulties mainly relate to the information available, as the types of drugs used, their duration of use and the outcome of pregnancies were not well recorded in many reports. One proposal associating the use of drug-induced ovulation and potential malignant transformation was seen in the increased ovarian cellular dyplasia in ovaries removed from women with a history of in-vitro fertilization treatment (Chene et al 2009). However, further larger longitudinal studies are needed to confirm the situation regarding infertility and ovarian cancer.

Endometriosis

Endometriosis affects approximately one in eight women. The notable tumours associated with endometriosis are ovarian clear cell carcinomas. Endometrioid tumours are also known to have a relationship with endometriosis, but this association is weaker. An interesting fact is that clear cell tumours are most prevalent in Japan, despite the fact that Japan has the lowest incidence of ovarian cancer in the world. The concept that endometriosis is a premalignant condition has been proposed, based on the ability of endometriosis to metastasize, and also as it is found in association with ovarian malignancies. There is a need for further work in this area, but it is interesting to note that women with endometriosis also have a higher relative risk of developing other cancers (Melin et al 2007).

DOI: 10.1016/B978-0-7020-3120-5.00045-X

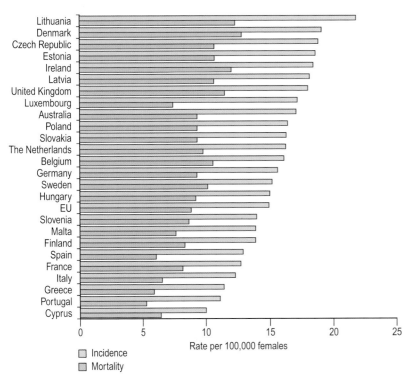

Figure 45.1 Age-standardized incidence and mortality rates for ovarian cancer, European Union, 2002 estimates.

Genetic factors

It is estimated that approximately 10% of all ovarian malignancies are hereditary, and the potential genetic factors in tubal malignancies are becoming increasingly recognized. The latter are rare, but represent sufficient reason to recommend removal of the fallopian tubes when undertaking prophylactic surgery. The two main mutations are *BRCA1* and *BRCA2*. These mutations interfere with the efficacy of p53, and thus permit progression of the malignant process. The greater risk is in women with *BRCA1* who have up to a 40% lifetime risk, compared with 20–25% in those with *BRCA2*. When considering prophylactic surgery, this should be performed before 40 years of age to gain a real benefit. Understandably, if the familial pattern is for a younger age group to develop the disease, siblings will often wish for earlier intervention. The only other familial association is with Lynch type 2 syndrome, with mutations on chromosome 5. In these patients, the family history mainly relates to bowel carcinoma, although the incidence of ovarian cancer is approximately 12% compared with a lifetime risk of approximately 2%. These patients do have a high risk for endometrial cancer, and thus will require the uterus to be removed at the same time if prophylactic surgery is deemed appropriate.

Molecular biology

One aspect of ovarian cancer is the somewhat limited understanding of the tumour biology and the natural history of the condition itself. Most patients present with advanced disease and it is often considered that ovarian cancer has a rapid growth phase, hence the late presentation with a short history of symptoms. Some work on symptoms in ovarian cancer suggests that these may be present some time prior to diagnosis (Goff et al 2007), and the natural progression of the disease may be different to previous assumptions. However, this requires further research before becoming acceptable.

In ovarian cancer, molecular markers have been researched although there is a lack of true understanding of tumour biology. Tumour vascular proteins (Buckanovich et al 2007) have been shown to have different expression in ovarian malignancies compared with normal, and with the development of antivascular endothelial growth factor therapies with a spectrum of tumour vascular proteins now recognized, further therapies may be developed. Serum mesothelin level is another marker noted to be elevated in ovarian cancer and to have a direct correlation with disease stage, and this could have potential use in screening (Huang et al 2006). Proteomic studies are used increasingly and should yield some valuable information to facilitate the understanding of ovarian cancer (Boyce and Kohn 2005).

Classification of ovarian tumours

Ovarian tumours can be solid or cystic. They may be benign or malignant. In addition, there are those which, while having some features of malignancy, lack any evidence of stromal invasion. These are called 'borderline tumours'.

The most commonly used classification of ovarian tumours was defined by the World Health Organization (Scully 1999). This is a morphological classification that attempts to relate the cell types and patterns of the tumour to tissues normally present in the ovary. The primary tumours are thus divided into those that are of epithelial type (implying an origin from surface epithelium and the adjacent ovarian stroma), those that are of sex cord gonadal type (also known as sex cord stromal type or sex cord mesenchymal type, and originating from sex cord mesenchymal elements) and those

Table 45.1 FIGO staging for ovarian cancer

Stage I	Growth limited to the ovaries
Stage IA	Growth limited to one ovary, no ascites, no tumour on external surface, capsule intact
Stage IB	Growth limited to both ovaries, no ascites, no tumour on external surface, capsule intact
Stage IC	Tumour as for stage IA or B, but tumour on surface of one or both ovaries or capsule ruptured or positive ascites/peritoneal washings
Stage II	Tumour as for stage IC, but growth involving one or both ovaries with pelvic extension
Stage IIA	Extension and/or metastases to the uterus and/or tubes
Stage IIB	Extension to other pelvic tissue
Stage IIC	Tumour as for stage IIA or B, but tumour on surface of one or both ovaries or capsule ruptured or positive ascites/peritoneal washings
Stage III	Tumour involving one or both ovaries with peritoneal implants outside the pelvis and/or positive retroperitoneal or inguinal nodes. Includes superficial liver metastases or histologically proven malignant extension to small bowel/omentum
Stage IIIA	Tumour grossly limited to true pelvis with negative nodes, but histologically confirmed microscopic seeding of abdominal peritoneal surfaces
Stage IIIB	Tumour involving one or both ovaries with histologically confirmed implants of abdominal peritoneal surfaces, none exceeding 2 cm in diameter
Stage IIIC	Abdominal implants greater than 2 cm in diameter and/or positive retroperitoneal or inguinal nodes
Stage IV	Growth of one or both ovaries with distant metastases, e.g. parenchymal liver metastases, or cytologically proven pleural effusion

Table 45.2 Simplified classification of ovarian cancers

Epithelial origin	Serous
	Mucinous
	Endometrioid
	Clear cell
	Papillary serous
	Brenner cell
	Undifferentiated adenocarcinomas and sarcomas
Germ cell origin	Teratomas
	Mature teratomas
	Immature teratomas
	Struma ovarii
	Carcinoid
	Dysgerminoma
	Embryonal cell carcinoma
	Endodermal sinus
	Primary choriocarcinoma
	Gonadoblastoma
Others	Stromal cell cancers
	Granulosa cell
	Theca cell
	Sertoli-Leydig cell

that are of germ cell type (originating from germ cells). A simplified classification is given in Table 45.2.

Pathology of epithelial tumours

Epithelial tumours are derived from the ovarian surface epithelium, which is a modified mesothelium with a similar origin and behaviour to the Müllerian duct epithelium, and from the adjacent distinctive ovarian stroma. They are subclassified according to epithelial cell type (serous, mucinous, endometrioid, clear, transitional, squamous); the relative amount of epithelial and stromal component (when the stromal is larger than the cystic epithelial component, the suffix 'fibroma' is added); and the macroscopic appearance (solid, cystic, papillary). They account for 50–55% of all ovarian tumours, but their malignant forms represent approximately 90% of all ovarian cancers in the Western world (Koonings et al 1989). Well-differentiated epithelial carcinomas are more often associated with early-stage disease, but the degree of differentiation does correlate with survival, except in the most advanced stages. Diploid tumours

tend to be associated with earlier stage disease and a better prognosis. Histological cell type is not in itself prognostically significant.

Comparing patients stage for stage and grade for grade, there is no difference in survival in different epithelial types. However, mucinous and endometrioid lesions are likely to be associated with earlier stage and lower grade than serous cystadenocarcinomas.

Serous carcinoma

Gross features

The majority of serous carcinomas show a mixture of solid and cystic elements, although a significant minority are predominantly cystic. Serous carcinomas have a propensity to bilaterality, ranging from 50% to 90%, but in only 25–30% of stage I cases.

Microscopic features

The better differentiated tumours have an obvious papillary pattern with unequivocal stromal invasion, and psammoma bodies (calcospherules) are often present. A highly differentiated form of serous papillary carcinoma called 'psammocarcinoma' contains large numbers of psammoma bodies surrounded by no more than 15 well to moderately differentiated serous cells, and has a favourable prognosis despite the fact that most lesions are found in stage III. None of these features are diagnostic of serous tumours alone. Endometrioid and clear cell carcinomas and, to a lesser extent, mucinous carcinomas may all form papillary structures. The term 'papillary carcinoma of the ovary' should not, therefore, be used as a diagnosis.

At the other end of the spectrum is the anaplastic tumour composed of sheets of undifferentiated neoplastic cells in masses within a fibrous stroma. Occasional glandular structures may be present to enable a diagnosis of adenocarcinoma. All gradations between these two are seen, sometimes in the same tumour.

Mucinous carcinoma

Gross features

Malignant mucinous tumours comprise approximately 12% of malignant tumours of the ovary. They are typically multilocular, thin-walled cysts with a smooth external surface and contain mucinous fluid. The locules vary in size and the tumour is often composed of one major cavity with many smaller daughter cysts apparently within its wall. Mucinous tumours are amongst the largest tumours of the ovary and may reach enormous dimensions; a cyst diameter of 25 cm is quite commonplace.

A mucinous cystadenocarcinoma may look the same as a benign tumour. Some malignant tumours may exhibit obvious solid areas, perhaps with necrosis and haemorrhage. The more advanced carcinomas will show the stigmata of ovarian malignancy, with adhesions to adjacent viscera and malignant ascites.

Microscopic features

Mucinous adenocarcinomas present a variety of histological appearances. They may contain endocervical-like cells alone, intestinal-type cells alone or a combination of the two, but are more often composed of mucinous cells without distinguishing features. The better differentiated examples are composed of cells that retain a resemblance to the tall, picket-fence cells of the benign tumour, although stromal invasion is present. As differentiation is lost, the cells become less easily recognizable as being of mucinous type and their mucin content diminishes.

Endometrioid carcinoma

Endometrioid carcinomas are ovarian tumours that resemble the malignant neoplasia of epithelial, stromal and mixed origin that are found in the endometrium (Czernobilsky et al 1970). They account for 2–4% of all ovarian tumours. They are accompanied by ovarian or pelvic endometriosis in 11–42% of cases, and a transition to endometriotic epithelium can be seen in up to 30% of cases. The pathologist must distinguish metaplastic and reactive changes in endometriosis from true neoplastic changes.

Gross features

There is little to characterize an ovarian tumour as being of endometrioid type by naked-eye examination. Most are cystic, often unilocular and contain turbid brown fluid. The internal surface of the cyst is usually rough with rounded, polypoid projections and solid areas, the appearances of which are usually distinct from those of the papillary excrescences seen in serous tumours.

Microscopic features

Endometrioid carcinomas resemble the endometrioid carcinomas of the endometrium. The pattern is predominantly tubular and may resemble proliferative endometrium. The epithelium is tall and columnar, with a high nuclear:cytoplasmic ratio. Endometrioid carcinomas of the ovary are more likely to be papillary than primary endometrial carcinomas. Five to 10% of cases are seen in continuity with recognizable endometriosis. Ovarian adenoacanthoma, with benign-appearing squamous elements, account for almost 50% in some series of endometrioid tumours.

Associated endometrial carcinoma

It is important to note that 15% of endometrioid carcinomas of the ovary are associated with endometrial carcinoma in the body of the uterus. Although this is sometimes due to a primary tumour in one site and a secondary tumour at the other, these are usually two separate primary tumours.

Clear cell carcinoma

Clear cell carcinomas are the least common of the malignant epithelial tumours of the ovary, accounting for 5–10% of ovarian carcinomas (Anderson and Langley 1970).

Gross features

There is nothing characteristic about the gross appearance of clear cell tumours to distinguish them from other cystadenocarcinomas of the ovary. Most are thick-walled, unilocular cysts containing turbid brown or bloodstained fluid, with solid, polypoid projections arising from the internal surface. Approximately 10% are bilateral.

Microscopic features

Clear cell carcinomas of the ovary are characterized by the variety of architectural patterns, which may be found alone or in combination in any individual tumour. The appearance from which the tumours derive their name is the clear cell pattern but, in addition, some areas show a tubulocystic pattern with the characteristic 'hob-nail' appearance of the lining epithelium. The third major pattern is papillary.

Association with endometriosis and endometrioid tumours

As there is a very strong association between clear cell tumours of the ovary and ovarian endometriosis, and because clear cell and endometrioid tumours frequently coexist, it has been suggested that clear cell tumours may be a variant of endometrioid tumours.

Transitional cell tumours

Transitional cell tumours represent 1–2% of all ovarian tumours and most are benign. The epithelial component resembles urothelium, which may undergo cystic, mucinous or serous metaplasia. The stromal component resembles that of fibromas in benign or borderline lesions, and the malignant counterpart resembles a transitional cell carcinoma.

Borderline epithelial tumours

Approximately 10% of all epithelial tumours of the ovary are borderline tumours, of which 30% are of the mucinous type, followed by the serous type. Other borderline tumours are rare. The histological diagnosis of borderline malignancy can be difficult, particularly in mucinous tumours. These show varying degrees of nuclear atypia and an increase in mitotic activity, multilayering of neoplastic cells and formation of cellular buds, but no invasion of the stroma. Most borderline tumours remain confined to the ovaries and this may account for their much better prognosis.

Peritoneal lesions are present in some cases and although a few are true metastases, many do not grow and even regress after removal of the primary tumour. Surgical pathological stage and subclassification of extraovarian disease into invasive and non-invasive implants are the most important prognostic indicators for serous borderline tumours, with survival for advanced-stage serous tumours with non-invasive implants being 95.3% compared with 66% for tumours with invasive implants (Seidman and Kurman 2000).

Diagnosis

The symptoms associated with ovarian cancer have come under particular scrutiny over the last few years. The main symptoms are abdominal pain, bloating, postmenopausal bleeding, weight loss and loss of appetite (Bankhead et al 2005, Goff et al 2007). In approximately 10% of cases, there are no symptoms and the disease is found serendipitously, such as following a scan for back pain. Once there is a clinical suspicion of ovarian cancer, investigations can facilitate in defining the risk of malignancy, which will ensure the patient is referred appropriately. This is important as the expertise of the operator will influence the outcome and success of achieving tumour clearance (Junor et al 1999, Tingulstad et al 2003, Earle et al 2006).

The main primary investigations are serum CA125 and abdominal/pelvic ultrasound. These, in conjunction with the menopausal status of the patient, enable calculation of the risk of malignancy. Table 45.3 shows one form of calculation employed. Thus, a high risk of malignancy index (RMI) will capture most advanced ovarian cancers (Jacobs et al 1990). It must be remembered that not all ovarian cancers produce CA125, and mucinous cancers, in particu-

lar, can often have a normal CA125. Equally, a high RMI is not itself diagnostic, and the system is far from perfect. However, it is the only available mechanism at present to triage patients to appropriate specialist centres of care.

In younger patients, the sensitivity of these tests is less as CA125 may be elevated due to menstruation, and scans will find ovulatory cysts which can further confound matters. As well as CA125, serum β-human chorionic gonadotrophin and α-fetoprotein should also be measured in women under 40 years of age as this age group contains most of the germ cell tumours which cause elevation of these markers. Serum carcinoembryonic antigen (CEA) can be useful when there is doubt regarding whether the primary disease originates from the colon. In cases where the CEA level is high, bowel investigations, such as colonoscopy, may be warranted.

Other investigations include computed tomography (CT) of the abdomen and pelvis, which can be used with CA125 to calculate the potential chance of achieving optimum debulking surgery. Magnetic resonance imaging is mainly used in defining the ovarian mass where there is some doubt on CT or ultrasound regarding the origin of the pelvic mass. Chest X-rays are used to detect any metastatic disease, in accordance with the staging recommendations of the International Federation of Gynecology and Obstetrics (FIGO).

Surgery

Surgery remains the main and internationally agreed primary intervention in suspected ovarian cancer. The objectives of surgery are manifold: to obtain a histological diagnosis, to undertake correct staging of the disease, to remove all or as much tumour as possible, and to alleviate symptoms. The procedures commonly undertaken are hysterectomy, bilateral salpingo-oophorectomy, omentectomy, retroperitoneal lymph node sampling, sampling of peritoneal fluids and other biopsies as deemed necessary. Whilst removing all visible disease seems logical, optimum debulking is also undertaken. This surgery is performed to ensure that no residual disease left *in situ* is greater than 1 cm in diameter. This is a unique approach for an intra-abdominal carcinoma and the historic reason is interesting.

In the 1970s, Griffiths published a paper relating survival in ovarian cancer to the amount of residual tumour left in the abdominal cavity. The original publication related to a retrospective series of just over 100 women, which indicated the preferable survival pattern in women with tumour residuum of less than 1.6 cm in diameter compared with those with great tumour loads. The premise for this was the report by Magrath et al (1974) on a similar finding with intra-abdominal Hodgkin's lymphoma. A subsequent prospective study on 26 patients was published, some of whom had undergone primary surgery previously, and some who had also been exposed to chemotherapy (Griffiths et al 1979). Following aggressive surgery, the preferable survival pattern was associated with those who had the lesser tumour residuum. Thus, the optimum debulking procedure became embedded within clinical practice, and many subsequent reports have confirmed this association. Notably, no prospective randomized trials were ever performed to ascertain the validity of this approach, and debate continues about whether those amenable to optimum

---

Table 45.3 Risk of malignancy estimate

RMI = Ultrasound score × Menopausal status × Serum CA125

Ultrasound score (U)
Score one point for each of the following:
– Multilocular cyst
– Evidence of solid areas
– Evidence of metastases
– Presence of ascites
– Bilateral lesions
U = 0 (0 points)
U = 1 (1 point)
U = 3 (2–5 points)

Menopausal status
– Premenopausal: score 1
– Postmenopausal: score 3

RMI	Risk of cancer (%)
<25	<3
25–250	20
>250	75

RMI, risk of malignancy index.

debulking are also those with the most chemosensitive tumours. Some meta-analyses have been published with variable results. Hunter et al (1992) reported on a cohort of over 6000 women with ovarian cancer, and concluded that the use of platinum agents rather than surgery was a more important factor in enhancing survival outcome. The more recent meta-analysis by Bristow et al (2002) associated the residuum of tumour with survival, and showed that each 10% increase in maximal cytoreductive surgery was associated with a 4.1% increase in median survival time. In Bristow et al's study, unlike that of Hunter et al, all patients were exposed to platinum therapies. Of course, the strength of meta-analyses based on essentially large non-randomized series does permit some questioning of the weight of the final conclusions. Interestingly, a recent randomized trial of complete para-aortic and pelvic lymphadenectomy in advanced ovarian cancer compared with excision of enlarged nodes alone did not reveal any survival benefit (Panici et al 2005).

Nowadays, there is a new approach of supraradical surgery in order to achieve total macroscopic clearance, and these operations can include resection of diaphragmatic lesion, hepatic and splenic metastases, and multiple bowel resections. Patients are carefully selected for these operations, and it remains to be proven whether this radical surgery enhances outcome. Prospective randomized trials are awaited.

An evidence base for practice is always welcome as this can at least attempt to ensure best practice and indeed facilitate patient counselling. Regarding primary surgical intervention, two trials have been undertaken, namely EORTC 55971 and CHORUS. These studies compared standard upfront surgery followed by platinum-based chemotherapy (six cycles) with neoadjuvant chemotherapy (three cycles) then surgery and then a further three cycles of platinum. The EORTC study has only been reported at meetings; peer-reviewed publications are awaited. The CHORUS study is ongoing. These studies are the first randomized trials to address the primary interventions in ovarian cancer (www.eortc.be/protoc/listprot.asp, www.ctu.mrc.ac.uk/studies/).

Fertility-sparing procedures

Whilst radical surgery does relate to the majority of situations, fertility-sparing surgery is advocated in younger women (<40 years) or women who have not completed their families. There are many reasons for this, but primarily younger patients tend to have the rarer ovarian tumours, such as borderline or germ cell tumours (the latter of which are very chemosensitive). In this situation, the affected ovary/cystic areas should be removed and a formal staging procedure — with preservation of fertility — should be undertaken. Naturally, if a standard tumour is found histologically, the option of further surgery can be discussed with the patient.

Surgery for borderline tumours

Specific mention must be made regarding borderline tumours. These are more common in younger patients, and are often only diagnosed at histopathology as the appearances can often be similar to benign ovarian cysts. The outcome for these tumours is excellent, and radical surgery is not required in most cases, with an estimated relapse rate of 10–15% in 10–15 years. The relapse rate in women who only have a cystectomy is estimated to be approximately 25%, but if a full oophorectomy has been performed, the relapse rate falls to 10–15%. When the patient has completed her family, the role of further surgery is unclear. The relapse rate is small, and there is no evidence that completion surgery would reduce this further. However, there are many 'unknowns' regarding borderline tumours, and a case could be made for completion surgery. It is probably best that expert counselling of patients is undertaken and each case should be managed individually.

Interventional debulking surgery

When optimum debulking is not achieved at the primary operation, a second attempt may be worthwhile. With this objective, three prospective randomized trials were developed. The smallest trial (Redman et al 1994) was stopped prematurely as no advantage was noted at the interim analysis. In this study, optimum debulking was defined as less than 2 cm in diameter. The second study (van der Burg et al 1995) randomized over 300 women who had primary suboptimal surgery (>1 cm residuum) and were chemosensitive to platinum. Optimum in this study was defined as tumour less than 1 cm in diameter. The study showed a 6 month improvement in median survival in those having a second operation (performed after three of six cycles of platinum treatment). This was the first randomized study published supporting the concept of optimum debulking as a procedure influencing survival in ovarian cancer. The Gynecologic Oncology Group (GOG) (Rose et al 2004) published a similar trial which did not reveal any survival difference with interventional debulking surgery. The trials differed in a few aspects: firstly, paclitaxel was included in the GOG study (not available in van de Burg et al's study), and secondly, more patients in the GOG study had primary surgery by trained gynaecological oncologists, thus influencing the primary optimum debulking rates. The conclusions are therefore conflicting: in European practice, interventional debulking surgery may have a role, but in present-day US practice, it does not seem to have a role if managed by gynaecological oncologists.

Second-look surgery

Second-look laparotomy (SLL) was introduced so that a thorough evaluation of tumour response was possible, and thus ongoing therapy could cease. This was during an era when therapy was continued for over 12 months, and it became evident that iatrogenic malignancies were developing with long-term treatment. The original SLL was performed after 12 months of cytotoxic therapy (Smith et al 1976). In present practice, there are many other non-invasive methods to determine tumour response, but SLL has remained part of routine practice in some countries. One randomized trial has been performed assessing the impact of SLL on survival outcome (Luesley et al 1988), and this did not reveal any benefit. As such, SLL should remain within the context of any relevant clinic trials, rather than part of routine care.

Surgery at relapse

With disease persisting after chemotherapy, or occurring within 6 months of completion of chemotherapy, such disease is deemed resistant and surgery has little role, other than palliation of symptoms. Outside this range, there may be a beneficial effect of further surgery. A series of retrospective studies have identified a group of women in whom surgery at relapse may prolong survival (Jänicke et al 1992, Zang et al 2004, Salani et al 2007). These patients had optimum debulking at primary surgery, a disease-free interval of 12 months and were less than 60 years of age. In this population, there was a greater chance of achieving optimum debulking at second surgery. The most comprehensive study (DESKTOP study) was a multinational study identifying predictive factors for complete tumour clearance in women presenting with relapsed ovarian cancer (Harter et al 2006). From this cohort of 267 women, a 79% prediction rate was achieved with the following variables: good performance status, original optimum debulking, early stage of disease at presentation and no ascites at relapse. In those who had complete resection at second surgery, median survival was 45.2 months compared with 19.7 months in those left with any visible disease. With good predictive models, individuals who may gain survival advantages with surgery at relapse can be identified and will require chemotherapy in conjunction with surgery. It is also well recognized that chemotherapy is more effective for longer disease-free intervals (Blackledge et al 1989); hence, tumour biology, not just surgery, may play an important role. Only a prospective trial will determine the true influence of surgery in this context.

Chemotherapy

Chemotherapy is administered to nearly all women suffering from ovarian cancer. The ICON 1 study (Colombo et al 2003), comparing adjuvant platinum-based chemotherapy with observation in mainly early-stage disease, did note benefits, even in those with early-stage disease, but no benefit was seen for those with well to moderately differentiated epithelial tumours. It is important that disease staging is performed correctly, as in a cohort from a similar type study (ACTION), it was noted that survival was improved in those receiving adjuvant chemotherapy who were not appropriately staged but assumed to have early-stage disease (Trimbos et al 2003).

The mainstay of therapy remains platinum based, with paclitaxel used in combination in many countries. This would be deemed standard in some countries following a series of studies reporting a superior survival pattern with the addition of paclitaxel to platinum agents in first-line therapy studies (McGuire et al 1996, Piccart et al 2000, Ozols et al 2003). However, in the UK, where ICON 4 (Parmar et al 2003) did not show a benefit associated with the addition of palitaxel, the guidance of the National Institute for Health and Clinical Excellence (2003) remains open in this regard.

Intraperitoneal therapy

Some years ago, intraperitoneal therapy was used, in that cyclophosphamide was administered into the peritoneal cavity at surgery. Subsequently, it was recognized that to become active, cyclophosphamide required liver metabolism. Hence the practice ceased. Advocates of the possible survival benefits remained, and in 1996, Alberts et al reported on an randomized controlled trial whereby intraperitoneal cisplatin was given in conjunction with intravenous therapy, and the median survival was increased from 40 to 48 months. There were known side-effects and there was no general acceptance of this type of therapy, mainly due to this and the more complicated manner of administration of cytotoxics compared with intravenous access. However, two further trials (Markman et al 2001, Armstrong et al 2006) which incorporated paclitaxel into the therapy showed increased median survival rates of over 10 months in the intraperitoneal arm. There has been some debate about these trials, in particular that the overall doses employed in the control arms could be considered suboptimal compared with more modern doses, and thus impacting on the survival differences noted (Swart et al 2008).

The issue regarding toxicity also arises, although one study showed that neurotoxicity remained the only variable worse in patients treated with intraperitoneal therapy, compared with intravenous therapy, at 1 year after treatment (Wenzel et al 2007). The recent Cochrane review on this topic concludes that intraperitoneal therapy does afford better survival patterns, but this needs to be measured carefully against toxicity (Jaaback and Johnson 2006) (Table 45.4).

Novel approaches

The approaches to ovarian cancer care are beginning to change, with neoadjuvant chemotherapy increasingly reported (Steed et al 2006). However, the more exciting approaches relate to using a greater number of molecular targets, and indeed developing studies which are more tumour specific. There are ongoing studies for ovarian clear cell tumours, and a study for mucinous tumours is in development. The main molecular targets of therapy are poly(ADP-ribose) polymerase inhibitors, used in *BRCA* mutational tumours such as breast and ovarian cancer (Drew and Calvert 2008). Equally, the results of large trials on targeting vascular endothelial growth factor are awaited with interest, and should hopefully add another approach to therapy (Table 45.5).

Carcinoma of the Fallopian Tube

Fallopian tube malignancies are very rare, although notably there is increasing interest in the proposal that many ovarian serous carcinomas are actually primary fallopian tube carcinomas. However, by virtue of the disease extent at surgery, it is impossible to distinguish the primary source of the cancer. The finding that women with fallopian tube cancers have a 15.9% prevalence of *BRCA1* or *BRCA2* mutations or family histories of early-onset breast or ovarian cancer (Aziz et al 2001) also suggests that some advanced 'ovarian' cancers may actually have originated from the fallopian tubes. Supporting this possibility is the fact that microscopic fallopian tube cancers are found in women undergoing prophylactic surgery for ovarian cancer, indicating a possible hereditary factor (Hirst et al 2009).

Cancers of the fallopian tube can be either primary or secondary. Most tumours involving the fallopian tube are

Table 45.4 The three main phase III intraperitoneal therapy studies

Study	Number	Drugs	Median survival (months)	P-value
Alberts et al	546	IV cisplatin 100 mg/m^2 and IV cyclophosamide	40	<0.02
		IP cisplatin 100 mg/m^2 and IV cyclophosamide	48	
Markman et al	462	IV cisplatin 75 mg/m^2 and IV paclitaxel 135 mg/m^2	52	<0.05
		IV carboplatin (AUC = 9), IV paclitaxel 135 mg/m^2 and IP cisplatin100 mg/m^2	63	
Armstrong et al	415	IP cisplatin 100 mg/m^2 and IV paclitaxel 135 mg/m^2	49.7	<0.03
		IP cisplatin 100 mg/m^2 and IP paclitaxel 60 mg/m^2	65.6	

IV, intravenous; IP, intraperitoneal; AUC, area under the curve.

Table 45.5 Randomized phase III surgical trials in ovarian cancer

Reference	Aim	Number	Conclusion
Luesley et al	SLL	166	No difference in survival
van der Burg et al	IDS	278	Median survival with IDS increased by 6 months
Rose et al	IDS	424	No difference in survival
EORTC	Neoadjuvant chemotherapy vs primary surgery	720	Awaited
CHORUS	Neoadjuvant chemotherapy vs primary surgery	Recruiting	Ongoing
Panici et al	Radical retroperitoneal lymphadenectomy vs none	427	No difference in survival

SLL, second-look laparotomy (after completion of chemotherapy); IDS, interventional debulking surgery (after three cycles of chemotherapy).

metastatic from ovarian cancer, but secondary spread from the breast and gastrointestinal tract also occurs. Primary carcinoma is usually unilateral. It is thought to be extremely rare, comprising only 0.3% of gynaecological malignancies. However, only early fallopian tube carcinomas can be distinguished with certainty from ovarian disease. Most present after the menopause, with the mean age of patients being 56 years. Many cases are nulliparous (45%) and infertility is reported in up to 71% of these women. Tumour spread is identical to that of ovarian cancer, and metastases to pelvic and para-aortic nodes are common.

Pathology

Due to the histological similarity between serous ovarian carcinoma and primary tubal carcinoma, strict criteria must be applied before a diagnosis of tubal carcinoma can be made. Carcinoma of the fallopian tube usually distends the lumen with tumour. The tumour may protrude through the fimbrial end and the tube may be retort shaped, resembling a hydrosalpinx. Histologically, tubal carcinoma is typically very similar to serous adenocarcinoma of the ovary. The predominant pattern is papillary, with a gradation through alveolar to solid as the degree of differentiation decreases.

Staging

The FIGO clinical staging for cancer of the fallopian tube is similar to that used for ovarian cancer. Probably because of the difficulty in distinguishing between advanced ovarian and advanced fallopian tube carcinoma, 74% of fallopian

tube carcinomas are diagnosed at stage I–IIA, while the remaining 26% are diagnosed at stage IIB–IV (Hellström et al 1994).

Clinical presentation and management

Most cases of cancer of the fallopian tube are diagnosed at laparotomy. The diagnosis is seldom considered before surgery. The usual presenting symptom is postmenopausal bleeding, and the diagnosis should be considered particularly if the patient also complains of a watery discharge and lower abdominal pain. Unexplained postmenopausal bleeding or abnormal cervical cytology without an obvious cause demands a careful bimanual examination and pelvic ultrasound. Laparoscopy may be required in doubtful cases.

The management of cancer of the fallopian tube is as for cancer of the ovary, with surgery to remove gross tumour. This will almost always involve a total abdominal hysterectomy and bilateral salpingo-oophorectomy. Omentectomy should be performed. Postoperative chemotherapy will be required with platinum analogues for all but the earliest cases. The treatment of carcinoma metastatic to the fallopian tube is determined by management of the primary tumour.

Results

The overall 5-year survival rate for carcinoma of the fallopian tube is approximately 35%. The prognosis is improved if the tumour is detected at an early stage. The 5-year survival rate for stage I is in the region of 70%, as is that for stage

IA cases. However, survival falls to 25–30% in stages IB–IIIC (Hellström et al 1994). Chemotherapy with platinum agents improves survival.

Conclusions

The management of ovarian and fallopian tube carcinomas involves surgery followed by adjuvant therapy in most cases, which is platinum based. The addition of paclitaxel has improved survival prospects for some patients with advanced disease. The absolute role of primary surgery and whether or not primary chemotherapy is preferable is being addressed in randomized controlled trials, and some prospective non-randomized trials have also been undertaken in the relapsed setting. Importantly, the greater individualization of therapy and the advent of therapies targeting tumours in a more specific molecular manner means that more sophisticated therapeutic options should become more common in the future.

KEY POINTS

1. Epithelial ovarian cancer usually occurs between the ages of 45 and 65 years. The disease is usually advanced at presentation. It has a poor prognosis except in cases when the disease is confined to the ovaries and is well or moderately well differentiated.

2. Use of oral contraceptives protects against the development of ovarian cancer.

3. Inheritance plays a significant role in approximately 5% of epithelial ovarian cancers. The *BRCA1* gene is associated with 80% of families with both breast and ovarian cancer, but the risk of ovarian cancer alone is variable. *BRCA1* does not appear to be responsible for many sporadic cases of ovarian cancers.

4. Population screening for ovarian cancer is not justified with the techniques evaluated to date.

5. Standard treatment at the present time is surgery followed by a platinum drug-based chemotherapy regimen. This approach allows many women to lead a relatively symptom-free life for periods of up to 2–3 years.

6. Chemotherapy of epithelial ovarian tumours with platinum agents, either alone or in combination, will prolong the patient's life but is unlikely to result in improved long-term survival. Combinations of platinum drugs with paclitaxel may not offer as great an advantage as first appeared to be the case.

7. At present, the biological factors inherent in each tumour, rather than treatment, determine survival.

8. Germ cell tumours occur in young women. They have a much better prognosis than epithelial tumours. Chemotherapy for germ cell tumours is effective even in advanced and recurrent cases, and fertility can be preserved. A young woman with a solid ovarian tumour should be referred to a gynaecological oncologist. If the diagnosis is made postoperatively, she should always be referred to a specialist team.

9. Primary carcinoma of the fallopian tube is treated like ovarian carcinoma.

References

Alberts DS, Liu PY, Hannigan EV et al 1996 Intraperitoneal cisplatin plus intravenous cyclophosphamide versus intravenous cisplatin plus intravenous cyclophosphamide for stage III ovarian cancer. New England Journal of Medicine 335: 1950–1955.

Anderson MC, Langley FA 1970 Mesonephroid tumours of the ovary. Journal of Clinical Pathology 23: 210–218.

Armstrong DK, Bundy B, Wenzel L, Huang HQ, Baergen R, Lele S Intraperitoneal cisplatin and paclitaxel in ovarian cancer. Gynecologic Oncology Group. New England Journal of Medicine 354: 34–43.

Aziz S, Kuperstein G, Rosen B et al 2001 A genetic epidemiological study of carcinoma of the fallopian tube. Gynecologic Oncology 80: 341–345.

Bankhead CR, Kehoe ST, Austoker J 2005 Symptoms associated with diagnosis of ovarian cancer: a systematic review. BJOG: an International Journal of Obstetrics and Gynaecology 112: 857–865.

Benedet JL, Sergio Pecorelli S, Ngan HYS et al 2006 Staging Classifications and Clinical Practice: Guidelines for Gynaecological Cancers. pp 95–117. www.figo.org/docs/staging_booklet.pdf.

Blackledge G, Lawton F, Redman C, Kelly K 1989 Response of patients in phase II studies of chemotherapy in ovarian cancer: implications for patient treatment and the design of phase II trials. British Journal of Cancer 59: 650–653.

Boyce EA, Kohn EC 2005 Ovarian cancer in the proteomics era: diagnosis, prognosis, and therapeutics targets. International Journal of Gynecological Cancer 15 (Suppl 3): 266–273.

Bristow RE, Tomacruz RS, Armstrong DK, Trimble EL, Montz FJ 2002 Survival effect of maximal cytoreductive surgery for advanced ovarian carcinoma during the platinum era: a meta-analysis. Journal of Clinical Oncology 20: 1248–1259.

Bristow RE, Eisenhauer EL, Santillan A, Chi DS 2007 Delaying the primary surgical effort for advanced ovarian cancer: a systematic review of neoadjuvant chemotherapy and interval cytoreduction. Gynecologic Oncology 104: 480–490.

Buckanovich RJ, Sasaroli D, O'Brien-Jenkins A et al 2007 Tumor vascular proteins as biomarkers in ovarian cancer. Journal of Clinical Oncology 25: 852–861.

Chene G, Penault-Liorca F, LeBoudedec G et al 2009 Ovarian epithelial dysplasia after ovulation induction: time and dose effect. Human Reproduction 24: 132–138.

Czernobilsky B, Silverman BB, Mikuta JJ 1970 Endometrioid carcinoma of the ovary. A clinicopathologic study of 75 cases. Cancer 26: 1141–1152.

Colombo N, Guthrie D, Chiari S et al 2003 International Collaborative Ovarian Neoplasm trial 1: a randomized trial of adjuvant chemotherapy in women with early-stage ovarian cancer. International Collaborative Ovarian Neoplasm (ICON) collaborators. Journal of the National Cancer Institute 95: 125–132.

Drew Y, Calvert H 2008 The potential of PARP inhibitors in genetic breast and ovarian cancers. Annals of the New York Academy of Sciences 1138: 136–145.

Earle CC, Schrag D, Neville BA et al 2006 Effect of surgeon specialty on processes of care and outcomes for ovarian cancer patients. Journal of the National Cancer Institute 98: 172–180.

Goff BA, Mandel LS, Drescher CW et al 2007 Development of an ovarian cancer symptom index: possibilities for earlier detection. Cancer 109: 221–227.

Griffiths CT 1975 Surgical resection of tumor bulk in the primary treatment of ovarian carcinoma. National Cancer Institute Monograph 42: 101–104.

Griffiths CT, Parker LM, Fuller AF Jr 1979 Role of cytoreductive surgical treatment in the management of advanced ovarian cancer. Cancer Treatment Reports 63: 235–240.

Gynecologic Oncology Group Phase II double blind randomized trial evaluating the biologic effect of levonorgestrel on the ovarian epithelium in women at high risk for ovarian cancer (IND# 79,610). http://www.cancer.gov/clinicaltrials/

Harter P, Bois A, Hahmann M et al 2006 Surgery in recurrent ovarian cancer: the Arbeitsgemeinschaft Gynaekologische Onkologie (AGO) DESKTOP OVAR trial. Arbeitsgemeinschaft Gynaekologische Onkologie Ovarian Committee; AGO Ovarian Cancer Study Group. Annals of Surgical Oncology 13: 1702–1710.

Hellström A-C, Silfverswärd C, Nilsson B, Pettersson F 1994 Carcinoma of the fallopian tube. A clinical and histopathological review. The Radiumhemmet series. International Journal of Gynecological Cancer 4: 395–400.

Hirst JE, Gard GB, McIllroy K, Nevell D, Field M 2009 High rates of occult fallopian tube cancer diagnosed at prophylactic bilateral salpingo-oophorectomy. International Journal of Gynecological Cancer 19: 826–829.

Hunter RW, Alexander ND, Soutter WP 1992 Meta-analysis of surgery in advanced ovarian carcinoma: is maximum cytoreductive surgery an independent determinant of prognosis? American Journal of Obstetrics and Gynecology 166: 504–511.

Huang CY, Cheng WF, Lee CN et al 2006 Serum mesothelin in epithelial ovarian carcinoma: a new screening marker and prognostic factor. Anticancer Research 26: 4721–4728.

Jaaback K, Johnson N 2006 Intraperitoneal chemotherapy for the initial management of primary epithelial ovarian cancer. Cochrane Database of Systematic Reviews 1: CD005340.

Jacobs I, Oram D, Fairbanks J, Turner J, Frost C, Grudzinskas JG 1990 A risk of malignancy index incorporating CA 125, ultrasound and menopausal status for the accurate preoperative diagnosis of ovarian cancer. BJOG: an International Journal of Obstetrics and Gynaecology 97: 922–929.

Jänicke F, Hölscher M, Kuhn W et al 1992 Radical surgical procedure improves survival time in patients with recurrent ovarian cancer. Cancer 70: 2129–2136.

Jensen A, Sharif H, Frederiksen K, Kjaer SK 2009 Use of fertility drugs and risk of ovarian cancer: Danish population based cohort study. BMJ (Clinical Research Ed.) 338: a3075.

Junor EJ, Hole DJ, McNulty L, Mason M, Young J 1999 Specialist gynaecologists and survival outcome in ovarian cancer: a Scottish national study of 1866 patients. BJOG: an International Journal of Obstetrics and Gynaecology 106: 1130–1136.

Koonings PP, Campbell K, Mishell DR, Grimes DA 1989 Relative frequency of primary ovarian neoplasms: a 10 year review. Obstetrics and Gynecology 74: 921–926.

Luesley D, Lawton F, Blackledge G et al 1988 Failure of second-look laparotomy to influence survival in epithelial ovarian cancer. The Lancet 2: 599–603.

Maggioni A, Benedetti Panici P, Dell'Anna T et al 2006 Randomised study of systematic lymphadenectomy in patients with epithelial ovarian cancer macroscopically confined to the pelvis. British Journal of Cancer 95: 699–704.

Mahdavi A, Pejovic T, Nezhat F 2006 Induction ovulation and ovarian cancer: a critical review of the literature. Fertility and Sterility 85: 819–826.

Markman M, Bundy BN, Alberts DS et al 2001 Phase III trial of standard-dose intravenous cisplatin plus paclitaxel versus moderately high-dose carboplatin followed by intravenous paclitaxel and intraperitoneal cisplatin in small-volume stage III ovarian carcinoma: an intergroup study of the Gynecologic Oncology Group, Southwestern Oncology Group, and Eastern Cooperative Oncology Group. Journal of Clinical Oncology 19: 1001–1007.

McGuire WP, Hoskins WJ, Brady MF et al 1996 Cyclophosphamide and cisplatin compared with paclitaxel and cisplatin in patients with stage III and stage IV ovarian cancer. New England Journal of Medicine 334: 1–6.

Magrath IT, Lwanga S, Carswell W, Harrison N 1974 Surgical reduction of tumour bulk in management of abdominal Burkitt's lymphoma. BMJ (Clinical Research Ed.) 2: 308–312.

Melin A, Sparén P, Bergqvist A 2007 The risk of cancer and the role of parity in women with endometriosis. Human Reproduction 22: 3021–3026.

National Institute for Health and Clinical Excellence 2003 Guidance on the Use of Paclitaxel in the Treatment of Ovarian Cancer. NICE, London. http://www.nice.org.uk/pdf/55_Paclitaxel_ovarianreviewfullguidance.pdf

Ozols RF, Bundy BN, Greer BE et al 2003 Phase III trial of carboplatin and paclitaxel compared with cisplatin and paclitaxel in patients with optimally resected stage III ovarian cancer: a Gynecologic Oncology Group study. Journal of Clinical Oncology 21: 3194–3200.

Panici PB, Maggioni A, Hacker N et al 2005 Systematic aortic and pelvic lymphadenectomy versus resection of bulky nodes only in optimally debulked advanced ovarian cancer: a randomized clinical trial. Journal of the National Cancer Institute 97: 560–566.

Parmar MK, Ledermann JA, Colombo N et al 2003 Paclitaxel plus platinum-based chemotherapy versus conventional platinum-based chemotherapy in women with relapsed ovarian cancer: the ICON4/AGO-OVAR-2.2 trial. The Lancet 361: 2099–2106.

Piccart MJ, Bertelsen K, James K et al 2000 Randomized intergroup trial of cisplatin-paclitaxel versus cisplatin-cyclophosphamide in women with advanced epithelial ovarian cancer: three-year results. Journal of the National Cancer Institute 92: 699–708.

Redman CWE, Warwick J, Luesley DM, Varma R, Lawton FG, Blackledge GPR 1994 Intervention debulking surgery in advanced epithelial ovarian cancer. BJOG: an International Journal of Obstetrics and Gynaecology 101: 142–146.

Rose PG, Nerenstone S, Brady MF et al 2004 Secondary surgical cytoreduction for advanced ovarian carcinoma. Gynecologic Oncology Group. New England Journal of Medicine 351: 2489–2497.

Salani R, Santillan A, Zahurak ML et al 2007 Secondary cytoreductive surgery for localized, recurrent epithelial ovarian cancer: analysis of prognostic factors and survival outcome. Cancer 109: 685–691.

Scully RE 1999 WHO International Histological Classification of Tumor. Histologic Typing of Ovarian Tumours. Springer, Heidelberg.

Seidman JD, Kurman RJ 2000 Ovarian serous borderline tumors: a critical review of the literature with emphasis on prognostic indicators. Human Pathology 31: 539–556.

Smith JP, Delgado G, Rutledge F 1976 Second-look operation in ovarian carcinoma: postchemotherapy. Cancer 38: 1438–1442.

Steed H, Oza AM, Murphy J et al 2006 A retrospective analysis of neoadjuvant platinum-based chemotherapy versus up-front surgery in advanced ovarian cancer. International Journal of Gynecological Cancer 16 (Suppl 1): 47–53.

Swart AM, Burdett S, Ledermann J, Mook P, Parmar MK 2008 Why i.p. therapy cannot yet be considered as a standard of care for the first-line treatment of ovarian cancer: a systematic review. Annals of Oncology 19: 688–695.

Tingulstad S, Skjeldestad FE, Hagen B 2003 The effect of centralization of primary surgery on survival in ovarian cancer patients. Obstetrics and Gynecology 102: 499–505.

Trimbos JB, Vergote I, Bolis G et al 2003 Impact of adjuvant chemotherapy and surgical staging in early-stage ovarian carcinoma: European Organisation for Research and Treatment of Cancer-Adjuvant ChemoTherapy in Ovarian Neoplasm trial. EORTC-ACTION collaborators. European Organisation for Research and Treatment of Cancer-

Adjuvant ChemoTherapy in Ovarian Neoplasm. Journal of the National Cancer Institute 95: 94–95.

van der Burg ME, van Lent M, Buyse M et al 1995 The effect of debulking surgery after induction chemotherapy on the prognosis in advanced epithelial ovarian cancer. Gynecological Cancer Cooperative Group of the European Organization for Research and Treatment of Cancer. New England Journal of Medicine 332: 629–634.

Wenzel LB, Huang HQ, Armstrong DK, Walker JL, Cella D 2007 Health-related quality of life during and after intraperitoneal versus intravenous chemotherapy for optimally debulked ovarian cancer: a Gynecologic Oncology Group Study. Journal of Clinical Oncology 25: 437–443.

Zang RY, Li ZT, Tang J et al 2004 Secondary cytoreductive surgery for patients with relapsed epithelial ovarian carcinoma: who benefits? Cancer 100: 1152–1161.

CHAPTER 46

Benign disease of the breast

Paul TR Thiruchelvam, William E. Svensson and John Lynn

Chapter Contents

STAGES OF HUMAN BREAST DEVELOPMENT	689		PROLIFERATIVE STROMAL LESIONS	697
CONGENITAL ABNORMALITIES	689		BREAST DISORDERS RELATED TO PREGNANCY AND LACTATION	697
ABERRATIONS OF NORMAL DEVELOPMENT AND INVOLUTION	690		NON-LACTATIONAL INFECTIONS	700
NIPPLE DISCHARGE	692		BENIGN NEOPLASMS OF THE BREAST	700
MASTALGIA	694		OTHER BREAST MASSES	702
FIBROCYSTIC CHANGE	695		KEY POINTS	703

More than 90% of women presenting to a breast clinic will have benign breast disease (BBD), a heterogeneous condition consisting of a large number of pathophysiological lesions of the different components of the breast (stromal, epithelial, vascular or adipocytes). BBD can be divided into congenital abnormalities, aberrations of normal breast development and involution (ANDI), and conditions secondary to another extrinsic factor. The ANDI classification (1987) of BBD enables a framework and states that breasts are under endocrine control and have a wide range of appearances during reproductive life. The incidence of BBD is difficult to estimate, as women with BBD are often not symptomatic and many do not present for a consultation. However, the incidence of BBD can be estimated by the prevalence in post-mortem examinations and cohort studies.

Stages of Human Breast Development

The lifecycle of the breast involves three main stages: development (and early reproductive life), mature reproductive life and involution. The mammary buds develop during the sixth week as outgrowths of epidermis into the underlying mesenchyme. These mammary buds develop as downgrowths from mammary crests, which are thickened strips of ectoderm extending from the axilla to the inguinal region. During the fourth week, the mammary crests appear and persist in humans in the pectoral region where the breasts develop (Sandler 2006). Several mammary buds developing from each primary bud eventually form lactiferous ducts, and by gestation 15–20 lactiferous ducts are formed. The adipose tissue and fibrous connective tissue of the breast develop from the surrounding mesenchyme. In the late fetal period, the epidermis at the origin of the mammary gland forms a shallow mammary pit, from which the nipples arise soon after birth due to epithelial proliferation of the surrounding connective tissue of the areola. At birth, the mammary glands of males and females are identical, enlarged and, on occasion, may produce a secretion called 'witch's milk'. The mammary gland remains undeveloped until puberty, with only the main lactiferous duct formed.

Breast development proceeds identically in boys and girls until puberty. During puberty, the female breast enlarges rapidly. The elevated level of circulating oestrogens causes growth of the ductal system; however, progesterones, growth hormone, prolactin and corticoids also play a role. During pregnancy, an increase in the number of lobules and a loss of fat occurs due to raised oestrogen levels and a sustained increase in the level of progesterone. The intralobular ducts form buds that become acini; the lactating breast is composed of dilated acini that contain milk. During weaning, following the suckling stimulus, the breast involutes and the secretory cells are removed by apoptosis and phagocytosis (Howard and Gusterson 2000). The two-layer epithelium of the breast is reformed following weaning. Following successive pregnancies and periods of involution, the terminal duct lobular units (the functional unit of the breast) increase and decrease in size, with an increase and decrease in the number of acini. During involution, the breast stroma is replaced by fat and, as a result, the breast becomes less radiodense, softer and more ptotic (Dixon 1994).

Congenital Abnormalities

These disorders are not uncommon referrals at breast clinics and can cause considerable concern.

DOI: 10.1016/B978-0-7020-3120-5.00046-1

Accessory breast tissue and supernumerary nipples

Accessory breast tissue consists of ectopic breast tissue resulting from the failure of the embryonic mammary ridge to regress, commonly found in the anterior axillary line (Qian et al 2008). This occurs in 0.4–0.6% of the population, although is more common in Asian women, and is bilateral in one-third of cases. Accessory breast tissue can cause discomfort, cosmetic problems and restriction in arm movement. This breast tissue may become prominent during pregnancy, and both benign and malignant conditions may occur within this tissue. An explanation of the 'abnormality' and reassurance is often all that is required, and surgical excision should be reserved for symptomatic patients as a good cosmetic outcome is difficult and associated with significant morbidity.

The nipple is normally positioned slightly inferomedial to the centre of the breast. The nipple areola complex is composed of pigmented squamous epithelium, but also contains a layer of circumferential smooth muscle and sebaceous glands which open through small prominences (Montgomery tubercles) surrounding the periphery of the areola. Common congenital malformations, including supernumerary nipple or nipples, may be found along the milk-line extending bilaterally from the axilla to the groin. Most commonly, these supernumerary or accessory nipples are found below the breast and above the umbilicus, with the most inferior location being the proximal medial thigh. Should an accessory nipple become irritating, excision can be offered.

Breast hypoplasia and Poland syndrome

Breast hypoplasia is failure of a breast to fully develop, which is usually unilateral but may be bilateral. Breast asymmetry usually only requires reassurance, but if asymmetry is significant, augmentation of the affected side with or without the contralateral breast may be required. Breast hypoplasia may be associated with tubular breasts; a deformity that can affect one or both breasts as a result of constriction at the base of the breasts, limiting growth. Surgical intervention in this group is often difficult and unsatisfactory.

Poland syndrome is a group of conditions in which amastia develops with varying degrees of absence of the pectoralis muscles and syndactyly, affecting one in 30,000 live births (Figure 46.1). It was first described by Alfred Poland in 1841, whilst he was a medical student at Guys Hospital, London (Ram and Chung 2009). Subsequent reports have added numerous additional components to the syndrome including mammary hypoplasia, costal cartilage defects and rib defects. One study evaluating 75 patients showed 100% with an absence or hypoplasia of the pectoralis major, 67% with a hand abnormality, and 49% with athelia (congenital absence of one or both nipples) and/or amastia (breast tissue, nipple and areola is absent; differs from amazia which only involves the absence of breast tissue, and the nipple and areola remain present) (Katz et al 2001). The syndrome is almost always unilateral, with the right side more often affected than the left side, and is more common in men than women (3:1). Patients with Poland syndrome often request reconstruction of the muscular

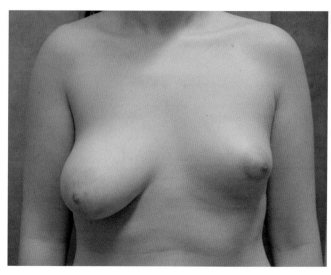

Figure 46.1 Poland syndrome (right side).
Image courtesy of Jacqueline Lewis, Imperial College NHS Trust, London, UK.

defect, producing symmetry and improving psychological well-being. This can be performed with an ipsilateral latissimus dorsi pedicled flap with or without an implant.

Aberrations of Normal Development and Involution

Most BBD arises from normal physiological processes, ranging from mild abnormality (aberration) to severe abnormality (disease). The breast passes through three phases relating to circulating hormone levels: development, cyclical change and involution.

Juvenile hypertrophy

Generalized hypertrophy of the adolescent breast is known as 'juvenile hypertrophy' and, in some cases, 'juvenile gigantomastia'. It can be bilateral or unilateral and is characterized by diffuse enlargement of the breast without nodularity or discrete masses. Growth of the breast is usually rapid and can be significant. Breasts can grow to be as large as 13–23 kg. The pathophysiology is thought to involve an abnormal response of the breast to hormonal stimulation, but the exact mechanism is not known. Hypertrophy is not associated with elevation in serum oestrogen, progesterone, prolactin or gonadotropins, and evidence is lacking for an increased number of oestrogen receptors in the breast. The weight of the breasts can cause back and neck pain, shoulder grooving, poor posture and an inability to perform daily tasks.

Psychological stress and social embarrassment are also common in these young women in whom body image is developing. Histologically, the breast shows stromal and ductal hyperplasia with dilated ducts. The treatment in most cases is reduction mammaplasty, for which there are a number of techniques. Depending on the timing of the operation in relation to puberty, there is a risk of recurrent hypertrophy of the remaining breast tissue, which may require further surgery. The closer surgery is to the end of puberty, the greater the chance of a permanent reduction in size. Hypertrophy of remaining breast tissue can occur with pregnancy. Several reports have shown that giving danazol during rapid breast enlargement has some benefit.

Premature breast development between the age of 6 months and 9 years requires investigation for signs of precocious puberty. Pubic hair, accelerated bone growth and genital development may be signs of an ovarian or adrenal tumour. Isolated thelarche [first stage of secondary (postnatal) breast development] can be observed, but patients should undergo careful physical examination every 6–12 months to look for other signs of puberty. Isolated breast development in the prepubertal child should regress within 1–2 years. Persistent or progressive development in the prepubertal child that does not regress requires endocrine assessment.

Fibroadenoma

Fibroadenomas are classified as an aberration of normal development, arising from the hormone-sensitive terminal ductal lobular unit, typically composed of stromal and epithelial cells. The stromal element defines its behaviour and classification.

Simple fibroadenoma

These are discrete, firm, highly mobile, benign breast masses which may present symptomatically or as an incidental screening finding. Fibroadenomas usually present unilaterally; however, in 20% of cases, multiple lesions may present in the same breast or bilaterally. They are found most commonly at the time of greatest lobular development in women aged 15–35 years. The encapsulation explains the motility of the masses, making them appear more superficial than they truly are (Figure 46.2). Fibroadenomas develop from the special stroma of the lobule. They are hormone dependent, lactate during pregnancy and involute with the rest of the breast in the perimenopause (Hughes et al 1987). A direct association has been reported between use of the oral contraceptive pill before the age of 20 years and risk of fibroadenoma. The Epstein–Barr virus is thought to play a causative role in the development of this tumour in immunosuppressed patients (Kleer et al 2002). Observation of fibroadenomas in younger women showed that 55% do not change size, 37% get smaller and 8% increase in size. Fifty percent of fibroadenomas contain other proliferative changes such as adenosis, sclerosing adenosis and duct epithelial hyperplasia; these are known as 'complex fibroadenomas'. Complex fibroadenomas, but not simple fibroadenomas, are associated with an increased risk of breast cancer (Carter et al 2001). Fibroadenomas in older women or in women with a family history of breast cancer have a higher risk of associated breast cancer (Dupont et al 1994, Shabtai et al 2001).

Fibroadenomas over 5 cm in size are known as 'giant fibroadenomas', and are seen more commonly in women of African origin. Cancers rarely appear within a fibroadenoma. Patients with a histologically confirmed fibroadenoma can be managed conservatively, with follow-up imaging at 6 months to confirm that the lesion is not increasing in size. Excision is recommended if the mass increases in size, if it

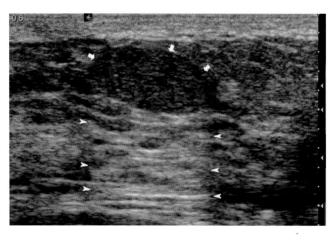

Figure 46.2 Fibroadenoma. Oval area of reduced echogenicity (arrows) with bright up due to good through transmission of sound and brighter echos deep to the fibroadenoma (arrow heads).
Image courtesy of Dr William E. Svensson, Consultant Radiologist, Imperial College NHS Trust, London, UK.

is larger than 3–4 cm or at the patient's request. Recurrence is rarely due to incomplete excision, and is often due to an undiagnosed adjacent mass. A minimally invasive technique, such as ultrasound-guided cryoablation, is a treatment option for fibroadenomas in women who do not wish to have surgery (Caleffi et al 2004). Rapid growth of a fibroadenoma can occur in adolescence (juvenile fibroadenoma) or in women of perimenopausal age. Juvenile fibroadenomas usually present as painless, solitary unilateral masses over 5 cm in size (reaching up to 15–20 cm). Although benign, surgical excision of these masses is advised (Wechselberger et al 2002).

Phyllodes tumour

Johannes Muller (1838) first described a large mammary tumour with a cystic appearance and leaf-like growth pattern; he named this 'cystosarcoma phyllodes'. Treves and Sunderland (1951) proposed that benign, premalignant and malignant forms of this disease existed. The term 'phyllodes tumour' (PT) was adopted by the World Health Organization in 1981 to describe this rare fibroepithelial lesion, which accounts for less than 1% of all breast neoplasms. They are less common than fibroadenomas (ratio 1:40), from which they need to be distinguished. PTs can present in women of any age, including adolescents and the elderly, but the majority occur in women aged 35–55 years; the median age of presentation is 45 years. PTs present clinically as a well-circumscribed, mobile mass which may be growing rapidly. The size of presentation of PTs is larger than that for fibroadenomas, although with increased breast awareness and the advent of breast screening, there has been a trend towards smaller tumours. Other signs and symptoms include dilated skin veins, blue skin discolouration, nipple retraction, fixation to the skin or pectoralis muscle, and pressure necrosis of the skin. Palpable axillary lymphadenopathy has been identified in up to 20% of patients, but axillary metastatic involvement is rare. PTs are more commonly found in the upper outer quadrant of the breast. Prevalence is higher in Latin American White and Asian populations. Certain clinical features may raise the index of suspicion, including a sudden increase in a longstanding breast mass, a fibroadenoma over 3 cm in size in a patient aged over 35 years, lobulated appearance on mammography, cystic areas within a solid mass on ultrasonography, and indeterminate features on fine needle aspiration cytology (FNAC) (Jacklin et al 2006). PTs are often not clinically distinguishable from fibroadenomas.

PTs often mimic fibroadenomas at mammography, appearing as large, well-circumscribed, oval or lobulated masses with rounded borders, and a radiolucent halo or coarse microcalcifications. Ultrasonography often shows a non-homogeneous, solid mass, with low-level internal echoes and smooth walls. Discovery of a cyst within a solid mass is highly suggestive of a PT. Dynamic enhancement patterns on magnetic resonance imaging may be useful for the diagnosis of tumours over 3 cm in size, although the role has not been fully elucidated.

Diagnosis of PTs by FNAC is associated with a high false-positive rate due to the heterogeneity of the tumours. The risk of sampling error is reduced following a core biopsy. Criteria have been formulated to help physicians to select patients for core biopsy — the Paddington Clinicopathologic Suspicion Score (Jacklin et al 2006). Twenty-five percent of PTs are categorized as malignant and more than 50% are categorized as benign, with a number of prognostic factors implicated in the risk of local and distant recurrence including tumour size, grade and margin status. Benign PTs have the potential to recur locally, and rarely present at distant sites. Despite having an increased risk of distant spread (20%), malignant lesions have a 15-year survival rate of 89%.

Wide local excision with margins over 1 cm is the preferred primary treatment of PTs, as microprojections of tumour frequently extend into the pseudocapsule of normal tissue surrounding the lesion. One study in which 99% of the patients had histologically negative margins still reported an 8% local recurrence rate, suggesting that risk of recurrence can be reduced with negative margins but not eliminated completely. Adjuvant chemotherapy and hormonal therapy has no role in the treatment of PTs, and there is no high-level evidence to support the role of radiotherapy in these lesions. Local recurrence will occur in 15% of patients with PTs, mostly within 2 years of initial surgery (range 1 month–17 years). These tumours generally present with the same histology, and guidelines advise re-excision with wide margins; the role of adjuvant radiotherapy is controversial. Metastatic lesions often develop within 3 years at sites including the lung, bone and abdominal viscera, with a poor prognosis and average survival of less than 2 years.

Nipple Discharge

Nipple discharge accounts for approximately 5% of breast clinic referrals. Important features to determine include whether the discharge is from one duct or several, is spontaneous or induced, and affects one or more breasts. It is important to note the colour, frequency and consistency of the discharge, with the aim of determining whether the cause of the discharge is physiological or pathological. Fluid can be elicited from the nipple by gentle manipulation in the majority of women (85%) regardless of age or health. Should the nipple discharge present with a mass, the management is directed to the diagnosis of the breast mass. Although nipple discharge usually has a benign aetiology, some studies have shown that the incidence of breast cancer is between 9.3% and 21.3% in women with pathological nipple discharge.

Assessment includes a thorough breast examination to ascertain whether a breast lump is present. Firm areola pressure can identify a dilated duct (and pressure over the duct can produce discharge). Firm digital pressure of the nipple can elicit fluid, and the site and character of the discharge can be noted. The presence of blood can be determined by testing the discharge for haemoglobin; however, only 10% of patients with bloodstained discharge will have an underlying malignancy. The sensitivity of Hemoccult (a guaiac reagent strip test for occult blood) has been shown to be only 50%. Mammography should be performed in women over 35 years of age as part of the assessment, with a sensitivity of 57% in this group. Ultrasonography can identify malignant lesions and papillomas. If no abnormality is found, any patient presenting with spontaneous single duct discharge should undergo surgery if it is associated with a mass, bloodstained or persistent (more than twice per week). Postmenopausal women with new serosanguineous discharge should also undergo surgery.

Ductoscopy allows direct visualization of the discharging duct, and biopsy, by a microendoscope, was investigated by Okazaki in the early 1990s. The procedure is carried out using local anaesthesia (topical local anesthetic cream plus intradermal local anesthetic injection at the areolar margin) and has no significant complications (Escobar et al 2006). An endoscope is inserted through the duct opening on the nipple surface after dilating the duct with a probe (e.g. lacrimal dilator), and saline solution is injected into the duct through the channel to widen it and facilitate the passage of the endoscope, enabling visualization of the intraductal space (Escobar et al 2006). Whilst ductoscopy can be used as a diagnostic and therapeutic addition in patients with nipple discharge, there is no evidence to support its use in the management or early detection of breast cancer.

A major limitation of nipple aspirate fluid is that insufficient material is present for cytology, which prompted the development of ductal lavage. By cannulating and irrigating a discharging duct, ductal lavage fluid can be sent for cytology (increasing cell yield by 100 times compared with ductal discharge). Ductal lavage is not sufficiently accurate for the assessment of patients with known breast cancers. One study has reported sensitivity of 17% for the diagnosis of breast cancer in the setting of a known malignancy. A number of groups are using a genomic approach to investigate nipple aspirate for malignant potential. Methylation of promoter regions of tumour suppressor genes is common in breast cancer, resulting in silencing of tumour suppressor genes. Promoter hypermethylation has been demonstrated in nipple aspirate fluid of patients with ductal carcinoma in situ (DCIS) and invasive ductal carcinoma. Nipple aspirate may become a surrogate for breast tissue, enabling many types of cellular and genomic assessment without a biopsy. Further advances in intraduct technology and techniques may add to our understanding of the biological progression of breast cancer, its prevention and treatment.

The aetiology of non-surgically-treated nipple discharge can be grouped into four categories:

- Physiological — includes lactation in the peripartum period, normal breast secretions which may be elicited by manual stimulation of the breast (note: all spontaneous discharge must be fully assessed by a clinician).
- Pathological endocrine causes (increased prolactin secretion or failure of normal prolactin inhibition) — prolactinomas are the most common secretory tumours of the anterior pituitary causing unilateral/bilateral galactorrhoea. Primary hypothyroidism can cause hyperprolactinaemia; rarely, bronchogenic carcinomas may result in ectopic production of prolactin. Other causes of increased prolactin include head trauma, encephalitis and hypothalamic infiltration (sarcoid/tumour).
- Pharmacological — several drugs can increase prolactin and galactorrhoea including: (1) psychoactive medication (e.g. phenothiazines, tricyclic antidepressants, selective serotonin reuptake inhibitors, haloperidol and anxiolytics), (2) antihypertensives (e.g. calcium channel blockers, methyldopa, reserpine), (3) gastrointestinal medication (e.g. metoclopramide, cimetidine, rantidine), (4) oestrogens (conjugated oestrogen and medroxyprogesterone acetate), (5) anaesthetics and (6) amphetamines and marijuana.
- Idiopathic — galactorrhoea is a bilateral, copious milky-white discharge from multiple ducts. If the prolactin level is raised (>1000 mIU/l), the cause may be secondary to medication or a primary tumour. If the prolactin level is normal, the patient can be reassured. Excision of the subareola ducts may be required in the case of persistent symptoms.

Duct ectasia

Duct ectasia is characterized by dilatation and shortening of the terminal ducts within 3 cm of the nipple. It is a common condition, increasing with age; post-mortem findings have reported duct ectasia in 24% of all women and in 43% of women over 60 years of age. It may present as a white or green viscous discharge, occasionally bloodstained. The colour of discharge varies significantly and can differ between ducts in the same breast. The nipple discharge may be either spontaneous or expressed by the patient. It typically comes from two or three ducts and may be bilateral. It is not known whether the primary event is inflammatory in origin, or whether lactation and stagnation of secretions leads to a secondary inflammation.

Intraductal papilloma and papillomatosis

Intraductal papillomas are benign intraductal proliferations, usually found in the major ducts beneath the nipple (lactiferous sinuses); however, they can be found anywhere in the breast. The term 'papilloma' describes the fibrovascular cores covered by a double layer of cells comprising an outer myoepithelial layer and an inner luminal cell layer (Mallon et al 2000). The cells are cytologically benign. Squamous and apocrine metaplasia are common findings. There are three types of intraduct papilloma: solitary, multiple or juvenile papillomas. Solitary duct papillomas are the most common; these occur in large ducts (within 5 cm of the nipple) and present with either bloody or a serous single duct discharge (Figure 46.3). Two studies have demonstrated a correlation between the presence of atypical ductal hyperplasia (ADH) in a papillary lesion on needle core biopsy and the presence of invasive or in-situ carcinoma of the breast in the excisional biopsy (Agoff and Lawton 2004, Ivan et al 2004). It has been suggested that the risk of recurrence of papilloma is related to the presence of proliferative breast lesions in the surrounding breast tissue (MacGrogan and Tavassoli 2003). Papillomatosis (multiple intraductal papillomas; 10% of intraductal papilloma) is defined as a minimum of five discrete papillomas within a localized segment of breast tissue. Papillomatosis tends to occur in younger patients and is less often associated with nipple discharge. Multiple papillomas are more frequently peripheral, bilateral, present as a palpable mass and have a higher probability of having an in-situ or invasive carcinoma than central papilloma. Thorough radiological imaging of the contralateral breast is required

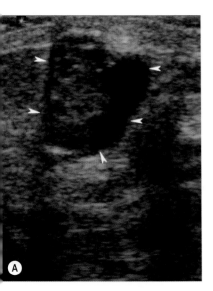
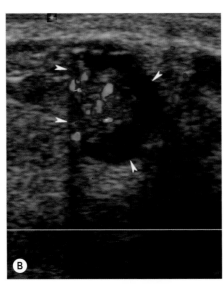

Figure 46.3 Intraduct papilloma. (A) The intraduct papilloma can be seen within the slightly dilated duct (arrow heads) allowing it to be differentiated from other lesions of reduced heterogeneous echogenicity. Intraduct papillomas are often quite vascular, which can be demonstrated with colour Doppler (B).

to exclude malignancy (Ali-Fehmi et al 2003). Multiple papillomas are associated with an increased risk of developing subsequent breast cancer (Krieger and Hiatt 1992, Page et al 1996, Levshin et al 1998). Juvenile papillomatosis is a rare condition defined as severe ductal papillomatosis occurring in women under 30 years of age (median age 20 years). It often presents as a discrete mass up to 8 cm in diameter, and consists of a mixture of cysts, nodules of sclerosing adenosis and complex intraduct proliferations containing myoepithelial cells and luminal cells. Due to the holes seen in the cut surface of the tumour, it has been called 'Swiss cheese disease'. A number of studies have suggested an association between juvenile papillomatosis and familial breast cancer; therefore, long-term follow-up is advised (Bazzocchi et al 1986).

Bloody nipple discharge in pregnancy

Bloody nipple discharge during pregnancy or lactation is a common finding. It occurs in 20% of women who present with nipple discharge during pregnancy, and is likely to be due to the increased vascularity of the developing tissue. It is benign and requires no specific treatment.

Ductal carcinoma *in situ*

Approximately one-third of symptomatic ductal carcinomas present with nipple discharge, and invasive cancers rarely cause nipple discharge in the absence of a mass. DCIS is thought to be responsible for approximately 10% of cases of unilateral nipple discharge.

Surgical treatment of nipple discharge

Historically, all patients with pathological nipple discharge are offered an operation. Patients with surgically significant nipple discharge aged 40 years or more are recommended to undergo Hadfield's procedure (radical subareolar duct excision). Patients under 40 years of age with persistant discharge are given the option of microdocectomy, particularly if they are intending to breast feed.

Microdocectomy

Microdocectomy involves the removal of a single duct through a circumareolar incision. Expression of nipple discharge is performed when the patient is in theatre, and the duct is then cannulated with a lacrimal probe. The probe aids identification of the discharging duct and enables the surgeon to dissect it from the surrounding tissue. At least 2–3 cm of duct should be removed and the excised duct should be opened and the distal remnant inspected. The procedure should not damage the surrounding ducts and should therefore allow subsequent breast feeding.

Total duct excision (Hadfield's operation)

In women of non-childbearing age, total/major duct excision is a surgical option for single duct discharge, multiple duct discharge and periductal mastitis. The procedure involves division of ducts underneath the nipple and removing the breast tissue to a depth of 2 cm under the nipple–areolar complex through a circumareolar incision. Complications include nipple necrosis, nipple inversion and reduced nipple sensation. Recurrence of periductal mastitis may occur if all of the ducts are not removed during the operation. The procedure can also be performed in women having a cosmetic nipple eversion procedure.

Mastalgia

The majority of women will suffer from mastalgia (breast pain) at some point in their lives. It is important to differentiate true mastalgia (originating from the breast) from referred pain. Referred pain is often unilateral, reproduced by pressure on the chest wall and associated with activity. Non-steroidal anti-inflammatory drugs, either orally or topically, can improve these symptoms. True breast pain is associated with swelling and nodularity, and can resolve spontaneously. This pain is often worse before menstruation and is relieved after the cessation of menstruation. It is not important to differentiate between non-cyclical and cyclical mastalgia as the treatment is the same. Symptoms may be exacerbated by exogenous hormones (hormone replacement therapy or oral contraceptive pill) and the perimenopausal state. The cause of mastalgia is unknown, but a number of theories have been postulated including excess oestrogen or prolactin, and low progesterone.

Assessment includes history, examination and, in women over 35 years of age, mammography. Five percent of women with breast cancer complain of pain, whilst only 2.7% of women with breast pain as their only complaint will have an underlying breast cancer. A pain chart can allow better interpretation of the pattern of pain and gives an objective evaluation of treatment.

The majority of patients can be managed by exclusion of cancer and reassurance. Evening primrose oil (EPO) was previously used in the treatment of mastalgia, but has recently been withdrawn from prescription by the Medicines Control Agency. A recent randomized, double-blind controlled trial of 121 women comparing EPO and fish oil with control oils in the treatment of mastalgia showed no clear benefit from either EPO or fish oils (Blommers et al 2002). This study showed that 33% of women with cyclical mastalgia and 17% of women with non-cyclical mastalgia showed an improvement in symptoms with EPO compared with the control group (46% and 17% improvement, respectively). Other agents have shown some benefit, including phytoestrogens (soya milk) and *Vitex agnus-castus* (a fruit extract). A reduction in dietary fat intake has also been shown to improve symptoms. Second-line treatments include tamoxifen 10 mg daily and danazol 200 mg daily. Tamoxifen given in the luteal phase of the menstrual cycle controlled mastalgia in 85% of women, with recurrent pain noted in 25% of patients at 1 year. Tamoxifen has been found to be superior to danazol with a better toxicity profile. Fifty-three percent of patients receiving tamoxifen compared with 37% of patients receiving danazol were pain-free after 1 year. It is important to note that tamoxifen is not licenced for use in mastalgia. Due to the high toxicity rate (80%), bromocriptine is no longer used in the treatment of mastalgia.

Fibrocystic Change

Fibrocystic change (FCC; also called fibrocystic disease, cystic mastopathy, chronic cystic disease, mazoplazia, Reculus's disease) is the most common benign disorder of the breast, affecting women between 20 and 50 years of age (Cole et al 1978, Hutchinson et al 1980, Cook and Rohan 1985, La Vecchia et al 1985, Bartow et al 1987, Sarnelli and Squartini 1991, Fitzgibbons et al 1998). FCC is observed in approximately 50% of women clinically and in 90% histologically (Love et al 1982). The most common symptoms of FCC are breast pain and tender nodularity. FCC is thought to be due to a hormonal imbalance, particularly the predominance of oestrogen over progesterone; however, the pathogenesis is not completely understood (Dupont and Page 1985). FCC is made up of cystic lesions (macrocystic and microcystic) and solid lesions, and includes adenosis, epithelial hyperplasia with or without atypia, apocrine metaplasia, papilloma and radial scar. FCC can be classified into non-proliferative lesions, and proliferative lesions with or without aytpia (atypical hyperplasia) (Dupont and Page 1985).

- Non-proliferative lesions — cysts, papillary apocrine change, epithelial-related calcifications, duct ectasia, non-sclerosing adenosis, periductal fibrosis and mild epithelial hyperplasia.
- Proliferative lesions without atypia — moderate/florid ductal hyperplasia of usual type, sclerosing adenosis, intraduct papilloma, papillomatosis and radial scar.
- Proliferative changes with atypia — ADH and lobular hyperplasia.

Non-proliferative lesions are not associated with an increased risk of developing breast cancer; however, women with proliferative disease without atypia and with atypia are at greater risk of breast cancer (relative risk 1.3–1.9 and 3.9–13.0, respectively) (Dupont and Page 1985, Palli et al 1991, Dupont et al 1993, Marshall et al 1997). Age is thought to play a key role, with the risk of breast cancer in young women with a diagnosis of atypical epithelial proliferation twice that of a women over 55 years of age with a similar diagnosis (Hartmann et al 2005).

Breast cysts

Breast cysts are fluid-filled, ovoid/round structures affecting one-third of women between 35 and 50 years of age. The majority are subclinical 'microcysts', but approximately 20–25% are palpable 'macrocysts' which are a common presentation at breast clinics (Haagenson 1986). Macrocysts are often multiple and appear in the fifth decade. Cysts are derived from the terminal duct lobular unit, and in most cysts, the epithelial lining is either flattened or absent (non-apocrine cysts). In a few cysts, the apocrine epithelial lining can be observed (apocrine cysts). Apocrine cysts have a higher recurrence rate than non-apocrine cysts (Dixon et al 1999). Breast cysts have mammographically characteristic halos, but cannot be reliably distinguished from solid masses; therefore, ultrasonography and fine needle aspiration (if indicated) are used for diagnosis (Figure 46.4). Ultrasonography can also distinguish between simple and complex cysts, and a cyst wall with any projections may

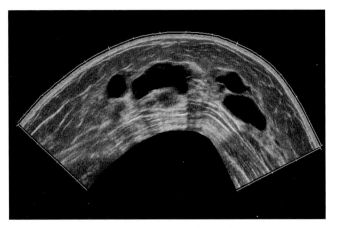

Figure 46.4 Multiple breast cysts within the breast demonstrated on an extended field to view ultrasound image. Cysts contain fluid and are usually anechoic and exhibit marked bright up (increased echogenicity) deep to them.

Image courtesy of Dr William E. Svensson, Consultant Radiologist, Imperial College NHS Trust, London, UK.

indicate carcinoma or an intracystic papilloma which necessitates either a core needle biopsy or a surgical excision biopsy (Vargas et al 2004, Houssami et al 2005). Complex (complicated/atypical) cysts, reported in approximately 5% of all breast ultrasounds, are characterized by internal echoes or thin septations, thickened and/or irregular wall, and absent posterior enhancement (Houssami et al 2005). Asymptomatic cysts are left alone but large painful cysts can be aspirated to dryness. Any bloodstained fluid should be sent for histology, and if a palpable mass is still evident after aspiration, further investigations are indicated. Cysts may recur following aspiration. There is a slightly increased relative risk of breast cancer in women with cysts.

Adenosis

Adenosis of the breast is characterized by an increase in either the number or size of glandular components, usually involving the lobular units. Sclerosing adenosis is a benign lesion of disordered acinar, myoepithelial and connective tissue which can mimic carcinoma (Jensen et al 1989). It can present as a palpable mass or as a suspicious finding at mammography, and is associated with other proliferative lesions including epithelial hyperplasia, papillomas, complex sclerosing lesions, apocrine changes and calcification. A number of studies have shown that it is a risk factor for invasive cancer. Microglandular adenosis is characterized by a proliferation of small, round glands distributed irregularly within dense fibrous and/or adipose tissue. Notably, microglandular adenosis lacks the outer layer of myoepithelia seen in other tissue types of adenosis. This lack of myoepithelial layer makes it difficult to differentiate from tubular carcinoma (Eusebi et al 1993). The absence of epithelial membrane antigen staining in the luminal epithelial cells, and the presence of basal lamina encircling glandular structures demonstrated by laminin or type IV collagen immunostaining distinguishes between microglandular adenosis and tubular carcinoma (Eusebi et al 1993). Microadenosis has a tendency to recur if not completely excised, and although it is defined as benign, there is growing evidence of the potential of this lesion to become invasive carcinoma (Acs et al 2003). Apocrine (adenomyoepithelial) adenosis is a variant of microglandular adenosis. Apocrine adenosis describes a wide spectrum of lesions, and in this case describes apocrine changes in the specific underlying lesion (deformed lobular unit, sclerosing adenosis, radial scars and complex sclerosing lesions) (O'Malley and Bane 2004). Tubular adenosis is a rare variant of microglandular adenosis that can be distinguished from tubular carcinoma by the presence of an intact myoepithelial layer around the tubules (Lee et al 1996).

Metaplasia

Apocrine metaplasia is characterized by columnar cells with granular, eosinophilic cytoplasm and luminal cytoplasmic projections (Guray and Sahin 2006). These cells line dilated ducts and are more frequently seen in younger women. When the nuclei of the apocrine cells display significant atypia, this is known as 'atypical apocrine metaplasia'. Clear cell metaplasia of the breast is morphologically similar to clear cell carcinoma; however, its immunohistochemical staining is similar to an 'eccrine' sweat gland (Vina and Wells 1989).

Epithelial hyperplasia

Epithelial hyperplasia is the most common form of proliferative breast disease. There are two types of epithelial hyperplasia — ductal and lobular epithelial hyperplasia — and these can be difficult to distinguish. It can also be difficult to distinguish between usual ductal/lobular hyperplasia and atypical ductal/lobular hyperplasia.

Ductal hyperplasia

Normal breast ducts are lined by two layers of cuboidal cells with specialized luminal borders and basal contractile myoepithelial cells. Epithelial hyperplasia is defined as an increase in cells within the ductal space. The degree of architectural and cytological features of the proliferating cells further classifies hyperplasia. Usual ductal hyperplasia has an increase in the number of cells without architectural distortion, and is not associated with an increased risk of breast cancer. Mild hyperplasia of usual type denotes a three- to four-cell layer of proliferating cells, whereas moderate hyperplasia describes a proliferating layer more than four cells thick. In florid hyperplasia, the lumen is distended and may be obliterated. The most important cytological feature of mild, moderate and florid hyperplasia is the mixture of cell types and variation in appearance of epithelial cells and their nuclei (Koerner 2004).

ADH is a type of hyperplasia that mimics low-grade DCIS. It is a rare condition seen in 4% of symptomatic benign biopsy lesions, and is often small and focal, involving a small part of the duct or a few ducts (Guray and Sahin 2006). More ADH lesions are being detected with the increased use of mammography. Thirty-one percent of biopsies due to microcalcifications show ADH (Pinder and Ellis 2003). Patients with ADH have a four to five times increased risk of developing breast cancer compared with the general population, and the risk is 10 times greater compared with the general population if the patient has a first-degree relative

with breast cancer. The increased risk of breast cancer is higher in both the ipsilateral and contralateral breasts (Page et al 1985, Tavassoli and Norris 1990). Women with ADH have an increased risk of developing cancer within 10–15 years of diagnosis, with this risk declining after 15 years (Page et al 1985, Dupont and Page 1989). Premenopausal women with ADH have a significantly higher risk of developing breast cancer than postmenopausal women. Routine follow-up of women with ADH is recommended.

Lobular hyperplasia

Atypical lobular hyperplasia and lobular in-situ neoplasia are collectively termed 'lobular neoplasia' because, unlike ductal lesions (which are heterogeneous), the histological features of lobular epithelial proliferations are very similar. The significant difference between lobular in-situ neoplasia and atypical lobular hyperplasia is the degree and extent of epithelial proliferation. Lobular neoplasia is a rare breast condition more prevalent in perimenopausal women, which rarely presents clinically and is often found as an incidental finding on biopsy. Both atypical lobular hyperplasia and lobular in-situ neoplasia increase the risk for development of invasive carcinoma (four- and 10-fold, respectively). Subsequent invasive carcinoma after atypical lobular hyperplasia is three times more likely to occur in the ipsilateral breast (Page et al 2003). Carcinoma may arise 15–20 years after the initial diagnosis. The risk of developing subsequent invasive carcinoma after a diagnosis of lobular in-situ neoplasia is similar in both the ipsilateral and contralateral breasts.

Columnar cell lesions

Columnar cell lesions can be classified as either columnar cell change or columnar cell hyperplasia with or without atypia (Schnitt and Vincent-Salomon 2003). Atypical columnar cell lesions (also called flat epithelial atypia, blunt duct adenosis, columnar alteration of lobules, hypersecretory hyperplasia with atypia, pretubular hyperplasia, and columnar alteration with prominent snouts and secretions) have a low local recurrence rate and a low risk of progressing to invasive carcinoma. Some columnar cell lesions may represent a precursor of low-grade DCIS or invasive carcinoma, especially tubular carcinoma (Schnitt 2003). Columnar cell lesions diagnosed by needle core biopsy are advisedly excised to exclude in-situ or invasive cancer. Close follow-up of the patient is advised following excision (Nasser 2004). The radiological features of radial scars can mimic carcinomas, and the role of FNAC in diagnosis is limited. As malignancy cannot be excluded following needle core biopsy, excision biopsy of these lesions is advised.

Complex sclerosing lesion and radial scar

Stromal involution can produce areas of fibrosis. Radial scars are benign pseudoinfiltrative lesions of unknown significance, characterized by a fibroelastic core with entrapped ducts surrounded by radiating ducts and lobules showing variable epithelial hyperplasia, adenosis duct ectasia and papillomatosis. Radial scars and 'complex sclerosing lesions' (CSL) are usually asymptomatic and discovered through mammographic screening, but may present as a palpable mass. The term 'radial scar' has been used for lesions measuring less than 1 cm, whereas CSL is reserved for those lesions over 1 cm in size (Kennedy et al 2003, Patterson et al 2004). Radial scars have been shown to be associated with BBD and a doubling of the risk of developing breast cancer (Nielsen et al 1987, Jacobs et al 1999). This risk is increased in women with larger and/or multiple radial scars.

Proliferative Stromal Lesions

Diabetic fibrous mastopathy

This is a rare form of lymphocytic mastitis and stromal fibrosis which can occur in patients with longstanding type 1 diabetes who have severe diabetic microvascular complications. It occurs in premenopausal women and, rarely, in men. It is known as 'diabetic mastopathy' or sclerosing lymphocytic lobulitis which does not predispose to breast carcinoma or lymphoma (Kudva et al 2003). Clinically, it is characterized by solitary or multiple ill-defined, painless, immobile, discrete lesions in one or both breasts. Mammographic and sonographic findings of these lesions are very suspicious for carcinoma; therefore, needle core biopsy is essential for diagnosis (Camuto et al 2000, Haj et al 2004). The pathogenesis of diabetic mastopathy is unknown, but it is thought to be an immune reaction to the abnormal accumulation of altered extracellular matrix in the breast, which occurs to connective tissue following hyperglycaemia (Haj et al 2004, Baratelli and Riva 2005). Annual follow-up is recommended in patients with diabetic fibrous mastopathy.

Pseudoangiomatous stromal hyperplasia of the breast

Pseudoangiomatous stromal hyperplasia (PASH) is a benign myofibroblastic proliferation of non-specialized mammary stroma. Clinicopathologically, it ranges from incidental, microscopic foci to mammographic and clinically palpable breast masses (Castro et al 2002, Guray and Sahin 2006). PASH is more common in premenopausal women and older women taking hormone replacement therapy; as a result, it was thought to be due to hormone stimulation, particularly progesterone. More recent studies have shown that only a small percentage of patients with PASH express either the oestrogen or progesterone receptor (Pruthi et al 2001, Castro et al 2002). PASH may present clinically as a well-circumscribed, dense rubbery mass mimicking a fibroadenoma or PT. As the mammographic and sonographic findings of PASH are non-specific, a needle core biopsy is required to exclude malignancy (Pruthi et al 2001, Mercado et al 2004). Wide local excision is the recommended treatment for PASH. It may recur but the prognosis is good (Castro et al 2002).

Breast Disorders Related to Pregnancy and Lactation

Pregnancy and lactation induce notable changes to the breasts in response to hormonal stimulation. Most of the tumours and disorders affecting the breasts are the same in pregnant/lactating women as in women who are not pregnant; however, some are unique to pregnancy and lactation. The majority of disorders related to pregnancy and lactation are benign, but pregnancy-associated breast cancer accounts for approximately 3% of all breast malignancies. All breast masses discovered during pregnancy and lactation require careful evaluation.

Lactogenesis

During pregnancy, the breast undergoes a number of changes in response to an increase in circulating hormones (oestrogen, progesterone and prolactin) beginning in the second month of the first trimester. Lactogenesis is a series of cellular changes whereby mammary epithelial cells are converted from a non-secretory state to a secretory state. This process is normally associated with the end of pregnancy and around the time of parturition.

Ultrasound is the most appropriate radiological investigation to evaluate breast disorders in women during pregnancy and lactation. The use of magnetic resonance imaging in the evaluation and treatment of pregnant women should be avoided, and only used where the risk:benefit ratio is clear (Talele et al 2003, Espinosa et al 2005). There is no conclusive evidence that magnetic resonance imaging has a toxic effect on the developing embryo, and the use of gadolinium-based contrast during pregnancy is probably safe as the quantity of gadolinium crossing the placenta is low and is rapidly excreted by the kidneys (Nagayama et al 2002, De Wilde et al 2005, Webb et al 2005). The use of mammography during pregnancy remains controversial, but it should be performed if malignancy is suspected as it is particularly effective in detection of microcalcifications and subtle areas of distortion, which may not be detected on ultrasound. The impact of prenatal exposure to ionizing radiation depends on three factors: the stage of fetal development at the time of exposure, the anatomical distribution of the radiation and the radiation dose. The fetus is most susceptible to radiation-induced malformations in the first 2 months of pregnancy (organogenesis). These malformations are believed to occur with exposure to more than 0.005 Gy of radiation (Greskovich and Macklis 2000). Two-view mammography of each breast performed with abdominal shielding exposes the fetus to 0.004 Gy of radiation; therefore, mammography with abdominal shielding can be performed should it be required during pregnancy. Recommendations are to avoid mammography in the first trimester; ultrasonography is preferable (Osei and Faulkner 1999, Sabate et al 2007).

Gestational and secretory hyperplasia

Microcalcifications following pregnancy or lactation are detectable by mammography, and it is important to distinguish these from pregnancy-like hyperplasia which manifests with similar findings in non-pregnant, non-lactating women (Sabate et al 2007).

Bloody spontaneous nipple discharge

This is an uncommon condition during pregnancy and lactation, but does occasionally occur in the third trimester when the vascularity of the breast is increased and changes in the epithelium are more marked. Bloody spontaneous nipple discharge usually resolves with nursing, but can persist in severe cases. Nipple discharge is an uncommon symptom of pregnancy-associated breast cancer, but carcinoma must be excluded (Kline and Lash 1964, O'Callaghan 1981, Lafreniere 1990).

Galactocele

Galactoceles are the most common benign lesions in lactating women; however, they actually occur more frequently following cessation of breast feeding when the milk is retained (Scott-Conner 1997, Son et al 2006). Galactoceles are cuboidal or flat epithelium-lined cysts containing fluid resembling milk and inflammatory debris (Figure 46.5). The cysts form as a result of duct dilatation, and aspiration of the cyst is both therapeutic and diagnostic, producing milk during lactation and a more thickened milky fluid after lactation has ceased (Gomez et al 1986). Infection remains a common complication of galactoceles, and is easily confirmed with fine needle aspiration by a mixed purulent–milky material (Sabate et al 2007).

Pseudolipoma

Pseudolipoma occurs when the fat content of the breast is very high, and is a radiolucent mass.

Pseudohamartoma

Pseudohamartoma occurs when galactoceles contain variable proportions of old milk and water. The mass resembles a hamartoma as the high viscosity of old milk does not allow the separation of milk and water (Gomez et al 1986).

Gigantomastia

Gestational gigantomastia complicates between 1:28,000 and 1:118,000 deliveries (Lewison et al 1960, Beischer et al 1989). Gestational gigantomastia is a common phenotypic outcome from one or more aberrant growth-related pathways resulting in massive breast enlargement (Swelstad et al 2006). The diagnosis is one of exclusion. Medical management is usually ineffective but remains first-line therapy in the hope of avoiding surgery during pregnancy. Bromocriptine is the most common medical regimen, resulting in mild regression or arrest in breast hypertrophy. Effects are variable, usually temporary and do not restore breast volume to normal. If the quality of a woman's life suffers significantly or endangers fetal viability, surgical management (reduction mammoplasty or simple mastectomy) should be utilized (Swelstad et al 2006). Bilateral mastectomy with delayed reconstruction provides the smallest risk of recurrence should the woman become pregnant again (Wolf et al 1995, Swelstad et al 2006).

Puerperal mastitis

Infection of the breast is uncommon during pregnancy, but affects between 5% and 33% of women at some point during lactation (World Health Organization 2000). A study following up 1075 breastfeeding women in Australia reported a 20% incidence of mastitis (Kinlay et al 1998). The wide variation in rates is probably because there is no standard definition of mastitis. The clinical spectrum of lactational mastitis (an acute inflammation of the interlobular connective tissue within the mammary gland, which may or may not be infective) ranges from focal inflammation to abscess with septicaemia. It most commonly develops in the early stages of feeding, with 74–95% of cases observed within the first 3 months of breast feeding (Devereux 1970, Marshall et al 1975, Foxman et al 2002). Cases have been reported as long as the woman is breast feeding. Three studies of breast-feeding women reported recurrent episodes of mastitis in 4–14.4% of cases (Fetherston 1997, Vogel et al 1999, Foxman et al 2002).

Mastitis is diagnosed on clinical symptoms and signs, and patients often present with pain, erythema and swelling. This can spread to affect the whole breast, with the patient becoming septic. It is usually unilateral and rarely presents at weaning. Breast examination often reveals oedema, erythema in a wedge-shaped distribution and tenderness (Bedinghaus 1997). If an abscess is present, a fluctuant mass may be palpable with overlying erythema. There are a number of predisposing factors for developing lactational mastitis including milk stasis [insufficient drainage of the breast, rapid weaning, oversupply of milk, pressure on breast (e.g from poorly fitting bra)], a blocked duct and skin breakdown of the nipple (e.g. fissure, cracks or blisters). Infections developing within the first few months are often due to organisms transmitted in hospital, and are therefore resistant to most commonly used antibiotics. One study has demonstrated that in the first month of breast feeding, more than half of women have nipples colonized with *Staphylococcus aureus* (Livingstone and Stringer 1999). Eczema is a risk factor for infection, as women with eczema are more likely to harbour *S. aureus* (Noble 1998, Amir 2002). Additional risk factors for colonization with meticillin-resistant *S. aureus* include caesarean birth, administration of antibiotics during labour or the early postpartum period, and multiple gestations (Morel et al 2002). Another potential risk factor is in-vitro fertilization, which requires mothers to return to hospital on numerous occasions. Maternal stress, fatigue, poor nutrition, and maternal or infant illness have been associated with mastitis, although the evidence is inconclusive.

When infectious mastitis does occur, the organisms most often cultured from breast milk include *S. aureus* and coagulase-negative staphylococci (Lawrence 2005). Streptococcal infection should be suspected whenever bilateral mastitis presents in the postpartum period (Mead 1992). Delayed care or inadequate treatment can lead to abscess formation. Breast abscess is seen in 0.4–0.5% of lactating women, rarely occurring after the first 6 weeks of lactation. A 2004 study of more than 1000 women showed that 3% of women with breast inflammation will develop an abscess (Amir et al 2004). Abscesses can result in a functional mastectomy (defined as a breast that is unable to effectively lactate) in 10% of women (World Health Organization 2000). Ultrasound plays an important role in the diagnosis and treatment of mastitis if abscess formation is suspected. Abscesses can be treated successfully with needle aspiration to dryness under ultrasound guidance. The cavity is often irrigated with local anaesthetic to reduce pain followed by saline solution

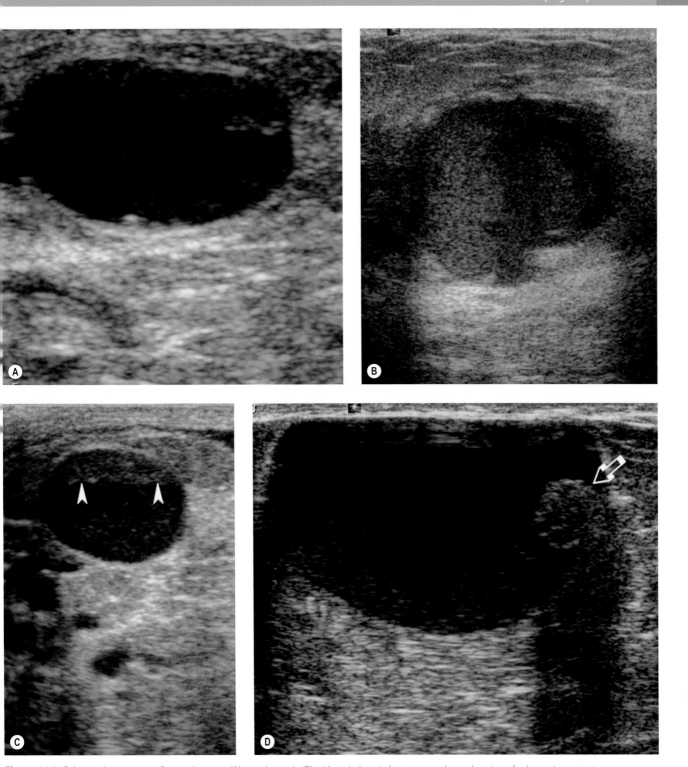

Figure 46.5 Galactoceles can range from echo-poor (A) to echogenic (B) with variations in between, such as a layering of echogenic contents (C, arrowheads) or even apparent solid areas (D). The open arrow points to a small area of cream which was mobile within the galactocele; aspiration confirmed its nature.

(Karstrup et al 1993, Ulitzsch et al 2004, Eryilmaz et al 2005).

The primary goal of treatment is to facilitate recovery and prevent complications. There is a consensus that lactation should be continued, allowing proper drainage of the breast. Early exclusive breast feeding (eight to 12 times per day) will reduce the risk of milk stasis and maintain adequate drainage. Regular and frequent drainage of the breast, either by the infant, hand expression and/or pumping, is vital. Correct positioning of the infant and an assessment of infant latching and sucking is necessary. Close attention to regular drainage of the breast is important, even if the mother is extremely unwell or the milk is contaminated. If direct breast feeding is not possible, regular bilateral pumping should be done with a hospital grade pump eight to 12 times per day for 15–20 min. Mothers require a lot of encouragement and emotional support to maintain breast feeding. As an adjunct to milk removal, a hot compress and gentle massage can also be used.

Promoting milk flow by continuing to breast feed from both breasts and the early use of appropriate antibiotics markedly reduces the rate of abscess formation. Culture of the milk organisms should ideally be performed before any antibiotics are commenced. Co-amoxiclav or flucloxacillin are the antibiotics of choice, or cephalexin and clindamycin in women allergic to penicillin. Tetracycline or ciprofloxacin should not be used in breastfeeding mothers as these medications enter the breast milk and may be harmful to the newborn child. Although there is no standard treatment length, a course of 10–14 days is often advised. Recurrent infective mastitis should be treated with antibiotics for no less than 14 days. Should recurrences occur two or three times in the same place, the breast should be further evaluated for an underlying aetiology such as a breast mass.

A number of complementary therapies for puerperal mastitis are available. These include herbal homeopathic options such as high-potency belladonna, Hepar sulph, *Bellis perennis* and Phytolacca (Barbosa-Cesnik et al 2003, Kvist et al 2007a). Midwives in Sweden use acupuncture needles placed at the heart 3, gallbladder 21, and spleen 6 (Kvist et al 2007b). They also use oxytocin nasal spray to improve the milk ejection reflex, which may have become distended from milk stasis (Kvist et al 2007).

Associated conditions include:

- Blocked ducts — usually present as hard lumps and can be an underlying aetiology of mastitis. Prevention of milk stasis is important, with other treatments including hot compresses and gentle massage over the blocked area. Recurrent blocked ducts may be prevented by manually expressing milk before feeding, limiting saturated fat intake, allowing for adequate rest and using a well-fitted bra.
- Nipple blebs — commonly associated with blocked ducts and manifest as a white spot on the nipple. They are treated by opening the pore with a sterile needle (Lawrence 2005). A galactocele may develop from a blocked duct, and infection should be suspected (particularly with *Candida* spp.) if the blocked ducts are persistent.
- Ductal infections —women often complain of a deep burning, aching or shooting pain in the breast during and after feeding (Amir and Pakula 1991). Should the nipple become involved, the mother may complain of itching. *S. aureus* and *Candida albicans* are the most commonly involved pathogens (Amir and Pakula 1991).

Non-Lactational Infections

These infections can be grouped into peripheral or periareolar. Periareolar infections are seen in young women, and are often secondary to periductal mastitis (associated with cigarette smoking) (Schafer et al 1988, Bundred et al 1993). It is thought that particulates in cigarette smoke may indirectly or directly damage the wall of the subareolar ducts. Metabolites such as epoxides, nicotine, cotinine and lipid peroxidise have been shown to accumulate in smokers within 15 min of a woman starting to breast feed (Petrakis et al 1980). Smoking may affect normal bacterial flora, leading to a proliferation of pathogenic aerobic and anaerobic Gram-negative bacteria. Microvascular changes may also lead to local ischaemia. Patients with periareolar inflammation often present with a mass. Very rarely, the infection is due to underlying comedo necrosis in DCIS. It is advisable to perform a mammogram for all women over 35 years of age after resolution of the inflammation. The rate of recurrence is high for periareolar infections. Peripheral non-lactational breast abscesses are three times more common in premenopausal women than peri-/postmenopausal women. Some of these infections are most commonly caused by *S. aureus* and may be associated with diabetes, rheumatoid arthritis, exogenous steroid use and trauma.

All breast infections are treated with broad-spectrum antibiotics and clinical/ultrasound-guided drainage of any collections of pus (Hayes et al 1991). Aspiration has now become the standard of treatment superseding open drainage (Dixon 1988, 1992, O'Hara et al 1996). Patients should be reviewed every 2–3 days and any further collections aspirated. Periareolar non-lactational abscesses can be treated by repeated aspiration; however, persistent abscesses are common. Mammary duct fistula occurs in one-third of patients following incision and drainage of periareolar abscesses (Bundred et al 1987). These are definitively managed by excising the entire fistula tract with primary closure and antibiotic cover. Laying open of a mammary fistula leaves an unsightly scar across the nipple.

HIV infections

Immunocompromised patients (men and women) are particular susceptible to breast infections.

Hidradenitis suppurativa

Hidradenitis suppurativa is an infection associated with the apocrine glands, affecting the axilla, perineum and breast. It is increasingly common in smokers, and treatment in the acute setting is as discussed above. Excision of the affected area with or without skin grafting is effective in 50% of patients.

Granulomatous mastitis

Granulomatous mastitis is a rare condition characterized by non-caseating granulomas and microabscesses confined to a breast lobule. Patients may present with recurrent/multiple abscesses or a hard, tender mass. Granulomatous mastitis occurs most commonly in parous, young women. Many different organisms can cause granulomatous mastitis, but a recent study isolated corynebacteria in nine out of 12 women with the condition (Erhan et al 2000, Paviour et al 2002, Diesing et al 2004). This condition is treated with broad-spectrum antibiotics.

Tuberculosis of the breast

Tuberculous mastitis is a rare breast condition in which the clinical and radiological features can be easily confused with carcinoma or pyogenic breast abscess. Diagnosis is based on identification of typical histological features under microscopy or the detection of tubercule bacilli (Tewari and Shukla 2005).

Foreign body reactions

Silicone and paraffin, both used in breast augmentation and reconstructive surgery, can cause a granulomatous reaction in the breast. Silicone granulomas (siliconomas) usually occur following direct injection of silicone into the breast tissue or following an extracapsular rupture of a silicone implant (van Diest et al 1998). Fibrosis and contraction may lead to the development of firm, tender nodules in the breast.

Recurring subareolar abscess (Zuska's disease)

This is a rare bacterial infection characterized by a triad of: (1) draining cutaneous fistula, (2) chronic, thick discharge from the nipple, and (3) recurrent mammary abscess (Passaro et al 1994). This is caused by squamous metaplasia of one or more lactiferous ducts, often induced by smoking. Keratin plugs obstruct and dilate the proximal duct, resulting in infection and rupture. An abscess may form which requires complete excision of the affected duct and the sinus tract for successful treatment.

Mastitis of infancy

During the last few uterine weeks, the fetus is subject to stimulation by placental and maternal hormones. Physiological hypertrophy of the breasts is a common feature in full-term neonates. On occasion, the swelling is more marked and may be accompanied by discharge from the nipple ('witch's milk'). The breast enlargement declines completely and the discharge resolves spontaneously. Occasionally, infants can present with a tender, erythematous breast mass accompanied by fever that requires intervention. Mastitis in early infancy is a rare, infectious complication of an otherwise physiological feature of postnatal breast hypertrophy.

Peak occurrence is reported between the second and fifth weeks of life (Rudoy and Nelson 1975, Walsh and McIntosh 1986, Efrat et al 1995, Stricker et al 2005). Females are more often involved than males (ratio 3.5:1). A possible explanation for the predominance of females is the tendency of breast hypertrophy in female newborns to persist longer than in males. The majority of cases are caused by S. aureus. The choice of antibiotic should be guided by Gram stain when possible, and otherwise should consist of an agent effective against S. aureus which is responsible for most cases. All patients require close monitoring for progression, and whilst there is no optimal duration of treatment, one study required treatment of patients for no longer than 14 days. In the case of abscess formation, incision and drainage under general anaesthetic combined with antibiotics is indicated.

Benign Neoplasms of the Breast

Adenoma

Adenoma is a pure epithelial neoplasm of the breast, and is subdivided into tubular, lactating, apocrine, ductal and pleomorphic adenomas. Lactating and tubular adenomas are more common in women of reproductive age. Lactating adenoma is the most common breast mass during pregnancy and puerperium, presenting as a solitary/multiple, discrete, palpable mobile mass, often less than 3 cm in size. The lesion is well circumscribed and lobulated, and acini are lined with actively secreting cuboidal cells. Lactating adenoma can occur in areas such as the axilla, chest wall or vulva (Reeves and Tabuenca 2000, Baker et al 2001). The tumour does not generally recur locally and there is no evidence of malignant potential.

Tubular adenoma of the breast (pure adenoma) presents as a solitary, well-circumscribed, firm mass. Radiologically, it may resemble a calcified fibroadenoma (Soo et al 2000). Lactating and tubular adenomas can be distinguished from fibroadenomas by the presence of scant stroma in the former.

Nipple adenoma

Nipple adenoma is a benign tumour that can clinically mimic Paget's disease. It presents as a discrete, palpable tumour of the papilla of the nipple. Nipple erosion and discharge are usually observed. It is treated by excision biopsy, but recurrences have been reported in incompletely excised lesions (Montemarano et al 1995).

Hamartoma

Hamartoma is an uncommon lesion also known as a 'fibroadenolipoma', 'lipofibroadenoma' or 'adenolipoma', consisting of varying amounts of glandular, adipose and fibrous tissue. Clinically, a hamartoma may present as a painless, discrete encapsulated mass, and although the pathogenesis is not certain, it is thought to develop as a result of dysgenesis. Mammographically, it is well circumscribed, consisting of both lipomatous and soft tissue elements (Herbert et al 2002, Gatti et al 2005). Histologically, the appearance is of normal breast and fat tissue distributed in a nodular fashion within a fibrotic stroma that extends between individual lobules and destroys the normal interlobular specialized loose stroma (Tse et al 2002). Hamartomas are managed by surgical excision.

Lipoma

Lipoma of the breast is a benign, often solitary tumour composed of mature fat cells that tends to present in the fifth decade. Clinically, it may present as a well-circumscribed, smooth or lobulated mass that is soft and non-tender. Imaging shows a radiolucent mass on mammography and either normal or echogenic fat on ultrasonography (Figure 46.6), and FNAC often reveals fat cells with or without normal epithelial cells. If the diagnosis is uncertain, surgical excision is recommended (Lanng et al 2004). Liposarcoma of the breast is very rare (Blanchard et al 2003). Pseudolipoma of the breast may present clinically as a lipoma, but is actually a small cancer that produces compressed fat lobules as the suspensory ligaments of the breast shorten.

Granular cell tumour

This is an uncommon benign tumour that arises from the Schwann cells of the peripheral nervous system. It occurs frequently in the head and neck (particularly the oral cavity), and occurs in the breast in 5–6% of cases (Montagnese et al 2004). Clinically and mammographically, it can mimic carcinoma (Ilvan et al 2005). These tumours are generally small (<3 cm) and well circumscribed; however, in some cases, infiltrative margins have been reported. S100 immunostaining supports the derivation of this tumour from Schwann cells (Balzan et al 2001). Most granular cell tumours are benign, but some malignant cases have been reported. Suspicious features for malignancy include size over 5 cm, cellular and nuclear pleomorphism, prominent nucleoli, increased mitotic activity, presence of necrosis and local recurrence

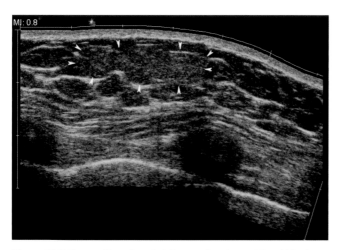

Figure 46.6 Lipoma. Note the subtle increase in echogenicity within the fat (arrow heads). The fibrous margins of the lipoma are only obvious where its capsule is near to right angles with the insinuating beam. The extended field to view image means that the capsule appears incomplete, but this is because the sound is only reflected when the capsule is at right angles to the insonating beam.

(Adeniran et al 2004). These tumours are treated with wide local excision, with incomplete margins resulting in local recurrence.

Other Breast Masses

Montgomery's glands

These are blind-ending ducts distributed throughout the areola which produce fluid to lubricate the areola during breast feeding. They were named after William Fetherstone Montgomery (1797–1859), an Irish obstetrician who was the first to describe them. These glands can become blocked, forming hard nodules on the periphery of the areola, which can occasionally become infected. The management of these prominent glands is reassurance unless the patient becomes symptomatic.

Fat necrosis

Fat necrosis is a benign non-suppurative inflammatory condition affecting the adipose tissue of the breast. It can occur secondary to trauma (accidental/surgical) or may be associated with carcinoma, duct ectasia and fibrocystic disease. Clinically, it can mimic carcinoma if it appears as an ill-defined or dense speculated mass, associated with skin retraction (Kinoshita et al 2002). Imaging may not always be able to distinguish between fat necrosis and carcinoma (Pullyblank et al 2001). Excision biopsy is required if malignancy cannot be excluded on needle core biopsy.

Mondor's disease

This is spontaneous superficial thrombophlebitis of a breast vein. It is often painful, and clinically, there may be a thick palpable cord with associated erythema. The aetiology includes surgery, trauma and infection. It is a self-limiting condition that resolves in a couple of weeks.

Oil cysts

This benign condition can be identified mammographically if the cysts have a calcified rim or lie within parenchyma.

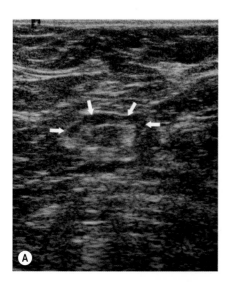

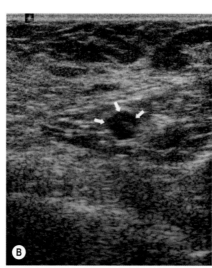

Figure 46.7 (A) A normal lymph node which is almost isoechoic with the axillary tissues, which are a mixture of fat and connective tissue. The arrows point to the outer edges of the cortex, which is of reduced echogenicity. This is an approximate 'C' shape, with a central medullary area of increased echogenicity within the 'C' shape. (B) An abnormal lymph node in the axilla of the same patient. Arrows point to an area of reduced echogenicity which has loss of the normal corticomedullary differentiation. Although this is a smaller lymph node, fine needle aspiration confirmed the presence of tumour.

Within the fat, they often cannot be identified because of the lack of difference in density. On ultrasound, it may not be possible to differentiate oil cysts from ordinary cysts because they may be echo-free or contain echoes, and have an appearance similar to fluid-filled cysts. If there is an oil/water mixture, the fluid level is easily identified on ultrasound or mammography.

Sebaceous cysts

Sebaceous cysts are easily identified on ultrasound due to their position, the fact that they are well defined, and because the internal echoes are usually increased due to the lipid content.

Lymph nodes

Lymph nodes may be isoechoic with the surrounding fat in a mainly fatty breast. They usually have an oval shape, with a slightly more translucent cortex and a slightly increased echogenic medulla (Figure 46.7). The vessels entering the hilum of the cortex can frequently be demonstrated with the aid of colour Doppler. Reactive, hypertrophied lymph nodes retain their anatomical structure and appearance, whereas lymph nodes that have been invaded by the tumour from a breast primary are usually masses of reduced echogenicity, often with a similar echogenicity to the tumour. As in other parts of the body, it is not always possible to exclude the presence of tumour from a node which appears to be hypertrophied with a normal architecture.

KEY POINTS

1. If possible, imaging of the breast should precede FNAC or core biopsy to avoid difficulties in interpretation due to the changes caused by these procedures.

2. Ultrasound can now diagnose many benign lesions with a high degree of certainty, and is the imaging method of choice for women under 35 years of age.

3. Mammography is not recommended for women under 35 years of age except if it is required to evaluate a known carcinoma.

4. Cyclical breast pain is very common and 85% of patients are satisfied with explanation alone. The remainder may be treated with gamolenic acid, danazol, bromocriptine or tamoxifen.

5. Women with multiple breast cysts have an increased risk of breast cancer.

6. Approximately 5% of what are thought clinically to be fibroadenomas are, in fact, malignant. Investigation with ultrasound and fine needle aspiration or core biopsy is required.

7. Breast abscesses can usually be treated with repeated needle aspiration.

References

Acs G, Simpson JF, Bleiweiss IJ et al 2003 Microglandular adenosis with transition into adenoid cystic carcinoma of the breast. American Journal of Surgical Pathology 27: 1052–1060.

Adeniran A, Al-Ahmadie H, Mahoney MC, Robinson-Smith TM 2004 Granular cell tumor of the breast: a series of 17 cases and review of the literature. The Breast Journal 10: 528–531.

Agoff SN, Lawton TJ 2004 Papillary lesions of the breast with and without atypical ductal hyperplasia: can we accurately predict benign behavior from core needle biopsy? American Journal of Clinical Pathology 122: 440–443.

Ali-Fehmi R, Carolin K, Wallis T, Visscher DW 2003 Clinicopathologic analysis of breast lesions associated with multiple papillomas. Human Pathology 34: 234–239.

Amir L 2002 Breastfeeding and Staphylococcus aureus: three case reports. Breastfeeding Review 10: 15–18.

Amir LH, Pakula S 1991 Nipple pain, mastalgia and candidiasis in the lactating breast. Australian and New Zealand Journal of Obstetrics and Gynaecology 31: 378–380.

Amir LH, Forster D, Mclachlan H, Lumley J 2004 Incidence of breast abscess in lactating women: report from an Australian cohort. BJOG: an International Journal of Obstetrics and Gynaecology 111: 1378–1381.

Baker TP, Lenert JT, Parker J et al 2001 Lactating adenoma: a diagnosis of exclusion. The Breast Journal 7: 354–357.

Balzan SM, Farina PS, Maffazzioli L, Riedner CE, Guedes Neto EP, Fontes PR 2001 Granular cell breast tumour: diagnosis and outcome. European Journal of Surgery 167: 860–862.

Baratelli GM, Riva C 2005 Diabetic fibrous mastopathy: sonographic–pathologic correlation. Journal of Clinical Ultrasound 33: 34–37.

Barbosa-Cesnik C, Schwartz K, Foxman B 2003 Lactation mastitis. Journal of the American Medical Association 289: 1609–1612.

Bartow SA, Pathak DR, Black WC, Key CR, Teaf SR 1987 Prevalence of benign, atypical, and malignant breast lesions in populations at different risk for breast cancer. A forensic autopsy study. Cancer 60: 2751–2760.

Bazzocchi F, Santini D, Martinelli G et al 1986 Juvenile papillomatosis (epitheliosis) of the breast. A clinical and pathologic study of 13 cases. American Journal of Clinical Pathology 86: 745–748.

Bedinghaus JM 1997 Care of the breast and support of breast-feeding. Primary Care 24: 147–160.

Beischer NA, Hueston JH, Pepperell RJ 1989 Massive hypertrophy of the breasts in pregnancy: report of 3 cases and review of the literature, 'never think you have seen everything'. Obstetrical and Gynecological Survey 44: 234–243.

Blanchard DK, Reynolds CA, Grant CS, Donohue JH 2003 Primary nonphyllodes breast sarcomas. American Journal of Surgery 186: 359–361.

Blommers J, De Lange-De Klerk ES, Kuik DJ, Bezemer PD, Meijer S 2002 Evening primrose oil and fish oil for severe chronic mastalgia: a randomized, double-blind, controlled trial. American Journal of Obstetrics and Gynecology 187: 1389–1394.

Bundred NJ, Dixon JM, Chetty U, Forrest AP 1987 Mammillary fistula. British Journal of Surgery 74: 466–468.

Bundred NJ, Dover MS, Aluwihare N, Faragher EB, Morrison JM 1993 Smoking and periductal mastitis. BMJ (Clinical Research Ed.) 307: 772–773.

Caleffi M, Filho DD, Borghetti K et al 2004 Cryoablation of benign breast tumors: evolution of technique and technology. Breast 13: 397–407.

Camuto PM, Zetrenne E, Ponn T 2000 Diabetic mastopathy: a report of 5 cases and a review of the literature. Archives of Surgery 135: 1190–1193.

Carter BA, Page DL, Schuyler P et al 2001 No elevation in long-term breast carcinoma risk for women with fibroadenomas that contain atypical hyperplasia. Cancer 92: 30–36.

Castro CY, Whitman GJ, Sahin AA 2002 Pseudoangiomatous stromal hyperplasia of the breast. American Journal of Clinical Oncology 25: 213–216.

Cole P, Mark Elwood J, Kaplan SD 1978 Incidence rates and risk factors of benign breast neoplasms. American Journal of Epidemiology 108: 112–120.

Cook MG, Rohan TE 1985 The patho-epidemiology of benign proliferative epithelial disorders of the female breast. Journal of Pathology 146: 1–15.

De Wilde JP, Rivers AW, Price DL 2005 A review of the current use of magnetic resonance imaging in pregnancy and safety implications for the fetus. Progress in Biophysics and Molecular Biology 87: 335–353.

Devereux WP 1970 Acute puerperal mastitis. Evaluation of its management. American Journal of Obstetrics and Gynecology 108: 78–81.

Diesing D, Axt-Fliedner R, Hornung D, Weiss JM, Diedrich K, Friedrich M 2004 Granulomatous mastitis. Archives of Gynecology and Obstetrics 269: 233–236.

Dixon J 1994 ABC of Breast Diseases. BMJ Publishing Group, London.

Dixon JM 1988 Repeated aspiration of breast abscesses in lactating women. BMJ (Clinical Research Ed.) 297: 1517–1518.

Dixon JM 1992 Outpatient treatment of non-lactational breast abscesses. British Journal of Surgery 79: 56–57.

Dixon JM, Mcdonald C, Elton RA, Miller WR 1999 Risk of breast cancer in women with palpable breast cysts: a prospective study. Edinburgh Breast Group. The Lancet 353: 1742–1745.

Dupont WD, Page DL 1985 Risk factors for breast cancer in women with proliferative breast disease. New England Journal of Medicine 312: 146–151.

Dupont WD, Page DL 1989 Relative risk of breast cancer varies with time since diagnosis of atypical hyperplasia. Human Pathology 20: 723–725.

Dupont WD, Parl FF, Hartmann WH et al 1993 Breast cancer risk associated with proliferative breast disease and atypical hyperplasia. Cancer 71: 1258–1265.

Dupont WD, Page DL, Parl FF et al 1994 Long-term risk of breast cancer in women with fibroadenoma. New England Journal of Medicine 331: 10–15.

Efrat M, Mogilner JG, Iujtman M, Eldemberg D, Kunin J, Eldar S 1995 Neonatal mastitis — diagnosis and treatment. Israel Journal of Medical Science 31: 558–560.

Erhan Y, Veral A, Kara E et al 2000 A clinicopathologic study of a rare clinical entity mimicking breast carcinoma: idiopathic granulomatous mastitis. Breast 9: 52–56.

Eryilmaz R, Sahin M, Hakan Tekelioglu M, Daldal E 2005 Management of lactational breast abscesses. Breast 14: 375–379.

Escobar PF, Crowe JP, Matsunaga T, Mokbel K 2006 The clinical applications of mammary ductoscopy. American Journal of Surgery 191: 211–215.

Espinosa LA, Daniel BL, Vidarsson L, Zakhour M, Ikeda DM, Herfkens RJ 2005 The lactating breast: contrast-enhanced MR imaging of normal tissue and cancer. Radiology 237: 429–436.

Eusebi V, Foschini MP, Betts CM et al 1993 Microglandular adenosis, apocrine adenosis, and tubular carcinoma of the breast. An immunohistochemical comparison. American Journal of Surgical Pathology 17: 99–109.

Fetherston C 1997 Characteristics of lactation mastitis in a Western Australian cohort. Breastfeeding Review 5: 5–11.

Fitzgibbons PL, Henson DE, Hutter RV 1998 Benign breast changes and the risk for subsequent breast cancer: an update of the 1985 consensus statement. Cancer Committee of the College of American Pathologists. Archives of Pathology and Laboratory Medicine 122: 1053–1055.

Foxman B, D'Arcy H, Gillespie B, Bobo JK, Schwartz K 2002 Lactation mastitis: occurrence and medical management among 946 breastfeeding women in the United States. American Journal of Epidemiology 155: 103–114.

Gatti G, Mazzarol G, Simsek S, Viale G 2005 Breast hamartoma: a case report. Breast Cancer Research and Treatment 89: 145–147.

Gomez A, Mata JM, Donoso L, Rams A 1986 Galactocele: three distinctive radiographic appearances. Radiology 158: 43–44.

Greskovich JF Jr, Macklis RM 2000 Radiation therapy in pregnancy: risk calculation and risk minimization. Seminars in Oncology 27, 633–645.

Guray M, Sahin AA 2006 Benign breast diseases: classification, diagnosis, and management. The Oncologist 11: 435–449.

Haagenson C 1986 Diseases of the Breast. WB Saunders, Philadelphia.

Haj M, Weiss M, Herskovits T 2004 Diabetic sclerosing lymphocytic lobulitis of the breast. Journal of Diabetes and its Complications 18: 187–191.

Hartmann LC, Sellers TA, Frost MH et al 2005 Benign breast disease and the risk of breast cancer. New England Journal of Medicine 353: 229–237.

Hayes R, Michell M, Nunnerley HB 1991 Acute inflammation of the breast — the role of breast ultrasound in diagnosis and management. Clinical Radiology 44: 253–256.

Herbert M, Sandbank J, Liokumovich P et al 2002 Breast hamartomas: clinicopathological and immunohistochemical studies of 24 cases. Histopathology 41, 30–34.

Houssami N, Irwig L, Ung O 2005 Review of complex breast cysts: implications for cancer detection and clinical practice. Australian and New Zealand Journal of Surgery 75: 1080–1085.

Howard BA, Gusterson BA 2000 Human breast development. Journal of Mammary Gland Biology and Neoplasia 5: 119–137.

Hughes LE, Mansel RE, Webster DJ 1987 Aberrations of normal development and involution (ANDI): a new perspective on pathogenesis and nomenclature of benign breast disorders. The Lancet 2: 1316–1319.

Hutchinson WB, Thomas DB, Hamlin WB, Roth GJ, Peterson AV, Williams B 1980 Risk of breast cancer in women with benign breast disease. Journal of the National Cancer Institute 65: 13–20.

Ilvan S, Ustundag N, Calay Z, Bukey Y 2005 Benign granular-cell tumour of the breast. Canadian Journal of Surgery 48: 155–156.

Ivan D, Selinko V, Sahin AA, Sneige N, Middleton LP 2004 Accuracy of core needle biopsy diagnosis in assessing papillary breast lesions: histologic predictors of malignancy. Modern Pathology 17: 165–171.

Jacklin RK, Ridgway PF, Ziprin P, Healy V, Hadjiminas D, Darzi A 2006 Optimising preoperative diagnosis in phyllodes tumour of the breast. Journal of Clinical Pathology 59: 454–459.

Jacobs TW, Byrne C, Colditz G, Connolly JL, Schnitt SJ 1999 Radial scars in benign breast-biopsy specimens and the risk of breast cancer. New England Journal of Medicine 340: 430–436.

Jensen RA, Page DL, Dupont WD, Rogers LW 1989 Invasive breast cancer risk in women with sclerosing adenosis. Cancer 64: 1977–1983.

Karstrup S, Solvig J, Nolsoe CP et al 1993 Acute puerperal breast abscesses: US-guided drainage. Radiology 188: 807–809.

Katz SC, Hazen A, Colen SR, Roses DF 2001 Poland's syndrome and carcinoma of the breast: a case report. The Breast Journal 7: 56–59.

Kennedy M, Masterson AV, Kerin M, Flanagan F 2003 Pathology and clinical relevance of radial scars: a review. Journal of Clinical Pathology 56: 721–724.

Kinlay JR, O'Connell DL, Kinlay S 1998 Incidence of mastitis in breastfeeding women during the six months after delivery: a prospective cohort study. Medical Journal of Australia 169: 310–312.

Kinoshita T, Yashiro N, Yoshigi J, Ihara N, Narita M 2002 Fat necrosis of breast: a potential pitfall in breast MRI. Clinical Imaging 26: 250–253.

Kleer CG, Tseng MD, Gutsch DE et al 2002 Detection of Epstein–Barr virus in rapidly growing fibroadenomas of the breast in immunosuppressed hosts. Modern Pathology 15: 759–764.

Kline TS, Lash SR 1964 The bleeding nipple of pregnancy and postpartum period; a cytologic and histologic study. Acta Cytologica 8: 336–340.

Koerner FC 2004 Epithelial proliferations of ductal type. Seminars in Diagnostic Pathology 21: 10–17.

Krieger N, Hiatt RA 1992 Risk of breast cancer after benign breast diseases. Variation by histologic type, degree of atypia, age at biopsy, and length of follow-up. American Journal of Epidemiology 135: 619–631.

Kudva YC, Reynolds CA, O'Brien T, Crotty TB 2003 Mastopathy and diabetes. Current Diabetes Reports 3: 56–59.

Kvist LJ, Hall-Lord ML, Larsson BW 2007a A descriptive study of Swedish women with symptoms of breast inflammation during lactation and their perceptions of the quality of care given at a breastfeeding clinic. International Breastfeeding Journal 2: 2.

Kvist LJ, Hall-Lord ML, Rydhstroem H, Larsson BW 2007b A randomised-controlled trial in Sweden of acupuncture and care interventions for the relief of inflammatory symptoms of the breast during lactation. Midwifery 23: 183–195.

La Vecchia C, Parazzini F, Franceschi S, Decarli A 1985 Risk factors for benign breast disease and their relation with breast cancer risk. Pooled information from epidemiologic studies. Tumori 71: 167–178.

Lafreniere R 1990 Bloody nipple discharge during pregnancy: a rationale for conservative treatment. Journal of Surgical Oncology 43: 228–230.

Lanng C, Eriksen BO, Hoffmann J 2004 Lipoma of the breast: a diagnostic dilemma. Breast 13, 408–411.

Lawrence RA 2005 Breastfeeding. A Guide for the Medical Profession. Mosby, St Louis.

Lee KC, Chan JK, Gwi E 1996 Tubular adenosis of the breast. A distinctive benign lesion mimicking invasive carcinoma. American Journal of Surgical Pathology 20: 46–54.

Levshin V, Pikhut P, Yakovleva I, Lazarev I 1998 Benign lesions and cancer of the breast. European Journal of Cancer Prevention 7 (Suppl 1): S37–S40.

Lewison EF, Jones GS, Trimble FH, da Lima LC 1960 Gigantomastia complicating pregnancy. Surgery, Gynecology and Obstetrics 110: 215–223.

Livingstone V, Stringer LJ 1999 The treatment of Staphyloccocus aureus infected sore nipples: a randomized comparative study. Journal of Human Lactation 15: 241–246.

Love SM, Gelman RS, Silen W 1982 Sounding board. Fibrocystic 'disease' of the breast — a nondisease? New England Journal of Medicine 307: 1010–1014.

MacGrogan G, Tavassoli FA 2003 Central atypical papillomas of the breast: a clinicopathological study of 119 cases. Virchows Archiv: an International Journal of Pathology 443: 609–617.

Mallon E, Osin P, Nasiri N, Blain I, Howard B, Gusterson B 2000 The basic pathology of human breast cancer. Journal of Mammary Gland Biology and Neoplasia 5: 139–163.

Marshall BR, Hepper JK, Zirbel CC 1975 Sporadic puerperal mastitis. An infection that need not interrupt lactation. Journal of the American Medical Association 233: 1377–1379.

Marshall LM, Hunter DJ, Connolly JL et al 1997 Risk of breast cancer associated with atypical hyperplasia of lobular and ductal types. Cancer Epidemiology, Biomarkers and Prevention 6: 297–301.

Mead PB 1992 Infectious Protocols for Obstetrics and Gynecology. Medical Economics Publishing, Montvale.

Mercado CL, Naidrich SA, Hamele-Bena D, Fineberg SA, Buchbinder SS 2004 Pseudoangiomatous stromal hyperplasia of the breast: sonographic features with histopathologic correlation. The Breast Journal 10: 427–432.

Montagnese MD, Roshong-Denk S, Zaher A, Mohamed I, StarenStaren ED 2004 Granular cell tumor of the breast. The American Surgeon 70: 52–54.

Montemarano AD, Sau P, James WD 1995 Superficial papillary adenomatosis of the nipple: a case report and review of the literature. Journal of the American Academy of Dermatology 33: 871–875.

Morel AS, Wu F, Della-Latta P, Cronquist A, Rubenstein D, Saiman L 2002 Nosocomial transmission of methicillin-resistant Staphylococcus aureus from a mother to her preterm quadruplet infants. American Journal of Infection Control 30: 170–173.

Muller J 1838 Ueber den feineran Bau und die Forman der Krankhaften Geschwulste. G Reimer, Berlin.

Nagayama M, Watanabe Y, Okumura A, Amoh Y, Nakashita S, Dodo Y 2002 Fast MR imaging in obstetrics. Radiographics 22: 563–580; discussion 580–582.

Nasser SM 2004 Columnar cell lesions: current classification and controversies. Seminars in Diagnostic Pathology 21: 18–24.

Nielsen M, Christensen L, Andersen J 1987 Radial scars in women with breast cancer. Cancer 59: 1019–1025.

Noble WC 1998 Skin bacteriology and the role of Staphylococcus aureus in infection. British Journal of Dermatology 139 (Suppl 53): 9–12.

O'Callaghan MA 1981 Atypical discharge from the breast during pregnancy and/or lactation. Australian and New Zealand Journal of Obstetrics and Gynaecology 21: 214–216.

O'Hara RJ, Dexter SP, Fox JN 1996 Conservative management of infective mastitis and breast abscesses after ultrasonographic assessment. British Journal of Surgery 83: 1413–1414.

O'Malley FP, Bane AL 2004 The spectrum of apocrine lesions of the breast. Advances in Anatomic Pathology 11: 1–9.

Osei EK, Faulkner K 1999 Fetal doses from radiological examinations. British Journal of Radiology 72: 773–780.

Page DL, Dupont WD, Rogers LW, Rados MS 1985 Atypical hyperplastic lesions of the female breast. A long-term follow-up study. Cancer 55: 2698–2708.

Page DL, Salhany KE, Jensen RA, Dupont WD 1996 Subsequent breast carcinoma risk after biopsy with atypia in a breast papilloma. Cancer 78: 258–266.

Page DL, Schuyler PA, Dupont WD, Jensen RA, Plummer WD Jr, Simpson JF 2003 Atypical lobular hyperplasia as a unilateral predictor of breast cancer risk: a retrospective cohort study. The Lancet 361: 125–129.

Palli D, Rosselli Del Turco M, Simoncini R, Bianchi S 1991 Benign breast disease and breast cancer: a case–control study in a cohort in Italy. International Journal of Cancer 47: 703–706.

Passaro ME, Broughan TA, Sebek BA, Esselstyn CB Jr 1994 Lactiferous fistula. Journal of the American College of Surgeons 178: 29–32.

Patterson JA, Scott M, Anderson N, Kirk SJ 2004 Radial scar, complex sclerosing lesion and risk of breast cancer. Analysis of 175 cases in Northern Ireland. European Journal of Surgical Oncology 30: 1065–1068.

Paviour S, Musaad S, Roberts S et al 2002 Corynebacterium species isolated from patients with mastitis. Clinical Infectious Diseases 35: 1434–1440.

Petrakis NL, Maack CA, Lee RE, Lyon M 1980 Mutagenic activity in nipple aspirates of human breast fluid. Cancer Research 40: 188–189.

Pinder SE, Ellis IO 2003 The diagnosis and management of pre-invasive breast disease: ductal carcinoma in situ (DCIS) and atypical ductal hyperplasia (ADH) — current definitions and classification. Breast Cancer Research 5: 254–257.

Pruthi S, Reynolds C, Johnson RE, Gisvold JJ 2001 Tamoxifen in the management of pseudoangiomatous stromal hyperplasia. The Breast Journal 7: 434–439.

Pullyblank AM, Davies JD, Basten J, Rayter Z 2001 Fat necrosis of the female breast — Hadfield re-visited. Breast 10: 388–391.

Qian JG, Wang XJ, Yu AR, Zhou FH 2008 Surgical correction of axillary accessory breast tissue: 12 cases with emphasis on treatment option. Journal of Plastic, Reconstructive and Aesthetic Surgery 61: 968–970.

Ram AN, Chung KC 2009 Poland's syndrome: current thoughts in the setting of a controversy. Plastic and Reconstructive Surgery 123: 949–953; discussion 954–955.

Reeves ME, Tabuenca A 2000 Lactating adenoma presenting as a giant breast mass. Surgery 127: 586–588.

Rudoy RC, Nelson JD 1975 Breast abscess during the neonatal period. A review. American Journal of Diseases of Children 129: 1031–1034.

Sabate JM, Clotet M, Torrubia S et al 2007 Radiologic evaluation of breast disorders related to pregnancy and lactation. Radiographics 27 (Suppl 1): S101–S124.

Sandler TW ed 2006 Langman's Medical Embroyology, 10th ed. Lippincott Williams & Wilkins, Philadelphia, 337–338.

Sarnelli R, Squartini F 1991 Fibrocystic condition and 'at risk' lesions in asymptomatic breasts: a morphologic study of postmenopausal women. Clinical and Experimental Obstetrics and Gynecology 18: 271–279.

Schafer P, Furrer C, Mermillod B 1988 An association of cigarette smoking with recurrent subareolar breast abscess. International Journal of Epidemiology 17: 810–813.

Schnitt SJ 2003 The diagnosis and management of pre-invasive breast disease: flat epithelial atypia — classification, pathologic features and clinical significance. Breast Cancer Research 5: 263–268.

Schnitt SJ, Vincent-Salomon A 2003 Columnar cell lesions of the breast. Advances in Anatomic Pathology 10: 113–124.

Scott-Conner CEH 1997 Diagnosing and managing breast disease during pregnancy and lactation. Medscape Women's Health 2: 1.

Shabtai M, Saavedra-Malinger P, Shabtai EL et al 2001 Fibroadenoma of the breast: analysis of associated pathological entities — a different risk marker in different age groups for concurrent breast cancer. Israel Medical Association Journal 3: 813–817.

Son EJ, Oh KK, Kim EK 2006 Pregnancy-associated breast disease: radiologic features and diagnostic dilemmas. Yonsei Medical Journal 47: 34–42.

Soo MS, Dash N, Bentley R, Lee LH, Nathan G 2000 Tubular adenomas of the breast: imaging findings with histologic correlation. AJR American Journal of Roentgenology 174: 757–761.

Stricker T, Navratil F, Sennhauser FH 2005 Mastitis in early infancy. Acta Paediatrica 94: 166–169.

Swelstad MR, Swelstad BB, Rao VK, Gutowski KA 2006 Management of gestational gigantomastia. Plastic and Reconstructive Surgery 118: 840–848.

Talele AC, Slanetz PJ, Edmister WB, Yeh ED, Kopans DB 2003 The lactating breast: MRI findings and literature review. The Breast Journal 9: 237–240.

Tavassoli FA, Norris HJ 1990 A comparison of the results of long-term follow-up for atypical intraductal hyperplasia and intraductal hyperplasia of the breast. Cancer 65: 518–529.

Tewari M, Shukla HS 2005 Breast tuberculosis: diagnosis, clinical features & management. Indian Journal of Medical Research 122: 103–110.

Treves N, Sunderland DA 1951 Cystosarcoma phyllodes of the breast: a malignant and a benign tumor; a clinicopathological study of seventy-seven cases. Cancer 4: 1286–1332.

Tse GM, Law BK, Ma TK et al 2002 Hamartoma of the breast: a clinicopathological review. Journal of Clinical Pathology 55: 951–954.

Ulitzsch D, Nyman MK, Carlson RA 2004 Breast abscess in lactating women: US-guided treatment. Radiology 232: 904–909.

van Diest PJ, Beekman WH, Hage JJ 1998 Pathology of silicone leakage from breast implants. Journal of Clinical Pathology 51: 493–497.

Vargas HI, Vargas MP, Gonzalez KD, Eldrageely K, Khalkhali I 2004 Outcomes of sonography-based management of breast cysts. American Journal of Surgery 188: 443–447.

Vina M, Wells CA 1989 Clear cell metaplasia of the breast: a lesion showing eccrine differentiation. Histopathology 15: 85–92.

Vogel A, Hutchison BL, Mitchell EA 1999 Mastitis in the first year postpartum. Birth 26: 218–225.

Walsh M, McIntosh K 1986 Neonatal mastitis. Clinical Pediatrics 25: 395–399.

Webb JA, Thomsen HS, Morcos SK 2005 The use of iodinated and gadolinium contrast media during pregnancy and lactation. European Radiology 15: 1234–1240.

Wechselberger G, Schoeller T, Piza-Katzer H 2002 Juvenile fibroadenoma of the breast. Surgery 132: 106–107.

World Health Organization 2000 Mastitis: Causes and Management. WHO, Geneva.

Wolf Y, Pauzner D, Groutz A, Walman I, David MP 1995 Gigantomastia complicating pregnancy. Case report and review of the literature. Acta Obstetricia et Gynecologica Scandinavica 74: 159–163.

CHAPTER 47

Malignant disease of the breast

Paul TR Thiruchelvam, William E. Svensson and John Lynn

Chapter Contents

INTRODUCTION	707
TRENDS IN BREAST CANCER INCIDENCE AND PREVALENCE	707
RISK FACTORS	709
QUANTITATIVE RISK ASSESSMENT	711
SCREENING, GENETIC TESTING AND RISK REDUCTION	712
PATHOLOGY	712
PRESENTATION	716
DIAGNOSIS	717
IMAGE-GUIDED BIOPSY	721
STAGING INVESTIGATIONS	721
TREATMENT PLANNING AND PATIENT COMMUNICATION	722
SURGERY AND RADIOTHERAPY	722
PERI- AND POSTOPERATIVE CARE	725
ENDOCRINE THERAPY	725
TARGETED THERAPIES	727
ADJUVANT CHEMOTHERAPY	728
NEOADJUVANT MEDICAL THERAPY	728
TRIPLE-NEGATIVE BREAST CANCERS	729
PROGNOSTIC FACTORS	729
GENOMICS AND PROTEOMICS	730
MICROMETASTASES IN BREAST CANCER	730
GENE EXPRESSION SIGNATURES	730
ADJUVANT ONLINE	731
METASTATIC BREAST CANCER	731
PRESERVATION OF FERTILITY IN BREAST CANCER PATIENTS	733
PREGNANCY-ASSOCIATED BREAST CANCER	734
BREAST CANCER IN THE ELDERLY	735
CLINICAL FOLLOW-UP	735
BREAST RECONSTRUCTION AFTER SURGERY FOR BREAST CANCER	735
ONLINE RESOURCES	737
KEY POINTS	737

Introduction

Breast cancer is one of the most common malignancies afflicting women, and is the leading cause of cancer-related mortality (Hortobagyi et al 2005). Worldwide, more than 1.2 million women are diagnosed with breast cancer each year, affecting 10–12% of the female population and resulting in 500,000 deaths per year. In the UK in 2005, there were 45,947 new cases: 45,660 (over 99%) in women and 287 (<1%) in men, causing approximately 14,000 deaths per year (Information Statistics Division Online 2008, Office for National Statistics 2008, Northern Ireland Cancer Registry 2008, Welsh Cancer Intelligence and Surveillance Unit 2008). The lifetime risk of a women being diagnosed with breast cancer is one in nine (Health Statistics Quarterly 1999, Information Statistics Division Online 2008, Welsh Cancer Intelligence and Surveillance Unit 2008). Whilst it is impossible to predict who will develop breast cancer, it is possible to identify those women who are at increased risk for breast cancer and provide options for reducing the risk.

Trends in Breast Cancer Incidence and Prevalance

More than 80% of cases of breast cancer occur in women over 50 years of age, with the highest incidence in women aged 50–69 years. The incidence of breast cancer has been increasing for many years in economically developed countries. The UK age-standardized incidence of breast cancer per 100,000 women increased from 74 in 1975 to 123 in 2005 (Coleman 2000). The introduction of a national screening programme in the UK in 1988 led to a transient increase in breast cancer incidence in women aged 50–64 years, as early undiagnosed cancers were detected. This increase lasted for the first 4–7 years of the programme. However, an underlying increase in incidence predating screening continues

DOI: 10.1016/B978-0-7020-3120-5.00047-3

today and is particularly evident in older age groups. Mortality rates for breast cancer have fallen in many developed countries since 1990, having been previously stable/increasing for several decades (Beral et al 1995, Peto et al 2000, Jatoi and Miller 2003). This reduction has been attributed to earlier detection following the implementation of breast screening, decreased use of exogenous hormones and the use of adjuvant therapies such as tamoxifen (Berry et al 2005).

As the incidence of breast cancer is high and the 5-year survival rate is approximately 80%, many women are alive who have been diagnosed with breast cancer. An estimated 550,000 women are alive in the UK who have received a diagnosis of breast cancer (Maddams et al 2008).

Risk Factors

Many factors are associated with an increased risk of developing breast cancer; however, only 25% of women with a sporadic case of breast cancer will have an identifiable risk factor.

Age

Age is the single most important risk factor for the development of breast cancer (Colditz and Rosner 2000). The incidence of breast cancer increases with age, doubling every 10 years to the menopause, and then the rate of increase slows, levelling to a plateau after 80 years (Anderson et al 2005). This creates a point of inflection in the age-specific incidence curve known as 'Clemmensen's hook' (Clemmensen 1948). The incidence of oestrogen-receptor-alpha (ERα)-negative tumours rises rapidly to 50 years and then flattens out/ decreases, whereas the incidence of ERα-positive tumours is similar up to the age of 50 years but then continues to increase, albeit at a slower pace. As a result, ERα-negative tumours tend to occur earlier in life and ERα-positive tumours are more common in older women. The peak age of onset for these two tumour phenotypes is 50 years and 70 years, respectively.

Ethnicity changes the effect of age on breast cancer risk. African-American women under 50 years of age have a higher age-specific incidence of breast cancer than their Caucasian counterparts (Vogel 1998). However, the incidence of breast cancer is higher in Caucasian women after 50 years of age. The difference in age-adjusted breast cancer mortality rates between African-American and Caucasian women in the 1980s was probably due to the greater incidence of ERα-negative tumours in African-American women, who will not have benefited from the introduction of adjuvant hormonal therapy (Jatoi et al 2005).

Geographical variation

Worldwide, more than 1 million women are diagnosed with breast cancer every year, accounting for 10% of all cancer cases and 23% of all female cancer cases (Ferlay et al 2004). Incidence rates for breast cancer are six times greater in the Western world than in underdeveloped countries. Approximately 430,000 new cases of breast cancer occur each year in Europe and an estimated 212,920 in the USA. The lowest rates in Europe are found in Romania and Latvia, and the highest rates are found in Northern and Western Europe. The incidence of breast cancer in American Hispanic women is 40–50% that of non-Hispanic White women.

Migrants from low-risk countries to high-risk countries have been shown to acquire the risk of the 'host nation' within two generations (Tominaga 1985, Ziegler et al 1993). Japanese migrants to the USA acquire an increased breast cancer risk compared with the population in Japan, and there is increasing evidence that the earlier in life a woman takes up residence in a 'high-risk' country, the higher the risk of breast cancer compared with the country of origin (Shimizu et al 1991, Ziegler et al 1993).

Ovulatory cycles

Events in a woman's life that alter her lifetime ovulatory cycles appear to correlate with the risk of breast cancer. Women who start menstruating early or have a late menopause have a 30–50% increase in risk of developing breast cancer. Similarly, late menarche and an early menopause lead to an equivalent reduction in breast cancer risk. The risk of developing breast cancer is doubled in those women who have a natural menopause after 55 years of age compared with those who experience the menopause before 45 years of age. A menopause induced before 40 years of age reduces the risk of breast cancer by almost two-thirds (Hankinson et al 2004).

Age at first pregnancy

Late age at first birth and nulliparity increase the lifetime risk of breast cancer. Nulliparity has been a well-known risk factor for developing breast cancer since Ramizzini described *horrendis mammarium canceris* in Catholic nuns (Ramazzini 1713).The risk of breast cancer in women who have their first child after 30 years of age is double that of women who have their first child before 20 years of age. The group at highest risk are those women who have their first child after 35 years of age. These women have a greater risk than nulliparous women. An early age of birth of a second child confers a reduced risk. The protective effects of an early full-term pregnancy have been observed in a number of ethnic groups and geographic locations, suggesting that the parity-induced protection results from biological changes in the breast rather than environmental factors.

Benign breast disease

Prospective and retrospective studies have shown a relative risk of breast cancer of 1.5–1.6 for women with benign breast disease compared with the general population (Hartmann et al 2005). This increased risk has been shown to persist for 25 years after biopsy. The relative risk of proliferative changes with atypia was 4.24 compared with a relative risk of 1.88 for those without atypia and 1.27 for non-proliferative lesions. The age at diagnosis of the benign breast disease appears to modify the risks related to the histological appearance of benign breast disease. The presence of atypia in women under 45 years of age conveys twice the risk observed among women over 55 years of age. The Breast Cancer Detection and Demonstration Project showed that the risk of breast cancer among premenopausal women with atypia was elevated by a factor of 12.0, compared with 3.3 for postmenopausal women with aytpia (London et al 1992, Dupont et al 1993). An increase in breast cancers has been demonstrated in the same breast during the first 5 years of follow-up following a diagnosis of benign breast disease, particularly in women with atypia.

Ionizing radiation exposure

The understanding of radiation-related breast cancer in women derives from epidemiological studies of patients exposed to diagnostic or therapeutic medical radiation (mantle irradiation for lymphoma) and of the Japanese atomic bomb survivors (United Nations Scientific Committee on the Effects of Atomic Radiation 2000). The breast tissue of young women is highly sensitive to the carcinogenic action of ionizing radiation. Only the bone marrow and the infant thyroid gland are more sensitive to the cancer-causing effects of radiation. Ionizing radiation is an established breast cancer risk factor and this risk has been shown to increase linearly with dose. Age at exposure directly affects radiation-related breast cancer risk, with the greatest risk seen in women exposed before 20 years of age and a significantly reduced risk seen for postmenopausal women. Periods of enhanced cell proliferation, namely *in utero*, puberty and pregnancy, have been proposed to represent windows of increased susceptibility for mammary carcinogenesis (Ronckers et al 2005).

A two-view mammogram results in a breast tissue dose of approximately 0.3 cGy (annual exposure from all sources of natural 'background' radiation being approximately 0.1 cGy). Therefore, with a woman receiving 10 mammograms as a young woman, the total dose would be approximately 3 cGy to each breast. Bearing in mind that epidemiological studies have not detected statistically significant increases below a dose of approximately 20 cGy, and knowing that 100 cGy increases risk by approximately 40%, one can estimate that 3 cGy from periodic mammography screenings would increase the risk by approximately 1.2% or a relative risk of 1.012. Such low risks are not detectable in human studies. Nonetheless, all unnecessary radiation should be avoided and although the presumed risk is very small, it should be clear that the benefit from the medical exposure would far outweigh it.

Oral contraceptive pill

Use of the oral contraceptive pill slightly increases the risk of breast cancer in current and recent users (1–4 years following cessation) with relative risks of 1.24 and 1.16, respectively (Collaborative Group on Hormonal Factors in Breast Cancer 2002). This risk diminishes after discontinuing use and returns to normal after 10 years.

These estimates are based on the Collaborative Group on Hormonal Factors in Breast Cancer study; a collaborative meta-analysis of 54 studies in 25 countries with data on over 50,000 women with breast cancer (Anonymous 1996). Cancers diagnosed in women who have used the oral contraceptive pill tend to be less clinically advanced than those detected in women who have never used it. Users of the oral contraceptive pill are generally younger women whose breast cancer risk is comparatively low, so the small excess in current users will result in a relatively small number of additional cases. Other findings of the study were:

- protective effect against benign breast disease;
- no duration-of-use effect, no pill-type effect and no effect of age at first use;
- no increased risk in women aged over 45 years; and
- the risk of using the oral contraceptive pill was similar regardless of a woman's family history, ethnic origin, age at menarche, height, weight, menopausal status and alcohol consumption.

A large case–controlled study of 4575 women aged 35–64 years showed that current or former use of the oral contraceptive pill was not associated with a significantly increased risk of breast cancer (Marchbanks et al 2002).

Hormone replacement therapy

Hormone replacement therapy (HRT) use increases the risk of breast cancer and reduces the sensitivity of mammography. The risk of breast cancer for current or recent users of HRT increases by 2.3% per year of use. For women who have used HRT for at least 5 years (average 11 years), the increased risk was 35% (Anonymous 1997a). The effect is substantially greater for oestrogen–progesterone combinations than for oestrogen-only HRT. Risk increases with duration of use; the risk for current users of oestrogen–progesterone combinations for more than 10 years was 2.31 compared with 1.74 for 1–4 years of use. Risk decreases with cessation of use; past users (>5 years following cessation) have a similar risk to those who have never taken HRT. One recent study reported that current users of combined HRT had a 2.7-fold elevated risk of lobular cancer and a 3.3-fold risk of ductal cancer. The risk of lobular cancer was only raised in women who had used HRT for 3 years or more.

In the UK over the past 10 years, it is estimated that 20,000 extra breast cancer cases have occurred among women aged 50–64 years as a result of HRT use, and three-quarters (15,000) of these additional breast cancers are due to the use of oestrogen–progesterone HRT. HRT is used by over 20 million women in Western countries for the alleviation of perimenopausal and postmenopausal symptoms, and is an important source of exogenous oestrogen and, in some cases, progesterone exposure. A recent review concluded that the excess incidence of breast cancer, stroke and pulmonary embolism in postmenopausal women who use HRT for 5 years was greater than the reduction in incidence of colorectal cancer and hip fracture (Beral et al 2002). The risks and benefits for treating menopausal symptoms should be evaluated on an individual basis.

A decrease in the incidence of breast cancer among postmenopausal women in the UK may be linked to a decrease in the use of HRT. Researchers calculated that between 1999 and 2005, the risk of the disease fell by 14% in women in their 50s, representing 1400 fewer cases in 2005, and 3300 fewer over the period (Parkin 2009). They suggest that the decrease in breast cancer since 1999 in women aged 50–59 years and since 2003 in women aged 60–64 years is a consequence of the reduced use of HRT. The use of HRT began to fall after the Million Women Study in the UK and the Women's Health Initiative Study in the USA showed that HRT could increase the risk of breast cancer. In women aged

45–69 years, the use of HRT increased from 1992 to reach a peak of 25% in 2000–2001, before falling to approximately half that by 2006.

Hormone therapy after breast cancer is becoming an increasingly relevant problem as more women survive breast cancer. The HABITS (Hormonal Replacement Therapy After Breast Cancer — Is It Safe?) trial was designed to confirm the efficacy of HRT given to women after treatment for breast cancer (Holmberg and Anderson 2004). The trial confirmed an unacceptably high risk in women allocated to receive HRT compared with those receiving best symptomatic treatment, and as a result was terminated. Analysis of women in the HABITS trial after a median follow-up of 4 years showed that 17.6% in the HRT treatment arm had developed breast cancer recurrence or a new breast cancer, compared with 7.7% in the control arm. The estimated 5-year cumulative rate for disease recurrence was 22.2% in the HRT arm and 9.5% in the control arm.

Endogenous hormones

Higher levels of endogenous hormones have been hypothesized to increase breast cancer risk. A pooled analysis of nine prospective cohort studies found a statistically significant increased risk of breast cancer in postmenopausal women with higher levels of sex hormones (Key et al 2002). The risk for women whose oestradiol levels were in the top quintile was approximately twice that compared with women whose oestradiol levels were in the bottom quintile. Evidence in premenopausal women was inconclusive.

Body weight

Increased weight and obesity, as measured by high body mass index (BMI), has been shown to moderately increase the risk of postmenopausal breast cancer and is one of the few modifiable risk factors. It is thought that between 7% and 15% of breast cancers in developed countries may be attributable to obesity. Two large studies — the EPIC study (European Prospective Investigation into Cancer and Nutrition) and the Million Women Study — have found that obese women have a 30% higher risk of postmenopausal breast cancer than women of a healthy weight. That means that if the average lifetime risk of breast cancer is one in nine, an obese woman's lifetime risk is one in seven. An increase in weight over time can also increase the risk of breast cancer.

Diet

A high-fat diet has been positively associated with breast cancer in a number of animal and case–control studies. Pooled analysis of cohort studies found no significant association between fat intake and breast cancer risk, whilst a meta-analysis found an association between higher total and saturated fat intake and an increased risk of breast cancer. A recent prospective study confirmed a significant association between saturated fat and breast cancer risk (Bingham et al 2003).

Alcohol intake

A significant association between alcohol intake and breast cancer has been found, with an increased risk of 7% for each 10 g alcohol/day (Hamajima et al 2002, Baan et al 2007). Approximately 4% of breast cancers in women from developed countries may be attributable to alcohol. In a recent large cohort of middle-aged women in the UK, a population with low-to-moderate alcohol consumption [10 g alcohol (one drink)/day] has shown a statistically increased risk of breast cancer; they also showed an increase in cancers of the oral cavity, pharynx, oesophagus, larynx, rectum and liver (Allen et al 2009). They calculated that the increased risk accounted for an additional 11 breast cancers per 1000 women up to 75 years of age. Although alcohol and tobacco are closely related social habits, there is no direct association between tobacco and breast cancer.

Height

Taller women have an increased risk of breast cancer (Hunter and Willett 1993). A pooled analysis estimated that the relative risk for women over 1.75 m tall compared with women under 1.6 m tall was 1.22 for all women and 1.28 for postmenopausal women (van den Brandt et al 2000).

Physical activity

A report from the International Agency for Research on Cancer concluded that physical activity has a preventive effect on breast cancer. This may be an indirect effect as exercise lowers BMI, or a direct effect on hormonal and growth factor levels. This varies between studies, with one showing a 30–40% reduction in the risk of breast cancer with a few hours of vigorous activity per week versus none (Monninkhof et al 2007).

Socioeconomic status

Breast cancer has a higher incidence in higher social classes. The age-standardized incidence rate is 115.1 per 100,000 women in the least deprived quintile compared with 97.3 per 100,000 women in the most deprived quintile. This is likely to be a reflection of other factors including reproductive history and early nutritional intake.

Mammographic density

There is extensive evidence that mammographic density is a risk factor for breast cancer, independent of other risk factors, and is associated with large relative and attributable risks for the disease. Women with increasingly dense breasts have two to six times the risk of breast cancer compared with women with less dense breasts (Boyd et al 1995). Parity, menopause and other risk factors only explain 20–30% of the variance in mammographic density (Boyd et al 2002). Early studies of mother–daughter sets and small twin studies suggested that genetic factors might explain a proportion of the variation of breast tissue patterns within a given population (Boyd et al 2002, Stone et al 2006). The genetic factors that influence mammographic density may also explain variations in breast tissue involution.

Previous history of breast cancer

If a woman has had breast cancer previously, the risk of developing a second primary breast cancer is two to six times greater compared with the the risk of the general population of developing a primary breast cancer (Chen and Thompson 1999).

Family history

A family history of breast cancer, particularly in first-degree relatives, is a well-known risk factor for the development of breast cancer. The past few years have seen a significant increase in knowledge of inherited breast cancer. Approximately 80% of breast cancers are sporadic, and the other 20% are familial, occurring within the context of a positive family history. Twin studies have shown that inherited factors may account for up to 25–30% of all breast cancers (Lalloo et al 2003). These cancers are the result of a combination of genetic and environmental factors that cause acquired genetic mutations over time (Vogel and Bevers 2003). A woman with one first-degree relative has approximately double the risk of breast cancer of a woman with no family history of the disease. The risk is greater if two (or more) relatives are affected. Multiple primary cancers in one individual or related early-onset cancers in a family pedigree are highly suggestive of a predisposing gene.

The first two major susceptibility genes for breast cancer, *BRCA1* and *BRCA2*, were identified in 1994 and 1995, respectively. Mutations and genomic rearrangements within the *BRCA1* and *BRCA2* genes have been clearly associated with breast cancer. The inherited mutation of these genes represents the first hit of Knudson's two-hit model of tumorigenesis. *BRCA* gene mutations interfere with the DNA-repair function of the normal gene, resulting in the accumulation of chromosomal abnormalities and an increased susceptibility to develop malignancy.

BRCA1 and *BRCA2* account for the largest proportion of familial breast cancer cases. It is thought that 20–25% of familial breast cancer cases are due to mutations or genomic rearrangements within these genes. The frequency of these mutations is rare, occurring in 0.1–0.5% of the general population, compared with 2% in Ashkenazi Jews (Rebbeck et al 2002). The breast cancer risk attributable to *BRCA1* and *BRCA2* mutations in Ashkenazi Jews is as high as 15–30% (FitzGerald et al 1996, Abeliovich et al 1997, Struewing et al 1997, Metcalfe et al 2004). A recent analysis of 22 studies showed that carrying a deleterious *BRCA1* or *BRCA2* mutation confers an estimated lifetime risk for developing breast cancer of 65% and 45%, respectively (Antoniou et al 2003). By the age of 40 years, carrying a deleterious *BRCA1* mutation confers a 20% chance of developing breast cancer, and the risk increases with age (Kauff et al 2002). Mutations in *BRCA1* are strongly associated with ovarian and fallopian tube cancers (Antoniou et al 2003). The risk of ovarian carcinoma for *BRCA1* carriers is 17%, 39% and 54% at 40, 70 and 80 years, respectively (Antoniou et al 2003). Penetrance of *BRCA1* with respect to ovarian, fallopian and breast cancer is greater than that for *BRCA2*.

Tumours associated with *BRCA1* carriers are more frequently grade 3, and ERα-negative and ovarian carcinomas, which occur in *BRCA1/2* families, are mostly non-mucinous epithelial cancers (Lakhani et al 2002). No single technique is able to detect all mutations, and even by sequencing the entire gene, the detection rate is only 85% (Evans et al 2003). Once a mutation has been identified in a family, definitive genetic testing can inform women more accurately

of their risks and give them an informed choice of their options. Mutational analysis of an unaffected individual is problematic without checking an affected relative. Identification of a mutation will confirm an increased risk; however, the absence of a mutation does not exclude the possibility of a refractory mutation of another gene. Where there is not a dominant family history or a *BRCA1/2* mutation is not identified, risk estimation gives a 1.5–3 fold relative risk with a family history of a single first-degree relative affected (Newman et al 1988, Claus et al 1994).

Quantitative Risk Assessment

A number of models are available to calculate a woman's risk of developing breast cancer. These utilize different combinations of risk factors derived from different data sets, and vary in the age to which they calculate cumulative risk of breast cancer. As a result, they may generate different risk estimates for a given patient.

The Gail model

The Gail model quantifies a woman's lifetime risk of developing breast cancer by incorporating patient age, age at menarche, age at first birth/nulliparity, number of breast biopsies, ethnic origin and history of breast cancer in first-degree relatives (Gail et al 1989, Costantino et al 1999). It does not, however, consider the ages of first-degree relatives with breast cancer, and overlooks a family history of bilateral breast disease, second-degree relatives with breast cancer and a family history of ovarian cancer. Also, the model does not account for a personal history of atypical hyperplasia and lobular carcinoma *in situ*, previous radiation therapy to the chest for the treatment of Hodgkin's lymphoma, or recent migration from a region of low breast cancer risk (e.g. rural China) to a high-risk region. The Gail model remains the most frequently used in defining eligibility for risk reduction trials.

The Claus model

The Claus model provides breast cancer risk estimates based on which relatives were diagnosed with breast cancer and at what age their diagnosis was made. Initially, only data from mothers and sisters were included, but second-degree relatives were included subsequently (Claus et al 1994).

BRCAPRO

BRCAPRO was developed by statisticians at Duke University to calculate age-specific probabilities of developing breast and ovarian cancer, based on the probability that the individual carries a mutation on one of the *BRCA* genes (Berry et al 1997). The model uses the observed incidences of breast and ovarian cancer among *BRCA* gene mutation carriers and non-carriers to calculate the probability that a given individual is a mutation carrier based on his/her family history.

The Tyrer–Cuzick model

The Tyrer–Cuzick model identifies the risk of breast cancer in unaffected women by taking into account their probability of carrying genetic risk factors, namely a *BRCA1/BRCA2* mutation; a notional common, low-penetrance dominant susceptibility allele that stands for all other genetic risk factors; and a number of other individual factors known to influence risk, such as age at menopause and menarche, weight, height, age, use of HRT, previous benign breast biopsies and parity (Tyrer et al 2004).

Future developments

The Breast Cancer Prevention Collaborative Group has advised that the following risk factors should be further examined by multivariate analysis in future studies: mammographic density, plasma hormone levels, bone density and fracture history, history of weight gain, BMI and hip–waist ratio (Santen et al 2007). It is thought that the addition of these risk factors will lead to a more accurate quantitative risk assessment model for use in future breast cancer prevention trials. Whilst breast cancer risk assessment using mathematical models based on epidemiological data is valid, no one model integrates benign breast disease, oestrogen exposure and family history in a comprehensive fashion. Therefore, it is important to use a variety of models in a specialized risk assessment clinic.

Screening, Genetic Testing and Risk Reduction

Identification of candidates for genetic counselling and genetic testing remains important as only a small fraction of the estimated carriers have been identified. There is growing evidence that high-penetrance germline mutations in genes such as *BRCA1* and *BRCA2* account for a small proportion of familial risk of breast cancer, and the majority of the remaining risk is likely to be caused by combinations of more common, lower penetrance variants.

Breast cancer family history clinics are well established in the UK, and are run by medical oncologists, clinical geneticists, nurse specialists and breast surgeons in a multidisciplinary approach with close involvement of radiologists and psychologists (Evans et al 1994, 1996). After a risk assessment, women are divided into three risk groups: average, moderate and high risk. Patients should undergo pretest counselling to ensure understanding of the implications of a positive test. This should also include the risks and benefits of early cancer detection and the prevention modalities available. Counselling following testing should be available to help patients to cope with their test results and review prevention modalities. Once advised of their risk, women deciding to pursue risk reduction therapy can be presented with their management options.

Surgical management

Prophylactic/risk-reducing mastectomy (RRM) is an option for breast cancer risk reduction in high-risk women. The significant psychological and physical burden associated with RRM is reserved for those women whose lifetime risk of developing breast cancer is high. High-risk women are classified as those with a lifetime risk above 25%. This risk is the equivalent of having one first-degree relative with breast cancer diagnosed below the age of 50 years, or three affected relatives (first-degree) diagnosed under the age of 60 years. The efficacy of RRM is controversial and depends on the amount of residual tissue following the procedure. A retrospective study of 639 women with a family history of breast cancer suggests that RRM is associated with a 90% reduction in risk (Hartmann et al 1999). One small prospective study investigating the efficacy of prophylactic mastectomy in *BRCA1/2* carriers with a mean follow-up of 3 years showed that those women undergoing mastectomy had a significant reduction in the incidence of breast cancer (0 of 76 women) compared with the surveillance group (eight of 63 women) (Meijers-Heijboer et al 2001).

The use of RRM is increasing, with women often choosing to have breast reconstruction surgery either immediately or delayed. The timing of the reconstruction is controversial, with immediate reconstruction appropriate in the majority of women. It is now felt that the psychological benefit of emerging from a mastectomy with a breast mound far outweighs the need for a waiting period (Kronowitz 2007). The process from first consultation to surgery takes 6–12 months; this delay deliberately allows women enough time for the decision-making process.

Bilateral prophylactic oophorectomy

Studies have shown a significant reduction in the incidence of breast cancer in women with *BRCA1/2* mutations that have undergone prophylactic bilateral oophorectomy (Rebbeck et al 2002). Before undergoing the procedure, the patient should take into account how long she wishes to maintain her fertility, and should receive counselling about the risks and benefits of prophylactic oophorectomy. Opinion is divided on the use of HRT following prophylactic oophorectomy, with some centres routinely recommending HRT for all patients up to 50 years of age; the decision to use oestrogens should be based on a consideration of symptoms affecting future health and quality of life.

Chemoprevention

Chemoprevention provides a non-invasive option for breast cancer risk reduction for many high-risk women. Tamoxifen, a selective oestrogen receptor modulator (SERM) well known for its antioestrogenic effects in breast tissue, was the first agent used in breast cancer risk reduction after it was found to reduce the incidence of all breast cancers by 38% and ER-positive tumours by 48% (Cuzick et al 2003).

Pathology

The World Health Organization's classification of breast tumours organizes both benign and malignant lesions by histological pattern. Epithelial tumours comprise the largest group, including intraductal papilloma, adenomas, intraductal and lobular carcinoma *in situ*, invasive (ductal and lobular) carcinoma, and Paget's disease of the nipple. Invasive ductal carcinoma is by far the most common type.

In-situ carcinoma

These are preinvasive carcinomas. The proliferation of epithelial cells remains confined by an intact basement membrane, with no invasion into the surrounding stroma.

Ductal carcinoma *in situ*

Breast screening has resulted in a marked increase in the detection of ductal carcinoma *in situ* (DCIS), accounting for 25–30% of all screen-detected tumours (Schwartz et al 2000). Over 90% of DCIS is impalpable, asymptomatic and often detected by screening as microcalcifications (Figure 47.1). The remaining 10% are symptomatic, presenting with nipple discharge, a palpable mass or Paget's disease of the breast. When diagnosed clinically, DCIS is often extensive or associated with a concurrent invasive tumour. Postmortem studies have shown prevalence of DCIS from 0.2% to 14% (Bartow et al 1987, Nielsen et al 1987). Risk factors for DCIS include older age at first childbirth, nulliparity and a family history of breast cancer (Raktovich 2000). Retrospective studies of cases of low-grade DCIS misdiagnosed as benign showed that 20 years after local excision, approximately 33% had developed invasive disease (Page et al 1995). DCIS is classified into two major subtypes according to the presence/absence of comedo necrosis (atypical cells with abundant luminal necrosis that fill at least one duct) (Silverstein et al 1996). A system of low, intermediate and high nuclear grade is used to classify DCIS.

- Low-grade DCIS: evenly spaced cells with centrally placed small nuclei, few mitoses and the nucleoli are not well seen.
- High-grade DCIS: pleomorphic irregularly spaced cells, with large irregular nuclei, frequent mitoses and prominent nucleoli. Often solid with comedo necrosis and calcification.
- Intermediate-grade DCIS: features between high- and low-grade DCIS.

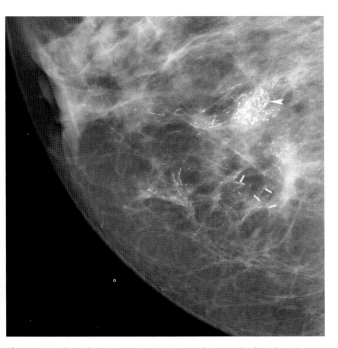

Figure 47.1 Ductal carcinoma *in situ*. Intermediate-grade ductal carcinoma *in situ* (DCIS) exhibiting classical comedo-type casting calcification within the ducts. The linear branching pattern is very typical of DCIS. Small arrows demonstrate the casting branching pattern of DCIS. The more density clustered area of calcification is associated with a local area of invasive ductal carcinoma (arrow head).

Most cases of DCIS are unicentric, with only 1% showing multicentric disease (Holland et al 1990b).

Multicentric tumour is defined as separate foci of tumour found in more than one breast quadrant or more than 5 cm from the primary tumour. Multifocal tumour is defined as more than one tumour foci in the same quadrant (Anonymous 1998c).

The spread of DCIS locally is along the branching ducts that form the glandular breast, and explains why most DCIS recurrences occur at or near the site of the initial tumour (Holland et al 1998). Micro-invasion is uncommon in DCIS, but confers a 2% risk of lymph node metastasis (van Dongen et al 1989). Studies have shown that poorly differentiated, high-grade comedo DCIS has low ER expression, high rates of cell proliferation, and overexpression of c-erbB2 (HER-2/neu) and epidermal growth factor receptor (EGFR) (Millis et al 1996). Low-grade lesions have high ER expression, lower rates of cell proliferation and rarely express HER-2 (Millis et al 1996, Boland et al 2002). Small, localized areas of DCIS (<4 cm) should be treated with breast-conserving surgery (BCS) with or without radiotherapy, and larger lesions need to be treated with mastectomy (Schwartz et al 2000).

The incidence of macroscopic nodal involvement in DCIS is less than 1%; however, nodal micrometastases have been reported in 5–14% of patients (Schuh et al 1986, Kitchen et al 2000). Two small, single-institution studies have reported a 3.1% rate of sentinel lymph node involvement in 223 patients with pure DCIS. Sentinel lymph node biopsy (SNB) for DCIS is not currently indicated but is under investigation, and may have a role in mastectomy for DCIS (Intra et al 2003). SNB should only be considered in those patients with a higher likelihood of underlying, undetected invasive disease (i.e. younger patients, DCIS >4 cm, high-grade DCIS and patients undergoing mastectomy). Twenty-five percent of cases recur within 8 years of BCS alone, 50% of which will present with invasive disease (Fisher et al 1999, Julien et al 2000, Ottesen et al 2000, Chan et al 2001); the recurrence rate for DCIS following mastectomy is 1% (Silverstein et al 1995). The key factor for recurrence is a clear margin at the time of surgery, and poor prognostic indicators include younger age at diagnosis (<40 years), poorly differentiated/high-grade tumours, presence of comedo necrosis, ER negativity and HER-2 positivity (Yen et al 2005).

The NSABP-B17, EORTC 10853 and UK/ANZ DCIS trials evaluated the value of radiotherapy following BCS for DCIS (Fisher et al 1999, Julien et al 2000, Houghton et al 2003). All of the trials reported a significant reduction in ipsilateral recurrence following radiotherapy. The EORTC trial showed a reduction in recurrence of DCIS from 8% to 5%, and a reduction in invasive recurrence from 8% to 4% at 5 years.

Lobular in-situ neoplasia

Lobular in-situ neoplasia (LISN; formerly known as lobular carcinoma *in situ*) is not itself a premalignant lesion but is a high-risk marker of invasive cancer. It is often an incidental finding during breast biopsy, and accounts for 0.5% of symptomatic and 1% of screen-detected tumours. Patients with LISN are younger, premenopausal with bilateral and multicentric disease of lower grade. Almost all patients express ER (Akashi-Tanaka et al 2000). If LISN is detected at core biopsy, the area should be subjected to excision biopsy to confirm the diagnosis and exclude an invasive focus. The NSABP P-1 prevention trial reported a 56% risk reduction of developing subsequent invasive cancer with tamoxifen in patients with a history of LISN (Dunn and Ford 2000).

Invasive carcinoma

Invasive ductal carcinoma

Approximately 80% of breast cancers are invasive (infiltrating) ductal carcinoma (IDC), not otherwise specified; a generic term used to distinguish between these tumours and other specific forms of ductal carcinoma, such as tubular, medullary, metaplastic and adenoid cystic carcinomas. IDC includes a subset of tumours that express, in part, characteristics of one of the specific types of breast carcinoma but do not constitute pure examples of the individual tumours. IDC invariably form a solid tumour, and cystic change in this group of lesions is extremely uncommon but may be a manifestation of necrosis.

Invasive lobular carcinoma

Invasive lobular carcinoma (ILC) is the second most common type of invasive breast cancer accounting for 8–14% of all invasive breast cancers (Arpino et al 2004). ILC clinically presents as a poorly defined thickening of the breast rather than a dominant mass. This makes the extent of the disease difficult to estimate on clinical examination, and difficult to visualize on mammography. Ultrasonography is more sensitive than mammography in detecting ILC, but may significantly underestimate the size of the lesions (Pritt et al 2004, Selinko et al 2004). Magnetic resonance imaging (MRI) is more accurate than either mammography or ultrasonography in defining the extent of the disease but is less widely available (Weinstein et al 2001). Due to the infiltrative growth pattern, there is a higher incidence of resection margin involvement than for IDC and a higher conversion rate to mastectomy (Yeatman et al 1995). ILC has a higher incidence of being bilateral, multifocal and multicentric than IDC (Figure 47.2) (Ashikari et al 1973). Axillary lymph nodes in ILC may remain impalpable even when extensively involved (Grube et al 2002). A large study from the National Cancer Database to examine treatment and outcomes in patients with ILC showed a similar 5-year survival rate between patients with ILC and IDC, and between those ILC patients receiving breast-conserving therapy and those receiving mastectomy (Winchester et al 1998).

Paget's disease of the breast

Sir James Paget (1874) described 'an eczematous change in the skin of the nipple preceding an underlying mammary cancer', now known as Paget's disease (Paget 1874). More than 95% of women with Paget's disease of the nipple have an underlying malignancy, although 50% are clinically and mammographically undetectable (Vielh et al 1993). Paget's disease accounts for 0.7–4.9% of all breast malignancies, and misdiagnosis as eczema and treatment with topical steroids explains an average 10–12-month delay in diagnosis

(Kister and Haagensen 1970, Lagios et al 1984, Chaudary et al 1986, Dixon et al 1991, Kothari et al 2002). The first symptoms include burning, itching and change in sensation of the nipple–areola complex; raised skin lesions follow this, with a clear demarcation from the surrounding skin. Rarely, nipple deformity and retraction may occur if there is tethering from an underlying malignancy. Characteristically, it starts on the nipple and spreads to the areola and then surrounding skin, and in the later stages may present with ulceration and bleeding. Differential diagnoses include chronic eczema, benign papilloma of the nipple, basal cell carcinoma, Bowen's disease and malignant melanoma (Jamali et al 1996).

A full-thickness punch biopsy of the nipple should be performed to confirm the diagnosis (Rosen 1996). Mammography, ultrasonography and MRI can be used to detect an underlying mass, as well as assessing the contralateral breast. Paget's disease often presents with multicentric disease (75%); therefore, mastectomy is advocated as the procedure of choice (Kothari et al 2002). However, several small studies of BCS and radiotherapy for Paget's disease have shown low rates of recurrence (Fourquet et al 1987, Dixon et al 1991, Kollmorgen et al 1998, Bijker et al 2001, Fu et al 2001, Marshall et al 2003). Attempts to preserve uninvolved areas of the nipple are associated with high rates of local recurrence (Stockdale et al 1989, Fu et al 2001). Staging by SNB or axillary dissection is required for all patients with invasive disease.

Inflammatory breast cancer

Inflammatory breast cancer (IBC) was first coined by Lee and Tannenbaum at the Memorial Hospital, New York in 1924 to describe an aggressive form of breast cancer with an incidence of 1–6% (Lee and Tannenbaum 1924, Levine et al 1985). A higher incidence is reported in African-Americans than in Caucasians and other ethnic groups (10.1%, 6.2% and 5.1%, respectively). Women with IBC often present at a younger age than women with non-IBC (NIBC) (Chang et al 1998, Anderson et al 2003, Charafe-Jauffret et al 2004). The 10-year survival rate of patients with IBC is 26.7%, compared with 44.8% for those with NIBC (Low et al 2002). A recent review of 635 patients at the M.D. Anderson, Texas (IBC, n = 214; stage III NIBC, n = 421) demonstrated a significantly reduced progression-free survival for IBC compared with NIBC (24 months and 35 months, respectively), and of overall survival for IBC compared with NIBC (42 months and 60 months, respectively).

The criteria for diagnosis was described by Haagensen including erythema, oedema involving more than two-thirds of the breast, tenderness, induration, warmth, enlargement, peau d'orange and diffuseness of the tumour on palpation (Haagensen 1971). These symptoms progress rapidly. At diagnosis, most patients (55–85%) have axillary lymph node involvement and up to 30% have distant metastases (Jaiyesimi et al 1992, Hance et al 2005). Pathology shows extensive lymphovascular invasion by tumour emboli, involving the superficial dermal plexus of vessels in the papillary and high reticular dermis (Taylor and Meltzer 1938). Primary IBC is the development of carcinoma and skin changes in a previously healthy breast, and secondary IBC is the development of inflammatory IBC in a breast

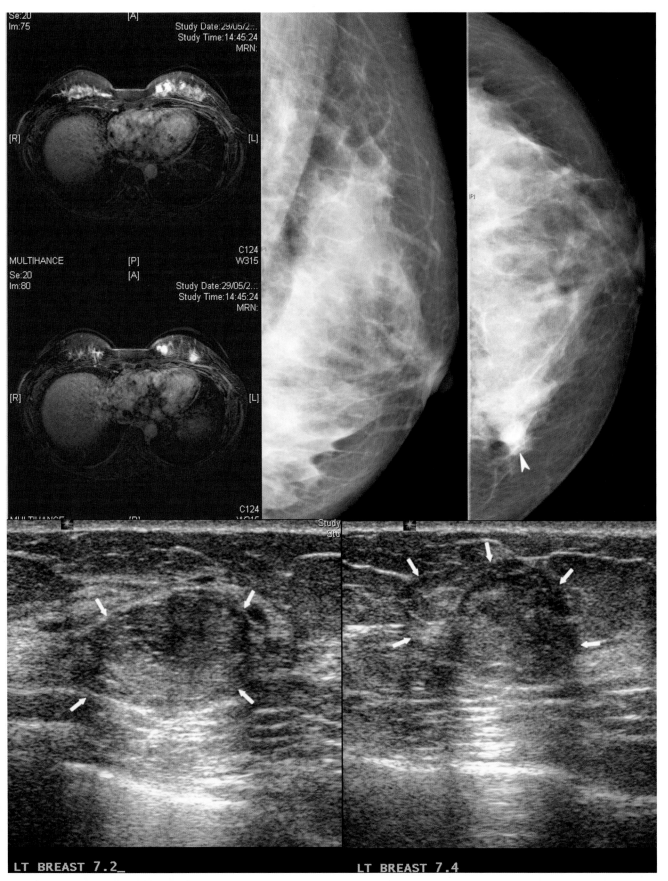

Figure 47.2 Multifocal breast cancer. Most commonly seen in invasive lobular cancer. The left mammogram images [mediolateral oblique (MLO) and craniocaudal (CC)] have dense parenchyma and only show a single subtle mass with slight distortion (arrowhead) on the MLO view. Ultrasound shows two subtle lesions (arrowed) close to each other (LT BREAST 7.2 and 7.4). Contrast-enhanced subtraction magnetic resonance shows multiple enhancing lesions (arrow heads) in the left breast on different slices.

that has had a previous malignancy or changes caused by irradiation.

One treatment protocol from the M.D. Anderson advises initial treatment with neoadjuvant sequential taxane (paclitaxel/docetaxel) and an anthracycline-based regimen (5-fluorouracil + epirubicin + cyclophosphamide) (Cristofanilli et al 2002). Patients who show a partial or complete response undergo surgery (mastectomy and axillary dissection) followed by adjuvant radiotherapy and hormonal therapy (if ERα-positive). For those patients who do not respond, radiotherapy to the breast and axilla is recommended, followed by surgery, if feasible, and adjuvant hormonal therapy (if ERα-positive) (Singletary 2008). SNB is not recommended in patients with IBC as the identification rate is only 70% and the false-negative rate is 40% (Stearns et al 2002). Currently, most practitioners recommend a delayed reconstruction after completion of therapy. Most local recurrences occur in the mastectomy flap.

A number of studies have reported a higher incidence of c-erbB2 (HER-2) in patients with IBC (Turpin et al 2002, Parton et al 2004). One small study (n = 22, IBC = 9, NIBC = 13) combining docetaxel with trastuzumab as part of the primary systemic therapy observed a complete response in 40% of patients (van Pelt et al 2003). Lapatinib (reversible inhibitor of c-erbB1 and c-erbB2) has shown partial responses in women with IBC who have been extensively pretreated (Burris et al 2005, Spector et al 2006). The combination of lapatinib with paclitaxel in a cohort of 21 chemotherapy-naïve IBC patients overexpressing HER-2 showed a clinical response rate of 95% (Cristofanilli et al 2006).

Other breast malignancies

Primary cutaneous melanoma of the skin of the breast is very rare, accounting for 0.28% of all cases of melanoma (Ariel and Caron 1972). It is more commonly found as a result of a distant metastasis from a primary elsewhere. A full history and physical examination for the presence of other melanomas should be performed. A core or surgical biopsy of the thickest portion of the melanoma will determine the depth of invasion. Immunostaining for HMB-45 and S100 enables differentiation of melanoma from other cutaneous masses. Staging is with computed tomography (CT) or positron emission tomography (PET), and lactate dehydrogenase levels should be measured. Wide local excision is recommended with margins dependent upon the depth of invasion, and SNB performed at the time of excision. Complete axillary dissection should be performed for those patients with clinically suspicious lymphadenopathy and those with melanomas larger than 4 mm (Essner et al 2002). Adjuvant therapy is similar to that for melanoma elsewhere in the body.

Radiation-induced primary angiosarcoma of the breast, first reported in 1981, is extremely rare (Maddox and Evans 1981). Approximately 60 cases have been reported, although the incidence is rising (Rao et al 2003). It presents as violet, blue, red or black skin nodules in a multifocal pattern, and is diagnosed by a punch, incisional or excisional biopsy (Fineberg and Rosen 1994). Fine needle aspiration, mammography and ultrasonography are often not helpful. Factor VIII-related antigen is positive in most angiosarcomas, dis-

tinguishing it from other sarcomas (Stokkel and Peterse 1992). Staging is based on the size, grade and depth of the tumour, with grade being the most important prognostic indicator. Most angiosarcomas are high grade and are treated with mastectomy (Fineberg and Rosen 1994). Axillary staging is not required, as most sarcomas do not metastasize to regional lymph nodes. The recurrence rate is 40% and prognosis is poor.

Primary breast lymphoma (PBL) is defined as a lymphoma localized to the breast and its draining basins, arising from lymphoid tissue in the breast (Smith et al 1987, Kuper-Hommel et al 2003). It accounts for 0.14% of all breast malignancies and 0.65% of all non-Hodgkin's lymphomas, with the most common type being diffuse large B-cell lymphoma (Ha et al 1998, Kuper-Hommel et al 2003). PBL arises most commonly in the seventh decade as a painless, enlarged rubbery mass. Mammographic and ultrasound findings are non-specific, and PBL is categorized according to the Ann Arbor classification of lymphomas. Diagnosis is by core biopsy, and the patient is staged by CT of the neck, chest, abdomen and pelvis, and bone marrow biopsy. Surgery with adjuvant radiotherapy is no longer advocated due to the high incidence of local and disseminated recurrence (Kuper-Hommel et al 2003). Treatment of PBL is now with chemotherapy, followed by targeted radiotherapy, with a 2-year survival rate of 63% (Ha et al 1998, Brogi and Harris 1999).

Metastasis to the breast

This is uncommon and accounts for 0.5–6.6% of breast malignancies, with the contralateral breast being the most common site of metastatic malignancy (Bohman et al 1982, Paulus and Libshitz 1982, Amichetti et al 1990). Other malignancies that metastasize to the breast include lymphoma, melanoma, rhabdomyosarcoma and small cell lung cancer (Bartella et al 2003). These lesions are indistinguishable from primary breast cancers by examination and imaging. Core biopsy is preferable as immunohistochemistry plays an important role in diagnosis and prognosis is poor, with a 1-year survival rate of 20% (Bartella et al 2003).

Presentation

Breast cancers may present symptomatically or through screening.

Breast screening

Breast screening aims to reduce mortality through early detection. A number of trials carried out between the 1960s and 1980s showed that population screening by mammography can be expected to reduce breast cancer mortality by 25% (Olsen and Gotzsche 2001, Tabar et al 2001, Anonymous 2002b, Duffy et al 2002, Nystrom et al 2002). The benefit of screening is greatest in women aged 55–70 years (Anonymous 2002b, Nystrom et al 2002). There is no mortality benefit of screening women under 40 years of age, and the mortality benefit of those aged between 40 and 55 years is 20% (Anonymous 2002b, Nystrom et al 2002). Breast screening has been introduced in many countries over the past 20 years. In some countries, screening is advised in all women over 40 years of age; however, in countries providing population-based screening, women over 50 years of age are targeted.

The UK National Breast Screening Programme (NHSBSP) was set up by the Department of Health in 1988 in response to the recommendations of a working group, chaired by Professor Sir Patrick Forrest, which had been set up to consider whether or not to implement a population screening programme in the UK. The report 'Breast Cancer Screening' was published in 1986, and became known as 'The Forrest Report' (Forrest 1986). The NHSBSP was the first of its kind in the world. It began inviting women for screening in 1988, and national coverage was achieved by the mid 1990s. It provides screening by invitation, free at the point of delivery to all women between 50 and 70 years of age (initially 50–64 years, age range increased in 2004). Women over 70 years of age can attend but are not invited, and more than 70% of the invited population are required to attend in order to obtain an overall mortality benefit. The screening method is two-view mammography (craniocaudal and medio-lateral oblique views) every 3 years. Approximately 5% of women screened are recalled for further assessment of a problem identified at screening. Three-quarters of women recalled simply require further imaging (ultrasound and/or mammography) and clinical assessment before being reassured and discharged. The remaining 25% will undergo a needle biopsy procedure in order to diagnose six cancers per 1000 women screened. Despite advances in needle biopsy techniques, 0.25% of all women screened will require an open surgical biopsy. Mammography can be expected to detect breast cancer 2 years before it becomes clinically apparent, and the frequency of mammography is determined by the lead time of breast cancer. Mammographic screening intervals, based on average growth time of breast cancer to age, should be yearly for women between 40 and 50 years of age, every 2 years in women between 50 and 60 years of age, and every 3 years thereafter. However, the Breast Screening Frequency trial did not show a significant benefit for women aged 50–64 years screened yearly compared with those screened every 3 years (Anonymous 2002a). One-third of breast cancers will present in the interval between screens, called 'interval cancers', and half of these will present in the third year after screening.

Screening high-risk young women

A national study evaluating mammographic screening for young women with a family history of breast cancer is being conducted (FH01 study), comparing screening in women aged 40–44 years with a moderate risk with a control arm; this study is currently unreported. Mammography has a higher predictive value in young women at high risk compared with age-matched controls, but is not sensitive, particularly in women with BRCA1 mutations (Chang et al 1999, Brekelmans et al 2001, Goffin et al 2001, Tilanus-Linthorst et al 2002, Hamilton et al 2004, Robson 2004, Warner et al 2004). Women with BRCA1 rarely present with associated DCIS, and the mammographic features are therefore usually of a mass lesion with no microcalcifications and no architectural distortion.

These often present as interval cancers. BRCA2 cancers present similarly to sporadic cancers, and are more likely to be detected by mammography. Ultrasonographic features in BRCA1 cancers are often indeterminate or benign.

MRI is the most sensitive imaging modality in young women (Kriege et al 2004, Robson 2004). Genetically predisposed women commonly develop breast cancer when young and when dense breast tissue reduces the sensitivity of mammography. The Magnetic Resonance Imaging for Breast Screening (MARIBS) study compared the performance of contrast-enhanced MRI with mammography in this group of women (Leach et al 2005). It confirmed that contrast-enhanced MRI was significantly more sensitive than mammography in cancer detection for the entire cohort, but especially in the subgroup of BRCA1 carriers. Specificity for both procedures was acceptable. In spite of a high proportion of grade 3 tumours, the tumours were small and few women were node positive. These findings confirm those from the Netherlands six-centre MRI Screening (MRISC) study and a single-centre study from Toronto (Warner et al 2004, Kriege et al 2007). These reports support a policy of annual screening combining contrast-enhanced MRI and mammography, which would detect most tumours. These studies show evidence of effective small cancer detection, but do not have sufficient power to show whether mortality is reduced, for which there is no current evidence. Age for starting screening must be based on age rather than age of affected relatives. For women at moderate risk, screening should be started at 40 years of age, and for those at high risk, screening may be started at 30–35 years of age. High risk can be described as more than 8% by 50 years or more than 25% for lifetime. It is important that these women be followed-up in a specialist centre.

Symptomatic disease

Approximately 60% of breast cancers present symptomatically with a discrete mass, skin changes (ulceration/dimpling), nipple changes or, rarely, pain (mastalgia). In the UK, guidelines have been issued by the Department of Health informing family practitioners of the suspicious symptoms which warrant urgent referral to a breast clinic. Referral must be within 24 h of seeing their general practitioner, and women should be seen by a specialist in a breast clinic within 2 weeks of referral. 'One-stop' clinics, where all the necessary tests required to make a diagnosis are performed, are recommended.

Diagnosis

The management of women with breast cancer should be undertaken in a specialist breast multidisciplinary unit, with members of the breast team divided into two separate but interdependent groups:

- Diagnostic team, including breast specialist clinician (normally a consultant breast surgeon), specialist radiographer and radiologist, pathologist (histopathologist/cytopathologist), breast care nurses, nurse practitioners, clinical staff, administrative staff and a dedicated multidisciplinary team (MDT) coordinator.

- Cancer treatment team, including members of the diagnostic team and clinical/medical oncologist, oncoplastic/plastic surgeon, medical geneticist, research/ward/breast care nurses, lymphoedema specialist, clinical psychologist, palliative care team and data management personnel.

Triple assessment

Patients undergo a triple assessment, which is a combination of clinical examination, imaging (mammography for women >35 years and ultrasonography for women <35 years) and cytology (fine needle aspiration) with or without needle core biopsy (both guided by either X-ray or ultrasonography). Triple assessment has a high positive predictive value and a low false-positive rate. The aim of triple assessment is to make a diagnosis prior to counselling and definitive treatment.

Mammography

X-ray mammography has been the basis of breast imaging for more than 30 years. The sensitivity of mammography for breast cancer is dependent on age, as the denser the breast tissue, the less effective it is in detection (Figure 47.3). Breast tissue is more dense in younger women and whilst the sensitivity of mammography for breast cancer in women over 60 years of age approaches 95%, detection rates are less than 50% in women under 40 years of age (Kolb et al 2002). Mammography uses ionizing radiation and should only be used where a clinical benefit is likely. The benefits of mammography in women over 40 years of age is likely to outweigh the oncogenic effects of repeated exposure. There is rarely an indication for performing mammography in women under 35 years of age unless there is a strong clinical suspicion of malignancy. The false-negative rate for mammography has been reported to be between 10% and 30%. Although many cancers are mammographically occult, especially in dense breasts, a large number of these are visible retrospectively. These oversights can be reduced by double reading, improving sensitivity by up to 15% (Skaane et al 2007). Computer-aided design (CAD) programmes are available to assist radiologists to detect potentially suspicious abnormalities.

Ultrasound

High-frequency ultrasound (>10 MHz) is a highly effective diagnostic tool in the investigation of focal breast symptoms (Wilson and Teh 1998). Ultrasound does not use ionizing radiation and has a very high sensitivity for breast pathology (Lister et al 1998). High-resolution ultrasonography can easily distinguish between most solid and cystic lesions, and can differentiate between benign and malignant lesions with a high degree of accuracy (Figure 47.4). It is the technique of choice for further investigation of focal symptomatic breast abnormalities for women under 35 years of age, and is used in conjunction with mammography in those over 35 years of age. Ultrasound is being used increasingly to assess the axilla in women with breast cancer. Those nodes with an abnormal morphology can be accurately sampled by fine needle aspiration.

Elastography ultrasound is a new adjunct to conventional B-mode ultrasound imaging, and uses the differences in tissue deformation to create an image of relative tissue stiffness (Wakeham et al 2006). Objects in the breast of different stiffness will displace different amounts, creating an image of relative stiffness (Svensson and Amiras 2006). Research into elasticity ultrasound has been ongoing for over 20 years, but it is only more recently with advances in computing power that commercial development of the potential clinical applications has become possible. A recent study has shown that benign lesions have a smaller size image on strain ultrasound than B-mode imaging, whilst malignant lesions usually have a larger strain image (Hall et al 2003). Malignant lesions mainly appear as stiff throughout, and strain imaging can reveal lesions that are occult on B-mode imaging, allowing accurate diagnostic biopsy. It may be that knowledge of the typical strain appearances may obviate the need to fine needle aspirate/biopsy certain benign lesions.

Magnetic resonance imaging

MRI of the breast is an important new investigation to evaluate breast cancer. Studies have shown almost 100% sensitivity in detecting invasive breast cancers, although most show poor specificity. Diagnostic breast MRI should be performed with a high field strength (>1.5 tesla) magnet with a dedicated breast radiofrequency coil. Contrast enhancement with gadopenate dimeglumine (Gd-DTPA) is essential in identifying breast cancers and distinguishing malignancies from benign masses. The role of MRI is evolving, and one of its most widely used indications is in preoperative evaluation of known tumours for size, extent of disease, multicentricity and multifocality (especially invasive lobular carcinoma). Few centres offer magnetic-resonance-guided breast biopsy, but most breast lesions over 10 mm seen on MRI can be visualized by ultrasound.

A Memorial Sloan-Kettering Cancer Center study of patients with invasive lobular cancer showed that MRI iden-

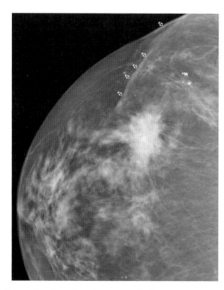

Figure 47.3 Invasive ductal carcinoma grade II mammogram. Irregular dense mass with a spiculated margin and fine spiculations extending out into the surrounding breast tissue. The spiculations are causing distortion and skin thickening (open arrows).

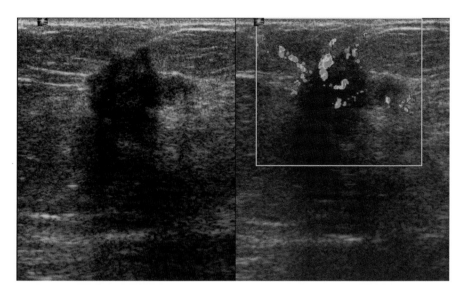

Figure 47.4 Invasive ductal carcinoma grade II ultrasound. This is the same tumour as shown in Figure 47.3. On the greyscale image, there is an irregular mass of reduced echogenicity which has posterior shadowing. The colour Doppler image shows surround vascularity which has a radial distribution feeding the cancer. Slight overlying skin thickening can be seen on the greyscale image.

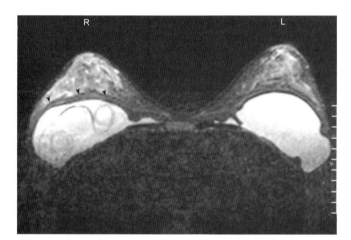

Figure 47.5 Magnetic resonance of ruptured prosthesis. Note the prosthesis lies behind the pectoral muscle (arrow heads). The right prosthesis has ruptured, and the curvilinear shape of the envelope of the prosthesis lying free within the silicone is clearly visible.

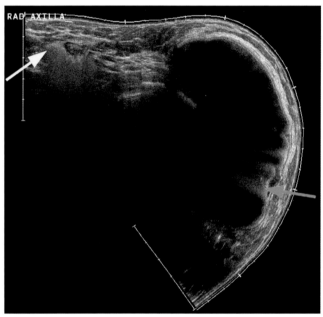

Figure 47.6 Leaking silicone breast prosthesis. Extended field of view image of a leaking prosthesis. The blue arrow shows free silicone outside the envelope of the prosthesis. There is increased echogenicity with a comet's tail of reverberation echogenicity deep to it. In the axilla, free silicone is demonstrated by the white arrow; again, there is increased echogenicity with a comet's tail of reverberation deep to it.

tified 27% more sites of cancer in the ipsilateral breast. Of these, 42% had DCIS and 58% had an infiltrating cancer (Quan et al 2003). Of the 62 women studied, multifocal cancer was present in 20%, multicentric cancer in 4%, and multifocal and multicentric cancer in 3%. Therefore, approximately one-quarter of additional ipsilateral cancers occur within the same quadrant. A recent multi-institutional study of women recently diagnosed with breast cancer showed that 3.1% had a cancer detected by MRI in an apparently uninvolved contralateral breast (Lehman et al 2007). MRI has been shown to accurately distinguish between scarring and tumour recurrence, provided that the scan is performed more than 18 months after surgery. The value of MRI screening in high-risk patients has been discussed previously. MRI is used to evaluate the integrity of saline and silicone implants (Figure 47.5), to discern extracapsular rupture from intracapsular rupture, and to identify silicone within the breast parenchyma (Holmich et al 2005). It is superior to

ultrasonography (Figure 47.6) in detecting implant ruptures in patients with both double and single lumen implants (Di Benedetto et al 2008).

Positron emission tomography

Most breast malignancies have greater metabolism and concentrate 18F-fluorodeoxyglucose (FDG), the agent most frequently used in clinical PET. PET and PET/CT the latter of which combines anatomical and physiological imaging are increasingly used in oncology (Figure 47.7). However, it is

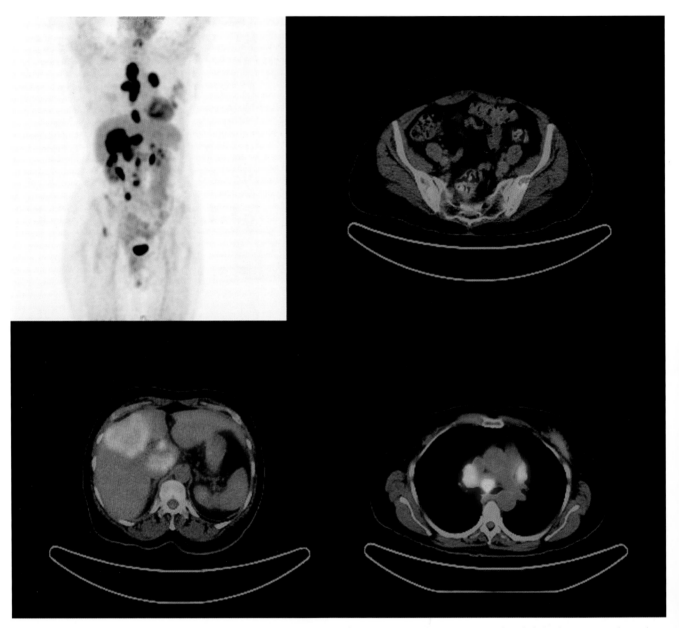

Figure 47.7 Positron emission tomography (PET)/computed tomography (CT) of breast carcinoma liver metastases. The whole-body PET image shows the extent of metastatic disease because of increased metabolic activity in the metastases demonstrated by the uptake of fluorodeoxyglucose, labelled with fluorine-18 (a positron emitter). The fused PET/CT images show the exact anatomical location of the metastases in mediastinal nodes, liver and left ilium adjacent to the anterior part of the sacroiliac joint. The colour denotes the increased metabolic activity which can be measured. The standard uptake value allows changes in metabolism to be detected, enabling assessment of whether or not metastases are responding to chemotherapy regimes before anatomical change occurs.

widely agreed that FDG-PET does not have a role in the detection of primary breast cancer.

FDG-PET and FDG-PET/CT can improve staging by detecting otherwise occult disease, particularly in the locoregional and mediastinal nodal basins (Eubank et al 2004, Eubank and Mankoff 2005). Eubank et al showed that FDG-PET detected more widespread disease changes, affecting treatment in up to 44% of patients thought to have locoregional recurrence. Skeletal metastases account for 90% of all metastatic lesions, as well as being the most common site of initial metastatic involvement. A number of studies have shown that FDG-PET is superior to bone scintigraphy in

detecting intramedullary and lytic lesions, but often fails to demonstrate blastic lesions, which are readily detected by bone scintigraphy (Cook et al 1998, Moon et al 1998, Kim et al 2001, Even-Sapir et al 2004, Isasi et al 2005, Nakai et al 2005, Tatsumi et al 2006).

Recently, a study of FDG-PET/CT evaluating asymptomatic breast cancer patients with rising tumour markers demonstrated 90% sensitivity for diagnosing recurrent tumour, affecting the clinical management in 51% of patients (Radan et al 2006). A number of studies have demonstrated the accuracy of FDG-PET in depicting response to treatment (Wahl et al 1993, Schelling et al 2000, Smith et al 2000,

Chen et al 2004, Mankoff and Eubank 2006, Rousseau et al 2006). More recently, a decline in FDG uptake of more than 50% indicated a good response to treatment in the metastatic setting (Gennari et al 2000). One study demonstrated a change in FDG uptake after one cycle of chemotherapy, and an absence of FDG uptake following completion of treatment predicted a better survival than in those patients with residual FDG-positive disease (Cachin et al 2006).

Image-Guided Biopsy

Fine needle aspiration cytology

Fine needle aspiration cytology (FNAC) of breast lumps is an important part of the triple assessment of the palpable breast lump. FNAC of breast masses has been shown to be a simple and safe diagnostic procedure. However, diagnostic failure of aspiration cytology has been attributed to a high unsatisfactory aspirate rate. This may be due to either insufficient epithelial cells present, equivocal smears or unrepresentative aspirates resulting in false-negative diagnoses. However, some patients find FNAC painful; it can be associated with haematoma formation; and, if performed before mammography or ultrasound, it can make radiological assessment of the breast more difficult.

Needle core biopsy

Automated core biopsy (14 G, 22 mm) provides significantly better sensitivity, specificity and positive predictive value than FNAC (Teh et al 1998, Britton 1999, Britton and McCann 1999, Vargas et al 2000). Most units in the NHSBSP now perform automated core biopsy as the primary diagnostic tool. Ultrasound provides real-time visualization of the biopsy procedure, and confirmation of sampling. Between 80% and 90% of breast abnormalities can be visualized on ultrasound, with the rest being performed under stereotactic X-ray guidance. Needle core biopsy is highly accurate in determining the nature of most breast lesions, and women with benign lesions can avoid unnecessary surgery. For those with breast cancer, needle biopsy provides an accurate diagnosis enabling physicians to make informed management decisions. Needle biopsy provides histology and tumour grade. A non-operative diagnosis should be possible in more than 90% of invasive cancers and 85% of non-invasive cancers.

Some lesions only visible on MRI may require MRI guidance for biopsy. The likelihood that a clinically palpable lesion which cannot be visualized on mammography and ultrasonography is malignant is less than 1%. In these circumstances, it is important to carry out a freehand biopsy to exclude the possibility of a diffuse malignant mass such as lobular carcinoma. The number of core specimens obtained should reflect the nature of the abnormality being sampled. For a suspicion of a carcinoma, it is recommended that at least two core specimens should be taken. For a stereotactic biopsy, a minimum of five core biopsies should be taken. In the event of a sampling error, either a repeat biopsy or an open excision biopsy can be performed.

Vacuum-assisted mammotome

When there is diagnostic uncertainty, 8 G vacuum-assisted mammotome can be used to obtain larger tissue volumes (approximately 300 mg/core) (Heywang-Kobrunner et al 1998, Brem et al 2001, Parker et al 2001). This is very successful for improving the diagnostic accuracy of borderline breast lesions and at sites where it is difficult to biopsy using other techniques. Indications for use include: small mass lesions, architectural distortions, failed needle biopsy, small clusters of microcalcifications, excision of small benign lesions and diffuse non-specific lesions. Two other types of vacuum-assisted core biopsy systems include minimally invasive breast biopsy and automated tissue excision and collection (an MRI-guided vacuum-assisted breast biopsy system).

Advanced breast biopsy instrumentation

Advanced breast biopsy instrumentation (ABBI) is used for surgical stereotactic biopsy of non-palpable breast lesions under radiographic guidance. This biopsy was developed for both diagnosis and therapy. ABBI requires an incision of 5–20 mm, is restricted to use on a prone table and requires the insertion of a localizing T-wire. This vacuum-assisted biopsy obtains a large cylinder of tissue from the subcutaneous tissue down to and beyond the lesion with an electrocautery snare. ABBI removes a larger volume of tissue, theoretically increasing the diagnostic accuracy of the biopsy. Failure rates of up to 31.5% have been reported due to poor patient selection, technical problems with the T bar and failure to remove tissue. Complication rates of ABBI procedures requiring intervention are significantly higher than those of core biopsy (1.1% and 0.2%, respectively). Complete removal of small lesions does occur and positive margins of 19–100% have been reported (Leibman et al 1999, Matthews and Williams 1999). ABBI is more expensive than any other percutaneous needle biopsy technique.

Open surgical biopsy

Diagnostic excision biopsy is now uncommon but is still required for definitive histology of some breast lesions graded B3/4 or C3/4. To minimize patient anxiety, an operation for diagnostic purposes should be performed within 2 weeks of the decision to operate. For patients having surgical removal of a proven benign lesion in the National Health Service (UK), an 18-week waiting time applies. Any benign diagnostic resection specimen weighing more than 40 g should be discussed at the postoperative MDT meeting and any mitigating reasons should be recorded.

Staging Investigations

Staging investigations in the absence of specific symptoms are not performed when patients have been diagnosed with breast cancer. Breast cancer is staged by the Tumour, Node, Metastasis system based on the International Union against Cancer criteria. This enables comparison of results of trials worldwide and provides information that can be used to inform treatment regimens. There is a degree of bias depending on the extent of axillary surgery, completeness of excision and staging investigations performed.

Treatment Planning and Patient Communication

The management of breast cancer within the context of an MDT of specialists facilitates rapid and accurate diagnosis as well as selection of appropriate treatment for all stages of disease. The specialist breast care team includes research nurses and specialist nurses that have a vital role in support and counselling patients. Breaking bad news requires time, patience, sensitivity and compassion. It is important to create an environment in which a patient can secure the information, autonomy and support that suits their need. Patients must be given adequate time, information and support in order to make a fully informed decision concerning their treatment.

A preoperative search for occult metastases by bone scan and liver ultrasound does not yield useful information in patients with operable primary breast cancer (Bishop et al 1979). Preoperative chest X-ray and relevant blood tests (full blood count, liver function tests and routine biochemistry) are agreed by local protocol.

Surgery and Radiotherapy

Surgery

The breast

The aim of breast cancer surgery is to achieve long-term local disease control with the minimum of morbidity. The majority of women diagnosed with breast cancer will have small breast cancers, suitable for BCS. The aims of BCS are to produce an acceptable cosmetic appearance and lower psychological morbidity (improved body image, sexuality and esteem) compared with mastectomy. Two studies have shown equivalence in terms of outcome for BCS compared with mastectomy (Anonymous 1995, Morris et al 1997). Meta-analysis of five trials comparing BCS with mastectomy involving 3006 women found no significant difference in the risk of death at 10 years (Anonymous 1995). It is important to ensure that only appropriate patients are selected for BCS, with the aim of minimizing local recurrence whilst achieving a good cosmetic outcome. Single cancers less than 4 cm in size can usually be managed by BCS. Many units have a 3-cm cut-off and lying more than 2 cm from the nipple–areolar complex for considering BCS, but it is the balance between tumour size and breast volume which determines whether or not a patient is suitable for BCS. For patients with large tumours, neoadjuvant chemotherapy can be considered.

Patients with multiple tumours in the same breast should not be considered for BCS as they have a high incidence of recurrence so are best treated with mastectomy with or without reconstruction (Fisher et al 1986, Kurtz et al 1990). Patients with two tumours in close proximity can be candidates for BCS provided that all disease is excised with clear margins. The aim of wide local excision is to remove all invasive and in-situ carcinoma with a 1-cm macroscopic margin of normal surrounding tissue. Incomplete excision rates should be approximately 10–25% and the most common problem following surgery is poor cosmetic result.

Women having more than 10–20% of breast volume removed are likely to have a poor cosmetic result (Cochrane et al 2003). Factors influencing local recurrence include young age (<40 years), tumour grade, presence of an extensive in-situ component and lymphovascular invasion (Holland et al 1990a, Anonymous 1991). More than 80% of local recurrences will occur at the site of previous cancer. Local recurrence following BCS is usually best treated with mastectomy, although re-excision is possible should the recurrence occur more than 5 years after initial treatment, as these are classified as a second primary cancer rather than recurrent disease. Local recurrence after 5 years is associated with a much better prognosis than recurrence within 5 years. The recently reported UK Standardisation of Breast Radiotherapy Trial (START) has demonstrated low rates of recurrence (3.5% at 5 years) following BCS (Dewar et al 2007). Local recurrence rates for invasive cancer after BCS should be less than 5% at 5 years with a target of less than 3% at 5 years.

The axilla

Management of the axilla is a subject of great debate. Surgical treatment of the axilla is two-fold, firstly in disease control and secondly in staging. Surgical staging of the axilla is by axillary lymph node dissection (ALND) for the majority of women, with data regarding nodal status being the most powerful variable in the prognosis for primary breast cancer. Disease-free interval and overall survival are directly related to the number of axillary nodes that contain metastases (Fisher et al 1984, Carter et al 1989). ALND provides the most accurate qualitative and quantitative assessment of the axilla, with the probability of lymph node involvement related to the size of the primary tumour. In small tumours with a size of approximately 10 mm, the risk of nodal metastases is 10% (Baxter et al 1996, Kollias et al 1999). Recurrence rates of 3–5% at 5 years have been reported following ALND, and it has been suggested that the axillary node recurrence rate should be less than 5% with a target of less than 3% (Fowble et al 1989, Siegel et al 1990, Halverson et al 1993, Forrest et al 1995).

Routine histological examination of dissected axillary lymph nodes may be inadequate in identifying the presence of small metastatic tumour deposits or 'micrometastases'. This has been described as a small cluster of cells measuring 0.2–2 mm. Studies have shown that it is possible to identify micrometastases in 50% of 'negative' lymph node cases using serial axillary sections, immunohistochemistry and polymerase chain reaction to detect mRNA transcripts (Trojani et al 1987, Hainsworth et al 1993, Mann et al 2000). Recent studies have shown that cases initially deemed to be 'node negative' but subsequently shown to have micrometastases are associated with a worse outcome (Huvos et al 1971, Fisher et al 1978, Rosen et al 1981, Friedman et al 1988, Anonymous 1990, Clayton and Hopkins 1993, McGuckin et al 1996, Dowlatshahi et al 1997).

Significant morbidity is associated with axillary dissection, including seroma, wound infection, reduced shoulder mobility, motor nerve damage (median pectoral nerve, long thoracic nerve of Bell, thoracodorsal nerve), numbness and paraesthesia (80%), and lymphoedema (Siegel et al 1990, Shaw and Rumball 1990, Hladiuk et al 1992, Lin et al 1993). Lymphoedema incidence has been reported to be between 10% and 25%, with hypertension and BMI being risk factors. A 40% incidence of lymphoedema has been reported in those patients undergoing ALND and radiotherapy to the axilla.

Cabanas first proposed the concept of SNB for penile cancer in 1977, followed by Morton for melanoma in 1992 (Cabanas 1977, Cochran et al 1992, Morton 1997). Krag et al first published the use of SNB in breast cancer in 1993 (Krag et al 1993). SNB is based on the knowledge that for any given tumour-bearing site, there is orderly progression of lymph drainage to a draining lymph node (sentinel node). It relies on the premise that skip metastases do not occur, and that the absence of tumour of the sentinel lymph node implies that the entire lymphatic bed is clear of metastatic disease. The aim of SNB is to provide accurate axillary staging by use of a minimally invasive surgical procedure and significantly reduced morbidity. The sentinel lymph nodes are identified using a radioisotope (Figures 47.8 and 47.9), injected on the day of surgery, and a coloured patent blue dye injected peritumorally or interdermally in the peri- and subareolar region 5–10 min before surgery with the breast gently massaged; this leads to an identification rate of 97% (Albertini et al 1996, Veronesi et al 1997, Cody 1999). Intraoperative identification of the sentinel lymph node is confirmed by a hand-held gamma probe, and visually by blue staining of the node. Risk factors of the procedure include allergic and anaphylactic reactions to the blue dye (Mullan et al 2001). Exposure to clinical staff from the radioisotope is negligible.

One disadvantage of SNB is that women with a positive sentinel node will require a second operation to clear the axilla. Intraoperative frozen section and imprint cytology have been used to assess the status of the sentinel nodes; however, neither procedure has proved acceptable. A small trial evaluating intraoperative reverse-transcriptase polymerase chain reaction (assay time 20–30 min) for epithelial markers mammaglobin and cytokeratin 19 has shown sensitivity of 96%, specificity of 100% and a positive predictive value of 100% for sentinel node detection (Cutress et al

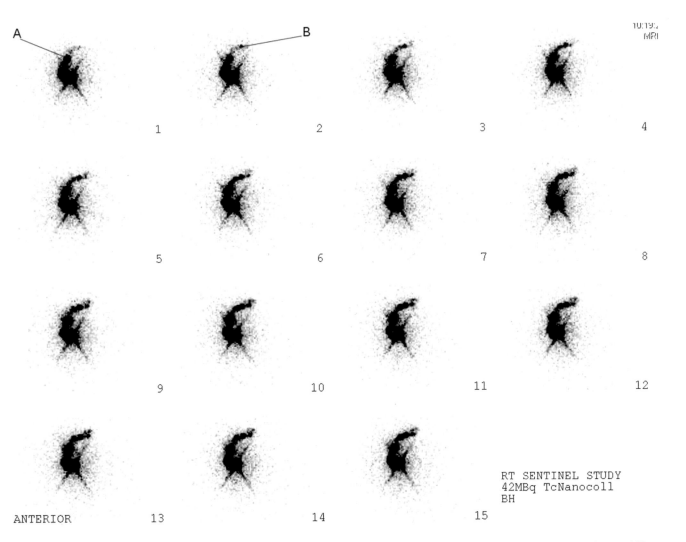

Figure 47.8 Axillary sentinel lymph node dynamic study. Images taken at 1-min intervals showing initial drainage through the draining lymphatic and filling of the (A) sentinel node with uptake into the second-order nodes (B) on subsequent images.

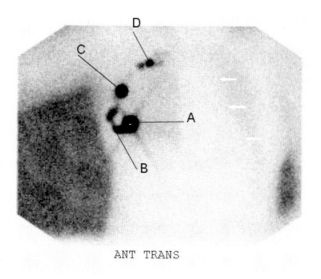

ANT TRANS

Figure 47.9 Axillary sentinel lymph node. Anterior view of breast sentinel lymph node imaging. A, periareolar injection site where technetium-99m radiolabelled macroaggregated albumin has been injected; B, draining lymphatic; C, sentinel lymph node at level 1; D, two second-order lymph nodes which have filled after the sentinel lymph node and lie at level 2. There is a radioactive flood source behind the patient to outline the anatomy. The white arrows point to the left mediastinal and cardiac border.

2008). In most studies, the number of sentinel lymph nodes identified ranged from 1.5 to 4.0, and recent studies have shown that, in a small number of cases, the sentinel lymph node was beyond the first two lymph nodes removed (McCarter et al 2001, Zervos et al 2001, Kennedy et al 2003). McCarter et al claimed that at least three nodes are required to identify 99% of node-positive patients, and the false-negative rate is significantly higher (16.5%) when only one lymph node is removed (McCarter et al 2001). Goyal has shown that 99.6% of metastases from node-positive tumours are found within the first four nodes, suggesting that between two and four nodes should be removed for optimum staging of the axilla (Goyal et al 2005).

Multifocality and multicentricity, once thought to be a relative contraindication to SNB, now appears to be feasible and accurate with an acceptably low false-negative rate, and can be used in patients presenting with a clinically negative axilla (Kumar et al 2003, Goyal et al 2004). Currently, there are no randomized controlled trials addressing the feasibility, accuracy or timing of SNB in neoadjuvant chemotherapy. A meta-analysis assessing the reliability of SNB in patients following neoadjuvant chemotherapy reported sensitivity of 88% (Xing et al 2006). Some centres advocate SNB at diagnosis, prior to initiation of neoadjuvant chemotherapy.

The increase in BCS for early breast cancer has resulted in a 10-year risk of ipsilateral recurrent breast cancer of 10–20% (Fisher et al 1989a, van Dongen et al 2000). This has resulted in an increasing population with ipsilateral tumour recurrence with prior axillary surgery, who were traditionally treated with salvage mastectomy and axillary node dissection. However, emerging data indicate that there may be a role for SNB in identifying aberrant lymphatic drainage patterns in recurrent breast cancer (Intra et al 2005, Roumen

et al 2006, Taback et al 2006). The incidence of axillary disease in patients with DCIS (6–9%) is greater in a subset of patients with microinvasion, younger patients, DCIS (>4 cm) and those with high-grade disease (Silverstein et al 1991, Cox et al 2000, Pendas et al 2000, Leonard and Swain 2004, Yen et al 2005). Current guidelines from the American Society of Clinical Oncology (ASCO) only recommend SNB in those patients undergoing mastectomy for DCIS, as an incidental invasive component is seen in 20% of these patients (Meyer et al 1999, Lyman et al 2005).

Internal mammary nodes (IMN) have been shown to have prognostic significance (Lacour et al 1983). IMN have been successfully biopsied in 60–85% of cases, with a prevalence of metastases in 5–27% of cases, resulting in upstaging and/or a change in management in 2–8% of patients. Whilst not standard practice, sentinel biopsy of IMN requires further investigation to determine efficacy and safety.

SNB is a new procedure, so long-term follow-up for axillary recurrence will be the ultimate measurement of its success. To date, the rate of axillary recurrence is lower than anticipated given the average false-negative rate of 5–6%. Non-operative staging of the axilla remains elusive. Clinical examination is unreliable, with sensitivity varying from 30% to 75% and specificity approaching 50%. Ultrasound in combination with FNAC can identify 40–45% of patients with involved nodes. PET has shown some promising early results, with sensitivity of 75% and specificity of 90%. Some Italian centres are using PET to assess the need for SNB in low-risk, clinically node-negative patients with a low probability of nodal involvement (Greco et al 2001).

Radiotherapy/radiation therapy

Breast radiotherapy

Multiple randomized trials have shown that radiotherapy substantially reduces the risk of local recurrence following BCS. Adjuvant radiotherapy aims to reduce the risk of locoregional recurrence and improve overall survival. Radiotherapy is not routinely given after mastectomy but tends to be reserved for those with large (>4 cm), high-grade tumours, direct invasion of the skin or pectoral fascia, and extensive nodal involvement who are at high risk of local recurrence. The 1995 Early Breast Cancer Trialists' Collaborative Group confirmed that locoregional recurrence was reduced by 66% with postmastectomy radiotherapy (Anonymous 1995). This trial confirmed a reduced risk of breast cancer with radiotherapy, but an increased risk of death from other causes (cardiac deaths). Recent randomized trials of women treated with more modern radiotherapy have confirmed that postmastectomy radiotherapy will prevent one death for every 11 women treated, and one locoregional recurrence for every three to five women treated (Ragaz et al 1997, Overgaard et al 1999).

It is important to define the group of patients in whom radiotherapy is required and the group in whom it is not. One recent trial showed no increase in survival on addition of radiotherapy to women over 70 years of age being treated with tamoxifen who were ERα positive with no nodal involvement and tumours less than 2 cm in size (Hughes et al 2004, Bentzen et al 2008).

Hypofractionation radiotherapy aims to deliver an increased dose of radiotherapy over a reduced time frame. The START trial has demonstrated equivalent recurrence rates at 5 years for patients with early-stage breast cancer. The Faster Radiotherapy for Breast Cancer Patients (FAST) trial is currently comparing larger doses (5.7–6 Gy) of radiotherapy given once weekly for 5 weeks with the standard daily 2-Gy treatment (Yarnold et al 2004).

The Targeted Intraoperative Radiotherapy Trial (TARGIT) is evaluating single-dose intraoperative radiotherapy using a low-energy X-ray source (50 kV) as an alternative to conventional postoperative radiotherapy for treatment of early-stage invasive breast cancer. The single-day targeted intraoperative radiotherapy is designed to administer the highest dose of radiotherapy to a distance of 1 cm surrounding the lumpectomy cavity, while sparing the nearby normal breast, chest and shoulder from the effects of radiation.

Axillary radiotherapy

Irradiation of lymph glands is advised if there is nodal involvement on sampling, SNB and level 1 dissection, and no further surgery is planned. Supraclavicular fossa irradiation is indicated in patients with more than four involved axillary lymph nodes and if the axillary has been cleared. Irradiation of a fully dissected axilla should be avoided unless there is extensive extracapsular tumour extension. The risk of lymphoedema following a full axillary dissection is increased to 40%.

Peri- and Postoperative Care

Patients should be supported by a breast care nurse who must have good links with outpatient, ward and community nurses to assist in continuity of care. Breast care nurses should assist in the fitting of breast prostheses following mastectomy, inform patients about the range of services available and provide them with literature including details of local self-help groups. The breast care team should ensure that primary care practitioners have a clear understanding of the diagnosis, care plan and toxicity profile of any proposed treatment. Following surgery, all patients with breast cancer should have their results discussed at an MDT meeting, where postoperative histology can be discussed and the need for further surgical treatment and/or adjuvant treatment discussed and recorded.

Endocrine Therapy

Breast cancer was the first malignancy for which systemic therapy was developed. The link between hormones and breast cancer growth and development has been recognized for more than a century. In 1896, George Beatson reported that removal of the ovaries from premenopausal women with advanced breast cancer produced a dramatic decrease in tumour size and improved the patient's prognosis (Beatson 1896). In 1900, Stanley Boyd at Charing Cross Hospital accumulated the national case reports of oophorectomy, and noted that only one-third of patients responded to ovarian ablation and responses lasted, on average, for 1–2 years (Boyd 1900).

Discovery that oestrogenic hormones were produced in the ovary prompted the search for therapeutic antagonists to reduce the incidence of breast cancer in individuals predisposed to the disease by their sensitivity to oestrogenic hormones (Allen and Doisy 1923). Subsequent laboratory, epidemiological and clinical studies have established that oestrogens stimulate the growth of breast cancers (Lacassagne 1936). Oestrogen actions are mediated by two oestrogen receptors, ERα and ERβ, which are members of the nuclear receptor superfamily of transcription factors that regulate the expression of responsive genes upon binding to their cognate ligand (Chawla et al 2001). Whilst the importance of ERβ in breast cancer is at present unresolved, ERα is expressed in the majority of breast cancers and its presence correlates with response to endocrine therapies (Fuqua et al 2003). Thus, current clinical practice involves determination of the ERα status of the malignant cells, followed by adjuvant treatment of ERα-positive cases with endocrine agents that inhibit ERα activity.

Inhibition of ERα activity is achieved with two main strategies: using antioestrogens, primarily tamoxifen, that bind to ERα to inhibit its activity; or by blocking oestrogen synthesis, such that ERα is not activated. Peripheral oestrogen synthesis is the main source of oestrogens in postmenopausal women, and drugs that reduce peripheral oestrogen synthesis, by blocking the activity of the aromatase enzyme, are being used as second- and third-line agents in hormone-sensitive disease once resistance to tamoxifen has developed (Johnston and Dowsett 2003).

Tamoxifen

Tamoxifen, a non-steroidal antioestrogen, is currently the most common form of endocrine therapy for women with ERα-positive breast cancer. Tamoxifen is a selective estrogen receptor modulator (SERM) which has partial agonist activity in some tissues, including bone, lipids and endometrium, but antagonist activity in breast tissue. The antitumour effect of tamoxifen is mediated via competitive inhibition of oestrogen binding to ERs. In women with ERα-positive breast cancer, 5 years of tamoxifen results in a 41% relative risk reduction of recurrence and a 34% relative risk reduction of death (Anonymous 2005). The National Surgical Adjuvant Breast and Bowel Project (NSABP) B-14 trial and the Scottish Adjuvant Tamoxifen trial demonstrated no benefit in taking tamoxifen for more than 5 years; in contrast, the Eastern Cooperative Oncology Group (ECOG) trial studying indefinite tamoxifen therapy in node-positive patients showed a statistically significant improvement in disease-free survival with extended tamoxifen (Tormey et al 1996, Fisher et al 2001, Stewart et al 2001). The adjuvant Tamoxifen Treatment — Offer More? (ATTOM) and Adjuvant Tamoxifen — Longer against Shorter (ATLAS) trials examining the efficacy of long-term tamoxifen had consistent findings, reporting increased disease-free survival but no overall survival advantage for long-term tamoxifen.

Tamoxifen is generally well tolerated, with the most common side-effects being hot flushes (50% of women), vaginal discharge and irregular menses (Fisher et al 1989b, 1996, Love et al 1991). These side-effects occur more often in pre-/perimenopausal women. The most important side-effect of tamoxifen is an increased risk of endometrial cancer, which equates to 80 extra cases per 10,000 women treated with tamoxifen at 10 years. The Early Breast Cancer Trialists' Collaborative Group (EBCTCG) analysing data from 37,000 women demonstrated a two-fold increase in endometrial cancer in women taking tamoxifen for 1–2 years and a four-fold increase in those taking it for 5 years (Anonymous 1998b). Tamoxifen is also associated with an increase in endometrial polyps, ovarian cysts and endometrial hyperplasia (Kedar et al 1994). The overall reduction of risk in developing breast cancer outweighs the risk of developing endometrial cancer. In postmenopausal women, tamoxifen increases bone mineral density of the axial skeleton; however, in premenopausal women, there may be a decrease in bone density (Love et al 1992, Kristensen et al 1994, Powles et al 1996). Tamoxifen has been shown to reduce total cholesterol and low-density lipoproteins, which explains the reduction in cardiovascular deaths in those taking tamoxifen (Rutqvist and Mattsson 1993, Costantino et al 1997).

Aromatase inhibitors

Aromatase inhibitors (AIs) significantly reduce oestrogen production in postmenopausal women by inhibiting aromatase, a cytochrome P-450 enzyme found in adipose tissue, liver, muscle, the brain and breast cancer tissue (Miller 2003b). In premenopausal women, AIs are ineffective as they produce an increase in gonadotrophin secretion, which results in reduced feedback of oestrogen on the pituitary and hypothalamus. AIs present an alternative to tamoxifen for antagonizing oestrogenic effects on the breast in postmenopausal women. In the 1990s, third-generation AIs were developed which included two subgroups: a steroidal analogue exemethstane, which binds irreversibly to aromatase and is an enzyme inactivator (type 1 inhibitor); and non-steroidal inhibitors that bind reversibly to the haem group of the enzyme (type 2 inhibitor), of which the main agents are anastrozole and letrozole.

Two randomized trials compared initial adjuvant therapy with tamoxifen with an AI. The Arimidex, Tamoxifen Alone or Combination (ATAC) trial showed a significantly improved disease-free survival, time to recurrence and incidence of contralateral breast cancer for arimidex compared with tamoxifen (median follow-up 68 months) (Baum et al 2002, 2003, Howell et al 2005). There were significantly fewer disease recurrences in the arimidex group, but no difference was seen in overall survival. Similar results were seen in the Breast International Group (BIG) 1-98 study comparing letrozole with tamoxifen upfront (Thurlimann et al 2005). In both the ATAC and BIG 1-98 studies, more fractures, fewer thromboembolic events and fewer endometrial cancers were seen in those taking an AI compared with tamoxifen.

A number of trials have looked at sequential endocrine treatment (tamoxifen → AI) including Arimidex, Tamoxifem Alone or together (ATAC), Mayo Clinic-17 (MA-17), the Intergroup Exemethstane Study (IES), Arimidex-Nolvadex-95 (ARNO-95) and Austrian Breast and Colorectal Cancer Study Group (ABCSG) (Goss et al 2003, 2005, Coombes et al 2004, Boccardo et al 2005, Howell et al 2005, Jakesz et al 2005). The IES showed a 24% improvement in disease-free survival in women taking tamoxifen for 2–3 years followed by exemethstane compared with 5 years of tamoxifen (Coombes et al 2004). This trial demonstrated an improvement in overall survival in the sequential group, which was significant in the node-positive patients. These trials clearly demonstrate an improvement in disease-free survival, and ASCO advises that AIs should be part of the adjuvant treatment of early-stage breast cancer in postmenopausal women.

AIs have a different side-effect profile compared with tamoxifen; these include hot flushes, vaginal dryness, musculoskeletal pain and headache. AIs are not associated with an increase in thromboembolic disease or endometrial carcinoma, but are associated with an increase in bone fractures and osteoporosis (BIG 1-98 and ATAC trials). Bone monitoring, using dual energy X-ray absorptiometry scanning, should be available for patients taking AIs. All women that start an AI should be advised about calcium and vitamin D supplementation, smoking cessation and the importance of exercise (Hillner et al 2003). It is advised that bone mineral density should be obtained at baseline and monitored annually for all women taking an AI. The Zometa/Femara Adjuvant Synergy trial suggests that treatment with a bisphosphonate at initiation of an AI may prevent a decline in bone health (Brufsky et al 2005).

Faslodex (Fulvestrant or ICI 182,780)

Faslodex is a pure steroidal antioestrogen that binds with 100 times greater affinity to ERs than tamoxifen (Wakeling and Bowler 1992, Rajah et al 1996). It is licensed for use in postmenopausal women with hormone-receptor-positive advanced breast cancer failing on prior antioestrogen therapy. It has a distinct mechanism of action, differing from that of tamoxifen or the AIs, which may help to delay the development of resistance.

Ovarian ablation

There are many methods for suppressing ovarian function in premenopausal women, including surgical oophorectomy, radiation-induced ovarian ablation and gonadotrophin-releasing hormone (GnRH) agonists. GnRH agonists are increasingly being used to achieve ovarian suppression. They overstimulate and subsequently downregulate GnRH receptors. Their effect is to produce an initial rise in luteinizing hormone and follicle-stimulating hormone in the first 7–10 days of treatment, followed by a decrease after 14–21 days that leads to postmenopausal oestrogen and progesterone levels (Williams et al 1986, Cockshott 2000). After 7.3 years of follow-up, the Zoladex Early Breast Cancer Research Association (ZEBRA), randomizing 1640 lymph node-negative, premenopausal ER-positive women, demonstrated no difference in disease-free survival, overall survival or quality of life between the GnRH agonist goserelin (Zoladex) and cyclophosphamide, methotrexate and 5-fluorouracil (CMF) chemotherapy (Jonat et al 2002, Kaufmann et al 2003). A number of trials are investigating the role of GnRH agonists in adjuvant treatment of premenopausal, early-stage breast cancer — Suppression of Ovarian Function Trial (SOFT), Tamoxifen and Exemethstane Trial (TEXT), and the Premenopausal Endocrine Responsive Chemotherapy (PERCHE) trial.

Raloxifene

Raloxifene, initially studied as an osteoporotic drug, is a second-generation SERM that has oestrogen antagonist properties on the breast and endometrium, and oestrogenic effects on lipid metabolism, bone and blood clotting. The Multiple Outcomes of Raloxifene Evaluation (MORE) trial confirmed a significant reduction in vertebral fractures in patients taking raloxifene, and as a secondary outcome reduced the incidence of breast cancer in ER-positive patients by 90% but had no effect on ERα-negative patients (Cummings et al 2002). The prospective, randomized controlled Study of Tamoxifen and Raloxifene (STAR) showed no significant difference in the incidence of invasive breast cancer in either group after 3.2 years; however, fewer uterine cancers were reported in the raloxifene group (not statistically significant) (Vogel 2009).

Targeted Therapies

Systemic therapies for breast cancer classically belonged to one of two categories: cytotoxic chemotherapy or hormonal therapy. Recently, a third category, biological/targeted therapy, has emerged. Targeted therapy is a type of medical therapy which blocks the growth of cancer cells by interfering with specific targeted molecules needed for carcinogenesis and tumour growth.

Targeting the epidermal growth factor receptor

The human EGFR-2 (HER-2)/neu (c-erbB-2) gene is localized to chromosome 17q and encodes a family of four transmembrane tyrosine kinase receptor proteins which are members of the EGFR or HER family (Ross et al 2003). These receptor tyrosine kinases provide a binding site for various ligands or proteins, which in turn activate downstream signalling pathways which are essential for cell proliferation and survival. Overexpression of the HER-2 protein occurs in 20–25% of breast cancers and is associated with a worse prognosis (disease-free survival and overall survival) (King et al 1985a, Slamon et al 1987, 1989). The most commonly used test for determining HER-2 protein overexpression is an immunohistochemical (IHC) assay scored from 0 to +3, with 0/+1 representing negative, +2 weakly positive and +3 positive. HER-2 can be measured quantitatively by fluorescence in-situ hybridization (FISH), which provides a direct measure of gene amplification (Perez et al 2002, Hicks and Tubbs 2005). FISH is currently the gold standard for evaluating HER-2 overexpression, and provides the best correlation with clinical response to trastuzumab. IHC3+ correlates well with FISH positivity, but only 20–24% of IHC2+ tumours are also FISH positive (Owens et al 2004).

A new method, chromogenic in-situ hybridization (CISH), has been approved by the US Food and Drug Administration for determining HER-2 status, as an alternative to FISH. CISH has several advantages over FISH in that it produces cheaper and permanent staining, allowing samples to be archived indefinitely (FISH signals are labile and fade over time). CISH is based on bright field microscopy and does not require an expensive fluorescence microscope with multiband pass filters. It allows concurrent analysis of morphological features of the tumours/cells and gene copy numbers, making the identification of components of interest easier. Tumour heterogeneity can be readily identified at low magnification (Tanner et al 2000, Zhao et al 2002, Arnould et al 2003).

Trastuzumab (Herceptin), a monoclonal antibody that targets HER-2, achieves tumour regression in some patients with HER-2-positive metastatic breast cancer (mBC). Patients with mBC taking trastuzumab in combination with chemotherapy have a longer time to progression (7.4 vs 4.6 months), a higher objective response rate (50% vs 32%), and a longer survival (25.2% vs 20.3%) than chemotherapy alone (Slamon et al 2001). A number of trials have been conducted investigating the role of trastuzumab in the adjuvant setting for HER-2-positive breast cancer. The Herceptin Adjuvant (HERA) trial compared 1–2 years of adjuvant trastuzumab with observation in HER-2-positive women who had completed adjuvant or neoadjuvant chemotherapy, surgery and/or radiotherapy (Piccart-Gebhart et al 2005). Analysis revealed a significant improvement in disease-free survival and overall survival in those taking trastuzumab, and this has become the standard of care for patients with HER-2-positive breast cancer.

Clinical benefit and response rates depend on the intensity of HER-2 overexpression (2+ or 3+), with response rates of 35% seen in grade 3+ but only minimal benefit seen in grade 2+ (Vogel et al 2002). Trastuzumab is well tolerated with side-effects including hypersensitivity and cardiotoxicity; the incidence of class III/IV congestive heart failure ranges from 0.4% to 3.8% (Adamo et al 2007, Anonymous 2008, Perez 2008).

Pertuzumab is a monoclonal antibody that prevents the formation of heterodimers between HER-2 and other members of the HER family (Nahta et al 2004). Pertuzumab localizes to a different domain of the HER-2 protein than trastuzumab. A synergistic interaction between pertuzumab and trastuzumab is being explored.

Dual tyrosine kinase inhibition

Lapatinib is an orally active dual erbB-1/2 tyrosine kinase inhibitor that blocks signalling of both epidermal growth factor (EGFR/erbB-1) and HER-2/neu (erbB-2). Lapatinib binds reversibly to the cytoplasmic ATP-binding site of the kinase and blocks receptor phosphorylation and activation, thereby preventing subsequent downstream signalling events, namely simultaneous activation of extracellular signal-related kinase-1/2 and phosphatidylinositol 3-kinase/Akt.

Lapatinib is active in refractory mBC patients and as a first-line metastatic treatment, with potential benefit in patients with brain metastases. Efficacy of lapatinib has been demonstrated in combination with capecitabine in patients with refractory erbB-2-overexpressing breast cancer (Geyer et al 2006). Lapatinib appears to have either very low or no incidence of cardiotoxicity. The most frequently reported adverse events include nausea, fatigue, itching, rash, diarrhoea, acne and dry skin. There are a number of ongoing phase III trials evaluating the role of lapatinib in the adjuvant setting, including the Tykerb Evaluation After Chemotherapy (TEACH) trial (Moy and Goss 2006).

Targeting the vascular endothelial growth factor pathway

Metastasis of all solid tumours requires angiogenesis (formation of new blood vessels). A number of agents have been developed that target the vascular endothelial growth factor (VEGF) pathway. Breast cancers that overexpress VEGF have a worse disease-free survival and overall survival. Bevacizumab (Avastin) is a human monoclonal antibody that recognizes all isoforms of VEGF-A. In the metastatic setting, bevacizumab has been shown to significantly increase response rates and progression-free survival when given in combination with paclitaxel (E2100 and Avastin and Docetaxel (AVADO) trials) (Miller 2003a, Miles et al 2008, Baar et al 2009). The Ribbon 1 and Ribbon 2 studies are currently investigating the combination of bevacizumab with a number of standard chemotherapy regimens for mBC.

Other targeted therapies

Other targeted therapies currently being evaluated include sunitinib (SU11248), an oral tyrosine kinase inhibitor which blocks a number of signalling pathways including VEGF receptor, platelet-derived growth factor receptor, kit and flt-3 (Miller and Burstein 2005). Rapamycin is an antibiotic that has demonstrated antitumour activity through cell cycle arrest resulting from inhibition of mammalian target of rapamycin (mTOR). Temsirolimus (CCI-779), an mTOR inhibitor, inhibited the proliferation of breast cancer cell lines in preclinical studies but has not entered routine clinical use (Yu et al 2001, Campbell et al 2004). Overexpression of insulin-like growth factor-1 receptor (IGF-1R) is associated with a poor prognosis and resistance to a number of therapies, including hormonal therapy and trastuzumab (Nahta et al 2005). A number of therapies are targeting IGF-1R, including the small molecule tyrosine kinase inhibitor (BMS-536924; Bristol-Myers Squibb) and monoclonal antibodies (CP-751,871; Pfizer).

Adjuvant Chemotherapy

Systemic chemotherapy has been an important part of the adjuvant treatment strategy for many women with early-stage breast cancer since reports of improved outcomes with single-agent chemotherapies following radical mastectomy in the 1970s. The recommendation for the use of chemotherapy is made within a multidisciplinary setting, and is supervised by a clinical or medical oncologist. The efficacy of each treatment is balanced against its specific toxicity profile. Chemotherapy is used primarily in the adjuvant setting for women thought to be at high risk of systemic disease; however, it is now being used increasingly in the neoadjuvant setting. Neoadjuvant chemotherapy is used in patients with large breast cancers to avoid mastectomy and is also the standard of care for inflammatory breast cancer.

Combination chemotherapy has a more prolonged benefit than single-agent chemotherapy, and is usually given in six cycles over a period of 4–6 months. The first adjuvant chemotherapy for breast cancer (CMF) was developed in the late 1970s, and was the mainstay of treatment for many years, significantly reducing risk of recurrence and death (Bona-donna et al 1976, 1985, Anonymous 1998a). CMF had a significant effect regardless of ER status, tamoxifen use and nodal status, but was influenced by age and menopausal status. Recent meta-analyses have confirmed the benefit of combination chemotherapy over monochemotherapy, with a greater benefit seen in younger patients (Anonymous 2005). For women under 50 years of age, chemotherapy significantly improved 10-year survival by over 10% for those with node-positive disease (53% vs 42%) and by 6% for those with node-negative disease (78% vs 71%). The National Cancer Institute of Canada MA.5 study confirmed the superiority of anthracyclines [six cycles of 5-fluorouracil, epirubicin, cyclophosphamide (FEC)] over CMF, and now anthracycline-based chemotherapy regimens are the standard of care (Levine et al 1998). The potential importance of taxanes (either paclitaxel or docetaxel) as adjuvant chemotherapy is emphasized by a large number of trials (Cancer and Leukemia Group (CALGB) 9344, National Surgical Adjuvant Breast and Bowel Project (NSABP) B-28, Breast Cancer International Research Group (BCIRG) and PACS01) (Henderson et al 2003, Mamounas et al 2003, Martin et al 2003). This body of evidence now supports the use of taxanes in high-risk women in the adjuvant setting (Goldhirsch et al 2005).

Neoadjuvant Medical Therapy

Neoadjuvant (preoperative) therapy is used increasingly with the major aim being to downstage large tumours, thereby avoiding mastectomy and allowing BCS to be performed. This has also enabled earlier assessment of chemosensitivity versus identification of patients with resistant disease. Several studies have documented the finding that response in the breast correlates with survival, demonstrating that downstaging is an excellent surrogate for systemic effectiveness. The decision to proceed with neoadjuvant chemotherapy is associated with several special considerations involving the pretreatment/diagnostic phase (percutaneous needle core biopsy preferable), preoperative planning (insertion of radio-opaque clips to mark the tumour bed prior to completion of chemotherapy; careful imaging to determine the extent of disease), and final surgical decision making (preoperative imaging in order to decide between lumpectomy and mastectomy).

Neoadjuvant endocrine therapy

The use of primary tamoxifen in older women as an alternative to surgery has demonstrated short-term tumour regression but unsatisfactory long-term local control (Cheung et al 2000). Higher response rates have been seen in older women treated with neoadjuvant anastrozole, letrozole and exemethstane compared with tamoxifen. Letrozole is currently the only AI licensed for use in the neoadjuvant setting.

Neoadjuvant chemotherapy

Neoadjuvant chemotherapy has significant activity in early breast cancer, with overall objective response rates of 70–90%, which is higher than response rates seen in patients with metastatic disease. Complete remission rates of approximately 20% are seen in patients receiving neoadjuvant chemotherapy (Smith and Lipton 2001).

Triple-Negative Breast Cancers

These are defined as the 10–15% of breast cancers (an increasing percentage of which occur in premenopausal African and African-American women) which do not express the ER, progesterone receptor (PgR) or erb-B2 receptor (Slamon et al 1989, Konecny et al 2003, Carey et al 2006, Dawood et al 2009). This disease is resistant to existing targeted treatments and hormonal therapies, and associated with a high risk of local and systemic relapse (van de Rijn et al 2002, Abd El-Rehim et al 2004, 2005, Foulkes et al 2004, Nielsen et al 2004). These tumours are often poorly differentiated, the majority of which are in the basal group of breast cancers. This basal group stains positively for the basal cell cytokeratins 5/6 and 17, has an increased proliferative rate, develops central necrosis, and does not stain for ERα, PgR or HER-2 receptors (Livasy et al 2006).

Limited clinical data suggest that these cancers are chemosensitive, although it is unclear which regimen provides the best response rates. Triple-negative breast cancers often overexpress EGFR, and as a result may be targeted by EGFR-directed antibodies such as cetuximab or inhibitors of receptor phosphorylation such as gefitinib and erlotinib (Mendelsohn and Baselga 2006). The efficacy of cetuximab alone or in combination with carboplatin is being investigated in the metastatic setting. Other therapies such as imatinib, lapatinib, dasatinib, poly (ADP-ribose) polymerase inhibitors, survivin inhibitors and pertuzumab are being evaluated in the treatment of this subgroup of breast cancers (Agus et al 2005, Burris et al 2005, Modi et al 2005).

Prognostic Factors

Adjuvant systemic therapy is an important component of breast cancer treatment, aiming to extend disease-free survival and overall survival. When considering which patients are suitable for treatment, systemic risk is assessed based on a number of prognostic factors (Box 47.1).

The Nottingham Prognostic Index (NPI) was developed in 1982 as an aid to the management of breast cancer. By using multivariate analysis, three factors were found to be significant: tumour grade, number of lymph nodes involved and size of the tumour. NPI is calculated using the following formula:

$$\text{NPI} = \text{pathological tumour size (cm)} \times 0.2 + \text{lymph node stage (1,2,3)} + \text{histological grade (1,2,3)}$$

where lymph node stage is scored 1 (no nodes affected), 2 (up to three glands affected) or 3 (more than three glands affected); and tumour grade is scored 1 (for grade I), 2 (for grade II) or 3 (for grade III). Cut-off points of 2.4, 3.4, 4.4, 5.4 and 6.4 are used to divide the patients into six prognostic

---

Box 47.1 Prognostic factors in breast cancer

Axillary lymph node status

Involvement of local and regional lymph nodes is one of the most important prognostic factors in breast cancer (Galea et al 1992). The 10-year survival reduces from 75% to 25–30% in women with nodal involvement compared with women with no nodal involvement, and the greater the number of nodes, the worse the prognosis (Neville et al 1992). Metastatic involvement to a higher axillary level, particularly those in the apex, carries a worse prognosis (Bedwani et al 1981, Rosen and Groshen 1990).

Tumour size

Smaller tumours (<15 mm) have been shown to have a 'better prognosis' than larger tumours (>15 mm), with a risk of axillary lymph nodal involvement of 40% compared with 12–20%, respectively (Carter et al 1989, Henson et al 1991, O'Dwyer 1991, Galea et al 1992, Neville et al 1992).

Differentiation

Juan Hassiman was the first to suggest a correlation between the microscopic appearance of tumours and their degree of malignancy in the 19th century (Carstens et al 1985). Certain types of invasive breast cancer (tubular, mucinous, cribriform, medullary and lobular) carry a more favourable prognosis than invasive cancer of no special type (Carstens et al 1985, Eichhorn 2004, Sullivan et al 2005, Gatti et al 2006, Tan et al 2008, Contreras and Sattar 2009). Bloom and Richardson (1957) developed a numerical grading system assigned by pathologists to invasive breast cancers. It is the most common type of cancer grading system currently used, based on three morphological features of invasive breast cancers: (1) the degree of tumour tubule formation (percentage cancer composed of tubular structures); (2) the mitotic activity of the tumour (rate of cell division); and (3) the nuclear pleomorphism of tumour cells (nuclear grade, change in cell size and uniformity). Each of these features is assigned a score ranging from 1 to 3. The scores are then added together for a final score ranging from 3 to 9. This value is then used to grade the tumour as follows: 3–5, grade 1 tumour (well differentiated); 6–7, grade 2 tumour (moderately differentiated); and 8–9, grade 3 tumour (poorly differentiated).

Lymphovascular invasion

The presence of lymphovascular invasion closely correlates with local and regional lymph node involvement (Ejlertsen et al 2009).

ER /PgR status

A response to endocrine therapy is seen in 50–60% of patients with ERα-positive tumours, compared with a minimal response seen in ERα-negative patients (Horwitz and McGuire 1975, Hunt 2001). In patients with ERα-/PgR-positive tumours, the response rate increases to 78%.

Histopathology of *BRCA1* mutations

Cancers associated with *BRCA1* mutations have a significantly higher mitotic rate, are less likely to be ERα-/PgR-positive, more aneuploid and have greater lymphocytic infiltration than sporadic cancers (Marcus et al 1996, Anonymous 1997b, Karp et al 1997, Armes et al 1998, Robson et al 1998).

Expression of growth factor receptors

Expression of EGFR is inversely correlated with ERα positivity, and therefore may be associated with endocrine resistance (Nicholson et al 1994). Slamon et al (1987) showed that *HER-2* gene amplification independently predicted poorer overall survival and disease-free survival in a multivariate analysis in node-positive patients. Larger tumour size and higher grade (poor prognostic factors) have been also correlated with HER-2 overexpression (Rilke et al 1991, Pietras et al 1995).

groups (excellent, good, moderate I and II, poor and very poor), giving 10-year survival rates of 96%, 93%, 82%, 75%, 53% and 39%, respectively.

Genomics and Proteomics

Genomics (study of the human genome) and proteomics (analysis of the protein component of the gene) are two branches of molecular biology that will have a major role in understanding, diagnosing and potentially providing therapeutic targets in breast cancer. Gene expression cDNA arrays in the landmark study by Perou et al identified five distinct gene expression patterns — two ERα-positive groups referred to as luminal subtypes (A and B) as they share features with luminal epithelial cells arising from the inner layer of the duct lining, another group that overexpresses HER-2, and a normal breast gene expression group characterized by elevated expression of basal epithelial cell genes and reduced expression of basal epithelial cell genes (Perou et al 2000). The final group was a basal-like subgroup which shares features with normal basal epithelial cells (ERα, PgR and HER-2 negative). cDNA arrays have also distinguished cancers associated with *BRCA1/BRCA2* mutations, ERα expression and prognostic subgroups in node-negative breast cancer. In the future, it is envisaged that gene expression profiles may guide decisions on the choice of adjuvant therapy for individual patients. Proteomics has already assumed a role in the monitoring of response and prediction of both resistance and relapse in patients treated with novel targeted therapies (van de Vijver et al 2002, McClelland and Gullick 2003).

Micrometastases in Breast Cancer

Disseminated tumour cells (DTCs) in the bone marrow of breast cancer patients are an independent predictor of poor prognosis. A number of studies have detected DTCs in 13–42% of patients without overt distant metastases (stage M0) (Schlimok et al 1987, Cote et al 1991, Harbeck et al 1994, Diel et al 1996, Molino et al 1997, Mansi et al 1999, Braun et al 2000b, Gebauer et al 2001, Gerber et al 2001, Wiedswang et al 2003, Braun et al 2005). The prognostic relevance of detecting DTCs has an impact on breast-cancer-specific survival, disease-free survival, distant disease-free survival and overall survival. In one multivariate analysis, bone marrow status was the most important independent factor for disease-free and overall survival. Several studies have shown that the presence of DTCs in bone marrow following adjuvant therapy is a predictor of poor prognosis (Braun et al 2000a, Wiedswang et al 2004, Janni et al 2005). Bone marrow analysis of high-risk patients (more than three involved axillary nodes), before and after receiving adjuvant taxane or anthracycline therapy, demonstrated that the presence of tumour cells was associated with an extremely poor prognosis and a heterogeneous response to treatment (Braun et al 2000a).

Circulating tumour cells (CTCs) are defined as micrometastases detected in peripheral blood. CTCs have been detected in 10–60% of primary breast cancer patients with no signs of overt metastases, depending on the detection technique used (Kraeft et al 2000, Witzig et al 2002). Several studies have used CTCs as a tool to assist breast cancer diagnosis (Reinholz et al 2005, Chen et al 2006). The majority of studies reporting on the prognostic significance of CTCs in patients with mBC use the Cell-Search (Veridex LLC) system. The presence of more than five CTCs per 7.5 ml of whole blood in patients with mBC before a new treatment was an independent predictor of overall survival and progression-free survival (Cristofanilli et al 2004). The presence of CTCs was also shown to be a better surrogate endpoint than current radiological imaging for assessing response to treatment (Budd et al 2006). The Southwest Oncology Group has launched a phase III trial (NCT00382018) evaluating a change in chemotherapy regimen in those mBC patients with elevated CTCs following the first follow-up assessment.

It is likely that the future role of minimal residual disease (DTCs/CTCs) will increase in the diagnosis, prognosis and treatment decision making of breast cancer patients.

Gene Expression Signatures

Decisions for treating patients with adjuvant therapy in locally advanced breast cancer have relied on assessing both patient-related and tumour-related prognostic markers providing valuable information on risk of relapse. Through use of gene expression microarray technology, studies in gene expression profiling have improved upon these traditional prognostic tools and enabled a risk prediction for an individual patient.

Gene expression signatures as predictors of recurrence

In the top-down approach, a gene expression signature is derived by seeking profiles that are correlated with clinical outcome without a previous biological assumption (Loi et al 2005).

The 70-gene prognostic signature (MammaPrint)

The Netherlands Cancer Institute in Amsterdam and Rossetta were the first to conduct a comprehensive genomewide assessment of gene expression identifying broadly applicable prognostic markers. This signature outperformed the St Gallen and National Institutes of Health criteria in being the strongest predictor for distant metastases free survival, independent of adjuvant treatment, tumour size, grade and age in both node-positive and node-negative patients. These findings suggest that MammaPrint could potentially increase the detection rate of those patients with a good prognosis, thereby decreasing the use of chemotherapy in these patients. In 2007, the US Food and Drug Administration cleared the MammaPrint test for use for node-negative breast cancer patients under 61 years of age with small tumours (<5 cm).

The Microarray In Node-negative Disease may Avoid Chemotherapy Trial (MINDACT) (EORTC 10041/BIG 03/04) is evaluating the gene expression signature MammaPrint. This trial is setting out to see whether it may be possible to distinguish between patients with a high risk of developing metastatic disease and patients who could be spared chemotherapy as their distant metastases risk is low so adjuvant chemotherapy would offer minimal benefit (Cardoso et al 2008). The trial is enrolling node-negative breast cancer patients who will have their risk assessed through both traditional clinicopathological factors (using Adjuvant Online; http://www.cancerscreening.nhs. uk/breastscreen/index.html) and MammaPrint. If the main hypothesis of the MINDACT is validated, it will be the first study to provide level I evidence for a decrease in the indications of adjuvant chemotherapy.

The 76-gene prognostic signature

Using a different microarray platform (Affymetrix), the Erasmus Medical Centre, Rotterdam in collaboration with Veridex LL identified a 76-gene prognostic signature that could be used to predict the development of distant metastases within 5 years in node-negative primary breast cancer patients ($n = 15$, irrespective of age and tumour size) who did not receive systemic treatment. Independent validation of both the 70-gene and 76-gene prognostic signatures has been conducted by TRANSBIG, a Translational Research Network associated with the Breast International Group.

Oncotype DX

Several signatures have been generated to predict prognosis in patients treated with endocrine therapy. Paik et al, in collaboration with Genomic Health Inc., developed a recurrence score based on 21 genes that appeared to accurately predict the likelihood of distant recurrence in tamoxifen-treated patients with node-negative, ER-positive breast cancer (Paik et al 2004). The process of clinical validation to achieve level I evidence is ongoing for Oncotype DX in the clinical trial TAILORx [Trial Assigning IndividuaLized Options for Treatment (Rx)]. This trial will evaluate whether women with node-negative, ERα-positive breast cancer need chemotherapy based on their recurrence score. The US Intergroup launched the trial in May 2006 and is expected to accrue over 10,000 patients, of which 29% will be low risk, 44% intermediate risk and 27% high risk.

In the bottom-up approach, a set of genes is generated from specific biological assumptions of cellular mechanisms, before being correlated with clinical outcome to assess relevance.

Wound-response signature

Chang et al derived a wound-response signature with prognostic potential by examining the processes involved in wound healing and then drawing similarities with the oncogenic process (Chang et al 2004).

Invasiveness gene signature

Lui et al generated a 186-gene 'invasiveness' signature (IGS) by using gene expression profiling of tumorigenic breast cancer cells compared with normal breast epithelium (Liu et al 2007). The IGS is significantly associated with overall and metastases-free survival independent of established pathological and clinical variables.

Gene expression signatures as predictors for drug sensitivity

Some gene signatures have been developed to identify patients who are sensitive to specific therapies; this is known as 'pharmacogenomics'. Markers predicting treatment response could ultimately lead to individualization of adjuvant therapy.

Gene signatures clearly represent a major step forward in the molecular prediction of drug sensitivity and patient outcomes. Trials such as MINDACT and TAILORx are still required to prove that clinical benefit can be derived from this new technology. This shift in emphasis towards molecular profiling represents a significant revolution in the management of breast cancer patients. It is likely that gene expression profiles will become part of an integrated decision-making model, but for the time being, the treatment guidelines of theNational Comprehensive Cancer Network, National Institutes of Health and St Gallen will continue to be used.

Adjuvant Online (http://www.adjuvantonline.com)

'The purpose of Adjuvant is to help health professionals and patients with early cancer discuss the risks and benefits of getting additional therapy (adjuvant therapy: usually chemotherapy, hormone therapy, or both) after surgery. The goal is to help health professionals make estimates of the risk of negative outcome (cancer-related mortality or relapse) without systemic adjuvant therapy, estimates of the reduction of these risks afforded by therapy, and risks of side-effects of the therapy. These estimates are based on information entered about individual patients and their tumours (e.g. patient age, tumour size, nodal involvement, histological grade, etc.) These estimates are then provided on printed sheets in simple graphical and text formats to be used in consultations.'

Metastatic Breast Cancer

Although survival from breast cancer has been improving, approximately 40% of women with early-stage breast cancer will develop metastatic disease. Median survival time following relapse is 18–24 months, but many live for several years and a few for a decade or more. The treatment of mBC patients is to prolong life, maintain a good quality of life and relieve symptoms. The goals for treatment are dependent upon a number of variables including patient-related factors such as comorbidities and age, and tumour related factors including hormone receptor status, tumour grade and site of metastasis. The recommended radiological tests routinely employed in the staging work-up for mBC include bone scintigraphy and contrast-enhanced CT of the chest, abdomen and pelvis (Figures 47.10 and 47.11). Treatment options include endocrine therapy with tamoxifen, AI, GnRH analogues and chemotherapy. Approximately 50% of patients achieve tumour regression with duration of less than 1 year.

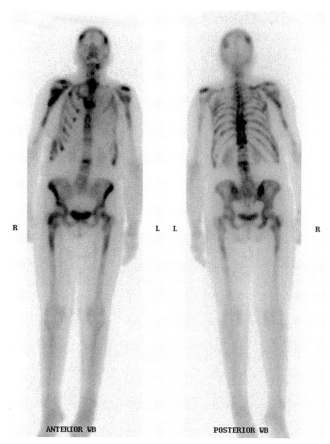

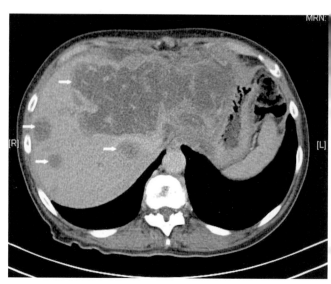

Figure 47.11 Computed tomography (CT) of liver breast metastases. Contrast-enhanced study of the liver showing lower attenuation of metastases which have not enhanced, like the surrounding liver, with contrast (white arrows). CT allows accurate measurement of metastatic deposits for assessing change in size response to chemotherapy and hormonal therapy regimes.

Figure 47.10 Bone scan breast metastases. Multiple areas of increased activity (black) are due to multiple bone metastases. The bisphosphonates used for bone scanning are labelled with technetium-99m. The tracer is taken up by osteoblasts within the bone.

Chemotherapy in metastatic breast cancer

Studies have shown that 24–30% of women with node-negative breast cancer and 50–60% of those with node-positive disease at diagnosis will relapse (Honig 1996). Approximately 6–10% of patients will present with de-novo metastatic disease at diagnosis (Honig 1996, Cardoso et al 2002). The median survival for women presenting with de-novo mBC is 2–4 years, although an increased survival is seen in a small percentage of patients (Falkson et al 1995, Greenberg et al 1996, Honig 1996). Despite the many new options for the treatment of mBC, mortality rates have only shown a small decline from 1930 to 1998 (1.6% annually from 1989 to 1995, and 3.4% more recently) (Jemal et al 2002).

The chemotherapy regimen selected will depend on previous adjuvant therapies received, and is chosen not just on the basis of efficacy, but also with the aim of minimizing toxicity. Anthracycline-based chemotherapy is well established as the first-line option for women with mBC, when this has not been used previously in the adjuvant setting. Both paclitaxel and docetaxel have been evaluated in mBC after anthracycline use. Recent meta-analysis has shown a significantly increased overall survival, time to progression and response rates in taxane-containing chemotherapy regimens compared with non-taxane-containing regimens.

Combination of the orally bioavailable prodrug capecitabine with docetaxel has shown greater response rates, time to disease progression and overall survival compared with docetaxel alone. Other agents include the semisynthetic vinca alkaloid vinorelbine, gemcitabine and the platinum salts cisplatin and carboplatin. There has been some evidence to suggest that sequential single agents may be equally effective in terms of survival, with reduced toxicity compared with combination chemotherapy. There appears to be little survival benefit in giving chemotherapy for more than 6 months. There is an underlying assumption that improvements in overall response rates translate into long-term survival benefit (Greenberg et al 1996, Fossati et al 1998, Pierga et al 2001, Bruzzi et al 2005).

Trastuzumab in metastatic breast cancer

Trastuzumab is effective in those women with mBC over-expressing HER-2 (only IHC3+ or FISH-positive patients benefit). Slamon et al (2001) were the first to show that addition of trastuzumab to chemotherapy in patients with HER-2-positive mBC was associated with a longer time to progression (7.4 months vs 4.6 months), higher response rate (50% vs 32%) and longer survival (25.1 vs 20.3 months). Combining trastuzumab with docetaxel has shown significantly greater response rates (61% vs 36%) and overall survival (24.1% vs 13.2 months) compared with single-agent docetaxel (Marty et al 2005). The duration of treatment with trastuzumab is unknown; however, this is being addressed by a large randomized study.

Other agents used in metastatic breast cancer

Epithilones are macrolide antibiotics isolated from the myxobacterium *Sorangium cellulosum*, which promote microtubule stabilization via a similar mechanism to that of the taxanes (Bollag et al 1995, Wartmann and Altmann 2002). Epithilones are associated with a lower susceptibility to drug resistance and greater efficacy in taxane-resistant tumours. Recently, the epithilone ixabepilone (Ixempra, Bristol-Myers Squibb) has been approved for use by the US Food and Drug Administration after having shown activity in chemotherapy-sensitive and chemotherapy-resistant tumour models, and synergistic activity with other chemotherapeutic and targeted agents. Randomized trials in patients with bony metastatic disease have shown that bisphosphonates can significantly reduce skeletal-related events, including pathological fractures, spinal cord compression, hypercalcaemia and the need for intervention with radiotherapy by 30–50%. They have also been shown to reduce bony pain, but have not shown any improvement in survival (Paterson et al 1993, van Holten-Verzantvoort et al 1993, Lipton et al 2000, Rosen et al 2001). The dual tyrosine kinase inhibitor lapatinib has shown significant efficacy in refractory metastatic HER-2-positive breast cancer patients (previously treated with trastuzumab) and as a first-line metastatic treatment, with potential benefit in patients with brain metastases.

Preservation of Fertility in Breast Cancer Patients

Breast cancer is the most common cancer affecting women of reproductive age, and approximately 13% of all breast cancer diagnoses are made in women aged under 45 years (Gloeckler Ries et al 2003). Many breast cancer patients may not have completed their family planning, and may wish to have children after their breast cancer treatment. Options for fertility preserving should be discussed before starting treatment in some patients. Standard regimens of radiation therapy for breast cancer do not affect the ovaries significantly; however, internal scatter radiation can reach the pelvis and ovaries. As a result, in-vitro fertilization (IVF) and egg harvesting should not be performed during treatment and pregnancy should be prevented (Arnon et al 2001, Falcone et al 2004, Jeruss and Woodruff 2009). Indirect evidence supports a delay of antioestrogen treatment to allow for pregnancy after surgery and radiotherapy are completed (Gradishar and Hellmund 2002, Goss 2007). As a result, the threat to fertility for a patient not receiving chemotherapy, whose baseline fertility is within the normal range, is small. Breast cancer treatments are well known to affect menstrual status and fertility among premenopausal women diagnosed with breast cancer (Lobo 2005). Amenorrhoea following systemic breast cancer treatment may result in loss of fertility, onset of menopausal symptoms, problems with sexual functioning, and exposure to the long-term health risks of an early menopause.

Risk of chemotherapy-related amenorrhoea and menopause

The risk of chemotherapy-related amenorrhoea depends on the patient's age, the type of chemotherapeutic agents used and the total dose administered. Older women have a higher incidence of complete ovarian failure and permanent infertility compared with younger women (Minton and Munster 2002, Maltaris et al 2007). This higher incidence is explained by the greater primordial follicle reserve (ovarian reserve) in younger women, which decreases with age. The degree of damage will determine whether the amenorrhoea is permanent or temporary; should no oocytes remain viable, menses may cease altogether and menopause will follow. Menstrual function may resume months or occasionally years after treatment; however, the majority of women who remain amenorrhoeic 1 year after treatment will not regain ovarian function. Assessment of the ovarian reserve in patients treated with chemotherapy includes serum measurements of anti-Müllerian hormone, follicle-stimulating hormone, inhibin B and oestrogen levels (Lutchman Singh et al 2007, van Beek et al 2007). An ultrasound-guided antral follicle count can also be useful for assessing ovarian reserve (Lutchman Singh et al 2007).

Chemotherapy can cause ovarian damage by a number of mechanisms. Dividing cells are vulnerable to most cytotoxic agents; however, alkylating agents such as cyclophosphamide present the greatest potential for ovarian failure among all chemotherapeutic agents (Meirow 1999). Alkylating agents are not cell cycle specific and may affect cells not actively dividing, including the pregranulosa cells of the primordial follicles and oocytes. The higher the cumulative dose of cyclophosamide, the greater the observed incidence of menopause. It has been reported that with the classic CMF regimen, the incidence of amenorrhoea was 61% in women under 40 years of age and 95% in women over 40 years of age (Goldhirsch et al 1990). The regimen of six cycles of FEC induces menopause in 60% of patients (Venturini et al 2005). A prospective cohort study evaluating 595 women aged 25–40 years treated for early breast cancer with a number of different chemotherapy regimens showed that menstrual cycles were more likely to persist in women treated with regimens containing less cumulative cyclophosamide (Petrek et al 2006). Those patients on a CMF regimen were more likely than women on other regimens to bleed within the first month of chemotherapy, but were less likely to commence menses 1 year later. The study also showed that tamoxifen accounted for a 15% decrease in menstrual cycling at 1 and 2 years, regardless of chemotherapy regimen. Most premenopausal women will continue to menstruate whilst taking tamoxifen, although their menses may become irregular. One study has shown no effect of trastuzumab on fertility (Abusief et al 2006).

Strategies to preserve fertility in women with breast cancer

The ASCO and UK National Health Service guidelines recommend that the implications of oncological treatment for fertility should be discussed with patients. If sufficient time exists before a woman is about to start chemotherapy or radiotherapy, she may undergo IVF to cryopreserve embryos or an embryo (Falcone et al 2004, Roberts and Oktay 2005, Agarwal and Chang 2007, West et al 2007). This technique requires a delay in cancer treatment for up to 1 month, which may not be an option for some patients. Cryopreservation remains the most effective approach to preserve fertility; however, post-thaw survival rates of embryos are in the range of 35–90%, and implantation rates are between 8% and 30%. If multiple embryos are available, cumulative pregnancy rates can be more than 60% (Seli and Tangir 2005). Delivery rates per embryo transfer using cryopreserved embryos are in the range of 18–20%. This approach requires IVF and a male partner.

Oocyte banking is more difficult than embryo cryopreservation, as oocyte cooling and exposure to cryopreservation agents affects the cytoskeleton and causes hardening of the zona pellucida. The success is dependent upon the number of eggs harvested (<10 oocytes = very low chance of pregnancy). The overall livebirth rate per preserved oocyte is approximately 3%, which is much lower than that for IVF using fresh oocytes (Gosden 2005). Several studies are evaluating the use of GnRH analogues to preserve ovarian function during cytotoxic treatment. Research in a population of older women of reproductive age has suggested that addition of a GnRH analogue to treatment may increase a woman's likelihood of remaining premenopausal after chemotherapy; however, the reproductive outcome was poor (Fox et al 2003).

It has been suggested that IVF could accelerate the disease process in women with ERα-positive breast cancer by increasing the oestrogen concentration. In one study of 100 patients, ovarian stimulation with concurrent administration of an AI or tamoxifen demonstrated no increase in recurrence and no effect on the IVF cycle (Oktay et al 2005, Azim et al 2008). Another technique whereby immature oocytes are collected and matured in vitro, avoiding ovarian stimulation, has been used in women with polycystic ovary syndrome (Lee 2007, Reinblatt and Buckett 2008). Oocyte donation is a well-established form of assisted reproduction, with 20% of replaced embryos resulting in a live birth. The harvesting of ovarian tissue is less established; this involves the removal of the ovarian cortex by laparoscopy, which is cryopreserved for later reimplantation. Only small numbers of women have had thawed ovarian tissue reimplanted, and only five live births have resulted to date (Donnez et al 2004, Meirow et al 2005, Demeestere et al 2007, Andersen et al 2008). The incidence of occult ovarian cancer in *BRCA1/BRCA2* carriers is low, but the potential for development of ovarian cancer in the transplanted tissue makes it a poor option in this subgroup (Colgan et al 2001).

Pregnancy-Associated Breast Cancer

Pregnancy-associated breast cancer (PBAC) is defined as breast cancer diagnosed during pregnancy or lactation or 1 year post partum (Petrek 1991). After cervical cancer, breast cancer is the second most common malignancy in pregnant women (Antonelli et al 1996). The diagnosis is often delayed due to physiological and anatomical changes in the breast, and a low index of suspicion of breast cancer in these patients. The average age of patients with PABC is 32–38 years. The estimated incidence of PBAC is 0.2–3.8% of all breast cancers, and it is reported to occur in one in 3000–10,000 pregnancies (Anderson 1979, Gemignani et al 1999). Women are three times more likely to have a family history of breast cancer than age-matched, non-pregnant/non-lactating women (Ishida et al 1992). Carriers of the *BRCA1/BRCA2* mutation who have had a full-term pregnancy are more likely to develop breast cancer before 40

years of age than nulliparous women with the *BRCA1/BRCA2* mutation (Jernstrom et al 1999).

PABC often presents as a painless mass, although clinical examination of the breast may be increasingly difficult because of increased nodularity (King et al 1985b, Ribeiro et al 1986). During pregnancy, oestrogen, progesterone, prolactin and chorionic gonadotrophin rise, and the breasts undergo marked ductal and lobular proliferation with blood flow increasing by 180% and weight doubling (Scott-Conner and Schorr 1995). A study of 63 women with PABC showed that less than 20% were diagnosed prior to delivery and the median size of the tumour was 3.5 cm. Sixty-two percent of patients were found to have nodal involvement compared with 39% of matched non-pregnant controls (Petrek 1991). PABC is more likely to present with larger tumours, vascular invasion and distant metastases (Guinee et al 1994).

Between 70% and 80% of breast biopsies performed during pregnancy are benign (Woo et al 2003). A dominant mass presenting during pregnancy must be formally investigated by 'triple assessment'. Mammography during pregnancy is not advised, and ultrasound can identify cystic lesions and help to characterize solid masses (Liberman et al 1994, Ahn et al 2003). Bone scans for metastatic disease are generally not recommended, and MRI can be used to evaluate liver and bony metastases (Baker et al 1987). PABC tends to present with ERα-/PgR-negative tumours, and appears to have a worse 5-year survival in women presenting with nodal involvement compared with non-pregnant matched controls (47% vs 59%) (Petrek 1991, Bonnier et al 1997). There appears to be an increased relative risk of dying from breast cancer if it develops within 4 years of giving birth, compared with age-matched women who have never been pregnant and who develop breast cancer (Duncan et al 1986, Guinee et al 1994).

Treatment of PABC should not be delayed because of pregnancy. Surgery can be performed during all trimesters of pregnancy with no effect on the fetus. Surgery is tailored to the gestation and the breast cancer stage. BCS is generally not recommended during the first trimester because of the need to delay radiotherapy and an increase in local risk of recurrence. Mastectomy can be performed during all trimesters of pregnancy, although immediate reconstruction is not recommended due to difficulty in achieving symmetry.

Chemotherapy is contraindicated in the first trimester because of an increased risk of spontaneous abortion and a teratogenic risk of 14–19%, falling to 1.4% by the second trimester (Ebert et al 1997). Chemotherapy can cross the placenta and, if given up to 15 weeks of gestation, has been shown to interfere with cell differentiation leading to permanent organ malformation. Administration of FEC chemotherapy during the second and third trimesters in a study of 24 women showed no congenital malformations, although chemotherapy should be stopped 3 weeks before delivery (Berry et al 1999, Keleher et al 2002). Women with node-positive PABC are advised to start chemotherapy after the first trimester. Tamoxifen is associated with an increased risk of congenital malformations and spontaneous abortion, and therefore endocrine therapy is not recommended during pregnancy (Isaacs et al 2001).

The use of radiotherapy in women with PABC poses a particular dilemma. During the first trimester, the fetus is outside the radiation field of the chest wall but is still exposed to scatter radiation; however, during the later stages of pregnancy, the fetus lies outside the pelvis and is closer to the radiation field, but will have completed organogenesis and the effects of radiation will be reduced (Saunders 2001). There have been anecdotal reports of fetal malformations as well as normal pregnancy outcomes in pregnant women receiving radiotherapy for breast cancer. Therefore, the teratogenic effects of radiotherapy need to be weighed up against the improvement in disease-free survival.

In women with metastatic PABC, the risk for quick treatment must be balanced against the risk to the fetus. No significant difference in survival is seen in women opting to continue pregnancy with an associated breast cancer and those opting for a termination of pregnancy. There is no time interval known to be safe for becoming pregnant after PABC. Some advocate 2 years following treatment for women with 'low-risk' PABC and longer for those with high-risk tumours.

Breast Cancer in the Elderly

Forty percent of breast cancers occur in women over 70 years of age. Historically, these women have been treated by hormone manipulation alone, but local control was frequently unsatisfactory, necessitating surgical intervention or radiotherapy at a later stage. Since the biology of cancers in this age group is similar to that in younger women, the majority of elderly patients presenting with breast cancer should be managed in the standard way. Primary hormonal treatment should be reserved for those women who decline surgical intervention or in whom comorbidity is such that their disease is unlikely to progress significantly within their natural lifetime.

Clinical Follow-Up

Most follow-up protocols are not evidence based and have evolved over time. In practice, the majority of recurrences are detected by patients themselves or by mammography. The aims of follow-up are: (1) early detection of local recurrence, (2) early detection of metastatic disease, (3) screening for new primary breast cancer, (4) detection of treatment-related toxicities, and (5) provision of psychological support. Two-thirds of local recurrences after mastectomy occur in the first 5 years, but after BCS, there is a steady relapse rate. Women with a history of invasive breast cancer have a five-fold increased risk of developing a second primary with an annual risk of contralateral breast cancer of 0.6%.

Patients continuing active treatment should be followed-up until such treatment has been completed. Follow-up should be stratified according to disease, with high-risk patients followed-up more closely with joint care by surgeons and oncologists according to agreed local protocols. Mammography is an important component of follow-up, and the current guidelines from the Royal College of Radiologists advise performing annual mammography for the first 5–10 years.

Breast Reconstruction after Surgery for Breast Cancer

Most healthy patients under the age of 70 years with a non-inflammatory or locally advanced tumour undergoing a skin-sparing mastectomy should be offered immediate breast reconstruction.

The surgical treatment for patients with breast cancer will involve either BCS or mastectomy, both of which will result in considerable asymmetry of the breasts. Improved survival as a result of earlier detection of breast cancers means that women will live for much longer with the psychological problems and physical defects of surgery. Mastectomy affects body image and can lead to depression, anxiety and poor self-esteem. Breast reconstruction offers restoration of breast symmetry to women by creating a breast which is similar in shape, size, contour and position to the opposite breast. It plays a significant role in the women's physical, psychological and emotional recovery from breast cancer.

Breast reconstruction has become an integral part in the management of women with breast cancer. Candidates for breast reconstructive surgery are those who have considerable asymmetry following tumour removal. The majority of reconstructions are performed in patients undergoing mastectomy, and reconstructive options should be discussed prior to surgery. The process of breast reconstruction involves:

- reconstruction of the breast mound (excision of breast tissue results in reduction in breast volume); and
- reconstruction of the skin (using local skin or by transferring skin from a distant site).

Further surgery may involve nipple–areola reconstruction and, in some cases, surgery to the contralateral breast to achieve symmetry. The process of breast reconstruction requires highly motivated surgical staff and patients, as many stages are involved. Skin-sparing mastectomy has significantly improved aesthetic outcomes with breast reconstruction. It allows mastectomy, with preservation of the breast skin and inframammary fold, with breast tissue excised through small skin incisions (Cunnick and Mokbel 2004). This technique produces excellent cosmetic results, particularly when combined with immediate reconstruction.

Breast reconstruction can be performed immediately at the time of mastectomy, or delayed following adjuvant therapy. Immediate reconstruction is advantageous as it results in reduced cost (single operation and hospital stay), superior cosmetic result (surgeon works with good-quality skin that is unscarred and not suffering from the effects of radiotherapy) and reduced psychological morbidity (Kroll et al 1995, Khoo et al 1998, Al-Ghazal et al 2000). The disadvantages of immediate reconstruction include limited time for patient decision making, increased operative time and the detrimental effect that chemotherapy and radiotherapy can have on some types of reconstruction (Kronowitz and Robb 2004). There are no significant differences in survival between immediate and delayed reconstruction. Delayed reconstruction allows the patient unlimited time for decision making, avoids adjuvant therapy delay and

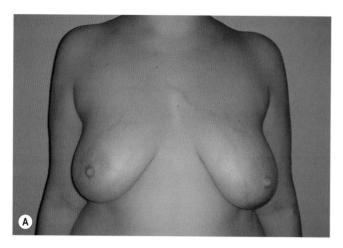

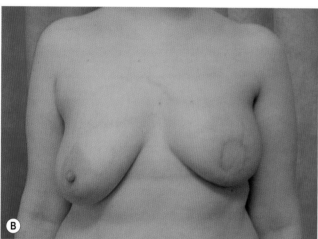

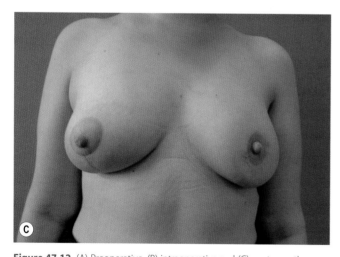

Figure 47.12 (A) Preoperative, (B) intraoperative and (C) postoperative latissimus dorsi (LD) reconstruction. Left breast skin-sparing mastectomy and immediate autologous LD flap breast reconstruction, right mastopexy and left nipple–areola reconstruction with a small local flap and tattoo. *Images courtesy of Miss Jacqueline Lewis, Consultant Oncoplastic Surgeon, Imperial College NHS Trust, London, UK.*

Box 47.2 Oncoplastic breast reconstructive techniques

Non-autologous methods

- Fixed volume breast implants
- Breast expanders

Autologous methods (using patient's own tissue)

- Extended latissimus dorsi flap
- Transverse rectus abdominis myocutaneous flap
- Deep inferior epigastric artery perforator flap
- Superior gluteal artery perforator flap

Combination of non-autologous and autologous methods

- Latissimus dorsi flap with breast implants (Figure 47.12)

Oncoplastic methods

- Breast reconstruction techniques
- Breast lift techniques

Box 47.3 Online breast cancer resources

- www.Imaginis.com — an independent American resource providing information and news on breast cancer and related women's health topics.
- www.y-me.org — a charitable, national voluntary health organization set up by breast cancer sufferers.
- www.mskcc.org — website for the Memorial Sloan-Kettering Cancer Center, New York offering a balanced and unbiased overview of the breast reconstruction options available to patients, and addressing the risk–benefit balance of each.
- www.cancerbackup.org.uk — a charitable resource that offers cancer patients and their families up-to-date information, practical advice and support on all cancers, including breast.
- www.cancer.gov — the National Cancer Institute is a component of the US National Institutes of Health, and is the Federal Government's principal agency for cancer research and training. This resource offers information for both medical professionals and patients.
- www.breastcancer.org — a non-profit organization dedicated to providing the most reliable, complete and up-to-date information about breast cancer.
- www.cancer.org — website of the American Cancer Society, a nationwide, community-based health organization dedicated to eliminating cancer as a major health problem and eliminating suffering due to cancer.
- http://qap.sdsu.edu/ — Cancer Clinical Services Quality Assurance Project and the Center for Health Professional Education and Training (the training centre provides this resource for healthcare providers involved in the early detection of breast and cervical cancers).
- www.breasthealth.com.au — official website of the National Breast Cancer Center, which was set up in 1955 by the Australian Government as a means to support patients and their families through comprehensive information on breast and ovarian cancer.
- www.breastcenter.com — official web page of the Center for Restorative Breast Surgery, founded by Dr Frank DellaCroce and Dr Scott Sullivan.
- www.mayoclinic.com — the official website of the Mayo Clinic has a page dedicated to breast reconstruction.

excludes the detrimental effects of adjuvant therapy. The mastectomy flaps, however, may be thin, scarred and contracted, resulting in a less pleasant aesthetic appearance. There are a number of contraindications to breast reconstruction including non-resectable chest wall disease, progressive systemic disease, patients with significant comorbidities and those felt to be unsuitable psychologically (Box 47.2 and Figure 47.12).

Oncoplastic techniques

A tumour may be excised within an area normally removed during a mastopexy (breast lift) or reduction, thereby achieving wide local excision of the mass and reconstruction of the breast. Symmetry can be achieved by contralateral breast reduction or mastopexy.

Nipple–areola reconstruction

Some patients are content with a prosthetic nipple, but all should have the opportunity to have a nipple–areola reconstruction. This is often performed 6 months after the reconstruction by a number of techniques including nipple sharing and use of local flaps. These procedures can be performed under local anaesthetic, and the areola is now reconstructed with a dermal tattoo using a three-dimensional colour chart to achieve a good colour match.

Online Resources

There are a host of online resources (Box 47.3) with an interest in breast cancer and reconstruction (Leff and Kinross 2007).

KEY POINTS

1. Breast cancer is common and is the cause of significant morbidity and mortality worldwide.
2. The incidence of breast cancer is increasing, but mortality is decreasing.
3. The incidence of breast cancer increases with age.
4. There is a small increased risk of breast cancer diagnosis in women taking HRT, but this needs to be balanced against the benefits of treatment.
5. Familial breast cancer accounts for only 5% of cases and nearly half of these are due to mutations in BRCA1 and BRCA2.
6. Breast cancer may present as symptomatic or screen-detected disease.
7. The diagnosis and management of breast cancer should be undertaken by an MDT of specialists.
8. Diagnosis is based on triple assessment — clinical examination, radiological imaging and cytology/histology.
9. The aim of primary surgical treatment is complete removal and hence control of local disease.
10. DCIS is treated by complete surgical excision. Axillary surgery is not required. The role of adjuvant treatments is uncertain.
11. Women undergoing mastectomy should be offered breast reconstruction.
12. Radiotherapy to the breast is standard after BCS for invasive disease to minimize the risk of local recurrence.
13. Patients with axillary node disease should have axillary clearance or radiotherapy.
14. All ER-positive patients should receive adjuvant tamoxifen for 5 years.
15. Adjuvant chemotherapy is offered to patients deemed to be at high risk of systemic relapse.
16. Metastatic disease is incurable and treatment is palliative.
17. Breast cancer in pregnancy usually presents at a more advanced stage, but the prognosis stage for stage is the same.
18. New hormonal and biological therapies for breast cancer are becoming available.

References

Abd El-Rehim DM, Ball G, Pinder SE et al 2005 High-throughput protein expression analysis using tissue microarray technology of a large well-characterised series identifies biologically distinct classes of breast cancer confirming recent cDNA expression analyses. International Journal of Cancer 116: 340–350.

Abd El-Rehim DM, Pinder SE, Paish CE et al 2004 Expression of luminal and basal cytokeratins in human breast carcinoma. Journal of Pathology 203: 661–671.

Abeliovich D, Kaduri L, Lerer I et al 1997 The founder mutations 185delAG and 5382insC in BRCA1 and 6174delT in BRCA2 appear in 60% of ovarian cancer and 30% of early-onset breast cancer patients among Ashkenazi women. American Journal of Human Genetics 60: 505–514.

Abusief ME, Missmer SA, Ginsburg ES, Weeks JC, Winer EP, Partridge AH 2006 Chemotherapy-related amenorrhea in women with early breast cancer: the effect of paclitaxel or dose density. ASCO annual meeting proceedings (post-meeting edition). Journal of Clinical Oncology 24: 105–106.

Adamo V, Franchina T, Adamo B et al 2007 Safety and activity of trastuzumab-containing therapies for the treatment of metastatic breast cancer: our long-term clinical experience (GOIM study). Annals of Oncology 18 (Suppl 6): vi11–vi15.

Agarwal SK, Chang RJ 2007 Fertility management for women with cancer. Cancer Treatment and Research 138: 15–27.

Agus DB, Gordon MS, Taylor C et al 2005 Phase I clinical study of pertuzumab, a novel HER dimerization inhibitor, in patients with advanced cancer. Journal of Clinical Oncology 23: 2534–2543.

Ahn BY, Kim HH, Moon WK et al 2003 Pregnancy- and lactation-associated breast cancer: mammographic and sonographic findings. Journal of Ultrasound in Medicine 22: 491–497; quiz 498–499.

Akashi-Tanaka S, Fukutomi T, Nanasawa T, Matsuo K, Hasegawa T, Tsuda H 2000 Treatment of noninvasive carcinoma: fifteen-year results at the National Cancer Center Hospital in Tokyo. Breast Cancer 7: 341–344.

Al-Ghazal SK, Sully L, Fallowfield L, Blamey RW 2000 The psychological impact of immediate rather than delayed breast reconstruction. European Journal of Surgical Oncology 26: 17–19.

Albertini JJ, Lyman GH, Cox C et al 1996 Lymphatic mapping and sentinel node biopsy in the patient with breast cancer. Journal of the American Medical Association 276: 1818–1822.

Allen E, Doisy E 1923 An ovarian hormone: preliminary report on its localization, extraction and partial purification and action in test animals. Journal of the American Medical Association 81: 819–821.

Allen NE, Beral V, Casabonne D et al 2009 Moderate alcohol intake and cancer incidence in women. Journal of the National Cancer Institute 101: 296–305.

Amichetti M, Perani B, Boi S 1990 Metastases to the breast from extramammary malignancies. Oncology 47: 257–260.

Andersen CY, Rosendahl M, Byskov AG et al 2008 Two successful pregnancies following autotransplantation of frozen/thawed ovarian tissue. Human Reproduction 23: 2266–2272.

Anderson JM 1979 Mammary cancers and pregnancy. BMJ (Clinical Research Ed.) 1: 1124–1127.

Anderson WF, Chu KC, Chang S 2003 Inflammatory breast carcinoma and noninflammatory locally advanced breast carcinoma: distinct clinicopathologic entities? Journal of Clinical Oncology 21: 2254–2259.

Anderson WF, Jatoi I, Devesa SS 2005 Distinct breast cancer incidence and prognostic patterns in the NCI's SEER program: suggesting a possible link between etiology and outcome. Breast Cancer Research and Treatment 90: 127–137.

Anonymous 1990 Occult axillary lymph-node micrometastases in breast cancer. The Lancet 336: 434–435.

Anonymous 1991 NIH consensus conference. Treatment of early-stage breast cancer. Journal of the American Medical Association 265: 391–395.

Anonymous 1995 Effects of radiotherapy and surgery in early breast cancer. An overview of the randomized trials. Early Breast Cancer Trialists' Collaborative Group. New England Journal of Medicine 333: 1444–1455.

Anonymous 1996 Breast cancer and hormonal contraceptives: collaborative reanalysis of individual data on 53 297 women with breast cancer and 100 239 women without breast cancer from 54 epidemiological studies. Collaborative Group on Hormonal Factors in Breast Cancer. The Lancet 347: 1713–1727.

Anonymous 1997a Breast cancer and hormone replacement therapy: collaborative reanalysis of data from 51 epidemiological studies of 52,705 women with breast cancer and 108,411 women without breast cancer. Collaborative Group on Hormonal Factors in Breast Cancer. The Lancet 350: 1047–1059.

Anonymous 1997b Pathology of familial breast cancer: differences between breast cancers in carriers of BRCA1 or BRCA2 mutations and sporadic cases. Breast Cancer Linkage Consortium. The Lancet 349: 1505–1510.

Anonymous 1998a Polychemotherapy for early breast cancer: an overview of the randomised trials. Early Breast Cancer Trialists' Collaborative Group. The Lancet 352: 930–942.

Anonymous 1998b Tamoxifen for early breast cancer: an overview of the randomised trials. Early Breast Cancer Trialists' Collaborative Group. The Lancet 351: 1451–1467.

Anonymous 1998c The management of ductal carcinoma in situ (DCIS). The Steering Committee on Clinical Practice Guidelines for the Care and Treatment of Breast Cancer. Canadian Association of Radiation Oncologists. Canadian Medical Association Journal 158 (Suppl 3): S27–S34.

Anonymous 2002a The frequency of breast cancer screening: results from the UKCCCR Randomised Trial. United Kingdom Co-ordinating Committee on Cancer Research. European Journal of Cancer 38: 1458–1464.

Anonymous 2002b WHO Handbook on Cancer Prevention, 7th edn. IARC Press, Lyon.

Anonymous 2005 Effects of chemotherapy and hormonal therapy for early breast cancer on recurrence and 15-year survival: an overview of the randomised trials. The Lancet 365: 1687–1717.

Anonymous 2008 Herceptin. Summary of Product Characteristics. Updated February 2009. www.medicines.org.uk.

Antonelli NM, Dotters DJ, Katz VL, Kuller JA 1996 Cancer in pregnancy: a review of the literature. Part II. Obstetrical and Gynecological Survey 51: 135–142.

Antoniou A, Pharoah PD, Narod S et al 2003 Average risks of breast and ovarian cancer associated with BRCA1 or BRCA2 mutations detected in case series unselected for family history: a combined analysis of 22 studies. American Journal of Human Genetics 72: 1117–1130.

Ariel IM, Caron AS 1972 Diagnosis and treatment of malignant melanoma arising from the skin of the female breast. American Journal of Surgery 124: 384–390.

Armes JE, Egan AJ, Southey MC et al 1998 The histologic phenotypes of breast carcinoma occurring before age 40 years in women with and without BRCA1 or BRCA2 germline mutations: a population-based study. Cancer 83: 2335–2345.

Arnon J, Meirow D, Lewis-Roness H, Ornoy A 2001 Genetic and teratogenic effects of cancer treatments on gametes and embryos. Human Reproduction Update 7: 394–403.

Arnould L, Denoux Y, Macgrogan G et al 2003 Agreement between chromogenic in situ hybridisation (CISH) and FISH in the determination of HER2 status in breast cancer. British Journal of Cancer 88: 1587–1591.

Arpino G, Bardou VJ, Clark GM, Elledge RM 2004 Infiltrating lobular carcinoma of the breast: tumor characteristics and clinical outcome. Breast Cancer Research 6: R149–R156.

Ashikari R, Huvos AG, Urban JA, Robbins GF 1973 Infiltrating lobular carcinoma of the breast. Cancer 31: 110–116.

Azim AA, Costantini-Ferrando M, Oktay K 2008 Safety of fertility preservation by ovarian stimulation with letrozole and gonadotropins in patients with breast cancer: a prospective controlled study. Journal of Clinical Oncology 26: 2630–2635.

Baan R, Straif K, Grosse Y et al 2007 Carcinogenicity of alcoholic beverages. The Lancet Oncology 8: 292–293.

Baar J, Silverman P, Lyons J et al 2009 A vasculature-targeting regimen of preoperative docetaxel with or without bevacizumab for locally advanced breast cancer: impact on angiogenic biomarkers. Clinical Cancer Research 15: 3583–3590.

Baker J, Ali A, Groch MW, Fordham E, Economou SG 1987 Bone scanning in pregnant patients with breast carcinoma. Clinical Nuclear Medicine 12: 519–524.

Bartella L, Kaye J, Perry NM et al 2003 Metastases to the breast revisited: radiological–histopathological correlation. Clinical Radiology 58: 524–531.

Bartow SA, Pathak DR, Black WC, Key CR, Teaf SR 1987 Prevalence of benign, atypical, and malignant breast lesions in populations at different risk for breast cancer. A forensic autopsy study. Cancer 60: 2751–2760.

Baum M, Budzar AU, Cuzick J et al 2002 Anastrozole alone or in combination with tamoxifen versus tamoxifen alone for adjuvant treatment of postmenopausal women with early breast cancer: first results of the ATAC randomised trial. The Lancet 359: 2131–2139.

Baum M, Buzdar A, Cuzick J et al 2003 Anastrozole alone or in combination with tamoxifen versus tamoxifen alone for adjuvant treatment of postmenopausal women with early-stage breast cancer: results of the ATAC (Arimidex, Tamoxifen Alone or in Combination) trial efficacy and safety update analyses. Cancer 98: 1802–1810.

Baxter N, McCready D, Chapman JA et al 1996 Clinical behavior of untreated axillary nodes after local treatment for primary breast cancer. Annals of Surgical Oncology 3: 235–240.

Beatson G 1896 On the treatment of inoperable cases of carcinoma of the mamma: suggestions for a new method of treatment with illustrative cases. The Lancet 2: 104–107.

Bedwani R, Vana J, Rosner D, Schmitz RL, Murphy GP 1981 Management and survival of female patients with 'minimal' breast cancer: as observed in the long-term and short-term surveys of the American College of Surgeons. Cancer 47: 2769–2778.

Bentzen SM, Agrawal RK, Aird EG et al 2008 The UK Standardisation of Breast Radiotherapy (START) Trial B of radiotherapy hypofractionation for treatment of early breast cancer: a randomised trial. The Lancet 371: 1098–1107.

Beral V, Hermon C, Reeves G, Peto R 1995 Sudden fall in breast cancer death rates in England and Wales. The Lancet 345: 1642–1643.

Beral V, Banks E, Reeves G 2002 Evidence from randomised trials on the long-term effects of hormone replacement therapy. The Lancet 360: 942–944.

Berry DA, Parmigiani G, Sanchez J, Schildkraut J, Winer E 1997 Probability of carrying a mutation of breast–ovarian cancer gene BRCA1 based on family history. Journal of the National Cancer Institute 89: 227–238.

Berry DA, Cronin KA, Plevritis SK et al 2005 Effect of screening and adjuvant therapy on mortality from breast cancer. New England Journal of Medicine 353: 1784–1792.

Berry DL, Theriault RL, Holmes FA et al 1999 Management of breast cancer during pregnancy using a standardized protocol. Journal of Clinical Oncology 17: 855–861.

Bijker N, Rutgers EJ, Duchateau L, Peterse JL, Julien JP, Cataliotti L 2001 Breast-conserving therapy for Paget disease of the nipple: a prospective European Organization for Research and Treatment of Cancer study of 61 patients. Cancer 91: 472–477.

Bingham SA, Luben R, Welch A, Wareham N, Khaw KT, Day N 2003 Are imprecise methods obscuring a relation between fat and breast cancer? The Lancet 362: 212–214.

Bishop HM, Blamey RW, Morris AH et al 1979 Bone scanning: its lack of value in the follow-up of patients with breast cancer. British Journal of Surgery 66: 752–754.

Bloom HJ, Richardson WW 1957 Histological grading and prognosis in breast cancer; a study of 1409 cases of which 359 have been followed for 15 years. British Journal of Cancer 11: 359–377.

Boccardo F, Rubagotti A, Puntoni M et al 2005 Switching to anastrozole versus continued tamoxifen treatment of early breast cancer: preliminary results of the Italian Tamoxifen Anastrozole Trial. Journal of Clinical Oncology 23: 5138–5147.

Bohman LG, Bassett LW, Gold RH, Voet R 1982 Breast metastases from extramammary malignancies. Radiology 144: 309–312.

Boland GP, Knox WF, Bundred NJ 2002 Molecular markers and therapeutic targets in ductal carcinoma in situ. Microscopy Research and Technique 59: 3–11.

Bollag DM, Mcqueney PA, Zhu J et al 1995 Epothilones, a new class of microtubule-stabilizing agents with a taxol-like mechanism of action. Cancer Research 55: 2325–2333.

Bonadonna G, Brusamolino E, Valagussa P et al 1976 Combination chemotherapy as an adjuvant treatment in operable breast cancer. New England Journal of Medicine 294: 405–410.

Bonadonna G, Valagussa P, Rossi A et al 1985 Ten-year experience with CMF-based adjuvant chemotherapy in resectable breast cancer. Breast Cancer Research and Treatment 5: 95–115.

Bonnier P, Romain S, Dilhuydy JM et al 1997 Influence of pregnancy on the outcome of breast cancer: a case–control study. Societe Francaise de Senologie et de Pathologie Mammaire Study Group. International Journal of Cancer 72: 720–727.

Boyd NF, Byng JW, Jong RA et al 1995 Quantitative classification of mammographic densities and breast cancer risk: results from the Canadian National Breast Screening Study. Journal of the National Cancer Institute 87: 670–675.

Boyd NF, Dite GS, Stone J et al 2002 Heritability of mammographic density, a risk factor for breast cancer. New England Journal of Medicine 347: 886–894.

Boyd S 1900 On oophorectomy in cancer of the breast. BMJ (Clinical Research Ed.) 2: 1161–1167.

Braun S, Kentenich C, Janni W et al 2000a Lack of effect of adjuvant chemotherapy on the elimination of single dormant tumor cells in bone marrow of high-risk breast cancer patients. Journal of Clinical Oncology 18: 80–86.

Braun S, Pantel K, Muller P et al 2000b Cytokeratin-positive cells in the bone marrow and survival of patients with stage I, II, or III breast cancer. New England Journal of Medicine 342: 525–533.

Braun S, Vogl FD, Naume B et al 2005 A pooled analysis of bone marrow micrometastasis in breast cancer. New England Journal of Medicine 353: 793–802.

Brekelmans CT, Seynaeve C, Bartels CC et al 2001 Effectiveness of breast cancer surveillance in BRCA1/2 gene mutation carriers and women with high familial risk. Journal of Clinical Oncology 19: 924–930.

Brem RF, Schoonjans JM, Sanow L, Gatewood OM 2001 Reliability of histologic diagnosis of breast cancer with stereotactic vacuum-assisted biopsy. The American Surgeon 67: 388–392.

Britton PD 1999 Fine needle aspiration or core biopsy? Breast 8: 1–4.

Britton PD, McCann J 1999 Needle biopsy in the NHS Breast Screening Programme 1996/7: how much and how accurate? Breast 8: 5–11.

Brogi E, Harris NL 1999 Lymphomas of the breast: pathology and clinical behavior. Seminars in Oncology 26: 357–364.

Brufsky A, Harker W, Beck J 2005 Zoledronic acid (ZA) effectively inhibits cancer treatment-induced bone loss (CTIBL) in postmenopausal women (PMW) with early breast cancer (BCa) receiving adjuvant letrozole (Let): 12 mos BMD results of the Z-FAST trial. ASCO Annual Meeting Proceedings. 23 (No. 16S, Pt I) (Suppl): 533.

Bruzzi P, Del Mastro L, Sormani MP et al 2005 Objective response to chemotherapy as a potential surrogate end point of survival in metastatic breast cancer patients. Journal of Clinical Oncology 23: 5117–5125.

Budd GT, Cristofanilli M, Ellis MJ et al 2006 Circulating tumor cells versus imaging — predicting overall survival in metastatic breast cancer. Clinical Cancer Research 12: 6403–6409.

Burris HA 3rd, Hurwitz HI, Dees EC et al 2005 Phase I safety, pharmacokinetics, and clinical activity study of lapatinib (GW572016), a reversible dual inhibitor of epidermal growth factor receptor tyrosine kinases, in heavily pretreated patients with metastatic carcinomas. Journal of Clinical Oncology 23: 5305–5313.

Cabanas RM 1977 An approach for the treatment of penile carcinoma. Cancer 39: 456–466.

Cachin F, Prince HM, Hogg A, Ware RE, Hicks RJ 2006 Powerful prognostic stratification by [18F]fluorodeoxyglucose positron emission tomography in patients with metastatic breast cancer treated with high-dose chemotherapy. Journal of Clinical Oncology 24: 3026–3031.

Campbell IG, Russell SE, Choong DY et al 2004 Mutation of the PIK3CA gene in ovarian and breast cancer. Cancer Research 64: 7678–7681.

Collaborative Group on Hormonal Factors in Breast Cancer 2002 Breast cancer and breastfeeding: collaborative reanalysis of individual data from 47 epidemiological studies in 30 countries, including 50 302 women with breast cancer and 96 973 women without the disease. The Lancet 360: 187–195.

Cardoso F, Di LA, Lohrisch C, Bernard C, Ferreira F, Piccart MJ 2002 Second and subsequent lines of chemotherapy for metastatic breast cancer: what did we learn in the last two decades? Annals of Oncology 13: 197–207.

Cardoso F, van't Veer L, Rutgers E, Loi S, Mook S, Piccart-Gebhart MJ 2008 Clinical application of the 70-gene profile: the MINDACT trial. Journal of Clinical Oncology 26: 729–735.

Carey LA, Perou CM, Livasy CA et al 2006 Race, breast cancer subtypes, and survival in the Carolina Breast Cancer Study. Journal of the American Medical Association 295: 2492–2502.

Carstens PH, Greenberg RA, Francis D, Lyon H 1985 Tubular carcinoma of the breast. A long term follow-up. Histopathology 9: 271–280.

Carter CL, Allen C, Henson DE 1989 Relation of tumor size, lymph node status, and survival in 24,740 breast cancer cases. Cancer 63: 181–187.

Chan KC, Knox WF, Sinha G et al 2001 Extent of excision margin width required in breast conserving surgery for ductal carcinoma in situ. Cancer 91: 9–16.

Chang HY, Sneddon JB, Alizadeh AA et al 2004 Gene expression signature of fibroblast serum response predicts human cancer progression: similarities between tumors and wounds. PLoS Biology 2: E7.

Chang J, Yang WT, Choo HF 1999 Mammography in Asian patients with BRCA1 mutations. The Lancet 353: 2070–2071.

Chang S, Parker SL, Pham T, Buzdar AU, Hursting SD 1998 Inflammatory breast carcinoma incidence and survival: the surveillance, epidemiology, and end results program of the National Cancer Institute 1975–1992. Cancer 82: 2366–2372.

Charafe-Jauffret E, Tarpin C, Bardou VJ et al 2004 Immunophenotypic analysis of inflammatory breast cancers: identification of an 'inflammatory signature'. Journal of Pathology 202: 265–273.

Chaudary MA, Millis RR, Lane EB, Miller NA 1986 Paget's disease of the nipple: a ten year review including clinical, pathological, and immunohistochemical findings. Breast Cancer Research and Treatment 8: 139–146.

Chawla A, Repa JJ, Evans RM, Mangelsdorf DJ 2001 Nuclear receptors and lipid physiology: opening the X-files. Science 294: 1866–1870.

Chen CC, Hou MF, Wang JY et al 2006 Simultaneous detection of multiple mRNA markers CK19, CEA, c-Met, Her2/neu and hMAM with membrane array, an innovative technique with a great potential for breast cancer diagnosis. Cancer Letters 240: 279–288.

Chen X, Moore MO, Lehman CD et al 2004 Combined use of MRI and PET to monitor response and assess residual disease for locally advanced breast cancer treated with neoadjuvant chemotherapy. Academic Radiology 11: 1115–1124.

Chen Y, Thompson W 1999 Epidemiology of contralateral breast cancer. Cancer Epidemiology, Biomarkers and Prevention 8: 855–861.

Cheung KL, Howell A, Robertson JF 2000 Preoperative endocrine therapy for breast cancer. Endocrine-related Cancer 7: 131–141.

Claus EB, Risch N, Thompson WD 1994 Autosomal dominant inheritance of early-onset breast cancer. Implications for risk prediction. Cancer 73: 643–651.

Clayton F, Hopkins CL 1993 Pathologic correlates of prognosis in lymph node-positive breast carcinomas. Cancer 71: 1780–1790.

Clemmensen J 1948 Carcinoma of the breast; results from statistical research. British Journal of Radiology 21: 583–590.

Cochran AJ, Wen DR, Morton DL 1992 Management of the regional lymph nodes in patients with cutaneous malignant melanoma. World Journal of Surgery 16: 214–221.

Cochrane RA, Valasiadou P, Wilson AR, Al-Ghazal SK, Macmillan RD 2003 Cosmesis and satisfaction after breast-conserving surgery correlates with the percentage of breast volume excised. British Journal of Surgery 90: 1505–1509.

Cockshott ID 2000 Clinical pharmacokinetics of goserelin. Clinical Pharmacokinetics 39: 27–48.

Cody HS 3rd 1999 Management of the axilla in early stage breast cancer: will sentinel node biopsy end the debate? Journal of Surgical Oncology 71: 137–139.

Colditz GA, Rosner B 2000 Cumulative risk of breast cancer to age 70 years according to risk factor status: data from the Nurses' Health Study. American Journal of Epidemiology 152: 950–964.

Coleman MP 2000 Trends in breast cancer incidence, survival, and mortality. The Lancet 356: 590–591; author reply 593.

Colgan TJ, Murphy J, Cole DE, Narod S, Rosen B 2001 Occult carcinoma in prophylactic oophorectomy specimens: prevalence and association with BRCA germline mutation status. American Journal of Surgical Pathology 25: 1283–1289.

Contreras A, Sattar H 2009 Lobular neoplasia of the breast: an update. Archives of Pathology and Laboratory Medicine 133: 1116–1120.

Cook GJ, Houston S, Rubens R, Maisey MN, Fogelman I 1998 Detection of bone metastases in breast cancer by 18FDG PET: differing metabolic activity in osteoblastic and osteolytic lesions. Journal of Clinical Oncology 16: 3375–3379.

Coombes RC, Hall E, Gibson LJ et al 2004 A randomized trial of exemestane after two to three years of tamoxifen therapy in postmenopausal women with primary breast cancer. New England Journal of Medicine 350: 1081–1092.

Costantino JP, Gail MH, Pee D et al 1999 Validation studies for models projecting the risk of invasive and total breast cancer incidence. Journal of the National Cancer Institute 91: 1541–1548.

Costantino JP, Kuller LH, Ives DG, Fisher B, Dignam J 1997 Coronary heart disease mortality and adjuvant tamoxifen therapy. Journal of the National Cancer Institute 89: 776–782.

Cote RJ, Rosen PP, Lesser ML, Old LJ, Osborne MP 1991 Prediction of early relapse in patients with operable breast cancer by detection of occult bone marrow micrometastases. Journal of Clinical Oncology 9: 1749–1756.

Cox CE, Bass SS, McCann CR et al 2000 Lymphatic mapping and sentinel lymph node biopsy in patients with breast cancer. Annual Review of Medicine 51: 525–542.

Cristofanilli M, Kau SW, Budzar AU 2002 Paclitaxel significantly improves the prognosis in ER-negative inflammatory breast cancer (IBC): The M.D. Anderson Cancer Center Experience (1974–2000).

Breast Cancer Research and Treatment 76 (Suppl 1): S158a.

Cristofanilli M, Budd GT, Ellis MJ et al 2004 Circulating tumor cells, disease progression, and survival in metastatic breast cancer. New England Journal of Medicine 351: 781–791.

Cristofanilli M, Boussen H, Baselga J 2006 A phase II combination study of lapatinib and paclitaxel as a neoadjuvant therapy in patients with newly diagnosed inflammatory breast cancer (IBC). Breast Cancer Research and Treatment (Suppl 1): S5 (abstract 1), 100.

Cummings SR, Duong T, Kenyon E, Cauley JA, Whitehead M, Krueger KA 2002 Serum estradiol level and risk of breast cancer during treatment with raloxifene. Journal of the American Medical Association 287: 216–220.

Cunnick GH, Mokbel K 2004 Skin-sparing mastectomy. American Journal of Surgery 188: 78–84.

Cutress R, Agrawal A, Etherington A et al 2008 Intra-operative assessment of axillary sentinel lymph nodes (SLN) using an RT-PCR based assay for Mammaglobin (MG) and cytokeratin 19 (CK19). European Journal of Surgical Oncology 34: 1159.

Cuzick J, Powles T, Veronesi U et al 2003 Overview of the main outcomes in breast-cancer prevention trials. The Lancet 361: 296–300.

Dawood S, Broglio K, Kau SW et al 2009 Triple receptor-negative breast cancer: the effect of race on response to primary systemic treatment and survival outcomes. Journal of Clinical Oncology 27: 220–226.

Demeestere I, Simon P, Emiliani S, Delbaere A, Englert Y 2007 Fertility preservation: successful transplantation of cryopreserved ovarian tissue in a young patient previously treated for Hodgkin's disease. The Oncologist 12: 1437–1442.

Dewar J, Havilland J, Agrawal R et al 2007 Hypofractionation for early breast cancer: first results of the UK standardisation of breast radiotherapy (START) trials. Journal of Clinical Oncology 25: LBA518.

Di Benedetto G, Cecchini S, Grassetti L et al 2008 Comparative study of breast implant rupture using mammography, sonography, and magnetic resonance imaging: correlation with surgical findings. The Breast Journal 14: 532–537.

Diel IJ, Kaufmann M, Costa SD et al 1996 Micrometastatic breast cancer cells in bone marrow at primary surgery: prognostic value in comparison with nodal status. Journal of the National Cancer Institute 88: 1652–1658.

Dixon AR, Galea MH, Ellis IO, Elston CW, Blamey RW 1991 Paget's disease of the nipple. British Journal of Surgery 78: 722–723.

Donnez J, Dolmans MM, Demylle D et al 2004 Livebirth after orthotopic transplantation of cryopreserved ovarian tissue. The Lancet 364: 1405–1410.

Dowlatshahi K, Fan M, Snider HC, Habib FA 1997 Lymph node micrometastases from breast carcinoma: reviewing the dilemma. Cancer 80: 1188–1197.

Duffy SW, Tabar L, Chen HH et al 2002 The impact of organized mammography service screening on breast carcinoma mortality in seven Swedish counties. Cancer 95: 458–469.

Duncan PG, Pope WD, Cohen MM, Greer N 1986 Fetal risk of anesthesia and surgery during pregnancy. Anesthesiology 64: 790–794.

Dunn BK, Ford LG 2000 Breast cancer prevention: results of the National Surgical Adjuvant Breast and Bowel Project (NSABP) breast cancer prevention trial (NSABP P-1: BCPT). European Journal of Cancer 36 (Suppl 4): S49–S50.

Dupont WD, Parl FF, Hartmann WH et al 1993 Breast cancer risk associated with proliferative breast disease and atypical hyperplasia. Cancer 71: 1258–1265.

Ebert U, Loffler H, Kirch W 1997 Cytotoxic therapy and pregnancy. Pharmacology and Therapeutics 74: 207–220.

Eichhorn JH 2004 Medullary carcinoma, provocative now as then. Seminars in Diagnostic Pathology 21: 65–73.

Ejlertsen B, Jensen MB, Rank F et al 2009 Population-based study of peritumoral lymphovascular invasion and outcome among patients with operable breast cancer. Journal of the National Cancer Institute 101: 729–735.

Essner R, Chung MH, Bleicher R, Hsueh E, Wanek L, Morton DL 2002 Prognostic implications of thick (> or = 4-mm) melanoma in the era of intraoperative lymphatic mapping and sentinel lymphadenectomy. Annals of Surgical Oncology 9: 754–761.

Eubank WB, Mankoff D, Bhattacharya M et al 2004 Impact of FDG PET on defining the extent of disease and on the treatment of patients with recurrent or metastatic breast cancer. AJR American Journal of Roentgenology 183: 479–486.

Eubank WB, Mankoff DA 2005 Evolving role of positron emission tomography in breast cancer imaging. Seminars in Nuclear Medicine 35: 84–99.

Evans DG, Fentiman IS, Mcpherson K, Asbury D, Ponder BA, Howell A 1994 Familial breast cancer. BMJ (Clinical Research Ed.) 308: 183–187.

Evans DG, Cuzick J, Howell A 1996 Cancer genetics clinics. European Journal of Cancer 32A: 391–392.

Evans DG, Bulman M, Young K, Gokhale D, Lalloo F 2003 Sensitivity of BRCA1/2 mutation testing in 466 breast/ovarian cancer families. Journal of Medical Genetics 40: e107.

Even-Sapir E, Metser U, Flusser G et al 2004 Assessment of malignant skeletal disease: initial experience with 18F-fluoride PET/CT

and comparison between 18F-fluoride PET and 18F-fluoride PET/CT. Journal of Nuclear Medicine 45: 272–278.

Falcone T, Attaran M, Bedaiwy MA, Goldberg JM 2004 Ovarian function preservation in the cancer patient. Fertility and Sterility 81: 243–257.

Falkson G, Holcroft C, Gelman RS, Tormey DC, Wolter JM, Cummings FJ 1995 Ten-year follow-up study of premenopausal women with metastatic breast cancer: an Eastern Cooperative Oncology Group study. Journal of Clinical Oncology 13: 1453–1458.

Ferlay J, Bray F, Pisani P, Parkin DM 2004 Cancer Incidence Mortality and Prevalence Worldwide, Version 2. Lyon, IARC Press.

Fineberg S, Rosen PP 1994 Cutaneous angiosarcoma and atypical vascular lesions of the skin and breast after radiation therapy for breast carcinoma. American Journal of Clinical Pathology 102: 757–763.

Fisher B, Redmond C, Poisson R et al 1989a Eight-year results of a randomized clinical trial comparing total mastectomy and lumpectomy with or without irradiation in the treatment of breast cancer. New England Journal of Medicine 320: 822–828.

Fisher B, Redmond C, Wickerham DL et al 1989b Systemic therapy in patients with node-negative breast cancer. A commentary based on two National Surgical Adjuvant Breast and Bowel Project (NSABP) clinical trials. Annals of Internal Medicine 111: 703–712.

Fisher B, Dignam J, Bryant J et al 1996 Five versus more than five years of tamoxifen therapy for breast cancer patients with negative lymph nodes and estrogen receptor-positive tumors. Journal of the National Cancer Institute 88: 1529–1542.

Fisher B, Dignam J, Bryant J, Wolmark N 2001 Five versus more than five years of tamoxifen for lymph node-negative breast cancer: updated findings from the National Surgical Adjuvant Breast and Bowel Project B-14 randomized trial. Journal of the National Cancer Institute 93: 684–690.

Fisher ER, Swamidoss S, Lee CH, Rockette H, Redmond C, Fisher B 1978 Detection and significance of occult axillary node metastases in patients with invasive breast cancer. Cancer 42: 2025–2031.

Fisher ER, Fisher B, Sass R, Wickerham L 1984 Pathologic findings from the National Surgical Adjuvant Breast Project (Protocol No. 4). XI. Bilateral breast cancer. Cancer 54: 3002–3011.

Fisher ER, Sass R, Fisher B, Wickerham L, Paik SM 1986 Pathologic findings from the National Surgical Adjuvant Breast Project (protocol 6). I. Intraductal carcinoma (DCIS). Cancer 57: 197–208.

Fisher ER, Dignam J, Tan-Chiu E et al 1999 Pathologic findings from the National Surgical Adjuvant Breast Project (NSABP) eight-year update of Protocol B-17:

intraductal carcinoma. Cancer 86: 429–438.

FitzGerald MG, MacDonald DJ, Krainer M et al 1996 Germ-line BRCA1 mutations in Jewish and non-Jewish women with early-onset breast cancer. New England Journal of Medicine 334: 143–149.

Forrest AP, Everington D, McDonald CC, Steele RJ, Chetty U, Stewart HJ 1995 The Edinburgh randomized trial of axillary sampling or clearance after mastectomy. British Journal of Surgery 82: 1504–1508.

Forrest P 1986 Breast Cancer Screening. Department of Health and Social Security, London.

Fossati R, Confalonieri C, Torri V et al 1998 Cytotoxic and hormonal treatment for metastatic breast cancer: a systematic review of published randomized trials involving 31,510 women. Journal of Clinical Oncology 16: 3439–3460.

Foulkes WD, Brunet JS, Stefansson IM et al 2004 The prognostic implication of the basal-like (cyclin E high/p27 low/p53+/ glomeruloid-microvascular-proliferation+) phenotype of BRCA1-related breast cancer. Cancer Research 64: 830–835.

Fourquet A, Campana F, Vielh P, Schlienger P, Jullien D, Vilcoq JR 1987 Paget's disease of the nipple without detectable breast tumor: conservative management with radiation therapy. International Journal of Radiation Oncology, Biology, Physics 13: 1463–1465.

Fowble B, Solin LJ, Schultz DJ, Goodman RL 1989 Frequency, sites of relapse, and outcome of regional node failures following conservative surgery and radiation for early breast cancer. International Journal of Radiation Oncology, Biology, Physics 17: 703–710.

Fox KR, Scialla J, Moore H 2003 Preventing chemotherapy-related amenorrhea using leuprolide during adjuvant chemotherapy for early-stage breast cancer [abstract 50]. Proceedings of the American Society of Clinical Oncology 22: 13.

Friedman S, Bertin F, Mouriesse H et al 1988 Importance of tumor cells in axillary node sinus margins ('clandestine' metastases) discovered by serial sectioning in operable breast carcinoma. Acta Oncologica 27: 483–487.

Fu W, Mittel VK, Young SC 2001 Paget disease of the breast: analysis of 41 patients. American Journal of Clinical Oncology 24: 397–400.

Fuqua SA, Schiff R, Parra I et al 2003 Estrogen receptor beta protein in human breast cancer: correlation with clinical tumor parameters. Cancer Research 63: 2434–2439.

Gail MH, Brinton LA, Byar DP et al 1989 Projecting individualized probabilities of developing breast cancer for white females who are being examined annually. Journal of the National Cancer Institute 81: 1879–1886.

Galea MH, Blamey RW, Elston CE, Ellis IO 1992 The Nottingham Prognostic Index in primary breast cancer. Breast Cancer Research and Treatment 22: 207–219.

Gatti G, Pruneri G, Gilardi D, Brenelli F, Bassani G, Luini A 2006 Report on a case of pure cribriform carcinoma of the breast with internal mammary node metastasis: description of the case and review of the literature. Tumori 92: 241–243.

Gebauer G, Fehm T, Merkle E, Beck EP, Lang N, Jager W 2001 Epithelial cells in bone marrow of breast cancer patients at time of primary surgery: clinical outcome during long-term follow-up. Journal of Clinical Oncology 19: 3669–3674.

Gemignani ML, Petrek JA, Borgen PI 1999 Breast cancer and pregnancy. Surgical Clinics of North America 79: 1157–1169.

Gennari A, Donati S, Salvadori B et al 2000 Role of 2-[18F]-fluorodeoxyglucose (FDG) positron emission tomography (PET) in the early assessment of response to chemotherapy in metastatic breast cancer patients. Clinical Breast Cancer 1: 156–161; discussion 162–163.

Gerber B, Krause A, Muller H et al 2001 Simultaneous immunohistochemical detection of tumor cells in lymph nodes and bone marrow aspirates in breast cancer and its correlation with other prognostic factors. Journal of Clinical Oncology 19: 960–971.

Geyer CE, Forster J, Lindquist D et al 2006 Lapatinib plus capecitabine for HER2-positive advanced breast cancer. New England Journal of Medicine 355: 2733–2743.

Gloeckler Ries LA, Reichman ME, Lewis DR, Hankey BF, Edwards BK 2003 Cancer survival and incidence from the Surveillance, Epidemiology, and End Results (SEER) program. Oncologist 8: 541–552.

Goffin J, Chappuis PO, Wong N, Foulkes WD 2001 Re: Magnetic resonance imaging and mammography in women with a hereditary risk of breast cancer. Journal of the National Cancer Institute 93: 1754–1755.

Goldhirsch A, Gelber RD, Castiglione M 1990 The magnitude of endocrine effects of adjuvant chemotherapy for premenopausal breast cancer patients. The International Breast Cancer Study Group. Annals of Oncology 1: 183–188.

Goldhirsch A, Glick JH, Gelber RD, Coates AS, Thurlimann B, Senn HJ 2005 Meeting highlights: international expert consensus on the primary therapy of early breast cancer 2005. Annals of Oncology 16: 1569–1583.

Gosden RG 2005 Prospects for oocyte banking and in vitro maturation. Journal of the National Cancer Institute Monographs 34: 60–63.

Goss PE 2007 Letrozole in the extended adjuvant setting: MA.17. Breast Cancer Research and Treatment 105 (Suppl 1): 45–53.

Goss PE, Ingle JN, Martino S et al 2003 A randomized trial of letrozole in postmenopausal women after five years of tamoxifen therapy for early-stage breast cancer. New England Journal of Medicine 349: 1793–1802.

Goss PE, Ingle JN, Martino S et al 2005 Randomized trial of letrozole following tamoxifen as extended adjuvant therapy in receptor-positive breast cancer: updated findings from NCIC CTG MA.17. Journal of the National Cancer Institute 97: 1262–1271.

Goyal A, Newcombe RG, Mansel RE et al 2004 Sentinel lymph node biopsy in patients with multifocal breast cancer. European Journal of Surgical Oncology 30: 475–479.

Goyal A, Newcombe RG, Mansel RE 2005 Clinical relevance of multiple sentinel nodes in patients with breast cancer. British Journal of Surgery 92: 438–442.

Gradishar WJ, Hellmund R 2002 A rationale for the reinitiation of adjuvant tamoxifen therapy in women receiving fewer than 5 years of therapy. Clinical Breast Cancer 2: 282–286.

Greco M, Crippa F, Agresti R et al 2001 Axillary lymph node staging in breast cancer by 2-fluoro-2-deoxy-D-glucose-positron emission tomography: clinical evaluation and alternative management. Journal of the National Cancer Institute 93: 630–635.

Greenberg PA, Hortobagyi GN, Smith TL, Ziegler LD, Frye DK, Buzdar AU 1996 Long-term follow-up of patients with complete remission following combination chemotherapy for metastatic breast cancer. Journal of Clinical Oncology 14: 2197–2205.

Grube BJ, Hansen NM, Ye X, Giuliano AE 2002 Tumor characteristics predictive of sentinel node metastases in 105 consecutive patients with invasive lobular carcinoma. American Journal of Surgery 184: 372–376.

Guinee VF, Olsson H, Moller T et al 1994 Effect of pregnancy on prognosis for young women with breast cancer. The Lancet 343: 1587–1589.

Ha CS, Dubey P, Goyal LK, Hess M, Cabanillas F, Cox JD 1998 Localized primary non-Hodgkin lymphoma of the breast. American Journal of Clinical Oncology 21: 376–380.

Haagensen C 1971 Diseases of the Breast. WB Saunders, Philadelphia.

Hainsworth PJ, Tjandra JJ, Stillwell RG et al 1993 Detection and significance of occult metastases in node-negative breast cancer. British Journal of Surgery 80: 459–463.

Hall T, Svensson W, Behren PV et al 2003 Lesion size ratio for differentiating breast masses. Ultrasonics 2003 IEEE Symposium on Ultrasound, 5–8 October.

Halverson KJ, Taylor ME, Perez CA et al 1993 Regional nodal management and patterns of failure following conservative surgery and radiation therapy for stage I and II breast cancer. International Journal of Radiation Oncology, Biology, Physics 26: 593–599.

Hamajima N, Hirose K, Tajima K et al 2002 Alcohol, tobacco and breast cancer — collaborative reanalysis of individual data from 53 epidemiological studies, including 58,515 women with breast cancer and 95,067 women without the disease. British Journal of Cancer 87: 1234–1245.

Hamilton LJ, Evans AJ, Wilson AR et al 2004 Breast imaging findings in women with BRCA1- and BRCA2-associated breast carcinoma. Clinical Radiology 59: 895–902.

Hance KW, Anderson WF, Devesa SS, Young HA, Levine PH 2005 Trends in inflammatory breast carcinoma incidence and survival: the surveillance, epidemiology, and end results program at the National Cancer Institute. Journal of the National Cancer Institute 97: 966–975.

Hankinson SE, Colditz GA, Willett WC 2004 Towards an integrated model for breast cancer etiology: the lifelong interplay of genes, lifestyle, and hormones. Breast Cancer Research 6: 213–218.

Harbeck N, Untch M, Pache L, Eiermann W 1994 Tumour cell detection in the bone marrow of breast cancer patients at primary therapy: results of a 3-year median follow-up. British Journal of Cancer 69: 566–571.

Hartmann LC, Schaid DJ, Woods JE et al 1999 Efficacy of bilateral prophylactic mastectomy in women with a family history of breast cancer. New England Journal of Medicine 340: 77–84.

Hartmann LC, Sellers TA, Frost MH et al 2005 Benign breast disease and the risk of breast cancer. New England Journal of Medicine 353: 229–237.

Health Statistics Quarterly 1999 Office for National Statistics. Registrations of Cancers Diagnosed in 1993–1996, England and Wales.

Henderson IC, Berry DA, Demetri GD et al 2003 Improved outcomes from adding sequential paclitaxel but not from escalating doxorubicin dose in an adjuvant chemotherapy regimen for patients with node-positive primary breast cancer. Journal of Clinical Oncology 21: 976–983.

Henson DE, Ries L, Freedman LS, Carriaga M 1991 Relationship among outcome, stage of disease, and histologic grade for 22,616 cases of breast cancer. The basis for a prognostic index. Cancer 68: 2142–2149.

Heywang-Kobrunner SH, Schaumloffel U, Viehweg P, Hofer H, Buchmann J, Lampe D 1998 Minimally invasive stereotaxic vacuum core breast biopsy. European Radiology 8: 377–385.

Hicks DG, Tubbs RR 2005 Assessment of the HER2 status in breast cancer by fluorescence in situ hybridization: a technical review with interpretive guidelines. Human Pathology 36: 250–261.

Hillner BE, Ingle JN, Chlebowski RT et al 2003 American Society of Clinical Oncology

2003 update on the role of bisphosphonates and bone health issues in women with breast cancer. Journal of Clinical Oncology 21: 4042–4057.

Hladiuk M, Huchcroft S, Temple W, Schnurr BE 1992 Arm function after axillary dissection for breast cancer: a pilot study to provide parameter estimates. Journal of Surgical Oncology 50: 47–52.

Holland PA, Gandhi A, Knox WF, Wilson M, Baildam AD, Bundred NJ 1998 The importance of complete excision in the prevention of local recurrence of ductal carcinoma in situ. British Journal of Cancer 77: 110–114.

Holland R, Connolly JL, Gelman R et al 1990a The presence of an extensive intraductal component following a limited excision correlates with prominent residual disease in the remainder of the breast. Journal of Clinical Oncology 8: 113–118.

Holland R, Hendriks JH, Vebeek AL, Mravunac M, Schuurmans Stekhoven JH 1990b Extent, distribution, and mammographic/histological correlations of breast ductal carcinoma in situ. The Lancet 335: 519–522.

Holmberg L, Anderson H 2004 HABITS (hormonal replacement therapy after breast cancer — is it safe?) a randomised comparison: trial stopped. The Lancet 363: 453–455.

Holmich LR, Vejborg I, Conrad C, Sletting S, McLaughlin JK 2005 The diagnosis of breast implant rupture: MRI findings compared with findings at explantation. European Journal of Radiology 53: 213–225.

Honig S 1996 Treatment of Metastatic Disease. Lippincott-Raven, Philadelphia.

Hortobagyi GN, de la Garza Salazar J, Pritchard K et al 2005 The global breast cancer burden: variations in epidemiology and survival. Clinical Breast Cancer 6: 391–401.

Horwitz KB, McGuire WL 1975 Predicting response to endocrine therapy in human breast cancer: a hypothesis. Science 189: 726–727.

Houghton J, George WD, Cuzick J, Duggan C, Fentiman IS, Spittle M 2003 Radiotherapy and tamoxifen in women with completely excised ductal carcinoma in situ of the breast in the UK, Australia, and New Zealand: randomised controlled trial. The Lancet 362: 95–102.

Howell A, Cuzick J, Baum M et al 2005 Results of the ATAC (Arimidex, Tamoxifen, Alone or in Combination) trial after completion of 5 years' adjuvant treatment for breast cancer. The Lancet 365: 60–62.

Hughes KS, Schnaper LA, Berry D et al 2004 Lumpectomy plus tamoxifen with or without irradiation in women 70 years of age or older with early breast cancer. New England Journal of Medicine 351: 971–977.

Hunt KK 2001 Breast Cancer. Springer-Verlag, New York.

Hunter DJ, Willett WC 1993 Diet, body size, and breast cancer. Epidemiologic Reviews 15: 110–132.

Huvos AG, Hutter RV, Berg JW 1971 Significance of axillary macrometastases and micrometastases in mammary cancer. Annals of Surgery 173: 44–46.

Information Statistics Division Online 2008 Information and Statistics Division, NHS Scotland. Department of Health, UK.

Intra M, Veronesi P, Mazzarol G et al 2003 Axillary sentinel lymph node biopsy in patients with pure ductal carcinoma in situ of the breast. Archives of Surgery 138: 309–313.

Intra M, Trifiro G, Viale G et al 2005 Second biopsy of axillary sentinel lymph node for reappearing breast cancer after previous sentinel lymph node biopsy. Annals of Surgical Oncology 12: 895–899.

Isaacs RJ, Hunter W, Clark K 2001 Tamoxifen as systemic treatment of advanced breast cancer during pregnancy — case report and literature review. Gynecology and Oncology 80: 405–408.

Isasi CR, Moadel RM, Blaufox MD 2005 A meta-analysis of FDG-PET for the evaluation of breast cancer recurrence and metastases. Breast Cancer Research and Treatment 90: 105–112.

Ishida T, Yokoe T, Kasumi F et al 1992 Clinicopathologic characteristics and prognosis of breast cancer patients associated with pregnancy and lactation: analysis of case–control study in Japan. Japanese Journal of Cancer Research 83: 1143–1149.

Jaiyesimi IA, Buzdar AU, Hortobagyi G 1992 Inflammatory breast cancer: a review. Journal of Clinical Oncology 10: 1014–1024.

Jakesz R, Jonat W, Gnant M et al 2005 Switching of postmenopausal women with endocrine-responsive early breast cancer to anastrozole after 2 years' adjuvant tamoxifen: combined results of ABCSG trial 8 and ARNO 95 trial. The Lancet 366: 455–462.

Jamali FR, Ricci A Jr, Deckers PJ 1996 Paget's disease of the nipple–areola complex. Surgical Clinics of North America 76: 365–381.

Janni W, Rack B, Schindlbeck C et al 2005 The persistence of isolated tumor cells in bone marrow from patients with breast carcinoma predicts an increased risk for recurrence. Cancer 103: 884–891.

Jatoi I, Miller AB 2003 Why is breast-cancer mortality declining? The Lancet Oncology 4: 251–254.

Jatoi I, Anderson WF, Rao SR, Devesa SS 2005 Breast cancer trends among black and white women in the United States. Journal of Clinical Oncology 23: 7836–7841.

Jemal A, Thomas A, Murray T, Thun M 2002 Cancer statistics 2002. CA: a Cancer Journal for Clinicians 52: 23–47.

Jernstrom H, Lerman C, Ghadirian P et al 1999 Pregnancy and risk of early breast cancer in carriers of BRCA1 and BRCA2. The Lancet 354: 1846–1850.

Jeruss JS, Woodruff TK 2009 Preservation of fertility in patients with cancer. New England Journal of Medicine 360: 902–911.

Johnston SR, Dowsett M 2003 Aromatase inhibitors for breast cancer: lessons from the laboratory. Nature Reviews Cancer 3: 821–831.

Jonat W, Kaufmann M, Sauerbrei W et al 2002 Goserelin versus cyclophosphamide, methotrexate, and fluorouracil as adjuvant therapy in premenopausal patients with node-positive breast cancer: the Zoladex Early Breast Cancer Research Association Study. Journal of Clinical Oncology 20: 4628–4635.

Julien JP, Bijker N, Fentiman IS et al 2000 Radiotherapy in breast-conserving treatment for ductal carcinoma in situ: first results of the EORTC randomised phase III trial 10853. EORTC Breast Cancer Cooperative Group and EORTC Radiotherapy Group. The Lancet 355: 528–533.

Karp SE, Tonin PN, Begin LR et al 1997 Influence of BRCA1 mutations on nuclear grade and estrogen receptor status of breast carcinoma in Ashkenazi Jewish women. Cancer 80: 435–441.

Kauff ND, Satagopan JM, Robson ME et al 2002 Risk-reducing salpingo-oophorectomy in women with a BRCA1 or BRCA2 mutation. New England Journal of Medicine 346: 1609–1615.

Kaufmann M, Jonat W, Blamey R et al 2003 Survival analyses from the ZEBRA study. Goserelin (Zoladex) versus CMF in premenopausal women with node-positive breast cancer. European Journal of Cancer 39: 1711–1717.

Kedar RP, Bourne TH, Powles TJ et al 1994 Effects of tamoxifen on uterus and ovaries of postmenopausal women in a randomised breast cancer prevention trial. The Lancet 343: 1318–1321.

Keleher AJ, Theriault RL, Gwyn KM et al 2002 Multidisciplinary management of breast cancer concurrent with pregnancy. Journal of the American College of Surgeons 194: 54–64.

Kennedy RJ, Kollias J, Gill PG, Bochner M, Coventry BJ, Farshid G 2003 Removal of two sentinel nodes accurately stages the axilla in breast cancer. British Journal of Surgery 90: 1349–1353.

Key T, Appleby P, Barnes I, Reeves G 2002 Endogenous sex hormones and breast cancer in postmenopausal women: reanalysis of nine prospective studies. Journal of the National Cancer Institute 94: 606–616.

Khoo A, Kroll SS, Reece GP et al 1998 A comparison of resource costs of immediate and delayed breast reconstruction. Plastic and Reconstructive Surgery 101: 964–968; discussion 969–970.

Kim TS, Moon WK, Lee DS et al 2001 Fluorodeoxyglucose positron emission tomography for detection of recurrent or metastatic breast cancer. World Journal of Surgery 25: 829–834.

King CR, Kraus MH, Aaronson SA 1985a Amplification of a novel v-erbB-related gene in a human mammary carcinoma. Science 229, 974–976.

King RM, Welch JS, Martin JK Jr, Coulam CB 1985b Carcinoma of the breast associated with pregnancy. Surgery, Gynecology and Obstetrics 160: 228–232.

Kister SJ, Haagensen CD 1970 Paget's disease of the breast. American Journal of Surgery 119: 606–609.

Kitchen PR, Cawson JN, Krishnan CM, Barbetti TM, Henderson MA 2000 Axillary dissection and ductal carcinoma in situ of the breast: a change in practice. Australian and New Zealand Journal of Surgery 70: 419–422.

Kolb TM, Lichy J, Newhouse JH 2002 Comparison of the performance of screening mammography, physical examination, and breast US and evaluation of factors that influence them: an analysis of 27,825 patient evaluations. Radiology 225: 165–175.

Kollias J, Murphy CA, Elston CW, Ellis IO, Robertson JF, Blamey RW 1999 The prognosis of small primary breast cancers. European Journal of Cancer 35: 908–912.

Kollmorgen DR, Varanasi JS, Edge SB, Carson WE 3rd 1998 Paget's disease of the breast: a 33-year experience. Journal of the American College of Surgeons 187: 171–177.

Konecny G, Pauletti G, Pegram M et al 2003 Quantitative association between HER-2/neu and steroid hormone receptors in hormone receptor-positive primary breast cancer. Journal of the National Cancer Institute 95: 142–153.

Kothari AS, Beechey-Newman N, Hamed H et al 2002 Paget disease of the nipple: a multifocal manifestation of higher-risk disease. Cancer 95: 1–7.

Kraeft SK, Sutherland R, Gravelin L et al 2000 Detection and analysis of cancer cells in blood and bone marrow using a rare event imaging system. Clinical Cancer Research 6: 434–442.

Krag DN, Weaver DL, Alex JC, Fairbank JT 1993 Surgical resection and radiolocalization of the sentinel lymph node in breast cancer using a gamma probe. Surgical Oncology 2: 335–339; discussion 340.

Kriege M, Brekelmans CT, Boetes C et al 2004 Efficacy of MRI and mammography for breast-cancer screening in women with a familial or genetic predisposition. New England Journal of Medicine 351: 427–437.

Kriege M, Brekelmans CT, Peterse H et al 2007 Tumor characteristics and detection method in the MRISC screening program for the early detection of hereditary breast

cancer. Breast Cancer Research and Treatment 102: 357–363.

Kristensen B, Ejlertsen B, Dalgaard P et al 1994 Tamoxifen and bone metabolism in postmenopausal low-risk breast cancer patients: a randomized study. Journal of Clinical Oncology 12: 992–997.

Kroll SS, Coffey JA Jr, Winn RJ, Schusterman MA 1995 A comparison of factors affecting aesthetic outcomes of TRAM flap breast reconstructions. Plastic and Reconstructive Surgery 96: 860–864.

Kronowitz SJ 2007 Immediate versus delayed reconstruction. Clinics in Plastic Surgery 34: 39–50; abstract vi.

Kronowitz SJ, Robb GL 2004 Breast reconstruction with postmastectomy radiation therapy: current issues. Plastic and Reconstructive Surgery 114: 950–960.

Kumar R, Jana S, Heiba SI et al 2003 Retrospective analysis of sentinel node localization in multifocal, multicentric, palpable, or nonpalpable breast cancer. Journal of Nuclear Medicine 44: 7–10.

Kuper-Hommel MJ, Snijder S, Janssen-Heijnen ML et al 2003 Treatment and survival of 38 female breast lymphomas: a population-based study with clinical and pathological reviews. Annals of Hematology 82: 397–404.

Kurtz JM, Jacquemier J, Amalric R et al 1990 Breast-conserving therapy for macroscopically multiple cancers. Annals of Surgery 212: 38–44.

Lacassagne A 1936 Hormonal pathogensis of adenocarcinoma of the breast. American Journal of Cancer 27: 217–225.

Lacour J, Le M, Caceres E, Koszarowski T, Veronesi U, Hill C 1983 Radical mastectomy versus radical mastectomy plus internal mammary dissection. Ten year results of an international cooperative trial in breast cancer. Cancer 51: 1941–1943.

Lagios MD, Westdahl PR, Rose MR, Concannon S 1984 Paget's disease of the nipple. Alternative management in cases without or with minimal extent of underlying breast carcinoma. Cancer 54: 545–551.

Lakhani SR, van de Vijver MJ, Jacquemier J et al 2002 The pathology of familial breast cancer: predictive value of immunohistochemical markers estrogen receptor, progesterone receptor, HER-2, and p53 in patients with mutations in BRCA1 and BRCA2. Journal of Clinical Oncology 20: 2310–2318.

Lalloo F, Varley J, Ellis D et al 2003 Prediction of pathogenic mutations in patients with early-onset breast cancer by family history. The Lancet 361: 1101–1102.

Leach MO, Boggis CR, Dixon AK et al 2005 Screening with magnetic resonance imaging and mammography of a UK population at high familial risk of breast cancer: a prospective multicentre cohort study (MARIBS). The Lancet 365: 1769–1778.

Lee B, Tannenbaum N 1924 Inflammatory carcinoma of the breast: a report of

twenty-eight cases from the breast clinic of Memorial Hospital. Surgery, Gynecology and Obstetrics 39: 580.

Lee D 2007 Ovarian tissue cryopreservation and transplantation: banking reproductive potential for the future. Cancer Treatment and Research 138: 110–129.

Leff DR, Kinross J 2007 Breast reconstruction. Annals of the Royal College of Surgeons of England 89: 445–446.

Lehman CD, Gatsonis C, Kuhl CK et al 2007 MRI evaluation of the contralateral breast in women with recently diagnosed breast cancer. New England Journal of Medicine 356: 1295–1303.

Leibman AJ, Frager D, Choi P 1999 Experience with breast biopsies using the Advanced Breast Biopsy Instrumentation system. AJR American Journal of Roentgenology 172: 1409–1412.

Leonard GD, Swain SM 2004 Ductal carcinoma in situ, complexities and challenges. Journal of the National Cancer Institute 96, 906–920.

Levine MN, Bramwell VH, Pritchard KI et al 1998 Randomized trial of intensive cyclophosphamide, epirubicin, and fluorouracil chemotherapy compared with cyclophosphamide, methotrexate, and fluorouracil in premenopausal women with node-positive breast cancer. National Cancer Institute of Canada Clinical Trials Group. Journal of Clinical Oncology 16: 2651–2658.

Levine PH, Steinhorn SC, Ries LG, Aron JL 1985 Inflammatory breast cancer: the experience of the Surveillance, Epidemiology, and End Results (SEER) program. Journal of the National Cancer Institute 74: 291–297.

Liberman L, Giess CS, Dershaw DD, Deutch BM, Petrek JA 1994 Imaging of pregnancy-associated breast cancer. Radiology 191: 245–248.

Lin PP, Allison DC, Wainstock J et al 1993 Impact of axillary lymph node dissection on the therapy of breast cancer patients. Journal of Clinical Oncology 11: 1536–1544.

Lipton A, Theriault RL, Hortobagyi GN et al 2000 Pamidronate prevents skeletal complications and is effective palliative treatment in women with breast carcinoma and osteolytic bone metastases: long term follow-up of two randomized, placebo-controlled trials. Cancer 88: 1082–1090.

Lister D, Evans AJ, Burrell HC et al 1998 The accuracy of breast ultrasound in the evaluation of clinically benign discrete, symptomatic breast lumps. Clinical Radiology 53: 490–492.

Liu R, Wang X, Chen GY et al 2007 The prognostic role of a gene signature from tumorigenic breast-cancer cells. New England Journal of Medicine 356: 217–226.

Livasy CA, Karaca G, Nanda R et al 2006 Phenotypic evaluation of the basal-like subtype of invasive breast carcinoma. Modern Pathology 19, 264–271.

Lobo RA 2005 Potential options for preservation of fertility in women. New England Journal of Medicine 353: 64–73.

Loi S, Desmedt C, Cardoso F, Piccart M, Sotiriou C 2005 Breast cancer gene expression profiling: clinical trial and practice implications. Pharmacogenomics 6: 49–58.

London SJ, Connolly JL, Schnitt SJ, Colditz GA 1992 A prospective study of benign breast disease and the risk of breast cancer. Journal of the American Medical Association 267: 941–944.

Love RR, Cameron L, Connell BL, Leventhal H 1991 Symptoms associated with tamoxifen treatment in postmenopausal women. Archives of Internal Medicine 151: 1842–1847.

Love RR, Mazess RB, Barden HS et al 1992 Effects of tamoxifen on bone mineral density in postmenopausal women with breast cancer. New England Journal of Medicine 326: 852–856.

Low JA, Berman AW, Steinberg SM 2002 Long-term follow-up for inflammatory (IBC) and non-inflammatory (NIBC) stage III breast cancer patients treated with combination chemotherapy. Proceedings of the American Society of Clinical Oncology 21: 63a.

Lutchman Singh K, Muttukrishna S, Stein RC et al 2007 Predictors of ovarian reserve in young women with breast cancer. British Journal of Cancer 96: 1808–1816.

Lyman GH, Giuliano AE, Somerfield M et al 2005 American Society of Clinical Oncology guideline recommendations for sentinel lymph node biopsy in early-stage breast cancer. Journal of Clinical Oncology 23: 7703–7720.

Maddams J, Moller H, Devane C 2008 Cancer Prevalance in the UK 2008. Thames Cancer Registry and Macmillan Cancer Support.

Maddox JC, Evans HL 1981 Angiosarcoma of skin and soft tissue: a study of forty-four cases. Cancer 48: 1907–1921.

Maltaris T, Seufert R, Fischl F et al 2007 The effect of cancer treatment on female fertility and strategies for preserving fertility. European Journal of Obstetrics, Gynecology and Reproductive Biology 130: 148–155.

Mamounas E, Bryant J, Lembersky BC et al 2003 Paclitaxel (T) following doxorubicin/ cyclophosphamide (AC) as adjuvant chemotherapy for node-positive breast cancer: results from NSABP B-28. ASCO Annual Meeting Proceedings. Proceedings of the American Society of Clinical Oncology 22: abstract 12.

Mankoff DA, Eubank WB 2006 Current and future use of positron emission tomography (PET) in breast cancer. Journal of Mammary Gland Biology and Neoplasia 11: 125–136.

Mann BG, Buchanan M, Collins PJ, Lichtenstein M 2000 High incidence of micrometastases in breast cancer sentinel nodes. Australian and New Zealand Journal of Surgery 70: 786–790.

Mansi JL, Gogas H, Bliss JM, Gazet JC, Berger U, Coombes RC 1999 Outcome of primary-breast-cancer patients with micrometastases: a long-term follow-up study. The Lancet 354: 197–202.

Marchbanks PA, McDonald JA, Wilson HG et al 2002 Oral contraceptives and the risk of breast. New England Journal of Medicine 346: 2025–2032.

Marcus JN, Watson P, Page DL et al 1996 Hereditary breast cancer: pathobiology, prognosis, and BRCA1 and BRCA2 gene linkage. Cancer 77: 697–709.

Marshall JK, Griffith KA, Haffty BG et al 2003 Conservative management of Paget disease of the breast with radiotherapy: 10- and 15-year results. Cancer 97: 2142–2149.

Martin M, Pienkowski T, Mackey J et al 2003 TAc improves disease free survival and overall survival over FAC in node positive early breast cancer patients. BCIRG 001: 55 month follow-up (abstract). Breast Cancer Research and Treatment 82 (Suppl. 1): abstract 43.

Marty M, Cognetti F, Maraninchi D et al 2005 Randomized phase II trial of the efficacy and safety of trastuzumab combined with docetaxel in patients with human epidermal growth factor receptor 2-positive metastatic breast cancer administered as first-line treatment: the M77001 study group. Journal of Clinical Oncology 23: 4265–4274.

Matthews BD, Williams GB 1999 Initial experience with the advanced breast biopsy instrumentation system. American Journal of Surgery 177: 97–101.

McCarter MD, Yeung H, Fey J, Borgen PI, Cody HS 3rd 2001 The breast cancer patient with multiple sentinel nodes: when to stop? Journal of the American College of Surgeons 192: 692–697.

McClelland CM, Gullick WJ 2003 Identification of surrogate markers for determining drug activity using proteomics. Biochemical Society Transactions 31: 1488–1490.

McGuckin MA, Cummings MC, Walsh MD, Hohn BG, Bennett IC, Wright RG 1996 Occult axillary node metastases in breast cancer: their detection and prognostic significance. British Journal of Cancer 73: 88–95.

Meijers-Heijboer H, van Geel B, van Putten WL et al 2001 Breast cancer after prophylactic bilateral mastectomy in women with a BRCA1 or BRCA2 mutation. New England Journal of Medicine 345: 159–164.

Meirow D 1999 Ovarian injury and modern options to preserve fertility in female cancer patients treated with high dose radio-chemotherapy for hemato-oncological neoplasias and other cancers. Leukemia and Lymphoma 33: 65–76.

Meirow D, Levron J, Eldar-Geva T et al 2005 Pregnancy after transplantation of cryopreserved ovarian tissue in a patient with ovarian failure after chemotherapy. New England Journal of Medicine 353: 318–321.

Mendelsohn J, Baselga J 2006 Epidermal growth factor receptor targeting in cancer. Seminars in Oncology 33: 369–385.

Metcalfe K, Lynch HT, Ghadirian P et al 2004 Contralateral breast cancer in BRCA1 and BRCA2 mutation carriers. Journal of Clinical Oncology 22: 2328–2335.

Meyer JE, Smith DN, Lester SC et al 1999 Large-core needle biopsy of nonpalpable breast lesions. Journal of the American Medical Association 281: 1638–1641.

Miles D, Chan A, Romieu G et al 2008 Randomized, double-blind, placebo-controlled, phase III study of bevacizumab with docetaxel or docetaxel with placebo as first-line therapy for patients with locally recurrent or metastatic breast cancer (mBC): AVADO. Journal of Clinical Oncology 26 (Suppl): abstract LBA1011.

Miller K, Burstein A 2005 Phase II study of SU11248, a multitargeted tyrosine kinase inhibitor in patients with previously treated metastatic breast cancer. 28th Annual San Antonio Breast Cancer Symposium, December 8–11.

Miller KD 2003a E2100: a phase III trial of paclitaxel versus paclitaxel/bevacizumab for metastatic breast cancer. Clinical Breast Cancer 3: 421–422.

Miller WR 2003b Aromatase inhibitors: mechanism of action and role in the treatment of breast cancer. Seminars in Oncology 30: 3–11.

Millis R, Bobrow L, Barnes D 1996 Immunohistochemical evaluation of biological markers in mammary carcinoma in situ: correlation with morphological features and recently proposed schemes for histological classification. Breast 5: 113–122.

Minton SE, Munster PN 2002 Chemotherapy-induced amenorrhea and fertility in women undergoing adjuvant treatment for breast cancer. Cancer Control 9: 466–472.

Modi S, Seidman AD, Dickler M et al 2005 A phase II trial of imatinib mesylate monotherapy in patients with metastatic breast cancer. Breast Cancer Research and Treatment 90: 157–163.

Molino A, Pelosi G, Turazza M et al 1997 Bone marrow micrometastases in 109 breast cancer patients: correlations with clinical and pathological features and prognosis. Breast Cancer Research and Treatment 42: 23–30.

Monninkhof EM, Elias SG, Vlems FA et al 2007 Physical activity and breast cancer: a systematic review. Epidemiology 18: 137–157.

Moon DH, Maddahi J, Silverman DH, Glaspy JA, Phelps ME, Hoh CK 1998 Accuracy of whole-body fluorine-18-FDG PET for the detection of recurrent or metastatic breast carcinoma. Journal of Nuclear Medicine 39: 431–435.

Morris AD, Morris RD, Wilson JF et al 1997 Breast-conserving therapy vs mastectomy in early-stage breast cancer: a meta-analysis of 10-year survival. Cancer Journal from Scientific American 3: 6–12.

Morton DL 1997 Sentinel lymphadenectomy for patients with clinical stage I melanoma. Journal of Surgical Oncology 66: 267–269.

Moy B, Goss PE 2006 Lapatinib: current status and future directions in breast cancer. The Oncologist 11: 1047–1057.

Mullan MH, Deacock SJ, Quiney NF, Kissin MW 2001 Anaphylaxis to patent blue dye during sentinel lymph node biopsy for breast cancer. European Journal of Surgical Oncology 27: 218–219.

Nahta R, Hung MC, Esteva FJ 2004 The HER-2-targeting antibodies trastuzumab and pertuzumab synergistically inhibit the survival of breast cancer cells. Cancer Research 64: 2343–2346.

Nahta R, Yuan LX, Zhang B, Kobayashi R, Esteva FJ 2005 Insulin-like growth factor-I receptor/human epidermal growth factor receptor 2 heterodimerization contributes to trastuzumab resistance of breast cancer cells. Cancer Research 65: 11118–11128.

Nakai T, Okuyama C, Kubota T et al 2005 Pitfalls of FDG-PET for the diagnosis of osteoblastic bone metastases in patients with breast cancer. European Journal of Nuclear Medicine and Molecular Imaging 32: 1253–1258.

Neville AM, Bettelheim R, Gelber RD et al 1992 Factors predicting treatment responsiveness and prognosis in node-negative breast cancer. The International (Ludwig) Breast Cancer Study Group. Journal of Clinical Oncology 10: 696–705.

Newman B, Austin MA, Lee M, King MC 1988 Inheritance of human breast cancer: evidence for autosomal dominant transmission in high-risk families. Proceedings of the National Academy of Sciences USA 85: 3044–3048.

Nicholson RI, McClelland RA, Gee JM et al 1994 Epidermal growth factor receptor expression in breast cancer: association with response to endocrine therapy. Breast Cancer Research and Treatment 29: 117–125.

Nielsen M, Thomsen JL, Primdahl S, Dyreborg U, Andersen JA 1987 Breast cancer and atypia among young and middle-aged women: a study of 110 medicolegal autopsies. British Journal of Cancer 56: 814–819.

Nielsen TO, Hsu FD, Jensen K et al 2004 Immunohistochemical and clinical characterization of the basal-like subtype of invasive breast carcinoma. Clinical Cancer Research 10: 5367–5374.

Northern Ireland Cancer Registry 2008 Cancer Incidence and Mortality, Department of Health, UK.

Nystrom L, Andersson I, Bjurstam N, Frisell J, Nordenskjold B, Rutqvist LE 2002 Long-term effects of mammography screening: updated overview of the Swedish randomised trials. The Lancet 359: 909–919.

O'Dwyer PJ 1991 Axillary dissection in primary breast cancer. BMJ (Clinical Research Ed.) 302: 360–361.

Office for National Statistics 2008 Cancer Statistics Registrations: Registrations of Cancer Diagnosed in 2005, England. Series MB1 No. 36. Department of Health, London.

Oktay K, Buyuk E, Libertella N, Akar M, Rosenwaks Z 2005 Fertility preservation in breast cancer patients: a prospective controlled comparison of ovarian stimulation with tamoxifen and letrozole for embryo cryopreservation. Journal of Clinical Oncology 23: 4347–4353.

Olsen O, Gotzsche PC 2001 Cochrane review on screening for breast cancer with mammography. The Lancet 358: 1340–1342.

Ottesen GL, Graversen HP, Blichert-Toft M, Christensen IJ, Andersen JA 2000 Carcinoma in situ of the female breast. 10 year follow-up results of a prospective nationwide study. Breast Cancer Research and Treatment 62: 197–210.

Overgaard M, Jensen MB, Overgaard J et al 1999 Postoperative radiotherapy in high-risk postmenopausal breast-cancer patients given adjuvant tamoxifen: Danish Breast Cancer Cooperative Group DBCG 82c randomised trial. The Lancet 353: 1641–1648.

Owens MA, Horten BC, Da Silva MM 2004 HER2 amplification ratios by fluorescence in situ hybridization and correlation with immunohistochemistry in a cohort of 6556 breast cancer tissues. Clinical Breast Cancer 5: 63–69.

Page DL, Dupont WD, Rogers LW, Jensen RA, Schuyler PA 1995 Continued local recurrence of carcinoma 15–25 years after a diagnosis of low grade ductal carcinoma in situ of the breast treated only by biopsy. Cancer 76: 1197–1200.

Paget J 1874 On disease of the mammary areola preceding cancer of the mammary gland. St. Bartholomew's Hospital Reports 10: 87–89.

Paik S, Shak S, Tang G et al 2004 A multigene assay to predict recurrence of tamoxifen-treated, node-negative breast cancer. New England Journal of Medicine 351: 2817–2826.

Parker SH, Klaus AJ, Mcwey PJ et al 2001 Sonographically guided directional vacuum-assisted breast biopsy using a handheld device. AJR American Journal of Roentgenology 177: 405–408.

Parkin DM 2009 Is the recent fall in incidence of post-menopausal breast cancer in UK related to changes in use of hormone replacement therapy? European Journal of Cancer 45: 1649–1653.

Parton M, Dowsett M, Ashley S, Hills M, Lowe F, Smith IE 2004 High incidence of HER-2 positivity in inflammatory breast cancer. Breast 13: 97–103.

Paterson AH, Powles TJ, Kanis JA, McCloskey E, Hanson J, Ashley S 1993 Double-blind controlled trial of oral clodronate in patients with bone metastases from breast cancer. Journal of Clinical Oncology 11: 59–65.

Paulus DD, Libshitz HI 1982 Metastasis to the breast. Radiologic Clinics of North America 20: 561–568.

Pendas S, Dauway E, Giuliano R, Ku N, Cox CE, Reintgen DS 2000 Sentinel node biopsy in ductal carcinoma in situ patients. Annals of Surgical Oncology 7: 15–20.

Perez EA 2008 Cardiac toxicity of ErbB2-targeted therapies: what do we know? Clinical Breast Cancer 8 (Suppl 3): S114–S120.

Perez EA, Roche PC, Jenkins RB et al 2002 HER2 testing in patients with breast cancer: poor correlation between weak positivity by immunohistochemistry and gene amplification by fluorescence in situ hybridization. Mayo Clinic Proceedings 77: 148–154.

Perou CM, Sorlie T, Eisen MB et al 2000 Molecular portraits of human breast tumours. Nature 406: 747–752.

Peto R, Boreham J, Clarke M, Davies C, Beral V 2000 UK and USA breast cancer deaths down 25% in year 2000 at ages 20–69 years. The Lancet 355: 1822.

Petrek JA 1991 Pregnancy-associated breast cancer. Seminars in Surgical Oncology 7: 306–310.

Petrek JA, Naughton MJ, Case LD et al 2006 Incidence, time course, and determinants of menstrual bleeding after breast cancer treatment: a prospective study. Journal of Clinical Oncology 24: 1045–1051.

Piccart-Gebhart MJ, Procter M, Leyland-Jones B et al 2005 Trastuzumab after adjuvant chemotherapy in HER2-positive breast cancer. New England Journal of Medicine 353: 1659–1672.

Pierga JY, Robain M, Jouve M et al 2001 Response to chemotherapy is a major parameter-influencing long-term survival of metastatic breast cancer patients. Annals of Oncology 12: 231–237.

Pietras RJ, Arboleda J, Reese DM et al 1995 HER-2 tyrosine kinase pathway targets estrogen receptor and promotes hormone-independent growth in human breast cancer cells. Oncogene 10: 2435–2446.

Powles TJ, Hickish T, Kanis JA, Tidy A, Ashley S 1996 Effect of tamoxifen on bone mineral density measured by dual-energy x-ray absorptiometry in healthy premenopausal and postmenopausal women. Journal of Clinical Oncology 14: 78–84.

Pritt B, Ashikaga T, Oppenheimer RG, Weaver DL 2004 Influence of breast cancer histology on the relationship between ultrasound and pathology tumor size measurements. Modern Pathology 17: 905–910.

Quan ML, Sclafani L, Heerdt AS, Fey JV, Morris EA, Borgen PI 2003 Magnetic resonance imaging detects unsuspected disease in patients with invasive lobular cancer. Annals of Surgical Oncology 10: 1048–1053.

Radan L, Ben-Haim S, Bar-Shalom R, Guralnik L, Israel O 2006 The role of FDG-PET/CT in suspected recurrence of breast cancer. Cancer 107: 2545–2551.

Ragaz J, Jackson SM, Le N et al 1997 Adjuvant radiotherapy and chemotherapy in node-positive premenopausal women with breast cancer. New England Journal of Medicine 337: 956–962.

Rajah TT, Dunn ST, Pento JT 1996 The influence of antiestrogens on pS2 and cathepsin D mRNA induction in MCF-7 breast cancer cells. Anticancer Research 16: 837–842.

Raktovich E 2000 Epidemiology of ductal carcinoma in situ. Current Problems in Cancer 24: 100–111.

Ramazzini B 1713 De Morbis Artificum, Ultrajecti: Apud Guilielmum van der Water Academiae Typographum.

Rao J, Dekoven JG, Beatty JD, Jones G 2003 Cutaneous angiosarcoma as a delayed complication of radiation therapy for carcinoma of the breast. Journal of the American Academy of Dermatology 49: 532–538.

Rebbeck TR, Lynch HT, Neuhausen SL et al 2002 Prophylactic oophorectomy in carriers of BRCA1 or BRCA2 mutations. New England Journal of Medicine 346: 1616–1622.

Reinblatt SL, Buckett W 2008 In vitro maturation for patients with polycystic ovary syndrome. Seminars in Reproductive Medicine 26: 121–126.

Reinholz MM, Nibbe A, Jonart LM et al 2005 Evaluation of a panel of tumor markers for molecular detection of circulating cancer cells in women with suspected breast cancer. Clinical Cancer Research 11: 3722–3732.

Ribeiro G, Jones DA, Jones M 1986 Carcinoma of the breast associated with pregnancy. British Journal of Surgery 73: 607–609.

Rilke F, Colnaghi MI, Cascinelli N et al 1991 Prognostic significance of HER-2/neu expression in breast cancer and its relationship to other prognostic factors. International Journal of Cancer 49: 44–49.

Roberts JE, Oktay K 2005 Fertility preservation: a comprehensive approach to the young woman with cancer. Journal of the National Cancer Institute Monographs 34: 57–59.

Robson M 2004 Breast cancer surveillance in women with hereditary risk due to BRCA1 or BRCA2 mutations. Clinical Breast Cancer 5: 260–268; discussion 269–271.

Robson M, Gilewski T, Haas B et al 1998 BRCA-associated breast cancer in young women. Journal of Clinical Oncology 16: 1642–1649.

Ronckers CM, Erdmann CA, Land CE 2005 Radiation and breast cancer: a review of current evidence. Breast Cancer Research 7: 21–32.

Rosen LS, Gordon D, Kaminski M et al 2001 Zoledronic acid versus pamidronate in the treatment of skeletal metastases in patients with breast cancer or osteolytic lesions of multiple myeloma: a phase III, double-blind, comparative trial. Cancer Journal 7: 377–387.

Rosen P 1996 Paget's disease of the nipple. In: Rosen P (ed) Rosen's Breast Pathology. Lippincott-Raven, Philadelphia.

Rosen PP, Saigo PE, Braun DW, Weathers E, Fracchia AA, Kinne DW 1981 Axillary micro- and macrometastases in breast cancer: prognostic significance of tumor size. Annals of Surgery 194: 585–591.

Rosen PP, Groshen S 1990 Factors influencing survival and prognosis in early breast carcinoma (T1N0M0–T1N1M0). Assessment of 644 patients with median follow-up of 18 years. Surgical Clinics of North America 70: 937–962.

Ross JS, Fletcher JA, Linette GP et al 2003 The Her-2/neu gene and protein in breast cancer 2003: biomarker and target of therapy. The Oncologist 8: 307–325.

Roumen RM, Kuijt GP, Liem IH 2006 Lymphatic mapping and sentinel node harvesting in patients with recurrent breast cancer. European Journal of Surgical Oncology 32: 1076–1081.

Rousseau C, Devillers A, Sagan C et al 2006 Monitoring of early response to neoadjuvant chemotherapy in stage II and III breast cancer by [18F] fluorodeoxyglucose positron emission tomography. Journal of Clinical Oncology 24: 5366–5372.

Rutqvist LE, Mattsson A 1993 Cardiac and thromboembolic morbidity among postmenopausal women with early-stage breast cancer in a randomized trial of adjuvant tamoxifen. The Stockholm Breast Cancer Study Group. Journal of the National Cancer Institute 85: 1398–1406.

Santen RJ, Boyd NF, Chlebowski RT et al 2007 Critical assessment of new risk factors for breast cancer: considerations for development of an improved risk prediction model. Endocrine-related Cancer 14: 169–187.

Saunders C 2001 Breast cancer and pregnancy. In: Tobias J, Houghton J, Henderson I (eds) Breast Cancer — New Horizons in Research and Treatment. Arnold, London.

Schelling M, Avril N, Nahrig J et al 2000 Positron emission tomography using [(18)F]fluorodeoxyglucose for monitoring primary chemotherapy in breast cancer. Journal of Clinical Oncology 18: 1689–1695.

Schlimok G, Funke I, Holzmann B et al 1987 Micrometastatic cancer cells in bone marrow: in vitro detection with anti-cytokeratin and in vivo labeling with anti-17-1A monoclonal antibodies. Proceedings of the National Academy of Sciences USA 84: 8672–8676.

Schuh ME, Nemoto T, Penetrante RB, Rosner D, Dao TL 1986 Intraductal carcinoma. Analysis of presentation, pathologic findings, and outcome of disease. Archives of Surgery 121: 1303–1307.

Schwartz GF, Solin LJ, Olivotto IA, Ernster VL, Pressman PI 2000 Consensus conference on the treatment of in situ ductal carcinoma of the breast, April 22–25 1999. Cancer 88: 946–954.

Scott-Conner CE, Schorr SJ 1995 The diagnosis and management of breast problems during pregnancy and lactation. American Journal of Surgery 170: 401–405.

Seli E, Tangir J 2005 Fertility preservation options for female patients with malignancies. Current Opinion in Obstetrics and Gynecology 17: 299–308.

Selinko VL, Middleton LP, Dempsey PJ 2004 Role of sonography in diagnosing and staging invasive lobular carcinoma. Journal of Clinical Ultrasound 32: 323–332.

Shaw JH, Rumball EM 1990 Complications and local recurrence following lymphadenectomy. British Journal of Surgery 77: 760–764.

Shimizu H, Ross RK, Bernstein L, Yatani R, Henderson BE, Mack TM 1991 Cancers of the prostate and breast among Japanese and white immigrants in Los Angeles County. British Journal of Cancer 63: 963–966.

Siegel BM, Mayzel KA, Love SM 1990 Level I and II axillary dissection in the treatment of early-stage breast cancer. An analysis of 259 consecutive patients. Archives of Surgery 125: 1144–1147.

Silverstein MJ, Gierson ED, Colburn WJ, Rosser RJ, Waisman JR, Gamagami P 1991 Axillary lymphadenectomy for intraductal carcinoma of the breast. Surgery, Gynecology and Obstetrics 172: 211–214.

Silverstein MJ, Barth A, Poller DN et al 1995 Ten-year results comparing mastectomy to excision and radiation therapy for ductal carcinoma in situ of the breast. European Journal of Cancer 31A: 1425–1427.

Silverstein MJ, Lagios MD, Craig PH et al 1996 A prognostic index for ductal carcinoma in situ of the breast. Cancer 77: 2267–2274.

Singletary SE 2008 Surgical management of inflammatory breast cancer. Seminars in Oncology 35: 72–77.

Skaane P, Kshirsagar A, Stapleton S, Young K, Castellino RA 2007 Effect of computer-aided detection on independent double reading of paired screen-film and full-field digital screening mammograms. AJR American Journal of Roentgenology 188: 377–384.

Slamon DJ, Clark GM, Wong SG, Levin WJ, Ullrich A, Mcguire WL 1987 Human breast cancer: correlation of relapse and survival with amplification of the HER-2/neu oncogene. Science 235: 177–182.

Slamon DJ, Godolphin W, Jones LA et al 1989 Studies of the HER-2/neu proto-oncogene in human breast and ovarian cancer. Science 244: 707–712.

Slamon DJ, Leyland-Jones B, Shak S et al 2001 Use of chemotherapy plus a monoclonal antibody against HER2 for metastatic breast cancer that overexpresses HER2. New England Journal of Medicine 344: 783–792.

Smith IC, Welch AE, Hutcheon AW et al 2000 Positron emission tomography using [(18)F]-fluorodeoxy-D-glucose to predict the pathologic response of breast cancer to primary chemotherapy. Journal of Clinical Oncology 18: 1676–1688.

Smith IE, Lipton L 2001 Preoperative/neoadjuvant medical therapy for early breast cancer. The Lancet Oncology 2: 561–570.

Smith MR, Brustein S, Straus DJ 1987 Localized non-Hodgkin's lymphoma of the breast. Cancer 59: 351–354.

Spector NL, Blackwell K, Hurley J 2006 EGF103009, a phase II trial of lapatinib monotherapy in patients with relapsed/refractory inflammatory breast cancer (IBC): clinical activity and biologic predictors of response. Journal of Clinical Oncology 24 (Suppl 18S): 502.

Stearns V, Ewing CA, Slack R, Penannen MF, Hayes DF, Tsangaris TN 2002 Sentinel lymphadenectomy after neoadjuvant chemotherapy for breast cancer may reliably represent the axilla except for inflammatory breast cancer. Annals of Surgical Oncology 9: 235–242.

Stewart HJ, Prescott RJ, Forrest AP 2001 Scottish adjuvant tamoxifen trial: a randomized study updated to 15 years. Journal of the National Cancer Institute 93: 456–462.

Stockdale AD, Brierley JD, White WF, Folkes A, Rostom AY 1989 Radiotherapy for Paget's disease of the nipple: a conservative alternative. The Lancet 2: 664–666.

Stokkel MP, Peterse HL 1992 Angiosarcoma of the breast after lumpectomy and radiation therapy for adenocarcinoma. Cancer 69: 2965–2968.

Stone J, Dite GS, Gunasekara A et al 2006 The heritability of mammographically dense and nondense breast tissue. Cancer Epidemiology, Biomarkers and Prevention 15: 612–617.

Struewing JP, Hartge P, Wacholder S et al 1997 The risk of cancer associated with specific mutations of BRCA1 and BRCA2 among Ashkenazi Jews. New England Journal of Medicine 336: 1401–1408.

Sullivan T, Raad RA, Goldberg S et al 2005 Tubular carcinoma of the breast: a retrospective analysis and review of the literature. Breast Cancer Research and Treatment 93: 199–205.

Svensson WE, Amiras D 2006 Ultrasound elasticity imaging. Breast Cancer Online 9: e24.

Taback B, Nguyen P, Hansen N, Edwards GK, Conway K, Giuliano AE 2006 Sentinel lymph node biopsy for local recurrence of breast cancer after breast-conserving therapy. Annals of Surgical Oncology 13: 1099–1104.

Tabar L, Vitak B, Chen HH, Yen MF, Duffy SW, Smith RA 2001 Beyond randomized controlled trials: organized mammographic screening substantially reduces breast carcinoma mortality. Cancer 91: 1724–1731.

Tan PH, Tse GM, Bay BH 2008 Mucinous breast lesions: diagnostic challenges. Journal of Clinical Pathology 61: 11–19.

Tanner M, Gancberg D, Di Leo A et al 2000 Chromogenic in situ hybridization: a practical alternative for fluorescence in situ hybridization to detect HER-2/neu oncogene amplification in archival breast cancer samples. American Journal of Pathology 157: 1467–1472.

Tatsumi M, Cohade C, Mourtzikos KA, Fishman EK, Wahl RL 2006 Initial experience with FDG-PET/CT in the evaluation of breast cancer. European Journal of Nuclear Medicine and Molecular Imaging 33: 254–262.

Taylor G, Meltzer A 1938 Inflammatory carcinoma of the breast. American Journal of Cancer 33: 33–49.

Teh WL, Evans AJ, Wilson AR 1998 Definitive non-surgical breast diagnosis: the role of the radiologist. Clinical Radiology 53: 81–84.

Thurlimann B, Keshaviah A, Coates AS et al 2005 A comparison of letrozole and tamoxifen in postmenopausal women with early breast cancer. New England Journal of Medicine 353: 2747–2757.

Tilanus-Linthorst M, Verhoog L, Obdeijn IM et al 2002 A BRCA1/2 mutation, high breast density and prominent pushing margins of a tumor independently contribute to a frequent false-negative mammography. International Journal of Cancer 102: 91–95.

Tominaga S 1985 Cancer incidence in Japanese in Japan, Hawaii, and western United States. Journal of the National Cancer Institute Monographs 69: 83–92.

Tormey DC, Gray R, Falkson HC 1996 Postchemotherapy adjuvant tamoxifen therapy beyond five years in patients with lymph node-positive breast cancer. Eastern Cooperative Oncology Group. Journal of the National Cancer Institute 88: 1828–1833.

Trojani M, de Mascarel I, Coindre JM, Bonichon F 1987 Micrometastases to axillary lymph nodes from invasive lobular carcinoma of breast: detection by immunohistochemistry and prognostic significance. British Journal of Cancer 56: 838–839.

Turpin E, Bieche I, Bertheau P et al 2002 Increased incidence of ERBB2 overexpression and TP53 mutation in inflammatory breast cancer. Oncogene 21: 7593–7597.

Tyrer J, Duffy SW, Cuzick J 2004 A breast cancer prediction model incorporating familial and personal risk factors. Statistics in Medicine 23: 1111–1130.

United Nations Scientific Committee on the Effects of Atomic Radiation 2000 Report to the General Assembly, with Annexes. Ionizing Radiation: Sources and Biological Effects. United Nations, New York.

van Beek RD, van den Heuvel-Eibrink MM, Laven JS et al 2007 Anti-Müllerian hormone is a sensitive serum marker for gonadal function in women treated for Hodgkin's lymphoma during childhood. Journal of Clinical Endocrinology and Metabolism 92: 3869–3874.

van de Rijn M, Perou CM, Tibshirani R et al 2002 Expression of cytokeratins 17 and 5 identifies a group of breast carcinomas with poor clinical outcome. American Journal of Pathology 161: 1991–1996.

van de Vijver MJ, He YD, van't Veer LJ et al 2002 A gene-expression signature as a predictor of survival in breast cancer. New England Journal of Medicine 347: 1999–2009.

van den Brandt PA, Spiegelman D, Yaun SS et al 2000 Pooled analysis of prospective cohort studies on height, weight, and breast cancer risk. American Journal of Epidemiology 152: 514–527.

van Dongen JA, Fentiman IS, Harris JR et al 1989 In-situ breast cancer: the EORTC consensus meeting. The Lancet 2: 25–27.

van Dongen JA, Voogd AC, Fentiman IS et al 2000 Long-term results of a randomized trial comparing breast-conserving therapy with mastectomy: European Organization for Research and Treatment of Cancer 10801 trial. Journal of the National Cancer Institute 92: 1143–1150.

van Holten-Verzantvoort AT, Kroon HM, Bijvoet OL et al 1993 Palliative pamidronate treatment in patients with bone metastases from breast cancer. Journal of Clinical Oncology 11: 491–498.

van Pelt AE, Mohsin S, Elledge RM et al 2003 Neoadjuvant trastuzumab and docetaxel in breast cancer: preliminary results. Clinical Breast Cancer 4: 348–353.

Vargas HI, Agbunag RV, Khaikhali I 2000 State of the art of minimally invasive breast biopsy: principles and practice. Breast Cancer 7: 370–379.

Venturini M, Del Mastro L, Aitini E et al 2005 Dose-dense adjuvant chemotherapy in early breast cancer patients: results from a randomized trial. Journal of the National Cancer Institute 97: 1724–1733.

Veronesi U, Paganelli G, Galimberti V et al 1997 Sentinel-node biopsy to avoid axillary dissection in breast cancer with clinically negative lymph-nodes. The Lancet 349: 1864–1867.

Vielh P, Validire P, Kheirallah S, Campana F, Fourquet A, Di Bonito L 1993 Paget's disease of the nipple without clinically and radiologically detectable breast tumor. Histochemical and immunohistochemical study of 44 cases. Pathology Research and Practice 189: 150–155.

Vogel CL, Cobleigh MA, Tripathy D et al 2002 Efficacy and safety of trastuzumab as a single agent in first-line treatment of HER2-overexpressing metastatic breast cancer. Journal of Clinical Oncology 20: 719–726.

Vogel VG 1998 Breast cancer risk factors and preventative approaches to breast cancer. In: Kavanagh J, Singletary SE (eds.) Cancers in Women. Blackwell Scientific Publications, Cambridge, MA.

Vogel VG 2009 The NSABP study of tamoxifen and raloxifene (STAR) trial. Expert Review of Anticancer Therapy 9: 51–60.

Vogel VG, Bevers T 2003 Handbook of Breast Cancer Risk Assessment. Evidence-based Guidelines for Evaluation, Prevention, Counselling and Treatment. Jones and Bartlett, Sudbury, MA.

Wahl RL, Zasadny K, Helvie M, Hutchins GD, Weber B, Cody R 1993 Metabolic monitoring of breast cancer chemohormonotherapy using positron emission tomography: initial evaluation. Journal of Clinical Oncology 11: 2101–2111.

Wakeham N, Svensson W, Zaman N et al 2006 P 19 Elasticity Ultrasound Appearances of Benign and Malignant Breast Disease. Royal College of Radiologists Breast Group, London.

Wakeling AE, Bowler J 1992 ICI 182,780, a new antioestrogen with clinical potential. Journal of Steroid Biochemistry and Molecular Biology 43: 173–177.

Warner E, Plewes DB, Hill KA et al 2004 Surveillance of BRCA1 and BRCA2 mutation carriers with magnetic resonance imaging, ultrasound, mammography, and clinical breast examination. Journal of the American Medical Association 292: 1317–1325.

Wartmann M, Altmann KH 2002 The biology and medicinal chemistry of epothilones. Current Medicinal Chemistry and Anticancer Agents 2: 123–148.

Weinstein SP, Orel SG, Heller R et al 2001 MR imaging of the breast in patients with invasive lobular carcinoma. AJR American Journal of Roentgenology 176: 399–406.

Welsh Cancer Intelligence and Surveillance Unit 2008 Cancer Incidence in Wales. Department of Health, UK.

West ER, Shea LD, Woodruff TK 2007 Engineering the follicle microenvironment. Seminars in Reproductive Medicine 25: 287–299.

Wiedswang G, Borgen E, Karesen R et al 2003 Detection of isolated tumor cells in bone marrow is an independent prognostic factor in breast cancer. Journal of Clinical Oncology 21: 3469–3478.

Wiedswang G, Borgen E, Karesen R et al 2004 Isolated tumor cells in bone marrow three years after diagnosis in disease-free breast cancer patients predict unfavorable clinical outcome. Clinical Cancer Research 10: 5342–5348.

Williams MR, Walker KJ, Turkes A, Blamey RW, Nicholson RI 1986 The use of an LH-RH agonist (ICI 118630, Zoladex) in advanced premenopausal breast cancer. British Journal of Cancer 53: 629–636.

Wilson ARM, Teh W 1998 Mini symposium: imaging of the breast. Ultrasound of the breast. Imaging 9: 169–185.

Winchester DJ, Chang HR, Graves TA, Menck HR, Bland KI, Winchester DP 1998 A comparative analysis of lobular and ductal carcinoma of the breast: presentation, treatment, and outcomes. Journal of the American College of Surgery 186: 416–422.

Witzig TE, Bossy B, Kimlinger T et al 2002 Detection of circulating cytokeratin-positive cells in the blood of breast cancer patients using immunomagnetic enrichment and digital microscopy. Clinical Cancer Research 8: 1085–1091.

Woo JC, Yu T, Hurd TC 2003 Breast cancer in pregnancy: a literature review. Archives of Surgery 138: 91–98; discussion 99.

Xing Y, Foy M, Cox DD, Kuerer HM, Hunt KK, Cormier JN 2006 Meta-analysis of sentinel lymph node biopsy after preoperative chemotherapy in patients with breast cancer. British Journal of Surgery 93: 539–546.

Yarnold J, Bloomeld D, Levay J 2004 Prospective randomized trial testing 5.7 Gy and 6.0 Gy fractions of whole breast radiotherapy in women with early breast cancer (FAST) trial. Journal of Clinical Oncology 16: S30.

Yeatman TJ, Cantor AB, Smith TJ et al 1995 Tumor biology of infiltrating lobular carcinoma. Implications for management. Annals of Surgery 222: 549–559; discussion 559–561.

Yen TW, Hunt KK, Ross MI et al 2005 Predictors of invasive breast cancer in patients with an initial diagnosis of ductal carcinoma in situ: a guide to selective use of sentinel lymph node biopsy in management of ductal carcinoma in situ. Journal of the American College of Surgeons 200: 516–526.

Yu K, Toral-Barza L, Discafani C et al 2001 mTOR, a novel target in breast cancer: the effect of CCI-779, an mTOR inhibitor, in preclinical models of breast cancer. Endocrine-related Cancer 8: 249–258.

Zervos EE, Badgwell BD, Abdessalam SF et al 2001 Selective analysis of the sentinel node in breast cancer. American Journal of Surgery 182: 372–376.

Zhao J, Wu R, Au A, Marquez A, Yu Y, Shi Z 2002 Determination of HER2 gene amplification by chromogenic in situ hybridization (CISH) in archival breast carcinoma. Modern Pathology 15: 657–665.

Ziegler RG, Hoover RN, Pike MC et al 1993 Migration patterns and breast cancer risk in Asian-American women. Journal of the National Cancer Institute 85: 1819–1827.

CHAPTER 48

Supportive care for gynaecological cancer patients: psychological and emotional aspects

Karen Summerville

Chapter Contents

INTRODUCTION	750
SPIRITUAL AND EMOTIONAL PAIN	750
QUALITY OF LIFE	751
PSYCHOSOCIAL ISSUES AND RETURNING TO NORMALITY	754
SEXUALITY AND PSYCHOSEXUAL ISSUES RELATING TO GYNAECOLOGICAL CANCER	754
BREAKING 'BAD NEWS'	757
TALKING TO CHILDREN ABOUT CANCER	759
RECURRENCE OF DISEASE AND CESSATION OF ACTIVE THERAPY	760
NEEDS OF THE WOMAN WHO IS DYING	763
BEREAVEMENT	763
SOURCES OF SUPPORT	764
KEY POINTS	764

Introduction

The patient

The aim of this chapter is to identify and discuss the psychological, psychosocial, psychosexual, emotional and practical needs of women affected by a gynaecological cancer. It considers ways in which we can provide care and support to meet the needs of patients and their families throughout their cancer journey. The role of the professional carer, and the knowledge and skills required to assess the individual needs of these women will be explored, and recommendations for practical interventions aimed at providing support will be discussed. These issues affect both cancer survivors and those in the palliative stage of their disease process.

When a woman is diagnosed with gynaecological cancer, it affects her life in many ways. At the time of diagnosis, it may feel like an emotional onslaught and the effects can be both abrupt and long lasting. Sometimes, issues and feelings remain long after the cancer has gone. The challenge is how best to help the woman to cope with the knowledge of her disease and its implications for herself and her family. Support may be required for an extended period of time, in a variety of forms and from a number of different people. This should not be seen as a task that is the sole responsibility of one individual, but will inevitably involve 'the team'. This is best managed by a multidisciplinary team approach, within a designated gynaecological oncology centre, where all members of the specialist support team are available (Improving Outcomes Guidance 1999) and with strong links to both hospital and community palliative care services.

The carers

The needs of the carers will also be addressed. In order to deal effectively and sensitively with the emotional and practical challenges with which they are confronted through caring for these women, healthcare professionals must understand their own feelings and develop insight into their reactions and coping mechanisms. They themselves may need to explore strategies in order to improve their ability to cope more effectively with the emotional onslaught to which they too are exposed through their own personal experience of care-giving.

Spiritual and Emotional Pain (Box 48.1)

Spiritual well-being has several components: a sense of purpose and meaning in life; a sense of relationship with self, others and a supreme being; and a feeling of hope (Moberg 1982, Miller 1985, Clark et al 1991). Both Clinebell (1966) and Ellison (1983) have identified four categories of basic spiritual needs: meaning; challenge in life; a reason for being; and continuing in the face of adversity. A person's spiritual outlook makes a tremendous difference to the process of both living and dying (Moberg 1982). Spirituality functions as a resource during multiple losses and change (Reed 1987).

DOI: 10.1016/B978-0-7020-3120-5.00048-5

Box 48.1 Three steps in the spiritual growth of both doctors and nurses

- Developing a 'greater awareness of the spirit within self' in order to be a better listener for the patient
- Opening the 'self' by being totally present with the patient
- Allowing the patient to share her feelings and emotions without reserve on the health professional's part

Source: From Lane J, The care of the human spirit, Journal of Professional Nursing 1987;3: 332–337.

Box 48.2 The changes in sexuality and their effects

- Reduced physical contact
- Loss of intimacy
- Loss of sex drive and desire disorders
- Early menopause
- Infertility
- Reduced human warmth

The diagnosis of cancer changes the patient's life forever, causing her to confront her own mortality. The doctor or nurse who cares for these women confronts his or her own mortality an equal number of times (Pace 2000).

If we are able to understand and learn to accept that mental pain is inevitable for both the patient and the carer, we may be freed from feelings of inadequacy and futility, which inhibit important discussion of the woman's hopes and fears.

In order to be effective in these painful situations, doctors and nurses must understand their own feelings and be aware of the natural devices they might use to avoid what may often be a difficult situation and one for which they have received no formal training. Saunders and Baines (1989) use the concept of 'staff pain'. They emphasize the need for staff to grieve the loss of a patient, and the importance of group support for staff and 'debriefing' sessions to allow opportunities to express these feelings in a safe and supportive environment.

Recognition of our own feelings of pain, and acceptance of help from others within the team and/or from a trained external facilitator is the only way to retain the resilience, sense of oneself and the humanity required in order to continue to 'care'.

Times of crisis can usually be turned into opportunities, and the intimacy of such moments between the woman and the doctor or nurse can produce deep feelings, sometimes tears. At times, it is appropriate to sit in silence and just the sense of being there can be recognition enough (Pace 2000). The most important point of all, at the core of every nursing or medical care situation, is the woman's need for someone who is genuine. They need the honest truth, not evasion or empty reassurances. If the healthcare professional has not questioned and analysed his or her own beliefs for the reassurance, doubts and answers they provide, there may be little of value to offer the patient who is forced to confront the ultimate truths and uncertainties of all that comes thereafter.

Care that integrates the spiritual dimensions creates a nurse or doctor who is actually involved in a human relationship. Qualities that demonstrate the ability to provide better spiritual care include a supportive approach to the patient; what has been termed a 'sense of benevolence' to the patient; awareness of the patient, self and the impact of family and significant others; empathy; and non-judgemental understanding (Dickenson 1975).

It takes more than just education for a nurse or doctor to feel comfortable with spiritual issues. Introspection and an awareness of their own personal spiritual journey are required to integrate the spiritual domain into patient care (Pace 2000).

It is emphasized that healthcare professionals need to take care of their own spiritual needs. Failure to do so will lead to emotional exhaustion (Lane 1987).

Quality of Life

What is quality of life?

Quality of life was broadly defined as early as 1947, when the World Health Organization described it as 'a state of complete physical, mental and social well-being, and not merely absence of disease and infirmity' (King et al 1997).

Quality of life is a complex phenomenon that affects an individual's personality and lifestyle. It is developed over time with physical, psychological, sociocultural, sexual and spiritual effects (Woods 1975). It is affected by change in appearance, mental states, personal and social factors and, in the case of cancer, the effects of disease process and treatments. It is tied closely to the concept of body image, self-esteem and self-concept, and is affected by attitudes, beliefs and behaviours (Penson et al 2000).

Poor body image can result in the patient feeling worthless as a person; physically unattractive or even repulsive; and unable to feel valued, loved or able to express themselves sexually (Box 48.2) (Dudas 1992). For some women, quality of life means feeling alive. It is personal and individual, and what is considered normal or acceptable to one person or couple may be unacceptable to another.

Effects of gynaecological cancer

The patient

Both the diagnosis and management of gynaecological cancer can have a major impact on every aspect of a woman's quality of life (Donovan et al 1989). It can be an overwhelming experience for a woman and her family, Then, before the woman has had time to work through her feelings of shock and grief relating to the diagnosis, she must begin treatment. There is no doubt that a diagnosis of gynaecological cancer can potentially compromise the key elements described for quality of life: body image, sexual health and relationships (Auchinloss 1989, Colyer 1996). Women of childbearing age experience sadness and anger at the loss of fertility, and women of all ages may view the loss of female organs as a loss of femininity (Steginga and Dunn 1997).

The short- and long-term side-effects of treatment may also affect a woman's self-worth, self-esteem and confidence, and have potential or actual psychosocial and psychosexual

> **Box 48.3** Physical effects of gynaecological cancer and its treatment
>
> - Pain
> - Fatigue and lethargy
> - Weight loss and anorexia
> - Weight gain (steroids, ascites, lymphoedema)
> - Skin irration
> - Odour, fistula, stomas
> - Discharge, bleeding
> - Vaginal change (stenosis, scarring, dryness)
> - Abdominal distension (bowel obstruction, ascites)

implications (Box 48.3) (Anderson 1985, Sacco Ezzell 1999). For example, a premature menopause, hair loss, lymphoedema, a stoma or a surgical scar may impact further on the reaction to the actual cancer (Anderson 1993).

However, it is also important to remember that body image may be altered and affect sexual health and quality of life without any change in appearance, function or control (Price 1990). Being told the diagnosis of cancer may alter body image, as this new knowledge of change may affect the woman's perception of herself and her health. This perception of change can lead to a distortion of body image; the woman may sense that something in herself or in her way of relating to others has changed, even before cancer or treatment have any physical effect. Smithman (1981) points out: 'Some changes in function can be purely psychological, and yet the potential for disturbed self-concept is great'. It is therefore widely accepted that body image, sexual health and overall quality of life are affected by physical factors, physical sensations, and emotional and social reactions.

The partner

It is also important to assess the partner's understanding and needs, as the effect of the cancer is on the relationship as a result of change to either individual. A needs assessment among cancer patients and their partners showed that 63% of the participants would have liked to receive more information about sexual functioning after treatment, and that 64% would participate in a specific counselling programme on the quality-of-life changes if this was offered (Bullard et al 1980).

Model (1990) examined reactions to body image change following surgery in some depth, and linked these to concepts of grief and loss. This is useful as it considers how nurses support both patients and their partners psychologically. Model suggests that we are far from doing this successfully, and that it is important to create an atmosphere in which patients and their partners feel accepted and understood if they experience anxiety, anger or grief, and to provide a medium through which they can express, share and clarify their feelings. Model recommends that the whole healthcare team should work together to do this, which does indeed seem vital, given that many patients and their partners express feelings of isolation following discharge from treatment and for some time thereafter (Colyer 1996).

A high proportion of women are anxious (31%) and depressed (41%) after surgery for gynaecological cancer

(Corney et al 1992). The majority have chronic sexual problems and a high proportion would like further information on after-effects: physical, sexual and emotional. Fifty per cent of young women would have liked their partners to be involved, and 25% of the 40 partners who were involved would have preferred further information.

Ten years on from the publication of these studies, there remains a lack of consistency within both nursing and the medical professions in the ongoing assessment process used to identify change and impact on quality of life for both women and their partners.

What we must try to achieve

The specialist multidisciplinary gynaecological oncology support team has an important role in patient education and management of side-effects, aimed at maintaining or improving quality of life.

Faced with multiple adjustment demands relating to the cancer, the treatments, survivorship issues or palliation of disease and its symptoms, it is important that the couple are encouraged to prioritize what is important to them and have ownership over agreed interventions. It is essential that this assessment not only covers the cancer diagnosis and treatment, but takes into account what life was like for the woman and her partner/family before the cancer (Box 48.4).

It is important that we view the woman as much more than a 'cancer diagnosis' and consider her uniqueness by asking ourselves 'Who is this woman we are trying to help?'. In this way, we can establish how actual or potential change may impact on her current measures for her quality of life. Roles, identity and relationships such as being a wife/partner, lover, mother, daughter, sister, employee or employer, friend and carer may be challenged, threatened and even altered either temporarily or permanently. Issues such as housing, transport, finances, insurance and ongoing responsibilities for paying the bills and child care, along with the challenge of a cancer diagnosis and treatment, may affect her ability to cope. Her usual resources and coping mechanisms and strategies may be challenged to the limit and all this will impact on her quality of life.

Assessing the needs

The effects of both the cancer and treatments have the potential to be both abrupt and long lasting, even when the goal is cure. The impact of altered body image resulting from treatments and/or surgical procedures for chronic illness extends beyond the immediate patient (Wilson and Williams 1988). Therefore, the need for individualized assessment on how this will impact on quality of life, both before and following cancer treatment, is fundamental (Box 48.5). Assessment must be as specific as possible (Box 48.6) and address the woman's concerns by self-assessment techniques.

The changing focus of need

Typically, the focus both before and following cancer treatment is on physical need. However, issues such as being unable to continue to work and the consequent reduced income or transport issues due to reduced mobility

Box 48.4 Aspects of quality of life that may change

- Altered body image
- Low self-confidence
- Low self-esteem
- Unable to deal with losses, i.e. fertility/premature menopause
- Loss of self-concept
- Loss of self-perception
- Loss of femininity
- Loss of control

Emotional impact (grieving scenario)

- Anxiety
- Fear
- Powerlessness
- Anger
- Depression
- Guilt
- Feelings of isolation

Social impact

- Feeling of isolation from:
  - partner/children
  - family
  - friends
  - work colleagues
- Changes in roles/relationships with:
  - partner
  - family/mother
  - work
  - sociocultural
- Impact on resources/finances
  - Unable to work—reduces income
  - Unable to afford to socialize
  - Transport (reduced mobility/isolation)
  - Unable to afford new clothes/extra laundry bills
  - Equipment issues/extra bedding

Box 48.5 The assessment process

- Listening to how patients talk about their body, in positive or negative terms
- Observation of how patients behave towards damaged body parts
- Listening to relatives'/visitors' reports about the woman and her methods of coping — is this typical coping behaviour?
- Observing for social withdrawal
- Identify social network/support
- Listening to patients' verbal accounts about how they anticipate life will be beyond the stay in hospital, e.g. how they anticipate others may react to their appearance or body function

Box 48.6 Evaluating adaptation to the cancer and treatment effects

- Has resumed former lifestyle
- Can verbalize concerns over changes in body image
- Demonstrates healthy coping abilities
- Can touch and look at body and accept change due to any scars, stomas or body shape
- Can incorporate necessary change to allow enjoyable activity
- Has incorporated altered body image as part of 'self'
- Shows evidence of high self-esteem
- Is willing to resume sexual relations/intimacy
- Can discuss and consider reconstruction of lifestyle

preventing use of public transport may be paramount, and need to be given priority for the woman and her family. In the initial stages of diagnosis and treatment for a gynaecological cancer, quality-of-life issues may not seem so important and the focus of concern may be on the tremendous physiological demands that occur as a result of coping with the disease process and treatments. However, as the illness trajectory lengthens, previously held notions may change as a woman adjusts to a new identity as a person with cancer.

Quality-of-life assessment and issues relating to the impact of actual or potential change require reassessment during treatment, at follow-up and as part of the long-term rehabilitation process. In women where the cancer progresses or recurs, the goals may change from cure to prolongation of life with the best possible quality for the woman and her family. Criteria for futility must be established to guide the transition from active to palliative management.

Rehabilitation and palliation both begin at diagnosis and continue throughout treatment and follow-up. They address the specific desires of each person and it is recommended

that they incorporate the contribution of every member of the multidisciplinary healthcare team.

The challenge facing all healthcare professionals is to achieve improvement in the quality of the patient's life by reducing dysfunction and disruption, and providing support with physical, psychological, social and spiritual aspects. In order to achieve this, it is important to identify information needs and individual coping strategies, explore issues identified as important to the patients themselves, and set realistic and achievable goals.

Whilst families are often the primary source of ongoing support to female cancer patients, women also derive considerable support from other patients and from healthcare professionals. The medical team should aim to develop psychological and psychosexual skills to cope with this important area of care. Further research is also needed into how support groups may best meet patients' needs (Veronesi et al 1999) and those of the care providers.

What we must learn

The following are essential in empowering both nurses and doctors to undertake their role: a comprehensive understanding of the aetiology of the gynaecological cancer and the effects of both the disease and treatment; knowledge of the ways of minimizing adverse problems; and assisting the woman and her partner in managing their needs.

Healthcare professionals must develop an appreciation of the wider issues and literature surrounding sexual health, altered body image, gender identity, role identity, cultural issues, religious beliefs, and how all the factors can influence self-esteem and body image and impact on quality of life in either a positive or negative way (Masters et al 1995).

Concern is often expressed in clinical practice that healthcare professionals lack the time and skills to deal with psychological and quality-of-life issues, although the literature suggests that giving patients the opportunity to express such concerns can be preventive of problems as well as therapeutic (Auchinloss 1989).

Despite its importance, quality of life is rarely a reported outcome in randomized clinical trials in cancer patients. Gynaecological oncology nurses, clinicians, educators and researchers must continue to work collaboratively to enhance the knowledge base regarding quality-of-life issues and to improve care provided to women with gynaecological cancer (King et al 1997). The impact of a gynaecological cancer on a woman's quality of life is an important outcome parameter that may be measured as survival without significant morbidity (Anderson and Lutgendorf 1997).

Psychosocial Issues and Returning to Normality

The woman may have undertaken several different roles and responsibilities prior to the cancer diagnosis and treatments. She may have been the central supporting figure in a household of some complexity, and may have provided the economic support, as well as the responsibilities of a mother, a partner, a lover and a homemaker. The very act of returning to any or all of these roles is often a significant milestone in recovery.

Apart from the obvious anxieties about her prognosis and family relationships, financial worries and change in role can be an immense source of stress for the patient and partner. The potential for this needs to be assessed prior to treatment and at subsequent follow-up.

Often practical help can be offered, such as a letter to the employer or facilitating the intervention of social services, and giving information on benefit entitlements and grants (e.g. Macmillan) where patients are unaware of possible financial assistance, and help in dealing with transport problems.

For patients living with severe ongoing disability due to the cancer or its treatment, or those with progressive disease where the aim is no longer cure but palliation, additional grants such as disability living allowance, attendance allowance and 'special rules' or palliative care funding may be applied for. The benefits helpline should be contacted to clarify eligibility.

The issues that must be addressed (Box 48.7) may be ongoing, and follow-up appointments provide an opportunity to assess how the woman and her family are readjusting to life following cancer.

Sexuality and Psychosexual Issues Relating to Gynaecological Cancer

In 1986, the World Health Organization stated that key elements of sexual health were:

Box 48.7 Issues that must be resolved

- Childcare issues
- Relationship dynamics
- Work-related responsibilities
- Housing needs
- Transport, travel, parking and fares
- Finances and adequate social resources
- Loss of fertility and premature menopause issues

- a capacity to enjoy and control sexual and reproductive behaviour in accordance with a social and personal ethic;
- freedom from fear, shame, guilt, false beliefs and other psychological factors inhibiting sexual response and impairing sexual relationships; and
- freedom from organic disorders, diseases and deficiencies that interfere with sexual and reproductive function

A gynaecological cancer diagnosis and treatment may threaten or actually change the key elements described for sexual health, and are associated with considerable sexual dysfunction (IOG 1999).

The background

A woman's physical genital development, her attitudes and security about being a woman, and her view of herself in relation to others, especially in intimate relationships, are all part of her uniqueness. Sexual functioning and concerns vary throughout one's lifespan and cannot be assumed for any age group or extent of disease. A woman's genital region may be perceived as psychologically very special, being both exquisitely sensitive and primal in sexual arousal. A malignancy in this area may be especially disturbing and significantly different in its emotional effects from cancer in other parts of the body. Reactions may vary according to feelings of the individual woman about her genitalia prior to developing a gynaecological cancer. However, there is no doubt that cancer of the vulva, which necessitates very evident vulval mutilation as a consequence of surgical treatment, can produce severe problems with psychosexual function (IOG 1999).

The quality of a woman's life needs to be considered and assessed in relation to what it was before she became ill. An unsatisfactory relationship prior to a cancer diagnosis may be improved by a couple having to cope and coming closer together. Alternatively, poor relationships may continue to be devoid of intimacy and affection. How the effects of the cancer and its treatment impact on either of these scenarios needs ongoing assessment.

Effects of gynaecological cancer

A study by Cull et al (1993) included 83 women with early-stage cervical cancer, half of whom had received surgery and half of whom had received radiotherapy. They were studied by standard self-report questionnaires and semi-structured interview. Over half reported deterioration in sexual function, and the irradiated women suffered more with loss of sexual pleasure. Many women felt that their psychological needs were not being met adequately.

A similar UK study included 105 women who had undergone radical pelvic surgery, of whom 65% had been treated for primary cervical cancer (Corney et al 1993). The mean time since treatment was 2 years. Of 73 women in whom the vagina had been preserved and who were in a sexual relationship, 16% never resumed intercourse. Two-thirds were experiencing sexual difficulties and around half reported a deterioration in their sexual relationship. However, this study highlights the need to never 'assume' as, interestingly, around one-third of these couples felt that their marital relationship had actually improved.

The need to provide information

The inadequate information about the effects of disease and its therapeutic interventions on people's sexual function and alterations in their quality of life is also reflected in the scarce amount of empirical research available on these issues. All oncology professionals should be aware of the importance of recognizing and addressing issues of sexual function as an integral aspect of quality of life for people with cancer and their partners (Gallo-Silver 2000), and both nurses and doctors need to develop skills in talking to patients and partners about sexual concerns and in taking a sexual history (Smith 1989, Green 1999).

Sexual function is an essential and fundamental area of the assessment process and should be discussed in a continuous fashion, rather than a haphazard or one-off fashion. A woman diagnosed with a gynaecological cancer and needing to undergo any form of treatment may have concerns relating to potential change in her sexuality or sexual function. However, she may be too embarrassed to ask and may worry or fear that it may be perceived as inappropriate to ask or discuss.

In a society that has moved rapidly towards an awareness of sexuality of all ages, these patients will demand, not without justification, that medical science passes both appreciation and expertise concerning this dimension of their disease.

They will require and expect therapeutic interventions which will assist them in becoming psychosexually as well as physically rehabilitated (Derogatis 1980).

The goal of intervention

The goal of sexual rehabilitation is to restore the patient's ability to engage in intimate interpersonal relationships, and incorporates the restoration of self-esteem and bodily function or adaption to change (Bancroft 1989). When appropriate and desired, sexual rehabilitation includes restoring physical ability to engage in sexual activity. Sexuality is an important aspect of quality of life and has a tremendous impact on an individual, their partner and families (Rutter 2000).

Listening and asking

Loss of sex drive may arise from an altered body image or there may be unresolved feelings such as guilt or fear of an association between sexual intercourse and cancer. Full assessment, discussion and information about the facts, in order to remove any misconceptions, are essential. The effect of the diagnosis on the partner is often overlooked, but it cannot be emphasized too strongly that preparation for the couple is the key to preventing avoidance or silence. The partner may fear that he could hurt or harm the woman, and other misconceptions that he can 'catch' cancer himself through being intimate may cause a barrier between them. Simple explanations and reassurance both before and following treatment, involving both partners if possible, can prevent problems arising or minimize problems by recognizing the important issues early.

Sexual functioning should be enquired into at the early follow-up visits and assessed continually, so that if any changes or difficulties occur, they can be recognized, support can be offered and appropriate interventions or specialist psychosexual referrals can be made as appropriate.

Sexuality may be expressed in a multitude of ways so it is imperative that healthcare professionals do not make assumptions about sexual behaviour, and understand that information assists women in regaining a sense of control over their behaviour and destiny (Burke 1996). This applies just as much to the late stages of the disease as to the early phases of the journey.

When physical love and intimacy have been important and are suddenly withdrawn, their loss is felt. Even when they have not been important, their need may now be recognized. We cannot assume. However, loving touch in the palliative stage of the disease process may be avoided for fear that it may lead to more sexual intimacy. This may be overcome if both partners are able to discuss their anxieties, either with each other or facilitated by a healthcare professional.

The woman may not touch her partner or avoid closeness for fear that it might lead to physical sex. The man may be just as fearful that coitus would damage or hurt his partner, and consequently keeps his distance. Both should be reassured that sexual intercourse is 'acceptable' at any stage of the disease process if there is sexual desire and drive on both sides and if it is physically possible. However, when coitus is not physically possible, methods of mutual masturbation can be explored, and sexual expression using sensate focus techniques can be explained (see below).

Communicating a willingness to assist women to ways to express their sexuality in spite of the cancer and consequences of treatment can be a challenge (MacElveen-Hoehn and McCorkle 1985). Basic counselling skills such as listening, a non-judgemental approach, and an open and accepting attitude with clear boundaries help to legitimize concerns as normal and valid (Lamb 1985, Laurent 1994).

Intervention

Both cognitive and behavioural sexual rehabilitation interventions have been suggested to assist women and their partners to adjust to the physical, psychological and psychosexual changes due to cancer and their impact on the relationship (Gallo-Silver 2000). The interventions described aim to increasing understanding and gradual adjustment, allowing the woman and her partner to have 'ownership' over the interventions chosen and to regain control.

Understanding and familiarity of appropriate use of the following interventions can prepare healthcare professionals to assist patients and their partners with sexual needs and concerns:

- educating patients about the phases of sexual functioning and the impact of treatment;
- giving permission to explore their ability to respond to sexual stimulation by using self-pleasuring exercises; and
- teaching sensate focus exercises that structure non-coital foreplay and suggesting changes in coital positions to increase both access and comfort.

The P-LI-SS-IT model (Box 48.8) (Royal College of Nursing 2000) is a framework for assessment of sexual need and can be useful as part of the multidisciplinary team approach to assessment of sexuality in women with cancer.

Box 48.8 Outline of P-LI-SS-IT model

Level 1: Permission (P)

The challenge for all healthcare professionals at level 1 is to create a comfortable environment that gives patients permission to discuss concerns and problems related to their sexuality and sexual health by:

- ensuring the physical environment is comfortable and private;
- communicating to the patient using acceptable counselling skills such as openness, reflection and paraphrasing;
- using cue questions to give the patient the opportunity to raise any sexuality and sexual health concerns;
- giving reassurance, where required, that the patient's current sexual practices are appropriate and healthy or that experimentation is appropriate;
- having a range of information available that is educational and non-personal;
- knowing where to get further information from and routes of referral for the patient;
- acknowledging the needs of sexual partners; and
- acknowledging the sexuality and sexual health needs of patients in relation to their cultural background.

Level 2: Limited information (LI)

This is where healthcare professionals provide non-expert or limited information relating to sexuality and sexual health. For example, a woman receiving pelvic radiotherapy will need to know about vaginal dryness and possible implications for her future fertility.

Level 3: Specific suggestions (SS)

To provide specific suggestions to help patients with sexuality and sexual health needs, healthcare professionals complete training at specialist practitioner level.

Level 4: Intensive therapy (IT)

The most advanced level of addressing sexuality and sexual health care involves complex interpersonal and psychological issues and is used with patients who have specific sexual problems such as dyspareunia or vaginismus. Relationship counselling falls into this category. Further training is needed in psychosexual medicine and relationship therapy to undertake this stage.

Source: Royal College of Nursing 2000 P-LI-SS-IT model. In: Sexuality and Sexual Health in Nursing Practice. RCN, London.

All patients need permission and limited information, frequently dispelling myths and eliminating ignorance about the disease and treatment effects on their sexuality. This is often enough to enable patients to resume sexual expression and intimacy. Specific suggestions can help patients whose radical surgery or radiotherapy treatment has resulted in physiological or anatomical alterations, such as a stoma formation or vaginal stenosis, or when the mechanisms of sexual response have been affected.

Despite careful assessment and interventions, problems may still arise and expectations may not be met. The need for the skills and expertise to provide in-depth assessment of need and intensive structured therapy in the form of marital or sexual counselling is recognized in the P-LI-SS-IT model (Bancroft 1989, Penson et al 2000). Doctors and nurses need to be secure in the knowledge that it is appropriate to refer to a sexual therapist as the need is identified with the patient or couple.

Behavioural therapy

Direct behavioural approaches for treating sexual dysfunction due to performance anxiety are advocated (Masters and Johnson 1970). Sensate focus may be useful as it is aimed at regaining intimacy within the relationship through mutual touching and physical sexual sensation and stimulation of each other's body parts, while not necessarily needing to involve the genitals or the act of intercourse. It is essentially about being able to communicate and relax with their partner, and developing a sense of trust and closeness which may have been lost (Leiblum and Rosen 1989). The sensate focus method restructures and reorientates how couples may ordinarily approach sexual interactions, allowing them to move away from old familiar habits and reinvent the physical side of their relationship. It is about touching and being touched. However, at the heart of the programme is an initial ban on sexual intercourse, particularly genital contact and penetration, until performance anxiety and fear of failure have subsided and trust within the relationship has been re-established.

Finally

For a woman to be sexually complete, she must feel secure and this is a fundamental need for a woman facing the future, especially when she is terminally ill. Respect, trust and love are needed in order to establish security. Fear, distrust and anger need to be dispelled. Respect includes self-respect and this may have been absent even before the occurrence of cancer. Altered body image may exacerbate already fragile and vulnerable emotions around oneself. To acknowledge the hurt and pain of emaciation, hair loss, discharge, bleeding, abdominal distension, colostomy or urostomy is difficult, and it can help to share this difficulty by not avoiding the important issues for the woman. Love of the person rather than the body must be constantly reinforced. There is an opportunity to engender new self-respect and trust, in discussing openly and honestly the issues that may be painful but most important to the woman at that time.

Breaking 'Bad News'

'Bad news' can be defined as any information that dramatically alters a patient's view of her future for the worse (Kay 1996). The way in which bad news is delivered affects both the patient's and the family's ability to cope, and should therefore be done in a sensitive and, where possible, planned and supportive way.

It is in the nature of gynaecological malignancies that the possibility of cancer is uppermost in the patient's mind even before the investigations that confirm her worst fear. Most studies in which patients with cancer have been asked how much information they want report that over 90% want all the information available, good or bad.

Bad news may be broken in the following circumstances:

- at the point of diagnosis;
- at the point of recurrence; and
- when entering the terminal phase of illness.

The manner in which this responsibility is undertaken determines the subsequent relationship between the patient and the healthcare professional. Trust and respect established at this time will ease future care and the relationship between them.

Breaking bad news well is important for the following reasons:

- to maintain trust which enables the relationship between the patient and healthcare professional to be based on openness and honesty;
- truthfulness about the disease allows open communication with the patient and fosters discussion about the disease process and its management;
- uncertainty may be reduced;
- to prevent the demoralization caused by unrealistic hope;
- to allow appropriate adjustment of the patient and her family, empowering them to make informed decisions about their future care;
- to prevent collusion with family members which destroys family communication and prevents mutual support; and
- information/bad news given to the patient and her family must be communicated to the patient's primary, secondary or tertiary care team to allow open and sensitive communication between care settings.

Standards of care suggested for breaking bad news

The specialist in charge must ensure that members of the multidisciplinary team have appropriate training and skills in breaking bad news. The patient's autonomy must be respected when making management plans. In this way, the patient will be given the option of involving a family member or carer to support her at the time of breaking of bad news. The doctor or specialist should plan, whenever possible, how this will be done, the setting and with a specialist nurse or appropriate member of the team present. It is the responsibility of the specialist team to ensure swift communication and liaison between the hospital-based team and the primary care services when bad news is broken.

The actual process of breaking bad news

Preparation

- Ensure all information is available (e.g. diagnostic information, knowledge of all the facts).
- Have a defined treatment plan/options available prior to the interview.
- Give the woman notice of the interview to enable her to invite a family member or friend.
- Invite a specialist nurse/support nurse to be with you whilst breaking bad news.
- Ensure that privacy is maintained with no interruptions; no telephones, bleeps or pagers; and an 'engaged' or 'do not disturb' sign on the door.
- Set time aside, indicate how long and indicate that arrangements can be made to meet again if needed.
- Book an interpreter if needed. Do not use a family member to break bad news.

The doctor's role in the breaking of bad news

- Give time, do not appear to hurry. Sit down facing the patient and her family (if present).
- Make any necessary introductions, including the family members and specialist/support nurse.
- Make eye contact.
- Find out the patient's perception of the situation.
- Ask if the patient wants more information (e.g. 'I have the results of your tests, would you like me to explain them to you now?').
- Avoid the use of medical jargon, use the patient's language. Be honest and clear.
- Give a warning shot (e.g. 'I'm afraid it looks rather serious'), followed by a simple, sensitive explanation, avoiding too much detail at this stage, unless the patient asks, as she will not remember everything that is said because of the shock process.
- Be optimistic and maintain realistic hope (e.g. 'There are things we can do to help you').
- Use the word 'cancer' and avoid the use of euphemisms.
- Stop at this point. Allow the patient time for expressions of feelings or stunned silence.
- At this point, check the patient's understanding of her situation now.
- Continue at the patient's pace with information-giving.
- Expect expression of feelings and sometimes angry questions.
- Be prepared to repeat yourself as details will not be remembered.
- Discuss treatment plan, time scales and other written information.
- Ensure the interview is closed sensitively and inform the woman when she will see you next or how to contact you if necessary.
- Offer to meet other members of family separately.
- Bad news will always be bad and will always be remembered, as will empathy and simple, clear, well-planned, sensitive and honest explanation.

The nurse's role in the breaking of bad news

- Be prepared to co-ordinate the process.
- Ensure a quiet room is available or screen off the bedside; no interruptions, bleeps, pagers or telephones.
- Make sure the patient and family are comfortable and all seated.
- Ensure the doctor is able to sit down comfortably to enable him/her to maintain eye contact throughout.
- The nurse's role is to support the patient, the family and the doctor.
- Ensure the patient's dignity is maintained at all times (e.g. dressed/covered before the consultation begins).
- If the woman is an outpatient, ensure that if she is alone, there are transport arrangements home and someone to collect her if in shock.
- It is necessary to ask the patient's permission to contact her general practitioner (GP) and any community support service (e.g. Macmillan).
- Stay with the patient and family following the interview. Allow time for them to compose themselves and the opportunity to ask questions.
- Offer relevant written information and contact numbers for the patient and family to access further information or advice (e.g. Macmillan nurse/support groups).

After the consultation

- The nurse should be available to the patient and family for as long as necessary.
- Ensure that the next appointment is made for further investigations, treatment, symptom review and follow-up.
- Offer nurse-led follow-up in the form of personal or telephone contact.
- Ensure that the GP is informed, and local community support as appropriate (e.g. Macmillan team/district nurses), as soon as possible by either telephone or fax regarding the bad news given, treatment plan and how the patient and family received the news. Indicate the name and contact number of the support/specialist nurse involved.

Dealing with collusion and the conspiracy of silence

Family distress at anticipated bad news can lead to collusion which, in turn, leads to poor communication between the family, patient and healthcare team. Some patients may not wish to have detailed information, and elect to permit their information to be discussed with the family or a carer.

To prevent collusion occurring, the following should be addressed.

- Deal with the patient's main concerns first.
- Ask the patient's permission to see the family/carer.
- Talk to the family/carer. Gain their trust to enable them to give 'permission' to talk openly and honestly.
  - Acknowledge that they know the patient best.
  - Check the family's understanding of the illness.
  - Check why the family do not want information given to the patient.
  - Indicate potential difficulties the family may experience if the patient is not told the information if she asks.
  - Ask permission to talk to the patient alone to elicit what she would like to know.
- Talk with the patient.
- Talk with the patient and family together.
- Document the outcome of discussions.

Relatives often ask that the patient should not be told the diagnosis. This wish can sometimes be very strongly stated, and may be driven by a strong desire to protect the patient. It is important to discover whether this is because their own fears are too great to face.

If the opportunity is given to discuss the woman's illness, with care and support for the whole family to cope, a very positive outcome can result. The alternative is that the strain of pretence will undermine patient and family alike, with both sides usually being unaware of the reality of the situation, even if this is not admitted (Twycross and Lack 1983).

Modern cancer treatment, often involving radical complex surgery, chemotherapy and radiotherapy, can hardly be carried out without the patient realizing she has cancer. Even if the medical and nursing staff collude with relatives to conceal the diagnosis, day-to-day discussion and comparison of treatments with other patients will usually result in her guessing the truth.

If an open, honest approach is not adopted from the onset of the relationship with the healthcare team, it imposes an almost intolerable burden on the person who is fully informed. There is a tragic irony in the situation where the nearest relative has been told the diagnosis but tries to preserve a façade, while the patient who has guessed the truth attempts to maintain a brave face for the benefit of her relatives. They are each left to face alone the prospect of uncertainty around the diagnosis of cancer, and the relatives are separated from the woman by this conspiracy of silence. It is far more constructive to be able to discuss their fears with each other, and to provide the close emotional support that they both need and deserve.

Giving the patient opportunities to ask and replying honestly

Simple questions such as 'Have I made myself clear?' or 'Is there anything I have not yet explained that you wish to know?' will give the woman a cue to discuss concerns. It is important to be aware of body language, both our own and the patient's, as this can speak volumes. Try to sit at the same level as the patient and maintain eye contact. Avoid any obstacles to open communication such as lack of privacy, constant interruptions, telephone calls or even interposing large desks. If an authoritarian posture is avoided, patients will be more likely to express their fears and feelings around what is always going to be a difficult subject.

Letting the news sink in

Patients' frequent dissatisfaction with the explanations given to them may not be due solely to a failure of communication or lack of time. They may not retain the information or may even suppress it when the content of the conversation is emotionally distressing and too painful to absorb.

Women often report that they 'shut off' and 'could no longer bear to listen'. Hogbin and Fallowfield (1989) have suggested that tape recording 'bad news' consultations and giving the tape to the patient to take away with them may help them to understand the problem, overcome failures of recall, and explain the diagnosis and any treatment plan to their relatives.

However, this approach may not suit every patient and may create further obstacles to communication by preventing the interview from achieving the degree of privacy and intimacy which is necessary for two-way open interaction.

Another suggestion is to write down the facts from the information given verbally following the consultation in which bad news is broken, and allow the patient an opportunity to absorb the information at her own pace over time and once the shock process has started to shift. Once the reality of her new situation has sunk in, the need for more factual information and exploration of the options in order to take back some control often takes over from initial fear, shock and stunned silence (IOG 1999). Written information following the breaking of bad news can then be extremely useful in helping the patient and family to formulate their questions prior to their next consultation with the specialist team.

Many areas also have local cancer support groups and there are national cancer helplines which may also be useful in helping patients to come to terms with the 'bad news' given (see Sources of support below).

Being realistic

It is important to be realistic at all times and to avoid giving false reassurance. At the same time, it is important not to deny the patient all hope. Encouraging a positive but realistic attitude will help. The importance of this stage cannot be emphasized too strongly. If the multidisciplinary care team forms an open and honest relationship when there is hope for cure, this will be far easier for the woman to accept if disease recurs or her condition does not respond to treatment and she enters the palliative stage of her journey. Some women will choose to cope with the news by denial. They should not be assaulted with the truth but allowed to come to terms with the situation in their own time. No response is needed other than gentle reiteration of the truth, relating the known facts when requested. Denial may, in part, be responsible for a woman's apparent lack of understanding after the initial interview. In this case, it should be carefully noted for use in further meetings, in order to manage her care in a professional, sensitive and individualized manner.

Talking to Children about Cancer

What makes cancer especially difficult are the many unknowns. Living with uncertainty is part of having cancer. There are some questions that cannot be answered. Helping the patient and her partner to accept that fact and to find out all they can to make the unknown more familiar to them is the first step in allowing them to be able to talk to their children and help them to accept the fact too.

Children need to be given information about their mother's condition, to a degree dependent on their maturity, in order to understand and cope with what is happening. Honesty is very important when communicating with children. The best person to give children information is the parent or another close family member. If they feel unable to do this, they can enlist the help of a professional; for example, a member of the multidisciplinary specialist cancer care team, a counsellor or social worker. However, it is important that the parent is present when the child is told bad news so that they know exactly what has been said and can comfort them with their immediate reaction to it.

Everyone who has a relationship with the patient will be affected by the cancer diagnosis, even if they do not show their feelings. If their mother is frequently absent or not well enough to care for and play with them as she did prior to her illness, children may feel inexplicably rejected. Without reassurance, a child may feel responsible for his or her mother's illness or subsequent death.

A child's understanding of illness and death, although not the same as an adult's, is often underestimated. Children can often accept the inevitable more easily than their elders. Sometimes all that is needed is time to adjust and the maintenance of some routine and stability. However, there are things that parents can say or do to help their children to cope with change and uncertainty.

Children need to be given information in a way they can understand. It is important that jargon and excessive medical details are avoided. Tell children what has happened, explain what will happen next and be prepared to repeat the information and to ask children questions to check whether they have understood what they have been told. The use of drawings or story books can help younger children to understand. Children need accurate information about cancer, not fears and assumptions gleaned from other sources.

It is important to ask children whether they have any questions and to let them know it is all right to ask anything they want. Children often take a long time to process information and may need to come back much later and ask more. As well as telling them about changes, it is important for them to know what will stay the same. Reassurance that they will always be looked after and loved in spite of the illness will help maintain feelings of security. However, false promises must be avoided, as cancer involves great uncertainty.

It is important to listen to children, as they will let us know what they can cope with. Honesty about what adults do not know is as important as sharing what we do know if children are to continue to trust. A child has a right to know anything that affects the family, as cancer does. Not telling them may feel like a breach of trust and children usually know when something is wrong. If parents try to protect them by saying nothing, they may actually develop fears which are worse than the real situation. Children can be left feeling isolated if they are not told the truth. Attempts to protect them may enhance their anxiety. Children have an amazing ability and capacity to deal with truth. Even sad truths can relieve the anxiety of too much uncertainty. Through sharing their feelings and being prepared to acknowledge and express sadness, the parents can offer support for their children.

Coping with cancer in the family can be an opportunity for children to learn about the body, cancer, treatment and healing. They can also learn about feelings and the strength of the human spirit in difficult times. Telling children means that they can share significant emotions with their parents and siblings. Children need to be given permission to feel sad, angry or scared. Children are very resilient. They can cope with difficult information if they are supported with it, left with a feeling of hope and assurance that they will still be loved and cared for.

It is important to talk to children individually as children's understanding and their concerns differ with age.

Children aged 3–7 years

Young children need very simple explanations of the cancer. The use of drawings will help to explain it to them, and will also help parents to understand their worries and feelings. At this age, children are very wrapped up in their own world and will be concerned about whether their needs will be met in this frightening situation. This anxiety may be expressed through regressive behaviour (showing the behaviour of a younger child) such as tantrums and bedwetting.

It is important that parents maintain their usual routine to provide reassurance, enlisting the help of other relatives and the child's school to do this. Discipline needs to be consistent, rewarding good behaviour and providing extra affection. Difficult behaviour should settle down in time as it is a normal reaction to stress and change.

Major fears for children of this age will be change in a parent; this may be frightening, such as hair loss, sickness and separation from the mother if she has to be admitted to hospital. Children will need a lot of reassurance from the mother and their well caregiver in order to cope with this change. Things that may help are simple information, use of calendars to help them understand time scales, reading them books about hospitals, explanations of how equipment works, creating a child-friendly environment in the hospital as much as possible, frequent visits to the ill parent, making cards and tapes for them, and speaking frequently to their mother on the telephone. For younger children especially, it is important to use the correct language and explain things literally as they may not understand what cancer, illness or death means. Using vague explanations about a mother's death, such as 'Mummy has gone to sleep', should be avoided as it may leave a young child confused when their mother does not wake up, or lead to fear of going to sleep themselves and nightmares.

Children aged 7–11 years

At this age, children have a more complex understanding of the situation. They will very often worry greatly about their mother and what will happen in the future. This may lead them to protect her by not asking questions or raising their fears. Keeping communication open and encouraging the children to do the same can be positive. It is important to let the school know so that they have alternative sources of support if they need it. Again, behaviour may be affected; children may become more aggressive or more withdrawn. Schoolwork may be affected. It is important that parents provide a lot of reassurance and support, as well as maintaining firm boundaries with regards to discipline.

Teenagers

Adolescents have a particularly difficult time, as they are already struggling with all kinds of development issues. They are trying to find a new identity and balance between dependence and independence. A mother's illness will challenge this balance and may promote resentment and anger in the child, which ultimately leads to guilt. They may rebel to a greater degree, exhibiting a lot of anger, or alternatively they may mature too quickly and take on a lot of responsibility.

After treatment, it is important that parents continue to keep children informed of what is going on and to balance hope with reality. If the mother's cancer recurs, children will need to know this. There may come a time when the reality is that the mother is not going to recover. This will be an incredibly difficult time for the parents and it may seem even harder to discuss this awful reality with children. Death and dying are not talked about openly in our culture, and it may be difficult for the mother to face the knowledge that she is going to die. It will be difficult for the whole family, including the children; facing it together and allowing them to be part of that process is likely to help them face the future.

It is vital that parents are honest and discuss the reality with children, as it makes it harder for everyone to cope if they are kept in the dark. Like adults, children need to prepare for loss and have the opportunity to say or do important things for their mother.

Children often know much more than we imagine and need to be given permission to talk about it. It is important to use language that they will understand, avoid jargon and use open, honest and direct communication. Most importantly, children need to be listened to. Parents can help their children face life afterwards by preparing them for the future without their mother. This is never going to be an easy process but however long a mother may have to live, time with her children can be precious. The whole family may discover reserves of love and inner strength that will enhance the rest of their life together.

Emotional difficulties linked to cancer are not always easy to talk about and are often difficult to share with those to whom we are closest, especially when children are involved. Trained counsellors in cancer care use their skills to help people talk about their thoughts, feelings and ideas, and may help in the process of untangling some of the difficulties and confusion that living with or dying from cancer can bring.

Recurrence of Disease and Cessation of Active Therapy

For the woman who hopes to be cured, the discovery of the recurrence of cancer is a time of great despair, rage and fear. This is often worse than the time of initial diagnosis and can be devastating. The three causes of anguish and anger described most commonly by patients are: delay in diagnosis; not being told the diagnosis until they were too ill to complete unfinished business; and return of the cancer when they felt they had been assured of cure.

The resentment at having been cheated can be great. For some, it is simply having cancer; for others, the word 'cure' has probably been 'heard' rather than said, but all feel that false hope has been given. The balance between false hope and no hope is difficult to achieve but is important (Saunders and Baines 1989). Anger may also be accompanied by spiritual pain. If this anger is accepted and understood, the path to acceptance is cleared. If it is not understood, and especially if it is met by a defensive attitude, it may increase as unresolved or unexpressed anger and may lead to depression (Massie and Holland 1989). Permanent, intermittent or transitory denial of the prognosis represents a necessary defence mechanism against a massive assault on the mind and emotions, and should be treated as such; the patient should be allowed to accept her situation at her own pace (Kay 1996). Cessation of active therapy means that the woman may now be facing the terminal stage of her journey. This knowledge is accompanied by new fears: the course of the disease, disfigurement, dependency, loss of self-respect and dignity, dying and the manner of dying.

Open discussion, honesty and acknowledgement of these anxieties with all concerned will help towards emotional security. Stopping treatment need not remove all hope. The nature of hope is to be flexible: hope for cure can be replaced with hope for time, and an opportunity to complete unfinished business or to aim for a particular personal milestone. Loneliness and a feeling of isolation are not only hard to bear in themselves but also heighten other symptoms of advanced disease. The isolation is sometimes imposed by the woman herself when the thought of parting becomes intolerable (Maguire 1993).

It is impossible to overestimate the benefits of an offer of palliative care; Macmillan nursing support, both community and hospital based; cancer counsellors and the specialist gynaecological cancer nurses. Even if little physical help is needed, the psychological support and ongoing relationship with the specialist multidisciplinary support team cannot be introduced too early. Palliative care support begins at the time of diagnosis, when there is uncertainty, and provides a natural link for the woman throughout her cancer journey. It is an important role for her and her family in providing reassurance that she will not be abandoned when there is cessation of active treatment. The focus of care will now be on her symptoms, psychological support and individual needs rather than her tumour. It is vital to watch and listen with care and to respond to what is seen and heard.

Now the patient has to face the more immediate prospect of death, it is possible to deal honestly with her without moving into stark truth (Saunders and Baines 1989). The immediate reaction may be disbelief or denial (Faulkner and Maguire 1994, Kay 1996). She may react with anger, either immediately or at a later stage. Depression is common and these different emotions may occur at any time; daily alterations between one and another are possible. The depression which may follow the woman's realization of the severity of her illness should not be confused with endogenous depression. When an individual is faced with the imminent prospect of death, depression and grief are appropriate, not pathological reactions (Massie and Holland 1989).

Although most patients welcome the truth, it may take some time and much discussion on several occasions for her to face her situation fully. She needs to feel she can survive as a fully integrated person, whatever length of time she has and however the disease process or treatment affects her.

There needs to be room for hope and for denial (Pace 2000). A scientific approach often suggests that we must give patients 'the facts' and help them to 'accept the truth', but denial may be a functional and appropriate coping skill at that particular time (Corless 1992). As the old hospice adage goes, unless something is terribly wrong with where the patient is, that is perhaps where the patient needs to be.

Reactions of partner, family and close friends

The partner, family members and close friends often exhibit similar reactions of grief, anger and denial. However, this is unpredictable, as is each person's individual reaction to a natural process of loss and change.

How each deals with that experience will be different depending on their individual relationship and their usual personal coping mechanisms. Feelings of loneliness and isolation are particularly difficult to endure for both the patient and those close to her, and are not helped by mere physical proximity to each other. They each need time and space to express themselves and what they are really feeling.

Family and friends who do not express their emotions or acknowledge either their own or the patient's pain may simply not know what to do or say, and it may be sufficient to show them that simple, truthful exchange is not damaging. The thought of loss may be unbearable and may be managed by assuming a routine and not facing up to the reality of change for both the woman and those close to her. This can be painful for the patient and cause anger and resentment unless its cause is understood. The partner may also feel isolated, emotionally and physically impotent, fearful of not being adequate and unable to bear the thought of any loss or death.

Close involvement in emotional support and practical care may ease the burden if sufficient confidence and professional help is provided. Trained cancer counsellors, Macmillan nurses and specialist gynaecological cancer nurses offer a service aimed at psychological support for the partner and family from diagnosis and throughout the journey, and either provide or refer on the appropriate bereavement services.

Fear of symptoms in advanced stage of disease

The patient's mental state will profoundly affect her symptomatology (Faulkner and Maguire 1994; Twycross 1997a). Fear of symptoms causes anxiety in the palliative stage, not only for themselves but for the significance they bear. If this is discussed fully with the patient and relatives, the anxiety can be diminished and the future can be faced with confidence that problems will be taken seriously.

The symptom most feared by patients and their families is pain. It was Cicely Saunders who first discussed the concept of 'total pain', which includes psychological, emotional, social and spiritual components as well as physical pain. Mental pain may present as physical pain or contribute to the extent of existing symptoms. Even mild pain should be taken seriously, so that confidence is established that pain can be treated quickly and effectively. When psychological adjustment and acceptance are achieved, the quantity of analgesia required may be reduced markedly.

Saunders and Baines (1989) have stressed the role of symptom control, but also point out that this requires time and close contact with the woman to give her the confidence to impart her deeper feelings, whether they be of anger, depression, guilt or regret. Guilt, anger and grief all need to be expressed, understood and acknowledged as valid, even if answers cannot be offered.

Factors that lower the pain threshold include fear, anger, sadness and boredom. Sympathy, understanding, companionship, diversional activity and elevation of mood raise the pain threshold (Twycross and Lack 1983).

Good communication which allows expression of fears and anxiety, and that conveys understanding and support can be a powerful means of alleviating pain. In some instances, the relief of persistent pain may require no more than providing the honest communication that has previously been denied to the patient (Lichter 1987).

It is a feature of all aspects of modern life that inadequate attention is given to spiritual needs. The effect on both the dying and those caring for them is 'spiritual pain'. Religion is a component of spirituality but is not always the total whole.

Man is not destroyed by suffering, he is destroyed by meaningless suffering (Frankl 1987).

Symptom control

The psychological and emotional aspects of care cannot be adequately assessed and managed if a woman is experiencing uncontrolled physical symptoms. Moreover, the patient's mental state will affect her symptoms profoundly.

The aim of symptom control is to release the woman from physical distress so that she can focus on important issues, such as:

- rehabilitation;
- changes in role;
- emotional adjustment;
- focus on relationships;
- unfinished business;
- meaning of life (Kay 1994).

Treatment goals must be realistic. The aim is to free the woman from the limitations imposed upon her life by the symptoms, as far as possible. This needs to be approached by a specialist multidisciplinary team wherever the woman chooses to be looked after (i.e. home, hospital, hospice or nursing home). Expert nursing care needs to be offered, including gynaecological cancer nurses, palliative care nurses and community Macmillan support and district nurses; counselling; palliative care doctors; rehabilitation services, including physiotherapists, occupational therapists, social workers and complementary therapists; spiritual support; family support; terminal care and bereavement services.

Physical, social, emotional and spiritual needs are often combined and can be complex. They will require time and sensitivity from a team approach in order to manage care.

Principles of symptom control

- Listen to the details.
- Ask about all symptoms.
- Detailed drug history.
- Ask why the symptom is occurring. Look for reversible factors.
- Interlace questions about physical symptoms with questions about feelings; this greatly increases the effectiveness of the consultation and the quality of the information.
- Treat promptly: symptoms have no more diagnostic usefulness in a situation of advanced disease.
- Make one change at a time (as far as possible).
- Explain changes.
- Include the patient in decision-making.
- Involve the relatives.
- Skilful prescribing.
- Use a drug card.
- Make a plan (e.g. What if she vomits?).
- Monitor regularly (until symptom free).
- Remember emotional factors.
- Reduce or stop drugs whenever possible (Kay 1994).

Pain control

This is managed best by following some simple general rules. First, it is important to try to establish the cause of the pain. Not all pains are due to cancer itself; previous treatment and incidental causes are also important. Investigations may be appropriate, although very ill patients should only be subjected to even simple investigation if it is clear that different results will lead to differences in management.

Assessment of pain

Clear assessment of the pain is required based on the patient's verbal reports. A history of the site/s, area of radiation, duration, aggravating and relieving factors, as well as relevant clinical examination is needed. It is important because continuous pain (visceral and soft tissue) responds to morphine, whereas other types of pain (bone, nerve, colic or non-cancer-related pain, e.g. migraine, angina) need other approaches (Kay 1994).

The pain must be approached with analgesia and with measures designed to improve the woman's ability to endure the pain by restoring her sense of personal worth, and by providing her with opportunities for creative and meaningful activity for as long as possible. Assessment tools may be useful in the assessment of complex or multiple types or sites of pain.

A body chart may be useful for initial assessment because it serves as a communication tool by making the pain 'visible'. It demonstrates the sites of pain, as 80% of patients are thought to have two or more pains (Kay 1994). It should be drawn with or by the patient herself.

Recording pain scores is another simple way to monitor difficult, complex pain control. The woman is asked three times a day to rate the severity of her pain on a scoring system of 0–10, where 0 is no pain at all and 10 is the worst pain imaginable. The scores are reproduced on a pain chart or kept in a patient diary. They may be useful to monitor responses to different treatments, are subjective to the woman's individual experience and allow early changes in pain management to be considered. It is important to remember that pain is whatever the patient says it is (Twycross 1997b).

Route and frequency of drug administration

When possible, analgesia should be given by mouth. Adequate analgesia is obtained by regular administration of an adequate dose of an appropriate drug at the time intervals which take into account the compound's pharmacokinetics and the individual woman's routine, i.e. time of waking, meal times and sleeping. This reduces the risk of breakthrough pain, but alternative or additional analgesics must be considered and prescribed for breakthrough pain before it actually occurs. Persistent pain requires preventative therapy; analgesics should be given regularly and prophylactically (Twycross 1997b).

Choosing the correct analgesia

The World Health Organization (1986) has suggested a three-stage analgesic ladder for the management of pain. This involves the choice of non-opioid analgesics, mild opioids and strong opioids, each stage involving appropriate use of other non-opioid or adjuvant drugs which may relieve pains of varying type and cause. If a drug fails to relieve the pain, it is important to move up the ladder or/and consider adjuvant drugs, but not to move laterally in the same efficacy group.

The right dose of analgesia for an individual woman is the dose which relieves the pain at night, at rest, during the day and on movement, although this may not be completely possible (Twycross 1997b).

The response to the analgesia must be monitored to ensure that benefits of treatment are maximized and adverse effects (e.g. drowsiness, nausea and constipation) are minimized.

Needs of the Woman Who is Dying

The question most frequently asked is when death will occur. An accurate answer cannot be given and any attempt to do so should be avoided because it causes distress, whether the predicted time is too short or longer than expected. It may be helpful to acknowledge to the patient how hard it must be to accept that healthcare professionals cannot really predict when death will occur.

When death is thought to be imminent, it is important that the patient and carers are kept adequately informed at all times. They may not only wish to know how long it is going to be, but also need to understand what might happen both before, during and after the event.

How people die remains in the memory of those who live on (Saunders and Baines 1989).

A peaceful death is important for the relatives as well as the patient. Families often find it comforting if carers continue to talk to the patient even after unconsciousness. Sedation for terminal agitation or distress should be prompt. It can be allowed to wear off once the patient is settled and any reversible causes have been treated to see if sedation is still necessary (Kay 1996).

As healthcare professionals, we should strive not just for death with dignity but for death with style. For both medical and nursing professionals, this suggests two things: first, that death should not be seen as a failure of medicine; and second, that each doctor and nurse becomes acquainted with death and comfortable in its presence, thus allowing them to participate fully in the patient's experience of death, whatever that means to that particular woman at the time.

The aim is to allow the woman to die as the person she has always been. Sensitive nursing and medical care can give great comfort, and anxieties which may seem too trivial to show to others may be expressed, as nurses and doctors often have great insight into the woman's need; time to share this insight is important.

The terminal phase is characterized by day-to-day deterioration. The common symptoms in the terminal 48 h are shown in Box 48.9. It is beyond the scope of this chapter to discuss the management of each individually.

Bereavement

Bereavement is the complex of emotions felt by those close to the person who is dying or who has died.

Grieving for the loss of someone that we love can be a lonely and frightening experience. Although many people talk about stages of grief, it is actually an unpredictable experience. Feelings can come and go in waves, taking the person forward and then pulling them back. Each person's experience of grief is different, although there are certain thoughts and emotions common to most people.

There is no fixed time scale for grieving; it is a natural process and varies from person to person. However, as an individual gradually faces up to and experiences the pain of grieving, the intensity of feelings will lessen with time and become more bearable. They may always miss the person they have lost and have special memories of them, but it will eventually become possible to live with the loss.

Numbness, shock and disbelief are common in the early days of bereavement. There may be displaced anger, which may be directed inappropriately towards the staff, especially if there appear to have been delays in diagnosis or problems with treatment. The best preparation for bereavement is sympathetic handling of the patient's and family's problems throughout their cancer journey. If anger is displayed, a

---

Box 48.9 Common symptoms in the last 48 h of life

- Pain
- Incontinence of urine
- Dyspnoea
- Retention
- Nausea and vomiting
- Sweating
- Jerking, twitching
- Plucking
- Confusion

Source: Lichter I, Hunt M 1990 Journal of Palliative Care 6: 7–15. Copyright: Institut universitaire de gériatrie de Montréal.

---

confrontational or authoritarian approach should be avoided. Questions should be answered honestly and often the real cause of the anger will eventually become apparent.

Immediate expressions of grief vary but the bereaved person may:

- experience numbness and shock at their loss — they may not be able to believe that the person is gone, particularly in the first few weeks;
- think that they have seen or heard the deceased person;
- feel guilty for things done or not done when the person was alive;
- feel angry with the deceased, medical profession or God;
- be relieved that the deceased's suffering is over;
- feel anxious, lonely, exhausted, depressed or despairing;
- search for reasons why they have lost their loved one;
- feel that they are 'going mad' because of the strength of their feelings;
- feel disappointed and/or cheated about plans and expectations that will never be fulfilled;
- have difficulties eating, concentrating and sleeping (due to persistent thoughts of the deceased or nightmares);
- feel unwell or generally run down;
- find everyday situations and relationships difficult to deal with;
- feel that no one understands how they feel;
- find it impossible to think about the future or believe that they could ever be happy again; and
- find that they have changes in sexual drive and desire.

Suggested 'dos' and 'do nots' that may help the bereaved person and their family in their grief are shown below:

Do

- Remember that grief is a normal process.
- Talk about your feelings.
- Resume a normal routine 2–3 weeks after the death.

- Allow children to go back to school and keep their normal activities, such as hobbies or playing sport.
- Allow children to share the grief by expressing their feelings and asking questions. Allow them to attend the funeral if they want to.
- Accept support, both practical and emotional, from family and friends.
- Take care of yourself — eat a balanced diet and take plenty of rest. Illness and accidents are more common when people are going through a traumatic time.
- Allow yourself time to grieve. When you are feeling low, take one day at a time. Grief cannot be hurried or avoided.

Do not

- Cut yourself off from sources of support.
- 'Bottle up' feelings and emotions.
- Dispose of the deceased's belongings until you are ready.
- Make major life decisions or changes in the first year of a bereavement if it can be avoided
- Turn to drugs, alcohol or heavy smoking.

Sources of Support

The bereaved person may feel that they have enough support from family, friends, the church or other organizations. However, feelings may sometimes seem too intense to cope with, or the bereaved may feel that they have no one to talk to who understands. They may find it helpful to talk about their feelings to someone outside their family and friends, or to meet people in a similar situation. This will not take away the pain of their loss, but may help them to cope better.

There are many national support organizations who help and support bereaved individuals.

KEY POINTS

1. Most patients prefer to be told the truth about their condition.
2. Supportive care is not the sole responsibility of one person but the onus lies with the doctor.
3. Staff need to be aware of their own feelings and attitudes to illness and death.
4. Staff must watch and listen carefully and respond to what they observe, rather than have any preconceived ideas about the woman's feelings and needs.
5. Time with the patient must be protected from interruption, and adequate time must be allocated.
6. Accepting the inevitability of mental pain in the patient frees the physician from feelings of inadequacy.
7. There must be no conspiracy of silence in the family, and children need to be included.
8. Many sexual problems can be avoided by simple discussion and encouragement.
9. Analgesia should usually be given orally in regular doses.
10. Intravenous fluids should be avoided in obstruction unless it is clear that surgical correction is a feasible option.
11. Cyclizine and haloperidol are very useful for controlling nausea in obstruction.
12. The GP can play a central role in mobilizing local help.
13. Bereavement affects both family and staff. Both need to mourn.

References

Anderson BL 1985 Sexual functioning and morbidity among cancer survivors: patient status and future research directions. Cancer 55: 1835–1842.

Anderson BL 1993 Predicting sexual and psychological morbidity and improving the quality of life for women with gynaecology cancer. Cancer 71: 1678–1690.

Anderson B, Lutgendorf S 1997 Quality of life in gynaecologic cancer survivors. Cancer: a Journal for Clinicians 47: 218–225.

Auchinloss C 1989 Sexual dysfunction in cancer patients: issues in evaluation and treatment. In: Holland J, Rowland J (eds) Handbook of Psycho-oncology. Oxford University Press, New York.

Bancroft J 1989 Human Sexuality and its Problems, 2nd edn. Churchill Livingstone, Edinburgh.

Bullard D, Causey G, Newman A 1980 Sexual health care and cancer: a needs assessment. In: Vaeth J (ed) Frontiers of Radiation Therapy in Oncology. Karger, Basel.

Burke LM 1996 Sexual dysfunction following radiotherapy for cervical cancer. British Journal of Nursing 4: 239–244.

Clark C, Cross J, Deane D, Lowry L 1991 Spirituality: integral to quality care. Holistic Nursing Practice 5: 67–76.

Clinebell HJJ 1966 Basic Types of Pastoral Counselling. Abington Press, Nashville, TN.

Colyer H 1996 Women's experiences of living with cancer (body image and sexuality in gynaecological cancer patients, focusing on three patient histories). Journal of Advanced Nursing 23: 496–501.

Corless I 1992 Hospice and hope: an incompatible duo. American Journal of Hospice and Palliative Care 9: 10–12.

Corney R, Everett H, Howells A, Crowther M 1992 The care of patients undergoing surgery for gynaecological cancer, the need for information, emotional support and counselling. Journal of Advanced Nursing 17: 667–671.

Corney RH, Crowther ME, Everett H et al 1993 Psychosexual dysfunction in women with gynaecological cancer following radical pelvic surgery. British Journal of Obstetrics and Gynaecology 100: 73–78.

Cull A, Cowie VJ, Farquharson D et al 1993. Early stage cervical cancer: psychosocial and sexual outcomes of treatment. British Journal of Cancer 68: 1216–1220.

Derogatis L 1980 Breast and gynaecological cancers: their unique impact on body image and sexual identity in women. In: Vaeth J (ed) Frontiers of Radiation Therapy and Oncology. Karger, Basel.

Dickenson C 1975 The search for spiritual meaning. American Journal of Nursing 75: 1789–1793.

Donovan K, Sanson-Fisher RW, Redman S 1989 Measuring quality of life in cancer patients. Journal of Clinical Oncology 7: 959–968.

Dudas S 1992 Manifestations of cancer treatment. In: Groenwold S, Hanson-Frogge M, Goodman M, Henke-Yarbo C (eds) Cancer Symptom Management. Jones and Bartlett, Boston.

Ellison E 1983 Spiritual well-being: conceptualization and measurement. Journal of Psychology and Theology 11: 330–340.

Faulkner A, Maguire P 1994 Talking to Cancer Patients and their Relatives. Oxford Medical Publications, Oxford.

Frankl VE 1987 Man's Search for Meaning, 50th edn. Hodder and Stoughton, London.

Gallo-Silver L 2000 The sexual rehabilitation of persons with cancer. Cancer Practice 8: 10–15.

Green J 1999 Taking a sexual history. Trends in Urology/Gynaecology and Sexual Health 31–33.

Hogbin B, Fallowfield L 1989 Getting it taped: the 'bad news'. Consultation with cancer patients. British Journal of Hospital Medicine 41: 330–333.

Kay P 1994 A–Z Pocket Book of Symptom Control. EPL Publications, London.

Kay P 1996 Breaking Bad News. EPL Publications, London.

Improving Outcome Guidance 1999 Guidelines on Commissioning Cancer Services. Improving Outcomes in Gynaecological Cancers. Department of Health, UK.

King CR, Harman M, Berry DL et al 1997 Quality of life and the cancer experience: the state of the knowledge. Oncology Nursing Forum 24: 27–41.

Lamb M 1985 Sexual dysfunction in gynaecology oncology patients. Seminars in Oncology Nursing 1: 9–17.

Lane J 1987 The care of the human spirit. Journal of Professional Nursing 3: 332–337.

Laurent M 1994 Talking treatment: nursing counsellor's role in helping patients deal with the psychosocial and sexual problems of treatment for cervical cancer. Nursing Times 10: 14–15.

Leiblum SR, Rosen RC (eds) 1989 Principles and Practice of Sex Therapy. Guilford Press, New York.

Lichter I 1987 Communication in Cancer Care. Churchill Livingstone, Edinburgh.

MacElveen-Hoehn P, McCorkle R 1985 Understanding sexuality in progressive disease. Seminars in Oncology Nursing 1: 56–62.

Maguire P 1993 Handling the withdrawn patients — a flow diagram. Palliative Medicine 7: 333–338.

Massie MJ, Holland JC 1989 Overview of normal reactions and prevalence of psychiatric disorders. In: Holland JC, Rowlands JH (eds) Handbook of Psycho-oncology. Oxford Medical Press, Oxford.

Masters WH, Johnson VE 1970 Human Sexual Inadequacy. Churchill, London.

Masters W, Johnson V, Kolodny R 1995 Human Sexuality. Harper Collins, New York.

Miller J 1985 Assessment of loneliness and spiritual well-being in chronically ill and healthy adults. Journal of Professional Nursing 1: 79–85.

Moberg D 1982 Spiritual well-being of the dying. In: Lesnoff-Caravaglia G (ed) Aging and the Human Condition. Human Sciences Press, Springfield, IL.

Model G 1990 A new image to accept: psychological aspects of stoma care. Professional Nurse 3: 10–16.

Pace JC 2000 Spirituality issues. Women and Cancer: a Gynaecological Oncology Nursing Perspective 15: 579–598.

Penson RT, Gallagher J, Giorella M et al 2000 Sexuality and cancer: conversation comfort zone. The Oncologist 5: 336–344.

Price B 1990 Body Image: Nursing Concepts and Care. Prentice Hall, London.

Royal College of Nursing 2000 P-LI-SS-IT model. In: Sexuality and Sexual Health in Nursing Practice. RCN, London.

Reed P 1987 Spirituality and well-being in terminally ill hospitalized adults. Research in Nursing and Health 10: 335–344.

Rutter M 2000 The impact of illness on sexuality. In: Wells D (ed) Caring for Sexuality in Health and Illness. Churchill Livingstone, Edinburgh.

Sacco Ezzell P 1999 Managing the effects of gynaecological cancer treatment on quality of life and sexuality. Society of Gynaecological Nursing Oncologists 8: 23–26.

Saunders C, Baines M 1989 Living with Dying. Oxford Medical Publications, Oxford.

Smith DB 1989 Sexual rehabilitation of the cancer patient. Cancer Nursing 12: 10–15.

Smithman C 1981 Nursing Actions for Health Care Promotion. FA Davis, Philadelphia.

Steginga K, Dunn J 1997 Women's experiences following treatment for gynaecological cancer. Oncology Nurses Forum 24: 1403–1407.

Twycross R 1997a Symptom Management in Advanced Cancer, 2nd edn. Radcliffe Medical Press, Oxford.

Twycross R 1997b Introductory Palliative Care, 2nd edn. Radcliffe Medical Press, Oxford.

Twycross R, Lack S 1983 Symptom Control in Far Advanced Cancer: Pain Relief. Pitman Medical, Tunbridge Wells.

Veronesi U, ven Kleist S, Redmond K et al 1999 Caring about women and cancer (CAWAC): a European survey of the perspectives and experiences of women with female cancers. European Journal of Cancer 35: 1667–1675.

Wilson E, Williams H 1988 Oncology nurses' attitudes and behaviours related to sexuality of patients with cancer. Oncology Nursing Forum 15: 49–53.

Woods N 1975 Human Sexuality in Health and Illness. CV Mosby, St Louis.

World Health Organization 1986 Concepts for Sexual Health. WHO Regional Office for Europe, Copenhagen.

Further Reading

Hammersmith Hospital Trust 2001 Breaking Bad News: Guidelines for Staff. HHT Palliative Care Team, London.

Hammersmith Hospital Trust 2001 Talking to Children about Cancer: Guidelines. HHT Palliative Care Team, London.

Classification of urogynaecological disorders

Stuart L. Stanton and Ash Monga

Chapter Contents

INTRODUCTION	767	CONCLUSION	769
TERMINOLOGY	767	KEY POINTS	769
CLASSIFICATION	768		

Introduction

If the body was divided into specialties by physiological rather than anatomical boundaries, there would be no need for an explanation of urogynaecology. As it is, this specialty represents an interface between gynaecologist and urologist. Physiological events or disease affecting gynaecological organs invariably affect the urinary tract, as they will also sometimes affect the adjacent alimentary system.

It is increasingly recognized that colorectal surgeons have an important role in the management of pelvic floor disorders. The studies of Snooks et al (1984a,b) and Sultan et al (1993) show the traumatic effects of vaginal delivery on the pelvic floor and anal sphincters. Wall and de Lancey (1991) succinctly summarized the need for a holistic approach involving gynaecologists, urologists and colorectal surgeons in the management of pelvic floor disorders.

Following the introduction of subspecialization by the American College of Obstetricians and Gynecologists, the Royal College of Obstetricians and Gynaecologists considered and then recommended subspecialization in 1982. Four subspecialties were created, among them urogynaecology. This comprised the following disorders: congenital anomalies, incontinence, voiding difficulties, urinary fistulae, bladder neuropathy, genital prolapse, urgency and frequency, and urinary tract infection. By common consent, all 'supravesical' conditions and neoplasia arising anywhere in the urinary tract belong to the realm of urology.

To these might now be added disordered bowel motility, descending perineum and rectal prolapse, anal sphincter injuries, rectovaginal fistula, perineal hernia, and faecal and flatal incontinence.

Terminology

As in any developing branch of medicine and science, old terms and definitions have become inadequate. To provide a common language for both clinician and researcher, the International Continence Society's (1973) Standardization Committee drew up standards of terminology of lower urinary tract function.

Nine reports have now been published, as follows.

1. Standardization of terminology of lower urinary tract dysfunction (Abrams et al 1988).
2. Lower urinary tract rehabilitation techniques: seventh report on the standardization of terminology of lower urinary tract function (Anderson et al 1992).
3. Standardization of terminology of female pelvic organ prolapse and pelvic floor dysfunction (Bump et al 1996).
4. Standardization of terminology and assessment of functional characteristics of intestinal urinary reservoirs (Thuroff et al 1996).
5. Standardization of terminology of lower urinary tract function: pressure–flow studies of voiding, urethral resistance and urethral obstruction (Griffiths et al 1997).
6. Standardization of outcome studies in patients with lower urinary tract dysfunction: a report on general principles from the Standardization Committee of the International Continence Society (Mattiasson et al 1998).
7. Outcome measures for research in adult women with symptoms of lower urinary tract dysfunction (Lose et al 1998).
8. Outcome measures for research of lower urinary tract dysfunction in frail older people (Fonda et al 1998).
9. Standardization of terminology in neurogenic lower urinary tract dysfunction (Stöhrer et al 1999).

The term 'stress incontinence' was coined by Sir Eardley Holland in 1928 and meant the loss of urine during physical effort. It came to be used not only as a symptom and sign, but also as a diagnostic term. As the pathophysiology of urinary incontinence became more clearly understood, it was apparent that the term 'stress incontinence' was ambiguous as it could be applied to a symptom, a sign and a diagnosis; indeed, the symptoms and sign of stress incontinence can be found in most types of incontinence.

Nowadays, the term 'stress incontinence' is retained for the symptom of involuntary loss of urine on physical exertion and the sign of urine loss from the urethra immediately on increase in abdominal pressure. The term 'genuine stress incontinence' was proposed by the International Continence Society in 1976 (Bates et al 1976) to mean the condition of involuntary loss of urine when 'the intravesical pressure exceeds the maximum urethral pressure in the absence of a detrusor contraction'. This condition has a number of synonyms: urethral sphincter incompetence, stress urinary incontinence and anatomical stress incontinence. The authors prefer the term 'urethral sphincter incompetence' because this accurately describes the pathophysiology of this condition.

In a similar way, the term 'dyssynergic detrusor dysfunction' was introduced by Hodgkinson et al in 1963 and other synonyms followed: urge incontinence, uninhibited bladder, bladder instability/unstable bladder and, more recently, overactive bladder. In 1979, the International Continence Society defined an unstable bladder as one 'shown objectively to contract, spontaneously or on provocation during the filling phase, while the patient is attempting to inhibit micturition. Unstable contractions may be asymptomatic and do not necessarily imply a neurological disorder.' The contractions are phasic. Another term, 'low compliance', is used to mean a gradual increase in detrusor pressure without a subsequent decrease during bladder filling. The term 'neurogenic detruser overactivity' is used for phasic uninhibited contractions when there is objective evidence of a relevant neurological disorder. Terms to be avoided include 'hypertonic', 'spastic' and 'automatic'.

Classification

Congenital anomalies (see Chapter 1)

The subject of congenital anomalies reaffirms the principle that a lesion affects multiple systems. These often present to the urologist as a primary urological problem (e.g. bladder exstrophy, horseshoe kidney). The gynaecologist's expertise lies in the area of diagnosis and management of dubious sexuality or later, when reconstructive surgery may be required for epispadias or haematocolpos.

Incontinence

Urinary incontinence forms the major proportion of urogynaecology. It is defined by the International Continence Society as 'an involuntary loss of urine which is objectively demonstrable and a social or hygienic problem'.

Incontinence is considered to be involuntary; for two categories of patients, further explanation is needed. In a child under 3 years of age, control of continence has not yet developed; however, careful observation shows that the normal child is dry between involuntary voids, whereas the incontinent child is wet the whole time. On the other hand, the mentally frail or elderly demented patient may be incontinent because she has lost her social consciousness and appreciation of the need to be dry.

The social isolation caused by incontinence is demonstrated by 25% of patients delaying for more than 5 years before seeking advice, owing to embarrassment (Norton et al 1988). Ostracism and rejection by relatives may lead to an elderly patient being institutionalized solely because of incontinence; paradoxically, some allegedly 'caring' institutions will not accept an elderly patient if she is incontinent.

It is now accepted that incontinence should be objectively demonstrable using urodynamic studies, which will define the cause and detect other conditions such as voiding disorders and overactive bladder.

The hygienic aspect of incontinence occupies some 25% of nursing time in hospitals. Unless managed, urinary odour is offensive to both patient and relatives alike.

Incontinence may be divided into urethral and extraurethral conditions (Figure 49.1).

Urethral conditions

Urethral sphincter incompetence (urodynamic stress incontinence)

This is the most common urethral condition, has several causes and can present from childhood (see Chapter 52). The original classification of type 1, 2 and 3 is facile. It is realistic to acknowledge that whilst only some patients have 'urethral hypermobility', all will have some degree of sphincter incompetence, otherwise they would not leak. Type 3 is gross incontinence with a maximum urethral closure pressure below 20 cmH$_2$O (more usefully termed 'intrinsic sphincter defect'). Conventional bladder neck elevating surgery or even midurethral support surgery is unlikely to succeed in type 3 patients; what is required is something to restore urethral pressure, such as an artificial urinary sphincter. For the vast majority (i.e. old type 1 and 2), either a bladder neck elevating procedure, such as a colposuspension or sling, or a midurethral support procedure, such as a

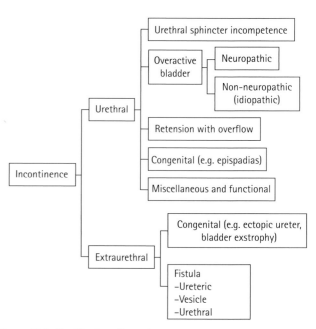

Figure 49.1 Classification of incontinence.

tension-free vaginal tape procedure, will likely suffice. The latter has shown that lack of midurethral support is a significant cause of sphincter incompetence.

Overactive bladder (see Chapter 53)

Depending on its cause, this may be subdivided into neuropathic or idiopathic. Some patients with overactive bladder and a competent sphincter mechanism may remain dry. If, however, there is coexistent sphincteric incompetence ('mixed incontinence'), the patient may complain of stress incontinence and urge incontinence.

Urinary retention and overflow (see Chapter 54)

This may be acute or chronic; the former is usually sudden in onset and painful. There may be an obvious cause, such as an impacted pelvic mass. Chronic retention, on the other hand, is often painless, insidious and frequently undetected, so errors in diagnosis are often made. It occurs more commonly in the elderly as a result of neuropathy (e.g. peripheral diabetic neuropathy or stenosis of the lumbar spinal canal).

Congenital disorders

Epispadias is usually detected during childhood, but occasionally it is not diagnosed until adult life.

Miscellaneous

These causes include urethral diverticulum, urinary tract infection (temporary and most common in the elderly), faecal impaction, drugs (such as α-adrenergic blocking agents) and functional disorders. These are rare; the patient should be fully investigated and all the above causes excluded before this diagnosis is made. The loss of social awareness of the need to be continent is usually associated with dementia or a space-occupying lesion of the frontal cortex.

Extraurethral conditions

These may be divided into congenital and acquired. Extraurethral conditions may be distinguished from urethral conditions by the symptom of continuous incontinence. The congenital disorders include ectopic ureter and bladder exstrophy. Acquired conditions include urinary fistulae, which in the Western world are largely iatrogenic, the majority occurring after abdominal hysterectomy for benign conditions (see Chapter 57). Other causes include pelvic carcinoma and its attendant surgery or radiotherapy. In the developing world, obstetrical causes such as obstructed labour with an impacted vertex are more common. If the fistula is small, skill and patience are required to detect it.

Voiding difficulties (see Chapter 54)

These are uncommon in the female and are frequently undiagnosed. If untreated, they can lead to recurrent urinary tract infection, or acute or chronic retention following otherwise successful bladder neck surgery for incontinence.

Urinary fistulae

These have already been referred to and are dealt with at length in Chapter 57.

Bladder neuropathy

This is rightfully dealt with by the urologist, but it is important for the gynaecologist to be aware of and to recognize these disorders.

Genital prolapse

Prolapse should not be considered in isolation as it is sometimes associated with urethral sphincter incompetence, or with perineal descent and faecal incontinence (see Chapter 55). The latter conditions represent an important interface with the colorectal surgeon.

Urgency and frequency

These symptoms can, of course, be part of a urinary disease process, such as urinary tract infection or overactive bladder, but can often present as single or combined symptoms in the absence of an obvious pathology (see Chapter 56).

Urinary tract infection (see Chapter 58)

This is of common interest to the obstetrician/gynaecologist, urologist and nephrologist, and the experience of all three may be required for difficult cases. However, the majority of patients are treated by the general practitioner without referral to hospital, although urinary tract infection is frequently unproven. Inadequate treatment during pregnancy can lead to acute pyelonephritis and abortion, and if neglected in later life, can lead to chronic pyelonephritis, hypertension and later renal failure.

Conclusion

This classification is an introduction to urogynaecology and the ensuing chapters will provide more detail. For more specialized reading, a list of selected books is given after the references.

KEY POINTS

1. Trauma, denervation and the menopause affect the whole of the pelvic floor.
2. Urogynaecology needs to include rectal prolapse, anal sphincter injury and rectovaginal fistula.
3. Standardized terminology and methodology, as suggested by the International Continence Society, should be used.
4. Incontinence has a variety of causes which need urodynamic studies for their accurate diagnosis.
5. Stress incontinence is a symptom and a sign, not a diagnosis.

References

Abrams P, Blaivas J, Stanton SL, Andersen J 1988 Standardization of terminology of lower urinary tract function. International Continence Society. Scandinavian Journal of Urology and Nephrology 114 (Suppl): 5–19.

Anderson JT, Blaivas JG, Cardozo L, Thüroff J 1992 Lower urinary tract rehabilitation techniques: seventh report on the standardisation of terminology of lower urinary tract function. International Urogynecology Journal 3:75–80.

Bates P, Bradley W, Glen E et al 1976 First report on standardization of terminology of lower urinary tract function. International Continence Society. British Journal of Urology 48: 39–42.

Bump R, Mattiasson A, Bo K et al 1996 Standardization of terminology of female pelvic organ prolapse and pelvic floor dysfunction. ICS Committee on Standardization of Terminology. American Journal of Obstetrics and Gynecology 175: 10–17.

Fonda D, Resnick NM, Colling J, Burgio K et al 1998 Outcome measures for research of lower urinary tract dysfunction in frail older people. Neurourology and Urodynamics 17: 173–281.

Griffiths D, Hofner K, van Mastrigt R et al 1997 Standardization of terminology of lower urinary tract function: pressure flow studies of voiding, urethral resistance and urethral obstruction. Neurourology and Urodynamics 16: 1–18.

Hodgkinson CP, Ayers M, Drukker B 1963 Dyssynergic detrusor dysfunction in the apparently normal female. American Journal of Obstetrics and Gynecology 87: 717–730.

Lose G, Fantl JA, Victor A et al 1998 Outcome measures for research in adult women with symptoms of lower urinary tract dysfunction. Neurourology and Urodynamics 17: 255–262.

Mattiasson A, Djurhuus JC, Fonda D et al 1998 Standardization of outcome studies in patients with lower urinary tract dysfunction: a report on general principles from the Standardisation Committee of the International Continence Society. Neurourology and Urodynamics 17: 249–253.

Norton P, MacDonald L, Sedgwick P, Stanton SL 1988 Distress and delay associated with urinary incontinence, frequency and urgency in women. BMJ (Clinical Research Ed.) 297: 1187–1189.

Snooks S, Barnes P, Swash M 1984a Damage to innervation of the voluntary anal and periurethral sphincter musculature in incontinence: an electrophysiological study. Journal of Neurology, Neurosurgery and Psychiatry 47: 1269–1273.

Snooks S, Swash M, Henry M, Setchell M 1984b Injury to innervation of pelvic floor sphincter musculature in childbirth. The Lancet ii: 546–550.

Stöhrer M, Goepel M, Kondo A et al 1999 The standardisation of terminology in neurogenic lower urinary tract dysfunction. Neurourology and Urodynamics 18: 139–158.

Sultan A, Kamm M, Hudson C, Thomas J, Bartram C 1993 Anal sphincter disruption during vaginal delivery. New England Journal of Medicine 329: 1905–1911.

Thuroff J, Mattiasson A, Anderson JT et al 1996 Standardization of terminology and assessment of functional characteristics of intestinal urinary reservoirs. Neurourology and Urodynamics 15: 499–511.

Wall LL, de Lancey J 1991 The politics of prolapse: a revisionist approach to disorders of the pelvic floor in women. Perspectives in Biology and Medicine 34: 486–496.

Further Reading

Cardozo L, Staskind D 2001 Textbook of Female Urology and Urogynaecology. Martin Dunitz, London.

Lentz G 2000 Urogynecology. Arnold, London.

Mundy A, Stephenson T, Wein A 1994 Urodynamics: Principles, Practice and Application, 2nd edn. Churchill Livingstone, Edinburgh.

Ostergard D, Bent A 1996 Urogynecology and Urodynamics: Theory and Practice, 4th edn. Williams and Wilkins, Baltimore.

Sand P, Ostergard D 1995 Urodynamics and Evaluation of Female Incontinence. Springer-Verlag, London.

Stanton SL, Tanagho E 1986 Surgery of Female Incontinence, 2nd edn. Springer-Verlag, Heidelberg.

Stanton SL, Monga A 2000 Clinical Urogynaecology, 2nd edn. Churchill Livingstone, London.

Stanton SL, Owyer PL 2000 Urinary Tract Infection in the Female. Martin Dunitz, London.

Stanton SL, Zimmern P 2002 Female Pelvic Reconstructive Surgery. Springer-Verlag, London.

Wall L, Norton P, de Lancey J 1993 Practical Urogynaecology. Williams and Wilkins, Baltimore.

Walters M, Karram M 1999 Urogynecology and Reconstructive Surgery, 2nd edn. Mosby, St Louis.

Zacharin RF 1988 Obstetric Fistula. Springer-Verlag, Vienna.

CHAPTER 50

The mechanism of continence

Ash Monga and Abdul Sultan

Chapter Contents

URINARY INCONTINENCE	771	CONCLUSIONS	781
ANAL INCONTINENCE	776	KEY POINTS	781
COMPARISON BETWEEN BLADDER AND BOWEL	781		

Urinary Incontinence

Introduction

Urinary incontinence may be defined as a condition in which an involuntary loss of urine is a social or hygienic problem and is objectively demonstrable. Therefore, continence is the ability to retain urine within the bladder between voluntary acts of micturition. In order to fully comprehend the pathological processes which lead to the development of urinary incontinence, a clear understanding of normal mechanisms for the maintenance of continence is fundamental.

Anatomy of the lower urinary tract

The bladder

The bladder consists of three layers of smooth muscle, known collectively as the 'detrusor', which functions as one syncytial mass with the exception of the trigone. The outer smooth muscle layer is oriented longitudinally, the middle layer is oriented circularly and the inner layer is oriented longitudinally.

Histochemically, the detrusor muscle has been shown to be rich in acetylcholinesterase by virtue of its rich cholinergic parasympathetic nerve supply. In contrast, the trigone only comprises two layers of smooth muscle. The inner layer is similar to the rest of the detrusor, but the outer layer consists of smooth muscle bundles with a sparse parasympathetic nerve supply. The outer layer extends to, and is continuous with, the proximal urethra and the distal portion of the ureter, where it may have a role in preventing ureteric reflux. The smooth muscle that forms the bladder neck is separate from the detrusor, with little or no sphincteric effect. Two or three layers of transitional epithelia cover the detrusor and secrete a protein on to their luminal surface that forms a watertight blood–bladder barrier. When empty, the urothelium relaxes into numerous folds or rugae.

The urethra

The normal female urethra is 30–50 mm in length. It comprises smooth and striated muscle. The smooth muscle is continuous with that of the detrusor, but has minimal parasympathetic innervation and little sphincteric effect in contrast to the profusion of acetylcholinesterase within the detrusor cells. The external urethral sphincter (rhabdosphincter) is one of two striated muscle components surrounding the urethra. Its fibres are bulked anteriorly at the midurethral level, are slow twitch in nature and are involved in maintaining continence at rest. The second striated muscle component is the periurethral portion of the levator ani, which is separated from the external urethral sphincter by a connective tissue septum. The fibres are bulked anterolaterally at a lower level than the external urethral sphincter, are fast twitch in nature and are involved in maintaining continence under stress.

The mucosa of the urethra is lined by pseudostratified transitional epithelia proximally, changing to non-keratinized stratified squamous epithelia distally. The junction between the two cell types alters with age and oestrogenic status, which may affect urinary symptoms. In young females, the submucosa has a rich venous supply which engorges the tissues, helping to close the urethra. This ceases after the menopause, and may be involved in the development of stress incontinence later in life due to poor urethral closure.

The pelvic floor

For the context of this chapter, the pelvic floor structures that will be described are the levator ani muscles, the endopelvic fascia and condensations of this fascia which form the ligaments. The levator ani muscles are often described as funnel-shaped structures, but in-vivo imaging has revealed that they are, in fact, more horizontal. The fibres of each side pass downwards and inwards. The two muscles, one on each side, constitute the pelvic diaphragm. Defects in the levator ani allow the urethra, vagina and

DOI: 10.1016/B978-0-7020-3120-5.00050-3

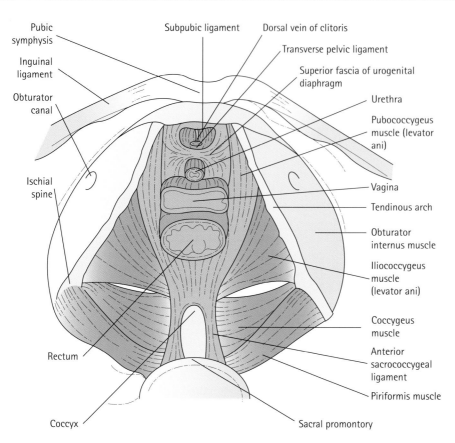

Pubic symphysis
Inguinal ligament
Obturator canal
Ischial spine
Rectum
Coccyx

Subpubic ligament
Dorsal vein of clitoris
Transverse pelvic ligament
Superior fascia of urogenital diaphragm
Urethra
Pubococcygeus muscle (levator ani)
Vagina
Tendinous arch
Obturator internus muscle
Iliococcygeus muscle (levator ani)
Coccygeus muscle
Anterior sacrococcygeal ligament
Piriformis muscle
Sacral promontory

Figure 50.1 The pelvic floor musculature and ligaments.

rectum to pass. The levator ani is subdivided into the pubococcygeus, iliococcygeus and coccygeus. The pubococcygeus arises anteriorly from the posterior aspect of the pubic bone and from the anterior portion of the arcus tendineus (white line), which is a condensation of the obturator internus fascia. The medial fibres of the pubococcygeus merge with the fibres of the vagina and perineal body, and have been given various names such as puborectalis, pubourethralis and pubovaginalis. The iliococcygeus arises from the remainder of the arcus tendineus, partly overlapping the pubococcygeus on its perineal surface and extending to the medial surface of the ischial spine. The coccygeus or ischiococcygeus is a rudimentary muscle arising from the tip of the ischial spine, and quite often constitutes only a few muscle fibres on the sacrospinous ligament. Posteriorly, the muscles of the levator ani or pelvic diaphragm insert into the sides of the coccyx and the anococcygeal raphe, which is formed by the interdigitation of muscle fibres from either side. The most medial fibres of the pubococcygeus that pass round the rectum at the anorectal junction form the puborectalis muscle (Figure 50.1).

The endopelvic fascia invests all the structures that lie within the pelvis and is mainly composed of loose areolar tissue, although smooth muscle cells have been identified. The layer between the bladder, urethra and vagina is termed the 'vesicovaginal fascia', and the layer between the vagina and rectum is known as the 'rectovaginal fascia' or 'rectovaginal septum'. Laterally, both these layers attach to a condensation of fascia known as the 'arcus tendineus fasciae pelvis'. This is a condensation of the endopelvic fascia which runs from the posterior part of the pubic ramus to the ischial

spine, and attaches to the stronger underlying obturator internus muscle fascia. The urethra has an intimate attachment to the lower one-third of the vagina, and therefore the supports for these structures are identical. The urethra has a further condensation of the endopelvic fascia which attaches to the symphysis pubis. These are known as the 'pubourethral ligaments' and lie at the midportion of the urethra. They are fairly loose attachments, and allow movement of the bladder neck during straining and also by voluntary contraction of the levator ani muscles.

The uterus, cervix and upper third of the vagina are attached to the pelvic side wall by broad condensations of endopelvic fascia with a high content of smooth muscle cells, known as the 'cardinal and uterosacral ligaments'. These ligaments originate from the region of the greater sciatic foramen and the lateral aspects of the sacrum. In the erect position, these ligaments run almost vertically and suspend their attached structures.

The levator ani muscles, ligaments and endopelvic fascia work in synergy. If any of these structures is not intact, the mechanisms of support and continence may be affected.

Innervation of the bladder and urethra

The bladder has a rich parasympathetic nerve supply (Figure 50.2). The postganglionic cell bodies lie either in the bladder wall or pelvic plexuses, innervated by preganglionic fibres that originate from cell bodies in the grey columns of S2–4. There is little sympathetic innervation of the bladder, although greater quantities of noradrenergic terminals can be detected in the bladder neck or trigone. Noradrenergic

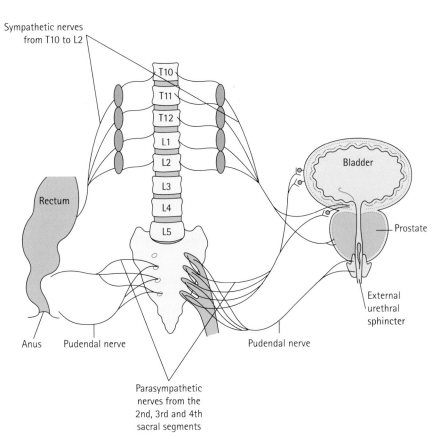

Figure 50.2 The major innervation pathways at the pelvic level that are basic to control of micturition and continence.

effects can be either inhibitory or excitatory, depending on the receptor type present.

- α-Receptors, located predominantly in the bladder base, cause detrusor contraction. They can be manipulated with limited success with α-adrenergic agonists to treat mild stress incontinence.
- β-Receptors which cause detrusor relaxation are found in the dome of the bladder.

The cell bodies of the sympathetic nerves originate in the grey matter of T10–L2, and pass through the sympathetic chain via the lumbar splanchnic nerve and left and right hypogastric nerves to the pelvic plexus. It is thought that the sympathetic nervous system exerts its effects by inhibiting the parasympathetic nervous system rather than by direct action. The visceral nerve afferents pass along the sacral and thoracolumbar visceral efferents, relaying sensations of touch, pain and distension. However, transection has little or no effect on micturition. The urethra possesses similar autonomic innervation. Parasympathetic efferents cause contraction but the functional significance of this remains in doubt. There is no obvious sphincteric function, but contraction produces shortening and widening of the urethra along with detrusor contraction during micturition. Sympathetic efferents innervate the predominantly α-adrenoreceptors.

Innervation of striated muscle

The rhabdosphincter muscle is supplied via the pelvic splanchnic nerves travelling with the parasympathetic fibres to the intrinsic smooth muscle of the urethra. This is analogous to the puborectalis muscle.

The extrinsic periurethral muscle of the levator ani is innervated by motor fibres of the perineal branch of the pudendal nerve. This is in common with the external anal sphincter (EAS). The pudendal nerve also supplies the striated elements of the levator ani on both sides, and there are associated somatic afferent fibres which travel with the pudendal nerves. They ascend via the dorsal columns to convey proprioception from the pelvic floor.

Central nervous control of continence

The connections of the lower urinary tract within the central nervous system are complex (Figure 50.3). There are many discrete areas which influence micturition, and these have been identified within the cerebral cortex, in the superior frontal and anterior cingulate gyri of the frontal lobe and the paracentral lobule; within the cerebellum, in the anterior vermis and fastigial nucleus; and in subcortical areas, including the thalamus, the basal ganglia, the limbic system, the hypothalamus and discrete areas of the mesencephalic pontine medullary reticular formation. The full function and interactions of these various areas are incompletely understood, although the effects of ablation and tumour growth in humans and stimulation studies in animals have given some insights.

The centres within the cerebral cortex are important in the perception of sensation in the lower urinary tract, and the inhibition and subsequent initiation of voiding. Lesions in the superior frontal gyrus and the adjacent anterior cin-

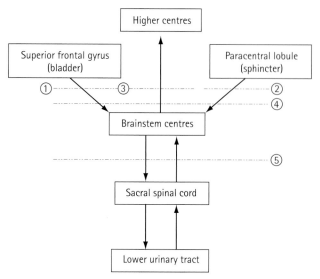

Figure 50.3 The interaction of the nervous system in micturition. Locations of possible nervous lesions are denoted by numbers. 1, lesions isolating superior frontal gyrus will prevent voluntary postponement of voiding; 2, lesions isolating paracentral lobule, often with hemiparesis, will cause spasticity of urethral sphincter and retention; 3, pathways of sensation are not known accurately; in theory, isolated lesion of sensation above brainstem would lead to unconscious incontinence, and defective conduction of sensory information would explain enuresis; 4, lesions above brainstem centres lead to involuntary voiding that is coordinated with sphincter relaxation; 5, lesions below brainstem centres but above the sacral spinal cord lead, after a period of bladder paralysis, to involuntary 'reflex' voiding that is not coordinated with sphincter relaxation.

gulate gyrus reduce or abolish both the conscious and unconscious inhibition of the micturition reflex. The bladder tends to empty at low functional capacity. Sometimes, the patient is aware of the sensation of urgency; sometimes, micturition may be entirely unconscious. These areas, which have been localized by functional magnetic resonance imaging (MRI), are supplied by the anterior cerebral and pericallosal arteries; spasm or occlusion of these arteries produces incontinence.

Localized lesions more posteriorly in the paracentral lobule may produce retention rather than incontinence because of the combination of impaired sensation and spasticity of the pelvic floor.

The thalamus is the principal relay centre for pathways projecting to the cerebral cortex, and ascending pathways activated by bladder and urethral receptors synapse on neurones in specific thalamic nuclei which have reciprocal connections with the cortex. Electrical stimulation of the basal ganglia in animals leads to suppression of the detrusor reflex, whereas ablation has resulted in detrusor hyper-reflexia; patients with Parkinsonism are commonly shown to have detrusor instability on cystometric examination.

Within the pontine reticular formation are two closely related areas with inhibitory and excitatory effects on the sacral micturition centre in the conus medullaris. Lesions of the cord below this level always lead to incoordinate voiding with a failure of urethral relaxation during detrusor contraction; lesions above this level may be associated with normal although involuntary micturition.

The mechanism of urinary continence

The mechanism of urinary continence is a complex dynamic process which relies on intact fascia, ligaments and muscles with their accompanying nerve and vascular supply. It relies on maximum urethral pressure being higher than maximum detrusor pressure. There are special features of physiology and anatomy that contribute to the maintenance of a low detrusor pressure, and adequate urethral closure and positioning. These features are discussed below.

Bladder

An intravesical pressure that exceeds urethral pressure will lead to incontinence. There are a number of factors which maintain a low intravesical pressure.

The hydrostatic pressure at the bladder neck

Any fluid within the bladder will itself have a pressure. This is due to a vertical gravitational pressure gradient. For clinical purposes, the intravesical pressure defines the pressure in the bladder with respect to atmospheric pressure measured at the level of the upper border of the symphysis pubis. This pressure works against the mechanisms that produce urethral closure, and very rarely amounts to more than 10 cmH_2O.

Transmission of intra-abdominal pressure

The bladder is normally an intra-abdominal organ and is subject to the pressures of adjacent organs and abdominal pressure. The pressures are normally equally transmitted to the bladder, the bladder neck and proximal areas of the urethra, and this helps to maintain continence.

Tension in the bladder wall

Due to higher control of the basic visceral reflexes, the bladder does not contract in response to stretch receptors within the bladder wall. This and the actual ability of the bladder to be compliant (i.e. to allow for a large rise in volume and little rise in pressure) make it an ideal storage organ.

Urethra

There are several components of urethral function that are necessary to maintain good urethral closure.

The hermetic seal

The vascularity in the submucosal urethral plexuses has been mentioned above, and there are also secretions that allow this seal to be maintained. This may fail after the menopause.

The intrinsic smooth and striated muscles and the extrinsic striated muscles

The intrinsic smooth and striated muscles exert a constant pressure from their constant tone, and the extrinsic striated muscle contracts during moments of stress to maintain urethral closure. It has been estimated from urethral pressure studies that resting urethral pressure is one-third due to external striated muscle effects, one-third due to smooth muscle effects and one-third due to its vascular supply. The highest pressure is found at the midurethral point.

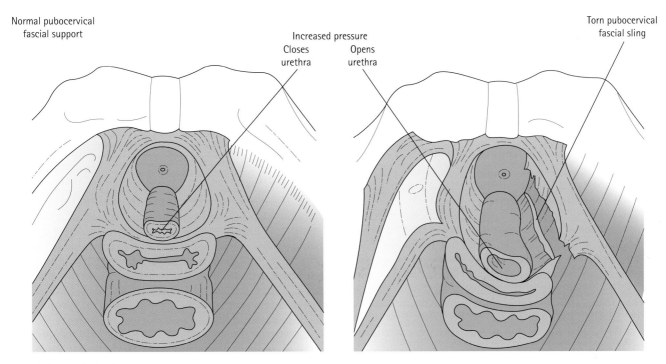

Normal pubocervical
fascial support

Increased pressure
Closes
urethra

Opens
urethra

Torn pubocervical
fascial sling

Figure 50.4 Fascial breaks.

Urethral support

From cadaveric studies, ultrasound and MRI, it is postulated that the urethra is supported by a hammock (Figure 50.4). This hammock is contributed to by its immediate intimate relationship with the vagina, and the pubocervical fascia that lies between them and attaches laterally to the arcus tendineus fascia pelvis, which attaches to muscle fascia and which are in connection with the levator ani muscles themselves. During any rise in abdominal pressure, these may cause compression of the urethra against the anterior vaginal wall. In this model, it is the stability of the supporting structures rather than the height of the urethra that determines stress continence. In an individual with a firm supportive layer, the urethral compression can be compared with the way that the flow of water through a garden hose can be stopped by stepping on it and compressing it against concrete. The pubourethral ligaments also contribute to midurethral support.

Normal micturition cycle

Filling and storage phase

The bladder normally fills with urine by a series of peristaltic contractions at a rate of between 0.5 and 5 ml/min. Under these conditions, the bladder pressure only increases minimally. Urethral closure is maintained by the three mechanisms mentioned above. During the early stages of bladder filling, proprioceptive afferent impulses from the stretch receptors within the bladder wall pass via the pelvic nerves to sacral dorsal roots S2–4. These impulses ascend in the cord via the lateral spinothalamic tracts, and any detrusor motor response is inhibited by descending impulses from higher centres. As bladder filling continues, further afferent impulses ascend to the cerebral cortex, and eventually a first

sensation to desire is appreciated. This is usually at approximately half of functional bladder capacity. The impulses increase as volume increases and reinforce conscious inhibition; micturition occurs when a suitable site and posture for micturition is found. At this time, in addition to the cortical suppression of detrusor activity, there may also be a voluntary pelvic floor contraction in an attempt to improve urethral closure.

Initiation phase

When a suitable time, site and posture for micturition have been selected, the process of voiding commences. Relaxation of the pelvic floor occurs early in the process of initiation and micturition. This can be observed radiologically and also by performing electromyography where an electrical silence is recorded. It is likely that a simultaneous relaxation of the intrinsic striated muscle also occurs, since a marked decrease in intraurethral pressure is seen before the intravesical pressure rises. A few seconds later, the descending inhibitory influences are suppressed, allowing rapid discharge of efferent parasympathetic impulses via the pelvic nerves to cause detrusor contraction at the bladder neck. In addition, there is probably efferent sympathetic discharge encouraging urethral relaxation.

Voiding phase

When the decreasing urethral pressure and increasing intravesical pressure equate, urine flow will commence. As bladder emptying occurs, the radius of the bladder decreases. However, the pressure remains constant during voiding, and therefore it is likely that the tension of the wall decreases as voiding continues. If micturition is voluntarily interrupted midstream by contraction of the periurethral striated muscle, the urethral pressure rises rapidly and urine flow stops. The detrusor is much slower to relax and therefore goes on contracting against the sphincter, and an isometric contraction occurs. At the end of micturition, the intravesical pressure gradually decreases as urine flow diminishes. The pelvic floor and intrinsic striated muscle are contracted, flow is interrupted in the mid urethra, and a process of milkback occurs where a few drops of urine are forced back into the bladder as urethral closure occurs in a cephalad direction.

Pathophysiology of urinary incontinence

The pathophysiology of major causes of incontinence is discussed in some detail in the following chapters. A few general principles are considered here.

If the lower urinary tract is intact, urine flow can only occur when the intravesical pressure exceeds the maximum urethral pressure or when the maximum urethral pressure becomes negative. Causes of this are discussed in later chapters but may be largely due to childbirth, with direct mechanical injury to the supports including muscle and connective tissue, and following denervation injury to those muscles. Ageing also plays a part, as does pelvic floor surgery and radiotherapy. Incontinence, therefore, may occur as a result of:

- a decrease in urethral pressure associated with an increase in intravesical pressure. This can occur during normal voiding or in cases of detrusor instability (Figure 50.5A);
- an increase in intravesical pressure associated with an increase in urethral pressure where the latter rise is insufficient to maintain a positive closure pressure. This may be the case in detrusor instability with associated detrusor sphincter dyssynergia (Figure 50.5B);
- an abnormally steep rise in detrusor pressure during bladder filling, suggesting impaired bladder compliance. This can occur after pelvic irradiation or with conditions that cause chronic inflammation such as tuberculosis or interstitial cystitis (Figure 50.5C);
- loss of urethral pressure alone. This can occur in urethral instability and also in women who have urethral insufficiency or, as it is otherwise termed, 'intrinsic sphincter deficiency'. This can commonly occur in the menopause, or after radiotherapy or surgery (Figure 50.5D); or
- during periods of stress, the intravesical pressure rises to a greater extent than the intraurethral pressure. This is usually due to a lack of urethral support, or an abnormally positioned bladder neck and proximal urethra where equal pressure transmission does not occur (Figure 50.5E).

Effect of continence surgery on mechanisms of continence

There are many operations for stress incontinence and the mechanism of their actions is debated. Operations such as the Burch colposuspension and Marshall–Marchetti–Krantz elevate the bladder neck, and this is assumed to restore it to its zone of equal pressure transmission. This has been shown using pressure transmission ratios, where increased pressure is transmitted to the proximal quartile of the urethra, but there are obviously obstructive components that also con-

tribute. Bladder neck injectables have been used to increase urethral length, allowing better transmission to the proximal urethra. Finally, tension-free vaginal tape and its evolutionary descendants obturator and single incision tapes are thought to work by increasing the support of the urethra in the midurethral zone, rather than influencing bladder neck position.

Anal Incontinence

Definition

Faecal incontinence is defined as 'the involuntary or inappropriate passage of faeces' (Royal College of Physicians 1995). This definition, however, is incomplete as it may not include incontinence to flatus. Therefore, many adopt the term 'anal incontinence' to include flatus. Furthermore, this definition includes transient episodes of incontinence that may be experienced following a bout of gastrointestinal upset, and therefore a definition similar to that proposed by the International Continence Society for urinary incontinence may be more appropriate; namely, anal incontinence is the involuntary loss of flatus or faeces that is a social or hygienic problem.

Prevalence of anal incontinence

The estimated community prevalence of faecal incontinence is 4.2 per 1000 in men aged 15–64 years, 10.9 per 1000 in men aged 65 years or over, 1.7 per 1000 in women aged 15–64 years and 13.3 per 1000 in women aged 65 years or over. In residential homes for the elderly, the incidence was found to be 10.3% but may approach 60% in the elderly. Although the incidence of faecal incontinence in 45-year-old women is eight times higher than that in men of the same age, its prevalence has not been accurately assessed in the younger age groups. Even a minor degree of faecal incontinence can be very distressing and is a cause of great embarrassment; therefore, very few admit to it and seek medical assistance. In one study, half the patients referred to a gastrointestinal clinic complaining of diarrhoea were incontinent, but less than half of them volunteered this information. Moreover, clinicians may not enquire or document this symptom, and therefore the true prevalence of faecal incontinence can be grossly underestimated. A validated scoring system would therefore be more representative for epidemiological and research purposes. The Wexner scoring system is very popular and includes the need to wear a pad and alteration in lifestyle (Table 50.1). A modified version of the Wexner score has also been introduced to include faecal urgency, the ability to defer defaecation and the use of antidiarrhoeal medications.

The anal sphincter mechanism

The puborectalis and the external anal sphincter

Proximally, the EAS lies in contiguity with the posterior half of the puborectalis; distally, it merges with the perianal skin. Like the levator ani, it is primarily composed of striated muscle. There is lack of consistency in the literature with regard to the structural subdivisions of the EAS.

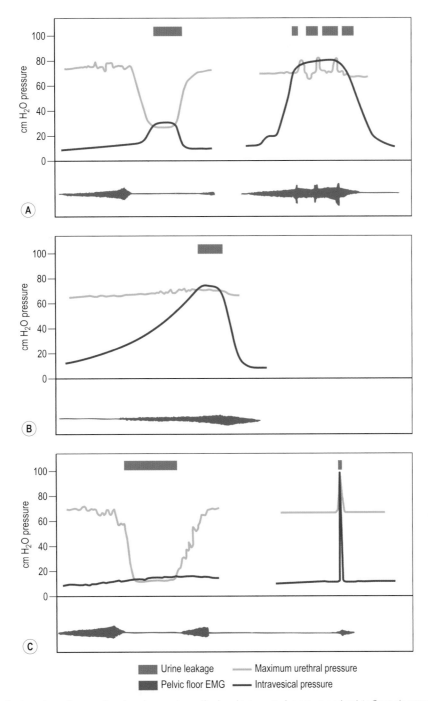

Urine leakage   Maximum urethral pressure
Pelvic floor EMG   Intravesical pressure

Figure 50.5 Mechanisms of urinary incontinence showing changes in urethral and intravesical pressure and pelvic floor electromyogram (EMG) at various stages of bladder filling in different types of incontinence. (A) Normal voiding or detrusor instability. (B) Detrusor instability with detrusor sphincter dyssynergia. (C) Impaired bladder compliance. (D) Urethral instability. (E) Genuine stress incontinence.

Some authors describe it as one structure, while others have subdivided it into two or even three components: the subcutaneous and deep EAS as annular muscles not attached to the coccyx, and the superficial EAS (middle layer) as being elliptical with fibres running anteroposteriorly from the perineal body to the coccyx and the anococcygeal raphe (Figure 50.6). The deep EAS has anterior fibres which cross over to the opposite side and combine with the superficial transverse perinei attaching to the ascending ramus of the ischium. Electrophysiological techniques have shown that the motor supply of the puborectalis is via direct branches of the sacral nerves (S3 and S4), and that of the EAS is via the pudendal nerve (S2–4). This supports the contention that the puborectalis is part of the levator ani and separate from the anal sphincter. Nevertheless, close cohesion between these muscles would seem to be essential because without it, peristalsis would pull the rectum upwards and over its contents without expelling them through the anus. Frustration in attempts to identify these subdivisions of the EAS led some authors to propose that the EAS is, in fact, a single structure with no real subdivision. As these subdivisions are not identified during surgery, they do not appear

Table 50.1 The Wexner score

Type of incontinence	Frequency				
	Never	**Rarely**	**Sometimes**	**Usually**	**Always**
Solid	0	1	2	3	4
Liquid	0	1	2	3	4
Gas	0	1	2	3	4
Wears pad	0	1	2	3	4
Lifestyle alteration	0	1	2	3	4

Never: 0.
Rarely: <1/month.
Sometimes: <1/week, ≤1/month.
Usually: <1/day, ≤1/week.
Always: ≤1/day.
0 = perfect continence.
20 = complete incontinence.

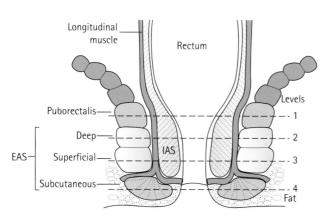

Figure 50.6 The anal sphincter mechanism showing the puborectalis and external anal sphincter (EAS), the longitudinal muscle, and the internal anal sphincter (IAS).

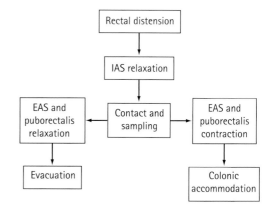

Figure 50.7 The mechanism of defaecation. EAS, external anal sphincter; IAS, internal anal sphincter.

to be clinically relevant. However, a clear understanding of normal anatomy and variants is important during imaging (ultrasound and MRI) of the anal sphincter in order to avoid misinterpretation.

The longitudinal muscle

The longitudinal muscle of the anal canal is a direct continuation of the smooth longitudinal muscle of the rectum. Between the lower border of the internal anal sphincter (IAS) and the upper border of the subcutaneous EAS, it attaches to the anal skin to form the anal intermuscular septum. Many of the fibres then pass outwards, traversing the subcutaneous EAS to insert into the perianal skin to form the corrugator cutis ani. The functional significance of this muscle is unknown.

The internal anal sphincter

The IAS is continuous with the inner circular smooth muscle of the rectum, and terminates in a sharply defined, thickened, rounded lower margin, separated from the subcutane-

ous EAS by the anal intermuscular septum. The IAS measures approximately 3 mm in length and 5 mm in thickness. It is tonically active and under autonomic control, namely excitatory (sympathetic L1–2) and inhibitory (parasympathetic S2–4).

The defaecation cycle

The main reservoir for faeces is the transverse colon, and the rectum is usually empty. Although the rectum has a poor supply of intraepithelial receptors, it is sensitive to distension. The first sensation of rectal filling occurs at a volume of 50 ml, with a maximum tolerated volume of 200 ml. Depending on various factors such as gut motility and stool consistency, colonic contents are delivered at a variable rate to the rectum.

Following rectal distension with either faeces or flatus, the internal sphincter relaxes to allow sampling of rectal contents to take place by the specialized sensory epithelium of the anal canal (Figure 50.7). This relaxation is mediated via myenteric connections modulated by the autonomic nervous system, and is known as the 'rectoanal inhibitory reflex'

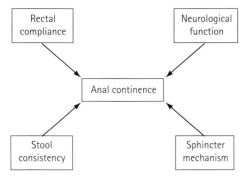

Figure 50.8 The mechanism of anal continence.

RAIR). If it is socially convenient, the puborectalis and external sphincter relax and evacuation occurs. If the time for evacuation is inappropriate, EAS contraction extends the period of continence to allow the compliance mechanisms within the colon to make adjustments in order to accommodate the increased rectal volume. Thereafter, the stretch receptors are no longer activated and afferent stimuli are abolished, together with the sensation of faecal urgency.

The factors contributing to the mechanism of incontinence will be discussed in detail below.

Anal continence mechanisms

The mechanism that maintains continence is complex and affected by various factors such as mental function, lack of a compliant rectal reservoir, changes in stool consistency and volume, diminished anorectal sensation and enhanced colonic transit (Figure 50.8). However, analogous to urinary continence, anal continence can be maintained provided that the anal pressure exceeds the rectal pressure. As shown in Figure 50.6, the ultimate barrier to rectal contents is provided by the puborectalis sling and anal sphincters. An increased volume of liquid stool coupled with rapid colonic transit may overwhelm the compliant rectal reservoir. Therefore, if the rectum is able to function effectively as a rectal reservoir and in the presence of normal stool consistency, faecal incontinence can usually be attributed to defective function of the anal sphincter complex.

The physiological role of various components of this complex in maintaining continence will be considered separately.

The puborectalis muscle and the anorectal angle

The anorectal angle is formed by the anteriorly directed pull of the puborectalis. The angle varies from 60° to 105° at rest; during defaecation, the angle straightens, allowing the rectum to empty. Two theories have been proposed to explain how the anatomical angulation at the anorectal junction may contribute to maintain continence. The first is the 'flutter' valve, which is created as the rectum passes through the slit-like aperture in the pelvic floor caused by the forward pull of the puborectalis; a rise in intra-abdominal pressure would create a high-pressure zone and result in apposition of the rectal walls at the anorectal junction. The second is the flap valve theory; contraction of the puborectalis creates an acute anorectal angle, and intra-abdom-

inal forces compress the anterior rectal wall against the upper anal canal. However, both these theories have lost credibility; for a flutter valve to produce such a high-pressure zone, intra-abdominal forces would have to be applied below the pelvic floor. Moreover, both theories would account for rectal pressures in excess of anal canal pressures without evacuation of rectal contents. As rectal pressures have been shown to be consistently lower than anal pressures in healthy subjects, continence must be sphincteric and not valvular.

The puborectalis is considered by some to be the most important muscle in maintaining continence. In children with congenital anomalies and absence of the anal sphincter, a high degree of continence can be maintained with the puborectalis. However, posterior division of the puborectalis in the treatment of chronic constipation made no difference to the anorectal angle, and was not associated with incontinence of solid stool. Furthermore, following successful postanal repair for faecal incontinence, no significant change was observed in the anorectal angle. The role of the anorectal angle in maintaining continence therefore remains controversial.

The puborectalis muscle functions in concert with the EAS, and it is probable that if damage occurs to one muscle, the other may compensate functionally. Faecal incontinence may ensue if, in addition, other factors in the continence mechanism (see below) are compromised or if the remaining muscle cannot compensate adequately.

Internal anal sphincter

There are conflicting opinions on the role of the IAS in maintaining continence. As 70% of the resting tone is contributed by the IAS, it is a major factor in keeping the anal canal closed at rest. This is supported by the finding that symptoms of incontinence can develop in up to 40% of cases following lateral internal anal sphincterotomy. Faecal incontinence has also been reported following anal dilatation, with sonographic evidence of internal sphincter disruption and a reduced resting pressure.

Ultrastructural changes have been identified in the morphology of the internal sphincter of patients suffering from neurogenic faecal incontinence. Although these changes are probably not the primary cause of faecal incontinence, they may have some relevance to IAS function. In addition, abnormalities of adrenergic innervation with a diminished sensitivity of the IAS to α-adrenergic agents *in vitro* have been demonstrated in patients with idiopathic faecal incontinence. These changes could be attributed to an intrinsic degeneration of the muscle and its receptors, or to simultaneous direct injury to the striated muscle of the pelvic floor.

The rectoanal inhibitory reflex

The RAIR or rectosphincteric reflex is a transient relaxation of the IAS when the rectum is distended. This response has been shown to persist in patients with cauda equina lesions and after complete transection of the spinal cord, indicating that it occurs independently of central control. It appears that the RAIR is mediated by intramural myenteric neurones because topical anaesthesia of the rectal mucosa blocks the reflex, and it is absent in patients with Hirschsprung's disease.

The RAIR causes equalization of rectal and upper canal resting pressures, and allows rectal contents to enter the anal canal. The contents are then analysed by the specialized sensory epithelium in the anal canal (sampling reflex). This is accompanied by a reflex contraction of the external sphincter and puborectalis (inflation reflex), which temporarily maintains the high-pressure zone in the anal canal until either evacuation occurs or the anal contents are pushed back into the rectum. The sampling reflex occurs as a normal physiological process about seven times per hour. The absence of the reflex in patients with faecal incontinence would indicate a weakness of the IAS, whereas in Hirschsprung's disease (segmental aganglionosis), it would be associated with obstructive defaecation rather than faecal incontinence. However, the value of this test is limited as the RAIR may be difficult to elicit consistently, even in healthy subjects.

The external anal sphincter

The EAS is inseparable from the puborectalis posteriorly, and both muscles appear to function as a single unit electrophysiologically. It has been shown that while contraction of the puborectalis accentuates the anorectal angle, it does not increase the intraluminal pressure of the anal canal.

The EAS, similar to the IAS, is in a state of tonic contraction, even at rest, and the activity is reflexly raised when intra-abdominal pressure is increased (e.g. when coughing, laughing or lifting). Activity is maximally raised when the EAS is contracted voluntarily, but contraction can only be maintained for 1–2 min. Stimulation of the perianal skin also results in a reflex EAS contraction via the pudendal nerve, called the 'cutaneo-anal reflex'. Electrical activity usually decreases during straining and when defaecation is attempted, although this is described as a variable response in some subjects.

The EAS contributes up to 30% of the resting pressure, and the increment of the squeeze pressure above the resting pressure predominantly reflects EAS function. The maintenance of tone is, however, also dependent on a sensory input, as it is lost if the sensory roots are destroyed (e.g. tabes dorsalis).

The response to changes in intra-abdominal pressure suggests that the EAS is actively involved in the preservation of continence. Further support for this hypothesis is that division of the internal sphincter alone can be associated with minor degrees of incontinence to flatus and liquid stool, but not usually to solid stool. These properties of the EAS may be diminished either by denervation, mechanical trauma or a combination of factors.

The anal cushions

The anal cushions, consisting of epithelium, subepithelium and the underlying haemorrhoidal plexuses, can contribute up to 15% of resting pressure. The anal sphincters cannot obliterate the lumen completely without the sealing effect of the anal cushions. The thickened cushions may account for the increased resting pressures seen in patients with haemorrhoids. The decrease in resting pressure following haemorrhoidectomy may explain the development of minor anal incontinence, although inadvertent damage to the sphincter, particularly the internal sphincter, has been observed using anal endosonography.

Rectal compliance

A compliant rectal reservoir that can accommodate large volumes of stool without significant increases in pressure is an important prerequisite for the effective function of barrier mechanisms of continence. Patients who have a reduction in rectal capacity, as occurs in colitis and radiation proctitis, often suffer from faecal urgency and incontinence.

Anorectal sensation

The epithelium of the anal canal is richly supplied with sensory nerve endings, exquisitely sensitive to pain, heat and cold. The afferent nerve pathways for anal canal sensation is via the posterior inferior haemorrhoidal branches of the pudendal nerve and anterior haemorrhoidal branches of the perineal nerve to the sacral roots of S2, S3 and S4, but in addition, direct anal and urethral branches arise from S4 and S5. Sampling has been shown to occur less frequently in incontinent patients compared with controls.

Central control of anal continence

The upper motor neurones for the voluntary sphincter muscles lie close to those of the lower limb musculature in the parasagittal motor cortex. They communicate by a fast conducting oligosymptomatic pathway, with the Onuf nucleus situated in the sacral ventral grey matter, mainly S2 and S3. The frontal cortex is important for the conscious awareness of the need to defaecate and appropriate social behaviour. Disease affecting the upper neurone motor pathway usually results in urgency and urge incontinence and provided the lower motor pathway is still intact, reflex defaecation will still be possible. Neurological diseases such as multiple sclerosis, Parkinson's disease and disorders of the spinal cord or cauda equina can be accompanied by incontinence because the central pathways which control sphincter function are located in the vicinity of the corticospinal tracts. Patients suffering with diabetes mellitus can have an autonomic neuropathy and this can also lead to faecal incontinence.

The lower motor neurones innervating the striated pelvic floor and urethral and anal sphincters arise from the Onuf nucleus. The most common cause of a lower motor neurone lesion in the adult is chronic stretching of the pudendal nerve, usually as a result of chronic straining at stool and/or childbirth. Damage to the pudendal nerve results in progressive denervation and reinnervation of the pelvic floor–anal sphincter complex, causing weakness and atrophy of these muscles.

Pathophysiology of anal incontinence

The development of anal incontinence may be due to either mechanical disruption or neuropathy, but sometimes both coexist. Obstetric trauma is a major cause of such injury although the peak incidence appears to be in the perimenopausal years. The development of anal endosonography has revolutionized our understanding of anal incontinence, and it has now been demonstrated that approximately one-third of primiparous women develop anal sphincter injury that is not recognized during vaginal delivery. However, even when it is recognized and repaired, the outcome is suboptimal as one-third continue to suffer impaired continence. Attention is now being focused on improved training in anatomy and repair techniques. However, there are other factors such as the effect of ageing, collagen weakness, progression of pelvic neuropathy, oestrogen deficiency, concurrent irritable bowel syndrome, primary degeneration of the IAS, severe constipation and uterovaginal/rectal prolapse that may contribute to a deterioration in anorectal function.

Effects of continence surgery on mechanisms of continence

The most common operation for faecal incontinence is an overlap anterior sphincteroplasty which serves to re-establish the continuity of the anal sphincter muscle ring in patients with a sphincter defect. In addition, some surgeons perform a levatoroplasty while others imbricate the internal sphincter. This operation has a success rate of 70–80%, although this can deteriorate to nearer 50% by 5 years. Anal pressures, particularly the voluntary squeeze pressure, increase. Pelvic neuropathy can cause atrophy of the sphincter muscles and hence have an adverse outcome. Some studies have suggested that a prolonged pudendal nerve latency prognosticates a poor outcome, but other studies have failed to identify a correlation. An abnormally prolonged latency of >2.4 ms in isolation correlates poorly with anal squeeze pressures, and therefore some neurophysiologists believe that this is not a good test of neuropathy as it is only a measure of conduction in the fastest conducting motor fibres of the pudendal nerve.

The postanal repair is performed when faecal incontinence is due to a neurogenic cause leading to pelvic floor atrophy. The intention is to recreate the anorectal angle by placating the levators at the back of the rectum. However, current evidence indicates that this operation does not have a significant effect on the anorectal angle, but appears to increase the functional length of the anal canal and may improve anal canal sensation.

Other surgical options include stimulated gracilis muscle neoplasty and artificial anal sphincter.

Table 50.2 Comparison of bladder and bowel conditions

Bladder	Bowel
Detrusor overactivity	Irritable bowel syndrome
Urodynamic stress incontinence	Faecal incontinence
Detrusor sphincter dyssynergia	Anismus
Urgency	Urgency
Hypotonic bladder	Constipation

Sacral nerve modulation is a relatively new technique that has added a new dimension to the management of faecal incontinence and defaecatory disorders. Short-term results are very encouraging with minimal morbidity. This technique provides new hope to women who otherwise would be left with no option but a stoma.

Comparison between Bladder and Bowel

Reflex adaptation of the rectum and bladder in response to filling are fairly analogous. There is an inverse relationship between distension and compliance. The 'irritable bladder' is more often found in patients with irritable bowel syndrome. The aetiology of faecal and urinary incontinence may also be comparable, and Table 50.2 compares bladder and bowel conditions.

Conclusion

An understanding of the mechanisms of urinary and anal continence is essential before one can discuss incontinence. Furthermore, if treatment is to be appropriately targeted, one must understand the anatomical deficiencies as repair of these often results in correction of function without causing new dysfunction. In the light of this type of knowledge, meaningful investigations can be carried out and treatment modalities selected on an individual basis.

KEY POINTS

1. The muscular, connective tissue and nerve components of the urethral and anal sphincter continence mechanisms are very similar. The levator ani and their contribution by means of the pubourethralis and puborectalis muscles play an important extrinsic striated muscle role for continence. Both mechanisms have smooth muscle components and a nerve supply largely from the pudendal nerves.

2. The bladder and urethra and the rectum and anal sphincter have complex autonomic innervation in addition to the somatic innervation that allows reflex interplay with the spinal cord and higher centres that provide proprioreceptive information from either **bladder, bowel or rectum.** Closure of the urethra and the anal canal is vital in maintaining continence, and the ability to choose the time to relax these mechanisms is essential for normal control of both continence mechanisms.

3. Mechanical damage to both the fascia and muscles is thought to be the most important factor in the aetiology of both urinary and faecal incontinence, and anal sphincter defects have been shown to correlate with anal incontinence.

4. Successful repair for both urinary and faecal incontinence is aimed at restoring anatomy and function; imaging methods are useful in the identification of defects, which can subsequently be appropriately repaired.

Further Reading

Royal College of Physicians 1995 Clinical Audit Scheme for the Management of Urinary and Faecal Incontinence. RCP, London (out of print; ISBN 9781860160530).

Urinary continence

Abrams P, Blaivas J, Stanton SL, Anderson J 1990 The standardisation of terminology of lower urinary tract function. International Urogynaecology Journal 1: 45–58.

Asmussen M, Ulmsten U 1983 On the physiology of continence and pathophysiology of stress incontinence in the female. In: Umsten U (ed) Contributions to Gynaecology and Obstetrics. Volume 10, Female Stress Incontinence. Karger, Basel, pp 32–50.

Bradley WE, Timm TW, Scott FB 1974 Innervation of the detrusor muscle and urethra. Urological Clinics of North America 1: 3–27.

Constantinou CE 1985 Resting and stress urethral pressures as a clinical guide to the mechanism of continence. Clinics in Obstetrics and Gynaecology 12: 343–356.

Coolsaet B 1984 Cystometry. In: Stanton SL (ed) Clinical Gynaecological Urology. CV Mosby, St Louis, pp 59–81.

DeLancey JO 1988 Structural aspects of the extrinsic continence mechanism. American Journal of Obstetrics and Gynecology 72: 296–301.

Gosling JA, Dixon J, Critchley HOD, Thompson SA 1981 A comparative study of human external sphincter and periurethral levator ani muscle. British Journal of Urology 53: 35–41.

Griffiths DJ 1980 Urodynamics. Adam Hilger, Bristol.

Hilton P 2000 Mechanism of continence. In: Stanton SL, Monga AK (eds) Clinical Urogynaecology. Churchill Livingstone, pp 31–40.

Kapoor D, Thakar R, Sultan AH 2005 Combined urinary and fecal incontinence. International Urogynaecology Journal and Pelvic Floor Dysfunction 16: 321–328.

Monga AK, Phillips C 1999 Structural urogynaecology. In: Thomas E, Stones RW (eds) Gynaecology Highlights. Health Press, Oxford, pp 43–52.

Wein A 1986 Physiology of micturition. Clinics in Geriatric Medicine 2: 689–699.

Zacharin RF 1963 The suspension mechanism of the female urethra. Journal of Anatomy 97: 423–427.

Anal continence

Matzel KE 2007 Sacral nerve stimulation for fecal disorders: evolution, current status, and future directions. Acta Neurochirurgica Supplement 97: 351–357.

Pemberton JH, Swash M Henry MM, (eds) 2002 The Pelvic Floor — its Function and Disorders. WB Saunders, London.

Sultan AH, Kamm MA, Hudson CN, Thomas JM, Bartram CI 1993 Anal sphincter disruption during vaginal delivery. USA Journal of Medicine 329: 1905–1911.

Sultan AH, Nugent K 2004 Pathophysiology and non-surgical treatment of anal incontinence. BJOG: an International Journal of Obstetrics and Gynaecology 111 (Suppl 1): 84–90.

Sultan AH, Thakar R, Fenner D 2007 Perineal and Anal Sphincter Trauma. Springer, London.

CHAPTER 51

Urodynamic investigations

Philip Toozs-Hobson and Matthew Parsons

Chapter Contents

INTRODUCTION	783		CONCLUSION	794
URODYNAMIC INVESTIGATIONS	784		KEY POINTS	795

Introduction

Evaluation of lower urinary tract dysfunction

Symptoms of lower urinary tract dysfunction are common amongst women of all ages and are the cause of significant impairment of quality of life (QoL). The Leicestershire Medical Research Council study (Perry et al 2000) estimates that up to 26% of community-dwelling adults have clinically significant symptoms, and up to 2.4% have significant bothersome and socially disabling symptoms, which equates to more than 40 patients per general practitioner in the UK. A thorough assessment of the symptoms, their impact and the cause is key to their successful treatment. The current guidelines of the National Institute for Health and Clinical Excellence (NICE) suggest that the initial assessment must categorize incontinence based on symptoms, and that all patients should be assessed using a 3-day diary along with a urine dipstick (National Institute for Health and Clinical Excellence 2006). Initial treatment should be conservative, with urodynamics reserved for refractory or complicated symptoms.

The term 'urodynamics' refers to a variety of tests ranging from a simple flow rate to complex tests performed in specialized units. The role of tests is to determine the cause objectively and to quantify the severity of urinary symptoms.

Normal assessment prior to urodynamics includes clinical history in isolation or the additional use of structured questioning or standardized symptom questionnaires. The utility of an accurate history (primarily categorizing incontinence as stress, urge or mixed incontinence) has been confirmed as part of a health technology assessment in the UK (Martin et al 2006), and was subsequently endorsed by NICE (National Institute for Health and Clinical Excellence 2006). These guidelines also highlight the role of disease-specific QoL questionnaires which may allow assessment of bothersomeness of symptoms, and these are increasingly used for the assessment of patients with urinary tract dysfunction in both clinical practice and clinical trials. The International Continence Society's (ICS) standardization document of 2002 also states that subjective, objective and QoL endpoints should be used as three separate measures of outcome (Abrams et al 2002). Ward and Hilton (2008) demonstrated that cure rates varied from 40% to 90% depending on the definition used, highlighting the importance of defining outcome measures accurately.

Urinary symptoms

The relationship between urinary symptoms, urodynamic investigations and QoL impairment is often complex. Weak correlations have been found between the presence of lower urinary tract symptoms and clinical measures such as urodynamics. Although urodynamic investigations determine the cause of urinary symptoms, they do not quantify their impact on women's QoL; therefore, all three components offer utility in the assessment of a patient.

Urinary symptoms may not consistently reflect the cause of lower urinary tract dysfunction, and hence there is a need for urodynamic investigations (Cundiff et al 1997). Jarvis et al (1980) compared the results of clinical and urodynamic diagnoses for 100 women referred for investigation of lower urinary tract disorders. There was agreement in 68% of cases of urodynamic stress incontinence, but only 51% of cases of overactive bladder. Although nearly all of the women with urodynamic stress incontinence complained of symptoms of stress incontinence, 46% also complained of urgency. Of the women with overactive bladder, 26% also had symptoms of stress incontinence.

Versi et al (1991), using an analysis of symptoms for the prediction of urodynamic stress incontinence in 252 patients, achieved a correct classification of 81% with a false-positive rate of 16%. Lagro-Jansson et al (1991) showed that symptoms of stress incontinence in the absence of symptoms of urge incontinence had a sensitivity of 78%, specificity of 84% and a positive predictive value of 87%. Where stress incontinence is the only symptom reported, urodynamic stress incontinence is likely to be present in over 90% of cases (Farrar et al 1975, Hastie and Moisey 1989). Even when women who only complain of stress incontinence and who have a normal frequency/volume chart are investigated,

DOI: 10.1016/B978-0-7020-3120-5.00051-5

65% have urodynamic stress incontinence and 8% have overactive bladder (James et al 1997).

The severity of urinary symptoms is often used as a measure of the impact of lower urinary tract dysfunction in both clinical practice and clinical trials. At its simplest, severity may reflect symptom frequency (e.g. the number of incontinent episodes, the number of daily voids or the number of episodes of nocturia). Measuring symptom frequency is relatively easy but offers little insight into their impact.

Quality-of-life assessment

Incontinence research requires that morbidity is measured by endpoints that assess different aspects and are not always independent, such as the number of micturitions and volume voided. The relationship of these endpoints to the lives of women is not well understood. For example, do fewer incontinent episodes or reduced volume of an incontinent episode improve QoL? There are probably individual factors involved which are centred around personal psychology, such as measures of hardiness or personal construct (Toozs-Hobson and Loane 2008). QoL measurement makes an attempt to standardize assessment of many aspects of these, including areas such as social, psychological, occupational, domestic, physical and sexual domains.

Wyman et al (1987) used the Incontinence Impact Questionnaire to show that women with overactive bladder experienced greater psychosocial dysfunction as a result of their urinary symptoms than women with urodynamic stress incontinence, although no relationship was found between the questionnaire score and the urinary diary or pad test results. Kobelt et al (1999) showed that the severity of symptoms of incontinence as expressed as frequency of voids and leakage correlates well with the patient's QoL and health status, as well as the amount that they are willing to pay for a given percentage reduction in their symptoms.

Symptoms may change over time as patients adapt. It is accepted that patients with stress incontinence may develop frequency in order to limit stress leakage, and that these symptoms may be more problematic than the stress urinary leakage itself. Irritative symptoms and voiding dysfunction can follow surgery for urodynamic stress incontinence, and voiding dysfunction and distressing antimuscarinic side-effects can follow drug treatment of overactive bladder. Such changes can have a negative impact on the overall QoL of patients.

The King's Health Questionnaire is a good example of a disease-specific QoL questionnaire which incorporates questions about both bothersomeness of symptoms and QoL (Kelleher et al 1997). It was specifically designed for the assessment of women with urinary symptoms, and has been shown to have good sensitivity to clinically relevant improvement in urinary symptoms in clinical practice and clinical trials (Kobelt et al 1999). In one study, the King's Health Questionnaire was used to assess the outcome of surgery (colposuspension) for the treatment of urodynamic stress incontinence. There was broad general agreement between objective urodynamic changes demonstrating continence as a result of surgery and symptom and QoL score improvements (Bidmead et al 2001). More recently, there have been attempts to integrate and standardize questionnaires with the International Consultation on Incontinence Modular Questionnaire (http://www.iciq.net/, Avery et al 2004) and the Electronic Personal Assessment Questionnaire (www.epaq-online.co.uk), which have the advantage of being computer based and giving an instant result.

Urodynamic Investigations

QoL measures have been used to compare impact and also populations, but not to direct treatment. There is still a need to include a diagnosis in treatment options.

Midstream urine specimen

Urinary symptoms can be caused by a urinary tract infection and treatment may resolve symptoms. A significant bacteriuria is growth of 10^5 organisms/ml of urine and is usually associated with pyuria. The presence of epithelial cells, erythrocytes and casts is also noted. Urine can be screened for infection using Multistix strips which test for nitrites, blood and leukocytes. This has been shown to pick up 95% of urinary tract infections.

Urodynamic studies are associated with a 1% risk of urinary tract infection (Coptcoat et al 1988), based on the risk of catheterization, so there is no need for women to have routine prophylactic antibiotics. However, women with particular risk factors, such as diabetes, or voiding difficulties should be given prophylactic antibiotics.

Urinary diary

A urinary diary is a simple paper record of when and how much fluid a woman drinks and voids (Figure 51.1). The diary should be completed for a minimum of 3 days (National Institute for Health and Clinical Excellence 2006). Leakage episodes are recorded and (ideally) the precipitating event is also noted. The documented record is more accurate than memory alone, having reasonable test–retest reliability, particularly for incontinence episodes (Wyman et al 1991).

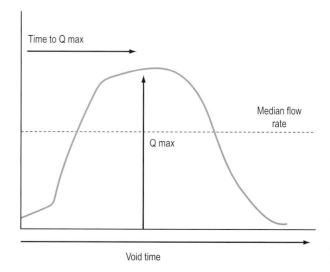

Figure 51.1 Diagrammatic representation of a urinary flow rate.

The functional capacity of the bladder is obtained and polydipsia, as a cause of polyuria, can be excluded. Unfortunately, the diary does not differentiate between the different urodynamic diagnoses (Larsson et al 1991, Larsson and Victor 1992). The urinary diary can also be used as a baseline for monitoring women undergoing bladder retraining. More recently, an electronic version has been launched commercially which ranks bladder capacity as a centile, matched for age and fluid intake (Amundsen et al 2007). This has the added advantage of an inbuilt character-recognition programme to combine the cheap cost of a paper diary with the rapid and accurate data manipulation of a computer system, and makes possible more quantitative clinical measures than are currently feasible.

Pad test

Pad tests differ according to the length of the test and the volume of fluid within the bladder. The ICS has defined a standard 1-h pad test with a 500 ml oral fluid load (Abrams et al 1988). This involves wearing a weighed towel and drinking 500 ml of water 15 min prior to starting the test. The woman performs 30 min of gentle exercise, such as walking and climbing stairs, followed by 15 min of more provocative exercise, including bending, standing and sitting, coughing, hand washing and running, if possible. The towel is then removed and reweighed. An increase in weight of more than 1 g is considered significant. Limitations of the 1-h pad test and an oral fluid load is that it is not reliable unless a fixed bladder volume is used (Lose et al 1988), with other authors suggesting that it has a poor predictive value (Constanti et al 2008) A 24-h pad test correlates well with symptoms of incontinence, has good reproducibility and is positive if the weight gain is over 4 g (Lose et al 1989, Martin et al 2006). The extended pad test is a more lengthy and objective measurement of leakage, and can be used to confirm or refute leakage in those women complaining of stress incontinence which has not been demonstrated on cystometry.

Uroflowmetry

Uroflowmetry is a simple non-invasive investigation and can be easily performed as an outpatient. Flow meters are relatively inexpensive and give a permanent graphic record.

Indications

Measurement of the flow rate is indicated in women with complaints of difficulty in voiding, neuropathy, a past history of urinary retention and prior to continence surgery. It is advisable for any incontinent woman to exclude voiding difficulties.

Measurements

The flow rate is defined as the volume of urine (in ml) expelled from the bladder each second. The flow time is the total duration of the void and includes interruptions in a non-continuous flow. The maximum flow rate is the maximum measured rate of flow, and the average flow is the volume voided divided by the flow time. The total

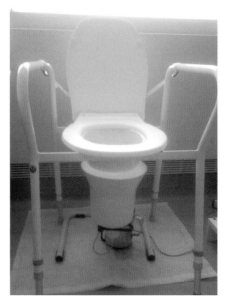

Figure 51.2 Gravimetric urinary flow meter.

volume voided can be calculated from the area under the flow curve. The two most useful parameters are the maximum flow rate and the voided volume, which should ideally be greater than 150 ml. However, the Liverpool nomograms (Haylen et al 1989) will allow assessment of flow rates at a lower volume. In women with intermittent flow, the same parameters can be used but time intervals between flow episodes must be discounted. Lower volumes at presentation are more likely in the elderly and those of lower parity with a diagnosis of sensory urgency or detrusor overactivity (Haylen et al 2009).

Equipment

There are three main types of flow meter. The gravimetric transducer measures the weight of urine voided over time and this is converted to a flow rate (Figure 51.2). The rotating disc flow meter has a disc spinning at a constant speed. The voided urine slows the rotating disc. The flow rate is calculated from the amount of power needed to maintain the disc spinning at a constant speed. The capacitance flow meter has a metal strip capacitor attached to a plastic dipstick inserted vertically into the jug containing the voided urine. The rate and volume changes are measured by a change in electrical conductance across the capacitor. This is the most expensive type of flow meter, but is robust and very reliable.

Abnormal flow rates

Nomograms for peak and average urine flow rates in women have been constructed from flow rates of 249 normal women (Haylen et al 1989). These allow comparison of a single value with a standard flow rate. A flow rate below 15 ml/s on more than one occasion is taken as abnormal when the voided volume is above 150 ml as flow rates on smaller volumes are less reliable.

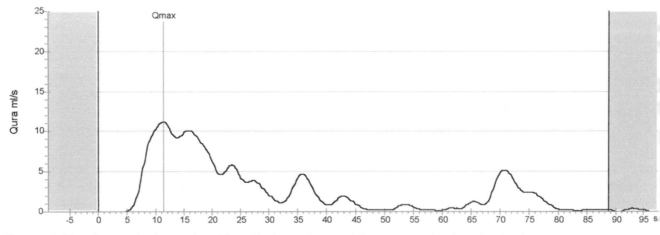

Figure 51.3 Urinary flow rate showing a prolonged flow with a low maximum peak flow rate suggestive of a voiding disorder.

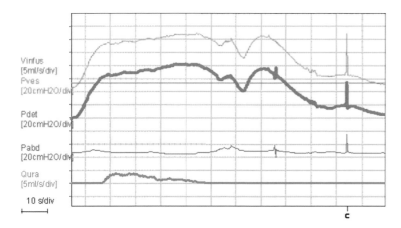

Figure 51.4 A high-pressure, low-flow pattern suggesting a voiding disorder.

A low peak flow rate and a prolonged voiding time suggest a voiding disorder (Figure 51.3). Straining can give abnormal pressure flow patterns (Figure 51.4) showing a high-pressure, low-flow pattern suggestive of obstruction. The cause of voiding dysfunction may be determined by measuring intravesical pressure simultaneously.

Cystometry

Cystometry involves measurement of the pressure/volume relationship of the bladder during filling and voiding, and is the most useful test of bladder function. It is a simple and accurate investigation, and is easy to perform.

Indications

Cystometry is indicated in patients with symptoms refractory to conservative or simple treatments, or patients with complex symptoms (National Institute for Health and Clinical Excellence 2006). However, the validity of the conclusions of NICE have been challenged and management without cystometry may be less accurate (Agur et al 2009).

Equipment

Twin-channel cystometry requires two transducers (external or microtip), a recorder and an amplifying unit (Figure 51.5). Bladder pressure is measured using a fluid-filled line attached to an external pressure transducer or a solid-state microtip pressure catheter. A rectal catheter is required to measure abdominal pressure; this is a fluid-filled, 2-mm-diameter catheter covered with a rubber finger cot to prevent blockage with faeces when the catheter is inserted into the rectum (Figure 51.6). The upper edge of the pubic symphysis is the zero reference for all measurements, which are made in centimetres of water (cmH₂O). External transducers are cheaper and less fragile, but the microtip transducer does not suffer from movement artefact.

The bladder is filled using a 12F catheter with a continuous infusion of normal saline at room temperature. The standard filling rate is between 10 and 100 ml/min and is provocative for overactive bladder. Slow-fill cystometry at a rate of 10–20 ml/min is indicated in women with neuropathic bladders. Rapid filling at over 100 ml/min is rarely used, but can be a further provocative test for overactive bladder. There is now an ICS standard for manufacturers to adhere to, and most modern equipment will easily meet this standard. Choice of equipment must be on personal requirements.

Measurements

The parameters measured are the intravesical pressure (measured with the bladder transducer) and the intra-abdominal pressure (measured with the rectal line). The detrusor pressure is obtained by subtracting the abdominal pressure from the intravesical pressure, and is displayed simultaneously. The flow rate, filling and voided volumes are also displayed.

Method

Women attend having completed a bladder diary with a comfortably full bladder. The woman then voids on the flow meter. The woman is then examined and the residual volume is noted on catheterization. During filling, the woman is asked to indicate her first desire to void and the maximal desire to void, and the volumes of these events are noted. There is evidence that women with overactivity may experience different sensations during filling compared with their stress-incontinent comparators (Digesu et al 2009). Systolic detrusor contractions and their association with urgency are noted. Precipitating factors, such as coughing or running water, are also noted. Any symptomatic detrusor pressure rise on standing is again recorded.

At the end of filling, the filling line is removed and the woman stands up. She is asked to cough and leakage is noted. Care must be taken to avoid artefact from the pressure lines moving. Provocative tests for overactive bladder, such as listening to running water and hand washing, are performed at this stage. The woman then transfers to the commode and voids with the pressure lines still in place.

Normal cystometry

The following are parameters of normal bladder function.

- Residual urine of less than 50 ml or 10% of voided volume.
- First desire to void between 150 and 200 ml.
- Capacity (taken as strong desire to void) of greater than 400 ml.
- Detrusor pressure rise on filling of less than 15 mmH$_2$O per 500 ml infused.
- Absence of systolic detrusor contractions.
- No leakage on coughing.
- No significant pain on filling.
- A detrusor pressure rise on voiding (maximum voiding pressure) of less than 50 cmH$_2$O, with a peak flow rate of more than 15 ml/s for a voided volume over 150 ml.

Abnormal cystometry

Urodynamic stress incontinence is defined by the ICS as leakage on coughing in the absence of a rise in detrusor pressure (Figure 51.7). It is therefore a diagnosis of

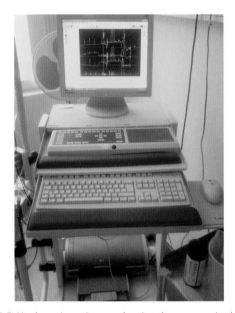

Figure 51.5 Urodynamic equipment showing the computerized cystometry unit.

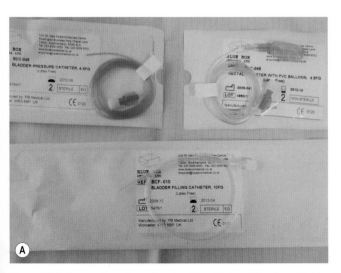
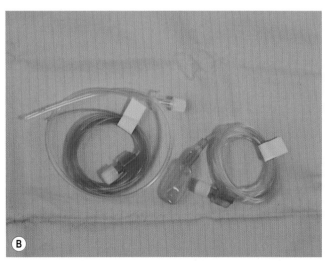

Figure 51.6 Pressure lines for cystometry. Clear bladder filling line with blue bladder pressure and red rectal pressure lines.

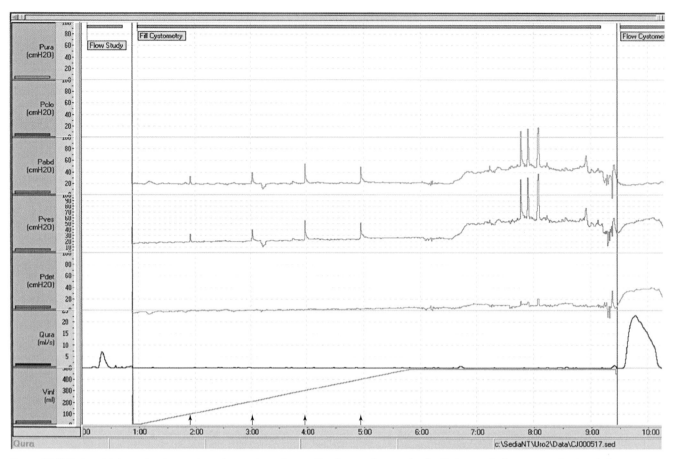

Figure 51.7 Cystometric trace showing urodynamic stress incontinence. The detrusor line remains flat. Each arrow indicates a cough, when leakage occurred.

exclusion, as cystometry by itself cannot determine bladder neck or urethral function; radiographic imaging or the addition of urethral function tests is required. Urodynamic detrusor overactivity is diagnosed during the filling phase if spontaneous or provoked detrusor contractions occur while the woman is attempting to inhibit micturition (Figure 51.8). Low compliance is diagnosed when the pressure rise is more than 15 cmH$_2$O on filling the bladder with 500 ml of fluid and does not settle after filling is stopped. These parameters are all given in the ICS good practice document (www.icsoffice.org).

Laboratory urodynamics does not provide a diagnosis in 15–25% of symptomatic women. If a laboratory test fails to answer the framed question, the investigator may feel that there is a need to request a further test. A recent study has reaffirmed the importance of urodynamics in women with symptomatic prolapse where 33% had their management changed as a result of urodynamics, including 7% having their surgery changed (Jha et al 2008).

Ambulatory monitoring

Standard twin-channel cystometry is carried out in an artificial environment over a short time frame with a filling rate that is not physiological. The test also renders the woman immobile, and bladder abnormalities produced by movement may be missed. Ambulatory urodynamic monitoring was introduced to avoid these problems, using portable digital data storage units attached to the woman for periods of several hours (van Waalwijk van Doorn et al 1991, Webb et al 1991, Anders et al 1997).

Technique

The woman wears her normal outdoor clothing and has a digital recording system (Figure 51.9). Intravesical and rectal pressures are recorded using microtip pressure transducers at a rate of 1 Hz. The ambulatory recording device can be used in conjunction with an electronic leakage detection system, and when the woman wishes to void, she connects the recorder to a flow meter and then voids. The test can last up to 6 h in clinical practice. The women are encouraged to mobilize and continue normal daily activities, including gentle exercise. Fluids should be encouraged and a minimum intake of 180 ml every 30 min is requested (Salvatore et al 1999). Antibiotic cover is not given as infection rates are less than 1%. At the end of the test, the woman is requested to attend with a full bladder and various provocative manoeuvres are carried out (similar to a standardized pad test). The woman will also keep a diary of events during the investigation, and the analysis occurs with the patient present referencing events recorded in the diary.

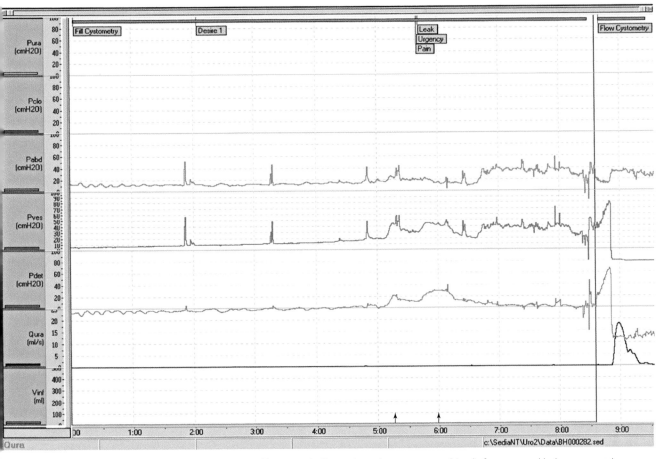

Figure 51.8 Cystometric trace showing detrusor overactivity. The arrows indicate where the woman complained of urgency and leakage occurred.

This investigation is available in specialist units and tends to be reserved for women in whom routine cystometry gives conflicting or unexpectedly negative results and where simple treatments have failed. This technique is more sensitive to the detection of abnormal overactive bladder in symptomatic women who had previously not been found to have an abnormality on laboratory urodynamics (Webb et al 1991, van Waalwijk van Doorn et al 1996). High rates of overactive bladder have been reported in asymptomatic controls (van Waalwijk et al 1992, Robertson et al 1994, Heslington and Hilton 1996). However, using a strict protocol for investigation and reporting, the high false-positive detection of overactive bladder in asymptomatic women is corrected (Salvatore et al 1996). There is some evidence that overactive bladder which develops after colposuspension may be occult and can be detected before surgery using ambulatory urodynamics (Khullar et al 1995). Ambulatory monitoring is time consuming and sometimes technically difficult. The equipment is expensive and fragile, which is important when women are being discharged home with the equipment *in situ*. Discomfort is a problem but is usually mild and more common in male than female patients. However, its utility has recently been reaffirmed (Pannek and Pieper 2008).

Radiology

General radiology

A plain abdominal X-ray is useful when symptoms suggest bladder calculi. Osteitis pubis is a rare complication of the Marshall–Marchetti–Krantz procedure, presenting with suprapubic pain, and is diagnosed on an anteroposterior pelvic X-ray. Sacral and lumbar spine X-rays are indicated if a congenital abnormality is suspected; for example, spina bifida and meningomyelocoele, which are important causes of neuropathic bladder disorders in children. Spinal cord trauma and tumours can also cause disturbances of micturition. Disc prolapse is common and is demonstrated on a myelogram.

Intravenous urography and computed tomography urogram

Intravenous urography is not indicated in most women with lower urinary tract symptoms unless for neuropathic bladder, suspected ureterovaginal fistula or haematuria. More commonly, a computed tomography urogram would be performed; whilst having a higher radiation dose, this also has a higher sensitivity for extrinsic pathology.

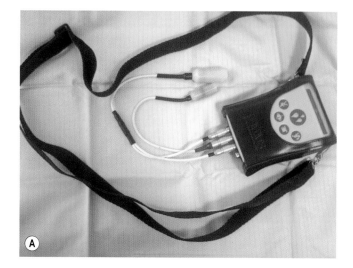

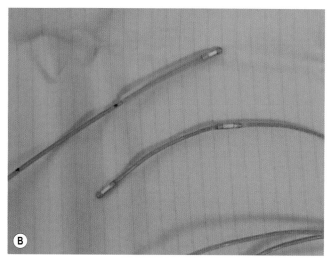

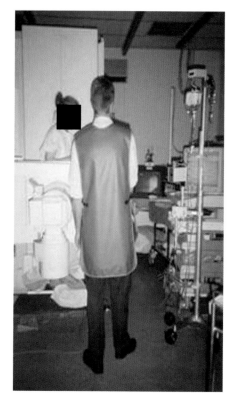

Figure 51.10 Woman undergoing a videocystourethrogram.

Figure 51.9 (A) Ambulatory recording box. (B) Microtip pressure transducers.

Videocystourethrography

Videocystourethrography (VCU) is radiological screening of the bladder synchronized with pressure studies of the bladder, recorded with a sound commentary on video (Figure 51.10). Stanton (1988) reviewed 200 cases of urinary incontinence following failed surgery, and concluded that VCU only had an advantage over cystometry in a few selected groups of women. VCU was indicated in women complaining of postmicturition dribble, which may be due to diverticulum (although magnetic resonance imaging is the gold standard for this diagnosis) (Figure 51.11).

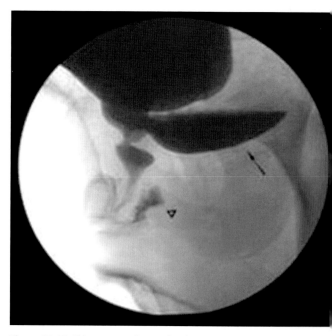

Figure 51.11 Videocystourethrography showing a urethral diverticulum.

Technique

The procedure is the same as for cystometry except the filling medium is Urografin 35% and the test is performed in a X-ray screening room. The main differences from cystometry are that the woman is tilted upright and positioned in the erect lateral oblique position. She is asked to cough and strain. Leakage, bladder neck opening and bladder base descent are all noted with X-ray screening. Any ureteric reflux and detrusor contractions are also noted. The woman commences voiding and is screened simultaneously; once the flow is established, she is asked to interrupt it. The ability of the urethra to milk contrast back into the bladder is noted.

All data are recorded and displayed at the same time as the bladder image. A sound commentary can also be recorded simultaneously.

Micturating cystogram

This investigation also involves radiological screening of the bladder but without pressure or flow measurements, and is therefore less useful in the investigation of incontinence. Its main value is to demonstrate vesicoureteric reflux, and abnormalities of bladder and urethral anatomy (e.g. diverticula, and bladder and urethral fistulae). It is not useful for the assessment of incontinence.

Ultrasound

Ultrasound is becoming more widely used in urogynaecology. Its most simple use is in the estimation of postmicturition residual urine volume and to assess the bladder neck and surrounding area.

Postmicturition urine estimation

This useful technique obviates the need for urethral catheterization with its risk of introducing infection. It is indicated in the investigation of women with voiding difficulties, either idiopathic or before surgery, and also following postoperative catheter removal. The bladder is scanned in two planes and three diameters are measured. As the bladder only approaches a spherical shape when it is full, a correction factor has to be applied. Several different formulae have been devised, and the most common is to multiply the product of three diameters (height × width × depth) by a figure of 0.625 (Hakenberg et al 1983). This has an error rate of 21%, which is acceptable. Ultrasound machines are expensive and not always available in the community setting, in clinics or on the postoperative ward where residual volumes often need to be measured. The bladder scan is a portable ultrasound device designed for the measurement of bladder volume (Figure 51.12). The machine calculates the urine volume using preconfigured settings without the operator needing to perform any mathematical calculations, and results are similar to those obtained with complex ultrasound technology for the assessment of residual urine assessment. These become inaccurate at higher volumes, but this is not of clinical significance as the relevance of a high residual, regardless of the amount, remains. The role of this technique is limited in the immediate postoperative period in a woman with an abdominal wound, and also post partum where lochia can lead to a false-positive result.

Bladder neck position

Ultrasound scanning of the bladder neck has been used as an alternative to radiological screening, and has been reported to give equivalent information to the clinician (Brown et al 1985, Richmond et al 1986).

Ultrasound of the bladder neck has been performed using the transabdominal (White et al 1980), rectal (Shapeero et al 1983), vaginal (Hol et al 1995) and transperineal (Khullar et al 1994a) routes. The transabdominal view of the

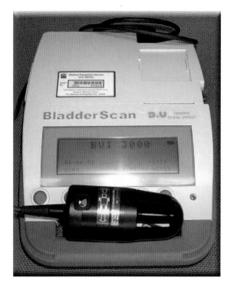

Figure 51.12 Portable ultrasound scanner used for detecting postvoid urinary residuals.

bladder neck is difficult in obese women, and there is no fixed reference point when assessing bladder neck movement. Transperineal measurement of bladder neck excursion with a specific Valsalva pressure in the antenatal period appears to predict the development of postnatal stress incontinence (King and Freeman 1998).

Vaginal, rectal and perineal probes use the lower border of the public symphysis as a fixed reference. The rectal probe is less acceptable to women, and difficulties arise with rotation of the probe, causing loss of the image.

Transvaginal ultrasound

The vaginal probe has been used successfully to image the bladder neck. Descent of the bladder base, together with bladder neck opening, has been demonstrated in a majority of women with stress incontinence but not in controls (Quinn 1990). However, bladder neck opening also occurs with overactive bladder, and this may be difficult to distinguish from stress incontinence unless there is a concomitant bladder pressure recording. The bladder neck can be compressed by the transvaginal ultrasound probe, preventing urinary leakage (Wise et al 1992). The potential for distortion of the bladder neck by the probe has not been fully assessed. Transvaginal ultrasonography has been used to measure bladder wall thickness (Khullar et al 1994b, 1996a) (Figure 51.13). Women with urodynamically diagnosed overactive bladder were found to have significantly thicker bladder walls than women with urodynamic stress incontinence, and this has been proposed as a screening and diagnostic test. However, the role of this has been challenged recently (Lekskuichai and Dietz 2008).

Perineal ultrasound

Perineal scanning is the most readily available and least expensive technique. It is less likely to cause pelvic

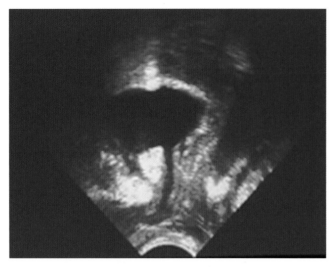

Figure 51.13 Transvaginal ultrasound picture showing measurement of bladder wall thickness in a woman with a diagnosis of detrusor overactivity.

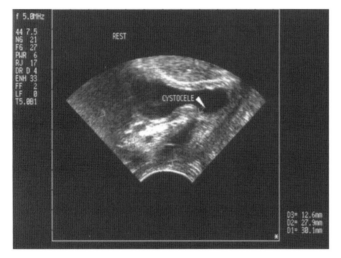

Figure 51.14 Transperineal two-dimensional ultrasound scan of the bladder neck.

distortion, is more acceptable to women and is feasible in obese women (Figure 51.14). The technique has been shown to be as accurate as lateral chain urethrocystography in the assessment of women with failed continence surgery. The equipment is accurate, portable and available in most gynaecology departments (Gordon et al 1989). It may be of use in the determination of causes of failed continence surgery (Creighton et al 1994).

Urethral ultrasound

Urethral cysts and diverticula can be examined using ultrasound. The disadvantage of this method is that unless the opening of the diverticulum is seen directly, the two cannot be differentiated. Intraurethral ultrasonography of the urethral sphincter has been described (Schaer et al 1998) and shows an association between decreased sphincter cross-sectional area and urodynamic stress incontinence. This is not used clinically at present.

Three-dimensional ultrasound of the urethra and urethral sphincter has been described (Khullar et al 1994c). This uses a perineal probe which records 150 ultrasound 'slices' as the probe scans 90° on its axis. A three-dimensional image is reconstructed, giving views of the urethra and rhabdosphincter (Figure 51.15). The volume of the urethral sphincter is larger in continent women compared with women diagnosed with urodynamic stress incontinence (Athanasiou et al 1995, Khullar et al 1996b). Evidence of damage to the rhabdosphincter is present in some women with severe urodynamic stress incontinence.

Investigations of urethral function

Urethral pressure measurement

Continence is maintained if the urethral pressure is higher than the intravesical pressure. Many methods of measuring urethral pressure have been used. It is usually measured with a catheter-tip dual-sensor microtransducer, although in the past, infusion catheters using fluid or gas and intraluminal balloons have been tried. The microtransducer system has two transducers which are 6 cm apart, 12 mm long and 1.6–2.3 mm in diameter, mounted on a 7F catheter. These catheters are easy to use but fragile and expensive.

Technique

The bladder is filled with 250 ml of physiological saline, and the catheter is passed so that both sensors are within the bladder. The catheter is then connected to a catheter withdrawal mechanism set at a standard speed of 5 cm/min and a chart recorder. The static urethral pressure is the urethral intraluminal pressure along its length with the bladder at rest. The dynamic urethral pressure (the urethral closure pressure) is the difference between the maximal urethral pressure and the intravesical pressure while the woman gives a series of coughs. Women with stress incontinence have a lower urethral closure pressure than continent women, and this is directly proportional to the severity of their incontinence (Hilton and Stanton 1983).

Clinical value

Urethral pressure measurements are useful in defining physical properties; however, their value in clinical practice is not certain, with some suggesting that this offers little added value in the prediction of outcome with contemporary sling surgery (Wadie and El-Hefnawy 2009). The static urethral pressure profile is useful to detect a low-pressure urethra where the urethral pressure is less than 20 cmH$_2$O, as these women have a 50% failure rate with conventional continence surgery. It has been suggested that they would benefit from a more obstructive procedure (Sand et al 1987).

The dynamic urethral pressure profile more closely approximates the clinical problem, but there is a large overlap for both the functional urethral length and the urethral closure pressure between normal and stress-incontinent women, and it is not possible to separate the two groups on urethral pressure profile alone. Versi (1990) compared the urethral

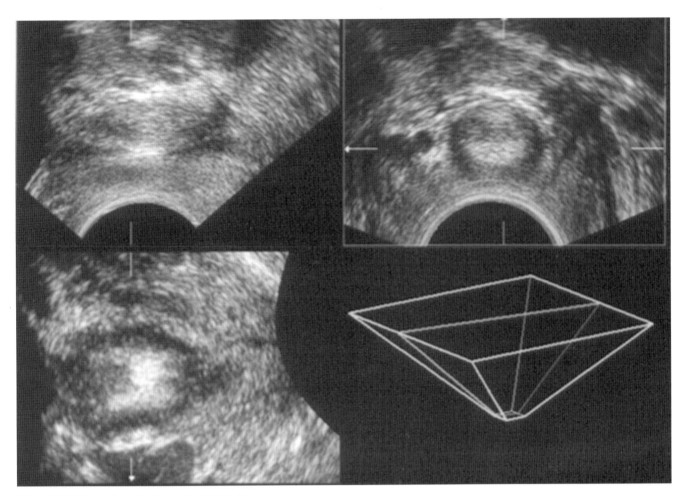

Figure 51.15 Three-dimensional scan of a rhabdosphincter.

pressure profile with VCU as the 'gold standard' investigation, and found that accurate diagnosis was not possible with the urethral pressure profile alone.

Urethral pressure measurements may be of value for the assessment of women following failed surgery and for the study of urethral diverticula or strictures.

Leak point pressure

Leak point pressures can be detrusor or abdominal. The detrusor leak point pressure is indicated in women who have incontinence and a neuropathic condition, or those who are unable to empty their bladders (McGuire and Brady 1979).

Abdominal leak point pressure is the pressure at which leakage occurs during either a cough or a Valsalva manoeuvre. The pressure can be measured using pressure catheters in the bladder, vagina or rectum. It has been proposed as a measure of urethral resistance of the urethral sphincter to increased intra-abdominal pressure (Robinson and Brocklehurst 1983). It is highly reproducible with a strong correlation with maximum urethral closure pressure. It is not clear whether this test is useful in the evaluation of urinary incontinence.

Cystourethroscopy

Cystoscopy allows the urethra and bladder to be visualized optically. It is indicated in a small group of women with incontinence, but is not a part of the routine investigation of incontinence as it gives little information about function.

Indications

- Reduced bladder capacity at cystometry.
- Recent (<6 months) history of irritative urinary symptoms (e.g. frequency and urgency).
- Suspected urethrovaginal or vesicovaginal fistula or other anatomical abnormality.
- Suspected foreign body (e.g after mesh surgery).
- Suspicion of interstitial cystitis.
- Haematuria unrelated to urinary tract infection.
- Need to exclude neoplasm in the presence of persistent urinary infection.

Cystoscopy comprises part of the operative technique in continence operations, such as the tension-free vaginal tape (TVT) procedure, to ensure that the TVT introducer needle has not passed through the bladder or in assisting in the

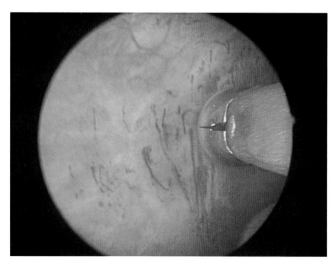

Figure 51.16 Cystoscopy with petechial haemorrhage and a Hunner's ulcer.

placement of injectables such as GAX collagen (Bard) or Macroplastique (Uroplasty).

Technique

Cystoscopy is a sterile technique performed under general or local anaesthetic. If it is used to assess reduced bladder capacity during urodynamic studies, it must be performed under general anaesthetic. The urethra is difficult to examine in women, and this is best done by withdrawing the cystoscope and using a urethroscope sheath. Residual urine should be noted, although it is not always accurate if the woman has not voided recently.

Bladder capacity is the volume at which filling usually stops using a 1-l bag of fluid under gravity feed. Using a 30° or 70° cystoscope, the mucosa should be inspected for abnormalities, such as signs of infection or tumour. A note is made on the state of the bladder and urethral mucosa, and the presence of normally situated ureteric orifices. Interstitial cystitis may be suggested by the presence of splits which bleed on decompression and a reduced capacity (Figure 51.16). If diverticula are present, an attempt must be made to see inside to exclude carcinoma and calculi. Bladder calculi may be present, particularly in women with neuropathic bladder and/or indwelling catheters. Abnormal areas must be biopsied.

Most makes of cystoscope are similar and, as they are often not interchangeable, it is preferable to stick to one type. A standard set should include a cystoscope, urethroscope sheath, 0°, 30° and 70° telescopes, a catheterizing bridge and a fibreoptic light. A set of biopsy forceps is essential, as is a method for dilating the urethra, such as a set of Hegar dilators or an Otis urethrotome. Flexible cystoscopes are more suitable for cystoscopy under local anaesthetic. If flexible cystoscopy has proven suboptimal, a formal rigid cystoscopy should be performed.

Electrophysiological tests

Electromyography

Electromyography is the study of bioelectrical potentials generated by smooth and striated muscles, and can be used to evaluate pelvic floor damage in women with urinary or faecal incontinence and prolapse. A motor unit comprises a motor nerve and the fibres it innervates. The electrical potential generated during a contraction is called the 'motor nerve unit action potential' and this can be measured using electromyography. If denervation occurs, the remaining nerves sprout collaterals to reinnervate the muscle fibres, thus increasing the dispersion of the motor unit so that more fibres of a particular unit will fire together at one time. This is seen on electromyography as an increase in the amplitude, duration and number of phases of the action potential. If reinnervation is present, polyphasic potentials are seen.

Partial denervation has been proposed as the mechanism by which childbirth contributes to the aetiology of stress incontinence. Allen et al (1990) performed transvaginal electromyography on primiparous women before and after delivery, and detected a highly significant increase in mean motor unit potential duration which was positively associated with birth weight and length of the second stage of labour. Smith et al (1989) studied anal sphincter fibre density in women with stress incontinence and/or prolapse, and found an increased fibre density in all groups compared with normal controls.

Electromyography can be performed using surface electrodes, such as anal or vaginal plugs, and ring electrodes mounted on a urethral catheter, or it can be performed using needle electrodes inserted into the external anal sphincter or periurethral muscles. Single-fibre needles give more selective recordings and allow measurement of motor unit fibre density. A single-fibre reading is more difficult to obtain than concentric needle signals as the sampling area of the needle is less (Kreiger et al 1988), but it can be improved using ultrasound (Fischer et al 2000).

Sacral reflexes

Sacral reflexes indicate the integrity of the sacral reflex arc by measuring the conduction time between a stimulus and an evoked muscle contraction. Electrical stimuli can be applied to the skin over the clitoris while recording from the pelvic floor muscle using an electromyography needle, a ring electrode on a Foley catheter or an anal plug electrode. This technique has been used in the investigation of neurogenic bladder disorders, although its usefulness in the detection of 'lower motor neurone' bladder disorders is not clear.

Conclusion

Urinary symptoms cause significant morbidity. Evaluation requires detailed symptom, QoL and urodynamic assessment. Whilst understanding the nature of urinary symptoms and their impact on patients' lives is important, determining their cause requires simple and sometimes complex urodynamic investigations. Only by fully understanding the cause of lower urinary tract pathology can we hope to improve our understanding of lower urinary tract dysfunction and provide appropriate treatment. Future developments may include non-invasive cystometry using techniques such as near-infrared spectrometry to detect contractions (Macnab and Stothers 2008).

KEY POINTS

1. Urinary infection must be excluded before any urodynamic investigation takes place.
2. Clinical history may not be a universally good predictor of urodynamic findings.
3. Peak urinary flow rate measurement is indicated in all women with voiding difficulty, particularly prior to continence surgery, which may aggravate this.
4. Stress incontinence diagnosed on cystometry is a diagnosis of exclusion; it is assessed by leakage in the absence of detrusor contractions.
5. Cough-induced detrusor overactivity may clinically mimic urodynamic stress incontinence.
6. Women undergoing repeat continence surgery should have urodynamic studies (VCU) performed.
7. Intravenous urography is not indicated in the routine investigation of incontinent women.
8. Ultrasound and magnetic resonance imaging are more widely used in assessment of the incontinent woman, with the advantage that radiological screening can be avoided.
9. Cystoscopy must be performed in the case of recurrent or persistent irritative urinary tract symptoms to exclude malignancy.
10. Partial denervation of the pelvic floor following childbirth contributes to the development of both incontinence and vaginal prolapse.

References

Abrams P, Blaivas JG, Stanton SL, Andersen JT 1988 The standardisation of terminology of lower urinary tract function. Scandinavian Journal of Nephrology Supplement 114: 5–19.

Abrams P, Cardozo L, Fall M et al 2002 The standardisation of terminology of lower urinary tract function: report from the Standardisation Sub-Committee of the International Continence Society. Neurourology and Urodynamics 21: 167–178.

Agur W, Housami F, Drake M, Abrams P 2009 Could the National Institute for Health and Clinical Excellence guidelines on urodynamics in urinary incontinence put some women at risk of bad outcome from stress incontinence surgery? BJU International 103: 635–639.

Allen RE, Hosker GL, Smith AR, Warrell DW 1990 Pelvic floor damage and childbirth: a neurophysiological study. British Journal of Obstetrics and Gynaecology 97: 770–779.

Amundsen CL, Parsons M, Tissot B, Cardozo L, Diokno A, Coats AC 2007 Bladder diary measurements in asymptomatic females: functional bladder capacity, frequency and 24 hour volume. Neurourology and Urodynamics 26: 341–349.

Anders K, Khullar V, Cardozo LD et al 1997 Ambulatory urodynamic monitoring in clinical urogynaecological practice. Neurourology and Urodynamics 16: 510–512.

Athanasiou S, Hill S, Cardozo LD et al 1995 Three dimensional ultrasound of the urethra, periurethral tissues and pelvic floor. International Urogynaecology Journal 6: 239.

Avery K, Donovan J, Peters TJ, Shaw C, Gotoh M, Abrams P 2004 ICIQ: a brief and robust measure for evaluating the symptoms and impact of urinary incontinence. Neurourology and Urodynamics 23: 322–330.

Bidmead J, Cardozo L, McLellan A, Khullar V, Kelleher CJ 2001 A comparison of the objective and subjective outcomes of colposuspension for stress incontinence in women. BJOG: an International Journal of Obstetrics and Gynaecology 108: 408–413.

Brown MC, Suthurst JR, Murray A, Richmond DH 1985 Potential use of ultrasound in place of X-ray fluoroscopy in urodynamics. British Journal of Urology 57: 88–90.

Constanti E, Lazzeri M, Bini V, Gianantoni A, Mearini L, Porena M 2008 Sensitivity and specificity of one hour pad test as a predictive value for female urinary incontinence. Urology International 81: 153–159.

Coptcoat MJ, Reed C, Cumming J, Shah PJR, Worth PHL 1988 Is antibiotic prophylaxis necessary for routine urodynamics? British Journal of Urology 61: 302–303.

Creighton SM, Clark A, Pearce JM, Stanton SL 1994 Perineal bladder neck ultrasound: appearances before and after continence surgery. Ultrasound in Obstetrics and Gynecology 14: 428–433.

Cundiff GW, Harris RL, Coates KW, Bump RC 1997 Clinical predictors of urinary incontinence in women. American Journal of Obstetrics and Gynecology 177: 262–266.

Digesu GA, Basra R, Khullar V, Hendricken C, Camarata M, Kelleher C 2009 Bladder sensations during filling cystometry are different according to urodynamic diagnosis. Neurourology and Urodynamics 28: 191–196.

Farrar DJ, Whiteside CG, Osborne JL, Turner-Warwick RT 1975 A urodynamic analysis of micturition symptoms in the female. Surgery in Gynecology and Obstetrics 141: 875–881.

Fischer JR, Heit MH, Clark MH, Benson JT 2000 Correlation of intraurethral ultrasonography and needle electromyography of the urethra. Obstetrics and Gynecology 95: 156–159.

Gordon D, Pearce M, Norton P, Stanton SL 1989 Comparison of ultrasound and lateral chain urethrocystography in the determination of bladder neck descent. American Journal of Obstetrics and Gynecology 160: 182–185.

Hakenberg OW, Ryall RL, Langlois SL, Marshal VR 1983 The estimation of bladder volume by sonocystography. Journal of Urology 130: 249–251.

Hastie KJ, Moisey CU 1989 Are urodynamics necessary in female patients presenting with stress incontinence. British Journal of Urology 63: 155–156.

Haylen BT, Ashby D, Sutherst JR, Frazer MI, West CR 1989 Maximum and average flow rates in normal male and female populations — the Liverpool nomograms. British Journal of Urology 64: 30–38.

Haylen BT, Yang V, Logan V, Husselbee S, Law M, Zhou J 2009 Does the presenting bladder volume at urodynamics have any diagnostic relevance? International Urogynecology Journal and Pelvic Floor Dysfunction 20: 319–324.

Heslington K, Hilton P 1996 Ambulatory monitoring and conventional cystometry in asymptomatic female volunteers. British Journal of Obstetrics and Gynaecology 103: 434–441.

Hilton P, Stanton SL 1983 Urethral pressure measurement by microtransducer: the results in symptom-free women and in those with genuine stress incontinence. British Journal of Obstetrics and Gynaecology 90: 919–933.

Hol M, van Bolhuis C, Vierhout ME 1995 Vaginal ultrasound studies of bladder neck mobility. British Journal of Obstetrics and Gynaecology 102: 47–53.

James MC, Jackson SL, Shepherd AM et al 1997 Can overactive bladder really be discounted with a history of pure stress urinary incontinence. International Urogynecology Journal 8: S53.

Jarvis GJ, Hall S, Stamp S, Millar DR, Johnson A 1980 An assessment of urodynamic examination in incontinent women. British

Journal of Obstetrics and Gynaecology 87: 893–896.

Jha S, Toozs-Hobson P, Parsons M, Gull F 2008 Does preoperative urodynamics change the management of prolapse? Journal of Obstetrics and Gynecology 28: 320–322.

Kelleher CJ, Cardozo LD, Khullar V, Salvatore S 1997 A new questionnaire to assess the quality of life of urinary incontinent women. British Journal of Obstetrics and Gynaecology 104: 1374–1379.

Khullar V, Abbott D, Cardozo LD et al 1994a Perineal ultrasound measurement of the urethral sphincter in women with urinary incontinence: an aid to diagnosis. British Journal of Radiology 54: 134–135.

Khullar V, Salvatore S, Cardozo LD, Kelleher CJ, Bourne TH 1994b A novel technique for measuring bladder wall thickness in women using transvaginal ultrasound. Ultrasound in Obstetrics and Gynaecology 14: 220–223.

Khullar V, Salvatore S, Cardozo LD et al 1994c Three dimensional ultrasound of the urethra and urethral pressure profiles. International Urogynaecology Journal 5: 319.

Khullar V, Salvatore S, Cardozo L, Yip A, Kelleher CJ, Hill S 1995 Prediction of the development of overactive bladder after colposuspension. Neurourology and Urodynamics 14: 486.

Khullar V, Cardozo L, Salvatore S, Hill S 1996a Ultrasound: a noninvasive screening test for overactive bladder. British Journal of Obstetrics and Gynaecology 103: 904–908.

Khullar V, Athanasiou S, Cardozo L, Salvatore S, Kelleher CJ 1996b Urinary sphincter volume and urodynamic diagnosis. Neurourology and Urodynamics 15: 334–336.

King JK, Freeman RM 1998 Is antenatal bladder neck mobility a risk factor for postpartum stress incontinence? British Journal of Obstetrics and Gynaecology 105: 1300–1307.

Kobelt G, Kirchberger I, Malone-Lee J 1999 Review. Quality-of-life aspects of the overactive bladder and the effect of treatment with tolterodine. British Journal of Urology 83: 583–590.

Krieger MS, Gordon D, Stanton SL 1988 Single fibre EMG — a sensitive tool for evaluation of the urethral sphincter. Neurourology and Urodynamics 7: 239–240.

Lagro-Jansson AL, Debruyne FM, van Weel C 1991 Value of patient's case history in diagnosing urinary incontinence in general practice. British Journal of Urology 67: 569–572.

Larsson G, Abrams P, Victor A 1991 The frequency/volume chart in overactive bladder. Neurourology and Urodynamics 10: 533–543.

Larsson G, Victor A 1992 The frequency/volume chart in genuine stress incontinent women. Neurourology and Urodynamics 11: 23–31.

Lekskulchai O, Dietz H 2008 Detrusor wall thickness as a test for detrusor overactivity in women. Ultrasound in Obstetrics and Gynecology 32: 535–539.

Lose G, Rosenkilde P, Gammelgaard J, Schroeder T 1988 Pad-weighing test performed with standardised bladder volume. Urology 32: 78–80.

Lose G, Jorgensen L, Thunedborg P 1989 24 hour home pad weighing test versus 1 hour ward test in the assessment of mild stress incontinence. Acta Obstetrica et Gynecologica Scandinavica 68: 211–215.

Macnab AJ, Stothers L 2008 Development of near-infrared spectroscopy instrument for applications in urology. Canadian Journal of Urology 15: 4233–4240.

Martin JL, Williams KS, Abrams KR et al 2006 Systematic review and evaluation of methods of assessing urinary incontinence. Health Technology Assessment 10: 1–132, iii–iv.

McGuire EJ, Brady S 1979 Detrusor sphincter dyssynergia. Journal of Urology 21: 774–777.

National Institute for Health and Clinical Excellence 2006 Urinary Incontinence: the Management of Urinary Incontinence in Women. Clinical Guideline 40. NICE, London.

Pannek J, Pieper P 2008 Clinical usefulness of ambulatory urodynamics in the diagnosis and treatment of lower urinary tract dysfunction. Scandinavian Journal of Urology and Nephrology 42: 428–432.

Perry S, Shaw C, Assassa P et al 2000 An epidemiological study to establish the prevalence of urinary symptoms and felt need in the community: the Leicestershire MRC Incontinence Study. Leicestershire MRC Incontinence Study Team. Journal of Public Health Medicine 22: 427–434.

Quinn MJ 1990 Vaginal ultrasound and urinary stress incontinence. Contemporary Reviews in Obstetrics and Gynaecology 2: 104–110.

Richmond DH, Sutherst JR, Brown MC 1986 Screening of the bladder base and urethra using linear array transrectal ultrasound scanning. Journal of Clinical Ultrasound 14: 647–651.

Robertson AS, Griffiths CJ, Ramsden PD, Neal DE 1994 Bladder function in healthy volunteers: ambulatory monitoring and conventional urodynamic studies. British Journal of Urology 73: 242–249.

Robinson JM, Brocklehurst JC 1983 Emepronium bromide and flavoxate hydrochloride in the treatment of urinary incontinence associated with overactive bladder in elderly women. British Journal of Urology 55: 371.

Salvatore S, Khullar V, Cardozo L et al 1996 Controlling for artefacts on ambulatory urodynamics. Neurourology and Urodynamics 15: 272–273.

Salvatore S, Khullar V, Cardozo L, Anders K, Digesu GA, Bidmead J 1999 Ambulatory urodynamics: do we need it? Neurourology and Urodynamics 18: 257–258.

Sand PK, Bowen LW, Panganiban R, Ostergard DR 1987 The low pressure urethra as a factor in failed retropubic urethropexy. Obstetrics and Gynecology 69: 399–402.

Schaer GN, Schmid T, Peschers U, Delancey JO 1998 Intraurethral ultrasound correlated with urethral histology. Obstetrics and Gynecology 91: 60–64.

Shapeero IG, Friedland GW, Perkash I 1983 Transrectal sonographic voiding cystourethrography: studies in neuromuscular bladder dysfunction. American Journal of Roentgenology 141: 83–90.

Smith AR, Hosker GL, Warrell DW 1989 The role of partial denervation of the pelvic floor in the aetiology of genitourinary prolapse and stress incontinence of urine. A neurophysiological study. British Journal of Obstetrics and Gynaecology 96: 24–28.

Stanton SL 1988 Videocystourethrography: its role in the assessment of incontinence in the female. Neurourology and Urodynamics 7: 172–173.

Toozs-Hobson P, Loane K 2008 Why successful treatments fail. Journal of the Association of Chartered Physiotherapists in Women's Health 102: 4–7.

van Waalwijk van Doorn ES, Remmers A, Janknegt RA 1991 Extramural ambulatory urodynamic monitoring during natural filling and normal daily activities: evaluation of 100 patients. Journal of Urology 146: 124–131.

van Waalwijk van Doorn ES, Remmers A, Janknegt RA 1992 Conventional and extramural ambulatory urodynamic testing of the lower urinary tract in female volunteers. Journal of Urology 47: 1319–1326.

van Waalwijk van Doorn ES, Meier AH, Ambergen AW, Janknegt RA 1996 Ambulatory urodynamics: extramural testing of the lower and upper urinary tract by Holter monitoring of cystometrogram, uroflowmetry, and renal pelvic pressures. Urologic Clinics of North America 23: 345–371.

Versi E 1990 Discriminant analysis of urethral pressure profilometry data for the diagnosis of genuine stress incontinence. British Journal of Obstetrics and Gynaecolology 97: 251–259.

Versi E, Cardozo L, Anand D, Cooper D 1991 Symptoms analysis for the diagnosis of genuine stress incontinence. British Journal of Obstetrics and Gynaecology 98: 815–819.

Wadie BS, El-Hefnawy AS 2009 Urethral pressure measurement in stress incontinence: does it help? International Urology and Nephrology 41: 491–495.

Ward KL, Hilton P 2008 Tension-free vaginal tape versus colposuspension for primary urodynamic stress incontinence: 5-year follow up. BJOG: an International Journal of Obstetrics and Gynaecology 115: 226–233.

Webb RJ, Ramsden PD, Neal DE 1991 Ambulatory monitoring and electronic measurement of urinary leakage in the diagnosis of overactive bladder and incontinence. British Journal of Urology 68: 148–152.

White RD, McQuown D, McCarthy TA, Ostergard DR, 1980 Real-time ultrasonography in the evaluation of urinary stress incontinence. American Journal of Obstetrics and Gynecology 138: 235–237.

Wise BG, Burton G, Cutner A, Cardozo LD 1992 Effect of vaginal ultrasound probe on lower urinary tract function. British Journal of Urology 70: 12–16.

Wyman JF, Harkins SW, Choi SC, Taylor JR, Fantl JA 1987 Psychosocial impact of urinary incontinence in women. Obstetrics and Gynecology 70: 378–381.

Wyman JF, Elswick RK, Wilson MS, Fantl JA 1991 Relationship of fluid intake to voluntary micturitions and urinary incontinence in women. Neurourology and Urodynamics 10: 132–143.

CHAPTER 52

Urethral sphincter incompetence: stress incontinence

Fiona Reid and Anthony RB Smith

Chapter Contents

TERMINOLOGY AND DEFINITIONS	798		EXAMINATION	800
EPIDEMIOLOGY	798		INVESTIGATIONS	801
PATHOPHYSIOLOGY	799		TREATMENT	802
AETIOLOGY	799		KEY POINTS	809
ASSESSMENT	800			

Terminology and Definitions

Good urogynaecological practice is dependent on the accurate definition of conditions. Any condition can be described in terms of symptoms, signs, and/or urodynamic or non-urodynamic observations. A symptom is the subjective indicator of a disease or change in condition as perceived by the patient and may lead them to seek help. A sign is any abnormality indicative of disease or a health problem, discoverable on examination of the patient; an objective indication of disease or a health problem.

The symptom of incontinence is the complaint of involuntary loss of urine (Abrams et al 2002). However, there are several types of incontinence symptoms. These have been defined by the International Continence Society's Standardization of Terminology Committee and are shown in Box 52.1. This chapter will focus on 'stress' urinary incontinence.

Stress incontinence is a well-recognized and familiar term; however, it can be misinterpreted by patients. Some patients make the assumption that 'stress' refers to their psychological state. In an attempt to reduce this confusion, other terms have been suggested such as 'activity incontinence' or 'urethral sphincter incompetence'.

The sign of stress incontinence is the observation of involuntary leakage from the urethra synchronous with effort or physical exertion, or on sneezing or coughing.

However, the urodynamic observation of stress incontinence is defined as the involuntary leakage of urine during filling cystometry, associated with increased intra-abdominal pressure, in the absence of a detrusor contraction.

The variation in prevalence of women in the population with stress incontinence partly depends on whether the presence of a symptom, sign or urodynamic observation is measured. This makes it difficult to be certain of the true prevalence of stress and other types of incontinence.

Epidemiology

The prevalence of incontinence is defined as the probability of being incontinent within the defined population group at a defined time point. The incidence of incontinence is the probability of developing incontinence during a defined period.

Almost all epidemiological studies of incontinence are cross-sectional and assess prevalence. There is a need for longitudinal studies to assess the risk factors, incidence, remission and impact of preventative strategies.

In the epidemiological assessment of the prevalence of incontinence, it is important to define the population because incontinence has been shown to vary with age and race. The prevalence of incontinence in an institutional elderly care setting is much higher than in a community-dwelling young population. Prevalence estimates for the most inclusive definitions of incontinence (e.g. 'have you ever experienced urinary incontinence') vary greatly from 5% (van Oyen and van Oyen 2002) to 69% (Swithinbank et al 1999); however, most studies fall within the range of 25–45% (Thomas et al 1980, Yarnell et al 1981, Holst and Wilson 1988, Rekers et al 1992, Lara and Nacey 1994, Hannestad et al 2000).

There is evidence that the prevalence varies depending on the methodology of the questionnaire, such as whether the survey was conducted by telephone or post.

Another factor which greatly impacts on the prevalence of urinary incontinence is bothersomeness. Swithinbank et al (1999) demonstrated that although urinary symptoms are common among the female population, they are not always perceived as a problem. Stress incontinence was experienced, at least occasionally, by 60% of the women, but only half of them felt that it was a problem.

There is less variation when studies asked about daily incontinence. Three studies conducted in women under 60

DOI: 10.1016/B978-0-7020-3120-5.00052-7

Box 52.1 International Continence Society's (ICS) standardization of terminology

Stress urinary incontinence: involuntary leakage on effort or exertion, or on sneezing or coughing.

Urge urinary incontinence: involuntary urinary leakage accompanied by or immediately preceded by urgency.

Mixed urinary incontinence: involuntary urinary leakage associated with urgency and also with effort or exertion, or on sneezing or coughing.

Enuresis: any involuntary loss of urine. If it is used to denote incontinence during sleep, it should be qualified by the adjective 'nocturnal'.

Continuous urinary incontinence: continuous leakage.

Other types of incontinence (not specifically defined by the ICS)

Situational incontinence: e.g. during sexual intercourse (during penetration, during intercourse or at orgasm) or when giggling.

Postural incontinence: involuntary loss of urine associated with change of body position, e.g. rising from a seated or lying position.

Insensible or unconscious loss: leakage that patients are unaware of as it occurs and which therefore is not associated with any trigger.

Box 52.2 Traditional risk factors for stress urinary incontinence

Parturition
Age
Oestrogen deficiency
Obesity
Pelvic support defects

years of age reported a prevalence of 4–7% (Burgio et al 1991, Miller et al 2000, Samuelson et al 2000), whilst the prevalence in women over 65 years of age was 4–14% (median 9%) (Wetle et al 1995, Nakanishi et al 1997, Brown et al 1999).

Most epidemiological studies assess all types of urinary incontinence, and few have attempted to assess the prevalence of stress incontinence. Overall, approximately half of all incontinent women have stress incontinence. Hannestad et al (2000) demonstrated that there is a regular rise in the proportion of cases of urge incontinence compared with stress incontinence from the age of 40 years. Hunskaar et al (2004), in a large epidemiological study of 29,500 women in four European countries, demonstrated a similar change in the prevalence of different types of incontinence with age. The relative prevalence of mixed urinary incontinence increased with age and that of stress incontinence decreased.

Pathophysiology

Stress incontinence occurs when the intravesical pressure overcomes the closure forces of the urethra. The factors which are necessary for the urethra to remain closed include:

- pudendal innervation;
- a well-vascularized urethral mucosa and submucosa;
- urethral smooth muscle mass;
- urethral striated muscle mass; and
- intact vaginal support of the urethra from levator ani, ligaments and fascia.

Possible variations in pathophysiology of incontinence can be made considering each of these components of continence (see Chapter 49).

However, in clinical practice, it has not been possible to accurately assess the individual components of the con-

tinence mechanism. Instead, a more simplistic approach has been adopted, categorizing stress incontinence into the dichotomous groups: intrinsic sphincter deficiency (ISD) and urethral hypermobility. The pathophysiology of stress incontinence is probably a continuum of the five factors listed above, and until they can be individually quantified, it will remain difficult to predict which specific treatment is most appropriate for an individual patient.

Aetiology

The possible risk factors for stress incontinence are shown in Box 52.2.

Some studies have demonstrated age as a significant risk factor for stress incontinence (Goldberg et al 2003), whilst others have only shown age to be significant in urge incontinence (Nygaard and Lemke 1996, Hannestad et al 2000, Samuelson et al 2000).

There are factors associated with age which may be responsible for incontinence rather than age alone. Resnick (1996) describes these using the mnemonic 'DIAPERS': Delerium, Infection, Atrophic changes, Pharmacological, psychological, Excess urine output, Restricted mobility and Stool impaction. Certainly, pharmacological agents such as α-blockers (e.g. doxazosin, an antihypertensive) can cause stress incontinence, and angiotensin-converting enzyme inhibitors can cause chronic cough which may aggravate stress incontinence.

Atrophic changes due to a lack of oestrogen may affect incontinence by decreasing urethral resistance and decreasing α-adrenoreceptor sensitivity in urethral smooth muscle.

There has been controversy about the role of oestrogens in the treatment of stress urinary incontinence, and a meta-analysis concluded that oestrogen did not improve the symptoms of stress incontinence (Ahmed Al-Badr Ross et al 2003).

Pregnancy, regardless of the mode of delivery, is associated with an increase in the prevalence of incontinence, although the majority of cases improve in the puerperium. Burgio et al (2003) found that 60% of women experienced urinary leakage during pregnancy, but this decreased to 11% by 6 weeks post partum. However, women who experience incontinence during pregnancy, even if it resolves in the puerperium, are more likely to experience incontinence in later life than those who have not had incontinence in pregnancy (Viktrup and Lose 2001).

In a large study involving over 15,000 women, Rortveit et al (2003) demonstrated that women who had a vaginal delivery were at greater risk of developing stress incontinence in later life compared with women who delivered by caesarean section (odds ratio 2.4). The evidence regarding the impact of other obstetric factors is less clear; however, there is some evidence that use of forceps increases the risk of urinary incontinence (Farrell et al 2001, Nelson et al 2001).

There is good evidence that obesity has a causal role in the development of stress incontinence. Several studies have demonstrated an association between obesity and stress incontinence (Brown et al 1999, Hannestad et al 2000, Viktrup and Lose 2001, Goldberg et al 2003), which has been confirmed by intervention studies of bariatric surgery (Deitel et al 1988, Bump et al 1992) and weight loss programmes (Auwad et al 2008). In the treatment group, there was a reduction of stress incontinence from 61% to 12% (Deitel et al 1988).

Epidemiological studies have demonstrated that the prevalence of stress incontinence is lower in Black African women (27%) compared with White women (61%) (Bump 1993). Thom et al (2006) found similar differences when comparing Black American women with White American women, and they adjusted for age, parity, hysterectomy, oestrogen use, body mass, menopausal status and diabetes. They suggested the presence of a protective factor in Black women.

Inherent differences in connective tissue may predispose to stress incontinence. Young nulliparous premenopausal women with stress incontinence had a decreased collagen I:III ratio compared with controls (Keane et al 1997).

Assessment

The assessment involves history, examination and investigations.

A detailed history is required using language that the patient understands. The International Continence Society has produced a document which standardizes the terminology of lower urinary tract symptoms (Abrams et al 2002), although these are not terms which patients will necessarily understand. The confusion caused by the term 'stress incontinence' has been highlighted. It is preferable to use a standardized validated symptom questionnaire to elicit the patient's symptoms. Terms which are not well understood are usually removed in the validation process. Such tools can be completed by the physician or the patient. They ensure that symptoms are not missed and may help patients to describe symptoms which they find embarrassing.

It is important to ask about the impact of stress incontinence on sexual function. In one study, 68% of women stated that their sex life was affected by their urinary symptoms (Ward and Hilton 2002).

Several validated symptom questionnaires exist, and the main differences are content. Some only address symptoms of stress incontinence; for example, the Severity of Symptoms Index developed by Black et al (1996). Others, such as the Kings Health Questionnaire (Kelleher et al 1997) and the Bristol Female Lower Urinary Tract Symptom (BFLUTS) Questionnaire (Jackson et al 1996), assess all lower urinary tract symptoms, and some assess all pelvic floor symptoms (Barber et al 2001, Radley et al 2006).

Recently published national guidelines in the UK (National Institute for Health and Clinical Excellence 2006) and the USA (Agency for Health Care Policy and Research 1992, 1996) even suggested that patients who only had the symptoms of pure stress incontinence could be treated surgically without the need for twin channel cystometry.

Harvey and Versi (2001) evaluated the symptoms and signs of stress incontinence in predicting the presence of urodynamic stress incontinence, and found that the isolated symptom of stress incontinence had a positive predictive value of only 56% for the diagnosis of pure urodynamic stress incontinence. This implies that history alone is not reliable in establishing a diagnosis. In practice, most urogynaecologists and urologists still perform urodynamics prior to surgery. If a detailed symptom questionnaire is used to elicit the history, few patients have 'pure' stress incontinence alone.

Some symptom questionnaires, such as BLFUTS and ePAQ (Electronic Personal Assessment Questionnaire), separately assess the degree of bother that each symptom causes and the severity of the symptom (Jackson et al 1996, Radley et al 2006). Epidemiological studies have shown that although symptoms of leakage are very common, occurring in up to 60% of the population, less than half of women are bothered by them (Swithinbank et al 1999). Hence, an assessment of bother is important. The degree to which a symptom causes bother may be specific to the patient's lifestyle and personality. Each individual patient will have their own expectations about treatment and goals which they hope to achieve. In clinical practice, it is important to establish whether or not the patient's goals are attainable.

In research or audit, a formal assessment of the impact of incontinence on a patient's quality of life can be made using a quality-of-life questionnaire. There are a large number of validated quality instruments available. The International Consultation on Incontinence (ICI) has appraised and rated the existing instruments (Donovan and Bosch 2005).

When taking a history of urinary symptoms, it is also important to consider past medical and surgical history which impacts on the diagnosis. Vesicovaginal fistulae following hysterectomy are uncommon but may be missed and diagnosed as stress incontinence.

Previous continence surgery may produce new urinary symptoms including voiding dysfunction, and may decrease the success rates of future surgery.

Examination

Physical examination of all patients with stress incontinence is important. Body mass index (BMI; kg/m^2) should be recorded because there is good evidence that links incontinence with high BMI (Hannestad et al 2000). General abdominal examination may reveal striae suggestive of underlying collagen disorders. There may also be evidence of benign joint hypermobility with hyperextension of joints. A general assessment of the patient's mobility and dexterity should be made with a view to considering if they would be capable of performing self-catheterization post operatively if necessary. A general neurological assessment should be performed because the presence of neurological disease may indicate an early need for urodynamics instead of conservative treatment.

Pelvic examination is performed to assess:

- urinary leakage;
- urethral mobility;

- bladder volume;
- assessment of levator ani;
- vaginal discharge;
- oestrogenization;
- perineum;
- prolapse; and
- pelvic mass.

Urinary leakage can be observed during a cough test which is normally performed in dorsal lithotomy with a comfortably full bladder. Stress incontinence is the observation of involuntary leakage from the urethra, synchronous with coughing or straining. A cough may induce a detrusor contraction which then causes leakage, but this can only be distinguished during cystometry. It is important to establish that leakage is not extraurethral from a urinary fistula or ectopic ureter.

Urethral mobility can be assessed visually. The patient is asked to cough or perform a Valsalva manoeuvre; if hypermobility is present, the anterior vaginal wall will rotate outwards and the urethral meatus towards the ceiling. Many clinicians will select the type of surgical intervention depending on the presence or absence of urethral mobility.

The levator ani can be assessed digitally just inside the posterior forchette on the left and right of the midline. The Modified Oxford Scale (Laycock and Jerwood 2001) (Table 52.1) provides a useful grading scale of the muscle, and has been shown to correlate well with surface electromyography and manometry (Haslam 1999).

It is always important to perform a visual inspection of the cervix because, occasionally, the leakage is due to copious vaginal discharge not urine. If there is doubt, an agent such as Pyridium can be used to stain urine.

The perineal skin should be assessed since it may be excoriated from inappropriate pad use, atrophy and ammoniacal dermatitis.

The presence of prolapse should be documented using a standardized assessment such as the pelvic organ quantification system (POP-Q) (Bump et al 1996). The advantage of POP-Q is that it has been shown to be reproducible.

Investigations

Pad tests

The main use of pad tests is to assess the outcome of treatment or to demonstrate urine loss. There are two types of pad test: short (≤ 2 h in duration) and long (>24 h). Although the only standardized test is the International Continence Society's 1-h pad test, its use as an outcome measure is limited due to its poor reliability. Simons et al (2001) demonstrated that test–retest reliability of the 1-h pad test over a period of 3–10 days, even when similar bladder volumes were used, was clinically inadequate as the first and second pad test could differ by −44 to +66 g.

The report from the second ICI (Artibani and Cerruto 2005) concluded that 24-, 48- and 72-h pad tests had better reproducibility than the 1-h test. Compliance decreases with increasing duration of the test, and for this reason, extending the test beyond 24 h was not recommended. A pad weight gain of 1.3 g or more was considered a positive test. Attempts have been made to objectively quantify the severity

Table 52.1 The Modified Oxford Scale for pelvic floor muscles (PFM)

Muscle grade	External observation	Internal examination
0	No indrawing movement of perineal body	No activity detected
1		A mere flicker of activity
2		A weak contraction but no PFM lift
3	An indrawing movement of perineal body	A moderate PFM lift but without resistance
4		A good PFM lift against some resistance
5		An ability to lift PFM against more resistance with strong grip of examing finger

of incontinence using pad tests, but there was poor correlation between the short duration tests and subjective assessments of severity (Reid et al 2007). Correlation with the 24-h pad test was only moderate (Sandvik et al 2006). Pad tests cannot be used to diagnose the type of incontinence.

Pyridium pad test

Pyridium (phenozopyridine hydrochloride) is a compound which, when ingested, causes urine to be dyed a bright yellow/orange colour. This test can be useful to determine if the leakage experienced is urine. The test needs to be performed very carefully due to the high risk of false-positive results from perineal staining after voiding. Nygaard and Zmolek (1995) reported nearly 100% Pyridium staining in asymptomatic women during exercise; however, the mean stained area was only 2.6 mm. Some women who have excessive vaginal discharge perceive this to be urine. A Pyridium test can be useful to distinguish the two conditions.

Urodynamics

Urodynamics are discussed in detail in Chapter 51. It has not yet been proven that preoperative evaluation of women with stress urinary incontinence improves the outcome of surgery. Despite this, urodynamic studies are regularly used to assess women with stress urinary incontinence in an attempt to identify preoperative risk factors for failure or postoperative voiding dysfunction. The presence of detrusor overactivity, ISD and voiding dysfunction are theoretically associated with lower cure rates. However, the ability to measure these parameters reliably using current urodynamic techniques remains debatable, and there is little robust evidence that diagnosis of these factors should alter surgical management. There is no agreed definition of ISD. Two commonly used definitions are a maximum urethral closure pressure (MUCP) of less than 20 cmH$_2$O and Valsalva leak point pressures (VLPP) of less than 60 cmH$_2$O; however, both have limitations. MUCP is a measurement made at rest, not during the dynamic stress phase. Although VLPP is a measure of pressure in the dynamic phase during 'stress', there is variation in the pressures recorded depending on catheter size, patient position and bladder volume. Another significant problem with VLPP is that up to 66% of women with stress incontinence experience leakage on coughing but do not leak with Valsalva (Sinha et al 2006).

There are no agreed definitions of significant postvoid residuals or voiding dysfunction in women, although many surgeons regard a preoperative flow rate less than 20 ml/s and a detrusor pressure at maximum flow of less than 20 cmH$_2$O as indications of higher risk of postsurgical voiding problems.

Treatment

Conservative treatment

Patients with stress incontinence may benefit from lifestyle advice. They should be encouraged to maintain a normal BMI. There is evidence that obesity is an independent risk factor for incontinence, and that weight loss in the morbidly (Deitel et al 1988, Bump et al 1992) and moderately (Subak et al 2002, Auwad et al 2008) obese will improve incontinence.

Patient are encouraged to cease smoking, reduce their caffeine intake and ensure that their fluid intake is within a normal range of 1–1.5 l/day.

There is some evidence of an association between chronic straining due to constipation and pelvic floor damage which increases the risk of incontinence (Diokno et al 1990, Spence-Jones et al 1994). However, there have been no intervention trials of the treatment of straining and urinary incontinence.

Pelvic floor muscle training

Pelvic floor muscle training (PFMT) was introduced by Kegel in the 1950s to address urinary incontinence in women (Kegel 1951). Patient education is a vital component to PFMT. The strength of pelvic floor muscle contraction should be assessed at the time of pelvic examination. On simple verbal command to squeeze their pelvic floor muscles around the examiner's fingers, many women are unable to do so, or they inadvertently contract their abdominal or gluteal muscles. Some women will even perform a Valsalva manoeuvre when asked to perform pelvic floor exercises. The pelvic examination provides an opportunity to teach the patient which muscles she needs to strengthen. Bump et al (1991) underscored the importance of education in a study in which women were given only verbal or simple written instructions to perform PFMT; 50% of the subjects were unable to perform a correct pelvic floor contraction despite their perception that they were doing so.

A large randomized controlled trial of PFMT vs no treatment in women with urodynamic stress incontinence demonstrated that self-reported cure is more likely following PFMT than no treatment (relative risk 16.8, 95% confidence interval 2.37–119.04) (Bo et al 1999).

There are very few long-term follow-up studies of PFMT. However, Lagro-Janssen and van Weel (1998) reported 5-year follow-up data on 101 of 110 women. Seven women had undergone surgery, five declined further follow-up and one had become pregnant. The results showed that the proportion of women who were dry (25%) was similar after 5 years, although the number with severe incontinence increased from 3% to 18%. Sixty-seven per cent of women remained satisfied with the outcome of treatment and did not want further treatment. Women with urge or mixed incontinence were less likely to be satisfied than women with stress urinary incontinence. Nearly half of the women (43%) who had received PFMT were no longer training at all. Logistical regression was used at 5 years to determine the relationship between age, parity, anxiety, incontinence severity, adherence to PFMT and treatment success. The only factor significantly associated with better outcome at 5 years was continued PFMT.

A Cochrane review published in 2006 investigated the effects of pelvic floor muscle training for women with urinary incontinence in comparison with no treatment, placebo or sham treatments, or other inactive control treatments (Hay-Smith and Dumoulin 2006). Six trials were included in the review, involving 403 women. The review concluded that there was some support for the widespread recommendation that PFMT be included in first-line conservative management programmes for women with not only stress urinary incontinence but also urge or mixed incontinence.

Some women are unable to isolate their pelvic floor muscles to perform PFMT, and others may perform incorrect contractions which may do more harm than good.

Biofeedback can be used to maximize rehabilitation in patients who have difficulty in performing pelvic floor contractions. Biofeedback is any signal, auditory or visual, which tells the patient that she is contracting the correct muscles. Simple verbal affirmation of a good pelvic floor muscle contraction at the time of pelvic examination is a form of biofeedback. More sophisticated forms include perineometers that consist of a rectal or vaginal probe, a visual or auditory analogue signal and abdominal electromyography electrodes. When the patient correctly contracts her pelvic floor, an analogue signal through the probe tells her she is utilizing the proper muscles. Similarly, an auditory signal via the electromyogram tells her to what degree, if any, she is recruiting her abdominal muscles. Biofeedback in addition to PFMT has been shown to be no more effective than PFMT on its own (Castleden et al 1984, Burns et al 1993); however, the group sizes were small and no trials specifically addressed the use of biofeedback in patients who could not perform a pelvic floor contraction at initial assessment.

Weighted vaginal cones represent another form of biofeedback (Figure 52.1). In theory, when a weighted cone is inserted into the vagina, the pelvic floor needs to contract to prevent it from slipping out. The patient places the lightest cone in the vagina for 15 min twice daily and goes about her normal activities. She has to contract her pelvic floor muscles to keep the cone from falling out of her vagina. When this weight becomes easy to manage, she exchanges this cone for the next heaviest. The weight of the cone is gradually increased.

A Cochrane review concluded that although limited evidence is available, it suggests that cones benefit women with stress urinary incontinence compared with no active treatment. Meta-analysis of eight trials found cones and PFMT to be no different in terms of subjective cure or improvement, pad test or pelvic muscle strength; however, PFMT was associated with a significantly greater reduction in the number of leakage episodes per day (Herbison et al 2002).

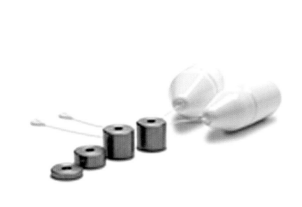

Figure 52.1 Vaginal cones.
Courtesy of Colgate Medical.

Patients who are unable to perform pelvic floor contractions despite biofeedback may be candidates for functional electrical stimulation. Direct mechanical stimulation of the pudendal nerve is delivered by either vaginal or rectal probe, causing contraction of the pelvic floor musculature. There is no robust evidence that electrical stimulation is better than PFMT alone.

Devices

The use of mechanical devices to control incontinence has been recorded since ancient Egyptian times; various elaborate but cumbersome and uncomfortable devices have been developed (Edwards 1970, Bonnar 1977). Most devices either occlude the urethra, being placed either within the urethra or over the external meatus, or are inserted into the vagina, and provide occlusive pressure against the urethra.

A Cochrane review of mechanical devices reported on six randomized controlled trials. These assessed three intravaginal and three intraurethral devices. Five of the six included studies had a very small sample size and were not large enough to detect a difference reliably. There was a lack of evidence to suggest that the use of mechanical devices is better than no treatment. There was insufficient evidence to favour one device over another, and no evidence to compare mechanical devices with other forms of treatment (Shaikh et al 2006).

Pharmacotherapy

The only pharmacological agent recommended for use in the management of stress urinary incontinence by the ICI in 2005 was duloxetine, a serotonin and noradrenaline reuptake inhibitor. Duloxetine inhibits the presynaptic reuptake of serotonin and noradrenaline in the motor neurones of the pudendal nerve, which increases the amount of these transmitters in the synapse which, in turn, increases pudendal nerve stimulation of the striated urethral sphincter. A systematic review by Mariappan et al (2007) describes the nine randomized controlled trials published comparing duloxetine with placebo. All nine trials were supported by the manufacturer of duloxetine, Eli Lilly. A total of 3066 women were randomized to duloxetine ($n = 1712$) and placebo ($n = 1354$). Subjective cure and improvement of incontinence were higher in the duloxetine arms than the placebo arms, but the differences were small and only three additional patients per 100 treated were improved. The withdrawal rate was 17% in the duloxetine group and 4% in the placebo group, and approximately 75% of withdrawals were directly attributable to duloxetine. The most commonly reported side-effects were nausea, fatigue, dry mouth, insomnia, constipation, dizziness and somnolence.

Vella et al (2008) studied a group of 228 women for up to 1 year after they were commenced on duloxetine for moderate stress incontinence. After 4 weeks, only 31% were continuing with duloxetine, 45% had discontinued it due to side-effects, and 24% had discontinued it due to lack of efficacy. At 12 months, only 9% remained on treatment. Another interesting finding of this study was that 5% of women stopped taking duloxetine after 6–12 months and remained dry. This could be due to increased bulk or strength of striated muscle, or spontaneous improvement which may reflect the natural history of incontinence.

Surgical treatment

Importance of evidence-based practice: an historical perspective

Surgical procedures to treat urinary incontinence have been reported for nearly 150 years. Initially, new operations were published as single case reports. These usually included a description of the operation and the surgeon's opinion of the value of the procedure. If an outcome was assessed, it was frequently prior to discharge, invariably successful and there were no reported complications (Brown 1864, Gilliam 1896).

In 1914, Kelly and Dumm reviewed the literature on surgery for urinary incontinence; 14 studies were included in the review. There was no documented evidence of the failure of any of the procedures. Kelly and Dumm described a new operative procedure, stating that it was more successful than any proposed previously (Kelly and Dumm 1914). The study represented a significant advancement in the reporting of the outcome of surgery for incontinence. Not only did it report a greater number of cases, a series of 20, but failures were also reported. Another notable change was the reporting of both short- and long-term outcomes. Follow-up was greater than 1 year in 13 of the 20 cases. The results of this series are shown in Table 52.2 and suggest that the operation's efficacy decreased with time. Although this trend was not noted in the report, Kelly and Dumm (1914) did criticize the short follow-up period of 5 months in a series of five patients reported by Dudley in 1895, possibly indicating a recognition that failure increases with time after surgery.

In view of the high success rates that had been reported by all surgeons up until this time, it is not surprising that Kelly and Dumm's anterior repair procedure was adopted as one of the most popular operations for urinary incontinence for the next 60 years. This suggests that contemporary operations may have had significant complications or failures that were not reported in the literature.

Other factors may have influenced the widespread adoption of Kelly and Dumm's operation; it may have been related to the relative simplicity of the procedure, or due to Kelly's general credibility, high standing and influence in the field of urology and gynaecology. Possibly, his charismatic championing of the procedure promoted its adoption (Nation 1997).

In 2009, the ICI report stated that there was enough evidence from randomized controlled trials to indicate that anterior colporrhaphy should not be used in the management of stress urinary incontinence alone (Grade A) (Smith et al 2009).

Over the last 10 years, there has been a significant change in the types of operation performed for urodynamic stress incontinence. Midurethral slings have become the most frequently performed procedure. Furthermore, the overall number of continence procedures performed in the UK has increased by 25%, from approximately 8000 per annum in 1994 to 10,000 in 2005 (Hilton 2008). The reason for this is unknown but it may be due to increased awareness among women and healthcare professionals that incontinence can be treated. However, it could be that the relative technical simplicity of midurethral slings has reduced clinicians' threshold for surgical intervention.

It is important that new procedures are assessed using robust scientific evidence. The 2008 ICI report reviewed surgical intervention for stress incontinence. The categorization of levels of evidence used by the ICI was the International Consultation on Urological Disease (ICUD) modification of the Oxford System summarized in Box 52.3. A summary of the recommendations for each operation is given in Table 52.3.

Burch colposuspension

In 1949, Marshall et al reported the empirical observation that suturing the periurethral tissues to the pubic bone alleviated stress urinary incontinence (Marshall et al 1949; Figure 52.2). The Burch procedure was developed as a modification of the Marshall–Marchetti–Krantz (MMK) procedure in 1961 (Burch 1961). The purpose is to return the bladder neck to an intra-abdominal location so that it encounters the same transmural pressure as the bladder during rises in intra-abdominal pressure.

The patient is placed in the dorsal lithotomy position to permit access to the vagina. A transverse suprapubic incision

is made and the rectus abdominis is divided along its midline raphe. The surgeon's hand is then passed beneath the rectus muscles above the peritoneum in the direction of the pubic symphysis; blunt dissection in this fashion opens the retropubic space. The operation can be performed with the peritoneum opened or closed. Once the retropubic space is exposed, the bladder neck is identified with the operator's non-dominant hand in the vagina using a Foley balloon as a guide. A swab on a stick is then used to sweep the fatty and vascular tissue off the periurethral fascia, while the vaginal fingers elevate the anterior vagina (Figure 52.3A). Keeping the vaginal fingers elevated, the surgeon is then able to take a full-thickness bite of tissue, excluding the vaginal mucosa if possible. At least two sutures are placed on both

---

Box 52.3 Modified Oxford System

Levels of evidence

1. Meta-analysis of RCTs or a good-quality RCT
2. Low-quality RCT or good-quality prospective cohort
3. Good-quality retrospective case-control and case series
4. Expert opinion without evidence

Grades of recommendation (positive or negative)

A. Usually consistent Level 1 evidence
B. Usually consistent Level 2 or 3 or 'majority evidence' from RCTs
C. Usually Level 4 or 'majority evidence' 2/3, Delphi processed expert opinion
D. Evidence is inadequate or conflicting; if expert opinion, delivered without a formal analytical process

RCT, randomized controlled trial.

Table 52.3 2009 International Consultation on Incontinence recommendations for surgery for stress urinary incontinence

Procedure	Recommended	Not recommended
Burch: open	A	
Burch: laparoscopic	B	
Tension-free vaginal tape	A	
Transobturator tapes	A	
Bladder neck sling: autologous fascia	A	
Bulking agents	B	
Anterior colporrhaphy		A
Transvaginal bladder neck sling (needle)		B
Paravaginal		B
MMK		B
Bladder neck sling: other	D	D

MMK, Marshall–Marchetti–Krantz.

Table 52.2 Case series of repairs

Outcome	At discharge	Follow-up (1–12 years)
Cured	15	4
Improved	4	6
Failed	1	3
Lost to follow-up	–	3
Total	20	16

Source: Kelly H, Dumm W 1914 Urinary incontinence in women, without manifest injury to the bladder. Surgery, Gynecology and Obstetrics 18:444–450.

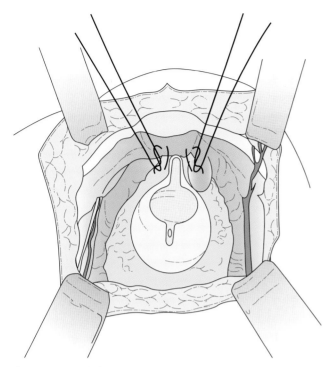

Figure 52.2 Marshall–Marchetti–Krantz procedure. One suture is placed bilaterally at the level of the bladder neck and then into the periosteum of the pubic symphysis.

Source: Karram MM, Baggish MS (eds) 2001 Atlas of Pelvic Anatomy and Gynecologic Surgery. Harcourt, New York.

sides of the bladder neck, one 2 cm lateral to the urethrovesical junction and the other 2 cm lateral to the proximal urethra. Each suture is then passed through the ipsilateral iliopectineal ligament (Cooper's ligament) on the posterolateral surface of the pubic bone (Figure 52.3B). Care should be taken not to overelevate the urethrovesical junction.

In the original MMK operation, the sutures were inserted into the periosteum which caused overelevation of the urethrovesical junction. The MMK was also associated with a 2.5% incidence of osteitis pubis.

Evidence of the effectiveness of Burch colposuspension

Burch colposuspension became the gold standard against which other procedures were compared. The outcome following open colposuspension is comparable with midurethral slings [evidence level (EL) 1], bladder neck slings (EL 1/2) and transobturator slings (EL 2).

The risk of voiding dysfunction following open colposuspension is greater than following the tension-free vaginal tape (TVT) procedure (EL 1); however, it is less than following a bladder neck sling procedure (EL 1). There is a higher incidence of pelvic organ prolapse after colposuspension compared with the TVT procedure (EL 1). The 2008 ICI report stated that open colposuspension can be recommended as an effective treatment for primary stress incontinence which has longevity (Grade A).

Evidence of the effectiveness of laparoscopic colposuspension

In 1991, Vancaillie described a laparoscopic approach for Burch colposuspension (Vancaillie and Schuessler 1991).

Laparoscopic colposuspension is comparable with open colposuspension when performed by experienced laparoscopic surgeons (EL 1/2). Studies demonstrate equal or higher cure rates with the TVT procedure (EL 1/2), and the operation time for the TVT procedure is shorter and the recovery is faster (EL 1/2). The 2008 ICI report recommended that laparoscopic colposuspension was an option for the treatment of stress incontinence (Grade B), but added the caveat that it should only be performed by experienced laparoscopic surgeons (Grade D).

Tension-free vaginal tape procedure

The TVT procedure was developed by Petros and Ulmstem (1993) and Ulmstem et al (1996) (Figure 52.4). The TVT was designed to place the sling around the midurethra, where the pubourethral ligaments are assumed to insert, rather than at the bladder neck where previous slings (e.g. Aldridge slings) were placed.

Ulmstem et al (1996) described insertion under sedation, with a premedication of 5 mg ketobemidone i.m., 0.05 mg fentanyl i.m. at the start of surgery and then prior to insertion of the sling. Up to 5 mg of midazolam i.v. was used during the operation. The bladder was emptied with a Foley catheter. Close to the superior rim of the pubic bone, two 1-cm-long transverse incisions 3 cm either side of the midline are made after injection of local anaesthetic. Between 60 and 70 ml of local anaesthetic (prilocaine and adrenaline 0.25%) is injected in the abdominal skin just above the symphysis pubis and down along the back of the pubic bone to the space of Retzius. Vaginally, 40 ml of prilocaine and adrenaline 0.25% is injected into the vaginal wall sub- and paraurethrally. An incision up to 1.5 cm long is made in the midline of the suburethral vaginal wall, starting 0.5 cm from the outer urethral meatus. Laterally from this incision, a blunt dissection 0.5–1 cm long is made with the scissors either side of the urethra to allow introduction of the TVT needle. A stent is inserted into the Foley catheter to deviate the urethravesical junction away from the path of the needle. The TVT needle perforates the urogenital diaphragm and is brought up to the abdominal incision, 'shaving' the back of the pubic bone. The procedure is then repeated on the other side, and then a cystoscopy is performed to exclude perforation; with 300 ml of saline in the bladder, the patient is asked to cough vigorously to ensure that she is dry. Importantly, the sling is only loosely placed without elevation. The plastic sheath which covers the tape is then removed, the tape is trimmed at the abdominal incisions and the incisions are closed. Ulmsten et al (1996) recommended that a size 7 Hegar dilator should be inserted into the urethra to check that the 'proximal urethra and bladder neck has an acceptable lumen and mobility'.

Evidence of the effectiveness of the tension-free vaginal tape procedure

The TVT prodecure is as effective as colposuspension and traditional sling operations (EL 1/2). Operation time, hospital stay and return to normal activity are shorter with the TVT procedure than with colposuspension (EL 1/2). Postoperative voiding problems and need for prolapse surgery are more common after colposuspension (EL 1/2).

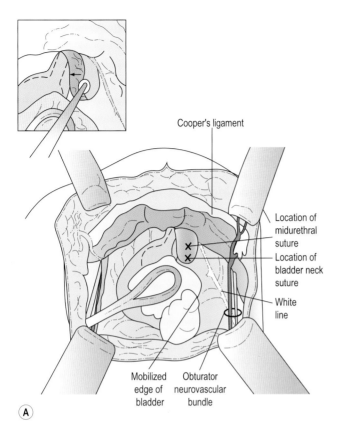

Cooper's ligament

Location of midurethral suture

Location of bladder neck suture

White line

Mobilized edge of bladder

Obturator neurovascular bundle

(A)

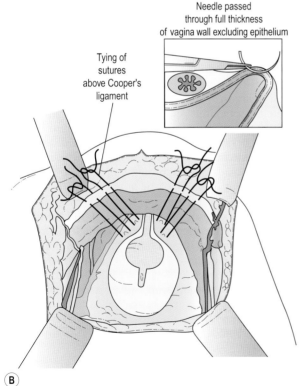

Needle passed through full thickness of vagina wall excluding epithelium

Tying of sutures above Cooper's ligament

(B)

Figure 52.3 (A) Burch colposuspension. The bladder is gently mobilized to the opposite side utilizing sponge sticks. The anterior vaginal wall is elevated by the middle finger of the surgeon's non-dominant hand. The position of the sutures should be at least 2 cm lateral to the proximal urethra and bladder neck. Xs mark the ideal placement of the Burch colposuspension sutures. Inset: The anterior vaginal wall on the right side is being elevated by a vaginal finger. A Kitner is passed on top of the finger mobilizing the fat medially. (B) Sutures have been appropriately placed on each side of the proximal urethra and bladder neck. Note: figure-of-eight bites are taken through the vagina. Double-armed sutures are utilized so the end of each suture can be brought up through the ipsilateral Cooper's ligament, thus allowing the sutures to be tied above the ligament. Inset: Detail of the suture being placed over the surgeon's vaginal finger. Note: suture should include full-thickness vaginal wall excluding the epithelium. *Source: Karram MM, Baggish MS (eds) 2001 Atlas of Pelvic Anatomy and Gynecologic Surgery. Harcourt, New York.*

The TVT procedure is more effective than the SupraPubic ARC (SPARC) procedure (EL 2), and the intravaginal sling-plasty procedure is comparable to the TVT procedure in terms of efficacy but has a higher complication rate (EL 2) (Smith et al 2008).

Transobturator tape procedure

In 2001, Delorme described a new procedure using transobturator tape based on the principles of the TVT procedure, but designed to avoid the risk of bladder perforation (Ward and Hilton 2002) and the rare complication of bowel perforation (Leboeuf et al 2003). Instead of passing the tape through the retropubic space, it is inserted via the obturator foramen. Delorme described an outside-in technique in which the tape is introduced through the skin of the groin, obturator foramen and out of the vaginal incision (Delorme 2001) (Figure 52.5).

Evidence of the effectiveness of the transobturator tape procedure

To date, two meta-analyses of transobturator tape procedures have been published and both concluded that there was limited evidence (Latthe et al 2007, Sung et al 2007). No objective outcomes were reported in the meta-analysis because these were only reported in one randomized controlled trial. The analysis by Latthe et al (2007) considered the two different routes of transobturator tapes and excluded SPARC retropubic tapes. When compared with the TVT procedure, the subjective cure of stress urinary incontinence was slightly worse in the TVT obturator procedure, inside-to-out group (odds ratio 0.69, 95% confidence interval 0.42–1.14), although this was not statistically significant. The transobturator tape procedures were associated with fewer bladder injuries and voiding difficulty than the TVT procedure, but more groin pain and vaginal mesh erosion (Latthe et al 2007).

The 2008 ICI report concluded that retropubic and transobturator tape procedures perform equally at a short-term follow-up of 6–12 months, and overall reported complication rates are comparable (EL 1/2).

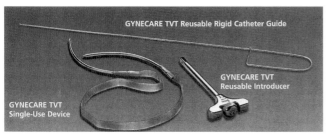

Figure 52.4 Tension-free vaginal tape. The needles are passed to either side of the midurethra with the help of the removable handle. Also shown is the catheter guide that is used during passing of the tape to divert the bladder neck away from the path of the needle.
Courtesy of Ethicon Inc.

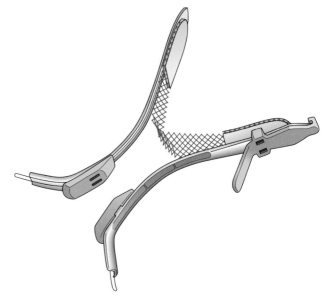

Figure 52.6 The TVT Secur.
Courtesy of Gynecare/Ethicon.

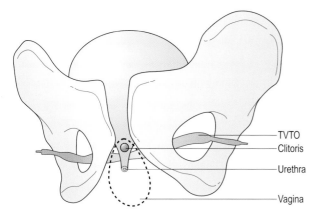

Figure 52.5 The outside-in technique in which the transobturator tape (TVTO) is introduced through the skin of the groin, obturator foramen and out of the vaginal incision.

Minitape procedures

A number of manufacturers have developed minitapes or single incision slings (SISs). They only require a vaginal incision. Potentially these SISs could be inserted under local anaesthetic as an office procedure; however, there is currently inadequate data to use these tapes outside of a research setting. Figure 52.6 shows the TVT Secur, the first of these minitapes.

Bladder neck sling procedures

Slings are performed with the patient in the dorsolithotomy position. A horizontal incision is made approximately 2 cm above the pubic symphysis. The subcutaneous fat is dissected, providing visualization of the rectus fascia. If rectus fascia is to be harvested from the patient, the incision may need to be longer. An alternative source of sling material is fascia lata that is obtained from the patient's thigh by excision or the use of a fascial stripper (Figure 52.7A). Once a 4 × 4 cm piece (for a patch-type sling) or two 2 × 8 cm portions (which are sewn end to end to create a long enough graft for a full-length sling) of fascia have been excised, the defect is closed with delayed absorbable suture. If the patient permits, cadaveric donor fascia can be used. It saves time, is

abundant and risk is minimal. The fascia is kept in saline until it is required.

Attention is then turned to the vagina where a midline anterior vaginal incision is made. The vaginal wall is dissected off the underlying bladder and urethra. This dissection is continued laterally to both sides of the bladder neck until the underside of the pubic symphysis is encountered. At this point, a curved instrument such as a Kelly clamp or Stamey needle is passed from the abdominal incision, through the rectus fascia just above the symphysis. It traverses through the retropubic space by keeping the instrument in constant contact with the back of the pubic bone, finally emerging into the vagina where the vaginal dissection is carried to the underside of the pubic bone. The entry of the instrument into the vaginal dissection is assisted by placing a vaginal finger lateral to the bladder neck along the underside of the symphysis. The instrument is aimed at this finger and guided into the vagina. The same procedure is repeated on the other side.

When placing a full-length sling, the central portion of the graft is sewn in place at the level of the bladder neck with an absorbable suture. Each end of the sling is then pulled up through the retropubic space using the previously passed instruments (Figure 52.7B). Once the end of the graft is above the level of the abdominal rectus fascia, it is either sewn to the fascia on either side or in the midline to the other end of the graft. For patch slings, the tissue is folded or trimmed to the correct size then sewn in place at the bladder neck (Figure 52.7C). A permanent suture is then fixed to either side of the patch and the ends are pulled up through the retropubic space to the abdominal incision, as described for the full-length sling. Similarly, the ends of the permanent suture can be tied to one another across the midline. Alternatively, the Stamey needle can be passed through the rectus fascia in two different locations on both

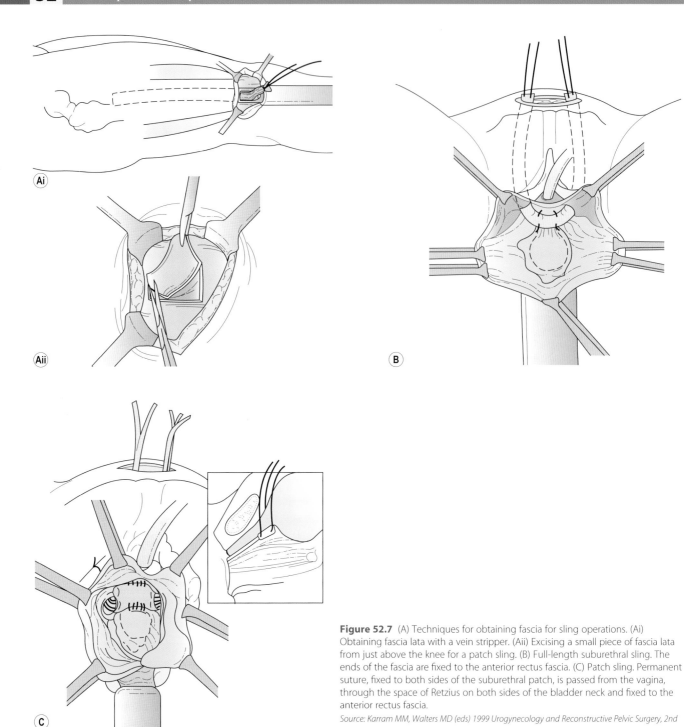

(Ai)

(Aii)

(B)

(C)

Figure 52.7 (A) Techniques for obtaining fascia for sling operations. (Ai) Obtaining fascia lata with a vein stripper. (Aii) Excising a small piece of fascia lata from just above the knee for a patch sling. (B) Full-length suburethral sling. The ends of the fascia are fixed to the anterior rectus fascia. (C) Patch sling. Permanent suture, fixed to both sides of the suburethral patch, is passed from the vagina, through the space of Retzius on both sides of the bladder neck and fixed to the anterior rectus fascia.

Source: Karram MM, Walters MD (eds) 1999 Urogynecology and Reconstructive Pelvic Surgery, 2nd edn. Mosby, St Louis.

sides (a total of four passes), and each end of the permanent suture can be brought up through its own tract. The two left ends are tied to one another on the left side and the two right ends are tied on the right.

The most challenging part of a sling procedure is determining the correct amount of tension to apply. The balance one tries to obtain is continence without creating postoperative voiding dysfunction. In general, the sling should be tied under as little tension as possible. This can be accomplished by placing a right-angle clamp between the sling and the bladder neck at the time when the abdominal portion of the

graft is being tied. Some advocate using a Q-tip to assist in tightening the sling until an angle of 0° to +10° is achieved. Others perform this portion of the procedure with a cystoscope in place, and some simply fill the bladder and adjust the sling until there is no leakage.

Evidence of the effectiveness of bladder neck sling procedures

The 2009 ICI report stated that rectus sheath fascial slings are effective (EL 1). There was no high-level evidence comparing autologous, biological and synthetic slings, although

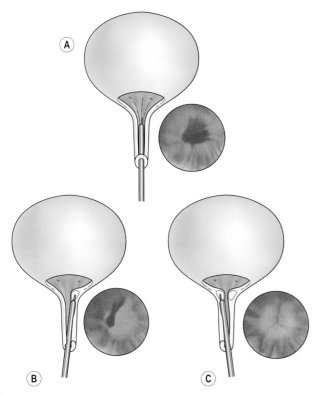

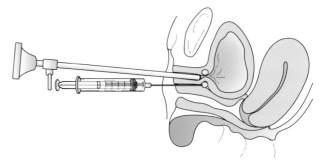

Figure 52.9 Technique for periurethral injection of urethral bulking agents.
Source: Karram MM, Walters MD (eds) 1999 Urogynecology and Reconstructive Pelvic Surgery, 2nd edn. Mosby, St Louis.

Figure 52.8 Technique for transurethral injection of urethral bulking agents. (A) Bladder neck open prior to injection. (B) Submucosal placement of needle at one site partially closes bladder neck. (C) Complete closure of bladder neck at completion of the procedure.
Source: Karram MM, Walters MD (eds) 1999 Urogynecology and Reconstructive Pelvic Surgery, 2nd edn. Mosby, St Louis.

autologous slings may be more effective (EL 2) and adverse events may be more common with alternative materials (EL 3). The ICI recommended that the autologous fascial sling procedure is an effective treatment for stress urinary incontinence which has longevity (Grade A). However, further research is required to compare autologous sling procedures with other sling materials.

Urethral bulking agents

For over 70 years, urethral bulking agents have been used for the treatment of stress urinary incontinence. They are injected transurethrally (Figure 52.8) or periurethrally (Figure 52.9) under direct cystoscopic guidance or through a guidance device.

The ideal urethral bulking agent has not yet been identified, nor has the injection route, location for injection or the optimal number of injection sites.

The mechanism of action is not fully understood, but it may be an obstructive effect. The long-term success may not correlate with the endoscopic appearance at the conclusion of the injection.

A variety of substances have been reported to be safe and effective. These include bovine glutaraldehyde cross-linked bovine collagen (Contigen®), polytetrafluoroethylene (Teflon®), polydimethyl-siloxane elastomer (Macroplastique®), porcine dermal implant (Permacol®), carbon-coated zirconium beads (Durasphere®), non-animal stabilized hyaluronic acid/dextranomer NASHA/Dx (Zuidex®), calcium hydroxyapatite (Coaptite®), ethylene vinyl alcohol (Uryx®, Tegress®) and, most recently, polyacrylamide hydrogel (Bulkamid®).

Evidence of the effectiveness of periurethral injection therapy

A Cochrane review in 2007 stated that the evidence was inadequate to inform practice; however, injection therapy may represent a useful option for short-term symptomatic relief amongst selected women with comorbidity that precludes anaesthesia (Keegan et al 2007).

With regard to urethral bulking agents, the 2008 ICI report concluded that the evidence of benefit from urethral bulking agents is limited, and appears to be short term.

There is no evidence that any one bulking agent has an advantage over any other (EL 2). Conventional surgery appears to provide a greater cure rate; however, the risk of complications may be greater (EL 2). There are no studies comparing urethral bulking agents with non-surgical treatments. The ICI recommended that when urethral bulking agents are to be used, women should be made aware that repeat injections are likely to be required to achieve efficacy, that efficacy diminishes with time, and efficacy is inferior to that of conventional surgical techniques; they should also be made aware of alternative minimally invasive procedures (Grade B).

KEY POINTS

1. Stress urinary incontinence (SUI) is the complaint of involuntary leakage on effort or exertion, or on sneezing or coughing.

2. The term stress incontinence can be misinterpreted by patients. Some make the assumption that 'stress' refers to their psychological state.

3. Prevalence depends on the population studied, the definition of incontinence used and the degree of bother assessed.

4. Between 4% and 7% of women under 60 years old experience daily incontinence.

5. There are multiple risk factors for the development of SUI, including parturition, advanced age, oestrogen deficiency, obesity and loss of pelvic tissue support.

6. Taking a good history is paramount because there has been a move to initiate conservative treatments prior to urodynamic assessment.

7. The ICI, NICE and Cochrane reviews provide up-to-date evidence about the efficacy of treatments.

8. All patients should be given a trial of conservative measures. These interventions may improve symptoms in up to 75% of patients.

9. The risks and untoward effects of the surgical options must be discussed in detail with the patient.

10. Patients with persistent recurrent SUI must be evaluated thoroughly to rule out complications of their prior incontinence operation.

References

Abrams P, Cardozo L, Fall M et al 2002 The standardisation of terminology of lower urinary tract function. The International Continence Society Committee on Standardisation of Terminology. Neurourology and Urodynamics 21: 167–178.

Agency for Health Care Policy and Research 1992 Clinical Practice Guideline: Urinary Incontinence in Adults. No. 92-0682. US Department of Health and Human Services, Rockville, MD.

Agency for Health Care Policy and Research 1996 Clinical Practice Guideline: Urinary Incontinence in Adults. No. 96-0682. US Department of Health and Human Services, Rockville, MD.

Ahmed Al-Badr Ross S, Soroka D, Durtz H 2003 What is the available evidence for hormone replacement therapy for women with stress incontinence? Journal of Obstetrics and Gynaecology Canada 25: 567–574.

Artibani W, Cerruto M 2005 Imaging and other investigations. International Consultation on Incontinence, Monaco. Health Publication Ltd, Plymouth, MA.

Auwad W, Steggles P, Bombieri L, Waterfield M, Wilkin T, Freeman R 2008 Moderate weight loss in obese women with urinary incontinence: a prospective longitudinal study. International Urogynecology Journal and Pelvic Floor Dysfunction 19: 1251–1259.

Barber M, Kuchibhatla MN, Pieper CF, Bump RC 2001 Psychometric evaluation of 2 comprehensive condition specific quality of life instruments for women with pelvic floor disorders. American Journal of Obstetrics and Gynecology 185: 1388–1395.

Black N, Griffiths J, Pope C 1996 Development of a symptom severity index and a symptom impact index for stress incontinence in women. Neurourology and Urodynamics 15: 630–640.

Bo K, Taleth T, Holme I 1999 Single blind RCT of pelvic floor exercises, electrical stimulation, vaginal cones and no treatment in the management of genuine stress incontinence in women. BMJ (Clinical Research Ed.) 318: 487–493.

Bonnar J 1977 Silicone vaginal appliance for control of stress spincontinence. The Lancet 2: 1161.

Brown B 1864 Clinical lectures on diseases of women remediable by operation. The Lancet 83(2114): 263–266.

Brown JS, Grady D, Ouslander JG, Herzog AR, Varner RE, Posner SF 1999 Prevalence of urinary incontinence and associated risk factors in postmenopausal women. Heart & Estrogen/Progestin Replacement Study (HERS) Research Group. Obstetrics and Gynecology 94: 66–72.

Bump RC 1993 Racial comparisons and contrasts in urinary incontinence and pelvic organ prolapse. Obstetrics and Gynecology 81: 421–425.

Bump RC, Hurt WG, Fantl JA, Wyman JF 1991 Assessment of Kegel pelvic muscle exercise performance after brief verbal instruction. American Journal of Obstetrics and Gynecology 165: 322–327.

Bump RC, Sugerman HJ, Fantl JA, McClish DK 1992 Obesity and lower urinary tract function in women: surgically induced weight loss. American Journal of Obstetrics and Gynecology 167: 392–397.

Bump R, Mathiasson A, Bo K 1996 The standardization of terminology of female pelvic organ prolapse and pelvic floor dysfunction. American Journal of Obstetrics and Gynecology 175: 10–17.

Burch J 1961 Urethrovaginal fixation to Cooper's ligament for correction of stress incontinence, cystocele and prolapse. American Journal of Obstetrics and Gynecology 81: 281–290.

Burgio K, Matthews K, Engel B 1991 Prevalence, incidence and correlates of urinary incontinence in healthy middle age women. Journal of Urology 146: 1255–1259.

Burgio KL, Zyczynski H, Locher JL, Richter HE, Redden DT, Wright KC 2003 Urinary incontinence in the 12-month postpartum period. Obstetrics and Gynecology 102: 1291–1298.

Burns PA, Pranikoff K, Nochajski TH, Hadley EC, Levy KJ, Ory MG 1993 A comparison of effectiveness of biofeedback and pelvic muscle excercise treatment of stress incontinence in older community dwelling women. Journal of Gerontology 48: M167–M174.

Castleden C, Duffin H, Mitchell E 1984 The effect of physiotherapy on stress incontinence. Age and Ageing 13: 235–237.

Deitel M, Stone E, Kassam HA, Wilk EJ, Sutherland DJ 1988 Gynecologic-obstetric changes after loss of massive excess weight following bariatric surgery. Journal of the American College of Nutrition 7: 147–153.

Delorme E 2001 Transobturator urethral suspension: mini-invasive procedure in the treatment of stress incontinence in women. Progres en Urologie 11: 1306–1313.

Diokno AC, Brock BM, Herzog AR, Bromberg J 1990 Medical correlates of urinary incontinence in the elderly. Urology 36: 129–138.

Donovan JL, Bosch R 2005 Symptom and quality of life assessment. International Consultation on Incontinence, Monaco. Health Publication Ltd, Plymouth, MA.

Dudley E 1895 Transactions of the American Gynecological Society xxx: 3.

Edwards L 1970 Mechanical and other devices. In: Urinary Incontinence. Academic Press, London, pp. 115–127.

Farrell S, Allen V, Baskett T 2001 Parturition and urinary incontinence in primiparas. Obstetrics and Gynecology 97: 350.

Gilliam T 1896 An operation for the cure of incontinence of urine in the female. American Journal of Obstetrics 33: 177–182.

Goldberg RP, Kwon C, Gandhi S, Atkuru LV, Sorensen M, Sand PK 2003 Urinary incontinence among mothers of multiples: the protective effect of cesarean delivery. American Journal of Obstetrics and Gynecology 188: 1447–1450.

Hannestad YS, Rortveit G, Sandvik H, Hunskaar S 2000 A community based epidemiological survey of female urinary incontinence: the Norwegian EPINCORT study. Journal of Clinical Epidemiology 53: 1150–1157.

Harvey M, Versi E 2001 Predictive value of clinical evaluation of stress urinary incontinence: a summary of the published literature. International Urogynaecology Journal 12: 31–37.

Haslam J 1999 Evaluation of Pelvic Floor Muscle Assessment: Digital, Manometric and Surface Electromyography in Females. MPhil Thesis, University of Manchester, Manchester.

Hay-Smith E, Dumoulin C 2006 Pelvic floor muscle training versus no treatment or inactive control treatments, for urinary incontinence in women. Cochrane Database of Systematic Reviews 1: CD005654.

Herbison P, Plevnik S, Mantle J 2002 Weighted vaginal cones for urinary incontinence. Cochrane Database of Systematic Reviews CD002114(1).

Hilton P 2008 Long-term follow-up studies in pelvic floor dysfunction: the Holy Grail or a realistic aim? BJOG: an International Journal of Obstetrics and Gynecology 115: 135–143.

Holst K, Wilson P 1988 The prevalence of urinary incontinence and reasons for not seeking treatment. New Zealand Medical Journal 101: 756–758.

Hunskaar S, Lose G, Sykes D, Voss S 2004 The prevalence of urinary incontinence in women in four European countries. BJU International 93: 324–330.

Jackson S, Donovan J, Brookes S, Eckford S, Swithinbank L, Abrams P 1996 The Bristol Female Lower Urinary Tract Symptoms questionnaire: development and psychometric testing. BJU International 77: 805–812.

Karram MM, Walters MD (eds) 1999 Urogynecology and Reconstructive Pelvic Surgery, 2nd edn. Mosby, St Louis.

Karram MM, Baggish MS (eds) 2001 Atlas of Pelvic Anatomy and Gynecologic Surgery. Harcourt, New York.

Keane DP, Sims TJ, Abrams P, Bailey AJ 1997 Analysis of collagen status in premenopausal nulliparous women with genuine stress incontinence. BJOG: an International Journal of Obstetrics and Gynaecology 104: 994–998.

Keegan PE, Atiemo K, Cody J, McClinton S, Pickard R 2007 Periurethral injection therapy for urinary incontinence in women. Cochrane Database of Systematic Reviews 3: CD003881.

Kegel A 1951 Physiological therapy for urinary stress incontinence. Journal of the American Medical Association 146: 915–917.

Kelleher CJ, Cardozo LD, Khullar V, Salvatore S 1997 A new questionnaire to assess the quality of life of urinary incontinent women. BJOG: an International Journal of Obstetrics and Gynaecology 104: 1374–1379.

Kelly H, Dumm W 1914 Urinary incontinence in women, without manifest injury to the bladder. Surgery, Gynecology and Obstetrics 18: 444–450.

Lagro-Janssen T, van Weel C 1998 Long term effect of treatment of female incontinence in general practice. British Journal of General Practice 48: 1735–1738.

Lara C, Nacey J 1994 Ethnic differences between Maori, Pacific Island and European New Zealand women in prevalence and attitudes to urinary incontinence. New Zealand Medical Journal 107: 374–376.

Latthe P, Foon R, Toozs-Hobson P 2007 Transobturator and retropubic tape procedures in stress urinary incontinence: a systematic review and a metaanalysis of effectiveness and complications. BJOG: an International Journal of Obstetrics and Gynaecology 114: 522–531.

Laycock J, Jerwood D 2001 Pelvic floor assessment: the PERFECT scheme. Physiotherapy 87: 631–642.

Leboeuf L, Tellez CA, Ead D, Gousse AE 2003 Complication of bowel injury perforation during insertion of tension-free vaginal tape. Journal of Urology 170: 1310.

Mariappan P, Alhasso A, Ballantyne Z, Grant A, N'Dow J 2007 Duloxetine, a serotonin and noradrenaline reuptake inhibitor (SNRI) for the treatment of stress urinary incontinence: a systematic review. European Urology 51: 67–74.

Marshall V, Marchetti A, Krantz K 1949 The correction of stress incontinence by simple vesicourethral suspension. Surgery, Gynecology and Obstetrics 88: 509–518.

Miller L, Lose G, Jorgensen T 2000 The prevalence and bothersomeness of lower urinary tract symptoms in women 40–60 years of age. Acta Obstetricia et Gynecologica Scandinavica 79: 298–305.

Nakanishi N, Tatara K, Naramura H, Fujiwara H, Takashima Y, Fukuda H 1997 Urinary and faecal incontinence in a community-residing older population in Japan. Journal of the American Geriatric Society 45: 215–219.

Nation E 1997 Howard Atwood Kelly (1858–1943). Journal of Pelvic Surgery 3: 71–74.

Nelson R, Furner S, Jesudason V 2001 Urinary incontinence in Wisconsin skilled nursing facility: prevalence and associations in common with fecal incontinence. Journal of Aging and Health 13: 539–547.

National Institute for Health and Clinical Excellence 2006 Urinary Incontinence: the Management of Urinary Incontinence in Women. NICE, London. Available at: http://www.nice.org.uk/CG040/.

Nygaard I, Lemke J 1996 Urinary incontinence in rural older women; prevalence, incidence and remission. Journal of the American Geriatric Society 44: 1049–1054.

Nygaard I, Zmolek G 1995 Exercise pad testing in continent exercisers: reproducibility and correlation with voided volume, pyridium staining and type of excercise. Neurourology and Urodynamics 14: 125–129.

Petros P, Ulmstem U 1993 An integral theory and its method for the diagnosis and management of female urinary incontinence. Scandinavian Journal of Urology and Nephrology 153: 1–93.

Radley SC, Jones GL, Tanguy EA, Stevens VG, Nelson C, Mathers NJ 2006 Computer interviewing in urogynaecology: concept, development and psychometric testing of an electronic pelvic floor assessment questionnaire (ePAQ) in primary and

secondary care. BJOG: an International Journal of Obstetrics and Gynaecology 113: 231–238.

Reid F, Smith A, Dunn G 2007 Which questionnaire? A psychometric evaluation of three patient-based outcome measures used to assess surgery for stress urinary incontinence. Neurourology and Urodynamics 26: 123–128.

Rekers H, Drogendijk AC, Valkenburg H, Riphagen F 1992 Urinary incontinence in women 35 to 79 years of age: prevalence and consequences. European Journal of Obstetrics, Gynecology and Reproductive Biology 43: 229–234.

Resnick N 1996 Geriatric incontinence. Urologic Clinics of North America 23: 55–74.

Rortveit G, Daltveit AK, Hannestad YS, Hunskaar S; Norwegian EPINCONT Study 2003 Urinary incontinence after vaginal delivery or cesarean section. New England Journal of Medicine 348: 900–907.

Samuelson E, Victor F, Svardsudd K 2000 Five year incidence and remission rates of female urinary incontinence in Swedish population less than 65 years old. American Journal of Obstetrics and Gynecology 183: 568–574.

Sandvik H, Espuna M, Hunskaar S 2006 Validity of incontinence severity index: comparison with pad-weighing tests. International Urogynecology Journal and Pelvic Floor Dysfunction 17: 520–524.

Shaikh S, Ong EK, Glavind K, Cook J, N'Dow JM 2006 Mechanical devices for urinary incontinence in women. Cochrane Database of Systematic Reviews 3: CD001756.

Simons AM, Yoong WC, Buckland S, Moore KH 2001 Inadequate repeatability of the one hour pad test; the need for a new incontinence outcome measure. BJOG: an International Journal of Obstetrics and Gynaecology 108: 315–319.

Sinha D, Nallaswamy V, Arunkalaivanan A 2006 Value of leak point pressure study in women with incontinence. Journal of Urology 176: 186–188.

Smith A et al 2009 Surgery for urinary incontinence in women. International Consultation on Incontinence, 2008. Health Publication Ltd, Plymouth, MA.

Spence-Jones C, Kamm MA, Henry MM, Hudson CN 1994 Bowel dysfunction: a pathogenic factor in uterovaginal prolapse and urinary stress incontinence. BJOG: an International Journal of Obstetrics and Gynaecology 101: 147–152.

Subak LL, Johnson C, Whitcomb E et al 2002 Does weight loss improve incontinence in moderately obese women? International Urogynecology Journal and Pelvic Floor Dysfunction 13(1): 40–43.

Sung VW, Schleinitz MD, Rardin CR, Ward RM, Myers DL 2007 Comparison of retropubic vs transobturator approach to midurethral slings: a sytematic review and meta-analysis. American Journal of Obstetrics and Gynecology 197: 3–11.

Swithinbank LV, Donovan JL, du Heaume JC et al 1999 Urinary symptoms and incontinence in women: relationship between occurrence, age and perceived impact. British Journal of General Practice 49: 897–900.

Thom DH, Van Den Eeden SK, Ragins AI et al 2006 Differences in prevalence of urinary incontinence by race/ethnicity 6. Journal of Urology 175: 259–264.

Thomas TM, Plymat KR, Blannin J, Meade TW 1980 Prevalence of urinary incontinence. BMJ (Clinical Research Ed.) 281: 1243–1245.

Ulmsten U, Henriksson L, Johnson P, Varhos G 1996 An ambulatory surgical procedure under local anesthesia for treatment of female urinary incontinence. International Urogynecology Journal and Pelvic Floor Dysfunction 7: 81–85.

van Oyen H, van Oyen P 2002 Urinary incontinence in Belgium; prevalence, correlates and psychological consequences. Acta Clinica Belgica 57: 207–218.

Vancaillie T, Schuessler W 1991 Laparoscopic bladderneck suspension. Journal of Laparoendoscopic Surgery 1: 169–173.

Vella M, Dukkett J, Basu M 2008 Duloxetine 1 year on: the long term outcome of women prescribed duloxetine. International Urogynecology Journal and Pelvic Floor Dysfunction 19: 961–964.

Viktrup L, Lose G 2001 The risk of stress incontinence 5 years after first delivery.

American Journal of Obstetrics and Gynecology 185: 82–87.

Ward K, Hilton P 2002 Prospective multicentre randomised trial of tension free vaginal tape and colposuspension as primary treament for stress incontinence. BMJ (Clinical Research Ed.) 325: 67–70.

Wetle T, Scherr P, Branch LG et al 1995 Difficulty with holding urine among older persons in a geographically defined community: prevalence and correlates. Journal of the American Geriatric Society 43: 349–355.

Yarnell JW, Voyle GJ, Richards CJ, Stephenson TP 1981 The prevalence and severity of urinary incontinence in women. Journal of Epidemiology and Community Health 35: 71–74.

CHAPTER 53

The overactive bladder syndrome

Dudley Robinson and Linda Cardozo

Chapter Contents

INTRODUCTION	813	PHARMACOLOGY	820
OVERACTIVE BLADDER	813	OESTROGENS IN THE MANAGEMENT OF OVERACTIVE BLADDER	826
DETRUSOR OVERACTIVITY	813	INTRAVESICAL THERAPY	827
INCIDENCE	813	BEHAVIOURAL THERAPY	827
AETIOLOGY	814	NEUROMODULATION	828
MUSCARINIC RECEPTORS	814	SURGERY	829
PATHOPHYSIOLOGY	814	NATIONAL INSTITUTE FOR HEALTH AND CLINICAL EXCELLENCE GUIDELINES	829
CLINICAL PRESENTATION	815	CONCLUSION	830
QUALITY OF LIFE	816	KEY POINTS	830
INVESTIGATIONS	816		
TREATMENT	819		

Introduction

The normal adult human bladder is under voluntary control and does not contract, except during micturition. Conversely, an overactive bladder is one which contracts involuntarily or can be provoked to do so. Raised bladder pressure was first reported in certain neurological conditions over 70 years ago (Rose 1931, Langworthy et al 1936), but its clinical significance was not appreciated until 1963 when Hodgkinson et al demonstrated urinary incontinence as a result of detrusor contractions in 64 neurologically normal women. They called this condition 'dyssynergic detrusor dysfunction'. Various other names have been used, including 'detrusor instability', 'detrusor reflex instability', 'overactive bladder' and 'detrusor hyperreflexia'. The terminology of lower urinary tract dysfunction has been revised and standardized by the International Continence Society in order to clarify understanding of patient symptoms and diagnosis (Abrams et al 2002).

Overactive Bladder

The term 'overactive bladder' (then 'unstable bladder') was first used by Bates et al (1970) to describe 'the objectively measured loss of ability to inhibit detrusor contraction even when it is provoked to contract by filling, change of posture, coughing, etc.' More recently, overactive bladder has been redefined as the symptom-based diagnosis of 'urgency, with or without urge incontinence usually with frequency and nocturia' (Abrams et al 2002).

Detrusor Overactivity

The symptoms of overactive bladder are due to involuntary contractions of the detrusor muscle during the filling phase of the micturition cycle. These involuntary contractions are termed 'detrusor overactivity' (Abrams et al 2002) and are mediated by acetylcholine-induced stimulation of bladder muscarinic receptors (Andersson 1997). However, overactive bladder is not synonymous with detrusor overactivity, as the former is a symptom-based diagnosis whilst the latter is a urodynamic diagnosis. It has been estimated that 64% of patients with overactive bladder have urodynamically proven detrusor overactivity, and 83% of patients with detrusor overactivity have symptoms suggestive of overactive bladder (Hashim and Abrams 2006).

Incidence

Epidemiological studies have reported the overall prevalence of overactive bladder in women to be 16.9%, suggesting that there could be 17.5 million women in the USA who suffer from the condition. The prevalence increases with age,

DOI: 10.1016/B978-0-7020-3120-5.00053-9

being 4.8% in women under 25 years of age and 30.9% in those over 65 years of age (Stewart et al 2001). This is supported by recent prevalence data from Europe in which 16,776 interviews were conducted in a population-based survey (Milsom et al 2001). The overall prevalence of overactive bladder in individuals aged 40 years and above was 16.6%, and this increased with age. Frequency was the most commonly reported symptom (85%), whilst 54% complained of urgency and 36% complained of urge incontinence. When considering management, 60% had consulted a physician, although only 27% were currently receiving treatment.

More recently, a further population-based survey of lower urinary tract symptoms in Canada, Germany, Italy, Sweden and the UK has reported on 19,165 men and women over the age of 18 years (Irwin et al 2006). Overall, 11.8% were found to complain of symptoms suggestive of overactive bladder and 64.3% reported at least one urinary symptom. Nocturia was the most prevalent lower urinary tract symptom, being reported by 48.6% of men and 54.5% of women.

Aetiology

No specific underlying cause for overactive bladder has been identified, but possible aetiologies include idiopathic, psychosomatic and neurogenic causes in addition to incontinence surgery and outflow obstruction (men).

During infancy, prior to toilet training, it is normal for the bladder to contract uninhibitedly at a critical volume, and overactive bladder may be the result of poorly learnt bladder control. Zoubek et al (1990) studied 46 toilet-trained children, all of whom developed isolated urinary frequency. In 40% of cases, a 'trigger' was identified prior to the onset of symptoms. This often involved problems at school. All cases were self-limiting or resolved following counselling or removal of the 'trigger'. In addition, there is a strong association between childhood nocturnal enuresis and overactive bladder presenting in adult life (Whiteside and Arnold 1975).

The psychoneurotic status of women with overactive bladder has been assessed by several authors, with conflicting results. Walters et al (1990) evaluated 63 women with incontinence and 27 continent controls using formal psychometric testing. They reported no difference in the test results between women with urodynamic stress incontinence and those with overactive bladder. Women with overactive bladder scored significantly higher than controls on the hypochondriasis, depression and hysteria scales. They concluded that these abnormalities may be related to incontinence in general and not to the specific diagnosis. Norton et al (1990) psychiatrically assessed 117 women prior to urodynamic investigation. There was no increased psychiatric morbidity in women with detrusor overactivity compared with women with urodynamic stress incontinence. Interestingly, women in whom no urodynamic abnormality could be detected had the highest scores for anxiety and neuroticism. These levels were comparable with those of psychiatric outpatients.

Neurological lesions such as multiple sclerosis and spinal cord injuries may cause uninhibited bladder contractions, which play an aetiological role in a small group of women with neurogenic detrusor overactivity.

In addition, following incontinence surgery, there is an increased incidence of detrusor overactivity (Cardozo et al 1979, Steel et al 1985, Brown and Hilton 1999) for which no specific cause has been found, but it may be due to extensive dissection around the bladder neck as it is more commonly seen after multiple previous operations. Alternatively, it may be failure to diagnose the abnormality prior to surgery or relative outflow obstruction caused by the operation itself. Outflow obstruction is rare in women and does not seem to cause detrusor overactivity in the same way that prostatic hypertrophy does in men. The increased incidence of detrusor overactivity in the elderly may be due to the onset of occult neuropathy (e.g. senile atherosclerosis or dementia).

Muscarinic Receptors

Molecular cloning studies have revealed five distinct genes for muscarinic acetylcholine receptors in rats and humans, and it has been shown that five receptor subtypes (M_1–M_5) correspond to these gene products (Caulfield and Birdsall 1998). In the human bladder, the occurrence of mRNA encoding M_2 and M_3 subtypes has been demonstrated, although not for M_1 (Yamaguchi et al 1996). The M_3 receptor is thought to cause a direct smooth muscle contraction (Harris et al 1995). Whilst the role of the M_2 receptor has not yet been clarified, it may oppose sympathetically mediated smooth muscle relaxation (Hegde et al 1997) or result in the activation of a non-specific cationic channel and inactivation of potassium channels (Hegde and Eglen 1999). In general, it is thought that the M_3 receptor is responsible for the normal micturition contraction, although in certain disease states, such as neurogenic bladder dysfunction, the M_2 receptors may become more important in mediating detrusor contractions (Braverman and Ruggieri 1998).

Pathophysiology

A detrusor contraction is initiated in the rostral pons. Efferent pathways emerge from the sacral spinal cord as the pelvic parasympathetic nerves (S2, 3 and 4) and run forwards to the bladder. Whilst preganglionic neurotransmission is predominantly mediated by acetylcholine acting on nicotinic receptors, transmission may also be modulated by adrenergic, muscarinic, purinergic and peptidergic presynaptic receptors.

Acetylcholine is released by the postganglionic nerves at the neuromuscular junction, and results in a coordinated detrusor contraction mediated through muscarinic receptors. However, adenosine triphosphate (ATP) also has a role (Burnstock 2001) mediated through non-adrenergic, noncholinergic receptors (O'Reilly et al 2002).

Conversely, sympathetic innervation is from the hypogastric and pelvic nerves acting on β-adrenoreceptors causing relaxation of the detrusor muscle. Thus, a balance between sympathetic and parasympathetic stimulation is required for normal detrusor function.

The pathophysiology of detrusor overactivity remains unclear. In-vitro studies have shown that in cases of idiopathic detrusor overactivity, the detrusor muscle contracts more than normal. These detrusor contractions are not nerve mediated and can be inhibited by the neuropeptide vasoactive intestinal polypeptide (Kinder and Mundy 1987). Other studies have shown that increased α-adrenergic activity causes increased detrusor contractility (Eaton and Bates 1982). There is evidence to suggest that the pathophysiology of idiopathic and obstructive overactive bladder is different. From animal and human studies on obstructive overactivity, it seems that the detrusor develops postjunctional supersensitivity, possibly due to partial denervation (Sibley 1997), with reduced sensitivity to electrical stimulation of its nerve supply but greater sensitivity to stimulation with acetylcholine (Sibley 1985). If outflow obstruction is relieved, the detrusor can return to normal behaviour and reinnervation may occur (Speakman et al 1987).

Relaxation of the urethra is known to precede contraction of the detrusor in a proportion of women with detrusor overactivity (Wise et al 1993a). This may represent primary pathology in the urethra which triggers a detrusor contraction, or may merely be part of a complex sequence of events which originate elsewhere. It has been postulated that incompetence of the bladder neck, allowing passage of urine into the proximal urethra, may result in an uninhibited contraction of the detrusor. However, Sutherst and Brown (1978) were unable to provoke a detrusor contraction in 50 women by rapidly infusing saline into the posterior urethra using modified urodynamic equipment.

Brading and Turner (1994) suggest that the common feature in all cases of detrusor overactivity is partial denervation of the detrusor, which may be responsible for altering the properties of the smooth muscle, leading to increased excitability and increased ability of activity to spread between cells, resulting in coordinated myogenic contractions of the whole detrusor (Brading 1997). They dispute the concept of neurogenic detrusor overactivity (i.e. increased motor activity to the detrusor) as the underlying mechanism in detrusor overactivity, proposing that there is a fundamental abnormality at the level of the bladder wall, with evidence of altered spontaneous contractile activity consistent with increased electrical coupling of cells, a patchy denervation of the detrusor and a supersensitivity to potassium (Mills et al 2000). Charlton et al (1999) suggest that the primary defect in the idiopathic and neuropathic bladders is a loss of nerves accompanied by hypertrophy of the cells, and an increased production of elastin and collagen within the muscle fascicles.

Clinical Presentation

Symptoms and signs

Overactive bladder usually presents with a multiplicity of symptoms. Those most commonly seen are urgency, daytime frequency, nocturia, urge incontinence, stress incontinence, nocturnal enuresis and often coital incontinence. However, it is important to remember that there are numerous other causes of urgency and frequency (Box 53.1).

Iatrogenic frequency and polyuria due to numerous cups of tea or coffee and fizzy drinks should be detected by means of a frequency/volume chart. Most women who are incontinent develop voluntary frequency, initially in order to try to reduce leakage. Nocturia is also a common symptom in overactive bladder, occurring in almost 70% of cases (Cardozo and Stanton 1980). However, being woken from sleep for some other reason and voiding because one is awake does not constitute nocturia. There is an increasing incidence of nocturia with increasing age, and it is normal for women over 70 years of age to void twice during the night, and women over 80 years of age to void three times during the night.

Urge incontinence is usually preceded by urgency (a sudden compelling desire to pass urine which is difficult to defer) and is due to an involuntary detrusor contraction. However, some women are unaware of any sensation associated with their detrusor contractions, and just notice that they are wet. There seems to be a strong correlation between

---

Box 53.1 Common causes of frequency and urgency of micturition

Urological
Urinary tract infection
Detrusor overactivity
Small-capacity bladder
Interstitial cystitis
Chronic urinary retention/chronic urinary residual
Bladder mucosal lesion (e.g. papilloma)
Bladder calculus
Urethral syndrome
Urethral diverticulum
Urethral obstruction

Gynaecological
Pregnancy
Genuine stress incontinence
Cystocoele
Pelvic mass (e.g. fibroids)
Previous pelvic surgery
Radiation cystitis/fibrosis
Postmenopausal urogenital atrophy
Sexual
Coitus
Sexually transmitted disease
Contraceptive diaphragm

Medical
Diuretic therapy
Upper motor neurone lesion
Impaired renal function
Congestive cardiac failure (nocturia)
Hypokalaemia
Endocrine
Diabetes mellitus
Diabetes insipidus
Hypothyroidism
Psychological
Excessive drinking
Habit
Anxiety

nocturnal enuresis, either childhood or current, and idiopathic detrusor overactivity (Whiteside and Arnold 1975). Some women complain of incontinence during sexual intercourse, and they can be broadly divided into two groups: those who leak during penetration and tend to have urodynamic stress incontinence, and those who leak at orgasm who tend to have detrusor overactivity (Hilton 1988).

The most noticeable feature of the symptomatology of overactive bladder is its infinite variability. Some patients may be severely incapacitated when at work but virtually asymptomatic when they go on holiday. Others complain of severe urgency and frequency in the mornings but void normally during the rest of the day, and others say that they are incontinent when they do the washing up or put the door key in the lock ('latch-key incontinence').

There are no specific clinical signs in women with overactive bladder, but it is always important to look for vulval excoriation, urogenital atrophy, a urinary residual and stress incontinence. Occasionally, an underlying neurological lesion such as multiple sclerosis will be discovered by examining the cranial nerves and S2, 3 and 4 outflow.

Quality of Life

Quality of life (QoL) has been defined as including 'those attributes valued by patients including their resultant comfort or sense of well being; the extent to which they were able to maintain reasonable physical, emotional, and intellectual function; the degree to which they retain their ability to participate in valued activities within the family and the community' (Naughton and Shumaker 1996). This helps to emphasize the multidimensional nature of QoL, and the importance of considering the patient's perception of their own situation with regard to non-health-related aspects of their life (Gill and Feinstein 1974).

QoL is assessed by the use of questionnaires completed by the patient alone or as part of the consultation, and its measurement allows the quantification of morbidity and the evaluation of treatment efficacy. It also acts as a measure of how lives are affected and coping strategies adopted. It is estimated that 20% of adult women suffer some degree of life disruption secondary to lower urinary tract dysfunction (Burgio et al 1991).

Generic questionnaires, such as the Short Form 36 (Jenkinson et al 1993), are general measures of QoL and are therefore applicable to a wide range of populations and clinical conditions, whilst disease-specific questionnaires have also been designed to focus on lower urinary tract symptoms. Generic questionnaires are not specific to a particular disease, treatment or age group and hence allow broad comparisons to be made. Consequently, they lack sensitivity when applied to women with lower urinary tract symptoms, and may be unable to detect clinically important improvement.

The King's Health Questionnaire is a reliable, validated, disease-specific tool used to assess women with lower urinary tract dysfunction (Kelleher et al 1997a). Experience using this questionnaire has shown that incontinence impact scores were significantly worse for women with detrusor overactivity than for those with urodynamic stress incontinence, and significantly better in women with normal urodynamics.

Investigations

Urine culture

A midstream specimen of urine should be sent for microscopy, culture and sensitivity in all cases of incontinence. An infection may contribute to the symptomatology, and investigations, which are mainly invasive, may exacerbate this. Such investigations are certainly uncomfortable when an infection is present and the results may be inaccurate.

Frequency/volume chart

It is the authors' practice to send all patients a frequency/volume chart with their appointment for urodynamic investigations, so that their fluid intake and voiding pattern can be evaluated. As well as the number of voids and incontinence episodes, the mean volume voided over a 24-h period can also be calculated as well as the diurnal and nocturnal volumes. They are asked to complete the chart (Figure 53.1) for 5 days, but are told that they need not measure their

KINGS COLLEGE HOSPITAL
FREQUENCY VOLUME CHART

Time	Day 1 In	Out	Wet	Day 2 In	Out	Wet	Day 3 In	Out	Wet	Day 4 In	Out	Wet	Day 5 In	Out	Wet
6 am		75		180	50		180	125					240	300	✓
7 am	180									125	225	✓			
8 am	180	150	✓	360	125		360	125			50 60		360	125	
9 am		100					180	350	✓	320	100			100	
10 am	360	75		180	250	✓					100 75	✓		125	✓
11 am							180	200	✓	180	50		180	100	✓
12 pm	180	225	✓	180	325	✓		100							
1 pm		100		180			180	75		180	300 75	✓	180	125	✓
2 pm	100	50			100						200				
3 pm		25 75		180	25 75		220	220	✓	160	100	✓	240		
4 pm	240	100	✓				75	90		75			180	320	✓
5 pm				220	200	✓					100			100	
6 pm	180	220	✓	220	50		100	125		120			180	100	
7 pm	180				50			200			100	✓			
8 pm		225						200			240			75	
9 pm				180	100			150	✓					360	
10 pm	180	100		180	75		180	100		190	225	✓		150	
11 pm								75 25		180	150		180	200	✓
12 am	240	100		180	150	✓	240				100		180	225	
1 am								100	✓						
2 am				180	125	✓				180	100			350	✓
3 am	180	300	✓											220	
4 am					300	✓		225	✓	180	100			100	✓
5 am													180		

Figure 53.1 Frequency/volume chart from a woman with overactive bladder.

oided volumes when at work if this proves difficult. In addition, there is now evidence that 3- and 4-day frequency/ volume charts are as accurate as 7-day diaries (Brown et al 2003). Some women find that this is a useful exercise, similar to home bladder drill.

Uroflowmetry

Although voiding difficulties are uncommon in women, a large chronic urinary residual may present with symptoms of urgency and frequency of micturition, so it is relevant to measure the urine flow rate prior to urodynamic assessment. In uncomplicated idiopathic detrusor overactivity, the flow rate is usually high and the voiding time short, with only a small volume being passed each time.

Cystometry

The urodynamic diagnosis of detrusor overactivity is made when detrusor contractions are seen on a cystometrogram. Detrusor overactivity is defined as 'a urodynamic observation characterised by involuntary detrusor contractions during filling which may be spontaneous or provoked' (Abrams et al 2002). The recorded detrusor pressure rise may take different forms on the cystometrogram trace. Most commonly, uninhibited systolic contractions occur during bladder filling (Figures 53.2 and 53.3). Not all cases of detrusor overactivity will be diagnosed on supine filling alone (Turner-Warwick 1975). Some show an abnormal detrusor pressure rise on a change of posture and may void precipitately on standing (Figure 53.4), or there may be detrusor contractions provoked by coughing which manifest as stress incontinence. Sometimes, a steep detrusor pressure rise occurs during bladder filling. This usually represents low compliance of the detrusor, but may be due to involuntary detrusor activity in some cases. It can be difficult to differentiate between systolic (phasic) detrusor overactivity and low compliance, which may coexist. Both conditions usually produce similar symptoms.

During the cystometrogram, it is important to ask the patient about her symptoms and relate them to the recorded changes. Most patients will complain of urgency when a detrusor contraction occurs, or urge incontinence if the detrusor pressure exceeds the urethral pressure. Thus, in order to diagnose or exclude detrusor overactivity, subtracted provocative cystometry must be employed. Other common, although not universal, features of the cystometrogram in women with detrusor overactivity are early first sensation,

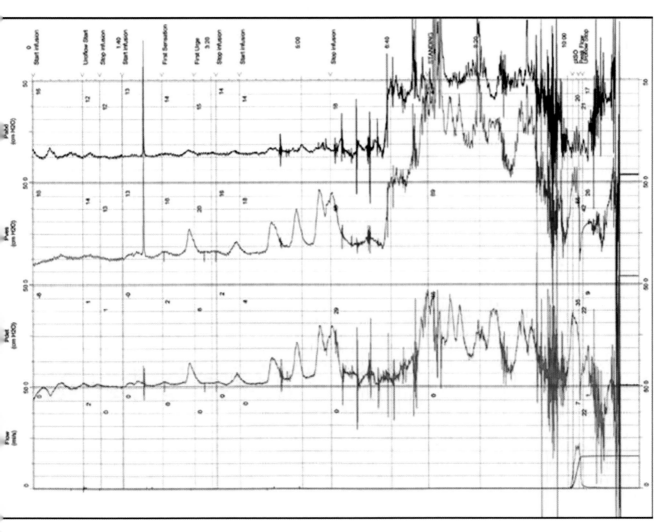

Figure 53.2 Cystometrogram showing severe systolic and provoked detrusor contractions during filling.

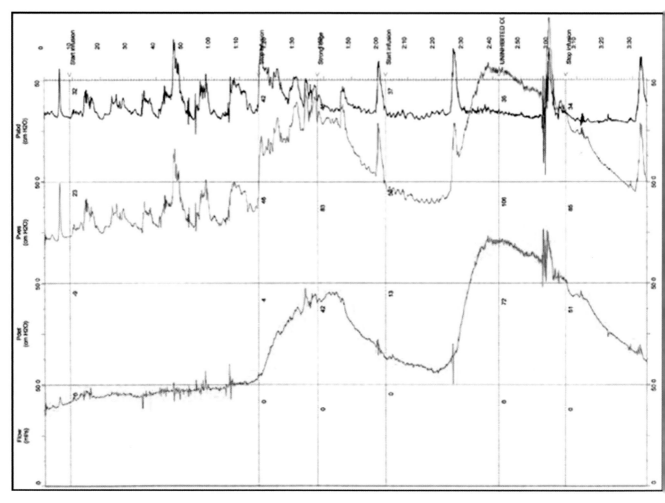

Figure 53.3 Cystometrogram showing neurogenic detrusor overactivity during filling in a patient with multiple sclerosis.

small bladder capacity and inability/or difficulty in interrupting the urinary stream. The latter may be associated with a high isometric detrusor contraction (Figure 53.4) or, if videocystourethrography is performed, slow or absent 'milkback' of contrast medium from the proximal urethra into the bladder.

Ambulatory urodynamics

There are three main components to an ambulatory urodynamic system: the transducers, the recording unit and the analysing system. The transducers are solid state and are mounted on 5 French and 7 French bladder and rectal catheters. It is the authors' practice to use two bladder transducers in order to reduce artifact. The recording system should be portable in order to allow freedom of movement, with a digital memory aiding compression and expansion of the traces which are obtained. An event marker is attached to the recording unit allowing the patient to mark episodes of urgency and also to document voids. In addition, the recording unit is attached to an electronic (Urilos) pad to document episodes of leakage during the study, and should have the facility to attach to a flow meter in order to record pressure flow voiding studies. The ambulatory protocol at Kings College Hospital consists of a 4-h period during which time

the patient is asked to drink 200 ml of fluid every 30 min and also to keep a diary of events and symptoms. On completion of the test, the trace is analysed with the patient using a personal computer and the urinary diary. Detrusor overactivity should only be diagnosed if there is a detrusor contraction noted on both bladder lines in the presence of symptoms (Figure 53.5).

The clinical usefulness of ambulatory urodynamics is limited by the high prevalence of abnormal detrusor (38–69%) contractions in asymptomatic volunteers (van Waalwijk van Doorn et al 1992, Robertson et al 1994, Heslington and Hilton 1996). However, the diagnosis of detrusor overactivity is highly dependent on interpretation of the results; in a prospective study of 26 asymptomatic women, the incidence of detrusor overactivity varied from 11.5% to 76.9% depending on the criteria used (Salvatore et al 1998, 2001). If the criteria for defining abnormal detrusor contractions are a simultaneous pressure rise on both bladder lines in addition to patient-reported symptoms of urgency or urge incontinence, the findings are normal in 90% of women; this is similar to that reported in laboratory urodynamics. In order to improve the diagnostic discrimination of ambulatory urodynamic studies, a standardization document has been published (van Waalwijk van Doorn et al 2000).

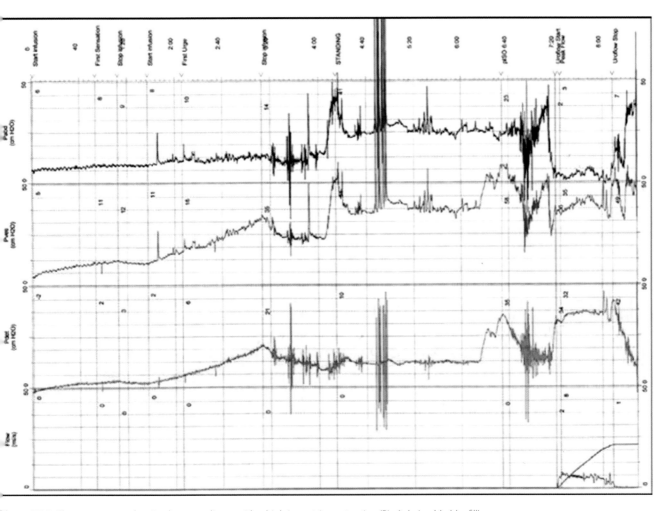

Figure 53.4 Cystometrogram showing low compliance with a high isometric contraction (Piso) during bladder filling.

Cystourethroscopy

Endoscopy is not helpful in diagnosing detrusor overactivity but may be used to exclude other causes for the symptoms, such as a bladder tumour or calculus. Coarse trabeculation and diverticulae of the bladder may be noted in longstanding cases of detrusor overactivity.

Videocystourethrography

Additional information may be acquired by undertaking videocystourethrography with pressure and flow studies, rather than subtracted cystometry, and this may also increase the diagnostic accuracy. Bladder diverticulae (Figure 53.6) and trabeculation (Figure 53.7) may be observed during videocystourethrography, and vesicoureteric reflux may be observed when severe detrusor overactivity has caused upper urinary tract damage.

Treatment

Not all women with overactive bladder require treatment. Once the problem has been explained to them, some will be able to control their own symptoms by behavioural modification, such as drinking less and avoiding tea, coffee and alcohol (which are bladder stimulants).

However, most women with overactive bladder request treatment, and although many different therapies have been tried, none have proved universally satisfactory. The major therapeutic interventions which are currently in use attempt to either improve central control, as in behavioural intervention, or alter detrusor contractility using drugs or surgical denervation techniques. When these measures fail to control the patient's symptoms adequately over a long period of time, more invasive treatment may be employed. Conventional bladder neck surgery (as is used to treat urodynamic stress incontinence) rarely cures women with detrusor overactivity and may make the symptoms of urgency and frequency worse.

Methods of treatment currently employed are behavioural intervention, drug therapy, intravesical botulinum toxin and neuromodulation. For patients with intractable overactive bladder who are resistant to therapy, surgical procedures such as augmentation cystoplasty and urinary diversion may have a role.

Historically, other types of treatment which have been tried include vaginal denervation (Hodgkinson and Drukker

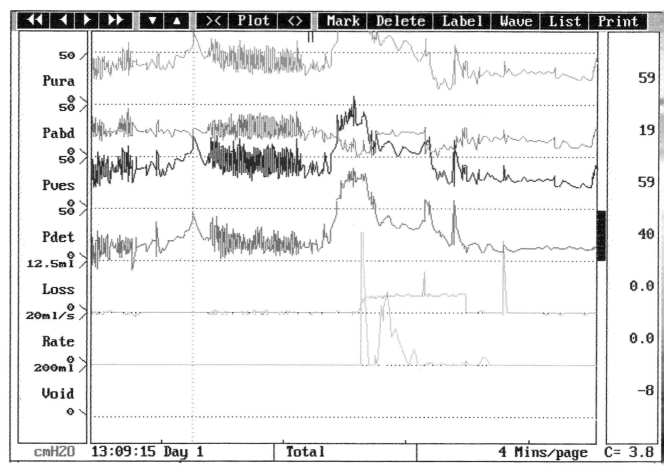

Figure 53.5 Cystometrographic recording obtained during ambulatory monitoring. A detrusor contraction (Pdet) is associated with pressure rises in both bladder lines (Pves, Pura) and leakage of urine (loss).

1977, Warrell 1977, Ingleman-Sundberg 1978), caecocysto-plasty, selective sacral neurectomy (Torrens and Griffiths 1974), cystodistension (Ramsden et al 1976, Higson et al 1978, Pengelly et al 1978) and bladder transection (Mundy 1983). All give some short-term benefit in carefully selected cases, but may produce significant morbidity. None have stood the test of time.

General management

All incontinent women benefit from advice regarding simple measures which they can take to help alleviate their symptoms. Many patients drink too much and they should be told to reduce their fluid intake to between 1 and 1.5 l/day (Swithinbank et al 2005), and to avoid tea, coffee and alcohol if these exacerbate their problem. In addition, there is also increasing evidence to suggest that weight loss may improve symptoms of urinary incontinence (Subak et al 2009). The use of drugs which affect bladder function, such as diuretics and α-adrenreceptor antagonists, should be reviewed and stopped if possible. If there is coexistent urodynamic stress incontinence, pelvic floor exercises may also be helpful.

It is usually preferable, in cases of mixed incontinence, to treat the overactive bladder prior to resorting to surgery for urethral sphincter incompetence. Such treatment may obviate the need for surgery (Karram and Bhatia 1989). In addition, there is always the risk that the incontinence operation may exacerbate the symptoms of overactive bladder.

For a peri- or postmenopausal woman, local oestrogen replacement therapy is unlikely to cure the problem, but may improve urogenital atrophy and increase the sensory threshold of the bladder, and may also make urinary symptoms easier to cope with. The most degrading aspect of urinary incontinence for many patients is the odour and staining of their clothes, and this can be helped by good advice regarding incontinence pads and garments.

Pharmacology

Drug therapy has an important role in the management of women with urinary symptoms caused by overactive bladder, although there are no drugs which act specifically on the bladder and urethra and do not have systemic effects. The large number of drugs available is indicative of the fact that none are ideal, and it is often their systemic adverse effects which limit their use in terms of efficacy and compliance (Kelleher et al 1997b). The pharmacology of drugs and recommendations for usage have been reviewed recently by the 4th International Consultation on Incontinence (Andersson et al 2009) (Table 53.1).

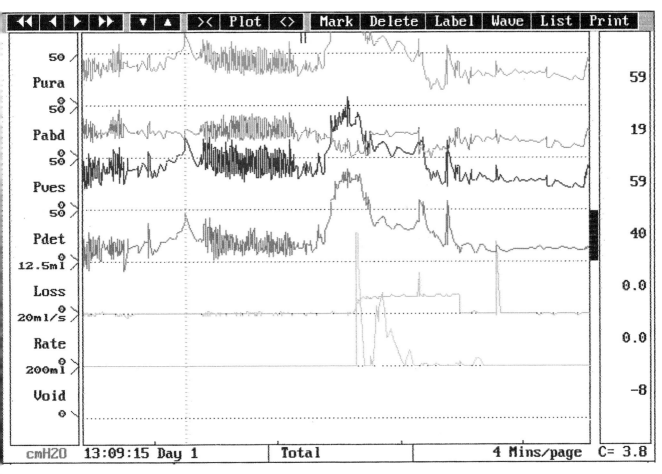

Figure 53.6 Multiple bladder diverticulae.

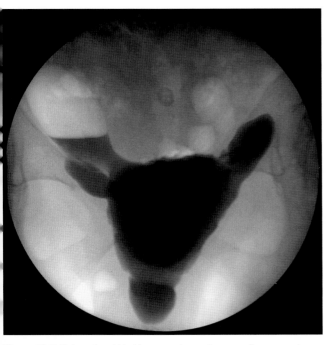

Figure 53.7 Trabeculated bladder secondary to longstanding overactive bladder, with bladder diverticulae and bilateral vesicoureteric reflux. The bladder neck is open during a detrusor contraction with associated leakage.

Antimuscarinic drugs

The detrusor is innervated by the parasympathetic nervous system (pelvic nerve), the sympathetic nervous system (hypogastric nerve) and by non-cholinergic, non-adrenergic neurones. The motor supply arises from S2, 3 and 4 and is conveyed by the pelvic nerve. The neurotransmitter at the neuromuscular junction is acetylcholine, which acts upon muscarinic receptors. Antimuscarinic drugs should therefore be of use in the treatment of detrusor overactivity. Atropine is the classic non-selective anticholinergic drug with antimuscarinic activity; however, its non-specific mode of action makes it unacceptable for clinical use because of the high incidence of side-effects. All antimuscarinic agents produce competitive blockade of acetylcholine receptors at postganglionic parasympathetic receptor sites. They all, to a lesser or greater extent, have the typical side-effects of dry mouth, blurred vision, tachycardia, drowsiness and constipation. Unfortunately, virtually all the drugs which are truly beneficial in the management of overactive bladder produce these unwanted systemic side-effects.

Tolterodine

Tolterodine is a competitive muscarinic receptor antagonist with relative functional selectivity for bladder muscarinic

Table 53.1 Drugs used in the treatment of overactive bladder

	Level of evidence*	Grade of recommendation#
Antimuscarinic drugs		
Tolterodine	1	A
Trospium	1	A
Solifenacin	1	A
Darifenacin	1	A
Fesoterodine	1	A
Propantheline	2	B
Atropine, hyoscamine	3	C
Drugs acting on membrane channels		
Calcium-channel antagonists	2	D
Potassium-channel openers	2	D
Drugs with mixed actions		
Oxybutynin	1	A
Propiverine	1	A
Flavoxate	2	D
α Antagonists		
Alfuzosin	3	C
Doxazosin	3	C
Prazosin	3	C
Terazosin	3	C
Tamsulosin	3	C
β Agonists		
Terbutaline	3	C
Salbutamol	3	C
Antidepressants		
Imipramine	3	C
Duloxetine	2	C
Prostaglandin synthesis inhibitors		
Indomethacin	2	C
Flurbiprofen	2	C
Vasopressin analogues		
Desmopressin	1	A
Other drugs		
Baclofen	3	C (intrathecal)
Capsaicin	2	C (intravesical)
Resiniferatoxin	2	C (intravesical)
Botulinum toxin (idiopathic)	3	B (intravesical)
Botulinum toxin (neurogenic)	2	A (intravesical)

Source: Andersson KE, Chapple CR, Cardozo L et al 2009 Pharmacological treatment of urinary incontinence. In: Abrams P, Cardozo L, Khoury S, Wein A (eds) Incontinence, 4th edn. Health Publication Ltd, Paris, pp 631–700.
*#See Appendix.

receptors (Ruscin and Morgenstern 1999). Whilst it shows no specificity for receptor subtypes, it does target the muscarinic receptors in the bladder rather than those in the salivary glands (Nilvebrant et al 1997). Several randomized, double-blind, placebo-controlled trials have demonstrated a significant reduction in incontinent episodes and micturition frequency (Jonas et al 1997, Hills et al 1998, Millard et al 1999), whilst the incidence of adverse effects has been shown to be no different to placebo (Rentzhog et al 1998). When compared with oxybutynin in a randomized, double-blind, placebo-controlled, parallel-group study, it was found to be equally efficacious and to have a lower incidence of side-effects, notably dry mouth (Abrams et al 1998). A pooled analysis of the safety, efficacy and acceptability of tolterodine in 1120 patients in four randomized, double-blind, parallel, multicentre trials found that both tolterodine and oxybutynin decreased incontinent episodes significantly, although tolterodine was associated with fewer adverse events, dose reductions and patient withdrawals than oxybutynin (Appell 1997).

Tolterodine has also been developed as an extended-release, once-daily preparation. A double-blind, multicentre trial of 1235 women compared extended-release tolterodine with immediate-release tolterodine and placebo. Whilst both formulations were found to reduce the mean number of urge incontinence episodes per week, the extended-release preparation was found to be significantly more effective (Swift et al 2003). In addition to increased efficacy, extended-release tolterodine has been shown to have better tolerability. In a double-blind, multicentre, randomized placebo-controlled trial of 1529 patients, extended-release tolterodine was found to be 18% more effective in the reduction of episodes of urge incontinence, whilst having a 23% lower incidence of dry mouth (van Kerrebroeck et al 2001).

Extended-release oxybutynin and extended-release tolterodine were compared in the OPERA (Overactive bladder: Performance of Extended Release Agents) study, which involved 71 centres in the USA. Improvements in episodes of urge incontinence were similar for the two drugs, although extended-release oxybutynin was significantly more effective than extended-release tolterodine in reducing the frequency of micturition. Significantly more women taking oxybutynin were also completely dry (23% vs 16.8%; $P = 0.03$), although dry mouth was significantly more common in the oxybutynin group (Diokno et al 2003).

In summary, the available evidence suggests that tolterodine is as effective as oxybutynin; in addition, as it has fewer adverse effects, patient tolerability and compliance are improved.

Trospium chloride

Trospium chloride is a quaternary ammonium compound which is non-selective for muscarinic receptor subtypes and shows low biological availability (Schladitz-Keil et al 1986). It crosses the blood–brain barrier to a limited extent and hence appears to have few cognitive effects (Fusgen and Hauri 2000). A placebo-controlled, randomized, double-blind, multicentre trial has shown trospium to increase cystometric capacity and bladder volume at the first unstable contraction, leading to significant clinical improvement without an increase in adverse effects over placebo (Cardozo et al 2000). When compared with oxybutynin, it has been found to have comparable efficacy but was associated with a lower incidence of dry mouth (4% vs 23%) and patient withdrawal (6% vs 16%) (Madersbacher et al 1995). At present, trospium chloride appears to be as effective as oxybutynin and may be associated with fewer adverse effects. More recently, an extended-release preparation (Dmochowski et al 2008) has been introduced in the USA and is soon to be licensed in the UK.

Solifenacin

Solifenacin is a potent M_3 receptor antagonist that has selectivity for M_3 receptors over M_2 receptors, and has much higher potency against M_3 receptors in smooth muscle than against M_3 receptors in salivary glands.

The clinical efficacy of solifenacin has been assessed in a multicentre, randomized, double-blind, parallel group, placebo-controlled study of solifenacin 5 mg and 10 mg once daily in patients with overactive bladder (Cardozo et al 2004a). The primary efficacy analysis showed a statistically significant reduction of micturition frequency following treatment with both 5-mg and 10-mg doses compared with placebo, although the largest effect was with the higher dose. In addition, solifenacin was found to be superior to placebo with respect to the secondary efficacy variables of mean volume voided per micturition, episodes of urgency per 24 h, number of incontinence episodes and episodes of urge incontinence. The most frequently reported adverse events leading to discontinuation were dry mouth and constipation. These were also found to be dose related. In order to assess the long-term safety and efficacy of solifenacin (5 mg and 10 mg once daily), a multicentre, open-label, long-term follow-up study has been reported. This was essentially an extension of two previous double-blind, placebo-controlled studies in 1637 patients (Haab et al 2005). Overall, the efficacy of solifenacin was maintained in the extension study with a sustained improvement in symptoms of urgency, urge incontinence, frequency and nocturia over the 12-month study period. The most commonly reported adverse events were dry mouth (20.5%), constipation (9.2%) and blurred vision (6.6%), and these were the primary reason for discontinuation in 4.7% of patients.

More recently, solifenacin 5 mg and 10 mg od have been compared with extended-release tolterodine 4 mg od (Chapple et al 2005). This was a prospective, double-blind, double-dummy, two-arm, parallel-group, 12-week study of 1200 patients with the primary aim of demonstrating non-inferiority of solifenacin to extended-release tolterodine. Solifenacin was not inferior to extended-release tolterodine with respect to change from baseline in the mean number of micturitions per 24 h (reduction of 2.45 micturitions/24 h vs 2.24 micturitions/24 h; $P = 0.004$). In addition, solifenacin resulted in a statistically significant improvement in urgency ($P = 0.035$), urge incontinence ($P = 0.001$) and overall incontinence compared with extended-release tolterodine. In addition, 59% of solifenacin-treated patients who were incontinent at baseline became continent by the study endpoint compared with 49% of patients on extended-release tolterodine ($P = 0.006$).

Darifenacin

Darifenacin is a tertiary amine with moderate lipophilicity, and is a highly selective M_3 receptor antagonist which has been found to have a 5-fold higher affinity for the human M_3 receptor relative to the M_1 receptor (Alabaster 1997).

A review of the pooled darifenacin data from the three Phase III, multicentre, double-blind clinical trials in patients with overactive bladder has been reported in 1059 patients (Chapple et al 2004a). Darifenacin resulted in a dose-related significant reduction in median number of incontinence episodes per week. Significant decreases in the frequency and severity of urgency, micturition frequency and number of incontinence episodes resulting in a change of clothing or pads were also apparent, along with an increase in bladder capacity. Darifenacin was well tolerated. The most common treatment-related adverse events were dry mouth and constipation, although these resulted in few discontinuations. The incidence of central nervous system and cardiovascular adverse events were comparable with placebo.

Fesoterodine

Fesoterodine is a new and novel derivative of 3,3-diphenyl-propyl-amine, which is a potent antimuscarinic agent that has recently been developed for the management of overactive bladder. A Phase II dose-finding study was conducted in 728 patients (Chapple 2004b). Fesoterodine 4 mg, 8 mg and 12 mg were all found to show significantly greater decreases in micturition frequency than placebo. The most commonly reported side-effect was dry mouth, with an incidence of 25% in the 4-mg group rising to 34% in the 12-mg group. Subsequently, a Phase III randomized placebo-controlled trial has been reported comparing fesoterodine 4 mg and 8 mg with extended-release tolterodine 4 mg in 1135 patients complaining of overactive bladder (Chapple et al 2006a, 2008). Both doses of fesoterodine demonstrated significant improvements over placebo in reduction of daytime frequency and number of urge incontinence episodes per day, and were found to be superior to tolterodine. The current evidence suggests that fesoterodine may offer some advantages over tolterodine in terms of efficacy and flexible dosing regimens.

Drugs that have a mixed action

Oxybutynin

Oxybutynin is a tertiary amine that undergoes extensive first-pass metabolism to an active metabolite, N-desmethyl oxybutynin (Waldeck et al 1997), which occurs in high concentrations (Hughes et al 1992) and is thought to be responsible for a significant part of the action of the parent drug. It has a mixed action consisting of both an antimuscarinic and a direct muscle relaxant effect in addition to local anaesthetic properties. The latter is important when given intravesically but probably has no effect when given systemically. Oxybutynin has been shown to have a high affinity for muscarinic receptors in the bladder (Nilvebrant et al 1985), and has a higher affinity for M_1 and M_3 receptors than M_2 receptors (Nilvebrant and Sparf 1986).

The effectiveness of oxybutynin in the management of patients with detrusor overactivity is well documented. A double-blind, placebo-controlled trial found oxybutynin to be significantly better than placebo in improving lower urinary tract symptoms, although 80% of patients complained of significant adverse effects, principally dry mouth or dry skin (Cardozo et al 1987). The antimuscarinic adverse effects of oxybutynin are well documented and are often dose limiting (Baigrie et al 1988), with 10–23% of women discontinuing medication (Kelleher et al 1994a). Using an intravesical route of administration, higher local levels of oxybutynin can be achieved whilst limiting the systemic adverse effects. Using this method, oxybutynin has been shown to increase bladder capacity and lead to a significant clinical improvement (Weese et al 1993). Intravesical administration of oxybutynin is an effective and useful alternative for patients with neurogenic detrusor overactivity who need to self-catheterize or who suffer from 'bypassing' an indwelling catheter (Madersbacher and Jilg 1991). Rectal administration has also been shown to be associated with fewer adverse effects compared with oral administration (Collas and Malone-Lee 1997).

A controlled-release oxybutynin preparation using an osmotic system has been developed which has been shown to have comparable efficacy when compared with immediate-release oxybutynin, and which is associated with fewer adverse effects (Anderson et al 1999). In order to maximize efficacy and minimize adverse effects, alternative delivery systems are currently under evaluation. An oxybutynin transdermal delivery system has been developed and compared with extended-release tolterodine in 361 patients with mixed urinary incontinence. Both agents significantly reduced incontinence episodes, increased volume voided and led to an improvement in QoL compared with placebo. The most common adverse event in the oxybutynin arm was application site pruritus (14%), although the incidence of dry mouth was reduced to 4.1% compared with 7.3% in the tolterodine arm (Dmochowski et al 2003).

More recently, a large prospective, multicentre, randomized, double-blind, placebo-controlled study has been reported investigating the use of oxybutynin gel in the management of overactive bladder in 704 patients (Staskin et al 2009). Overall, there was a significant reduction in urge incontinence episodes in the gel arm compared with the placebo arm (−3.0 vs −2.5/day; $P<0.0001$), a significant reduction in daytime frequency (−2.7, $P = 0.0017$) and an increase in volume voided. When considering adverse events, dry mouth was more common in the treatment arm compared with the placebo arm (6.9% vs 2.8%), and skin site reactions were infrequent in both arms (5.4% and 1.0%, respectively). Consequently, oxybutynin gel may represent an important development over the oxybutynin patch in terms of patient acceptability.

In summary, the efficacy of oxybutynin is well documented, although its clinical usefulness is very often limited by adverse effects. Alternative routes and methods of administration may produce better patient acceptability and compliance.

Propiverine

Propiverine has both antimuscarinic and calcium-channel-blocking actions (Haruno et al 1989). Open studies have demonstrated a beneficial effect in patients with overactive bladder (Mazur et al 1995) and neurogenic detrusor overactivity (Stoher et al 1999). Dry mouth was experienced by 37% in the treatment group as opposed to 8% in those taking placebo, with dropout rates of 7% and 4.5%, respectively. Propiverine has also been compared with oxybutynin in the management of neurogenic detrusor overactivity in children and adolescents (Madersbacher et al 2009). Overall, propiverine was found to have comparable efficacy to oxybutynin but was better tolerated in terms of adverse effects.

The efficacy and cardiac safety of propiverine has been assessed in a double-blind, multicentre, placebo-controlled, randomized study in 98 elderly patients suffering from urgency, urge incontinence or mixed urge/stress incontinence. After a 2-week placebo run-in period, the patients received propiverine (15 mg tds) or placebo (tds) for a 4-week period. Propiverine caused a significant reduction in micturition frequency and a significant decrease in episodes of incontinence. Only 2% of patients complained of dry mouth, and resting and ambulatory electrocardiograms showed no significant changes (Dorschner et al 2000).

More recently, extended-release propiverine has been introduced and been shown to be as effective as the immediate-release preparation in the management of overactive bladder (Jünemann et al 2006).

Tricyclic antidepressants

These drugs have a complex pharmacological action. Imipramine has antimuscarinic, antihistaminic and local anaesthetic properties. It may increase outlet resistance by peripheral blockage of noradrenaline uptake and it also acts as a sedative. The side-effects are antimuscarinic, together with tremor and fatigue. Imipramine is particularly useful for the treatment of nocturia and nocturnal enuresis (Castleden et al 1981), although other studies have reported little effect (Diokno et al 1972). Other tricyclic antidepressants such as amitriptyline may be substituted for imipramine if specific side-effects are a problem, whilst doxepin has been found to be more potent in its musculotropic relaxant and antimuscarinic activity (Lose et al 1989). A tricyclic antidepressant given prophylactically before sexual intercourse may be of benefit to patients with coital incontinence at orgasm (Cardozo 1988).

In light of relatively poor evidence and the serious adverse effects associated with tricyclic antidepressants, their role in detrusor overactivity remains of uncertain benefit although they are often useful in patients complaining of nocturia or bladder pain.

Calcium-channel antagonists

Contractile activity in the bladder smooth muscle is activated by the movement of extracellular calcium into the cell. Spontaneous and evoked contractile activity are mediated by membrane depolarization and the movement of calcium into the smooth muscle cell through L-type Ca^{2+} channels (Brading 1997). Inhibition of the entrance of Ca^{2+} can prevent spontaneous and evoked contractile activity (Levin et al 1991) with L-type Ca^{2+} blocking agents, such as nifedipine, inhibiting the entry of extracellular calcium.

At present, there is insufficient evidence to suggest that calcium-channel-blocking agents are effective in the treatment of detrusor overactivity, although the development of a selective calcium-channel-blocking agent which eliminates spontaneous contractions without affecting micturition may prove to be of use in the treatment of detrusor overactivity.

Potassium-channel-opening drugs

The opening of K^+ ion channels in the membrane of the detrusor muscle cell leads to an increase in K^+ movement out of the cell, resulting in membrane hyperpolarization (Andersson 1997). This reduces the opening probability of ion channels involved in membrane depolarization and hence excitability is reduced (Andersson 1992). These agents act during the filling phase and, whilst abolishing spontaneous detrusor contractions, are not thought to affect normal bladder contractions. Their clinical usefulness is limited by significant cardiovascular effects, with cromakalin and pinacidil being found to be up to 200 times more potent as inhibitors of vascular preparations than of detrusor muscle (Edwards et al 1991). At present, none are commercially available, although the development of subtype-selective drugs may lead to a role in the management of overactive bladder (Lawson 1996).

More recently, newer drugs with K_{ATP}-channel-opening properties have been described (Andersson and Arner 2004). These may be useful for the treatment of bladder overactivity, although there is no evidence at present to suggest that potassium channel openers represent a viable treatment alternative. This is supported by a recently reported randomized, double-blind, placebo-controlled Phase II study evaluating the efficacy and safety of a novel ATP-sensitive potassium channel opener in 299 patients with detrusor overactivity. Whilst treatment was safe and well tolerated, there was no difference over placebo in mean volume voided per micturition and micturition frequency (Chapple et al 2006b).

Antidiuretic agents

Desmopressin

Synthetic vasopressin (desmopressin) has been shown to reduce nocturnal urine production by up to 50%. It can be used for children or adults with nocturia or nocturnal enuresis (Norgaard et al 1989), but must be avoided in patients with hypertension, ischaemic heart disease or congestive cardiac failure (Hilton and Stanton 1982). There is good evidence to show that it is safe to use in the long term (Knudsen et al 1989, Rew and Rundle 1989), and it may be given orally or as a buccal preparation.

Desmopressin has also been used as a 'designer drug' for daytime incontinence (Robinson et al 2004), and also in the treatment of overactive bladder (Hashim et al 2009).

Desmopressin is safe for long-term use; however, the drug should be used with care in the elderly due to the risk of hyponatraemia. The current recommendations are that serum sodium should be checked in the first week following the start of treatment. To identify the safety of desmopressin, a recent systematic review and meta-analysis has been performed of cohort studies and randomized controlled trials using the oral and intranasal preparations in the treatment of nocturia. In total, 75 papers were identified of which seven reported the incidence of hyponatraemia, giving an overall pooled estimate of 7.6% (95% confidence interval 3.7–15.1). The authors concluded that hyponatraemia is a relatively common adverse event associated with the use of desmopressin, and regular monitoring should be used, particularly in the elderly (Weatherall 2004)

Prostaglandin synthetase inhibitors

Bladder mucosa has been shown to have the ability to synthesize eicosanoids (Jeremy et al 1987), although it is uncertain whether they contribute to the pathogenesis of overactive detrusor contractions. However, they may have a role in sensitizing sensory afferent nerves, increasing the afferent input produced by a given bladder volume. A double-blind controlled study of flurbiprofen in women with detrusor overactivity was shown to have an effect, although it was associated with a high incidence of adverse effects (43%) including nausea, vomiting, headache and gastrointestinal symptoms (Cardozo et al 1980). Indomethacin has also been reported to give symptomatic relief, although the incidence of adverse effects was also high (59%) (Cardozo et al 1980). At present, this evidence does not support the use of prostaglandin synthetase inhibitors in detrusor overactivity.

α-Adrenoreceptor antagonists

The lower urinary tract is innervated by both the parasympathetic and the sympathetic nervous systems, which act via muscarinic and adrenergic receptors, respectively. During the storage phase, continence is maintained by inhibition of the parasympathetic system and by activation of the sympathetic system, which lead to bladder relaxation and urethral sphincter contraction by acting on β_2- and α-adrenergic receptors, respectively. Conversely, during voiding, the pontine micturition centre inhibits the sympathetic system and activates the parasympathetic system, resulting in urethral relaxation and a sustained bladder contraction.

The adrenergic receptors found at the bladder neck are α_1 adrenergic, and three subtypes have been identified: α_{1A}, α_{1B} and α_{1D} (Malloy et al 1998). Those receptors present in the bladder are predominantly α_{1A} and α_{1D}, whilst α_{1B} receptors are found in the vasculature and are involved in blood pressure control. Consequently, α_1-adrenergic blocking agents with subselectivity for α_{1A} and α_{1D} may be most useful in the management of lower urinary tract dysfunction, and it has been speculated that the α_{1D} receptor may mediate the overactive symptoms of overactive bladder while the α_{1A} receptor mediates the obstructive symptoms (Schwinn 2000). Anecdotal evidence has demonstrated that tamsulosin, a selective α_1-adrenoceptor antagonist, may improve urinary symptoms secondary to detrusor overactivity in men, and it has been used 'off label' in women with symptoms of overactive bladder for some time.

A randomized, double-blind, placebo-controlled study evaluating the efficacy of tamsulosin in the management of women complaining of overactive bladder has been reported recently (Robinson et al 2007). Overall, 364 women (53.3% treatment naïve) were randomized to receive one of four doses of tamsulosin (0.25 mg, 0.5 mg, 1.0 mg or 1.5 mg), extended-release tolterodine 4 mg or placebo for 6 weeks. The primary efficacy analysis showed that the difference from placebo in the mean number of micturitions/24 h was not statistically significant for tamsulosin 1.5 mg (P = 0.189). Interestingly, no statistically significant difference was observed for extended-release tolterodine 4 mg (P = 0.353). Similarly, when considering the secondary outcome parameters, there was no statistically significant difference between tamsulosin and placebo. Although women taking extended-release tolterodine 4 mg od demonstrated a consistently greater increase in mean volume voided and consistent decreases in incontinence episodes/24 h, urgency episodes/24 h and episodes of nocturia/24 h, this was not statistically significant compared with placebo. In addition, there was no significant improvement in QoL scores across the treatment groups. The results from this study suggest that α-adrenoreceptor antagonists alone are not clinically useful in the management of overactive bladder in women.

Oestrogens in the Management of Overactive Bladder

Oestrogens have been used in the treatment of urinary urgency and urge incontinence for many years, although there have been few controlled trials to confirm their efficacy. A double-blind, placebo-controlled, crossover study using oral oestriol in 34 postmenopausal women produced subjective improvement in eight women with mixed incontinence and 12 women with urge incontinence (Samsicoe et al 1985). However, a double-blind, multicentre study of the use of oestriol (3 mg/day) in postmenopausal women complaining of urgency has failed to confirm these findings (Cardozo et al 1993), showing both subjective and objective improvement but not significantly better than placebo. The use of sustained-release 17β-oestradiol vaginal tablets has also been examined in postmenopausal women with urgency and urge incontinence or a urodynamic diagnosis of sensory urgency or detrusor overactivity. These vaginal tablets have been shown to be well absorbed from the vagina and to induce maturation of the vaginal epithelium within 14 days (Nilsson and Heimer 1992). However, following a 6-month course of treatment, the only significant difference between active and placebo groups was an improvement in the symptom of urgency in those women with a urodynamic diagnosis of sensory urgency (Benness et al 1992). A further double-blind, randomized, placebo-controlled trial of vaginal 17β-oestradiol vaginal tablets has shown lower urinary tract symptoms of frequency, urgency, urge and stress incontinence to be significantly improved, although no objective urodynamic assessment was performed (Eriksen and Rasmussen 1992). In both of these studies, the subjective improvement in symptoms may simply represent local oestrogenic effects reversing urogenital atrophy rather than a direct effect on bladder function.

A randomized, parallel group, controlled trial has been reported, comparing the oestradiol-releasing vaginal ring with oestriol vaginal pessaries in the treatment of postmenopausal women with bothersome lower urinary tract symptoms (Lose and Englev 2000). Low-dose vaginally administered oestradiol and oestriol were found to be equally efficacious in alleviating lower urinary tract symptoms of urge incontinence (58% vs 58%), stress incontinence (53% vs 59%) and nocturia (51% vs 54%), although the vaginal ring was found to have greater patient acceptability.

A meta-analysis of the use of oestrogen in women with symptoms of overactive bladder has been reported by the Hormones and Urogenital Therapy Committee to try and clarify the role of oestrogen therapy in the management of women with urge incontinence (Cardozo et al 2004b). In a review of 10 randomized placebo-controlled trials, oestrogen was found to be superior to placebo when considering symptoms of urge incontinence, frequency and nocturia, although vaginal oestrogen administration was found to be superior for symptoms of urgency. In those taking oestrogens, there was also a significant increase in first sensation and bladder capacity compared with placebo.

Intravesical Therapy

Capsaicin

Capsaicin is the pungent ingredient found in red chillies and is a neurotoxin of substance-P-containing (C) nerve fibres. Patients with neurogenic detrusor overactivity secondary to multiple sclerosis appear to have abnormal C fibre sensory innervation of the detrusor, which leads to premature activation of the holding reflex arc during bladder filling (Fowler et al 1992). Intravesical application of capsaicin dissolved in 30% alcohol solution can be effective for up to 6 months. The effects are variable (Chandiramani et al 1994) and the long-term safety of this treatment has not yet been evaluated.

Resiniferatoxin

Resiniferatoxin is a phorbol-related diterpene isolated from the cactus, and is a potent analogue of capsaicin that appears to have similar efficacy but fewer side-effects of pain and burning during intravesical instillation (Kim and Chancellor 2000). It is 1000 times more potent than capsaicin at stimulating bladder activity (Ishizuka et al 1995). As with capsaicin, the currently available evidence does not support the routine clinical use of the agents, although they may prove to have a role as an intravesical preparation in neurological patients with neurogenic detrusor overactivity.

Botulinum toxin

Clostridium botulinum produces its effect by production of a neurotoxin; different strains produce seven distinct serotypes designated A–G. All seven have a similar structure and molecular weight, consisting of a heavy and a light chain joined by a disulphide bond (Dolly 1997). They interfere with neural transmission by blocking the calcium-dependent release of neurotransmitter (acetylcholine), causing the affected muscle to become weak and atrophic. The affected nerves do not degenerate, but as the blockage is irreversible, only the development of new nerve terminals and synaptic contacts allows recovery of function.

The use of intravesical botulinum toxin was first described in the treatment of intractable neurogenic detrusor overactivity in 31 patients with traumatic spinal cord injury (Schurch et al 2000). Subsequently, a larger European study has reported on 231 patients with neurogenic detrusor overactivity (Reitz et al 2004). All were treated with 300 units of botulinum-A toxin which was injected cystoscopically into the detrusor muscle at 30 different sites, sparing the trigone. At 12- and 36-week follow-up, there was a significant increase in cystometric capacity and bladder compliance. Patient satisfaction was high, the majority stopped taking antimuscarinic medication and there were no significant complications. More recently, the first randomized placebo-controlled trial has been reported in 59 patients with neurogenic detrusor overactivity (Schurch et al 2005). At 6 months, there was a significant reduction in incontinence episodes in the botox group compared with the placebo group, and a corresponding improvement in QoL evaluation.

Whilst the role of botulinum toxin has been established in the treatment of neurogenic detrusor overactivity, the data regarding its use in intractable idiopathic detrusor overactivity is less robust. A prospective open-label study has recently been reported assessing the use of botulinum-A toxin in both neurogenic (300 units) and idiopathic (200 units) detrusor overactivity in 75 patients (Popat et al 2005). When considering urodynamic outcome parameters in both groups, there was a significant increase in cystometric capacity and a decrease in maximum detrusor pressure during filling in both groups. Clinically, there was also a significant reduction in frequency and episodes of urge incontinence. Interestingly, however, 69% of patients with neurogenic detrusor overactivity required self-catheterization following treatment compared with 19.3% of those with idiopathic detrusor overactivity.

At present, the evidence suggests that intravesical administration of botulinum toxin may offer an alternative to surgery in those women with intractable detrusor overactivity, although the effect is only temporary and there is little long-term data regarding the efficacy and complications associated with repeat injections (Grosse et al 2005).

Behavioural Therapy

As continence is normally learned during infancy, it is logical to suppose that it can be relearned during adult life. Bladder re-education includes bladder drill, biofeedback and hypnotherapy. Bladder discipline was first described as a method of treating urgency incontinence by Jeffcoate and Francis (1966) in the belief that it was exacerbated or even caused by underlying psychological factors. Since then, Frewen (1970) has shown that many women with overactive bladder are able to correlate the onset of their symptoms with some untoward event, which can be identified by taking a careful history. He showed that both inpatient and outpatient bladder drill can be effective forms of treatment for many such women.

The technique for performing inpatient bladder drill has been established by Jarvis (1989) and is shown below. It may be performed either in the inpatient or outpatient setting.

Technique for bladder drill

- Exclude pathology and admit to hospital (if possible).
- Explain rationale to patient.
- Instruct patient to void every 1.5 h during the day (either she waits or is incontinent).
- When 1.5 h is achieved, increase by 30 min and continue with 2-h voiding, etc.
- Allow normal fluid intake (1500 ml/24 h).
- Patient keeps a fluid balance chart.
- Patients meets a successful patient.
- Patient receives encouragement from patients, nurses and doctors.

Jarvis and Millar (1980) performed a controlled trial of bladder drill in 60 consecutive incontinent women with idiopathic overactive bladder. They showed that following inpatient treatment, 90% of the bladder drill group were continent and 83.3% remained symptom-free after 6 months. In the control group, 23.2% were continent and symptom-free due to the placebo effect. Despite the excellent early results, it has been shown that up to 40% of patients relapse within 3 years (Holmes et al 1983).

Biofeedback

Biofeedback is a form of learning or re-education in which the patient is given information about a normally unconscious physiological process in the form of an auditory, visual or tactile signal. The objective effects of biofeedback in the treatment of detrusor overactivity can be recorded on a polygraph trace, but the subjective changes may be difficult to separate from the placebo effect. This technique was originally described by Cardozo et al (1978a). Thirty women aged between 16 and 65 years suffering from idiopathic overactive bladder which was resistant to conventional therapy were treated in two centres (Cardozo et al 1978b). Some 80% of the women were cured or significantly improved subjectively, and 60% were cured or improved objectively. Long-term follow-up revealed a relatively high relapse rate (Cardozo and Stanton 1984) consistent with the long-term effects of bladder drill. Other reports suggest that bladder training with or without biofeedback can be effectively used to treat incontinence due to overactive bladder (Millard and Oldenberg 1983, Burgio et al 1986). However, this type of treatment is time-consuming and requires trained personnel. At present, biofeedback is used almost exclusively to treat children with maladaptive voiding problems.

Hypnotherapy

Hypnotherapy can be used in one of two ways: either symptom removal by suggestion alone, or by attempting to help the patient to disclose hidden emotions or memories which may be pathogenic. Freeman and Baxby (1982) treated 61 women with idiopathic overactive bladder using 12 sessions of hypnosis over a period of 1 month. They achieved an overall improvement rate of over 80%, but unfortunately only nine of the women remained symptom-free at 2-year follow-up (Freeman 1989). Consequently, this type of treatment is not currently employed in the management of overactive bladder.

Acupuncture

Acupuncture is thought to act by increasing levels of endorphins and encephalins in the cerebrospinal fluid. Encephalins are known to inhibit detrusor contractility *in vitro* (Klarskov 1987). Naloxone, an opiate antagonist, conversely causes decreased bladder capacity and increased detrusor pressure (Murray and Feneley 1982). Several studies have shown symptomatic improvement (Philp et al 1988) or decreased frequency and urinary leakage (Pigne et al 1985) in patients with overactive bladder treated with acupuncture. Gibson et al (1990) utilized infra-red low-power laser on acupuncture points with initial success, but unfortunately there was a high relapse rate at 6 months. Acupuncture is as effective as oxybutynin in the treatment of symptoms associated with idiopathic low compliance, and it is acceptable to patients but time-consuming for the operator (Kelleher et al 1994b). Acupuncture has also been compared with placebo treatment in a randomized controlled trial of 85 women (Emmons and Otto 2005). Overall, there was a greater reduction in incontinence episode frequency in the acupuncture arm compared with the placebo arm (59% vs 40%; $P > 0.05$), with a significant reduction in frequency (14%; $P = 0.013$) and improvement in QoL ($P < 0.001$).

All forms of bladder retraining in the treatment of overactive bladder are advantageous because there are few unpleasant side-effects and no patient is ever made worse. Mild-to-moderate overactive bladder can be cured or improved significantly by re-educating the bladder. However, the relapse rate is very high, and although this type of treatment avoids the morbidity associated with surgery and the side-effects of drug therapy, it requires skilled personnel and is time-consuming for both the patient and the operator. A meta-analysis has concluded that bladder retraining is more effective than placebo and medical therapy, although there is insufficient evidence to support the effectiveness of electrical stimulation and too few studies to evaluate the effect of pelvic floor exercises and biofeedback in women with urinary urge incontinence (Berghmans et al 2000).

Neuromodulation

Sacral neuromodulation

Stimulation of the dorsal sacral nerve root using a permanent implantable device in the S3 sacral foramen has been developed for use in patients with overactive bladder and neurogenic detrusor overactivity. Prior to implantation, temporary cutaneous sacral nerve stimulation is performed to check for a response; if successful, a permanent implant is inserted under general anaesthesia. Initial studies in patients with overactive bladder refractory to medical and behavioural therapy have demonstrated that after 3 years, 59% of 41 urinary urge incontinent patients showed greater than 50% reduction in incontinence episodes, with 46% of patients being completely dry (Seigel et al 2000).

Whilst neuromodulation remains an invasive and expensive procedure, it does offer a useful alternative to medical and surgical therapies in patients with severe, intractable overactive bladder prior to considering reconstructive surgery, although technical failure may often necessitate surgical revisions.

Peripheral neuromodulation

Stimulation of the posterior tibial nerve in patients with urge incontinence was first reported in 1983 (McGuire et al 1983), and has also been proposed for pelvic floor dysfunction (Stoller 1999). The tibial nerve is a mixed nerve containing L4–S3 fibres and originates from the same spinal cord segments as the innervation to the bladder and pelvic floor. Consequently, peripheral neural modulation may have a role in the management of urinary symptoms.

In a prospective multicentre study, 35 patients with urge incontinence underwent 12 weekly sessions of posterior tibial nerve stimulation (PTNS), with 70% of patients reporting a greater than 50% reduction in urinary symptoms and 46% being completely cured (Vandoninick et al 2003). More recently, a prospective, randomized, multicentre North American study has been reported comparing PTNS with extended-release tolterodine 4 mg in 100 patients. Overall, there was an improvement in 75% of patients with PTNS compared with 55.8% with extended-release tolterodine, and there was a significant improvement in QoL in both groups (Peters et al 2008).

Consequently, peripheral neuromodulation may offer an alternative therapeutic option for those patients with intractable overactive bladder who have failed to respond to medical therapy.

Surgery

Approximately 10% of women with overactive bladder remain refractory to medical and behavioural therapy, and may be considered for surgery. Various different surgical techniques have been developed, although augmentation is currently the most commonly performed technique using a clam cystoplasty, or autoaugmentation using detrusor myectomy.

Clam cystoplasty

In clam cystoplasty (Bramble 1990, Mast et al 1995), the bladder is bisected almost completely and a patch of gut (usually ileum) equal in length to the circumference of the bisected bladder (approximately 25 cm) is sewn in place. This often cures the symptoms of overactive bladder (McRae et al 1987) by converting a high-pressure system into a low-pressure system, although inefficient voiding may result. Patients have to learn to strain to void or may have to resort to clean intermittent self-catheterization, sometimes permanently. In addition, mucus retention in the bladder may be a problem, but this can be partially overcome by ingestion of 200 ml of cranberry juice each day (Rosenbaum et al 1989) in addition to intravesical mucolytics such as acetylcysteine. The chronic exposure of the ileal mucosa to urine may lead to malignant change (Harzmann and Weckerman 1992). There is a 5% risk of adenocarcinoma arising in ureterosigmoidostomies, where colonic mucosa is exposed to N-nitrosamines found in both urine

and faeces, and a similar risk may apply to enterocystoplasty. Biopsies of the ileal segment taken from patients with clam cystoplasties show evidence of chronic inflammation of villous atrophy (Nurse and Mundy 1987), and diarrhoea due to disruption of the bile acid cycle is common (Barrington et al 1995). This may be treated using cholestyramine. In addition, metabolic disturbances such as hyperchloraemic acidosis, B_{12} deficiency and, occasionally, osteoporosis secondary to decreased bone mineralization may occur.

Detrusor myectomy

Detrusor myectomy offers an alternative to clam cystoplasty by increasing functional bladder capacity without the complications of bowel interposition. In this procedure, the whole thickness of the detrusor muscle is excised from the dome of the bladder, thereby creating a large bladder diverticulum with no intrinsic contractility (Cartwright and Snow 1989). Whilst there is a reduction in episodes of incontinence, there is little improvement in functional capacity and thus frequency remains problematic (Kennelly et al 1994, Snow and Cartwright 1996).

Urinary diversion

As a last resort, for those women with severe overactive bladder or neurogenic detrusor overactivity who cannot manage clean intermittent catheterization, it may be more appropriate to perform a urinary diversion. Usually, this will utilize an ileal conduit to create an incontinent abdominal stoma for urinary diversion. An alternative is to form a continent diversion using the appendix (Mitrofanoff) or ileum (Koch pouch), which may then be drained using self-catheterization.

National Institute for Health and Clinical Excellence Guidelines

The medical management of overactive bladder has been reviewed recently by the National Institute for Health and Clinical Excellence (2006). In the first instance, bladder retraining lasting for a minimum of 6 weeks should be offered to all women with mixed or urge incontinence. In those women who do not achieve satisfactory benefit from bladder retraining alone, an antimuscarinic agent in addition to bladder retraining should be considered.

When considering drug therapy, immediate-release nonproprietary oxybutynin should be offered to women with overactive bladder or mixed urinary incontinence as first-line drug treatment if bladder retraining has been ineffective. If immediate-release oxybutynin is not well tolerated, darifenacin, solifenacin, tolterodine, trospium or an extended-release or transdermal formulation of oxybutynin should be considered as alternatives. In addition, women should be counselled regarding the adverse effects of antimuscarinic drugs.

Propiverine should be considered as an option to treat the frequency of micturition, but this is not recommended for the treatment of urinary incontinence. Flavoxate, propantheline and imipramine should not be used for the treatment of overactive bladder. Whilst desmopressin may be considered specifically to reduce nocturia in women, this is currently outside the marketing authorization; hence, informed consent must be obtained.

When considering the role of oestrogens, the recommendations are that systemic hormone replacement therapy should not be recommended, although intravaginal oestrogens are recommended for the treatment of overactive bladder in postmenopausal women with urogenital atrophy.

Conclusion

Overactive bladder is a common and distressing condition, affecting people of all ages. It is characterized by multiple symptoms which, although not life-threatening, may cause much embarrassment and a very restricted lifestyle. Lack of understanding of the underlying pathology of overactive bladder is reflected in the numerous different methods of treatment which are currently employed, none of them wholly satisfactory. Conventional bladder neck surgery is not useful in the treatment of overactive bladder unless there is concomitant urethral sphincter incompetence; therefore, it is important to make an accurate diagnosis before treatment is commenced.

Behavioural intervention seems to be the best type of treatment of idiopathic overactive bladder because it may produce a permanent cure without any significant morbidity or side-effects. However, the majority of patients are still treated with drug therapy, which they may need to take indefinitely as symptoms usually return once the tablets are discontinued. Surgical procedures such as augmentation cystoplasty are reserved for women with severe symptoms in whom other forms of treatment have been tried and failed.

Fortunately, overactive bladder is a disease of spontaneous exacerbations and remissions. Therefore, short courses of drug therapy, when symptoms are at their worst, may be sufficient for the sufferer to maintain a normal lifestyle. Although it is rare to cure a patient completely with any form of treatment, most can have their symptoms reduced significantly. The elucidation of the patient's main complaints is therefore of great importance. As the pathophysiology of the condition becomes clearer, leading to the development of new drugs offering greater efficacy and improved compliance, significant advances in the management of overactive bladder can be expected.

KEY POINTS

1. Overactive bladder is a symptomatic diagnosis.
2. Detrusor overactivity is a urodynamic-based diagnosis.
3. Detrusor overactivity may occur in 10% of the normal population and be asymptomatic.
4. The incidence of overactive bladder increases with age.
5. Whilst neurogenic detrusor overactivity is associated with neurological disease, the cause of idiopathic detrusor overactivity remains unknown.
6. The diagnosis of overactive bladder can be suggested by symptoms, but a diagnosis of detrusor overactivity can only be confirmed on cystometry.
7. Bladder retraining and behaviour modification are important primary treatments which can be augmented by antimuscarinic drug therapy.
8. Most antimuscarinic drugs need to be given at a dosage which will produce parasympathetic side-effects.
9. Mild overactivity can be cured or improved by bladder retraining but the relapse rate is high.
10. Where detrusor overactivity and urethral sphincter incompetence coexist (mixed incontinence), it is preferable to treat the detrusor overactivity prior to considering continence surgery.

Appendix

Levels of evidence

I   Systematic review of all relevant randomized controlled trials

IIA   One randomized controlled trial — low probability of bias and high probability of causal relationship

IIB   One randomized controlled trial

IIIA   Well-designed controlled trials (no randomization)

IIIB   Cohort or case–control studies

IIIC   Multiple time series or dramatic results in uncontrolled experiments

IV   Expert opinion (traditional use)

Grades of recommendations

A   A systematic review of randomized controlled trials or a body of evidence consisting principally of studies rated as 1 directly applicable to the target population and demonstrating overall consistency of results

B   A body of evidence including studies rated as 2A directly applicable to the target population and demonstrating overall consistency of results or

   Extrapolated evidence from studies rated as 1

C   A body of evidence including studies rated as 2B directly applicable to the target population and demonstrating overall consistency of results or

   Extrapolated evidence from studies rated as 2

D   Evidence level 3 or 4 or

   Extrapolated evidence from studies rated as 2

Sources: Hadom DC, Baker D, Hodges JS, Hicks N 1996 Journal of Clinical Epidemiology 49: 749–754. Harbour R, Miller J 2001 BMJ (Clinical Research Ed) 323: 334–336.

References

Abrams P, Freeman R, Anderstrom C, Mattiasson A 1998 Tolterodine, a new antimuscarinic agent: as effective but better tolerated than oxybutynin in patients with an overactive bladder. British Journal of Urology 81: 801–810.

Abrams P, Cardozo L, Fall M et al 2002 The standardisation of terminology of lower urinary tract function. Report from the Standardisation Committee of the International Continence Society. Neurourology and Urodynamics 21: 167–178.

Alabaster VA 1997 Discovery and development of selective M3 antagonists for clinical use. Life Science 60: 1053–1060.

Anderson RU, Mobley D, Blank B, Saltzstein D, Susset J, Brown JS 1999 Once daily controlled versus immediate release oxybutynin chloride for urge urinary incontinence. OROS Oxybutynin Study Group. Journal of Urology 161: 1809–1812.

Andersson KE 1992 Clinical pharmacology of potassium channel openers. Pharmacology and Toxicology 70: 244–245.

Andersson KE 1997 The overactive bladder: pharmacologic basis of drug treatment. Urology 50: 74–89.

Andersson KE, Arner A 2004 Urinary bladder contraction and relaxation: physiology and pathophysiology. Physiological Reviews 84: 935–986.

Andersson KE, Chapple CR, Cardozo L et al 2009 Pharmacological treatment of urinary incontinence. In: Abrams P, Cardozo L, Khoury S, Wein A (eds) Incontinence, 4th edn. Health Publication Ltd, Paris, pp 631–700.

Appell RA 1997 Clinical efficacy and safety of tolterodine in the treatment of overactive bladder: a pooled analysis. Urology 50: 90–96.

Baigrie RJ, Kelleher JP, Fawcett DP, Pengelly AW 1988 Oxybutynin: is it safe? British Journal of Urology 62: 319–322.

Barrington JW, Fern Davies H, Adams RJ, Evans WD, Woodcock JP, Stephenson TP 1995 Bile acid dysfunction after clam enterocystoplasty. British Journal of Urology 76: 169–171.

Bates CP, Whiteside CG, Turner-Warwick RT 1970 Synchronous cine-pressure-flow cystourethrography with special reference to stress and urge incontinence. British Journal of Urology 50: 714–723.

Benness C, Wise BG, Cutner A, Cardozo LD 1992 Does low dose vaginal oestradiol improve frequency and urgency in postmenopausal women. International Urogynecology Journal 3: 281.

Berghmans LC, Hendricks HJ, de Bie RA, van Waalwijk van Doorn ES, Bo K, van Kerrebroeck PE 2000 Conservative treatment of urge urinary incontinence in women: a systematic review of randomized clinical trials. BJU International 85: 254–263.

Brading AF 1997 A myogenic basis for the overactive bladder. Urology 50: 57–67.

Brading AF, Turner WH 1994 The unstable bladder: towards a common mechanism. British Journal of Urology 73: 3–8.

Bramble FJ 1990 The clam cystoplasty. British Journal of Urology 66: 337–341.

Braverman AS, Ruggieri MR 1998 The M_2 receptor contributes to contraction of the denervated rat urinary bladder. American Journal of Physiology 275: 1654.

Brown JS, McNaughton KS, Wyman JF et al 2003 Measurement characteristics of a voiding diary for use by men and women with overactive bladder. Urology 61: 802–809.

Brown K, Hilton P 1999 The incidence of overactive bladder before and after colposuspension: a study using conventional and ambulatory urodynamic monitoring. BJU International 84: 961–965.

Burgio KL, Robinson JC, Engel BT 1986 The role of biofeedback in Kegel exercise training for stress incontinence. American Journal of Obstetrics and Gynecology 154: 64–88.

Burgio KL, Matthews KA, Engel BT 1991 Prevalence, incidence and correlates of urinary incontinence in healthy, middle-aged women. Journal of Urology 146: 1255–1259.

Burnstock G 2001 Purinergic signaling in lower urinary tract. In: Abbracchio MP, Williams M (eds) Purinergic and Pyrimidinergic Signalling I: Molecular, Nervous and Urogenitary System Function. Springer, Berlin, pp 151: 423–515.

Cardozo LD 1988 Sex and the bladder. BMJ (Clinical Research Ed.) 296: 587–588.

Cardozo LD, Stanton SL, Allan V 1978a Biofeedback in the treatment of overactive bladder. British Journal of Urology 50: 250–254.

Cardozo LD, Abrams PH, Stanton SL, Feneley RCL 1978b Idiopathic overactive bladder treated by biofeedback. British Journal of Urology 50: 521–523.

Cardozo LD, Stanton SL, Williams JE 1979 Detrusor instability following surgery for urodynamic instability. British Journal of Urology 51: 204–207.

Cardozo LD, Stanton SL 1980 Genuine stress incontinence and overactive bladder: a review of 200 cases. BJOG: an International Journal of Obstetrics and Gynaecology 87: 184–190.

Cardozo LD, Stanton SL, Robinson H, Hole D 1980 Evaluation on flurbiprofen in detrusor instability. BMJ (Clinical Research Ed.) 280: 281–282.

Cardozo LD, Stanton SL 1984 Biofeedback: a five year review. British Journal of Urology 56: 220.

Cardozo LD, Cooper D, Versi E 1987 Oxybutynin chloride in the management of idiopathic overactive bladder.

Neurourology and Urodynamics 6: 256–257.

Cardozo LD, Rekers H, Tapp A et al 1993 Oestriol in the treatment of postmenopausal urgency: a multicentre study. Maturitas 18: 47–53.

Cardozo LD, Chapple CR, Toozs-Hobson P et al 2000 Efficacy of trospium chloride in patients with overactive bladder: a placebo-controlled, randomized, double-blind, multicentre clinical trial. BJU International 85: 659–664.

Cardozo L, Lisec M, Millard R et al 2004a Randomised, double blind placebo controlled trial of the once daily antimuscarinic agent solifenacin succinate in patients with overactive bladder. Journal of Urology 172: 1919–1924.

Cardozo L, Lose G, McClish D, Versi E 2004b A systematic review of the effects of oestrogens for symptoms suggestive of overactive bladder. Acta Obstetricia et Gynecologica Scandinavica 83: 892–897.

Cartwright PC, Snow BW 1989 Bladder autoaugmentation: partial detrusor excision to augment the bladder without use of bowel. Journal of Urology 142: 1050–1053.

Castleden CM, George CF, Renwick AG, Asher MJ 1981 Imipramine — a possible alternative to current therapy for urinary incontinence in the elderly. Journal of Urology 125: 318–320.

Caulfield MP, Birdsall NJ 1998 International Union of Pharmacology XVII. Classification of muscarinic acetylcholine receptors. Pharmacological Reviews 50: 279.

Chandiramani VA, Peterson T, Beck RO, Fowler CJ 1994 Lessons learnt from 44 intravesical instillations of capsaicin. Neurourology and Urodynamics 13: 348–349.

Chapple CR 2004a Darifenacin is well tolerated and provides significant improvement in the symptoms of overactive bladder: a pooled analysis of phase III studies. European Urology 171 (Suppl): 130 (abstract).

Chapple C 2004b Fesoterodine: a new effective and well tolerated antimuscarinic for the treatment of urgency–frequency syndrome: results of a phase II controlled study. Neurourology and Urodynamics 23: 598–599.

Chapple CR, Martinez-Garcia R, Selvaggi L et al; STAR study group 2005 A comparison of the efficacy and tolerability of solifenacin succinate and extended release tolterodine at treating overactive bladder syndrome: results of the STAR trial. European Urology 48: 464–470.

Chapple C, van Kerrebroeck P, Tubaro A, Millard R 2006a Fesoterodine in non-neurogenic voiding dysfunction — results on efficacy and safety in a phase III trial. European Urology 5 (Suppl): 117.

Chapple C, Patroneva A, Raines S 2006b Effect of an ATP-sensitive potassium channel opener in subjects with overactive bladder: a randomized double-blind placebo controlled study (ZD09471L/0004). European Urology 49: 879–886.

Chapple CR, van Kerrebroeck PE, Junemann KP, Wang JT, Brodsky M 2008 Comparison of fesoterodine and tolterodine in patients with overactive bladder. BJU International 102: 1128–1132.

Charlton RG, Morley AR, Chambers P, Gillespie JI 1999 Focal changes in nerve, muscle and connective tissue in normal and unstable human bladder. BJU International 84: 953–960.

Collas D, Malone-Lee J 1997 The pharmacokinetic properties of rectal oxybutynin — a possible alternative to intravesical administration. Neurourology and Urodynamics 16: 346–347.

Diokno AC, Hyndman CW, Hardy DA, Lapides J 1972 Comparison of action of imipramine (Tofranil) and propantheline (Probanthine) on detrusor contraction. Journal of Urology 107: 42–43.

Diokno AC, Appell RA, Sand PK et al; OPERA Study Group 2003 Prospective, randomised, double blind study of the efficacy and tolerability of the extended-release formulations of oxybutynin and tolterodine for overactive bladder: results of the OPERA trial. Mayo Clinic Proceedings 78: 687–695.

Dmochowski RR, Sand PK, Zinner NR, Gittelman MC, Davila GW, Sanders SW; Transdermal Oxybutynin Study Group 2003 Comparative efficacy and safety of transdermal oxybutynin and oral tolterodine versus placebo in previously treated patients with urge and mixed urinary incontinence. Urology 62: 237–242.

Dmochowski RR, Sand PK, Zinner NR, Staskin DR 2008 Trospium 60 mg once daily for overactive bladder syndrome: results from a placebo controlled interventional study. Urology 71: 449–454.

Dolly JO 1997 Therapeutic and research exploitation of botulinum neurotoxins. European Journal of Neurology 4 (Suppl 2): S5–S10.

Dorschner W, Stolzenburg JU, Griebenow R et al 2000 Efficacy and safety of propiverine in elderly patients — a double blind, placebo controlled clinical study. European Urology 37: 702.

Eaton AC, Bates CP 1982 An in vitro physiological, study of normal and unstable human detrusor muscle. British Journal of Urology 54: 653–657.

Edwards G, Henshaw M, Miller M, Weston WH 1991 Comparison of the effects of several potassium-channel openers on rat bladder and rat portal vein in vitro. British Journal of Pharmacology 102: 679–686.

Emmons SL, Otto L 2005 Acupuncture for overactive bladder: a randomised controlled trial. Obstetrics and Gynecology 106: 138–143.

Eriksen PS, Rasmussen H 1992 Low dose 17β-oestradiol vaginal tablets in the treatment of atrophic vaginitis: a double-blind placebo controlled study. European Journal of Obstetrics, Gynaecology and Reproductive Biology 44: 137–144.

Fowler CJ, Jewkes D, McDonald WI, Lynn B, DeGroat WC 1992 Intravesical capsaicin for neurogenic bladder dysfunction. The Lancet 339: 1239.

Freeman RM 1989 Hypnosis and psychomedical treatment. In: Freeman RM, Malvern J (eds) The Unstable Bladder. Wright, Bristol, pp 73–80.

Freeman RM, Baxby K 1982 Hypnotherapy for incontinence caused by the unstable detrusor. BMJ (Clinical Research Ed.) 284: 1831–1834.

Frewen WK 1970 Urge and stress incontinence: fact and fiction. Journal of Obstetrics and Gynaecology of the British Commonwealth 77: 932–934.

Fusgen I, Hauri D 2000 Trospium chloride: an effective option for medical treatment of bladder overactivity. International Journal of Clinical Pharmacology and Therapeutics 38: 223–234.

Gibson JS, Pardley J, Neville J 1990 Infra-red low power laser therapy on acupuncture points for treatment of the unstable bladder. Proceedings of the 20th Meeting of the International Continence Society, Aarhus, Denmark, pp 146–147.

Gill TM, Feinstein AR 1974 A critical appraisal of the quality of life measurements. Journal of the American Medical Association 272: 619–626.

Grosse J, Kramer G, Stoher M 2005 Success of repeat detrusor injections of botulinum-A toxin in patients with severe neurogenic detrusor overactivity and incontinence. European Urology 47: 653–659.

Haab F, Cardozo L, Chapple C, Ridder AM; Solifenacin Study Group 2005 Long-term open label solifenacin treatment associated with persistence with therapy in patients with overactive bladder syndrome. European Urology 47: 376–384.

Hadom DC, Baker D, Hodges JS, Hicks N 1996 Rating the quality of evidence for clinical practice guidelines. Journal of Clinical Epidemiology 49: 749–754.

Harbour R, Miller J 2001 A new system for grading recommendations in evidence based guidelines. BMJ (Clinical Research Ed.) 323: 334–336.

Harzmann R, Weckerman D 1992 Problem of secondary malignancy after urinary diversion and enterocystoplasty. Scandinavian Journal of Urology and Nephrology 142 (Suppl): 56.

Haruno A, Yamasaki Y, Miyoshi K et al 1989 Effects of propiverine hydrochloride and its metabolites on isolated guinea pig urinary bladder. Folia Pharmacologica Japonica 94: 145–150.

Harris DR, Marsh KA, Birmingham AT et al 1995 Expression of muscarinic M_3 receptors coupled to inositol phospholipid hydrolysis in human detrusor cultured smooth muscle cells. Journal of Urology 154: 1241.

Hashim H, Abrams P 2006 Is the bladder a reliable witness for predicting detrusor overactivity? Journal of Urology 175: 191–195.

Hashim H, Malmberg L, Graugaard-Jensen C, Abrams P 2009 Desmopressin as a 'designer-drug' in the treatment of overactive bladder syndrome. Neurourology and Urodynamics 28: 40–46.

Hegde SS, Chopin A, Bonhaus D et al 1997 Functional role of M_2 and M_3 muscarinic receptors in the urinary bladder of rats in vitro and in vivo. British Journal of Pharmacology 120: 1409.

Hegde SS, Eglen RM 1999 Muscarinic receptor subtypes modulating smooth muscle contractility in the urinary bladder. Life Sciences 64: 419.

Heslington K, Hilton P 1996 Ambulatory urodynamic monitoring. BJOG: an International Journal of Obstetrics and Gynaecology 103: 393–399.

Higson RH, Smith JC, Whelan P 1978 Bladder rupture: an acceptable complication of distension therapy. British Journal of Urology 50: 529–534.

Hills CJ, Winter SA, Balfour JA 1998 Tolterodine. Drugs 55: 813–820.

Hilton P 1988 Urinary incontinence during sexual intercourse: a common but rarely volunteered symptom. BJOG: an International Journal of Obstetrics and Gynaecology 95: 377–381.

Hilton P, Stanton SL 1982 Use of desmopressin (DDAVP) in nocturnal urinary frequency in the female. British Journal of Urology 54: 252–255.

Hodgkinson CP, Ayers MA, Drukker BH 1963 Dyssynergic detrusor dysfunction in the apparently normal female. American Journal of Obstetrics and Gynecology 87: 717–730.

Hodgkinson CP, Drukker BH 1977 Infravesical nerve resection for detrusor dyssynergia (the Ingleman-Sundberg operation). Acta Obstetricia et Gynecologica Scandinavica 56: 401–408.

Holmes DM, Stone AR, Barry PR, Richards CJ, Stephenson TP 1983 Bladder training — years on. British Journal of Urology 55: 660–664.

Hughes KM, Lang JCT, Lazare R et al 1992 Measurement of oxybutynin and its N-desethyl metabolite in plasma, and its application to pharmacokinetic studies in young, elderly and frail elderly volunteers. Xenobiotica 22: 859–869.

Ingleman-Sundberg A 1978 Partial bladder denervation for detrusor dyssynergia. Clinical Obstetrics and Gynaecology 21: 797–805.

Irwin DE, Milsom I, Hunskaar S et al 2006 Population-based survey of urinary incontinence, overactive bladder and other lower urinary tract symptoms in five countries; results of the EPIC study. European Urology 50: 1306–1315.

Ishizuka O, Mattiasson A, Andersson K-E 1995 Urodynamic effects of intravesical resiniferatoxin and capsaicin in conscious rats with and without outflow obstruction. Journal of Urology 154: 611–616.

Jarvis GT 1989 Bladder drill. In: Freeman R, Malvern J (eds) The Unstable Bladder. Wright, Bristol, pp 55–60.

Jarvis GT, Millar DR 1980 Controlled trial of bladder drill for overactive bladder. BMJ (Clinical Research Ed.) 281: 1322–1323.

Jeffcoate TNA, Francis WJA 1966 Urgency incontinence in the female. American Journal of Obstetrics and Gynecology 94: 604–618.

Jenkinson C, Coulter A, Wright L 1993 Short Form 36 (SF-36) health survey questionnaire. Normative data for adults of working age. BMJ (Clinical Research Ed.) 306: 1437–1440.

Jeremy JY, Tsang V, Mikhailidis DP, Rogers H, Morgan RJ, Dandona P 1987 Eicosanoid synthesis by human urinary bladder mucosa: pathological implications. British Journal of Urology 59: 36–39.

Jonas U, Hofner K, Madesbacher H, Holmdahl TH 1997 Efficacy and safety of two doses of tolterodine versus placebo in patients with detrusor overactivity and symptoms of frequency, urge incontinence, and urgency: urodynamic evaluation. World Journal of Urology 15: 144–151.

Jünemann KP, Hessdörfer E, Unamba-Oparah I et al 2006 Propiverine hydrochloride immediate and extended release: comparison of efficacy and tolerability in patients with overactive bladder. Urology International 77: 334–349.

Karram MM, Bhatia NW 1989 Management of coexistent stress and urge urinary incontinence. Obstetrics and Gynecology 73: 4–7.

Kelleher CJ, Cardozo LD, Khullar V, Salvatore S, Hill S 1994a Anticholinergic therapy: the need for continued surveillance. Neurourology and Urodynamics 13: 432–433.

Kelleher CJ, Filsche J, Burton G, Cardozo LD 1994b Acupuncture and the treatment of irritative bladder symptoms. Acupuncture in Medicine 12: 9–12.

Kelleher CJ, Cardozo LD, Khullar V, Salvatore S 1997a A new questionnaire to assess the quality of life of urinary incontinent women. BJOG: an International Journal of Obstetrics and Gynaecology 104: 1374–1379.

Kelleher CJ, Cardozo LD, Khullar V, Salvatore S 1997b A medium-term analysis of the subjective efficency of treatment for women with detrusor instability and low bladder compliance. BJOG: an International Journal of Obstetrics and Gynaecology 104: 988–993.

Kennelly MJ, Gormley EA, McGuire EJ 1994 Early clinical experience with adult bladder autoaugmentation. Journal of Urology 152: 303–306.

Kim DY, Chancellor MB 2000 Intravesical neuromodulatory drugs: capsaicin and resiniferatoxin to treat the overactive bladder. Journal of Endourology 14: 97–103.

Kinder RB, Mundy AR 1987 Pathophysiology of idiopathic overactive bladder and detrusor hyperreflexia — an in vitro study of human detrusor muscle. British Journal of Urology 60: 509–515.

Klarskov P 1987 Gukephaline inhibits presynaptically the contractility of urinary tract smooth muscle. British Journal of Urology 59: 31–35.

Knudsen UB, Rittig S, Pedersen JP, Norgaard JP, Djurhuus JC 1989 Long-term treatment of nocturnal enuresis with desmopressin — influence on urinary output and haematological parameters. Neurourology and Urodynamics 8: 348–349.

Langworthy DR, Kolb LG, Dees JE 1936 Behaviour of the human bladder freed from cerebral control. Journal of Urology 36: 577–597.

Lawson K 1996 Is there a therapeutic future for 'potassium channel openers'? Clinical Science 91: 651–663.

Levin RM, Kitada S, Hayes L et al 1991 Experimental hyperreflexia: effect of intravesical administration of various agents. Pharmacology 42: 54.

Lose G, Jorgensen L, Thunedborg P 1989 Doxepin in the treatment of female detrusor overactivity: a randomized double-blind crossover study. Journal of Urology 142: 1024–1027.

Lose G, Englev E 2000 Oestradiol-releasing vaginal ring versus oestriol vaginal pessaries in the treatment of bothersome lower urinary tract symptoms. BJOG: an International Journal of Obstetrics and Gynaecology 107: 1029–1034.

Madersbacher H, Jilg S 1991 Control of detrusor hyperreflexia by the intravesical instillation of oxybutynin hydrochloride. Paraplegia 29: 84–90.

Madersbacher H, Stoher M, Richter R et al 1995 Trospium chloride versus oxybutynin: a randomised, double-blind multicentre trial in the treatment of detrusor hyperrflexia. British Journal of Urology 75: 452–456.

Madersbacher H, Murtz G, Alloussi S et al 2009 Propiverine vs oxybutynin for treating neurogenic detrusor overactivity in children and adolescents: results of a multicentre observational cohort study. BJU International 103: 776–781.

Malloy BJ, Price DT, Price RR et al 1998 α_1 Adrenergic receptor subtypes in human detrusor. Journal of Urology 160: 937–943.

Mast P, Hoebeke P, Wyndale JJ, Oosterlinck W, Everaert K 1995 Experience with clam cystoplasty. A review. Paraplegia 33: 560–564.

Mazur D, Wehnert J, Dorschner W, Schubert G, Herfurth G, Alken RG 1995 Clinical and urodynamic effects of propiverine in patients suffering from urgency and urge incontinence. Scandinavian Journal of Urology and Nephrology 29: 289–294.

McGuire EJ, Shi-Chun Z, Horwinski ER et al 1983 Treatment of motor and sensory detrusor instability by electrical stimulation. Journal of Urology 129: 78.

McRae P, Murray KH, Nurse DE, Stephenson JP, Mundy AR 1987 Clam entero-cystoplasty in the neuropathic bladder. British Journal of Urology 60: 523–525

Millard RJ, Oldenberg BF 1983 The symptomatic, urodynamic and psycho-dynamic results of bladder re-education programmes. Journal of Urology 130: 717–719.

Millard R, Tuttle J, Moore K et al 1999 Clinical efficacy and safety of tolterodine compared to placebo in detrusor overactivity. Journal of Urology 161: 1551–1555.

Mills IW, Greenland JE, McMurray G et al 2000 Studies of the pathophysiology of idiopathic overactive bladder: the physiological properties of the detrusor smooth muscle and its pattern of innervation. Journal of Urology 163: 646–651.

Milsom I, Abrams P, Cardozo L, Roberts RG, Thuroff J, Wein AJ 2001 How widespread are the symptoms of overactive bladder and how are they managed? A population-based prevalence study. BJU International 87: 760–766.

Mundy AR 1983 The long-term results of bladder transection for urge incontinence. British Journal of Urology 55: 642–644.

Murray KH, Feneley RCL 1982 Endorphins — a role in lower urinary tract function The effect of opioid blockade on the detrusor and urethral sphincter mechanism. British Journal of Urology 54: 638–640.

Naughton MJ, Shumaker SA 1996 Assessment of health related quality of life. In: Furberg CD, DeMets DL (eds) Fundamentals of Clinical Trials, 3rd edn. Mosby Press, St Louis, p 185.

National Institute for Health and Clinical Excellence 2006 The Management of Urinary Incontinence in Women. NICE Guideline 40. Department of Health, London. Available at: www.nice.org.uk.

Nilsson K, Heimer G 1992 Low dose oestradiol in the treatment of urogenital oestrogen defiiciency — a pharmacokinetic and pharmacodynamic study. Maturitas 15: 121–127.

Nilvebrant L, Andersson KE, Mattiasson A 1985 Characterization of the muscarinic cholinoreceptors in the human detrusor. Journal of Urology 134: 418–423.

Nilvebrant L, Sparf B 1986 Dicyclomine, benzhexol and oxybutynin distingush between subclasses of muscarinic binding sites. European Journal of Pharmacology 123: 133–143.

Nilvebrant L, Andersson K-E, Gillberg P-G, Stahl M, Sparf B 1997 Tolterodine — a new bladder selective anti-muscarinic agent. European Journal of Pharmacology 327: 195–207.

Norgaard JP, Rillig S, Djurhuus JC 1989 Nocturnal enuresis: an approach to treatment based on pathogenesis. Journal of Pediatrics 114: 705–709.

Norton KRW, Bhat AV, Stanton SL 1990 Psychiatric aspects of urinary incontinence in women attending an outpatient clinic. BMJ (Clinical Research Ed.) 31: 271–272.

Nurse DE, Mundy AR 1987 Cystoplasty infection and cancer. Neurourology and Urodynamics 6: 343–344.

O'Reilly BA, Kosaka AH, Knight GF et al 2002 P2X receptors and their role in female idiopathic detrusor instability. Journal of Urology 167: 157–164.

Pengelly AW, Stephenson TP, Milroy EJG, Whiteside CG, Turner-Warwick R 1978 Results of prolonged bladder distension as treatment for overactive bladder. British Journal of Urology 50: 243–245.

Peters KM, Leong FC, Shoberi SA et al 2008 A randomised multicentre study comparing percutaneous tibial nerve stimulation with pharmaceutical therapy for the treatment of overactive bladder. Poster Presentation. American Urological Association, Orlando, FL.

Philp T, Shah PJR, Worth PHL 1988 Acupuncture in the treatment of bladder instability. British Journal of Urology 61: 490–493.

Pigne A, Degansac C, Nyssen C, Barratt J 1985 Acupuncture and the unstable bladder. In: Proceedings of the 15th International Continence Society Meeting, pp 186–187.

Popat R, Apostolidis A, Kalsi V, Gonzales G, Fowler CJ, Dasgupta P 2005 A comparison between the response of patients with idiopathic detrusor overactivity and neurogenic detrusor overactivity to the first intradetrusor injection of botulinum-A toxin. Journal of Urology 174: 984–989.

Ramsden PD, Smith JC, Dunn M, Ardran GM 1976 Distension therapy for the unstable bladder: late results including an assessment of repeat distensions. Journal of Urology 48: 623–629.

Reitz A, Stroher M, Kramer G et al 2004 European experience of 200 cases treated with botulinum-A toxin injections into the detrusor muscle for urinary incontinence due to neurogenic detrusor overactivity. European Urology 45: 510–515.

Rentzhog L, Stanton SL, Cardozo LD, Nelson E, Fall M, Abrams P 1998 Efficacy and safety of tolterodine in patients with overactive bladder: a dose ranging study. British Journal of Urology 81: 42–48.

Rew DA, Rundle JSH 1989 Assessment of the safety of regular DDAVP therapy in primary nocturnal enuresis. British Journal of Urology 63: 352–353.

Robertson AS, Griffiths CJ, Ramsden PD, Neal DE 1994 Bladder function in healthy volunteers: ambulatory monitoring and conventional urodynamic studies. British Journal of Urology 73: 242–249.

Robinson D, Cardozo L, Akeson M, Hvistendahl G, Riis A, Norgaard J 2004 Anti-diuresis — a new concept in the management of daytime urinary

incontinence. BJU International 93: 996–1000.

Robinson D, Cardozo L, Terpstra G, Bolodeoku J 2007 A randomised double blind placebo controlled study to evaluate the efficacy of tamsulosin OCAS in the management of women with overactive bladder. BJU International 100: 840–845.

Rose DK 1931 Clinical application of bladder physiology. Journal of Urology 26: 91–105.

Rosenbaum TP, Shah PJR, Rose GA, Lloyd-Davies RW 1989 Cranberry juice helps the problem of mucus production in enterouroplasties. Neurourology and Urodynamics 8: 344–345.

Ruscin JM, Morgenstern NE 1999 Tolterodine use for symptoms of overactive bladder. Annals of Pharmacotherapy 33: 1073–1082.

Salvatore S, Khullar V, Anders K, Cardozo LD 1998 Reducing artifacts in ambulatory urodynamics. British Journal of Urology 81: 211–214.

Salvatore S, Khullar V, Cardozo L, Anders K, Zocchi G, Soligo M 2001 Evaluating ambulatory urodynamics: a prospective study in asymptomatic women. BJOG: an International Journal of Obstetrics and Gynaecology 108: 107–111.

Samsicoe G, Jansson I, Mellstrom D, Svanberg A 1985 Urinary incontinence in 75 year old women. Effects of oestriol. Acta Obstetricia et Gynecologica Scandinavica 1985; 93: 57.

Schladitz-Keil G, Spahn H, Mutschler E 1986 Determination of bioavailability of the quaternary ammonium compound trospium chloride in man from urinary excretion data. Arzneimittel Forschung/Drug Research 36: 984–987.

Schurch B, Stohrer M, Kramer G, Schmid DM, Gaul G, Hauri D 2000 Botulinum-A toxin for treating detrusor hyperreflexia in spinal cord injured pateints: a new alternative to anticholinergic drugs? Preliminary results. Journal of Urology 164: 692–697.

Schurch B, de Seze M, Denys P et al; Botox Detrusor Hyperreflexia Study Team 2005 Botulinum toxin type a is a safe and effective treatment for neurogenic urinary incontinence: results of a single treatment, randomized, placebo controlled 6-month study. Journal of Urology 174: 196–200.

Schwinn DA 2000 Novel role for alpha 1-adrenergic receptor sub-types in lower urinary tract symptoms. BJU International 86 (Suppl 2): 11–20.

Seigel SW, Cantanzaro F, Dijkema HE et al 2000 Long term results of a multicentre study on sacral nerve stimulation for treatment of urinary urge incontinence, urgency–frequency and retention. Urology 56: 87–91.

Sibley GN 1985 An experimental model of overactive bladder in the obstructed pig. British Journal of Urology 57: 292–298.

Sibley GN 1997 Developments in our understanding of overactive bladder. British Journal of Urology 80: 54–61.

Snow BW, Cartwright PC 1996 Bladder autoaugmentation. Urologic Clinics of North America 23: 323–331.

Speakman MJ, Brading AF, Gilpin CJ, Dixon JS, Gilpin SA, Gosling JA 1987 Bladder outflow obstruction — cause of denervation supersensitivity. Journal of Urology 183: 1461–1466.

Staskin DR, Dmochowski RR, Sand PK et al 2009 Efficacy and safety of oxybutynin chloride topical gel for overactive bladder: a randomised double-blind, placebo controlled, multicentre study. Journal of Urology 181: 1764–1772.

Steel SA, Cox C, Stanton SL 1985 Long-term follow-up of overactive bladder following the colposuspension operation. British Journal of Urology 58: 138–142.

Stewart WF, Corey R, Herzog AR et al 2001 Prevalence of overactive bladder in women: results from the NOBLE program. International Urogynecology Journal 12: S66.

Stoher M, Madersbacher H, Richter R, Wehnert J, Dreikorn K 1999 Efficacy and safety of propiverine in SCI-patients suffering from detrusor hyperreflexia: a double-blind, placebo-controlled clinical trial. Spinal Cord 37: 196–200.

Stoller ML 1999 Afferent nerve stimulation for pelvic floor dysfunction. European Urology 135: 32.

Subak LL, Wing R, West DS et al; PRIDE Investigators 2009 Weight loss to treat urinary incontinence in overweight and obese women. New England Journal of Medicine 360: 481–490.

Sutherst JR, Brown M 1978 The effect on the bladder pressure of sudden entry of fluid into the posterior urethra. British Journal of Urology 50: 406–409.

Swift S, Garely A, Dimpfl T, Payne C; Tolterodine Study Group 2003 A new once-daily formulation of tolterodine provides superior efficacy and is well tolerated in women with overactive bladder. International Urogynecology Journal and Pelvic Floor Dysfunction 14: 50–54.

Swithinbank L, Hashim H, Abrams P 2005 The effect of fluid intake on urinary symptoms in women. Journal of Urology 174: 187–189.

Torrens MJ, Griffiths HB 1974 The control of the uninhibited bladder by selective sacral neurectomy. British Journal of Urology 46: 639–644.

Turner-Warwick RT 1975 Some clinical aspects of detrusor dysfunction. Journal of Urology 113: 539–544.

Vandoninck V, van Balken MR, Finazzi Agro E et al 2003 Posterior tibial nerve stimulation in the treatment of urge incontinence. Neurourology and Urodynamics 22: 17–23.

van Ermenegen E 1897 Uber einen neuen anaeroben Bacillus und seine Beziehungen zum Botulismus. Zeitschrift fuer Hygiene und Infektionskrankheiten 26: 1–56.

van Kerrebroeck P, Kreder K, Jonas U, Zinner N, Wein A; Tolterodine Study Group 2001 Tolterodine once-daily: superior efficacy and tolerability in the treatment of overactive bladder. Urology 57: 414–421.

van Waalwijk van Doorn ESC, Remmers A, Janknegt RA 1992 Conventional and extramural ambulatory urodynamic testing of the lower urinary tract in female volunteers. Journal of Urology 47: 1319–1326.

van Waalwijk van Doorn ESC, Anders K, Khullar V et al 2000 Standardisation of ambulatory urodynamic monitoring: report of the Standardisation Sub-committee of the ICS for Ambulatory Urodynamic Studies. Neurourology and Urodynamics 19: 113–125.

Waldeck K, Larsson B, Andersson KE 1997 Comparison of oxybutynin and its active metabolite, N-desmethyl-oxybutynin, in the human detrusor and parotid gland. Journal of Urology 157: 1093–1097.

Walters MD, Taylor S, Schoenfeld LS 1990 Psychosexual study of women with overactive bladder. Obstetrics and Gynecology 75: 22–26.

Warrell DW 1977 Vaginal denervation of the bladder nerve supply. Urology International 32: 114–116.

Weatherall M 2004 The risk of hyponatraemia in older adults using desmopressin for nocturia: a systematic review and meta-analysis. Neurourology and Urodynamics 23: 302–305.

Weese DL, Roskamp DA, Leach GE, Zimmern PE 1993 Intravesical oxybutynin chloride: experience with 42 patients. Urology 41: 527–530.

Whiteside CG, Arnold GP 1975 Persistent primary enuresis: a urodynamic assessment. BMJ (Clinical Research Ed.) 1: 364–369.

Wise BG, Cardozo LD, Cutner A, Benness CJ, Burton G 1993a The prevalence and significance of urethral instability in women with overactive bladder. British Journal of Urology 72: 26–29.

Wise BG, Benness CJ, Cardozo LD, Cutner A 1993b Vaginal oestradiol for lower urinary tract symptoms in post-menopausal women. A double blind placebo-controlled study. In: Proceedings of the 7th International Congress on the Menopause, Stockholm, 1993, p 15.

Yamaguchi O, Shisida K, Tamura K et al 1996 Evaluation of mRNAs encoding muscarinic receptor subtypes in human detrusor muscle. Journal of Urology 156: 1208.

Zoubek J, Bloom D, Sedman AB 1990 Extraordinary urinary frequency. Pediatrics 85: 1112–1114.

CHAPTER **54**

Voiding difficulty

L. Bombieri and Robert Freeman

Chapter Contents

INTRODUCTION	836	INVESTIGATIONS	841
DEFINITIONS	836	MANAGEMENT	843
INCIDENCE	837	PREVENTION	845
SYMPTOMS AND CLINICAL EFFECTS	837	KEY POINTS	846
CAUSES	838		

Introduction

Normal voiding occurs when tension receptors in the bladder sense fullness and stimulate a sacral reflex of somatically mediated relaxation of the pelvic floor and urethra, and parasympathetically mediated detrusor contraction. In the adult, this simple reflex is under voluntary control via a set of complex pathways which run from the cerebral cortex to the pontine micturition centre and the sacral spinal cord via the lateral spinothalamic tracts and the posterior columns. The sacral micturition centre is located at S2–4 level. Peripheral innervation to the bladder and urethral sphincter is supplied by the pelvic, hypogastric and pudendal nerves.

Imaging studies on normal women have shown that the bladder base and the upper urethra move downwards, the lower urethra remains fixed, the bladder as a whole becomes more ovoid in shape, the posterior urethrovesical angle becomes obliterated, funnelling occurs at the bladder neck, and the whole urethra dilates as the fluid passes.

Studies on detrusor pressure during voiding in normal women suggest that most void with a detrusor contraction greater than 15 cmH$_2$O (mean detrusor pressure at maximum flow 23–28 cmH$_2$O, maximum detrusor pressure 20–36 cmH$_2$O) (Figure 54.1). Detrusor pressure during voiding is generally lower in women than in men. A few normal women have been reported to void with a low pressure detrusor contraction of less than 15 cmH$_2$O, but no normal women void with no contraction at all; such an event may indicate low urethral closure pressure.

There are variations in the way that women void. Some women, in addition to pelvic relaxation and detrusor contraction, may strain by an unconscious but sustained Valsalva manoeuvre (Figure 54.2). The contribution of abdominal pressure to the voiding process varies considerably between individuals and within the same individual during consecutive voids.

The 'normal' voiding curve in women has a single peak, with a fast crescendo and a relatively slow diminuendo, with minimal fluctuations. However, an interrupted pattern can be seen repeatedly in a minority of normal women. Studies of flow rates suggest that most normal women void with a peak flow rate greater than 15 ml/s, with mean values of 23–27 ml/s (Figure 54.1). Peak flow rate values are generally higher in women than in men. The main variable affecting flow rates in normal women is bladder volume, with greater flow rates seen with increasing volumes. Parity, weight and height have no influence on flow rates.

In this chapter, deviations from this pattern of normality will be presented and discussed, particularly with reference to clinical situations relevant to urogynaecological practice.

Definitions

Voiding difficulty

A joint International Urogynecological Association/International Continence Society (ICS) Report on terminology for female pelvic floor dysfunction defines 'voiding difficulty' as 'abnormally slow and/or incomplete micturition' (Haylen et al 2010). The diagnosis is obtained by symptoms (see below) and urodynamic investigations, and should be based on repeated measurements to confirm abnormality.

Abnormally slow urine flow rates, as determined by uroflowmetry, are best referenced to nomogram charts which provide a range of normality for urinary flow rates in relation

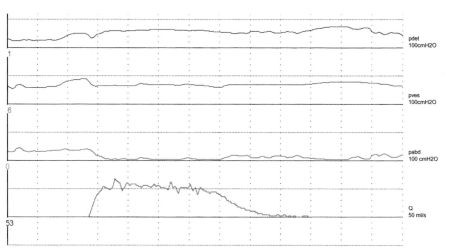

Figure 54.1 Normal voiding.

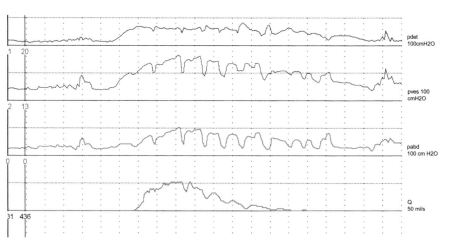

Figure 54.2 Voiding with detrusor contraction supplemented with abdominal straining.

to volume voided; abnormal flow is defined as flow under the 10th centile (Haylen et al 1989). To encourage the use of these charts, a larger version of the original charts has been republished recently (Haylen et al 2008a).

Abnormally high postvoid residuals (i.e. volume left in the bladder at the completion of micturition) depend on the method used for measurement and the timing of the measurement after micturition, taking into account renal input of 1–14 ml urine/min (Haylen et al 2010).

Upper limits of postvoid residuals of 30 ml (using immediate ultrasound assessment) and 50–100 ml (using urethral catheterization) have been proposed (Haylen et al 2010).

Acute retention of urine

This is defined as a generally, but not always, painful, palpable or percussable bladder, when the patient is unable to pass any urine when the bladder is full (Haylen et al 2010).

Chronic retention of urine

This is defined as a non-painful bladder where there is a chronic high postvoid residual (Haylen et al 2010).

Incidence

Depending on definition and type of clinic, voiding difficulty in women presenting to a urology or urogynaecology clinic has a variable prevalence ranging from 14% (when using a strict definition based on multiple variables including low flow, high pressure and increased postvoid residual) (Massey and Abrams 1988) to 39% (using a postvoid residual of 30 ml or more) (Haylen et al 2007).

Symptoms and Clinical Effects

When present, symptoms of voiding difficulty are non-specific and include hesitancy, slow stream, straining to void, feeling of incomplete bladder emptying, spraying, need to immediately revoid, position-dependent micturition (e.g. leaning forwards or backwards, semi-erect), and dysuria.

Women with voiding dysfunction may present with urinary incontinence; this is often unconscious leakage due to 'overflow incontinence', although this term lacks a precise definition. Recurrent urinary tract infections (UTI) and 'irritative' bladder symptoms such as frequency and urgency, with and without coexistent detrusor overactivity, may be reported.

Inability to void usually leads to prolonged use of urinary catheters and an increased incidence of UTI. The risk of acquiring bacteriuria relates to the duration of catheterization, and ranges from 4% to 7.5%/day over the first 10 days of catheterization (Schaeffer 1986). The majority of patients on long-term clean catheterization have bacteriuria, and about one-third of them require intermittent treatment with antibiotics due to symptomatic infection (Lapides et al 1976). Catheter-related UTI is an important cause of hospital-acquired infections, morbidity (e.g. pyelonephritis) and, in the elderly, mortality.

When voiding difficulty develops after surgery, hospital stay is often prolonged. When patients are discharged with a catheter, daily nursing care in the community is required. This can lead to an escalation in costs.

In the long term, inability to void may lead to profound alterations in quality of life and have serious psychological effects.

Causes

The causes of voiding difficulty are shown in Box 54.1.

Effects of age on voiding function

The incidence of voiding dysfunction in women increases with age (Haylen et al 2008b), and the process of ageing may decrease detrusor contractility and increase urethral rigidity.

Urodynamic studies have shown that both peak flow rate and detrusor pressure during voiding decrease with advancing age. Older women are also more likely to strain abdominally during voiding and to have higher residual urine volumes (Malone-Lee and Wahedna 1993).

With advancing age, anatomical changes occur in the bladder wall leading to reduced bladder contractility (e.g. increased collagen content in the detrusor muscle, reduction in the number of cholinergic nerves, dedifferentiation of detrusor muscle cells). Changes leading to urethral atrophy and increased rigidity also occur (e.g. reduced striated muscle and vessel content, increased connective tissue).

Box 54.1 Causes of voiding difficulty

- Age
- Postoperative: pelvic surgery, incontinence surgery, prolapse surgery
- Post partum
- Neurological disease
- Psychogenic
- Pelvic organ
- Prolapse
- Idiopathic bladder neck obstruction
- Bladder overdistension/infrequent voiding
- Drugs
- Infection
- Pelvic mass
- Urethral or bladder pathology
- Detrusor myopathy/acontractility
- Iatrogenic

While it is not clear whether voiding dysfunction is due to 'normal' ageing of the lower urinary tract or to the presence of disease processes, age is the only risk factor that has been consistently associated with the development of postoperative voiding dysfunction after anti-incontinence surgery. Increased urethral rigidity may increase the likelihood of causing obstruction, and reduced detrusor contractility may reduce the ability to cope with it.

It is not clear whether the menopause has an effect on voiding which is distinct from age. There are no studies showing that the menopause *per se* has a deleterious effect on voiding function. However, the distal urethra is oestrogen dependent and therefore susceptible to postmenopausal atrophic changes; the reduction in urethral functional length seen after the menopause is likely to be a manifestation of this process. There is evidence that these changes are more pronounced in a minority (18%) of postmenopausal women (Smith 1972). These women may have increased urethral rigidity and may be predisposed to the development of voiding dysfunction should they undergo pelvic or anti-incontinence surgery.

Postoperative voiding dysfunction

Pelvic surgery

Temporary voiding difficulty is commonly observed after pelvic surgery. In the immediate postoperative period, many reversible factors are likely to play a role. Atropine and other anaesthetic reversal agents with anticholinergic effects (some with a half-life of 3–4 days) may reduce detrusor contractility. Opiates might reduce bladder sensation, pain might inhibit perineal relaxation, and bladder overfilling might depress detrusor contractility. In addition, bruising and oedema can also depress bladder contractility and cause temporary obstruction. Spinal anaesthesia depresses voiding function for up to 4–8 h, depending on whether short- or long-acting agents are used. Epidural anaesthesia may depress voiding function for 14–16 h, especially when supplemented by opioids in the epidural space.

With regards to specific procedures, clinical and urodynamic studies have found no evidence of increased voiding dysfunction in the short term after vaginal hysterectomy with anterior colporrhaphy performed at the same time (Stanton et al 1982), and after abdominal hysterectomy (Wake 1980). Also, no differences in bladder function were observed in a randomized study comparing total with subtotal hysterectomy (Thakar et al 2002). However, a history of previous hysterectomy has been associated with increased risk of voiding difficulty, possibly due to nerve dysfunction (Dietz et al 2002).

Extensive pelvic surgery might lead to denervation and prolonged or permanent voiding difficulty. Radical hysterectomy has been shown to lead to prolonged voiding difficulty in one-quarter of patients (Scotti et al 1986) due to neuropathic dysfunction.

Surgery for stress incontinence

Surgery for stress incontinence is an important cause of impaired bladder emptying in women. There is no universally accepted definition of voiding dysfunction after

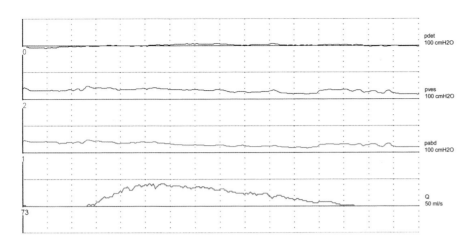

Figure 54.3 Voiding without detrusor contraction (pelvic relaxation alone).

incontinence surgery, and voiding function is often reported empirically in studies (e.g. as 'time required for resumption of voiding' or 'time of catheter removal'). In most cases, postoperative voiding problems are short term, but they can persist in the long term and lead to profound alterations in quality of life. Prolonged or 'late' voiding dysfunction after incontinence surgery may also affect patients who did not have 'early' dysfunction in the immediate postoperative period. This may be due to failure to obtain an early diagnosis, progressive effects of scarring or onset of new pathology.

Women with stress incontinence may already have some impairment of voiding function, which may make them more vulnerable to the obstructive effects of surgery. This is suggested by differences in several urodynamic (voiding) variables noted in these women. For example, in contrast with normal women, women with stress incontinence are more likely to strain during voiding, and to initiate voiding with a Valsalva manoeuvre as opposed to pelvic relaxation. They also void with significantly lower detrusor pressures, and up to 15% have been shown to void without a contraction (Figure 54.3; Karram et al 1997). It is not clear whether this is due to the lower mean urethral pressure of women with urodynamic stress incontinence, or whether there is a real impairment of detrusor muscle function in these women.

Postoperative voiding disorders have been reported to occur after most operations for stress incontinence. Prolonged voiding dysfunction is uncommon after urethral injectables, although an incidence of 5% has been reported (Khullar et al 1997). The colposuspension operation leads to postoperative voiding dysfunction in a mean of 12.5% of patients (Jarvis 1994). Laparoscopic and open colposuspension have the same incidence of postoperative voiding difficulty (Carey et al 2006). Results of a randomized study comparing the tension-free vaginal tape (TVT) procedure with colposuspension suggest that the incidence of voiding difficulty at 6 months is similar after both operations (7%), although patients experience earlier voiding in the immediate postoperative period after the TVT procedure (Ward and Hilton 2002). After the TVT procedure, 11% of women have been reported to need a catheter for more than 24 h (Vervest et al 2007), with only 2% needing

tape release for prolonged difficulty (Kuuva and Nilsson 2002, Karram et al 2003, Vervest et al 2007). The transobturator tape (TOT) procedure has been shown to have a lower incidence of postoperative voiding difficulty than the TVT, possibly as it is less obstructive (Latthe et al 2007).

Voiding difficulty after incontinence surgery is multifactorial. In addition to temporary factors, as detailed above, permanent factors might be relevant from the outset. Some factors are obstructive and relate to the operative technique (e.g. excessive tape tension when using midurethral slings, or excessive bladder neck elevation at colposuspension), while others relate to the patient and her capacity to deal with obstruction (e.g. age and poor detrusor contractility). An intrinsically weak detrusor may be unable to cope with even the slightest increase in outflow resistance.

Prolapse surgery

Short-term voiding difficulty is common after vaginal surgery for prolapse. In a large series of women undergoing such surgery, urinary retention (defined as a postvoid residual of ≥200 ml after removal of the catheter the day after the operation) occurred in 29% of women, with 9% experiencing retention for more than 3 days (Hakvoort et al 2009). In another study, 11% of women required catheterization at home after discharge from hospital (Vierhout 1998). However, no patients experienced long-term voiding difficulty (Vierhout 1998, Hakvoort et al 2009). Performing a levator muscle plication (as part of a posterior colporrhaphy) and a Kelly suburethral plication (as part of an anterior colporrhaphy) can increase the risk of postoperative retention (Hakvoort et al 2009).

A policy of early catheter removal, the day after vaginal surgery seems preferable to routine prolonged catheterization (4 days) as it is associated with a lower incidence of UTI and a shorter duration of hospital stay (Hakvoort et al 2004). However, early catheter removal increases the risk of recatheterization: 40% in the 'early' removal group vs 9% in the 'late' removal group (Hakvoort et al 2004). Prolonged catheterization may therefore be preferable in individual cases when there is an increased risk of postoperative voiding difficulty.

Postpartum voiding difficulty

Prolonged voiding difficulty in the postpartum period requiring self-catheterization is uncommon and has been reported to occur after less than 1% of deliveries (Glavind and Bjørk 2003). However, when using strict criteria [similar to those proposed recently by the International Urogynecological Association/International Continence Society (2010)], up to 43% of women have been shown to have some degree of voiding difficulty after delivery (Ramsay and Torbet 1993). Recognized risk factors for voiding difficulty in the immediate postpartum period are primiparity, instrumental delivery, epidural analgesia, prolonged labour, perineal trauma and poor bladder management resulting in overdistension. In addition to temporary factors (e.g. epidural, morphine, anaesthetic), other factors causing prolonged voiding dysfunction may be present (e.g. trauma to the bladder, pelvic floor muscles and nerves).

Neurological disease

The effects of neurological disease on bladder function and the upper renal tracts depend on the site of the lesion(s). Interruption of the mainly inhibitory pathways from the cerebral cortex to the pontine micturition centre (e.g. stroke, tumour, trauma, Parkinson's disease) is likely to result in uninhibited detrusor contraction and incontinence. Interruption of the neural pathways from the pontine to the sacral centres [e.g. spinal cord injury, multiple sclerosis (MS)] may also lead to uninhibited contractions (neurogenic detrusor overactivity) with or without failure of relaxation of the urethral sphincter (detrusor sphincter dyssynergia). Interruption of the sacral reflex arc (e.g. diabetic neuropathy, low spinal cord tumours, lumbar disc prolapse) may lead to acontractility of the detrusor muscle (atonic bladder), with voiding difficulty and retention.

Impaired voiding function (e.g. detrusor sphincter dyssynergia) can potentially lead to high detrusor pressure, reflux and upper tract changes (e.g. hydronephrosis), resulting in renal failure.

Specific neurological conditions are discussed below.

Lumbar intervertebral disc prolapse

Lumbar disc prolapse is extremely common, with approximately 30% of adults without back pain having evidence of a protruded disc on magnetic resonance imaging (MRI) (Jarvik and Deyo 2007). In patients with symptomatic lumbar disc prolapse, urodynamic studies have shown voiding difficulty due to reduced detrusor contractility in approximately one-quarter of cases (Bartolin et al 1998). The most common sites of lumbar disc prolapse are L4–5 and L5–S1. Compression occurs more often in a posterolateral direction but may also be central. Patients may report a long history of low back pain, or voiding difficulty may be the first or only symptom. Compression of the sacral nerves can lead to cauda equina syndrome, characterized by voiding difficulty, saddle anaesthesia, bilateral sciatica and low back pain. Physical examination in these cases shows reduced sensation in the saddle and perianal area. If nerve compression is seen on MRI, urgent surgical treatment, usually laminectomy, is indicated. Despite this, voiding

function often fails to improve after surgery (Bartolin et al 1999).

The lithotomy position commonly used to perform gynaecological procedures can potentially precipitate lumbar disc prolapse (Choudhari et al 2000). It has been suggested that flexion and hyperabduction of the hips may stretch nerve roots already compromised by a partial 'occult' disc prolapse (Choudhari et al 2000). When no other explanation can be found, this possibility should always be considered and investigated by MRI should a patient develop prolonged voiding difficulty after a gynaecological procedure.

Parkinson's disease

Parkinson's disease typically affects the basal ganglia where loss of the substantia nigra results in dopamine deficiency. This has a profound effect on the extrapyramidal system. However, other 'Parkinsonian' syndromes (e.g. multiple system atrophy) are associated with lesions in other areas of the central and peripheral nervous systems. The majority of women with these conditions have urinary symptoms. These may be due to detrusor overactivity (more common in Parkinson's disease) or detrusor underactivity (more common in multiple system atrophy). Coexistent urethral sphincter dysfunction is common, with poor sphincter coordination with voiding (more frequent in Parkinson's disease) and intrinsic sphincter deficiency (more frequent in multiple system atrophy).

Multiple sclerosis

MS plaques are common along the spinal cord in a variety of locations. Lower urinary tract dysfunction is therefore present in the majority of women affected by MS. Reported symptoms include frequency, urgency, urge incontinence and voiding difficulty. In a small minority of women, bladder symptoms are the presenting manifestation of the disease.

Functional effects are various and may change during the course of the disease. They include neurogenic detrusor overactivity (with or without detrusor sphincter dyssynergia) and, less frequently, detrusor acontractility.

In the past, the death of MS patients could often be attributed to urological complications (e.g. upper tract changes and infection). Prompt recognition and management of voiding dysfunction in these patients has made this a rare occurrence.

Diabetes

Bladder dysfunction is relatively common in diabetic women and has been reported in 22% of women attending a diabetic clinic (Yu et al 2004). It is due to peripheral and autonomic neuropathy, leading to reduced bladder sensation and contractility. The classical features of diabetic cystopathy are an insidious onset with impaired bladder sensation and progressive voiding difficulty. Recurrent UTIs are common. Detrusor overactivity also occurs frequently, perhaps as a sign of cortical or spinal involvement.

Psychological factors

Psychological factors may cause or contribute to voiding dysfunction by centrally mediated, unconscious inhibition of either detrusor contraction, pelvic floor relaxation or both. This is confirmed by the inability of many individuals to void when there is a lack of privacy (so-called 'paruresis' or 'shy bladder syndrome').

True psychogenic urinary dysfunction is uncommon but is usually accompanied by obvious psychological or psychiatric features, such as conversion disorder (hysteria) and anxiety. There is often a precipitating stressful 'trigger' event. A history of sexual abuse may be present.

Idiopathic bladder neck obstruction

This is a poorly defined, infrequent condition characterized by failure of the urethral sphincter to relax, and possibly hypertrophy, with urodynamic variables showing high pressure and low flow in the absence of neurological or urological abnormality. It was originally described in a cohort of young women with polycystic ovaries and voiding difficulty (Fowler's syndrome; Fowler et al 1988). The cause is unknown. There is a suggestion that α-blockers may be beneficial in these patients (Athanasopoulos et al 2009).

Pelvic organ prolapse

Although the majority of women with pelvic organ prolapse (POP) can void effectively, there is an association between POP and voiding dysfunction (Coates et al 1997, Haylen et al 2008b). Symptoms of voiding difficulty (Digesu et al 2005) and high postvoid residuals (Haylen et al 2008b) are more common in women with POP. Urodynamic evidence of voiding difficulty has been found to correlate with POP severity, with high-grade cystocoele being the most common anatomical defect leading to voiding difficulty (Romanzi et al 1999). Severe prolapse of the posterior vaginal compartment has also been shown to have a negative effect on voiding function (Myers et al 1998, Dietz et al 2002). Kinking of the urethra (by a prolapse of the anterior vaginal compartment) or direct pressure on the urethra and bladder neck (by a prolapsing uterus or posterior vaginal compartment) are possible mechanisms of obstruction, leading to voiding difficulty.

Overactive bladder symptoms and occult stress incontinence often coexist with voiding difficulty in women with pelvic organ prolapse (Romanzi et al 1999).

Prolapse correction with a pessary has been shown to improve voiding function in the majority of women with both pathologies (Romanzi et al 1999). In most women with severe prolapse and voiding difficulty, corrective surgery restores voiding successfully (Fitzgerald et al 2000, Liang et al 2008).

Bladder overdistension

Bladder overdistension can be iatrogenic (i.e. the result of a delay in the diagnosis of voiding difficulty, with delayed catheterization), and this event *per se* can also lead to further and sometimes prolonged voiding difficulty. Studies of bladder function after overdistension, mostly in animal models and in men with retention associated with prostatic hypertrophy, have shown reduced bladder contractility. This is probably due to denervation, stretch damage to the detrusor muscle, and metabolic injury due to ischaemia and reperfusion. The time of recovery after such injury has not been investigated in women, but is likely to depend on the cause of the bladder overdistension, the amount of fluid retained and the time of retention.

Infrequent voiding can lead to chronic bladder overdistension and voiding difficulty, but evidence for this is lacking.

Others

In addition to anaesthetics and analgesics, drugs with anticholinergic action (e.g. antidepressants, antipsychotics, oxybutinin etc.) can potentially worsen voiding function and precipitate retention in individual cases. However, antimuscarinic therapy was not found to worsen voiding function in a series of women with overactive bladder and mild voiding difficulty (postvoid residuals of ≥100 ml) (Robinson et al 2003).

Intravesical Botox for treatment of the overactive bladder has been shown to increase postvoid residuals, but retention requiring self-catheterization is uncommon (Duthie et al 2007), with one large series reporting an incidence of 4% (Schmid et al 2006).

Pelvic masses (e.g. fibroids, retroverted gravid uterus, ovarian cysts, faecal impaction, haematocolpos) can cause voiding difficulty due to a direct pressure effect.

Infections (e.g. urethritis, cystitis, vulvovaginitis) can cause acute retention due to inflammation and pain, with genital herpes and sacral herpes zoster possibly also due to nerve impairment.

Urethral pathology, other than the effects of incontinence surgery (e.g. tumours, strictures, diverticulae, foreign bodies and stones), may rarely cause voiding difficulty.

Lichen's sclerosus can cause complete fusion of the labia and closure over the urethral meatus, resulting in voiding difficulty.

Investigations

Uroflowmetry

In practical terms, most women with voiding difficulty require simple flow studies with measurement of post void residual urine with catheters or ultrasound. Features include changes in the normal bell-shaped curve, with intermittent or multiple peaked flow (suggestive of abdominal straining or unsustained bladder contractions) (Figure 54.4), and/or low flow rates. Although there are no clear-cut values, low peak flow rates of less than 12–20 ml/s have been used traditionally, with voided volumes of 150–200 ml. Postvoid residual urine volumes of more than 50–100 ml were arbitrarily considered abnormal.

It is now suggested that volume-specific nomograms should be used, with abnormal flow defined as under the 10th centile (International Urogynecological Association/International Continence Society 2010). Repeated measurements are necessary to confirm abnormality.

Upper limits of postvoid residuals of 30 ml using immediate ultrasound assessment and 50–100 ml using urethral catheterization have been proposed, taking into account renal input of 1–14 ml urine/min (International Urogynecological Association/International Continence Society 2009).

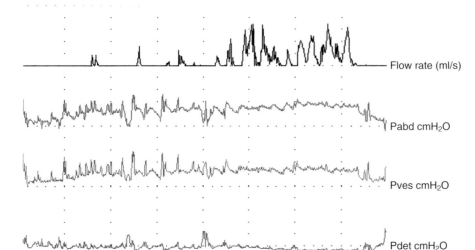

Flow rate (ml/s)

Pabd cmH$_2$O

Pves cmH$_2$O

Pdet cmH$_2$O

An alternative screening method, using a peak flow rate of less than 15 ml/s and/or postvoid residual urine volume greater than 50 ml with a minimum total bladder volume of 150 ml before voiding, has been shown to correlate well with the Liverpool nomograms (Haylen et al 1989), and could be used if nomogram charts are not available (Costantini et al 2003).

Uroflowmetry, however, is only a screening test. More complex urodynamic studies are advisable in the presence of coexistent overactive bladder symptoms, neurological disease or when the cause of voiding difficulty is unclear.

Pressure–flow studies

The assessment of voiding difficulty in the female, as in the male, relies on pressure–flow studies. In men, low flow in the presence of high detrusor pressure usually signifies obstruction (using nomograms), but this is less clear in women.

In an attempt to obtain cut-off values for the definition of obstruction in women, urodynamic studies have been performed in obstructed patients and compared with controls. For example, in repeated non-invasive flow studies, the presence of a peak flow rate of less than 12 ml/s, with a detrusor pressure at maximum flow of more than 20 cmH$_2$O (Figure 54.5), has been considered to be suggestive of obstruction and used to construct female nomograms (Blaivas and Groutz 2000). The practical value of these observations remains unclear, as the clinical and radiological criteria used to define obstruction are arbitrary. Symptoms are often non-specific, and anatomical evidence of obstruction is often missing using videourodynamics or cystourethroscopy (Groutz et al 2000).

In contrast, other authors do not rely heavily on strict urodynamic criteria for the diagnosis of obstruction, and suggest that relative obstruction can exist in the presence of normal or low detrusor pressures (Foster and McGuire 1993, Carr and Webster 1997). Obstruction after incontinence surgery is therefore diagnosed purely on the basis of a clear-cut temporal relationship between surgery and the onset of persistent voiding difficulty. Successful urethrolysis has even been performed on women who had acontractile bladders after stress incontinence surgery (Figure 54.6; Foster and McGuire 1993, Carr and Webster 1997), thus challenging the concept that obstruction only exists in the presence of high pressures.

Videourodynamics

More detailed studies on patients with prolonged postoperative voiding difficulty can be performed using videourodynamics. However, anatomical abnormalities (e.g. a narrowed or deviated urethra) leading to obstruction are only detected in a minority of patients (Groutz et al 2000).

Cystourethroscopy

This has been reported to reveal urethral strictures or fibrosis in approximately half of women who had suspected obstruction during pressure–flow studies (Groutz et al 2000).

Electromyography

Surface or needle electrodes can be used to evaluate distal urethral sphincter function. Failure of the sphincter to relax can be documented in cases of Fowler's syndrome (Fowler et al 1988). When used with urodynamics, simultaneous detrusor contraction and failure of relaxation of the sphincter can be observed in neuropathic patients (detrusor sphincter dyssynergia).

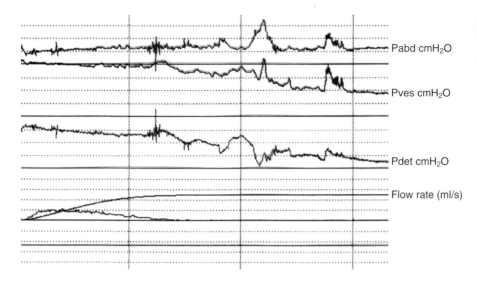

Figure 54.5 Voiding difficulty with obstruction due to urethral diverticulum (peak flow rate 10 ml/s, maximum detrusor pressure 80 cmH$_2$O, postvoid residual 600 ml).

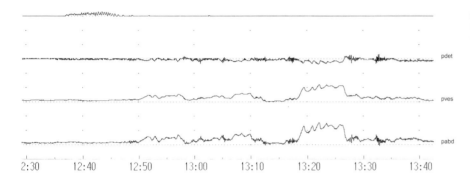

Figure 54.6 Voiding difficulty with acontractile bladder after colposuspension (volume voided 7 ml, postvoid residual 350 ml).

Management

Short-term management

Voiding difficulty is usually managed with indwelling urethral catheters (e.g. Foley catheters). These are generally well tolerated but have been reported to be unpleasant by more than one-third of patients (Vierhout 1998). Catheters come in a variety of sizes and are made with a variety of materials (e.g. latex, silicone, polyvinyl chloride). Specialized catheters, impregnated with silver or antibiotics, have been developed to reduce the risk of infection, with evidence that they reduce the risk of bacteriuria by one-third to one-half in the short term (Schumm and Lam 2008). There is weak evidence that antibiotic prophylaxis reduces the rate of symptomatic UTI in patients using a urethral catheter in the short term (Niel-Weise and van den Broek 2005).

Suprapubic catheters may be preferred when surgery has greater potential for obstruction (e.g. colposuspension) or when patients undergoing surgery are already known to have voiding difficulty. They are more practical and allow patients to attempt voiding without needing recatheterization. The residual urine volume can be measured easily. Compared with urethral catheters, they have a lower incidence of sig-nificant bacteriuria, voiding occurs earlier and patient acceptability is higher.

Early clean intermittent self-catheterization (CISC) has advantages compared with suprapubic bladder drainage in terms of hospital stay and sepsis. When considering potentially obstructive stress incontinence surgery, particularly in patients at high risk of voiding difficulty (see below), CISC should be discussed and taught beforehand as it is easier for patients to learn before rather than after surgery.

Long-term management

Indwelling urethral catheters are often used for chronic voiding difficulty, particularly in long-term care settings. While a variety of different catheters exist, insufficient evidence exists to recommend one over another (Jahn et al 2007).

Suprapubic catheterization is a better option than urethral catheterization. Epithelium will form in the tract in 6–8 weeks. A size 14F catheter should be used to keep the tract open and changed every 8–12 weeks. Vitamin C can acidify urine and prevent crust formation. There is usually no need for prophylactic antibiotics.

Indwelling catheters (urethral or suprapubic) are not ideal in the long term as they are conspicuous and demoralizing.

Urethral catheters interfere with coitus and ambulation, and can be associated with incontinence due to bypass. They are associated with recurrent UTI, stones, strictures and urethral erosion, and need to be changed frequently or irrigated due to blockage.

Rather than indwelling catheters, the preferred treatment for chronic voiding difficulty is CISC. This is based on the principle that retention rather than catheterization is the cause of infection. The advantages over an indwelling catheter are lower incidence of UTI and improved mental status.

The frequency of catheterization depends on severity of the voiding difficulty and residual urine volume. Old age and disability are not necessarily an impediment, but motivation and manual dexterity are essential. Most patients performing CISC have bacteriuria not requiring antibiotics, and treatment is only required in those with symptoms. More frequent catheterization and an increased fluid intake may be helpful if symptomatic infections occur. At present, there is no evidence that the incidence of UTI in patients performing CISC is affected by variables such as the type of catheter (coated or uncoated) or the technique used (single/sterile or multiple use/clean) (Moore et al 2007).

CISC has been shown to be effective in the long term. Two-thirds of patients available for follow-up 10 years after commencing treatment were satisfied and still performing the procedure, with no evidence of renal impairment (Diokno et al 1983). Although long-term follow-up studies may suffer from selection bias — most available responders are treatment 'successes' — up to 80% of patients find CISC easy, with only a minority reporting severe pain (Kessler et al 2009).

General measures may also be helpful in individual patients. These include standing or leaning forwards during voiding, abdominal straining, double voiding, voiding at regular intervals and treating constipation.

Women who experience voiding difficulty after surgery or post partum should be reassured that voiding function often improves with time. A positive view of CISC should be given, with support from continence advisors.

Role of drug therapy

The effect of drugs for the treatment of voiding difficulty has been disappointing. α-Adrenoreceptor antagonists to relax the urethra (e.g. phenoxybenzamine hydrochloride, alfuzosin), detrusor-stimulating drugs such as cholinergic agents (e.g. bethanechol chloride), anticholinesterase (e.g. distigmine bromide) and prostaglandins have been used with inconsistent results. Due to their inconsistent effect and unproven value, drugs are not currently recommended for the prevention and treatment of voiding difficulty in women.

Oestrogen may be of benefit for women with genital atrophy causing obstruction and voiding difficulty.

Role of surgery

Urethral dilatation and urethrotomy may be effective in patients with voiding difficulty due to urethral narrowing, particularly after anti-incontinence procedures. However, the benefit seems to be short lived as scarring is likely to recur and may even result in worsening obstruction. In addition, stress incontinence has been reported to reappear (Delaere et al 1983). When this method is deemed necessary (e.g. for a traumatic stricture), repeated catheterization (e.g. CISC) is advisable to maintain patency.

Suprapubic and vaginal 'take-down' procedures involving urethrolysis, with or without additional resuspension procedures, have been described after retropubic procedures (e.g. colposuspension) (Foster and McGuire 1993, Carr and Webster 1997). Symptoms of voiding difficulty in these patients are usually combined with urgency symptoms. Despite the lack of uniformity with regards to patient selection, definition of obstruction, surgical treatment and outcome measures, it would appear that urethrolysis is a possible alternative to CISC. It may be suitable for patients who are unwilling or unable to perform the technique. However, the reported success rate is variable and unpredictable, and there is a risk of recurrent stress incontinence.

When voiding difficulty occurs after midurethral sling procedures, release of the tape can be performed. Loosening the tape by applying downward traction is usually possible in the immediate postoperative period (2–3 weeks), producing immediate symptomatic relief in most cases. Later, if scarring does not allow tape descent, transection of the tape (laterally or in the midline) has been described (Rardin et al 2002, Laurikainen and Kiiholma 2006, Segal et al 2006). While voiding function has been reported to improve in most women after late tape revisions, coexistent overactive bladder symptoms often remain unchanged (Segal et al 2006, McCrery 2007). The reported risk of recurrent stress incontinence after tape revision ranges from 5% to 50% (Klutke et al 2001, Rardin et al 2002, Karram et al 2003). Urethral injury may occur due to the formation of dense scarring between tape and urethra (Klutke et al 2001, Laurikainen and Kiiholma 2006).

Role of nerve stimulation

Unobstructive voiding difficulty can respond to techniques of nerve stimulation. The sacral nerves can be stimulated indirectly (posterior tibial nerve stimulation) or directly (sacral nerve stimulation). The precise mode of action is not known, and it is also not clear why the same techniques can help patients with an overactive detrusor muscle as well as an underactive detrusor muscle.

Posterior tibial nerve stimulation involves the placement of needle electrodes above the medial malleolus to stimulate the posterior tibial nerve, which contains mixed fibres from L5–S3. Early reports show objective improvement in voiding function, with approximately 60% of patients willing to continue treatment (Vandoninck et al 2004). However, the technique is time consuming and requires repeat stimulation.

Sacral nerve stimulation is a promising technique that uses an implantable system (Interstim device) to stimulate the pelvic nerves (at S3 level). An initial test procedure is performed to assess response, positioning a temporary electrode with an external stimulator. If appropriate, a permanent lead is then inserted and connected to a pulse generator positioned in the upper buttocks or anterior abdominal wall. In addition to unobstructed voiding difficulty, indications for sacral nerve stimulation include faecal incontinence, bladder overactivity and interstitial cystitis. A recent review reports a response rate for voiding difficulty of 38–68%, with good medium-term results in 58–76% of responders (Bosch 2006). Technical problems and adverse events are unfortunately common (e.g. pain at the stimulator site, new pain, pain at the lead site, lead migration, infection, transient electric shock, changes in bowel function), with a reoperation rate of approximately 50% (Bosch 2006). There are no reports of long-lasting neurological complications.

Other treatments

A suprapubic vibration device (Queen Square bladder stimulator) has been shown to improve voiding in some patients with neurogenic bladders (Dasgupta et al 1997). The device was only effective in patients with a postvoid residual of less than 400 ml, reducing the postvoid residual from a mean of 175 ml to a mean of 68 ml (Dasgupta et al 1997). However, there is no evidence of benefit in other types of voiding difficulty.

Urinary diversion can be considered in selected cases as a last resort (e.g. ileal conduit or Indiana pouch).

Prevention

The early diagnosis of voiding difficulty and avoidance of bladder overdistension is crucial in order to reduce the risk of prolonged bladder dysfunction. As acute retention can be insidious and occur in women who appear to be voiding, close attention to bladder function after surgery or after delivery is important. This relies on good nursing care, ward protocols on bladder function, and easy access to portable bladder ultrasound to check postvoid residuals. Equally, bowel function should be taken into account as constipation can have a negative effect on voiding function.

Regular bladder emptying during labour, the use of catheters in women at risk (e.g. after instrumental deliveries, epidural, perineal trauma, etc.) and careful monitoring of voiding function after delivery or after catheter removal are considered essential preventative measures to avoid overdistension.

Appropriate placement of patients on the operating table may help to prevent postoperative voiding difficulty associated with the exacerbation of lumbar intervertebral disc prolapse.

Although urodynamics are not considered essential prior to stress incontinence surgery in all women (National Institute for Health and Clinical Excellence 2006), pressure–flow studies may help to identify women with existing or borderline voiding difficulty. Preoperative urodynamic variables (e.g. straining during voiding, voiding with low or absent detrusor contraction, low peak flow rate) may be predictive of postoperative voiding difficulty (Figures 54.2, 54.3 and 54.7), although the reported evidence is inconsistent. If urodynamics are not performed routinely, screening of women prior to surgery in order to identify those with voiding difficulty is simple and non-invasive (e.g. using uroflowmetry and/or ultrasound to check postvoid residual urine volumes). Elderly women and patients undergoing multiple procedures at the same time (e.g. midurethral slings combined with POP surgery) may be at increased risk of postoperative voiding difficulty. Patients at risk should be managed by experienced clinicians. Careful counselling is important in all cases. In women with existing voiding difficulty, consideration should be given to teaching CISC.

During surgery for urinary incontinence, excessive elevation should be avoided during colposuspension. For women undergoing midurethral sling procedures, it has been suggested that the cough test, with the observation of a reduction in leakage after tensioning the tape, can reduce the risk of postoperative voiding difficulty (Ulmsten et al 1996). However, the evidence for this is inconclusive, and in practice, the cough test is often poorly reproducible and influenced by the type of anaesthetic used. Consideration should be given to use of the TOT procedure in women at risk, as this is shown to be less likely to cause voiding difficulty (Latthe et al 2007).

A potentially difficult group of patients are those with intrinsic sphincter deficiency, as shown by reduced urethral closure pressures using urethral pressure profilometry. The TOT procedure has been shown to have a lower success rate than the TVT procedure in these patients (Schierlitz et al 2008). This is because the TOT procedure is less obstructive, and successful treatment of stress incontinence in such

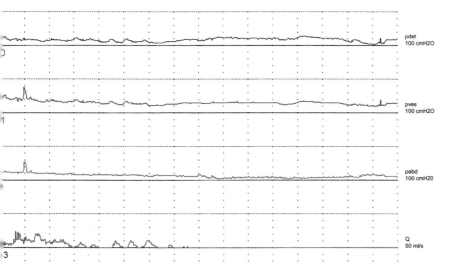

Figure 54.7 Voiding with low peak flow rate and low detrusor pressure (12 ml/s at 9 cmH$_2$O for 414 ml volume and no residual).

patients often entails urethral support with an additional element of obstruction and the placement of a tighter tape; minimal degrees of tension can be crucial to achieve success without causing voiding difficulty. These women should be managed by experienced surgeons. A cough test in these circumstances may be useful as a measure of tension. The use of adjustable tapes has been proposed in patients with intrinsic sphincter deficiency, as well as in those at risk of voiding difficulty, as the tension can be modified in the postoperative period (Araco et al 2008, Romero Maroto et al 2008).

When voiding difficulty arises after midurethral sling procedures, early revision (within 2–3 weeks) is likely to be appreciated by patients, and loosening of the tape is usually possible. Urethral injury is unlikely to occur at this stage as there is minimal scarring.

Box 54.2 shows the key points for prevention.

Box 54.2 Prevention: key points

- Key times for prevention: labour, post partum and after surgery
- Avoidance of bladder overdistension: prophylactic use of catheters, surveillance and early diagnosis of voiding difficulty
- Screening and identification of patients at risk prior to surgery using flow studies and postvoid scan
- Pressure–flow studies in selected cases, if not routinely available
- Avoidance of bladder neck overelevation at colposuspension
- TVT procedure when using midurethral slings
- TOT procedure in women at risk but with no evidence of urethral sphincter deficiency
- Possibly cough test or adjustable tapes in women with urethral sphincter deficiency
- If voiding difficulty occurs, early tape revision is easier and less traumatic than later intervention

---

KEY POINTS

1. Normal voiding in the female occurs by detrusor contraction and pelvic floor relaxation, with or without abdominal straining. A minority of women with stress incontinence void without a detrusor contraction, possibly due to low urethral resistance.
2. When strict diagnostic criteria are applied (postvoid residual urine volume >30 ml), up to 39% of women attending a urogynaecology clinic have been found to have voiding difficulty.
3. Symptoms of voiding difficulty are non-specific.
4. Screening and diagnosis of voiding difficulty are based on uroflowmetry and measurement of the postvoid residual urine volume. Repeat measures are required to make a diagnosis. Urodynamics are useful in individual cases, although obstruction in women may not always lead to a detrusor pressure rise.
5. Attention to bladder care at key times (labour, post partum, after surgery) is essential to avoid bladder overdistension and prolonged voiding difficulty.
6. Surgery for POP and stress incontinence are common causes of voiding difficulty. Counselling before surgery is essential. Management after surgery mainly relies on the use of catheters. When obstruction is suspected, early relief (e.g. loosening of a midurethral tape) usually leads to resolution.

References

Araco F, Gravante G, Dati S, Bulzomi V, Sesti F, Piccione E 2008 Results 1 year after the Reemex system was applied for the treatment of stress urinary incontinence cause by intrinsic sphincter deficiency. International Urogynecology Journal and Pelvic Floor Dysfunction 19: 783–786.

Athanasopoulos A, Gyftopoulos K, Giannitsas K, Perimenis P 2009 Effect of alfuzosin on female primary bladder neck obstruction. International Urogynecology Journal and Pelvic Floor Dysfunction 20: 217–222.

Bartolin Z, Gilja I, Bedalov G, Savic I 1998 Bladder function in patients with lumbar intervertebral disk protrusion. Journal of Urology 159: 969–971.

Bartolin Z, Vilendecic M, Derezic D 1999 Bladder function after surgery for lumbar intervertebral disk protrusion. Journal of Urology 161: 1885–1887.

Blaivas JG, Groutz A 2000 Bladder outlet obstruction nomogram for women with lower urinary tract symptomatology. Neurourology and Urodynamics 19: 553–564.

Bosch JL 2006 Electrical neuromodulatory therapy in female voiding dysfunction. BJU International 98 (Suppl 1): 43–48.

Carey MP, Goh JT, Rosamilia A et al 2006 Laparoscopic versus open Burch colposuspension: a randomised controlled study. BJOG: an International Journal of Obstetrics and Gynaecology 113: 999–1006.

Carr LK, Webster GD 1997 Voiding dysfunction following incontinence surgery: diagnosis and treatment with retropubic or vaginal urethrolysis. Journal of Urology 157: 821–823.

Choudhari K, Choudhari Y, Fannin T 2000 Acute lumbar intervertebral disc prolapse: a complication of the lithotomy position. BJOG: an International Journal of Obstetrics and Gynaecology 107: 1519–1521.

Coates KW, Harris RL, Cundiff GW, Bump RC 1997 Uroflowmetry in women with urinary incontinence and pelvic organ prolapse. British Journal of Urology 80: 217–221.

Costantini E, Mearini E, Pajoncini C, Biscotto S, Bini V, Porena M 2003 Uroflowmetry in female voiding disturbances. Neurourology and Urodynamics 22: 569–573.

Dasgupta P, Haslam C, Goodwin R, Fowler CJ 1997 The 'Queen Square bladder stimulator': a device for assisting emptying of the neurogenic bladder. British Journal of Urology 80: 234–237.

Delaere KPJ, Debruyne FMJ, Moonen WA 1983 Bladder neck incision in the female: a hazardous procedure? British Journal of Urology 55: 283–286.

Dietz HP, Haylen BT, Vancaillie TG 2002 Female pelvic organ prolapse and voiding dysfunction. International Urogynecology Journal and Pelvic Floor Dysfunction 13: 284–288.

Digesu GA, Chaliha C, Salvatore S, Hutchings A, Khullar V 2005 The relationship of vaginal prolapse severity to symptoms and quality of life. BJOG: an International Journal of Obstetrics and Gynaecology 112: 971–976.

Diokno AC, Sonda P, Hollander JB, Lapides J 1983 Fate of patients started on clean intermittent catheterisation therapy 10 years ago. Journal of Urology 129: 1120–1121.

Duthie J, Wilson DI, Herbison GP, Wilson D 2007 Botulinum toxin injections for adults with overactive bladder syndrome. Cochrane Database of Systematic Reviews 3: CD005493.

Fitzgerald MP, Kulkami N, Fenner D 2000 Postoperative resolution of urinary retention in patients with advanced pelvic organ prolapse. American Journal of Obstetrics and Gynecology 183: 1361–1364.

Foster HE, McGuire EJ 1993 Management of urethral obstruction with transvaginal urethrolysis. Journal of Urology 150: 1448–1451.

Fowler CJ, Christmas TJ, Chapple CR, Parkhouse HF, Kirby RS, Jacobs HS 1988 Abnormal electromyographic activity of the urethral sphincter, voiding dysfunction and polycystic ovaries: a new syndrome? BMJ (Clinical Research Ed.) 297: 1436–1438.

Glavind K, Bjørk J 2003 Incidence and treatment of urinary retention postpartum. International Urogynecology Journal and Pelvic Floor Dysfunction 14: 119–121.

Groutz A, Blaivas JG, Chaikin DC 2000 Bladder outlet obstruction in women: definition and characteristics. Neurourology and Urodynamics 19: 213–220.

Hakvoort RA, Elberink R, Vollebregt A, Ploeg T, Emanuel MH 2004 How long should urinary bladder catheterisation be continued after vaginal prolapse surgery? A randomised controlled trial comparing short term versus long term catheterisation after vaginal prolapse surgery. BJOG: an International Journal of Obstetrics and Gynaecology 111: 828–830.

Hakvoort RA, Dijkgraaf MG, Burger MP, Emanuel MH, Roovers JP 2009 Predicting short-term urinary retention after vaginal prolapse surgery. Neurourology and Urodynamics 28: 225–228.

Haylen BT, Ashby D, Sutherst JR, Frazer MI, West CR 1989 Maximum and average urine flow rates in normal male and female populations — the Liverpool nomograms. British Journal of Urology 64: 30–38.

Haylen BT, Krishnan S, Schulz S et al 2007 Has the true prevalence of voiding dysfunction in urogynecology patients been underestimated? International Urogynecology Journal and Pelvic Floor Dysfunction 18: 53–56.

Haylen BT, Yang V, Logan V 2008a Uroflowmetry: its current clinical utility for women. International Urogynecology Journal and Pelvic Floor Dysfunction 19: 899–903.

Haylen BT, Lee J, Logan V, Husselbee S, Zhou J, Law M 2008b Immediate postvoid residual volumes in women with symptoms of pelvic floor dysfunction. Obstetrics and Gynecology 111: 1305–1312.

Haylen BT, de Ridder D, Freeman RM et al 2010 An International Urogynecological Association (IUGA)/International Continence Society (ICS) Joiunt Report on the Terminology of Remale Pelvic Floor Dysfunction. International Urogynecology Journal and Pelvic Floor Dysfunction 21: 5–26.

Jahn P, Preuss M, Kernig A, Seifert-Huhmer A, Langer G 2007 Types of indwelling catheters for long-term bladder drainage in adults. Cochrane Database of Systematic Reviews 3: CD004997.

Jarvik JG, Deyo RA 2007 Diagnostic evaluation of low back pain with emphasis on imaging. Annals of Internal Medicine 147: 478–491.

Jarvis JG 1994 Surgery for genuine stress incontinence. BJOG: an International Journal of Obstetrics and Gynaecology 101: 371–374.

Karram MM, Partoll L, Bilotta V, Angel O 1997 Factors affecting detrusor contraction strength during voiding in women. Obstetrics and Gynecology 90: 723–726.

Karram MM, Segal JL, Vassallo BJ, Kleeman SD 2003 Complications and untoward effects of the tension-free vaginal tape procedure. Obstetrics and Gynecology 101: 929–932.

Kessler TM, Ryu G, Burkhard FC 2009 Clean intermittent self-catheterization: a burden for the patient? Neurourology and Urodynamics 28: 18–21.

Khullar V, Cardozo LD, Abbott D, Anders K 1997 GAX collagen in the treatment of urinary incontinence in elderly women: a two year follow-up. BJOG: an International Journal of Obstetrics and Gynaecology 104: 96–99.

Klutke C, Siegel S, Carlin B, Paszkiewicz E, Kirkemo A, Klutke J 2001 Urinary retention after tension-free vaginal tape procedure: incidence and treatment. Urology 58: 697–701.

Kuuva N, Nilsson CG 2002 A nationwide analysis of complications associated with the tension-free vaginal (TVT) procedure. Acta Obstetricia et Gynecologica Scandinavica 81: 72–77.

Lapides J, Diokno AC, Gould FR, Lowe BS 1976 Further observations on self catheterisation. Journal of Urology 116: 169–171.

Latthe PM, Foon R, Tooz-Hobson P 2007 Transobturator tape procedures in stress urinary incontinence: a systematic review and meta-analysis of effectiveness and complications. BJOG: an International Journal of Obstetrics and Gynaecology 114: 522–531.

Laurikainen E, Kiiholma P 2006 A nationwide analysis of transvaginal tape release for urinary retention after tension-free vaginal tape procedure. International Urogynecology Journal and Pelvic Floor Dysfunction 17: 111–119.

Liang CC, Tseng LH, Chang SD, Chang YL, Lo TS 2008 Resolution of elevated postvoid residual volumes after correction of severe pelvic organ prolapse. International Urogynecology Journal and Pelvic Floor Dysfunction 19: 1261–1266.

Malone-Lee J, Wahedna I 1993 Characterisation of detrusor contractile function in relation to old age. British Journal of Urology 72: 873–880.

Massey JA, Abrams PH 1988 Obstructed voiding in the female. British Journal of Urology 61: 36–39.

McCrery R 2007 Transvaginal urethrolysis for obstruction after anti-incontinence surgery. International Urogynecology Journal and Pelvic Floor Dysfunction 18: 627–633.

Moore KN, Fader M, Getliffe K 2007 Long-term bladder management by intermittent catheterisation in adults and children. Cochrane Database of Systematic Reviews 4: CD006008.

Myers DL, Lasala CA, Hogan JW, Rosenblatt PL 1998 The effect of posterior wall support defects on urodynamic indices in stress urinary incontinence. Obstetrics and Gynecology 1998; 91: 710–714.

National Institute for Health and Clinical Excellence 2006 Urinary Incontinence. NICE Clinical Guideline No. 40. NICE, London. Available at: www.nice.org.uk.

Niel-Weise BS, van den Broek PJ 2005 Antibiotic policies for short-term catheter bladder drainage in adults. Cochrane Database of Systematic Reviews 3: CD005428.

Ramsay IN, Torbet TE 1993 Incidence of abnormal voiding parameters in the immediate postpartum period. Neurourology and Urodynamics 12: 179–183.

Rardin CR, Rosenblatt PL, Kohli N, Miklos JR, Heit M, Lucente VR 2002 Release of tension-free vaginal tape for the treatment of refractory postoperative voiding dysfunction. Obstetrics and Gynecology 100: 898–902.

Robinson D, Dixon A, Cardozo L, Anders K, Balmforth J, Parsons M 2003 Does antimuscarinic therapy exacerbate voiding difficulties? Neurourology and Urodynamics 22: 535–536.

Romanzi LJ, Chaikin DC, Blaivas JG 1999 The effect of genital prolapse on voiding. Journal of Urology 161: 581–586.

Romero Maroto J, Ortiz Gorraiz M, Prieto Chaparro L, Pacheco Bru J, Miralles Bueno J, Lopez Lopez C 2008 Transvaginal adjustable tape: an adjustable mesh for surgical treatment of female stress urinary incontinence. International Urogynecology Journal and Pelvic Floor Dysfunction 19: 1109–1116.

Schaeffer AJ 1986 Catheter-associated bacteriuria. Urologic Clinics of North America 13: 735–747.

Schierlitz L, Dwyer PL, Rosamilia A et al 2008 Effectiveness of tension-free vaginal tape compared with transobturator tape in women with stress urinary incontinence and intrinsic sphincter deficiency: a randomised controlled trial. Obstetrics and Gynecology 112: 1253–1261.

Schmid DM, Sauerman P, Werner M et al 2006 Experience with 100 cases treated with botulinum-A toxin injections in the detrusor muscle for idiopathic overactive bladder syndrome refractory to anticholinergics. Journal of Urology 176: 177–185.

Schumm K, Lam TBL 2008 Types of urethral catheters for management of short-term voiding problems in hospitalised adults: a short version Cochrane review. Neurourology and Urodynamics 27: 738–746.

Scotti RJ, Bergman A, Bhatia NN, Ostergard DR 1986 Urodynamic changes in urethrovesical function after radical hysterectomy. Obstetrics and Gynecology 68: 111–120.

Segal J, Steele AC, Vassallo BJ et al 2006 Various surgical approaches to treat voiding dysfunction following anti-incontinence surgery. International Urogynecology Journal and Pelvic Floor Dysfunction 17: 372–377.

Smith P 1972 Age changes in the female urethra. British Journal of Urology 44: 667–676.

Stanton SL, Norton C, Cardozo L 1982 Clinical and urodynamic effects of anterior colporrhaphy and vaginal hysterectomy for prolapse with and without incontinence. BJOG: an International Journal of Obstetrics and Gynaecology 89: 459–463.

Thakar R, Ayers S, Clarkson P, Stanton S, Manyonda I 2002 Outcomes after total versus subtotal abdominal hysterectomy. New England Journal of Medicine 347: 1318–1325.

Ulmsten U, Henriksson L, Johnson P, Varhos G 1996 An ambulatory surgical procedure under local anesthesia for treatment of female urinary incontinence. International Urogynecology Journal and Pelvic Floor Dysfunction 7: 81–86.

Vandoninck V, van Balken MR, Finazzi Agrò E et al 2004 Posterior tibial nerve stimulation in the treatment of voiding dysfunction: urodynamic data. Neurourology and Urodynamics 23: 246–251.

Vervest HA, Bisseling TM, Heintz AP, Schraffordt Koops SE 2007 The prevalence of voiding difficulty after TVT, its impact on quality of life and related risk factors. International Urogynecology Journal and Pelvic Floor Dysfunction 18: 173–182.

Vierhout ME 1998 Prolonged catheterisation after vaginal prolapse surgery. Acta Obstetricia et Gynecologica Scandinavica 77: 997–999.

Wake CR 1980 The immediate effect of abdominal hysterectomy on intravesical pressure and detrusor activity. BJOG: an International Journal of Obstetrics and Gynaecology 87: 901–902.

Ward K, Hilton P 2002 Prospective multicentre randomised trial of tension-free vaginal tape and colposuspension as primary treatment for stress incontinence. BMJ (Clinical Research Ed.) 325: 67–70.

Yu HJ, Lee WC, Liu SP, Tai TY, Wu HP, Chen J 2004 Unrecognized voiding difficulty in female type 2 diabetic patients in the diabetes clinic: a prospective case–control study. Diabetes Care 27: 988–989.

CHAPTER 55

Pelvic organ prolapse

Colin A. Walsh and Mark Slack

Chapter Contents

INTRODUCTION	849		INVESTIGATION	854
PREVALENCE	849		PREVENTATIVE STRATEGIES/NATURAL HISTORY	855
AETIOLOGY	849		TREATMENT	856
CLASSIFICATION	850		CONCLUSIONS	860
PELVIC ANATOMY	851		KEY POINTS	860
CLINICAL PRESENTATION	852			

Introduction

Pelvic organ (urogenital) prolapse (POP) is a disorder unique to women and describes the herniation of one of the pelvic organs (uterus, vaginal apex, bladder, rectum) from its normal anatomical position into or beyond the vagina. Although women with asymptomatic POP can often be managed expectantly, current treatment options for symptomatic women are limited to vaginal pessaries and surgery. Surgical repair of POP is a rapidly evolving field, and the optimal reconstructive procedure for prolapse is one of the most debated issues in contemporary gynaecological practice.

Prevalence

Pelvic organ prolapse is very common. In the Women's Health Initiative (WHI), 41% of 27,342 women aged 50–79 years showed some degree of POP (Hendrix et al 2002, Figure 55.1). Indeed, with both life expectancy and rates of obesity increasing, the prevalence of POP is likely to rise. However, the majority of such women are symptom free and much of this prolapse is not considered clinically significant. Large cross-sectional studies have demonstrated rates of symptomatic POP of 3–11% (Tegerstedt et al 2005, Nygaard et al 2008, Fritel et al 2009). Women whose prolapse extends beyond the hymenal remnants are more likely to be symptomatic (Swift et al 2003). Although POP is rarely life threatening, it has a substantial impact on quality of life, such that 6.7% of women in the USA will undergo a surgical procedure for prolapse by 80 years of age (Olsen et al 1997).

Aetiology

The aetiology of POP is poorly understood, which is remarkable given the magnitude of the problem. Although multifactorial in nature, vaginal birth has emerged as the principal risk factor (Mant et al 1997). Avulsion injury to the levator ani during childbirth and, less commonly, pudendal neuropathy and fascial damage appear to be the most common causes (Dietz 2008a, Figure 55.2). Unsurprisingly, therefore, increasing parity, fetal macrosomia and perineal trauma increase the odds of subsequent POP, although the much-quoted link to instrumental vaginal delivery is not borne out in all studies (Uma et al 2005, Tegerstedt et al 2006).

Nulliparous women may also develop prolapse, and various non-obstetric aetiological factors have been identified (Miedel et al 2009). A number of reports, including the WHI, have demonstrated increasing rates of POP with advancing age (Hendrix et al 2002, Handa et al 2004), although a simple linear relationship is not universally accepted (Dietz 2008b). Some studies have shown an impact of ethnicity on POP, with lower rates of POP among Black women and higher rates among Hispanic women compared with White women (Hendrix et al 2002, Rortveit et al 2007). An association with body mass index (BMI) is generally agreed (Whitcomb et al 2009), and is of particular concern given the global rise in obesity. In addition, twin studies have demonstrated a clear genetic component to the disorder (Altman et al 2008), supported by stronger family histories among affected women (McLennan et al 2008).

The evidence directly linking hysterectomy and POP is not compelling and is potentially confounded by the

DOI: 10.1016/B978-0-7020-3120-5.00055-2

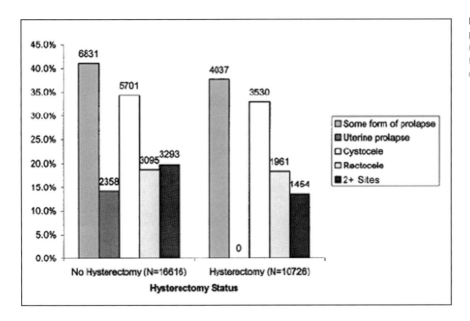

Figure 55.1 Prevalence of pelvic organ prolapse from the Women's Health Initiative. *Redrawn from Hendrix et al. Pelvic organ prolapse in the Women's Health Initiative: gravity and gravidity. Am J Obstet Gynecol 2002;186:1160–6.*

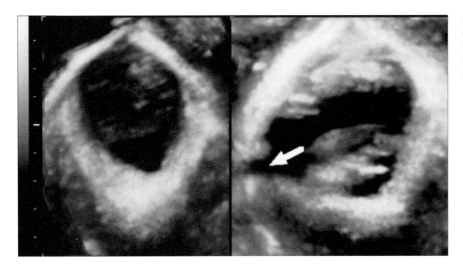

Figure 55.2 Translabial pelvic floor ultrasound demonstrating right-sided avulsion of the puborectalis at 3 months post partum. *Source: Dietz HP 2005 Best Practice and Research Clinical Obstetrics and Gynaecology 19: 913–924.*

indication for the original hysterectomy. Among 384 women undergoing surgery for POP/incontinence, 60% had a previous hysterectomy and/or pelvic floor repair, suggesting a potential aetiological role (Olsen et al 1997). Despite this, the cumulative probability of requiring a POP repair 20 years following hysterectomy for non-prolapse is only 0–2%, raising the possibility that it is the history of prolapse and not the hysterectomy *per se* which is the dominant risk factor (Blandon et al 2007). Finally, conditions associated with increased intra-abdominal pressure (constipation, cough, heavy lifting) are generally considered to be risk factors for prolapse (Rortveit et al 2007).

Classification

Management of POP is determined primarily by the findings on physical examination; thus, a standardized and reproducible classification system is crucial. Initially, POP is classified by vaginal compartment into (Figure 55.3):

- anterior compartment prolapse (cystocele, urethrocele);
- posterior compartment prolapse (rectocele, enterocele); or
- apical prolapse (prolapse of uterus/vaginal vault).

The anterior compartment is the most common site of POP, although in most cases, there will be evidence of prolapse in more than a single compartment (Hendrix et al 2002). In addition to classifying POP by anatomical compartment, an assessment of prolapse severity (stage) is undertaken. A variety of systems to stage POP have been described (Figure 55.4). However, in 1996, the Pelvic Organ Prolapse Quantification (POP-Q) system was developed by consensus of international expert groups (Bump et al 1996). It is a more objective, site-specific system for staging pelvic support with proven inter- and intraobserver reliability (Hall et al 1996). The POP-Q system references nine vaginal points (two anterior, two posterior, two superior, two frontal and total vaginal length) to the plane of the hymen during Valsalva strain to create a 'topographic' map of the vagina (Figure 55.5). These anatomical points are measured follow

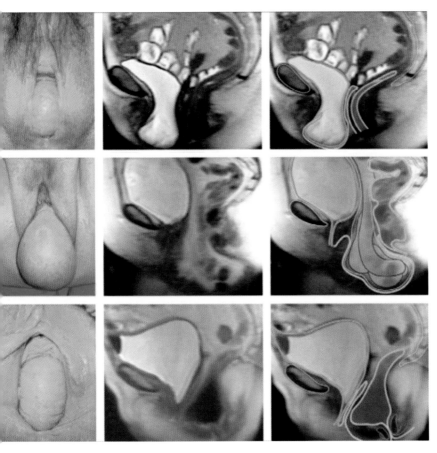

Figure 55.3 Photographs in lithotomy position and sagittal magnetic resonance image showing vaginal wall prolapse. Prolapse might include (top to bottom): bladder (cystocele), small bowel (enterocele) or rectum (rectocele). Colour codes include purple (bladder), orange (vagina), brown (colon and rectum) and green (peritoneum). *Jelovsek JE, Maher C, Barber MD (2007) Pelvic organ prolapse. Lancet 369:1027–38.*

ng demonstration of the maximum extent of the prolapse o determine the stage. Typically, the nine-point findings are ranslated into an ordinal staging system (stage 0–IV) to aid omparative analyses and facilitate more practical commu-ication (Figure 55.4).

Pelvic Anatomy

upport of the pelvic organs is achieved through a complex nterplay between the pelvic ligaments, muscles and endo-elvic fascia which attach the pelvic organs to the bony elvis to form a continuous support structure. The levator ni muscle group is the major structural component of the elvic floor, and in practical terms, the pelvic floor is syn-nymous with the levator ani. Laterally, the levator is com-osed of iliococcygeus, a thin muscle layer originating from he arcus tendineus levator ani, a fascial condensation over-ying the obturator internus muscle. The medial portion of he levator ani (pubococcygeus and puborectalis) arises rom the pubic bone (lateral to the pubic symphysis) and orms a sling around the bladder, urethra, vagina and ectum. The obturator internus and piriformis muscles form he pelvic sidewall. The obturator internus is a large fan-haped muscle which can be palpated vaginally. Another rominent connective tissue structure, the arcus tendineus ascia pelvis ('white line'), passes from the pubic tubercle to he ischial spine and provides lateral pelvic support to the nterior vaginal wall (analogous to the cable of a suspension ridge). The urethra and vagina pass through the urogenital

hiatus in the levator ani, and it is through this opening that POP occurs. The levator ani muscles, together with coccy-geus and the overlying superior and inferior fascia, form the pelvic diaphragm.

On each side of the pelvis, a dense layer of connective tissue, the endopelvic fascia, envelops the uterus and cervix and attaches to the pelvic sidewall. As well as providing support, the endopelvic fascia also serves as a neurovascular conduit and is composed of collagen, smooth muscle, blood vessels and nerves. In certain areas, thickened condensations of this fascia form pelvic 'ligaments' which add support. The clinically important ligaments include the uterosacral ligaments (extending laterally from the posterior cervix to the anterior sacrum), the cardinal ligaments (transverse cervical/Mackenrodt's ligaments, extending from the lateral cervix and upper vagina to the pelvic sidewall) and the round ligament (extending from the uterine cornu to the labia majora as the superior part of the broad ligament) (Raizada and Mittal 2008).

DeLancey introduced the concept of three levels of con-nective tissue support in the anterior pelvis. Level I (apical vaginal) support is via the uterosacral/cardinal ligament complex, and damage at this level results in uterine/vaginal vault prolapse (DeLancey 1992). Level II (midvaginal) support is achieved via the endopelvic fascia and its lateral insertion into the white line. Level III (distal vaginal) support incorporates the endopelvic fascia anteriorly and the peri-neal body posteriorly. Anterior and posterior compartment prolapse result from damage to level II/III support, respec-tively. Although DeLancey's system creates artificial divides

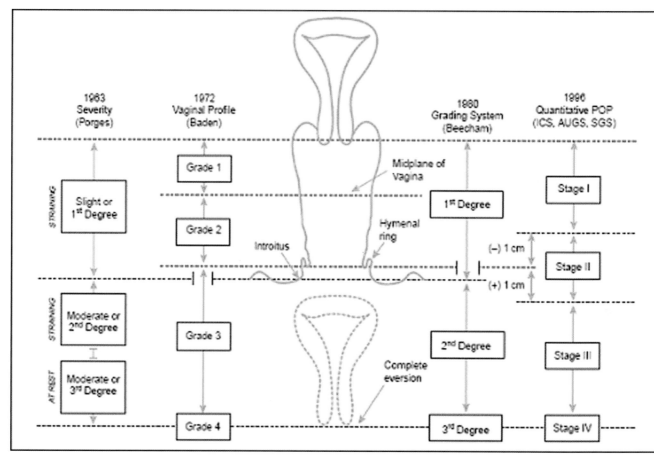

Figure 55.4 Comparison of commonly used grading systems. POP, pelvic organ prolapse; ICS, International Continence Society; AUGS, American Urogynecological Society; SGS, Society of Gynecologic Surgeons.

Mouritsen L (2005) Classification and evaluation of prolapse. Best Pract Res Clin Obstet Gynaecol. 19(6):895–911.

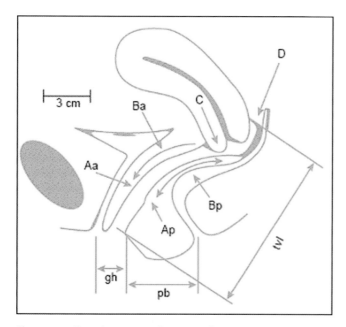

Figure 55.5 The pelvic organ prolapse quantification (POPQ) system. gh, genital hiatus; pb, perineal body; tvl, total vaginal length.

Bump R et al (1996) The standardization of terminology of female pelvic organ prolapse and pelvic floor dysfunction. Am J Obstet Gynecol. 1996 Jul;175(1):10–7.

in what is essentially a continuous connective tissue structure, it does aid understanding of how loss of support correlates with clinical findings, and is widely reproduced in the gynaecological literature.

Clinical Presentation

Patients who seek medical care have a wide range of symptoms (Table 55.1). Women frequently present with a sensation of 'something coming down' or of 'something falling out of the vagina'. Other women may see or feel a vaginal bulge or they may complain of less specific herniation symptoms, such as pelvic pressure or heaviness. As might be expected, a visible vaginal bulge correlates better with objective evidence of POP on examination than the more general complaint of pelvic heaviness or discomfort (Miedel et al 2008).

Urinary symptoms

Among 237 women with symptomatic POP, 87% reported frequency/urgency, 73% reported urinary incontinence and 50–60% reported symptoms of voiding dysfunction (Ellerkmann et al 2001). A complex relationship exists

Table 55.1 Common symptoms associated with pelvic organ prolapse

Vaginal symptoms
Sensation of pressure ('something coming down')
Seeing or feeling a bulge
Dyspareunia

Urinary symptoms
Urinary incontinence
Frequency
Incomplete emptying
Hesitancy
Poor stream
Digitation/positional change needed to void

Bowel symptoms
Incontinence of flatus/faeces
Straining to defaecate
Sensation of incomplete emptying
Faecal urgency
Vaginal/anal digitation to defaecate
Splinting perineum to defaecate

between POP and stress urinary incontinence, and may result from shared risk factors rather than a direct causal link (Smith and Appell 2005). In practice, many women present with both cystocele and stress incontinence, and loss of the anterior vaginal wall support is thought to contribute to urethral hypermobility and subsequent stress incontinence (DeLancey 2002). However, the relationship is not linear and some studies have demonstrated lower rates of stress leakage in more advanced POP (Yalcin et al 2001, Burrows et al 2004). This is likely due to a direct compressive effect or a urethral kinking mechanism, and is important given the risk of hidden or 'occult' stress incontinence manifesting once the prolapse is reduced (see 'Investigation' section). Interestingly, posterior vaginal wall prolapse has recently been linked to stress incontinence (Miedel et al 2008). More advanced POP can produce obstructive voiding symptoms or, rarely, urinary retention. The need to manually reduce a bulge to void is progressively linked to more severe POP (Burrows et al 2004, Miedel et al 2008). The relationship between POP and overactive bladder symptoms has not been studied as extensively. Analysis of 330 women undergoing surgery for POP or incontinence found that urgency/urge incontinence occurred more often in women with less advanced prolapse (Burrows et al 2004). Other studies, however, have shown a positive association between urge incontinence and both anterior and posterior compartment prolapse (Miedel et al 2008). This is supported by short-term improvements in overactive bladder symptoms following prolapse repair (Nguyen and Bhatia 2001, Digesu et al 2007).

Bowel symptoms

Bowel symptoms and difficulty with defaecation are common symptoms among women with POP. These include straining, sensation of incomplete emptying and the need to manually assist defaecation (digital pressure to the vagina or perineum). Among 280 women with symptomatic POP, almost three-quarters (73%) reported at least one bowel symptom (Miedel et al 2008). The most consistently reported prevalence of faecal incontinence associated with POP ranges from 14% to 19% (Jackson et al 1997, Burrows et al 2004, Jelovsek et al 2005, Miedel et al 2008). The extent of POP does not appear to predict bowel symptoms (Jelovsek et al 2005), although the need to manually assist defaecation has been associated with more severe prolapse (Burrows et al 2004). Much has been written about the relationship between posterior compartment prolapse and constipation, and it has been suggested that constipation contributes to the development of rectocele and vice versa. However, the exact nature of the association remains uncertain. It is notable that several studies have failed to identify a relationship between constipation and POP (Samuelsson et al 1999, Jelovsek et al 2005).

Sexual dysfunction

Sexual dysfunction is very common in women attending urogynaecology clinics (Pauls et al 2006), although it may not be volunteered due to patient embarrassment or poor history taking. Sexual satisfaction is a complex issue and studies examining the association between POP and sexual dysfunction have yielded conflicting results. Although high rates of satisfaction have been reported in women with POP (Barber et al 2002, Burrows et al 2004), other data have shown POP to have an adverse effect on sexual function (Rogers et al 2001, Novi et al 2005). It appears that women with POP are more likely to complain of problems with sexual function than those with urinary incontinence (Barber et al 2002). Weber found no differences in measures of sexual function in women with POP and incontinence compared with continent women without prolapse (Weber et al 1995). Furthermore, the benefits of pelvic floor surgical repair on sexual function have not been consistent (Thakar 2009).

Prediction of symptoms

Attempts have been made to correlate the severity (stage) of POP with the likely development of symptoms. Consistently strong correlations between increasing severity of POP and the development of symptoms have not been demonstrated (Burrows et al 2004). Many studies indicate a lower rate of stress incontinence in more severe anterior compartment prolapse. Miedel et al (2008) showed that most urinary and bowel symptoms associated with POP lack stage dependency, although there was correlation between a vaginal bulge and more advanced prolapse in all compartments. However, a large prospective study of 477 patients suggested that women whose prolapse extends beyond the hymenal remnants are more likely to be symptomatic (Swift et al 2003).

Physical examination

All women who present with symptoms consistent with POP should undergo a physical examination, including pelvic examination. Although some authorities advocate the need for physical examination in the standing position for all patients, use of the dorsal lithotomy position with Valsalva has been shown to be as good (Swift and Herring 1998). In practice, many clinicians examine women lying supine during resting and straining, and it is reasonable to reserve the standing position for women who feel that their prolapse is not being seen at its worst extent in that position (American College of Obstetricians and Gynecologists 2007). Conventionally, prolapse is examined while asking the woman to perform a Valsalva or cough stress test so that the maximum extent of the prolapse can be appreciated. A Sim's speculum (or the posterior blade of a bivalve speculum) is inserted into the vagina to retract the posterior wall and allow visualization of the anterior wall; the extent of any prolapse is noted while the woman strains. The process is repeated for the posterior wall with the speculum retracting anteriorly. Sometimes, an anterior wall prolapse may be better appreciated with the woman in the left lateral position and her right hip flexed. Finally, the cervix or vaginal vault is assessed either through visualization or with gentle traction from a ring forceps, although, in practice, many women find the latter uncomfortable. Areas of bleeding/ulceration, which can be seen in prolapse extending past the introitus in particular, should be noted (Figure 55.6). Women with recurrent prolapse should have a meticulous examination to assess previous surgical repair and plan future management. Staging of the prolapse should be recorded for all compartments using the practitioner's chosen method, although the POP-Q system is the internationally accepted standard (Figure 55.5, see 'Classification' section).

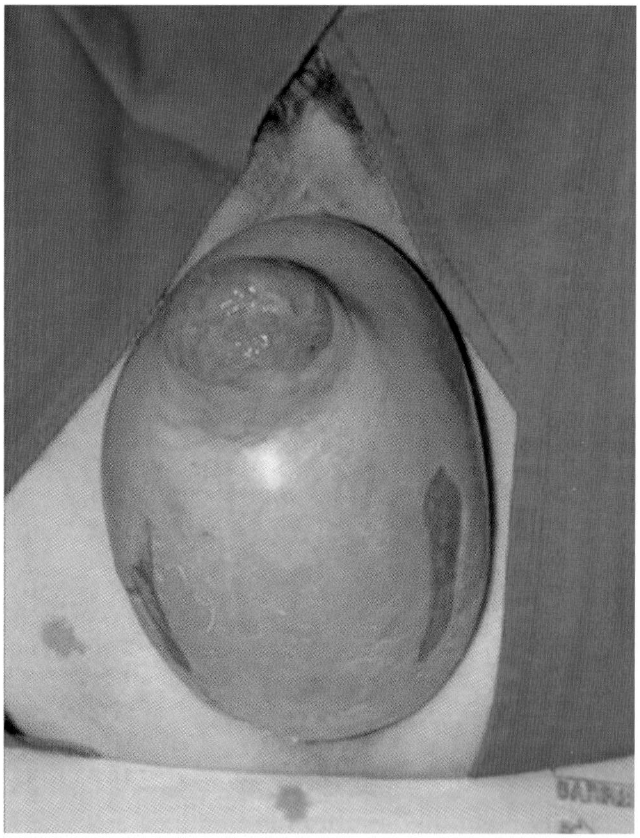

In addition to staging POP, a number of other features of the physical examination are noteworthy. Abdominal palpation and a bimanual pelvic examination should be performed in these patients as, occasionally, a large pelvic mass, such as a fibroid uterus or ovarian mass, may be detected. Although routine rectal examination for all patients is unnecessary, it can be useful in defining a posterior compartment prolapse, particularly where there is suspicion of an enterocele (which can be felt between a thumb placed in the vagina and a finger placed in the rectum). In addition, it can be useful to look for stress urinary incontinence on provocation by asking the patient to cough, assuming the bladder has not been emptied recently. Furthermore, in cases of advanced anterior compartment prolapse in women who do not complain of urinary leakage, there is concern that prolapse reduction may unmask 'occult' stress incontinence. Therefore, a cough test following temporary reduction of the prolapse into a more anatomical position (manually or with a cotton swab or ring forceps) may be useful (Fatton 2009). In a large randomized trial, reduction using a cotton swab most closely reproduced postoperative status following sacrocolpopexy compared with other reduction techniques (Visco et al 2008). Finally, digital assessment of the strength of the patient's pelvic floor muscle contraction is beneficial in women with concomitant stress urinary incontinence.

Investigation

A thorough physical examination is the cornerstone of POP management, and further investigations are usually second line. In women with urinary symptoms, a midstream specimen of urine should be cultured to exclude infection. Additionally, where there is suspicion of a voiding problem, women should undergo a voiding study with measurement of the residual volume using an ultrasound scan. If one is not available, the postvoid residual volume can be assessed using an in–out catheter.

The most contentious issue in the investigation of POP is the need for preoperative urodynamic testing. Women with POP without stress leakage have a 10–50% chance of developing de-novo ('occult') stress incontinence post repair (Fatton 2009). An anti-incontinence procedure may be performed concomitantly but will likely overtreat a proportion of women, and increases postoperative voiding problems and overactive bladder symptoms (de Tayrac et al 2004). Alternatively, a two-stage strategy can be adopted, where an interval continence procedure is reserved for patients with troubling stress urinary incontinence following prolapse repair. The use of preoperative urodynamics to better stratify patients into those who may or may not benefit from concomitant continence surgery has been suggested. However, there is little evidence that preoperative urodynamics improves the outcome of prolapse surgery (Roovers and Oelke 2007). The CARE (Colpopexy and Urinary Reduction Efforts) trial did show that women with POP and preoperative urodynamic stress incontinence during reduction testing had a higher rate of stress leak following abdominal sacrocolpopexy without the conti-

Figure 55.6 Complete uterovaginal prolapse. Note the linear erosions on the posterior vaginal mucosa.

Jelovsek JE, Maher C, Barber MD (2007) Pelvic organ prolapse. Lancet 369:1027–38.

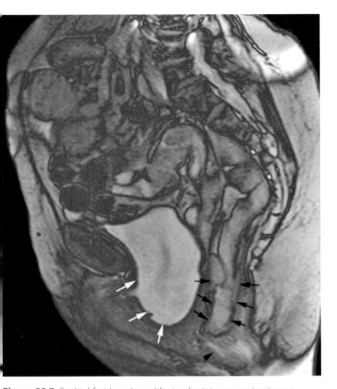

Figure 55.7 Sagittal fast imaging with steady state precession image though the midline of the pelvis in a female patient during magnetic resonance imaging proctography. A loop of small bowel has descended anterior to the rectum to form a large enterocoele (black arrows). Note the coexistent cystocoele (white arrows) and small collapsed rectocoele (arrow head).

Taylor SA (2009) Imaging pelvic floor dysfunction. Best Practice & Research Clinical Gastroenterology 23:487–503.

nence procedure. It is notable that even with optimal prolapse reduction during preoperative urodynamics (by cotton swab), one-third of women who were dry before surgery developed postoperative stress incontinence (Visco et al 2008).

Various radiographic modalities have been proposed to further define the extent of POP, although none are in mainstream clinical use. Dynamic magnetic resonance imaging (MRI) is the most commonly described technique (Law and Fielding 2008, Taylor 2009). Dynamic MRI offers excellent anatomical detail and allows visualization of all three compartments together (Figure 55.7), but is expensive and dispute remains over the appropriate radiological landmarks for staging POP (Broekhuis et al 2009). Transperineal ultrasound (TPUS), and increasingly three- and four-dimensional TPUS, have also been used in staging POP radiologically (Dietz 2004). Recently, moderate-to-good correlation was demonstrated between three-dimensional TPUS and defaecography (traditionally the gold standard investigation) in the assessment of posterior compartment prolapse (Steensma et al 2009). However, TPUS does not appear to be superior to clinical assessment of POP (Kluivers et al 2008). Finally, anorectal physiology studies (including anal manometry and pudendal nerve latency) and endoanal ultrasound should be considered in women with symptoms of bowel dysfunction, particularly faecal incontinence.

Preventative Strategies/Natural History

POP and surgical prolapse repair place a significant demand on healthcare resources. Therefore, strategies to minimize POP and reduce the resultant disease burden are vital (Subramanian et al 2009).

Lifestyle modification

Four-year prospective results from one of the WHI study centres have confirmed that progression of POP over time is not inevitable; in some cases, POP can regress. Specifically, among 259 non-hysterectomized postmenopausal women undergoing serial POP-Q assessments, the maximum vaginal descent increased by ≥2 cm in 11% and regressed by this amount in 2.7% (Bradley et al 2007). POP progression was more likely in obese women, of higher parity (particularly for five children or more) and with more severe baseline degrees of prolapse. Progression was less likely in smokers, although this may be related to a lower BMI in women who smoked rather than a genuine protective effect. Another large secondary analysis from the WHI study confirmed a higher rate of progression in women with raised BMI, but found that weight loss was not associated with regression of POP, suggesting irreversible pelvic floor changes secondary to obesity (Kudish 2009). Therefore, although weight loss forms part of the standard advice given to overweight women with POP, highlighting the importance of avoiding weight gain in women of normal BMI may be more valuable. Pelvic floor muscle (Kegel) exercises are frequently recommended for women with POP. Although they are an effective therapy in stress urinary incontinence (which may coexist), pelvic floor exercises are of no proven benefit in the prevention of POP, although studies are lacking (Bø 2006).

Obstetric risk

Given the clear aetiological link between vaginal childbirth and POP, the role of caesarean delivery as a strategy to prevent POP is debated (Richter 2006, Weber 2007). The relative contributions made by the pregnancy, labour and mode of delivery itself are difficult to tease out. Based on POP-Q assessments on 94 primigravidae at 36 weeks of gestation and again at 6 weeks post partum, intrapartum caesarean section performed during the first stage of labour has not been shown to protect against POP compared with women undergoing vaginal delivery (Sze et al 2002). A similar study of 135 primigravidae involved POP-Q assessments on women from each trimester and post partum (O'Boyle et al 2005). POP was significantly more common in both the third trimester and post partum compared with the first trimester. Forty percent of women examined in the third trimester had stage II POP or worse. Among postpartum women, there was a higher incidence of stage II POP in the vaginal birth group compared with those who delivered by intrapartum caesarean. Although this finding contrasts with that of Sze et al (2002), the role of elective caesarean delivery was not examined and both studies were underpowered to determine the impact of mode of delivery on POP. A survey of 4458 women showed POP to be three times more common among vaginally parous women compared with nulliparous women [adjusted odds ratio (AOR) 3.2]. A history of caesarean delivery alone was protective (AOR 1.6 compared with nulliparous). However, elective prelabour caesarean conferred a higher benefit than caesarean in labour, suggesting that intrapartum events and not simply mode of delivery contribute to POP (Lukacz et al 2006).

Hysterectomy

The precise incidence of posthysterectomy POP is difficult to determine. A recent case–control study demonstrated a cumulative incidence of vaginal vault prolapse repair of 0.5% at 3–23 year follow-up (Dällenbach et al 2008). Overall, rates of pelvic floor repair are higher in women whose original hysterectomy was performed for prolapse compared with other clinical indications (Mant et al 1997, Blandon et al 2007). Numerous surgical strategies to prevent posthysterectomy vault prolapse have been described. The McCall and modified McCall culdoplasty techniques involve various means of anchoring the uterosacral pedicles to the vaginal vault during vaginal hysterectomy. Many studies have reported success rates in excess of 90% in preventing enterocele/vault prolapse at 12–108 months (Chene et al 2008). These techniques are superior to the Moschcowitz procedure in this regard (Cruikshank and Kovac 1999). Some authorities recommend prophylactic sacrospinous ligament suspension at the time of vaginal hysterectomy if the vault descends to the introitus during closure (Royal College of Obstetricians and Gynaecologists 2007), but there is no evidence to support this practice.

Treatment

Many women with POP, particularly those with minor degrees of prolapse not extending past the hymenal remnants, complain of little or no discomfort. Adopting a policy of expectant management is entirely appropriate in such cases. Indeed, these women are often relieved to be told that surgery is not always warranted for POP. However, more proactive treatment may be necessary if problems, such as urinary obstruction, chronic vaginal ulceration or worsening POP symptoms, arise.

Non-surgical treatment

Pelvic floor muscle training

As has been noted above, the effectiveness of pelvic floor exercises in the treatment of POP remains unproven. Although pelvic floor muscle training is unlikely to cause harm and may benefit stress urinary incontinence, there are associated cost implications. An international, multicentre, randomized controlled trial to assess the role of physiotherapy in prolapse is currently recruiting (http://www.charttrials.abdn.ac.uk/poppy/index.php). A pilot study of 47 women with stage I or II POP showed improvement in both subjective and objective measures of POP in women treated with pelvic floor muscle training and lifestyle advice compared with lifestyle advice alone (Hagen et al 2009).

Weight loss

A large population-based study of almost 5500 Swedish women showed that women who are overweight (BMI 26–30) are twice as likely to complain of symptomatic POP as women of normal weight (BMI 20–24, Miedel et al 2009). Weight loss should be encouraged in the management of POP for all women as it does not cause harm, reduces perioperative complication rates if surgery is later contemplated, and is of proven benefit in treating stress urinary incontinence, which often coexists (Subak et al 2009).

Vaginal pessaries

Vaginal pessaries represent the only proven non-surgical option for women who require treatment for POP. Although all women can be offered a trial of pessary use, they are particularly useful for women who decline surgery or are medically unsuitable for surgery, during pregnancy, and as an interim measure prior to surgery or for those who desire future childbearing. Pessary materials have evolved and are now made predominantly from non-reactive silicone, which is non-allergenic, durable and autoclavable (Shah et al 2006). A wide range of styles and shapes is available, and the ring pessary, which permits sexual intercourse, is the most widely used (Cundiff et al 2000, Figure 55.8). Some styles are also useful in the treatment of urinary incontinence. Pessaries are valid treatment options for advanced POP, although sturdier, 'space-filling' designs, such as the Gelhorn pessary, may be required (Powers et al 2006). In advanced POP, double pessaries are occasionally used (Singh and Reid 2001).

Fitting a pessary is based on a clinical assessment of vaginal length, introital size and severity of POP, and is often a process of trial and error. A pessary which is too small will not be retained, whereas one that is too large will be uncomfortable. The aim should be to place the largest size of which the patient is unaware. Most women will require trials of more than one option (Hanson et al 2006), and it is good practice to schedule a return appointment to the clinic 1–2

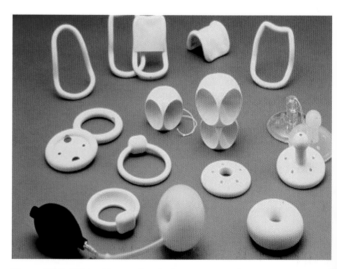

Figure 55.8 Different types of vaginal support pessaries.
Elneil S (2009) Complex pelvic floor failure and associated problems. Best Practice & Research Clinical Gastroenterology 23: 555–573.

weeks following the initial fitting to assess discomfort and the development of vaginal bleeding or de-novo incontinence. Results from multiple studies suggest that pessaries can be successfully fitted in approximately two-thirds of candidates. Reported predictors of an unsuccessful fitting include prior prolapse surgery or hysterectomy, younger age, higher parity and obesity (Mutone et al 2005, Nguyen and Jones 2005). Local oestrogen cream improves the success rate, even for patients taking systemic hormone replacement, and should be offered to all women (Hanson et al 2006). Women in whom pessaries are successfully fitted usually require assessment, vaginal examination and pessary removal/cleaning/reinsertion every 4–6 months, although there is no clear consensus on the most appropriate follow-up protocol. For those who can be taught self-removal, less frequent visits are reasonable. Prolonged use can lead to vaginal erosion with subsequent granulation formation. This can cause vaginal discharge and bleeding, which are common reasons for discontinuation. However, serious complications such as fistula, and urinary and bowel obstruction are rare and are usually limited to pessaries that have been neglected (Arias et al 2008).

Surgery

Women with symptomatic POP who decline or fail pessary management require surgical intervention. The surgical procedures and approaches available to women are rapidly evolving, due primarily to concerns about the longevity of more traditional prolapse repairs. The aims of surgical intervention are to restore anatomy, relieve symptoms, and preserve or restore urinary, bowel and sexual function. Among US women undergoing prolapse surgery, 20% will have a concomitant anti-incontinence procedure (Brown et al 2002).

In patients considering surgical management of POP, a fastidious preoperative work up is essential as a number of these patients have significant comorbidities. During surgery, the use of Allen legs in the vaginal and laparoscopic procedures will reduce iatrogenic injury to the patient and allow safer manipulation of the legs. The use of self-retaining retractors, such as the ReeTrakt (Insightra Medical, Irvine, CA, USA), will aid vaginal surgery significantly (Figure 55.9).

Following surgery, attention should be paid to thromboprophylaxis and prophylactic antibiotic coverage. Appropriate dietary advice, fluid intake and, if necessary, stool softeners should be given to avoid the woman straining at stool in the immediate postoperative period.

Options for surgical repair of POP can be classified by compartment and further subdivided into vaginal and abdominal approaches. However, it is important to remember that prolapse of a single compartment is rare, and failure to repair all defects may result in higher recurrence rates. Level I evidence supports a superior restoration of anatomy via the abdominal route, which may be offset partly by higher short-term morbidity associated with a more invasive approach (Maher et al 2007, Brubaker et al 2009). Comparison of different surgical techniques for POP is made difficult by the lack of consensus on outcome measures, which include subjective cure by symptoms, anatomical cure by examination and/or the need for reoperation for recurrent POP.

Surgery for apical prolapse

The apex is the cornerstone of good pelvic organ support, and if the uterus or vaginal vault is poorly supported, the posterior and, in particular, the anterior vaginal wall are exposed to intra-abdominal forces (Lowder et al 2008). Optimal surgical repair of advanced anterior compartment prolapse will often necessitate an apical support procedure (Rooney et al 2006). Abdominal sacrocolpopexy and vaginal sacrospinous ligament suspension are the two most common procedures performed for apical prolapse. Abdominal sacrocolpopexy involves suspending the vaginal apex to the anterior longitudinal ligament of the sacrum using an intervening material, typically a synthetic mesh. Traditionally, this is performed via a Pfannenstiel incision, and reported anatomical success rates range from 74% to 100% (Hilger et al 2003, Nygaard et al 2004). Laparoscopic sacrocolpopexy aims to minimize the morbidity while retaining the benefits associated with abdominal sacrocolpopexy (Figure 55.10).

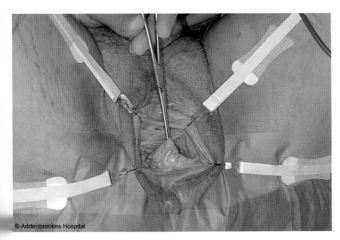

© Addenbrookes Hospital

Figure 55.9 ReeTrakt (Insightra Medical, Irvine, CA, USA).

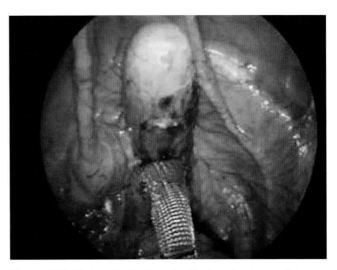

Figure 55.10 Mesh applied to the perineal body and on to part of the vaginal vault during a laparoscopic sacrocolpopexy procedure.
Elneil S (2009) Complex pelvic floor failure and associated problems. Best Practice & Research Clinical Gastroenterology 23: 555–573.

Although no randomized trials comparing these two approaches with sacrocolpopexy have been published, medium-term observational data from more than 1000 patients have shown a 94% satisfaction rate and 6% need for reoperation (Ganatra et al 2009).

Sacrospinous ligament suspension (sacrospinous colpopexy) suspends the vaginal apex to the lateral aspect of the sacrospinous ligament using permanent suture material. Typically, the sacrospinous ligament suspension uses an extraperitoneal approach to the right sacrospinous ligament, although bilateral fixation may be performed. Reported anatomical cure rates following sacrospinous fixation range from 63% to 97% (Sze and Karram 1997, Maher et al 2004). Meta-analysis comparing abdominal sacrocolpopexy with sacrospinous ligament suspension found lower rates of recurrent vault prolapse [relative risk (RR) 0.23] and dyspareunia (RR 0.39), but a longer operating time (on average 21 min), increased cost and increased risk of mesh erosion in women undergoing abdominal sacrocolpopexy (Maher et al 2007). Mesh erosion complicates 2–11% of sacrocolpopexies (Nygaard et al 2004), with higher rates among smokers and, in some studies, women undergoing concomitant hysterectomy (Cundiff et al 2008). It may be reasonable to offer younger women the higher success rate with sacrocolpopexy; in older, frailer patients, the reduced morbidity and quicker return to daily activities associated with sacrospinous ligament suspension may be more appropriate. In addition to abdominal sacrocolpopexy and sacrospinous ligament suspension, a number of other procedures for apical prolapse have been described. Iliococcygeus suspension involves suspension of the vaginal vault to the iliococcygeus fascia over the levator plate. Theoretically, this is meant to reduce anterior wall recurrence and pudendal neurovascular injury compared with sacrospinous ligament suspension, although data are sparse and limited to case series (Meeks et al 1994, Maher et al 2001). Uterosacral ligament suspension is also performed vaginally and, although originally described 80 years ago (Miller 1927), attention has once again started to focus on the uterosacral ligament as a potential site for apical suspension (Shull et al 2000, Silva et al 2006), although ureteric injury remains a concern and randomized trials are needed.

Surgery for anterior compartment prolapse

The traditional procedure for anterior compartment prolapse has been the anterior colporrhaphy (Kelly 1913). Many variations have been described, involving midline plication of the vaginal muscularis and adventitia followed by excision and/or plication of redundant vaginal wall mucosa. Case series have reported success rates of 80–100% for anterior colporrhaphy; however, prospective randomized trials have shown the success of anterior colporrhaphy alone to be only 37–57% (Sand et al 2001, Weber et al 2001). It is likely that such variable rates of success result from the heterogeneous nature of anterior compartment prolapse and different surgical techniques. In addition to midline defects of the endopelvic fascia, lateral or paravaginal defects resulting from detachment of the lateral vaginal wall from the arcus tendineus fascia pelvis ('white line') can also give rise to anterior support abnormalities. This concept of 'site-specific' anterior vaginal wall defects was introduced by George White 100 years ago (White 1909), and subsequently

repopularized by Cullen Richardson in the 1970s (Richardson et al 1976). Originally, this procedure was described as a treatment for stress urinary incontinence, but significant benefits for anterior wall support were demonstrated. Paravaginal repair can be approached both transabdominally and transvaginally, which largely depends on surgeon preference as no direct comparison has been performed. The procedure involves reapproximating the white line with the thickened lateral portion of the fascia overlying the obturator internus muscle. Similar success rates have been reported from both abdominal paravaginal repair (76–97%) and vaginal paravaginal repair (67–100%), although the transvaginal approach is technically more difficult (Brubaker et al 2009). Currently published data on laparoscopic paravaginal repair are sparse; of the studies reported, many include a concomitant Burch colposuspension (Diwadkar et al 2008). In one prospective study, the objective cure rate of laparoscopic paravaginal repair at 14 months was 74% (Behnia-Willison et al 2007).

Given the relatively high failure rate for anterior colporrhaphy and following on from the successful use of grafts in abdominal hernia repair and tension-free vaginal tape, there has been a recent trend towards the use of graft materials in prolapse surgery to augment more traditional repairs (Sung et al 2008, Jakus et al 2008). However, the overall advantage of mesh and other graft materials has not been definitively proven, as the potential benefit in reducing failure rates must be balanced against the risk of mesh-related complications. Indeed, the appropriate use of reconstructive materials in prolapse surgery has become one of the most debated issues in contemporary gynaecological practice, with most authorities acknowledging the risk of adverse events and the lack of data on long-term functional outcomes (Murphy 2008, Brubaker et al 2009). Grafts may be biological (allograft, autograft or xenograft) or synthetic in nature. Synthetic materials are further subclassified as absorbable or non-absorbable and by pore size [macroporous (>75 μm) or microporous (<75 μm)]. A meta-analysis of ten randomized controlled trials found that at 1 year post-operatively, women who had anterior repair with graft use had a lower rate of recurrence than women undergoing standard 'native tissue' repair (odds ratios 0.56 and 0.44 for biological and absorbable synthetic mesh, respectively) (Foon et al 2008).

The risk of mesh-related complications — predominantly mesh erosion, infection, mesh shrinkage and fibrosis — remains a concern (Bako and Dhar 2009, Figure 55.11). Additionally, since 2004, trocar-guided transvaginal surgical mesh 'kits' have gained rapid widespread acceptance due to the suggestion that reconstructive materials in prolapse surgery require 'anchoring' outside of the affected tissues (Elmér et al 2009). A variety of armed mesh kits are currently available, including the Perigee/Apogee (American Medical Systems), the Prolift (Johnson & Johnson) and the Posterior Intravaginal Slingplasty (Tyco Healthcare).

However, randomized data to support the use of mesh kits are sparse. Furthermore, in addition to the risk of 'mesh-related' complications noted above, these kits also have the added risk of 'trocar-related' complications, including bladder/rectal perforation and vascular injury (Feiner et al 2009). A different procedure, using a trocarless mesh and a silicone vaginal device to support the graft during tissue ingrowth, has been described (Carey et al 2008, Figure 55.12).

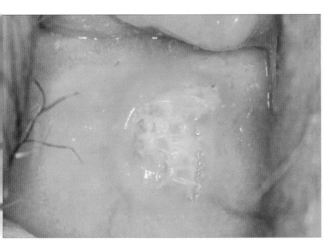

Figure 55.11 Mesh erosion seen on posterior vaginal wall.
Jelovsek JE, Maher C, Barber MD (2007) Pelvic organ prolapse. Lancet 369:1027–38.

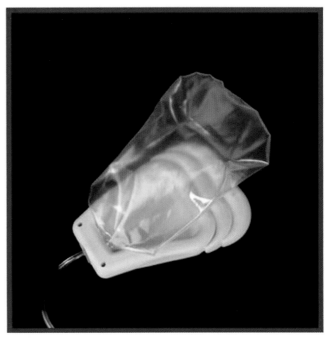

Figure 55.13 Gynecare Prosima, Ethicon, Somerville, NJ, USA.

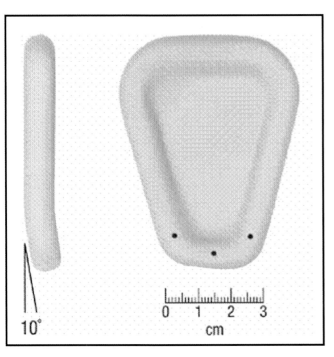

Figure 55.12 Silicone vaginal support device.
Carey M et al. (2008) Vaginal surgery for pelvic organ prolapse using mesh and a vaginal support device. BJOG 115:391–7.

The same authors recently reported a modification of this technique, which uses a silicone device and inflatable balloon to support the mesh repair (Gynecare Prosima, Ethicon, Somerville, NJ, USA; Figure 55.13). A recent multi-centre study described an 88% success rate at 1 year for women with stage II and III prolapse following this procedure. The vaginal support device was shown to be well tolerated (Slack et al 2009).

Surgery for posterior compartment prolapse

The standard surgical procedure for posterior compartment prolapse is the posterior colporrhaphy, involving midline plication of the rectovaginal fascia. The traditional description of this procedure also involves midline plication of the levator ani muscles (Francis and Jeffcoate 1961), although

this can result in high rates of postoperative dyspareunia among sexually active women. Analogous to the anterior compartment, site-specific repair of posterior defects has also been described (Richardson 1993), whereby rectovaginal defects are identified by a rectal finger. A prospective randomized trial found higher anatomical cures at 1 year in the colporrhaphy group (86%) compared with the site-specific repair group (78%) (Paraiso et al 2006). In addition, modification of the standard sacrocolpopexy to include extension of the posterior mesh to the rectovaginal septum or perineal body can also benefit posterior prolapse.

Although gynaecologists conventionally repair posterior compartment prolapse transvaginally in the lithotomy position, the colorectal surgeon typically performs a transanal repair. Level I evidence to support the superiority of the transvaginal repair over the transanal approach has been published (Nieminen et al 2004). There is currently no evidence to support the routine use of graft augmentation in the surgical repair of posterior compartment prolapse (Brubaker et al 2009).

Laparoscopic/robotic pelvic floor repair

A variety of laparoscopic reconstructive procedures have been described which aim to improve anatomical detail, minimize surgical morbidity and reduce hospital stay, while retaining the advantages of the abdominal operation. Paravaginal repair, sacrocolpopexy, enterocele repair and uterosacral ligament suspension have all been described laparoscopcially (Paraiso et al 2006, Behnia-Willison et al 2007). However, in many cases, direct comparison with the gold standard has not been performed, and the efficacy of a standard surgical technique should not be compromised simply so that the procedure can be completed laparoscopically.

To date, robotic surgery has been most widely accepted in urological oncology. Recently, a limited number of publications have described the use of robotic systems in achieving sacrocolpopexy, with 95% success at 24 months, albeit with small numbers (Elliott et al 2006, Akl et al 2009). Robotic-assisted laparoscopic hysterectomy has also been reported (Reynolds and Advincula 2006). It is unlikely, however, that robotics will significantly impact pelvic reconstructive surgery, at least in the short term.

Obliterative surgical procedures

In addition to the reconstructive surgical procedures outlined above, women who do not wish to preserve coital function may be suitable for a vaginal obliterative procedure. Colpocleisis is a relatively straightforward surgery associated with high cure rates and fast recovery times (Hullfish et al 2007). It may be performed in women with or without a uterus, and involves excision of rectangular pieces of vaginal epithelium anteriorly and posteriorly, vaginal inversion and closure with sutures, thus obliterating the vaginal space. Among appropriately selected women, studies have demon-strated low rates of regret for loss of sexual function (Wheeler et al 2005). There is a risk of stress urinary incontinence developing after colpocleisis, and a concomitant midure-thral tape may be appropriate in selected cases.

Conclusions

POP is a significant cause of morbidity among women. It presents a huge disease burden to society which, given the ageing population, is unlikely to abate. Although many women with POP are symptom free, the optimal management of women who desire treatment continues to generate considerable debate among gynaecologists. The appropriate use of graft materials to augment traditional surgical techniques and the role of laparoscopic pelvic floor repair are particular sources of controversy. Good quality, randomized studies to guide practitioners and answer these uncertainties are urgently needed.

KEY POINTS

1. Prolapse is a common condition with a long-term cure rate which may not exceed 70%.
2. Vaginal delivery is the most common cause.
3. Prolapse may affect all compartments and both urinary and anal sphincters, and therefore examination and investigation must include all of these.
4. Validated outcome measures, rather than terms such as 'slight' or 'moderate', should be used.
5. Preventive measures include avoidance of unnecessary lifting, straining at stool and a prolonged second stage of labour.
6. A variety of pessaries are available and should be used when appropriate.
7. Urinary incontinence may be masked by prolapse, and urodynamic studies are advised before prolapse surgery.
8. Surgery for recurrent prolapse may need mesh reinforcement.
9. Complex prolapse should only be attempted by those familiar with, and trained in, prolapse surgery.

References

American College of Obstetricians and Gynecologists 2007 ACOG Practice Bulletin No. 85. Pelvic Organ Prolapse. ACOG, Washington, DC.

Altman D, Forsman M, Falconer C, Lichtenstein P 2008 Genetic influence on stress urinary incontinence and pelvic organ prolapse. European Urology 54: 918–922.

Akl MN, Long JB, Giles DL, et al 2009 Robotic-assisted sacrocolpopexy: technique and learning curve. Surgical Endoscopy 23: 2390–2394.

Arias BE, Ridgeway B, Barber MD 2008 Complications of neglected vaginal pessaries: case presentation and literature review. International Urogynecology Journal and Pelvic Floor Dysfunction 19: 1173–1178.

Bako A, Dhar R 2009 Review of synthetic mesh-related complications in pelvic floor reconstructive surgery. International Urogynecology Journal and Pelvic Floor Dysfunction 20: 103–111.

Barber MD, Visco AG, Wyman JF, Fantl JA, Bump RC 2002 Sexual function in women with urinary incontinence and pelvic organ prolapse. Obstetrics and Gynecology 99: 281–289.

Behnia-Willison F, Seman EI, Cook JR, O'Shea RT, Keirse MJ 2007 Laparoscopic paravaginal repair of anterior compartment prolapse. Journal of Minimally Invasive Gynecology 14: 475–480.

Blandon RE, Bharucha AE, Melton LJ 3rd et al 2007 Incidence of pelvic floor repair after hysterectomy: a population-based cohort study. American Journal of Obstetrics and Gynecology 197: 664.e1–664.e7.

Bø K 2006 Can pelvic floor muscle training prevent and treat pelvic organ prolapse? Acta Obstetricia et Gynecologica Scandinavica 85: 263–268.

Bradley CS, Zimmerman MB, Qi Y, Nygaard IE 2007 Natural history of pelvic organ prolapse in postmenopausal women. Obstetrics and Gynecology 109: 848–854.

Broekhuis SR, Fütterer JJ, Barentsz JO, Vierhout ME, Kluivers KB 2009 A systematic review of clinical studies on dynamic magnetic resonance imaging of pelvic organ prolapse: the use of reference lines and anatomical landmarks. International Urogynecology Journal and Pelvic Floor Dysfunction 20: 721–729.

Brown JS, Waetjen LE, Subak LL, Thom DH, Van den Eeden S, Vittinghoff E 2002 Pelvic organ prolapse surgery in the United States, 1997. American Journal of Obstetrics and Gynecology 186: 712–716.

Brubaker L, Glazener C, Jacquetin B et al 2009 Surgery for pelvic organ prolapse. In: Abrams P, Cardozo L, Koury S et al (eds) 4th International Consultation on Incontinence, Paris, pp 1273–1320.

Bump RC, Mattiasson A, Bø K et al 1996 The standardization of terminology of female pelvic organ prolapse and pelvic floor dysfunction. American Journal of Obstetrics and Gynecology 175: 10–17.

Burrows LJ, Meyn LA, Walters MD, Weber AM 2004 Pelvic symptoms in women with pelvic organ prolapse. Obstetrics and Gynecology 104: 982–988.

Carey M, Slack M, Higgs P, Wynn-Williams M, Cornish A 2008 Vaginal surgery for pelvic organ prolapse using mesh and a vaginal support device. BJOG: an International

Journal of Obstetrics and Gynaecology 115: 391–397.

Chene G, Tardieu AS, Savary D et al 2008 Anatomical and functional results of McCall culdoplasty in the prevention of enteroceles and vaginal vault prolapse after vaginal hysterectomy. International Urogynecology Journal and Pelvic Floor Dysfunction 19: 1007–1011.

Cruikshank SH, Kovac SR 1999 Randomized comparison of three surgical methods used at the time of vaginal hysterectomy to prevent posterior enterocele. American Journal of Obstetrics and Gynecology 180: 859–865.

Cundiff GW, Varner E, Visco AG et al 2008 Risk factors for mesh/suture erosion following sacral colpopexy. American Journal of Obstetrics and Gynecology 199: 688.e1–688.e5.

Cundiff GW, Weidner AC, Visco AG, Bump RC, Addison WA 2000 A survey of pessary use by members of the American Urogynecologic Society. Obstetrics and Gynecology 95: 931–935.

Dällenbach P, Kaelin-Gambirasio I, Jacob S, Dubuisson JB, Boulvain M 2008 Incidence rate and risk factors for vaginal vault prolapse repair after hysterectomy. International Urogynecology Journal and Pelvic Floor Dysfunction 19: 1623–1629.

DeLancey JO 1992 Anatomic aspects of vaginal eversion after hysterectomy. American Journal of Obstetrics and Gynecology 166: 1717–1724.

DeLancey JO 2002 Fascial and muscular abnormalities in women with urethral hypermobility and anterior vaginal wall prolapse. American Journal of Obstetrics and Gynecology 187: 93–98.

de Tayrac R, Gervaise A, Chauveaud-Lambling A, Fernandez H 2004 Combined genital prolapse repair reinforced with a polypropylene mesh and tension-free vaginal tape in women with genital prolapse and stress urinary incontinence: a retrospective case–control study with short-term follow-up. Acta Obstetricia et Gynecologica Scandinavica 83: 950–954.

Dietz HP 2004 Ultrasound imaging of the pelvic floor. Part II: three-dimensional or volume imaging. Ultrasound in Obstetrics and Gynecology 23: 615–625.

Dietz HP 2005 Childbirth and pelvic floor trauma. Best Practice and Research Clinical Obstetrics and Gynaecology 19: 913–924.

Dietz HP 2008a The aetiology of prolapse. International Urogynecology Journal and Pelvic Floor Dysfunction 19: 1323–1329.

Dietz HP 2008b Prolapse worsens with age, doesn't it? Australian and New Zealand Journal of Obstetrics and Gynaecology 48: 587–591.

Digesu GA, Salvatore S, Chaliha C, Athanasiou S, Milani R, Khullar V 2007 Do overactive bladder symptoms improve after repair of anterior vaginal wall prolapse? International Urogynecology Journal and Pelvic Floor Dysfunction 18: 1439–1443.

Diwadkar GB, Chen CC, Paraiso MF 2008 An update on the laparoscopic approach to urogynecology and pelvic reconstructive procedures. Current Opinion in Obstetrics and Gynecology 20: 496–500.

Ellerkmann RM, Cundiff GW, Melick CF, Nihira MA, Leffler K, Bent AE 2001 Correlation of symptoms with location and severity of pelvic organ prolapse. American Journal of Obstetrics and Gynecology 185: 1332–1337.

Elliott DS, Krambeck AE, Chow GK 2006 Long-term results of robotic assisted laparoscopic sacrocolpopexy for the treatment of high grade vaginal vault prolapse. Journal of Urology 176: 655–659.

Elmér C, Altman D, Engh ME, Axelsen S, Väyrynen T, Falconer C 2009 Trocar-guided transvaginal mesh repair of pelvic organ prolapse. Obstetrics and Gynecology 113: 117–126.

Elneil S 2009 Complex pelvic floor failure and associated problems. Best Practice and Research Clinical Gastroenterology 23: 555–573.

Fatton B 2009 Is there any evidence to advocate SUI prevention in continent women undergoing prolapse repair? An overview. International Urogynecology Journal and Pelvic Floor Dysfunction 20: 235–245.

Feiner B, Jelovsek JE, Maher C 2009 Efficacy and safety of transvaginal mesh kits in the treatment of prolapse of the vaginal apex: a systematic review. BJOG: an International Journal of Obstetrics and Gynaecology 116: 15–24.

Foon R, Toozs-Hobson P, Latthe PM 2008 Adjuvant materials in anterior vaginal wall prolapse surgery: a systematic review of effectiveness and complications. International Urogynecology Journal and Pelvic Floor Dysfunction 19: 1697–1706.

Francis WJ, Jeffcoate TN 1961 Dyspareunia following vaginal operations. Journal of Obstetrics and Gynaecology of the British Commonwealth 68: 1–10.

Fritel X, Varnoux N, Zins M, Breart G, Ringa V 2009 Symptomatic pelvic organ prolapse at midlife, quality of life, and risk factors. Obstetrics and Gynecology 113: 609–616.

Ganatra AM, Rozet F, Sanchez-Salas R et al 2009 The current status of laparoscopic sacrocolpopexy: a review. European Urology 55: 1089–1130.

Hagen S, Stark D, Glazener C, Sinclair L, Ramsay I 2009 A randomized controlled trial of pelvic floor muscle training for stages I and II pelvic organ prolapse. International Urogynecology Journal and Pelvic Floor Dysfunction 20: 45–51.

Hall AF, Theofrastous JP, Cundiff GW et al 1996 Interobserver and intraobserver reliability of the proposed International Continence Society, Society of Gynecologic Surgeons, and American Urogynecologic Society pelvic organ prolapse classification system. American Journal of Obstetrics and Gynecology 175: 1467–1470.

Handa VL, Garrett E, Hendrix S, Gold E, Robbins J 2004 Progression and remission of pelvic organ prolapse: a longitudinal study of menopausal women. American Journal of Obstetrics and Gynecology 190: 27–32.

Hanson LA, Schulz JA, Flood CG, Cooley B, Tam F 2006 Vaginal pessaries in managing women with pelvic organ prolapse and urinary incontinence: patient characteristics and factors contributing to success. International Urogynecology Journal and Pelvic Floor Dysfunction 1: 155–159.

Hendrix SL, Clark A, Nygaard I, Aragaki A, Barnabei V, McTiernan A 2002 Pelvic organ prolapse in the Women's Health Initiative: gravity and gravidity. American Journal of Obstetrics and Gynecology 186: 1160–1166.

Hilger WS, Poulson M, Norton PA 2003 Long-term results of abdominal sacrocolpopexy. American Journal of Obstetrics and Gynecology 189: 1606–1610.

Hullfish KL, Bovbjerg VE, Steers WD 2007 Colpocleisis for pelvic organ prolapse: patient goals, quality of life, and satisfaction. Obstetrics and Gynecology 110: 341–345.

Jackson SL, Weber AM, Hull TL, Mitchinson AR, Walters MD 1997 Fecal incontinence in women with urinary incontinence and pelvic organ prolapse. Obstetrics and Gynecology 89: 423–427.

Jakus SM, Shapiro A, Hall CD 2008 Biologic and synthetic graft use in pelvic surgery: a review. Obstetrical and Gynecological Survey 63: 253–266.

Jelovsek JE, Barber MD, Paraiso MF, Walters MD 2005 Functional bowel and anorectal disorders in patients with pelvic organ prolapse and incontinence. American Journal of Obstetrics and Gynecology 193: 2105–2111.

Jelovsek JE, Maher C, Barber MD 2007 Pelvic organ prolapse. The Lancet 369: 1027–1038.

Kelly HA 1913 Incontinence of urine in women. Urologic and Cutaneous Review 17: 291–293.

Kluivers KB, Hendriks JC, Shek C, Dietz HP 2008 Pelvic organ prolapse symptoms in relation to POPQ, ordinal stages and ultrasound prolapse assessment. International Urogynecology Journal and Pelvic Floor Dysfunction 19: 1299–1302.

Kudish BI, Iglesia CB, Sokol RJ et al 2009 Effect of weight change on natural history of pelvic organ prolapse. Obstetrics and Gynecology 113: 81–88.

Law YM, Fielding JR 2008 MRI of pelvic floor dysfunction: review. AJR American Journal of Roentgenology 191: S45–S53.

Lowder JL, Park AJ, Ellison R et al 2008 The role of apical vaginal support in the appearance of anterior and posterior vaginal prolapse. Obstetrics and Gynecology 111: 152–157.

Lukacz ES, Lawrence JM, Contreras R, Nager CW, Luber KM 2006 Parity, mode of delivery, and pelvic floor disorders. Obstetrics and Gynecology 107: 1253–1260.

Maher CF, Murray CJ, Carey MP, Dwyer PL, Ugoni AM 2001 Iliococcygeus or sacrospinous fixation for vaginal vault prolapse. Obstetrics and Gynecology 98: 40–44.

Maher CF, Qatawneh AM, Dwyer PL, Carey MP, Cornish A, Schluter PJ 2004 Abdominal sacral colpopexy or vaginal sacrospinous colpopexy for vaginal vault prolapse: a prospective randomized study. American Journal of Obstetrics and Gynecology 190: 20–26.

Maher C, Baessler K, Glazener CM, Adams EJ, Hagen S 2007 Surgical management of pelvic organ prolapse in women. Cochrane Database of Systematic Reviews 18: CD004014.

Mant J, Painter R, Vessey M 1997 Epidemiology of genital prolapse: observations from the Oxford Family Planning Association Study. BJOG: British Journal of Obstetrics and Gynaecology 104: 579–585.

McLennan MT, Harris JK, Kariuki B, Meyer S 2008 Family history as a risk factor for pelvic organ prolapse. International Urogynecology Journal and Pelvic Floor Dysfunction 19: 1063–1069.

Meeks GR, Washburne JF, McGehee RP, Wiser WL 1994 Repair of vaginal vault prolapse by suspension of the vagina to iliococcygeus (prespinous) fascia. American Journal of Obstetrics and Gynecology 171: 1444–1452.

Miedel A, Tegerstedt G, Maehle-Schmidt M, Nyrén O, Hammarström M 2008 Symptoms and pelvic support defects in specific compartments. Obstetrics and Gynecology 112: 851–858.

Miedel A, Tegerstedt G, Maehle-Schmidt M, Nyrén O, Hammarström M 2009 Nonobstetric risk factors for symptomatic pelvic organ prolapse. Obstetrics and Gynecology 113: 1089–1097.

Miller N 1927 A new method of correcting complete inversion of the vagina. Surgery, Gynecology and Obstetrics 44: 550–554.

Mouritsen L 2005 Classification and evaluation of prolapse. Best Practice and Research Clinical Obstetrics and Gynaecology 19: 895–911.

Murphy M 2008 Clinical practice guidelines on vaginal graft use from the society of gynecologic surgeons. Obstetrics and Gynecology 112: 1123–1130.

Mutone MF, Terry C, Hale DS, Benson JT 2005 Factors which influence the short-term success of pessary management of pelvic organ prolapse. American Journal of Obstetrics and Gynecology 193: 89–94.

Nguyen JK, Bhatia NN 2001 Resolution of motor urge incontinence after surgical repair of pelvic organ prolapse. Journal of Urology 166: 2263–2266.

Nguyen JN, Jones CR 2005 Pessary treatment of pelvic relaxation: factors affecting

successful fitting and continued use. Journal of Wound Ostomy and Continence Nursing 32: 255–261.

Nieminen K, Hiltunen KM, Laitinen J, Oksala J, Heinonen PK 2004 Transanal or vaginal approach to rectocele repair: a prospective, randomized pilot study. Diseases of the Colon and Rectum 47: 1636–1642.

Novi JM, Jeronis S, Morgan MA, Arya LA 2005 Sexual function in women with pelvic organ prolapse compared to women without pelvic organ prolapse. Journal of Urology 173: 1669–1672.

Nygaard IE, McCreery R, Brubaker L et al 2004 Abdominal sacrocolpopexy: a comprehensive review. Obstetrics and Gynecology 104: 805–823.

Nygaard I, Barber MD, Burgio KL et al 2008 Prevalence of symptomatic pelvic floor disorders in US women. Journal of the American Medical Association 300: 1311–1316.

O'Boyle AL, O'Boyle JD, Calhoun B, Davis GD 2005 Pelvic organ support in pregnancy and postpartum. International Urogynecology Journal and Pelvic Floor Dysfunction 16: 69–72.

Olsen AL, Smith VJ, Bergstrom JO, Colling JC, Clark AL 1997 Epidemiology of surgically managed pelvic organ prolapse and urinary incontinence. Obstetrics and Gynecology 89: 501–506.

Paraiso MF, Barber MD, Muir TW, Walters MD 2006 Rectocele repair: a randomized trial of three surgical techniques including graft augmentation. American Journal of Obstetrics and Gynecology 195: 1762–1771.

Pauls RN, Segal JL, Andre Silva W, Kleeman SD, Karram MM 2006 Sexual function in patients presenting to a urogynecology practice. International Urogynecology Journal and Pelvic Floor Dysfunction 17: 576–580.

Powers K, Lazarou G, Wang A et al 2006 Pessary use in advanced pelvic organ prolapse. International Urogynecology Journal and Pelvic Floor Dysfunction 17: 160–164.

Raizada V, Mittal RK 2008 Pelvic floor anatomy and applied physiology. Gastroenterology Clinics of North America 37: 493–509.

Reynolds RK, Advincula AP 2006 Robot-assisted laparoscopic hysterectomy: technique and initial experience. American Journal of Surgery 191: 555–560.

Richardson AC 1993 The rectovaginal septum revisited: its relationship to rectocele and its importance in rectocele repair. Clinical Obstetrics and Gynecology 36: 976–983.

Richardson AC, Lyon JB, Williams NL 1976 A new look at pelvic relaxation. American Journal of Obstetrics and Gynecology 126: 568–573.

Richter HE 2006 Cesarean delivery on maternal request versus planned vaginal delivery: impact on development of pelvic organ prolapse. Seminars in Perinatology 30: 272–275.

Rogers GR, Villarreal A, Kammerer-Doak D, Qualls C 2001 Sexual function in women with and without urinary incontinence and/or pelvic organ prolapse. International Urogynecology Journal and Pelvic Floor Dysfunction 12: 361–365.

Rooney K, Kenton K, Mueller ER, FitzGerald MP, Brubaker L 2006 Advanced anterior vaginal wall prolapse is highly correlated with apical prolapse. American Journal of Obstetrics and Gynecology 195: 1837–1840.

Roovers JP, Oelke M 2007 Clinical relevance of urodynamic investigation tests prior to surgical correction of genital prolapse: a literature review. International Urogynecology Journal and Pelvic Floor Dysfunction 18: 455–460.

Rortveit G, Brown JS, Thom DH, Van Den Eeden SK, Creasman JM, Subak LL 2007 Symptomatic pelvic organ prolapse: prevalence and risk factors in a population-based, racially diverse cohort. Obstetrics and Gynecology 109: 1396–1403.

Royal College of Obstetricians and Gynaecologists 2007 Green-Top Guideline No. 46. The Management of Post-hysterectomy Vaginal Vault Prolapse. RCOG, London.

Samuelsson EC, Arne Victor FT, Tibblin G, Svardsudd KF 1999 Signs of genital prolapse in a Swedish population of women 20 to 59 years of age and possible related factors. American Journal of Obstetrics and Gynecology 180: 299–305.

Sand PK, Koduri S, Lobel RW et al 2001 Prospective randomized trial of polyglactin 910 mesh to prevent recurrence of cystoceles and rectoceles. American Journal of Obstetrics and Gynecology 184: 1357–1362.

Shah SM, Sultan AH, Thakar R 2006 The history and evolution of pessaries for pelvic organ prolapse. International Urogynecology Journal and Pelvic Floor Dysfunction 17: 170–175.

Shull BL, Bachofen C, Coates KW, Kuehl TJ 2000 A transvaginal approach to repair of apical and other associated sites of pelvic organ prolapse with uterosacral ligaments. American Journal of Obstetrics and Gynecology 183: 1365–1373.

Singh K, Reid WM 2001 Non-surgical treatment of uterovaginal prolapse using double vaginal rings. BJOG: an International Journal of Obstetrics and Gynaecology 108: 112–113.

Silva WA, Pauls RN, Segal JL, Rooney CM, Kleeman SD, Karram MM 2006 Uterosacral ligament vault suspension: five-year outcomes. Obstetrics and Gynecology 108: 255–263.

Slack M, Zyczynski H, Reisenauer C et al 2009 A new operation for vaginal prolapse repair using mesh and a vaginal support device: 1 year anatomic and functional results of an international multicentre study. International Urogynecology Journal and Pelvic Floor Dysfunction 20 (Suppl): S157–S158.

Smith PP, Appell RA 2005 Pelvic organ prolapse and the lower urinary tract: the relationship of vaginal prolapse to stress urinary incontinence. Current Urology Reports 6: 340–347.

Steensma AB, Oom DM, Burger CW Rudolph Schouten W 2009 Assessment of posterior compartment prolapse; a comparison of evacuation proctography and 3D transperineal ultrasound. Colorectal Disease 12: 533–539.

Subak LL, Wing R, West DS et al 2009 Weight loss to treat urinary incontinence in overweight and obese women. New England Journal of Medicine 360: 481–490.

Subramanian D, Szwarcensztein K, Mauskopf JA, Slack MC 2009 Rate, type, and cost of pelvic organ prolapse surgery in Germany, France, and England. European Journal of Obstetrics, Gynecology and Reproductive Biology 144: 177–181.

Sung VW, Rogers RG, Schaffer JI et al 2008 Graft use in transvaginal pelvic organ prolapse repair: a systematic review. Obstetrics and Gynecology 112: 1131–1142.

Swift SE, Herring M 1998 Comparison of pelvic organ prolapse in the dorsal lithotomy compared with the standing position. Obstetrics and Gynecology 91: 961–964.

Swift SE, Tate SB, Nicholas J 2003 Correlation of symptoms with degree of pelvic organ support in a general population of women: what is pelvic organ prolapse? American Journal of Obstetrics and Gynecology 189: 372–377.

Sze EH, Karram MM 1997 Transvaginal repair of vault prolapse: a review. Obstetrics and Gynecology 89: 466–467.

Sze EH, Sherard GB 3rd, Dolezal JM 2002 Pregnancy, labor, delivery, and pelvic organ prolapse. Obstetrics and Gynecology 100: 981–986.

Taylor SA 2009 Imaging pelvic floor dysfunction. Best Practice and Research Clinical Gastroenterology 23: 487–503.

Tegerstedt G, Maehle-Schmidt M, Nyrén O, Hammarström M 2005 Prevalence of symptomatic pelvic organ prolapse in a Swedish population. International Urogynecology Journal and Pelvic Floor Dysfunction 16: 497–503.

Tegerstedt G, Miedel A, Maehle-Schmidt M, Nyrén O, Hammarström M 2006 Obstetric risk factors for symptomatic prolapse: a population-based approach. American Journal of Obstetrics and Gynecology 194: 75–81.

Thakar R 2009 Review of current status of female sexual dysfunction evaluation in urogynecology. International Urogynecology Journal and Pelvic Floor Dysfunction 20 (Suppl 1): S27–S31.

Uma R, Libby G, Murphy DJ 2005 Obstetric management of a woman's first delivery and the implications for pelvic floor surgery in later life. BJOG: an International Journal of Obstetrics and Gynaecology 112: 1043–1046.

Visco AG, Brubaker L, Nygaard I et al 2008 The role of preoperative urodynamic testing in stress-continent women undergoing sacrocolpopexy: the Colpopexy and Urinary Reduction Efforts (CARE) randomized surgical trial. International Urogynecology Journal and Pelvic Floor Dysfunction 19: 607–614.

Weber AM 2007 Elective cesarean delivery: the pelvic perspective. Clinical Obstetrics and Gynecology 50: 510–517.

Weber AM, Walters MD, Schover LR, Mitchinson A 1995 Vaginal anatomy and sexual function. Obstetrics and Gynecology 86: 946–949.

Weber AM, Walters MD, Piedmonte MR, Ballard LA 2001 Anterior colporrhaphy: a randomized trial of three surgical techniques. American Journal of Obstetrics and Gynecology 185: 1299–1304.

Wheeler TL 2nd, Richter HE, Burgio KL et al 2005 Regret, satisfaction, and symptom improvement: analysis of the impact of partial colpocleisis for the management of severe pelvic organ prolapse. American Journal of Obstetrics and Gynecology 193: 2067–2070.

Whitcomb EL, Lukacz ES, Lawrence JM, Nager CW, Luber KM 2009 Prevalence and degree of bother from pelvic floor disorders in obese women. International Urogynecology Journal and Pelvic Floor Dysfunction 20: 289–294.

White GR 1909 Cystocele: a radical cure by suturing lateral sulci of vagina to white line of pelvic fascia. Journal of the American Medical Association 21: 1707–1710.

Yalcin OT, Yildirim A, Hassa H 2001 The effects of severe cystocele on urogynecologic symptoms and findings. Acta Obstetricia et Gynecologica Scandinavica 80: 423–427.

CHAPTER 56

Frequency, urgency and the painful bladder

Michelle M. Fynes and Stergios K. Doumouchtsis

Chapter Contents

INTRODUCTION	864		ASSESSMENT	865
DEFINITIONS	864		TREATMENT	868
PREVALENCE	865		SUMMARY	872
AETIOLOGY	865		KEY POINTS	872

Introduction

'Cystitis' is a term used for irritative urinary symptoms of frequency, urgency, suprapubic pain and dysuria. These symptoms of altered lower urinary tract sensation may be of recent onset (acute), longstanding (chronic) or recurrent. They may be caused by a variety of intravesical pathology such as infection, calculi, drug-induced inflammation, non-infective inflammatory processes due to local [e.g. painful bladder syndrome (PBS)] or systemic conditions (e.g. sarcoidosis), benign or malignant lower urinary tract tumours, or extravesical pelvic pathology such as pelvic masses (e.g. fibroids, endometriosis). Accurate diagnosis, appropriate intervention and therapy requires careful patient evaluation and a sound understanding of the differential causes (Figure 56.1).

Women with longstanding or recurrent chronic symptoms are often treated as recurrent bacterial cystitis. Often, it is only after a poor response to antibiotics or failure to culture uropathogens that an alternative diagnosis is considered. It is essential that these women have a thorough evaluation to exclude any serious underlying pathology (e.g. carcinoma) so that effective treatment can be commenced. Women with chronic irritative symptoms frequently have conditions such as PBS (formerly known as 'interstitial cystitis') or urethral syndrome. The pathogenesis for these conditions is poorly understood, and response to current therapy is often unsatisfactory.

Definitions

The Standardisation Sub-committee of the International Continence Society (ICS) published a terminology statement on lower urinary tract function in 2002 (Abrams et al 2002a,b). The majority of the following definitions are based on this statement.

Urgency is the complaint of a sudden compelling desire to pass urine which is difficult to defer. Overactive bladder (OAB) syndrome, urge syndrome or urge-frequency syndrome is characterized by urgency with or without urge incontinence, usually with frequency and nocturia. These symptom combinations are suggestive of urodynamically demonstrable detrusor overactivity, but may be due to other forms of urethrovesical dysfunction. These terms can be used in the absence of proven infection or other obvious pathology.

Daytime frequency is the number of voids recorded during waking hours, and includes the last void before sleep and the first void after waking and rising in the morning. Increased daytime frequency is the complaint by the patient who considers that he/she voids too often during the day.

Nocturia is the complaint that the individual has to wake at night, once or more, to void. In other words, it is the number of voids recorded during a night's sleep; each void is preceded and followed by sleep.

24-h frequency is the total number of daytime voids and episodes of nocturia during a 24-h period.

Bladder pain can be severe and frequently ill defined with radiation to the vagina and rectum. It is often aggravated by bladder distension, sexual intercourse, spicy foods, alcohol and caffeine, and relieved by voiding.

Dysuria is urethral pain during micturition and may be secondary to obvious pathology such as infection or a urethral diverticulum, or less clear causes such as atrophic urethritis or urethral syndrome.

Haematuria is an important symptom that requires urgent evaluation to exclude carcinoma.

PBS is the complaint of suprapubic pain related to bladder filling accompanied by other symptoms such as increased daytime and night-time frequency, in the absence of proven urinary infection or other pathology. The ICS believes this to be a preferable term to 'interstitial cystitis'. Interstitial

DOI: 10.1016/B978-0-7020-3120-5.00056-4

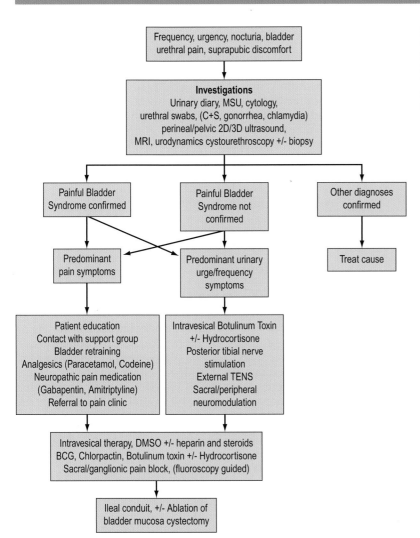

Figure 56.1 **Figure 56.1** Management strategy for women presenting with intractable lower urinary tract symptoms. MSU, midstream urine sample; 2D, two dimensional; 3D, three dimensional; MRI, magnetic resonance imaging; TENS, transcutaneous electrical nerve stimulation; BCG, bacillus Calmette-Guérin; DMSO, dimethyl sulfoxide; C+S, culture and sensitivity.

cystitis is a specific diagnosis requiring confirmation by the typical cystoscopic and histological features.

Urethral pain syndrome is recurrent episodic urethral pain, usually on voiding, with daytime frequency and nocturia in the absence of proven infection or other pathology.

Prevalence

A population-based study on the prevalence of lower urinary tract symptoms showed that the most commonly reported storage symptom in women is nocturia (54.5%). Urgency occurs in 12.8% and frequency in 7.4% of women. If nocturia is defined as two or more nocturnal micturitions per night, instead of one or more, the prevalence is decreased to 24% (Irwin et al 2006). PBS is a common condition in women, with reported prevalence of 1.7% in those aged under 65 years and 4% in those aged over 80 years. The vast majority of women with PBS have moderate or severe symptoms (Lifford and Curhan 2009).

Aetiology

Irritative bladder symptoms can be caused by a number of conditions originating within the lower urinary tract (Box

56.1). Infection and functional disorders, such as detrusor overactivity or voiding dysfunction, may cause urge symptoms and should be excluded. These conditions should be differentiated from more generalized systemic disorders (e.g. pregnancy, diabetes mellitus, renal disease), pelvic inflammatory disease or gynaecological surgery. A pelvic mass may cause urge-frequency symptoms due to bladder compression.

The aetiology of PBS is poorly understood. Several theories have been proposed over the years, including infection, immunological factors, leaky urothelium due to glycosaminoglycan deficiency, mast cell activation and altered neural function. Consensus is developing regarding epithelial dysfunction, mast cell activation and neurogenic inflammation; all part of a possible inflammatory response (Elgavish 2009).

Assessment

History

A detailed history should include specific questions regarding gynaecological and urinary symptoms. Frequency, urgency and nocturia in association with incontinence are likely to reflect underlying detrusor overactivity. In contrast,

Box 56.1 Non-infective sensory disorders of the lower urinary tract

Inflammatory bladder conditions

- PBS/interstitial cystitis
- Drug-induced cystitis
- Chemical cystitis
- Eosinophilic cystitis
- Granulomatous cystitis
- Radiation cystitis

Non-malignant conditions affecting the lower urinary tract

- Proliferative
  - Cystitis cystica
  - Cystitis glandularis
- Metaplastic
  - Keratinizing and non-keratinizing squamous metaplasia
  - Intestinal metaplasia
- Other
  - Endometriosis
  - Nephrogenic adenomatosis
  - Amyloidosis

Benign and malignant bladder and urethral tumours

- Papillomas
- Polyps
- Carcinoma *in situ*
- Bladder and urethral carcinoma (primary or secondary)
- Benign and malignant non-epithelial tumours

Miscellaneous

- Bladder or urethral calculi
- Urethrovesical foreign bodies (e.g. sutures, mesh erosion)
- Urethral diverticulum
- Atrophic urethritis
- Urethral mucosal prolapse
- Urethral caruncle
- Acute and chronic urethral syndromes
- Reiter's syndrome

chronic severe urgency and bladder pain without incontinence are likely to be secondary to intravesical pathology such as infective or non-infective cystitis. A history of present and past medications [e.g. diuretics, tiaprofenic acid (Surgam) and cyclophosphamide], previous urinary tract infection (UTI) and pelvic surgery should be sought. Predisposing or exacerbating factors may include sexual intercourse (e.g. 'honeymoon cystitis'), barrier contraception (e.g. diaphragm, condoms) and contact irritants (e.g. vaginal douches, spermicidal agents). More general irritant factors can include washing powder, soaps and gels.

Voiding dysfunction should be suspected with symptoms of hesitancy, poor urinary stream, straining and incomplete bladder emptying. Impaired bladder emptying due to detrusor underactivity or urethral obstruction may be idiopathic or secondary to neurological disease, pelvic surgery or uterovaginal prolapse.

Examination

Abdominal examination may reveal a palpable bladder secondary to urinary retention, pelvic mass or bladder tenderness from cystitis. Neurological examination with directed assessment of the S2–4 nerve roots, which innervate the bladder, should be performed. Vaginal examination using a Sims speculum allows visualization of the anterior and posterior walls, and may reveal genital prolapse, atrophy, inflammation or infection. Urethral inspection may reveal a mass, mucosal prolapse or caruncle. Paraurethral masses can be identified on bimanual examination by compressing the urethral and paraurethral tissues against the back of the pubic symphysis; expression of urethral pus suggests a urethral diverticulum.

Investigations

Urinary diary

A detailed 3-day urinary frequency–volume diary is an important part of the initial and ongoing assessment (Figure 56.2). These diaries are more accurate than patient recall, allowing rapid and accurate diagnosis of urinary frequency, nocturia, estimation of voided volumes, functional bladder capacity, and assessment of episodes of urgency, pain and incontinence as well as their temporal relationship. A diary will also educate the patient regarding voiding habits, and is essential for bladder retraining.

Microbiology

Midstream urine sample (MSU) for microscopy, culture and sensitivity, and cytology will diagnose a UTI, confirming or excluding the presence of leukocytes, nitrites, red blood cells and any abnormal tumour cells shed from a bladder cancer. Isolated haematuria with a negative MSU may be caused by inflammatory cystitis or carcinoma, and is an indication for cystoscopy.

Urethral swabs are indicated where the MSU is negative and there is urethral tenderness, discharge or the patient is sexually active. In these cases, appropriate culture media should also be used for *Chlamydia trachomatis* and *Neisseria gonorrhoeae*. Other organisms commonly identified include coliforms and *Staphylococcus saprophyticus*. Tuberculosis is still prevalent, especially in developing countries, and should be considered with persistent sterile cystitis and pyuria. Diagnosis is based on a positive Lowernstein–Jensen culture using three early morning urine specimens.

Urodynamics

Urodynamic studies should be considered once infection has been excluded and symptoms have not responded to conservative treatment, especially if urinary incontinence is an associated problem. Uroflowmetry measures the voided volume, and maximum and average flow rates, and also records the voiding pattern. Filling cystometry gives information on bladder sensation, compliance and detrusor contractility, and may identify underlying stress incontinence, detrusor overactivity or voiding dysfunction. A diagnosis of bladder hypersensitivity is based on the following findings at urodynamics: stable bladder, capacity less than 350 ml

URODYNAMIC UNIT

Dept. of Obstetrics & Gynaecology
St. George's Hospital,

Cranmer Terrace
London, SW17 0RE
Telephone: 081-672 1255 Ext.55981

URINARY DIARY

NAME..........................

UNIT NO ....

WEEK BEGINNING ..JANUARY 2009....

CHART NO............................

Instructions

This chart is designed to help us assess and treat your urinary problems. It will only help us to help you if you take time to fill it in accurately.

Please enter the amount each time you pass urine (measured by jug) or drink any liquid.

e.g. 1 cupful = 6 oz. or 175 ml
      1 tumblerful = 7 oz. or 200 ml
      1 soupbowl = 11 oz. or 300 ml

If you leak urine try to estimate the amount (1 = few drops; 2 = soaked underwear; 3 = emptied bladder). Also note whether you had any warning or urge to pass urine at that time.

Use a blue pen for daytime records and a red pen after you retire to bed.

DAY:

TIME	INTAKE (ml)	OUTPUT (ml)	ACTIVITY	Amount	Urge	Wet Bed
03:00		200	~~crossed out~~			
05:30		250				
06:00	250					
07:00		200	WALKING	++	✓	
07:30	200					
08:30	200					
09:00		100	SHOPPING	+	✓	
10:30	200					
11:00		150	WORKING	+	✓	
12:30	300					
13:30		250	GARDENING	++	✓	
16:00	200					
16:30		200				
18:00		150				
18:30	250					
19:30	250					
20:30	200					
21:00		300	BATHING	+	✓	
22:00		150				

DAY:

TIME	INTAKE (ml)	OUTPUT (ml)	ACTIVITY	Amount	Urge
04:00	100	150			
06:00	250				
06:10		300			
08:00	250				
08:30		200	WALKING	+	✓
09:30		100			
10:30	250				
11:30	250				
12:00		300			
13:00	250				
13:30		150	WALKING	++	✓
16:00		250			
16:30	250				
18:00		150			
18:40	250				
20:00	250				
21:00		250			
21:30	250				
22:00		150			
24:00	100	150	SLEEPING	+	✓
04:00	100	300			

Figure 56.2 Urinary frequency–volume diary.

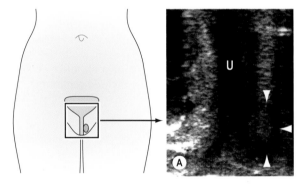

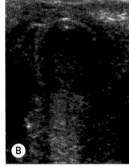

Figure 56.3 Transperineal high-frequency ultrasound and corresponding line diagram demonstrating a large urethral diverticulum. U, urethra. (A) The arrows indicate the paraurethral lesion (diverticulum. (B) Enlarged ulltrasound image of the diverticulum in (A) demonstrating mixed reflective echogenic pattern.

and urgency at less than 150 ml. Both urodynamic assessment and a urinary diary will give an indication of functional bladder capacity and the severity of bladder hypersensitivity. Women with severe PBS/interstitial cystitis are frequently unable to hold more than 50–100 ml.

Imaging

Imaging of the urinary tract can be performed using ultrasound or contrast radiography, either alone or synchronously with urodynamic assessment [videocystourethrography (VCU)]. VCU demonstrates voiding function and can identify urethral obstruction, a urethral diverticulum or external compression due to fibroids or prolapse. Haematuria in the absence of identifiable uropathogens, negative cystoscopy or recurrent UTI is an indication for assessment of the upper urinary tract using contrast intravenous urography or urinary tract ultrasound. Ultrasound can also determine bladder residual volume and bladder wall thickness, and identify any structural abnormalities, including urethral diverticulae (Figure 56.3) (Doumouchtsis et al 2008).

In women with recurrent UTI, 5% have an abnormality of the urinary tract (e.g. calculus, duplex system, tumour). In women with irritative lower urinary tract symptoms and a paraurethral mass, a micturating cystogram or double balloon contrast urethrogram may identify a communicating tract with a urethral diverticulum. Transperineal ultrasound provides comparable information, is less invasive and allows differentiation between solid (e.g. fibroid, lipoma), cystic lesions (diverticulum, Skene's cyst or abscess, Gartner's duct cyst) and vascular lesions (haemangioma, fibroid). Mixed echogenic contents suggest an infected diverticulum or paraurethral abscess.

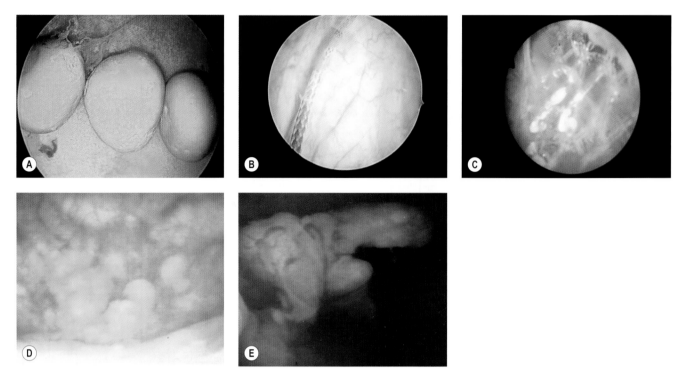

Figure 56.4 Cystoscopy. (A) Bladder calculi. (B) Suture material in bladder. (C) Urethral mesh erosion. (D) Postmenopausal recurrent bacterial cystitis. Squamous metaplasia/cystitis cystica involving trigone and above (benign). Treated with topical oestrogens and rotational antibiotic prophylaxis. (E) Trabeculation, bladder tumour of the right side of bladder wall (malignant). Transurethral resection of bladder tumour undertaken.

Plain abdominal X-ray will demonstrate 90% of calculi present in the kidney, ureters or bladder due to the presence of calcium or cystine. Computed tomography (urogram or magnetic resonance imaging) may be required to provide accurate imaging of upper and lower urinary tract pathology. The automated bladder ultrasound machine is a simple, inexpensive tool used to measure urinary residual volume. However, it does have relatively poor sensitivity for volumes of less than 100 ml or more than 400 ml. In addition, artefacts may be introduced by the presence of pelvic pathology (e.g. uterine fibroids, pelvic haematoma, ovarian cysts) (Cooperberg et al 2000). The automated bladder ultrasound machine is a useful screening tool in older women with urge-frequency syndrome and/or recurrent cystitis with suspected voiding difficulty.

Cystourethroscopy

Evaluation of the lower urinary tract by cystourethroscopy is an essential skill for all gynaecological surgeons, not only in the assessment of urinary symptoms and pain but during pelvic surgery for the prevention and early treatment of bladder and urethral injury. Cystoscopy is undertaken in an inpatient or outpatient setting using a flexible or rigid system. Rigid cystosocopy is well tolerated by women under local anaesthetic in an outpatient setting (Lee et al 2009). Cystoscopy is indicated for haematuria, abnormal urinary cytology, recurrent UTI or persistent symptoms despite conservative treatment. At cystourethroscopy, the lower urinary tract should be carefully visualized using a 70° or 30° scope for the bladder and a 0° scope with Sasche sheath for the urethra. Features such as mucosal trabeculation, bladder diverticula, tumours, squamous metaplasia, bladder calculi

and foreign bodies are readily identifiable (Figure 56.4). Women with misplaced intravesical sutures (e.g. colposuspension), eroded mesh following slings for incontinence or grafts for prolapse surgery, exposed urethral bulking agents or sterile abscess (e.g. Zuidex) may present with urgency, bladder pain and/or recurrent UTI. A biopsy should be taken of any suspicious localized lesions to exclude carcinoma.

Miscellaneous

Renal function, endocrine profile, glucose tolerance test, serum calcium or urinary osmolality tests may be indicated, especially in the presence of polyuria and polydipsia. This is usually detected by a urinary diary. If any of these investigations are positive, referral to an appropriate specialist for further investigation is necessary.

Treatment

For women with idiopathic urge-frequency syndrome, simple patient education with reduction of caffeine, fluid or alcohol intake, adjustment of diuretic or other medications, and bladder retraining with or without anticholinergic agents is effective (50–70%). The aim of bladder retraining is to normalize voiding habits by encouraging increased voided volumes and time between micturitions. If symptoms are severe or do not respond to conservative treatment, further evaluation, particularly with cystourethroscopy, is warranted to identify treatable causes. Cystodistension is not effective in the longer term and may cause bladder perforation. Women with frequency, urgency and bladder pain with reduced functional bladder capacity on urinary diary and urodynamic assessment may have PBS. Typically, these women will have changes at cystoscopy (petechial haemorrhages on empty and refill, erythema, fissuring).

Painful bladder syndrome/interstitial cystitis

The European Society for the Study of Interstitial Cystitis (ESSIC) recently proposed the term 'bladder pain syndrome/interstitial cystitis' (van de Merwe et al 2008). Guy Hunner first described this condition in 1914, and the mucosal tearing and fissuring which he described as an 'ulcer' carries his name. PBS/interstitial cystitis is a chronic bladder condition seen mainly in women (10:1 female:male ratio). The main presenting symptoms are frequency, urgency, nocturia and bladder pain, which often increase as the bladder fills and reduce after micturition. Pain may be experienced in the urethra, loin area and/or perineum. Chronic pelvic pain, dyspareunia and dysmenorrhoea are also common symptoms, and coexistence with other causes of pelvic pain (e.g. endometriosis) is well recognized. There are cystoscopic and histological features which are considered typical, but in many cases, the diagnosis is one of exclusion, having ruled out specific causes such as infection and malignancy.

OAB shows some similarity in its clinical presentation but without the pain, which is the defining symptom of PBS/interstitial cystitis.

The reported prevalence of PBS/interstitial cystitis varies widely due to different diagnostic criteria. It has been estimated at 18 per 100,000 women in Finland (Oravisto 1975), eight to 16 per 100,000 in the Netherlands (Bade et al 1995), 30 per 100,000 in 1987 in the USA, and 865 per 100,000 women in 1994 in the USA (Rosamilia 2005). Delay between onset of symptoms and diagnosis can be 5–7 years. Leppilahti et al (2005) found that the prevalence of clinically confirmed probable interstitial cystitis in women was 230/100,000 and the prevalence of possible/probable interstitial cystitis was 530/100,000.

The pathophysiology is poorly understood and the condition is considered multifactorial (Nickel 2002). Proposed aetiologies include an infective agent, allergic or autoimmune conditions, 'leaky' urothelium secondary to a defective glycosaminoglycan layer, urinary toxins, lymphatic or vascular abnormalities and neurogenic inflammation. Any of these pathological changes may be a result rather than cause of the disease process. Loss of integrity at the epithelial surface of the bladder, secondary to an infective or other inflammatory insult, has been implicated along with sensory nerve upregulation and enhanced mast cell activation (Sant 2002), resulting in regional neuropathy. Other gynaecological and gastrointestinal manifestations may be present, including pain and voiding symptoms (Nickel 2002).

The ESSIC group (van de Merwe et al 2008) proposed that a diagnosis of PBS should be made on the basis of exclusion of confusable diseases and by the recognition of the specific combination of symptoms and signs of PBS. Confusable diseases include carcinoma, infection, urethral diverticulum, prolapse, endometriosis, OAB and pudendal nerve entrapment. Symptoms and signs for use in diagnostic criteria do not need to be specific. On the contrary, if a specific symptom or sign existed for the target disease, a diagnosis would only require the presence of the specific feature, and diagnostic criteria would not be necessary. PBS should be diagnosed on the basis of chronic (>6 months) pelvic pain, pressure or discomfort perceived to be related to the urinary bladder, accompanied by at least one other urinary symptom such as persistent urge to void or frequency. Further classification of PBS is based on findings at cystoscopy using hydrodistension and bladder biopsies. Cystoscopic features accepted as positive signs are glomerulations, Hunner's lesions or both (Figure 56.5). Hunner's lesion is 'a circumscript, reddened mucosal area with small vessels radiating towards a central scar, with a fibrin deposit or coagulum attached. This site ruptures with increasing bladder distension, with petechial oozing of blood from the lesion and mucosal margins in a waterfall manner. A rather typical, slightly bullous edema develops post-distension with varying peripheral extension'. Biopsy findings accepted as positive signs of PBS are inflammatory infiltrates and/or granulation tissue and/or detrusor mastocytosis and/or intrafascicular fibrosis (van de Merwe et al 2008). Only 50% of cases have positive histopathology findings, and the purpose of biopsy is often to exclude malignancy.

As the aetiology of the syndrome is multifactorial, treatment efficacy may vary among different patients, and multiple treatment modalities are often necessary, directed at different disease processes (e.g. bladder retraining, neuromodulation, polypharmacy), if a successful outcome is to be achieved. Although many options are available for controlling symptoms, cures are rare and relapse is common. Sympathetic support by family, medical staff and self-help groups are invaluable. In order to identify the most effective treatment for a patient, they should be tried one at a time. Limited evidence is available from randomized controlled trials. A placebo effect is probably significant in these treatment modalities.

A simple treatment is dietary manipulation. Eliminating substances that may cause bladder inflammation can help some patients (e.g. caffeine, spicy foods). Other non-invasive measures include bladder retraining and relaxation techniques in order to gradually prolong the time periods between voids.

There are several oral or intravesical options with variable efficacy, and to date there is no consensus regarding which treatment is best. Pentosan polysulfate sodium (Elmiron) is a polysaccharide which decreases urothelial permeability by substituting for a defect in the glycosaminoglycan layer. The recommended oral dose is 100 mg three times a day between meals. Response to treatment is likely to be slow, and patients may not notice any benefit until several months of treatment. Antihistamines prevent activation of mast cells. Cimetidine, an H_2 receptor antagonist, has also been tried with variable results. Tricyclic antidepressants have anticholinergic, analgesic and sedative effects on the bladder. Amitriptyline has also shown some benefit. The dose can be increased up to 100 mg. Anticholinergic drugs may be effective, especially if frequency and urgency are predominant symptoms. Oxybutynin has been used orally as well as intravesically. Dimethyl sulfoxide is a chemical solvent that is used intravesically. It penetrates cell membranes and has anti-inflammatory, analgesic and muscle-relaxant properties. It is thought to inhibit mast cells and dissolve collagen. The treatment is repeated at intervals of 2 weeks. Over 50% symptom improvement is common with this

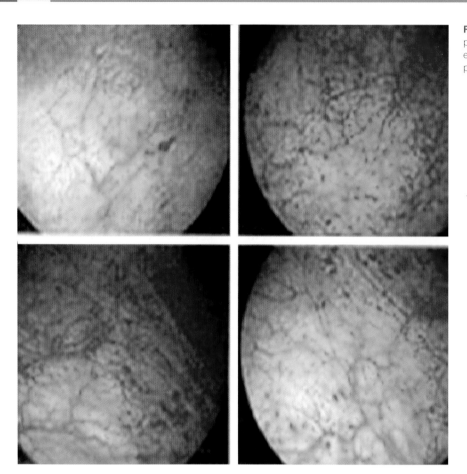

Figure 56.5 Cystoscopic images demonstrating progressive petechial haemorrhaging on bladder emptying under direct vision in a patient with painful bladder syndrome/interstitial cystitis.

treatment, which may be long lasting. Intravesical heparin instillation has also been used, but the evidence for its efficacy is poor. Other medications include bacillus Calmette-Guérin (BCG), hyaluronic acid, chondroitin sulphate and resiniferatoxin.

Botulinum toxin A has been used in the treatment of PBS with variable results. A Cochrane review on intravesical therapy showed that BCG and oxybutynin are reasonably well tolerated, and evidence is most promising for these. Resiniferatoxin has limited efficacy and causes pain, reducing treatment compliance (Dawson and Jamison 2007). Major urological surgery involving ulcer resection, bladder denervation, and partial or total cystectomy with urinary diversion should be considered as a last resort.

Drug-induced cystitis

The bladder is susceptible to the adverse effects of drugs because of the excretion of several drug metabolites in the urine. A history of present and past medications is important as drug-induced cystitis can occur immediately following administration or may manifest many years later. The term 'drug-induced cystitis' is therefore dependent on evidence of the onset of irritative symptoms and inflammatory changes at cystoscopy following drug administration, resolution following withdrawal, and recurrence with readministration of the drug. Implicated drugs include cyclophosphamide, tiaprofenic acid (Surgam), sulphasalazine, fenfluramine, fluoxetine, simvastatin, danazol and a number of non-

steroidal anti-inflammatory drugs. Drugs that cause cystitis should be withdrawn if a patient develops irritative symptoms or haematuria. Adverse effects of cyclophosphamide can be reduced with prophylactic administration of Mesna (2-meracaptoethane sulfonate sodium) and adequate hydration. Mitomycin, doxorubicin or BCG instilled locally to treat bladder tumours can also cause cystitis, contracture and calcification. Their administration should therefore be limited to 1 h/week for a maximum of 8 weeks (Drake et al 1998).

Radiation cystitis

Radiation cystitis may occur as an early or late complication. The bladder can be irradiated intentionally for the treatment of bladder cancer, or incidentally for the treatment of pelvic malignancies. Radiation cystitis is characterized by dysuria and increased urinary frequency (Chuang et al 2008). Acute cystitis is caused by the inflammatory response to radiation, and consists of urgency, frequency, dysuria and haematuria. Chronic cystitis is the end result of the inflammatory process. Ischaemia and fibrosis may result in a small contracted nonfunctional bladder with severe frequency, urgency and incontinence. Radiation cystitis can range from minor temporary irritative voiding symptoms to severe haematuria, incontinence, fistula formation, necrosis and death. The total single dose, duration of radiotherapy, treatment cycle, preceding surgery, pre-existent infection and previous radiotherapy all influence the risk of radiation cystitis.

Eosinophilic cystitis

Eosinophilic cystitis is a rare inflammatory condition of the bladder which has been associated with allergy, bladder tumours, bladder injury, infections and drugs. It is characterized by the antigen–antibody reaction and probably represents a type 1 hypersensitivity reaction to exogenous allergens. Transmural inflammation of the bladder, predominantly with eosinophils, is followed by fibrosis in the chronic phase. Affected individuals typically have a history of atopy and present with frequency, dysuria, suprapubic pain, haematuria, proteinuria and pyuria. Eosinophiluria occurs in 30% of cases, but up to 50% will have a raised serum eosinophil count. Cystoscopy and biopsy are the gold standard for diagnosis. Medical therapy, such as non-steroidal anti-inflammatory agents or steroids, may provide symptomatic relief, but long-term follow-up is mandatory as the lesion tends to recur (Teegavarapu et al 2005).

Granulomatous cystitis

This condition may arise following bladder resection, bladder biopsy, bacterial infection or BCG instillation, and should be distinguished from tuberculosis. The patient may be asymptomatic or present with haematuria, frequency, urgency and pain. Discrete plaques or nodules may be evident at cystoscopy. At histology, diffuse granulomas or histiocytic inflammation are usually identified.

Proliferative and metaplastic lesions of the bladder

'Brunn's nests', cystitis cystica, cystitis glandularis and squamous metaplasia are common findings at cystoscopy, which are likely to represent normal histological variants. They are usually located on the trigone and anterior wall of the female bladder. Coexistent symptoms of frequency, urgency or bladder pain are more likely to be associated with infection or other inflammatory pathology.

Proliferative cystitis typically starts with 'Brunn's nests', which are clusters of pale yellow cells, 1–5 mm in diameter, within the lamina propria. These lesions are usually confined to the trigone but may be diffuse; differentiation from carcinoma requires biopsy for histological analysis. Cystitis cystica is a result of dilatation of the Brunn's nests within the lamina propria, which are lined by stratified or squamous epithelium, and in cystitis glandularis by columnar epithelium.

Squamous metaplasia is a well-delineated 'white patch' confined to the trigone, and is present in oestrogen-producing women. Keratinizing squamous metaplasia is also known as 'leukoplakia'. It is generally diffuse and associated with recurrent infection and chronic irritation. It often occurs in association with bladder calculi, urethral diverticula or a foreign body. Macroscopically, the affected areas of the bladder have a thickened white and shiny appearance interspersed with areas of bladder inflammation. Bladder biopsies typically demonstrate mature keratinized stratified squamous epithelium. Its clinical significance remains unclear, but has been linked to the development of invasive squamous cell carcinoma. Both synchronous diagnosis of urothelial tumour and subsequent tumour development on follow-up have been identified. The risk of malignancy is increased in cases with dysplasia as well as extensive keratinization. Lesions should be treated with local transurethral resection. Although dysplasia is considered to be a premalignant condition, there is not enough evidence to identify keratinizing squamous metaplasia of the bladder as premalignant. However, all patients should undergo regular surveillance (Ahmad et al 2008).

Lower urinary tract tumours

Carcinoma *in situ* (CIS) may be asymptomatic or present with microscopic or gross haematuria, urgency, frequency and dysuria. Diagnosis is often delayed because symptoms are attributed to UTI. More than 50% of patients with CIS have coexistent papillary cancer. Cystoscopic appearance varies from normal to erythema or oedema. Histology usually demonstrates abnormal pleomorphic transitional cells confined to the urothelium. Investigation includes urine cultures for fungi and tuberculosis, and cytology studies. Urine cytology is positive in 80–90% of cases. Intravesical BCG instillation is considered the preferred treatment. Surgical resection with radical cystectomy or ablation using transvesical laser or diathermy are indicated for persistent disease, but recurrence or progression to muscle invasion will occur in more than 40% of these women. Chemotherapy, α-interferon and photodynamic therapy are other treatment options for BCG-refractory cases. Outcomes vary and depend on whether CIS is *de novo*, secondary or concomitant to papillary bladder cancer (Nese et al 2009).

The majority of primary invasive lower urinary tract tumours present with painless haematuria or irritative bladder symptoms. UTI is a frequent association. The most common histological type of primary bladder carcinoma is transitional cell (>90%). In the developing world, however, schistosomiasis is associated with an increased incidence of squamous carcinoma. Adenocarcinoma is uncommon but may arise in the embryological remnants of the urachus.

Lower urinary tract calculi

Bladder and urethral calculi in women often arise secondary to a foreign body (e.g. suture material, mesh erosion) or structural abnormalities such as a bladder or urethral diverticulum. They commonly present with recurrent UTI or irritative bladder symptoms. Treatment is directed at removal of the calculus by cystoscopy or lithotripsy, and correction of the underlying abnormality.

Urethral diverticulum

Female urethral diverticula are an uncommon variable in presentation, and the diagnosis is sometimes difficult and delayed. They represent an outpouching of the urethral mucosa through a defect of the periurethral fascia, and may be congenital (embryonic cystic remnants) or more commonly acquired. Obstruction of the periurethral glands, infection and subsequent rupture into the urethral lumen may lead to a urethral diverticulum. Weakening of the periurethral fascia following intraurethral trauma (urethral dilatation), continence surgery or childbirth may result in a diverticulum. Diverticula may be asymptomatic or present with a variety of symptoms, including urgency, recurrent cystitis, haematuria, urethral discharge, vaginal pain or dyspareunia (Romanzi et al 2000). Depending on the patency of the diverticular ostium, contents may stagnate, predisposing to infection or abscess in up to 30% of cases (El-Mekresh 2000), calculi in 1.5–10% of cases or metaplasia leading to malignancy. Investigations include cystourethroscopy, retrograde urethrography, magnetic resonance imaging, and high-resolution transvaginal or transperineal ultrasound (Rovner 2007).

Urethral pressure profilmetry may demonstrate a bifid profile where the urethral diverticular ostium crosses the high-pressure urethral zone.

Surgical excision is necessary in symptomatic women. The aim of surgical repair is to excise the diverticular wall, close the ostium and repair the periurethral fascial defect in layers without tension to reduce the risk of recurrence or fistula formation. In the presence of a large defect or poor tissue integrity, reinforcement of the repair is required. Autologous pubovaginal slings with rectus abdominis fascia or local vaginal, labial or bladder wall flaps have been used. The Martius labial fat graft uses a sleeve of adipose tissue mobilized from the labia majora, still attached to its vascular pedicle. This is rotated and tunnelled under the skin into the vagina (Leach 1991). Complications of diverticulectomy include stricture or scarring, recurrence, stress incontinence, fistula, sloughing, urethral pain and dyspareunia. Stress incontinence is more common where the diverticular ostium crosses the urethral sphincter.

Urethral syndrome

Urethral syndrome is a non-specific group of lower urinary tract symptoms, which include pain (suprapubic or urethral) with urinary frequency and urgency. The pain is typically exacerbated by micturition. The diagnosis is one of exclusion. Investigations should exclude infectious and non-infectious causes of cystitis, inflammation secondary to trauma, foreign bodies, contact irritation or localized paraurethral lesions (Skene's abscess, urethral stricture, diverticulum, tumour), and urethral manifestations of systemic disorders (Reiter's syndrome, Stevens–Johnson syndrome). Cystourethroscopy is necessary to exclude local pathology. An MSU and urethral swab should be performed for microscopy and culture. In women with recent-onset dysuria and frequency (acute urethral syndrome), and an MSU specimen demonstrating pyuria with less than 10^5 micro-organisms/ml, an infective cause is often identified (Stamm et al 1980). The most common organisms isolated on culture of urinary specimens or urethral swabs include coliforms, *C. trachomatis*, *S. saprophyticus* and *N. gonorrhoeae*. If cultures are negative, empirical antibiotic therapy with doxycycline alone or in combination with a sulphonamide should be considered, and is frequently associated with symptomatic resolution (Latham and Stamm 1984).

In women with chronic urethral symptoms, an infective cause is less likely. In the past, urethral dilatation was frequently performed based on the assumption that the condition was due to urethral obstruction, with 80% of women reporting symptom improvement. Symptomatic improvement is also noted following cystoscopy alone, and urethral dilatation may be associated with urethral fibrosis or damage to the urethral sphincter with secondary stress incontinence. Pharmacological agents (e.g. benzodiazepines) have also been used. Their presumed effect is to reduce urethral spasm, although there is no evidence to support this hypothesis.

Urethral syndrome may represent another variation of chronic pain syndromes which are complex and poorly understood (e.g. PBS, vulvodynia). There is no consensus on appropriate management of this condition. Amitriptyline, used for the treatment of other chronic pain syndromes, is often helpful and also has a beneficial anticholinergic effect. Pharmacological therapy should be combined with education and psychological counselling.

Summary

Sensory disorders of the lower urinary tract are common and frequently unrecognized. This often leads to many years of suffering before an accurate diagnosis is made. This is distressing for both the affected individual and their family, and may be potentially serious. A sound working knowledge of the clinical presentation, differential diagnoses and diagnostic criteria for these conditions is essential for all practising gynaecologists. While some of these disorders have specific and effective therapeutic options, others remain poorly understood. Further research is required to evaluate the pathogenesis of these conditions, as it is likely that effective therapeutic protocols will only be developed when the disease process itself is understood.

KEY POINTS

1. Urge-frequency syndrome is common and caused by a wide variety of localized and systemic conditions. A detailed history, examination and sound basic knowledge are required to provide an accurate diagnosis and therapy.
2. Frequency–volume diaries are an inexpensive and accurate way to assess symptom severity and response to behavioural therapy.
3. Cystoscopic evaluation of the lower urinary tract is an essential skill for all gynaecological surgeons, not only in the assessment of urinary symptoms and pain but during pelvic surgery for the prevention and early treatment of bladder and urethral injury.
4. Patient education and access to support networks are important aspects in the management of PBS and other chronic pain syndromes.
5. Bladder retraining, and oral and intravesical drug therapy are effective treatments for the management of PDS or urge-frequency syndrome. The role of botulinum toxin A is unclear.
6. Where urinary cultures are negative, empirical therapy with antibiotics may result in symptom resolution in women with 'urethral syndrome'.

References

Abrams P, Cardozo L, Fall M et al 2002a The standardisation of terminology of lower urinary tract function: report from the Standardisation Sub-committee of the International Continence Society. American Journal of Obstetrics and Gynecology 187: 116–126.

Abrams P, Cardozo L, Fall M et al 2002b The standardisation of terminology of lower urinary tract function: report from the Standardisation Sub-committee of the International Continence Society. Neurourology and Urodynamics 21: 167–178.

Ahmad I, Barnetson RJ, Krishna NS 2008 Keratinizing squamous metaplasia of the bladder: a review. Urology International 81: 247–251.

Bade JJ, Rijcken B, Mensink HJ 1995 Interstitial cystitis in The Netherlands: prevalence, diagnostic criteria and therapeutic preferences. Journal of Urology 154: 2035–2037; discussion 2037–2038.

Chuang YC, Kim DK, Chiang PH, Chancellor MB 2008 Bladder botulinum toxin A injection can benefit patients with radiation and chemical cystitis. BJU International 102: 704–706.

Cooperberg MR, Chambers SK, Rutherford TJ, Foster HE Jr 2000 Cystic pelvic pathology presenting as falsely elevated post-void residual urine measured by portable ultrasound bladder scanning: report of 3 cases and review of the literature. Urology 55: 590.

Dawson TE, Jamison J 2007 Intravesical treatments for painful bladder syndrome/ interstitial cystitis. Cochrane Database of Systematic Reviews 4: CD006113.

Doumouchtsis SK, Jeffery S, Fynes M 2008 Female voiding dysfunction. Obstetrical and Gynecological Survey 63: 519–526.

Drake MJ, Nixon PM, Crew JP 1998 Drug-induced bladder and urinary disorders. Incidence, prevention and management. Drug Safety 19: 45–55.

El-Mekresh M 2000 Urethral pathology. Current Opinion in Urology 10: 381–390.

Elgavish A 2009 Epigenetic reprogramming: a possible etiological factor in bladder pain syndrome/interstitial cystitis? Journal of Urology 181: 980–984.

Irwin DE, Milsom I, Hunskaar S et al 2006 Population-based survey of urinary incontinence, overactive bladder, and other lower urinary tract symptoms in five countries: results of the EPIC study. European Urology 50: 1306–1314; discussion 1314–1315.

Latham RH, Stamm WE 1984 Urethral syndrome in women. Urologic Clinics of North America 11: 95–101.

Leach GE 1991 Urethrovaginal fistula repair with Martius labial fat pad graft. Urologic Clinics of North America 18: 409–413.

Lee JW, Doumouchtsis SK, Jeffery S, Fynes MM 2009 Evaluation of outpatient cystoscopy in urogynaecology. Archives of Gynecology and Obstetrics 279: 631–635

Leppilahti M, Sairanen J, Tammela TL, Aaltomaa S, Lehtoranta K, Auvinen A 2005 Prevalence of clinically confirmed interstitial cystitis in women: a population based study in Finland. Journal of Urology 174: 581–583.

Lifford KL, Curhan GC 2009 Prevalence of painful bladder syndrome in older women. Urology 73: 494–498.

Nese N, Gupta R, Bui MH, Amin MB 2009 Carcinoma in situ of the urinary bladder: review of clinicopathologic characteristics with an emphasis on aspects related to molecular diagnostic techniques and prognosis. Journal of the National Comprehensive Cancer Network 7: 48–57.

Nickel JC 2002 Interstitial cystitis: characterization and management of an enigmatic urologic syndrome. Reviews in Urology 4: 112–121.

Oravisto KJ 1975 Epidemiology of interstitial cystitis. Annales Chirurgiae et Gynaecologiae Fenniae 64: 75–77.

Romanzi LJ, Groutz A, Blaivas JG 2000 Urethral diverticulum in women: diverse presentations resulting in diagnostic delay and mismanagement. Journal of Urology 164: 428–433.

Rosamilia A 2005 Painful bladder syndrome/ interstitial cystitis. Best Practice and Research in Clinical Obstetrics and Gynaecology 19: 843–859.

Rovner ES 2007 Urethral diverticula: a review and an update. Neurourology and Urodynamics 26: 972–977.

Sant GR 2002 Etiology, pathogenesis, and diagnosis of interstitial cystitis. Reviews in Urology 4 (Suppl 1): S9–S15.

Stamm WE, Wagner KF, Amsel R et al 1980 Causes of the acute urethral syndrome in women. New England Journal of Medicine 303: 409–415.

Teegavarapu PS, Sahai A, Chandra A, Dasgupta P, Khan MS 2005 Eosinophilic cystitis and its management. International Journal of Clinical Practice 59: 356–360.

van de Merwe JP, Nordling J, Bouchelouche P et al 2008 Diagnostic criteria, classification, and nomenclature for painful bladder syndrome/interstitial cystitis: an ESSIC proposal. European Urology 53: 60–67.

CHAPTER 57

Fistulae

Paul Hilton

Chapter Contents

INTRODUCTION	874	INVESTIGATIONS	882
AETIOLOGY AND EPIDEMIOLOGY	874	MANAGEMENT	885
PREVALENCE	879	PROGNOSIS	891
CLASSIFICATION	880	PREVENTION	893
PRESENTATION	881	KEY POINTS	893

Introduction

A fistula may be defined as an abnormal communication between two or more epithelial surfaces. In the context of gynaecology, we are concerned primarily with fistulae between the genital tract (vagina, cervix, uterus or perineum, in decreasing order of frequency) and either the urinary tract (bladder, urethra or ureter) or the gastrointestinal tract (rectum, colon, anal canal or small bowel).

Multiple or complex fistulae are common, particularly after attempts at surgical repair. Dual involvement of the bowel and urinary tract is regularly seen, and concurrent involvement of, for example, ureter and bladder, or bladder and urethra is often seen in strategically placed or large urinary fistulae. They may also involve an intervening cavity so that the fistulous nature of an inflammatory mass may not be immediately obvious.

Rarer forms may occur, such as a salpingocolic fistula in association with actinomycosis or tuberculosis. Whilst such pathologies are interesting and important as causes of diagnostic confusion and therapeutic difficulty, they are not considered further in this chapter due to their rarity.

Aetiology and Epidemiology

The aetiology of urogenital fistulae is varied, and may be broadly categorized into congenital or acquired, the latter being divided into obstetric, surgical, radiation, malignant and miscellaneous causes. The same factors may be responsible for intestinogenital fistulae, although inflammatory bowel disease is an additional important aetiological factor here. In most developing countries, over 90% of fistulae are of obstetric aetiology, whereas in the UK, approximately 70% follow pelvic surgery (Table 57.1).

Congenital fistulae are strictly outside the scope of this chapter, and readers are advised to refer to Chapter 13 for further information. Some cases of ectopic ureter may discharge into the vagina, and their presentation may be delayed into teens or adult life, hence leading to confusion with acquired fistulae or other causes of incontinence. This occurs particularly if the abnormal ureter is only draining a small or poorly functioning part of the renal tissue. Under these circumstances, the abnormal tissue may be insufficient to show up as a soft tissue shadow on a plain X-ray, and so poorly functional that it is not easily seen on excretion urography. A high index of clinical suspicion is required if the diagnosis is not to be overlooked (Figure 57.1A,B).

Obstetric

The underlying factors responsible for the development of obstetric fistulae may be considered in physical, biosocial, cultural, and geographical or political terms. The basic physical factors responsible for obstetric fistula development include obstructed labour, accidental injury at the time of caesarean section, forceps delivery, craniotomy, symphysiotomy, traditional surgical practices including circumcision and 'gishiri', and complications of criminal abortion.

The overwhelming majority are complications of neglected obstructed labour. During normal labour, the bladder is displaced upwards and the anterior vaginal wall, bladder base and urethra are compressed between the fetal head and the posterior surface of the pubis. No harm results if this occurs for a short time, but in prolonged obstructed labour, the intervening tissues are devitalized by ischaemia. Usually, the anterior vaginal wall and underlying bladder neck are affected, although the area of necrosis is sometimes higher, in which case the anterior lip of the cervix and underlying trigone are involved. Compression of the soft tissues between the sacral promontory and the presenting part may occur at the same time, with necrosis at the posterior vaginal wall and underlying rectum. The devitalized

DOI: 10.1016/B978-0-7020-3120-5.00057-6

Table 57.1 Aetiology of urogenital fistulae in two series from the north-east of England (Hilton unpublished) and from south-east Nigeria (Hilton and Ward 1998)

Aetiology	North-east England ($n = 300$)	South-east Nigeria ($n = 2389$)	Aetiology	North-east England ($n = 300$)	South-east Nigeria ($n = 2389$)
Obstetric			**Surgical**		
Obstructed labour	2	1918	Total abdominal hysterectomy and colposuspension	1	
Caesarean section	13	165	Laparoscopic oophorectomy	1	
Ruptured uterus	8	119	Sling	2	
Forceps/ventouse	5		Partial vaginectomy	3	
Breech extraction	1		Periurethral bulking agents	1	
Placental abruption	1		Needle suspension	1	
Caesarean hysterectomy	3		Subtrigonal phenol injection	1	
Symphysiotomy	2		Lithocast	1	
Obstetric subtotal (% of total)	35 (11.7%)	2202 (92.2%)	Ileoanal pouch	1	
Surgical			Sacrospinous fixation	1	
Abdominal hysterectomy	120	33	Unknown surgery in childhood	1	
Radical hysterectomy	15		Suture to vaginal laceration		12
Urethral diverticulectomy	15		Surgical subtotal (% of total)	207 (69.0%)	105 (4.4%)
Colectomy	9		**Radiation**		
Colporrhaphy	9	35	Radiation subtotal (% of total)	28 (9.3%)	0
Vaginal hysterectomy	5	25	**Malignancy**		
Midurethral tape procedures	4		Malignancy subtotal (% of total)	2 (0.7%)	42 (1.8%)
Laparoscopically assisted vaginal hysterectomy	3		**Miscellaneous**		
Cystoplasty and colposuspension	2		Vaginal pessary	8	
Colposuspension	2		Infection	5	7
Cervical stumpectomy	2		Congenital	5	
Large loop excision of the transformation zone	2		Foreign body	4	
Nephroureterectomy	2		Catheter induced	3	
Subtotal hysterectomy	2		Trauma	2	11
Total abdominal hysterectomy and colporrhaphy	1		Coital injury	1	22
			Miscellaneous subtotal (% of total)	28 (9.3%)	40 (1.7%)

Sources: Hilton (unpublished).
Hilton P, Ward A 1998 Epidemiological and surgical aspects of urogenital fistulae: a review of 25 years experience in south-east Nigeria. International Urogynecology Journal and Pelvic Floor Dysfunction 9: 189–194.

area separates as a slough usually between the third and 10th day of the puerperium, with resulting incontinence (Figure 57.2).

Accidental injury to the vaginal wall during a difficult operative delivery may involve damage to the underlying bladder wall, particularly if the tissues are devitalized by prolonged pressure. Forcible rotation of the head with Kielland's forceps is particularly liable to produce such an injury by shearing stresses. The bladder is particularly exposed to injury following symphysiotomy if the pubic bones are too widely separated by forced abduction of the thighs. In these circumstances, the unsupported bladder neck is very likely to be damaged, especially if the head is rotated and extracted with forceps. The posterior wall of the bladder may be accidentally incised during lower segment caesarean section or repair of ruptured uterus, particularly if the bladder is not reflected sufficiently far downwards before the lower segment is opened. During the reflection itself, the bladder may be torn, especially if a previous operation has made it densely adherent to the lower segment. If the bladder injury goes

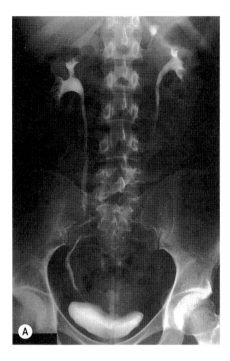
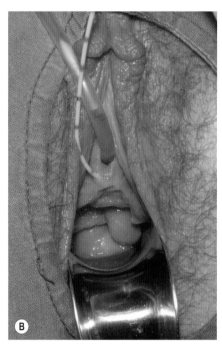

Figure 57.1 (A) Intravenous urogram from patient presenting with continuous urinary incontinence; a small discrete upper pole element is visible, although the upper pole ureter is not clearly seen. (B) Appearance of vulva with urethral catheter in place, and a ureteric catheter placed in the ectopic ureteric opening just below the external urethral meatus.

undetected at the time, urinary leakage through the abdominal wound soon develops. This is usually followed by incontinence vaginally when the urine finds its way through the uterine incision. The abdominal leakage then dries up as the bladder drains through the resulting vesicocervical fistula. Alternatively, sutures may be passed through the posterior bladder wall during repair of the uterine incision. The appearance of urinary incontinence in these cases is delayed until the intervening bladder tissue caught up in the suture sloughs.

The perineum and posterior vaginal wall are, of course, at risk from even the most straightforward delivery, although primiparity, forceps delivery, birth weight over 4 kg and occipitoposterior position have been found to be significant risk factors associated with third-degree tears (Sultan et al 1994). Even when identified and repaired, this increases the risk of rectovaginal fistula.

Traditional surgical practices are undertaken in up to 98% of women in some parts of Africa (United Nations Population Fund 2007, World Health Organization 2008), and may play a role in the aetiology of both direct 'surgical' and obstetric fistulae. The practices of 'angurya' and 'gishiri' cutting [female genital mutilation (FGM) type IV] (World Health Organization 2008) are commonly employed to treat a wide variety of conditions including obstructed labour, infertility, dyspareunia, dysuria, amenorrhoea, goitre, backache and presumed tumour. The traditional cut made with a razor blade or knife through the vaginal introitus is sometimes superficial, but may result in fistula formation (Figure 57.3). Since cuts are usually made by linear incision into healthy tissues, repair is often much easier than for those resulting from pressure necrosis. Tahzib (1983, 1985) reported on the epidemiological determinants of vesicovaginal fistulae in northern Nigeria. In 84% of cases, obstructed labour was the major aetiological factor, 33% had undergone 'gishiri', and this was felt to be the main aetiological factor in 15%.

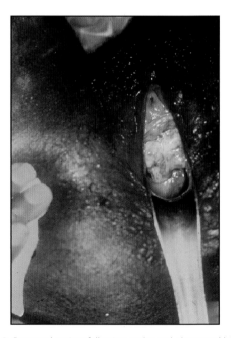

Figure 57.2 Puerperal patient following prolonged obstructed labour. An area of devitalized tissue is seen on the anterior vaginal wall, about to slough with resultant fistula formation.

Female circumcision has been practised in various forms in much of North Africa, being most prevalent in Ethiopia, Eritrea, Sudan, Egypt, Mali and Guinea, where currently over 75% of women are affected (World Health Organization 2008). The more extreme forms (previously referred to as 'pharaonic circumcision') involve removal of the labial minora (FGM type IIa), and may include removal of the clitoris (FGM type IIb) and labia majora (FGM type IIc) (see Figure 57.4). In FGM type III, the introitus may be reduced to pin-hole size by excision and apposition of the cut edges

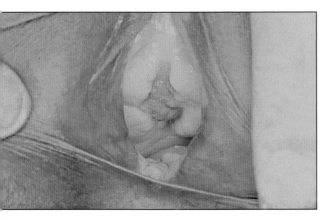

Figure 57.3 Vesicovaginal fistula resulting from 'gishiri' cutting (female genital mutilation type IV).

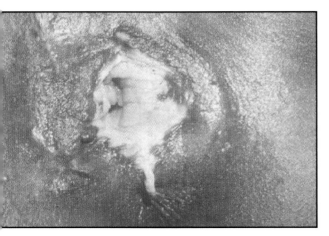

Figure 57.4 Excisional type of female genital mutilation, with excision of labia minora and most of clitoris and labia majora (female genital mutilation type IIc).

of the labia minora or majora (infibulation) (World Health Organization 2008). Whilst an association between FGM and both vesicovaginal and rectovaginal fistula is recognized (Lovel et al 2000), the strength of the association and the exact mechanisms are less certain and are currently under investigation (World Health Organization 2008).

In considering obstetric fistulae, it is important to consider the social, cultural and geographical influences just as much as the direct physical injury to the lower urinary tract. Obstructed labour is most often due to a contracted pelvis. This usually results from stunting of growth by malnutrition and untreated infections in childhood and adolescence. Where women retain a subservient role in society and standards of education are limited, early marriage and the absence of family planning services result in an early start to childbearing; where first pregnancies occur soon after the menarche, before growth of the pelvis is complete, this also contributes to obstruction in labour.

The influence of these factors is illustrated in the epidemiological studies alluded to earlier. Tahzib (1983) reported that over 50% of the cases of vesicovaginal fistulae seen in northern Nigeria were under 20 years of age, over 50% were in their first pregnancy, and only one in 500 had received any formal education. From the same area, Murphy (1981)

reported that 88% of patients had married at 15 years of age or less, and 33% had delivered their first child before the age of 15 years. However, in different developing world societies, these factors do seem to have variable influence. For example, in south-east Nigeria (Hilton and Ward 1998) and the north-west frontier of Pakistan (World Health Organization 1989), fistula patients seem to be somewhat older and of higher parity; they also appear to have a higher literacy rate, and to be more likely to remain in a married relationship after the development of their fistula (Hilton and Ward 1998). It is likely that the development of fistulae here reflects other biosocial variations (Table 57.2). It is clear that in these populations, even where skilled maternity care is available, uptake may be poor. Mistrust of hospitals is commonplace, antenatal care is poorly attended, and delivery is commonly conducted at home by elderly relatives or unskilled traditional birth attendants. Where labour is prolonged, transfer to hospital may only be used as a last resort.

Surgical

Genital fistula may occur following a wide range of surgical procedures within the pelvis (Table 57.1, Figure 57.5A–F). It is often supposed that this complication results from direct injury to the lower urinary tract at the time of operation. Certainly, on occasions, this may be the case; careless, hurried or rough surgical technique makes injury to the lower urinary tract much more likely. However, of 300 fistulae referred to the author in the UK over the last 20 years, 207 have been associated with pelvic surgery and 147 followed hysterectomy; of these, only seven presented with leakage of urine on the first postoperative day. In other cases, compromise to the blood supply may result in tissue necrosis and subsequent leakage; alternatively, a small pelvic haematoma may develop in association with the vaginal vault, which subsequently becomes infected and discharges with the characteristic puff of haematuria 5–10 days later, with incontinence following shortly thereafter. Recent animal studies suggest that the inadvertent placement of vault sutures into the bladder wall at hysterectomy may not carry as great a risk of fistula formation as previously thought (Meeks et al 1997).

Although it is important to remember that the majority of surgical fistulae follow apparently straightforward hysterectomy in skilled hands, several risk factors may be identified that make direct injury more likely (Table 57.3). Obviously, anatomical distortion within the pelvis by ovarian tumour or fibroid will increase surgical difficulty, and abnormal adhesions between bladder and uterus or cervix following previous surgery or associated with previous sepsis, endometriosis or malignancy may make fistula formation more likely. Preoperative or early postoperative radiotherapy may decrease vascularity, and make the tissues generally less forgiving of poor technique.

Issues of training and surgical technique are, of course, also important. The ability to locate and, if necessary, dissect out the ureter must be part of routine gynaecological training, as should the first aid management of lower urinary tract injury when it arises. The use of gauze swabs to separate the bladder from the cervix at caesarean section or hysterectomy should be discouraged; sharp dissection with knife or scissors does less harm, especially where the tissues are abnormally adherent.

Table 57.2 Epidemiological aspects of obstetric fistula as illustrated in five studies from Nigeria, Ethiopia and Pakistan

	Northern Nigeria (Murphy 1981) $n = 100$	**Northern Nigeria (Tahzib 1983)** $n = 1443$	**Ethiopia (Kelly and Kwast 1993)** $n = 309$	**South-east Nigeria (Hilton and Ward 1998)** $n = 2389$	**Pakistan (World Health Organization 1989)** $n = 325$
Mean age (years)	20	21	22	28	32
Mean parity	?	1.6	2.1	3.5	?
First pregnancy (%)	65	52	63	31	15
Divorced/deserted (%)	54% divorced/separated	?	52% deserted	10% divorced/separated	?
Literacy (%)	8	0.2	?	29	?
Delivered at home (%)	?	64	58	27	?

Sources: Hilton P, Ward A 1998 Epidemiological and surgical aspects of urogenital fistulae: a review of 25 years experience in south-east Nigeria. International Urogynecology Journal and Pelvic Floor Dysfunction 9:189–194.
Kelly J, Kwast B 1993 Epidemiologic study of vesico-vaginal fistula in Ethiopia. International Urogynecology Journal 4: 278–281.
Murphy M 1981 Social consequences of vesico-vaginal fistula in Northern Nigeria. Journal of Biosocial Sciences 13: 139–150.
Tahzib F 1983 Epidemiological determinants of vesicovaginal fistulas. British Journal of Obstetrics and Gynaecology 90:387–391.
World Health Organization 1989 The Prevention and Treatment of Obstetric Fistulae: a Report of a Technical Working Group. WHO, Geneva.

It has recently been shown that there is a high incidence of abnormalities of lower urinary tract function in fistula patients (Hilton 1998); whether these abnormalities antedate the surgery, or develop with or as a consequence of the fistula, cannot be answered from this data. However, it is likely that patients with a habit of infrequent voiding, or with inefficient detrusor contractility, may be at increased risk of postoperative urinary retention; if this is not recognized early and managed appropriately, the risk of fistula formation may be increased.

Radiation

As noted above, preoperative pelvic irradiation increases the risk of postoperative fistula development, but irradiation itself may be a cause of fistula (Figure 57.5G). The obliterative endarteritis associated with ionizing radiation in therapeutic dosage proceeds over many years, and may be aetiological in fistula formation long after the primary malignancy has been treated. Of the 28 radiation fistulae in the author's series, the fistulae developed at intervals between 1 and 30 years following radiotherapy. Not only does this ischaemia produce the fistulae, it also causes significant damage in the adjacent tissues, so ordinary surgical repair has a high likelihood of failure and modified surgical techniques are required.

Malignancy

The treatment of pelvic malignancy by either surgery or radiotherapy is associated with a risk of fistula development, but tissue loss associated with malignant disease itself may result in genital tract fistula. Carcinoma of cervix, vagina and rectum are the most common malignancies to present in this way. It is relatively unusual for urothelial tumours to present with fistula formation, other than following surgery or radiotherapy. The development of a fistula may be a distressing part of the terminal phase of malignant disease; it

is, nevertheless, one deserving not simply compassion but full consideration of the therapeutic or palliative possibilities.

Inflammatory bowel disease

Inflammatory bowel disease is the most significant cause of intestinogenital fistulae in the UK, although these rarely present directly to the gynaecologist. Crohn's disease is by far the most important, and appears to be increasing in frequency in the Western world. A total fistula rate approaching 40% has been reported, and the involvement of the genital tract in females may be up to 7%.

Ulcerative colitis has a small incidence of low rectovaginal fistulae. Diverticular disease can produce colovaginal fistulae and, rarely, colouterine fistulae, with surprisingly few symptoms attributable to the intestinal pathology. The possibility should not be overlooked if an elderly woman complains of feculent discharge or becomes incontinent without concomitant urinary problems (Figure 57.6).

Miscellaneous

Among other miscellaneous causes of fistulae in the genital tract, the following should be considered.

- Infection
  - Lymphogranuloma venereum
  - Schistosomiasis
  - Tuberculosis
  - Actinomycosis
  - Measles
  - Noma vaginae
- Other
  - Penetrating trauma
  - Coital injury
  - Neglected pessary
  - Other foreign body
  - Catheter-related injury

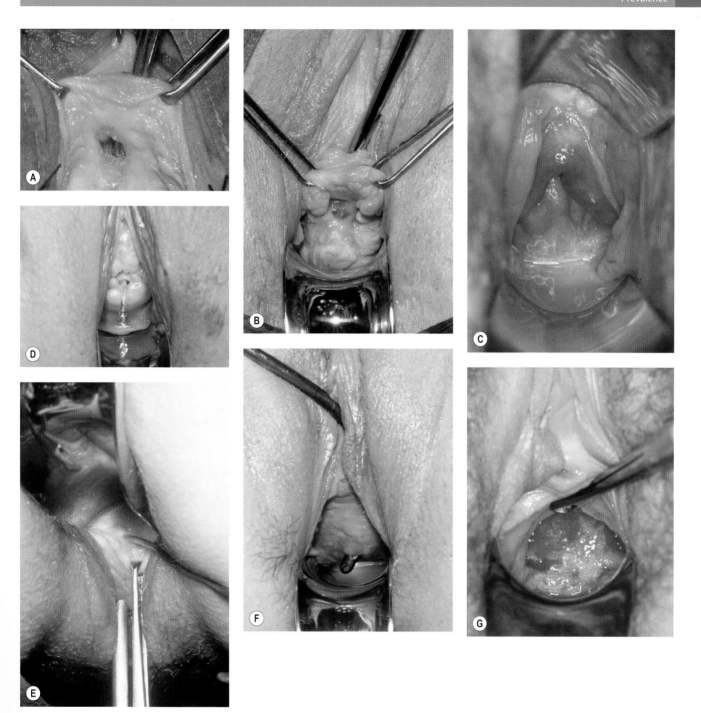

Figure 57.5 Urogenital fistulae of varying aetiologies: (A) following anterior colporrhaphy, (B) urethral diverticulectomy, (C) radical hysterectomy, (D) midurethral tape procedure for stress incontinence, (E) colposuspension (the fistula in the latter case was fixed retropubically in the midline at the bladder neck, and the photograph shows the patient prone, in the reverse lithotomy position), (F) subtrigonal phenol injection, (G) radiotherapy for carcinoma of cervix.

Prevalence

United Kingdom

The prevalence of genital fistulae obviously varies from country to country and continent to continent as the main causative factors vary. Accurate figures are impossible to obtain since those areas with the highest overall prevalence are also those with the poorest systems of health data col-

lection. UK National Health Service data reported approximately 150 operations for vesicovaginal and urethrovaginal fistula per year in England and Wales in the early 1990s (Hilton 1997). The most recent data from Health Episode Statistics for England suggest an average of 95 operations for vesicovaginal fistula and 10 operations for urethrovaginal fistula per year in England (Department of Health 2009). It is tempting to suggest that this apparent reduction in incidence of fistulae may reflect changes in the practice of

Table 57.3 Risk factors for postoperative fistulae

Risk factor	Pathology	Specific example
Anatomical distortion		Fibroids
		Ovarian mass
Abnormal tissue adhesion	Inflammation	Infection
		Endometriosis
	Previous surgery	Caesarean section
		Cone biopsy
		Colporrhaphy
	Malignancy	
Impaired vascularity	Ionizing radiation	Preoperative radiotherapy
	Metabolic abnormality	Diabetes mellitus
	Radical surgery	
Compromised healing		Anaemia
		Nutritional deficiency
Abnormality of bladder function		Voiding dysfunction

Sources: Hilton P, Ward A 1998 Epidemiological and surgical aspects of urogenital fistulae: a review of 25 years experience in south-east Nigeria. International Urogynecology Journal and Pelvic Floor Dysfunction 9: 189–194.
Kelly J, Kwast B 1993 Epidemiologic study of vesico-vaginal fistula in Ethiopia. International Urogynecology Journal 4: 278–281.
Murphy M 1981 Social consequences of vesico-vaginal fistula in Northern Nigeria. Journal of Biosocial Sciences 13: 139–150.
Tahzib F 1983 Epidemiological determinants of vesicovaginal fistulas. British Journal of Obstetrics and Gynaecology 90: 387–391.
World Health Organization 1989 The Prevention and Treatment of Obstetric Fistulae: a Report of a Technical Working Group. WHO, Geneva.

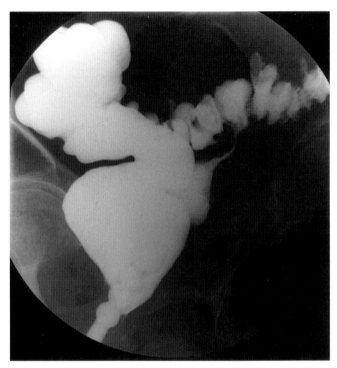

Figure 57.6 Barium enema from patient complaining of vaginal discharge; demonstrates extensive diverticular disease and obvious colovaginal fistula.

hysterectomy. However, assuming that 50% of urogenital fistulae in the UK follow hysterectomy (as in the author's series), the rate of fistula formation following hysterectomy seems, if anything, to be increasing; from approximately one in 1200 hysterectomies in the period 1990–1991 to 1994–1995 to approximately one in 750 in 2003–2004 to 2007–2008 (Department of Health 2009). Whilst there are other possible explanations, it may be that as fewer hysterectomies are undertaken, those that remain are the more difficult procedures. Studies from Finland suggest a similar rate of posthysterectomy fistulae overall, with approximately one per 1000 abdominal hysterectomies and one per 450 laparoscopic hysterectomies (Harkki-Siren et al 1998). Similarly, ureteric injury may be up to six times as common following laparoscopic hysterectomy compared with open hysterectomy (Harkki-Siren et al 1998), and two to 10 times as common following radical hysterectomy and exenteration (Averette et al 1993, Bladou et al 1995, Emmert and Köhler 1996). Sultan et al (1994) reported that third-degree tears followed 0.6% of vaginal deliveries, and a rectovaginal fistula resulted in 6% of these (one in 3000 deliveries overall).

Developing world

In the developing world, many fistula cases are unknown to medical services, being separated from their husbands and ostracized from society. Although the true prevalence in the developing world is unknown, particularly high prevalence rates are reported in Nigeria, Ethiopia, Sudan and Chad. The estimated prevalence in the developing world is one to two per 1000 deliveries, with perhaps 50,000–100,000 new cases each year. Although several units exist in Nigeria, Ethiopia and Sudan, which deal with 100–700 cases per year, this does not come close to meeting the demand, and there are estimated to be perhaps 500,000 to 2 million untreated cases worldwide (Waaldijk and Armiya'u 1993).

Classification

Many different fistula classifications have been described in the literature on the basis of anatomical site or position in relation to meatus or sphincter mechanism; these are often subclassified into simple cases (where the tissues are healthy and access is good) (Figure 57.7A,B) or complicated cases (where there is tissue loss, scarring, impaired access, involvement of the ureteric orifices, or the presence of coexistent rectovaginal fistula) (Figure 57.7C) (Lawson 1978, Waaldijk 1995, Goh 2004). Urogenital fistulae may be classified into urethral, bladder neck, subsymphysial (a complex form involving circumferential loss of the urethra with fixity to bone), midvaginal, juxtacervical or vault fistulae; massive fistulae extending from bladder neck to vault; and vesico-uterine or vesicocervical fistulae. It is interesting to note that whereas over 60% of fistulae in the developing world are

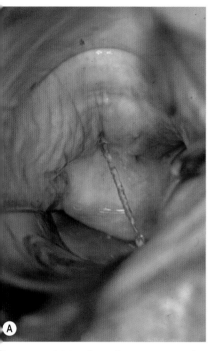
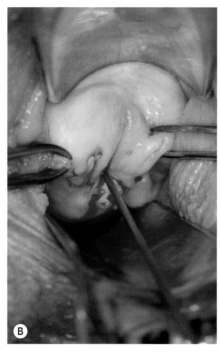
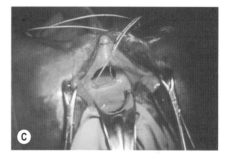

Figure 57.7 (A) Simple posthysterectomy vault vesicovaginal fistula. (B) Same case as in (A) illustrating tissue mobility and ease of access for repair per vaginam. (C) Complex obstetric fistula; a massive vesicovaginal fistula with involvement of both ureteric orifices and coexistent rectovaginal fistula.

midvaginal, juxtacervical or massive (reflecting their obstetric aetiology) (Hilton and Ward 1998), such cases are relatively rare in Western fistula practice; in contrast, 50% of the fistulae managed in the UK are situated in the vaginal vault reflecting their surgical aetiology). There have been recent calls for classification systems more predictive of outcome Arrowsmith 2007, Goh et al 2008).

Presentation

Fistulae between the urinary tract and the female genital tract are characteristically said to present with continuous urinary incontinence, both by day and night. In patients with large fistulae, the volume of leakage may be such that they rarely feel any sensation of bladder fullness, and normal voiding may be infrequent. Where there is extensive tissue loss, as in obstetric fistulae from obstructed labour or radiation fistulae, this typical history is usually present, the clinical findings gross, and the diagnosis rarely in doubt. With postsurgical fistulae, for example, the history may be atypical and the orifice small, elusive or occasionally completely invisible. Under these circumstances, the diagnosis can be much more difficult, and a high index of clinical suspicion must be maintained.

Occasionally, a patient with an obvious fistula may deny incontinence, and this is presumed to reflect the ability of the levator ani muscles to occlude the vagina below the level of the fistula. Some patients with vesicocervical or vesico-uterine fistula following caesarean section may maintain continence at the level of the uterine isthmus, and complain of cyclical haematuria at the time of menstruation, or menouria (Falk and Tancer 1956, Youssef 1957). In other cases, patients may complain of little more than a watery vaginal discharge, or intermittent leakage, which seems posturally related. Leakage may appear to occur specifically on standing or on lying supine, prone, or in left or right lateral positions, presumably reflecting the degree of bladder distension and the position of the fistula within the bladder; such a pattern is most unlikely to be found with ureteric fistulae.

Although in the case of direct surgical injury, leakage may occur from the first postoperative day, in most surgical and obstetric fistulae, symptoms develop between 5 and 14 days after the causative injury; however, the time of presentation may be quite variable. This will depend, to some extent, on the severity of symptoms, but as far as obstetric fistulae in the developing world are concerned, is determined more by access to health care. In a review of cases from Nigeria, the average time for presentation was over 5 years, and in some cases over 35 years, after the causative pregnancy (Hilton and Ward 1998).

Urethrovaginal fistulae distal to the sphincter mechanism will often be asymptomatic and require no specific treatment. Some may lead to obstruction, and are more likely to present with postmicturition dribbling than other types of incontinence; they can therefore be very difficult to recognize. More proximally situated urethral fistulae are perhaps most likely to present with stress incontinence, since bladder neck competence is frequently impaired.

Ureteric fistulae occur from similar aetiologies to bladder fistulae, and the causative mechanism may be one of direct injury by incision, division or excision, or of ischaemia from strangulation by suture, crushing by clamp or stripping by dissection (Yeates 1987). The presentation may therefore be similarly variable. With direct injury, leakage is usually apparent from the first postoperative day. Urine output may be physiologically reduced for some hours following surgery, and if there is significant operative or postoperative hypotension, oliguria may persist longer. However, once renal function is restored, leakage will usually be apparent promptly. With other mechanisms, obstruction is likely to be present to a greater or lesser degree, and the initial symptoms may be of pyrexia or loin pain, with incontinence only occurring after sloughing of the ischaemic tissue, from around 5 days up to 6 weeks later. On occasion, the reverse pattern may be seen, with apparent relief of leakage resulting from the development of obstruction as scarring in the ureter proceeds (Figure 57.8A).

With intestinal fistulae, the history may be much more misleading. A small communication with the large bowel may only cause an offensive discharge. Even fistulae of obstetric origin may be rendered relatively asymptomatic by the cicatrization of the vagina, which occurs following sloughing. A small high posterior horseshoe-shaped fistula may only become apparent during division of constricting bands for the repair of a vesicovaginal fistula. Most typically, however, patients will complain of incontinence of liquid stool, and flatus, and whilst they may often be unsure about whether stool is from the vagina or anus, the sensation of flatus from the vagina is rarely misinterpreted.

Investigations

If there is suspicion of a fistula but its presence is not easily confirmed by clinical examination with a Sims' speculum, further investigation will be necessary to confirm or fully exclude the possibility. Even where the diagnosis is clinically obvious, additional investigation may be appropriate for full evaluation prior to deciding treatment.

Microbiology

Urinary infection is surprisingly uncommon in fistula patients, although urine culture should be undertaken and appropriate antibiotic therapy instituted, especially where there have been previous attempts at surgery. Urine culture is not easily obtained when a fistula produces severe incontinence, but a pipette may be used to obtain a small intravesical sample for investigation.

Dye studies

When the diagnosis is in doubt, it is important to confirm that the discharge is urinary and that the leakage is extra-urethral rather than urethral, and to establish the site of leakage. Although other imaging techniques undoubtedly have a role (see below), carefully conducted dye studies remain the investigation of first choice.

Excessive vaginal discharge, or the drainage of serum from a pelvic haematoma following surgery, may simulate a urinary fistula. If the fluid is in sufficient quantity to be collected, biochemical analysis of its urea content in comparison to that of urine and serum will confirm its origin. Phenazopyridine is no longer available in the UK, although it has previously been used orally (200 mg tds) to stain the urine and hence confirm the presence of a fistula; alternatively, indigo carmine may be used intravenously for the same purpose. The identification of the site of a fistula

is best carried out by the instillation of coloured dye (methylene blue or indigo carmine) into the bladder via catheter with the patient in the lithotomy position. The traditional 'three swab test' has its limitations and is not recommended; the examination is best carried out with direct inspection, and multiple fistulae may be located in this way. It is important to be alert for leakage around the catheter, which may spill back into the vagina creating the impression of a fistula. It is also important to ensure that adequate distension of the bladder occurs, as some fistulae do not leak at small volumes; conversely, some fistulae with an oblique track through the bladder wall may leak at small volume but not at capacity. If leakage of clear fluid continues after dye instillation, a ureteric fistula is likely; previously, this could be confirmed by a 'two dye test', using phenazopyridine to stain the renal urine, and methylene blue to stain the bladder contents (Raghavaiah 1974). However, intravesical followed by intravenous injection of dye may be required nowadays.

Dye tests are less useful for intestinal fistulae, although a carmine marker taken orally may confirm their presence. Rectal distension with air via a sigmoidoscope may be of more value; if the patient is kept in a slight head-down position and the vagina filled with saline, the bubbling of any air leaked through a low fistula may be detected.

Imaging

Excretion urography

Although intravenous urography is a particularly insensitive investigation in the diagnosis of vesicovaginal fistula, knowledge of upper urinary tract status may have a significant influence on treatment measures applied, and intravenous urography or computed tomography urogram should be looked on as an essential investigation for any suspected or confirmed urinary fistula (Figure 57.8A,B). Compromise to ureteric function is a particularly common finding when a fistula occurs in relation to malignant disease or its treatment (by radiation or surgery).

Dilatation of the ureter is characteristic in ureteric fistula, and its finding in association with a known vesicovaginal fistula should raise suspicion of a complex ureterovesicovaginal lesion. Whilst essential for the diagnosis of ureteric fistula, urography is not completely sensitive, although the presence of a periureteric flare is highly suggestive of extravasation at this site (Figure 57.8B).

Retrograde pyelography

Retrograde pyelography is a more reliable way of identifying the exact site of a ureterovaginal fistula, and may be undertaken simultaneously with either retrograde or percutaneous catheterization for therapeutic stenting of the ureter (see below) (Figure 57.8C).

Cystography

Cystography is not particularly helpful in the basic diagnosis of vesicovaginal fistulae, and a dye test carried out under direct vision is likely to be more sensitive. It may, however, be useful in achieving a diagnosis in complex fistulae (Figure 57.8D), or vesicouterine fistulae, where a lateral view may

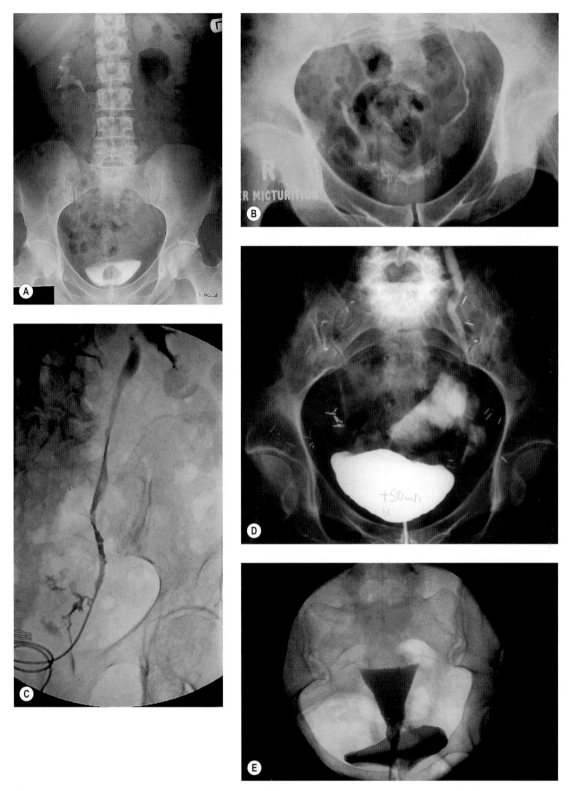

Figure 57.8 (A) Intravenous urogram in a patient who presented with incontinence following hysterectomy, presumed initially to be due to a vesicovaginal fistula. Apparent resolution of the leakage following catheterization was, in fact, due to progressive obstruction above the level of a ureterovaginal fistula. (B) Intravenous urogram showing periureteric flare typical of ureterovaginal fistula. (C) Retrograde pyelogram demonstrating ureterovaginal fistula. (D) Intravenous urogram (with simultaneous cystogram) demonstrating a complex surgical fistula occurring after radical hysterectomy. After further investigation including cystourethroscopy, sigmoidoscopy, barium enema and retrograde cannulation of the vaginal vault to perform fistulography, the lesion was defined as an ureterocolovesicovaginal fistula. (E) Hysterosalpinogram in patient with vesicocervical fistula following caesarean section.

show the cavity of the uterus filled with radiopaque dye behind the bladder.

Fistulography

This is a special example of the X-ray technique commonly referred to as 'sinography'. For small fistulae, a ureteric catheter is suitable, although if the hole is large enough a small Foley catheter may be used to deliver the radio-opaque dye; this is of particular value for fistulae for which there is an intervening abscess cavity. If a catheter will pass through a small vaginal aperture into an adjacent loop of bowel, its nature may become apparent from the radiological appearance of the lumen and haustrations, although further imaging studies are usually required to demonstrate the underlying pathology.

Colpography and hysterosalpingography

If a fistula opening cannot be identified directly, colpography or hysterography may occasionally be helpful. If a large Foley catheter with a large balloon is distended in the lower vagina, injection of a non-viscous opaque medium under pressure may outline a fistulous track to an adjacent organ. However, failure to demonstrate a fistula by this means does not exclude its presence. If a patient with a vesicouterine fistula has no history of incontinence but complains of cyclical haematuria, contrast studies carried out through the uterus (hysterosalpingography) may be more rewarding than cystography. Again, a lateral view is necessary to detect the anterior leak (Figure 57.8E).

Barium enema, barium meal and follow-through

Either or both of these may be required for evaluation of the intestinal condition when an intestinal fistula is present above the anorectum. Aside from confirming the presence of a fistula, evidence of malignant or inflammatory disease may be identified.

Ultrasound, computed tomography and magnetic resonance imaging

These may occasionally be appropriate for the complete assessment of complex fistulae. Endoanal ultrasound and magnetic resonance imaging are particularly useful in the investigation of anorectal and perineal fistulae.

Examination under anaesthesia

Careful examination, if necessary under anaesthetic, may be required to determine the presence of a fistula, and is deemed by several authorities to be an essential preliminary to definitive surgical treatment (Chassar Moir 1967, Lawson 1978, Jonas and Petri 1984, Lawson and Hudson 1987). A malleable silver probe is invaluable for exploration of the vaginal walls, and tissue forceps or plastic surgical skin hooks are helpful to put tension on the tissues for the identification of small fistulae. If the probe passes directly into the rectum, it may be felt digitally or seen via the proctoscope. In the bladder or urethra, it may be identified by a metallic click against a silver catheter, or seen by a cystoscope; in either case, the diagnosis is then obvious.

It is also important at the time of examination to assess the available access for repair vaginally, and the mobility of the tissues (Figure 57.7A,B). The decision between the vaginal and abdominal approaches to surgery is thus made; when the vaginal route is chosen, it may be appropriate to select between the more conventional supine lithotomy with a head-down tilt, and the prone (reverse lithotomy) with head-up tilt (Figure 57.9). This may be particularly useful in allowing the operator to look down on to bladder neck and subsymphysial fistulae, and is also of advantage in some massive fistulae in encouraging the reduction of the prolapsed bladder mucosa (Lawson 1967).

Endoscopy

Cystoscopy

Although some authorities suggest that endoscopy has little role in the evaluation of fistulae, it is the author's practice to perform cystourethroscopy in all but the largest defects (Figure 57.10). Although in some obstetric and radiation fistulae, the size of the defect and the extent of tissue loss and scarring may make it difficult to distend the bladder, much useful information is still obtained. The exact level and position of the fistula should be determined, and its relationship to the ureteric orifices and bladder neck are particularly important. With urethral and bladder neck fistulae, the failure to pass a cystoscope or sound may indicate that there has been circumferential loss of the proximal urethra; a circumstance which is of considerable importance in determining the appropriate surgical technique and the likelihood of subsequent urethral incompetence. Similar considerations may apply to investigation of the lower bowel following major obstetric injuries in which segmental circumferential loss of the upper rectum may have occurred.

The condition of the tissues must be assessed carefully. Persistence of slough means that surgery should be deferred, and this is particularly important in obstetric and postradiation cases. Biopsy from the edge of a fistula should be taken in radiation fistulae, if persistent or recurrent malignancy is suspected. Malignant change has been reported in a long-standing benign fistula, so where there is any doubt at all

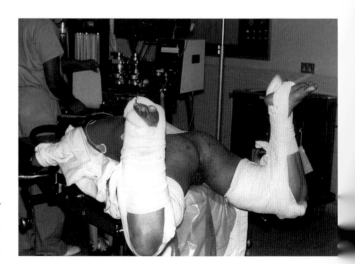

Figure 57.9 Patient in prone (reverse lithotomy) position with head-up tilt in preparation for repair of a fixed subsymphysial fistula.

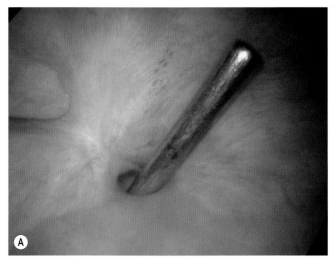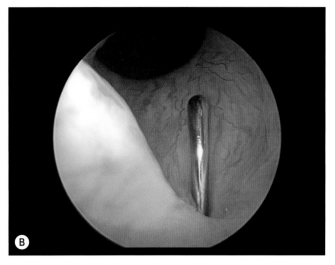

Figure 57.10 Endoscopic appearance of (A) vesicovaginal fistula following total abdominal hysterectomy, (B) urethrovaginal fistula following midurethral tape procedure.

about the nature of the tissues, biopsy should be undertaken (Hudson 1968). In areas of endemicity, evidence of schistosomiasis, tuberculosis and lymphogranuloma may become apparent in biopsy material, and again it is important that specific antimicrobial treatment is instituted prior to definitive surgery. If calculi are identified clinically, radiologically or endoscopically in the bladder, vaginal vault or diverticulum, their removal prior to any attempt at surgical correction is essential.

Sigmoidoscopy and proctoscopy

These examinations are important for the diagnosis of inflammatory bowel disease, which may not have been suspected before the occurrence of a fistula. Biopsies of the fistula edge or any unhealthy looking area should always be obtained.

Management

Immediate management

Before epithelialization is complete, an abnormal communication between viscera will tend to close spontaneously, provided that the natural outflow is unobstructed. Normal continence mechanisms, however, involve the intermittent physiological contraction of urethral and anal sphincters (see Chapter 50). As a result, although spontaneous closure of genital tract fistulae does occur, it is the exception rather than the rule. Bypassing the sphincter mechanisms, or diverting flow around the fistula (e.g. by urinary catheterization or defunctioning colostomy), may encourage closure.

The early management is of critical importance, and depends on the aetiology and site of the lesion. If surgical trauma is recognized within the first 24 h post operatively, immediate repair may be appropriate, provided that extravasation of urine into the tissues has not been great. The majority of surgical fistulae are, however, recognized between 5 and 21 days post operatively, and these should be treated with continuous bladder drainage. It is worth persisting with

this line of management in vesicovaginal or urethrovaginal fistulae for 6–8 weeks since spontaneous closure may occur within this period (Davits and Miranda 1991). Although only 8% of the fistulae in the author's series are known to have healed with catheter drainage, it is possible that the actual rate of spontaneous healing in surgical fistulae is as high as 20%.

Obstetric fistulae developing after obstructed labour should also be treated by continuous bladder drainage (Waaldijk 1994a), combined with antibiotics to limit tissue damage from infection. Indeed, if a patient is known to have been in obstructed labour for any significant length of time, or is recognized to have areas of slough on the vaginal walls in the puerperium, or has any indication of urine leakage, prophylactic catheterization should be undertaken; with this approach, spontaneous healing has been reported in up to 28% of cases (Waaldijk 1997). If sloughing of the rectal wall has also occurred, faecal discharge will adversely affect spontaneous healing, and temporary defunctioning colostomy should be performed.

The management of ureterovaginal fistulae is beyond the skill of most gynaecologists, and even those with specialist skills in urogynaecology are likely to liaise with urological and radiological colleagues in this situation. Whilst in the past, ureteric reimplantation has been looked on as the preferred approach in most cases, the use of stents inserted either in retrograde (endoscopically) or antegrade (percutaneously) fashion is successful in the majority of cases unless there is complete obstruction (Chang et al 1987, Schwartz and Stoller 2000). Where stenting cannot be achieved, or does not result in closure of the fistula, definitive surgery should be undertaken at 4–6 weeks, unless progressive calyceal dilatation or impairment of function demands earlier intervention.

The immediate management of obstetric third-degree tears has traditionally been thought to lead to good outcome. Recent data suggest that approximately half of patients sustaining such injuries will have subsequent defaecatory symptoms as a result of sphincter disruption rather than denervation, and 6% may end up with rectovaginal fistulae

(Sultan et al 1994). It has not been investigated whether primary repair by a more experienced surgeon or delayed repair would improve outcome.

It is important to appreciate that some fistulae may be associated with minimal symptoms, and even if persistent, these may not require surgical treatment. Small distal urethrovaginal fistulae, uterovesical fistulae with menouria and some low rectovaginal fistulae may fall into this category.

Palliation and skin care

During the waiting period between diagnosis and repair, incontinence pads should be provided in generous quantities so that patients can continue to function socially to some extent. Fistula patients usually leak much greater quantities of urine than those with urethral incontinence from whatever cause, and this needs to be recognized in terms of provision of supplies.

The vulval skin may be at considerable risk from ammoniacal dermatitis, and liberal use of silicone barrier cream should be encouraged. Steroid therapy has been advocated in the past as a means of reducing tissue oedema and fibrosis, although these benefits are refuted and there may be a risk of compromise to subsequent healing (Jonas and Petri 1984). Local oestrogen has been recommended by some authors (Kelly 1983, Jonas and Petri 1984), and whilst empirically, one might expect benefit in postmenopausal women or those obstetric fistula patients with prolonged amenorrhoea, the evidence for this is lacking.

Nutrition

Due to social ostracism and the effects of prolonged sepsis, patients with obstetric fistulae may also suffer from malnutrition and anaemia. To maximize the prospects for postoperative healing, it is essential that the general health of the patient should be optimized. Where there is severe inflammatory bowel disease, the question of an elemental diet or even total parenteral nutrition may need to be considered in consultation with the gastroenterologist involved.

Physiotherapy

Obstetric fistulae are commonly associated with lower limb weakness, foot drop and limb contracture. In a group of 479 patients studied prospectively, 27% had signs of peroneal nerve weakness at presentation, and a further 38%, whilst having no current signs, gave a history of relevant symptoms (Waaldijk and Elkins 1994). Early involvement of the physiotherapist in preoperative management and rehabilitation of such patients is essential.

Antimicrobial therapy

In tropical countries, the treatment of malaria, typhoid, tuberculosis and parasitic infections should be rigorously undertaken before elective surgery. There is no evidence of benefit from prophylactic antibiotics in the management of obstetric fistulae (Tomlinson and Thornton 1998). Opinions differ on the desirability of prophylactic antibiotic cover for surgery in the developed world, with some avoiding their use other than in the treatment of specific infection, and some advocating broad-spectrum treatment in all cases. The author's current practice is for single-dose prophylaxis with co-amoxiclav in urinary fistulae, and 5 days cover for intestinal fistulae using metronidazole and cefuroxime. Only symptomatic urinary tract infections need to be treated in the catheterized patient.

Bowel preparation

Although surgeons vary in the extent to which they prepare the bowel prior to rectovaginal fistula repair, it is the author's preference to carry out formal preparation in all cases of intestinogenital fistula, whatever the level of the lesion. A low-residue diet should be advised for 1 week prior to admission, followed by a fluid-only diet for 48 h before surgery. Polyethylene glycol 3350 (Kleneprep), four sachets in 4 l of water over a 4-h period, or sodium picosulphate (Picolax) 10 mg repeated after 6 h is given orally on the day before operation. Bowel wash-out should be carried out on the evening before surgery, and if bowel content is not completely clear, this should be repeated on the morning of surgery.

Counselling

Surgical fistula patients are usually previously healthy individuals who entered hospital for what was expected to be a routine procedure, and they end up with symptoms infinitely worse than their initial complaint. Obstetric fistula patients in the developing world are social outcasts. In both situations, therefore, these women are invariably devastated by their situation; significant impact on their mental health has been objectively confirmed (Browning et al 2007). It is vital that they understand the nature of the problem, why it has arisen, and the plan for management at all stages. Confident but realistic counselling by the surgeon is essential, and the involvement of nursing staff or counsellors with experience of fistula patients is also highly desirable. The support given by previously treated sufferers can also be of immense value in maintaining patient morale, especially where a delay prior to definitive treatment is required.

General principles of surgical treatment

Details of individual operations are outside the scope of this chapter, and readers wishing for further information about this aspect of fistula management are referred to operative surgical texts or more specific texts on the subject (Chassar Moir 1967, Lawson and Hudson 1987, Zacharin 1988, Mundy 1993, Waaldijk 1994b).

Timing of repair

The timing of surgical repair is perhaps the single most contentious aspect of fistula management. Whilst shortening the waiting period is of both social and psychological benefit to what are always very distressed patients, one must not trade these issues for compromise to surgical success. The benefit of delay is to allow slough to separate and inflammatory change to resolve. In both obstetric and radiation fistulae, there is considerable sloughing of tissues, and it is imperative that this should have settled before repair is undertaken

In radiation fistulae, it may be necessary to wait 12 months or more. In obstetric cases, most authorities suggest that a minimum of 3 months should be allowed to elapse, although Waaldijk (1994a) has advocated surgery as soon as slough is separated.

With surgical fistulae, the same principles should apply, and although the extent of sloughing is limited, extravasation of urine into the pelvic tissues inevitably sets up some inflammatory response. Although early repair is advocated by several authors (Iselin et al 1998), most would agree that 10–12 weeks after surgery is the earliest appropriate time for repair.

Pressure from patients to undertake repair at the earliest opportunity is always understandably great, but never more so than in the case of previous surgical failure. Such pressure must, however, be resisted, and 8 weeks is the minimum time that should be allowed between attempts at closure.

Route of repair

Many urologists advocate an abdominal approach for all fistula repairs, claiming the possibility of earlier intervention and higher success rates in justification. Others suggest that all fistulae can be successfully closed by the vaginal route (Waaldijk 1994b). Such arguments have little merit, and both approaches have their place. Surgeons involved in fistula management must be capable of both approaches, and have the versatility to modify their techniques to select that most appropriate to the individual case. Where access is good and the vaginal tissues are sufficiently mobile, the vaginal route is usually most appropriate. If access is poor and the fistula cannot be brought within reach, the abdominal approach should be used. Although such difficulties can sometimes be handled vaginally, an abdominal procedure may be used to advantage where there is concurrent involvement of ureter or bowel in a surgical fistula.

Overall, more surgical fistulae are likely to require an abdominal repair than obstetric fistulae, although in the author's series of cases from the UK, and those reviewed from Nigeria, two-thirds of cases were satisfactorily treated by the vaginal route, regardless of aetiology (Table 57.4).

Instruments

All operators have their own favoured instruments, although those described in the treatise by Chassar Moir (1967) and Lawson (1967) are eminently suitable for repair by any route (Figure 57.11).

Dissection

Great care must be taken over the initial dissection of the fistula, and one should probably take as long over this as over the repair itself. Preliminary infiltration with 1 : 200,000 solution of adrenaline may help to separate planes and reduce oozing. The fistula should be circumcised in the most convenient orientation, depending on size and access. All things being equal, a longitudinal incision should be made around urethral or midvaginal fistulae, so that during repair, sutures tend to close the bladder neck; conversely, vault fistulae are better handled by a transverse elliptical incision, so that sutures do not tend to approximate the ureters during repair (Figure 57.12A).

The tissue planes are often obliterated by scarring, and dissection close to a fistula should therefore be undertaken with a scalpel or scissors (Figure 57.12B). Sharp dissection is easier with counter traction applied by skin hooks, tissue forceps or retraction sutures. Blunt dissection with small

Table 57.4 Route of primary repair (i.e. first repair at referral centre) of urogenital fistulae in two series from the north-east of England (Hilton unpublished) and from south-east Nigeria (Hilton and Ward 1998)

Route of repair (primary procedure)	North-east England (*n* = 249) %	South-east Nigeria (*n* = 2485) %
Abdominal	**34.8**	**17.0**
Transperitoneal	18.6	13.4
Transvesical	6.5	
Ureteric reimplantation/ stenting	7.7	3.0
Ureterosigmoid transplantation	0	0.6
Ileal conduit	2.0	0
Vaginal	**64.4**	**80.0**
Layer dissection	40.5	80.0
Layer dissection + Martius graft	11.7	0
Urethral reconstruction	6.5	
Colpocleisis	5.3	0
Urethrocleisis + insertion of suprapubic catheter	0.4	
Vaginal, reverse lithotomy	**0.8**	**3.0**
Total	**100.0**	**100.0**

Sources: Hilton (unpublished).
Hilton P, Ward A 1998 Epidemiological and surgical aspects of urogenital fistulae: a review of 25 years experience in south-east Nigeria. International Urogynecology Journal and Pelvic Floor Dysfunction 9: 189–194.

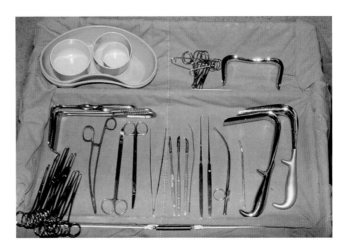

Figure 57.11 Fistula repair instruments.

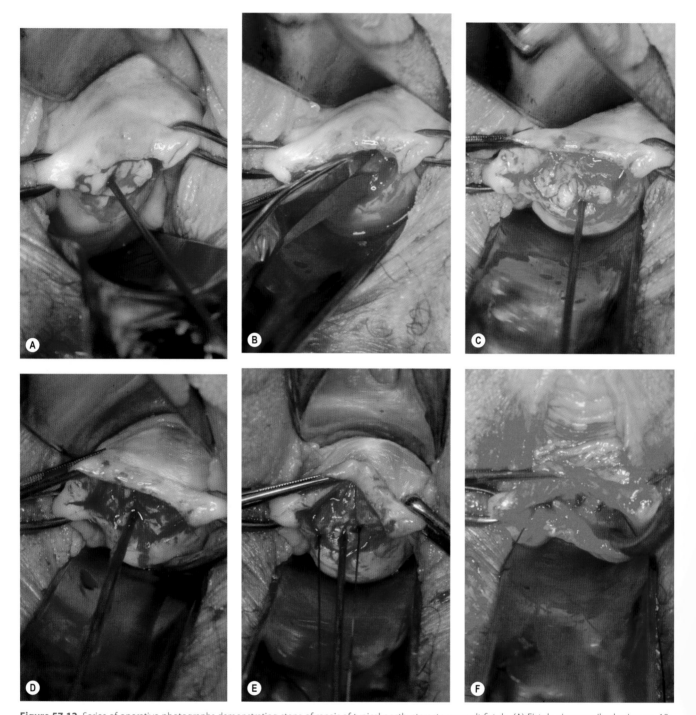

Figure 57.12 Series of operative photographs demonstrating steps of repair of typical posthysterectomy vault fistula. (A) Fistula circumscribed using no. 12 scalpel, (B) sharp dissection around fistula edge, (C) fistula fully mobilized, (D) vaginal scar edge trimmed, (E) first two sutures of first layer of repair in place lateral to the angles of the repair, (F) second layer completed, sutures catching back of vaginal flaps to close off dead space, (G) testing the repair with methylene blue dye instillation, (H) final layer of mattress sutures in the vaginal wall.

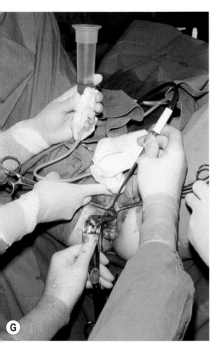 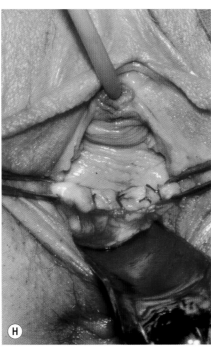

pledgets may be helpful once the planes are established, and provided one is away from the fistula edge. Wide mobilization should be performed, so that tension on the repair is minimized (Figure 57.12C).

There are arguments over the benefits of excision of the fistula track itself. Excision of the bladder walls is probably unwise, as it enlarges the defect and may increase the amount of bleeding into the bladder. However, limited excision of the scarred vaginal wall is usually appropriate (Figure 57.12D).

Bleeding is rarely troublesome with vaginal procedures, except occasionally with proximal urethrovaginal fistulae. Diathermy is best avoided to prevent further devascularization of tissues, and pressure or under-running sutures are preferred.

Suture materials

Although a range of suture materials have been advocated over the years, and a range of opinions still exist, the author's view is that absorbable sutures should be used throughout all urinary fistula repair procedures. Polyglactin (Vicryl) 2/0 suture on a 25-mm heavy tapercut needle is preferred for both the bladder and vagina, and polydioxanone (PDS) 4/0 on a 13-mm round-bodied needle is used for the ureter. 3/0 sutures on a 30-mm round-bodied needle are used for bowel surgery, polydioxanone (PDS) for the small bowel, and either PDS or braided polyamide (Nurolon) for large bowel reanastomosis.

Testing the repair

The closure must be watertight and should be tested at the end of vaginal repairs by the instillation of dye into the bladder under minimal pressure; a previously unsuspected second fistula is occasionally identified this way. Testing after abdominal procedures is impractical.

Specific repair techniques

Vaginal procedures

Dissection and repair in layers

There are two main types of closure technique applied to the repair of urinary fistulae: the classical saucerization technique described by Sims (1852), and the much more commonly used dissection and repair in layers. Sutures must be placed with meticulous accuracy in the bladder wall, with care being taken not to penetrate the mucosa, which should be inverted as far as possible. The repair should be started at either end, working towards the midline, so that the least accessible aspects are sutured first (Figure 57.12E). Interrupted sutures are preferred and should be placed approximately 3 mm apart, taking as large a bite of tissue as feasible. Stitches that are too close together, or the use of continuous or purse-string sutures, tend to impair blood supply and interfere with healing. Knots must be secure with three hitches, so that they can be cut short leaving the minimum amount of material within the body of the repair.

With dissection and repair in layers, the first layer of sutures in the bladder should invert the edges (Figure 57.12E); the second adds bulk to the repair by taking a wide bite of bladder wall, but also closes off dead space by catching the back of the vaginal flaps (Figure 57.12F). After testing the repair (Figure 57.12G) (see below), a third layer of interrupted mattress sutures is used to evert and close the vaginal wall, consolidating the repair by picking up the underlying bladder wall (Figure 57.12H).

Saucerization

The saucerization technique involves converting the track into a shallow crater, which is closed without dissection of bladder from vagina using a single row of interrupted sutures.

The method is only applicable to small fistulae and perhaps residual fistulae after closure of a larger defect; in other situations, the technique does not allow secure closure without tension.

Vaginal repair procedures in specific circumstances

The conventional dissection and repair in layers as described above is entirely appropriate for the majority of midvaginal fistulae, although modifications may be necessary in specific circumstances. In juxtacervical fistulae in the anterior fornix, vaginal repair may be feasible if the cervix can be drawn down to provide access. Dissection should include mobilization of the bladder from the cervix. The repair must be undertaken transversely to reconstruct the underlying trigone and prevent distortion of the ureteric orifices.

Vault fistulae, particularly those following hysterectomy, can usually be managed vaginally. The vault is incised transversely, and mobilization of the fistula is often aided by deliberate opening of the pouch of Douglas (Lawson 1972). The peritoneal opening does not need to be closed separately, but is incorporated into the vaginal closure.

With subsymphysial fistulae involving the bladder neck and proximal urethra as a consequence of obstructed labour, tissue loss may be extensive, and fixity to underlying bone is a common problem. The lateral aspects of the fistula require careful mobilization to overcome disproportion between the defect in the bladder and the urethral stump. A racquet-shape extension of the incision facilitates exposure of the proximal urethra. Although transverse repair is often necessary, longitudinal closure gives better prospects for urethral competence.

Where there is substantial urethral loss, reconstruction may be undertaken using the method described by Chassar Moir (1967) or Hamlin and Nicholson (1969). A strip of anterior vaginal wall is constructed into a tube over a catheter. Plication behind the bladder neck is probably important if continence is to be achieved. The interposition of a labial fat or muscle graft not only fills up the potential dead space, but also provides additional bladder neck support and improves continence by reducing scarring between bladder neck and vagina.

With very large fistulae extending from bladder neck to vault, the extensive dissection required may produce considerable bleeding. The main surgical difficulty is to avoid the ureters. They are usually situated close to the superolateral angles of the fistula, and if they can be identified, they should be catheterized (Figure 57.8). Straight ureteric catheters passed transurethrally or double pigtail catheters may be useful in directing the intramural portion of the ureters internally; nevertheless, great care must be taken during dissection.

Radiation fistulae present particular problems in that the area of devitalized tissue is usually considerably larger than the fistula itself. Mobilization is often impossible, and if repair in layers is attempted, the flaps are likely to slough; closure by colpocleisis is therefore required. Some have advocated total closure of the vagina, although it is preferable to avoid dissection in the devitalized tissue entirely and to perform a lower partial colpocleisis converting the upper vagina into a diverticulum of the bladder. It is usually necessary to fill the dead space below this with an interposition graft (see below).

Abdominal procedures

Transvesical repair

Repair by the abdominal route is indicated when high fistulae are fixed in the vault and are therefore inaccessible by the vaginal route. Transvesical repair has the advantage of being entirely extraperitoneal. It is often helpful to elevate the fistula site by a vaginal pack, and the ureters should be catheterized under direct vision. The technique of closure is similar to that of the transvaginal flap-splitting repair, except that for haemostasis, the bladder mucosa is closed with a continuous suture.

Transperitoneal repair

It is often said that there is little place for a simple transperitoneal repair, although a combined transperitoneal and transvesical procedure is favoured by urologists and is particularly useful for vesicouterine fistulae following caesarean section. A midline split is made in the vault of the bladder; this is extended downwards in a racquet shape around the fistula. The fistulous track is excised, and the vaginal or cervical defect is closed in a single layer. The bladder is then closed in two layers.

For ureteric fistulae not manageable by stenting, reimplantation is considered preferable to reanastomosis of the ureter itself, which carries a greater risk of stricture. Several techniques are described for ureteroneocystostomy, and the most appropriate will depend on the level of the fistula and the nature of the antecedent pathology. The most widely used techniques are direct reimplantation using a psoas hitch, or the creation of a flap of bladder wall (the Boari-Ockerblad technique). There are few lesions which are too high for this approach, although where there is significant deficiency, it may be necessary to perform an end-to-side anastomosis between the injured ureter and the good contralateral ureter (i.e. a ureteroureterostomy), or to interpose a loop of small bowel.

Interposition grafting

Several techniques have been described to support fistula repair in different sites, although the precise role of such grafts is unclear. Some claim that the interposed tissue may serve to create an additional layer in the repair, to fill dead space and to bring in new blood supply to the area, and hence may be of particular value where there is sphincter involvement, and in multiple or recurrent fistulae (Rangnekar et al 2000) or following radiotherapy (Kiricuta 1965). Others, however, have questioned their value (Browning 2006a). There are no randomized data establishing the role of interposition grafts. In retrospective, uncontrolled or non-randomized cohort studies, it is perhaps inevitable that surgeons will have employed grafting in their more complex cases, resulting in misleading conclusions regarding the value of the procedure. The tissues used include the following.

- Martius graft: labial fat and bulbocavernosus muscle passed subcutaneously to cover a vaginal repair; this is particularly appropriate to provide additional bulk in a colpocleisis, and in urethral and bladder neck fistulae may help to maintain competence of closure mechanisms by reducing scarring.

- Gracilis muscle passed either via the obturator foramen or subcutaneously (Hamlin and Nicholson 1969), or rectus abdominis muscle (Bruce et al 2000) may be used as above.
- Omental pedicle grafts (Kiricuta and Goldstein 1972, Turner-Warwick 1976) may be dissected from the greater curve of the stomach and rotated down into the pelvis on the right gastroepiploic artery; this can be used for any transperitoneal procedure, but has its greatest advantage in postradiation fistulae.
- Peritoneal flap graft (Jonas and Petri 1984) is an easier way of providing an additional layer at transperitoneal repair procedures, by taking a flap of peritoneum from any available surface, most usually the paravesical area.

Postoperative management

Fluid balance

Nursing care of patients who have undergone fistula repair is of critical importance, and obsessional postoperative management may do much to secure success. As a corollary, however, poor nursing may easily undermine what the surgeon has achieved. Strict fluid balance must be kept, and a daily fluid intake of at least 3 l and output of 100 ml/h should be maintained until the urine is clear of blood. Haematuria is more persistent following abdominal than vaginal procedures, and intravenous fluid is therefore likely to be required for longer in this situation.

Bladder drainage

Continuous bladder drainage in the postoperative period is crucial to success, and where failure occurs after a straightforward repair, it is almost always possible to identify a period during which free drainage was interrupted. Nursing staff should check catheters hourly throughout each day, to confirm free drainage and check output. Catheters should, of course, drain into a sterile closed drainage system with a non-return valve (Hilton 1987). In circumstances where supplies of sterile disposables are limited or where standards of nursing are poor, as in many developing countries, open drainage has been advocated with good success and low infection rates. Bladder irrigation and suction drainage are no longer recommended.

Views differ regarding the ideal type of catheter. The calibre must be sufficient to prevent blockage, although whether the suprapubic or urethral route is used is, to a large extent, a matter of individual preference. A urethral Foley catheter should probably be avoided following bladder neck fistulae, and either a suprapubic catheter or a non-balloon urethral catheter sutured in place would be preferred. The bladder should not be distended to insert a suprapubic catheter after a vaginal repair, although it could be inserted before surgery by the technique of cutting on to a sound. The author's usual practice is to use a 'belt and braces approach' of both urethral and suprapubic drainage initially, so that if one becomes blocked, free drainage is still maintained. The urethral catheter is removed first, and the suprapubic catheter retained and used to assess residual volume until the patient is voiding normally (Hilton 1987).

The duration of free drainage depends on the fistula type. Following repair of surgical fistulae, 12 days is adequate.

With obstetric fistulae, up to 21 days of drainage may be appropriate, although recent data suggest that this may not be necessary for less complicated cases (Nardos et al 2008). Following repair of radiation fistulae, 21–42 days of drainage may be appropriate. In any of these situations, it is wise to carry out dye testing (see above) prior to catheter removal if there is any doubt about the integrity of the repair. Where a persistent leak is identified, free drainage should be maintained for 6 weeks.

Bowel management

If patients are restricted to bed following urogenital fistula repair, a laxative should be administered to prevent excessive straining at stool. Traditionally, patients have been managed by nasogastric tube, by being kept nil by mouth until they are passing flatus, after abdominal repair of intestinovaginal fistulae; however, evidence that this approach is necessary is lacking. Once oral intake is allowed, or following vaginal repair of rectovaginal fistulae, a low-residue diet should be administered until at least the fifth postoperative day. Enemas and suppositories should be avoided, although a mild aperient such as dioctyl sodium (Docusate) is advised to ease initial bowel movements.

Subsequent management

On removal of catheters, most patients will feel the desire to void frequently since the bladder capacity will be functionally reduced having been relatively empty for so long. In any case, it is important that they do not become overdistended, and hourly voiding should be encouraged and fluid intake limited. It may also be necessary to wake them once or twice through the night for the same reason. After discharge from hospital, patients should be advised to gradually increase the period between voiding, aiming to be back to a normal pattern by 4 weeks after surgery. Tampons, pessaries, douching and penetrative sex should be avoided until 3 months after surgery.

Prognosis

Results

It is difficult to compare the results of treatment in different series since the lesions involved and the techniques of repair vary so greatly. Cure rates should be considered in terms of closure at first operation, and vary from 60% to 98% (Turner-Warwick et al 1967, Hamlin and Nicholson 1969, Chassar Moir 1973, Hudson et al 1975, Goodwin and Scardino 1979, Patil et al 1980, O'Conor 1980, Wein et al 1980, Elkins et al 1988, Lee et al 1988, World Health Organization 1989, Hilton 1995, Hilton and Ward 1998). In ideal circumstances, one might anticipate an 80% continence rate, 10% failures and, in the case of obstetric fistulae at least, 10% suffering from postfistula stress incontinence.

Of the 300 patients in the author's series managed in the UK, 25 (8.3%) healed without operation, 10 (3.3%) declined surgery, 12 (4.0%) were telephone referrals only and either healed spontaneously or were treated at their local hospital, five (1.7%) underwent primary urinary diversion, and four died from malignancy or the effects of radiation prior to

Table 57.5 Outcome of treatment in the author's series of urogenital fistulae treated in the north-east of England between 1987 and 2008

Aetiology		Surgical	Obstetric	Radiation/malignant	Miscellaneous	Total
Number		207	35	30	28	300
Healed spontaneously	n	18	4	0	3	25
	%	8.7	11.4	0	10.7	8.3
Deceased, declined surgery or referred for advice alone	n	8	3	10	5	26
	%	3.9	8.6	33.3	17.9	8.7
Primary urinary diversion	n	1	0	4	0	5
	%	0.5	0	13.3	0	1.7
Primary repair procedure	n	180	28	16	20	244
	%	87.0	80.0	53.3	71.4	81.3
Closed at first operation	n	174	25	14	19	232
	%	96.7	89.3	87.5	95.0	95.1

treatment. Of the remaining 244 who have undergone repair surgery, 232 (95.1%) were closed at their first operation, although of these, 12 (5.2%) have some residual incontinence. More specifically, the rate of closure at first operation in the author's series is 97% in surgical cases, 95% in miscellaneous cases, 89% in obstetric cases and 88% in radiotherapy cases. Of the 130 fistulae following simple hysterectomy undergoing surgical treatment in Newcastle, 128 (98.5%) were cured at their first operation (Table 57.5).

Long-term outcome has rarely been considered. Dolan et al (2008) reported a median 4 year follow-up of women undergoing fistula repair in the UK. Despite their fistulae being anatomically closed, most women reported one or more urinary symptoms in the long term, although only one in eight found these symptoms significantly problematic. Frequency, nocturia, and stress or urge incontinence were the most common troublesome symptoms, and there was no obvious trend to improvement over time.

Of the largely obstetric fistulae reviewed from Nigeria by Hilton and Ward (1998), 81.2% were cured by the first operation and 97.7% were eventually successfully anatomically repaired, with only 0.6% undergoing urinary diversion. It is commonly assumed that follow-up of obstetric fistula patients after discharge from hospital is not feasible; however, two recent studies have found this not to be the case (Browning and Menber 2008, Nielsen et al 2009). Both studies found fistula closure to be associated with improvement in quality of life and reintegration into society. In the longer-term follow-up study of Browning and Menber (2008), although incontinence persisted in some patients, there was a tendency to further improvement over time.

A law of diminishing returns has been reported previously (Lawson 1978). Although repeat operations are certainly justified, the success rate decreases progressively with increasing numbers of previous unsuccessful procedures. In the series reported from Nigeria, although the cure rate at first operation was 81.7%, the success rate for those patients requiring two or more procedures fell to 65% (Hilton and Ward 1998). It cannot be overemphasized that the best prospect for cure is at the first operation, and there is no place for the well-intentioned occasional fistula surgeon, be they gynaecologist or urologist.

Postfistula stress incontinence

Stress incontinence has long been recognized as a complication of vesicovaginal fistulae (Lawson 1967). It is most likely to occur in obstetric fistula patients when the injury involves the sphincter mechanism, particularly if there is tissue loss (Waaldijk 1989, Browning 2006b), although it has also been reported in a large proportion of surgical fistulae involving the urethra or bladder neck (Hilton 1998). It affects at least 10% of all fistula patients, and its impact in terms of the patient's quality of life and mental health may be as great as that of the fistula itself (Browning et al 2007).

The extent of scarring in the area means that conventional approaches to bladder neck elevation may be technically difficult and of limited success. The use of a labial musculo-fat graft in the initial repair may reduce the likelihood of the complication (Waaldijk 1994b), and a number of other techniques have been attempted (Hudson et al 1975, Waaldijk 1994b). The implantation of an artificial urinary sphincter or neourethral reconstruction may be appropriate from a theoretical point of view (Hilton 1990), but the former would be prohibitively expensive, and both would be excessively morbid, for use in the developing world. Periurethral injections hold promise as a minimally invasive technique particularly appropriate in the situation of urethral insufficiency with a relatively fixed immobile urethra. Although initial success has been reported in postfistula stress incontinent patients (Hilton et al 1998), the long-term outcomes are disappointing.

Subsequent pregnancy

Although many patients with obstetric vesicovaginal fistula will experience amenorrhoea for 2 years or more after the causative pregnancy (Hilton and Ward 1998), where tissue loss is not great, hypothalamic function often returns to normal immediately after successful repair, and fertility may be relatively normal. Kelly (1979) reported on 33 patients who became pregnant within 1 year of fistula repair, 12 of whom were delivered vaginally without damage to the repair. His criteria for attempting vaginal delivery were: that the fistula arose from a non-recurring cause (i.e. malpresentation as opposed to pelvic contraction), that an interposition graft had been utilized in the repair, and that the labour was conducted under skilled supervision in hospital (Kelly 1979). However, most other authorities have emphasized the need for caesarean section in any subsequent pregnancy (Lawson 1978). Most recently, in a study from Ethiopia, Browning (2009) described no recurrent fistulae, and 47 livebirths from 49 pregnancies delivered by a policy of elective caesarean section (in the rare cases where dates were certain) or emergency caesarean section at premature rupture of membranes or onset of labour.

Prevention

It has been estimated by the World Health Organization (WHO) that there are approximately 500,000 maternal deaths per year worldwide (World Health Organization 1989), and it is clear that the prevalence of obstetric fistulae and maternal mortality rates are closely related. Indeed, one might look on the vesicovaginal fistula patient as being the 'near-miss' maternal death. In recognition of this fact, WHO established, through their 'Safe Motherhood Initiative', a technical working group to investigate the problems of prevention and management of obstetric fistulae. The recommendations from that working group included the extension of antenatal and intrapartum care; the transfer of women in prolonged labour for delivery by skilled personnel; the identification of areas where fistulae are still prevalent, so that resources could be mobilized to deal with fistulae more effectively; and the creation of specialized centres for management, training and research, with a specific aim of treating existing cases within 5 years (World Health Organization 1989). One thousand years ago, Avicenna recognized the problems of early childbearing, saying: 'in cases where

women are married too young the physician should instruct the patient in the ways of prevent of pregnancy. In these patients the bulk of the fetus may cause a tear in the bladder which results in incontinence of urine which is incurable and remains until death' (Hilton 1995). Clearly, the achievement of WHO's aims and recommendations is critically dependent on major social change in areas of endemicity. Without improvement in the status of women, an extension of primary education, deferment of marriage and childbearing, improved nutritional status and contraceptive services, and skilled attendants in childbirth throughout the world, the problem of obstetric fistulae will remain with us well into the new millennium.

In the developed world, our concern must lie with the prevention and management of fistulae following gynaecological surgery. Primarily, we need to be aware of those factors increasing the likelihood of lower urinary tract injury during surgery, and must recognize the limits of our own, and perhaps more importantly our trainees', surgical skills. We should not expect staff in training to undertake surgery in cases where risk factors are known to be present without adequate supervision and support. We should be equally aware of the signs of injury in the postoperative period, and should have standard regimens for the management of patients with voiding difficulty in the postoperative period if bladder overdistension and risk of late damage is to be avoided. As indicated earlier, with advances in medical therapy for menorrhagia, and in minimally invasive surgery and techniques of endometrial resection/ablation, the need for hysterectomy is reducing considerably. However, hysterectomy will always be necessary for fibroids, endometriosis, sepsis and malignancy, and these carry the greatest risk of lower urinary tract injury. If these are the only cases on which our trainees can train, there is a danger that surgical skills, in general, may decline, in the same way that skills in vaginal breech delivery and rotational forceps delivery have declined with increasing use of caesarean section. Although the total number of fistulae seen in the UK is also reducing, the rate of urinary tract injury at hysterectomy seems, if anything, to be increasing.

KEY POINTS

1. In developing countries, over 90% of fistulae are of obstetric origin and are due to pressure necrosis from prolonged obstructed labour.

2. In the UK, approximately 70% of fistulae follow pelvic surgery, and 70% of these cases are associated with hysterectomy.

3. The characteristic presentation with continuous urinary leakage and reduced frequency and bladder sensation is not always present in patients with small fistulae, and a high index of suspicion must be maintained if the diagnosis is not to be missed. With intestinal fistulae, the history may be similarly misleading.

4. The upper urinary tracts should be assessed by intravenous or computed tomography urogram in all patients with urogenital fistulae.

5. The current best estimate is that urogenital fistula complicates one in 750 hysterectomies in the UK; this is rarely due to direct injury, and more often results from tissue ischaemia, adjacent sutures, haematoma or infection. Although poor surgical technique

increases the risk, the mere fact of fistula development following hysterectomy does not imply negligence.

6. Where bladder damage is suspected or fistula is confirmed following surgery or childbirth, catheterization should be undertaken and continuous drainage maintained; spontaneous healing may occur up to 8 weeks after the initiating event.

7. The possibility of inflammatory bowel disease should always be considered in patients with intestinogenital fistula, even in the absence of specific bowel symptoms. Of the inflammatory causes, Crohn's disease is the most important. Ideally, surgical treatment should only be undertaken when the bowel pathology is quiescent.

8. Biopsy of the fistula edge or any unhealthy looking local tissue should be undertaken before embarking on repair of radiation, inflammatory or potentially infective fistulae.

9. Malnutrition, anaemia and infection should be treated before attempting surgical closure; this applies most particularly in patients with obstetric fistulae in the developing world.

10. Surgery for urogenital or intestinogenital fistulae should only be undertaken by surgeons with the appropriate training and experience, and with the versatility to undertake the most appropriate operation by the most appropriate route.

11. Layered closure with avoidance of tension on the suture lines, good haemostasis and obliteration of dead space are important technical points for successful closure.

12. Interposition grafting with pedicled fat or muscle may be a useful adjunct in fistula surgery, by providing an additional layer to the repair, filling dead space, bringing new blood supply and encouraging tissue mobility.

13. Successful anatomical closure of a urinary or intestinal fistula is not necessarily associated with restoration of complete functional normality. Incompetence of sphincter mechanisms may occur, with residual stress urinary incontinence, faecal soiling or incontinence of flatus. Although patients should be made aware that some residual symptoms may persist after fistula repair, for the majority, successful closure is associated with marked improvement in quality of life. For obstetric fistula patients, this is associated with reintegration into normal society.

14. Diversion of urinary or faecal stream should rarely be required as definitive measures for the management of obstetric or surgical fistulae, although they have a small but important place in the management of postradiotherapy fistulae.

References

Arrowsmith S 2007 The classification of obstetric vesico-vaginal fistulas: a call for an evidence-based approach. International Journal of Gynecology and Obstetrics 99 (Suppl 1): S25–S27.

Averette HE, Nguyen HN, Donato DM et al 1993 Radical hysterectomy for invasive cervical cancer. A 25-year prospective experience with the Miami technique. Cancer 71: 1422–1437.

Bladou F, Houvenaeghel G, Delpero JR, Guerinel G 1995 Incidence and management of major urinary complications after pelvic exenteration for gynecological malignancies. Journal of Surgical Oncology 58: 91–96.

Browning A 2006a Lack of value of the Martius graft in obstetric fistula repair. International Journal of Gynecology and Obstetrics 93: 33–37.

Browning A 2006b Risk factors for developing residual urinary incontinence after obstetric fistula repair. BJOG: an International Journal of Obstetrics and Gynaecology 113: 482–485.

Browning A 2009 Pregnancy following obstetric fistula repair, the management of delivery. BJOG: an International Journal of Obstetrics and Gynaecology 116: 1265–1267.

Browning A, Fentahun W, Goh JT 2007 The impact of surgical treatment on the mental health of women with obstetric fistula. BJOG: an International Journal of Obstetrics and Gynaecology 114: 1439–1441.

Browning A, Menber B 2008 Women with obstetric fistula in Ethiopia: a 6-month follow up after surgical treatment. BJOG: an International Journal of Obstetrics and Gynaecology 115: 1564–1569.

Bruce RG, El-Galley RES, Galloway NTM 2000 Use of rectus abdominis muscle flap for the treatment of complex and refractory urethrovaginal fistulas. Journal of Urology 163: 1212–1215.

Chang R, Marshall F, Mitchell S 1987 Percutaneous management of benign ureteral strictures and fistulas. Journal of Urology 137: 1126–1131.

Chassar Moir J 1967 The Vesico-vaginal Fistula, 2nd edn. Baillière, London.

Chassar Moir J 1973 Vesico-vaginal fistulae as seen in Britain. Journal of Obstetrics and Gynaecology of the British Commonwealth 80: 598–602.

Davits R, Miranda S 1991 Conservative treatment of vesico-vaginal fistulas by bladder drainage alone. British Journal of Urology 68: 155–156.

Department of Health 2009 Hospital Episode Statistics. Department of Health. Available at: www.hesonline.nhs.uk.

Dolan L, Dixon W, Hilton P 2008 Urinary symptoms and quality of life following urogenital fistula repair: a long-term follow-up study. BJOG: an International Journal of Obstetrics and Gynaecology 115: 1570–1574.

Elkins TE, Drescher C, Martey JO, Fort D 1988 Vesicovaginal fistula revisited. Obstetrics and Gynecology 72: 307–312.

Emmert C, Köhler U 1996 Management of genital fistulas in patients with cervical cancer. Archives of Gynecology and Obstetrics 259: 19–24.

Falk F, Tancer M 1956 Management of vesical fistulas after caesarean section. American Journal of Obstetrics and Gynecology 71: 97–106.

Goh J 2004 A new classification for female genital tract fistula. Australian and New Zealand Journal of Obstetrics and Gynaecology 44: 502–504.

Goh JT, Browning A, Berhan B, Chang A 2008 Predicting the risk of failure of closure of obstetric fistula and residual urinary incontinence using a classification system. International Urogynecology Journal of Pelvic Floor Dysfunction 19: 1659–1662.

Goodwin WE, Scardino PT 1979 Vesicovaginal and ureterovaginal fistulas: a summary of 25 years of experience. Transactions of the American Association of Genitourinary Surgeons 71: 123–129.

Hamlin R, Nicholson E 1969 Reconstruction of urethra totally destroyed in labour. BMJ (Clinical Research Ed.) 2: 147–150.

Harkki-Siren P, Sjoberg J, Tiitinen A 1998 Urinary tract injuries after hysterectomy. Obstetrics and Gynecology 92: 113–118.

Hilton P 1987 Catheters and drains. In: Stanton S (ed) Principles of Gynaecological Surgery. Springer-Verlag, Berlin, pp 257–283.

Hilton P 1990 Surgery for genuine stress incontinence: which operation and for which patient? In: Drife J, Hilton P, Stanton S (eds) Micturition—Proceedings of the 21st RCOG Study Group. Springer-Verlag, London, pp 225–246.

Hilton P 1995 Sims to SMIS—an Historical Perspective on Vesico-vaginal Fistulae. The Yearbook of the RCOG, 1994. Royal College of Obstetricians and Gynaecologists, London, pp 7–16.

Hilton P 1997 Debate: 'Post-operative urinary fistulae should be managed by gynaecologists in specialist centres'. BJU International 80 (Suppl 1): 35–42.

Hilton P 1998 The urodynamic findings in patients with urogenital fistulae. British Journal of Urology 81: 539–542.

Hilton P, Ward A 1998 Epidemiological and surgical aspects of urogenital fistulae: a review of 25 years experience in south-east Nigeria. International Urogynecology Journal and Pelvic Floor Dysfunction 9: 189–194.

Hilton P, Ward A, Molloy M, Umana O 1998 Periurethral injection of autologous fat for the treatment of post-fistula repair stress incontinence: a preliminary report. International Urogynecology Journal and Pelvic Floor Dysfunction 9: 118–121.

Hudson C 1968 Malignant change in an obstetric vesico-vaginal fistula. Proceedings of the Royal Society of Medicine 61: 121–124.

Hudson C, Hendrickse J, Ward A 1975 An operation for restoration of urinary continence following total loss of the urethra. British Journal of Obstetrics and Gynaecology 82: 501–504.

Iselin CE, Aslan P, Webster GD 1998 Transvaginal repair of vesicovaginal fistulas after hysterectomy by vaginal cuff excision. Journal of Urology 160: 728–730.

Jonas U, Petri E 1984 Genitourinary fistulae. In: Stanton S (ed) Clinical Gynecologic Urology. CV Mosby, St Louis, pp 238–255.

Kelly J 1979 Vesicovaginal fistulae. British Journal of Urology 51: 208–210.

Kelly J 1983 Vesico-vaginal fistulae. In: Studd J (ed) Progress in Obstetrics and Gynaecology, 3rd edn. Churchill Livingstone, Edinburgh, pp 324–333.

Kelly J, Kwast B 1993 Epidemiologic study of vesico-vaginal fistula in Ethiopia. International Urogynecology Journal 4: 278–281.

Kiricuta I 1965 Use of the greater omentum in the treatment of vesicovaginal and rectovesicovaginal fistulae after radiotherapy and cystoplasties [in French]. Journal de Chirurgie 89: 477–484.

Kiricuta I, Goldstein A 1972 The repair of extensive vesicovaginal fistulas with pedicled omentum: a review of 27 cases. Journal of Urology 108: 724–727.

Lawson J 1967 Injuries to the urinary tract. In: Lawson J, Stewart D (eds) Obstetrics and Gynaecology in the Tropics and Developing Countries. Edward Arnold, London, pp 481–522.

Lawson J 1972 Vesical fistulae into the vaginal vault. British Journal of Urology 44: 623–631.

Lawson J 1978 The management of genito-urinary fistulae. Clinics in Obstetrics and Gynaecology 6: 209–236.

Lawson L, Hudson C 1987 The management of vesico-vaginal and urethral fistulae. In: Stanton S, Tanagho E (eds) Surgery for Female Urinary Incontinence. Springer-Verlag, Berlin, pp 193–209.

Lee R, Symmonds R, Williams T 1988 Current status of genitourinary fistula. Obstetrics and Gynecology 71: 313–319.

Lovel H, McGettigan C, Mohammed Z 2000 A Systematic Review of the Health Complications of Female Genital Mutilation Including Sequelae in Childbirth. World Health Organization, Geneva.

Meeks GR, Sams JO, Field KW, Fulp KS, Margolis MT 1997 Formation of vesicovaginal fistula: the role of suture placement into the bladder during closure of the vaginal cuff after transabdominal hysterectomy. American Journal of Obstetrics and Gynecology 177: 1298–1304.

Mundy A 1993 Urodynamic and Reconstructive Surgery of the Lower Urinary Tract. Churchill Livingstone, Edinburgh.

Murphy M 1981 Social consequences of vesico-vaginal fistula in northern Nigeria. Journal of Biosocial Sciences 13: 139–150.

Nardos R, Browning A, Member B 2008 Duration of bladder catheterization after surgery for obstetric fistula. International Journal of Gynecology and Obstetrics 103: 30–32.

Nielsen H, Lindberg L, Nygaard U et al 2009 A community based long-term follow-up of obstetric fistula patients in rural Ethiopia. BJOG: an International Journal of Obstetrics and Gynaecology 2009: 116: 1258–1264.

O'Conor VJ 1980 Review of experience with vesicovaginal fistula repair. Journal of Urology 123: 367–369.

Patil U, Waterhouse K, Laungani G 1980 Management of 18 difficult vesicovaginal and urethrovaginal fistulas with modified Ingelman-Sundberg and Martius operations. Journal of Urology 123: 653–656.

Raghavaiah N 1974 Double-dye test to diagnose various types of vaginal fistulas. Journal of Urology 112: 811–812.

Rangnekar NP, Imdad AN, Kaul SA, Pathak HR 2000 Role of the Martius procedure in the management of urinary-vaginal fistulas. Journal of the American College of Surgeons 191: 259–263.

Schwartz BF, Stoller ML 2000 Endourologic management of urinary fistulae. Techniques in Urology 6: 193–195.

Sims J 1852 On the treatment of vesico-vaginal fistula. American Journal of Medical Sciences XXIII: 59–82.

Sultan AH, Kamm MA, Hudson CN, Bartram CI 1994 Third degree obstetric and sphincter tears: risk factors and outcome of primary repair. BMJ (Clinical Research Ed.) 308: 887–891.

Tahzib F 1983 Epidemiological determinants of vesicovaginal fistulas. British Journal of Obstetrics and Gynaecology 90: 387–391.

Tahzib F 1985 Vesicovaginal fistula in Nigerian children. The Lancet 2: 1291–1293.

Tomlinson AJ, Thornton JG 1998 A randomised controlled trial of antibiotic prophylaxis for vesico-vaginal fistula repair. British Journal of Obstetrics and Gynaecology 105: 397–399.

Turner-Warwick R 1976 The use of the omental pedicle graft in urinary tract reconstruction. Journal of Urology 116: 341–347.

Turner-Warwick RT, Wynne EJ, Handley-Ashken M 1967 The use of the omental pedicle graft in the repair and reconstruction of the urinary tract. British Journal of Surgery 54: 849–853.

United Nations Population Fund 2007 A Holistic Approach to the Abandonment of Female Genital Mutilation/Cutting.

UNFPA, New York. Available at: www.unfpa.org/webdav/site/global/shared/documents/publications/2007/726_filename_fgm.pdf.

Waaldijk K 1989 The Surgical Management of Bladder Fistula in 775 Women in Northern Nigeria. MD Thesis, Amsterdam. Benda B.V., Nijmegen, The Netherlands.

Waaldijk K 1994a The immediate surgical management of fresh obstetric fistulas with catheter and/or early closure. International Journal of Gynecology and Obstetrics 45: 11–16.

Waaldijk K 1994b Step-by-step Surgery for Vesico-vaginal Fistulas. Campion, Edinburgh.

Waaldijk K 1995 Surgical classification of obstetric fistulas. International Journal of Gynaecology and Obstetrics 49: 161–163.

Waaldijk K 1997 Immediate indwelling bladder catheterisation at postpartum urine leakage—personal experience of 1200 patients. Tropical Doctor 27: 227–228.

Waaldijk K, Armiya'u Y 1993 The obstetric fistula: a major public health problem still unsolved. International Urogynecology Journal 4: 126–128.

Waaldijk K, Elkins T 1994 The obstetric fistula and perineal nerve injury: an analysis of 947 consecutive patients. International Urogynecology Journal 5: 12–14.

Wein AJ, Malloy TR, Carpiniello VL, Greenberg SH, Murphy JJ 1980 Repair of vesicovaginal fistula by a suprapubic transvesical approach. Surgery, Gynecology and Obstetrics 150: 57–60.

World Health Organization 1989 The Prevention and Treatment of Obstetric Fistulae: a Report of a Technical Working Group. WHO, Geneva.

World Health Organization 2008 Eliminating Female Genital Mutilation: an Interagency Statement: UNAIDS, UNDP, UNECA, UNESCO, UNFPA, UNHCHR, UNHCR, UNICEF, UNIFEM, WHO. WHO, Geneva. Available at: www.who.int/reproductive-health/publications/fgm/fgm_statement_2008.pdf.

Yeates W 1987 Uretero-vaginal fistulae. In: Stanton S, Tanagho E (eds) Surgery for Female Urinary Incontinence, 2nd edn. Springer-Verlag, Berlin, pp 211–217.

Youssef A 1957 'Menouria' following lower segment caesarean section: a syndrome. American Journal of Obstetrics and Gynecology 73: 759–767.

Zacharin R 1988 Obstetric Fistula. Springer-Verlag, Vienna.

CHAPTER 58

Urinary tract infection

Charlotte Chaliha and Michael R. Millar

Chapter Contents

INTRODUCTION	896	PHYSICAL SIGNS	899
TERMINOLOGY AND DEFINITIONS	896	MANAGEMENT	899
MICROBIOLOGY OF URINARY TRACT INFECTION	897	SPECIFIC CLINICAL SITUATIONS	903
PATHOGENESIS	897	CONCLUSIONS	904
NATURAL HISTORY	899	KEY POINTS	904
PRESENTATION	899		

Introduction

Urinary tract infections (UTIs) are a common cause of morbidity in women, affecting 50% of adult women at least once in their lives. In women aged 20–65 years, at least 20% will suffer an infection each year. Each year, approximately 5% of women will present to their general practitioners with dysuria and frequency (Hamilton-Miller 1994), and approximately half of these will have a UTI. It has been estimated that, on average, a case of uncomplicated acute cystitis results in 6.1 days of symptoms, 2.4 days of restriction of activities and 0.4 days in bed (Foxman and Frerichs 1985a). In women, the incidence of UTI increases with age and with the onset of sexual activity, and is highest amongst the elderly. In children under 1 year of age, the prevalence is higher in boys than girls, with a male:female ratio of 3:1–5:1. UTI in the neonate should be considered to be secondary to an underlying anatomical abnormality until proven otherwise (Kunin 1987).

The prevalence of UTI increases significantly with increasing age, and is higher in women than in men. In the elderly, the prevalence may be as high as 50%, especially if the woman is institutionalized (Boscia and Kaye 1987). This high prevalence in the elderly is thought to be secondary to cerebrovascular accidents, reduced mental and functional capacity, the use of bladder catheters and diabetes.

Approximately 25–30% of affected women will develop recurrent UTI that is not related to an underlying anatomical or functional abnormality of the urinary tract (Hooton 2001, Finer and Landau 2004).

This chapter will concentrate on UTI in the adult female and discuss strategies for treatment and prevention.

Terminology and Definitions

UTI is defined as inflammation of the urinary tract due to microbial invasion. There is considerable overlap in the clinical presentations of the various syndromes, including cystitis, pyelonephritis and urethritis. Complicated UTI is UTI associated with functional or anatomical abnormalities that increase the risk of serious complications or treatment failure, such as conditions which cause obstruction or relative stasis of urinary flow (Box 58.1).

Urine samples collected directly from the bladder, ureter or renal pelvis should be sterile. Urine passed through the urethra always contains some bacteria derived from the terminal urethra. Significant bacteriuria is defined by the culture of increased numbers of bacterial colony-forming units (CFUs). The absolute number needed to define significant bacteriuria depends on the sample type. The threshold of more than 10^5 CFU/ml has been a standard for the definition of significant bacteriuria using carefully collected midstream urine (MSU) since the 1950s (Kass 1956). A significant proportion of patients with UTI will have less than 10^5 CFU/ml (Johnson and Stamm 1987, 1989). Therefore, current recommendations (Warren et al 1999) suggest more than 10^3 CFU/ml for a diagnosis of cystitis, and more than 10^4 CFU/ml for a diagnosis of pyelonephritis. An important consideration with these diagnostic criteria is that they rely on careful collection of the MSU. This requires that care is taken in the instruction and support that patients are given to collect these samples. Bacteriuria is common in association with any long-term catheter and is not in itself an indication for treatment of UTI.

DOI: 10.1016/B978-0-7020-3120-5.00058-8

Box 58.1 Conditions associated with a complicated UTI

Obstruction/structural
- Presence of stones, catheters, stents or abnormalities, nephrostomy tubes
- Urinary tract malignancy
- Diverticuli
- Fistula
- Ileal conduits/urinary diversions
- Coexisting pelvic malignancy or inflammatory bowel conditions

Functional abnormality
- Neurogenic bladder
- Anticholinergic drugs (leading to incomplete bladder emptying)

Miscellaneous
- Diabetes mellitus
- Pregnancy
- Renal failure
- Immunosuppression
- Hospital-acquired/resistant infections

Asymptomatic bacteriuria is defined as the presence of more than 10^5 CFU/ml in two MSU samples in the absence of symptoms (Zhanel et al 1990). Cystitis is an inflammation of the bladder which may be due to infection or a variety of other causes. Urethritis is inflammation of the urethra and may be a consequence of a wide range of causes including UTI, sexually transmitted diseases such as chlamydia, vaginitis, trauma and allergy. Bacterial pyelonephritis is infection of the renal pelvices which may be acute or chronic.

Microbiology of Urinary Tract Infection

The majority of UTIs are caused by facultative bacteria and, occasionally, by fungi and viruses. *Escherichia coli* accounts for up to 70% of community-acquired infections (Grüneberg 1994), with the remainder predominantly caused by *Staphylococcus saprophyticus* and a variety of Gram-negative rods within the Enterobacteriaceae. In hospital-acquired infections, approximately 50% are caused by *E. coli*, 15% by *Enterococcus* spp. and the remainder by members of the Enterobacteriaceae, *Pseudomonas* spp., *Staphylococcus* spp. and yeasts (Bryan and Reynolds 1984). Hospital-acquired UTIs are frequently associated with iatrogenic risk factors such as instrumentation, and also with patient comorbidities. Antibiotic resistance is also much more likely to complicate hospital-acquired UTI.

Pathogenesis

There are host, iatrogenic and bacterial factors that contribute to the pathogenesis of UTI. Foreign bodies such as urinary catheters are major risk factors for infection through mechanisms that include trauma, compromise of local immunity, and by providing protected niche(s) for microbial proliferation and surfaces for biofilm production.

Bacterial virulence factors

The ability of bacteria to adhere to uroepithelial cells is a prerequisite for infection to occur, and reduces the chance of the bacteria being cleared from the urinary tract during voiding. There are various adherence factors, called 'adhesins'; *E. coli* possess surface organelles called 'pili' that act as adhesins. These adhesins attach to complementary structures on the uroepithelial cell wall, and act not only to promote infection but also to help promote growth and toxin production (Zafriri et al 1987). There are many different types of adhesins, such as type 4 pili, outer membrane proteins, curli, filamentous haemagglutinins and adhesive pili. Other virulence factors that may facilitate infection are specific to each pathogen. These include the surface antigens on *E. coli* and haemolysins that are produced to help degrade cells, and aerobactins that enhance iron uptake which encourages *E. coli* growth.

Much of our understanding of UTI comes from the study of uropathogenic *E. coli* (UPEC). The type of pili of the different strains of UPEC may determine the site of disease in the urinary tract as they have specific cell affinity (Gunther et al 2002). The virulence of UPEC has been attributed mainly to the presence of type 1 fimbriae, a mannose-binding adhesion protein called 'FimH' (Abraham et al 1988). Another pathogenic mechanism is the development of intracellular UPEC pods which act as a reservoir for infection (Anderson et al 2003). These pods contain bacteria that are encased in a polysaccharide matrix and protected by a uroplakin coating which help to evade host defence mechanisms and antimicrobials. This initiates the invasion into cells to develop intracellular bacterial communities. It is this reservoir that can serve as a source of bacteria that may reinitiate infection (Figure 58.1)

Host factors

Regular voiding flushes the urinary tract of pathogens and the acidity of urine inhibits bacterial growth. A healthy vaginal flora is thought to be essential in reducing infection. This flora is predominantly lactobacilli and this maintains an acidic pH in the vagina. Lactobacilli and uromucoid in the urine are thought to interfere with bacterial adherence and colonization. It is also thought that the composition of the flora is important as it provides a continuous microbial stimulus to the host immune system, such that it is primed to respond to pathogens. In women with recurrent UTI, the flora has reduced lactobacillus composition (Kirjavainen et al 2009). The glycosaminoglycan layer of the bladder also serves as a protective layer preventing bacterial adherence.

Factors that increase the risk of infection include:

- impaired bladder emptying which can occur with neurogenic disorders such as diabetes, multiple sclerosis, cerebrovascular events and anatomical abnormalities. Anticholinergic drugs may also impair bladder emptying;
- instrumentation of the urinary tract which may traumatize the urethra;
- foreign bodies such as catheters and stones increase the risk of infection as they are a focus for infection;

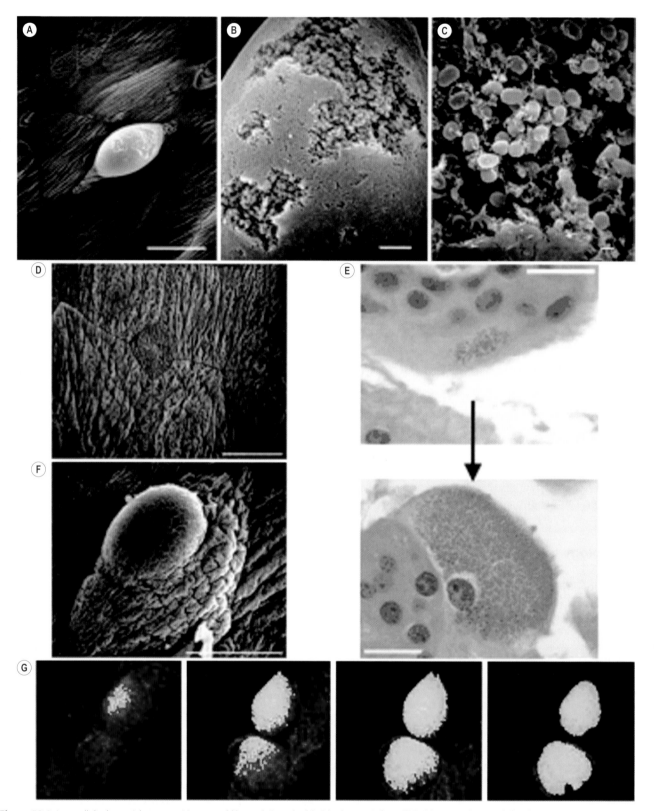

Figure 58.1 Intracellular bacterial communities extend like pods into the bladder lumen. Infected bladders were bisected, fixed and visualized by either scanning electron microscopy (SEM) or light microscopy [haematoxylin and eosin (H&E) staining]. (A–C) SEM images of a pod on the surface of a C3H/HeJ mouse bladder infected with UTI89 for 24 h show large intracellular communities of bacteria inside pods. Scale bars: 50 μm (A), 5 μm (B), 0.5 μm (C). (D) SEM revealed no pods in C3H/HeJ bladders infected with MG1655. Scale bar: 50 μm. (E) H&E-stained sections of UTI89-infected C3H/HeJ mouse bladders show a bacterial factory 6 h after inoculation (top panel) and a pod 24 h after inoculation (bottom panel). Bacteria in the pod were densely packed, shorter and completely filled the host cell. Video microscopy has shown that bacterial factories mature into pods. Scale bars: 20 μm. (F) Pods were evident in wild-type C3H/HeN bladders infected with UTI89. Scale bar: 50 μm. (G) Confocal Z-section series from whole-mounted bladder infected with UTI89 expressing green fluorescent protein from the plasmid pcomGFP and stained with antibody to uroplakin (primary antibody) and tetramethyl rhodamine isothiocyanate-labelled secondary antibody, showing uroplakin coating the surface of pods. The series depicts the lumenal surface on the left and progresses through the epithelium toward the right. Optical section thickness: 1 μm. All images are representative of the entire sample surface and are from bladders harvested 24 h after inoculation, unless otherwise indicated.

Source: Anderson GG, Palermo JJ, Schilling JD, Roth R, Heuser J, Hultgren SJ 2003 Intracellular bacterial biofilm-like pods in urinary tract infections. Science 301: 105–107.

- pelvic tumours and inflammatory bowel disorders may invade the bladder directly and also affect bladder emptying;
- glycosuria that occurs in diabetes mellitus is a potent culture medium for bacterial growth;
- genetic factors have been postulated to increase the risk of recurrent infection. Women with recurrent infection are more likely to be non-secretors of histo-blood group antigens, and *E. coli* is found to adhere better to uroepithelial cells of non-secretors than secretors (Lomberg et al 1986, Sheinfeld et al 1989). Further evidence for a genetic susceptibility is that female relatives of women with recurrent UTI are more likely to suffer from UTI as an adult (Hopkins et al 1999);
- in menopausal women, the lack of oestrogen reduces lactobacillus growth and, with the rise in vaginal pH, leads to a predisposition to growth of enterobacteria (Cardozo 1996); and
- sexual intercourse and contraception are strongly associated with the onset of UTI (Hooton et al 1996, Foxman et al 1997). Sexual intercourse not only results in trauma and disruption to the uroepithelial cells, but may also introduce rectal and vaginal bacteria into the urethra. In a woman who has had sex in the previous 48 h, the odds ratio for a UTI is increased 60 times over a woman who has not (Nicolle et al 1982). The use of spermicides with diaphragms alters vaginal flora, increases vaginal pH and decreases lactobacilli concentration, promoting colonization with *E. coli*.

In addition to all these factors, there is a well-developed and effective innate and adaptive host response to bacterial invasion. The mucosal lining of the urinary tract has a number of immune surveillance molecules that function to recognize invading pathogens. The best characterized of these is the Toll-like receptor (TLR) family (Samuelsson et al 2004, Zhang et al 2004, Anderson-Nissen et al 2007). These receptors function to initiate appropriate host immune defences when triggered by a pathogen. There are 11 TLRs; TLR4 is the best characterized and is present on the epithelial cells of the bladder and kidney, and promotes cytokine and chemokine responses to Gram-negative pathogens. This TLR4 response can still occur even once intracellular bacterial invasion has occurred. The importance of host-mediated immunity can be seen in women with recurrent UTI. A study comparing vaginal, urine and blood samples from 22 women wirh recurrent UTI and 17 controls showed an aberrant immune response. Women with recurrent UTI had defective T-cell activation and a lower concentration of tissue-repair-associated vascular endothelial growth factor (Kirjavainen et al 2009).

Natural History

In children up to 1 year of age, 1.1% of girls and 1.2% of boys may suffer a symptomatic UTI. In school-age children, a UTI has been reported in 8% of girls and 2% of boys (Hansson et al 1997). The sequelae of UTI in neonates and young children include pyelonephritis and renal scarring, especially if infection occurred before 5 years of age. Vesico-

ureteric reflux is a significant aetiological factor in the occurrence of UTI in the young.

In young women, UTI can result in asymptomatic bacteriuria, cystitis and pyelonephritis. These do not usually affect renal function, except in the elderly where bacteriuria has been associated with a decrease in glomerular filtration rate. In pregnancy, UTIs have been associated with an increased risk of prematurity, perinatal mortality and perinatal complications (Maclean 2000). The incidence of asymptomatic bacteriuria is similar to non-pregnant women (4–7%) (Patterson and Andriole 1997); however, in pregnancy the risk of developing a symptomatic UTI is much higher, and 10–30% of women with asymptomatic bacteriuria develop pyelonephritis.

Presentation

A UTI may present either as an asymptomatic bacteriuria, acute cystitis or, more seriously, as acute pyelonephritis, bacteraemia and renal failure. The classic symptoms of acute cystitis include dysuria, frequency, urgency and suprapubic pain. If the upper urinary tract is involved, haematuria, loin pain, renal angle tenderness and fever may also occur. In children and the elderly, the classic clinical features of a UTI may not be present. In young children, clinical features of a UTI may be failure to thrive or a non-specific abdominal pain. In the elderly, UTIs often present as confusion and general malaise.

Physical Signs

In cases of acute cystitis or urethritis, there is often suprapubic tenderness and, occasionally, fever. The clinical presentation of acute pyelonephritis is often much more florid, with the patient often looking unwell with pyrexia and tachycardia. There is usually loin tenderness and, if severe, features of septicaemia may be present. In young children and the elderly, as with symptoms, clinical signs may be non-specific and atypical in nature.

Other associated physical signs which may point to the aetiology are a sensory neuropathy or evidence of a spinal cord lesion in cases of a UTI secondary to a neuropathic bladder.

Management

History and examination

In many women, infection can be diagnosed on the basis of history and clinical examination alone. A history should be taken to identify any predisposing features, such as recent UTI, recent urinary tract operations, recent sexual intercourse and the use of the contraceptive diaphragm and condom. Poor bladder emptying secondary to neurological disorders or the use of anticholinergic therapy, pregnancy, the presence of pelvic tumours and diabetes mellitus may also predispose to infection.

Clinical examination should include a general systemic examination, especially if the patient is pyrexial. Examination of the renal angles is required to elicit signs of pyelonephritis. If a neuropathy is suspected, a neurological examination of the S2–4 nerve roots should be performed, assessing for sensation around the buttocks. A gynaecological examination should be performed to exclude residual urine, a pelvic mass or pregnancy. Differential diagnoses that should be considered include detrusor overactivity, cystitis, bladder stones or tumours, ovarian torsion or cysts, ectopic pregnancy and miscarriage.

Investigations

Investigations should be aimed to help select appropriate treatment and to exclude any underlying cause which may predispose to recurrence (Arnold 2000).

Urinalysis

Freshly voided urine may be cloudy if it contains large numbers of cells (e.g. bacteria, red or white blood cells). Urine which has been allowed to stand may also become cloudy as a result of the formation of crystals as the urine cools.

Commercial stick tests are available for detection of various urinary components. The tests which are most useful are those for the detection of white blood cell leukocyte esterase and nitrites (formed from the conversion of urinary nitrate by bacteria). A clear freshly voided urine with negative nitrite and leukocyte tests indicates that UTI is unlikely (a high negative predictive value). The stick tests are not reliable to exclude asymptomatic bacteriuria when the patient has recently received antibiotics, in the immunocompromised, if there are delays in testing the urine, or if the number of bacteria is less than 10^5 CFU/ml (Stevens 1989). Patients with suspected UTI should be treated empirically and promptly, even with negative stick test results. It is imperative that urine culture is performed in pregnancy, in the immunocompromised, in those with complicated infections, and where previous empirical therapy has failed.

Urine microscopy and culture

Urine culture has traditionally been the gold standard for the diagnosis of UTI. An MSU sample requires that the vulva is separated, the periurethral area cleaned with water, and a sample collected midstream. The quantitative criteria for diagnosis of bacteriuria or infection require that the sample is collected carefully. If a catheter is in place, the sample should be taken by syringe aspiration or via a drainage port. Samples should ideally be cultured within 4 h. Urine samples can be stored overnight at 4°C. Borate can be used as a preservative; however, if used, it is important that the container is filled to the correct level to ensure that the borate concentration is within the correct range to act as a preservative rather than a disinfectant.

There are a variety of methods in current use for urine microscopy, including automated image analysers, flow cytometry and manual light microscopy. It is important to be aware of normal ranges for the technology used, and also the relevant test performance measures such as positive and negative predictive values. An increase in the numbers of bacteria and white blood cells above the normal range has a high positive predictive value for UTI. Urine culture has the advantage of allowing detection of the organism and appropriate antibiotic sensitivities. Urine culture methods are designed to detect the bacterial species most frequently associated with UTI, and may not culture fastidious bacteria or those that grow slowly such as *Mycobacterium tuberculosis*. If tuberculosis is suspected, at least three early-morning urine specimens should be sent for culture using appropriate methods. Catheter urine samples frequently grow mixtures of bacteria, as do contaminated samples or following microbial proliferation following delays in sample transport.

Imaging studies

The majority of women with uncomplicated UTIs can be managed on the basis of a history, examination and basic laboratory investigations such as urinalysis and culture. In these situations, there should be a good response to antibiotics. Radiological evaluation may be useful to help direct treatment in those with complicated UTIs, such as those in whom there are features suggestive of obstruction, a fever that does not settle despite 48 h of intravenous therapy, or an uncommon infective agent. Imaging modalities that are available include ultrasound, intravenous urography, computed tomography (CT) and magnetic resonance imaging (MRI). Each has potential advantages and disadvantages to consider.

Intravenous urography

Intravenous urography has largely been superseded by ultrasound and isotope studies which do not utilize high-dose radiation and are free of the risk of allergy. It does, however, have the advantage that it delineates the anatomical relationships of the ureter, and can detect the level and severity of obstructive lesions. It is particularly indicated in the investigation of unexplained haematuria. It does, however, have lower sensitivity for detecting emphysema and perinephric abscesses compared with CT imaging.

Ultrasound

Ultrasound has the advantage of being easily accessible, cost-effective and free of radiation, and therefore can be used in childbearing women. It can be used to delineate the contours of the kidneys, and assess obstruction and bladder emptying. However, the use of ultrasound is limited in the visualization of the midportion of the urethra, which is often the site of obstructive lesions or stones. It may also be limited in patients of high body mass index. Ultrasound is useful for the detection of parenchymal tumours, but it has low specificity for the detection of urothelial tumours of the renal pelvis or urinary tract.

Ultrasound can also measure postvoid residual volume which may be useful if poor bladder emptying and a high residual urine is thought to be predisposing to infection.

Plain abdominal radiograph

Plain abdominal radiography can be used to supplement an ultrasound to detect stones or foreign bodies. If stones are present, 90% will be visualized as they contain calcium or cystine and so are radio-opaque. Calcification in lymph nodes or renal tumours may also be seen. In combination with ultrasound, it has been shown to be superior to an intravenous urogram and incurs less radiation exposure (Lewis-Jones et al 1989, Spencer et al 1990).

Micturating cystogram

A micturating cystogram is useful in the detection of vesico-ureteric reflux, particularly in children, which often results in renal damage. This investigation should also be considered in women with recurrent upper tract infection or evidence of upper tract damage.

Nuclear medicine scanning

Nuclear medicine scans are generally only of use in complicated infections. They can be used to detect obstruction and also to evaluate differential function within each kidney.

The DMSA (dimercaptosuccinate) nucleotide is retained in the renal tubules and therefore this scan delineates renal anatomy and function. In patients with acute pyelonephritis, the affected area or scarring may be seen, along with any deterioration in proximal function. It should be considered in women with severe or unresolving pyelonephritis. In children under 5 years of age, it is more sensitive than ultrasound and intravenous urography in detecting renal scars (Mansour et al 1987). If obstruction is suspected, a DTPA (diethylenetriamine penta-acetic acid) or MAG3 (mercaptoacetyl triglycerine) scan is useful, as obstruction will result in delayed washout of the isotope from the renal pelvis. It will also allow calculation of the glomerular filtration rate and assessment of the contribution of each kidney to total renal function. MAG3 scans are also useful in delineating areas of reduced uptake and renal scars.

Computed tomography

In the majority of cases, ultrasound and intravenous urography are sufficient to reach a diagnosis; however, CT scanning is a useful adjunctive test where ultrasound and intravenous urography fail to make a diagnosis. In many units, CT imaging is now readily available and used for its increased sensitivity. It also allows a more global assessment of the pelvis. CT allows detailed anatomical demonstration of the kidney, intrarenal collecting system, ureter and bladder (Silverman et al 2009). It can thus be used for the investigation of haematuria.

CT can be used without contrast; however, the use of contrast does allow better anatomical detail and may give functional information. Contrast is usually injected into the collecting system 2–3 min after injection, and imaging can be performed at different stages of contrast enhancement to delineate areas of low or abnormal attenuation, such as seen with damaged parenchyma (Kawashima et al 1997).

In acute pyelonephritis, CT can be used to delineate focal or diffuse changes in the renal architecture and define the extent of hydronephrosis (Talner et al 1994). Spiral CT scan images, which are very much faster, can also detect ureteric stones or abscesses.

Magnetic resonance imaging

MRI has the advantage over CT that it does not use ionizing radiation or iodinated contrast. However, it is generally more expensive, less accessible and may be less well tolerated by patients and sensitive to motion artefact. It is also less sensitive for detecting renal calculi (Silverman et al 2009).

Blood tests

If deterioration of renal function is suspected, plasma creatinine and urea estimation should be performed. If diabetes is suspected, a fasting glucose test or glucose toleration test should be performed.

Cystoscopy

Cystoscopy is rarely useful in the diagnosis of uncomplicated infection, but it is indicated in all cases of haematuria and may be considered in women with symptoms of recurrent cystitis or infection. It can be used to identify any predisposing factors for infection, such as a bladder tumour or stone.

Treatment

There are three principles in the management of infection. General supportive measures relieve symptoms and may help to eradicate infection. Antimicrobial therapy should be instituted appropriately, and if an underlying cause is found, such as obstruction, this should be treated. Finally, prevention of further infection will help to reduce recurrence.

General measures

Generally, patients are advised to maintain a high fluid intake of at least 2 l/day and to void regularly to ensure adequate bladder emptying. However, there is not much evidence that this practice improves outcomes over and above appropriate antibiotic therapy. If the patient is septicaemic, more intensive supportive measures and monitoring are required. Intravenous fluids, vasoactive drugs and treatment of the septicaemia should be considered.

Antimicrobial therapy

The aim of antimicrobial therapy is to eradicate pathogenic organisms with minimal local and systemic side-effects. A suitable antimicrobial agent should reach a suprainhibitory concentration in urine and have activity against the range of common causative agents of UTI. An ideal antibiotic would have a low potential to select for bacterial resistance and to give rise to side-effects, be inexpensive and easily administered. Selection of antibiotics for empirical treatment should take account of local resistance patterns, which may vary geographically and are also dependent on whether the infection is hospital or community acquired. Side-effects include anaphylaxis, skin rashes, gastrointestinal disturbances, fungal infection and *Clostridium difficile* colitis (particularly in the elderly). Multiresistant *E. coli* is becoming more commonly recognized as a cause of community-acquired as well as hospital-acquired infection, making the requirement to take account of local antibiotic resistance information increasingly important when designing treatment algorithms.

Many antibiotics administered systemically reach much higher concentrations in urine than in serum. These include β-lactams, aminoglycosides, fluoroquinolones and trimethoprim, so large doses of these agents are rarely required. Amoxycillin resistance is now so common in laboratory isolates in the UK that it is best avoided in the empirical treatment of UTI, and in some areas, trimethoprim resistance is reaching similar levels. The true level of antibiotic resistance amongst agents of community infection is not known. The levels of resistance in laboratory isolates from patients in the community may be an overestimate because of biases in the way in which laboratories are used. For example, samples may only be sent to the laboratory when patients return to a doctor after failure of empirical treatment. Estimates of the levels of antibiotic resistance for hospital infections may be more accurate because of the relative ease of use of the laboratory. Alternatives to amoxicillin or trimethoprim for oral use include nalidixic acid, penicillin/enzyme inhibitor combinations (such as amoxicillin with clavulanate), nitrofurantoin, oral cephalosporins and quinolones. The British National Formulary gives good advice on antibiotic selection and treatment durations for specific clinical scenarios. The duration of therapy has come under some debate with a move to shorter regimes to increase compliance, as these will have less effect on the faecal and vaginal flora and reduce the risk of resistant strains. Three-day regimes are as effective as 5- and 7-day regimes for those with uncomplicated UTI (Norrby 1990). Ideally, protocols should be developed with local microbiologists and/or infectious disease specialists that take account of local resistance information. Additional information on the use of antibiotics is provided in the section dealing with specific clinical presentations.

Prevention

For many women with recurrent infection, suggested preventive measures include maintaining a high fluid intake, instructions on perineal hygiene such that the perineum is wiped from front to back after defaecation and micturition (thus reducing the risk of faecal contamination of the urethra), and the avoidance of bubble baths, vaginal deodorants and specific underwear. The benefits of these practices are unclear and they have not been shown to reduce the frequency of infections in case–control studies (Foxman and Frerichs 1985b, Remis et al 1987).

There is, however, a strong association between sexual behaviour and contraceptive use (Foxman and Chi 1990). If sexual intercourse is a precipitating factor, postcoital treatment and voiding are recommended. In women using spermicides and diaphragms for contraception, alternative methods may be recommended.

The beneficial effects of cranberry juice are receiving increasing attention as a simple remedy that reduces the incidence of recurrent infection; however, most studies have been relatively small and inconclusive. There are two postulated mechanisms of action: competitive inhibition of the E. coli fimbrial subunit to the uroepithelial cells, or prevention of the expression of the normal fimbrial subunits (Patel and Daniels 2000). In a randomized double-blind trial to determine the effect of cranberry juice on bacteriuria and pyuria in 153 elderly women, there was reduced frequency of bacteriuria (15% vs 28%) with daily ingestion of 300 ml of cranberry juice (Avorn et al 1994). There was a decrease in the incidence of symptomatic UTI but this did not reach statistical significance; however, antibiotic use decreased by approximately 50% in the group who drank cranberry juice.

The Cochrane analysis of cranberries for prevention of UTI found that the studies assessed were flawed as the amount and type of cranberries given differed, and there was only weak evidence to support the use of cranberry juice for prevention (Jepson et al 2004).

In postmenopausal women, there is increased susceptibility to infection secondary to the changes in the vaginal flora and the uroepithelium secondary to oestrogen deficiency. There are few randomized trials of hormone replacement therapy in the prevention of UTI. In a double-blind, placebo-controlled trial of oestriol cream for the treatment of recurrent infection in 93 women, Raz and Stamm (1993) found that those on topical oestriol had a lower incidence of UTI (0.5 vs 5.9 episodes/patient-year). The decrease in UTI was seen together with a decrease in vaginal pH and recolonization with lactobacilli. In a later study by Cardozo et al (1998), daily use of oestriol cream was found to be superior to placebo in the treatment of recurrent UTI.

The recent Cochrane review (Perrotta et al 2008) of oestrogen use in postmenopausal women with recurrent UTI reviewed nine studies which included 3345 women. The data were difficult to summarize as studies were heterogeneous and used different application methods and doses. Pooled data from four studies showed that oral oestrogens did not reduce UTI compared with placebo. There were two small relevant studies comparing vaginal oestrogens which showed a reduction in UTI.

Low-dose prophylactic antibiotics can be considered if the frequency of attacks is two or more per 6 months or three or more over 12 months (Nicolle and Ronald 1987, Stamm and Hooton 1993). The aim of treatment is to eradicate urinary bacteria without affecting the healthy flora of the bowel and vagina, or causing the development of resistant strains. The usual suppressive dose is one-quarter to one-third of the antimicrobial dose required to treat an acute infection. This is usually prescribed at night to maintain a high antimicrobial concentration for as long as possible. The antibiotics of choice are trimethoprim, trimethoprim and sulphamethoxazole, nitrofurantoin, nalidixic acid and cephalexin (Harding et al 1982). In patients with neuropathic bladders, long-term indwelling catheters or ileal conduits who are at increased risk of recurrent infection, it is not advisable to begin long-term prophylaxis as this increases the risk of resistance and antimicrobial side-effects. In these cases, the patient should be advised to seek early treatment when a UTI is suspected.

Future approaches to treatment

The increasing problem of antimicrobial resistance and the lack of efficacy of conventional therapy in recurrent infection has led to new strategies to reduce bacterial penetration and alter the host innate or adaptive immunity.

There is much interest in the use of lactobacillus-containing probiotics for preventing recurrent infection. Probiotics are 'live micro-organisms' and the rationale for their use is that they restore the commensal flora of the genitourinary tract which inhibits colonization with uropathogens. Four randomized trials (Reid et al 1992, 1995, Baerheim et al 1994, Kontiokari et al 2001) have studied lactobacilli for the prevention of recurrent UTI; however, only one reported a reduction in episodes of recurrent UTI compared with the year prior to the study (Reid et al 1995). There are also concerns regarding the stability of probiotics and strain-specific effects.

The identification of various *E. coli* adhesins, including the type I and P fimbriae, has stimulated the search for vaccines against the development of UTI. Animal studies have shown that vaccination with antibodies to the FimH adhesin, which mediates binding to the bladder mucosa, reduces bacterial binding, bacteriuria and pyuria (Langermann et al 2000).

As the host immune response may determine susceptibility to infection, modulators of the immune system have been proposed as adjuvants to help boost the normal immunological mechanisms to vaccines (Ishii and Akira 2007, Parker et al 2007). Data from animal studies have shown a greater antigen-specific immune reponse and a reduced bacterial load when immunomodulators have been used (Bishop et al 2007, Huleatt et al 2007).

The clinical application and efficacy of these new strategies for treatment are still unclear; however, if found to be useful, they may act in combination or instead of antimicrobials to decrease recurrent infection and increase treatment efficacy.

Specific Clinical Situations

Asymptomatic bacteriuria

Asymptomatic bacteriuria is defined as the presence of increased numbers of bacterial CFUs in a urine sample in the absence of clinical signs or symptoms of UTI. In a carefully collected MSU sample, this number is more than 10^5 CFU/ml. If left untreated, 60–80% of patients will spontaneously clear the infection without long-term sequelae. However, there are several situations where treatment is advisable. In obstetric and gynaecological practice, these situations include pregnancy and urogenital surgery.

There has been much debate on the benefits and cost-effectiveness of screening pregnant women for asymptomatic bacteriuria. The prevalence of asymptomatic bacteriuria has been reported to range from 2% to 13% (Norden and Kass 1968). There is an association with premature birth and low birth weight (Andriole and Patterson 1991), as well as an increased risk of developing pyelonephritis. In a study of 5000 antenatal patients, it was reported that in women with asymptomatic bacteriuria in pregnancy, 36% progressed to acute pyelonephritis if untreated compared with 5% if treated (Little 1965). Current recommendations in the UK (National Institute for Health and Clinical Excellence 2008) support the screening of pregnant women for bacteriuria at the time of booking by urine culture, because treatment with antibiotics reduces the risk of pyelonephritis. Antibiotic choices should be based on the culture result and should take account of the safety profile of the selected agent in pregnancy. Tests for urinary nitrite and leukocyte esterase are unreliable for the diagnosis of asymptomatic bacteriuria (Tincello and Richmond 1998).

Recurrent infection

Up to 20% of women with acute cystitis develop recurrent UTI which is defined as three or more laboratory-confirmed infections per year. These occur due to either reinfection or a relapse of persistent infection. Risk factors such as atrophic vaginitis should be looked for and treated. Maintaining a good urine output is advisable to promote voiding and avoid urinary stasis. Prophylactic use of trimethoprim, nitrofurantoin or norfloxacin therapy may reduce the risk of recurrent attacks but may also select for antibiotic resistance. Cranberry juice may reduce the risk of recurrent UTI without the risk of antibiotic resistance (Kontiokari et al 2001).

Postcoital prophylaxis with a single dose of an antibiotic can be used if infection is related to intercourse. Alternatively, patients can be given antibiotics to use when symptoms occur, or daily prophylaxis with nitrofurantoin, trimethoprim, norfloxacin or cephalexin. A 6-month trial of prophylaxis is usually recommended, with the patient observed to see if infection recurs once the regime is discontinued. However, recurrence seems to occur and a longer period of prophylaxis is now advocated for at least 2 years. Antimicrobials such as trimethoprim have been effective and well tolerated for up to 5 years (Nicolle and Ronald 1987, Nicolle et al 1988).

Acute pyelonephritis

Prompt antimicrobial treatment reduces the risk of serious adverse outcomes, so treatment should be commenced as soon as a diagnosis of urosepsis is considered (clinical signs and symptoms of UTI such as dysuria or loin pain in association with systemic signs of infection such as fever, rigors, hypotension, tachypnoea and tachycardia) and prior to the results of urine culture. Potential complications of pyelonephritis include Gram-negative bacteraemia, endotoxic shock and disseminated intravascular coagulation. In general, acute pyelonephritis resolves without long-term renal damage in the majority of women. However, in the presence of obstruction, such as with stones, infection may result in papillary necrosis, renal or perinephric abscess, or xanthogranulomatous pyelonephritis (Cattell 1998). Treatment consists of aggressive supportive treatment including rehydration and intravascular volume expansion.

Drugs of choice for parenteral therapy include cephalosporins, fluoroquinolones or an aminoglycoside. After the culture results are available, treatment may be changed to the appropriate antibiotic if necessary in consultation with a microbiologist or infectious disease specialist. The duration of treatment is usually 10–14 days (Bailey 1998, Cattell 1998).

Imaging of the renal tract is not usually necessary unless there has been no response to antibiotics or if there is a strong clinical suspicion of renal tract obstruction. Intravenous urography will be normal in 75% of cases of uncomplicated acute pyelonephritis (Fraser et al 1995), as well as renal ultrasound. CT imaging is usually normal unless infection is severe, when changes include renal enlargement, focal swelling and parenchymal attenuation.

Catheter-associated infection

Urethral catheterization is a major risk factor for UTI and local trauma, so should not be undertaken lightly. Those who carry out urinary tract catheterization should have received appropriate training in technique and catheter type (Carter et al 1990). A UTI is reported to occur in approximately one-third of patients catheterized in hospital (Hayley et al 1985). The risk of a UTI after an in–out catheter is 1–2% (Turck et al 1962), but the risk is higher in pregnancy, with a high bladder residual and in the immunocompromised. Basic measures such as the use of a closed-drainage system and gravity-dependent drainage of urine decrease the risk of UTI, and a policy of expediting catheter removal as soon as clinically appropriate should be practised.

Long-term urinary catheters become colonized with bacteria, and UTI is a frequent complication. The underlying cause is the development of a pathogenic biofilm on the surface of an indwelling catheter. The rate of bacteriuria is 3–10%/day and approaches 100% in those with long-term catheters (Warren et al 1982, Saint et al 2002). Inhibiting biofilm formation is one mechanism to reduce UTI, and urinary catheters have been modified to promote this. Impregnation of catheters with antimicrobial agents such as silver have been shown to delay or reduce the onset of bacteriuria; however, there is the possibility of future resistance to silver (Brosnahan et al 2004). Treatment may be required when the patient develops systemic signs or symptoms of infection. Antibiotic treatment choice is best based on culture results.

Urinary tract tuberculosis

Urinary tract tuberculosis is usually caused by *M. tuberculosis* or, more rarely, *M. bovis* or *M. africanum*. Bloodborne spread occurs from the initial primary site, usually the lung but occasionally the gut. This form of tuberculosis tends to affect young adults and presents as a miliary tuberculosis or a nodular or cavitating tuberculosis affecting one kidney. Three early-morning specimens should be sent for Lowenstein-Jensen culture for acid-fast bacilli, as routine culture is sterile and usually reveals pyuria and haematuria alone. Renal function is usually normal unless there is widespread parenchymal damage. Therefore, urea and creatinine levels should be assessed in all patients, and renal imaging should be undertaken to reveal the extent of the disease. Intravenous urography and cystoscopy should also be performed to assess the presence of urethral strictures, pyocalyx, pyonephrosis or a non-functioning kidney. Characteristic appearances on intravenous urography and ultrasound include hydronephrosis and/or a small bladder. Bladder biopsies may be taken which culture more readily than urine; this can take up to 8 weeks until considered truly negative. A chest radiograph should also be performed.

After diagnosis, antituberculous therapy should be commenced. This consists of a four-drug treatment regime usually with isoniazid, rifampacin, ethambutol and pyrazinamide, modified to two drugs when the sensitivities of the tubercle bacilli are known. In total, if rifampacin is used, treatment should continue for 9 months.

Contact tracing should be performed as tuberculosis is a notifiable communicable disease and contacts need prophylaxis.

Urolithiasis

In the presence of a stone, a UTI must be treated and the urinary tract drained before removal of the stone. If a pyonephrosis or perirenal abscess is complicating the stone, immediate drainage using percutaneous nephrostomy is required. A xanthogranulomatous pyelonephritis is a rare complication of a UTI in the presence of a stone. This usually presents with loin pain, intermittent fever, anaemia and malaise. A palpable unilateral renal mass is usually present and, as well as a positive urine culture, liver function may be deranged. These cases are often resistant to antibiotics and a nephrectomy will be required.

Histologically, the affected kidney will show diffuse replacement of the renal parenchyma with lipid-filled macrophages, neutrophils, plasma cells and necrotic debris.

Conclusions

UTIs are the most common type of infection in women and a significant cause of distress and morbidity. The aetiology is multifactorial, and treatment strategies are based on identifying any predisposing causes and eradicating pathogenic organisms adequately to prevent recurrence of infection and long-term sequelae.

The management of women presenting with symptoms includes a detailed and stepwise diagnosis and investigation strategy with institution of appropriate antimicrobial treatment. Antimicrobial therapy should be tailored to the individual patient, accounting for local drug resistance patterns, antimicrobial sensitivities, and whether the infection is complicated or uncomplicated. All antimicrobial regimes should be combined with advice on preventing recurrence of infection. If treatment fails, further investigations and treatment should be considered.

KEY POINTS

1. Urinary infections are a significant cause of morbidity in women aged 20–65 years.
2. Infections can present with only 10^2 or 10^3 organisms/ml urine and even in the presence of sterile urine.
3. Up to 80% of recurrent infections are reinfection.
4. Approximately 25–30% of women will develop recurrent UTI not related to an underlying functional or anatomical abnormality.
5. The majority of UTIs are caused by facultative bacteria, and *E. coli* accounts for up to 70% of community-acquired infections.
6. Between 10% and 30% of women with asymptomatic bacteriuria develop acute pyelonephritis during pregnancy. This requires treatment as there is a risk of pregnancy-related complications.
7. Imaging should be considered in those with complicated infections and those whose temperatures do not resolve after 48 h of intravenous antibiotics.
8. Treatment should include advice on increasing fluid intake and perineal hygiene.

9. Symptomatic lower urinary infection requires at least a 3-day course of antibiotics.

10. UTI in a patient with a neuropathic bladder, indwelling catheter or ileal conduit should only be treated when it is symptomatic or if there is proven bacteriuria.

11. Training in catheter insertion and use should reduce the risk of catheter-associated infections. A closed-gravity-dependent drainage system should be employed.

References

Abraham SN, Sun D, Dale JB, Beachey EH 1988 Conservation of the D-mannose adhesion protein among type 1 fimbriated members of the family Enterobacteriaceae. Nature 336: 682–684.

Anderson GG, Palermo JJ, Schilling JD, Roth R, Heuser J, Hultgren SJ 2003 Intracellular bacterial biofilm-like pods in urinary tract infections. Science 301: 105–107.

Andersen-Nissen E, Hawn TR, Smith KD et al 2007 Cutting edge: TLr5-/- mice are more suspectible to Escherichia coli urinary tract infection. Journal of Immunology 178: 4717–4720.

Andriole VT, Patterson TF 1991 Epidemiology, natural history and management of urinary tract infections in pregnancy. Medical Clinics of North America 75: 359–373.

Arnold E 2000 Investigations. In: Stanton SL, Dwyer P (eds) Urinary Ttract Infections in the Female. Martin Dunitz, London, pp 35–59.

Avorn J, Monane M, Gurwitz JH, Glynn RJ, Choodnovskiy I, Lipsitz LA 1994 Reduction of bacteriuria and pyuria after ingestion of cranberry juice. Journal of the American Medical Association 271: 751–754.

Bailey RR 1998 Vesicoureteric reflux and reflux nephropathy. In: Schrier RW, Gootschalk GW (eds) Diseases of the Kidney, 4th edn. Little, Brown and Company, Boston, pp 748–783.

Baerheim A, Larsen E, Digranes A 1994 Vaginal application of lactobacilli in the prophylaxis of recurrent lower urinary tract infection in women. Scandinavian Journal of Primary Health Care 12: 239–243.

Bishop BL, Duncan MJ, Somg J, Li G, Zaas D, Abraham SN 2007 Cyclic AMP-regulated exocytosis of Escherichia coli from infected bladder epithelial cells. Nature Medicine 13: 625–630.

Boscia JA, Kaye D 1987 Asymptomatic bacteriuria in the elderly. Infectious Diseases Clinics of North America 1: 892–903.

Brosnahan J, Jull A, Tracy C 2004 Types of Urethral Catheters for the Management of Short-term Voiding Problems in Hospitalized Adults. Cochrane Library, Issue 2. Update Software, Oxford.

Bryan CS, Reynolds KL 1984 Hospital acquired bacteraemic urinary tract infection: epidemiology and outcome. Journal of Urology 132: 494–498.

Cardozo L 1996 Postmenopausal cystitis. BMJ (Clinical Research Ed.) 313: 129.

Cardozo L, Benness C, Abbott D 1998 Low dose oestrogen prophylaxis for recurrent tract infections in elderly women. British Journal of Obstetrics and Gynaecology 105: 403–407.

Carter R, Aitchison M, Mufti GR, Scott R 1990 Catheterisation: your urethra in their hands. BMJ (Clinical Research Ed.) 301: 905.

Cattell WR 1998 The patient with urinary tract infections. In: Davison AM, Cameron JS, Grunfeld J, Kerr DNS, Ritz E, Winearls CG (eds) Oxford Textbook of Clinical Nephrology, 2nd edn. Oxford University Press, New York, pp 1252–1259.

Ditchburn RK, Ditchburn JS 1990 A study of microscopical and chemical tests for the diagnosis of urinary tract infections in general practice. British Journal of General Practice 40: 241–243.

Finer G, Landau D 2004 Pathogenesis of urinary tract infections with normal female anatomy. The Lancet Infectious Diseases 4: 631–635.

Foxman B, Chi JW 1990 Health behavior and urinary tract infection in college-aged women. Journal of Clinical Epidemiology 43: 329–337.

Foxman B, Frerichs RR 1985a Epidemiology of urinary tract infection. I. Diaphragm use and sexual intercourse. American Journal of Public Health 75: 1308–1313.

Foxman B, Frerichs RR 1985b Epidemiology of urinary tract infections. II. Diet, clothing and urinary habits. American Journal of Public Health 75: 1314–1317.

Foxman B, Marsh J, Gillespie B et al 1997 Condom use and first-time urinary tract infection. Epidemiology 8: 637–641.

Fraser IR, Birch D, Fairley KF et al 1995 A prospective study of corticol scarring in acute febrile pyelonephritis in adults: clinical and bacteriological characteristics. Clinics in Nephrology 47: 13–18.

Gunther IN, Snyder JA, Lockatell V et al 2002 Assessment of virulence of uropathogenic Escherichia coli type 1 fimbrial mutants in which the invertible element is phase-locked on or off. Infection and Immunity 70: 3344–3354.

Grüneberg RN 1994 Changes in urinary pathogens and their antibiotic sensitivities, 1971–1992. Journal of Antimicrobial Chemotherapy 33 (Suppl A): 1–8.

Hamilton-Miller JMT 1994 The urethral syndrome and its management. Journal of Antimicrobial Chemotherapy 33 (Suppl A): 63–73.

Hansson S, Martinell J, Stokland E, Jodal U 1997 The natural history of bacteriuria in childhood. Infectious Diseases Clinics of North America 11: 499–512.

Harding GKM, Ronald AR, Nicolle LE, Thomson MJ, Gray GJ 1982 Long term antimicrobial prophylaxis for recurrent urinary infection in females. Review of Infectious Diseases 4: 438–443.

Hayley RW, Culver DH, Waite JW, Morgan WM, Emori TG 1985 The national nosocomial infection rate. A new need for new vital statistics. American Journal of Epidemiology 121: 159–167.

Hopkins WJ, Uehling DT, Wargowski DS 1999 Evaluation of a familial predisposition to recurrent urinary tract infections in women. American Journal of Medical Genetics 83: 422–424.

Hooton TM, Scholes D, Hughes JP et al 1996 A prospective study of risk factors for symptomatic urinary tract infection in young women. New England Journal of Medicine 335: 468–474.

Hooton TM 2001 Recurrent urinary tract infection in women. International Journal of Antimicrobial Agents 17: 259–268.

Huleatt JW, Jacobs AR, Tang J et al 2007 Vaccination with recombinant fusion proteins incorporating Toll-like receptor ligands induces rapid cellular and humoral immunity. Vaccine 25: 763–775.

Ishii KJ, Akira S 2007 Toll or Toll-free adjuvant path towatd the optimal vaccine development. Journal of Clinical Immunology 27: 363–371.

Jepson RG, Mihaljevic L, Craig J 2004 Cranberries for Preventing Urinary Tract Infections. The Cochrane Library, Issue 2. Update Software, Oxford.

Johnson JR, Stamm WE 1987 Diagnosis and treatment of acute urinary tract infections. Infectious Diseases Clinics of North America 1: 773–791.

Johnson JR, Stamm WE 1989 Urinary tract infections in women: diagnosis and treatment. Annals of Internal Medicine 111: 906–917.

Kass EH 1956 Asymptomatic infections of the urinary tract. Transactions of the

Association of American Physicians 69: 56–64.

Kawashima A, Sandler C, Goldman S, Raval B, Fishman E 1997 CT of renal inflammatory disease. Radiographics 17: 851–866.

Kirjavainen PK, Paulter S, Baroja ML et al 2009 Abnormal immunological profile and vaginal microbiota in women prone to urinary tract infections. Clinical Vaccine Immunology 16: 29–36.

Kontiokari T, Sundqvist K, Nuutinen M, Pokka T, Koskela M, Uhari M 2001 Randomised trial of cranberry–lingonberry juice and lactobacillus GG drink for the prevention of urinary tract infections in women. BMJ (Clinical Research Ed.) 322: 1571.

Kunin CM 1987 Detection, Prevention and Management of Urinary Tract Infections, 4th edn. Lea and Febiger, Philadelphia, pp 57–124.

Langermann S, Mollby R, Burlein JE et al 2000 Vaccination against FimH adhesin protects cynomolgus monkeys from colonisation and infection by uropathogenic Escherichia coli. Journal of Infectious Diseases 181: 774–778.

Lewis-Jones HG, Lamb GHR, Hughes PL 1989 Can ultrasound replace the intravenous urogram in the preliminary investigation of urinary tract disease? British Journal of Radiology 62: 977–980.

Little PJ 1965 Prevention of pyelonephritis of pregnancy. The Lancet i: 567–569.

Lomberg H, Cedergren B, Leffler H et al 1986 Influence of blood group on the availability of receptors for attachment of uropathogenic Escherichia coli. Infection and Immunology 51: 919–926.

Maclean A 2000 Pregnancy. In: Stanton SL, Dwyer PL (eds) Urinary Tract Infection in the Female. Martin Dunitz, London, pp 145–160.

Mansour M, Azmy AF, MacKenzie JR 1987 Renal scarring secondary to vesicoureteric reflux. Critical assessment and new grading. British Journal of Urology 70: 32–34.

National Institute for Health and Clinical Excellence 2008 Antenatal Care: Routine Care for the Healthy Pregnant Woman. Clinical Guideline 62. NICE, London.

Nicolle LE, Ronald AR 1987 Recurrent urinary infection in adult women: diagnosis and treatment. Infectious Diseases Clinics of North America 1: 793–806.

Nicolle LE, Harding GKM, Preiksaitis J, Ronald AR 1982 The association of urinary tract infection with sexual intercourse. Journal of Infectious Diseases 146: 579–584.

Nicolle LE, Harding GKM, Thomson M, Kennedy J, Urias B, Ronald AR 1988

Efficacy of five years of continuous, low-dose trimethoprim–sulfamethoxazole prophylaxis for urinary tract infection. Journal of Infectious Diseases 157: 1239–1241.

Norden CW, Kass EH 1968 Bacteriuria of pregnancy — a critical appraisal. Annual Reviews in Medicine 19: 431–470.

Norrby SR 1990 Short-term treatment of uncomplicated urinary tract infections in women. Review of Infectious Diseases 12: 458–467.

Parker LC, Prince LR, Sabroe I 2007 Translational mini-review series on Toll-like receptors: networks regulated by Toll-like receptors mediate innate and adaptive immunity. Clinical and Experimental Immunology 147: 199–207.

Patel N, Daniels IR 2000 Botanical perspectives on health: of cystitis and cranberries. Journal of the Royal Society of Health 120: 52–53.

Patterson JE, Andriole VT 1997 Bacterial urinary tract infections in diabetes. Infectious Disease Clinics of North America 11: 735–750.

Perrotta C, Aznar M, Mejia R, Albert X, Ng CW 2008 Oestrogens for preventing recurrent urinary tract infection in postmenopausal women. Cochrane Database of Systematic Reviews 2: CD005131.

Raz R, Stamm WE 1993 A controlled trial of intravaginal estriol in postmenopuasal women with recurrent urinary tract infections. New England Journal of Medicine 329: 753–756.

Reid G, Bruce AW, Taylor M 1992 Influence of 3-day antimicrobial therapy and lactobacillus vaginal suppositories on recurrence of urinary tract infections. Clinical Therapeutics 14: 11–16.

Reid G, Bruce AW, Taylor M 1995 Instillation of lactobacillus and stimulation of indigenous organisms to prevent recurrence of urinary tract infections. Microecology and Therapy 23: 32–45.

Remis RS, Gurwith MJ, Gurwith D, Hargett-Bean NT, Layde PM 1987 Risk factors for urinary tract infection. American Journal of Epidemiology 126: 685–694.

Saint S, Lipsky BA, Goold SD 2002 Indwelling urinary catheters: a one-point restraint? Annals of Internal Medicine 137: 125–128.

Samuelsson P, Hang L, Wullt B, Irjala H, Svanborg C 2004 Toll-like receptor 4 expression and cytokine responses in the human urinary tract mucosa 2004. Infection and Immunity 72: 3179–3186.

Sheinfeld J, Schaeffer AJ, Cordon-Cardo C, Rogatko A, Fair WR 1989 Association of Lewis blood-group phenotype with recurrent urinary tract infections in women. New England Journal of Medicine 320: 773–777.

Silverman SG, Leyendecker JR, Amis ES 2009 What is the current role of CT urography and MR urography in the evaluation of the urinary tract? Radiology 250: 309–323.

Spencer J, Lindsell D, Mastorakou I 1990 Ultrasonography compared with intravenous urography in the investigation of urinary tract infection in adults. BMJ (Clinical Research Ed.) 301: 221–224.

Stamm WE, Hooton TM 1993 Management of urinary tract infection in adults. New England Journal of Medicine 329: 1328–1334.

Stevens M 1989 Screening urine for bacteriuria. Medical Laboratory Science 46: 194–206.

Talner CB, Davidson AJ, Lebowitz RI, Dalla-Palma L, Goldman SM 1994 Acute pyelonephritis: can we agree on terminology? Radiology 192: 297–305.

Tincello DG, Richmond DH 1998 Evaluation of reagent strips in detecting asymptomatic bacteriuria in early pregnancy: prospective case series. BMJ (Clinical Research Ed.) 316: 435–437.

Turck M, Giffe B, Petersdorf RG 1962 The urethral catheter and urinary tract infection. Journal of Urology 88: 834–837.

Warren JW, Tenney JH, Hoopes JM et al 1982 A prospective study microbiologic study of bacteriuria in patients with chronic indwelling urethral catheters. Journal of Infectious Diseases 146: 719–723.

Warren JW, Abrutyn E, Hebel JR, Johnson JR, Schaeffer AJ, Stamm WE 1999 Guidelines for antimicrobial treatment of acute bacterial cystitis and acute pyelonephritis in women. Infectious Diseases Society of America (IDSA). Clinical Infectious Diseases 29: 745–758.

Zafriri D, Oron Y, Einenstein BI, Ofek I 1987 Growth advantages and enhanced toxicity of Escherichia coli adherent to tissue culture cells due to restricted diffusion of products secreted by cells. Journal of Clinical Investigation 79: 1210–1216.

Zhang D, Zhang G, Hayden MS et al 2004 A Toll-like receptor that prevents infection by uropathogenic bacteria. Science 303: 1148–1155.

Zhanel GG, Harding GKM, Guay DRP 1990 Asymptomatic bacteriuria: which patients should be treated. Archives of Internal Medicine 150: 1389–1396

CHAPTER 59

Lower intestinal tract disease

Karen Nugent

Chapter Contents

INTRODUCTION	907	SUMMARY	917
INVESTIGATIONS	907	KEY POINTS	917
COMMON CONDITIONS AND TREATMENTS	909		

Introduction

There is emerging evidence of the interdependence of pathology and function between anterior, middle and posterior compartments of the pelvic floor. Many patients presenting to a gynaecologist or a coloproctologist have a mixture of urological, gynaecological and colorectal symptoms. The close anatomical, physiological and functional relationship between these compartments is reflected by the overlapping symptoms. Interventions to any one compartment may have an effect on the other compartments and may unearth a variety of new symptoms.

These close relationships have led to joint working in outpatient clinics and operating lists, and also to the emergence of multidisciplinary meetings. These can be held locally and regionally. They provide education for the members into the understanding of symptoms and treatment within the multidisciplinary field; meetings can be used to plan treatment and joint procedures, as well as for education (Mirnezami et al 2008).

A basic understanding of the anatomy and physiology of the colon, rectum and anus is essential in order to understand the symptoms associated with the posterior compartment (see Chapter 50).

Investigations

A detailed history and examination is often adequate to initiate basic treatment. It is always important to exclude serious pathology, and patients may require full bowel imaging of some sort (colonoscopy, barium enema or computed tomography colonography). In recent years, measurement of patient benefit from treatment has led to the use of incontinence and constipation scores which can be recorded before and after treatment. The Cleveland Clinic Incontinence Score (Table 59.1) is most commonly used.

The Cleveland Clinic Incontinence Score does not include aspects of urgency, but the Vaizey score (Vaizey et al 1999) attempted to address this. Vaizey et al reported that urgency of less than 15 min is not usually a problem; however, when patients are not able to hold for more than 2 min, this has a significant impact on quality of life. A recent study (Cotterill et al 2008) took comments from a panel of seven clinical experts and from patients, and reported five key issues related to anal incontinence. These were unpredictability, toilet locations, coping strategies, embarrassment and restriction of social activities. This group are working on a new instrument to help validate treatments for anal incontinence based around quality of life as well as symptom severity.

Further investigations may be helpful to assess function and structure; they also provide essential evidence in some medicolegal cases.

Anorectal manometry

There are limitations to the reproducibility and reliability of anorectal manometry across institutions. However, a standardized protocol should be used within each institution. Tests are helpful in predicting realistic expectations from surgery and also in explaining the scope of problems to patients.

Anal manometry is not a single test but a series of measurements used to assess anal sphincter function, rectal sensation, rectoanal reflexes and compliance of the rectum (Kourakalis and Andromanakos 2004). The use of pull-through anal manometry allows assessment of the length of the functioning sphincter, resting pressures give a good estimation of internal sphincter function, and squeeze pressures assess external sphincter function. The patient is usually placed in the left lateral position, and manometry can be performed either using stationery pull-through or continuous pull-through techniques. Many catheters have four or eight channels, and these can therefore record different pressures in different parts of the external sphincter and internal sphincter at different levels. Using vector analysis, it is possible to look at the symmetry of the anal canal pressure, and

DOI: 10.1016/B978-0-7020-3120-5.00059-X

Table 59.1 Cleveland Clinic Incontinence Score

	Never	Rarely	Sometimes	Weekly	Daily
Incontinence: solid stool	0	1	2	3	4
Incontinence: liquid stool	0	1	2	3	4
Incontinence: gas	0	1	2	3	4
Lifestyle ateration	0	1	2	3	4
Wears pads	0	1	2	3	4

combining this with anal ultrasonography can show whether there is a structural as well as a functional problem in either of the sphincter muscles. The rectoanal inhibitory reflex is usually assessed during the physiology. Absence of this may indicate a longstanding problem such as Hirschsprung's disease. Rectal distension is assessed by inflating a balloon within the rectum; measurements are taken when the patient first feels the sensation of rectal filling, the feeling when there is maximum fullness, and then the feeling of urgent desire to defaecate. This can be extended to when the volume is unbearable. If the rectal threshold is low, even with a normal anal pressure, continence may be impaired.

Anal skin sensation is usually assessed by some form of electrical stimulation. Pudendal nerve terminal motor latencies are performed by stimulating the pudendal nerve transanally through the lateral wall of the rectum as the nerve transverses the ischial spine, using a St Mark's electrode on the tip of the examining finger. The normal delay between stimulation and recording is less than 2.2 ms and a longer delay suggests that there has been damage to the pudendal nerve. A lengthening of the pudendal nerve latency is often associated with poorer outcomes after surgery, and may suggest that the patient's incontinence is associated with nerve damage. An important outcome measure for sphincter repair is whether there is any pudendal neuropathy, as patients with pudendal neuropathy only have a 10% chance of success compared with 80% in patients without pudendal neuropathy (Laurberg et al 1988).

Ultrasound and dynamic imaging

The investigation of choice for structural abnormalities within the anal sphincter is a three-dimensional anal ultrasound. A data set can be captured and then manipulated at a later date to look at structural abnormalities throughout the anal canal (Figure 59.1).

Length of sphincter, damage to internal and external sphincters, and presence of sepsis or abnormalities can all be assessed.

Using the same anal probe transvaginally, it is possible to examine the levator plate and many other anatomical aspects of the pelvic floor. Asymmetry within the levator plate suggests damage during childbirth and often leads to the anus being diverted to the side of the damage (Figure 59.2).

Dynamic images of the bladder and rectum can be taken using an 8848 transvaginal scanner, looking for perineal descent as well as enteroceles, rectoceles and rectal intussusception.

Further assessment of the pelvic floor often requires some form of proctography. In order to assess the whole pelvic

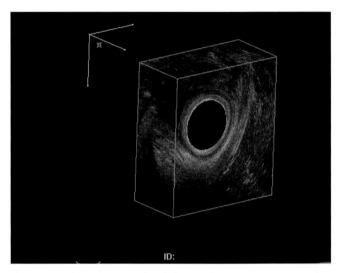

Figure 59.1 Three-dimensional anal ultrasound.

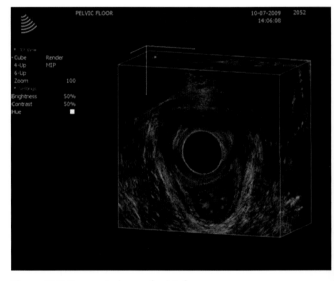

Figure 59.2 Transvaginal scan of pelvic floor.

floor using defaecating proctography, patients require not only contrast within the rectum but also in the small bowel, vagina and bladder. Defaecatory magnetic resonance imaging (Figure 59.3) can show all these parts of the pelvic floor. There are very few open magnets where a patient can sit and defaecate; therefore, the majority of these studies are performed with the patient lying prone.

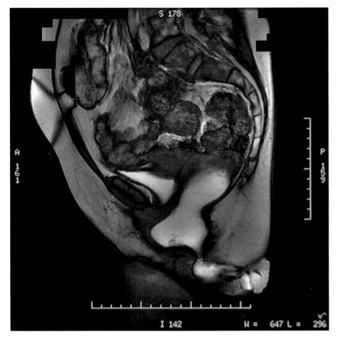

Figure 59.3 Rectocele seen on dynamic magnetic resonance imaging.

It has been shown that magnetic resonance proctography shows increased evidence of other pelvic floor abnormalities over defaecating proctography. However, it underestimates the size of rectoceles and intussusception (Pilkington et al 2009).

Shapes study

By marking and counting the passage of ingested radio-opaque markers on a plain abdominal X-ray, it is possible to make an estimate of segmental and total colonic transit times. In a simplified method, 20 radio-opaque markers are ingested and an X-ray is taken at 60 and 96 h. Transit through the whole colon of more than 67 h is considered abnormal. Transit time is prolonged in 80% of patients suffering from constipation.

It is essential that all of these investigations are taken into consideration along with a full pelvic floor history and diary of bowel habit problems. Discussion at a pelvic floor multi-disciplinary team (MDT) meeting allows every compartment to be assessed in equal relevance.

Common Conditions and Treatments

Haemorrhoids

The term 'haemorrhoids' (also known as 'piles') is generally used to describe enlarged anal cushions which become symptomatic through symptoms of either bleeding or prolapse. However, correlation between symptoms and the treatment of haemorrhoids is poor. Haemorrhoids and associated symptoms are an extremely common problem, presenting in patients at general practitioners' surgeries and coloproctology clinics. During their lifetime, many patients will present with symptoms of rectal bleeding and many of these will have bleeding secondary to piles. It is most impor-

tant to ensure that there is no other treatable or more serious problem relating to this bleeding, such as cancer, polyps or inflammatory bowel disease.

Piles often present with a combination of symptoms, including itching, soreness, postdefaecatory leakage and lumps around the anus. It is thought that the sliding anal canal theory proposed by Thompson (1975) is the most likely cause of piles, where Treitz's muscle is stretched repeatedly resulting in fragmentation of the connective tissue. Haemorrhoids may be small and highly symptomatic, or large and asymptomatic. This is especially so in elderly female patients where normal anal canal pressures are low, and this can result in prolapse but little in the way of symptoms. Several classifications of haemorrhoids have been used over time. Goligher's classification (Goligher 1976) describes the degree of prolapse and whether these reduce spontaneously (grade 2), require manual reduction (grade 3) or are permanently prolapsed (grade 4). However, although this is good for the description, it does not consider the symptoms of the piles. Work by Lunniss and Mann (2004) has produced a more accurate and useful classification of haemorrhoids, dividing them into non-prolapsing and prolapsing, looking at not only the morphological presentation but also any additional features such as pruritus or pain.

The diagnosis of haemorrhoids relies on a good history, exclusion of other possible causes of these problems and then a thorough clinical assessment. Anal pain may be associated not only with haemorrhoids but also abscesses, fistulae or fissures. Discharge and pruritus may be associated with warts, hypertrophied anal papillae or rectal prolapse. Anal incontinence is usually secondary to internal sphincter dysfunction and a lump or prolapse. Inspection of the perianal area may be done with the patient either lying in the left lateral position or with legs up in a gynaecology chair. The presence of anal skin tags is often suggestive of previous episodes of haemorrhoidal prolapse. If the haemorrhoids are associated with a predominant feature of itching, skin may be macerated or discoloured, and the presence or absence of scars or previous surgery should also be determined.

Second- or third-degree piles may become evident on asking the patient to bear down, and fourth-degree piles should be obvious at the time of examination. Palpation of the rectum is essential in order to exclude any other pathology, although the piles themselves are not easily examined as, by virtue of the nature of the anal canal and the soft tissues, no lumps will usually be felt. However, at the time of digital examination, it is also prudent to examine both the squeeze and the resting pressure associated with the anal canal. A proctoscopy is essential in examining for haemorrhoids, although internal haemorrhoids may be well visualized using an internal flexible sigmoidoscope.

Treatment of haemorrhoids

Estimates of the proportion of the UK population affected with haemorrhoids range from 4.4% to 24.5%. In 2004–2005, approximately 23,000 haemorrhoidal procedures were carried out, and approximately 8000 of these were excision haemorrhoidectomies (National Institute for Health and Clinical Excellence 2007a).

Treatment of haemorrhoids can be divided into internal haemorrhoids (i.e. those above the dentate line) and external haemorrhoids (i.e. those below the dentate line and therefore covered with sensate epithelium).

Medical treatment for haemorrhoids

Patients with symptomatic but small internal haemorrhoids are best treated with dietary management; increasing the intake of fluid and fibre is the mainstay of this treatment. The typical symptoms of internal haemorrhoids are rectal bleeding and, sometimes, prolapse; avoiding straining by these dietary methods usually improves the symptoms. Dietary manipulation also improves rectal bleeding alone from grade 1 and grade 2 haemorrhoids, and this has been proven in three randomized controlled trials (Cataldo et al 2005).

Patients with persistent symptoms from grade 1, 2 or 3 haemorrhoids may benefit from an outpatient procedure. The most common procedure used and probably the most effective is haemorrhoidal banding. Other procedures that may be offered include sclerotherapy, infrared coagulation and cryotherapy. All of these treatments are aimed at decreasing the haemorrhoidal tissue volume and fixing the anal cushion back to the rectal wall. A meta-analysis of outpatient treatment suggested that rubber band ligation was the most effective of all outpatient procedures and was associated with a lower recurrence rate (MacRae and McLeod 1995). It is, however, relatively painful and the pain associated with the procedure increases with the number of rubber bands that are used to treat these piles. It is essential that the bands are placed well above the dentate line, or the immediate pain felt from the sensate epithelium is excruciating and patients will need to have these bands removed. Rubber band ligation is associated with a success rate of 65–85%, but follow-up at 5 years shows a relatively high recurrence rate. Following outpatient procedures for haemorrhoids, approximately 2% of patients report pain and less than 1% report urinary retention. Major complications include significant haemorrhage, which may take place immediately or as a secondary haemorrhage between postoperative days 7 and 10.

Thrombosed external haemorrhoids

Thrombosed external haemorrhoids are extremely painful and the thrombosis will settle; however, patients sometimes need intervention prior to spontaneous resolution of symptoms. External haemorrhoids do thrombose spontaneously and the exact aetiology remains unclear. Patients may be treated conservatively, especially if they present more than 3 days after the thrombosis occurred; actulose, analgesia and ice packs on the perineum will often resolve the symptoms more quickly than a surgical procedure.

Operative procedures for haemorrhoids

Haemorrhoidectomy of any sort should only be offered to patients with large external haemorrhoids or significant prolapse, or those who have been resistant to outpatient procedures. Open haemorrhoidectomy is effective; however, it is associated with pain, infection and other complications, such as incontinence and stenosis of the anal canal. More recently, patients have been able to undertake a less painful form of surgical procedure called a 'stapled haemor-

rhoidopexy'. The evidence for this has been reviewed by the National Institute for Health and Clinical Excellence (NICE) (2007a). A stapled haemorrhoidopexy is an intrarectal procedure that aims to reduce the prolapse of haemorrhoidal tissue by excising a band of the prolapse anal mucosal membrane above the dentate line using a specific circular stapling device (PPH03 Ethicon). The procedure is thought to interrupt the blood supply to the haemorrhoids and reduce the potential continuing prolapse of mucosa. The NICE review studied 27 randomized controlled trials of stapled haemorrhoidopexy and found that the procedure was associated with less pain up to 14 days following surgery, shorter wound healing times and significantly less postoperative bleeding. On the basis of the evidence in the literature, it was felt that a stapled haemorrhoidopexy offered benefits over a conventional haemorrhoidectomy in the reduction of short- and medium-term postoperative pain. However, although stapled haemorrhoidopexy is associated with a higher rate of recurrent prolapse, the committee concluded that 'a stapled haemorrhoidopexy should be recommended as a treatment option for people in whom surgical intervention is considered appropriate for the treatment of prolapsed internal haemorrhoids'.

Surgical haemorrhoidectomy can be performed open (Milligan-Morgan) or closed (Ferguson). During an open procedure, the haemorrhoid is dissected and the pedicle is either ligated or cauterized with diathermy; the wounds are left to heal by secondary intention. This may result in extreme discomfort and postoperative morbidity. The closed technique involves greater dissection but the wound is closed with a running suture.

Anal fissures

Patients with pelvic floor straining and post childbirth often present with anal pain associated with an anal fissure. An anal fissure is a tear running longitudinally in the epithelium of the anal canal, the majority of which lie posteriorly in the midline. Acute fissures are usually superficial, whereas chronic fissures may be associated with secondary changes including a sentinel tag or hypertrophied anal papilla. As with all acute and chronic anal conditions, efforts should be made to identify any precipitating causes or associated diseases (Crohn's disease or anal carcinoma). A recent consensus statement from the Association of Coloproctology of Great Britain and Ireland covers aspects of diagnosis and treatment (Cross et al 2008). The most common presenting features are pain during defaecation which may last for several hours afterwards, as well as rectal bleeding. The most consistent finding on examination is spasm of the anal canal, and it is uncertain whether this is the result of or due to ischaemia. Many of the management options have been based around reducing the internal anal spasm, but as with many benign anal conditions, one of the most important measures is to increase dietary fibre and adequate fluid intake. The majority of fissures, especially posterior fissures, are associated with a high resting pressure and a low blood flow to the anoderm resulting from this spasm. However, postpartum fissures are usually anterior and may be associated with a rectocele. The scar formation may be associated with ischaemia; however, the resting pressures in these patients are usually low. If there are multiple fissures or the fissures are not in the midline, a differential diagnosis of Crohn's disease, ulcerative colitis, human immunodeficiency virus and associated infections as well as neoplasia should be considered. An anal fissure may occur at any time in life but is most common between the second and fourth decades, with an equal distribution between men and women and a lifetime incidence of just over 11%. Inspection of the anus will usually reveal the fissure, and it is not usually possible to carry out any further examination due to the pain associated with the fissure.

Treatment of anal fissures

Acute anal fissures are usually treated conservatively with stool softeners and topical analgesics. Recurrence rates are reduced from 68% to 16% after continuing conservative management (Jensen 1987).

Medical therapies

The majority of medical therapies are aimed at relaxation of the internal anal sphincter, and this can be achieved using glyceryl trinitrate (GTN) ointment, diltiazem ointment or botulinum toxin.

Glyceryl trinitrate

GTN is a widely used drug that works by vasodilating and relaxing smooth muscle. It is suggested that patients should be treated with 0.2% or 0.4% GTN two to three times per day, and healing will occur in approximately 60% of patients in the short term. Unfortunately, the side-effect of severe headaches often precludes usage, although these headaches do wear off with time (Cross et al 2008).

Calcium channel blockers

Diltiazem and nifedipine cause muscle relaxation and vascular dilatation by inhibiting the entry of calcium ions. Diltiazem 2% used topically is rarely associated with the GTN headache, and healing rates are similar to those seen with GTN.

Botulinum toxin

Botulinum toxin works by binding irreversibly to the presynaptic nerve terminals preventing acetylcholine release and resulting in hypotonia and a reduced resting anal pressure. The effects last for 2–3 months until the acetylcholine has reaccumulated in the nerve terminals (Jones et al 2003). The majority of people use 20 units of botulinum toxin, although the dosages reported in the literature vary between 10 and 100 units; healing rates of 40–100% have been reported. Botulinum toxin is given in two doses into the internal sphincter, and 75% of patients will be healed using this treatment.

Surgery

If these conservative and medical treatments have failed, patients may require surgery. Surgical options include lateral sphincterotomy which permanently divides the internal sphincter, fissurectomy and advancement procedures. Lateral sphincterotomy has a reported cure rate of approximately 85%; however, the downside of this procedure is a significant incontinence problem, with up to 30% of patients having difficulty in controlling wind and at least 3–5% of

people suffering from overt incontinence (Garcia-Aguilar et al 1996). If a sphincterotomy is performed, it should be limited to the length of the fissure as this almost certainly reduces the incontinence problems. If the patient has a short anus or has had previous anorectal surgery, extreme caution is advised.

Fissurectomy

Excising the fissure and the fibrotic edge may improve healing rates and can be used in association with botulinum toxin.

Anal advancement flap

In patients in whom the fissure is associated with a low pressure, any medical or surgical aims to reduce anal pressure are unlikely to cause healing. Therefore, these patients should usually have some form of V–Y advancement flap or rotational flap, and although the results can be good, there may be problems with infection and wound healing at the donor site.

Faecal incontinence

Faecal incontinence is a debilitating symptom or sign which occurs in 1–10% of adults. It is largely a hidden problem due to embarrassment, and may be a result of many contributing factors. Recent NICE guidelines recognized that the treatment of this problem should be patient centred, and will vary considerably between patients according to their lifestyle and culture (National Institute for Health and Clinical Excellence 2007b). One of the recommendations is that people who are reported to have faecal incontinence should be offered care which is managed by appropriate healthcare professionals, and these people should have relevant skills, training and experience. They should also work within an integrated continence service. Groups who are at very high risk of faecal incontinence include frail, older people; people with loose stools from any cause; women following childbirth, especially after a third- or fourth-degree tear; and patients with pelvic organ prolapse or rectal prolapse. Other groups include patients with cognitive impairment or learning difficulties, and those who have undergone pelvic radiotherapy. It is essential to be aware that faecal incontinence is a symptom, not a disease, and there are many contributing factors; there is not usually a primary diagnosis.

Assessment

The baseline assessment of these patients should include a relevant medical history, examination and anorectal examination. Once again, the focus should be on warning signs for a lower gastrointestinal cancer, prolapse, acute disc prolapse or cauda equina syndrome (which would be associated with anal sensation loss), and potentially treatable causes of diarrhoea. The long-term management of patients with incontinence should include a 6-monthly review of symptoms, and giving patients contact details of all relevant support groups as well as advice about continence products, skin care and how to communicate with their friends and families. It is of utmost importance to preserve dignity and offer emotional support as well as psychological support, as appropriate.

The history should focus on differentiation between urge, passive and postdefaecatory leakage. A full assessment of obstetric history, trauma and surgery to the perineum, previous pelvic surgery, back problems/surgery and medical conditions (diabetes and neurological conditions) is essential. Examination should focus on an abdominal examination and a full pelvic floor examination, including anterior and posterior compartment. Sigmoidoscopy and proctoscopy is essential to examine for rectal and anal pathology.

Investigations specific to incontinence include anorectal physiology, anal and perineal ultrasound, and sometimes magnetic resonance proctogram.

Initial management

It is important to explain to patients that there is no 'quick fix' for incontinence, and a range of treatments and interventions may be necessary. The mainstay of initial treatment is alteration of stool consistency in order to try to reduce wind and avoid soft bowel motions. Patients should still be encouraged to drink at least 1.5 l of fluid per day unless contraindicated, and one of the best routes for reducing bowel frequency is to limit wheat fibre or insoluble fibre intake, as well as reducing the intake of caffeine and fizzy drinks. It is often useful to get the patient to diary their problem (i.e. stool consistency, number and types of leakage or urge incontinence episodes), and to encourage them to alter one part of their diet or management at a time. It is then possible to decide whether this alteration has been appropriate or helped their incontinence problem. Patients who have urge incontinence with soft stools or even normal stools often do very well with a very low dose of loperamide hydrochloride. This comes in a syrup, which allows patients to closely titrate the amount of loperamide (2 teaspoons = 1 tablet). Occasionally, patients develop abdominal pain with this; these patients should be offered codeine phosphate or co-phenotrope instead. Patients should not be offered loperamide if they have an acute flare of ulcerative colitis, hard or infrequent stools, or diarrhoea without a diagnosed cause. It is usually beneficial to start the loperamide at 1 teaspoon or less, and to advise patients to use the loperamide to manipulate their bowel movements and consistency, rather than allowing their bowel movements to control their lifestyle.

Many of these patients who are post childbirth have poor pelvic floor muscles and a reduced rectoanal angle which contributes to their incontinence. These patients should be referred for physiotherapy, electrical stimulation and management within the continence advisory service. This gives them access to a group of professionals who are readily available to help manage their needs for pads and anal plugs, and who can then provide a link back into secondary health care when appropriate.

Patients who continue to have episodes of faecal incontinence after this initial management may need to be referred to a specialist continence service where they can undertake pelvic floor retraining, bowel retraining, biofeedback, electrical stimulation and rectal irrigation. Rectal irrigation is particularly beneficial for those who have poor emptying as well as incontinence, and two types of pumps are readily available: the Braun irrimatic pump and the Peristeen pump (Coloplast). In order for these systems to be useful, patients need to have the ability to insert a tube into the rectum and manage the irrigation system.

Further treatment

All patients with faecal incontinence who are being considered for surgery should be referred to a specialist colorectal surgeon, who can offer the surgical and non-surgical options and discuss the realistic and likely outcome of any surgical intervention. Patients with a full-length external anal sphincter defect (which can be assessed on three-dimensional ultrasound) which is 90° or greater may be considered for an overlapping sphincter repair. This is done through a transperineal incision (Figure 59.4), and good long-term results at 5 years of 70% improvement should be expected. However, results deteriorate with time (Table 59.2). Patients with a Cleveland Clinic Incontinence Score below 9 should not be offered this as there is also a 15–20% risk that these patients will remain the same or be made worse. If patients have an incomplete internal sphincter defect, pudendal neuropathy, loose stools or irritable bowel, these are likely to decrease the effectiveness of a sphincter repair.

Patients in whom sphincter surgery is deemed inappropriate (i.e. those who have an intact anal sphincter, those in whom sphincter disruption is small, or where there is an absence of much in the way of voluntary contraction) may be referred for sacral nerve stimulation.

Sacral nerve stimulation

Sacral nerve stimulators have revolutionized the treatment of anal incontinence, and probably work through stimulation of both the external sphincter and the pelvic floor. Patients with significant anal incontinence are asked to keep a 2-week diary (Figure 59.5) about their episodes of incontinence. They have a test or trial of a percutaneous nerve stimulator, placed through S3 (or S2 or S4), and are asked to rediary their bowel movements during the 2 weeks of stimulation.

Results suggest that 70–80% of incontinent patients (urge and passive) will benefit from sacral nerve stimulation. If the trial is successful, these patients should be offered a permanent sacral nerve stimulator. This process involves implantation of a battery connected to a tyned wire which is inserted through the sacral foramen under X-ray guidance. The wire is tunnelled back to the battery, which is placed in the buttock or, occasionally, on the abdominal wall. Between 90% and 95% of patients who have at least a 50% improvement in symptoms with a temporary wire have a benefit with the permanent sacral nerve stimulator. There is a risk of infection, lead displacement and non-functioning of the permanent wire. NICE guidelines (National Institute for Health and Clinical Excellence 2004) looked at the results in 266 patients who had a sacral nerve stimulator; complete continence was achieved in 41–75%, and 75–100% of patients experienced a decrease of 50% or more in the number of incontinence episodes. As well as the incontinence, there is an ability to defer defaecation, which was absent previously, and an improvement in general quality of life. Adverse events in the fitting of the permanent implant are low (13%), mostly involving infection (three out of 149), lead migration (seven out of 149) and pain

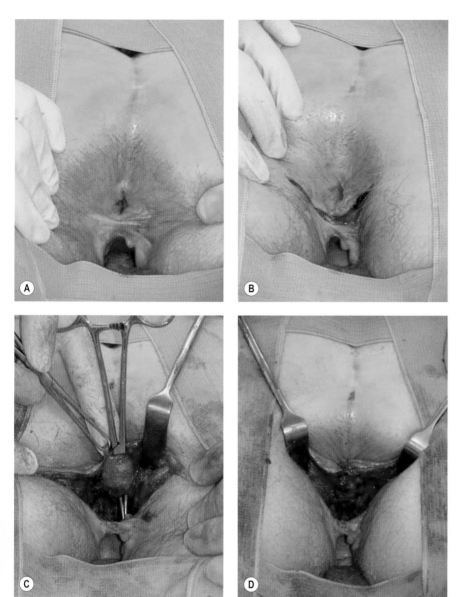

Figure 59.4 Overlapping sphincter repair. (A) Prone jack-knife position. (B) Curvilinear perineal incision to access ends of anal sphincter. (C) Sphincter muscle and scar tissue identified. (D) Overlapping repair with two layers of PDS (polydioxanone suture).

Table 59.2 Long-term results

Centre	Year	Patients (n)	Follow-up (months)	Full continence (%)	Success (%)
Malouf et al	2000	38	77	0	50
Zorcolo et al	2005	62	70	2	45
Maleskar et al	2007	64	84	20	80
Stikans et al	2007	34	41.5	7	73

(six out of 149) (National Institute for Health and Clinical Excellence 2004).

Gracioplasty and artificial bowel sphincter

If sphincter repair and sacral nerve stimulation have failed after full maximization of medical treatment, alternatives include a stimulated gracioplasty or an artificial bowel sphincter. Stimulated gracioplasty involves making a new anal sphincter using the gracilis muscle, which is transposed after dissecting it off its attachments on the medial aspects of the tibia. The muscle is then wrapped around the anus and reattached on to the ischial tuberosity. Electrodes are implanted into the transposed muscle and stimulated continuously in order to change the muscle fibres from type 2 to type 1 (smooth muscle).

In 2006, NICE looked at a systematic review of 37 studies of gracioplasty and found that 42–85% of patients are continent after the procedure (National Institute for Health and

Day	8	9	10	11	12	13	14
Controlled bowel movements (no incontinence: underwear, pads or pants remained clean)							
How many times did you go to the toilet (controlled)?							
How many times did you go in a rush to reach the toilet in time?							
Uncontrolled bowel movements (incontinence: underwear, pads or pants got dirty)							
How many times did you NOT make it in time to toilet (rush)?							
How many times did you not feel the bowel movement but only afterwards? (passive leakage)							
Staining/ minor soiling of underwear							
Did you stain/soil your underwear, pants or pad(s) today?	yes / no	yes / no	yes / no	yes / no	yes / no	yes / no	yes / no
Pad usage/ Enema/ Suppository							
Pad(s) used for incontinence?	yes / no	yes / no	yes / no	yes / no	yes / no	yes / no	yes / no
Enema/ Suppository administrated?	yes / no	yes / no	yes / no	yes / no	yes / no	yes / no	yes / no
Social functioning							
Did your (faecal) incontinence limit you in your daily activities (e.g. leaving the house, shopping etc)?	yes / no	yes / no	yes / no	yes / no	yes / no	yes / no	yes / no
Stool consistency							
What was your stool consistency today (circle one)	solid / mushy / liquid	solid / mushy / liquid	solid / mushy / liquid	solid / mushy / liquid	solid / mushy / liquid	solid / mushy / liquid	solid / mushy / liquid

Figure 59.5 Medtronic diary card for assessment of results from sacral nerve stimulation.

Clinical Excellence 2006). One case series reported a successful outcome in 72% of patients at 5-year follow-up. One of the most common complications of this procedure is wound infection (overall rate of 28%, with 15% requiring hospitalization). Electrical or technical problems also occur in 48% of patients; one of the side-effects of the procedure is problems with evacuation resulting in obstructive defaecation. The procedure is recommended but only if performed in specialist units and in carefully selected patients in whom other treatments have failed.

Artificial anal sphincters were adapted from approved urinary sphincters. They have been associated with high levels of infection and mechanical failure. Recently, in an attempt to avoid these septic complications, Finlay et al (2004) developed a transabdominal artificial bowel sphincter with a control balloon reservoir in the abdominal space. An inflatable cuff keeps the anal canal closed, and the patient presses a control pump in the abdominal wall which deflates the cuff in order to evacuate the bowel. Repressing the button closes the sphincter again by allowing the fluid to return into the cuff. In a series of 12 patients with follow-up of 59 months, 75% of patients had a functioning implant and the continence scores were improved from 16 to 3 after surgery. Three out of 12 patients had to have the device removed because of complications, and it is recommended that this procedure should only be performed under strict audit and clinical governance conditions and in units with specialist interest in faecal incontinence (National Institute for Health and Clinical Excellence 2008a). However, it may be a promising route for patients with severe faecal incontinence.

Injectable bulking agents

Few long-term data are available for the use of bulking agents in passive leakage or incontinence. Injections of a variety of bulking agents (collagen, carbon beads and silicon particles) have been used. They are usually injected submucosally in three or four places, just above the dentate line (where the anal canal is less sensate and therefore less painful), in order to try and reproduce the anal cushions and stop passive leakage. The largest case series has shown that 82 patients had significant continence score improvement in 6–12 months (Tjandra et al 2004). The largest case series showed that the most common complications are pain, minor ulceration and, occasionally, infection, as well as leakage of the substance from the anus. NICE guidance suggests that the evidence is not adequate for bulking agents to be used without special arrangements for consent, audit and research, and these procedures should only be performed in units specializing in faecal incontinence that have the ability to audit these results and inform patients of the potential lack of evidence (National Institute for Health and Clinical Excellence 2007c).

Stoma

Patients who fail all of the above procedures may require a stoma, and in many circumstances, colostomies can improve quality of life and decrease the amount of time organizing bowel care. Nowadays, An end colostomy can be performed laparoscopically. Although it is a relatively simple procedure, there are complication rates of between 25% and 75%. Often, patients experience problems with skin irritation, retraction and bleeding from the stoma, as well as problems with the bag sticking. However, the most common problems in the long term are parastomal hernias, stenosis and prolapse.

Rectal prolapse surgery for full-thickness rectal prolapse

A full-thickness rectal prolapse is an extremely distressing and uncomfortable condition. It occurs most frequently in elderly ladies, and the quality of life of these patients can be severely compromised. Occasionally, there are complications such as gangrene and perforation, but the majority of patients have symptoms of a heavy feeling, mucus leakage, bleeding and recurrent prolapse through the anus. This may be associated with other pelvic floor prolapses such as uterine prolapse. In younger age groups, full-thickness rectal prolapse may be associated with previous eating disorders and although the cause is not known, it is suspected that this may be due to a problem of collagen formation. The only possible curative treatment for a full-thickness rectal prolapse is surgery, but if a patient is relatively asymptomatic, surgery can be avoided and patients can have their constipation treated with a stool softener. Surgical interventions are based on either 'chopping off the prolapse' or 'hitching it up'. When hitching it up (rectopexy), a resection of the sigmoid may also be undertaken if there is associated constipation. A recent Cochrane analysis (Tou et al 2008) looked at a series of five different types of intervention, with the outcome measures being morbidity, length of stay and mortality. Unfortunately, the number of studies available was extremely small, and most of the randomized controlled trials included few patients. Twelve studies were included in this work with a total of 380 participants. Patients who are fit should be offered a laparoscopic or open rectopexy; these are associated with lower recurrence than a perineal procedure. Frail and unfit patients should have a perineal procedure (i.e. Altemeier operation or Delorme's procedure), the results of which suggest a recurrence rate of 25–40%. However, the morbidity and mortality associated with perineal procedures is low, and since many of these patients are over 80 years of age, this may make the recurrence rates relatively acceptable. If any form of prolapse is associated with a gynaecological prolapse, a combined procedure should be undertaken.

Altemeier operation

The design of this operation is to resect any prolapsing or redundant bowel and to attempt to recreate the pelvic floor by plicating the levators and reconnecting the sigmoid colon back to the anus with a coloanal anastomosis. However, there is no fixation of the rectum back up to the sacrum. The recurrence rate is approximately 16%, in comparison with 5% or less for an abdominal procedure (Tou et al 2008).

Delorme's procedure

The alternative perineal procedure is the Delorme's procedure, where the mucosa is resected off the bowel muscle tube. The bowel wall is then plicated and the mucosa of the anal canal is reanastomosed to the musosa high up within the anal canal. It is associated with a relatively high recurrence rate (up to 37%) (Tou et al 2008).

Rectopexy

The rectopexy has a much lower recurrence rate (<10%), and although mucosal prolapse is a relatively common form of recurrence, full thickness rarely occurs. The rectum is dissected down to the pelvic floor and then fixed up to the presacral fascia. Nowadays, this is mainly done laparoscopically and with sutures, but meshes and sponges were used for this fixation in the past.

In summary, healthy patients or patients with low comorbidity should probably have an abdominal or laparoscopic approach to treat their rectal prolapse with some sort of fixation. If there is any evidence of constipation, sigmoid resection with proctopexy is the preferred choice. However, there is a risk of an anastomosis and potential leak. In high-risk patients, a perineal approach should be offered and this varies culturally between an Altmeier's operation (often performed in the USA) and a Delorme's procedure (tends to be favoured in the UK).

Solitary rectal ulcer syndrome

This is a rare syndrome associated with rectal straining, resulting in an ischaemic, ulcerated wall of the rectum. This usually occurs anteriorly. The symptoms which then develop include further straining, a feeling of incomplete emptying, rectal bleeding and the passage of mucus as well as pain. On clinical examination, there is often a single or occasionally multiple ulcers, which are shallow. Occasionally, this may present as a polypoid lesion, which can be confused with the gross appearance of a carcinoma or a large polyp. A biopsy will confirm the diagnosis. Treatment is aimed at preventing straining and further chronic damage. Internal intussusception is found in a large number of these patients, but it is difficult to know whether this is related to solitary rectal ulcer formation or a result of the long-term straining. The mainstay of treatment is biofeedback aimed at reducing the length of time on the toilet. Straining patients are told how and where to sit and are given psychological support. They may require repeated courses of biofeedback as the results tend to fade after 2–3 years. Many people have tried a variety of surgical treatments for these ulcers, including local excision, rectopexy, stoma and even anterior resection. However, it has been found that resection is unlikely to improve the problem, and the majority of the surgical procedures result in less than 50% of the patients being cured. Even formation of a stoma may not relieve the symptoms. The patient will still have tenesmus and feel the need to defaecate continually.

Chronic constipation

Constipation in adults is extremely common and may be associated with a variety of abdominal symptoms as well as perineal discomfort.

Rome criteria for constipation

Constipation is defined as the presence of two or more of the following symptoms:

- Straining during at least 25% of defaecation.
- Lumpy or hard stools in at least 25% of defaecation.
- Sensation of incomplete emptying for at least 25% of defaecation.
- Sensation of anorectal obstruction blockage for at least 25% of defaecation.
- Manual manoeuvres to facilitate at least 25% of defaecation (such as digital evacuation support of the pelvic floor).
- Fewer than three bowel movements a week.
- Loose stools are rarely present without the use of laxatives.

Criteria have to have been met for the previous 3 months with the onset of symptoms 6 months prior to diagnosis.

Constipation occurs in up to 30% of the population (Garrigues et al 2004), and females have a higher incidence than males. Physical exercise and a high fibre diet are protective against constipation. Constipation can be divided into slow transit constipation, obstructive defaecation syndrome and irritable bowel syndrome (IBS).

Simple causes of constipation include a low fibre diet, dementia, depression and eating disorders. There are metabolic causes such as hypothyroidism, hypokalaemia, hypercalcaemia and diabetes mellitus (McCallum et al 2009). Neurological problems can include multiple sclerosis and Parkinson's disease, and there are a variety of drug-related causes for constipation. Patients with painful anorectal conditions such as fissures, haemorrhoids, fistulas etc. may develop constipation secondary to their painful anus. The majority of cases of constipation can be treated with basic dietary advice. Patients should sit on the toilet with their feet raised so that they sit in a semi-squatting position; this opens up the anorectal junction and allows them to defaecate more effectively. The use of abdominal massage and exercises which can be provided through a specialist nurse practitioner can help with the process of defaecation. Patients should ensure that they are well hydrated and take adequate amounts of fluid as well as exercise. Fibre may be beneficial, although patients with constipation related to IBS may find that their abdominal pain is increased with their intake of fibre. Preferred laxatives include movicol and magnesium hydroxide which do not rely on gut stimulation. However, stimulant laxatives are sometimes of use in patients who have poor colonic motility, especially secondary to opiates (McCallum et al 2009).

Obstructive defaecation

'Obstructive defaecation' is a term coined to indicate that a patient has stool in the rectum but is unable to evacuate it. The cause may be functional or anatomical. Anatomical problems include a rectocele, possibly an intussusception, enterocele, sigmoidocele and rectal prolapse. Functionally, patients may have paradoxical contractions of the pelvic floor or an inability to relax the anus which stops them from defaecating. Patients will complain of a feeling of incomplete evacuation, and will often need to digitate rectally or vaginally. A rectocele or pelvic floor weakness may be assessed clinically, but magnetic resonance defaecography is useful to see a non-emptying rectum. An additional investigation is colonic transit studies which may suggest that there is slow transit constipation.

Treatment of obstructive defaecation

Conservative treatment of obstructive defaecation includes bulking of the stools so that there is increased pressure of stools from above. Physical exercise and the use of suppositories or enemas may aid evacuation. More recently, rectal irrigation using either the Braun irrimatic pump or the Peristeen pump has been shown to aid patients who have both functional and structural problems within the pelvic floor. Behavioural therapy with biofeedback training teaches patients to coordinate the muscles required to defaecate. Rectoceles sometimes present to a coloproctologist along with a history of obstructive defaecation, and repairs may include the traditional transvaginal, transperineal or transanal route. More recently, coloproctologists have been using a stapled transanal rectal resection for patients with a combined rectocele and rectal intussusception. A British national database of these patients has shown that these procedures may improve functional results in up to 88% of patients. There have been some problems with urgency,

especially in patients who had a degree of incontinence prior to their surgery.

Slow transit constipation

Slow transit constipation is often idiopathic or may be associated with a neuropathy or recent or previous pelvic surgery. Patients with a megacolon associated with slow transit constipation and a normal functioning rectum may do well with a subtotal colectomy and ileorectal anastomosis; satisfaction rates of up to 90% have been reported (Lubowski et al 1996). Segmental resection appears to be unsatisfactory, and those patients who have an associated megarectum may be better treated with a ileoanal pouch (Gladman et al 2005). More recently, there have been some promising results using sacral nerve stimulators in patients with slow transit and combined causes of constipation. This seems to work by retrograde stimulation of the parasympathetic and sympathetic nerve chain.

Irritable bowel syndrome

IBS is one of the most common gastrointestinal disorders with an estimated prevalence of 10–20%. Patients present with a very wide range of symptoms, many of which overlap with other gastrointestinal disorders. It is essential, as always, to exclude any other significant pathology that may be causing these symptoms, but over-investigation is associated with a poorer outcome. A patient should present with symptoms for at least 6 months for a diagnosis of IBS to be made. They usually have a history of abdominal pain or discomfort associated with bloating, and often a change in bowel habit. In order to make a diagnosis of IBS, the pain or discomfort should be relieved by defaecation, or be associated with altered bowel frequency or stool form.

At least two of the following should also be associated:

- altered ability to defaecate including straining, urgency or incomplete evacuation;
- abdominal bloating and distension;
- symptoms made worse by eating; and
- passage of mucus.

Patients do not need investigation with invasive tests, but should have a full blood count, erythrocyte sedimentation rate, C-reactive protein (CRP) and antibody testing for coeliac disease. Patients should only be referred for secondary care if they have associated symptoms of unintentional or unexplained weight loss, associated rectal bleeding, a family history of any bowel or ovarian cancer, or are over 60 years of age with a change in bowel habit lasting more than 6 weeks with looser and/or more frequent stools. Additional 'red flags' are anaemia, abdominal masses, rectal masses or raised CRP (National Institute for Health and Clinical Excellence 2008b).

Patients should be treated for their IBS symptoms by self-help; this means looking at lifestyle, physical activity, diet and symptom-targeted medications. An essential part of treatment of IBS is assessing diet and nutrition (this includes fibre intake, which should usually be reduced). Insoluble fibre, especially wheat fibre, seems to exacerbate patients' symptoms by creating more wind; if more fibre is needed in order to treat constipation-related IBS, patients should ea

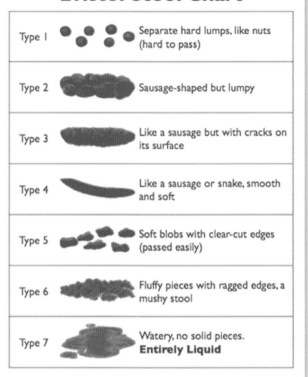

Bristol Stool Chart

Type 1		Separate hard lumps, like nuts (hard to pass)
Type 2		Sausage-shaped but lumpy
Type 3		Like a sausage but with cracks on its surface
Type 4		Like a sausage or snake, smooth and soft
Type 5		Soft blobs with clear-cut edges (passed easily)
Type 6		Fluffy pieces with ragged edges, a mushy stool
Type 7		Watery, no solid pieces. **Entirely Liquid**

Figure 59.6 Bristol stool chart.

foods high in soluble fibre (e.g. oat fibre). Other general dietary advice includes taking small meals regularly, eating meals slowly, avoiding missing meals and drinking at least eight cups of fluid per day, especially non-caffeinated drinks or water. Caffeine intake should be restricted, as should the intake of alcohol or fizzy drinks. Fresh fruit should be limited to three portions per day, and if IBS is associated with diarrhoea, artificial sweeteners should be avoided, as should diabetic insulin products. Other management can be by pharmacological intervention, and the decision regarding which drugs should be used should be tiered to the predominant symptom. If pain is a problem, patients should be offered antispasmodic agents. For patients with constipation, laxatives should be given but fybogel and lactulose should be avoided because of their wind and bloating aspects. If patients have diarrhoea-associated IBS, loperamide is the first-choice antimotility agent, and patients should be advised to adjust the dosage of laxative or antimotility agent to aim for a well-formed stool (type 4 on Bristol stool chart; Figure 59.6) (National Institute for Health and Clinical Excellence 2008b).

Second-line treatment, tricylic antidepressants, may be used for pain relief, starting with an extremely low dose (5–10 mg) of amitryptyline, taken once at night. A selective serotonin reuptake inhibitor may be used if a tricylic antidepressant is ineffective. Patients should be warned that side-effects of dry mouth and drowsiness may occur with these medications. Patients should not be referred to hospital or followed-up except on an annual basis unless symptoms change. NICE has published a full report of treatment options (National Institute for Health and Clinical Excellence 2008b).

Summary

In summary, there are many functional and structural bowel problems which occur alone and in combination with gynaecological and urological symptoms. Cancer and significant pathology should be excluded. A full history and examination, as well as some specific tests, will aid diagnosis and help to plan treatment. Patients should be assessed within a multidisciplinary team.

KEY POINTS

1. Anal manometry, electrophysiology and rectal sensation can provide valuable functional information on the anorectal complex. Combined with structural information from endoanal ultrasound, this allows the possibility of evidence-based management.

2. Evacuation proctography, isotope defaecography and colonic motility studies allow structural and functional assessment of defaecation which is vital for patient selection for surgery.

3. Faecal incontinence is an under-reported problem and there are multiple aetiologies. Obstetric injury is the most common cause of anal sphincter disruption, and although anal sphincter repair can be very successful, results are influenced by the extent of injury and the presence of pudendal neuropathy.

4. Assessment of constipation should include a detailed history and examination, combined with selective investigations. Management is predominantly conservative.

5. Joint assessment of patients with pelvic floor disorders in a combined pelvic floor clinic by a colorectal surgeon and a urogynaecologist is extremely valuable. Benefits include combined assessment, single hospital admission for complex joint surgery, and exchange of research ideas.

References

Cataldo P, Ellis CN, Gregorcyk S et al 2005 Practice parameters for the management of hemorrhoids (revised). Diseases of the Colon and Rectum 48: 189–194.

Cotterill N, Norton C, Avery KNL, Abrams P, Donovan JL 2008 A patient-centred approach to developing a comprehensive symptom and quality of life assessment of anal incontinence. Diseases of the Colon and Rectum 51: 82–87.

Cross KLR, Massey EJD, Fowler AL, Monson JRT 2008 The management of anal fissure: ACPGBI position statement. Colorectal Disease 10 (Suppl 3): 1–7.

Finlay IG, Richardson W, Hajivassiliou CA 2004 Outcome after implantation of a novel prosthetic anal sphincter in humans. British Journal of Surgery 91: 1485–1492.

Garcia-Aguilar J, Belmonte C, Wong WD, Lowry AC, Madoff RD 1996 Open vs. closed sphincterotomy for chronic anal fissure: long term results. Diseases of the Colon and Rectum 39: 440–443.

Garrigues V, Gálvez C, Ortiz V, Ponce M, Nos P, Ponce J 2004 Prevalence of constipation: agreement among several criteria and evaluation of the diagnostic accuracy of qualifying symptoms and self-reported definition in a population-based survey in Spain. American Journal of Epidemiology 159: 520–526.

Gladman MA, Scott SM, Lunniss PJ, Williams NS 2005 Systematic review of surgical options for idiopathic megarectum and megacolon. Annals of Surgery 241: 562–574.

Goligher JC 1976 Cryosurgery for haemorrhoids. Diseases of the Colon and Rectum 19 (3): 213–218.

Jensen SL 1987 Maintenance therapy with unprocessed bran in the prevention of acute anal fissure recurrence. Journal of the Royal Society of Medicine 80: 296–298.

Jones OM, Moore JA, Brading AF, Mortenesen NJ 2003 Botulinum toxin injection inhibits myogenic tone and sympathetic nerve function in the porcine internal anal sphincter. Colorectal Disease 5: 552–557.

Kourakalis G, Andromanakos N 2004 Evaluating patients with anorectal incontinence. Surgery Today 34: 304–312.

Laurberg S, Swash M, Henry MM 1988 Delayed external sphincter repair for obstetric tear. British Journal of Surgery 75: 786–788.

Lubowski DZ, Chen FC, Kennedy ML, King DW 1996 Results of colectomy for severe slow transit constipation. Diseases of the Colon and Rectum 39: 23–29.

Lunniss PJ, Mann CV 2004 Classification of internal haemorrhoids: a discussion paper. Colorectal Disease 6: 226–232.

MacRae HM, McLeod RS 1995 Comparison of haemorrhoidal treatment modalities. A meta-analysis. Diseases of the Colon and Rectum 38: 687–694.

Malouf AJ, Norton CS, Engel AF, Nicholls RJ, Kamm MA 2000 Long-term results of overlapping anterior anal-sphincter repair for obstetric trauma. The Lancet 355: 260–265.

Maslekar S, Gardiner AB, Duthie GS 2007 Anterior anal sphincter repair for fecal incontinence: good long term results are possible. Journal of the American College of Surgeons 204: 40–46.

McCallum IJD, Ong S, Mercer-Jones M 2009 Chronic constipation in adults. BMJ (Clinical Research Ed.) 338: 763–766.

Mirnezami A, Pilkington S, Monga A, Nugent KP 2008 Multidisciplinary team meetings for pelvic floor disorders. Colorectal Disease 10: 413.

National Institute for Health and Clinical Excellence 2004 Sacral Nerve Stimulation for Faecal Incontinence. IPG99. NICE, London.

National Institute for Health and Clinical Excellence 2006 Stimulated Graciloplasty for Faecal Incontinence. IPG159. NICE, London.

National Institute for Health and Clinical Excellence 2007a Stapled Haemorrhoidopexy for the Treatment of Haemorrhoids. TA128. NICE, London.

National Institute for Health and Clinical Excellence 2007b Faecal Incontinence: the Management of Faecal Incontinence in Adults. CG49. NICE, London.

National Institute for Health and Clinical Excellence 2007c Injectable Bulking Agents for Faecal Incontinence. IPG210. NICE, London.

National Institute for Health and Clinical Excellence 2008a Transabdominal Artificial Bowel Sphincter Implantation for Faecal Incontinence. IPG276. NICE, London.

National Institute for Health and Clinical Excellence 2008b Irritable Bowel Syndrome in Adults: Diagnosis and Management of Irritable Bowel Syndrome in Primary Care. CG61. NICE, London.

Pilkington SA, James A, Monga A, Dewbury K, Nugent K 2009 Comparing the diagnostic findings of dynamic MRI proctography and evacuating barium proctography for the assessment of patients with obstructive defaecation. Colorectal Disease 11: 662.

Stikans C, Pilkinton SA, Nugent 2009 Secondary repair of obstetric anal sphincter injury (OASIS). Colorectal Disease 11: 663.

Thompson WHF 1975 The nature of haemorrhoids. British Journal of Surgery 62: 542–552.

Tjandra JJ, Lim JF, Hiscock R, Rajendra P 2004 Injectable silicone biomaterial for fecal incontinence caused by internal anal sphincter dysfunction is effective. Diseases of the Colon and Rectum 47: 2138–2146.

Tou S, Brown SR, Malik AJ, Nelson RL 2008 Surgery for complete rectal prolapse in adults. Cochrane Database of Systematic Reviews Issue 4.

Vaizey CJ, Carapeti E, Cahill JA, Kamm MA 1999 Prospective comparison of faecal incontinence grading systems. Gut 44: 77–80.

Zorcolo L, Covotta L, Bartolo DC 2005 Outcome of anterior sphincter repair for obstetric injury: comparison of early and late results. Diseases of the Colon and Rectum 48: 524–531.

CHAPTER 60

Sexual dysfunction in urogynaecology

Ranee Thakar

Chapter Contents

INTRODUCTION	919
DEFINITION AND CLASSIFICATION	919
PREVALENCE OF SEXUAL DYSFUNCTION IN WOMEN WITH UROGYNAECOLOGICAL PROBLEMS	920
AETIOLOGY OF SEXUAL DYSFUNCTION IN WOMEN WITH PELVIC FLOOR DYSFUNCTION	920
RELATIONSHIP BETWEEN PELVIC ORGAN DYSFUNCTION AND SEXUAL FUNCTION	921
EFFECT OF TREATMENT OF PELVIC FLOOR DYSFUNCTION ON SEXUAL FUNCTION	922
EVALUATION	924
TREATMENT	925
KEY POINTS	926

Introduction

Sexuality and its expression contribute to some of the most complex aspects of human behaviour. The expression of sexuality and intimacy remains important throughout the lifespan of a woman, and hence needs to be understood in health as well as in illness. Although sexual problems are highly prevalent, a very small proportion of women consult a physician. In a UK- based survey, 54% of women reported at least one sexual problem lasting for at least 1 month during the previous year, which caused 62% of them to avoid sex. Only 21% with problems had sought help, of which 74% consulted their general practitioner (Mercer et al 2003). A web-based survey of 3807 women in the USA revealed that the most important barriers for women to seek help were embarrassment and feeling that the physician would not be able to provide help. Only 42% of this cohort sought help from their gynaecologist (Berman et al 2003). The high prevalence of sexual dysfunction and reluctance of women to seek help is a reflection on physicians' attitudes and ability to communicate with female patients about their sexual function.

Research into female sexuality has been a neglected area. It was Kinsey's research in the 1950s on sexual practices in men and women that helped to dispel the myth that women are not interested in sex. However, it has taken a long time to accept that women have a right to sexuality. The advent of new therapies for male sexual dysfunction has led to recent interest in these problems in women. There are a number of reasons why research in the past has focused more on male sexual problems than female. Firstly, it has been difficult to measure appropriate endpoints in clinical trials due to a lack of valid outcome measures. Secondly, the female sexual response is complex, as highlighted by current models (Figure 60.1) compared with the previously described linear models which were based on the relatively uncomplicated male sexual response cycle. The new, non-linear model of female sexual response considers emotional intimacy, sexual stimuli and relationship satisfaction (Basson 2001). This circular model demonstrates that many women initially begin a sexual encounter from a point of sexual neutrality. The decision to be sexual may come from a conscious wish for emotional closeness or as a result of seduction or suggestion from a partner. Women may have numerous reasons for engaging in sexual activity other than sexual drive. Sexual neutrality or being receptive to rather than initiating sexual activity is considered a normal variation of female sexual functioning. In addition, it is frequently the case that subjective and physiological sexual arousal precedes desire.

Definition and Classification

According to the World Health Organization's International Classification of Diseases (ICD-10) (World Health Organization 1992), the definition of sexual dysfunction includes 'the various ways in which an individual is unable to participate in a sexual relationship he or she would wish'. On the other hand, in the Diagnostic and Statistical Manual of Mental Disorders IV (DSM-IV) (American Psychiatric Association 1994), female sexual dysfunction (FSD) is defined as 'disturbances in sexual desire and in the psychophysiological changes that characterise the sexual response cycle and cause marked distress and interpersonal difficulty'. Although both systems recognize the need for a subjective distress criterion, these definitions rely on the linear human response cycle. Furthermore, both systems are based on conceptualization

DOI: 10.1016/B978-0-7020-3120-5.00060-6

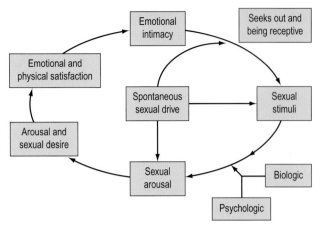

Figure 60.1 Female sexual response cycle.

Adapted from Kingsberg S, Janata JW (2007) Female Sexual Disorders: Assessment, Diagnosis and Treatment. Urol Clin N Am 34:497–506.

of sexual response as a 'psychosomatic process' involving psychological and somatic components. In 1998, the Sexual Function Health Council of the American Foundation devised the first consensus-based definition and classification system for FSD, which was further updated in 2003 (Basson et al 2004) (Box 60.1). FSD is best regarded as a spectrum of disorders with considerable overlap. Understanding this interplay of physical and psychosocial factors in context with illnesses, and medical and/or surgical interventions will help the clinician in managing FSD. Sexual dysfunction may arise because of an illness or disability, a medication or surgical procedure, changes accompanying the ageing process, relationship difficulties, abusive experiences, performance anxiety or any combination of factors such as these (Table 60.1).

Prevalence of Sexual Dysfunction in Women with Urogynaecological Problems

Sexual dysfunction occurs commonly in women attending urogynaecological services. Up to 64% of sexually active women attending a urogynaecology clinic suffer from FSD (Pauls et al 2006). Although it is a very common problem, a recent survey of members of the American Urogynecologic Society (AUGS) showed that only a minority of urogynaecologists screen all patients for FSD. Lack of time, uncertainty about therapeutic options and older age of the patient were cited as potential reasons for failing to address sexual complaints as part of routine history (Pauls et al 2005). A survey of the members of the British Urogynaecological Society (BSUG) using the same questionnaire with a few modifications reflected similar findings. Fifty percent of the BSUG members regularly screened for FSD at clinic visits and 49.5% after surgery, compared with 77% and 76% of AUGS members, respectively. The most important barrier for not enquiring about FSD was lack of time. Seventy-six percent found training for FSD to be unsatisfactory (Roos et al 2009). The similarity in trends between the UK and USA highlights that this may be a more global problem that needs wider exploration. Furthermore, the subject of FSD should be given more importance in the undergraduate and post-

graduate curriculum, so that clinicians enquire about this embarrassing problem.

Aetiology of Sexual Dysfunction in Women with Pelvic Floor Dysfunction

In a survey of 104 patients attending a urogynaecology clinic (Sutherst 1979), 46% admitted that their urinary disorder

---

Box 60.1 Definition and classification of FSD

Sexual interest/desire disorder

There are absent or diminished feelings of sexual interest or desire, absent sexual thoughts or fantasies, and a lack of responsive desire. Motivations (here defined as reasons/incentives) for attempting to have sexual arousal are scarce or absent. The lack of interest is considered to be beyond the normative lessening with lifecycle and relationship duration.

Arousal disorder

Subjective sexual arousal disorder

Absence of or markedly diminished feelings of sexual arousal (sexual excitement and pleasure) from any type of sexual stimulation. Vaginal lubrication or other physical response still occur.

Combined genital and subjective arousal disorder

Absence of or markedly diminished feelings of sexual arousal (sexual excitement and pleasure) from any type of sexual stimulation, as well as complaints of absent or impaired genital sexual arousal (vulval swelling, lubrication).

Genital sexual arousal disorder

Complaints of absent or impaired genital sexual arousal. Self-report may include minimal vulval swelling or vaginal lubrication from any type of sexual stimulation, and reduced sexual sensations from caressing genitalia. Subjective sexual excitement still occurs from non-genital stimuli.

Persistent sexual arousal disorder

Spontaneous intrusive and unwanted genital arousal (e.g. tingling, throbbing, pulsating) in the absence of sexual interest and desire. The arousal is unrelieved by one or more orgasms, and the feelings of arousal persist for hours or days.

Orgasmic disorder

Despite the self-report of high sexual arousal/excitement, there is either lack of orgasm, marked diminished intensity of orgasmic sensations or marked delay of orgasm from any kind of stimulation.

Sexual pain disorders

Dyspareunia

Recurrent or persistent pain with attempted or complete vaginal entry and/or penile vaginal intercourse.

Vaginismus

The persistent or recurrent difficulties of the woman to allow vaginal entry of a penis, a finger and/or any object, despite the woman's expressed wish to do so. There is often (phobic) avoidance and anticipation/fear/experience of pain, along with variable involuntary pelvic muscle contraction.

Other sexual pain disorders

Recurrent or persistent genital pain induced by non-coital sexual stimulation.

Table 60.1 Conditions that affect female sexual function and their effects

Condition	Effect(s)
Oestrogen deficiency e.g. menopause, secondary amenorrhea (binge-eating disorders, rigorous diet), puerperal amenorrhoea (lactational amenorrhoea), contraception with super-light pills, menopause	Decreased lubrication and arousal
Testosterone deficiency e.g. premature iatrogenic menopause	Decreased desire
Diabetes	Decreased lubrication
Hormonal disorders e.g. thyroid, pituitary, adrenal	Decreased lubrication and desire
Neurological disorders e.g. Parkinson's disease, multiple sclerosis	Decreased lubrication, arousal, desire and difficulty reaching orgasm
Genital prolapse	Decreased desire and arousal
Urinary incontinence	Decreased desire, arousal and pain
Atrophy, vaginitis, pelvic inflammatory disease, endometriosis, vestibulitis, cystitis	Pain and vaginismus
Arthritis	Limitation of movement
Trauma, sexual assault	Arousal disorder
Procedure	
Oophorectomy	Decreased desire and lubrication
Episiotomy and pelvic floor repairs	Pain
Drugs	
Antihypertensives e.g. β-blockers, α-blockers, diuretics	Decreased desire and difficulty reaching orgasm
Psychotherapeutic drugs e.g. tricyclic antidepressants, selective serotonin reuptake inhibitors, lithium, benzodiazepines	Difficulty reaching orgasm
Hormones e.g. oral contraceptives, oestrogens, progestins, gonadotrophin-releasing hormone agonists	Decreased desire
Cardiovascular agents e.g. lipid-lowering agents, digoxin	Decreased desire
Chemotherapeutic agents	Vaginal dryness, decreased desire and difficulty reaching orgasm

had an adverse effect on sexual relations. The reasons for reduced frequency of sexual intercourse were superficial or deep dyspareunia (most common), wetness at night and the need for protection of a towel all the time, leakage of urine during coitus, decreased libido, depression or embarrassment, marital discord and the need for separate beds.

Women with pelvic organ prolapse may have sexual dysfunction due to mechanical obstruction. However, the reasons probably extend beyond the local effects. It has been shown that women seeking treatment for advanced prolapse have poorer body image and quality-of-life scores compared with women with normal vaginal support (Jelovsek and Barber 2006). Using the female sexual response cycle, one can conceptualize how incontinence and prolapse may affect sexuality. Arousal may be reduced in a woman with coital incontinence or prolapse due to embarrassment. This, in turn, affects orgasm and can also lead to reduced lubrication. Sexual intercourse in this situation will cause the woman to experience pain, which may affect arousal (Figure 60.2).

Surgery for prolapse and urinary incontinence has a role in reconstructing the local anatomy and alleviating symptoms. This, however, does not necessarily ensure optimal sexual function. The cause of sexual dysfunction following vaginal surgery may be classified into organic and/or psychosocial. Organic causes are anatomical, physiological, vascular, neural and hormonal. It can be hypothesized that surgical disruption of the iliohypogastic and/or pudendal arterial blood may result in compromised blood flow, which may cause vaginal dryness and dyspareunia. The anterolateral vaginal walls are densely innervated by pelvic autonomic nerves which are critical for preserving sexual function. Surgery in this region for stress urinary incontinence and cystocele repair may affect this innervation and alter sexual experience. Damage to the dorsal nerve of the clitoris due to its close proximity while performing surgery in the anterior compartment (various sling procedures) may cause impairment of orgasmic function. Vaginal narrowing and shortening, especially following posterior repairs, may cause dysfunction. Concomitant procedures such as oophorectomy may cause loss of a physiological testosterone milieu with a subsequent decrease of sexual libido, pleasure and sense of well-being. In addition, coexisting psychosocial factors such as life stressors, anxiety and depression need to be borne in mind. Altered perception of genital health, both by the woman and her partner, after surgery with associated apprehension and fear of damage to the internal organs can also be contributory factors for a negative impact on sexual function.

Relationship between Pelvic Organ Dysfunction and Sexual Function

Evidence from large prospective studies has demonstrated that prolapse and/or incontinence have an adverse effect on sexual function (Rogers et al 2001a, Handa et al 2004, Novi et al 2005). Complaints of stress urinary incontinence, overactive bladder (OAB) and lower urinary tract symptoms have been shown to have a negative impact on all domains of sexual function (Salonia et al 2004, Aslan et al 2005). The most common sexual complaints in women with urinary incontinence are low desire, vaginal dryness and dyspareunia (Handa et al 2004). Amongst the different types of urinary incontinence, OAB has a particularly high association with sexual dysfunction, which could be indicative of an underlying psychosomatic disorder.

Using a validated questionnaire, Novi et al (2005) demonstrated significantly lower measures of sexual function in

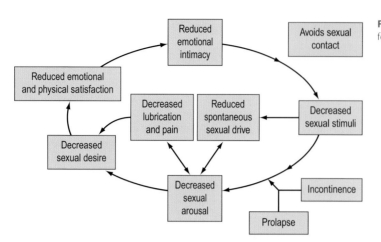

women with pelvic organ prolapse. Women with prolapse were more likely to have urinary and/or faecal incontinence during sexual activity, more dyspareunia and fewer orgasms. They were also more likely to report negative emotional reactions associated with sex, and higher rates of embarrassment leading to avoidance of sex. Presence of both prolapse and incontinence has a cumulative negative effect on sexual function, with libido, sexual excitement and orgasm being significantly affected (Ozel et al 2006). Increasing severity of prolapse is associated with symptoms related to urinary incontinence, voiding, and defaecatory and sexual dysfunction, which do not necessarily correlate with the location of prolapse and therefore are not compartment specific (Ellerkmann et al 2001).

Effect of Treatment of Pelvic Floor Dysfunction on Sexual Function

Assuming that the physical effect of prolapse and incontinence is one of the contributing factors for sexual dysfunction, one could logically assume that an intervention leading to their improvement should improve sexual function.

Urinary incontinence

Pelvic floor rehabilitation appears to positively influence female sexuality. Zahariou et al (2008) evaluated the effect of a programme of supervised pelvic floor muscle training on sexual function, in a group of women with urodynamically diagnosed stress urinary incontinence, using a validated questionnaire (Female Sexual Function Index, FSFI) 12 months after treatment. All domains of the FSFI improved significantly, with median total FSFI scores increasing from 20.3 to 26.8. The improvement in sexual function could be due to the improvement in strength of the pelvic floor muscles. Pelvic floor contraction plays an important role in female orgasmic response. Furthermore, the strength of the pelvic floor muscles probably affects the anatomical position of the clitoral erectile tissue, with consequences for sexual stimulation. In addition, muscle training improves muscle morphology and neuromuscular function. Although there are extensive data on the effect of various pharmaceutical agents in women with OAB, sexual function has only been evaluated in one study (Sand et al 2006). The Multicentre Assessment of Transdermal Therapy in Overactive Bladder with Oxybutynin study was an open-label, prospective trial of 2878 subjects with OAB, treated with transdermal oxybutynin for 6 months or less. The impact of OAB on sexual function before and after treatment was assessed via item responses from the King's Health Questionnaire and Beck Depression Inventory-II. At baseline, 23.1% of participants reported that OAB had an impact on their sex life. Coital incontinence in 22.8% of women decreased after treatment to 19.3%. The effects of OAB on subjects' sex lives improved in 19.1% of cases (worsened in 11.2%), and the effect on relationships with partners improved in 19.6% of cases (worsened in 11.9%). Reduced interest in sex, reported by 52.1% of women at baseline, improved significantly. Considering that sexual dysfunction is highly prevalent in women with OAB, it is surprising that such scarce data are available.

Prior to introduction of the minimally invasive sling suburethral procedures, the Burch colposuspension was regarded as the 'gold standard' surgical treatment option for stress urinary incontinence. Considering that the procedure was used for many decades, there are few data on the impact of colposuspension on sexual health. Moran et al (1999) evaluated 55 women with stress urinary incontinence who reported coital incontinence before undergoing colposuspension. Preoperative coital leakage occurred in 65% of women with penetration, 16% with orgasm and 18% with both. After surgery, 81% of the women reported no coital incontinence. Similarly, Baessler and Stanton (2004) showed that 6 months after colposuspension, while stress urinary incontinence improved in 77% of patients, coital incontinence was cured in 70% and improved in almost 7%, which suggests that coital incontinence is likely to be cured when urinary incontinence is successfully treated by Burch colposuspension.

Recent prospective studies of surgery for urinary incontinence using tension-free vaginal tape have found a positive impact on sexual function, primarily because of cure of coital incontinence with the associated emotional benefits of loss of fear and embarrassment due to leakage (Shah et al 2005, Ghezzi et al 2006). Causes of postoperative worsening of sexual function have been attributed to loss of libido, dyspareunia and partner discomfort. Cases of dysfunction due to vaginal erosion of the mesh and de-novo anorgasmia are infrequent. A recent study based on a postal questionnaire survey has shown that the transobturator tape (TOT) procedure can have a positive, but also a negative, outcome on female sexual function (Sentilhes et al 2008). Comparing the TOT procedure with the transvaginal approach, Elzevier et al (2008) found that both procedures had a positive effect on sexual function due to improvement in incontinence. However, pain due to vaginal narrowing was significantly more common in the TOT procedure group.

Prolapse

Sexual activity in women with pessaries *in situ* is poorly studied. It has been shown that long-term pessary use is acceptable to sexually active women. Using the FSFI questionnaire, Kuhn et al (2009) showed that desire, lubrication and sexual satisfaction improved significantly, and orgasm remained unchanged in women who used pessaries for pelvic organ prolapse and were sexually active.

Anterior repair does not seem to have an effect on sexual function unless it is combined with another procedure. Colombo et al (2000) reviewed 23 women who had an anterior repair for cystocele and stress urinary incontinence 8 years after surgery, and found that 56% had mild-to-severe postoperative dyspareunia. However, all patients in this study also had a posterior repair and perineorrhaphy. Most studies on vaginal surgery in the posterior compartment for rectocele repair have demonstrated improvement in sexual function, with a decrease in dyspareunia when only midline fascial plication or site-specific repair was done (Cundiff et al 1998, Kenton et al 1999, Porter et al 1999, Glavind and Tetsche 2004). However, when the repair involved levator plication, there was a significant increase in dyspareunia following surgery (Kahn and Stanton 1997).

Vaginal vault prolapse surgery is difficult to study as the problem usually involves multiple compartments of the pelvic floor. However, the Colpopexy and Urinary Reduction Efforts trial (Handa et al 2007) provided a unique opportunity to study sexual function in women undergoing sacrocolpopexy with and without colposuspension. Using a validated questionnaire [Pelvic Organ Prolapse/Urinary Incontinence Sexual Functioning Questionnaire (PISQ-12)] and telephone interviews 1 year after surgery, the authors found that, after surgery, fewer women reported sexual interference from 'pelvic or vaginal symptoms', fear of incontinence, vaginal bulging and pain. More women were sexually active after surgery. The addition of Burch colposuspension did not have an adverse effect on sexual function. Dyspareunia after sacrospinous fixation procedure may be attributable to either vaginal narrowing, pudendal injury, deviation of the vagina or excessive colpectomy during the concomitant repair procedure. The rates of postoperative dyspareunia are reported to be between 8% and 16% (Aslan et al 2005). Iliococcygeal fixation is another technique used to correct vault prolapse. In a matched case–control study comparing sacrospinous with iliococcygeal fixation, Maher et al (2004) found no significant difference in the percentage of women who were sexually active, or who had dyspareunia or buttock pain.

Meshes, both synthetic and biological, on their own or in the form of kits are used increasingly to reinforce vaginal repairs, with the purpose of improving long-term results and preventing recurrences. However, there is very little information about their influence on sexual function. Following repair of large or recurrent anterior and posterior compartment prolapse using an overlay graft (atrium polypropylene), Dwyer and O'Reilly (2004) showed a decrease in dyspareunia over a 24-month period after surgery. In contrast, Milani et al (2005) found a 20% increase in dyspareunia after anterior repair and a 63% increase after posterior repair reinforced by mesh. Neither of these studies assessed other aspects of sexual function. More recently, Novi et al (2007) compared sexual function of women undergoing rectocele repair with porcine dermis graft with site-specific repair of the rectovaginal fascia using a validated questionnaire (PISQ), and found that subjects undergoing porcine dermis graft scored significantly higher on the PISQ 6 months after surgery. There is an urgent need for proper evaluation of meshes in all forms before they are widely used.

Historically, the uterus has been regarded as the regulator and controller of important physiological functions, a sexual organ, a source of energy and vitality, and a maintainer of youth and attractiveness. It is logical to hypothesize that removal of such an organ would lead to sexual problems. However, there is evidence to the contrary. The largest prospective study to date is the Maryland Women's Health Study (Rhodes et al 1999), which enrolled 1299 women who were interviewed with validated questionnaires before and 6, 12, 18 and 24 months after hysterectomy for benign conditions. They found a significant increase in frequency of sexual activity, a decreased rate of frequent dyspareunia, a decrease in reduced orgasm and a reduction in low libido rates. The distribution of women not experiencing vaginal dryness improved significantly. Overall, this study found substantial improvements in sexual function after hysterectomy. An enduring debate in the late 1980s and the 1990s was whether subtotal hysterectomy might confer advantages over total hysterectomy with regard to sexual, urinary and bowel function, since the former entails minimal neuroanatomical disruption. However, a recent Cochrane review (Lethaby et al 2006) did not demonstrate any difference in pelvic organ dysfunction, quality of life and psychological function in women with and without conservation of the cervix 1 year after surgery, and this effect seems to persist on long-term follow-up (Thakar et al 2008). Roovers et al (2003), in a prospective, observational study over 6 months, found a reduction in sexual problems after vaginal, subtotal or total hysterectomy. However, the prevalence of one or more bothersome sexual problems 6 months after vaginal, subtotal or total hysterectomy was 43%, 41% and 39%, respectively, and new sexual problems developed in over 9% of cases. The authors acknowledged that the size of the study population might have been too small to detect slight differences.

Childbirth and puerperium

In the postpartum period, the combination of a new baby, fatigue, hormonal changes and a healing episiotomy scar may contribute to diminished frequency and enjoyment of sexual intercourse. Recent work on women's sexual health after childbirth has shown that sexual health problems are common in this period. In a cross-sectional study of 796 primiparous women over a 6-month period after delivery, Barrett et al (2000) found that 32% had resumed intercourse within 6 weeks of birth and 89% had resumed intercourse within 6 months. Sexual health problems, as recalled by the women, increased significantly after childbirth, with 83% experiencing sexual problems in the first 3 months, which declined to 64% at 6 months, although not reaching the prepregnancy levels of 38%. Dyspareunia at 6 months post partum was significantly associated with a previous experience of dyspareunia and current breast feeding. In a further analysis of the same cohort of women, it was found that women who were depressed were less likely than women who were not depressed to have resumed sexual intercourse and to report sexual health problems at 6 months post partum (Morof et al 2003) . However, sexual health problems were common after childbirth in both depressed and non-depressed women, and therefore the authors suggested that postnatal sexual morbidity cannot be assumed to be simply a product of depressed mental state. When the mode of delivery was analysed in this cohort of women, in comparison with vaginal delivery, the protective effect of caesarean section on sexual function was limited to the early postnatal period, primarily due to dyspareunia-related symptoms. At 6 months, differences in dyspareunia-related symptoms, sexual-response-related symptoms and postcoital problems between caesarean and vaginal delivery were much reduced or reversed, with none reaching statistical significance (Barrett et al 2005). van Brummen et al (2006) performed a prospective longitudinal study on 377 primiparous women using the Maudsley Marital Questionnaire to evaluate factors which determine sexual activity and sexual relationship 1 year after the first delivery. Not being sexually active in early pregnancy (up to 12 weeks of gestation), older maternal age at delivery and third/fourth degree anal sphincter tear were the main predictors of sexual inactivity and dissatisfaction with sexual relationship at 1 year post partum. Perineal trauma (second, third and fourth) and use of obstetric instrumentation were related to increased frequency and severity of dyspareunia at 6 months post partum.

Evaluation

Management of FSD begins with identification and diagnosis, and is based on the patient's self-report in conjunction with a clinical evaluation. It is important to make the environment conductive so that the patient feels at ease.

History

Presentation may be overt, wherein the woman presents with symptoms of lack of desire, orgasm and arousal, and/or pain. Sexual problems are often disguised and may present as unresolved complaints, requests for repeated investigations and multiple consultations, all of which should raise the suspicion of a hidden agenda. Removing the protective coat of the hidden agenda through listening, observing, feeling, interpretation and reflection of all the clues present in the consultation allows for its emergence

into the conscious. The hidden agenda of the patient needs to be acknowledged, the reason for the concealment needs to be respected, and the practitioner needs to provide an environment in which it can be expressed without fear. Thus, even taking a brief sexual history during a new patient visit is effective, and indicates to the patient that the discussion of sexual concerns is appropriate and a routine component of the consultation. For screening of sexual problems, simple questions are as effective as lengthy interviews and can be used in clinical settings (Roos et al 2009). Questions regarding the sexual problem should be asked to generate the full picture of current sexual response. The impact of the dysfunction on the patient's personal well-being and its significance should be quantified. In addition, the role of the partner, and the partner's sexual response and reaction to sexual problems should be ascertained where possible. As sexual functioning is multifactorial, a thorough medical, surgical, obstetric, gynaecological, psychiatric and social history should also be taken. History of cigarette smoking and alcohol and/or drug intake should be taken. Medications are an important part of the history, as many medications can have an adverse effect on sexual function. However, it should be noted that much of the available information is based on data from male subjects, and it is unknown whether dysfunctions noted in males will also exist in females. A history of sexual assault or trauma is a potential contributor to sexual and pelvic floor dysfunction.

With better understanding of the domains of female sexual function, there has been an increasing use of self-report questionnaires. The advantage of using these questionnaires, apart from the fact that they are valid and reliable measures of sexual function, is that they are easy to administer, relatively inexpensive and unobtrusive, and normative values are available for both clinical and non-clinical populations. Several generic questionnaires are available (e.g. the Brief Index for Sexual Function in Women, the Female Sexual Function Index and the Sexual Distress Scale). Recently, a condition-specific questionnaire has become available to evaluate sexual function in women with incontinence and prolapse — the PISQ. The PISQ was developed and validated in New Mexico in the USA. The PISQ has a long form and a short form. The long form contains 31 items, all with Likert scale responses, which are divided into three domains: behavioural-emotive (comprising 15 questions), physical (ten questions) and partner related (six questions). Higher PISQ scores indicate better sexual function (Rogers et al 2001b). The short form consists of 12 questions and is not divided into the three domains (Rogers et al 2003). The short form of the PISQ is useful in the clinical setting because it reduces the time and burden to the patient, and provides the clinician with objective means of evaluating functional outcomes of either medical or surgical interventions. In the research setting, the short form of the PISQ is useful when quality-of-life analysis is part of the armamentarium used to evaluate outcomes and compare results.

Other self-report measures, such as daily diaries and event logs, are also useful. These record sexual function variables such as the frequency of intercourse, quality of sexual encounter, satisfaction, medication use, etc. Diaries typically require the subject to record sexual activity on a daily basis, whereas event logs are only completed on days when sexual activity occurs. The advantage of diary or event log measures is that they provide quantitative data regarding the frequency of sexual activity, and the proportion of successful attempts at intercourse or other forms of sexual activity. However, they are highly restricted in the scope of measurement, as they do not provide the broad multidimensional assessment of response afforded by self-administered questionnaires and are subject to response bias. However, despite these limitations, daily diaries and event logs have been recommended by regulatory agencies as primary endpoints for clinical trials in FSD.

Physical examination

A general physical examination, with specific attention to the vascular and neurological systems, should be carried out. In addition to blood pressure and peripheral pulses, general appearance should be assessed for secondary sex characteristics, hirsutism and signs of virilization. The genitalia and perineum should be examined in detail where a physical cause is suspected. This includes inspection for any developmental anomalies, signs of vaginal atrophy, warts, infections and scarring. Cotton bud evaluation of the external genitalia may confirm vestibular vulvitis and neuropathies. Signs of urinary incontinence should be elicited by asking the patient to cough with a full bladder. Gentle digital examination to elicit tenderness and scarring may be undertaken and, if tolerated, followed by bimanual examination to assess the condition of the cervix, uterus and adnexa. Any tenderness, swelling and thickening should be noted. If the patient complains of pain, it is important to try and reproduce the complaint. Episiotomy and previous surgical incisions may be sites of tenderness as a result of vaginal narrowing, scarring and nerve entrapment. The tone of the pelvic floor muscles should be assessed and any prolapse should be documented. At this time, the presence of vaginismus may also be noted as an involuntary contraction of the outer third of the vagina, which may be severe enough to preclude speculum examination. Speculum examination should reveal the condition of the vagina and cervix; where appropriate, bacteriological and chlamydia swabs can be taken. Sometimes, a rectal examination may be indicated with specific attention to the anal reflex.

Laboratory testing

Laboratory testing may be needed in some patients depending on the underlying condition, although no test can be recommended routinely. Standard serum biochemistry, full blood count and lipid profiles may identify vascular risk factors, such as hypercholesterolaemia, diabetes mellitus and renal disease. A measurement of serum thyroid-stimulating hormone may also be indicated if thyroid dysfunction is suspected. If menopausal status is uncertain, oestradiol, follicle-stimulating hormone and luteinizing hormone testing are recommended. The consensus of opinion is that analogue assays for free testosterone should not be recommended.

Specialized diagnostic testing

Diagnostic methods such as vaginal photoplethysmography, duplex Doppler ultrasonography, vaginal and clitoral temperature, and vibratory sensory testing, as well as selective pudendal arteriography increase the clinician's and patient's understanding of the pathophysiological mechanisms of sexual dysfunction, but lack of normative data limits the use of specialized testing.

Treatment

When an obvious underlying cause is found, this should be treated. Successful management of FSD entails understanding where the break occurred in the sexual response cycle. As there are multiple factors associated with dysfunction, the traditional medical illness model of cause and effect does not apply in FSD. Often a multidisciplinary, collaborative approach is needed. Referral to a psychotherapist should be considered when no organic cause is found, when the patient does not respond or is not satisfied with the primary intervention provided, or when the clinician feels that specialist intervention may offer the diagnosis and treatment that is most appropriate. Once a diagnostic evaluation is carried out, the patient's dysfunction can be accurately classified. It is important to identify to the patient any obvious reversible causes for FSD, or potential lifestyle changes that may be beneficial to sexual function, such as stopping smoking, eating a healthy diet, regular exercise, improving partner communication and stress reduction. In liaison with the general practitioner, it may be necessary to change medications which may affect sexual function.

Especially in the elderly, vaginal dryness may be alleviated by use of water-soluble lubricants. Although current evidence does not suggest a role of systemic oestrogen or oestrogen/progestin therapy in women with reduced desire, they have been used effectively in FSD related to genitourinary atrophy. Low-dose vaginal oestrogens are minimally absorbed and are associated with fewer side-effects than systemic therapy, and are therefore preferred. Currently available vaginal oestrogen products include vaginal oestrogen creams that are effective in low doses (0.5 g twice weekly) and a vaginal oestradiol tablet (twice weekly).

Most trials of testosterone replacement therapy have shown statistically significant improvement in sexual function and well-being in women who have undergone oophorectomy. Transdermal testosterone therapy in the form of a patch or gel, which delivers physiological doses, has shown positive impacts on sexual function domains in postmenopausal and surgically menopausal women with hypoactive sexual desire disorder receiving concomitant oestrogen therapy in a recent randomized trial (Kingsberg et al 2007). However, at present, there are no safety and efficacy data for testosterone supplementation in oestrogen-deficient women, with even less support for women who are not oestrogen deficient and who have intact ovaries. Furthermore, the adverse effects of long-term use are largely unknown, with most studies having a follow-up duration of up to 2 years. Risks of androgen therapy include hirsutism, acne, adverse liver function and lipid profile changes, with a potential increase in insulin resistance and metabolic syndrome with long-term use. For surgically menopausal women who present with symptoms of reduced desire, low-dose testosterone can be started along with continuous oestrogen therapy. The response to treatment (both efficacy and side-effects) should be evaluated after 3–6 months. If the problem persists, the patient should be referred to a specialist clinic, or for relationship counselling, psychotherapy or lifestyle advice, as appropriate.

There are other agents in the experimental phase that deserve mention for their potential to improve symptoms. These include sildenafil (Viagra), L-arginine (a nitric oxide precursor), sublingual apomorphine (a dopamine agonist), prostaglandin E1 (applied topically to increase blood flow) and phentolamine (oral or vaginal application; an adrenergic receptor antagonist).

After vaginal delivery, the patient may experience persistent pain over the episiotomy or perineal trauma site. If localized tender scar tissue is identified, women can be advised to have sexual intercourse after application of lidocaine gel/ointment. If pain persists, perineal injections, consisting of a cocktail of 10 ml bupivacaine 0.5%, 1500 iu hyaluronidase and 1 ml Depo-Medrone, is injected into the site of maximal tenderness (Figure 60.3). Occasionally, a woman may present with a perineal skin web in the posterior fourchette or fusion of the labia. These can be divided after infiltrating the area with a local anaesthetic injection. In women who are breast feeding, dyspareunia may be due to vaginal dryness. New mothers could be alerted to this side-effect and given advice on the use of lubricants and oestrogen pessaries or creams if necessary, while being reassured about the benefits of breast feeding. In the absence of local pathology, if a psychosexual problem is suspected, referral to a psychosexual counsellor may be helpful (Thakar and Sultan 2007).

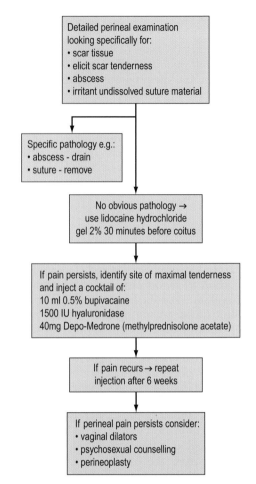

Figure 60.3 Suggested regime for management of perineal pain/dyspareunia.

Adapted from Thakar R and Sultan A (2007) Postpartum problems and the role of a perineal clinic. In: Sultan AH, Thakar R and Fenner D (eds) Perineal and anal sphicncter trauma. Springer-Verlag, London, with permission Springer Science+Business Media.

KEY POINTS

1. Sexual dysfunction is a highly prevalent condition in women attending urogynaecological services.
2. Only a minority of urogynaecologists screen all patients for FSD.
3. Lack of time, uncertainty about therapeutic options and older age of the patient have been cited as potential reasons for failing to address sexual complaints as part of routine history.
4. Evidence from large prospective studies has shown that prolapse and/or incontinence have an adverse effect on sexual function.
5. Current evidence of the effect of conservative and surgical management of pelvic floor disorders on sexual function is encouraging.
6. Referral to a psychotherapist should be considered when no organic cause is found, when the patient does not respond or is not satisfied with the primary intervention provided, or when the clinician feels that specialist intervention may offer the diagnosis and treatment that is most appropriate
7. While multiple tools are available for evaluation, assessment and therapy of FSD, a case-specific comprehensive and judicious approach works best.

References

American Psychiatric Association 1994 DSM-IV: Diagnostic and Statistical Manual of Mental Disorders, 4th edn. APA, Washington, DC.

Aslan G, Koseoglu H, Sadik O, Gimen S, Cihan A, Esen A 2005 Sexual function in women with urinary incontinence. International Journal of Impotence Research 17: 248–251.

Baessler K, Stanton SL 2004 Does Burch colposuspension cure coital incontinence? American Journal of Obstetrics and Gynecology 190: 1030–1033.

Barrett G, Pendry E, Peacock J, Victor C, Thakar R, Manyonda I 2000 Women's sexual health after childbirth. BJOG: an International Journal of Obstetrics and Gynaecology 107: 186–195.

Barrett G, Peacock J, Victor CR, Manyonda I 2005 Cesarean section and postnatal sexual health. Birth 32: 306–311.

Basson R 2001 Female sexual response: the role of drugs in the management of sexual dysfunction. Obstetrics and Gynecology 98: 350–353.

Basson R, Althof S, Davis S et al 2004 Summary of the recommendations on sexual dysfunctions in women. Journal of Sexual Medicine 1: 24–34.

Berman L, Berman J, Felder S et al 2003 Seeking help for sexual function complaints: what gynecologists need to know about the female patient's experience. Fertility and Sterility 79: 572–576.

Colombo M, Vitobello D, Proietti F, Milani R 2000 Randomised comparison of Burch colposuspension versus anterior colporrhaphy in women with stress urinary incontinence and anterior vaginal wall prolapse. BJOG: an International Journal of Obstetrics and Gynaecology 107: 544–551.

Cundiff GW, Weidner AC, Visco AG, Addison WA, Bump RC 1998 An anatomic and functional assessment of the discrete defect rectocele repair. American Journal of Obstetrics and Gynecology 179: 1451–1456.

Dwyer PL, O'Reilly BA 2004 Transvaginal repair of anterior and posterior compartment prolapse with atrium polypropylene mesh. BJOG: an International Journal of Obstetrics and Gynaecology 111: 831–836.

Ellerkmann RM, Cundiff GW, Melick CF, Nihira MA, Leffler K, Bent AE 2001 Correlation of symptoms with location and severity of pelvic organ prolapse. American Journal of Obstetrics and Gynecology 185: 1332–1337.

Elzevier HW, Putter H, Delaere KP, Venema PL, Nijeholt AA, Pelger RC 2008 Female sexual function after surgery for stress urinary incontinence: transobturator suburethral tape vs. tension-free vaginal tape obturator. Journal of Sexual Medicine 5: 400–406.

Ghezzi F, Serati M, Cromi A, Uccella S, Triacca P, Bolis P 2006 Impact of tension-free vaginal tape on sexual function: results of a prospective study. International Urogynecology Journal and Pelvic Floor Dysfunction 17: 54–59.

Glavind K, Tetsche MS 2004 Sexual function in women before and after suburethral sling operation for stress urinary incontinence: a retrospective questionnaire study. Acta Obstetricia et Gynecologica Scandinavica 83: 965–968.

Handa VL, Harvey L, Cundiff GW, Siddique SA, Kjerulff KH 2004 Sexual function among women with urinary incontinence and pelvic organ prolapse. American Journal of Obstetrics and Gynecology 191: 751–756.

Handa VL, Zyczynski HM, Brubaker L et al 2007 Sexual function before and after sacrocolpopexy for pelvic organ prolapse. American Journal of Obstetrics and Gynecology 197: 629.e1–e6.

Jelovsek JE, Barber MD 2006 Women seeking treatment for advanced pelvic organ prolapse have decreased body image and quality of life. American Journal of Obstetrics and Gynecology 194: 1455–1461.

Kahn MA, Stanton SL 1997 Posterior colporrhaphy: its effects on bowel and sexual function. BJOG: an International Journal of Obstetrics and Gynaecology 104: 82–86.

Kenton K, Shott S, Brubaker L 1999 Outcome after rectovaginal fascia reattachment for rectocele repair. American Journal of Obstetrics and Gynecology 181: 1360–1363.

Kingsberg S, Shifren J, Wekselman K, Rodenberg C, Koochaki P, DeRogatis L 2007 Evaluation of the clinical relevance of benefits associated with transdermal testosterone treatment in postmenopausal women with hypoactive sexual desire disorder. Journal of Sexual Medicine 4: 1001–1008.

Kingsberg S, Janata JW 2007 Female sexual disorders: assessment, diagnosis and treatment. Urologic Clinics of North America 34: 497–506.

Kuhn A, Bapst D, Stadlmayr W, Vits K, Mueller MD 2009 Sexual and organ function in patients with symptomatic prolapse: are pessaries helpful? Fertility and Sterility 91: 1914–1918.

Lethaby A, Ivanova V, Johnson NP 2006 Total versus subtotal hysterectomy for benign gynaecological conditions. Cochrane Database of Systematic Reviews 2: CD004993.

Maher CF, Qatawneh AM, Dwyer PL, Carey MP, Cornish A, Schluter PJ 2004 Abdominal sacral colpopexy or vaginal sacrospinous colpopexy for vaginal vault prolapse: a prospective randomized study. American Journal of Obstetrics and Gynecology 190: 20–26.

Mercer CH, Fenton KA, Johnson AM et al 2003 Sexual function problems and help seeking behaviour in Britain: national probability sample survey. BMJ (Clinical Research Ed.) 327: 426–427.

Milani R, Salvatore S, Soligo M, Pifarotti P, Meschia M, Cortese M 2005 Functional and anatomical outcome of anterior and posterior vaginal prolapse repair with prolene mesh. BJOG: an International Journal of Obstetrics and Gynaecology 112: 107–111.

Moran P, Dwyer PL, Ziccone SP 1999 Burch colposuspension for the treatment of coital urinary leakage secondary to genuine stress incontinence. Journal of Obstetrics and Gynaecology 19: 289–291.

Morof D, Barrett G, Peacock J, Victor CR, Manyonda I 2003 Postnatal depression and sexual health after childbirth. Obstetrics and Gynecology 102: 1318–1325.

Novi JM, Jeronis S, Morgan MA, Arya LA 2005 Sexual function in women with pelvic organ prolapse compared to women without pelvic organ prolapse. Journal of Urology 173: 1669–1672.

Novi JM, Bradley CS, Mahmoud NN, Morgan MA, Arya LA 2007 Sexual function in women after rectocele repair with acellular porcine dermis graft vs site-specific rectovaginal fascia repair. International Urogynecology Journal and Pelvic Floor Dysfunction 18: 1163–1169.

Ozel B, White T, Urwitz-Lane R, Minaglia S 2006 The impact of pelvic organ prolapse on sexual function in women with urinary incontinence. International Urogynecology Journal and Pelvic Floor Dysfunction 17: 14–17.

Pauls RN, Kleeman SD, Segal JL, Silva WA, Goldenhar LM, Karram MM 2005 Practice patterns of physician members of the American Urogynecologic Society regarding female sexual dysfunction: results of a national survey. International Urogynecology Journal and Pelvic Floor Dysfunction 16: 460–467.

Pauls RN, Segal JL, Silva WA, Kleeman SD, Karram MM 2006 Sexual function in patients presenting to a urogynecology practice. International Urogynecology Journal and Pelvic Floor Dysfunction 17: 576–580.

Porter WE, Steele A, Walsh P, Kohli N, Karram MM 1999 The anatomic and functional outcomes of defect-specific rectocele repairs. American Journal of Obstetrics and Gynecology 181: 1353–1358.

Rhodes JC, Kjerulff KH, Langenberg PW, Guzinski GM 1999 Hysterectomy and sexual functioning. Journal of the American Medical Association 282: 1934–1941.

Rogers GR, Villarreal A, Kammerer-Doak D, Qualls C 2001a Sexual function in women with and without urinary incontinence and/or pelvic organ prolapse. International Urogynecology Journal and Pelvic Floor Dysfunction 12: 361–365.

Rogers RG, Kammerer-Doak D, Villarreal A, Coates K, Qualls C 2001b A new instrument to measure sexual function in women with urinary incontinence or pelvic organ prolapse. American Journal of Obstetrics and Gynecology 184: 552–558.

Rogers RG, Coates KW, Kammerer-Doak D, Khalsa S, Qualls C 2003 A short form of the Pelvic Organ Prolapse/Urinary Incontinence Sexual Questionnaire (PISQ-12). International Urogynecology Journal and Pelvic Floor Dysfunction 14: 164–168.

Roos AM, Thakar R, Sultan AH, Scheer I 2009 Female sexual dysfunction: are urogynecologists ready for it? International Urogynecology Journal and Pelvic Floor Dysfunction 20: 89–101.

Roovers JP, van der Bom JG, van der Vaart CH, Heintz AP 2003 Hysterectomy and sexual wellbeing: prospective observational study of vaginal hysterectomy, subtotal abdominal hysterectomy, and total abdominal hysterectomy. BMJ (Clinical Research Ed.) 327: 774–778.

Salonia A, Zanni G, Nappi RE et al 2004 Sexual dysfunction is common in women with lower urinary tract symptoms and urinary incontinence: results of a cross-sectional study. European Urology 45: 642–648.

Sand PK, Goldberg RP, Dmochowski RR, McIlwain M, Dahl NV 2006 The impact of the overactive bladder syndrome on sexual function: a preliminary report from the Multicenter Assessment of Transdermal Therapy in Overactive Bladder with Oxybutynin trial. American Journal of Obstetrics and Gynecology 195: 1730–1735.

Sentilhes L, Berthier A, Caremel R, Loisel C, Marpeau L, Grise P 2008 Sexual function after transobturator tape procedure for stress urinary incontinence. Urology 71: 1074–1079.

Shah SM, Bukkapatnam R, Rodriguez LV 2005 Impact of vaginal surgery for stress urinary incontinence on female sexual function: is the use of polypropylene mesh detrimental? Urology 65: 270–274.

Sutherst JR 1979 Sexual dysfunctional and urinary incontinence. BJOG: an International Journal of Obstetrics and Gynaecology 86: 387–388.

Thakar R, Sultan A 2007 Postpartum problems and the role of a perineal clinic. In: Sultan AH, Thakar R, Fenner D (eds) Perineal and Anal Sphincter Trauma. Springer-Verlag, London, pp 65–79.

Thakar R, Ayers S, Srivastava R, Manyonda I 2008 Removing the cervix at hysterectomy: an unnecessary intervention? Obstetrics and Gynecology 112: 1262–1269.

van Brummen HJ, Bruinse HW, van de Pol G, Heintz AP, van der Vaart CH 2006 Which factors determine the sexual function 1 year after childbirth? BJOG: an International Journal of Obstetrics and Gynaecology 113: 914–918.

World Health Organization 1992 ICD-10: International Statistical Classification of Diseases and Related Health Problems. WHO, Geneva.

Zahariou AG, Karamouti MV, Papaioannou PD 2008 Pelvic floor muscle training improves sexual function of women with stress urinary incontinence. International Urogynecology Journal and Pelvic Floor Dysfunction 19: 401–406.

Chronic pelvic pain

William Stones

Chapter Contents

INTRODUCTION	929		CLINICAL ASSESSMENT	933
BIOLOGY OF PAIN	929		INVESTIGATIONS	934
EPIDEMIOLOGY OF PELVIC PAIN: POPULATIONS, CONSULTING AND REFERRAL PATTERNS	930		DIAGNOSIS AND TREATMENT: SPECIFIC CONDITIONS	934
PSYCHOLOGICAL FACTORS IN CHRONIC PELVIC PAIN	931		MANAGEMENT SETTINGS AND STRATEGIES	938
SOCIOCULTURAL FACTORS IN CHRONIC PELVIC PAIN	932		KEY POINTS	938

Introduction

Chronic pelvic pain is recognized as a difficult or unsatisfactory area of clinical practice by both patients and doctors. Women report problems in communicating the impact of their longstanding symptoms to their gynaecologist, and clinicians trained in a surgical model of care may feel frustrated at their inability to rapidly identify a causal pathological process and institute curative therapy. This chapter aims to draw together current knowledge on the condition. While it would be impossible to attempt comprehensive elucidation of all the related subject areas, the aim is to present an overview which at least acknowledges the key elements of an integrative biopsychosocial approach to understanding the pathophysiology and management of the condition.

Biology of Pain

Pain is defined by the International Association for the Study of Pain as 'an unpleasant sensory and emotional experience associated with actual or potential tissue damage, or described in terms of such damage' (IASP Task Force on Taxonomy 1994). The emphasis in this definition is that pain is an experience rather than a neurophysiological process, and is therefore subjective. There is no such thing as 'objective' pain. This does not mean, however, that pain cannot be studied or that reproducible experimental models cannot be devised. Neuroscience has advanced knowledge of the biological processes underlying pain. It is no longer appropriate to discuss the subject in terms of 'pain pathways', by analogy with a wiring diagram, or even to consider that the nervous system conveys perceptions such as touch or pain. Rather, the elements of the nervous system, comprising the 'different fibres, tracts, pathways and nuclei process and convey information about bodily stimulus

events' (Berkley and Hubscher 1995). In this model, pain is a central nervous system construct derived from the totality of sensory input rather than from the activation of a particular pathway. Even the anatomy of neural pathways in the adult cannot be considered immutable; plasticity of the central nervous system has been clearly demonstrated in reproducible animal experimental models, such that a nerve injury leads to sprouting of afferent fibres within the dorsal horn of the spinal cord (Woolf et al 1992).

Special features of chronic and visceral pain

The processes underlying the transition from a single or repeated acute painful episode to a chronic pain state are of great potential clinical significance. Patients often relate the onset of their chronic condition to an event such as an acute infection or surgical procedure. Moreover, visceral sensory mechanisms differ in certain respects from those found in cutaneous tissues. Key mechanisms potentially underlying the transition from acute to chronic visceral pain states are the activation of silent afferents in viscera (McMahon 1997) and central sensitization (Woolf 1983). There are certain similarities but also important differences in the context of visceral sensation between central sensitization and wind-up, where the response to repeated C-fibre stimulation is progressively augmented (Herrero et al 2000). It had been hoped that the development of central sensitization and/or wind-up could be modulated by analgesics or other agents using a therapeutic strategy of pre-emptive analgesia (Dickenson 1997), although clinical applications of this concept have been disappointing.

Vascular pain and pelvic congestion

By analogy with the pathogenesis of cerebral migraine, it has been suggested that pain associated with pelvic congestion

DOI: 10.1016/B978-0-7020-3120-5.00061-8

might arise through vascular perturbation at the ovarian or uterine arteriolar level, resulting in the release of endothelial factors such as ATP which act by exciting sensory nerves in the outer muscle coat of venules and veins, and which also cause vasodilatation through the release of nitric oxide (Stones 2000).

Sex differences in pain

There is a marked sex difference in the prevalence of a number of chronic painful conditions unrelated to the reproductive tract in the general population, such as irritable bowel syndrome (IBS), temporomandibular dysfunction and interstitial cystitis, which has prompted research on the potential underlying mechanisms using animal models such as bladder irritation (Bon et al 1997), and uterine and vaginal distension (Bradshaw et al 1999). Illustrating the complexity of the central mechanisms underlying nociception, vaginal hyperalgesia resulting from induced endometriosis in rats was exacerbated in the presence of increased oestradiol levels, whereas in ovariectomized animals, hyperalgesia was relieved by oestradiol (Berkley et al 2007).

Studies of human volunteers have investigated pain thresholds in women at different stages of the menstrual cycle using electrical stimulation, pressure dolorimetry on the skin, thermal stimulation and induced ischaemic pain. Patterns of variation in response seen in studies using these modalities were different, and a meta-analytical review of pain perception across the menstrual cycle (Riley et al 1999) estimated the effect size for menstrual cycle fluctuation of pain sensitivity between the most and least sensitive phase to be 0.40. The effect size for sex difference was approximately 0.55, indicating that hormone variability could account for a substantial proportion but not all of the observed differences.

Illustrating some of the possible underlying mechanisms, a study of the discrimination of thermal pain in male and female volunteers showed that women had a lower pain threshold and tolerance, as also noted in a number of other studies (Fillingim et al 1998). A further complexity to be considered when interpreting studies of human volunteers is that subjects may well have prior pain experience which could influence responses to experimental pain (Fillingim et al 1999). Finally, the potential influence on pain perception of exogenous hormone therapy needs to be considered. In 87 postmenopausal women consulting for chronic orofacial pain, hormone replacement therapy (HRT) was associated with greater reported levels of pain, with substantial effect sizes between 0.39 and 0.62 (Wise et al 2000). The possibility of increased pain as a result of HRT use has not been addressed prospectively but may be clinically important, especially in women with vulval pain where oestrogen deficiency changes are thought to coexist.

Genetic variation in susceptibility to pain

There is now evidence for a genetic basis for the variation in response to pain seen in human experimental studies. Shabalina et al (2009) studied polymorphisms of the 'mu' opioid receptor OPRM1 gene locus, and reported a strong association between the single nucleotide polymorphism rs563649 and individual variations in pain perception.

There are also relevant observations from clinical populations with gynaecological pain; for example, a twin study showed that while 39% of the variance in reported menstrual flow was accounted for by genetic factors, the corresponding figure for dysmenorrhoea was 55% and for functional limitation from menstrual symptoms was 77% (Treloar et al 1998).

Epidemiology of Pelvic Pain: Populations, Consulting and Referral Patterns

The first assessment of the prevalence and economic burden associated with chronic pelvic pain was based on extrapolation from hospital practice in the UK, and estimated the prevalence in women at 24.4 per 1000. The annual direct treatment cost was estimated at £158 million, with indirect costs of £24 million (Davies et al 1992). The above prevalence now appears an underestimate since data from population-based studies have become available. A telephone survey was undertaken in the USA using a robust sampling methodology (Mathias et al 1996). Women aged 18–50 years were interviewed about pelvic-pain-related symptoms. In total, 17,927 households were contacted, 5325 women agreed to participate and 925 reported pelvic pain of at least 6 months' duration, including pain within the past 3 months. Following exclusion of pregnant and postmenopausal women and those with pain that was solely cycle related, 773/5263 (14.7%) were identified as suffering from chronic pelvic pain. Direct costs of health care, estimated from Medicare tariffs and hence very conservative, were $881.5 million, patients' out-of-pocket expenses were estimated at $1.9 billion and indirect costs due to time off work were estimated at $555.3 million.

In the UK, the population perspective was provided by a postal survey of 2016 women selected at random from the Oxfordshire Health Authority register of 141,400 women aged 18–49 years (Zondervan et al 2001b). Chronic pelvic pain was defined as recurrent pain of at least 6 months' duration, unrelated to periods, intercourse or pregnancy. For the survey, a 'case' was defined as a women with chronic pelvic pain in the previous 3 months, and on this basis the prevalence was 483/2016 (24.0%). Among those with pelvic pain, dysmenorrhoea was reported by 81% of those who had periods, and dyspareunia was reported by 41% of those who were sexually active. Among women who did not have chronic pelvic pain as defined above, dysmenorrhoea was reported by 58% of those who had periods, and dyspareunia was reported by 14% of those who were sexually active.

An estimate of the consulting pattern associated with pelvic pain was obtained using a national database study of UK general practices (Zondervan et al 1999b). Data relating to 284,162 women aged 12–70 years who had a general practice contact in 1991 were analysed to identify subsequent contacts over the following 5 years. The monthly prevalence rate was 21.5/1000 and the monthly incidence rate was 1.58/1000. These prevalence rates are comparable with those for migraine, back pain and asthma in primary care. Older women had higher monthly prevalence rates; for example, the rate was 18.2/1000 in women aged 15–20 years and 27.6/1000 in women over 60 years of age. This association is thought to be due to persistence of symptoms

In older women, with the median duration of symptoms being 13.7 months in 13–20 year olds and 20.2 months in women over 60 years of age (Zondervan et al 1999a). It is clear that future population-based studies need to include older women.

Among 483 women with chronic pelvic pain participating in the Oxfordshire population study discussed above, 195 (40.4%) had not sought a medical consultation, 127 (26.3%) reported a past consultation and 139 (28.8%) reported a recent consultation for pain (Zondervan et al 2001b). Of those women identified as cases of pelvic pain in the national general practice database, 28% were not given a specific diagnosis and 60% were not referred to hospital (Zondervan et al 1999a). The US population-based study discussed above also drew attention to the large numbers of women who have troublesome symptoms but do not seek medical attention: 75% of this sample had not seen a healthcare provider in the previous 3 months. It might be thought that not seeking care would be an indicator of milder symptoms; indeed, in the US study, those who did seek medical attention had higher pain and lower general health scores than those who did not seek medical attention. However, among those not seeking help, scores for pain and functional impairment were still substantial. Lack of use of medical services might reflect sociocultural factors, but could equally reflect previous unsatisfactory experiences of investigation and treatment, as discussed later in this chapter.

Among women referred to a UK gynaecology outpatient clinic with chronic pelvic pain of at least 6 months' duration, the impact of the condition on quality of life was assessed using the Short Form-36 (SF-36) questionnaire (Stones et al 2000). Figure 61.1 shows a comparison of physical and mental component summary scores derived from the eight SF-36 subscales (Jenkinson et al 1996a) in this hospital population with the data from the Oxfordshire population study described above. These summary scores are adjusted such that 50 represents a normal population mean. It will be noted that, as might be expected, the hospital sample is consistent with the trend, evident in those who have previously or recently sought medical advice compared with those who have not, to greater impairment of function on both physical and mental components.

Psychological Factors in Chronic Pelvic Pain

Many writers on pelvic pain have attempted to characterize an adverse psychological profile which might help the clinician to distinguish between 'organic' and 'psychogenic' pain; a distinction not in keeping with current neurophysiological understanding as discussed above. It is likely that some of the psychological disturbance that can be identified in women with chronic pelvic pain is the result of longstanding pain symptoms and unsatisfactory treatment, rather than the cause of pain (Slocumb et al 1989). Pain may contribute to or confirm a sense of helplessness or a tendency to engage in catastrophic thoughts, and may itself be exacerbated by them (Horn and Munafo 1997). On the other hand, it is clear that concomitant mood disturbance or specific psychopathology may impair the patient's ability to cope with her symptoms and contribute to functional impairment, and recognition is important but often neglected in the hurried

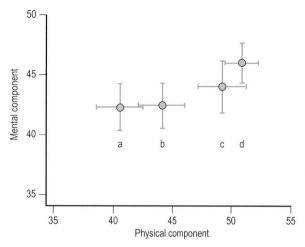

Figure 61.1 Means ± 95% confidence interval for the Short Form-36 mental component and physical component summary scales. Women with pelvic pain (a) seen in a general gynaecology clinic (Stones et al 2000), or in a postal survey (Zondervan et al 2001b) reporting (b) a recent consultation, (c) a previous consultation or (d) no medical consultation. Arbitrary units such that 50 represents the mean of a normal population. *From Stones RW, Selfe SA, Fransman S, Horn SA (2000) Psychosocial and economic impact of chronic pelvic pain. Baillière's Clinical Obstetrics and Gynaecology 14:27–43 and From Zondervan KT, Yudkin PL, Vessey MP et al (2001b) The community prevalence of chronic pelvic pain in women and associated illness behaviour. British Journal of General Practice 51(468):541–547.*

setting of a gynaecology clinic (Yonkers and Chantilis 1995). The presence of adverse psychological propensities such as catastrophizing is a factor affecting outcome of treatment for chronic pelvic pain (Weijenborg et al 2008).

Depression

Women presenting with multiple pain symptoms are at especially high risk for current mood disturbance; the likelihood of an associated mood disorder was increased six-fold in individuals with two pain complaints and eight-fold in those with three complaints (Dworkin et al 1990). In keeping with the irrelevance of the organic/psychogenic distinction for diagnosis, the absence of laparoscopically visible pathology was not associated with a higher probability of depression (Peveler et al 1995, Waller and Shaw 1995). In these studies, no differences in mood-related symptoms were identified in women with chronic pelvic pain with or without endometriosis. Antidepressant therapy may be indicated in order to alleviate depression, but sertraline was not effective for pelvic pain in a recent small but well-conducted randomized trial (Engel et al 1998).

Abuse and somatization

Child sexual or physical abuse may be an antecedent for chronic pelvic pain, but many individuals have suffered such abuse without this or other consequences in later life, and the research literature is beset with the problem of appropriate comparison groups. A study from a tertiary referral multidisciplinary clinic setting reported on the full assessment of psychological factors in three groups of 30 women with chronic pelvic pain, chronic pain of other types, or without pain identified from general practitioner records. Twelve (40%) of those with chronic pelvic pain reported sexual abuse, compared with five (17%) in each of the two comparison groups. Experience of physical violence was similar in the three groups, but women with chronic pelvic pain had higher scores for somatization, meaning the experience and communication of distress and physical symptoms without clear underlying pathology. In women with pelvic pain, abuse histories were evenly distributed among those with and without identified pelvic pathology such as endometriosis, but somatization scores were higher among those with identified pathology (Collett et al 1998). It has been suggested that the potential link between sexual abuse and pelvic pain might be that abuse is an observable marker for childhood neglect in general (Fry et al 1997), and this might explain the association in some studies with physical rather than sexual abuse (Rapkin et al 1990). With regard to mediators between abuse and pain experience, those who reported abuse were more likely to be distressed and anxious (Poleshuck et al 2005).

Identification of patients with features suggesting somatization disorder is important as failure to do so will lead to further inappropriate investigation, and treatment directed towards physical symptoms which are, in fact, manifestations of psychological distress. There are limited data regarding the prevalence of frank somatization disorder in clinic populations; in a study comparing the medical assessment with a standardized questionnaire, doctors identified 19% of patients as being potential somatizers, and approximately 5% met questionnaire criteria for overt somatization disorder (Peveler et al 1997). With regard to patients within the pelvic pain spectrum of conditions, the finding of Zolnoun et al (2008) of higher scores for somatization among patients with primary vulval vestibulitis compared with those with secondary vulval vestibulitis indicates a need for more detailed characterization of this propensity among the different clinical subpopulations.

Sociocultural Factors in Chronic Pelvic Pain

It could be argued that in life-threatening medical conditions or conditions where a technical solution gives excellent results, the patient's experience of care and the quality of doctor–patient communication are not critical to the outcome. In contrast, in ill-defined, chronic conditions where a technical solution is unlikely to provide relief, sociocultural factors have a major influence on the patient's decision to seek care and the referral pathway subsequently followed. The population-based studies cited above provide an indication of the size of the iceberg of symptoms below the waterline of care seeking. Similarly, in general practice, many women remain undiagnosed and unreferred. This is not necessarily inappropriate but the determinants of presentation and referral are unlikely to be disease factors alone. Once seen in a gynaecology clinic, the interaction between disease states and the consultation setting can be identified in statistical models; the presence of endometriosis was a factor predicting continuing pain 6 months after an initial hospital outpatient consultation, but so also were the patient's initial report of pain interfering with exercise, her rating of the initial medical consultation

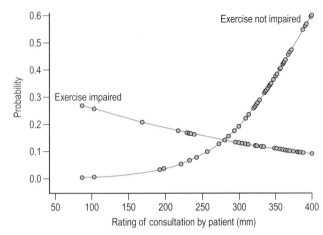

Figure 61.2 Fitted probabilities of complete pain resolution with and without exercise impairment in relation to the patient's rating of the initial hospital consultation. In women without exercise impairment, a favourable rating of the initial consultation is associated with a higher probability of pain resolution, but the consultation has no effect in those with impairment. *From Selfe SA, Matthews Z, Stones RW (1998) Factors influencing outcome in consultations for chronic pelvic pain. Journal of Women's Health 7:1041–1048.*

as less satisfactory (Figure 61.2) and the individual clinician undertaking the consultation (but not the doctor's grade or gender) (Selfe et al 1998a). The ability to establish a therapeutic rapport and meet the patient's expectations during consultations, rather than simply convey information, may be factors that favour a good outcome (Stones et al 2006).

These statistical observations are consistent with women's descriptions of their experiences during the referral and treatment process. Sometimes, news of the absence of specific pathology at laparoscopy is received not as reassurance but as a dismissal. The patient's loss of confidence is expressed in these words obtained during focus group interviews:

> Well — I suppose they must have done their job but they said to me that I probably had endometriosis and I felt all my symptoms related to that and that's what it was going to be — it seems strange that they don't actually find anything but obviously they're looking and they know what they can see …

Often, problems are encountered not just with a particular individual clinician or aspect of care, but tend to accumulate for some patients as they move through the system. This seems to be more of a problem for women of low socioeconomic status (Grace 1995). A solution to this mismatch between women's needs and the structures through which care is provided may be the multidisciplinary approach which at least works against the crude compartmentalized organic/psychological causation model, although it has been suggested that a more fundamental reconsideration of the medical paradigm is required (Grace 1998). Meanwhile, within the practical constraints of time, lack of continuity of care in the hospital setting and very limited access to multidisciplinary resources, gynaecologists can at least recognize the potential impact of their own attitudes and communication styles (Selfe et al 1998b).

Clinical Assessment

The conventional gynaecological history needs to be supplemented by additional information in consultations for chronic pelvic pain to aid understanding of the impact of symptoms and diagnosis.

Pain history

The history needs to include the onset and duration of symptoms, the location and radiation of pain, factors associated with exacerbation and relief, and the relationship of pain to the menstrual cycle. Dysmenorrhoea may be a separate or related symptom. Dyspareunia may include pain during intercourse but, for many women, a particularly unpleasant symptom is postcoital pain; specific enquiry should be made about this.

A number of validated pain assessment measures are available for use in research and clinical practice, the most convenient of which are the 10 cm visual analogue scale, the Brief Pain Inventory (BPI) and the McGill Short Form pain questionnaire. The McGill questionnaire is included in the International Pelvic Pain Society's assessment form, available for downloading at www.pelvicpain.org; the BPI may be downloaded at mdanderson.org/departments/PRG/. Patients' recall of pain symptoms over the previous month seems to be adequate, and it is probably unnecessary to ask for a daily pain diary: 10 cm visual analogue scales for 'usual' and 'most severe' intensity of pain recalled over the past 4 weeks correlated very well with mean and maximal diary records (Figure 61.3) (Stones et al 2001).

Impact on quality of life

At present, a validated illness-specific instrument is not available for assessing quality of life and functional impairment

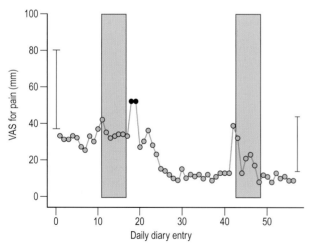

Figure 61.3 Visual analogue pain scores (circles) from a daily pain diary completed over 8 weeks by a patient undergoing treatment as part of a clinical trial. Vertical bars show the recalled 'usual' (lower end of bars) and 'most severe' (upper end of bars) pain scores from the previous 4 weeks. Shaded columns areas show days of menstruation and filled circles indicate days when intercourse occurred. VAS, visual analogue scale.
Source: Stones RW, Bradbury L, Anderson D 2001 Randomized placebo controlled trial of lofexidine hydrochloride for chronic pelvic pain in women. Human Reproduction 16: 1719–1721.

in women with pelvic pain. Simple questions about the effect of the pain on work, leisure, sleep and sexual relationships are nevertheless useful. A generic quality of life measure such as the SF-36 may be used for monitoring outcomes. The SF-36 is somewhat problematic when used in episodic conditions such as menorrhagia (Jenkinson et al 1996b), but has face validity and reliability in chronic pelvic pain (Stones et al 2000).

Sexual and physical abuse

The extent to which clinicians can or should attempt to elicit a history of sexual or physical abuse during a gynaecological consultation is a matter for judgement in relation to the setting, in particular the follow-up and support that are available to women following such disclosure. The history may be volunteered unprompted by the patient, particularly during a subsequent consultation when rapport has been established. Some women may even find it easier to raise the subject with an unfamiliar specialist than with a general practitioner with whom they have regular consultations for other matters. It may be useful to incorporate questions on abuse into a self-completion questionnaire, such as that provided by the International Pelvic Pain Society, or in a multidisciplinary clinic to address the topic during a consultation with the nurse or psychologist (see Chapter 65 for more information).

Systems review

The history should be thorough with regards to symptoms potentially indicative of IBS; the poor outcome of patients with IBS referred to gynaecology clinics has been emphasized (Prior and Whorwell 1989). It is unlikely that dyspareunia can be attributed to IBS; bowel spasm perhaps accounts for the experience of those patients who describe an interval between the end of intercourse and the onset of acute pain (Whorwell 1995) associated with the urge to defaecate and abdominal distension. Pain associated with micturition or a full bladder should be enquired about, as there may be some overlap between chronic pelvic pain and the interstitial cystitis spectrum discussed in Chapter 56.

Physical examination

Observing the patient as she walks may give an indication of a musculoskeletal problem, and examination of the back is relevant in those giving a history of pain radiating or originating in this area. Abdominal examination may reveal specific sites of tenderness. One-finger 'trigger point' tenderness will suggest a nerve entrapment, often involving the ilioinguinal or iliohypogastric nerves. These can develop spontaneously as well as following surgery. The diagnosis is confirmed after obtaining appropriate consent by infiltration of local anaesthetic into the tender area. 'Ovarian point' tenderness has been described as a feature of pelvic congestion syndrome (Beard et al 1988), but this sign is problematic in patients with IBS who often have similar abdominal tenderness. A general neurological examination is appropriate to exclude a systemic neuropathy or demyelination; if abnormalities are present, a neurology opinion should be sought.

Vaginal examination should commence with a careful inspection of the vulva and introitus, paying particular attention to the presence of erythema which might suggest primary vulval vestibulitis (Gibbons 1998) (see Chapter 40). More frequently, no erythema is evident but a gentle touch with a cotton-tipped swab in the area just external to the hymeneal ring elicits intense sharp pain, even in patients who do not complain of dyspareunia. This allodynia in the absence of visible erythema probably represents referred sensation from painful areas higher in the pelvis, but represents the primary problem for some women. Vulval varices may indicate incompetence of valves in the pelvic venous circulation; this subgroup of patients may benefit from radiological assessment and treatment (see below).

A gentle one-finger digital examination commences with palpation of the pelvic floor muscles. Focal tenderness may be present, indicating a primary musculoskeletal problem that should prompt referral to a pelvic floor physiotherapist for further assessment. As with 'vestibulitis', pelvic muscle tenderness may be a residual secondary response to pain from other parts of the pelvis; for example, a previous episode of pelvic infection. Further digital examination may reveal nodularity in the pouch of Douglas or restricted uterine mobility suggestive of endometriosis. Adenomyosis may be suggested by a bulky tender uterus. Uterine retroversion should be noted, although its relevance to dyspareunia is debatable. Adnexal rather than uterine tenderness may point to pelvic congestion syndrome. In the UK clinic setting, pelvic tenderness is unlikely to indicate chronic pelvic inflammatory disease (PID), although this diagnosis will be more likely among populations where early and appropriate antibiotic treatment for acute pelvic sepsis is less readily given.

Investigations

It is helpful to discount active pelvic infection, especially the presence of chlamydia, early in the assessment by taking endocervical swabs. Ultrasound examination may be useful in identifying uterine or adnexal pathology. The presence of dilated veins may indicate pelvic congestion (Stones et al 1990), but a recent study using power Doppler suggested that the primary value of sonography was to identify the characteristic multicystic ovarian morphology seen in this condition (Halligan et al 2000). Transuterine venography is of limited value in routine clinical practice, but is technically simpler than selective catheterization of the ovarian vein. Magnetic resonance imaging provides the opportunity to identify adenomyosis but is not indicated routinely.

Laparoscopy is commonly undertaken as the primary investigation for chronic pelvic pain in many countries. The aim of laparoscopy is to aid diagnosis but also, increasingly, to provide 'one-stop' treatment for endometriosis and adhesions where these are identified. This approach is cost-effective for endometriosis treatment, as the expense of a second procedure or hormonal treatment is obviated (Stones and Thomas 1995). However, given the potential for confusion arising from a 'negative' laparoscopy (Howard 1996) and the lack of a clear impact of recourse to laparoscopy on outcome at the referral population level (Peters et al 1991, Selfe et al 1998b), arguments in favour of deferring laparos-

copy, at least until initial symptomatic treatment has failed, take on some force. The impetus for treatment using gonadotrophin-releasing hormone (GnRH) agonists without laparoscopic diagnosis has emanated from the US-managed care environment (Winkel 1999), and from retrospective assessment of outcomes in the UK (Lyall et al 1999). For clinical practice, the timing of laparoscopy is a matter for discussion with the patient based on her needs for diagnosis and treatment, and the overall context of treatment modalities available.

Pain mapping by laparoscopy under conscious sedation can be a useful procedure, particularly where the site of pain is unilateral, allowing comparison with a 'control' area to assess the significance of adhesions, to identify unrecognized occult inguinal or femoral hernias, and in the negative sense to identify individuals with a generalized hyperalgesic chronic pain state for whom further surgical intervention would be hazardous. The choice of instrumentation represents a trade-off between the lower quality field of view available from a 2 mm laparoscope and patient discomfort associated with a larger trocar and cannula. In practice, a 5 mm laparoscope does not cause significantly more pain than the smaller instruments. Following early reports of experience (Howard 1999), there are indications that clinical outcomes can be improved for some patients where conventional approaches have not proved successful and the laparoscopic findings have been unclear (Swanton et al 2006).

Diagnosis and Treatment: Specific Conditions

There is limited evidence from randomized clinical trials on which to base treatment decisions for women with chronic pelvic pain (Stones et al 2005). An approach to specific conditions is outlined below.

Pelvic congestion syndrome

This condition may be considered a clinical syndrome based on the characteristic symptom complex described by Beard et al (1988). Pelvic congestion is typically a condition of the reproductive years and, in contrast to endometriosis, is equally prevalent among parous and nulliparous women. There may be an underlying endocrine dysfunction, although peripheral hormone levels are not abnormal. The associated ovarian morphology is characterized by predominantly atretic follicles scattered throughout the stroma, while in contrast to polycystic ovary syndrome, the volume of the ovary is normal. The thecal androstenedione response to luteinizing hormone was increased as in polycystic ovaries, but granulosa cell oestradiol production was reduced compared with normal tissue (Gilling-Smith et al 2000).

Symptoms include exacerbation of pain with prolonged standing, dyspareunia, postcoital aching and a fluctuating localization of pain. Patients may derive reassurance from being given the diagnosis as an explanation of their pain in terms of a functional condition similar to cerebral migraine. Therapy includes identification of stressors and the use of hormonal treatment in combination with stress and pain management, with the aim of encouraging the patient to make appropriate lifestyle changes so that her symptoms are less likely to recur on completion of a course of hormonal treatment. Medroxyprogesterone acetate 50 mg daily has been shown to be effective (Farquhar et al 1989), and GnRH agonists with oestrogen 'add-back' are increasingly used in this indication although randomized trial data are lacking to date. Hysterectomy and bilateral salpingo-oophorectomy followed by long-term oestrogen replacement therapy is an option for those who have extreme symptoms partially or temporarily relieved by hormonal therapy, but this is naturally a treatment of last resort (Beard et al 1991).

Patients with peripheral venous disease and vulval varicosities are probably manifesting a different clinical entity from those described above. A surgical approach involving extraperitoneal dissection of the ovarian veins has been described (Hobbs 1976), and this group of patients may benefit from current interventional radiology techniques for vein occlusion (Figure 61.4). However, the evidence for useful benefit in those without vulval or lower limb varices is restricted to series where definition of the case mix is not always clear.

Endometriosis

Endometriosis is discussed in detail in Chapter 33. From the perspective of clinical practice in chronic pelvic pain, endometriosis presents special problems at both ends of the spectrum of disease severity. Women with endometriosis have poor outcomes compared with those with other conditions in terms of pain relief (Selfe et al 1998a), and they require careful attention to the provision of effective pain relief. Many women have undergone laparoscopy with the expectation of endometriosis being confirmed, and have difficulty coming to terms with the lack of a positive diagnosis when endometriosis is not found, as illustrated in the extract from a patient's comments presented above.

Treatments which suppress or ablate endometriosis are, in general, associated with relief of pain. In the case of hormonal therapies, a major benefit is the suppression of menstruation, resulting in the prevention of dysmenorrhoea. Laparoscopic surgical ablation of deposits in stage I–III disease is associated with reduction in pain, as demonstrated in the single available randomized trial (Sutton et al 1994), and laparoscopic surgery for endometriosis also improves pain symptoms, quality of life and sexual function (Abbott et al 2004). There are insufficient data to make clear recommendations about the different available surgical approaches (e.g. laser vaporization vs excision and diathermy) with respect to pain outcomes.

The place of laparoscopic uterine nerve ablation, as opposed to ablation of visible deposits, remains unclear. More positive results have been reported for presacral neurectomy in primary dysmenorrhoea (Chen et al 1996, Nezhat et al 1998), which perhaps reflects the greater potential for interrupting sensory pathways to the uterus offered by this procedure. There is significant surgical risk associated with presacral neurectomy, and an incidence of complications, especially constipation, and the importance of high-level surgical skills has been emphasized (Perry and Perez 1993). In the light of the discussion of pain mechanisms earlier in this chapter, efforts to achieve pain relief by interruption of nerve pathways are probably naïve as they do not take into account the central nervous system contribution to the maintenance of chronic pain states following an initial inflammatory insult, of which endometriosis represents a good example.

Adhesions

Critical studies of the relationship between adhesions and pain suggest that they are often likely to be coincidental rather than causal (Rapkin 1986). Adhesiolysis by laparotomy was only effective for adhesions that were dense, vascularized or adherent to bowel (Peters et al 1992). Taking these findings together with those of Swank et al (2003) where laparoscopic treatment was employed, there is little evidence to support this approach (Stones et al 2005). As discussed above, pain mapping by laparoscopy under conscious sedation may be useful in identifying adhesions that are tender rather than asymptomatic, with due regard to the complexities of visceral sensory pathways previously reviewed and the sensitivity and discrimination of sensations from the pelvic organs under normal conditions (Koninckx and Renaer 1997). Laparoscopic adhesiolysis needs to be undertaken with particular care so as to avoid bowel injury, and with appropriate preoperative counselling and bowel preparation.

Chronic pelvic inflammatory disease

In UK clinical practice, chronic PID should be a laparoscopic diagnosis based on the finding of tubal damage and signs of active infection. The true prevalence will vary depending on the referral population, but a diagnosis based on a clinical impression of pelvic tenderness and partial response to repeated courses of antibiotics is likely to be incorrect. This observation is also relevant for regions with a higher background prevalence of PID such as sub-Saharan Africa (Kasule 1991). Apart from not resolving her problem, incorrect labelling of a patient as suffering from chronic PID may lead the patient to adopt an extremely negative self-image, and inflict on her inappropriate anxiety about future fertility.

Where the diagnosis is confirmed, surgery in the form of salpingectomy or salpingo-oophorectomy may well be indicated rather than conservative management. Efforts to prevent continuing pain from ovarian adhesions have included ovariopexy and the use of barrier films, but evidence in the literature of actual pain relief is scanty.

Nerve entrapment

The finding of abdominal wall tenderness which is consistently localized to a particular point should lead to consideration of a nerve entrapment. This predominantly involves the ilioinguinal and iliohypogastric nerves, the anatomy of which is illustrated in Figure 61.5, but genitofemoral nerve entrapment has also been described. A typical protocol for management includes establishing the diagnosis by infiltration of bupivacaine 0.25%, and demonstrating complete relief of pain and tenderness. This can be followed by one or two injections 1 month apart of bupivacaine and a long-acting corticosteroid such as Depo Medrone 40 mg. Surgical exploration and excision of the nerve can be undertaken with approximately 70% success (Hahn 1989, Lee and Dellon 2000). The response to an initial infiltration of bupivacaine is often much more prolonged than would be

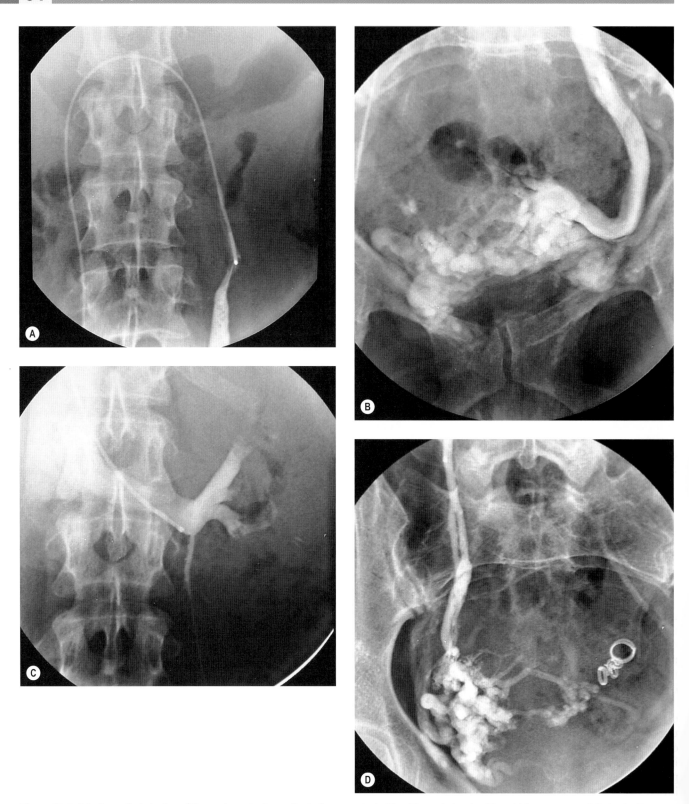

Figure 61.4 Selective catheterization of the ovarian veins in a patient who presented with aching vulval varicosities which were successfully treated by embolization. (A) Transfemoral approach to the proximal left ovarian vein. (B) Distal left ovarian vein. Note dilatation and extensive communications to the uterine veins despite previous left oophorectomy. (C) Transjugular approach 2 months post embolization. Note occluded left ovarian vein. (D) Right ovarian vein showing residual collaterals. Note embolization coils visible on the patient's left.

Images courtesy of Dr Nigel Hacking, Southampton General Hospital.

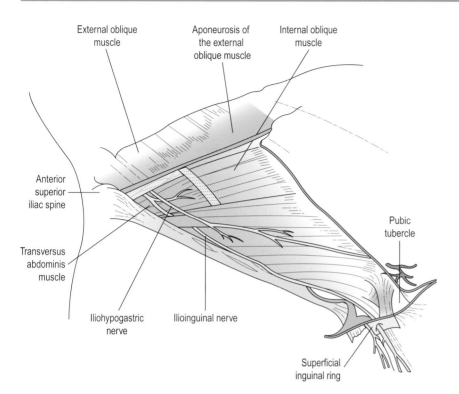

External oblique muscle

Aponeurosis of the external oblique muscle

Internal oblique muscle

Anterior superior iliac spine

Transversus abdominis muscle

Iliohypogastric nerve

Ilioinguinal nerve

Pubic tubercle

Superficial inguinal ring

Figure 61.5 Abdominal wall anatomy illustrating the course of the ilioinguinal and iliohypogastric nerves.
Source: von Bahr V 1979 Local anaesthesia for inguinal herniorrhaphy. In: Eriksson E (ed) Illustrated Handbook in Local Anaesthesia, 2nd edn. Lloyd-Luke, London, pp 52–54.

expected from the duration of action of the local anaesthetic, perhaps because minor perineural adhesions are broken down by the volume of the infiltration, or surrounding muscle spasm is relieved.

Neuropathic and postsurgical pelvic pain

Whereas abdominal nerve-related pain can often be clearly localized to a particular site, posthysterectomy pain at the vaginal vault and vaginal pain following childbirth may be more difficult to evaluate. It is likely that the nerves involved are small unmyelinated fibres travelling in the nervi erigentes to the sacral segments and branches of the pudendal nerve. While nerve latency studies may be of value in assessing injury to the pudendal nerve, local anaesthetic nerve blockade is singularly unsuccessful. There may be the potential for surgery to decompress Alcock's canal where this is identified as the specific area of nerve compression, but case definition remains controversial.

In posthysterectomy pain, pain mapping may be useful to delineate the extent of tenderness at the vaginal vault, but this is usually with a view to aiding acceptance of a multidisciplinary pain management approach to treatment including drugs such as gabapentin and cognitive–behavioural psychology (see below) rather than with an expectation of identifying a focal lesion amenable to surgery. Patients with more extensive neuropathy should be referred for a neurology opinion.

A special instance of postsurgical pain where further surgery is indicated is ovarian remnant syndrome, where a fragment of active ovarian tissue generates pain through continued ovulatory activity. The diagnosis can be made by withdrawing oestrogen replacement therapy and demonstrating endogeneous hormone production, and the lesion can be localized by the administration of clomiphene or human menopausal gonadotropin prior to imaging. The surgery is technically challenging and is best approached by laparotomy rather than laparoscopy (Richlin and Rock 2001).

Hernias

Occult inguinal hernias have been recognized in women presenting with pain but without the normal swelling or cough impulse (Herrington 1975), but surgeons have naturally been reluctant to operate in the absence of more definite physical signs. Current surgical thinking on inguinal and femoral hernias, and rarities such as spigelian and obturator hernias, is reviewed by Daoud (1998). Inguinal and femoral hernias can readily be evaluated during pain mapping laparoscopy, as the anatomy can be easily visualized, localized tenderness can be detected, and laparoscopic repair can subsequently be undertaken.

Diagnostic overlap and 'no diagnosis'

Despite the best efforts of clinicians to identify specific causes of pelvic pain, it will be unclear how to classify many patients. In a consecutive series of 98 patients referred for investigation by their general practitioner, diagnoses were endometriosis ($n = 12$), adhesions ($n = 10$) and other gross pathology ($n = 15$). No positive diagnosis could be established in 29 patients. Three or more IBS symptoms were present in 15 patients, but there was overlap with other diagnoses in 13 of these patients. A symptom complex suggestive of pelvic congestion syndrome was present in 57 patients, but this overlapped with seven cases of endometriosis, six cases of adhesions, eight cases of gross pathology and nine cases of IBS (Selfe et al 1998b). Similar findings of no positive diagnosis and diagnostic overlap were noted in women consulting in primary care (Zondervan et al 1999a), and self-reports of symptoms and received diagnoses in a population survey (Zondervan et al 2001a).

Management Settings and Strategies

The general approach to treatment of chronic pelvic pain needs to reflect the patient population and meet the different needs of individual women. Diagnostic and treatment plans need to be able to accommodate the spectrum of chronicity and severity of symptoms; it would probably be inappropriate to enrol every patient referred from general practice into a comprehensive multidisciplinary pain management programme, but it would be equally inappropriate to subject a patient who has undergone multiple previous investigations and treatments for longstanding disabling pain to a brief clinical encounter with an inconclusive outcome. If data from a UK hospital outpatient population can be regarded as typical, approximately 25% of women referred by general practitioners still had significant pain 6 months after an initial consultation; this may represent the scale of unmet need for a multidisciplinary service.

An important step in formulating a management plan for any patient is to establish her treatment goals, especially whether she is primarily concerned with identifying a cause for her pain or is less concerned with causation but desires rapid symptomatic relief. In the former instance, further investigation such as laparoscopy may help the patient towards her goal, whereas in the latter case, initial symptomatic treatment may be more appropriate. Further clarification may be required regarding the relative priority that the patient gives to pain relief and restoration of normal function. The impact of a well-conducted and sympathetic consultation may itself be therapeutic based on some of the research discussed above; indeed, ultrasonography has been used effectively as a means of providing reassurance (Ghaly 1994).

For patients at the more severe end of the illness spectrum, the elements of a pain management approach become more important; randomized trial evidence supports multidisciplinary care (Peters et al 1991). Multidisciplinary care may include contributions from other disciplines including anaesthesia, psychology, physiotherapy, nursing and liaison psychiatry. The analgesic regimen is optimized, bearing in mind that 6–10% of the Caucasian population are unable to metabolize codeine (Eckhardt et al 1998), and full use is made of adjunctive agents such as amitriptyline 10–50 mg at night or gabapentin in an incremental regimen from 400 to 3600 mg daily. The latter agent is indicated for neuropathic pain and does not interact with the oral contraceptive

pill, but has adverse effects of giddiness and drowsiness. Randomized trials have shown gabapentin to be of benefit for pain relief in diabetic neuropathy and trigeminal neuralgia (Backonja et al 1998, Rowbotham et al 1998).

Outcomes from non-randomized studies of multidisciplinary management in North Carolina were positive; 46% of 370 patients reported pain improvement after 1 year, with similar outcomes in those who had received primarily medical treatment (including psychological input) or primarily surgical treatment (Lamvu et al 2006). On the other hand, in Holland, 3-year follow-up of a cohort of 72 patients seen in a multidisciplinary clinic revealed a majority with continuing symptoms, pointing to the need for ongoing care for a chronic condition rather than a high expectation of cure (Weijenborg et al 2007).

Regular scheduled follow-up is an important element of a pain management programme, as distinct from pain-contingent consultations, and every effort must be made to provide continuity of care. Transcutaneous electrical nerve stimulation (TENS) can be offered in appropriate circumstances and advice given on its correct use. The neurophysiological basis for TENS is that transmission of impulses via unmyelinated C fibres is inhibited at the level of the dorsal horn of the spinal cord by the activation of cutaneous myelinated afferents using electrical stimulation. Evidence from randomized trials suggests that while ineffective in labour pain and acute postsurgical pain, there may well be benefit in dysmenorrhoea. Formal trials of TENS in the context of chronic pelvic pain are lacking.

Where mood disturbance is identified, concomitant antidepressant therapy should be suggested. Where there are indications of more complex psychopathology, particularly somatoform disorder, a liaison psychiatry opinion is appropriate. The rate of attendance by gynaecological patients referred to psychiatric departments is extremely low, and there are considerable advantages to service models which enable cross-referral on the same premises at short notice; however, these often present practical problems. Psychological assessment itself has therapeutic value (Price and Blake 1999), and a psychologist or psychotherapist can provide guidance on pain and/or stress management and motivate patients to move from passivity to active participation in their treatment. Wherever possible, patients should be offered the opportunity of a structured programme of cognitive–behavioural therapy (CBT), as evidence for the benefit of this approach is strong. Taking the rigorous approach of identifying 'clinically significant change' as an endpoint for outcomes in a routine clinical setting, between one in three and one in seven patients seen in a UK chronic pain clinic experienced useful benefits from CBT (Morley et al 2008).

KEY POINTS

1. Pain is a central nervous system construct.
2. The organic/psychogenic categorization is obsolete.
3. The central nervous system exhibits plasticity.
4. Hormonal, sex and genetic factors influence pain perception.
5. Chronic visceral pain may involve activation of silent afferents and hyperalgesia.
6. Chronic pelvic pain is common among the general population and those consulting general practitioners.
7. Consultation rates are influenced by social class.
8. Mood disturbance and sequelae of abuse may be associated factors.

9. Women with multiple unexplained physical symptoms may have somatoform disorder.

10. Women with pelvic pain often find their experience of care unsatisfactory.

11. Pelvic congestion symptoms include dyspareunia and postcoital aching.

12. Pain mapping may be useful in the assessment of adhesions.

13. Chronic PID should only be diagnosed at laparoscopy and is uncommon in UK practice.

14. In many women, the diagnosis is unclear or diagnoses overlap.

15. Multidisciplinary care is more effective than standard care.

16. The model of care needs to meet the individual needs of women.

17. Experience of care can influence clinical outcome.

18. Ultrasonography can be used to provide reassurance.

References

Abbott J, Hawe J, Hunter D, Holmes M, Finn P, Garry R 2004 Laparoscopic excision of endometriosis: a randomized, placebo-controlled trial. Fertility and Sterility 82: 878–884.

Backonja M, Beydoun A, Edwards K et al 1998 Gabapentin for the symptomatic treatment of painful neuropathy in patients with diabetes mellitus — a randomized controlled trial. JAMA: the Journal of the American Medical Association 280: 1831–1836.

Beard RW, Reginald PW, Wadsworth J 1988 Clinical features of women with chronic lower abdominal pain and pelvic congestion. British Journal of Obstetrics and Gynaecology 95: 153–161.

Beard RW, Kennedy RG, Gangar KF et al 1991 Bilateral oophorectomy and hysterectomy in the treatment of intractable pelvic pain associated with pelvic congestion. British Journal of Obstetrics and Gynaecology 98: 988–992.

Berkley K, Hubscher CH 1995 Are there separate central nervous system pathways for touch and pain? Nature Medicine 1: 766–773.

Berkley KJ, McAllister SL, Accius BE, Winnard KP 2007 Endometriosis-induced vaginal hyperalgesia in the rat: effect of estropause, ovariectomy, and estradiol replacement. Pain 132 (Suppl 1): S150–S159.

Bon K, Lanteri-Minet M, Menetrey D, Berkley KJ 1997 Sex, time-of-day and estrous variations in behavioral and bladder histological consequences of cyclophosphamide-induced cystitis in rats. Pain 73: 423–429.

Bradshaw HB, Temple JL, Wood E, Berkley KJ 1999 Estrous variations in behavioral responses to vaginal and uterine distention in the rat. Pain 82: 187–197.

Chen FP, Chang SD, Chu KK, Soong YK 1996 Comparison of laparoscopic presacral neurectomy and laparoscopic uterine nerve ablation for primary dysmenorrhea. Journal of Reproductive Medicine for the Obstetrician and Gynecologist 41: 463–466.

Collett BJ, Cordle CJ, Stewart CR, Jagger C 1998 A comparative study of women with chronic pelvic pain, chronic nonpelvic pain and those with no history of pain attending general practitioners. BJOG: an International Journal of Obstetrics and Gynaecology 105: 87–92.

Daoud I 1998 General surgical aspects. In: Steege JF, Metzger DA, Levy BS (eds) Chronic Pelvic Pain: an Integrated Approach. WB Saunders, Philadelphia, pp 329–336.

Davies L, Gangar KF, Drummond M, Saunders D, Beard RW 1992 The economic burden of intractable gynaecological pain. Journal of Obstetrics and Gynaecology 12 (Suppl 2): S54–S56.

Dickenson AH 1997 Plasticity: implications for opioid and other pharmacological interventions in specific pain states. Behavioral and Brain Sciences 20: 392–403.

Dworkin SF, Von-Korff M, LeResche L 1990 Multiple pains and psychiatric disturbance. An epidemiologic investigation. Archives of General Psychiatry 47: 239–244.

Eckhardt K, Li SX, Ammon S, Schanzle G, Mikus G, Eichelbaum M 1998 Same incidence of adverse drug events after codeine administration irrespective of the genetically determined differences in morphine formation. Pain 76: 27–33.

Engel CC, Walker EA, Engel AL, Bullis J, Armstrong A 1998 A randomized, double-blind crossover trial of sertraline in women with chronic pelvic pain. Journal of Psychosomatic Research 44: 203–207.

Farquhar CM, Rogers V, Franks S, Pearce S, Wadsworth J, Beard RW 1989 A randomized controlled trial of medroxyprogesterone acetate and psychotherapy for the treatment of pelvic congestion. BJOG: an International Journal of Obstetrics and Gynaecology 96: 1153–1162.

Fillingim RB, Edwards RR, Powell T 1999 The relationship of sex and clinical pain to experimental pain responses. Pain 83: 419–425.

Fillingim RB, Maixner W, Kincaid S, Silva S 1998 Sex differences in temporal summation but not sensory-discriminative processing of thermal pain. Pain 75: 121–127.

Fry RPW, Beard RW, Crisp AH, McGuigan S 1997 Sociopsychological factors in women with chronic pelvic pain with and without pelvic venous congestion. Journal of Psychosomatic Research 42: 71–85.

Ghaly AFF 1994 The psychological and physical benefits of pelvic ultrasonography in patients with chronic pelvic pain and negative laparoscopy. A random allocation trial. Journal of Obstetrics and Gynaecology 14: 269–271.

Gibbons JM 1998 Vulvar vestibulitis. In: Steege JF, Metzger DA, Levy BS (eds) Chronic Pelvic Pain: an Integrated Approach. WB Saunders, Philadelphia, pp 181–187.

Gilling-Smith C, Mason H, Willis D, Franks S, Beard RW 2000 In-vitro ovarian steroidogenesis in women with pelvic congestion. Human Reproduction 15: 2570–2576.

Grace VM 1995 Problems of communication, diagnosis, and treatment experienced by women using the New Zealand health services for chronic pelvic pain: a quantative analysis. Health Care for Women International 16: 521–535.

Grace VM 1998 Mind/body dualism in medicine: the case of chronic pelvic pain without organic pathology — a critical review of the literature. International Journal of Health Services 28: 127–151.

Hahn L 1989 Clinical findings and results of operative treatment in ilioinguinal nerve entrapment syndrome. BJOG: an International Journal of Obstetrics and Gynaecology 96: 1080–1083.

Halligan S, Campbell D, Bartram CI et al 2000 Transvaginal ultrasound examination of women with and without pelvic venous congestion. Clinical Radiology 55: 954–958.

Herrero JF, Laird JMA, Lopez-Garcia JA 2000 Wind-up of spinal cord neurones and pain sensation: much ado about something? Progress in Neurobiology 61: 169–203.

Herrington JK 1975 Occult inguinal hernia in the female. Annals of Surgery 181: 481–483.

Hobbs JT 1976 The pelvic congestion syndrome. The Practitioner 216: 529–540.

Horn S, Munafo M 1997 Pain Theory, Research, and Intervention. Open University Press, Buckingham.

Howard FM 1996 The role of laparoscopy in the evaluation of chronic pelvic pain:

pitfalls with a negative laparoscopy. Journal of the American Association of Gynecologic Laparoscopists 4: 85–94.

Howard FM 1999 Pelvic pain. In: Thomas EJ, Stones RW (eds) Gynaecology Highlights 1998–99. Health Press, Oxford, pp 53–63.

IASP Task Force on Taxonomy 1994 Classification of Chronic Pain, 2nd edn. IASP Press, Seattle.

Jenkinson C, Layte R, Wright L, Coulter A 1996a The UK SF-36: an Analysis and Interpretation Manual. Health Services Research Unit, University of Oxford, Oxford.

Jenkinson C, Peto V, Coulter A 1996b Making sense of ambiguity: evaluation of internal reliability and face validity of the SF-36 questionnaire in women presenting with menorrhagia. Quality in Health Care 5: 9–12.

Kasule J 1991 Laparoscopic evaluation of chronic pelvic pain in Zimbabwean women. East African Medical Journal 68: 807–811.

Koninckx PR, Renaer M 1997 Pain sensitivity of and pain radiation from the internal female genital organs. Human Reproduction 12: 1785–1788.

Lamvu G, Williams R, Zolnoun D, Wechter ME, Shortliffe A, flton G, Steege JF 2006 long-term outcomes after surgical and nonsurgical management of chronic pelvic pain: one year after evaluation in a pelvic pain specialty clinic. American Journal of Obstetrics and Gynecology 195: 591–598.

Lee CH, Dellon AL 2000 Surgical management of groin pain of neural origin. Journal of the American College of Surgeons 191: 137–142.

Lyall H, Campbell-Brown M, Walker JJ 1999 GnRH analogue in everyday gynecology: is it possible to rationalize its use? Acta Obstetrica et Gynecologica Scandinavica 78: 340–345.

Mathias SD, Kuppermann M, Liberman RF, Lipschutz RC, Steege JF 1996 Chronic pelvic pain: prevalence, health-related quality of life, and economic correlates. Obstetrics and Gynecology 87: 321–327.

McMahon SB 1997 Are there fundamental differences in the peripheral mechanisms of visceral and somatic pain? Behavioral and Brain Sciences 20: 381–391.

Morley S, Williams A, Hussain S 2008 Estimating the clinical effectiveness of cognitive behavioural therapy in the clinic: evaluation of a CBT informed pain management programme. Pain 137: 467–468.

Nezhat CH, Seidman DS, Nezhat FR, Nezhat CR 1998 Long-term outcome of laparoscopic presacral neurectomy for the treatment of central pelvic pain attributed to endometriosis. Obstetrics and Gynecology 91: 701–704.

Perry CP, Perez J 1993 The role for laparoscopic presacral neurectomy. Journal of Gynecologic Surgery 9: 165–168.

Peters AA, van Dorst E, Jellis B, van Zuuren E, Hermans J, Trimbos JB 1991 A randomized clinical trial to compare two different approaches in women with chronic pelvic pain. Obstetrics and Gynecology 77: 740–744.

Peters AAW, Trimbos-Kemper GCM, Admiraal C, Trimbos JB 1992 A randomized clinical trial on the benefit of adhesiolysis in patients with intraperitoneal adhesions and chronic pelvic pain. BJOG: an International Journal of Obstetrics and Gynaecology 99: 59–62.

Peveler R, Edwards J, Daddow J, Thomas EJ 1995 Psychosocial factors and chronic pelvic pain: a comparison of women with endometriosis and with unexplained pain. Journal of Psychosomatic Research 40: 305–315.

Peveler R, Kelkenny L, Kinmonth A-L 1997 Medically unexplained physical symptoms in primary care: a comparison of self-report screening questionnaires and clinical opinion. Journal of Psychosomatic Research 42: 245–252.

Poleshuck EL, Dworkin RH, Howard FM et al 2005 Contributions of physical and sexual abuse to women's experiences with chronic pelvic pain. Journal of Reproductive Medicine 50: 91–100.

Price JR, Blake F 1999 Chronic pelvic pain: the assessment as therapy. Journal of Psychosomatic Research 46: 7–14.

Prior A, Whorwell PJ 1989 Gynaecological consultation in patients with the irritable bowel syndrome. Gut 30: 996–998.

Rapkin AJ 1986 Adhesions and pelvic pain: a retrospective study. Obstetrics and Gynecology 68: 13–15.

Rapkin AJ, Kames LD, Darke LL, Stampler FM, Naliboff BD 1990 History of physical and sexual abuse in women with chronic pelvic pain. Obstetrics and Gynecology 76: 92–96.

Richlin SS, Rock JA 2001 Ovarian remnant syndrome. Gynaecological Endoscopy 10: 111–117.

Riley JL, Robinson ME, Wise EA, Price DD 1999 A meta-analytic review of pain perception across the menstrual cycle. Pain 81: 225–235.

Rowbotham M, Harden N, Stacey B, Bernstein P, Magnus Miller L 1998 Gabapentin for the treatment of postherpetic neuralgia — a randomized controlled trial. JAMA: the Journal of the American Medical Association 280: 1837–1842.

Selfe SA, Matthews Z, Stones RW 1998a Factors influencing outcome in consultations for chronic pelvic pain. Journal of Women's Health 7: 1041–1048.

Selfe SA, van Vugt M, Stones RW 1998b Chronic gynaecological pain: an exploration of medical attitudes. Pain 77: 215–225.

Shabalina SA, Zaykin DV, Gris P et al 2009 Expansion of the human mu-opioid receptor gene architecture: novel functional variants. Human Molecular Genetics 18: 1037–1051.

Slocumb JC, Kellner R, Rosenfeld RC, Pathak D 1989 Anxiety and depression in patients with the abdominal pelvic pain syndrome. General Hospital Psychiatry 11: 48–53.

Stones RW 2000 Chronic pelvic pain in women: new perspectives on pathophysiology and management. Reproductive Medicine Review 8: 229–240.

Stones RW, Rae T, Rogers V, Fry R, Beard RW 1990 Pelvic congestion in women: evaluation with transvaginal ultrasound and observation of venous pharmacology. British Journal of Radiology 63: 710–711.

Stones RW, Thomas EJ 1995 Cost-effective medical treatment of endometriosis. In: Bonnar J (ed) Recent Advances in Obstetrics and Gynaecology 19. Churchill Livingstone, Edinburgh, pp 139–152.

Stones RW, Selfe SA, Fransman S, Horn SA 2000 Psychosocial and economic impact of chronic pelvic pain. Baillière's Clinical Obstetrics and Gynaecology 14: 27–43.

Stones RW, Bradbury L, Anderson D 2001 Randomized placebo controlled trial of lofexidine hydrochloride for chronic pelvic pain in women. Human Reproduction 16: 1719–1721.

Stones RW, Cheong Y, Howard FM 2005 Interventions for treating chronic pelvic pain in women. Cochrane Database of Systematic Reviews 3: CD000387.

Stones RW, Lawrence WT, Selfe SA 2006 Lasting impressions: influence of the initial hospital consultation for chronic pelvic pain on dimensions of patient satisfaction at follow-up. Journal of Psychosomatic Research 60: 163–167.

Sutton JG, Ewen SP, Whitelaw N, Haines P 1994 Prospective, randomized, double-blind, controlled trial of laser laparoscopy in the treatment of pelvic pain associated with minimal, mild and moderate endometriosis. Fertility and Sterility 62: 696–700.

Swank DJ, Swank-Bordewijk SC, Hop WC et al 2003 Laparoscopic adhesiolysis in patients with chronic abdominal pain: a blinded randomised controlled multi-centre trial. The Lancet 361: 1247–1251.

Swanton A, Iyer L, Reginald PW 2006 Diagnosis, treatment and follow up of women undergoing conscious pain mapping for chronic pelvic pain: a prospective cohort study. BJOG: an International Journal of Obstetrics and Gynaecology 113: 792–796.

Treloar SA, Martin NG, Heath AC 1998 Longitudinal genetic analysis of menstrual flow, pain, and limitation in a sample of Australian twins. Behavior Genetics 28: 107–116.

von Bahr V 1979 Local anaesthesia for inguinal herniorrhaphy. In: Eriksson E (ed) Illustrated Handbook in Local Anaesthesia, 2nd edn. Lloyd-Luke, London, pp 52–54.

Waller KG, Shaw RW 1995 Endometriosis, pelvic pain, and psychological functioning. Fertility and Sterility 63: 796–800.

Weijenborg PT, Greeven A, Dekker FW, Peters AA, Ter Kuile MM 2007 Clinical course of chronic pelvic pain in women. Pain 132 (Suppl 1): S117–S123.

Weijenborg PT, Ter Kuile MM, Gopie JP, Spinhoven P 2008 Predictors of outcome in a cohort of women with chronic pelvic pain — a follow-up study. European Journal of Pain 13: 769–775.

Whorwell P 1995 The gender influence. Women and IBS 2: 2–3.

Winkel CA 1999 Modeling of medical and surgical treatment costs of chronic pelvic pain: new paradigms for making clinical decisions. American Journal of Managed Care 5: S276–S290.

Wise EA, Riley JL, Robinson ME 2000 Clinical pain perception and hormone replacement therapy in postmenopausal women experiencing orofacial pain. Clinical Journal of Pain 16: 121–126.

Woolf CJ 1983 Evidence for a central component of post-injury pain hypersensitivity. Nature 306: 686–688.

Woolf CJ, Shortland P, Coggeshall RE 1992 Peripheral nerve injury triggers central sprouting of myelinated afferents. Nature 355: 75–78.

Yonkers KA, Chantilis SJ 1995 Recognition of depression in obstetric/gynecology practices. American Journal of Obstetrics and Gynecology 173: 632–638.

Zolnoun D, Park EM, Moore CG, Liebert CA, Tu FF, As-Sanie S 2008 Somatization and psychological distress among women with vulvar vestibulitis syndrome. International Journal of Gynaecology and Obstetrics 103: 38–43.

Zondervan KT, Yudkin PL, Vessey MP, Dawes MG, Barlow DH, Kennedy SH 1999a Patterns of diagnosis and referral in women consulting for chronic pelvic pain in UK primary care. BJOG: an International Journal of Obstetrics and Gynaecology 106: 1156–1161.

Zondervan KT, Yudkin PL, Vessey MP, Dawes MG, Barlow DH, Kennedy SH 1999b Prevalence and incidence of chronic pelvic pain in primary care: evidence from a national general practice database. BJOG: an International Journal of Obstetrics and Gynaecology 106: 1149–1155.

Zondervan KT, Yudkin PL, Vessey MP et al 2001a Chronic pelvic pain in the community — symptoms, investigations, and diagnoses. American Journal of Obstetrics and Gynecology 184: 1149–1155.

Zondervan KT, Yudkin PL, Vessey MP et al 2001b The community prevalence of chronic pelvic pain in women and associated illness behaviour. British Journal of General Practice 51: 541–547.

CHAPTER 62

Pelvic inflammatory disease

Nazar N. Amso and Anthony Griffiths

Chapter Contents

INTRODUCTION	942	EVIDENCE-BASED MANAGEMENT	946
EPIDEMIOLOGY	942	LONG-TERM SOCIETAL AND GLOBAL HEALTH IMPACT	950
PATHOGENESIS AND PATHOGENS	943	PREVENTION	950
DIAGNOSIS	944	KEY POINTS	952

Introduction

Pelvic inflammatory disease (PID) refers to ascending infection of the upper genital tract affecting the uterus (endometritis), fallopian tubes and ovaries (salpingitis, oophoritis, salpingo-oophoritis, tubo-ovarian abscess), and neighbouring structures. Although the definition of PID is precise, its diagnosis is not. The acute onset of clinical symptoms and signs aids the diagnosis of PID, but it is often subclinical and is only manifested through its long-term sequelae such as pelvic pain, dyspareunia, infertility or ectopic pregnancy.

The World Health Organization (WHO) guide to essential practice, 'Integrating STI/RTI Care for Reproductive Health: Sexually Transmitted and Other Reproductive Tract Infections', defined reproductive tract infections (RTIs) as a broad term that includes sexually transmitted infections (STIs) as well as other infections that are not sexually transmitted (World Health Organization 2005). Not all STIs are RTIs, a reference to the location of the infection, and not all RTIs are STIs. In most instances, STIs have much more severe health consequences than other RTIs, and the terms 'STI' and 'RTI' are often used together to highlight the importance of STIs within RTIs.

This chapter will address PID as an upper genital tract infection that may be caused by organisms normally present in the reproductive tract (endogenous), or introduced from the outside during sexual contact (STI) or medical procedures (iatrogenic), and will outline its consequences and management as well as wider global prevention. Readers are also referred to Chapter 63 on non-HIV STIs.

Epidemiology

Epidemiological studies of PID are adversely affected by diagnostic and reporting uncertainties. The symptoms are often subtle and mild, and it is common that many cases of PID are missed because women or healthcare professionals fail to recognize mild or non-specific symptoms and their implications. As there are no simple, safe and specific diagnostic tests for PID, Simms et al (2003) proposed that it was time to rethink its diagnosis.

To complicate matters, adolescent and young adult women are reported to have anxiety surrounding pelvic examination (Millstein et al 1984), and in another study, over half of teens screened for STIs by urine testing and pelvic examination preferred the urine screening (Serlin et al 2002) for evaluating genitourinary (GU) symptoms without undergoing a speculum examination. Such new approaches may encourage young women who fear or otherwise avoid pelvic examinations to receive more timely evaluation, and could also result in access to diagnostic services in settings that do not currently provide them, such as school-based health centres, community centres and detention facilities, enabling clinicians to diagnose and treat many high-risk youth whose infections might otherwise go undetected (Burstein et al 1998, Pack et al 2000).

Estimates of prevalence

STI clinics are commonly viewed as the source for determining the prevalence and incidence of PID. However, an individual's attempt to seek medical advice following risk exposure is dependent on the individual's perception of risk level of concern, tendency to utilize such clinics, development of symptoms or fear of transmitting infection to their sexual partner. Furthermore, to determine the true prevalence or incidence, it is essential to have a clearly defined base population, be it 'at-risk' or 'general'; something that is inherently difficult and very complex.

Adolescent and young adult women account for nearly half of over 1 million cases of PID reported annually in the USA (Washington and Katz 1991). Chlamydia infection is the most common bacterial STI in the USA, with more than 2.8 million new cases estimated to occur each year (Weinstock et al 2004); this is the most common cause of PID

During 2007, approximately 1.1 million cases of chlamydia were reported to the Centers for Disease Control and Prevention (CDC); more than half of these were in females aged 15–25 years (Centers for Disease Control and Prevention 2009a).The annual incidence and prevalence of STIs is difficult to calculate. The incidence of STIs may be estimated on the bases of nationally notifiable diseases, national surveys, WHO reports and medical literature in this area. There is almost certainly under reporting due to the frequently asymptomatic nature of the disease, and the true annual incidence and prevalence are very likely to be much higher. A recent trend in developed countries highlights a shift in the microbial aetiology of PID, with an increasing role of chlamydia and a decreased role of gonococcal infection (van der Heyden et al 2000). Similarly, PID is now a disease that is mainly diagnosed in primary care or other similar outpatient environments. Since the advent of sensitive molecular amplification tests that permit non-invasive diagnosis of chlamydia, epidemiological evidence suggests that the proportion of chlamydial PID is increasing compared with other causative agents (Hughes et al 2001). There is also evidence that a significant number of chlamydial infections are asymptomatic, which allows silent cross-infection, and if untreated remains infectious in male and female hosts for months. Joyner et al (2002) demonstrated the persistence of chlamydia in 87% of men and women. WHO estimated 89 million new cases of genital chlamydial infections worldwide in 1995 and 92 million in 1999 (Peeling et al 1998, World Health Organization 2001).

In the UK, STI surveillance systems are based on data from GU medicine clinics and laboratory reports submitted to the Health Protection Agency Centre for Infections. However, this does not take into account the substantial number of relatively asymptomatic STIs that are diagnosed and treated in primary care settings. Simms et al (2006) examined the strengths and weaknesses of the Royal College of General Practitioners' (RCOG) Weekly Returns Service to determine the incidence of a range of STIs and associated clinical conditions. In their study, data were collated from 78 sentinel general practices in England and Wales between 1994 and 2001, covering a population of approximately 600,000. The authors reported that candidiasis was the most common condition reported in both men and women, followed by PID in women. The mean annual incidences per 100,000 women between 15 and 44 years of age were as follows: PID, 1787; vaginal discharge, 285; non-specific urethritis, 8.2; candidiasis, 4218; Trichomonas vaginalis, 28; genital herpes, 127; and genital warts, 184. Interestingly, the incidence of candidiasis and PID declined over this period in all groups, while the incidence of vaginal discharge doubled in 15–24 year olds over the same period. This decline in the incidence of PID is in marked contrast with the 148% increase in the diagnosis of chlamydial infections made in GU medicine clinics in the same period. The increase in diagnosis may have been brought about by an increase in case ascertainment, the increased availability of diagnostic facilities and an increase in disease incidence, while the decrease in PID probably reflects improved diagnosis and management of the syndrome. The aim of the National Chlamydia Screening Programme (NCSP) since its introduction in England in 2003 has been to control the infection through early detection and treatment of asymptomatic individuals. More than

one and a half million (1,673,276) tests were performed on 15–24 year olds by the NCSP between 2003 and the end of July 2009, and a further 376,966 non-NCSP, non-GU medicine tests were reported. Interestingly, the test-positive rate has declined steadily for both men and women since the programme started. The average test-positive rates for screened women and men were 8.38% and 6.78% for 2008–2009, and 7% and 6.3% for the first quarter of 2009–2010, respectively. In both durations, the highest rates were found in women aged 16–19 years and men aged 20–24 years (Figure 62.1). Other risk groups were those reporting behavioural risk factors and certain ethnic groups (National Chlamydia Screening Programme 2009).

Pathogenesis and Pathogens

The main causative agent of PID in the UK is *Chlamydia trachomatis*. Other less common causes include gonorrhoea, mycoplasma, gardnerella and Gram-negative rods (British

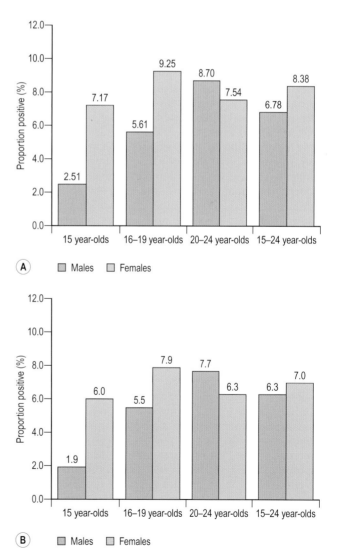

Figure 62.1 Proportion of positive cases of chlamydia by age and sex in England. (A) April 2008–March 2009. (B) April–June 2009.
Source: National Chlamydia Screening Programme 2009 Data accessed on NCSP website: www.chlamydiascreening.nhs.uk/ps/rd/lit.html (accessed 10/08/2009).

943

Association for Sexual Health and HIV 2005). *Trichomonas vaginalis* appears to have little, if any, role in the aetiology of PID. Bacterial vaginosis has been associated with PID, and the presence of bacterial vaginosis and leukocytes on vaginal slides is associated with a five-fold risk of PID (von Knorring and Wilson 2007). Other pathogens that should be considered, especially in immigrant women, include tuberculosis and schistosoma. Pelvic and genital tuberculosis is a blood-borne infection. Schistosoma infection should be considered in cases of granulomatous salpingitis (Kameh et al 2004). Actinomycosis is another causative agent of PID, and is often associated with intrauterine contraceptive device (IUCD) use.

Chlamydia

Chlamydia is a Gram-negative obligate intracellular parasite that can cause a variety of disease manifestations in humans. Chlamydia can be defined into different species depending upon its biochemical properties, although molecular analysis has led to further reclassification. In humans, serovars A–C cause conjunctivitis and resultant trachoma, whilst serovars D–K cause urethritis, cervicitis, ophthalmia noenatorum and neonatal pneumonia. LGV serovars produce a specific STI called lymphogranuloma venereum. Chlamydia has many features that are similar to a bacterium. It possesses a cell wall, hence it is sensitive towards penicillin, has the capacity to reproduce RNA and DNA, and is treatable with antibiotics. Unlike bacteria but like viruses, it must infect a host cell to reproduce. These characteristics initially made research difficult, but the application of genetic amplification tests resolved this problem. Chlamydia has a great affinity to adhere to the columnar epithelial cells of the endocervical canal, and also the epithelial cells of the endometrium and fallopian tube. Chlamydia is highly infectious in its extracellular state and consists of particles 0.2–0.4 μm in diameter, known as 'elementary bodies'. These elementary bodies enter the cell via phagocytosis, but have the capacity to avoid immunological destruction by inhibiting fusion with lysosomes. Over the following 24 h, the elementary bodies expand into larger reticulate bodies. These bodies rapidly divide by a process of binary fission to create several intracellular inclusion bodies, each of which is crammed with thousands of new reticulate bodies. These reticulate bodies condense to form new elementary bodies to complete the replication cycle, and upon lysis of the infected cell, thousands of new highly infectious elementary bodies are released. Host cell destruction is, of course, a byproduct of the replication process, but this is not enough tissue damage to explain the significant upper genital tract damage that occurs with chlamydial infection. This is likely to be due to the host humoral and cell-mediated immune response to infection, and would explain the differences in the effect of the host genetics upon the degree of clinical infection and the long-term sequelae. It is interesting to note that primary infection of chlamydia in monkeys in self-limiting but repeat exposure results in tubal damage, supporting a delayed immune response (Agrawal et al 2007).

Gonococcus

Gonococcal PID has decreased but is still a frequently encountered problem. Gonococcus, unlike chlamydia, is a true bacterium with an incubation period of 2–14 days. On light microscopy it can be seen as a Gram-negative diplococcus. It has the capacity to adhere selectively to non-ciliated secretory cells, including those lining the fallopian tubes, thanks to its cellular pili. These are fine protoplasmic projections that allow attachment to host cells. It is believed that gonococcal infection produces an acute polymorphonuclear reaction, and this generates a toxin that damages fallopian tube ciliated cells. Males tend to present with symptoms, while it is asymptomatic in at least 60% of infected women. Gonococcal infection should be considered in women who present with PID and concurrent dermatitis or new arthritis; rarely, it results in septicaemia or concurrent pharyngitis.

Other agents

Aerobic and anaerobic agents are also often associated with PID, and are believed to be secondary agents that have the capacity to cause symptomatic infection after primary damage by chlamydia or gonococcus. Aerobic bacteria include staphylococcus, group B and D streptococcus, coliforms and *Haemophilus influenzae*. Pneumococcus has also been recorded to occur, and this is believed to be due to orogenital contact. The anaerobic group includes bacteroides, fusobacterium, peptococcus and a variety of clostridium species. Often, a mixed growth is cultured. Hence, it is important to treat both aerobic and anaerobic infections, and in the case of true tubo-ovarian abscess, the growth tends to consist mainly of anaerobes.

Source of entry

The majority of acute PID are ascending infections through the genital tract to the endocervix, which can act as a reservoir and spread to the endometrium and the peritoneal cavity via the fallopian tubes (Figure 62.2). There is evidence to suggest that the actual degree of symptoms and long-term complications of such infection are greatly dependent upon the type of infection and the host's immune response. Once infection has gained access to the peritoneal cavity, it can cause a significant inflammatory response including the formation of pus and resultant abscess formation, especially the destructive tubo-ovarian abscess. In addition, pathogens can cause periappendicitis, perisplenitis and perihepatitis. A well-known but inadequately studied phenomenon is the perihepatic adhesions of Fitz–Hughes–Curtis syndrome. It is believed that chlamydia and gonococcus act as primary pathogens disrupting the normal protective barriers of infection, which then allows the clinical infection of other secondary pathogens including endogenous microbes, causing a polyinfection, frequently with anaerobic involvement.

Diagnosis

Symptoms and signs

Even the most experienced reflective clinician may face a dilemma in making a diagnosis of PID, or feel concerned about over- or underdiagnosing PID, primarily due to the lack of good evidence-based diagnostic criteria compounded by its polymicrobial aetiology. Common PID symptoms are outlined in Box 62.1.

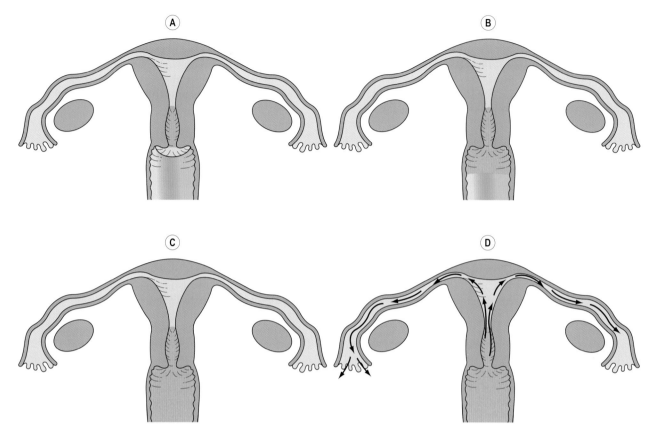

Figure 62.2 Pathogenesis of pelvic inflammatory disease (PID). PID begins with chlamydial and/or gonococcal cervicitis (A). This is followed by an alteration in the cervicovaginal microenvironment (B), leading to bacterial vaginosis (C). Finally, the original cervical pathogens, the flora causing vaginitis or both ascend into the upper genital tract (D). The grey shaded areas indicate the affected portions of the genital tract.
Modified from McCormack 1994 New England Journal of Medicine 330: 115–119.

The majority of women present with some but not all of these symptoms, which are not pathognomonic and account for the significant differences in determining PID rates among clinicians (Doxanakis et al 2008) and may result in failed treatments. In order to formulate an evidence-based approach to the diagnosis, several authors have attempted to generate a diagnostic scoring system to accept or refute the diagnosis of PID. A frequently used system is that published by Jacobson and Westrom (1969), whereby a diagnosis is made if acute lower abdominal/pelvic pain is accompanied by any two of the following features: abnormal vaginal bleeding, fever, vomiting, menstrual abnormalities, urinary symptoms, proctitis symptoms, marked pelvic tenderness, palpable mass or swelling, or erythrocyte sedimentation rate (ESR) >15 mm/h.

Although this is similar to the current guidelines of the RCOG, it remains a major concern that women with confirmed damaged fallopian tubes have no previous history of PID, mainly due to asymptomatic or atypical disease not being recognized (Sellors et al 1988). Munday's (2000) comprehensive review of the literature reported that many of the studies undertaken to estimate the accuracy of PID symptoms as a 'diagnostic test' had significant methodological flaws. Several used laparoscopy as a gold standard, which unfortunately may not be true, as it was reported to be of limited value with only 64% of suspected PID cases in one series being confirmed at laparoscopy (Sellors et al 1991).

Box 62.1 Symptoms and signs commonly associated with PID

- Bilateral lower abdominal tenderness (with occasional radiation to the legs)
- Abnormal vaginal or cervical discharge
- Fever (>38°C)
- Abnormal vaginal bleeding (intermenstrual, postcoital or breakthough)
- Deep dyspareunia
- Cervical motion tenderness on bimanual vaginal examination
- Adnexal tenderness or bimanual vaginal examination

Source: Royal College of Obstetricians and Gynaecologists 2009 Pelvic Inflammatory Disease. Green Top Guideline No. 32. RCOG Press, London.

Simms et al (2003) analysed the signs and symptoms of potential PID to generate likelihood ratios, and reported that abnormal vaginal bleeding, fever, vomiting, menstrual irregularity, ongoing bleeding, symptoms of urethritis, marked tenderness of pelvic organs on bimanual palpation, adnexal mass and ESR >15 mm in the first hour did not have significantly high sensitivity or specificity to be clinically valuable, and concluded that there was insufficient evidence to support existing diagnostic criteria for PID.

Current consensus suggests that the positive predictive value of a clinical diagnosis of PID is between 65% and 90%

when compared with laparoscopic findings, but this greatly depends upon the population studied (British Association for Sexual Health and HIV 2004). Adnexal tenderness has a particularly high sensitivity of 95%, but a very poor specificity of 22% (Peipert et al 2001).

The CDC factsheet (Centers for Disease Control and Prevention 2009b) indicates that the diagnosis is usually based on clinical findings, and if symptoms are present, a physical examination should be performed and further tests should be undertaken to identify the infection-causing organism. In view of the significant effects and long-term sequelae of untreated PID, it is wise to adopt a low threshold for treatment (Barrett and Taylor 2005) and to initiate early empirical treatment, although there is concern that this may lead to unnecessary treatment of women and there is no evidence to support or refute this strategy (Ross 2001a). With this in mind, clinicians should consider other risk assessments or investigations to improve diagnostic accuracy.

Risk assessment

Risk factors for STIs and PID are the same. In a longitudinal study, it was found that 39% of women with laparoscopically diagnosed PID were found to be infected with chlamydia and 14% with gonorrhoea (Bevan et al 1995). It is important to take a comprehensive sexual history from a patient with suspected PID. Risk factors include multiple sexual partners, lack of barrier contraception, young age and lower socioeconomic group. There is good evidence that anything that disrupts the cervical mucous barrier is a risk factor for PID. This includes uterine instrumentation, termination of pregnancy and insertion of an IUCD. There is significant evidence to support the fact that there are different levels of host susceptibility towards the development of PID, whereby polymorphism of mannose-binding lectin, an important component of the innate immune system and protector against chlamydial infection, may affect the extent of tubal damage in cases of chlamydial infection (Sziller et al 2008).

Evidence-Based Management

Investigations

Specific tests

Several tests may be employed for the diagnosis of PID, including microbiological swabs (endocervical, urinary, high and low vaginal swabs), inflammatory markers (C-reactive protein, ESR and differential white cell counts) and biophysical tests [transvaginal ultrasound scanning, Doppler scanning and magnetic resonance imaging (MRI) of the pelvis]. Microbiological tests remain the principal approach for the diagnosis of gonococcal and chlamydial infections, although the PID rate caused by the former is decreasing. Chlamydial tests have included cell culture, antibody tests and, more recently, nucleic acid amplification tests (NAAT), which allow greater accuracy at a relatively low cost. A recent meta-analysis suggested that pooled sensitivities for ligase chain reaction, polymerase chain reaction, gene probe and enzyme immunoassay of urine specimens were 96.5%,

85.6%, 92% and 38%, respectively, while on cervical swabs, the corresponding sensitivities were for PCR, gene probe and EIA 88.6%, 84% and 65%, respectively (Watson et al 2002). With any test, it is important to remember that the absence of lower genital tract infection does not exclude PID (Royal College of Obstetricians and Gynaecologists 2009).

Biochemical tests

Biochemical tests are often performed in suspected cases of PID. C-reactive protein is a non-specific acute phase inflammatory marker not normally found in serum. A cut-off value of 10 mg/l has a sensitivity of 93% and a specificity of 83% for acute PID. It responds more rapidly to therapy and thus is viewed as a better marker than ESR. C-reactive protein is also elevated in other infections, ovarian cyst accidents, ectopic pregnancies, malignancies, inflammatory bowel disease, appendicitis and endometriosis. ESR and differential white cell count are also non-specific and have a limited role in the diagnosis of PID.

Currently, it is recommended to perform endocervical swabs for chlamydia and gonorrhoea in suspected cases of PID (British Association for Sexual Health and HIV 2005). For chlamydia, NAAT performed on first-catch urine samples or vulvovaginal swabs are acceptable substitutes for endocervical swabs. Endocervical swabs for gonorrhoea should be sent in transport media and must arrive at the laboratory within 24 h. A positive NAAT for gonorrhoea should be confirmed by a positive culture test (British Association for Sexual Health and HIV 2005). Positive chlamydia and gonorrhoea tests (adjusted odds ratio 4.3, 95% confidence interval 2.89–2.63) are strongly associated with endometritis (Peipert et al 2001). Women with PID should be offered screening for other STIs (British Association for Sexual Health and HIV 2005).

A pregnancy test should also be performed to exclude ectopic pregnancy and to ensure that PID in pregnancy is treated promptly with inpatient management. It is also recommended to perform an urinanalysis and urine culture to exclude urinary tract infection.

Imaging tests

Advances in medical imaging technology [ultrasound, computed tomography (CT), MRI] have renewed interest in their use for the diagnosis of PID.

Ultrasound scanning, especially transvaginal scan (TVS) (Figure 62.3), is particularly helpful in the diagnosis of tubo-ovarian abscess, where thick-walled, pus-filled, inflamed tubes may be demonstrated, and also in diagnosing other pathologies (e.g. ovarian cyst torsion, cyst accidents). TVS may also be beneficial in the diagnosis of acute appendicitis. Ultrasound in the acute diagnostic setting has not been subjected to the rigours of a clinical trial. Preliminary data on its use as a follow-up tool reported that of 86 women followed-up 3 months after confirmed acute PID, five developed a hydrosalpinx (Taipale et al 2003). TVS has become a first-line investigative tool in emergency gynaecology, and at least 10% of all referrals for TVS are for the investigation of acute pelvic pain. TVS allows rapid assessment of pelvic anatomy with greater accuracy and diagnostic detail compared with that of a bimanual examination. Abdomina ultrasound can be used in cases of suspected appendicitis. Several other ultrasound features have been noted in cases of PID, including disruption of the normal pelvic anatomy, tenderness during TVS or the presence of free fluid in the pouch of Douglas. In a small study, the frequency of the ultrasound features of acute and chronic PID were assessed (Timor-Tritsch et al 1998). In the 14 patients with acute PID, a thickening of the fallopian wall was noted in all women, 12 demonstrated the 'cog wheel' sign and none of the patients demonstrated the 'beads on a string' sign. This was in marked contrast to women with chronic PID, where TVS could exclude other pathologies as well as distinguish between acute and chronic PID.

The addition of Doppler to grey-scale TVS may improve the sensitivity and specificity. Molander et al (2001) reported that an increase in the thickness of the fallopian tube walls was present in women with or without acute PID, but the application of Doppler ultrasound demonstrated the hyperaemia associated with acute PID. Pulsatility indices were significantly lower in women with acute PID compared with a control group. The use of power Doppler as a diagnostic

tool remains under investigation, and cannot yet be recommended to current practice. The application of percutaneous drainage with ultrasound imaging has been reported, but to date there have been no randomized controlled studies comparing percutaneous drainage with formal laparoscopic draining.

The evidence for the use of CT and MRI in suspected cases of acute PID is extremely limited, and their use is compounded by additional logistical problems and cost. CT imaging in PID may demonstrate thickening of the uterosacral ligaments, and the normally distinct pelvic floor fascial planes become obscured (Sam et al 2002). In more advanced disease, reactive inflammatory changes including large bowel ileus, hydroureter and even right upper quadrant inflammation consistent with Fitz–Hughes–Curtis syndrome may be noted. There is no comparative trial of CT in the diagnosis of PID. MRI has been compared with TVS and was reported to have greater sensitivity and specificity, but was limited by cost and accessibility (Tukeva et al 1999).

Laparoscopy

Diagnostic laparoscopy is often described as the diagnostic gold standard for PID; however, a negative laparoscopy does not exclude PID, and equally there is no evidence on the correlation between acute laparoscopic findings and the long-term sequelae of the disease. Its sensitivity is greatly dependent upon the diagnostic criteria used, and should be considered if there is a diagnostic dilemma or the presence of tubo-ovarian abscess is suspected. Features of PID seen at laparoscopy are shown in Figure 62.4.

Treatment

Treatment for suspected PID includes pain management, appropriate antibiotics, contact tracing, counselling and, occasionally, surgical intervention.

Outpatient care

Women with suspected mild-to-moderate PID can be effectively managed as an outpatient or within primary care provided that an ectopic pregnancy has been ruled out (Royal College of Obstetricians and Gynaecologists 2009). The Pelvic Inflammatory Disease Evaluation and Clinical Health (PEACH) randomized controlled trial ($n = 831$) reported that outpatient treatment of women with mild-to-moderate PID is as effective as inpatient treatment (Ness et al 2002). Short-term clinical and microbiological improvements were similar between the two groups, and after a mean follow-up period of 35 months, pregnancy rates were nearly equal (42.0% and 41.7%, respectively). There were also no differences in the time to pregnancy, chronic pelvic pain, ectopic pregnancy and recurrent PID rates between the two groups.

Inpatient care

Indications for hospital admission include severe symptoms and signs (nausea, vomiting and temperature >38°C), signs of peritonitis, pregnancy, suspected tubo-ovarian abscess, 'unwell patient' or uncertain diagnosis, poor compliance with an outpatient regimen, and suspected perihepatitis.

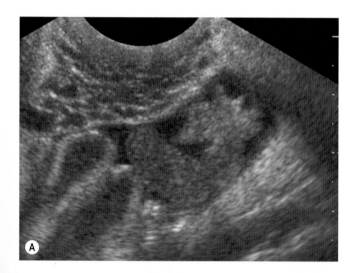

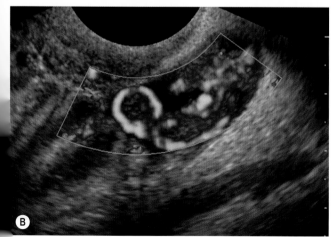

Figure 62.3 (A) Transvaginal scan showing fallopian tube fimbrial and ampullary sections, loops of bowel and pouch of Douglas fluid collection. (B) Power Doppler transvaginal scan image of acute salpingitis. The thickened fallopian tube is entirely visualized because of surrounding pouch of Douglas fluid. Note hyperaemia associated with acute inflammation.

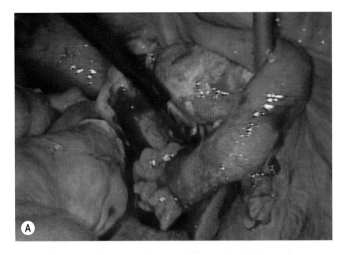

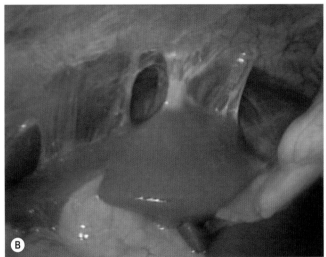

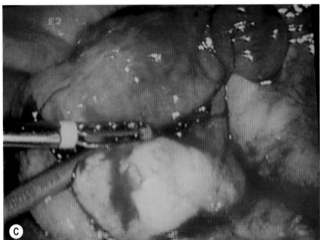

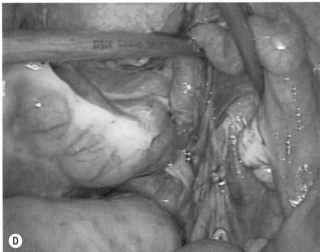

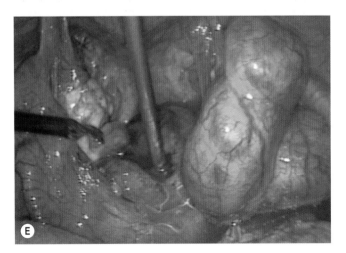

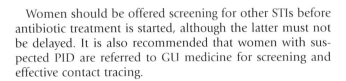

Figure 62.4 (A) Laparoscopic view of acute salpingitis. Note swollen hyperaemic fallopian tube next to a normal right ovary. The right tube has just been detached from the pelvic peritoneum. (B) Laparoscopic view of perihepatitis. Note perihepatic adhesions formed after chlamydial infection. The patient developed acute symptoms with severe pain in the right upper quadrant. (C) Laparoscopic view of severe pelvic inflammatory disease (PID). Note pyosalpinx formation with a phimotic fimbrial end. Normal ovary is visualized underneath the infected fallopian tube. (D) Laparoscopic view of severe PID. Note a unilateral left-sided tubo-ovarian abscess. (E) Laparoscopic view of severe PID. Note large bilateral pyosalpinx formation.

Women should be offered screening for other STIs before antibiotic treatment is started, although the latter must not be delayed. It is also recommended that women with suspected PID are referred to GU medicine for screening and effective contact tracing.

Analgesia

Analgesia should be started with ibuprofen or paracetamol; both should be combined if pain relief is unsatisfactory, or

one could consider adding codeine. If this is still unsatisfactory, it may be necessary to revise the diagnosis and treat as an inpatient (Ross 2001b). Drug interactions should be considered in women with medical problems such as epilepsy to avoid worsening of the primary illness.

Antibiotics

There is overall agreement that antibiotic therapy is appropriate for treating PID and conservative treatment cannot be recommended, although there has never been a trial comparing placebo with any antibiotic treatment as this would now be unethical. Choice of antibiotic options are dependent on whether there is a high or low risk of gonococcal infection.

Box 62.2 outlines the appropriate antibiotic options for outpatient treatment of mild-to-moderate PID. It is important to inform the patient verbally and in writing that if she is using the combined contraceptive pill, patch or vaginal ring, additional conception is required for the duration of the antibiotic treatment and also for 7 days afterwards. It is also important to enquire about alcohol use before prescribing metronidazole. Patients should be informed that there is a potential risk of flushing, nausea, headache and dizziness if alcohol is taken with metronidazole. The incidence of this reaction is unknown, but it has been reported to occur between 0% and 100% (Baxter 2006). If the patient is unable to tolerate metronidazole, it may be stopped in cases of mild-to-moderate PID as the evidence to support its addition is extremely limited (Royal College of Obstetricians and Gynaecologists 2009).

Regimens containing ofloxacin or azithromycin are not recommended for cases with a high potential for gonococcal infection, as there appears to be increased prevalence of gonococcal resistance in the UK. A large multinational randomized double-blinded study compared the treatment of PID with moxifloxacin alone or with a combination of ofloxacin and metronidazole in women with no evidence of tubo-ovarian abscesses. This study concluded that both treatment options had similar efficacy, but moxifloxacin had fewer side-effects. However, moxifloxacin-resistant gonococci appear to exist (Ross et al 2006). In animal studies, ofloxacin may have associated side-effects and is not currently recommended to patients under 18 years of age (Royal College of Obstetricians and Gynaecologists 2009). Moxiflaxacin is not licensed for the treatment of PID, and has been associated with an increased risk of life-threatening liver reaction (Medicines and Healthcare Products Regulatory Agency 2008).

There is better evidence to support the use of cefoxitin for the treatment of PID. However, it is often not widely available in the UK, and cefriaxone is a suitable third-generation cephalosporin substitute. Patients treated with doxycycline should be advised to avoid sunlamps or direct sunlight as there is a risk of photosensitivity reactions. A commonly used regimen for PID is still metronidazole and doxycycline, although there is no good evidence to support this, with a cure rate as low as 55% (Piyadigamage and Wilson 2005). In a systematic review of 39 studies, two trials evaluated treatment with metronidazole and doxycycline, and reported a clinical cure rate of 75% and a microbiological cure rate of 71% (Walker et al 1999). There is no evidence to support the use of a single dose of azithromycin alone, where better compliance might be an advantage (Bevan et al 2003).

PID in pregnancy

In early or potential early pregnancy, paracetamol is believed to be a safe analgesic, although the evidence for ibuprofen is weaker. The available evidence from the National Teratology Information Service has not noted any increase in congenital malformations before 30 weeks of gestation (National Teratology Information Service 2004). Current RCOG guidelines suggest that administering antibiotics in very early pregnancy is very unlikely to cause any fetal risks as significant drug toxicity would cause failed implantation. PID is very rare in later gestations. Tetracycline compounds should be avoided in pregnancy as they cause brown discoloration of the bone and teeth in fetuses exposed after 15 weeks of gestation, but this side-effect is not encountered with accidental exposure at earlier gestations (Schaefer et al 2007). Currently, the RCOG recommends treatment with cefotaxime, azithromycin and metronidazole for 14 days. No risk was associated with the use of metronidazole in pregnancy (National Teratology Information Service 2004), and no adverse effects were noted from the use of ceftriaxone on fetal development in animal studies. Similarly, azithromycin has very limited published data, but there does not seem to be an increase rate of fetal malformations following in-utero exposure.

PID and IUCDs

In women using an IUCD, it is appropriate to remove the device before treatment is started or if the symptoms have not resolved after 72 h. Clinicians should consider removing the IUCD in a patient with pelvic pain who has been noted to have actinomyces-like organisms previously. Where necessary, appropriate emergency contraception should be offered.

PID and HIV

In women with human immunodeficiency virus (HIV), treatment should be the same as for women without HIV (British Association for Sexual Health and HIV 2005). However, in clinically immunocompromised women or when there is failure to respond to standard treatment, advice from a HIV specialist team is recommended.

Compliance and partner screening

Women should be advised and counselled carefully about the implications of PID, the importance of compliance with treatment regimens, avoiding sexual intercourse until the

---

Box 62.2 Outpatient treatment for mild-to-moderate PID

Low-risk gonococcal infection

- Ofloxacin 400 mg orally twice daily and metronidazole 400 mg twice daily for 14 days.
- Ceftriaxone 250 mg as a single intramuscular dose plus oral doxycycline 100 mg twice daily and oral metronidazole 400 mg twice daily, both for 14 days.
- Ceftriaxone 250 mg as a single intramuscular dose followed by oral azithromycin 1 g per week for 2 weeks.

High-risk gonococcal infection

- Ceftriaxone 250 mg as a single intramuscular dose plus oral doxycycline 100 mg twice daily and oral metronidazole 400 mg twice daily, both for 14 days.

patient and her partner have completed the course of treatment to reduce the risk of reinfection, the advantages of screening for other STIs and the need for contact tracing. The patient may have to use barrier methods if intercourse is unavoidable (Royal College of Obstetricians and Gynaecologists 2009). Sexual partners within the preceding 6 months should be offered referral to a GU medicine clinic or be seen in primary care. The partner(s) should be tested for chlamydia, but empirical treatment would be recommended if this was not available. Gonorrhoea testing is only offered if the woman's or another partner's swab results are positive for gonococcus (Royal College of Obstetricians and Gynaecologists 2009).

Follow-up allows an assessment of compliance, encourages contact tracing, and is an opportunity to discuss the swab results, future prevention and health implications with patients. Acute PID managed on an outpatient basis should be reviewed within 72 h to assess the response and improvement of symptoms. If there is no benefit, it would be wise to consider reviewing the diagnosis and managing as an inpatient. Further follow-up may be arranged at 4 weeks to confirm that appropriate contact tracing has been carried out and to discuss PID implications. Generally, there is no need for further testing unless symptoms persist or there is a high risk of poor compliance.

Long-Term Societal and Global Health Impact

As indicated earlier, it is estimated that 8–10% of chlamydia infections and 8–20% of gonorrhoea infections progress to PID. In developing and low-resource communities, it is estimated that PID-related gynaecology admissions amount to 17–40% of all admissions in Africa, and 15–37% of all admissions in South-East Asia. After unsafe abortion, it is estimated that 10–23% of women with chlamydia and 15% of women with gonorrhoea will develop PID. This accounts for 7–29% of maternal deaths in developing regions. Equally, postpartum infection, which is rare with normal delivery if nothing is introduced into the vagina during labour, is up to 10 times more common in developing countries, accounting for up to 30% of maternal deaths (World Health Organization 2005).

A large ($n = 2501$) prospective cohort study between 1960 and 1984 reported an increase in infertility after PID (Westrom et al 1992). Sixteen percent of women with abnormal findings at laparoscopy (patients) and 2.7% of women with normal laparoscopy (control) failed to conceive. There was a higher rate of confirmed tubal factor in the women with abnormal findings at laparoscopy (10.8% and 0%, respectively). It was also noted that the incidence of tubal factor infertility increased with the number and severity of PID episodes. It was estimated that tubal factor infertility varied between 37% in developed countries and 85% in developing countries, which was very likely due to the effects of PID. Others have also reported a correlation between the severity of PID and the probability of infertility (Lepine et al 1998). After one episode of PID, the risk of infertility was estimated to be 15–25%, increasing to 50–60% after the third episode, and even higher rates where antibiotic treatment is not available. With this in mind, it is not surprising that there is a 10-fold increase in the incidence of ectopic

pregnancy (Westrom and Mardh 1983). In Africa, ectopic pregnancies occur in up to 32 per 1000 live births (World Health Organization 2005).

It is well established that communities with good access to effective prevention and treatment services have lower rates of STIs and associated complications. Thus, to broaden the benefits of prevention, active steps are required to overcome the challenges encountered in controlling STIs at community level by: (1) raising awareness; (2) promoting early use of clinic services and teaching people how to recognize symptoms and when to seek help; (3) promoting safer sexual practices when counselling clients (e.g. consistent use of condoms, fewer partners and delaying the age of first sexual intercourse); (4) detecting infections that are not obvious and screening for asymptomatic infection when possible; (5) preventing iatrogenic infection; (6) managing symptomatic STIs/RTIs effectively; and (7) counselling patients on staying uninfected after treatment.

Thailand demonstrated the success of prevention by greatly reducing the prevalence and transmission of common STIs/RTIs through addressing social and structural challenges. The incidence of the most common STIs was reduced by over 90% (Figure 62.5) through strong government commitment, the use of targeted strategies to reach the population where most STI transmission was taking place, better STI treatment and promoting increased use of condoms among commercial sex workers (World Health Organization 2005).

Chronic pelvic pain is common after acute PID and is often difficult to manage satisfactorily. Women with chronic pelvic pain after PID have a lower quality of life, may suffer work-related sequaele, are likely to experience adverse financial implications for treatment (Rein and Gift 2004), and frequently require operative interventions. It has been noted that hysterectomy and removal of adnexa is more common in women with a previous history of PID.

Prevention

Prevention of PID is most effectively achieved through avoiding exposure to STIs/RTIs, and endogenous or iatrogenic infections; equally, most of the serious health problems caused by STIs/RTIs are preventable. This section will assess options to prevent PID and its sequelae.

Prevention of sexually transmitted infections

Delaying sexual activity

Adolescents may come under significant peer pressure to become sexually active at an early age, when they are particularly vulnerable and at higher risk of STIs. Confidential support should be available for those who wish to delay sexual activity. Equally, adequate information should be available on safe sex, and prevention of STIs and pregnancy for those who decide to become sexually active.

Decreasing the number of sexual partners

Reducing the number of sexual partners reduces the risk of STIs and consequently PID. Partners in a longstanding monogamous relationship have an extremely low risk of

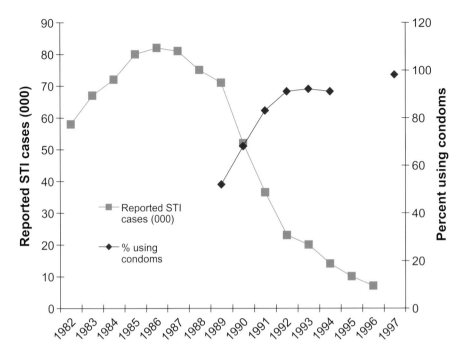

Figure 62.5 Reported cases of sexually transmitted infection (STI) and clients using condoms in Thailand 1982–1997.
Source: World Health Organization 2005 Integrating STI/RTI Care for Reproductive Health: Sexually Transmitted and Other Reproductive Tract Infections: a Guide to Essential Practice. WHO, Geneva.
Adapted from: Sentinel Serosurveillance, Division of Epidemiology, Ministry of Health, Thailand.

STIs. Rapid succession of monogamous relationships or a number of sexual partners increases the risk considerably. Couples separated from each other for long intervals (e.g. due to travel or business, migrant workers, military) are also at increased risk of STIs, and preventative measures should be employed.

Safe sex and barrier contraception

Male and female condoms are widely regarded as the most reliable methods for protection and prevention from STIs if used correctly and consistently. The latex male condom may fail if handled or stored incorrectly, or used with lubricants that may damage the material. The female condom, made of polyurethane plastic, is equally protective against STIs, empowers women to have control of their protection and can be used with any lubricants.

Contact prevention

A high index of suspicion for PID, prompt recognition of STIs and effective treatment reduces the probability of disseminating infection in the community. However, this is not always possible, and contact tracing protocols should be in place to screen and treat sexual partners.

Screening

Detection of asymptomatic lower genital tract infections is crucial to preventing PID. Screening may be undertaken at any time when a speculum examination is done for another reason, during pregnancy or targeted for at-risk populations such as 15–24 year olds, sex workers and others who are at higher risk of STIs. Similarly, when a women presents herself with vague symptoms of lower abdominal discomfort, intermenstrual bleeding or dyspareunia, tests should be undertaken to exclude the presence of genital infections, especially chlamydia or gonorrhoea. Screening may also be undertaken prior to transcervical interventions.

Screening programmes and identifying populations at risk

A screening programme is a control and prevention project usually targeted at the highest risk group in order to maximize benefit and be cost-effective. In 2003, two pilot chlamydia screening programmes in England demonstrated that opportunistic screening using urine samples is practical and acceptable, and that the frequency of chlamydia infection in women using these services (including non-GU medicine services) was substantial (Pimenta et al 2003a,b). Subsequently, the Chlamydia Screening Studies (ClaSS) project (Low et al 2007), which screened 19,773 women and men aged 16–39 years selected from general practice lists, used urine and (for women) vulvovaginal swab specimens self-collected at home and sent to a laboratory for chlamydia testing. This study demonstrated that chlamydia infection in the general population was highest in those under 25 years of age, with similar results in men and women. Furthermore, self-collected urine specimens and vulvovaginal swabs were found to be suitable for diagnostic testing using NAATs (Low et al 2007).

Evidence for the effectiveness of chlamydia screening emanates from randomized controlled trials that have demonstrated reductions in the risk of PID among women screened for chlamydia. In the USA, Scholes et al (1996) reported that, at 12 months, women screened for chlamydia had a reduced risk of PID (8/10,000 woman-months) compared with the usual care arm (18/10,000 woman-months), resulting in a relative risk reduction of 56% among those screened. In Denmark, Ostergaard et al (2000) showed that, at 12 months, women offered home-sample screening for chlamydia had reduced prevalence of infection and diagnoses of

PID (2.9%) compared with women offered clinic services (6.6%), and 2.1% of the home group were treated for PID compared with 4.2% of the control group. Additionally, it has been reported that the incidence of PID and ectopic pregnancy has declined in a number of countries conducting chlamydia screening, including Sweden, the USA and Canada (Hillis et al 1995, Kamwendo et al 1996, Egger et al 1998, Sutton et al 2005, Rekart et al 2009). Turner et al (2006), using mathematical modelling, estimated that annual screening of 30% of men and women under 25 years of age with 20% partner notification would reduce the population prevalence of chlamydia by 29% after 1 year, 68% after 5 years and 82% after 10 years. If screening coverage was increased to 50%, the estimated reductions in prevalence would be 40% after 1 year, 79% after 5 years and 89% after 10 years, with an even greater decline in prevalence if partner notification rates were higher. Such mathematical modelling estimates are not without limitations, and several important parameters such as the prevalence of undiagnosed/untreated chlamydia, patterns of sexual contacts and chlamydia transmission, and the rate of progression to PID may affect the ultimate effectiveness of screening (US Preventive Services Task Force 2007). In a meta-analysis, Low et al (2009) reported that register-based chlamydia screening of high-risk women and female and male high school students reduced the incidence of PID in women at 1 year, and that opportunistic screening in women undergoing surgical termination of pregnancy reduced postabortion rates of PID compared with no screening. Low et al (2009) concluded that there was no evidence to support opportunistic screening in the general population under 25 years of age. Evidence suggests that a screening programme may be cost-effective at prevalences of 3.1–10% (Honey et al 2002), and that as there is high prevalence of asymptomatic infection in men, efforts to screen them for chlamydia should be strengthened.

In 2009, among the UK home nations, only England has a national chlamydia screening programme. In Wales, Scotland and Northern Ireland, advice varies and individuals can request confidential screening from their general practitioners or GU medicine clinics. High-risk 15–24 year olds are offered testing when they attend healthcare institutions.

In Europe, chlamydia is one of the most common STIs, with rates among young sexually active people ranging between 5% and 10%. The number of diagnosed cases is increasing due to more cases being diagnosed and the use of more sensitive tests. The European Centre for Disease Control monitors chlamydia control activities in 29 European countries, including the 24 member states. In Canada, chlamydia is one of three nationally reportable STIs, and its infection rates have been increasing since 2007. There are national screening guidelines for sexually active and high-risk individuals. In the USA, chlamydia is the most frequently reported STI, and national chlamydia testing recommendations have been in place since 1993. In 2008, the CDC partnered with a number of non-profit organizations to form a 'US Chlamydia Coalition'. In Australia, chlamydia is the most commonly diagnosed STI, and the federal government has provided funding to increase chlamydia awareness, improve surveillance and undertake a pilot chlamydia testing programme as well as chlamydia prevention projects targeting high-risk groups.

Prevention of iatrogenic infections

PID due to iatrogenic infection is preventable by reducing the risks associated with vaginal or cervical interventions. Good antenatal care, safe delivery practices, good postabortion care and management of complications are accepted standards in developed countries, and have resulted in a dramatic decline in maternal morbidity; however, iatrogenic infection remains a major cause of PID in the developing world. Similarly, the risk of infection following transcervical procedures depends on the background STI prevalence, resource and capacity level, and conditions under which procedures are performed. Applying appropriate infection prevention measures, aseptic techniques and treating any existing cervical infection will reduce the risk of PID considerably.

Prevention of endogenous infections

Infections with bacterial vaginosis and *Candida albicans* are common and can be easily treated. However, their role in PID is debatable. Factors such as pregnancy, use of the oral contraceptive pill, chronic medical illnesses such as diabetes or HIV, and long-term use of steroids or antibiotics increase the risk of vaginal infections. Personal hygiene and elective treatment of high-risk patients will ensure the prevention of such infections.

KEY POINTS

1. Ascending chlamydial infection is the most common cause of PID.
2. Women under 25 years of age are the highest risk group.
3. Clinical presentation can range from no symptoms to very severe disease.
4. Delay in treatment increases the risk of long-term complications.
5. Treatment for suspected PID includes pain management, appropriate antibiotics, contact tracing, counselling and, occasionally, surgical intervention.
6. A screening programme is a control and prevention project, usually targeted at the highest risk group.
7. Prevention of PID is most effectively achieved through avoiding exposure to STIs/RTIs, and endogenous or iatrogenic infections.
8. Long-term sequelae include tubal factor infertility, ectopic pregnancy and chronic pelvic pain.
9. PID is a sexually transmitted infection with potentially harmful sequelae often managed suboptimally by physicians with little interest in the condition.
10. PID is the only preventable cause of infertility.
11. Screening for *Chlamydia trachomatis* is the most effective method of preventing PID.
12. The accuracy of syndrome diagnosis of PID should be improved by simple tests for the presence of lower genital tract infection.

References

Agrawal T, Vats V, Salhan S, Mittal A 2007 Mucosal and peripheral immune responses to chlamydial heat shock proteins in women infected with Chlamydia trachomatis. Clinical and Experimental Immunology 148: 461–468.

Barrett S, Taylor C 2005 A review on pelvic inflammatory disease. International Journal of STD and AIDS 16: 715–720.

British Association for Sexual Health and HIV 2004 Recommendations from the Bacterial Special Interest Group of BASHH: testing for sexually transmitted infections in primary care settings. BASHH, London.

British Association for Sexual Health and HIV 2005 UK National Guideline on the Management of Pelvic Inflammatory Disease. Clinical Effectiveness Group (Association for Genitourinary Medicine and the Medical Society for the Study of Venereal Diseases), London.

Baxter K 2006 Stockley's Drug Interactions: a Source Book of Interactions, their Mechanisms, Clinical Importance and Management, 7th edn. Pharmaceutical Press, London, pp 39–151.

Bevan CD, Johal BJ, Mumtaz G et al 1995 Clinical, laparoscopic and microbiological findings in acute salpingitis: a report on a United Kingdom cohort. British Journal of Obstetrics and Gynaecology 102: 407–414.

Bevan CD, Ridgway GL, Rothermel CD 2003 Efficacy and safety of azithromycin as monotherapy or combined with metronidazole compared with two standard multidrug regimens for the treatment of acute pelvic inflammatory disease. Journal of International Medical Research 31: 45–54.

Burstein G, Gaydos CA, Diener-West M et al 1998 Incident Chlamydia trachomatis infections among inner-city adolescent females. Journal of the American Medical Association 280: 521–526.

Centers for Disease Control and Prevention 1998 Guidelines for treatment of sexually transmitted diseases. MMWR Recommendations and Reports 47: 1–111.

Centers for Disease Control and Prevention 2009a Sexually Transmitted Disease Surveillance. US Department of Health and Human Services, Atlanta, GA. Available at: www.cdc.gov/std/stats07/toc.htm.

Centers for Disease Control and Prevention 2009b Pelvic Inflammatory Disease — the Facts. CDC Publication No. 99–8827.

Daling JR, Chow WH, Weiss NS et al 1985 Ectopic pregnancy in relation to previous induced abortion. Journal of the American Medical Association 15: 1005–1008.

Doxanakis A, Hayes RD, Chen MY et al 2008 Missing pelvic inflammatory disease? Substantial differences in the rate at which doctors diagnose PID. Sexually Transmitted Infections 84: 518–523.

Egger M, Low N, Smith GD et al 1998 Screening for chlamydial infections and the risk of ectopic pregnancy in a county in Sweden: ecological analysis. BMJ (Clinical Research Ed.) 316: 1776–1780.

Hillis SD, Nakashima A, Amsterdam L et al 1995 The impact of a comprehensive chlamydia prevention program in Wisconsin. Family Planning Perspective 27: 108–111.

Honey E, Augood C, Templeton A et al 2002 Cost effectiveness of screening for Chlamydia trachomatis: a review of published studies. Sexually Transmitted Infections 78: 406–412.

Hughes G, Brady AR, Catchpole MA et al 2001 Characteristics of those who repeatedly acquire sexually transmitted infections: a retrospective cohort study of attendees at three urban sexually transmitted disease clinics in England. Sexually Transmitted Diseases 28: 379–386.

Jacobson L, Westrom L 1969 Objectivized diagnosis of acute pelvic inflammatory disease. Diagnostic and prognostic value of routine laparoscopy. American Journal of Obstetrics and Gynecology 105: 1088–1098.

Joyner JL, Douglas JM, Foster M, Judson FN 2002 Persistence of Chlamydia trachomatis infection detected by polymerase chain reaction in untreated patients. Sexually Transmitted Diseases 29: 196–200.

Kameh D, Smith A, Brock MS 2004 Female genital schistosomiasis: case report and review of the literature. Southern Medical Journal 97: 525–527.

Kamwendo F, Forslin L, Bodin L, Danielsson D 1996 Decreasing incidences of gonorrhea- and chlamydia-associated acute pelvic inflammatory disease. A 25-year study from an urban area of central Sweden. Sexually Transmitted Diseases 23: 384–391.

Lepine LA, Hillis SD, Marchbanks PA et al 1998 Severity of pelvic inflammatory disease as a predictor of the probability of live birth. American Journal of Obstetrics and Gynecology 178: 977–981.

Low N, McCarthy A, Macleod J et al 2007 Epidemiological, social, diagnostic and economic evaluation of population screening for genital chlamydial infection. Health Technology Assessment 11: 1–165.

Low N, Bender N, Nartey L et al 2009 Effectiveness of chlamydia screening: systematic review. International Journal of Epidemiology 38: 435–448.

McCormack WM 1994 Pelvic inflammatory disease. New England Journal of Medicine 330: 115–119.

Medicines and Healthcare Products Regulatory Agency 2008 Moxifloxacin: restricted use. Drug Safety Update 2: 8.

Millstein SG, Adler NE, Irwin CE 1984 Sources of anxiety about pelvic examinations among adolescent females. Journal of Adolescent Health Care 5: 105–111.

Molander P, Sjöberg J, Paavonen J, Cacciatore B 2001 Transvaginal power Doppler findings in laparoscopically proven acute pelvic inflammatory disease. Ultrasound in Obstetrics and Gynecology 17: 233–238.

Munday PE 2000 Pelvic inflammatory disease— an evidence based approach to diagnosis. Journal of Infection 40: 31–41.

National Chlamydia Screening Programme 2009 Data accessed on NCSP website: www.chlamydiascreening.nhs.uk/ps/rd/lit.html (accessed 10/08/2009).

National Teratology Information Service 2004 Use of Ibuprofen in Pregnancy. TOXBASE, NTIS Regional Drug and Therapeutics Centre, Newcastle upon Tyne, UK.

Ness RB, Soper DE, Holley RL et al 2002 Effectiveness of inpatient and outpatient treatment strategies for women with pelvic inflammatory disease: results from the Pelvic Inflammatory Disease Evaluation and Clinical Health (PEACH) randomized trial. American Journal of Obstetrics and Gynecology 186: 929–937.

Ostergaard L, Andersen B, Møller JK, Olesen F 2000 Home sampling versus conventional swab sampling for screening of Chlamydia trachomatis in women: a cluster-randomized 1-year follow-up study. Clinical Infectious Diseases 31: 951–957.

Pack RP, DiClemente RJ, Hook EW, Oh MK 2000 High prevalence of asymptomatic STDs in incarcerated minority male youth: a case for screening. Sexually Transmitted Diseases 27: 175–177.

Peeling RW, Toye B, Jessamine P, Gemmill I 1998 Pooling of urine specimens for PCR testing: a cost saving strategy for Chlamydia trachomatis control programmes. Sexually Transmitted Infections 74: 66–70.

Peipert JF, Ness RB, Blume J et al 2001 Pelvic Inflammatory Disease Evaluation and Clinical Health Study Investigators. Clinical predictors of endometritis in women with symptoms and signs of pelvic inflammatory disease. American Journal of Obstetrics and Gynecology 184: 856–863.

Pimenta JM, Catchpole M, Rogers PA et al 2003a Opportunistic screening for genital chlamydial infection. I: Acceptability of urine testing in primary and secondary healthcare settings. Sexually Transmitted Infections 79: 16–21.

Pimenta JM, Catchpole M, Rogers PA et al 2003b Opportunistic screening for genital chlamydial infection. II: Prevalence among healthcare attenders, outcome, and evaluation of positive cases. Sexually Transmitted Infections 79: 22–27.

Piyadigamage A, Wilson J 2005 Improvement in the clinical cure rate of outpatient management of pelvic inflammatory disease following a change in therapy. Sexually Transmitted Infections 81: 233–235.

Rein DB, Gift TL 2004 A refined estimate of the lifetime costs of pelvic inflammatory disease. Sexually Transmitted Diseases 31: 325.

Rekart M, Gilbert M, Chang M et al 2009 Documenting the success of chlamydia control in British Columbia (BC). Abstract P4.64. 18th ISSTDR Conference, London, UK.

Ross JD 2001a European Branch of the International Union against Sexually Transmitted Infections and the European Office of the World Health Organization. European guideline for the management of pelvic inflammatory disease and perihepatitis. International Journal of STD and AIDS 21: 84–87.

Ross J 2001b Pelvic inflammatory disease. Extracts from clinical evidence. BMJ (Clinical Research Ed.) 17: 658–659.

Ross JD, Cronje HS, Paszkowski T et al 2006 Moxifloxacin versus ofloxacin plus metronidazole in uncomplicated pelvic inflammatory disease: results of a multicentre, double blind, randomised trial. Sexually Transmitted Infections 82: 446–451.

Royal College of Obstetricians and Gynaecologists 2009 Pelvic Inflammatory Disease. Green Top Guideline No. 32. RCOG Press, London.

Sam JW, Jacobs JE, Birnbaum BA 2002 Spectrum of CT findings in acute pyogenic pelvic inflammatory disease. Radiographics 22: 1327–1334.

Schaefer C, Peters P, Miller RK (eds) 2007 Drugs during Pregnancy and Lactation: Treatment Options and Risk Assessment, 2nd edn. Academic Press, Oxford.

Scholes D, Stergachis A, Heidrich FE et al 1996 Prevention of pelvic inflammatory disease by screening for cervical chlamydial infection. New England Journal of Medicine 334: 1362–1366.

Sellors JW, Mahony JB, Chernesky MA, Rath DJ 1988 Tubal factor infertility: an association with prior chlamydial infection and asymptomatic salpingitis. Fertility and Sterility 49: 451–457.

Sellors J, Mahony J, Goldsmith C et al 1991 The accuracy of clinical findings and laparoscopy in pelvic inflammatory disease. American Journal of Obstetrics and Gynecology 164: 113–120.

Serlin M, Shafer MA, Tebb K et al 2002 What sexually transmitted disease screening method does the adolescent prefer? Archives of Pediatric & Adolescent Medicine 156: 588–591.

Simms I, Warburton F, Weström L 2003 Diagnosis of pelvic inflammatory disease: time for a rethink. Sexually Transmitted Infections 79: 491–494.

Simms I, Fleming DM, Lowndes CM et al 2006 Surveillance of sexually transmitted diseases in general practice: a description of trends in the Royal College of General Practitioners Weekly Returns Service between 1994 and 2001. International Journal of STD and AIDS 17: 693–698.

Sutton MY, Sternberg M, Zaidi A et al 2005 Trends in pelvic inflammatory disease hospital discharges and ambulatory visits, United States, 1985–2001. Sexually Transmitted Diseases 32: 778–784.

Sziller I, Fedorcsák P, Csapó Z et al 2008 Circulating antibodies to a conserved epitope of the Chlamydia trachomatis 60-kDa heat shock protein is associated with decreased spontaneous fertility rate in ectopic pregnant women treated by salpingectomy. American Journal of Reproductive Immunology 59: 99–104.

Taipale P, Tarjanne H, Ylostalo P 2003 Transvaginal sonography in suspected pelvic inflammatory disease. Ultrasound in Obstetrics and Gynecology 6: 430–434.

Timor-Tritsch IE, Lerner JP, Monteagudo A et al 1998 Transvaginal sonographic markers of tubal inflammatory disease. Ultrasound in Obstetrics and Gynecology 12: 56–66.

Tukeva TA, Aronen HJ, Karjalainen PT et al 1999 MR imaging in pelvic inflammatory disease: comparison with laparoscopy and US. Radiology 210: 209–216.

Turner KM, Adams EJ, Lamontagne DS 2006 Modelling the effectiveness of chlamydia screening in England. Sexually Transmitted Infections 82: 496–502.

US Preventive Services Task Force 2007 Screening for chlamydial infection: US Preventive Services Task Force recommendation statement. Annals of Internal Medicine 147: 128–134.

van der Heyden JHA, Catchpole MA, Paget WJ, Stroobant A 2000 Trends in gonorrhoea in nine western European countries, 1991–1996. European Study Group. Sexually Transmitted Infections 76: 110–116.

von Knorring N, Wilson J 2007 Sorting out pelvic inflammatory disease. Trends in Urology, Gynaecology and Sexual Health 12: 31–36.

Walker CK, Workowski KA, Washington AE et al 1999 Anaerobes in pelvic inflammatory disease: implications for the Centers for Disease Control and Prevention's guidelines for treatment of sexually transmitted diseases. Clinical Infectious Diseases 28: S29–S36.

Washington AE, Katz P 1991 Cost of and payment source for pelvic inflammatory disease: trends and projections, 1983 through 2000. Journal of the American Medical Association 266: 2565–2569.

Watson EJ, Templeton A, Russell I et al 2002 The accuracy and efficacy of screening tests for Chlamydia trachomatis: a systematic review. Journal of Medical Microbiology 51: 1021–1031.

Weinstock H, Berman S, Cates W, Jr 2004 Sexually transmitted diseases among American youth: incidence and prevalence estimates, 2000. Perspectives in Sexual and Reproductive Health 36: 6–10.

Westrom LR 1980 Incidence, prevalence, and trends of acute pelvic inflammatory disease and its consequences in industrialized countries. American Journal of Obstetrics and Gynecology 138: 880–892.

Westrom L, Mardh PA 1983 Chlamydial salpingitis. British Medical Bulletin 39: 145–150.

Westrom LR, Joesoef R, Reynolds G et al 1992 Pelvic inflammatory disease and fertility. A cohort study of 1,844 women with laparoscopically verified disease and 657 control women with normal laparoscopic results. Sexually Transmitted Diseases 19: 185–192.

World Health Organization 2001 Global Prevalence and Incidence of Selected Curable Sexually Transmitted Infection. WHO, Geneva.

World Health Organization 2005 Integrating STI/RTI Care for Reproductive Health: Sexually Transmitted and Other Reproductive Tract Infections: a Guide to Essential Practice. WHO, Geneva.

CHAPTER 63

Non-HIV sexually transmitted infections

Daniel P. Hay and Eimear P. Kieran

Chapter Contents

INTRODUCTION	955	GONORRHOEA	966
EPIDEMIOLOGY	956	CHLAMYDIA	967
PRINCIPLES OF MANAGEMENT OF SEXUALLY TRANSMITTED INFECTIONS	957	*MYCOPLASMA GENITALIUM* AND *UREAPLASMA UREALYTICUM*	968
CLINICAL PRESENTATIONS	958	GENITAL WARTS (CONDYLOMATA ACCUMINATA)	969
GENITAL HERPES	958	MOLLUSCUM CONTAGIOSUM	971
SYPHILIS	961	VIRAL HEPATITIS	971
LYMPHOGRANULOMA VENEREUM	964	VAGINAL INFECTIONS	973
CHANCROID	965	ECTOPARASITIC INFESTATIONS	976
GRANULOMA INGUINALE (DONOVANOSIS)	965	KEY POINTS	978

Introduction

Sexually transmitted infections (STIs) are infections whose primary route of transmission is through sexual contact. They are common, often occult in nature, have serious sequelae and are synergistic with human immunodeficiency virus (HIV). In developing countries, they are the second most common cause of death amongst women aged 15–44 years, after maternal mortality. The serious nature of many of these conditions and the fact that the presence of one STI suggests the possibility of others is a caution to the gynaecologist to manage such patients with appropriate input from others, notably genitourinary physicians and microbiologists.

More than 20 pathogens are transmissible through sexual intercourse. Many are curable but, in spite of the availability of effective treatment, they remain a major public health concern in both industrialized and developing countries.

Globally, the exact prevalence of STIs is largely unknown. Surveillance systems exist in some countries but the data rendered are not always reliable or complete. The quality and completeness of the available data and estimates depend on the quality of STI services, the extent to which patients seek health care, the intensity of case finding and diagnosis, and the quality of reporting.

The completeness is further affected by the natural history of STIs, since a large number of infections are asymptomatic. Moreover, only part of the symptomatic population seeks health care and an even smaller number of cases are reported. The social stigma that is usually associated with STIs may result in people seeking care from alternative providers or not seeking care at all. As a result, report-based STI surveillance systems tend to underestimate the total number of new cases substantially.

World Health Organization (WHO) estimates suggest that more than 12 million new cases of syphilis, 62 million new cases of gonorrhoea, 92 million new cases of chlamydial infection and 174 million new cases of trichomoniasis occurred throughout the world in 1999 (World Health Organization 2001). Congenital syphilis, prevention of which is relatively easy and cost-effective, may still be responsible for as many as 14% of neonatal deaths. Up to 10% of women who are untreated, or inadequately treated, for chlamydial and gonococcal infections may become infertile as a consequence. On a global scale, up to 4000 newborn babies each year may become blind because of gonococcal and chlamydial ophthalmia neonatorum (note: ophthalmia neonatorum is a notifiable disease).

Both symptomatic and asymptomatic infections can lead to the development of serious complications with severe consequences. The most serious complications and

DOI: 10.1016/B978-0-7020-3120-5.00063-1

long-term consequences of untreated STIs tend to be in women and newborn babies. Sequelae in women include recurring herpes episodes, pelvic inflammatory disease (PID), ectopic pregnancy, spontaneous miscarriage, premature rupture of the membranes, puerperal sepsis, tubal factor infertility and cervical cancer consequent to human papilloma virus (HPV) infection. Neonates may be born premature or even stillborn. They may be born with infection or the consequences of congenital syphilis.

STIs also enhance the sexual transmission of HIV infection. The presence of an untreated STI can increase the risk of both acquisition and transmission of HIV by a factor of up to 10. Ulcerative STIs disrupt the integrity of the protective tegument and increase the presence of HIV-susceptible cells (e.g. CD4 lymphocytes). Non-ulcerative STIs similarly increase HIV-susceptible cells in the area. Moreover, improvement in the management of STIs can reduce the incidence of HIV-1 infection in the general population by approximately 40%. STI prevention and treatment are, therefore, important components in HIV prevention.

Guidelines covering the majority of STIs exist within the UK. They discuss aspects relating to screening, diagnostic criteria, management and prevention. Crucially, they also set standards for audit, providing a tool for improvement in all these aspects in all units across the UK. They will be quoted from heavily in this chapter in condensed form. The guidelines are not primarily directed *per se* at gynaecologists, but it is of vital importance that specialists in this area are aware of them.

Epidemiology

WHO estimated that 340 million new cases of STIs occurred worldwide in 1999. The largest number of new infections occurred in South and South-east Asia, followed by sub-Saharan Africa, Latin America and the Caribbean. However, the highest rate of new cases per 1000 population occurred in sub-Saharan Africa (World Health Organization 2001).

In developing countries, STIs and their complications are among the top five disease categories for which adults seek health care. In women of childbearing age, STIs (excluding HIV) are second only to pregnancy as causes of morbidity and mortality.

Globally, the highest rates of STIs are generally found in urban men and women aged 15–35 years. On average, women become infected at a younger age than men.

In the UK, peaks in STI diagnoses occurred in the mid-to-late 1940s (post World War II) and from the mid 1960s through to the early 1980s [from the age of sexual liberation to the advent of acquired immunodeficiency syndrome (AIDS)]. From 1998 to 2007, there was a substantial increase in diagnoses of most STIs (overall 6%). Cases of uncomplicated gonorrhoea increased by 42%, while chlamydia increased by 150%. Chlamydia has been the most commonly reported STI since 2001, overtaking genital warts (see Figure 63.1).

The rapid increase in reports of STIs is probably, in part, due to a general deterioration in sexual health amongst young people and men who have sex with men. However, the greater acceptability of using genitourinary medicine

(GUM) services and new campaigns to encourage testing have also made a contribution. In 2000, the UK survey of sexual attitudes and lifestyle over 10 years reported that 30% of 15-year-old girls were sexually active and half of all UK teenagers were sexually active before 17 years of age. Consistent condom usage decreased by 3% over the period of study. Male homosexual activity increased, as did the prevalence of unsafe sex in this group, especially in London. The number of heterosexual partners also increased, and more people were engaging in concurrent relationships.

Certain ethnic minority groups are disproportionately affected by some STIs. In 2005, the GRASP (Gonococcal Resistance to Antimicrobials Surveillance Programme) survey found that Black Caribbeans accounted for 18% of gonorrhoea diagnoses at the clinics studied.

The UK population is mobile and certain groups are at particular risk, including tourists, professional travellers, immigrants and members of the armed forces. In addition, poverty, urbanization, social migration and war often increase levels of prostitution.

The important features in maintaining an STI in a community have been factored into the following formula:

$$Ro = \beta cd$$

where Ro is the average number of new infections that result from one infection, β is transmissibility, c is the average rate of acquiring partners, and d is the duration of infection.

If Ro >1, the rate of spread in a community will rise; if Ro <1, the rate of spread will fall. This gives the principles behind effective STI control. β can be reduced by promoting condom use and vaccination, c can be reduced by encouraging behavioural change, and d can be reduced by encouraging diagnosis, treatment and contact tracing. These principles then translate into effective health education. d can also be reduced by screening.

Screening

There are guidelines for routine screening in pregnancy in the UK, and the current programme screens all pregnant women at booking for syphilis, hepatitis B and HIV after a pretest discussion. In addition, screening for hepatitis C should be undertaken in intravenous drug users. There is also a national screening programme for *Chlamydia trachomatis*.

In the UK, the National Institute for Health and Clinical Excellence (NICE) issued guidelines entitled 'Prevention of sexually transmitted infections and under 18 conceptions' in 2007. These guidelines were not specifically aimed at gynaecologists but more at primary care agencies. In summary, these guidelines set recommendations as follows.

Recommendations 1 and 2: for key groups at risk of STIs

- Identify individuals at high risk of STIs using their sexual history. Opportunities for risk assessment may arise during consultations on contraception, pregnancy or abortion, and when carrying out a cervical smear test, offering an STI test or providing travel immunization. Risk assessment can also be

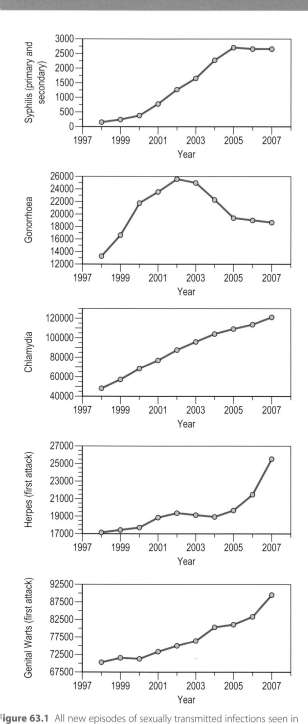

Figure 63.1 All new episodes of sexually transmitted infections seen in genitourinary medicine clinics 1998–2007.
Source: Health Protection Agency 2008 All new episodes seen at GUM clinics: 1998–2007. United Kingdom and country specific tables.

- When did she last have sexual intercourse?
- What is the nature of her sexual activity? (hetero-/homo-/bisexual) (oral/anal/vaginal)
- When did she last have sexual intercourse with anyone else other than that person?
- Was a barrier method of contraception used?
- Was any method of contraception used? (risk of pregnancy)
- Travel history (and that of the partner)
- History of intravenous drug abuse
- History of giving or accepting money for sex
- History of previous STIs

can help to reduce risk-taking and improve self-efficacy and motivation. Ideally, each session should last for at least 15–20 min. The number of sessions will depend on individual need.

Recommendation 3: patients with an STI

- Help patients with an STI to get their partners tested and treated (partner notification), when necessary. This support should be tailored to meet the patient's individual needs. If necessary, refer patients to a specialist with responsibility for partner notification. Partner notification may be undertaken by the health professional or by the patient.
- Provide the patient and their partners with infection-specific information, including advice about possible reinfection. For chlamydia infection, also consider providing a home sampling kit.

Information given to patients for any condition should be supported by written evidence-based information, in a clear, jargon-free format, to reinforce the message.

Principles of Management of Sexually Transmitted Infections

History

Whilst in the UK, STIs are principally managed by specialist clinics (GUM), STIs also commonly present to the gynaecologist. The threshold at which the gynaecologist should take a sexual history is correspondingly low. The essentials are establishment of a rapport, privacy and confidence in the manner of questioning. Embarrassment on the part of the patient is quite understandable and should be dealt with empathetically. Phrases can be couched in terms such as 'I am sorry to have to ask you this, please don't be offended, it is important'. Essential elements of the sexual history, taken in combination with a general gynaecological and medical history, are shown in Box 63.1.

One of the markers for women at risk of STIs is the age range (15–34 years). This takes the age range down to childhood, and these patients frequently present with a parent. It is highly unlikely that a girl will reveal all matters regarding

carried out during routine care or when a new patient registers.

Have one-to-one structured discussions with individuals at high risk of STIs (if trained in sexual health), or arrange for these discussions to take place with a trained practitioner. The discussions should be structured on the basis of behaviour change theories. They should address factors that her sexual activity in front of her mother. Such questions relating to this may be more profitably asked in the examination room with the mother back in the waiting room. In such cases, confidentiality should be emphasized and reassurance given that the information will not get back to her parents.

Examination

It is essential that a chaperone is present (irrespective of the gender of the examining doctor) and that consent has been obtained for intimate examination. Ideally, examination should be performed in lithotomy; in any case, there should be adequate exposure to allow thorough examination in good light of the external genitalia, mons pubis, perineum and perianal area. One should observe for *Pediculosis pubis* (crabs), scabies, *molluscum contagiosum*, warts, ulceration, excoriation, scars and any discharge from the introitus; and palpate for inguinal lymphadenopathy and tenderness. A bivalve speculum should be passed, gently, as the patient may find this uncomfortable. The cervix should be examined, looking for ectropion, warts, cervicitis and mucopurulent discharge. The vaginal walls should be observed for inflammation or warts. At this time, 'triple swabs' should be taken.

The first swab is taken from the posterior fornix and is placed into Stuart's transport medium (agar and charcoal). This swab essentially screens for *Trichomonas vaginalis*, bacterial vaginosis and *Candida* spp. The second swab is taken from the endocervix and is a screen for *Neisseria gonorrhoeae*; this is also placed into Stuart's transport medium. The third swab is also taken from the endocervix and is a screen for *C. trachomatis*. This last swab needs to be taken in a particular way as *C. trachomatis* is an obligate intracellular organism. Thus, to be sampled, the swab needs to pick up some cells from the sampled area. The swab should be rotated in the endocervix for at least a count of 10 and placed into chlamydia transport medium.

The speculum should then be removed and a digital examination performed. The patient should be examined for cervical excitation, uterine and adnexal tenderness, and adnexal masses.

Specialist clinic tests

In a GUM clinic, further refinements to this examination include a test of vaginal pH using narrow-range pH paper. The normal vaginal pH is 3.8–4.5. Bacterial vaginosis, trichomoniasis and atrophic vaginitis often cause a vaginal pH higher than 4.5. For a 'whiff test', several drops of a potassium hydroxide solution are added to a sample of the vaginal discharge. A strong fishy odour (ammonia) from the mix means that bacterial vaginosis is present. For a wet mount, a sample of the vaginal discharge is placed on a glass slide and mixed with a salt solution. The slide is looked at under a microscope (under dark ground illumination) for yeast cells, trichomoniasis and treponemes. A Gram stain is made of any discharge and examined for *N. gonorrhoeae* (Gram-negative diplococci) and the clue cells of bacterial vaginosis. Further swabs are frequently taken from the urethra, anus and throat, and sent in Stuart's transport medium for culture (looking for *N. gonorrhoeae*). Any woman

reporting anal intercourse will also undergo proctoscopy looking for warts.

If one STI is present, there may be others. In practice, a patient with an STI will be referred to a GUM clinic, counselled and offered a full screen including serological tests for syphilis, hepatitis B, HIV and hepatitis C, if indicated. The GUM clinic will also arrange for contact tracing to break the chain of infection. They may also arrange for a follow-up test of cure.

If drug treatment is given, it is better to use simple, if possible, single-dose regimes and advise the woman to abstain from intercourse during treatment to prevent reinfection until her partner is also treated. In practice, regimens are given that will cover *N. gonorrhoea*, *C. trachomatis*, *T. vaginalis* and bacterial vaginosis.

In the spirit of the NICE guidelines, time should be allocated to discuss modification of any high-risk activity to prevent reinfection (National Institute for Health and Clinical Excellence 2007). This should be non-judgmental and should be accompanied by written information on the subject to reinforce the message.

Clinical Presentations

Patients present with clinical syndromes rather than microbiological presentations. In fact, the most common presentation is none whatsoever! The patient is picked up on opportunistic screening, by partner notification or by chance when presenting with another condition. This emphasizes the importance of the NICE guidelines, especially in the light of increasing prevalences of STIs in the UK.

Vaginal infection and/or cervicitis may present with a discharge, and cervicitis may also present as postcoital bleeding. Endometritis may cause erratic bleeding and pelvic pain. Adnexitis is synonymous with acute PID and may produce dyspareunia and pelvic pain. Fitz–Hugh–Curtis syndrome consists of right upper quadrant pain resulting from ascending pelvic infection and inflammation of the liver capsule or diaphragm.

Genital Herpes

Genital ulcers have a broad differential diagnosis, but the most common cause of de-novo and recurring multiple painful ulceration is herpes simplex virus (HSV). The infection is lifelong and has the potential for recurrence. It can be managed but not eradicated. It is a disease that has long been in the public domain with varying levels of informed and misinformed knowledge. A patient with this diagnosis needs careful counselling, explanation and support. Between 1998 and 2007, diagnoses of genital herpes rose by 51% in the UK.

Aetiology

Herpes simplex virus 1 and 2 (HSV-1 and HSV-2) are species of *Herpesviridae*, which cause genital herpes. Herpes viruses are composed of relatively large double-stranded, linear DNA genomes encoding 100–200 genes encased within an icosahedral proteinaceous capsid which is wrapped in a lipid bilayer envelope. They are nuclear, replicating the viral DNA being transcribed to RNA within the infected cell's nucleus. HSV enters a latent phase within the neurones (local sensory ganglia) between active symptomatic episodes. Reactivation leads to production of virions, which may then be passed to a new host by sexual contact (in the case of genital herpes). Genital HSV-2 recurs and sheds more often than genital HSV-1; the converse is true for oral herpes.

Clinical features

Only about half those infected will get symptoms at the time of infection. Some may become symptomatic at a later date and some not at all. The seropositivity rates are 7% in the UK, 22% in the USA and 40% in 19-year-old females in Tanzania. In those cases that become symptomatic, the incubation period is 7–14 days.

The first episode presents with multiple painful genital ulcers (see Figure 63.2). It is less severe in those with a history of oral herpes. Typical lesions begin as vesicles, at any or all sites from the introitus to the cervix, which become superficial tender ulcers with an erythematous halo and a yellow or grey base (Figure 63.3). Immunocompromised patients may have an atypical appearance which is an elongated 'knife cut' ulcer. There may be bilateral inguinal lymphadenopathy. Viral shedding continues until the lesions crust over. One-third of patients have systemic symptoms of fever and general malaise. Ten percent will experience viral meningitis with photophobia and headache. A few patients experience retention of urine, either because of pain due to passing urine over the lesions (in which case, micturating in a bath may help) or because of a viral autonomic neuritis. Involvement of other nerves may lead to hyperaesthetic buttocks, thighs or perineum for a time. Severe encephalitis is rare but may be seen more frequently in immunocompromised patients. Without treatment, the first episode lasts for 3–4 weeks.

Complications of the first episode are common. There may be secondary bacterial infection of lesions. Autoinoculation may occur, often to fingers and eyes.

Recurrent episodes occur in approximately half of patients, tend to be less severe and are relatively less common after the first year. HSV-2 is more likely to become recurrent than HSV-1. There does not necessarily have to be a precipitating event, although stress, menstruation, trauma (sexual intercourse) and ultraviolet light are implicated. Immunosuppression increases the frequency and duration of episodes; herpetic ulceration persisting for over 1 month in a patient with HIV is AIDS defining.

Diagnosis

In the UK, guidelines for diagnostic criteria for herpes were drawn up by the British Association for Sexual Health and HIV (BASHH) in 2006. These are summarized below.

Screening of asymptomatic GUM clinic attendees by either HSV antibody testing or HSV detection in genital specimens is not recommended at present, although this area is under active review.

Virus detection and characterization

The confirmation and characterization of the infection and its type, by direct detection of HSV in genital lesions, are essential for diagnosis, prognosis, counselling and management. Methods should be used that directly demonstrate HSV in swabs taken from the base of the genital lesion. Virus typing to differentiate between HSV-1 and HSV-2 should be performed in all patients with newly diagnosed genital herpes. HSV isolation in cell culture is the current routine diagnostic method in the UK. Virus culture is slow, labour-intensive and expensive. Specificity is virtually 100%, but

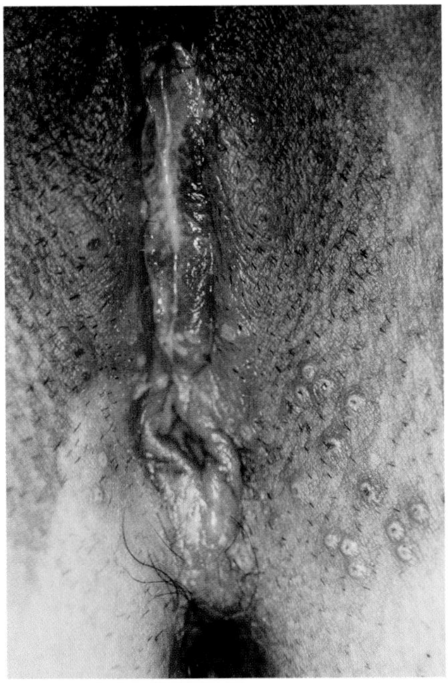

Figure 63.2 Primary genital herpes: multiple painful ulcers are present.
From Bolognia J et al, Dermatology 2e, with permission of Elsevier.

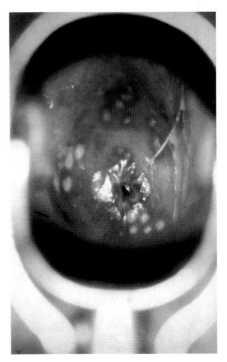

Figure 63.3 Primary genital herpes: ulcers on cervix.

levels of virus shedding, quality of specimens, and sample storage and transport conditions influence sensitivity. Delayed sample processing and lack of specimen refrigeration after collection and during transport significantly reduce the yield of virus culture at all stages of infection.

HSV DNA detection by polymerase chain reaction (PCR) increases HSV detection rates by 11–71% compared with virus culture. PCR-based methods allow less stringent conditions for sample storage and transport than virus culture, and new real-time PCR assays are rapid and highly specific. Real-time PCR is recommended as the preferred diagnostic method for genital herpes.

Serology

Testing for HSV type-specific antibodies can be used to diagnose HSV infection by the detection of HSV-1 IgG or HSV-2 IgG or both. It is difficult to say whether the infection is recent, as immunoglobulin M (IgM) detection is unreliable. Collection of serum samples a few weeks apart can be used to show seroconversion. HSV-2 antibodies are indicative of genital herpes, whereas HSV-1 antibodies do not differentiate between genital and oropharyngeal infection.

Western blot is the diagnostic gold-standard, but it is not commercially available. Several commercial assays, as well as validated in-house methods, are available which show 91–99% sensitivity and 92–98% specificity relative to Western blot in sexually active adults.

Caution is needed in interpreting serology results because even highly sensitive and specific assays have poor predictive values in low-prevalence populations. Local epidemiological data and patient demographic characteristics should guide testing and interpretation of results. In patients with a low likelihood of genital herpes, a positive HSV-2 antibody result should be confirmed in a repeat sample or by a different assay.

The differential diagnosis of vulval ulcers is shown in Table 63.1.

Treatment

First episode of genital herpes

Saline bathing should be advised and oral analgesia provided. Topical anaesthetic agents, such as 5% lidocaine (lignocaine) ointment, may be useful to apply, especially prior to micturition, but should be used with caution because of the risk of potential sensitization.

Oral antiviral drugs are indicated within 5 days of the start of the episode and while new lesions are still forming.

Aciclovir, valaciclovir and famciclovir all reduce the severity and duration of episodes. Antiviral therapy does not alter the natural history of the disease. Topical agents are less effective than oral agents. Combined oral and topical treatment is of no benefit. Intravenous therapy is only indicated when the patient cannot swallow or tolerate oral medication because of vomiting. There is no evidence for benefit from courses longer than 5 days. However, it may be prudent to review the patient after 5 days and continue therapy if new lesions are still appearing at this time.

Recommended regimens (all for 5 days)

- Aciclovir 200 mg five times daily.
- Aciclovir 400 mg three times daily.
- Valaciclovir 500 mg twice daily.
- Famciclovir 250 mg three times daily.

Hospitalization may be required for urinary retention, meningism and severe constitutional symptoms. If catheterization is required, suprapubic catheterization is preferred to prevent the theoretical risk of ascending infection, to reduce the pain associated with the procedure, and to allow normal micturition to be restored without multiple removals and recatheterizations.

Recurrent genital herpes

Recurrences are self-limiting and generally cause minor symptoms. Management decisions should be made in partnership with the patient. Strategies include supportive therapy alone, episodic antiviral treatments and suppressive antiviral therapy. The best strategy for managing an individual patient may change over time according to recurrence frequency, symptom severity and relationship status.

General advice includes saline bathing, Vaseline, analgesia and 5% lidocaine (lignocaine) ointment.

Episodic antiviral treatment (oral aciclovir, valaciclovir and famciclovir) reduces the duration (by median of 1–2 days) and severity of recurrent genital herpes. Patient-initiated treatment started early in an episode is most likely to be effective.

Recommended regimens (all for 5 days)

- Aciclovir 200 mg five times daily.
- Aciclovir 400 mg three times daily.
- Valaciclovir 500 mg twice daily.
- Famciclovir 125 mg twice daily.

Short-course therapies

- Aciclovir 800 mg three times daily for 2 days.
- Famciclovir 1 g twice daily for 1 day.
- Valaciclovir 500 mg twice daily for 3 days.

Suppressive antiviral therapy

Patients who have taken part in trials of suppressive therapy have had at least six recurrences per annum. Such patients have fewer or no episodes on suppressive therapy. Patients

Table 63.1 The differential diagnosis of genital ulcers

Infective	Non-infective
Herpes simplex virus	Aphthous ulcers
Primary syphilis	Trauma
Lymphogranuloma venereum	Skin disease (e.g. lichen sclerosis et atrophicus) Chancroid
Donovanosis	Behçet's syndrome
Human immunodeficiency virus	Other multisystem disorder (e.g. sarcoidosis)
	Dermatitis artefacta

with lower rates of recurrence will probably also have fewer recurrences with treatment.

Patient safety and resistance data for long-term suppressive therapy with aciclovir now extends to over 18 years of continuous surveillance.

Recommended regimens

- Aciclovir 400 mg twice daily.
- Aciclovir 200 mg four times daily.
- Famciclovir 250 mg twice daily.
- Valaciclovir 500 mg once daily.

If breakthrough recurrences occur on standard treatment, the daily dosage should be increased (e.g. aciclovir 400 mg three times daily). Suppressive therapy should be discontinued after a maximum of 1 year to reassess recurrence frequency. The minimum period of assessment should include two recurrences. Patients who continue to have unacceptably high rates of recurrence may restart treatment.

Condoms may be partially effective in preventing acquisition of HSV, especially in preventing transmission from infected males to their female sexual partners. The efficacy of male condoms in preventing transmission from infected females to uninfected male partners has not been demonstrated, and the efficacy of female condoms to reduce HSV transmission during intercourse has not been assessed.

Suppressive antiviral therapy with valaciclovir 500 mg once daily reduces the rate of acquisition of HSV-2 infection and clinically symptomatic genital herpes in serodiscordant couples. In a randomized trial involving 1484 patients treated for 8 months, 0.5% valaciclovir recipients developed symptomatic infection compared with 2.2% of placebo recipients (75% reduction); however, 60 people needed to be treated to prevent one transmission. Other antivirals may be effective but efficacy has not been proven in clinical trials.

Diagnosis often causes considerable distress. Counselling should be as practical as possible and should address particular personal situations. The Family Planning Association (FPA) produces a range of leaflets on sexual health for the UK National Health Service (NHS). Their leaflet on genital herpes provides comprehensive patient information based on the BASHH guidelines, and can be purchased or viewed as a non-printable PDF file on the FPA website.

No vaccines have been approved for prevention of genital herpes, although trials are ongoing. Published studies using the HSV-2 glycoprotein-D adjuvant vaccine have shown limited efficacy in preventing clinical disease, and only in women who were seronegative for both HSV-1 and HSV-2 at baseline. The guideline authors do not support the use of unauthorized or unlicensed vaccines outside of clinical trials.

Management of herpes in pregnancy and neonatal herpes prevention

Guidelines for genital herpes in pregnancy are categorized into management of first episodes and recurrent episodes. Accurate clinical classification is difficult. Viral isolation and typing and the testing of paired sera (if a booking specimen is available) may be helpful. Referral to a genitourinary physician for advice on management of women with suspected genital herpes is recommended.

First-episode genital herpes

First-episode genital herpes has been associated with first-trimester miscarriage; however, there is no conclusive evidence that it causes developmental abnormality if the pregnancy continues. The occurrence of first-episode genital herpes is not considered an indication for termination of pregnancy (TOP). An anomaly scan may be considered at 20–22 weeks of gestation where this is not routine. Management should be in line with the clinical condition, with the use of either oral or intravenous aciclovir. Although aciclovir is not licensed for use in pregnancy, there is substantial clinical experience supporting its safety. Vaginal delivery should be anticipated.

Daily suppressive aciclovir from 36 weeks of gestation may be considered for women who experience first-episode genital herpes in order to reduce the likelihood of HSV lesions at term, and negate an offer of caesarean section (CS) delivery. There are sound arguments for using aciclovir 400 mg three times daily because of the altered pharmacokinetics of the drug in late pregnancy.

Third-trimester acquisition

CS for the prevention of neonatal herpes has not been evaluated in randomized controlled trials. CS should be offered to all women presenting with first-episode genital herpes lesions at the time of delivery, or within 6 weeks of the expected date of delivery or onset of labour. However, CS may not be of benefit in reducing transmission for women presenting with ruptured membranes for greater than 4 h. In all these cases, the paediatricians should be informed. Continuous aciclovir in the last 4 weeks of pregnancy reduces the risk of both clinical recurrence at term and delivery by CS.

Recurrent genital herpes

Antiviral treatment is rarely indicated for treatment of recurrent episodes of genital herpes during pregnancy. Symptomatic recurrences during the third trimester are likely to be brief, and vaginal delivery is appropriate if no lesions are present at delivery.

CS should be considered for women with recurrent genital herpes lesions at the onset of labour. Recurrent genital herpes at any other time during pregnancy is not an indication for delivery by CS. The risks of vaginal delivery for the fetus are small and must be set against risks to the mother of CS.

Syphilis

There was a post World War II peak in the incidence of syphilis, but with the advent of penicillin, it became one of the less common STIs in the UK. However, infectious syphilis is reported to have increased by a factor of 19 between 1998 and 2007 (2680 new diagnoses in that year). To a large extent, this rise has been fuelled by syphilis outbreaks among male homosexuals.

Nevertheless, the most dramatic recent increases in syphilis cases have been among women and heterosexual men. Although the numbers involved are considerably lower than those for chlamydia, this is still a worrying trend as syphilis can have serious health implications (left untreated, syphilis can damage the heart, aorta, brain, eyes and bones, and can be fatal) and had been thought for years to be under control in the UK.

Globally, WHO estimates that there are 12 million new cases of syphilis each year, most of which occur in South and South-east Asia, and sub-Saharan Africa. Infectious syphilis is reaching epidemic proportions in states of the former Soviet Union, and is increasingly substantially in the USA, especially in the African-American population.

Aetiology

Treponema pallidum venereum or *Treponema pallidum pallidum* is a motile spirochaete, entering the host via breaches in epithelium. The organism can also be transmitted vertically to a fetus in the later stages of pregnancy, giving rise to congenital syphilis.

The subspecies of *T. pallidum* causing yaws (*pertenue*), pinta (*carateum*) and bejel or endemic syphilis (*endemicum*) are morphologically and serologically indistinguishable from *T. pallidum pallidum* (syphilis); however, their transmission is not venereal in nature and the course of each disease is significantly different. They are worthy of mention as they can cause diagnostic confusion. Yaws occurs in sub-Saharan Africa, the Caribbean and most of the humid tropics. Bejel occurs in desert regions, and pinta occurs in parts of Central and South America. If venereal syphilis cannot be excluded in someone originating from one of these areas, it is safest to treat.

Clinical features

Primary syphilis

The incubation period after inoculation is 9–90 days (mean 21 days). The lesions may be extragenital and may be multiple. Chancres are usually painless, raised, well-circumscribed ulcers (Figure 63.4). There is a non-tender regional lymphadenopathy. The lesion may well go unnoticed, especially if it is intravaginal or rectal. It will heal spontaneously in 3–10 weeks.

Secondary syphilis

The lesions of secondary syphilis usually manifest some 4–8 weeks after the appearance of the chancre, but sometimes up to 6 months later. In one-third of cases, the chancre is still there. There is a systemic eruption of a non-itchy maculopapular rash, symmetrical and involving the palms and soles (Figure 63.5). Papular lesions may coalesce into large fleshy wart-like lesions, condylomata lata, in areas such as the anus and the labia. Mucous patches and linear (snail-track) ulcers are seen on the mucosae. There may be a generalized lymphadenopathy. The secondary stage involves a bacteraemia with fever, headache, bone pain, alopecia, arthritis and meningitis. There may be hepatitis, optic neuritis and papilloedema. A sensorineural deafness can occur due to destruction of hair cells in the inner ear.

Without treatment, the lesions of secondary syphilis resolve. Approximately one-quarter of cases will have a recurrence of secondary syphilis; although unusual after 1 year, it can recur up to 2 years later, during which time the infection can be transmitted to a sexual partner.

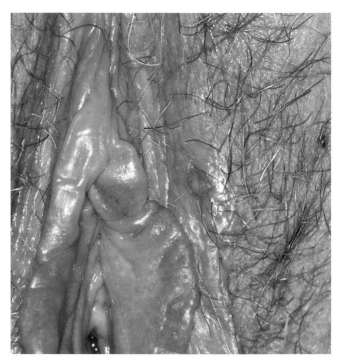

Figure 63.4 The chancre of primary syphilis.
From Morse S et al., Atlas of Sexually Transmitted Diseases and AIDS, 3e, with permission of Elsevier.

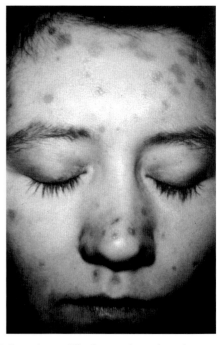

Figure 63.5 Secondary syphilis: the maculopapular rash.

Syphilis is transmissible to other adults through sexual contact in primary and secondary syphilis and, occasionally, in early latent syphilis.

Latent syphilis

- Early: the disease has been present for less than 2 years; this is the time when relapse into secondary syphilis may occur.
- Late: the disease has been present for more than 2 years.

Late sequelae

Approximately one-third of cases will go on to develop late clinical sequelae. Of all cases infected with syphilis who are untreated, 10% of men and 5% of women will develop neurosyphilis, sometimes within 5 years. Meningovascular syphilis presents most commonly with headache, and sometimes with signs akin to a stroke with palsies of cranial nerves III, VI, VII and VIII. Rarely, there may be hemiplegia. Argyll Robertson pupils are a manifestation; they accommodate but do not react to light. Parenchymatous neurosyphilis presents as general paresis of the insane or, as a consequence of degeneration of the posterior columns, tabes dorsalis. The latter presents with ataxia, failing vision, sphincter disturbances and attacks of severe pain. Approximately 20% of cases will develop cardiovascular syphilis; many years later, this may manifest as a thoracic aortic aneurysm or aortic regurgitation. Gummas develop 3–12 years later in 15% of cases. They may occur on the skin, mucous membranes and, more rarely, bone or viscera.

Diagnosis

Dark ground microscopy of a wet preparation scraped from the base of a chancre or a lesion of secondary syphilis will display the treponeme as a bluish-white thread-like organism with a coiled body, some 6–20 μm long (Figure 63.6). It is motile and displays three distinct movements: watchspring, corkscrew and jack-knife. Due to sensitivity and specificity issues with serological testing, this is by far the best chance of establishing a firm diagnosis.

Dark ground/dark field microscopy (DGM) of lesion exudate or lymph nodes should be performed by experienced clinicians because of interference from commensal spirochaetes that are found in the normal flora of the genital and rectal mucosae. DGM is considered to be less reliable in examining rectal and non-penile genital lesions, and is not suitable for examining oral lesions.

If the initial examination is negative, DGM should be repeated daily for at least 3 days. Antibiotics should be withheld during this period, and local saline lavage may be used to reduce local sepsis.

Testing of material submitted on dry swabs by PCR is recommended for oral or other lesions where contamination with commensal treponemes is likely.

PCR is also useful in the diagnosis of primary syphilis and is available via local laboratories sending samples to the Sexually Transmitted Bacteria Reference Laboratory at the Health Protection Agency.

Serological tests can be divided into non-specific tests [Venereal Disease Reference Laboratory (VDRL) and rapid plasmin reagin (RPR)] and specific tests [*T. pallidum* enzyme immunoassay (EIA), fluorescent treponemal antibody (FTA), *T. pallidum* haemagglutination assay (TPHA) and *T. pallidum* particle assay]. Non-specific tests usually become negative after successful treatment, whereas specific tests remain positive. All tests, specific or otherwise, are positive for bejel, yaws and pinta.

Non-specific tests become positive 3–5 weeks post inoculation, and as they are quantitative, they may be used to monitor treatment. However, they may also decay naturally, even yielding false-negative results. They may also

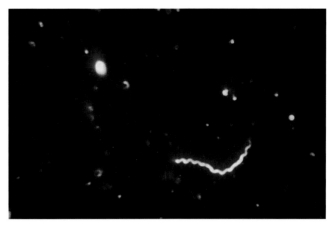

Figure 63.6 Dark ground microscopy showing bluish-white thread-like treponeme.
From Cohen J et al., Infectious Diseases, 3e, with permission of Elsevier.

Table 63.2 Diagnosis and serological interpretation

Results positive	Diagnosis
None	Syphilis not present or very early primary syphilis
All	Untreated, recently treated or latent syphilis
T. pallidum EIA (or FTA) and VDRL	Primary syphilis
T. pallidum EIA (or FTA) and TPHA	Treated syphilis or untreated late latent or late syphilis
T. pallidum EIA or FTA only	Early primary syphilis, untreated or recently treated early syphilis
VDRL/RPR only	False positive reaction

EIA, enzyme immunoassay; FTA, fluorescent treponemal antibody; VDLR, Venereal Disease Reference Laboratory; TPHA, *Treponema pallidum* haemagglutination assay; RPR, rapid plasmin reagin.

give false-positive results in the presence of active herpes, measles, mumps, chronic autoimmune disease and rheumatoid arthritis, and also after immunization for typhoid or yellow fever.

EIA tests become positive soon after infection (3–4 weeks, similar to the FTA) and have the advantage of being easy to automate.

A guide to interpretation of tests is given in Table 63.2.

The UK Department of Health has reviewed the current practice of offering syphilis testing routinely for pregnant women, and has recommended that screening for syphilis should continue. EIA is gradually replacing VDRL/RPR and TPHA as a screening tool by recommendation of the UK Public Health Laboratory Service.

Management

Box 63.2 shows the guidelines of therapeutic regimens approved by BASHH in 2008 for the treatment of syphilis.

With parenteral therapy with penicillin, the Jarisch–Herxheimer reaction is common in both primary and secondary

Box 63.2 Guidelines of therapeutic regimens approved by BASHH in 2008 for the treatment of syphilis

Incubating syphilis/epidemiological treatment

- Benzathine penicillin G 2.4 MU intramuscularly, single dose.
- Doxycycline 100 mg orally twice daily for 14 days.
- Azithromycin 1 g orally stat.

Early syphilis (primary, secondary and early latent)

- Benzathine penicillin G 2.4 MU intramuscularly, single dose.
- Procaine penicillin G 600,000 units intramuscularly once daily for 10 days.

Alternative regimens may be required for those with penicillin allergy or refusing parenteral treatment

- Doxycycline 100 mg orally twice daily for 14 days.
- Azithromycin 2 g orally stat or 500 mg once daily for 10 days.
- Erythromycin 500 mg orally four times daily for 14 days.
- Ceftriaxone 500 mg intramuscularly once daily for 10 days (if no anaphylaxis to penicillin).
- Amoxycillin 500 mg orally four times daily plus probenecid 500 mg four times daily for 14 days.

Early syphilis in pregnancy

- Benzathine penicillin G 2.4 MU intramuscularly single dose in the first and second trimesters. When maternal treatment is initiated in the third trimester, a second dose of benzathine penicillin G 2.4 MU intramuscularly should be given after 1 week.
- Procaine penicillin G 600,000 unit intramuscularly once daily for 10 days.

Alternative regimens

- Amoxycillin 500 mg orally four times daily plus probenecid 500 mg orally four times daily for 14 days.
- Ceftriaxone 500 mg intramuscularly daily for 10 days.
- Erythromycin 500 mg orally four times daily for 14 days or azithromycin 500 mg orally once daily for 10 days plus evaluation and treatment of neonates at birth with penicillin.

Late/latent syphilis in pregnancy

- Benzathine penicillin 2.4 MU intramuscularly weekly for 2 weeks (three doses).
- Procaine penicillin 600,000 units intramuscularly once daily for 17 days.

Alternative regimens

- Amoxycillin 2 g orally three times daily plus probenecid 500 mg four times daily for 28 days.

syphilis. Patients should be warned about the possibility of flu-like illness after the first injection. The chancre may become larger initially or the rash may become more widespread. Reassurance and therapy with paracetamol and non-steroidal anti-inflammatory drugs are usually all that is necessary.

Congenital syphilis is preventable. Antenatal testing has always been cost-effective, and this is even more so with the increase in the prevalence of syphilis in the UK. *T. pallidum* can infect the fetus transplacentally at any time. This is less likely in late or latent syphilis (5%), but is very common in the first two stages (50%). In sub-Saharan Africa, it is associated with 25% of all stillbirths.

Lymphogranuloma Venereum

Aetiology

Lymphogranuloma venereum (LGV) is a systemic disease caused by one of three invasive serovars (L1, L2 or L3) of *C. trachomatis*, but other strains may occasionally be involved

LGV has been a rare occurrence in industrialized countries since the mid-1960s. Since 2003, however, a series of LGV outbreaks have been reported in several European cities, starting in the Netherlands. In the UK, more than 290 cases had been confirmed by December 2005. The majority of cases have been diagnosed in GUM clinics in London. At that time, all new cases were among male homosexuals, the majority of whom were HIV positive.

LGV is endemic in several tropical areas, including East, West and Southern Africa; Madagascar; India; South-east Asia; Papua New Guinea; and some Caribbean islands. A large epidemic has been reported recently among crack cocaine users in the Bahamas.

Clinical features

The clinical course of LGV is classically divided into three stages.

Primary lesion

The incubation period is extremely variable (range 3–30 days) from the time of sexual contact with an infected individual. The primary lesion is transient and often imperceptible, in the form of a painless papule or pustule, or a shallow erosion. It is found on the coronal sulcus of males, and on the posterior vaginal wall, fourchette, vulva or, occasionally, cervix of females. Extragenital lesions have been reported, such as in the oral cavity (tonsil) and extragenital lymph nodes.

Secondary lesion, lymphadenitis, or lymphadenopathy or bubo

The most common clinical manifestation of LGV is tender inguinal and/or femoral lymphadenopathy that is typically unilateral (two-thirds of cases). It may involve one lymph node or the entire chain, which can become matted with considerable periadenitis and bubo formation, and may ulcerate and discharge pus from multiple points, creating chronic fistulae. When both inguinal and femoral lymph nodes are involved, they may be separated by the 'groove sign', separation of these two lymph node systems by the inguinal ligament. Lymphadenopathy commonly follows the primary lesion by a period of a few days to weeks (10–30 days, rarely months). The systemic spread of *C. trachomatis* may be associated with fever, arthritis, pneumonitis and, more rarely, perihepatitis.

Tertiary stage or the genito–ano–rectal syndrome

The vast majority of patients recover after the secondary stage without sequelae. A few patients develop proctitis, acute proctocolitis mimicking Crohn's disease, fistulae, strictures and a chronic granulomatous disfiguring condition of the vulva.

Long-term complications

The destruction of lymph nodes may result in lymphoedema of genitals (elephantiasis) with persistent suppuration and pyoderma.

Diagnosis

Positive diagnosis of LGV is difficult, requiring a combination of good clinical acumen and supportive investigations. LGV can be suspected on positive chlamydial serology, isolation of *C. trachomatis* from the infected site or histological identification of chlamydia in infected tissue. Traditional methods for LGV diagnosis have been reviewed based on nucleic acid amplification tests (NAATs).

Chlamydiae are intracellular organisms, so samples must contain cellular material which can be obtained from the ulcer base exudate or from rectal tissue, or by aspiration from fluctuant lymph nodes or buboes. A urethral swab or first-catch urine (FCU) sample can be used when lymphadenopathy is present and LGV is suspected as the cause.

Treatment

- First choice: doxycycline 100 mg twice daily orally for 21 days (or tetracycline 2 g daily or minocycline 300 mg loading dose followed by 200 mg twice daily).
- Second choice: erythromycin 500 mg four times daily orally for 21 days.

Chancroid

Aetiology

An infection caused by *Haemophilus ducreyi*, the global distribution is similar to that of LGV. Co-infections of *H. ducreyi* with *T. pallidum* or HSV are frequent and occur in over 10% of patients in many African studies. Chancroid is characterized by painful anogenital ulceration (multiple) and lymphadenitis with progression to bubo formation. The incubation period ranges between 3 and 10 days, and the initial lesion may progress rapidly to form an open sore. There are no prodromal symptoms.

In males, most ulcers are found on the prepuce near the frenulum or in the coronal sulcus. In females, most lesions are found at the entrance of the vagina, particularly the fourchette. Several lesions may merge to form gigantic ulcers.

Diagnosis

The main methods revolve around the identification of *H. ducreyi* by: culture of material obtained from the ulcer base on specialized agar; detection of nucleic acid (DNA) by amplification techniques such as PCR; using nested techniques; microscopy of a Gram-stained smear (or other stains) of material from the ulcer base or of pus aspirate from the bubo; or demonstration of characteristic Gram-negative coccobacilli, with occasional characteristic chaining. The test has low sensitivity and is not recommended as a diagnostic test.

Treatment

- Azithromycin 1 g orally in a single dose.
- Ceftriaxone 250 mg intramuscularly in a single dose.
- Ciprofloxacin 500 mg orally in a single dose.
- Ciprofloxacin 500 mg orally twice daily for 3 days.
- Erythromycin 500 mg orally four times daily for 7 days.

Granuloma Inguinale (Donovanosis)

The following is a condensation of the 2001 guidelines for the management of donovanosis (granuloma inguinale) from the Clinical Effectiveness Group (Association for Genitourinary Medicine and the Medical Society for the Study of Venereal Diseases). This can be found on the BASHH website (http://www.bashh.org).

Aetiology

Donovanosis is seen chiefly in small endemic foci in tropical countries. In recent years, active foci of disease have been described in India, Papua New Guinea, the Caribbean, Brazil, the Guyanas, South Africa, Zambia, Vietnam and in Australian aboriginals. The causative organism, formerly *Calymmatobacterium granulomatis*, has recently been officially redesignated *Klebsiella granulomatis*.

Clinical features

At the site of primary inoculation, one or more papules/nodules develop into friable ulcers or hypertrophic lesions which gradually increase in size. Lesions do not tend to be painful. Regional lymphadenopathy is followed by either abscess formation (pseudobubo) or ulceration of the overlying skin. Untreated infections may either resolve spontaneously or persist and slowly spread. Primary lesions of mouth and cervix occur, and the latter have often been mistaken for malignant lesions. Complications include haemorrhage, genital lymphoedema, genital mutilation and cicatrization, development of squamous carcinoma and, on rare occasions, haematogenous dissemination to bone and viscera (particularly during pregnancy). Rare cases of vertical transmission have been reported. Lesions of the ears of infants are characteristic in such cases.

Diagnosis

The main method of diagnosis is the demonstration of Donovan bodies (Figure 63.7) in cellular material taken by scraping/impression smear/swab/crushing of pinched off tissue fragments on to a glass slide, or a tissue sample collected by biopsy. Either can be stained by Giemsa.

Management

- Azithromycin 1 g weekly or 500 mg daily.
- Ciprofloxacin 750 mg twice daily.
- Doxycycline 100 mg twice daily.
- Gentamicin (recommended by the US Centers for Disease Control and Prevention (CDC) as an adjunct to therapy in patients whose lesions do not respond in the first few days to other agents).

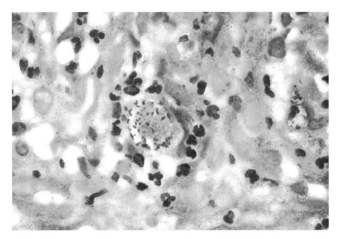

Figure 63.7 Granuloma inguinale: the histiocytes contain characteristic Donovan bodies (Warthin–Starry stain).
Image courtesy of W. Grayson MD, University of Witwatersrand, Johannesburg, South Africa.

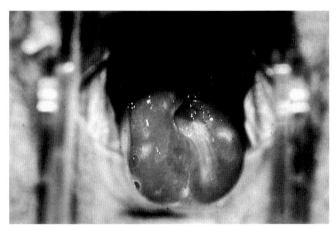

Figure 63.8 Gonococcal cervicitis: the purulent endocervical discharge.
From Cohen J et al., Infectious Diseases, 3e, with permission of Elsevier.

Treatment should continue until the lesions have healed. Healing times vary considerably between patients. The CDC recommends a minimum of 3 weeks.

Gonorrhoea

In the UK, cases of uncomplicated gonorrhoea increased by 42% between 1998 and 2007. Gonorrhoea is the clinical disease resulting from infection with the Gram-negative diplococcus *N. gonorrhoeae*. The primary sites of infection are the mucous membranes of the urethra, endocervix, rectum, pharynx and conjunctiva.

Clinical features

* Infection at the endocervix is frequently asymptomatic (up to 50%).
* Increased or altered vaginal discharge is the most common symptom (up to 50%).
* Lower abdominal pain may be present (up to 25%).
* Urethral infection may cause dysuria (12%) but not frequency.
* Gonorrhoea is a rare cause of intermenstrual bleeding or menorrhagia.
* Rectal infection more frequently develops by transmucosal spread of infected genital secretions than from anal intercourse, and is usually asymptomatic.
* Pharyngeal infection is usually asymptomatic (>90%).
* *N. gonorrhoeae* may coexist with other pathogens, notably *T. vaginalis*, *Candida albicans* and *C. trachomatis*. If symptoms are present, they may be attributable to the coinfecting pathogen.
* Mucopurulent endocervical discharge and easily induced endocervical bleeding (<50%) (see Figure 63.8).
* Pelvic/lower abdominal tenderness (<5%).
* Commonly, no abnormal findings are present on examination.

Transluminal spread of *N. gonorrhoeae* may occur from the urethra or endocervix to involve the epididymis and prostate

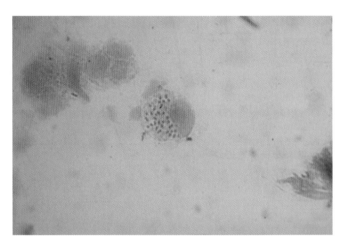

Figure 63.9 Gram-negative diplococci within polymorphonuclear leukocyte.

in men (≤1%), and the endometrium and pelvic organs in women (probably <10%). Haematogenous dissemination may also occur from infected mucous membranes, resulting in skin lesions, arthralgia, arthritis and tenosynovitis. Disseminated gonococcal infection is uncommon (<1%).

Diagnosis

The diagnosis is established by the identification of *N. gonorrhoeae* at an infected site. Culture offers a readily available, specific, sensitive and cheap diagnostic test that readily allows confirmatory identification and antimicrobial susceptibility testing. Alternative tests include NAATs and nucleic acid hybridization tests. NAATs are more sensitive than culture and can also be used as diagnostic/screening tests on non-invasively collected specimens (urine and self-taken vaginal swabs). The sensitivity of culture may be less than 75% for endocervical swabs.

Rapid diagnostic tests can be performed to facilitate immediate diagnosis and treatment. Microscopy (×1000) of Gram-stained genital specimens allows direct visualization of *N. gonorrhoeae* as Gram-negative diplococci within polymorphonuclear leukocytes (Figure 63.9).

Management

Referral to a GUM department for management is strongly encouraged. Patients should be given a detailed explanation of their condition with particular emphasis on the long-term implications for the health of themselves and their partner(s). This should be reinforced with clear and accurate written information. Patients should be advised to avoid unprotected sexual intercourse until they and their partner(s) have completed treatment.

Screening for coincident STIs should be performed routinely in patients with or at risk of gonorrhoea.

Treatment

- Ceftriaxone 250 mg intramuscularly as a single dose.
- Cefixime 400 mg orally as a single dose.
- Spectinomycin 2 g intramuscularly as a single dose.

Surveillance data for 2004 show significant levels of *N. gonorrhoeae* resistance to penicillin (11.2%), tetracyclines (44.5%) and ciprofloxacin (14.1%) in the UK. Most resistant infections are acquired in the UK. The following alternative regimens may be used when an infection is known to be sensitive to these antimicrobials or where the regional prevalence of resistance to them is less than 5%.

- Ciprofloxacin 500 mg orally as a single dose.
- Ofloxacin 400 mg orally as a single dose.
- Ampicillin 2 g or 3 g plus probenecid 1 g orally as a single dose.
- Cefotaxime 500 mg intramuscularly as a single dose.
- Cefoxitin 2 g intramuscularly as a single dose plus probenecid 1 g orally.

Clinicians using alternative regimens are recommended to review local antimicrobial sensitivity testing regularly with microbiology colleagues.

Pregnancy and breast feeding

Pregnant women should not be treated with quinolone or tetracycline antimicrobials.

Recommended regimes

- Ceftriaxone 250 mg intramuscularly as a single dose.
- Cefixime 400 mg orally as a single dose.
- Spectinomycin 2 g intramuscularly as a single dose.
- Amoxycillin 3 g.
- Ampicillin 2 g or 3 g plus probenecid 1 g orally as a single dose, where regional prevalence of penicillin-resistant *N. gonorrhoeae* is ≤5%.

Screening for *C. trachomatis* should be performed routinely on adults with gonorrhoea, or treatment should be given to eradicate possible coinfection. Combining effective antimicrobial therapy against *C. trachomatis* with single-dose therapy for gonococcal infection is particularly appropriate when there is doubt that a patient will return for follow-up evaluation.

Chlamydia

Chlamydia can have serious side-effects, one of which is PID which can lead to infertility and ectopic pregnancy in women. However, the disease can often be symptomless and therefore many people do not come forward to be tested.

New initiatives such as the National Chlamydia Screening Programme (NCSP) aim to control STIs through early detection and treatment. In particular, the NCSP targets sexually active people who might not normally have been tested for chlamydia. Nevertheless, there remains a vast number of people with chlamydia who do not know that they are infected.

Recent surveys of young women attending general practice clinics have reported prevalences of chlamydia of 8.1% among those under 20 years old and 5.2% among those aged 20–24 years. However, rates vary widely according to the setting in which the surveys take place. For example, among women under 20 years old, surveys have reported chlamydia prevalence of 17.3% in GUM clinics, 12.6% in antenatal clinics, 12.3% in TOP clinics, 10.7% in youth clinics, 10.0% in family planning clinics and 5.0% in the general population. In each setting, chlamydia prevalence is lower in higher age groups.

Between April 2005 and March 2006, the NCSP found chlamydia prevalences of 10.2% among women under 25 years old and 10.1% among men in the same age group. The NCSP uses a wide variety of non-GUM screening venues, including family planning clinics, general practice surgeries, prisons and military establishments. The rate peaked in the 16–19 years age group.

Aetiology

C. trachomatis is an obligate intracellular human pathogen. It is Gram-indeterminate (i.e. cannot be stained with the Gram stain), but structurally the organism is Gram-negative.

Chlamydia is the most common curable STI in the UK. It is frequently asymptomatic in both men and women, and ongoing transmission in the community is sustained by this unrecognized infection.

If untreated, infection may persist or resolve spontaneously. Two-thirds of sexual partners of chlamydia-positive individuals are also chlamydia-positive.

Clinical features

Chlamydia is asymptomatic in approximately 70% of infected women, but may cause any of the following: post-coital or intermenstrual bleeding, lower abdominal pain, purulent vaginal discharge, mucopurulent cervicitis (see Figure 63.10) and/or contact bleeding or dysuria. Rectal infections are usually asymptomatic, but may cause anal discharge and anorectal discomfort (proctitis).

Complications

In the absence of treatment, 10–40% of infected women will develop PID, with a significant proportion of these cases being asymptomatic or having mild, atypical symptoms. PID can result in tubal factor infertility, ectopic pregnancy and chronic pelvic pain. Other complications include Fitz–Hugh–Curtis syndrome (perihepatitis), transmission to neonate (neonatal conjunctivitis, pneumonia), epididymo-orchitis, adult conjunctivitis and sexually

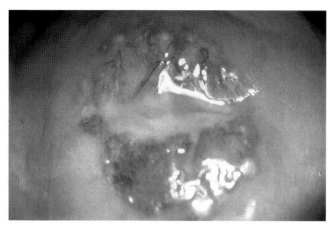

Figure 63.10 Chlamydia cervicitis: a purulent discharge and inflamed follicles are seen.

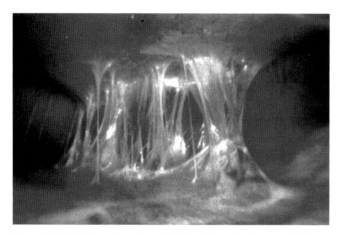

Figure 63.11 Chlamydia perihepatitis violin-string adhesions are visible.

acquired reactive arthritis/Reiter's syndrome (more common in men).

Diagnosis

Nucleic acid amplification technique

Although the technology for diagnosing chlamydia continues to be a rapidly developing field, the standard of care for all cases, including medicolegal cases, is a NAAT. NAATs are more sensitive and specific than EIAs. The Department of Health has advised that the use of suboptimal EIAs is no longer appropriate, and has provided funding to support laboratories moving from EIAs to NAATs. In general, NAATs are 90–95% sensitive.

If a speculum examination is not possible, urine samples can be utilized. Variable sensitivities (65–100%) have been reported using an FCU specimen. Patients should hold their urine for at least 1 h before providing an FCU specimen.

Cell culture

Sensitivity of 60–80%, specificity of 100% and expertise is essential. The routine use of cell culture is not recommended due to high cost and low sensitivity.

Enzyme immunoassays

The sensitivity of the majority of EIAs is probably only 40–70% and their use is not recommended.

Management

Uncomplicated genital tract infection with *C. trachomatis* is not an indication for removal of an intrauterine contraceptive device.

Recommended regimens

- Doxycycline 100 mg twice daily for 7 days (contraindicated in pregnancy).
- Azithromycin 1 g orally in a single dose.

Alternative regimens

For use if either of the above treatments are contraindicated.

- Erythromycin 500 mg twice daily for 10–14 days.
- Ofloxacin 200 mg twice daily or 400 mg once daily for 7 days.

Erythromycin is less efficacious than either azithromycin or doxycycline. When taken four times daily, 20–25% of cases may experience side-effects sufficient to cause the patient to discontinue treatment. Oxytetracycline 500 mg twice daily for 10 days has also been shown to be effective.

Pregnancy and breast feeding

- Erythromycin 500 mg four times daily for 7 days.
- Erythromycin 500 mg twice daily for 14 days.
- Amoxicillin 500 mg three times daily for 7 days.
- Azithromycin 1 g stat.

A test of cure is not routinely recommended but should be performed in pregnancy or if non-compliance or re-exposure is suspected. It should be deferred for 5 weeks (6 weeks if azithromycin given) after treatment is completed.

Mycoplasma genitalium and *Ureaplasma urealyticum*

Mycoplasma (including *Ureaplasma urealyticum*) are small and have no cell wall. They are Gram negative and are difficult to culture. There are no commercially available tests. PCR is sometimes used for their detection.

Aetiology

Mucopurulent cervicitis is the female equivalent of non-gonococcal urethritis (NGU), 40% of cases being due to infection with *C. trachomatis*. *Mycoplasma genitalium* is an unproven cause of PID.

There are a number of uncertainties with NGU in men. Urethral inflammation can occur without a known pathogen being isolated in the majority of patients, even using more sensitive detection methods. The most common organisms implicated are *C. trachomatis* and *M. genitalium*, with the latter perhaps causing more symptoms. In 30–80% of cases with NGU, neither *C. trachomatis* nor *M. genitalium* is detected. The exact role of ureaplasmas in NGU has been controversial due to the conflicting observations in clinical studies. Ureaplasmas are ubiquitous micro-organisms which have recently been divided into two biovars; *U. urealyticum* biovar 2 may account for 5–10% of cases of acute NGU. There is no clear indication for its treatment in women.

Management

The importance of evaluation and treatment of sexual partners is stressed in cases of NGU as *C. trachomatis* may be detected in the woman.

Treatment

Treatment as for *C. trachomatis* will eradicate *Mycoplasma* spp. including ureaplasma. However, it seems that resistant strains are emerging.

Genital Warts (Condylomata Accuminata)

Aetiology

The causative organism is the HPV (a DNA virus of the papovavirus group), especially types 6 and 11 (also 16, 18, 31, 33 and 35). Subclinical infection is extremely common, and trigger factors for an eruption of warts are not known. Occasionally in pregnancy, they may become very large and confluent. In men, similar giant and destructive warts may appear on the penis (Buschke–Löwenstein tumour) associated with types 6 and 11.

Cervical dysplasia and subsequent carcinoma is strongly associated with types 16 and 18; these types are associated with 70% of cervical cancers. Types 31, 33 and 35 represent the majority of other cases. Whilst cervical warts are seen in 10% of women with obvious warts elsewhere in the anogenital area, one-third will have evidence of wart infection on cytology or at colposcopic examination. In terms of risk for cervical cancer, the greatest threat seems to be from latent or subclinical infections with types 16 and 18.

Diagnosis

Between 1998 and 2007, the diagnosis of genital warts rose by 28%. The diagnosis is solely on clinical appearance. Warts in women are most commonly found on the vulva, but may appear anywhere in the anogenital area. They are usually painless. The presence of another STI is common (25%), and a full screen should be undertaken (see Figures 63.12 and 63.13).

Prevention

A decision by the UK Department of Health to introduce vaccination against HPV types 16 and 18 (Cervarix) was taken in October 2007. This decision follows the advice of the Joint Committee on Vaccination and Immunisation which, based on a detailed review of evidence surrounding HPV vaccination, recommended the routine vaccination of girls aged 12–13 years, recommended a catch-up programme of girls under the age of 18 years, and acknowledged that the evidence that a catch-up programme for all women aged 18–25 years was unlikely to be cost-effective but could benefit some individual women. The Department of Health will consider this further.

Two vaccines, Cervarix and Gardasil, were competing for the contract. Both vaccines demonstrate highly effective protection against HPV 16 and 18, which are responsible for the majority of cases of cervical cancer. However, only one of the vaccines, Gardasil, protects against HPV types 6 and 11, as well as 16 and 18.

Treatment

Surface applications

Treatment choice depends on the morphology, number and distribution of warts, and patient preference. The evidence base to direct first- and second-line treatments is not strong. All treatments have significant failure and relapse rates. Treatment may involve discomfort and local skin reactions. Written information on the management of treatment side-effects is recommended.

Soft non-keratinized warts respond well to podophyllin, podophyllotoxin and trichloroacetic acid (TCA). Keratinized lesions are better treated with physical ablative methods such as cryotherapy, excision or electrocautery. Imiquimod may be suitable for both keratinized and non-keratinized warts. People with a small number of low-volume warts, irrespective of type, are best treated with ablative therapy from the outset.

Practitioners should consider developing a treatment algorithm or protocol. This has been shown to improve clinical outcome significantly.

Podophyllin is a non-standardized cytotoxic compound and is no longer recommended for use. It has been associated with severe local reactions. Serious systemic adverse events have occurred when used outside guidelines. Best practice described in the British National Formulary recommends supervised application in GUM clinics or general practice by trained nurses after screening for other STIs. Animal experiments indicate teratogenic and oncogenic properties. It should be avoided in pregnancy and not used on the cervix or anal canal. A 15–25% solution can be carefully applied to lesions, in clinic, once or twice weekly and washed off 4 h later.

Podophyllotoxin, a purified extract of podophyllin in the form of a 0.5% solution or 0.15% cream, is suitable for home treatment; supervision by medical staff is recommended for larger lesions. Podophyllotoxin has a license for the treatment of genital warts, but not extragenital lesions such as anal warts. Treatment cycles consist of twice-daily application for 3 days, followed by 4 days of rest for four to five cycles. Unprotected sexual contact should be avoided soon after application because of a possible irritant effect on the partner. Podophyllotoxin should be avoided in pregnancy.

TCA 80–90% solution is suitable for weekly application in a specialist clinic setting only. It acts as a caustic agent, resulting in cellular necrosis. An intense burning sensation may be experienced for 5–10 min after application. Ulceration penetrating into the dermis may occur, and it is

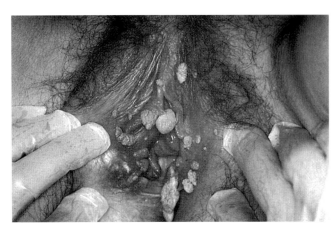

Figure 63.12 Vulval warts.
Courtesy of Dr I H Ahmed.

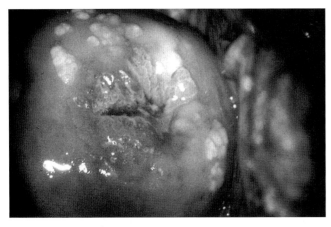

Figure 63.13 Cervical warts.

therefore not recommended for large-volume warts. TCA can be used at most anatomical sites.

TCA is extremely corrosive to the skin. Careful application and protection of the surrounding skin with petroleum jelly is recommended. A neutralizing agent (e.g. sodium bicarbonate) should always be available in case of excess application or spills.

5-Fluorouracil is a DNA antimetabolite, available in a 5% cream. Its use is limited by severe local side-effects, which may result in long-term problems such as neovascularization and vulval burning. It may be teratogenic and therefore should not be used in pregnancy. As satisfactory alternatives exist, this treatment is no longer recommended for the routine management of anogenital warts.

Various regimens have been described using interferons α, β and γ as creams and as intralesional or systemic injections. Their use is limited by expense, systemic side-effects and a variable response rate. Cyclical low-dose injection used as an adjunct to laser therapy has resulted in a lower relapse rate. Interferons are not recommended for routine management of anogenital warts and should only be used on expert advice.

Imiquimod is an immune response modifier. Available as a 5% cream, it induces a cytokine response when applied to skin infected with HPV. It is suitable for use on all external lesions, but is not recommended for use in pregnancy or

internally. It should be applied to lesions three times weekly and washed off 6–10 h later for up to 16 weeks. Unprotected sexual contact should be avoided soon after application because of a possible irritant effect on the partner. Latex condoms may be weakened if they come into contact with imiquimod.

Physical ablation

Removal of warts under local anaesthetic injection is particularly useful for pedunculated warts, and small numbers of keratinized warts at anatomically accessible sites. The use of an anaesthetic cream prior to injection is recommended. Treatment can be repeated as required. This is a good method of treatment for small numbers of warts and may be underused.

Cryotherapy using a liquid nitrogen spray or a cryoprobe causes cytolysis at the dermal epidermal junction resulting in necrosis. Treatment should be applied until a 'halo' of freezing has been established a few millimetres round the treated lesion. A freeze, thaw, freeze technique should be used and lesions held frozen for 10–30 s, depending upon size.

Electrocautery results in burning of the treatment site and surrounding tissue.

Hyfrecator acts by electrofulgaration resulting in superficial charring and little dermal damage or, for deeper tissue penetration, electrodessication. This can be followed by curettage.

For monopolar surgery, different waveforms can be generated allowing desiccation, cutting or coagulation. This results in a cleaner cut and less damage to surrounding tissue (note: skin bridges should be left between treatment sites to aid healing and minimize scarring).

Laser treatment

The carbon dioxide laser is especially suitable for large-volume warts and can be used at difficult anatomical sites, such as the urethral meatus or anal canal.

All electrosurgical and laser techniques result in a plume of smoke which has been shown to contain HPV DNA, which may potentially cause infection of the respiratory tract in operating personnel. Therefore, masks should be worn and adequate extraction should be provided during these procedures.

The NHS Cervical Screening Programme does not recommend colposcopy in women with genital warts, including those with cervical lesions, unless there is diagnostic uncertainty or clinical concern. Additional cervical cytology is not recommended.

Pregnancy

Podophyllin, podophyllotoxin and 5-fluorouracil should be avoided because of possible teratogenic effects. Imiquimod is not approved for use in pregnancy. Treatment aims to minimize the number of lesions present at delivery to reduce exposure of the neonate to the virus. Potential problems for offspring are the development of laryngeal papillomatosis and anogenital warts. Very rarely, a CS is indicated because of obstruction of the vaginal outlet with warts or the presence of gross cervical warts. CS is not indicated to prevent laryngeal papillomatosis/anogenital warts in the neonate, as both conditions are rare.

Immunosuppressed patients

People with impaired cell-mediated immunity (e.g. organ transplant patients or those with HIV infection) are likely to have poor treatment responses, increased relapse rates and an increased risk of developing anogenital intraepithelial neoplasia.

Molluscum Contagiosum

Aetiology and clinical features

Molluscum contagiosum is a benign viral skin infection most commonly seen in children. However, sexual contact in adults may lead to the appearance of lesions in the genital area. The condition is harmless.

Molluscum contagiosum is caused by a pox virus passed on by direct skin-to-skin contact, and may affect any part of the body. There is anecdotal evidence associating facial lesions with HIV-related immunodeficiency.

After an incubation period of 3–12 weeks, discrete, pearly, papular, smooth or umbilicated lesions appear (Figure 63.10). In immunocompetent individuals, the size of the lesions seldom exceeds 5 mm, and if untreated, there is usually spontaneous regression after several months. Secondary bacterial infection may result if lesions are scratched. In the immunocompromised, lesions may become large and exuberant, and secondary infection may be problematic. As other STIs may coexist, a full screen for these should be undertaken. HIV testing is recommended in patients presenting with facial lesions.

Treatment

Cryotherapy: liquid nitrogen should be applied until a halo of ice surrounds the lesion. Repeat applications may be necessary. The pearly core should be expressed either manually or using forceps, and the lesion can be pierced with an orange stick with or without the application of tincture of iodine or phenol. Curettage or diathermy may be carried out under local anaesthesia.

In patients with HIV infection, the introduction of highly active antiretroviral therapy may lead to resolution of lesions. Contact tracing of partners is unnecessary.

Viral Hepatitis

It should be noted that viral hepatitis is a notifiable disease in the UK, irrespective of the causative virus. Characteristics of the known hepatitis viruses are shown in Table 63.3.

Hepatitis A

Hepatitis A is caused by a picorna (RNA) virus, and is particularly common in areas of the world where sanitation is poor. It largely affects children, although 784 cases were reported in England and Wales in 2004.

Transmission can be oral (via food, water, close personal contact), by anal or digital-rectal contact, and via contaminated batches of factor VIII. The incubation period lasts 15–45 days. Most children and up to half of adults are asymptomatic or have mild non-specific symptoms with little or no jaundice. In clinical cases, there are two phases of symptoms: flu-like symptoms (malaise, myalgia, fatigue), often with right upper abdominal pain, which last for 3–10

Table 63.3 Characteristics of the known hepatitis viruses

Hepatitis virus	Transmission	Clinical features	Chronic infection
A	Faecal-oral	Silent in 90%	No
	Oroanal in homosexual men	Fulminant hepatitis very rare	
B	Parenteral	Silent in 90%	10% in adults
	Sexual	Children more often asymptomatic	90% in perinatal infection
	Vertical		
	Horizontal in endemic areas	Fulminant hepatitis in 1%	Can lead to: Chronic active hepatitis Cirrhosis Hepatocellular carcinoma
C	Parenteral	Silent in 95%	60%
	Sexual transmission uncommon	Fulminant hepatitis very rare	Chronic hepatitis Cirrhosis Hepatocellular carcinoma
D	Parenteral	Coinfection or superinfection with hepatitis B	60%
	Sexual		Effects as for HBV
	Only in those infected with HBV	Fulminant hepatitis 20%	
E	Faecal-oral	? limited to Africa/Asia	No
	Oroanal possible	Fulminant hepatitis common in pregnant women (10%)	

days; followed by anorexia, nausea and fatigue, which usually lasts for 1–3 weeks. It can persist for 12 or more weeks in a minority of patients who have cholestatic symptoms (itching and deep jaundice). Fever is not found in this phase. There may be jaundice with pale stools and dark urine. Liver enlargement/tenderness and signs of dehydration are also common.

Fifteen percent of patients may require hospital care, of whom one-quarter will have severe hepatitis (prothrombin time >3 s prolonged, or bilirubin >170 mmol/l). The infection does not have any teratogenic effects but there is an increased rate of miscarriage and premature labour, proportional to the severity of the illness. There have been case reports of possible vertical transmission.

Serology

Measurement of specific IgM (HAV-IgM) is best and remains positive for 6 months or more. HAV-IgG does not distinguish between current or past infection, and may remain positive for life.

Screening should be undertaken for other STIs in cases of sexually acquired hepatitis or if otherwise appropriate.

Hepatitis A vaccine may be given up to 14 days after exposure, providing exposure was within the infectious period of the source case (during the prodromal illness or first week of jaundice).

Hepatitis B

Hepatitis B is caused by an hepadna (DNA) virus. It is endemic worldwide with very high carriage rates (up to 20%), particularly in South and East Asia, but also in Southern Europe, Central and South America, Africa and Eastern Europe. In the UK, carriage varies from 0.01–0.04% in blood donors to more than 1% in intravenous drug users and homosexual men. In 2003, 1151 cases were notified in England and Wales. There are eight distinct genotypes (A–H) which vary in geographical distribution, pathogenicity and treatment susceptibility.

Transmission occurs in immune men who have sex with men and correlates with multiple partners, unprotected anal sex and oroanal sex. Transmission also occurs after heterosexual contact (e.g. 18% infection rates for regular partners of patients with acute hepatitis B). Sex workers are also at higher risk, as are intravenous drug users. Vertical transmis-

sion of infection occurs in 90% of pregnancies where the mother is hepatitis B e antigen positive, and in approximately 10% of surface-antigen-positive, e-antigen-negative mothers. Most (>90%) infected infants become chronic carriers. Infants born to infectious mothers are vaccinated from birth, usually in combination with hepatitis-B-specific immunoglobulin 200 iu intramuscularly; this reduces vertical transmission by 90%.

Asymptomatic infection is also found in 10–50% of adults in the acute phase and is especially likely in those with HIV coinfection. Chronic carriers are usually asymptomatic but may have fatigue or loss of appetite. The prodromal and icteric phases are very similar to hepatitis A, but may be more severe and prolonged.

Fulminant hepatitis occurs in less than 1% of symptomatic cases but carries a worse prognosis than that caused by hepatitis A. Concurrent hepatitis C infection can lead to fulminant hepatitis, more aggressive chronic hepatitis and increased risk of liver cancer.

If chronic infection occurs (as it does in 5–10% of symptomatic cases, higher in the immunocompromised), there are often no physical signs. After many years of infection, depending on the severity and duration, there may be signs of chronic liver disease including spider naevi, finger clubbing, jaundice and hepatosplenomegaly, and in severe cases, thin skin, bruising, ascites, liver flap and encephalopathy.

Mortality is less than 1% for acute cases. Between 10% and 50% of chronic carriers will develop cirrhosis, leading to premature death in approximately half. Ten percent or more of cirrhotic patients will progress to liver cancer.

Concurrent HIV infection increases the risk of progression to cirrhosis and death.

The serology profiles are shown in Table 63.4.

Patients should be advised to avoid unprotected sexual intercourse until they have become non-infectious or their partners have been successfully vaccinated. They should have a full STI screen. Further management is undertaken by hepatologists or physicians with experience in the management of hepatitis.

Hepatitis B testing in asymptomatic patients should be considered in men who have sex with men, sex workers (of either sex), injecting drug users, HIV-positive patients, sexual assault victims, people from countries where hepatitis B is common, and women attending antenatal clinics. If patients are non-immune, vaccination should be considered. If

Table 63.4 Hepatitis B serology: interpretation of common results

	HBsAg	Anti HBs	Anti HBc	Anti HBc-IgM	HBeAg	Anti HBe
Never infected	–	–	–			
Immune after vaccination	–	+	–			
Immune after infection	–	+	+			
Acute infection (early)	+	–	–	–	±	–
Acute infection (late)	+	–	+	+	+	–
Chronic infection (high infectivity)	+	–	+	±	+	–
Chronic infection (low infectivity)	+	–	+	–	–	+

Source: Gibson R 2004 Viral hepatitis. In: Adler M, Cowan F, French P, Mitchell H, Richens J (eds) ABC of Sexually Transmitted Infections, 5th edn. BMJ Books, London.

patients are found to be chronic carriers, referral for therapy should be considered. The simplest initial screening test in someone who is unvaccinated or is of unknown infection status is anti-hepatitis B core antigen, with the addition of other tests as necessary. Some also screen for hepatitis B surface antigen initially.

Hepatitis D

This is caused by a defective RNA virus which cannot thrive in the absence of chronic hepatitis B. In such patients, the clinical course is severe. Simultaneous coinoculation with hepatitis B usually resolves. Hepatitis D may be acquired sexually but the population at greatest risk is intravenous drug users. Diagnosis is by antibody assay. The management belongs properly in the hands of hepatologists.

Hepatitis C

Hepatitis C is another RNA virus causing chronic hepatitis. It may be transmitted sexually but this has proved inefficient with less than 5% of long-term partners becoming infected. Injecting drug users are the highest risk group. Vertical transmission is rare but the risk increases if there is coexisting HIV infection. Exposure to the virus from contaminated blood and blood products used in health care has been eliminated. There is no vaccine. Diagnosis is on serology; however, an antibody response may be delayed by up to 4 weeks so the test may need repeating. The management is undertaken by hepatologists and the virus may be cleared by combination therapy with interferon and ribavirin.

Hepatitis E

Hepatitis E is an RNA virus which usually causes an acute and self-limiting infection. It is spread by orofaecal transmission. It has a high mortality rate in pregnant women (17–30%). It causes sporadic cases and waterborne epidemics in the Indian subcontinent, South-east and Central Asia, Africa and North America. Cases in the UK are usually only seen in travellers returning from these areas. It is detected on serology.

Vaginal Infections

The acidic milieu of the vagina (pH 4.5) is maintained by lactobacilli (Döderlein's) which accounts for 95% of the bacteria found in the normal vaginal flora. This inhibits the overgrowth of other vaginal commensals under normal conditions. The substrate for lactic acid production is glycogen in the vaginal squamous cells, which is itself dependent upon the presence of oestrogen. Thus, prepubertal girls, pregnant women and postmenopausal women may have increased vaginal pH. Another more direct cause of increasing vaginal pH is the practice of douching, which should be discouraged. Smokers also have increased vaginal pH. The differential diagnoses of the common causes of vaginal discharge are summarized in Table 63.5.

Bacterial vaginosis

An elevation in pH may allow other commensals of the vagina to replicate in greater quantity and this may result in bacterial vaginosis. This is a common cause of attendance at GUM clincs, as it is mistaken by the woman as a possible STI, which it is not. The prevalence in the UK is of the order of 15% but it may be under-reported.

Bacterial vaginosis is characterized by an overgrowth of predominantly anaerobic organisms (*Gardnerella vaginalis*, *Prevotella* spp., *Mycoplasma hominis*, *Mobiluncus* spp.) in the vagina, leading to replacement of lactobacilli and an increase in pH from less than 4.5 to as high as 7.0.

Clinical features and complications

There is an offensive fishy smelling, thin, white vaginal discharge not associated with soreness, itching or irritation. However, in many women (approximately 50%), bacterial vaginosis is asymptomatic (see Figure 63.14).

The prevalence of bacterial vaginosis is high in women with PID, and it is common in some populations of women undergoing elective TOP, and associated with post-TOP endometritis and PID. In pregnancy, bacterial vaginosis is associated with late miscarriage, preterm birth, preterm premature rupture of the membranes and postpartum endometritis.

Diagnosis

Two approaches are available.

Amsel criteria

At least three of the following four criteria need to be present for the diagnosis to be confirmed.

Table 63.5 Differential diagnosis of the common causes of vaginal discharge

Symptoms and signs	Candidiasis	Bacterial vaginosis	Trichomoniasis	Cervicitis
Itching or soreness	++	–	+++	–
Smell	May be yeasty	Offensive, fishy	May be offensive	–
Colour	White	White or yellow	Yellow or green	Clear or coloured
Consistency	Curdy	Thin, homogeneous	Thin, homogeneous	Mucoid
pH	<4.5	4.5–7.0	4.5–7.0	<4.5
Confirmed by	Microscopy and culture	Microscopy	Microscopy and culture	Microscopy, tests for chlamydia and gonorrhoea

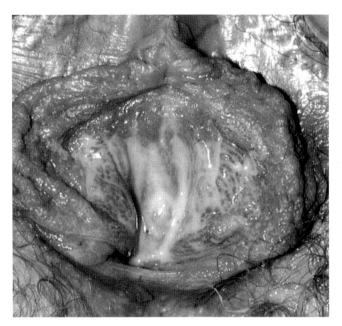

Figure 63.14 Bacterial vaginosis.

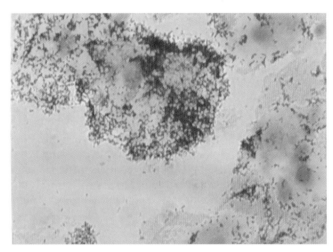

Figure 63.15 Clue cells: vaginal squamous cells covered in bacteria.
Image courtesy of Dr I.H. Ahmed, Nottingham University Hospitals, UK.

- Thin, white, homogeneous discharge.
- Clue cells (Figure 63.15) on microscopy of wet mount.
- pH of vaginal fluid >4.5.
- Release of a fishy odour on adding alkali (10% potassium hydroxide).

Gram-stained vaginal smear

This is evaluated with the Hay (note: not the author)/Ison criteria or the Nugent criteria. The Hay/Ison criteria are defined as follows.

- Grade 1 (normal): lactobacillus morphotypes predominate.
- Grade 2 (intermediate): mixed flora with some lactobacilli present, but gardnerella or mobiluncus morphotypes also present.

- Grade 3 (bacterial vaginosis): predominantly gardnerella and/or mobiluncus morphotypes. Few or absent lactobacilli.

Management

Patients should be advised to avoid vaginal douching, use of shower gel, and use of antiseptic agents or shampoo in the bath. Treatment is indicated for symptomatic women, and women undergoing some surgical procedures and women who do not volunteer symptoms may elect to take treatment if offered. They may report a beneficial change in their discharge following treatment. Metronidazole 400–500 mg twice daily for 5–7 days or 2 g as a single dose is most commonly prescribed. Alternative regimens are intravaginal metronidazole gel (0.75%) once daily for 5 days, intravaginal clindamycin cream (2%) once daily for 7 days, clindamycin 300 mg twice daily for 7 days or tinidazole 2 g single dose. All these treatments have been shown to achieve cure rates of 70–80% after 4 weeks.

Clindamycin cream can weaken condoms, which should not be used during such treatment. Symptomatic pregnant women should be treated as above. A test of cure is not required if symptoms resolve.

There are few published studies evaluating the optimal approach to women with frequent recurrences of bacterial vaginosis. Possible approaches being evaluated include metronidazole gel 0.75% twice weekly for 4–6 months to decrease symptoms, after an initial treatment daily for 10 days, or metronidazole orally 400 mg twice daily for 3 days at the start and end of menstruation, combined with fluconazole 150 mg as a single dose if there is also a history of candidiasis.

Small studies of live yoghurt or *Lactobacillus acidophilus* have not demonstrated benefit.

Candidiasis

This is a common non-STI cause of infective vaginal discharge that will affect approximately 75% of women at some stage during their reproductive life.

Aetiology and clinical features

The causative agent is *C. albicans* in 80–92% of cases. Non-albicans species (e.g. *C. glabrata*, *C. tropicalis*, *C. krusei*, *C. parapsilosis* and *Saccharomyces cerevisiae*) account for the remainder of cases.

Vulval itch and/or soreness, vaginal discharge (typically curdy but may be thin, non-offensive), superficial dyspareunia and external dysuria are common complaints. There may be erythema, fissuring, oedema, satellite lesions and excoriation. None of these symptoms or signs are pathognomonic for vulvovaginal candidiasis. Many women may have other conditions, such as dermatitis, allergic reactions and lichen sclerosus. In addition, symptoms/signs are no guide to species (see Figure 63.16).

Ten to twenty percent of women of reproductive age may be colonized with *Candida* spp. but have no clinical signs or symptoms. These women do not require treatment.

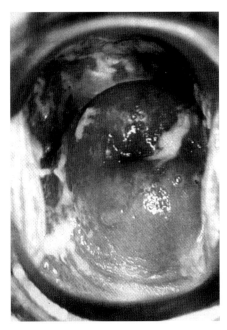

Figure 63.16 Candida vaginitis: note the thick adherent discharge.

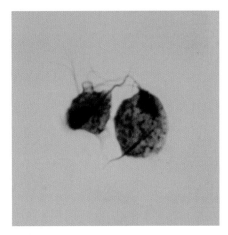

Figure 63.17 *Trichomonas vaginalis.*

Diagnosis

In the context of comprehensive sexual health services, routine microscopy and culture is the standard. A vaginal swab should be taken from the anterior fornix for a Gram or wet film examination. This should be directly plated to solid fungal media. Speciation is essential if complicated disease is present.

Since all topical and oral azole therapies give a clinical and mycological cure rate of over 80% in uncomplicated acute vulvovaginal candidiasis, choice is a matter of personal preference, availability and affordability. Topical azole therapies can cause vulvovaginal irritation, and this should be considered if symptoms worsen or persist. In pregnancy, oral azole therapy is contraindicated.

Recurrent vulvovaginal candidiasis (occurs in 5% of women of reproductive age) is defined as at least four documented episodes of symptomatic vulvovaginal candidiasis annually. Positive microscopy or a moderate/heavy growth of *C. albicans* should be documented on at least two occasions when symptomatic.

Candidiasis is usually caused by host factors (e.g. uncontrolled diabetes mellitus, immunosuppression, hyperoestrogenaemia (e.g. hormone replacement therapy) and the combined oral contraceptive pill) rather than a more virulent strain or reintroduction of the organism to the genital tract. Occasionally, it is due to disturbance of vaginal flora, such as through use of broad-spectrum antibiotics.

Vulval emollients may give symptomatic relief. High-oestrogen contraceptives should be avoided, or consideration given to changing to a non-oestrogenic form of contraception.

Fluconazole may be given to suppress recurrences in regimes up to and including once weekly for 6 months. Topical imidazole therapy can be increased to 10–14 days according to symptomatic response.

In general, longer courses may be needed for non-albicans infection although there are no data on optimum duration; 2 weeks is suggested. There is no comparative evidence for different treatments. A suggested alternative is nystatin (a polyene); these pessaries are the only licensed alternative to azole therapy, and are therefore the usual first-line treatment for non-albicans infection.

Trichomoniasis

Aetiology and clinical features

T. vaginalis is a flagellate protozoan (Figure 63.17). In women, the organism is found in the vagina, urethra and paraurethral glands. While the urinary tract is the sole site of infection in less than 5% of cases, urethral infection is present in 90% of episodes. In adults, transmission is almost exclusively sexual. Due to site specificity, infection can only follow intravaginal or intraurethral inoculation of the organism.

Ten to fifty percent of infected women are asymptomatic. In those with symptoms, these include vaginal discharge, vulval itching, dysuria or offensive odour. Occasionally, the presenting complaint is low abdominal discomfort.

Vaginal discharge occurs in up to 70% of cases, varying in consistency from thin and scanty to profuse and thick; the classical frothy yellow discharge occurs in 10–30% of women. Approximately 2% of patients will have strawberry cervix appearance to the naked eye. Higher rates are seen on colposcopic examination. No abnormalities will be seen in 5–15% of women on examination.

There is increasing evidence that *T. vaginalis* infection can have a detrimental outcome on pregnancy, and is associated with preterm delivery and low birth weight. However, further research is needed to confirm causality. Moreover, recent trials have found that treatment does not improve pregnancy outcome, and may be harmful. Screening of asymptomatic individuals for *T. vaginalis* infection is therefore not currently recommended (see Figure 63.18A,B).

Diagnosis

Direct observation by wet mount or acridine orange staining is approximately 70% sensitive compared with culture in

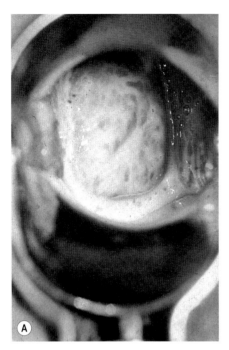
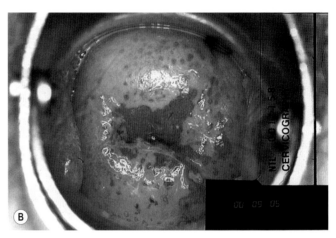

Figure 63.18 Trichomonas: (A) grey watery discharge, (B) strawberry cervix with petechial haemorrhage.

females. Microscopy for *T. vaginalis* should be performed as soon as possible after the sample is taken, as motility diminishes with time.

Culture techniques are still regarded as the most sensitive and specific. Culture media vary in efficiency, but Diamond's TYM medium (or modified version) is among the best.

PCR-based diagnostic tests have been developed recently, and sensitivities and specificities approaching 100% have been reported. No PCR assay for *T. vaginalis* is currently on the market.

Trichomonads are sometimes reported on cervical cytology; however, a meta-analysis has shown that while it has good specificity, the weighted mean sensitivity was only 58%. In such cases, it is prudent to confirm the diagnosis, preferably by culture of vaginal secretions.

Management and treatment

Sexual partner(s) should be treated simultaneously. Patients should be advised to avoid sexual intercourse (including oral sex) until they and their partner(s) have completed treatment and follow-up.

Screening for coexistent STIs should be undertaken in both men and women.

The frequency of infection of the urethra and paraurethral glands in females dictates that systemic chemotherapy should be given to effect a permanent cure. Most strains of *T. vaginalis* are highly susceptible to metronidazole and related drugs (approximately 95% cure rate). There is a spontaneous cure rate of the order of 20–25%.

Recommended regimens

- Metronidazole 2 g orally in a single dose.
- Metronidazole 400–500 mg twice daily for 5–7 days — most commonly prescribed with tinidazole

2 g orally in a single dose as an alternative regimen.

Patients should be advised not to take alcohol for the duration of treatment and for at least 48 h afterwards because of the possibility of a disulfiram-like (Antabuse effect) reaction.

The British National Formulary advises against high-dose regimens in pregnancy.

Patients who fail to respond to the first course of treatment often respond to a repeat course of standard treatment. Current partners should be screened for the full range of STIs and treated for *T. vaginalis* irrespective of the results of investigations.

Trichomonas infection may be acquired perinatally and occurs in approximately 5% of babies born to infected mothers. Infection beyond the first year of life should suggest sexual contact.

Ectoparasitic Infestations

Pediculosis pubis (Phthirus pubis)

Aetiology and clinical features

The crab louse *Phthirius pubis* (Figure 63.19) is transmitted by close body contact. The incubation period is usually between 5 days and several weeks, although occasional individuals appear to have more prolonged, asymptomatic infestation.

Adult lice infest coarse hairs of the pubic area, body hair and, rarely, eyebrows and eyelashes. Eggs (nits) are laid which adhere to the hairs. There may be no symptoms or there may be itching due to hypersensitivity to feeding lice. Blue macules (maculae caeruleae) may be visible at feeding sites.

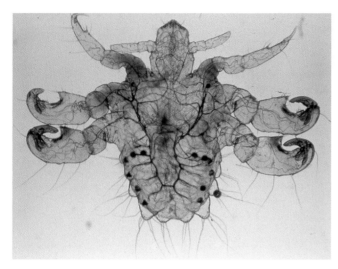

Figure 63.19 The crab louse: *Phthirius pubis* or *Pediculosis pubis*.
Source: World Health Organization.

Diagnosis

Diagnosis is based on finding adult lice and/or eggs. Examination under light microscopy can confirm the morphology if necessary.

Management and treatment

Patients should be advised to avoid close body contact until they and their partner(s) have completed treatment and follow-up. A full screen for other STIs should be undertaken.

Lotions are likely to be more effective than shampoos, and should be applied to all body hair including the beard and moustache if necessary. A second application after 3–7 days is advised.

Agents used

- Malathion 0.5%: apply to dry hair and wash out after at least 2 h, and preferably 12 h (i.e. overnight).
- Permethrin 1% cream rinse: apply to damp hair and wash out after 10 min.
- Phenothrin 0.2%: apply to dry hair and wash out after 2 h.
- Carbaryl 0.5 and 1% (unlicensed indication): apply to dry hair and wash out 12 h later.

Infestation of eyelashes can be treated with permethrin 1% lotion, keeping the eyes closed during the 10-min application. Alternatively, an inert ophthalmic ointment with a white or yellow paraffin base such as simple eye ointment BP may be applied to the eyelashes twice daily for 8–10 days. This works by suffocating lice and avoids any risk of eye irritation by topical insecticide.

Permethrin is safe during pregnancy and breast feeding

Current sexual partners should be examined and treated. Contact tracing of partners from the previous 3 months should be undertaken. Patients should be re-examined for absence of lice after 1 week. Treatment failures should be given an alternative from the above list. It should be explained to patients that dead nits may remain adherent to hairs. This does not imply treatment failure, and the nits can be removed with a comb designed specifically for the purpose.

Scabies

Aetiology and clinical features

The infestation is caused by the mite *Sarcoptes scabiei*. Mites burrow into the skin where they lay eggs, the resulting offspring crawl out on to the skin and make new burrows. Any part of the body may be affected, and transmission is by skin-to-skin contact. The absorption of mite excrement into skin capillaries generates a hypersensitivity reaction. The main symptom, which may take 4–6 weeks to develop, is generalized itch, especially at night.

Characteristic silvery lines may be seen in the skin where mites have burrowed. Classic sites include the interdigital folds, the wrists, elbows and around the nipples in women. Papules or nodules that may result from itching often affect the genital area. In HIV infection, crusted lesions that teem with mites (Norwegian scabies) pose a significant risk of transmission to others.

Secondary infection of the skin lesions can occur following repeated scratching. The clinical appearance is usually typical, but there may be diagnostic confusion with other itching conditions such as eczema. Scrapings taken from burrows may be examined under light microscopy to reveal mites.

Management and treatment

Patients should be advised to avoid close body contact until they and their partner(s) have completed treatment. A full screen for other STIs should be undertaken, as there is anecdotal evidence of rates of infection similar to other patients attending GUM clinics.

Two topical treatments are recommended in the UK. Benzyl benzoate is regarded as too irritant, and crotamiton is ineffective compared with the recommended options which are Permethrin 5% cream or Malathion 0.5% aqueous lotion. These should be applied to the whole body from the neck downwards, and washed off after 12 h, usually overnight. Itch may persist for several weeks. Application of crotamiton cream may give symptomatic relief, and antihistamines may also be helpful. Potentially contaminated clothes and bedding should be washed at a high temperature (>50°C) if possible. Mites separated from the human host die within 72 h. Permethrin is safe during pregnancy and breast feeding.

Current sexual partners as well as other members of the household should be examined and treated. An arbitrary time span is for contacts from the previous 2 months to be traced. No clear evidence exists regarding optimal follow-up. The appearance of new burrows at any stage following treatment is indicative of a need for further therapy, although in reinfection, symptoms of pruritus may recur before typical burrows have developed. Pruritus persisting for more than 2 weeks after treatment may reflect treatment failure, reinfection or drug allergy to antiscabetics.

Acknowledgements

The authors wish to thank Dr I.H. Ahmed, Consultant GU Physician, Nottingham University Hospitals and President of BASSH for help with the sourcing of images, and Dr J.J. Anson, Consultant Microbiologist at the Royal Liverpool University Hospital for assistance in discussing serology and NAAT techniques.

References

Health Protection Agency 2008 All new episodes seen at GUM clinics: 1998–2007. United Kingdom and country specific tables.

National Institute for Health and Clinical Excellence 2007 Prevention of Sexually Transmitted Infections and Under 18 Conceptions. NICE, London.

World Health Organization 2001 Global Prevalence and Incidence of Selected Curable Sexually Transmitted Infections. World Health Organization, Geneva, Switzerland.

Further Reading

Adler M, Cowan F, French P, Mitchell H, Richens J 2004 ABC of Sexually Transmitted Infections, 5th edn. BMJ Books, London.

Avert website: http://www.avert.org/

Department of Health 2005 National Chlamydia Screening Programme Phase 3 Guide. Department of Health, London.

Gibson R 2004 Viral hepatitis. In: Adler M, Cowan F, French P, Mitchell H, Richens J (eds) ABC of Sexually Transmitted Infections, 5th edn. BMJ Books, London.

Johnson AM, Mercer CH, Erens B et al 2001 Sexual behaviour in Britain: partnerships, practices, and HIV risk behaviours. The Lancet 358: 1835–1842.

Lewis DA, Latif AS, Ndowa F 2007 WHO global strategy for the prevention and control of sexually transmitted infections: time for action. Sexually Transmitted Infections 83: 508–509.

Wellings K, Nanchahal K, Macdowall W et al 2001 Sexual behaviour in Britain: early heterosexual experience. The Lancet 358: 1843–1850.

CHAPTER 64

Human immunodeficiency syndrome

Saurabh V. Phadnis and Margaret A. Johnson

Chapter Contents

INTRODUCTION	979	PREPARATION FOR GYNAECOLOGICAL SURGERY	985
BACKGROUND	979	NOSOCOMIAL TRANSMISSION	985
GYNAECOLOGICAL SYMPTOMATOLOGY	981	CONCLUSION	985
PREGNANCY	983	KEY POINTS	986
PREGNANCY CONTROL	984		

Introduction

Over 50% of all individuals infected with human immuno-deficiency virus (HIV) are women (Joint United Nations Programme on HIV/AIDS 2008). Whilst HIV itself has no major specific gynaecological manifestations, it does impinge heavily on gynaecological practice. Some problems, such as recurrent vaginal candidiasis, florid human papilloma virus (HPV) infection and an increased prevalence of cervical intraepithelial neoplasia (CIN), are the result of increasing immunosuppression. However, many of the current gynaecological issues encountered in the HIV-infected woman, such as contraception, pregnancy and infertility management, are a result of dramatic improvements in available therapy and consequent improvement in overall prognosis.

Background

HIV is a retrovirus, a double-stranded RNA virus that uses the enzyme reverse transcriptase to form DNA and integrate itself into the host cell which then becomes a 'factory' for producing more virus (Figure 64.1). T-cell helper lymphocytes bearing the CD4 receptor, pivotal in the cell-mediated immune response, are targeted by the virus and destroyed.

The natural history of HIV is characterized by gradual clinical deterioration. A decreasing CD4 lymphocyte count and increasing levels of virus in the blood plasma are used in monitoring the course of the disease in conjunction with clinical events. Most evidence regarding the natural history of HIV infection is based on studies of men, and it is not clear whether this is directly applicable to women. Seroconversion, the development of antibodies to HIV detectable in the serum, usually occurs soon after infection and the new fourth-generation combined antigen–antibody assays enable an accurate diagnosis to be made within 14 days of infection. Up to 50% of patients may experience an acute infectious mononucleosis-like syndrome, the 'primary HIV infection', at the time of seroconversion with rash, fever, myalgia, arthralgia, headache, diarrhoea and sore throat.

Acquired immunodeficiency syndrome (AIDS) diagnoses represent a range of disorders including infection and neoplasia (Centers for Disease Control and Prevention 1992). The risk of severe immunodeficiency and AIDS increases with the duration of infection. The median time to development of AIDS in untreated HIV-positive patients is approximately 7–10 years. Prior to the development of AIDS, patients may either be asymptomatic or experience persistent generalized lymphadenopathy (enlarged lymph nodes in at least two extrainguinal sites, lasting for at least 3 months and not attributable to any other cause) or symptoms due to immune deterioration that has many manifestations.

Early in the epidemic, before the widespread use of antiretroviral therapy and prophylaxis against opportunistic infections, median survival after an AIDS-defining illness was 11 months. Early studies did suggest a worse prognosis for women with HIV, although this finding is likely to have been the result of inequalities in access to care rather than biological gender differences. The course of infection varies between individuals, and there are 'long-term non-progressors' who are infected for long periods of time but manifest no evidence of immunocompromise in terms of either peripheral CD4 count or clinically detectable disease.

Treatment

In the last decade, widespread use of combination antiretroviral therapy in Europe and the USA has substantially reduced the rate of progression to AIDS and improved survival. Deaths that included AIDS-related causes decreased

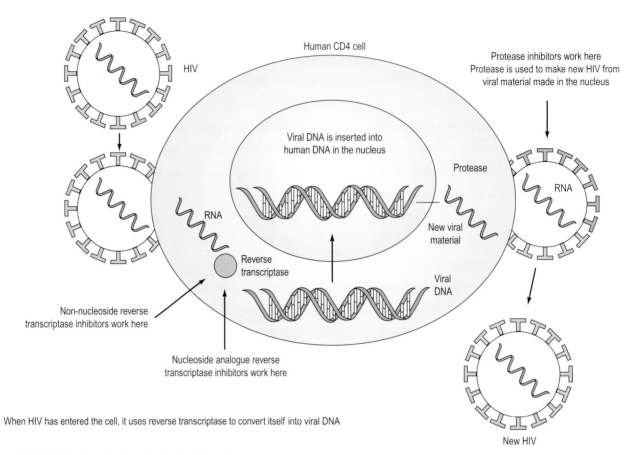

Figure 64.1 HIV lifecycle and action of antiretroviral agents.

from 3.79/100 person-years in 1996 to 0.32/100 person-years in 2004 (Palella et al 2006). Six classes of antiretroviral agents are now available — nucleoside reverse transcriptase inhibitors (NRTIs), non-nucleoside reverse transcriptase inhibitors (NNRTIs), protease inhibitors, integrase inhibitors, entry inhibitors (or fusion inhibitors) and maturation inhibitors — all of which interrupt the virus' lifecycle (Figure 64.1). The aim of highly active antiretroviral therapy (HAART), a combination of three or more drugs usually including a protease inhibitor or an NNRTI, is to slow progression of the disease by reducing viral load and thus increasing CD4 count. The British HIV Association has published guidelines on when to start HAART (British HIV Association Treatment Guidelines Writing Group 2008). Efavirenz should be considered as the first-line therapy in all patients, unless the patient is trying to conceive and has primary NRTI or NNRTI resistance. After treatment is commenced, viral load should reach 'undetectable' levels, usually less than 50 copies/ml. The CD4 count should rise, with levels below 200×10^6/l representing a significant risk of development of an opportunistic infection. Compliance with HAART regimes needs to be in excess of 95% (Paterson et al 2000) for treatment to be effective and to reduce the chance of emergence of resistant virus.

Transmission

HIV has been isolated in blood, seminal fluid, vaginal secretions, cerebrospinal fluid, saliva, lacrimal secretions and breast milk. The concentration in different body fluids varies.

The virus may be transmitted by sexual intercourse, intravenous drug use, transfusion, occupational exposure and vertically from mother to child. The predominant route of infection worldwide is heterosexual sex and, with the great majority of the affected population being in their reproductive years, vertical transmission is an increasing problem. Proper use of condoms is known to greatly reduce the risk of transmission (Heikinheimo and Lähteenmäki 2009). Male-to-female transmission is more efficient than female-to-male transmission, with the mucous membrane of the vagina being more permeable and the surface area being greater, although a partner receptive to anal intercourse is at greatest risk. It is difficult to quantify the risk of sexual transmission 'per act' as a constellation of factors are involved, although higher levels of viral load and intercurrent sexually transmitted infection (Wasserheit 1992), particularly ulcerative conditions, in either partner make transmission more likely. Use of barrier methods should also be encouraged in concordant HIV-positive couples to reduce the risk of transmission of resistant virus.

Although transmission of HIV between women who have sex with women (Monzon and Capellan 1987) is very rare, cases have occurred. Use of dental dams (latex barriers) should be encouraged to reduce oral contact with vaginal secretions, and shared sex toys should be cleaned appropriately. Salivary hypotonicity is thought to inactivate HIV-infected lymphocytes, and hence salivary transmission is almost certainly very rare. Oral sex, although less risky than vaginal or anal sex, may result in transmission and this may, in part, be the result of the isotonic nature of seminal fluid overcoming the inactivation of infected cells by hypotonic saliva.

In 2007, approximately 370,000 children under 15 years of age became infected with HIV, mainly through mother-to-child transmission (MTCT). Approximately 90% of infections due to MTCT occurred in Africa where AIDS is beginning to reverse decades of steady progress in child survival. In high-income countries, MTCT has been virtually eliminated thanks to effective voluntary testing and counselling, access to antiretroviral therapy, safe delivery practices, and the widespread availability and safe use of breast-milk substitutes.

HIV testing

HIV testing should be performed with the woman's consent, and needs only a pretest discussion and consent by a trained healthcare worker. Medical care and support for those diagnosed HIV positive should be arranged immediately after diagnosis. As with all medical care, patient confidentiality should be respected.

There are two methods in routine practice for testing for HIV: screening assay, where blood is sent to the laboratory for testing, or a rapid point of care test (UK National Guidelines for HIV Testing 2008). The recommended first-line assay is one which tests for HIV antibody and p24 antigen simultaneously. These are termed 'fourth-generation assays' and have the advantage of reducing the time between the infection and testing HIV positive to 1 month; this is 1–2 weeks earlier than with sensitive third-generation (antibody-only detection) assays. HIV RNA quantitative assays (viral load tests) are not recommended as screening assays because of the possibility of false-positive results, and because they only have a marginal advantage over the fourth-generation assays for the detection of primary infection. Laboratories undertaking screening tests should be able to confirm antibody and antigen/RNA. There is a requirement for three independent assays able to distinguish HIV-1 from HIV-2. These tests could be provided within the primary testing laboratory or by a referral laboratory. All new HIV diagnoses should be made following appropriate confirmatory assays and testing a second sample. Testing including confirmation should follow the standards laid out by the Health Protection Agency (2007).

Point of care tests offer the advantage of a result from either a finger prick or a mouth swab sample within minutes. They have advantages of ease of use when venepuncture is not possible (e.g. outside conventional healthcare settings) and where a delay in obtaining results is a disadvantage, but these must be weighed against the disadvantages of a test which has reduced specificity and reduced sensitivity compared with current fourth-generation assays. Point of care tests are therefore recommended in the following settings:

- clinical settings where rapid turnaround of testing results is desirable;
- community testing sites;
- urgent source testing in cases of exposure incidents; and
- circumstances where venepuncture is refused.

Although a cure for HIV remains elusive, the advent of effective treatment has resulted in a significantly more optimistic outlook for infected patients. There are clear advantages to knowledge of HIV status, not only in terms of accessing medical monitoring and treatment but also regarding protection of sexual partners and reduction of risk of MTCT. Antenatal testing, previously only offered to women deemed at high risk of infection, is now offered universally as part of routine investigations offered to women in early pregnancy (see below).

The HIV epidemic

More than 25 million people have died of AIDS since 1981. Globally, there were an estimated 33 million people living with HIV in 2007. The annual number of new HIV infections declined from 3 million in 2001 to 2.7 million in 2007. Overall, 2 million people died due to AIDS in 2007, compared with an estimate of 1.7 million in 2001. While the percentage of people living with AIDS has stabilized since 2000, the overall number of people living with HIV has increased steadily as new infections occur each year, HIV treatments extend life and new infections still outnumber AIDS deaths. Southern Africa continues to bear a disproportionate share of the global burden of HIV; 35% of HIV infections and 38% of AIDS deaths occurred in that subregion in 2007. Sub-Saharan Africa is home to 67% of people living with HIV (Joint United Nations Programme on HIV/AIDS 2008).

In 2007, there were an estimated 77,400 persons living with HIV (both diagnosed and undiagnosed), equivalent to 127 persons living with HIV per 100,000 population in the UK (170 per 100,000 men and 84 per 100,000 women). Among 73,300 persons aged 15–59 years living with HIV, 28% are unaware of their infection. A total of 7734 persons (4887 men and 2846 women) were diagnosed with HIV in 2007; a rate of 16 new diagnoses per 100,000 men and nine per 100,000 women. Seventy per cent of the 56,556 persons seen for HIV care were receiving antiretroviral therapy. However, almost one in five HIV-infected persons with severe immunosuppression were not on treatment (Health Protection Agency 2008).

Gynaecological Symptomatology

Women with HIV experience the same range of gynaecological symptoms as their HIV-negative counterparts. As with any woman, it is important that she is treated with compassion and understanding, and that investigation and treatment of gynaecological problems are thorough and tailored to the woman's individual situation. Problems that might, in the past, not have been of real significance to women coping with a terminal disease are now increasingly relevant, with women realistically expecting a near-normal lifespan. By and large, HIV status should not alter treatments available to women, although there are a few caveats to this which are discussed below. As with all medical care, good communication with accurate information is essential.

Menstrual cycle

Intuitively, it might be expected that women with HIV, as with any chronic disease, might experience menstrual irregularity or periods of ammenorhoea, perhaps associated with weight loss or deteriorating health. It is certainly true that associated medical problems such as thrombocytopenia may result in menorrhagia, while liver or renal insufficiency may cause amenorrhoea.

While, anecdotally, women with HIV are often said to suffer menstrual disturbance, evidence to support an effect of HIV itself on menstrual pattern is sparse and often conflicting. The consensus is that there is no direct effect of HIV on menstrual pattern, although increasingly disturbed cycles may occur in women with advanced HIV infection who are severely immunocompromised (CD4 count <200) (Harlow et al 2000).

The clinical impression of a high prevalence of an abnormal bleeding pattern may be biased in two ways:

- women with HIV routinely see their doctors at frequent (usually 3-monthly) intervals and so have more opportunity to consult their physicians regarding any perceived problem; and
- the majority of infected women are of Black African origin and are therefore more likely to have fibroids.

HIV shedding into cervical fluid is lowest in the follicular phase and peaks during menstruation (Reicheldorfer et al 2000), with obvious implications for sexual transmission.

Little information is available on endocrine function in females with HIV. In men, no striking differences have been found when the men are well, but hypogonadotrophic hypogonadism has been reported as a common feature in those who have AIDS. It has been suggested that this may relate to chronic ill health and weight loss rather than to HIV infection itself.

In general, menstrual abnormality should be investigated and treated as in the HIV-negative population, although caution should be exercised when intercurrent disease or treatment affects liver function and may alter metabolism of drug therapy or hormones. In severely immunocompromised patients, abnormal uterine bleeding may be a result of an HIV-related condition, opportunistic infection or neoplasm, and investigation should be tailored appropriately.

Vaginitis

Recurrent vaginal candidiasis is the most common initial clinical manifestation of HIV infection in women (Carpenter et al 1991), and is a problem even at relatively well-maintained CD4 counts. Imam et al (1990) suggested a hierarchy of risk of candidal infection, with recurrent vaginal candidiasis becoming more common with early systemic immunosuppression, oral candidiasis becoming more common with moderate immunosuppression, and oesophageal candidiasis (an AIDS-defining diagnosis) typically occurring with severe immunosuppression. Not only are HIV-infected women more prone to recurrence, but yeasts other than *Candida albicans* (e.g. *Torulopsis glabrata*) are isolated more frequently and there is a shorter time before recurrence (Spinollo et al 1994). Response to treatment is usually good, but relapses frequently require retreatment or maintenance therapy.

Pelvic sepsis

Studies of HIV-infected women show no significant difference in the prevalence rates of gonorrhoea and Chlamydia among HIV-positive and HIV-negative women (Minkoff et al 1999). Women with a concurrent sexually transmitted infection are more likely to have a higher viral load in vaginal secretions. Patients should be treated using standard therapy and referred to genitourinary medicine clinics for initiation of contact tracing and follow-up. Pelvic sepsis is probably more common in patients with HIV, but presentation can be varied with less severe symptoms and lesser rises in lymphocyte count, sometimes occurring at the lowest levels of immunocompetence (Korn et al 1993). In general terms, early treatment with standard antibiotics is appropriate and effective.

Syphilis

Syphilis should be treated similarly to HIV-negative patients, although some suggest a value in cerebrospinal fluid examinations before treatment or treatment that will cross the blood–brain barrier as HIV-positive patients may experience neurological manifestations earlier in the course of the disease.

Herpes simplex virus and genital ulceration

Frequency, duration and severity of herpes simplex virus attacks may be increased in HIV-positive women, particularly in immunocompromised women. Attacks may be avoided or treated with oral acyclovir, although resistance can occur, and culture and sensitivity testing is sometimes useful. In resistant cases of genital ulceration, directed biopsy may be necessary to exclude neoplasia.

Genital warts

Human papillomavirus (HPV), usually types 6–11, is common in HIV-infected women and may be more extensive and florid as compared to HIV-negative women. Treatment is along standard lines and, in those with severe immune compromise, resolution may be seen with increasing CD4 count resulting from systemic antiretroviral therapy.

Cervical intraepithelial neoplasia

CIN is common in women with HIV (Adachi et al 1993, Massad et al 1999), and prevalence increases with advancing immunosuppression (Schäfer et al 1991, Johnson et al 1992). HIV-positive women are more likely to be infected with HPV (Palefsky et al 1999), and more of this infection is the result of 'high-risk' HPV than in the HIV-negative population. Notably, HPV has been found in women who have sex exclusively with women; therefore, even this population must undergo cervical screening.

Data from the pre-HAART era suggested that CIN was more often of higher grade and more often aggressive in women with HIV compared with seronegative women, and that dysplasia was more likely to persist and progress than in seronegative women (Ahdieh et al 1999). Treatment with HAART may influence cervical dysplasia, although results are not consistent across studies, with some suggesting that women treated with HAART experience early regression of lesions (Heard et al 1998) and others showing no convincing evidence of an effect (Moore et al 2002).

There have been concerns about the usefulness of cervical cytology in HIV-infected women, and the optimal method and frequency of screening of this population remain unresolved. Larger studies have validated the use of cervical cytological screening combined with a low threshold for colposcopy and directed biopsy. The guidelines of the Royal College of Obstetricians and Gynaecologists advocate annual smears for women with HIV with no history of abnormality. Screening intensity should continue unaltered in women with excellent CD4 and viral load responses to HAART. High-grade cervical lesions should be treated appropriately, whilst women with low-grade abnormalities who are likely to adhere to follow-up may safely be monitored on a 6-monthly basis. The clinical usefulness and cost-effectiveness of HPV typing incorporated in routine clinical practice in women with HIV remains uncertain.

Cancer of the cervix

This diagnosis is a gender-specific AIDS diagnosis added to the AIDS definition in 1993. In the UK, there has not been a great rise in the number of cases of cervical carcinoma in HIV-positive women, and this may represent either effective screening or long latency of the disease, with more effective antiretroviral therapy likely to play a role. One study has shown that 2.5% of HIV-positive women aged 15–49 years in European countries have presented with this malignancy as a first AIDS-defining event (Serraino et al 2002).

Other genital neoplasias

Vulval and anal intraepithelial neoplasias have also been reported more commonly in HIV-infected women (Williams et al 1994), although the possible role of screening has not been evaluated.

Pregnancy

Fertility does not seem to be affected by HIV infection. Women (and men) with HIV are just as keen to pursue pregnancy as the HIV-negative population. Even before the advent of HAART, termination rates were no higher amongst those who were HIV-positive. Pregnancy does not appear to have a major effect on the rate of progression of HIV disease, and HIV infection itself (unless very advanced) does not affect pregnancy outcome. The main concern is the risk to the baby of becoming infected with HIV. Of infected babies, approximately one-third present early with symptoms and progress rapidly, one-third experience a relapsing–remitting course, and the remainder have more chronic infection and live well into their teenage years.

In order to prevent vertical transmission, the diagnosis of HIV must be made. The UK's record on antenatal diagnosis was extremely poor, and the majority of mothers of children vertically infected with HIV only discovered their own diagnosis when the child developed AIDS (Public Health Laboratory Service 1999). The Department of Health subsequently issued guidelines that all pregnant women should be offered an HIV test, with the aim that uptake of the test be 90% by the end of 2002 and the number of vertically HIV-infected babies reduced by 80% (Department of Health 1999). Great progress has already been made towards this goal, with more than 90% of HIV-infected women diagnosed before giving birth in 2007. This high rate of detection in pregnancy means that the estimated proportion of exposed infants who become infected also remained low, at less than 5% (Health Protection Agency 2008).

Factors known to be associated with increasing risk of MTCT are increasing viral load, decreasing CD4 count, increasing duration of rupture of membranes, vaginal route of delivery, younger gestational age at delivery, the presence of other sexually transmitted infections, invasive medical procedures such as amniocentesis, fetal blood sampling, assisted delivery and breast feeding.

Care of a pregnant, HIV-positive woman has two main aims: first, to ensure the good health of the mother; and second, to attempt to reduce the risk of transmission of HIV to the baby to a minimum.

Antiretroviral therapy

If the mother is not yet on HAART but requires antiretroviral therapy, this should be given in accordance with the British HIV Association guidelines for non-pregnant women. Some women choose to defer treatment until after the period of organogenesis after discussion with their HIV physician. Women already taking HAART will often choose to continue their therapy, although uncertainty regarding the long-term effects of intrauterine exposure to antiretrovirals at any gestation may be a cause for anxiety.

In developed countries, most studies have shown a transmission rate of 15–25% in the absence of treatment, but the use of antiretroviral therapy in pregnancy has reduced transmission rates significantly. Use of AZT (a nucleoside) monotherapy was a breakthrough in reducing vertical transmission (Connor et al 1994). AZT commenced prior to the third trimester, given to the mother intravenously during delivery and given to the neonate orally led to a decrease in transmission by 67% in a placebo-controlled trial. AZT monotherapy does not reduce viral load to undetectable levels, and so does not prevent vertical transmission solely by an effect on viral load. Its precise mechanism of action remains uncertain. For this reason, although AZT monotherapy is still a regime recommended by the British HIV Association, there is a trend towards use of short-term antiretroviral therapy (START) regimes (combination therapy taken from approximately 28 weeks of gestation for the duration of the pregnancy), even in mothers who do not require antiretroviral therapy for themselves (i.e. who have a CD4 count >350). Unlike AZT monotherapy, START regimes aim to reduce viral load to undetectable levels to reduce levels of transmission as much as possible.

The potential for simplified regimes has been assessed, and neviripine (an NNRTI) monotherapy given in two doses, one to the mother during labour and the other to the neonate at 48–72 h, has been shown to be more effective than a single dose of AZT in Africa (Guay et al 1999). However, evidence of subsequent neviripine resistance (which will compromise effective treatment regimes available to the mother) continues to emerge and use of neviripine monotherapy is generally not advised.

Obstetricians should be aware of possible side-effects occurring in women receiving antiretroviral therapy. Protease inhibitors may lead to glucose intolerance and an increasing likelihood of gestational diabetes, whilst two of the nucleoside agents (DD1 and D4t) have been associated with the development of lactic acidosis (three fatal cases), which may mimic the haemolysis–elevated liver enzymes–low platelets syndrome. These agents should probably be avoided if possible. Those women with greater immune compromise may be taking antibiotic prophylaxis against opportunistic infection. Septrin, the agent most commonly used, is a folate antagonist, and prescription of folate supplements should prevent developmental abnormalities.

All women should be registered prospectively on the Anti-retroviral Pregnancy Registry (managed by Glaxo-SmithKline), set up to monitor short- and long-term side-effects. Women and their children should also be registered with the Royal College of Obstetricians and Gynaecologists and the British Paediatric Surveillance Unit. Efavirenz (an NNRTI also known as DMP) has been shown to cause a range of defects of varying severity in cynomolgus monkeys, and its use should be avoided if at all possible. In counselling women in this area, it is important to weigh up the uncertainty regarding toxicity against the undisputed benefits of preventing vertical transmission.

Delivery route

In the majority of cases, transmission occurs at the time of delivery; however, this will occur *in utero* in a small percentage of cases. There is now conclusive evidence to recommend prelabour lower segment caesarean section. A meta-analysis of 15 prospective cohort studies showed a 50% reduction in transmission (International Perinatal HIV Group 1999), and a 70% reduction was found in the European controlled trial (European Mode of Delivery Collaboration 1999). There is uncertainty regarding whether there is a persistent benefit in caesarean section when the mother has an undetectable viral load (<50 copies/ml).

Breast feeding further increases the risk of transmission of HIV by between 7% and 22% (Dunn et al 1992). In the developed world, the majority of postpartum transmission is the result of breast feeding, and its avoidance significantly reduces rates of infection (Kreiss 1997). If a woman decides to breast feed despite this evidence, she should be advised to breast feed exclusively as transmission rates are highest when mixed feeding is employed. There may well be considerable cultural difficulties around not breast feeding, and women need support and advice regarding how to deal with this.

Transmission rates

Transmission rates of between 1% and 2% can be achieved by a combination of antenatal treatment with antiretrovirals, AZT infusion at a prelabour caesarean section, avoidance of breast feeding and infant antiretroviral therapy. Treatment and follow-up of the infant should be undertaken by a specialist paediatric team.

Pregnancy Control

Contraception

All patients should be advised to use barrier contraception to protect against transmission of HIV, transmission of resistant HIV, other infections and pregnancy. Many women decide to use a 'belt and braces' approach, using an additional method to reduce the risk of unplanned pregnancy further, although there is some evidence that condom use declines in HIV-positive women who use combined oral contraception (COC). Women taking antiretroviral therapy which may induce or suppress liver enzymes to varying degrees should be made aware of the possible risk of sub-therapeutic levels of their COC pill, and advice to use condoms as well should be reinforced. Those using depot injections and taking HAART should have injections every 10 weeks. HAART regimes containing protease inhibitors have been associated with elevations in blood triglycerides and cholesterol, which should be monitored closely in those taking COC.

Previous advice was for women with HIV to avoid use of intrauterine devices because of potential risks of infection and a possible increase in risk of transmission to male partners resulting from increased duration and heaviness of menses. This has not been substantiated (European Study Group on Heterosexual Transmission of HIV 1992), and this may well be a method of choice in carefully selected candidates (Sinei et al 1998). The progestogen intrauterine system is increasingly used for women with HIV, with the benefits of excellent contraception and a reduction in blood flow.

Sterilization should be undertaken following the same guidelines as apply to other women. However, care needs to be taken around the time of diagnosis of HIV, when women have not had sufficient opportunity to adjust to the diagnosis and may subsequently regret the procedure.

Spermicides, such as nonoxynol-9, appear to inactivate HIV *in vitro* but may not be so effective *in vivo*. Unfortunately, there is evidence that nonoxynol-9 may cause mucosal inflammation that might lead to an increased risk of HIV transmission. The contraceptive implant Implanon has not been evaluated in these women, although it is likely to play a role. All women should be aware of emergency contraception (Levonelle and emergency intrauterine device insertion) and where this can be accessed.

Termination of pregnancy

Women requesting termination of pregnancy should be referred to an appropriate clinic where both medical and surgical options may be offered as appropriate. As for HIV-negative women who have had unprotected sexual intercourse, sexually transmitted infection screening may also be appropriate at this time.

Planning pregnancy

Any woman planning pregnancy should be advised to stop smoking and reduce alcohol consumption, and folate supplements should be prescribed. It is sensible to assess the woman's overall state of health, and in the HIV-positive woman, this will include checking recent levels of viral load and CD4 count. HAART regimes containing a known teratogen such as efavirenz should be altered if possible.

Both partners may be HIV infected or only one. Where only the woman is infected, the entirely safe method of artificial insemination using the partner's semen can be employed. Advice should be given regarding the timing of ovulation and the optimum time of insemination, with some women preferring to buy commercially available ovulation predictor kits.

An HIV-negative woman may have an HIV-positive male partner. HIV does not appear to infect sperm directly. Therefore, if sperm can be isolated from the white blood cells and the seminal plasma in a 'sperm-washing' procedure, it should be possible to inseminate a woman safely. Semprini et al (1992), Gilling-Smith (2000) and Marina et al (1998) have experience of more than 3000 cycles of sperm washing and intrauterine insemination or in-vitro fertilization (resulting in 300 live births) with no reported seroconversions. The sperm-washing procedure is expensive and not currently freely available, and some couples may decide to pursue 'unsafe' insemination with unprocessed semen or to practice 'unsafe' sex. Mandelbrot et al (1997), however, have published results of a study of 92 HIV-negative women whose partners were HIV positive and who had 104 pregnancies. All couples had unprotected intercourse during the fertile period as determined with commercial ovulation predictor kits. There were only four seroconversions, all in couples who did not use condoms consistently during the rest of the cycles.

Even when both partners are infected with HIV, condom-free intercourse cannot be recommended because of the possibility of transmission of resistant virus. Couples may choose to perform, possibly less risky, home insemination.

Infertility

This has been a contentious but important area. Women and their partners should not automatically be denied access to treatment because of HIV infection. As with HIV-negative women with potentially life-shortening conditions such as complicated diabetes, post transplant or a history of cancer, HIV-infected women must be equipped with information and allowed to make their own reproductive decisions (Gilling-Smith et al 2001).

Continuing childlessness can be extremely distressing, and factors such as current state of health and long-term prognosis, support networks and motivation to pursue often stressful investigations and treatments should be discussed and counselling given. Advice regarding HIV, treatment and prevention of vertical transmission should be accurate, up to date and given in conjunction with expert HIV physicians.

Infertility may present in a number of different situations with one or both partners being infected with HIV. Where in-vitro fertilization is necessary, the possible emotional and financial costs should be discussed, and this treatment should only be carried out where there are provisions to perform treatment safely and without risk of infection to others.

Preparation for Gynaecological Surgery

Most HIV-infected women will tolerate surgery well, even if their CD4 count is low. Chest and wound infections are more common, but with the use of prophylactic antibiotics and physiotherapy, these will not usually present serious problems. Where surgery is indicated, HIV status itself should not affect the decision to operate.

Nosocomial Transmission

Occupational transmission to healthcare workers

Most occupational transmission has occurred following needlestick or other sharps injuries, and there have been a very few documented seroconversions after contamination of broken skin or mucous membranes. The risk of acquiring HIV from a single accidental parenteral exposure to infected blood has been estimated at approximately 0.3%. Those performing surgical procedures should employ universal precautions, bearing in mind the prevalence of undiagnosed HIV and hepatitis B and C infection. The last two conditions are much more readily transmitted than HIV. A woman with HIV should not be subjected to any unnecessary and discriminatory infection control procedures which could isolate her or draw attention to her before other patients or relatives.

Postexposure prophylaxis

Immediately after a percutaneous or mucous membrane exposure to potentially HIV-infected blood, thorough washing with warm running water and soap and clinical evaluation of the injury should be performed. Any bleeding should be encouraged. Consultation with local HIV experts should be as rapid as possible in order that appropriate prophylactic antiretroviral therapy can be commenced, preferably within 1 h, to reduce the risk of seroconversion (Department of Health 2000).

HIV-infected healthcare workers

The Department of Health (2000), Medical Defence Union and UKCC [United Kingdom Central Council for Nursing, Midwifery and Health Visiting (now Nursing and Midwifery Council, NMC)] are clear that HIV-positive health workers should not take part in invasive 'exposure-prone' procedures, and the individual should inform their occupational health department of their status. In addition, the General Medical Council recommends that staff who think they have been at risk should be tested confidentially.

Conclusion

The national strategy for sexual health and HIV (Department of Health 2001) aims to reduce the transmission of HIV, increase the diagnosis of prevalent cases, improve the health and social care of people with HIV, and reduce the stigma attached to the diagnosis. Rates of HIV infection continue to increase, and the number of woman affected is rising. Use of HAART has dramatically improved the prognosis for patients with HIV. Obstetricians and gynaecologists should be aware of the possibility of HIV infection in their patients, and should facilitate HIV testing in order that women are able to experience the benefits of therapy.

KEY POINTS

1. There is a steady increase in the prevalence of HIV infection in women.
2. Whilst HIV remains an incurable condition, advances in therapy have improved the prognosis dramatically.
3. Women with HIV experience the same range of gynaecological problems as their HIV-negative counterparts, and their HIV status itself should not influence the treatment they receive.
4. CIN is more common in this population and women should have an annual screen.

5. MTCT can be reduced to under 2% with appropriate intervention.
6. HIV infection should not influence the availability of fertility investigation and treatment.
7. Obstetricians and gynaecologists should be aware of the possibility of HIV in their patients, and should facilitate testing to monitor infection rates and to alert infected women to their need for treatment.

References

Adachi A, Fleming I, Burk RD, Ho CYF, Klein RS 1993 Women with human immunodeficiency virus infection and abnormal papanicolaou smears: a prospective study of colposcopy and clinical outcome. Obstetrics and Gynecology 81: 372–377.

Ahdieh L, Munoz A, Vlahov D et al 2000 Cervical neoplasia and repeated positivity of human papillomavirus infection in human immunodeficiency virus-seropositive and -seronegative women. American Journal of Epidemiology 151(12): 1148–1157.

British HIV Association Treatment Guidelines Writing Group 2008 British HIV Association guidelines for treatment of HIV-1-infected adults with anti-retroviral therapy 2008. HIV Medicine 9: 563–608.

Carpenter CC, Mayer KH, Stein MD, Leibman BD, Fisher A, Fiore TC 1991 Human immunodeficiency virus infection in North American women: experience with 200 cases and a review of the literature. Medicine 70: 307–325.

Centers for Disease Control and Prevention 1992 Revised classification system for HIV infection and expanded surveillance case definition for AIDS among adolescents and adults. Morbidity and Mortality Weekly Report 41: 1–19.

Connor EM, Sperling RS, Gelber R et al 1994 Reduction of maternal–infant transmission of human immunodeficiency virus type 1 with zidovudine treatment. New England Journal of Medicine 331: 1173–1180.

Department of Health 1999 Targets Aimed at Reducing the Numbers of Children Born with HIV. DOH, London.

Department of Health 2000 HIV Post-exposure Prophylaxis: Guidance from the UK Chief Medical Officer's Expert Advisory Groups on AIDS. DOH, London.

Department of Health 2001 The National Strategy for Sexual Health and HIV. DOH, London.

Dunn DT, Newell ML, Ades AE, Peckham C 1992 Estimates of the risk of HIV-1 transmission through breast feeding. The Lancet 320: 585–588.

European Mode of Delivery Collaboration 1999 Elective caesarean section versus vaginal delivery in prevention of vertical HIV-1 transmission: a randomised clinical trial. The Lancet 353: 1035–1039.

European Study Group on Heterosexual Transmission of HIV 1992 Comparison of female to male and male to female transmission of HIV in 563 stable couples. BMJ (Clinical Research Ed.) 304: 809–813.

Gilling-Smith C 2000 Assisted reproduction in HIV discordant couples. AIDS Reader 10: 581–587.

Gilling-Smith C, Smith JR, Semprini AE 2001 HIV and infertility: time to treat. There's no justification for denying treatment to parents who are HIV positive. BMJ (Clinical Research Ed.) 322: 566–567.

Guay LA, Musoke P, Fleming T et al 1999 Intrapartum and neonatal single-dose neviripine compared with zidovudine for prevention of mother-to-child transmission of HIV-1 in Kampala, Uganda: HIVNET 012 randomised trial. The Lancet 354: 795–802.

Harlow SD, Schuman P, Cohen M et al 2000 Effect of HIV infection on menstrual cycle length. Journal of Acquired Immune Deficiency Syndromes 24: 68–75.

Health Protection Agency 2007 Anti-HIV Screening — Minimum Testing Algorithm. National Standard Method VSOP 11(1). HPA, London. Available at: http://www.hpa-standardmethods.org.uk/documents/vsop/pdf/vsop11.pdf.

Health Protection Agency 2008 HIV in the United Kingdom 2008 Report. HPA, London. Available at: http://www.hpa.org.uk/webc/HPAwebFile/HPAweb_C/1227515298354.

Heard I, Schmitz V, Costagliola D, Orth G, Kazatchkine MD 1998 Early regression of cervical lesions in HIV-seropositive women receiving highly active antiretroviral therapy. AIDS 12: 1459–1464.

Heikinheimo O, Lähteenmäki P 2009 Contraception and HIV infection in women. Human Reproduction Update 15: 165–176.

Imam N, Carpenter CC, Mayer KH, Fisher A, Stein M, Danforth SB 1990 Hierarchical pattern of mucosal Candida infections in HIV-seropositive women. American Journal of Medicine 89: 142–146.

International Perinatal HIV Group 1999 Mode of delivery and vertical transmission of HIV-1: a meta-analysis from 15 prospective cohort studies. New England Journal of Medicine 340: 977–987.

Johnson JC, Burnett AF, Willet GD, Young MA, Doniger J 1992 High frequency of latent and clinical human papillomavirus cervical infections in immunocompromised human immunodeficiency virus infected women. Obstetrics and Gynecology 79: 321.

Joint United Nations Programme on HIV/AIDS 2008 Report on the Global HIV/AIDS Epidemic. UNAIDS, Geneva. Available at: http://www.unaids.org/en/KnowledgeCentre/HIVData/GlobalReport/2008/2008_Global_report.asp.

Korn AP, Landers DV, Green JR, Sweet RL 1993 Pelvic inflammatory disease in human immunodeficiency virus-infected women. Obstetrics and Gynecology 82: 765–768.

Kreiss J 1997 Breast feeding and vertical transmission of HIV-1. Acta Paediatrica 421 (Suppl): 113–117.

Mandelbrot L, Heard I, Henrion-Geant E, Henrion R 1997 Natural conception in HIV-negative women with HIV-infected partners. The Lancet 349: 850–851.

Marina S, Marina F, Alcolea R et al 1998 Human immunodeficiency virus type-1 serodiscordant couples can bear healthy children after undergoing intrauterine insemination. Fertility and Sterility 70: 35–39.

Massad LS, Riester KA, Anastos KM et al 1999 Prevalence and predictors of squamous cell abnormalities in Papanicolaou smears from women with HIV-1. Women's Interagency HIV Study Group. Journal of Acquired Immune Deficiency Syndromes 21(1): 33–41.

Minkoff HL, Eisenberger-Matityahu D, Feldman J, Burk R, Clarke L 1999 Prevalence and incidence of gynaecologic disorders among women infected with human immunodeficiency virus. American Journal of Obstetrics and Gynecology 180: 824–836.

Monzon OT, Capellan JMB 1987 Female-to-female transmission of HIV. The Lancet 2: 40–41.

Moore AL, Sabin CA, Madge S, Mocroft A, Reid W, Johnson MA 2002 Highly active antiretroviral therapy and cervical intraepithelial neoplasia. AIDS 16: 927–929.

Palefsky JM, Minkoff H, Kalish LA et al 1999 Cervicovaginal human papillomavirus infection in human immunodeficiency virus-1 positive and high risk HIV-negative women. Journal of the National Cancer Institute 91: 226–236.

Palella FJ Jr, Baker RK, Moorman AC et al; HIV Outpatient Study Investigators 2006 Mortality in the highly active antiretroviral therapy era: changing causes of death and disease in the HIV outpatient study. Journal of Acquired Immune Deficiency Syndromes 43: 27–34.

Paterson DL, Swindells S, Mohr J et al 2000 Adherence to protease inhibitor therapy and outcomes in patients with HIV infection. Annals of Internal Medicine 133: 21–30.

Public Health Laboratory Service 1999 Available at: http://www.phls.co.uk/facts/HIV/hiv.htm.

Reicheldorfer BA, Coombs R, Wright KD et al 2000 Effect of menstrual cycle on HIV-1 levels in the peripheral blood and genital tract. WHS 001 Study team. AIDS 14: 2101–2107.

Schäfer A, Friedmann W, Mielke M, Schwartländer B, Koch MA 1991 The increased frequency of cervical dysplasia-neoplasia in women infected with human immunodeficiency virus is related to the degree of immunosuppression. American Journal of Obstetrics and Gynecology 164: 593–599.

Semprini AE, Levi-Setti P, Bozzo M et al 1992 Insemination of HIV-negative women with processed semen of HIV-positive partners. The Lancet 340: 1317–1319.

Serraino D, Dal Maso L, La Vecchia C, Franceschi S 2002 Invasive cervical cancer as an AIDS-defining illness in Europe. AIDS 16: 781–786.

Sinei SK, Morrison CS, Sekadde-Kigondu C, Allen M, Kokonya D 1998 Complications of use of intrauterine devices among HIV-1 infected women. The Lancet 351: 1238–1241.

Spinollo A, Michelone G, Cavanna C et al 1994 Clinical and microbiological characterisation of symptomatic vulvovaginal candidiasis in HIV-seropositive women. Genitourinary Medicine 70: 268–272.

UK National Guidelines for HIV testing 2008 Joint BHIVA, BASHH and BIS Guidelines [Writing Committee (Palfreeman A, Fisher M, Ong E et al)], BHIVA, London, UK]. Available at: http://www.bhiva.org/files/file1031097.pdf.

Wasserheit JN 1992 Epidemiological synergy. Interrelationships between human immunodeficiency virus infection and other sexually transmitted diseases. Sexually Transmitted Diseases 19: 61–77.

Williams AB, Darragh TM, Vranizan K, Ochia C, Moss AR, Palefsky JM 1994 Anal and cervical human papillomavirus infection and risk of anal and cervical epithelial abnormalities in human immunodeficiency virus-infected women. Obstetrics and Gynaecology 83: 205–211.

CHAPTER 65

Forensic gynaecology

Helen Margaret Cameron

Chapter Contents

INTRODUCTION	988	ABSENCE OF GENITAL INJURY	996
SEXUAL ASSAULT REFERRAL CENTRES	989	THE STATEMENT	996
THE RECORD OF FORENSIC EXAMINATION	991	PATTERNS OF INJURY	997
INJURIES	994	VULNERABLE WOMEN	998
THE INFLUENCE OF ALCOHOL- AND DRUG-FACILITATED SEXUAL ASSAULT	994	COURT PROCEEDINGS	998
		CONCLUSION	1000
DESCRIPTION OF WOUNDS	995	KEY POINTS	1000

Introduction

There seems to be an escalating epidemic of rape globally, and it is known that the majority of sexual assaults are not reported to the police, and domestic or spousal rape is even less commonly reported. Sexual assault is not only a serious criminal justice problem but is also a major public health issue. In the UK, 'intimate violence' is a collective term used for partner abuse, family abuse and sexual assault, with 'sexual assault' being defined as indecent exposure, sexual threats and unwanted touching ('less serious'), rape or assault by penetration including attempts ('serious') by any person including a partner or family member (Roe 2008). Annual figures relating to crime in England and Wales are published as the Home Office Statistical Bulletin, reflecting not only the police recorded crime but also findings from the British Crime Survey (BCS) (Kershaw et al 2008). The BCS is a large victimization survey of approximately 47,000 adults living in private houses in England and Wales. Based on the 2006/07 BCS self-completion module on intimate violence, approximately 3% of women and 1% of men had experienced a sexual assault (including attempts) in the previous 12 months. The majority of these were less serious sexual assaults. A significant minority (40%) of victims of serious sexual assault had not told anyone about their most recent experience, with only 11% informing the police. A further worrying statistic is that for victims of serious sexual assault, 37% were repeat victims. In a three-city comparative study of client violence against prostitutes working from street and off-street locations, 28% of women involved in street-based prostitution reported attempted rape (Barnard et al 2002).

In a global context, it is known that conclusions drawn from crime statistics are virtually useless for estimating the incidence of sexual assault because women are universally reluctant to report rape to the authorities. In 2007, the Home Office in the UK produced the first cross-government action plan on sexual assault, which included a range of measures aimed at improving the criminal justice response to sexual violence.

Most rape allegations do not proceed to court; in 1982–1985, 20% of reported cases went to court in Oslo (Bang 1993). In the UK, the conviction rate for all reported cases is currently between 5.7% and 6.5% (Dyer 2008, Williams 2009). The Home Office figures suggest that actual numbers of convictions for rape are increasing year on year, but the increase in convictions is not keeping pace with the increased reporting, thus there is a high level of attrition or case drop-out. Victims who decline to complete the initial investigative process are more likely to do this in areas where there is no sexual assault referral centre (SARC) (Kelly et al 2005). SARCs are widely regarded as the ideal environment for quality forensic examination, ensuring that the victim has access to other services such as sexual health and professional counsellors.

Legal aspects

Under the UK Sexual Offences Act (SOA) 2003, a person can legally consent to sexual activity if he or she is aged 16 years or older. The SOA 2003 covers over 50 sexual offences, and sexual assault is defined as a non-consensual sexual offence, with consent being defined as having the freedom and capacity to choose.

The SOA 2003 was a significant overhaul of the UK law that dealt with sexual violence, and there are now new offences such as the offence of rape to include oral and anal penetration with a penis, and assault by penetration;

DOI: 10.1016/B978-0-7020-3120-5.00065-5

penetration may be by part of the defendant's body but not the penis, or penetration with an object (Rights of Women 2008).

Medical practitioners need to be aware of the legal context in which they gather evidence, and the forensic examination has a dual purpose: firstly, to address the immediate needs and concerns of women; and secondly, the justice system's need for the documentation of physical findings, the rigorous collection and preservation of evidence, an interpretation of the findings, and provision of expert opinion in legal proceedings (Kelly and Regan 2003).

Her Majesty's Government have indicated that they have strengthened the capacity of specialist rape prosecutors and rape coordinators to ensure that the best case is built, and expanded special measures to make it easier for vulnerable victims to give evidence (H.M. Government 2007). Indeed, the Youth Justice and Criminal Evidence Act 1999 legislation gives vulnerable and intimidated witnesses the opportunity to give evidence from behind screens, by video link or for the court to be cleared.

Reasons for failure to report sexual assault

The most important barriers to reporting rape and sexual assault are:

- ignorance about where to find help;
- fear of not being believed;
- fear of becoming involved in complicated police investigations and subsequent court proceedings;
- known low conviction rates;
- concerns about confidentiality;
- anxiety, guilt, shame, embarrassment and not wanting friends and family to know;
- fear of reprisal or retaliation by perpetrator; and
- cases involving a known perpetrator (Kelly et al 2005).

Attrition

Attrition in sexual offences cases refers to cases dropping out from the time of initial complaint to the trial. There is an increasing justice gap for victims as the increasing number of convictions for rape is not keeping pace with the increased reporting (H.M. Crown Prosecution Service Inspectorate 2007). Attrition during investigations begins early. Two significant factors were identified by the review of the handling of investigations by the police and Crown Prosecution Service Inspectorate, one of which is the decision by the victim not to complete the initial process. The other factor was the decision to withdraw support for the investigation or prosecution (H.M. Crown Prosecution Service Inspectorate 2007).

In 2005, Kelly et al pointed out that the majority of sexual assault incidents are reported to the police within 24 h, but that over half of cases lost at the investigative stage are due to evidential issues such as:

- complainant with learning difficulties or mental health problems, or victims who are otherwise unable to give a clear account;
- DNA testing not conducted; and
- an offender was identified but not traced.

Victim withdrawals occur primarily:

- when the victim declines to complete the initial investigative process;
- at the police stage, where over one-third of cases are lost; and
- where there is no SARC (Kelly et al 2005).

Sexual Assault Referral Centres

In early 2009, there were 24 SARCs in England and Wales, the main client group being complainants of recent sexual assault and where the victim has access to a range of agencies including health, the services of counsellors and trained volunteers (H.M. Crown Prosecution Service Inspectorate 2007). The UK Home Office has indicated that SARCs should have the infrastructure to support ongoing victim care, and there should be adequate training and development and quality assurance. There should also be evidence of operational and management policies and procedures (Home Office 2005). It is important that despite the need for cleanliness in the examination room, there are separate interview rooms with a calming and relaxing feel about them (Kelly and Regan 2003).

The services that SARCs provide include:

- experienced women doctors to conduct the medical examination in a purpose-built suite (Figure 65.1);
- confidential access to experienced counsellors regardless of whether the woman reports the assault to the police or not;
- for those women who wish to involve the police, specially trained women police officers to conduct the interview and take a statement; and
- referral may be through the police, general practitioner, hospital doctor or by self-referral without any involvement from the police.

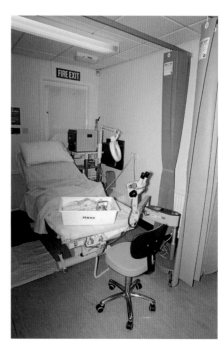

Figure 65.1 Examination suite.

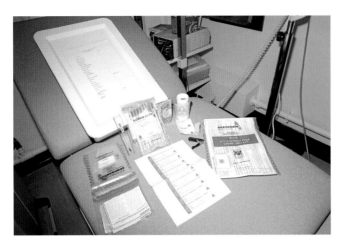

Figure 65.2 Evidence kit.

The clinical requirements of the SARC include:

- clinical and evidential protocols;
- evidence kits (Figure 65.2) which are applied flexibly to fit the nature of the case;
- examination suite with appropriate cleansing and decontamination services;
- first aid facilities;
- emergency contraception supplies and literature;
- access to services for the prevention and management of sexually transmitted infections (STIs); and
- access to psychosocial support.

Consenting to a medical and forensic examination

In achieving consent for a forensic examination, it is important to remember the principles of confidentiality. The General Medical Council (GMC) indicate that 'Patients have a right to expect that information about them will be held in confidence by their doctors', accepting that doctors may have contractual obligations to third parties, such as in their work as police surgeons, and in such circumstances, disclosure may be expected (General Medical Council 2006). In such circumstances, the GMC recommends that the doctor is 'satisfied that the patient has been told at the earliest opportunity about the purpose of the examination and/or disclosure, the extent of the information to be disclosed and the fact that relevant information cannot be concealed or withheld'.

Consent to forensic medical examination should include the nature of the medical examination, the collection of forensic evidence, that photography may form part of the record of the examination and report, and those details in the medical record may be disclosed to police and the Crown Prosecution Service (CPS) for use in evidence.

The woman should also be made aware that the examination can be discontinued at any stage if she so wishes. The stage of the examination reached and the time at which she decides against further examination should be recorded.

The complainant may agree to a 'qualified consent' (i.e. to the release of information to the prosecution without allowing scrutiny by the defence). If she does not consent to release of the medical details, the examiner may be ordered to disclose information by a judge, in which case the forensic physician (FP) should only disclose information relevant to the request for disclosure. In the 'Disclosures to courts or in connection with litigation' section of the GMC document 'Confidentiality: Protecting and Providing Information', it is stated 'You should object to the judge or the presiding officer if attempts are made to compel you to disclose what appear to you to be irrelevant matters' (General Medical Council 2004). The section continues, 'You must not disclose personal information to a third party such as a solicitor, police officer or officer of a court without the patient's express consent'.

If the woman is a non-police referral, she should be informed that she could pursue a formal complaint subsequently, at which stage additional consent should be sought.

Examination of the complainant of sexual assault

Forensic examination is only the first part of the immediate health-based response, the key elements of which include:

- treatment and documentation of injuries;
- collection of medicolegal evidence and maintaining the chain of evidence;
- treatment and evaluation of STIs;
- pregnancy risk evaluation and prevention; and
- crisis intervention and arrangements for counselling.

Forensic examination can provide relevant evidence up to 72 h after an assault, but can even be useful after that time (e.g. if a woman is bleeding or in pain, or if she has been subjected to a serious level of physical violence).

The forensic examination may provide vital evidence that identifies the assailant and/or supports the complainant's account should the case come to court. Not only does the forensic examination itself increase the likelihood of legal action, but having a forensic examination doubles the likelihood of prosecution (McGregor et al 2002, Kelly and Regan 2003).

Who should undertake the examination?

In ideal circumstances, the victim of sexual assault should be allowed to choose the gender of the examining doctor. In the 1980s, the gender of the examining physician was not always felt to be a factor affecting the victim's response to the medical examination (Hockbaum 1987), but recent evidence shows that most victims (male and female) prefer female staff; 43.5% of victims said that they would not continue the forensic examination if the doctor was male (Chowdhury-Hawkins et al 2008).

Training in sexual assault examination

Few doctors have received formal training in the principles of clinical forensic medicine.

To ensure optimal care for the victims of sexual assault, a coordinated multidisciplinary approach should be made to tackle the theoretical and practical training issues. Local and national programmes have been developed at all levels, from specialist registrars through to continuing medical education of those actively involved in rape examination. Subspecialist gynaecology trainees in sexual and reproductive health are expected to compete the forensic and domestic violence competencies module as part of their subspecialty training, which emphasizes the importance of preserving evidence and maintaining the evidence chain whilst providing appropriate sexual and reproductive health care for the complainants of sexual assault (Royal College of Obstetricians and Gynaecologists 2009).

Sexual assault victims may present to an accident and emergency (A&E) department and be seen by the on-call doctor, and whilst resuscitation and immediate clinical management are their prime concern, every A&E department should have a policy for the management of such women and training for first-line staff in the initial care of such vulnerable victims.

One area of training that is especially valuable is court witness skills, and it is vitally important to maintain one's skills in this field through continuing professional development programmes in forensic gynaecology.

Role of the police officer

The police officer has an important role in the rape victim's experience and decision to further pursue legal prosecution. Specially trained police officers not only gather evidence but also have a unique role in liaising with victims of sexual assault, offering advice and information about the criminal justice process as well as taking the formal, detailed statement. In addition, the officer accompanies the complainant to the examination centre, ensuring that she takes a change of clothes with her. The police officer is responsible for the 'Early Evidence Kit' collection of first (timed) urine sample for urine toxicology; it is particularly valuable where there is likely to be a delay before the medical examination. Where an oral sex allegation has been made, the police officer will ask the woman to use a mouth rinse as this is known to be more efficient at recovering semen from the oral cavity. Other early evidence samples include used sanitary wear and toothbrush where oral sex is being alleged and the complainant has cleaned her teeth.

Prior to the doctor taking a history of the assault, the officer provides a summary of the allegation for the doctor. During the examination, the officer may act as a chaperone for the examining doctor and assist in a discreet manner, ensuring that each forensic sample is correctly labelled and sealed. The forensic samples are then sent to a central submissions unit for later dispatch to the forensic science laboratory.

The examining doctor

The experienced clinician will realize that pre-existing diseases, mental health issues and previous trauma can affect the interpretation of the forensic examination findings. It is important to take an accurate account of the event to ensure that an appropriate examination is undertaken and that the collection of forensic evidence is complete. The use of a record of examination with checklists and body diagrams to illustrate the findings provides invaluable assistance to the examining doctor, who is not infrequently called to a complainant in the middle of the night.

The examining doctor must be objective and non-judgemental, and must avoid giving even the smallest cues of suspicion or disbelief which may heighten the victim's anxiety and emotional trauma, and cause a spiralling decline as her guilt and shame increase and her story is shaken (Dupré et al 1993).

Forensic examination is time-consuming and often lasts in excess of 2 h. A speedy response from the forensic examiner is, however, essential for evidential purposes and victim comfort. The importance of examination within 24 h was emphasized in a study on the outcome of sexual assault victims who pursue legal action (Wiley et al 2003). The characteristics positively associated with a legal outcome included:

- being examined within 24 h of assault;
- partner/spouse as an assailant;
- oral assault; and
- anogenital injury (AGI).

Cross-contamination is a major concern now that DNA can be detected in smaller and smaller quantities, and SARCs should have policies in place for cleansing of the medical suite as contaminated samples could have a significant impact on the investigation of the offence and might even result in the investigation being abandoned. FPs should have their DNA added to the police staff elimination database so that checks can be made if a cross-contamination issue arises.

The Record of Forensic Examination

Documentation

The record of the forensic examination should be seen as a confidential *aide memoire* for the clinician, and should contain the following sections.

Complainant and SARC personnel information
Consent

Details of consent to forensic medical examination include:

- medical examination: non-genital/genital;
- recording of the details of the examination;
- retention of relevant items of clothing for forensic examination;
- collection of forensic evidence;
- disclosure of details of the medical record and/or laboratory tests to police/Crown Court/CPS for use in evidence; and
- the taking of photographs which will be used as part of the medical record, may form part of the report based on the examination and may be revealed in subsequent court proceedings.

Medical details

It is the clinician's responsibility to obtain a pertinent medical history, remembering that pre-existing conditions may affect interpretation, such as scars from surgery.

The clinician should enquire about general health and current medical problems, current or recent genital symptoms, bladder or bowel symptoms, and relevant past medical history. Relevant obstetric details should include her parity and mode of delivery. Medication details should be sought, including prescribed and over-the-counter drugs, together with details of street drugs if this is thought to be relevant, as well as social and employment information.

It is essential to gather information about the last menstrual period, time interval since the last sexual intercourse if this is within 14 days, condom usage and any other contraception.

Account of the event

This is usually in the form of an account of events from the complainant and the police officer taking details of the sequence of events before, during and after the incident. Such an account allows the doctor to adapt the standard forensic examination according to the circumstances of the assault. The complainant may, however, be unable to recall the details of the assault, possibly due to the influence of alcohol/drugs at the time of the assault or subsequently. The victim may be naturally reticent, as in the elderly victim, or already suffering 'memory block' associated with rape-related post-traumatic stress disorder (PTSD). Hence it is safer practice to complete the full forensic sampling at this time, usually the only opportunity afforded to the doctor to collect evidence. Loss of evidence may be caused by a delay in presentation, so particular attention should be paid to the time interval since the incident.

Details of the complainant's actions taken since the incident should be recorded, such as specific details of genital cleansing and change of sanitary protection.

General medical examination

The details of the complainant's general appearance should be documented (e.g. build/body mass index, hygiene, demeanor, mood and details of any disability). In addition, it is important to comment upon her reaction to the examination. A sexual examination kit with all necessary equipment should be to hand. For complex injuries, it is very important to request the assistance of a female police photographer.

There are a number of key sites where injuries are most likely to be found during the examination of the victim of sexual assault (e.g. thighs, neck, inner aspect of upper arms and face). It is important that the medical record should contain a reference to any area that is omitted. All injuries should be drawn on body diagrams with corresponding measurements and description, each injury being numbered so that it can be cross-referenced in the statement. Each body diagram used should include a statement to say that the injuries are not drawn to scale.

The Faculty of Forensic and Legal Medicine (FFLM) has reminded forensic examiners about the importance of recording and measuring injuries caused by teeth, and that a full description and overall dimensions should be documented (Rowlinson et al 2008).

The severely injured patient

The medical needs of the victim must take priority over the need to achieve forensic samples, and urgent medical advice should be sought, where necessary, in an appropriately equipped setting (e.g. an A&E department). The reason for delay in undertaking the forensic examination should be carefully documented in the medical record. The sexual examination kit can be collected from the SARC for use in a hospital ward or outreach facility once the complainant's condition is deemed stable and she is willing and able to consent to forensic examination.

Genital examination

The genital examination should begin with a description of the external genital appearance and the presence of any anatomical variation or disease process. There should be a careful documentation of any injuries, using a standardized labelled diagram to record such findings. It can be helpful to use the analogy of a clock face to describe the site of an injury where the 12 o'clock position is anterior. The details of the internal examination (speculum and digital) should be documented next, describing the site and nature of any injuries, with an estimate of the dimensions and the nature of any discharge, blood or fluids seen.

Colposcopic examination

Colposcopic examination is known to increase the positive genital findings compared with inspection of the genitalia. A study of 200 cases of sexual assault examined with a colposcope revealed positive findings in 32% on inspection; however, the positive findings increased to 87% with colposcopic examination (Sommers 2006). Where forced digital penetration is alleged, colposcopy has been found to be particularly useful (Rossman et al 2004).

Questions have been raised regarding why photocolposcopic examination of AGI in a sexually assaulted child is considered the 'gold standard' of examination, yet gross visualization is the standard procedure in adult examination (Brennan 2006). A possible explanation is that colposcopy is seen as an invasive procedure which is ethically unacceptable.

The significance of some of the genital findings during the colposcopic examination remains controversial, especially when images are interpreted by inexperienced clinicians (Templeton and Williams 2006).

If the examiner is unable to carry out the internal examination, the reason should be documented, especially if this is due to client distress or consent being withdrawn. Where indicated, a meticulous description of the perianal and anal examination, and proctoscopy findings should be documented.

Forensic sampling

The forensic evidence collected during the examination is used to help to:

- confirm that sexual contact has taken place;
- establish the lack of consent on the part of the victim;
- establish the identity of the assailant;
- estimate the force used; and
- corroborate the complainant's account.

The FFLM has produced a guideline for good practice regarding collection of forensic specimens which is updated at 6-monthly intervals (Faculty of Forensic and Legal Medicine 2008a). Most SARCs/police forces will have access to a 'sample reference form' (Figure 65.3), with tables listing the forensic samples with their corresponding exhibit number, sample description etc. Recent evidence has shown that posi-

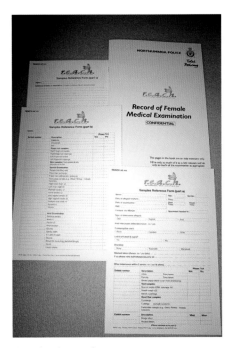

Figure 65.3 Sample reference forms.

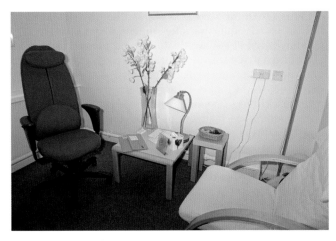

Figure 65.4 Counselling room.

tive forensic results are achieved in approximately 38% of forensic examinations (McGregor et al 2002).

Postexamination arrangements

Communication with the forensic science laboratory

The forensic examiner should complete a forensic specimen form and assist colleagues in the laboratory by providing a brief description of the facts of the case.

Photographs of injuries

Where there is complex skin trauma, photography may act as an adjunct to the description to the findings. It has been claimed that a carefully observed, well-documented description of any injury or group of injuries is worth many photographs (Bunting 1996). Others claim that a photograph can be worth a thousand words if the assailant is claiming consent and the attorney has pictures of the victim with a black eye or worse (Ledray 1993).

Re-examination

This is occasionally indicated if:

• genital injuries are not visible but were anticipated from the account of the incident;
• the examination took place shortly after the incident; or
• there is tenderness on examination.

Referral to counselling services

At best, a follow-up rate of 31% was achieved in a sexual assault follow-up evaluation clinic, despite efforts to encourage female victims to use the clinic (Holmes et al 1996) (Figure 65.4). Our ability to reduce the occurrence of the long-term effects of sexual assault is limited by the low rates of reporting and lack of focused follow-up for those who do report their assault. However, the doctor can significantly

enhance the uptake of counselling in the aftermath of an assault.

Emergency contraception

Hormonal pregnancy prevention is prescribed as soon as possible and up to 72 h after the incident (levonorgestrel 1.5 mg as a single dose), and an intrauterine contraceptive device with antibiotic cover can be inserted at any time up to 5 days after the incident.

Sexually transmitted infections

The frequency of STIs in victims of sexual assault is difficult to estimate due to the low reporting and follow-up of victims. In Mexico, the frequency of STIs was 20% amongst 213 patients (Martinez et al 1999).

Clients are offered referral to a genitourinary medicine (GUM) clinic, where they are seen for screening for STIs 10–14 days after the assault to allow for incubation of newly acquired infection (Home Office 2005). If, however, there are no SARC facilities for human immunodeficiency virus (HIV) and hepatitis screening, the client should be seen in the GUM clinic as soon as possible, preferably within 72 h. Where the complainant declines referral, the forensic examiner should recommend antibiotic prophylaxis against gonorrhoea and chlamydia.

HIV testing and hepatitis screening

The risk of acquiring HIV and hepatitis B following rape in the UK is rare and is estimated to be approximately 0.1–0.2% for vaginal rapes and 1–2% for anal rapes for HIV in developed countries (Kelly and Regan 2003). HIV risk assessment should be carried out, assessing the type of assault and enquiring about additional factors which increase or decrease risk (trauma, breech of hymen, condom usage), together with an appraisal of known or overt risk factors to do with the assailant (Home Office 2005).

Postexposure prophylaxis, if given, should be started as soon as possible after sexual assault as it is unlikely to be beneficial after 72 h. The Clinical Effectiveness Group of the British Association for Sexual Health and HIV have updated the UK guideline for the use of postexposure prophylaxis for

HIV after sexual exposure (PEPSE), facilitating calculation of the risk of HIV infection after potential exposure, recommending when PEPSE would and would not be considered. It is believed that transmission of HIV is likely to be increased following aggravated sexual intercourse (anal or vaginal) such as occurs during sexual assault, and the authors recommend that clinicians should consider recommending PEPSE more readily in such situations where the 'source' individual's HIV status is unknown (Fisher et al 2006).

Risk assessment for hepatitis B infection in sexual assault victims should be along the lines of the HIV assessment. Hepatitis B vaccination is recommended for all victims of sexual assault, and hepatitis B immunization should be considered for a non-immune contact after single unprotected forced sexual exposure if the assailant is known or is strongly suspected to be infectious as long as it is given within 7 days; it is, however, best given within 48 h of the contact.

Odontological examination

The FFLM recommend an odontologist for photography of injuries caused by teeth. Some injuries may become clearer with time, so repeat photography should be considered (Rowlinson et al 2008).

GP letter

A letter to the general practitioner should be supplied, with victim's consent, and take-home literature about local support networks given.

Injuries

Non-genital injury

The majority of female victims (40–88%) will have some form of physical injury, although most will be of a minor nature (Bowyer and Dalton 1997, McGregor et al 2002, Palmer et al 2004). Less than 5% of complainants attending SARCs require hospital admission for treatment (Home Office 2005). Where a clinical injury extent score was applied to rate the physical severity of the assault in 113 cases of sexual crime, the injuries were ranked as:

- 44% with light injury;
- 18% with moderate injury; and
- one victim with severe injury (Alempijevic et al 2007) (1%).

Also, 63.4% of victims had one or more injuries, whereas 35.6% had no injuries. Injuries, predominantly bruises, were located on limbs (32%), face (23%) and torso (7%).

Genital injury

The overall incidence of genital injury is of the order of 20–49% (McGregor et al 2002, Palmer et al 2004, Drocton et al 2008). Genital injury in the absence of non-genital injury is rare (3%) (Palmer et al 2004). Palmer et al also found that risk factors for genital injury were:

- the presence of non-genital injury [odds ratio (OR) 19, 95% confidence interval (CI) 6.0–63.0];
- threats of violence (OR 3.7, 95% CI 1.5–8.9); and
- being aged over 40 years (OR 5.6, 95% CI 1.6–20.3).

Clinical injury extent scoring

McGregor et al devised a clinical injury extent scoring, categorizing injuries as none, mild, moderate or severe, based upon observed genital and extragenital injury (McGregor et al 1999). Criteria for clinical injury scoring were devised; for example, one of the criteria for a moderate injury score was 'injury or injuries expected to have some impact on function'. The results supported the hypothesis that there is an association between the laying of charges and the presence of documented moderate or severe injury. These findings were supported by a subsequent study where a gradient association was found for genital injury extent score and charge filing, but an injury extent score defined as severe was the only variable significantly associated with conviction.

Genital trauma associated with forced digital penetration has been found in 81% of complainants (Rossman et al 2004). This retrospective study documented the frequency and type of injury in 53 women in whom forced digital penetration was the only reported type of assault. The mean number of genital injuries was 2.4, and 56% of the injuries occurred at four sites: the fossa navicularis, labia minora, cervix and posterior fourchette. The most common types of injury were erythema (34%), superficial tears (29%) and abrasions (21%).

Forensic examiners remain unsure about why some sexual victims display acute injury while others do not (Drocton et al 2008). The potential reasons for these differential findings among female victims were explored for 3356 complainants, of whom 49% displayed AGI. Significant increased risk for AGI was noted with vaginal penetration or attempted penetration using penis, finger or object, and anal-penile penetration. Victims less likely to display AGI were those with a longer postcoital interval and those with increased parity.

The Influence of Alcohol- and Drug-Facilitated Sexual Assault

The true extent of alcohol- and drug-facilitated sexual assault (DFSA) is not known and is difficult to estimate, but drugs and alcohol do impair the recollection of events surrounding the sexual assault, making identification and prosecution of the assailant even more difficult. The SOA 2003 states that voluntary intoxication affects a woman's capacity to choose. The BCS also noted that a significant minority of victims report that they were under the influence of drink in the most recent incident of sexual assault they had experienced (Kershaw et al 2008). Alcohol is also known to be a factor involved in 34% of rape cases reported to the police (Kelly et al 2005). The proportion of DFSA in four American localities was estimated with urine and hair specimens tested for 45 drugs (Juhascik et al 2007). Of 144 subjects, 43% were characterized as DFSA. There was considerable under-reporting of the use of drugs by the subjects.

A study into the nature of DFSA in England examined samples from 120 cases of sexual assault (Operation Matisse 2006). One hundred and nineteen of the 120 victims reported drinking alcohol; however, alcohol was only detected in 62 (52%) cases. In 22 of the 62 (35%) cases, blood alcohol at the time of the incident was estimated to be greater than or equivalent to 200 mg% (i.e. more than twice the driving limit of 80 mg%). The authors commented that a combination of drugs and alcohol exacerbates intoxication, and suggested that some of the cases could be opportunistic DFSA (i.e. where an assailant assaults a victim who is profoundly intoxicated by her own action), whereas other offenders facilitate sexual assault by administering drugs, including alcohol, to the victim.

Description of Wounds

The doctor examining a complainant of sexual assault may experience difficulty with the nomenclature when describing wounds, and may be daunted by the medicolegal significance of the lesions. Even more difficulty may be encountered when asked to give an opinion as to how they may have been caused. The following classification has been adapted from Crane (1996).

Bruises

A bruise is caused by the application of blunt force to the skin that damages small blood vessels beneath the skin surface. The blood then spreads through the tissue spaces. Bruises resolve over a variable period of time. On the whole, blue and black bruises are indicative of recent trauma, but estimating the age of a bruise is a risky undertaking and should be avoided at all costs, especially if one is asked to do so in court.

Petechiae

Petechiae are pinhead-sized haemorrhages within the skin caused by:

- mechanical trauma, with underlying clothing leaving an imprint of the material's texture as petechiae;
- sucking, as in 'love-bites'; and
- congestion/mechanical asphyxiation on face, upper neck, conjunctiva as in childbirth and strangulation.

Purpura

Purpura are larger haemorrhages within the skin, often seen in the elderly.

Haematoma

Haematomas are blood that collects as a mass beneath the skin.

Factors to remember about bruising

- May be delayed in appearance. Deep bruises can take 12–24 h to appear.
- May not reflect the size of the object impacting with the skin.
- May not represent the point of impact due to tracking along tissue planes.
- May not represent the severity of the blow due to age or frailty of tissues.
- Can vary according to the site (e.g. underlying bone).
- Appearance of a bruise can be affected by skin colour.

- Interpretation of bruises in hairy areas can be difficult.
- Can assist in interpretation of causation (e.g. finger-tip bruising on inner aspect of upper arms).
- There are considerable difficulties in timing injuries by the colour of a bruise.

A study into the ageing of bruises determined that the only reliable fact is that bruises with a yellow colour are more than 18 h old, and that the appearance of the other colours is less reliable (Langlois and Gresham 1991).

The following observations should be recorded for each bruise:

- dimensions;
- colour;
- pattern;
- site; and
- associated injuries.

The following observations should be recorded for each abrasion, laceration, incision and stab wound:

- nature and number of such injuries;
- site;
- dimensions including injury depth;
- pattern and shape of injury;
- whether injury is unilateral/bilateral;
- active bleeding;
- presence of foreign material in the wound;
- evidence of healing;
- suturing, dressing or plaster cast obscuring the injury;
- coexisting injury;
- associated injury; and
- whether there is any pre-existing injury.

Abrasions

Abrasions are also known as scratches or grazes, where a scratch is a linear abrasion and a graze is a 'brush-mark' abrasion. Abrasions are injuries involving only the outer layers of skin: partial-thickness tears. The skin injury of an abrasion is at the site of the impact with injuring force. Abrasions are usually linear in nature but may be curved due to fingernails or a human bite.

Lacerations

Lacerations, also known as cuts or tears, occur when the injuring blunt force causes full-thickness splitting of the skin in a ragged way. They are often associated with bruising and there may be flaps of skin due to a shearing force being applied.

Incisions

Incisions are caused by sharp cutting weapons and are seen less commonly in the genital injuries of rape and sexual assault, although the genitalia and breasts may be the target of the assailant wielding a knife or similar sharp weapon. The tissues are cleanly divided and the cut is long and less deep than a stab wound.

Stab wounds

A stab wound is a penetrating deep injury. With respect to transvaginal impalement, there is considerable risk of damage to extravaginal sites. Identification of possible extensive injury may be difficult and would require multi-disciplinary involvement.

Thermal injury

Thermal injuries are caused by dry heat sources such as chemicals, electricity, friction and lighted cigarettes. Moist heat injuries usually refer to injuries caused by scalds.

Fracture

Fractures need careful recording of site, whether open/closed, and need for fixation or treatment.

Organ rupture

Organ rupture is uncommon, but can be life-threatening if the liver or spleen is affected. It may not be visibly obvious, so needs to be remembered if patients develop signs of shock.

Absence of Genital Injury

The absence of genital injuries should not negate an allegation of sexual assault/rape, but the presence of genital injury is thought to carry more weight in obtaining a successful conviction. In a retrospective view of case records of women from Northumbria Police area, only 22 of 83 women had genital injuries (27%) (Bowyer and Dalton 1997). It was concluded that the 'absence of genital injury should not be used as pivotal evidence by the police or CPS'. Similar incidence of genital injury was reported in a study of 440 cases of reported sexual assault, where 16% of the victims had visible genital injury (Cartwright et al 1986). By the same token, absence of genital injury in no way implies consent by the victim nor the absence of vaginal penetration by the assailant (Cartwright et al 1986).

Reasons for absence of genital injury

Reasons for absence of genital injury may include:
- verbal threats to the victim, intimidation and threats that failure to comply with the assailant's demands will result in physical injury/death to herself or another person (e.g. child);
- coercion may play a significant role in marital rape;
- force used is insufficient to produce an injury (especially in sexually active parous women);
- use, or threat of use, of a weapon;
- complainant under the influence of drugs/alcohol;
- bruises may not become apparent for 48 h;
- delay in reporting assault, allowing healing of lesions;
- use of lubricant at time of rape; and
- false allegation.

The absence of injury must also make the forensic examiner consider and include a comment regarding whether the complainant could have been threatened.

A common tactic of the barrister defending a suspect in a rape trial is not to deny that sexual intercourse between their client and the complainant took place, but rather to claim that she consented to the encounter (Cartwright et al

1986). The defending barrister may also point out to the FP and jury that there are no injuries to the victim's genitalia, and may ask the doctor how a victim of an alleged rape could escape injury unless, of course, she actually consented to intercourse, highlighting how unimpressive a case may look where there is absence of injury. Cartwright et al found that 75 victims in a review of 440 cases of reported rape showed objective evidence of non-compliance (injuries to non-genital sites) and vaginal penetration (sperm in the vagina), and only 28% of these women had sustained genital injury.

The Statement

Medical witness statement

The minimum requirement for a doctor's (professional) statement is in the form of a 'witness to the fact' document providing a basic interpretation of the findings alone. The FFLM has recommended that all FPs should have training in the production of a factual statement, and should have ongoing support with writing statements from experienced FPs (Faculty of Forensic and Legal Medicine 2008b).

Timing of statement preparation

It is a wise practice to complete a statement as soon as possible after the examination, and include an interpretation and opinion at the end of the statement, either using lay terms where possible or including a glossary of the medical terminology.

The statement should contain core data such as the examiner's qualifications, relevant experience and number of cases examined, although this can be considered an optional field for new forensic examiners. This should be followed by a summary of the history of the incident. The findings, both normal and abnormal, must be documented.

Interpretation of findings

- Causation of injuries.
- Mechanisms leading to injury.
- Degree of force required to produce the injury.
- Other possible causes for findings.
- Exclusion of unlikely causes.
- Consistency of findings.
- Opinion — using a sliding scale to describe the degree of certainty.

Interpretation of the physical findings is one of the most difficult aspects of forensic gynaecology. The legal profession, in particular, has an unrealistic expectation regarding what conclusions can be reached following a forensic medical examination, and the unwary examiner may find themselves accused of bias.

It is important to comment upon whether appearances of the genital area are normal or abnormal.

In general, when considering bruises, one should assess the site of the bruising and how this may affect the appearance of the bruise, the causation and the force of impact that might have caused the bruising. It is helpful to use a scale to describe one's degree of certainty about the likely cause of the particular injuries.

Conclusions

In preparing the conclusions, the overall causation and consistency need to be addressed so that the following aspects are covered:

- the presence of signs that support the allegation;
- whether the signs are consistent with the allegation;
- the probable causation of the injuries;
- whether or not consensual sexual activity could explain the findings;
- the effect of age and hormonal status on the genital tissues;
- the presence of any unusual injuries and the implication of such injuries;
- reasons for absence of injury should be addressed;
- suggest realistic alternative causation such as an accidental injury (e.g. streaky, linear bruising due to a watchstrap or piece of jewellery, or an ovoid abrasion due to a fall against a similarly shaped object);
- the site of injuries is very important (e.g. accidental bruising on the inner aspect of the thighs or knees is very unlikely, a more likely cause being the blunt force of an assailant's knees or thumbs being applied to separate the legs); and
- inconsistencies — the possibility of a false allegation must be entertained when preparing the opinion. Also, in interpreting any injury, the doctor must consider whether it has any features suggestive of being self-inflicted. Clues that may assist in this assessment include location of the wound (accessibility), the direction of linear (often parallel) scratches, and the sparing of sensitive areas of the body.

The conclusion should end with a sentence indicating that the statement has been 'based on information given to me to date'. Also, there should be some indication that modification of the conclusions may be necessary if further, relevant information becomes available.

Use of relevant references

The absence of genital injuries should not negate an allegation of sexual assault or rape, but it does make it more difficult to prove to a jury as the presence of genital injury is thought to carry more weight in obtaining a successful conviction. With reported rates of visible genital injury being of the order of 20–49%, it is important that the examining doctor is able to quote published data to support the statement that the absence of genital injury does not imply consent by the complainant, and that the presence of genital injury should not be required to validate an allegation of sexual assault (Cartwright et al 1986, McGregor et al 2002, Palmer et al 2004, Drocton et al 2008).

Final reminders on statement presentation

The forensic examiner should ensure that the statement has a professional appearance, and having checked the document for errors, should also make a check for areas of vulnerability to criticism. In England and Wales, there is a statutory declaration to sign and date the beginning of the statement.

Patterns of Injury

Patterns

Some female survivors of sexual assault sustain more physical injuries than others, and factors influencing the type of injury include the complainant's skin fragility. Genital trauma is more common in older women (Ramin et al 1992). Where there are multiple bruises, it is essential to undertake a collective assessment of both the bruises and any other surrounding injury in an attempt to reconstruct events. It is also important to recognize particular patterns of injury (e.g. finger-tip bruising consisting of a row or a pair of circular or oval bruises, suggesting the blunt force of gripping associated with resistance in areas such as the upper arms, breasts and legs).

Postmenopausal women

One of the factors influencing the type of injury sustained is the victim's age. Postmenopausal women only represent a small percentage of the number reporting sexual assault: 2.2% in Dallas County between 1986 and 1991 (Ramin et al 1992). There was no significant difference in the relative proportion of women experiencing non-genital injuries; trauma in general occurred as frequently in the older woman (67%) as in the younger group. This was confirmed in a later study on the effects of age and ethnicity on physical injury from rape (Sommers et al 2006).

Genital trauma is more common: 43% in the postmenopausal group compared with 18% in younger women (Ramin et al 1992). Almost one in five older women had genital lacerations. Other authors have reported an increased frequency of genital injuries in the older victim of sexual assault, and being aged over 40 years has been identified as a risk factor for genital injury (Cartwright et al 1986, Palmer et al 2004). However, no significant association between age and genital injury was found by Sommers et al (2006).

Where there is an increased genital trauma rate, it is presumably due to postmenopausal atrophy causing increased genital tissue susceptibility. It is sad to reflect that older victims tend to live alone, are often robbed and are more likely to be raped by a stranger (Tyra 1993).

Adolescent victims

A pre-existing relationship between a victim and the assailant may explain other elements that distinguish an adolescent victim from her adult counterpart (Muram et al 1995). An assessment of the epidemiology and patterns of AGI in a group of adolescents (13–17 years old) compared with women over 17 years of age showed that adolescents were more likely to be assaulted by an acquaintance or relative (Jones et al 2003).

Weapons and physical force are used less frequently where adolescent victims are involved, but alcohol and drug use is prevalent in adolescent victims (47% of cases) (Muram et al 1995). There are conflicting opinions about the frequency of physical, non-genital injuries in adolescents compared with older victims of sexual assault, but a recent study showed that adolescent victims were less likely to experience non-genital injuries than adults but had a greater frequency of AGI (Jones et al 2003). Common sites of injury in adolescents were posterior, including fossa navicularis, labia minora, fourchette and hymen, whereas for adults, there was a less consistent pattern of AGI, although they did have fewer hymenal injuries and greater injury to the perianal area.

A significant association has been found between race (Black vs White) and genital injury, where Whites were four times as likely as Blacks to have genital injury (Sommers et al 2006). The reasons for this disparity appear to be complex, and the simple explanation of skin colour explaining race/ethnic difference in injury prevalence may suffice for the forensic examiner. However, health disparities may affect the reporting of genital injuries amongst women of colour in the USA.

Vulnerable Women

Mental health

It is important that all the professionals involved with victims of sexual assault recognize that the assault may be followed by rape-related PTSD. This is a debilitating psychiatric condition that can occur in people who experience extremely stressful or traumatic life events, and sexual assault is thought to be one of the most traumatic stressors in life. It is believed that victims attending for forensic examination may already be in the acute phase of PTSD, exhibiting shock, disbelief, anger and possibly memory blocking. The risk of PTSD among female victims of sexual assault is 2.9 times higher compared with women who reported no history of sexual assault, according to a cross-sectional telephone survey of 1769 adult female residents in Virginia (Masho and Ahmed 2007).

When attending a victim of recent sexual assault, the FP may question whether such a woman is able to give 'informed' consent to all aspects of the forensic medical examination. It may be appropriate, in this case, to complete the consent for examination and sample collection, and defer the consent to disclosure of the medical details until a later date.

A high background prevalence of mental health problems and deliberate self-harm was found in a study of 121 complainants of sexual violence at The Haven, Whitechapel (Campbell et al 2007). When mental health problems were identified, additional questions were asked. Of the female victims, 8% had learning difficulties, 21% had a past history of deliberate self-harm and 20% had a psychiatric history. Three percent of the female victims required immediate referral to the psychiatric liaison team. One must not forget that vulnerable people are at increased risk following sexual violence; indeed, a high frequency of PTSD is seen in female refugees who allege torture (Asgary et al 2006, Edston and Olsson 2007, Hooberman et al 2007).

Women with disabilities

Very few studies have examined how sexual assault patterns differ for women with disabilities, and whether a woman's disability status influences the degree and nature of the sexual violence. Study data derived from the initial encounter of 16,672 women survivors of sexual assault in Massa-chusetts from 1987 to 1995 showed that more than 10% of survivors reported one or more disability (Nannini 2006). Among women with a single disability, a survivor who delayed seeking services for 6 months or more was more likely to have a mental health disability. Women with disabilities have been shown to have four times the odds of experiencing sexual assault in the past year compared with women without disability, according to a study in North Carolina (Martin et al 2006). A retrospective longitudinal study of 6273 non-institutionalized women participating in the National Violence Against Women survey in the USA found that women with disabilities that severely limit activities of daily living are four times more likely to be sexually assaulted than women with no reported disability (Casteel et al 2008).

There are even fewer studies concerning refugees who allege that they have been sexually assaulted as victims of torture. In Sweden, the records of 63 female victims of torture were studied (Edston and Olsson 2007). Rape, often both anal and vaginal, several times and by different persons, was reported by 76% of the women. Physical abuse by use of blunt force was alleged by 95%. In a study in the USA, 89 asylum seekers/torture survivors from 30 countries were assessed in an urban primary care clinic, and 7% of cases alleged that rape was the means of abuse (Asgary et al 2006). The authors point out that physicians evaluating torture survivors should be trained in identification and documentation of torture. This is particularly important where sexual violence as a means of torture is alleged.

Migrant women

In the UK, migrant women may be reluctant to seek help and advice, or approach the criminal justice authorities if they perceive that their immigration status might be put at risk by coming forward. In addition, such women may not be aware of the interpreter services that exist for women seeking help with health-related problems. Worldwide, the higher vulnerability of migrant women to sexual abuse and violence is known to place them at risk of STIs and mental health problems associated with sexual violence. Migrant women face sexual abuse by employers in receiving countries, and from personnel in refugee camps (Carballo et al 1996). Migration also fuels the sex tourism industry in countries as diverse as the Netherlands and Thailand.

Court Proceedings

Victim in court

The victim may be called to give evidence as a witness at a Crown Court if the attacker pleads 'not guilty'. In addition to the support of the police officers and counsellors involved, they can also seek the support of the Crown Court Witness Service. Arrangements can be made for the complainant to visit the court before the trial, and information on police and court procedure, liaison with other organizations on behalf of the victim, and assistance in application for compensation from the Criminal Injuries Compensation Board can be provided.

Pretrial conference

The examining doctor will be expected to read through the notes carefully and should expect to be called to a pretrial discussion, in their capacity as a professional or an expert prosecution witness, with the reviewing lawyer, CPS caseworker, police officer and counsel for the prosecution (barrister). It is important that the examining doctor has access to the committal papers (witness statements, transcripts of taped interviews and the defence statement), the complainant's forensic test results and the defence medical expert's report, and is able to discuss this opinion with counsel.

Doctor in court

The doctor should be familiar with the courtroom lay-out (in particular, the location of the witness box, judge's bench and the jury) and the Crown Court etiquette, such as addressing the jury at all times, and should decide ahead of time whether to make a solemn affirmation or swear an oath.

The defence usually asks for an independent medical expert report and they will have access to copy statements from the complainant, the examining doctor and the defendant, and transcripts of interviews. The defence may also request the contemporaneous medical notes.

Examination-in-chief

The examining doctor may be called to court as a professional witness to help the court to establish the facts. The purpose of the examination-in-chief is for the FP to make their evidence clear to the judge and jury. The reviewing barrister establishes the professional witness's name, qualifications and expertise, and then asks for confirmation of the details of the statement. Addressing the jury, the doctor will be asked by the counsel for the prosecution (reviewing barrister) to describe what was found at the time of the examination. The doctor is usually asked to give an opinion regarding the possible causation for the findings.

Cross-examination

Counsel for the defence (opposing barrister) then conducts the cross-examination of the professional witness, asking questions to probe particular issues in the professional witness's statement in order to identify any contentious issues of fact or opinion. The defence barrister's role is to draw the professional witness's attention to any deficiencies in the evidence that will favour their client.

Re-examination

When cross-examination is complete, the prosecuting barrister has the opportunity to re-examine, clarifying any issues raised. No fresh material can be raised at this point. The judge, too, may wish to ask further questions or summarize what has been said.

Expert witnesses in sexual assault

Medical evidence is an important factor in the prosecution of rape offences, but it is felt that its evidential worth is not always properly understood by the prosecution. 'It is vital that the quality of the expert evidence relied upon to support the investigation and prosecution of rape is sound. If it is flawed then challenge by the Defence is inevitable' (H.M. Crown Prosecution Service Inspectorate 2007). The FFLM believes that expert evidence should only be sought from FPs who have gained a postgraduate qualification in clinical forensic medicine.

The GMC in 'Acting as an Expert Witness' emphasizes the importance of 'understanding and adhering to the laws and codes of practice that affect your work as an expert witness. In particular, you should make sure that you understand:

- how to construct a court-compliant report
- how to give oral evidence
- the specific framework of law and procedure within which you are working'.

Expert witness statement

The concept of a two-stage report in a single contact case of sexual assault/rape has been proposed, and the philosophy of such an approach is to improve the successful conviction rate and to provide a structure that is supportive to relatively inexperienced forensic examiners. The initial statement made by the examining doctor who is a professional witness is a factual account of the findings, and for those cases likely to proceed to court, a second 'expert' statement might be commissioned. The initial forensic examiner might wish to end their initial conclusion with the following comment: 'Should it appear likely that this case would proceed to court, a second, more detailed statement will be required. Either:

- I am prepared to provide that statement; or
- An expert forensic examiner will prepare this statement'.

The FFLM recommend that all FPs should annotate their professional statements with 'this is a professional witness statement of fact. I am able/unable to provide expert opinion evidence in relation to this matter/and would be happy to do so on supply of all relevant documents' (Faculty of Forensic and Legal Medicine 2008b).

As an expert, the doctor's legal position is one of an advisor to the prosecution on matters which are outside the experience of the general public. The expert should have access to the fullest possible picture in order to give the best advice and opinion. Accordingly, the expert should have sight of all relevant statements, a record of the defendant's interview, relevant medical records and the results of the scientific tests. An expert should prepare their statement based upon their analysis of the case, and provide an opinion with the assistance of the examining doctor.

It is recognized that an important factor in the development of expertise is the building of case experience, and so within the REACH organization, it has been established that an 'expert' forensic examiner is one who has examined 20 rape/sexual assault cases and has been actively involved as a FP for at least 2 years. In addition, the expert will have undertaken appropriate training and be an 'accredited' FP. The term 'accredited FP' implies that the doctor is willing and able to provide an expert statement. An 'accredited FP' is under no obligation and the provision of an expert opinion is optional to those experienced enough to do so. Such a two-tier system may prove costly, but with UK conviction rates running at approximately 6.5%, this novel approach may assist the CPS in their assessment of the strength of a particular case (McGregor et al 2002).

Conclusion

There is growing international concern about the low conviction rate for rape. Forensic examination services, clinicians and the judiciary are jointly involved in addressing the attrition rates in sexual assault cases in the UK. The reporting of rape can act as a gateway to other services, and this is particularly important for vulnerable women such as those with mental health problems. The criminal justice system has introduced initiatives in an attempt to improve the response to rape cases, but it is also important to recognize that there is a need for improvement in the clinical/forensic management of sexual assault cases including:

- improved levels of support for complainants at all stages;
- improved levels of communication between the FP, counsellors, police, CPS, general practitioner and complainant;
- continuing improvements in evidence gathering and report writing;
- recruitment to forensic gynaecological training programmes and hence to forensic examination teams; and
- continuing multidisciplinary education for all concerned in the care of rape victims.

In addition, it is very important that there is rapid implementation of the new laws that aim to protect the victims of sexual assault, especially vulnerable witnesses in rape trials, and that research programmes are established to gain a better understanding of why there is a high rate of charge reduction and why complainants withdraw their allegations.

KEY POINTS

1. There may be many reasons for failure to report sexual assault.
2. Consent to forensic medical examination differs from the standard consent forms and must accommodate details about disclosure of evidence.
3. The estimation of the age of a bruise should be avoided.
4. The absence of genital injury does not imply consent by the victim.

5. Following the examination, the victim should be offered appropriate medical advice, counselling and follow-up.
6. When interpreting the findings, the professional witness should comment upon whether the appearances are normal or abnormal, and describe their degree of certainty about the likely cause of any injuries.

References

Alempijevic D, Savic S, Pavlekic S, Jecmenica D 2007 Severity of injuries among sexual assault victims. Journal of Forensic and Legal Medicine 14: 266–269.

Asgary RG, Melatlios EE, Smith CL, Paccione GA 2006 Evaluating asylum seekers/torture survivors in urban primary care: a collaborative approach at the Bronx Human Rights Clinic. Health and Human Rights 9: 164–179.

Bang L 1993 Rape victims — assaults, injuries and treatment at a medical rape trauma service at Oslo Emergency Hospital. Scandinavian Journal of Primary Health Care 11: 15–20.

Barnard MA, Hurt G, Benson C, Church S 2002 Client Violence Against Prostitutes Working from Street and Off-street Locations: a Three-city Comparison. Economic and Science Research Council, Swindon.

Bowyer L, Dalton ME 1997 Female victims of rape and genital findings. BJOG: an International Journal of Obstetrics and Gynaecology 104: 617–620.

Brennan PA 2006 The medical and ethical aspects of photography in sexual assault examination: why does it offend? Journal of Clinical Forensic Medicine 13: 194–202.

Bunting R 1996 Clinical examination in the police context. In: McLay WDS (ed)

Clinical Forensic Medicine. Greenwich Medical Media, London, pp 59–73.

Campbell L, Keegan A, Cybulska D, Forster G 2007 Prevalence of mental health problems and deliberate self-harm in complainants of sexual violence. Journal of Forensic and Legal Medicine 14: 75–78.

Carballo M, Grocutt M, Hadzihasanovic A 1996 Women and migration: a public health issue. World Health Statistics Quarterly — Rapport Trimestriel de Statistiques Sanitaires Mondiales 49: 158–164.

Cartwright PS, Moore RA, Anderson JR, Brown DH 1986 Genital injury and implied consent to alleged rape. Journal of Reproductive Medicine 31: 1043–1044.

Casteel C, Martin SL, Gurka KK, Kupper LL 2008 National study of physical and sexual assault among women with disabilities. Injury Prevention 14: 87–90.

Chowdhury-Hawkins R, McLean I, Winterholler M, Welch J 2008 Preferred choice of gender of staff providing care to victims of sexual assault in sexual assault referral centres (SARCs). Journal of Forensic and Legal Medicine 15: 363–367.

Crane J 1996 Injury. In: McLay WDS (ed) Clinical Forensic Medicine. Greenwich Medical Media, London, pp 143–162.

Drocton P, Sachs C, Chu L, Wheeler M 2008 Validation set correlates of anogenital injury after sexual assault. Academic Emergency Medicine 15: 231–238.

Dupré AR, Hampton HL, Morrison H, Meeks GR 1993 Sexual assault. Obstetrical and Gynaecological Survey 48: 640–648.

Dyer C 2008 Rape cases: police admit failing victims. The Guardian. Available at: www.guardian.co.uk/uk/2008/mar/04/ukcrime.law.

Edston E, Olsson C 2007 Victims of torture. Journal of Forensic and Legal Medicine 14: 368–373.

Faculty of Forensic and Legal Medicine 2008a Guidelines for the Collection of Forensic Specimens from Complainants and Suspects. Available at: www.fflm.ac.uk.

Faculty of Forensic and Legal Medicine 2008b Forensic Physicians as Witnesses in Criminal Proceedings. Available at: www.fflm.ac.uk.

Fisher M, Benn P, Evans B, Poznaik A, Jones M, MacLean S, Davidson O, Summerside J, Hawkins D 2006 BASHH Guideline. UK Guideline for the use of post-exposure prophylaxis for HIV following sexual exposure. International Journal of STD and AIDS 17: 81–92.

General Medical Council 2004 Disclosures to courts or in connection with litigation. In:

Confidentiality: Protecting and Providing Information. GMC, London. Available at: www.gmc-uk.org/guidance/current/library/confidentiality.asp.

General Medical Council 2006 Relationships with patients — confidentiality. In: Good Medical Practice. GMC, London.

General Medical Council 2008 Acting as an Expert Witness. GMC, London. Available at: www.gmc-uk.org/guidance/ethical_ethicalguidance/expert_witness_guidance.asp.

H.M. Government 2007 Cross Government Action Plan on Sexual Violence and Abuse. Home Office, London.

H.M. Crown Prosecution Service Inspectorate 2007 Without Consent. A Report on the Joint Review of the Investigation and Prosecution of Rape Offence. HMIC, London.

Hockbaum SR 1987 The evaluation and treatment of the sexually assaulted patient. Emergency Medicine Clinics of North America 5: 601–622.

Holmes MM, Resnick HS, Kilpatrick DG, Best CL 1996 Rape-related pregnancy: estimates and descriptive characteristics from a national sample of women. American Journal of Obstetrics and Gynecology 175: 320–325.

Home Office 2005 Medical Care Following Sexual Assault: Guidelines for Sexual Assault Referral Centre. Home Office, London.

Hooberman JB, Rosenfeld B, Lhewa D, Rasmussen A, Keller A 2007 Classification of torture experiences of refugees living in US. Journal of Interpersonal Violence 22: 108–123. Available at: www.crimereduction.homeoffice.gov.uk/sexualoffences/sexual03.htm.

Jones JS, Rossman L, Wynn BN, Dunnock C, Schwatz N 2003 Comparative analysis of adult versus adolescent sexual assault: epidemiology and patterns of anogenital injury. Academic Emergency Medicine 10: 872–877.

Juhascik MP Negrusz A, Faugno D, Ledray L, Greene P, Lider A, Haner B, Gaensslen RE 2007 An estimate of the proportion of drug-facilitation of SA in 4 US localities. Journal of Forensic Sciences 52: 1396–1400.

Kelly L, Regan L 2003 Good Practice in Medical Responses to Recently Reported Rape, Especially Forensic Examinations. A Briefing Paper for the Daphne Strengthening the Linkage Project. Child and Woman Abuse Studies Unit, London Metropolitan University, London.

Kelly L, Lovett J, Regan L 2005 A Gap or a Chasm: Attrition in Reported Rape Cases. Home Office Research Study 293. Home Office, London.

Kershaw C, Nicholas S, Walker A (eds) 2008 Crime in England and Wales. Home Office Statistics Bulletin 07/08. Home Office Research Development and Statistics, Home Office, London.

Langlois NEI, Gresham GA 1991 The ageing of bruises: a review and study of the colour changes with time. Forensic Science International 50: 227–238.

Ledray L 1993 Sexual assault nurse clinician: an emerging area of nursing experience. AWHONN's Clinical Issues 4: 180–190.

Martin SL, Ray N, Sotres-Alvarez D, Kupper LL, Moracco KE, Dickens PA, Scandlin D, Gizlice Z 2006 Physical and sexual assault of women with disabilities. Violence against Women 12: 823–837.

Martinez AH, Villanueva LA, Torres C, Garcia LE 1999 Sexual aggression in adolescents. Epidemiologic study. Ginecologia y Obstetricia de Mexico 67: 449–453.

Masho SW, Ahmed G 2007 Age at sexual assault and posttraumatic stress disorder among women: prevalence, correlates and implications for prevention. Journal of Women's Health 16: 262–271.

McGregor MJ, Grace L, Marion SA, Wiebe E 1999 Examination for sexual assault: is documentation of physical injury associated with the laying of charges? A retrospective cohort study. Canadian Medical Association Journal 160: 1565–1569.

McGregor MJ, Du Mont J, Myhr TL 2002 Sexual assault forensic medical examination: is evidence related to successful prosecution? Annals of Emergency Medicine 39: 639–647.

Muram D, Hostetler BR, Jones CE, Speck PM 1995 Adolescent victims of sexual assault. Journal of Adolescent Health 17: 372–375.

Nannini A 2006 Sexual assault patterns among women with and without disabilities seeking survivor services. Women's Health Issues 16: 372–379.

Operation Matisse 2006 Investigating Drug Facilitated Sexual Assault. ACPO. Available at: www.acpo.police.uk/asp/policies/Data/operation%20Matisse.

Palmer CM, McNulty AM, D'Este C, Donovan B 2004 Genital injuries in women reporting sexual assault. Sexual Health 1: 55–59.

Ramin SM, Satin AJ, Stone IC, Wendel GD 1992 Sexual assault in postmenopausal women. Obstetrics and Gynecology 80: 860–864.

Rights of Women 2008 From Report to Court. A Handbook for Adult Survivors of Sexual Violence. Aldgate Press, London.

Roe S 2008 Intimate violence. In: Kershaw C, Nicholas S, Walker A (eds) Crime in England and Wales. Home Office Statistics Bulletin 07/08. Home Office Research Development and Statistics, Home Office, London.

Rossman L, Jones JS, Dunnock C, Wynn BN, Bermingham, M 2004 Genital trauma associated with forced digital penetration. American Journal of Emergency Medicine 22: 101–104.

Rowlinson C, Ritchie G, Nicholson F, Wall IF 2008 Faculty of Forensic and Legal Medicine in conjunction with the British Association for Forensic Odontology Recommendations. Management of Injuries Caused by Teeth. Available at: www.fflm.ac.uk.

Royal College of Obstetricians and Gynaecologists 2009 Sexual and Reproductive Health Subspecialty Curriculum Module 3. Forensic and Domestic Violence Competencies. RCOG. Available at: www.rcog.org.uk/curriculum-module/sexual-reproductive-health-srh-0.

Sommers MS, Zink T, Baker RB, Fargo JD, Porter J, Weybright D, Schafer JC 2006 Effects of age and ethnicity on physical injury from rape. Journal of Obstetric, Gynecologic and Neonatal Nursing 35: 199–207.

Templeton DJ, Williams A 2006 Current issues in the use of colposcopy for examination of sexual assault victims. Sexual Health 3: 5–10.

Tyra PA 1993 Older women: victims of rape. Journal of Gerontology Nursing 19: 7–12.

Wiley J, Sugar N, Fine D, Eckert LO 2003 Legal outcome of sexual assault. American Journal of Obstetrics and Gynecology 188: 1638–1641.

Williams R 2009 Conviction rates for rape remain appallingly low. The Guardian. Available at: www.guardian.co.uk/uk/2009/mar/27/rape-convictions-rates.

CHAPTER 66

Violence against women

Mary Hepburn and Kirstyn Brogan

Chapter Contents			
BACKGROUND	1002	MANAGEMENT OF PROBLEM SUBSTANCE USE	1006
PREVALENCE	1003	SEXUAL VIOLENCE IN WAR	1006
REPRODUCTIVE HEALTH CONSEQUENCES	1003	SUMMARY	1007
MANAGEMENT OF PROSTITUTION	1005	KEY POINTS	1007

Background

Violence against women is prevalent worldwide and is most commonly inflicted by men. Such violence takes many forms in different settings, sometimes legally sanctioned by the state and/or morally sanctioned by the society within which it occurs. However, while women can be at risk in many settings, the most common form of violence against women is domestic violence or abuse inflicted by the woman's partner or ex-partner, and the violence usually takes place in the home.

While the term 'domestic violence' could imply violence or abuse from either partner in a heterosexual or homosexual relationship, a United Nations report in 1995 recognized that the most common manifestation is violence against women by male partners (United Nations 1995). In the 1992 British Crime Survey (Mayhew et al 1993), domestic violence constituted the single largest category of assaults, with 80% directed against women. In the USA, it is estimated that 95% of battered partners are women (Jones 1997). The United Nations report highlighted the range of types of physical abuse suffered worldwide by women at the hands of their partners, including battering, marital rape, dowry violence, domestic murder, forced pregnancy, abortion, sterilization and forced prostitution. During pregnancy, violence may also cause miscarriage or fetal injury and/or death. Women also experience non-physical abuse in the form of psychological, emotional and economic abuse.

Domestic violence or abuse is difficult to define but a definition such as 'the psychological, emotional and economic as well as physical and sexual abuse of women by male partners or ex partners' (Scottish Needs Assessment Programme 1997) indicates the range of ways and circumstances in which women can be abused by their partners. Thus, while society's perception is that the greatest risk of violence comes from strangers outside the home, statistics confirm that this is not the case for women. Nevertheless, in addition to beating of a wife by her husband, violence against women includes other types of abuse such as abortion of female fetuses, female genital mutilation, forced prostitution by non-partners, rape (including rape and sexual violence as a war strategy) and murder. Women are also at risk of violence or abuse from any relationship or interaction with men in which sex is a factor; thus, while forced prostitution by a partner is itself a form of partner violence, women working as prostitutes, whether for a partner, another man or independently, are also at risk of violence from their clients. However, it is important to recognize that prostitution encompasses a wide spectrum of circumstances; while violence may occur as part of the practice of prostitution, it does not follow that all prostitution constitutes violence against women.

Violence against women is important to those providing reproductive health care. Women experiencing or at risk of violence are particularly vulnerable during pregnancy. Domestic violence often starts or escalates during pregnancy, and since the circumstances that drive a woman to commercial sex do not change because she has become pregnant, prostitution continues throughout pregnancy. Violence during pregnancy has obvious implications for the health of both mother and baby, and consequently has relevance for those providing maternity care (although recognition of this has been slow to develop). The relevance of violence to non-pregnant women is often only viewed in terms of rape. However, violence can cause or affect other gynaecological conditions, as well as having implications for other types of reproductive health care. It is therefore important to recognize that the entire spectrum of violence against women is of relevance to all aspects of reproductive health care.

The last 20 years has seen a worldwide increase in recognition of the health consequences of violence against women and the large spectrum of types of violence. This was accompanied by considerable research, the findings of which are

DOI: 10.1016/B978-0-7020-3120-5.00066-7

supported by ongoing work in this area (Tjaden and Thoennes 2000, Watts and Zimmerman 2003).

Prevalence

The true prevalence of violence against women is difficult to determine. This is largely because of underidentification, but also because prevalence will depend on the definition of violence adopted. Studies in many countries have produced a range of estimates of prevalence for various categories of domestic violence and/or abuse. While the figures vary according to the type of abuse recorded, all are likely to be underestimates. The World Health Organization's Multi-country Study on Women's Health and Domestic Violence Against Women (2005) surveyed 10 countries, representing diverse cultural settings including urban and rural areas within the same country. It obtained information from over 24,000 women. The prevalence of women who reported episodes of domestic violence ranged between 15% and 71%, with the greatest amount of violence being reported in provincial settings in Bangladesh and Peru. In countries where large cities and rural areas were studied, partner violence was consistently higher in provincial settings. Women's attitudes to violence and acceptance also varied; violence was condemned in urban areas, whereas in some rural areas, violence was accepted and justified, especially in situations such as female infidelity.

In the USA, estimates ranged between 2 million (United Nations 1995) and 4 million battered women, with 2000 women murdered each year (30% of female homicides) in association with battering (Jones 1997). In a Canadian survey of 12,300 women, 29% reported that they had experienced violence from a current or previous marital partner since 16 years of age (Johnson and Sacco 1995). In the UK, the Home Affairs Select Committee Report on Domestic Violence (1993) concluded that domestic violence is 'common'. While the 1992 British Crime Survey (Mayhew et al 1993) found that 11% of women reported physical violence in their relationships, a 1993 crime survey in Islington, London (Mooney 1994) found that one in four women reported a lifetime experience of domestic violence. In a study of 930 women in San Francisco, 12% reported rape by their husbands (Russell 1982), while in a UK study of 1000 women, one in four reported that they had experienced marital rape. The prevalence of violence to prostitutes from both clients and pimps (regardless of whether or not the latter is the regular sexual partner) is also difficult to assess. Nevertheless, its occurrence is well recognized by those who work with prostitutes, although not necessarily by the criminal justice system whose response has often been inappropriate (Kennedy 1993).

The abuser, the abused and patterns of abuse

Many of the forms of violence described above occur in the UK. It is widely believed that such violence is largely confined to the lower social classes, but this is a misconception. Domestic abuse occurs across the social spectrum, and is inflicted by men who are not necessarily mentally ill but who have a range of personality defects (Mezey 1997). Various factors may coexist with violence either as cause or effect. While abuse occurs throughout society, socioeconomic deprivation, unemployment and lack of education are cited as precipitating and perpetuating factors (Kennedy and Dutton 1989). Whatever the precise relationship, women from backgrounds of socioeconomic deprivation may have fewer resources and fewer options for dealing with the abuse.

Problem drug and alcohol use are often thought to be linked to abuse and are often offered as an excuse or justification. While men with substance misuse problems may be more likely to abuse their partners, this may not be because they are intoxicated, and they may do so while sober. The 1996 British Crime Survey showed that intoxication of the perpetrator with alcohol or drugs was less common in the case of domestic violence than in stranger and acquaintance violence (Mirrlees-Black et al 1996). Additionally, abusive men may cite substance misuse by the partner as the cause or justification for their abusive behaviour. While there is no evidence to support this, it is true that women suffering abuse may develop drug and/or alcohol problems as a consequence of the abuse (Stark and Flitcraft 1991, Plichta 1992).

Women working as prostitutes experience poverty and many have drug or alcohol problems. Many such women will have a history of abuse, including sexual abuse by a family member, partner or other person. Their partner may also have problem substance use financed by the prostitution. The more chaotic the woman's lifestyle, the greater her financial need, the less she is paid, the more clients she has to service to raise the necessary money, the more dangerous the circumstances in which she must work and the greater her exposure to the risk of violence.

However, while associations with various factors do exist and some groups of women are consequently at increased risk of violence, it is important to remember that these factors are not necessarily obvious. Moreover, there is no typical abuser and no typical abused woman.

Reproductive Health Consequences

Women who experience violence are more likely to suffer a number of consequences relevant to reproductive health services. More than 30% of domestic violence begins during pregnancy (CEMACH 2004), and more than 14% of maternal deaths occur in women who had told their health professional that they were in an abusive relationship (CEMACH 2007).

During pregnancy, the injury sites include breasts and abdomen with consequent risk of injury to the fetus, including miscarriage, premature delivery and fetal death (Mezey and Bewley 1997). Women who have experienced violence are more likely to suffer miscarriage (Stark and Flitcraft 1996). Pregnancy, genital tract infections and genital tract injury are possible consequences of sexual violence, while other persistent gynaecological problems, especially abdominal pain, may be the presentation of abuse. Such women may find it difficult to undergo pelvic examination.

Obviously, in all of these situations, the converse does not apply and not all women with such problems or difficulties have been abused. Equally, many women who have been abused demonstrate no obvious problems or stigmata which might indicate a history of abuse.

Presentation

Women may present because of violence in a number of ways. They may specifically report physical violence, including rape (see Chapter 65), or may present for treatment of physical injuries sustained (with or without admission of the circumstances), in which case the setting is most commonly the accident and emergency department or the general practitioner's surgery. Injuries sustained include bruises, cuts, fractured bones and internal injuries (Dobash and Dobash 1980). In pregnancy, injuries include maternal rupture of the uterus, spleen or liver; placental abruption; premature spontaneous rupture of the membranes; miscarriage and fetal death (James-Hanman and Long 1994). Other indicators of domestic abuse are late booking and poor or non-attendance at antenatal clinics, repeated attendance during pregnancy with minor ailments and unexplained admissions. Previous reports of maternal deaths involving domestic abuse recommend that all women attending maternity services should be asked specifically about domestic abuse and given the opportunity to disclose this information.

Abused women may present later with psychological problems such as anxiety, depression (including suicide attempts), and drug or alcohol problems (Stark et al 1979, Hillard 1985). They may present to reproductive health services, including obstetric and gynaecology departments, in various ways. Immediate problems prompting attendance include obstetric complications and injuries, including genital tract injuries. Women may present with clinical problems secondary to the violence, such as possible genital tract infection, the need for emergency contraception or subsequently with a pregnancy. Many women only present later with chronic gynaecological problems, such as chronic pelvic pain.

Violence, domestic or otherwise, may therefore be highly relevant to women's attendance at obstetric and/or gynaecology services. However, irrespective of the immediacy or directness of the association, and no matter how obvious the markers, the possibility will not necessarily be recognized. Moreover, women who present in these ways rather than with a specific complaint of violence and/or rape, whether or not the perpetrator is the partner, are unlikely to admit the abusive circumstances unless asked directly. Violence and/or abuse may therefore not be identified unless healthcare workers ask; since the occurrence of abuse is often not suspected in such situations, routine direct enquiry will be necessary for effective identification and management of this problem.

Identification

Violence against women is often not identified within healthcare services because women may not volunteer the information and they are often not asked about it. In one study of 290 pregnant women in which 23% reported past or present battering, none had been questioned about violence by any healthcare providers (Helton et al 1987). Many women do not want to involve authorities such as the police or law courts, and the authorities may not consider the

problem within their remit; indeed, they may not even consider it a problem at all. In the UK until 1829, a man had a right to 'chastise' his wife provided he used a stick 'no thicker than his thumb'. The possible existence of rape within marriage was only recognized in Scotland in 1989 and in England and Wales in 1991. Since commercial sex is widely viewed as voluntary, with the women morally responsible, violence against prostitutes is often considered an unavoidable risk of this activity that does not justify legal pursuit. Even when the violence extends to murder, this is seen as different from murder of a 'respectable' woman (Kennedy 1993).

Women who experience violence from a partner often feel ashamed. They also often feel that they are at least partly to blame, and must have deserved the abuse in some way. They are also afraid that if they disclose the abuse to a third party, their partner will find out and they will suffer even more violence. Similarly, women working as prostitutes are often ashamed of their involvement in prostitution and do not want to admit it. While not necessarily believing they deserve violence, they may feel that their activities invite it and they therefore bear some responsibility. Whatever their feelings, however, most prostitutes believe that a report of violence would not be received sympathetically by the relevant services, would not lead to an effective response and would therefore be pointless. Similarly, many women suffering partner violence do not expect a sympathetic or helpful response from services. Nevertheless, evidence shows that despite their reluctance to raise the subject and report the violence, and despite the inadequacy of responses, women who suffer violence or abuse want to be asked about it and to be given an opportunity to disclose it. In one American primary care survey, 75% of women favoured routine enquiry about physical abuse, and 97% of female and male respondents said that they would answer truthfully if asked directly. However, only 7% said that they had ever been asked (Friedman et al 1992).

There are various reasons why healthcare workers do not ask about violence (Sugg and Inui 1992). They may be unaware of the possibility of abuse or think it is rare; they may not perceive violence, domestic or otherwise, as their responsibility; or they may be unwilling to ask, either because they feel they lack the necessary skills, because they fear they may cause offence or because they are afraid of broaching a problem that they would not have the time or the knowledge to deal with. In many areas, there are insufficient or inadequately resourced support services to which women could be offered referral. The advice given is often limited to a recommendation to leave the batterer, and frustration is expressed when women do not follow this advice. Consequently, many healthcare workers feel unhappy asking about abuse and would only do so if there was obvious evidence of abuse. Any injury might be expected to raise suspicion, but injuries at various sites, of different ages and for which no good explanation is offered should indicate possible abuse. However, even in the presence of obvious markers of abuse, healthcare workers do not always make the connection and, whether consciously or unconsciously, do not recognize the possibility of abuse or enquire about it. Moreover, many abused women will not demonstrate any of the recognized markers, and not all women with these markers will have been abused.

Risk markers are therefore insufficiently sensitive or specific, and should not be used as a basis for selective enquiry. As well as being ineffective, selective enquiry (if obviously selective) can also be offensive regardless of whether or not the woman has suffered abuse. Any awkwardness on the part of the healthcare worker will be conveyed to the woman. The way the question is posed is therefore important. A statement such as 'I know this probably doesn't apply to you but we have to ask everyone' gives a clear indication of the 'correct' response and does not encourage disclosure. Identification of violence is important in reproductive health care; given the nature of services provided, it is entirely appropriate to take an adequate sexual and social history, including direct enquiry about violence and abuse in all cases.

Management of abuse

While all women should be asked about abuse, the circumstances must be conducive to disclosure. Privacy is essential and all women should have at least part of any reproductive health consultation conducted on a one-to-one basis with the doctor, nurse or midwife. The presence of a partner who is reluctant to leave will not only prevent enquiry but may be an indicator of abuse. There should be recognition that not all abused women will admit this on routine enquiry; a negative response will not preclude violence, and if there are strong suspicions, some support can often be provided in the absence of an explicit admission. Disclosure may then occur during a later consultation.

All women presenting in pregnancy should be asked about the circumstances of the pregnancy; whether the pregnancy is planned, intended and/or wanted; their relationship with their partner (or man who accompanies them) and whether he is the baby's father. In this context, it is simple to ask the woman about the quality of the relationship and specifically whether her partner has ever been violent to her. She should also be asked whether anyone else has ever been violent to her and whether she has ever been forced to have sex with someone against her wishes. Women presenting with a gynaecological problem should similarly have a full sexual history taken. All women, pregnant or non-pregnant, presenting for any type of reproductive health care should have a social history taken. This should include questions about lifestyle, including use of tobacco, alcohol and illicit drugs, all of which can directly affect reproductive health. Women who disclose illicit drug use should be asked how this is financed, including specific enquiry about involvement in commercial sex.

There are several important aspects to management (Heath 1992). It is important that a woman who discloses a history of violence is reassured that she is believed and that she is not responsible for nor deserving of the violence. In the reproductive health setting, management of the relevant injuries or medical problems with which she presents will be a priority (management of women presenting with a present history of rape or sexual abuse is described in Chapter 65), but the healthcare worker's responsibility does not end there. Details of the violence together with the woman's circumstances should be elicited, and an assessment should be made of immediate risk to the woman and/or her children or others in her immediate circle. The information she

provides should be documented accurately together with details of examination findings, including injuries if present and any treatment given. Such information may be required for future legal action. She should be reassured that any information she provides will be treated with confidentiality, but there should also be discussion about the meaning of and limits to confidentiality. Should the healthcare worker envisage having to disclose the information, such as to ensure child protection, this should be discussed with the woman at the outset.

There should be discussion with women experiencing domestic violence or abuse about the possibility of leaving the abuser. Information including contact telephone numbers should be provided about residential and non-residential services for women experiencing violence, as well as availability of any other alternative accommodation. However, it is important to recognize that it is often not feasible for women to remove themselves from the situation. For example, they may be financially, emotionally or otherwise dependent on the abuser, or it might not be possible for them to take their children with them for various reasons. Moreover, when the woman appears to be at significant and imminent risk of further violence, leaving the situation may increase that risk; women are especially likely to suffer significant injury or even be killed when they leave a violent domestic environment (Browne 1987, Geberth 1992). It is therefore essential that women are reassured that there is recognition of and sympathy for the limitations to their options, and are not given the impression that they are expected to leave or will be considered stupid or weak if they fail to do so.

Regardless of their circumstances or chosen action, women should be provided with information about services and also the offer of direct referral. Where specific problems (whether cause or effect) are identified, such as mental health or substance misuse problems, appropriate referral for specialist management will be helpful even if it does not resolve the problem of violence. Moreover, problem drug and/or alcohol use can have direct effects on reproductive health, which merit treatment of the problem in their own right. This is therefore discussed later.

Management of Prostitution

At present, approaches to legislation differ across countries with regards to prostitution. In the UK, a Home Office consultation paper, 'Paying the Price' (Home Office 2004), prioritized the needs of communities in preference to the health and safety of sex workers. This led to publication of the Coordinated Prostitution Strategy (Home Office 2006) that focuses on criminalization of prostitution. In a Canadian study, Lowman et al found that a criminalized system increased the risks to vulnerable women, and they were more likely to be vulnerable to predatory and premeditated forms of violence in comparison with women working within a legalized framework where violence was often situational (i.e regarding non-payment for services) (Lowman 2000).

In contrast to the UK, countries such as New Zealand and the Netherlands have focused on decriminalizing sex work; a decision based on a duty to protect sex workers. The

Prostitution Reform Act 2003 in New Zealand decriminalized sex work and improved workers' health, safety and job satisfaction. Women found that they could use the law to encourage condom use and reduce their risk of sexually transmitted infections, and were more confident at refusing clients who did not adhere to this.

Criminalizing prostitution forces the most vulnerable women away from health services, and increases the risk of violence and other health consequences.

Women experiencing violence in non-domestic settings receive similar support. Women seen at reproductive health services who admit involvement in commercial sex will invariably have attended for some other reason and the presenting problem will obviously need to be dealt with. Nevertheless, an admission of prostitution should prompt a full relevant history, including details of type of services offered and clients buying them. Sexual behaviour and consequent risks, together with relevant signs and symptoms, should be explored. In the obstetric context, women engaging in commercial sex will often claim that paternity is not in doubt and the pregnancy is definitely to their partner. However, clients often pay more for unprotected intercourse and a carefully taken sexual history may indicate that such confidence is misplaced. Nevertheless, such self-deception by a woman and/her partner, whether conscious or unconscious, is often an essential coping strategy, so it is not necessarily helpful to comment on it unless specifically asked to do so, when it should be discussed with the woman on her own. Even if not explicitly admitted, however, uncertainty or concern about paternity may increase the risk of violence to the woman from her partner. It is, of course, entirely reasonable and appropriate to discuss strategies for risk reduction in terms of sexually transmitted infections and unplanned/unwanted pregnancies with non-pregnant women involved in prostitution. In this context, it would also be appropriate to discuss possible paternity problems if the woman is not pregnant but keen to conceive to her partner. Preconception counselling about risks to a pregnancy from sexually transmitted infections (including bloodborne viruses such as human immunodeficiency virus) would also be desirable in this situation.

Women engaged in commercial sex will escape the consequent violence by ceasing prostitution. For those women whose prostitution is directed and controlled by their sexual partner, this may be achieved by leaving the partner as in other domestic abuse situations; however, for similar reasons, this may be difficult or impossible. In addition, some such women and many working independently will have to continue working because of their own financial needs. There is a social hierarchy of prostitution. At the upper end of the market, in saunas and other indoor settings, there is less risk, often less financial pressure but greater financial rewards. At the more risky, lower end of the market, financial need is often greater or more acute but income is lower. Amongst the most vulnerable women working on the streets, factors such as problem drug and/or alcohol use that necessitate prostitution are also much more common. Nevertheless, all women engaged in prostitution, regardless of the circumstances, are at risk of violence. An approach similar to that described for domestic abuse should be adopted. An adequate history and examination are essen-

tial, as is accurate documentation of relevant information. Immediate healthcare needs should be assessed and appropriate management instigated; in this situation, the presence of any genital tract trauma or infection, whether the woman is pregnant, and consequently whether she requires maternity care, a termination of pregnancy, effective contraception or preconceptual care.

While some women working as prostitutes might be able to leave the violent situation by leaving a violent partner or pimp for whom they were earning money, most would only be able to stop prostituting if their own financial needs were resolved. For many, this would require effective management of their drug or alcohol problem.

Management of Problem Substance Use

Problem drug and/or alcohol use is often associated with poor nutrition which, in turn, may cause amenorrhoea. Heroin use can also cause amenorrhoea with or without anovulation. Methadone substitution therapy improves social stability and general health, including nutrition; commencement of therapy is often followed by return of fertility which can precede return of menstruation.

Many drug-using women incorrectly assume that their amenorrhoea indicates infertility, but they must be warned this is not so and provided with effective contraception if they do not want to become pregnant. Conversely, however, drug-using women who experience difficulty in conceiving should be advised that stabilization of their drug use, and consequently their lifestyle, with methadone substitution therapy where appropriate will increase their chances of conception. Such measures would also improve the baby's health as well as the mother's parenting abilities. This advice also holds true for their partners, since reduced sperm motility is often observed in association with use of sedative drugs including benzodiazepines and opiates/opioids (including methadone). Although the precise functional significance of this is uncertain, in the absence of successful conception, it seems reasonable to give both partners general advice about reduction in levels of drug use, and for those on substitute medication, to recommend stabilization at the lowest level compatible with stability.

Management of the drug problem *per se* is obviously not the clinical responsibility of reproductive healthcare professionals. However, if such a problem is identified, whether incidentally or in association with prostitution, violence or reproductive health problems, women should be given appropriate information about possible effects on pregnancy, fertility and effective contraception if indicated. This should be provided together with information about specialist services and the offer of referral.

Sexual Violence in War

The use of sexual violence as a strategy in war has been observed and reported by healthcare workers, humanitarian organizations and others working in such settings (Shanks et al 2001). Women who have experienced such violence may move to other countries as refugees or asylum seekers, and may then present to healthcare workers who do not have direct experience of such problems. Refugees presenting for reproductive health care may have experienced violence; their trauma may be exacerbated by being in a culturally unfamiliar environment, possibly without the support of family or friends, often with language and communication difficulties, and encountering healthcare workers who are unaware of or have no understanding of their previous circumstances and experiences. Some such women may be in the country illegally or awaiting the outcome of an asylum application. They may consequently be unable or afraid to access services, or to admit or discuss their problems when they do so. Similarly, other Black or ethnic minority women may be reluctant to seek help because of previous experience of racism from public services or institutions (Mama 1989), and expectation of repetition and/or fear of deportation. They may also have problems in accessing services or obtaining financial support, making it even more difficult for them to leave an abusive partner.

Summary

There is now a wide range of literature on various aspects of domestic abuse. There is increasing recognition of the need to acknowledge the impact of abuse on health, the need to deal with the problem effectively and the need for adequate training to do so. There is also recognition that this requires a multidisciplinary approach. These issues have been addressed strategically at national level (Department of Health 2000, Scottish Executive 2000). The British Medical Association (1998) has considered the problem of domestic violence in relation to health and health care in general, while in common with many other professional bodies, the Royal College of Obstetricians and Gynaecologists has dealt with the issue from a specialty viewpoint and examined domestic violence in the context of reproductive health (Bewley et al 1997).

Violence against women is common and is relevant to all aspects of reproductive health care. Women are often reluctant to admit that they have experienced abuse, but most want to be asked about it and to have an opportunity to discuss it. While there are some indicators that indicate the possibility of abuse, they are insufficiently sensitive or specific to form the basis for selective enquiry. All women presenting for any type of reproductive health care, but especially pregnant women, should have a full sexual and social history taken which includes routine direct enquiry about violence or abuse from their partner or other individual.

Women who volunteer a history of abuse should have their experience validated. In addition to treatment of the immediate health consequences, they should have their current situation and level of risk assessed and be given information about available services, including the offer of direct referral. Limitations of options, including difficulties in removing themselves from the abusive situation, should be recognized. Careful documentation is essential for future use, including possible legal action. Effective management of this problem requires not only adequate availability of suitable services, but adequate training of healthcare professionals. Both require adequate resources.

KEY POINTS

1. Most violence against women is inflicted by men, most commonly partners or ex-partners, and usually occurs in the home.
2. Domestic abuse occurs throughout the social spectrum, but women from disadvantaged backgrounds may have fewer resources to deal with it.
3. Abuse experienced by women may be physical, psychological, emotional or economic.
4. Women are at risk of violence in any situation involving sex, including commercial sex which carries a risk of violence from both partners (and/or men controlling their prostitution) and clients.
5. Domestic abuse often begins or escalates during pregnancy.
6. Domestic abuse has gynaecological and obstetric consequences, and should therefore be addressed by those providing reproductive health care.
7. Mental health and behavioural problems, including depression and substance misuse, are more commonly effects of domestic abuse rather than causes.
8. Markers of abuse are insufficiently specific or sensitive to be used as indicators for enquiry, and all pregnant women should be asked routinely about domestic abuse.
9. Healthcare workers require training in social history taking, identification and management of domestic abuse.
10. The possibility that healthcare workers may themselves be experiencing domestic abuse must be borne in mind.

References

Bewley S, Friend J, Mezey G 1997 Violence Against Women. RCOG Press, London.

British Medical Association 1998 Domestic Violence: a Health Care Issue? BMA, London.

Browne A 1987 When Battered Women Kill. Collier Macmillan, London.

CEMACH 2004 Why Mothers Die 2000–2002. The Sixth Report of the Confidential Enquiries into Maternal Deaths in the United Kingdom. RCOG Press, London.

CEMACH 2007 Saving Mothers Lives 2003–2005. The seventh report of the confidential enquiries into maternal deaths in the United Kingdom. RCOG Press, London.

Department of Health 2000 Domestic Violence: a Resource Manual for Health Care Professionals. DoH, London.

Dobash RE, Dobash RP 1980 Violence Against Wives. Open Books, London.

Friedman LS, Samet JH, Roberts MS, Hudlin M, Hans P 1992 Inquiry about victimization experiences. A survey of patient preferences and physician practices. Archives of Internal Medicine 152: 1186–1190.

Geberth VJ 1992 Stalkers. Law and Order 140: 138–143.

Heath I 1992 Domestic violence: the general practitioner's role. In: Royal College of General Practitioners Members Reference Book. Sabrecrown, London.

Helton AS, McFarlane J, Anderson ET 1987 Battered and pregnant: a prevalence study. American Journal of Public Health 77: 1337–1339.

Hillard PJA 1985 Physical abuse in pregnancy. Obstetrics and Gynecology 66: 185–190.

Home Affairs Select Committee 1993 Domestic Violence. HMSO, London.

Home Office 2004 Paying the Price: a Consultation Paper on Prostitution. HMSO, London.

Home Office 2006 Coordinated Prostitution Strategy. HMSO, London.

James-Hanman D, Long L 1994 Crime prevention: an issue for midwives? British Journal of Midwifery 2: 29–32.

Johnson H, Sacco V 1995 Researching violence against women: Statistics Canada's national survey. Canadian Journal of Criminology 37: 281–304.

Jones RF 1997 Domestic violence — a physician's perspective. In: Bewley S, Friend J, Mezey G (eds) Violence Against Women. RCOG Press, London, p 84.

Kennedy H 1993 Eve was Framed. Vintage, London.

Kennedy LW, Dutton DG 1989 The incidence of wife assault in Alberta. Canadian Journal of Behavioural Sciences 21: 40–54.

Lowman J 2000 Violence and the outlaw status of (street) prostitution in Canada. Violence Against Women 6: 987–1011.

Mama A 1989 The Hidden Struggle: Statutory and Voluntary Responses to Violence Against Black Women in the Home. Runnymede Trust, London.

Mayhew P, Maung NF, Mirrlees-Black C 1993 The 1992 British Crime Survey. HMSO, London.

Mezey GC 1997 Perpetrators of domestic violence. In: Bewley S, Friend J, Mezey G (eds) Violence Against Women. RCOG Press, London.

Mezey GC, Bewley S 1997 Domestic violence and pregnancy. BMJ (Clinical Research Ed.) 314: 1295.

Mirrlees-Black C, Mayhew P, Percy A 1996 The 1996 British Crime Survey: England and Wales. HMSO, London.

Mooney J 1994 The Hidden Figure: Domestic Violence in North London. Islington Council, London.

Plichta S 1992 The effects of woman abuse on health care utilisation and health status: a literature review. Women's Health Issues 2: 154–163.

Prostitution Reform Act 2003 New Zealand.

Russell D 1982 Rape in Marriage. Indiana University Press, Bloomington.

Scottish Executive 2000 Scottish Partnership on Domestic Abuse: National Strategy to Address Domestic Abuse in Scotland. Scottish Executive, Edinburgh.

Scottish Needs Assessment Programme 1997 SNAP report on domestic violence. Scottish Forum for Public Health Medicine, Glasgow.

Shanks L, Ford N, Schull M et al 2001 Responding to rape. The Lancet 357: 304.

Stark E, Flitcraft A, Frazier W 1979 Medicine and patriarchal violence. The social construction of a private event. International Journal of Health Services 9: 41–93.

Stark E, Flitcraft AH 1991 Spouse abuse. In: Rosenberg M, Mercy J (eds) Violence in America: a Public Health Approach. Oxford University Press, New York.

Stark E, Flitcraft A 1996 Women at Risk. Sage, London.

Sugg NK, Inui T 1992 Primary care physicians' response to domestic violence: opening Pandora's box. JAMA: the Journal of the American Medical Association 267: 3194–3195.

Tjaden P, Thoennes N 2000 Extent, Nature, and Consequences of Intimate Partner Violence. US Department of Justice, Washington, DC.

United Nations 1995 Violence Against Women: a World-wide Report. United Nations, New York.

Watts C, Zimmerman C 2003 Violence against women: global scope and magnitude. The Lancet 359: 1232–1237.

World Health Organization 2005 Multi-country Study on Women's Health and Domestic Violence Against Women: Summary Report of Initial Results on Prevalence, Health Outcomes and Women's Responses. WHO, Geneva.

CHAPTER 67

Lesbian and bisexual women's health issues

Julie Fish and Susan Bewley

Chapter Contents

INTRODUCTION	1009	**EDUCATION AND RESEARCH**	1013
SOCIAL CHANGE	1009	**TOWARDS GOOD PRACTICE**	1014
THE MEDICAL MODEL	1010	**CONCLUSIONS**	1014
ATTITUDES IN HEALTH CARE	1010	**KEY POINTS**	1015
IMPLICATIONS FOR GYNAECOLOGICAL HEALTH	1010		
LESBIAN AND BISEXUAL WOMEN'S EXPERIENCES OF HEALTH CARE	1012		

Introduction

Lesbian and bisexual women come from all walks of life: they may be old or young, disabled, Black and minority ethnic, living in poverty or living in rural areas. Despite this, some health professionals continue to believe that they have no lesbian or bisexual patients. Recent government figures estimate that there are 1.6 million lesbian and bisexual women living in the UK, comprising 5% of the female population (Department of Trade and Industry 2004). Studies suggest that up to one-third of lesbian and bisexual women have children, they may be more likely to have had a university education, but there is conflicting evidence about their income relative to heterosexual women (Fish 2006).

It is increasingly recognized that obstetricians and gynaecologists know little of their distinctive health concerns. Although notions persist that homosexuality itself is a disease, many healthcare professionals otherwise believe that there are no differences in lesbian and bisexual women's health from that of women in general; there is often a perception that sexual orientation is a private matter which is irrelevant to the health consultation (McNair 2003). Over the past 20 years, research has suggested that the health of sexual minority women differs in key ways: in their health behaviour, health risks and experiences of health care. Lesbian and bisexual women are less prevention oriented and avoid routine screening tests, such as cervical cytology and mammograms. For these reasons, sexual orientation has been recognized by the Department of Health as a ground for health inequalities (Fish 2007). Sexual orientation is unique among the six equality strands (i.e. 'race', gender, age, disability and religion) in not being included in the UK census; this omission has contributed to a lack of research

in sexual orientation and health, and a dearth of statistics about their demographic characteristics. Healthcare professionals may also lack specific knowledge of lesbian and bisexual women's needs and be unable to provide relevant health information (Hughes and Evans 2003, McNair 2003).

Evidence suggests that discriminatory treatment is now less common in health care (Solarz 1999). Lack of understanding and the personal discomfort of health professionals, however, often mean that lesbian and bisexual women have a differential experience of health care. Doctors are sometimes uncomfortable in providing care to sexual minority patients or embarrassed to ask questions relating to sexual behaviour (Hinchliff et al 2005). Good medical practice (General Medical Council 2006) and the desire to provide optimal health care requires health professionals to be informed about the continued barriers to health care and of differences in health risks, to be sensitive to historical stigmatization, and to be aware of issues of cultural competence with sexual minority women (Mayer et al 2008).

This chapter aims to contribute to meeting the gap in the knowledge base about lesbian and bisexual women's obstetric and gynaecological concerns.

Social Change

The introduction of the 2007 Equality Act (Sexual Orientation) Regulations offers the protection of equal treatment in public services, including the National Health Service (NHS). Current policy offers possibilities for improvement in the health of lesbian and bisexual women as legislation prohibits discrimination in health services and means that they can neither be refused care nor receive a lower standard of care. The most common response has been to overlook lesbian and bisexual women as a patient group; they have often been

DOI: 10.1016/B978-0-7020-3120-5.00067-9

invisible patients within health services, and their needs have been poorly understood. However, increasingly, their health issues are receiving attention from clinicians, other health professionals and policy makers. The Department of Health in England and Wales is working to promote inclusive services and reduce health inequalities for lesbian, gay, bisexual and transgender people; sexual orientation is included in current efforts to mainstream equality and diversity in health care (e.g. the Pacesetters Programme), and the General Medical Council has published guidance for the protection of lesbian, gay and bisexual people as patients (General Medical Council and Stonewall 2007). However, these initiatives have not been consistently implemented or acknowledged across the NHS.

The Medical Model

In biomedical accounts, lesbian health has been located within a sickness paradigm (Burns 1992). The assumption that lesbianism itself was caused by a biological, hormonal or psychological deficiency meant that the principal concern of medical professionals was to find a cause or cure. The illness model in mental health derives from assumptions that heterosexuals are normal and mentally healthy, while lesbians are impaired or abnormal in their psychological functioning (Peplau and Garnets 2000).

The aetiology of lesbianism has been variously attributed to hormonal (Veniegas and Conley 2000), biological (Terry 1990) or mental health differences (Peplau and Garnets 2000). Studies have looked for a biological origin to sexual orientation (Bogaert and Friesen 2002). Other researchers have suggested deficiencies evident in a masculinized finger-length ratio (Williams et al 2000); cerebral functioning (Rahman et al 2006); inner ears, leading to hearing loss in comparison with heterosexual women (McFadden and Pasanen 1998); and impairments in psychological functioning (Garnets and Peplau 2000). Lesbianism was widely considered a pathological condition in need of treatment, and included as a mental disorder in the Diagnostic and Statistical Manual. Until the early 1970s, lesbians underwent electric shock aversion therapy, oestrogen treatment and psychoanalysis aimed at curing their homosexuality in NHS hospitals in the UK (Smith et al 2004). Following intensive lobbying by lesbian, gay and bisexual rights groups, being lesbian (or gay) was declassified as a mental disorder by the American Psychiatric Association in 1973, removed from the World Health Organization's International Classification of Diseases in 1992, and the recommendation to convert lesbians to heterosexuality was no longer included in the guidelines of the American Medical Association from 1996 (Council on Scientific Affairs, American Medical Association 1996).

Attitudes in Health Care

Sexual behaviour between women does not result in any unique health problems, and lesbian and bisexual women experience broadly the same range of obstetric and gynaecological conditions. However, the medical model had considerable influence upon the attitudes of healthcare professionals;

lesbian and bisexual women were often considered inferior. Many doctors believe that lesbian and bisexual women can be identified by their physical appearance; they sometimes assume that lesbian and bisexual women are masculine in their presentation and behaviour.

As any woman who comes to a gynaecologist may be a lesbian or bisexual, the quality of the history taking, the development of rapport and the appropriateness of the advice given will be affected if her experiences, needs and specific fears are not understood. The good health practitioner is aware of the reasons why a lesbian or bisexual woman might be reluctant to seek health care, has an understanding of the effect of homophobia and heterosexism on health, and is knowledgeable about her specific health concerns. Lesbian and bisexual women often seek 'gay-friendly' health professionals, i.e. those who are non-judgemental in their attitudes, have an understanding of health needs and are able to facilitate the disclosure of sexuality (McNair 2003).

Assumption of heterosexuality

Unless a woman discloses, or 'comes out', to a healthcare professional, it is usually assumed that she is heterosexual. Some professionals may suppose that enquiry about sexual orientation is only relevant to the provision of health care if the concern specifically relates to sexual health. However, being a lesbian or bisexual woman is more than mere sexual behaviour. It may impact on the whole of a woman's social, family and personal life.

The issue of whether or not a lesbian or bisexual woman comes out to a gynaecologist or other health professional has consequences for her health. A number of health benefits may be associated with disclosure. Lesbian and bisexual women are likely to experience greater ease in communicating with their doctor and are more likely to be satisfied and comfortable with the care they receive if they have been able to come out and receive a positive response to their disclosure. Disclosure also allows for the possibility of involving their partner in treatment decisions. Non-disclosure may mean inaccurate diagnoses, inappropriate questioning and irrelevant health information.

The meanings about sexual behaviour differ from those for heterosexual women. The gynaecologist may need to know when the patient last had intercourse, or to advise her on resuming sex after surgery or the likely effects of treatment on sexual sensation or function. Healthcare professionals usually only understand heterosexual sex when they use the terms 'sex' or 'sexual intercourse'. If the gynaecologist regards every patient as heterosexual, the advice offered will reflect this assumption (e.g. the advice to avoid having sex with her husband). The presumption of heterosexuality is implicit when discussing whether a woman may be pregnant without realizing it, or in relation to advice offered about contraception.

Implications for Gynaecological Health

Reproductive health

Increasingly, lesbian and bisexual women are choosing to have children within same-sex relationships; this may be by home conception using sperm from a man who is known to them, or through commercial networking agencies. Alternatively, they may choose to conceive at a licensed fertility clinic using a known sperm donor, or by using a sperm bank where the donor will remain anonymous to the mother (although the child may choose to know the identity of the father when they reach 18 years of age). If a woman is unable to conceive in these ways or has fertility problems, she may seek in-vitro fertilization (IVF) treatment.

A substantial amount of research exists about the parenting skills of lesbian couples. Research initially focused upon women who had started a family in a heterosexual relationship but who subsequently raised their children in a lesbian household. More recently, research has concentrated upon lesbian couples who seek to have a child through donor insemination at a licensed fertility clinic. Single women seeking fertility treatment with donor sperm have children who compare well emotionally and psychologically with children born by donor insemination to two heterosexual parents (Murray and Golombok 2005a,b). Social research on the children of lesbian parents has produced similar findings to those children born to single women. Their emotional and psychological development is comparable to that of children born of donor insemination to two heterosexual parents. In fact, the second female parent often has greater parent–child interaction than the father in heterosexual couples (Brewaeys et al 1997).

Until the amendments to the Human Fertility and Embryology Bill in 2008, fertility clinics had an obligation not to provide treatment unless account had been taken 'of the welfare of any child who may be born as a result of treatment (including the need for a father)'. This was used by many to refuse treatment for lesbian couples; the wording has been replaced in the new legislation by the 'need for supportive parenting'. There has been a four-fold increase in the number of lesbian couples receiving IVF treatment (Human Fertilisation and Embrylogy Authority 2009). The implications for gynaecologists include: involving all parties desired by patients, including partners, known sperm donors and coparents; enabling women to make informed choices about interventions that are consistent with their known or presumed fertility; offering fertility support that is specific to lesbian and bisexual women; and helping lesbian and bisexual women to access other relevant services (Ross et al 2006). They also need to be aware of the known quality of lesbian parenting and be prepared to judge individual cases on the facts and evidence.

Lesbian mothers' access to maternity services

In the past, lesbian couples have been considered less ideal parents than their heterosexual counterparts. Their children were said to have difficulty forming a normal heterosexual identity. It was also assumed that children without a father lack appropriate gender role models; in particular, that a boy brought up by lesbians would be effeminate. Notwithstanding the obvious argument that most homosexuals were born to heterosexual parents (and thus the likely disconnection between the parent's sexuality and child's sexual orientation), and that most boys in single mother families remain heterosexual, empirical evidence is now available. Comparisons of children's development in lesbian mother and heterosexual households show no difference in the likelihood

of growing up gay; boys growing up in families without a father showed no less masculine gender role behaviour than boys brought up by a woman and a man (MacCallum and Golombok 2004).

Attitudes can influence how lesbian mothers are treated in maternity services (i.e. with hostility, curiosity or respect). Responses from healthcare professionals have sometimes been inappropriate, such as prying into a lesbian's decision to become a mother. In other circumstances, lesbians have felt that their partner was invisible or merely tolerated (Wilton and Kaufmann 2001). The changing social climate may mean that lesbian and bisexual women may be more likely to 'come out' to health professionals in the expectation that their relationship will be acknowledged, their partner will be treated as a coparent and their support needs, including referral to appropriate parenting support groups, will be met.

Cervical screening and cancer

As the risk of cervical cancer is associated with sex with men, lesbian and bisexual women are sometimes mistakenly believed to be at no risk or substantially lower risk of cervical cancer than heterosexual women (Fish 2009).

Studies suggest that up to four-fifths of lesbians have had sex with men in their lifetime (Marrazzo et al 2001). Human papillomavirus (HPV) has a long latency period (Carroll et al 1997), and any previous heterosexual sex may contribute to lesbians' risk of cervical cancer.

Smoking is also a risk factor for cervical cancer; there is some evidence that lesbians are more likely to smoke than heterosexual women (Gruskin et al 2001).

Transmission of human papilloma virus between women

Potential routes of transmission between women include oral sex, vaginal penetration with the fingers, sharing sex toys or skin-to-skin contact (Marrazzo et al 2001).

Prevalence of human papilloma virus and cervical cancer in lesbian and bisexual women

Researchers have sought to identify prevalence rates because no surveillance data are available on the incidence of cervical abnormalities in lesbian and bisexual women. A case–control study of 1408 lesbian and bisexual women and 1423 heterosexual women found that cervical abnormalities [cervical intraepithelial neoplasia (CIN) 1, CIN 2–3] were equally prevalent in both groups (Fethers et al 2000). A US clinic study reported a prevalence of HPV in lesbian and bisexual women of 13%; among those with HPV detected, 74% had oncogenic types (Marrazzo et al 2001).

Furthermore, cervical abnormalities have been found in women who report that they have never had sex with men (Bailey et al 2000, Fethers et al 2000, Marrazzo et al 2001). Lesbians whose female sexual partners have had previous heterosexual sex may therefore remain at some risk. Cervical abnormalities (borderline, mild, moderate or severe dyskaryosis) were more common in women who had been sexually active with men than in 'exclusively' lesbian subjects (10.9% vs 4.9%) (Bailey et al 2000).

Uptake of cervical screening among lesbian and bisexual women

Studies have found that lesbians, but not bisexual women, were less likely than heterosexual women to have been screened routinely (Diamant et al 2000, Matthews et al 2004, Kerker et al 2006).

Women's screening behaviour differed significantly according to whether they reported having had sex with men (Marrazzo et al 2001). Lesbians who had never had sex with men were more likely to report no prior screening than those who had been sexually active with men (42% vs 12%, $P < 0.001$, Bailey et al 2000).

Advice from healthcare professionals

There is evidence that lesbians are deemed to be ineligible for screening because of their sexuality; notwithstanding their risk from prior heterosexual sex, they are often judged on their current activities. Marrazzo et al (2001) found that 10% had been told by a healthcare provider that they did not need to be screened because they were not sexually active with men. These providers were identified as doctors in all but one case. There is also some evidence to suggest that lesbian and bisexual women have been refused cervical screening when they requested a test (Hunt and Fish 2008).

Sexually transmitted infections

Sex between women is often considered a negligible risk for sexually transmitted infections (STIs) (Mercer et al 2007). However, studies suggest that women who report that they have only had sex with women are susceptible; in woman-to-woman transmission, a greater number of sexual exposures are needed, while in heterosexual transmission, a greater number of partners increased the risk of transmission (Bauer and Welles 2001). STIs are more common among women who have had previous heterosexual contact or whose female partners have had male sexual partners (Carroll et al 1997, Mercer et al 2007). Bacterial vaginosis is more common among lesbians than among heterosexual women; it is significantly associated with a larger number of female sexual partners and smoking (Skinner et al 1996, McCaffrey et al 1999). Genital warts, genital herpes and trichomoniasis have been diagnosed in lesbian and bisexual women; other STIs such as chlamydia, pelvic inflammatory disease and gonorrhoea are comparatively rare (Bailey et al 2004). Gynaecologists and other healthcare professionals may need to consider the potential risks for STI transmission in medical decision-making. STI testing should be offered to lesbian and bisexual women based on the number and gender of their sexual partners (Bauer and Welles 2001).

Breast cancer

Lesbian and bisexual women are believed to be at higher 5-year and lifetime risk for breast cancer in comparison to heterosexual women; they are more likely to report a diagnosis of breast cancer than heterosexual women (Valanis et al 2000). Studies have suggested that reproductive factors may play a role, as they may have fewer pregnancies and children (Dibble et al 2004, Brandenburg et al 2007). Other potential risks include increased alcohol consumption, a significantly greater number of breast biopsies and being overweight (Cochran et al 2001). Although the risks confuse behaviour (having children) with identity (being lesbian), some lesbians do have children while some heterosexual women do not; research suggests that the rates of nulliparity are higher among lesbians than heterosexual women (76% vs 22%) (Case et al 2004).

Breast awareness and screening behaviours

Key differences in breast health care between lesbians and heterosexual women may relate to breast awareness and screening behaviours. Despite controversy about the efficacy of breast self-examination, biomedical sources continue to advise women to be aware of changes in their breasts because as many as 90% of breast lumps are found by women themselves (Fish and Wilkinson 2003). Lesbians appear to be less likely to be 'breast-aware'; current health promotion emphasizes 'Touch, Look and Check'. Lesbians commonly said that they did not know what they were looking for or how to check their breasts (Fish and Wilkinson 2003). Although some studies find that lesbian and bisexual women attend for mammography at the same rates as heterosexual women (e.g. Fish and Anthony 2005), others suggest that relationships with health professionals and the anticipation of heterosexism may affect their experiences of mammography and their future reattendance (e.g. Lauver et al 1999).

Lesbian and Bisexual Women's Experiences of Health Care

The field of lesbian and bisexual women's experiences of health care is dominated by studies from North America and the quantitative research paradigm (Wilkinson 2002). Consequently, few studies have investigated sexual minority women's perceptions and experiences of health care. Recent government policy initiatives, the White Papers 'Choosing Health 2004' and 'Our Health, Our Care, Our Say 2006', seek to give patients greater choice about healthcare services and to consult with them about service delivery. There are a number of challenges, however, in eliciting the views of a hidden population. Although the following findings are derived from a non-random sampling survey, they represent the best-available data about lesbian and bisexual women's healthcare experiences in the UK (Hunt and Fish 2008). The questionnaire asked lesbian and bisexual women about how healthcare services can be improved. Analysis of the data identified three main themes: (i) assumption of heterosexuality, (ii) facilitating access and (iii) improving attitudes.

Assumption of heterosexuality

Although increasingly liberal social attitudes have meant that greater numbers of lesbian and bisexual women have 'come out' to their family, friends and work colleagues, health care is the environment where they are least likely to disclose their sexual orientation. Almost half of the lesbian and bisexual women in the study had not come out, or only to a few healthcare professionals (Hunt and Fish 2008). As one participant in the study said, receiving health care can make a patient feel vulnerable, and additional barriers, such as coming out, may add to an already stressful situation:

> Personally I have had very positive dealings with most GPs and hospital staff but there is this underlying assumption that when you bring your partner, you have either brought your sister or friend with you. Having to constantly out yourself to people who make this assumption, even when no malice is intended, is stressful when you're already in a stressful situation due to a health problem.

Some patients feel that they must make a choice between disclosing their sexual orientation or receiving a good service:

> I have felt frightened in health care of having to choose between a good service and coming out [especially in hospital]. Healthcare providers need to show openly their welcome and skills for dealing with lesbian patients — posters, asking open questions, mentioning 'partners', not assuming sex of partner [or if they have a partner or just one partner], the usual things about not assuming you need contraception.

Healthcare professionals can take steps to make it easier for a lesbian or bisexual woman to disclose her sexual orientation and to understand the potential health benefits of doing so.

Facilitating access

Since the introduction of the Civil Partnership Act 2004, women in same-sex relationships have the same rights and responsibilities as married heterosexual couples, including the right in health care to have their partner recognized as their next of kin. The legislation has implications for all documentation where 'marital status' is required. Research undertaken by the Royal College of Nursing (2003) suggests that some healthcare professionals refuse to acknowledge a same-sex partner, and deny the partner visiting rights and access to information. Participants in the study shared similar experiences:

> I feel that especially in hospitals, lesbian partners are not recognized immediately as next of kin and are subsequently overlooked and/or ignored when it comes to their spouse's treatment.

In contrast, other participants said that their relationship was acknowledged and that staff took steps to ensure that the patient could be visited by her partner without difficulty:

> I had a protracted stay at a small rural hospital and had been nervous about how they would respond but in the end needed to come out to enable my partner access to my bedside. In fact we were very pleasantly surprised and staff made a conscious effort, handing over to new staff each shift that my partner was female and should be allowed to visit, thus preventing any difficulties/ awkwardness.

Access to health care can also be facilitated by positive images, relevant health promotion materials, clearly dis-

played confidentiality policies and equal opportunity policies which include sexual orientation.

Improving attitudes and behaviours

The doctor–patient relationship is often said to be as important to a patient's experience as the treatment of disease (Wilton 2000). Skilled interviewing and positive attitudes are associated with good health care; doctors' values and attitudes are linked to patient satisfaction, the willingness of a patient to return to their health provider and improved heath outcomes (Gruskin 1999). Attitudes are also informed by knowledge about lesbian and bisexual women's communities and the ways in which their lives are organized:

> For the most part, my experience and my partner's experience have been extremely positive and we have generally encountered excellent care from healthcare professionals. However, it was really a problem for us, and more particularly for our children's father, that our local hospital was unable to accommodate our unusual family structure during the births of our children.

Conversely, poor attitudes have a potentially detrimental impact on health care:

> During a visit to [unnamed] Hospital in London for a gynaecological problem, the nurses were surprised to find out that I had two children. Health professionals must think I'm from another planet just because I'm a lesbian. It's a real shame that their experience of our community is still so very limited.

Education and Research

Undergraduate medical education

Studies point to the absence of lesbian and bisexual women's health concerns on undergraduate and postqualifying medical curricula, and highlight the need for cultural competence, including sensitive communication and informed values (Hutchinson et al 2006).

Research in lesbian and bisexual women's health

Unlike for heterosexual women, research in lesbian and bisexual women's health has been largely overlooked. A review of English language articles found that only 0.1% (n = 3777) of all articles cited in Medline addressed lesbian, gay, bisexual or transgender issues (Boehmer 2002). Almost two-thirds (61%) of these were disease specific, pointing to the continuing dominance of the biomedical paradigm, and most (80%) focused on gay men. These findings suggest that lesbian and bisexual women's concerns have been historically neglected in health research. In recent years, the research base has grown in the USA and this can be attributed to a number of factors, including increased access to research funding, the establishment of a lesbian health fund by the Gay and Lesbian Medical Association, the development of new methodologies in lesbian and bisexual women's health, and the inclusion of questions relevant to sexual minority women on population-based studies (Solarz 1999). However, there are continuing obstacles: research grants are relatively small, there are few available funding streams, and significant barriers to publication remain (Plumb 2001).

Towards Good Practice

This section identifies a number of pointers for good practice which can be incorporated into everyday healthcare interactions. What would a good gynaecologist provide for his or her lesbian patients?

Knowledge

Good gynaecologists provide high-quality, skilled medical care for all their patients, regardless of background. The well-trained gynaecologist would have awareness that any patient who attends (single, married, young, old, White or Black) might be lesbian or bisexual, and would not make assumptions on the basis of appearance or probability. He or she would be apprised of the health risks and health concerns that different sexual behaviours and identity might bring.

Having knowledge of appropriate services, support groups and referral networks would allow consultations to take place freely, as the doctor would be confident to cope with disclosure, distress or expectations of help.

Professionals need to be sensitive to historical stigmatization, and it is particularly important to understand the need for confidentiality when 'coming out' might be dangerous to self-esteem, family relationships or security at work.

A lesbian might have 'next of kin' issues in that her biological family and social network of good friends and support may be fully integrated or estranged, and this requires sensitivity, especially around visiting time and discussions about competence or end-of-life.

Communication skills

It is not very difficult to create a 'trusting' or 'distrusting' atmosphere with patients. Simple things, such as posters in the waiting room, wearing of lapel pins or badges, family photos in the surgery and the use of language, can create a very welcoming or potentially hostile environment even before a consultation starts. Contrary to popular belief, you cannot tell if a woman is a lesbian or bisexual from her appearance, but only if she tells you; this will be dependent on her working out what your reaction might be.

Questions that use inclusive terms will facilitate safe disclosure. Gender-neutral language such as 'Who do you live with? Have you a partner? Does he or she work', rather than 'What work does your husband do? Are you using contraception? Why not?', are more likely to put lesbian or bisexual patients at ease.

Attitudes

Good doctors, even those who have deep seated religious, political or personal beliefs that might conflict with their patients' beliefs or lifestyles were they to meet in a non-professional context, will put those aside in the consulting room as they recognize that prejudice will hamper their ability to do their best for all patients. An awareness of heterosexism and homophobia in health care and in everyday life would allow the doctor to empathize ('walk in another's shoes'), be non-judgemental and avoid stereotypes about lesbians (e.g. that they are all 'mannish' or 'man-haters'). Just as with heterosexuals, it is important to assess the quality of their social support and relationships, and preferably involve partners in treatment decisions.

Conclusions

Recommendations

Lesbian and bisexual women's health should be included in medical education programmes

The curriculum should include: (i) training in lesbian and bisexual women's needs and risks, and (ii) training in cultural competence by displaying the attitudes and values to promote health and wellbeing through appropriate communication with lesbian and bisexual women, taking sensitive sexual histories, and knowledge and understanding of sexual minority women's health concerns.

Avoid assumptions of heterosexuality

Healthcare professionals should take steps to facilitate disclosure, to ask questions in ways which do not presume heterosexuality and to understand differences in meanings (e.g. when referring to sexual activity). However, not all lesbian and bisexual women will choose to come out to their doctor.

Develop a welcoming environment

Reception staff should develop cultural competence; clinic waiting rooms should have written policies on sexual orientation antidiscrimination, clear confidentiality policies and relevant intake forms; and posters, brochures and other health promotion materials should be displayed or made available.

Competent gynaecologists will:

- be aware that any patient might be lesbian or bisexual, and will not make assumptions on the basis of appearance or probability;
- be aware of sexual orientation as a social determinant of health;
- be knowledgeable about the different health risks and health behaviours affecting sexual minority women;
- be aware of appropriate referral networks;
- be willing to facilitate the disclosure of sexual orientation by the use of inclusive terms such as 'partner';
- involve partners and/or friends as next of kin in medical decision-making; and
- facilitate access to health care by positive images, relevant health promotion materials, clearly displayed confidentiality policies and equal opportunity policies which include sexual orientation.

KEY POINTS

1. Any patient might be lesbian or bisexual.
2. Gynaecologists should not make assumptions on the basis of appearance or probability.
3. Sexual orientation is a social determinant of health.
4. There are some different reproductive health risks and health behaviours affecting sexual minority women.
5. Gynaecologists should be: (i) willing to facilitate the disclosure of sexual orientation by the use of inclusive terms such as 'partner';

(ii) willing to involve partners and/or friends as next of kin in medical decision-making; and (iii) be aware of appropriate referral networks. Access to health care is facilitated by positive images, relevant health promotion materials, clearly displayed confidentiality policies and equal opportunity policies which include sexual orientation

Acknowledgement

The authors wish to acknowledge the late Tamsin Wilton's contribution to the development of lesbian health as a research discipline, and to her particular influence in the writing of this chapter.

References

Bailey JV, Kavanagh J, Owen C, McClean KA, Skinner CJ 2000 Lesbians and cervical screening. British Journal of General Practice 50: 481–482.

Bailey JV, Farquhar C, Owen C, Mangtani P 2004 Sexually transmitted infections in women who have sex with women. Sexually Transmitted Infections 80: 244–246.

Bauer G, Welles S 2001 Beyond assumptions of negligible risk: sexually transmitted diseases and women who have sex with women. American Journal of Public Health 91: 1281–1286.

Boehmer U 2002 Twenty years of public health research: inclusion of lesbian, gay, bisexual, and transgender populations. American Journal of Public Health 92: 1125–1130.

Bogaert AF, Friesen C 2002 Sexual orientation and height, weight, and age of puberty: new tests from a British national probability sample. Biological Psychology 59: 135–145.

Brandenburg DL, Matthews AK, Johnson TP, Hughes TL 2007 Breast cancer risk and screening: a comparison of lesbian and heterosexual women. Women and Health 45: 109–130.

Brewaeys A, Ponjaert I, van Hall E, Golombok S 1997 Donor insemination: child development and family functioning in lesbian mother families. Human Reproduction 12: 1349–1359.

Burns J 1992 The psychology of lesbian health care. In: Nicolson P, Ussher J (eds) The Psychology of Women's Health Care. Macmillan, Basingstoke, pp 225–248.

Carroll N, Goldstein RS, Wilson L, Mayer K 1997 Gynecological infections and sexual practices of Massachusetts lesbian and bisexual women. Journal of the Gay & Lesbian Medical Association 1: 15–23.

Case P, Austin SB, Hunter DJ et al 2004 Sexual orientation, health risk factors, and physical functioning in the Nurses' Health Study II. Journal of Women's Health 13: 1033–1047.

Cochran SD, Mays VM, Bowen D et al 2001 Cancer-related risk indicators and preventive screening behaviors among lesbians and bisexual women. American Journal of Public Health 91: 591–597.

Council on Scientific Affairs, American Medical Association 1996 Health care needs of gay men and lesbians in the United States. JAMA: the Journal of the American Medical Association 275: 1354–1359.

Department of Trade and Industry 2004 Final Regulatory Impact Assessment: Civil Partnership Act 2004. DTI, London.

Diamant AL, Wold C, Spritzer K, Gelberg L 2000 Health behaviors, health status, and access to and use of health care: a population-based study of lesbian, bisexual, and heterosexual women. Archives of Family Medicine 9: 1043–1051.

Dibble SL, Roberts SA, Nussey B 2004 Comparing breast cancer risk between lesbians and their heterosexual sisters. Women's Health Issues 14: 60–68.

Fethers K, Maraks C, Mindel A, Estcourt CS 2000 Sexually transmitted infections and risk behaviours in women who have sex with women. Sexualy transmitted Infections 76(5): 345–349.

Fish J 2006 Heterosexism in Health and Social Care. Palgrave, Basingstoke.

Fish J 2007 Reducing Health Inequalities for LGBT People: Briefing Papers for Health and Social Care Staff. Department of Health, London.

Fish J 2009 Lesbians and Bisexual Women and Cervical Screening: a Review of the Literature Using Systematic Methods.

Report commissioned by the NHS Cervical Screening Programme, Sheffield.

Fish J, Anthony D 2005 UK National lesbians and health care survey. Women and Health 41: 27–45.

Fish J, Wilkinson S 2003 Understanding lesbians' healthcare behaviour: the case of breast self-examination. Social Science and Medicine 56: 235–245.

Garnets LD, Peplau LA 2000 Understanding women's sexualities and sexual orientations: an introduction. Journal of Social Issues 56: 181–192.

General Medical Council 2006 Good Medical Practice. http://www.gmc-uk.org/guidance/good_medical_practice/GMC_GMP.pdf (retrieved 03/02/2009).

General Medical Council, Stonewall 2007 Protecting Patients: your Rights as Lesbian, Gay and Bisexual People. GMC, Manchester.

Gruskin EP 1999 Treating Lesbians and Bisexual Women: Challenges and Strategies for Health Professionals. Sage Publications, Thousand Oaks, CA.

Gruskin EP, Hart S, Gordon N, Ackerson L 2001 Patterns of cigarette smoking and alcohol use among lesbians and bisexual women enrolled in a large health maintenance organization. American Journal of Public Health 91: 976–979.

Hinchliff S, Gott M, Galena E 2005 'I daresay I might find it embarrassing': general practitioners' perspectives on discussing sexual health issues with lesbian and gay patients. Health & Social Care in the Community 13: 345–353.

Human Fertilisation and Embryology Authority http://www.hfea.gov.uk/docs/ Figures for treatment of single women and lesbian couples 2000-2005.pdf (retrieved 03/02/2009)

Hughes C, Evans A 2003 Health needs of women who have sex with women. BMJ (Clinical Research Ed.) 327: 939–940.

Hunt R, Fish J 2008 Prescription for Change: Lesbian and Bisexual Women's Health Check. Stonewall, London.

Hutchinson MK, Thompson AC, Cederbaum JA 2006 Multisystem factors contributing to disparities in preventive health care among lesbian women. Journal of Obstetric, Gynecologic, and Neonatal Nursing 35: 393–402.

Kerker BD, Mostashari F, Thorpe L 2006 Health care access and utlitization among women who have sex with women: sexual behavior and identity. Journal of Urban Health 83: 970–979.

Lauver DR, Karon SL, Egan J et al 1999 Understanding lesbian's mammography utilization. Women's Health Issues 9: 264–274.

MacCallum F, Golombok S 2004 Children raised in fatherless families from infancy: a follow-up of children of lesbian and single heterosexual mothers at early adolescence. Journal of Child Psychology and Psychiatry and Allied Disciplines 45: 1407–1419.

Marrazzo JM, Koutsky LA, Kiviat NB, Kuypers JM, Stine K 2001 Papanicolaou test screening and prevalence of genital human papillomavirus among women who have sex with women. American Journal of Public Health 91: 947–952.

Matthews AK, Brandenburg DL, Johnson TP, Hughes TL 2004 Correlates of underutilization of gynecological cancer screening among lesbian and heterosexual women. Preventive Medicine 38: 105–113.

Mayer KH, Bradford J, Makadon HJ, Stall R, Goldhammer H, Landers S 2008 Sexual and gender minority health: what do we know and what needs to be done? American Journal of Public Health 98: 989–995.

McCaffrey M, Varney P, Evans B, Taylor-Robinson D 1999 Bacterial vaginosis in lesbians: evidence for lack of sexual transmission. International Journal of STD and AIDS 10: 305–308.

McFadden D, Pasanen EG 1998 Comparison of the auditory systems of heterosexuals and homosexuals: click-evoked otoacoustic emissions. Proceedings of the National Academy of Sciences 95: 2709–2713.

McNair RP 2003 Lesbian health inequalities: a cultural minority issue for health professionals. Medical Journal of Australia 178: 643–645.

Mercer CH, Bailey JV, Johnson AM et al 2007 Women who report having sex with women: British national probability data on prevalence, sexual behaviors, and health outcomes. American Journal of Public Health 97: 1126–1133.

Murray C, Golombok S 2005a Solo mothers and their donor insemination infants: follow-up at age 2 years. Human Reproduction 20: 1655–1660.

Murray C, Golombok S 2005b Going it alone: solo mothers and their infants conceived by donor insemination. American Journal of Orthopsychiatry 75: 242–253.

Peplau LA, Garnets LD 2000 A new paradigm for understanding women's sexuality and sexual orientation. Journal of Social Issues 56: 329–350.

Plumb M 2001 Undercounts and overstatements: will the IOM report on lesbian health improve research? American Journal of Public Health 91: 873–875.

Rahman Q, Cockburn A, Govier E 2006 A comparative analysis of functional cerebral asymmetry in lesbian women, heterosexual women, and heterosexual men. Archives of Sexual Behaviour 37: 566–571.

Ross LE, Steele LS, Epstein R 2006 Lesbian and bisexual women's recommendations for improving the provision of assisted reproductive technology services. Fertility and Sterility 86: 735–738.

Royal College of Nursing 2003 Lesbian, Gay, Bisexual and Transgender Patients or Clients. Guidance for Nursing Staff on Next of Kin Issues. RCN, London.

Skinner CJ, Stokes J, Kirlew Y, Kavanagh J, Forster GE 1996 A case–controlled study of the sexual health needs of lesbians. Genitourinary Medicine 72: 277–280.

Smith G, Bartlett A, King M 2004 Treatments of homosexuality in Britain since the 1950s — an oral history: the experience of patients. BMJ (Clinical Research Ed.) 328: 427.

Solarz A (ed) 1999 Lesbian Health: Current Assessment and Directions for the Future. National Academy Press, Washington, DC.

Valanis BG, Bowen DJ, Bassford T et al 2000 Sexual orientation and health: comparisons in the WHI sample. Archives of Family Medicine 9(9): 843–853.

Veniegas RC, Conley TD 2000 Biological research on women's sexual orientations: evaluating the scientific evidence. Journal of Social Issues 56: 267–282.

Wilkinson S 2002 Lesbian Health. In: Coyle A, Kitzinger C (eds) Lesbian & Gay Psychology: New Perspectives. BPS and Blackwell, Oxford, pp 117–134.

Williams TJ, Pepitone ME, Christensen SE et al 2000 Finger-length ratios and sexual orientation. Nature 404: 455–456.

Wilton T 2000 Sexualities in Health and Social Care: a Textbook. Open University Press, Buckingham.

Wilton T, Kaufmann T 2001 Lesbian mothers' experiences of maternity care in the UK. Midwifery 17: 203–211.

CHAPTER 68

Evidence-based care in gynaecology

Arri Coomarasamy and Siladitya Bhattacharya

Chapter Contents

INTRODUCTION	1017	CONCLUSION	1024
EVIDENCE-BASED MEDICINE PROCESSES	1017	KEY POINTS	1024

Introduction

Evidence-based medicine (EBM) has been defined as the 'conscientious, explicit and judicious use of current best evidence in making decisions about the care of individual patients' (Sackett et al 1996). It incorporates three fundamental elements: external research evidence, clinical expertise, and patients' views and values in the delivery of health care (Figure 68.1).

Although discussions about EBM generally revolve around acquisition and appraisal of external research evidence, the critical importance of the other two components cannot be overstated. Failure to elicit the right diagnosis or to communicate the management plan to a patient in a meaningful way is unlikely to lead to better clinical outcomes. Similarly, if a patient's beliefs, expectations and concerns are not explored and incorporated into the management plan, a well-laid-out course of therapy may fail due to lack of compliance. The ideal clinical decision is a product of complex personal characteristics as well as objective research evidence. Effective implementation of EBM is only possible if a proposed intervention has the support of health professionals and patients.

The aim of this chapter is to introduce the reader to the concept of EBM as applied to clinical gynaecology.

Evidence-Based Medicine Processes

The practice of EBM involves systematically identifying, appraising and applying contemporaneous research findings as the basis of clinical decisions. This process is often summarized by the four 'A's:

- Ask: formulate a structured question based on a clinical problem.
- Acquire: search the literature for relevant guidelines, reviews or primary article(s).
- Appraise: evaluate (critically appraise) the literature for validity and usefulness.
- Apply: implement useful relevant research findings in clinical practice, taking patient preferences into account.

A fifth 'A' for 'Audit' can be added to these steps to take EBM beyond the care of the individual patient (Figure 68.2).

Formulation of a structured question

A well-structured question is essential in order to get the right clinical answer. It also facilitates the process of searching for evidence. A suggested approach uses five components (PICOD: Population, Intervention, Comparison, Outcome(s) and Design), as shown in Table 68.1.

The purpose of this step is to get clarity regarding the clinical question. Writing down the question in free form often makes it possible to break it down into a PICOD format. In practice, this may not always be feasible for all clinical questions, and missing out some elements of PICOD is not necessarily a cause for concern.

Searching the literature

Approximately 17,000 journals collectively publish over 1 million biomedical articles each year. Identifying relevant articles will require the use of apposite keywords (and their combinations) to search appropriate databases. A hierarchical approach to literature searching is recommended (Figure 68.3).

The first step is to look for an up-to-date professional guideline that has been developed on the basis of systematic appraisal of available evidence. Table 68.2 lists some sources of guidelines and evidence summaries. The Royal College of Obstetricians and Gynaecologists (RCOG) has long acknowledged the need to update clinical practice on the basis of research findings. Since 1973, the RCOG has

DOI: 10.1016/B978-0-7020-3120-5.00068-0

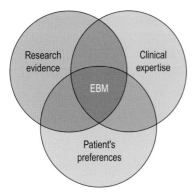

Figure 68.1 Evidence-based medicine (EBM) triad: the three components of EBM.

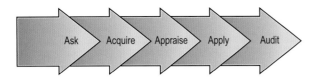

Figure 68.2 The five 'A's of evidence-based medicine.

Table 68.1 Components of structured clinical questions

Component	Example 1	Example 2
P: Population, patient or problem	In women suffering with heavy menstrual bleeding…	In postoperative women with swollen legs…
I: Intervention (test, medical or surgical treatment, or process of care)	… would treatment with norethisterone…	… would a Doppler ultrasound be accurate…
C: Comparison (placebo, another alternative treatment or the gold standard in a diagnostic accuracy study)	… compared with no treatment at all or alternative treatments (e.g. levonorgestrel IUS)…	… compared with venography as the gold standard…
O: Outcome(s)	… lead to an improvement in their symptoms?	… in diagnosing deep venous thrombosis?
D: Ideal design for the study	A randomized controlled trial	A test accuracy study

IUS, intrauterine system. Produced by Bob Phillips, Chris Ball, Dave Sackett, Doug Badenoch, Sharon Straus, Brian Haynes, Martin Dawes since November 1998. Updated by Jeremy Howick March 2009.

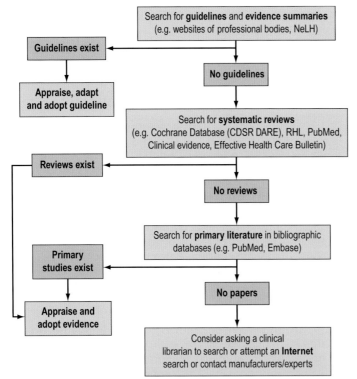

Figure 68.3 Hierarchical approach to literature searching. DARE, Database of Abstracts of Reviews of Effectiveness; RHL, Reproductive Health Library; NeLH, National electronic Library of Health. *Source: Khan and Coomarasamy (2003). NeLH, National electronic Library for Health; RHL, Reproductive Health Library.*

regularly convened study groups to address important growth areas within the specialty. These groups have met, evaluated the results of research and conducted in-depth discussions on a variety of topics. These discussions have shaped the development of clinical recommendations which were initially based on consensus. Over the years, this approach has been modified in order to produce genuine evidence-based guidelines. To be effective and relevant, guidelines must fulfil fthe following three essential criteria.

- They must be multidisciplinary: in other words, they must be developed by a multiprofessional working group including clinicians, nurses and other health professionals as well as users of health services (i.e. consumer representatives).

Table 68.2 Sources of guidelines and evidence summaries (relevant for gynaecology)

Sources of guidelines and evidence summaries	Website
Royal College of Obstetricians and Gynaecologists (RCOG)	www.rcog.org.uk
American College of Obstetricians and Gynecologists (ACOG)	www.acog.org
The Society of Obstetricians and Gynaecologists of Canada (SOGC)	www.sogc.org
The Royal Australian and New Zealand College of Obstetricians and Gynaecologists (RANZCOG)	www.ranzcog.edu.au
International Federation of Gynecology and Obstetrics (FIGO)	www.figo.org
Faculty of Sexual and Reproductive Healthcare (FFPRHC)	www.ffprhc.org.uk
British Fertility Society (BFS)	www.britishfertilitysociety.org.uk
British Gynaecological Cancer Society (BGCS)	www.bgcs.org.uk
British Society for Colposcopy and Cervical Pathology (BSCCP)	www.bsccp.org.uk
British Society of Urogynaecology (BSUG)	www.rcog.org.uk/bsug
British Society for Gynaecological Endoscopy (BSGE)	www.bsge.org.uk
The Association of Early Pregnancy Units (AEPU)	www.earlypregnancy.org.uk
The NHS National Library for Health (NLH)	www.library.nhs.uk
The National Institute for Health Clinical Excellence (NICE)	www.nice.org.uk
Scottish Intercollegiate Guideline Network (SIGN)	www.sign.ac.uk
NHS Clinical Knowledge Summaries (NHS CKS; formerly PRODIGY)	www.cks.library.nhs.uk
The National Guideline Clearing House (NGC, US)	www.guidelines.gov

Table 68.3 Sources of evidence

Systematic reviews	
Sources of systematic reviews	Website
The Cochrane Library	www.cochrane.org/reviews/
The CRD databases (including DARE)	www.crd.york.ac.uk/crdweb
The Pubmed Systematic Reviews Search Filter	www.ncbi.nlm.nih.gov/entrez/query/static/clinical.shtml
Bandolier	www.jr2.ox.ac.uk/bandolier
The WHO Reproductive Health Library (RHL)	www.rhlibrary.com
Health Technology Assessment (HTA) database	www.ncchta.org/project/htapubs.asp

Sources of primary literature		
Sources of primary literature	Subject matter	Website
Pubmed (Medline)	Medicine, bioscience	www.pubmed.gov
EMBASE	Medicine, pharmacology, nursing	www.embase.com
CINAHL	Nursing and allied health care	www.cinahl.com
AMED	Allied and alternative health care	www.bl.uk (search for 'AMED')
BNI (British Nursing Index)	Nursing	
HMIC (Health Management Information Consortium) database	Health management	

WHO, World Health Organization; CRD, Centre for Reviews and Dissemination; DARE, Database of Abstracts of Reviews of Effectiveness.

- They must be evidence based: guideline development must include a systematic search for and synthesis of all available research evidence.
- They must be evidence linked: individual recommendations within a guideline must be explicitly linked to the strength and quality of the evidence on which they are based, using a recognized grading scheme (Centre for Evidence-based Medicine, Oxford University, www.cebm.net) (see Appendix).

It is generally anticipated that national guidelines will, in turn, be used as a basis for the development of local protocols and guidelines in conjunction with local commissioners and providers of health care as well as service users. These should take into account the specific needs of local service provision and the preferences of the local population.

In the absence of credible evidence-based guidelines, the next step would be to search for an up-to-date, good-quality, systematic review. Some sources of systematic reviews are given in Table 68.3.

Apart from the traditional sources of systematic reviews, such as the Cochrane Library and DARE, MEDLINE and Pubmed have now become a rich source of systematic reviews. Pubmed contains a systematic review filter within Pubmed Clinical Queries (http://www.ncbi.nlm.nih.gov/entrez/query/static/clinical.shtml), and MEDLINE has the indexing term 'reviews, systematic' as a 'publication type'.

If no systematic reviews are identified, or if reviews are out-of-date, non-systematic or of marginal relevance to the clinical question, it is necessary to continue the literature search for primary studies. Table 68.3 provides a list of important sources of primary literature.

Efficient searching for primary literature requires training and practice, and input from an experienced librarian or information scientist. Careful selection of keywords for searching, matching these keywords to Medical Subject Heading terms, and combining the terms with 'AND' or 'OR' Boolean operators are necessary skills that are best learnt from librarians. Pubmed carries three tools that clinicians can employ to optimize their searches, and these are discussed below.

Pubmed 'clinical queries' (www.ncbi.nlm. nih.gov/entrez/query/static/clinical.shtml)

This has now established itself as the primary gateway for efficient literature searching to support evidence-based practice. 'Clinical queries' uses filters that allow retrieval of articles for the five main categories of clinical questions: therapy, diagnosis, aetiology, prognosis and clinical prediction. The option of 'sensitive search' in 'clinical queries' allows for a broad search that may identify many relevant articles, but also carries the risk of getting many irrelevant hits; the 'specific search', on the other hand, performs a narrow search and would retrieve fewer articles, but at the risk of missing some relevant articles. It is advisable to start with a sensitive search, and to move to a specific search if the number of hits is unmanageably large on the sensitive search.

Pubmed 'SLIM' (SLider Interface for Medline/Pubmed)

This exciting new development uses six different slider bars to control search variables, improving user control and the capability to instantly refine and refocus search strategies (https://pmi.nlm.nih.gov/slim/).

Pubmed 'related articles'

Once a relevant citation is found, clicking on the 'related articles' function to the right of the identified citation retrieves other similar articles.

Evaluation of the literature

Once relevant articles have been identified and retrieved, the next step is to select those which are appropriate and methodologically sound. Many papers published in medical journals have serious design flaws, and most are irrelevant for everyday clinical practice. Most clinicians are accustomed to functioning as 'users' when dealing with evidence to support practice, but the absence of up-to-date and valid preappraised evidence makes it necessary to switch to an 'appraiser' mode and evaluate articles in terms of validity (methodological soundness), importance {e.g. effect sizes [relative risks, odds ratio, numbers needed to treat (NNT) for therapy studies, and accuracy estimates (e.g. likelihood ratios)] for test accuracy studies}, and applicability of the results in practice.

In addition, an overall judgement on the quality of the evidence will need to take two other issues into account: consistency, the extent to which different studies found similar results; and robustness, the extent to which minor alterations in results do not change the conclusions drawn from those data.

Various checklists can be used to appraise different types of clinical questions. Checklists for therapeutic and diagnos-

Table 68.4 Research designs for specific clinical questions

Clinical question	Ideal research design
Effectiveness of therapy	RCT
Prevention	RCT
Screening	Cluster RCT
Diagnosis (accuracy)	Cross-sectional study (comparison of index test with reference standard test)
Prognosis	Cohort study
Aetiology	Case–control or cohort study
Adverse events	Case report, case series, case–control studies, cohort studies and RCTs
Economic assessment of medical interventions	Depending on the exact question: Cost-minimization study Cost-effectiveness study Cost–utility study Cost–benefit study

RCT, randomized controlled trial.

tic questions as well as systematic reviews are given in Tables 68.5, 68.7 and 68.10. In appraising a study, it is important to assess the suitability of the research design and methods used in the context of the specific clinical question. Randomized trials provide the best evidence for treatment, but valid evidence for diagnosis, prognosis and causation may be derived from publications based on other study designs (Table 68.4).

Appraising a paper on effectiveness of therapy (randomized controlled trial)

A randomized controlled trial reduces the risk of bias (systematic deviations or errors in the results) by minimizing the likelihood of important differences between the treatment and control arms of the study. If no randomized controlled trials are available, other research designs (e.g. a non-randomized controlled study or even a case–control study) may provide valuable information about therapy, although they may exaggerate the potential benefits of treatment and thus represent a lower grade of evidence (see evidence grades, Centre for Evidence-based Medicine, Oxford University, www.cebm.net) (see Appendix). A checklist can be used to appraise a therapy article (Table 68.5).

If the results for a randomized controlled trial are dichotomous (i.e. a 'yes/no' outcome), and there are two arms in the study, the findings can be presented and analysed in a 2×2 table, as shown in Table 68.6.

NNT is a particularly useful measure to express the magnitude of treatment benefit. NNT is defined as the number of patients that will need to be treated to achieve one additional good outcome. Thus, the lower the NNT, the greater the magnitude of the outcome, and an NNT below 10 is often (arbitrarily) regarded as a 'large effect size'. However, such arbitrary thresholds for defining benefit sizes should be used with caution, as a small effect size (with a correspondingly large NNT) can still be important if the outcome in question is serious (e.g. deaths prevented).

Table 68.5 Critical appraisal checklist for randomized controlled trials

I. Are the results valid?

1. Is the assignment of patients randomized? Appropriate methods are: random number tables and computer-generated random numbers
2. Is allocation of treatment concealed? Appropriate methods are: opaque envelopes, third party randomization, distant (telephone or Internet) allocation
3. Are patients, health workers and study personnel 'blinded' to the intervention?
4. Are patients analysed in the groups to which they were randomized? ('intention to treat' analysis)
5. Are all patients who entered the trial properly accounted for?
6. Is follow-up complete?
7. Are the randomized groups similar at the start of the trial? (normally presented in 'Table 1' of the article)
8. Apart from the experimental and control interventions, are the groups treated equally?
9. Was the study adequately powered?*
10. Was ethical approval obtained for the study?*

II. What are the results (i.e. importance of results)?

1. How large is the treatment effect? (reported as relative risks, odds ratios, absolute risks, numbers needed to treat or differences in means or medians)
2. How precise is the treatment effect? (95% confidence intervals around the above)

III. Will the results help me in caring for my patients (applicability)?

1. Can the results be applied to my patients?
2. Are all clinically important outcomes considered?
3. What are the likely benefits? Are they worth the potential harms and costs?

*These items do not strictly relate to 'validity'; nevertheless, they are important and should be part of the appraisal process.

Table 68.6 2 × 2 table to present the results of a two-arm trial with a dichotomous outcome

	Outcome (live birth)	
	Event	Non-event
Experimental group (surgery for endometriosis)	a	b
Control group (no surgery)	c	d

Risk in the experimental group (or experimental event rate) = a/(a+b)
Risk in the control group (or control event rate) = c/(c+d)
Relative risk (or risk ratio) = [a/(a+b)]/[c/(c+d)]
Absolute risk reduction (ARR) = [c/(c+d)] − [a/(a+b)]
Numbers needed to treat = 1/ARR
Odds in the experimental group = a/b
Odds in the control group = c/d
Odds ratio = (a/b)/(c/d)

Appraising a diagnostic article

The checklist shown in Table 68.7 can be used to appraise a diagnostic accuracy article. It should be noted that this checklist only applies to accuracy studies; there are other aspects of testing that may need to be judged on other crite-

Table 68.7 Critical appraisal checklist for diagnostic accuracy studies

I. Are the results valid?

1. Does the patient sample include an appropriate spectrum of patients to whom the test will be applied in clinical practice?
2. Are the test and reference (gold) standard results blinded?
3. Did everyone get both the test and the reference standard?
4. Is the test described fully?
5. Is the reference standard described fully?

II. What are the results?

1. What are the results? (sensitivity, specificity, predictive values or likelihood ratios)
2. What is their precision? (95% confidence intervals)

III. Will the results help me in caring for my patients?

1. Are the results applicable to my patients?
2. Will the results change my management?
3. Will patients be better off as a result of the test?

ria. For example, evaluating the inter- or intraobserver reliability or the clinical impact of testing will require designs other than the one employed for accuracy evaluation, and will often need to be judged by other criteria.

The sensitivity, specificity, predictive values and prevalence are defined in the marginal cells of Table 68.8. The sensitivities and specificities are often misinterpreted, and the mnemonics 'SnNout' and 'SpPin' are very useful to ensure correct interpretations.

- SnNout: when a test has high *Sensitivity*, a *Negative* test result rules *out* the diagnosis.
- SpPin: when a test has high *Specificity*, a *Positive* test result rules *in* diagnosis.

Thus, sensitivities relate to negative test results, whilst specificities relate to positive test results.

Likelihood ratios, which can be calculated from the 2 × 2 table, or derived from sensitivities and specificities as shown in the footnote of Table 68.8, are generally considered to be the most useful of all test accuracy summaries. The likelihood ratio indicates how much a given test result raises or lowers the probability of having the disease. The higher the likelihood ratio of an abnormal test, the greater the value of the test. Conversely, the lower the likelihood ratio of a normal test, the greater the value of the test. Although a guide to the interpretation of likelihood ratios is provided in Table 68.9, it should be noted that the value of a test may vary depending on the pretest probability and the consequences of having the condition.

Appraising a systematic reviews or meta-analysis

A systematic review aims to provide a complete exploration of evidence on a subject. It is an overview of studies using explicit, systematic and therefore reproducible methods to locate, select, appraise and synthesize relevant and reliable evidence. Although the terms 'systematic review' and 'meta-analysis' are often used interchangeably, the term 'meta-analysis' has a specific meaning; it is the mathematical pooling of numerical results from individual studies. All good systematic reviews have the following five features:

Table 68.8 2 × 2 table for test accuracy results

		Reference standard (e.g. venography to confirm or refute the diagnosis of DVT)		
		Disease present	Disease absent	
Index test (e.g. ultrasound Doppler to diagnose DVT)	Positive test	a (true positive)	b (false positive)	PPV= a/(a+b)
	Negative test	c (false negative)	d (true negative)	NPV=d/(c+d)
		Sensitivity = a/(a+c)	Specificity= d/(b+d)	Prevalence=(a+c)/(a+b+c+d)

DVT, deep venous thrombosis; PPV, positive predictive value; NPV, negative predictive value.
Likelihood ratio for positive test (LR+) = [a/(a+c)]/[b/(b+d)] = sensitivity/(1 − specificity)
Likelihood ratio for negative test (LR−) = [c/(a+c)]/[d/(b+d)] = (1 − sensitivity)/specificity

Table 68.9 Interpretation of likelihood ratios (LR)

LR for positive test	LR for negative test	Value of test
>10	<0.1	Very useful
5–10	0.1–0.2	Moderately useful
2–5	0.5–0.2	Somewhat useful
>1–2	0.5–<1	Little useful
1	1	Useless

- a clearly framed question;
- comprehensive literature search across multiple databases for published and often unpublished data;
- explicit inclusion and exclusion criteria for study selection;
- careful assessment of methodological quality of the included studies; and
- synthesis of the evidence (with quantitative synthesis, or meta-analysis when appropriate).

The checklist in Table 68.10 can be used to appraise a systematic review.

One needs to be mindful of the following three issues when interpreting the findings of systematic reviews and meta-analyses.

- 'Garbage in, garbage out': if the studies that make up a systematic review are flawed, the systematic review itself is likely to be unreliable.
- Publication bias: unfortunately, studies that show negative and/or statistically non-significant results are less likely to be published. This could be due to apathy or conflict of interest of the researchers or sponsors, or the disinterest of journal reviewers and editors. Although systematic reviewers are expected to make all efforts to locate published and unpublished data, it is possible that negative studies remain buried, thus biasing the findings of a review. Statistical tests such as funnel plot analysis can indicate the presence of publication and related biases.
- Heterogeneity: the degree to which the effect sizes from the various individual studies in a systematic review agree (homogeneity) or disagree (heterogeneity) has important implications for inferences. If the findings

Table 68.10 Critical appraisal of systematic reviews

I. Are the results valid?

1. Does the article address a clearly focused question? (i.e. are the PICOD elements defined clearly?)
2. Are the criteria used to select articles for inclusion appropriate?
3. Is the literature search comprehensive? (MEDLINE, EMBASE, Cochrane Library, CINAHL, searchers for abstracts, hand-searching etc.)
4. Is the validity of the included studies appraised? (using checklists or tables like those given in Tables 68.7 and 68.9)
5. Did two or more reviewers extract the data independently?
6. Are the results consistent from study to study?
7. Is there an assessment for publication bias? (e.g. funnel plot analysis)

II. What are the results?

1. What are the results of the study?
2. How precise are the results? (95% confidence intervals)

III. Will the results help me in caring for my patients?

1. Can the results be applied to my patient care?
2. Are all clinically relevant outcomes considered?
3. Are the benefits worth the harms and costs?

are homogeneous (i.e. the results of various studies agree with each other), one is more likely to believe the meta-analysed summary result. Heterogeneity can be assessed visually by examining the forest plot, or statistically using tests such as Chi-square, Cochran Q or I^2 statistics.

Findings of a meta-analysis are often presented as a forest plot (Figure 68.4). Forest plots can be used to plot relative risks, risk differences, odds ratios, mean differences or other summary estimates such as sensitivities, specificities and likelihood ratios. Each individual study in the systematic review is represented in a row, with its own point estimate (the 'box') and the 95% confidence interval (the 'whiskers'). The pooled summary estimate is shown as a diamond at the bottom of the chart. The centre of the diamond represents the pooled estimate and the ends of the diamond represent the 95% confidence interval for the pooled estimate.

Implementation of useful findings

The final step in EBM is implementation or incorporating the identified evidence in clinical practice. This may seem a

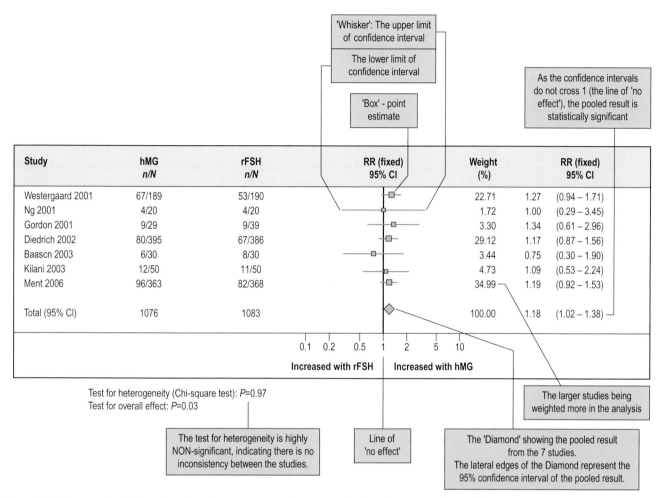

Figure 68.4 An example of a forest plot: urinary human menopausal gonadotrophin (hMG) versus recombinant follicle-stimulating hormone (rFSH) for controlled ovarian hyperstimulation in in-vitro fertilization (IVF) treatment for the outcome of live births per IVF cycle started. RR, relative risk. See the source reference for details of the individual study references.

Source: Coomarasamy A, Afnan M, Cheema D, van der Veen F, Bossuyt PM, van Wely M. Urinary hMG versus recombinant FSH for controlled ovarian hyperstimulation following an agonist long down-regulation protocol in IVF or ICSI treatment: a systematic review and meta-analysis. Hum Reprod. 2008 Feb;23(2):310–5.

deceptively simple step (e.g. a case of writing up a prescription), but in practice can be the most complex of all EBM steps. As a minimum, this requires careful consideration of the following issues.

How generalizable are the results of the study to your specific patient or patient group?

This issue is variously described as 'generalizability', 'applicability' or 'external validity', and requires the examination of study population (e.g. the inclusion and exclusion criteria) and study conduct to answer the question: 'Are there important reasons to believe that the results of this study may not apply to my patient(s)?' It is important not to be unreasonably stringent in this evaluation. For instance, if a US study recruiting women under the age of 40 years with severe endometriosis found that treatment X was effective in improving quality of life, would the evidence apply to a 42-year-old English woman with moderate endometriosis? Although this woman may not have been eligible for the trial, there is probably no reason to believe that the results of the study should not apply to her.

What is the balance between benefit and harm?

Many effective treatments come with their own set of problems, including adverse effects, toxicity and operative complications (for surgical interventions). Whilst a full and formal clinical decision analysis or other similar techniques to comprehensively analyse the net benefits and harm with their associated values and costs would be outside the scope (and perhaps need) of most clinicians and their patients, it is essential that an overall assessment of the net balance sheet is made. To make a reliable assessment on this issue, the identified studies need to have reported all clinically relevant outcomes over a reasonable period of time. Often, it is necessary to undertake separate literature searches to identify rarer or long-term adverse outcomes.

What does the patient think?

Eliciting ideas, concerns and expectations from the patient about the condition and the potential therapeutic interventions that are available is crucial to a successful consultation. Patients may place different values on various outcomes and adverse events; unless these are elicited and incorporated into the decision-making, satisfaction with the management plan and compliance with therapy are unlikely to ensue. Building a partnership with the patient, providing a balanced discussion about the risks and benefits, and seeking agreement and providing support are all essential to the 'Apply' step of EBM.

Despite being accessed and appraised systematically, most research findings are currently applied intuitively. If EBM is to be seen through to its logical conclusion involving a synthesis of empirical evidence and human values, the current conflict between the explicit collection of data and its implicit use must be addressed. This area is being investigated and possible options are being evaluated. These include decision analysis, which provides an intellectual framework for the development of an explicit decision-making algorithm (Lilford et al 1998), and computerized decision support systems. When there are several treatment options which may have different effects on a patient's life, there is a strong case for offering patients a number of choices. It is possible that their active involvement in the decision-making process may actually increase the effectiveness of the treatment (Coulter et al 1999).

Conclusion

The purpose of clinical research is to generate new knowledge on how to treat individual patients and how best to deliver healthcare services. The objective of EBM and its component activities is to maximize the extent to which clinical practice is based on research evidence, and consequently improve the net health gain for patients. Within gynaecology, the recent years have seen considerable progress in strategies aimed at seeking, appraising and applying evidence. A comprehensive approach towards getting research evidence into practice is promoted by National Health Service clinical effectiveness and clinical governance initiatives. What is being challenged is the way in which doctors make clinical decisions and the way in which patients respond to them.

KEY POINTS

1. Evidence-based medicine (EBM) involves the integration of best available research evidence with clinical expertise and patients' views and preferences.
2. EBM has four steps: (i) Ask a structured clinical question; (ii) Acquire the relevant literature; (iii) Appraise the literature for validity and usefulness; and (iv) Apply the findings.
3. Asking a structured clinical question involves breaking it down to PICOD: Population, Intervention, Comparison, Outcomes, and Desired study design.
4. Acquiring evidence involves taking a hierarchic approach to literature searching: look for evidence-based guidelines first, then for systematic reviews, and then for primary studies if no relevant guidelines or systematic reviews exist.
5. Good guidelines are evidence-based, evidence-linked and produced by a multidisciplinary team. They can often be found in various professional body websites.
6. Appraisal of literature involves assessment for validity, usefulness and applicability.
7. Strategies need to be developed to overcome existing barriers to the wider implementation of evidence-based care in gynaecology.

References

Coulter A, Entwistle V, Gilbert D 1999 Sharing decisions with patients: is the information good enough? BMJ (Clinical Research Ed.) 318: 318–322.

Coomarasamy A, Afnan M, Cheema D et al 2008 Urinary hMG versus recombinant FSH for controlled ovarian hyperstimulation following an agonist long down-regulation protocol in IVF or ICSI treatment: a systematic review and meta-analysis. Human Reproduction 23(2): 310–315.

Khan KS, Coomarasamy A 2003 Searching for evidence to inform clinical practice. Current Obstetrics and Gynaecology. Doi:10.1061/j.curobgyn.2003.12.006.

Lilford RJ, Pauker SG, Braunholtz DA, Chard J 1998 Decision analysis and the implementation of research findings. BMJ (Clinical Research Ed.) 317: 405–409.

Sackett DL, Rosenberg WM, Gray JA, Haynes RB, Richardson WS 1996 Evidence based medicine: what it is and what it isn't. BMJ 312: 71–72.

Further Reading

Guyatt G, Rennie D, O'Meade M, Cook DJ 2008 JAMA Users' Guide to the Medical Literature. A Manual for Evidence-based Clinical Practice. McGraw Hill, New York.

Haynes RB, Devereaux PJ, Guyatt GH 2002 Physicians' and patients' choices in evidence based practice. BMJ (Clinical Research Ed.) 324: 1350.

Khan KS, Coomarasamy A 2003 Searching for evidence to inform clinical practice. Current Obstetrics and Gynaecology Doi:10.1016/j.curobgyn.2003.12.006.

Straus SE, McAlister FA 2000 Evidence-based medicine: a commentary on common criticisms. CMAJ: Canadian Medical Association Journal 163: 837–841.

Straus SE, Richardson WS, Glasziou P, Haynes RB 2005 Evidence-based Medicine: How to Practice and Teach EBM, 3rd edn. Elsevier Churchill Livingstone, Edinburgh.

Useful Websites

Centre for Evidence-based Medicine, Oxford University, UK: http://www.cebm.net/

For an excellent website that brings together various resources relevant to evidence-based practice, visit: A ScHARR

Introduction to Evidence Based Practice on the Internet: http://www.shef.ac.uk/~scharr/ir/netting/

Index

NB: Page numbers followed by *f* indicate figures; *t* indicate tables; *b* indicate boxes. Entries beginning with Figures, e.g. 21, will be filed as if spelled out, e.g. twenty-one

A

Abagovomab, 559
Abberations of normal development and involution (ANDI), benign breast disease, 690–692
Abdomen, opening and closing, 105–107
Abdominal aorta, 11
Abdominal hysterectomy, 467
Abdominal pregnancy, 377
Ablation
  cervical premalignancy, 574, 574t
  endometrial techniques *see* Endometrial ablation techniques
  free fluid, 30, 30f
  genital warts, 970
  lasers, 463
  ovarian, 726
Abortion
  assessment of patient, 434
  cervical and vaginal lacerations, 437
  complications of, 436–437
  counselling, 434
  early-first-trimester, 435–436
  and ectopic pregnancy, 365
  follow-up, 436
  and HIV, 984
  incomplete, 436–437
  infertility, 437
  late complications, 437
  late-first-trimester, 436
  legal aspects, 433–434
  medical, 435–436
  mid trimester, 436
  minor complications, 437
  missed (early fetal demise), 340
  mortality risk, 436
  psychological aspects, 437
  service provision, 434
  subsequent pregnancy, 437
  surgical methods, 435
  techniques, 434–436
  see also Contraception/contraceptive advice; Pregnancy
Abrasions, 995
Abscess
  breast, 698–699
  hidradentitis, 607
  recurring subareolar, 701
  tubo-ovarian, 67f

Abuse
  abused victims, 1003
  management of, 1005
  patterns of, 1003
  pelvic pain, 931–932
  sexual and physical, 933
Aceclofenac, 456
Acetylcholine, 814, 821
Aciclovir, 960–961, 982
Acquired immunodeficiency syndrome (AIDS), 956, 979
  see also Human immunodeficiency syndrome (HIV)
Actinomycin D, 660–661
Activated protein C resistance, 346
Active Electrode Monitoring system, 52
Activin, 205
Actulose, 910
Acupuncture, overactive bladder syndrome, 828
Acute myocardial infarction, combined hormonal contraceptives, 425
Acute pylonephritis, 903
Acute urinary retention, 837
  ultrasound, 88
Adenoacanthoma (endometrial adenocarcinoma with squamous metaplasia), 632, 633f
Adenocarcinomas, 587, 633
Adenohypophysis, 197
Adenolipoma, 701
Adenoma, breast, 701
Adenomyosis
  dysmenorrhoea, 455
  fibroids, 477
  imaging techniques, 65–66, 65f–66f
Adenosis, 695–696
Adenosquamous carcinoma, 587, 632–633
Adhesion molecules and mucins, implantation, 271–272
Adiana procedure, hysteroscopy, 31, 31f
Adolescents *see* Children and young people
Adrenal cortex, 140
Adrenal gland, androgen-secreting tumours, 171
Adrenal hormones, 140–141
Adrenal hyperplasia, late-onset congenital, 385
Adrenal rest tumours
Adrenal steroid synthesis, endocrine control, 151–152
Adrenarche, 183
  premature, 188

Adrenocorticotrophic hormone (ACTH), 129, 151, 198–199
  and CAH, 169
  precocious puberty, 188
α-adrenoreceptor antagonists, 826, 844
Advanced breast biopsy instrumentation (ABBI), 721
α-fetoprotein (AFP), 142–143
Age factors
  age at first pregnancy, breast cancer risk, 708
  assisted reproduction treatments, 321–322
  breast cancer risk, 708
  hydatidiform mole, 652–653
  ovarian hyperstimulation syndrome, 244–245
  pelvic organ prolapse, 849
  preoperative assessment, 97
  voiding difficulties, 838
Age-related changes
  ovaries, 2
  uterus, 5
  vagina, 5
  vulva, 6–7
  see also Pubertal development
Agnus castus, premenstrual syndrome, 396
Alcohol intake
  breast cancer risk, 710
  violence against women, 1003
Alendronate, 413
Alimentary tract toxicity, chemotherapy, 552
Allergies
  assessment of allergic patients, 97
  chemotherapy effects, 552
  ovarian hyperstimulation syndrome, 245
Alloimmune factors, miscarriage, 346–347
Allopregnanolone, 394
Alopecia, chemotherapy, 552
Alpha folate receptor, 560
Alprazolam, 400
Alprostadil, 445
Altemeier operation, faecal incontinence, 915
Alternative therapies, premenstrual syndrome, 397, 398t
Alzheimer's disease, 408
Ambiguous genitalia, 170
Ambulatory Gynaecology Service, 80
Ambulatory monitoring
  overactive bladder syndrome, 818, 820f
  urethral sphincter incompetence, 788–789, 790f
Amenorrhoea, 204, 212, 223–224
  causes, 213–223, 214b
    anatomical, 213–214, 215b
    anti-Müllerian hormone

chemotherapy and ovarian reserve
  chronic illness, 218–219
  CNS-hypothalamic disturbance, 216–217
  endocrine, 214–215, 223
  exercise, 217–218
  hyperprolactinaemia, 219–220
  hypogonadotrophic hypogonadism, 216
  hypothalamic and pituitary lesions, 216
  idiopathic delayed puberty, 219
  Kallman's syndrome, 215–216
  measuring ovarian reserve, 222
  metabolic hormones regulating
    reproductive function, 218
  ovarian failure, 220–222
  physiological amenorrhoea, 213
  weight, 217
chemotherapy-related, in breast
  cancer, 733
chronic illness, 218–219
CNS-hypothalamic disturbance, 216–217
complete androgen insensitivity, 213–214
definitions, 212
diagnosis and management, 223–225
ectopic pregnancy, 366–367
endocrine causes, 214–215, 223
exercise-related, 217–218
follicle-stimulating hormone
hyperprolactinaemia, 219–220
hypogonadotrophic hypogonadism, 216,
  224–225
hypothalamic and pituitary lesions, 216
hypothalamic-pituitary dysfunction,
  214–215
impedance bipolar radiofrequency, 30
Kallman's syndrome, 215–216
ovarian failure, 220–223
phenotypes, 213–214
physiological, 213
substance abuse, 1006
ultrasound
weight-related, 217
American Society of Anesthesiologists, 97
Amino acid derivatives, 128
Aminoglycosides, 901–903
Amitryptyline, 606, 869–870, 938
Amoxycilin, 967–968
Ampicillin, 967
Ampulla, fallopian tubes, 3
Ampullary implantation, ectopic pregnancy,
  366
Amsel criteria, bacterial vaginosis, 973–974,
  974f
Anabolic steroids, 306
Anaemia, 540, 551–552
Anaesthesia
  fistulae, examining, 884, 884f
  hysteroscopy, 21
  and miscarriage, 339
Anal advancement flap, anal fissures,
  911
Anal canal, 9
Anal carcinoma, 910–911
Anal continence
  central control of, 780
  mechanisms, 779–780
Anal cushions, 780
Anal fissures, 910–911
Anal incontinence *see* Faecal incontinence

Anal skin sensation, assessment, 908
Anal sphincter and mechanisms, 776–778,
  778f, 908–909
  anal cushions, 780
  anorectal sensation, 780
  artificial sphincters, 914
  external anal sphincter, 773, 776–778, 780
  internal anal sphincter, 778–779
  longitudinal muscle, 778
  overlapping sphincter repair, 913f
  puborectalis muscle and external anal
    sphincter, 776–778
  rectal compliance, 780
  rectoanal inhibitory reflex, 779–780
  ultrasound and dynamic imaging, 908
  see also Faecal incontinence
Analgesia
  in cancer patients, 762–763
  chronic pelvic pain, 938
  endometriosis, 501
  haemorrhoids, 910
  PCA, 119
  pelvic inflammatory disease, 948
  postoperative care, 119
  and TVUS, 81
  World Federation of Societies of
    Anaesthesiologists' analgesic ladder,
    119, 119f
Anastamosis breakdown, bowel preparation,
  102
Anastrozole, 481
Anatomy
  bladder, 7–8
  fallopian tubes, 3
  hypothalamic-pituitary axis, 197–198
  ovaries, 1–3
  pelvic musculofascial support, 9–11
  pelvis, 851–852
  rectum, 8–9
  sigmoid colon, 8
  ureter, 5, 7, 107
  urethra, 8
  uterus, 3–5, 19f, 20
  vagina, 5, 599–600
  vulva, 5–7, 599–600
Androgen insensitivity syndrome, 193
  5α-reductase deficiency, 173
  complete insensitivity, 173–174, 213–214
  mixed, 213–214
  partial insensitivity, 174, 213–215
  target site, 173–174, 173t
Androgen receptors, 137
  androgen receptor blockade, 189
Androgen tests, polycystic ovary syndrome,
  384–385
Androgens
  classification of steroid hormones, 145
  therapeutic option, menopause, 409
Androgen-secreting tumours
  intersex disorders, 171
  ovarian cysts, 669, 675–676
  and premature adrenarche, 188
Aneuploidy, 168, 168b, 343
Angiogenesis inhibition, gynaecological
  cancers, 554–556
Angiography, 62
Angiomyofibroblastoma, 608
Angiomyxoma, 608

Angiopoietins, 452
Angiotensin, 151–152
Anorectal angle, puborectalis muscle, 779
Anorectal manometry, 907–908
Anorectal sensation, 780
Anorexia nervosa, 185, 204
Anovulation, 223, 225
Anteflexion, uterus, 4–5
Anterior colporrhaphy, 858
Anterior pituitary hormones, 139–140
Anteversion, uterus, 4–5
Anthracyclines, 551, 716
Antiacne agents, topical, 260
Anti-alpha inhibin, radionuclide imaging, 61
Antiandrogenic compounds, 388
  see also Systemic antiandrogen therapy
Antibiotic prophylaxis
  goal, 100
  preoperative care, 100–101
  urinary tract infections, 902–903
Antibiotic therapy
  breast infections, 700
  chancroid, 965
  chlamydia, 968
  gonorrhoea, 967
  granulomatous mastitis, 700
  hidradentitis, 607
  mastitis, 700
  pelvic inflammatory disease, 948–949
  urinary tract infections, 901–902
  vulval infections resulting from, 606
Anticholinergic drugs, 869–870
Anticholinesterase, 844
Anticoagulants, 102
Anticonvulsants, 306
Anti-D immunoglobulin use, 82, 376
Antidepressants
  bladder disorders, 869–870
  chronic pelvic pain, 938–939
  depression, 931
  irritable bowel syndrome, 917
  premature ejaculation, 445
  premenstrual syndrome, 399–400, 401t
Antidiuretic agents, 825–826
Antiemetics, 552–553
Antifibrinolytics, abnormal menstrual
  bleeding, 460
Antihistamines, 869–870
Antimetabolites, chemotherapy, 550–551
Antimicrobial therapy, 886, 901–902
Anti-Müllerian hormone (AMH)
  and amenorrhoea, 213–214
  assessment of ovarian reserve (inhibin B),
    314–315
  ovarian hormones, 141–142
Antimuscarinic drugs, 821–824
Antiobesity drugs, 259
Antioestrogens, 236–238, 261, 306
Antioxidants, 415
Antiphospholipid syndrome, miscarriage,
  345–346
Antiprogesterone treatment, fibroids,
  481–482
Anti-retroviral Pregnancy Registry, 984
Antiretroviral therapy, 979–981, 983–984
Antisperm antibodies, 304, 306, 433
Anti-vascular growth factor therapies, ovarian
  cancer, 679

Antral follicle count (AFC), 315
Antrum, 232
Anxiety, in PMS, 400
Anxiolytic agents, 400
AP23573, 558
AP23994, 560
Aplasia Ras homolog member 1 (*ARH!*), tumour suppressor gene, 532
Apocrine adenosis, 695–696
Apocrine metaplasia, 696
Apoptosis, 532
Appendices epipolicae, sigmoid colon, 8
Arginine vasopressin, 128
Argon lasers, 56
Argyll-Robertson pupils, syphilis, 963
Aromatase inhibitors
    breast cancer, 725–726
    endometriosis, 504
    fibroids, 481
    polycystic ovary syndrome, 261
Arterial disease, 425
Artificial insemination, 65
Arzoxifene, 414
Ascites, 670
Asherman's syndrome
    amenorrhoea, 214
    hysteroscopy, 18, 27
    and miscarriage, 341
Ashkenazi Jewish women, *BRCA* gene mutations in, 527
Asoprisnil, 481–482
Assessment, preoperative, 96–99
    accurate diagnosis, 96–97
    antibiotic prophylaxis, 100–101
    indications, 98t
    preparation, thromboprophylaxis, 99–100
    risk assessment *see* Risk assessment, preoperative
Assisted reproduction treatments, 312–334
    antenatal and intrapartum complications following, 191
    clinical management of treatment cycle, 316–318
    consents, 94
    ectopic pregnancy, 325–326, 365
    embryo transfer, 320–321, 324
    evaluation of male partner, 315
    evaluation of pelvis, 313–314
    female reproductive disorders, 289
    fibroids, 478–479
    future developments, 329–331
    health risks associated with treatment
        congenital anomalies, 327–328
        ectopic pregnancy, 325–326, 365
        genital and breast cancers, 327
        malignancy in children, 328
        malignancy in newborn, 327–328
        ovarian hyperstimulation syndrome, 326–327
    IVF/ICSI, problems with, 273
    laboratory techniques, 319–320
    male infertility and assisted conception, 302, 307–309
    obstetric and perinatal outcomes, 191–193
    oocyte retrieval, 318–319
    outcome measures/success rate factors
        duration of infertility, 323
        embryo cryopreservation, 324–325

endometrial thickness, 324
        female age, 321–322
        infertility causes, 322–323
        number of attempts, 324
        number of embryos transferred, 324
        obesity, 322
        oocyte donation, 325
        pregnancy, livebirth and miscarriage rates
    ovarian reserve, assessment, 314–315
    perinatal outcome of pregnancies, 328–329
    preimplantation genetic diagnosis/ screening, 329
    selection and evaluation of patients, 312–315
    technology, 273
    see also Fertilization; Infertility; Pregnancy
Asthenozoospermia, 301–302
Atrophy, 609
Atypical apocrine metaplasia, 696
Atypical ductal hyperplasia (ADH), 693–694, 696
Atypical hyperplasia, 577–579
Autoimmune disease, 345–346, 418, 433
Autonomic nerves, 13
Avastin, 555–556
Aversion disorder, 920
Axillary lymph node dissection (ALND), 722
Axillary surgery, breast cancer, 716, 722–724, 723f–724f
Azithromycin, 949, 965, 968
AZT monotherapy, HIV, 983

B

Bacterial vaginosis, 609, 973–974, 974f
    Amsel criteria, 973–974, 974f
    clinical features and complications, 973
    diagnosis, 973–974
    gram-stained vaginal smear, 974
    management, 974
    and miscarriage, 338, 344
'Bad news', breaking
    absorbing of news, 758–759
    asking/replying honestly, 758
    being realistic, 759
    circumstances, 757
    collusion, dealing with, 758
    conspiracy of silence, 758
    definition of 'bad news', 757
    desire for information, 757
    doctor's role, 757
    following consultation, 758
    importance, 757
    nurse's role, 758
    preparation, 757
    standards of care suggested, 757
Balanitis xerotica obliterans, 603
Bariatric surgery, 243, 259
Barium enema/meal, 884
Barrier contraceptive methods, 429–430, 951
Bartholinitis, 607
Bartholin's glands
    carcinoma, 622
    vestibule, 6
Basal body temperature (BBT), 281, 429
    charts, 234
Basal cell carcinoma, 623

Basal lamina, 232
Basement membrane zone antibodies, 603
Bazedoxifene, 414
BBD *see* Benign breast disease (BBD)
Beckwith–Wiedemann's syndrome, 651
Behavioural treatment methods
    overactive bladder syndrome, 827–828
    sexual problems, 446, 756
Behçet's syndrome, 606
Belinostat, 561
Benign breast disease (BBD), 689–706
    aberrations of normal development and involution, 690–692, 691f
    accessory breast tissue and supernumerary nipples, 690
    adenoma, 701
    adenosis, 695–696
    blocked ducts, 700
    breast cancer risk, 708–709
    columnar cell lesions, 696
    complex sclerosing lesions and radial scars, 696–697
    congenital abnormalities, 689–690, 690f
    cysts, 695, 695f, 702–703
    diabetic fibrous mastopathy, 697
    duct ectasia, 693
    ductal carcinoma in situ, 694, 712–714
    ductal hyperplasia, 696
    ductal infections, 700
    epithelial hyperplasia, 696
    fat necrosis, 702
    fibroadenoma, 691–692, 691f
    fibrocystic change, 695–697, 695f
    foreign body reactions, 701
    granular cell tumour, 702
    hamartoma, 701
    hidradentitis suppurativa, 700
    HIV infections, 700
    hyperplasia, 690
    hypertrophy, physiological, 701
    intraductal papilloma and papillomatosis, 693–694, 693f
    juvenile hypertrophy, 690–691
    lipoma, 701–702
    lobular hyperplasia, 696
    lymph nodes, 702f, 703
    mastalgia, 694
    metaplasia, 696
    microdocectomy, 694
    Mondors's disease, 702
    Montgomery's glands, 702
    neoplasms, 701–702
    nipple blebs, 700
    nipple discharge, 692–694, 693f
    oil cysts, 702–703
    Phyllodes tumour, 691–692
    Poland syndrome, 690, 690f
    pregnancy and lactation
        bloody nipple discharge, 694, 697–698
        galactocele, 698
        gestational and secretory hyperplasia, 697
        gigantomastia, 698
        lactogenesis, 697
        pseudohamartoma, 698
        pseudolipoma, 698
        puerperal mastitis, 698–700
    proliferative stromal lesions, 697

pseudoangiomatous stromal hyperplasia, 697
sebaceous cysts, 703
and stages of human breast development, 689
surgical treatment, 694
total duct excision, 694
tuberculosis of breast, 701
see also Breast cancer
Benign endometrioid tumours, 674–675
Benign germ cell tumours, 673–674
Benign mucinous tumours, 674
Benign mucous membrane pemphigoid, 606
Benzodiazepines, 1006
Benzyl benzoate, 977
Bereavement, 763–764
Beta-human chorionic gonadotrophin assays, 654
beta-human chorionic gonadotrophin as tumour marker, 654–655
see also Human chorionic gonadotrophin (hCG)
Bettochhi hysteroscope, 19f, 28f
Bevacizumab (Avastin), 555–556
Bilateral gonadectomy
Bilateral groin lymph node dissection, vulval cancer, 617–619
Bilateral oophorectomy
breast cancer prevention, 712
ovarian cancer, 682
premenstrual syndrome, 400
secondary premature ovarian failure, 418
Binding assays, 138–139
Bioassays, 138
Biochemical tests
ectopic pregnancy, 368–369
pelvic inflammatory disease, 946
Biofeedback
overactive bladder syndrome, 828
pelvic floor muscle training, 802
solitary rectal ulcer syndrome, 915
vulvodynia, 606
Bioidentical hormones, therapeutic option, menopause, 409
Biopsy
bladder disorders, 871
cervical cancer, 512
colposcopic, cervical cancer, 573–574, 588
endometrial cancer, 637–638
eosinophilic cystitis, 871
image-guided *see* Image-guided biopsy
of nipple, in Paget's disease, 714
ovarian cancer, 682
sentinel lymph node, cervical cancer, 592
solitary rectal ulcer syndrome, 915
testicular, 305
vulval cancer, 615
Bipolar diathermy, 48, 49f, 50, 430
Bipolar disorder, 218
Bipolar electrosurgery, hysteroscopy, 27, 28f
Birth control *see* Contraception/contraceptive advice
Bisexual women *see* Lesbian and bisexual women
Bisphosphonates, 413–414
Black cohosh, 416

Bladder, 771
anatomy/anatomical relations, 7–8, 109, 771
bowel compared, 781
conditions of *see* Bladder disorders
damage to, 109–112
avoiding damage, 109–110
drainage, fistulae surgery, 891
dynamic imaging, 908
hydrostatic pressure at neck of, 774
innervation, 772–774
intra-abdominal pressure, transmission of, 774
neck position, 791
normal capacity, 7
overdistension of, 841
postoperative care, routine, 117–118
postoperative complications, 123
repairing, 110–112
structure, 7–8
surgical injury, 8
tension in wall of, 774
urinary incontinence, mechanism, 774
see also Urinary incontinence
vesical interior, 7, 7f
Bladder disorders, 769, 864–873
aetiology, 865
assessment
cystourethroscopy, 793–794, 868
examination, 866
history, 865–866
imaging, 867–868
microbiology, 866
urinary diary, 784–785, 866
urodynamics, 866–867
benign and malignant bladder and urethral tumours, 866
cystitis *see* Cystitis
cystourethroscopy, 793–794, 868
definitions, 864–865
examination, 866
history, 865–866
imaging, 867–868
incontinence *see* Urinary incontinence
inflammatory conditions, 866
investigations, 866–868
lower urinary tract calculi, 871
lower urinary tract tumours, 871
microbiology, 866
miscellaneous conditions, 866
neuropathy, 769
non-infective sensory disorders of lower urinary tract, 866b
non-malignant conditions affecting lower urinary tract, 866
overactive bladder *see* Overactive bladder (OAB) syndrome
painful bladder syndrome, 869–870
prevalence, 865
proliferative and metaplastic lesions, 871
swabs, 866
treatment, 868–872
urethral diverticulum, 871–872
urethral syndrome, 872
urinary diary, 866
urinary retention and overflow, 88, 769
urodynamics, 866–867
Bladder drill technique, 828

Bladder neck sling procedures, 807–809, 808f
Bladder pain syndrome, 869
Bladder retraining, 868–869
Bleeding
abnormal menstrual
antifibrinolytics, 460
endometrial ablation techniques, 463–466
hysterectomy, 466–467
hysteroscopy, 33
acute, with negative pregnancy test, 89–90
angiography, 62
diagnostic indications, 17
ectopic pregnancy, 366–367
hysteroscopy complication, 33
hysteroscopy contraindicated for, 18
hysteroscopy indication for, 20–21
with positive pregnancy test, 83
postmenopausal, 90, 637
one-stop postmenopausal bleeding clinic, 638
recurrent, 638
vascular damage, 113
see also Haemorrhage
Bleomycin, 551–552
Blepharophimosis/ptosis/epicanthus (BEPS) syndrome, 418
Blighted ovum (early embryonic demise), 84
Blood karyotyping, 343
Blood products, refusal by Jehovah's Witnesses, 94
Blood tests, urinary tract infections, 901
Blood vessels, damage to, 114–115
Blood-testis barrier, 293
BMP15 gene, premature ovarian failure, 221
BMS-214662, 561
Boari flap, 109, 111f
Body image, 751–752
Body weight/BMI
breast cancer risk, 710
closed laparoscopy technique, 40
endometrial cancer, 629–630
in menopause, 407
pelvic organ prolapse, 849
see also Obese patients
Bone marrow suppression, chemotherapy, 551–552
Bone mineral density (BMD), 408, 427
Bonney's myomectomy lamp, 483, 484f
Botanical treatment, osteoporosis, 416–417
Botulinum toxin, 827, 870, 911
Bowel
bladder compared, 781
damage to, 112
laparoscopy, 40, 114
minor lacerations, 124
postoperative complications, 124
Veress needle puncture, 124
delayed presentation of postoperative complications, 124
disorders of *see* Intestinal tract disease
faecal fistula, 125
intraoperative detection of complications, 124
large *see* Large bowel
obstruction, 124

paralytic ileus, 124
postoperative complications, 124–125
  management of, 125
prolapse causing symptoms in, 853
repairing, 112
small see Small bowel
see also Anal continence, mechanisms; Anal
    sphincter mechanism; Faecal
    incontinence; Intestinal disorders
Bowel preparation, preoperative care, 102
Bowel sounds, absence, 670
Brachytherapy, 541, 544–546
  cervical cancer, 592–594
  delivery systems, 545
  dose rates, 544
  high-dose rate, 544
  image-guided adaptive, 546, 547f
  interstitial, 545–546
  intracavitary, 545, 545f
  moderate-dose rate, 544
  pulsed-dose rate, 544
  vaginal cancer, 624
  vaginal vault, 545
Braun irrimatic pump, rectal irrigation, 912
BRCA gene mutations, 684
  breast cancer, 711–712
  cDNA arrays, 730
  chromosome 13q (BRCA2), 527
  chromosome 17q (BRCA1), 527
  fallopian tube carcinoma, 684
  familial cancers, 527
  family history, 517
  ovarian cancer, 530–531, 679, 734
  peritoneal cancer, 530
  poly (ADP-Ribose) polymerase inhibitors,
    557–558
  prophylactic mastectomy, 712
  prophylactic oophorectomy, 712
  ultrasonographic features of BRCA1
    cancers, 717
BRCAPRO, breast cancer risk, 711
Breakthrough bleeding (BTB), 426
Breast cancer, 707–749
  advanced breast biopsy instrumentation
      (ABBI), 721
  assisted reproduction treatments risks, 327
  axillary surgery, 716, 722–724, 723f–724f
  bilateral oophorectomy, 712
  BRCAPRO, 711
  breast reconstruction, 735–737, 736b
  chemoprevention, 712
  chemotherapy
    adjuvant, 728
    amenorrhoea and menopause, 733
    metastatic disease, 732
    neoadjuvant medical therapy, 728
    preventive role, 712
  Claus model, 711
  clinical follow-up, 735
  Collaborative Group on Hormonal Factors
      in Breast Cancer study, 425–426, 709
  diagnosis, 717–721
    image-guided biopsy, 721
    magnetic resonance imaging, 718–719,
      719f
    mammography, 718
    positron emission tomography, 719–721,
      720f

triple assessment, 718
  ultrasound, 718, 719f
dual tyrosine kinase inhibitors, 727
ductal carcinoma in situ, 694, 712–714
  in elderly patients, 735
  endocrine therapy, 725–728
EPIC study, 710
epidermal growth factor receptor, targeting,
    727
fertility preservation in patients, 733–734
fine needle aspiration cytology, 721
Gail model, 711
gene expression signatures see Gene
    expression signatures
genetic factors, 653
genomics and proteomics, 730
HABITS trial, 710
high-risk young women, screening, 717
HRT risks, 411
image-guided biopsy, 721
incidence and prevalence trends, 707–708
inflammatory, 714–716
invasive carcinoma, 714–716, 715f
invasive ductal carcinoma, 714
in lesbian and bisexual women, 1012
lobular in-situ neoplasia, 713–714
magnetic resonance imaging, 718–719,
    719f
malignancy types, other, 716
mammography, 718
metastasis to breast, 716
metastatic, 731–733
micrometastases, 730
multifocal, 715f
needle core biopsy, 721
neoadjuvant medical therapy, 728
Nottingham Prognostic Index, 729
online resources, 737
open surgical biopsy, 721
Paget's disease, 714
pathology, 712–716, 715f
peri- and postoperative care, 725
polycystic ovary syndrome, 258
positron emission tomography, 719–
    721, 720f
pregnancy-related, 734–735
presentation, 716–717
prognostic factors, 729–730, 729b
quantitative risk assessment, 711–712
radiotherapy/radiation therapy, 724–725
risk factors, 708–711
  age, 708
  age at first pregnancy, 708
  alcohol intake, 710
  benign breast disease, 708–709
  body weight, 710
  dietary factors, 710
  endogenous hormones, 710
  family history, 711
  geographical variation, 708
  height, 710
  hormone replacement therapy, 411,
    709–710
  ionizing radiation exposure, 709
  mammographic density, 710
  oral contraception, 709
  ovolutory cycles, 708
  physical activity, 710

previous history, 710–711
  socioeconomic status, 710
risk-reducing mastectomy, 712
screening, 712, 716–717
  lesbian and bisexual women, 1012
skin of breast, 716
SNB use, 723–724
staging investigations, 716, 721–722
surgery, 712, 722–724, 723f–724f
symptomatic disease, 717
targeted therapies, 727–728
trastuzumab, 727, 732
treatment planning and patient
    communication, 722
triple negative, 729
Tyrer-Cuzick model, 711–712
ultrasound, 718, 719f
vacuum-assisted mammotome, 721
vascular endothelial growth factor
    pathway, 728
see also Benign breast disease (BBD)
Breast Cancer Prevention Collaborative
    Group, 712
Breast development stages, 184–185, 184f,
    186f
Breast hyperplasia, 690
Breastfeeding
  chlamydia treatment, 968
  gonorrhoea treatment, 967
  mastitis, 698–700
Breasts, benign disease of see Benign breast
    disease (BBD)
Brenner tumours, 675
Brief Pain Inventory (BPI), 933
Bristol stool chart, 917f
British Society for Antimicrobial
    Chemotherapy, 101
Bromocriptine, 698
  gigantomastia, 698
  male infertility, 306
  ovulation induction, 238
  premenstrual syndrome, 397
Brompheniramine maleate, 306–307
Brostacillin, 561
Bruises, 995
'Brunn's nests', bladder lesions, 871
Bulbospongiosus, 11
Bulking agents, 809–810, 809f, 914
Bupivacaine, 935–937
Burch colposuspension, 804–805, 806f

C

C. albicans, 606, 974–975
C. difficile, 101
C. trachomatis, 353–354, 967–968
Ca², second messenger pathways, 136
CA125 serum markers
  endometriosis, 287–288, 499, 670
  novel therapies, 559
  ovarian cancer, 75, 517, 580, 682
  ovarian cysts, 670–671
  pelvic inflammatory disease, 670
Cabergoline, 238
Caesarean scar ectopic pregnancy, 376–377
CAH see Congenital adrenal hyperplasia
    (CAH)
Calcitonin, 414

Calcitriol, 414
Calcium, 395–396, 414
Calcium channel blockers, 911
Calcium-channel antagonists, 825
Calvert formula, chemotherapy, 549
Camera and stack system, hysteroscopy, 19f, 20
Cancer predisposition genes, 526
Cancers
　assisted reproduction treatments risks, 191, 327
　breast see Breast cancer
　in children, risk of, 328
　choriocarcinoma see Choriocarcinoma
　colorectal see Colorectal cancer
　combined hormonal contraceptives see under Combined hormonal contraceptives
　fibroids, malignant transformation of, 479
　fistulae, 878
　gestational trophoblastic tumours see Gestational trophoblastic tumours (GTTs)
　gynaecological see Gynaecological cancers
　hysteroscopy, 18, 33
　in newborn, risk of, 327–328
　ovulation induction, risks, 247–248
　staging investigations, breast cancer, 721–722
　testicular, 309
　vasectomy, 433
　see also Chemotherapy; Premalignant disease of genital tract; Radiotherapy; Tumours
Candidiasis, 606, 974–975, 975f
Capacitative coupling, diathermy, 51
Capecitabine, 550, 552
Capsaicin, 827
Carbaryl, 977
Carbon dioxide laser, 54–55, 55f, 577
Carboplatin chemotherapy, 549–550, 561
　vs cisplatin, 552
Carcinoembryonic antigen (CEA), 682
Carcinoma in situ (CIS), 566, 582, 694, 871
　and breast cancer, 712–714
　ductal, 694, 712–714
　trials, 713
Carcinosarcoma, 631
Cardiopulmonary disorders, hysteroscopy contraindicated for, 18
Cardiovascular complications, postoperative care, 125–126
Cardiovascular disease, 407, 433
Carneous mole, 366
Carunculae myrtiformes, hymen, 5
Catastrophic thought patterns, 931
Catecholamines, 128
Catheter-associated infection, 903–904
Catheterization
　indwelling catheters, 609, 843–844
　prolonged, following surgery, 117
　suprapubic, 9, 117–118, 843
　tubal, 355, 359
Cauda equina lesions, 779
CD4 count, HIV, 979–980, 982–983, 985
CD99, radionuclide imaging, 61
CDNA microarrays, ovarian cancer, 533
Cediranib (AZD2171), 556

Cefixime, 967
Cefotaxime, 967
Cefoxitin, 949, 967
Ceftriaxone, 965, 967
Cell adhesion molecule (CAM), 271–272
Cell surface receptors
　availability of (up- and down regulation), 131–132
　binding of hormone to, 132–133, 134f
　Class 1, 132
　G-protein coupled, 135, 136f
　second messenger pathways, 135–136
　signal transduction, 133–135
　structure/actions, 131–136, 133f
　tyrosine kinase, 135
Cellular angiofibroma, 608
Cellular leiomyoma, 476, 476f
Centers for Disease Control and Prevention (CDC), 942–943
Cephalexin, 700
Cephalosporin, 901–903, 949
Cerazette, 427
C-erbB2 (HER-2) gene
　breast cancer, 716, 727
　endometrial cancer, 647
Cerebral metastases, management, 662
Cervarix, 583
Cervical cancer, 582–598
　adverse histological prognostic factors, 589t
　aetiology, 582–583
　assessing response and recurrence, 72
　brachytherapy, 592–594
　and CIN, 512–513
　clinical examination, 584
　clinical presentation, 584
　co factors, 583
　complications in advanced disease, management, 595–596
　cytology, cervical
　　detection, 569–570, 570f
　　and HPV, 570, 583
　descriptive epidemiology, 510–511
　diagnosis, 584–586, 585f
　disseminated recurrence, 595
　distant spread, 72
　epidemiology, 582
　follow-up following treatment, 595
　histology, 587, 589t
　and HIV, 511–512, 983
　human papilloma virus, 511, 582–583
　　prevalence in lesbian and bisexual women, 1011
　　transmission between women, 1011
　　vaccines, 513–514, 583
　hysteroscopy contraindicated for, 33
　imaging, 69–72, 71f, 584, 585f
　immunodeficiency, 583
　invasive/preinvasive phases, 510
　molecular genetics, 529–530
　multidisciplinary discussion, 584
　natural history, 512–513, 583
　nodal involvement, 71–72, 71f
　oral contraception, 583
　parametrium, 70–71
　pathology review, 584
　in pregnancy, 596
　prevalence in lesbian and bisexual women, 1011

prevention and screening, 513
radiotherapy, 592–594
　adjuvant, 594
　brachytherapy, 592–594
　complications, 594
　external beam, 592
　pelvic recurrence following, 594–595
　primary, 592–594
recurrent, 594–595
risk factors, 511–512
screening of lesbian and bisexual women, 1011–1012
sentinel lymph node biopsy, 592
smoking, 583
squamous cell carcinomas, 426, 587
staging, 584–586
　surgery (Stage 1A1), 588
　surgery (Stage 1A2), 588
　surgery (Stage 1B1 and IIA), 588
　surgery (Stage 1B2), 589
　surgery (Stage 11B-IVA), 589
structure of cervical epithelium, 509–510
surgical management, 587–589, 588t
　pelvic recurrence following, 594
　Stage 1A1, 588
　Stage 1A2, 588
　Stage 1B1 and 11A, 588
surgical techniques, 589–592
teletherapy, 592
trachelectomy see Trachelectomy
treatment, see surgical management above; surgical techniques above
see also Cervical premalignancy
Cervical fibroids, 476
Cervical glandular intraepithelial neoplasia (CGIN), 566–568, 567f
Cervical incompetence, recurrent miscarriage, 344
Cervical intraepithelial neoplasia (CIN)
　and cervical cancer, 510, 512–513, 588
　high-grade, 574–575
　and HIV, 982–983
　and lesbian and bisexual women, 1011
　malignant potential of lesions, 568–575
　pathology, 567
　risk factors, 568t
　terminology, 566
　treatment, 574t
　ultraviolet lasers, 56
　see also Cervical premalignancy
Cervical pregnancy, 376
Cervical premalignancy
　ablation, 574, 574t
　aetiology, 568–569
　behavioural changes to prevent, 569
　choice of treatment, 575
　CIN see Cervical intraepithelial neoplasia (CIN)
　colposcopy see Colposcopy
　cytology, 569–570, 570f
　detection, 569–570, 570f
　excision, 574–575, 574t
　histological problems, 567
　HPV detection assay, 570, 583
　immunization to prevent, 569
　malignant potential of lesions, 568–575
　pathogenesis, 567–568, 568t
　pathology, 567

prevention, 569
results of treatment, 575
terminology, 566–567
treatment, 574–575, 574t
see also Cervical cancer
Cervical Screening Programme (NHS), 970
Cervical smear, 442
Cervical stenosis, hysteroscopy
        contraindicated for, 18
Cervical warts, 970f
Cervix
    anatomy, 3–4
    imaging, 69–70
    postmenopausal women, 50
    sagittal view, 85f
Chancroid, 965
Chemical agents, and miscarriage, 339
Chemoprevention
    breast cancer, 712
    premalignant disease of genital
        tract, 580
Chemoradiation, 592
    concomitant, 540
Chemotherapy
    adjuvant, 547–548, 554
    administration routes, 548–549
    alkylating agents, 549–550
    antimetabolites, 550–551
    bleomycin, 551
    breast cancer
        adjuvant treatment, 728
        amenorrhoea and menopause, 733
        metastatic, 732
        neoadjuvant medical therapy, 728
        in pregnancy, 734
        preventive role, 712
    Calvert formula, 549
    classification, 549–551
    combination, 728
    combination therapy principles, 549
    dose calculation, 549
    drug discovery/clinical trials, 548
    drug resistance, 549
    duration of therapy, 549
    endometrial cancer, 644–645, 645t
    gestational trophoblastic tumours
        (GTTs), 658–660
        follow-up, 663
    and hormones, 552–553
    intraperitoneal, 548–549
    lower urinary tract disorders, 871
    metronomic, 555
    and miscarriage, 339
    ovarian cancer, 684
    and ovarian reserve
    pharmacology, 548–549
    Phase I and II studies, 548, 555
    Phase III trials, 548–549
    placental-site trophoblastic tumour, 663
    platinum agents, ovarian cancer, 516,
        682–684
    secondary premature ovarian
        failure, 418
    single-agent, 549
    systemic, 548
    taxanes, 551, 560, 716
    in terminal cases, 547–548
    topoisomerase inhibitors, 551

toxic effects
    alimentary tract, 552
    allergic reactions, 552
    alopecia, 552
    bone marrow suppression, 551–552
    on heart, 552
    on kidneys, 552
    on lungs, 552
    on nervous system, 552
    on reproductive system, 552
    on skin, 552
    vinca alkaloids, 551
    vulval cancer, 621
    see also individual drugs
Cherney incision, abdominal procedures, 106
Chest X-ray, 656–657, 682
Childbirth
    maternal age at, and trachelectomy,
        591–592
    pelvic floor dysfunction, 923–924
    tearing of perineal body during, 6
Children and young people
    bladder training, 814
    cancer, talking to about, 759–760
        children aged 3-7 years, 760
        children aged 7-11 years, 760
        teenagers, 760
    consent issues, 96
    mastitis of infancy, 701
    risk of malignancy in assisted reproduction
        treatments treatment, 191
    sexual assault of adolescents, 997–998
Chlamydia, 967–968
    aetiology, 967
    alternative regimens, 968
    cell culture, 968
    chronic pelvic pain, 934
    clinical features, 967, 968f
    complications of, 967–968, 968f
    diagnosis, 968
    enzyme immunoassays, 968
    epidemiology, 956
    initiatives, 967
    management, 968
    nucleic acid amplification technique, 968
    pelvic inflammatory disease, 943f, 944
    and PID, 942–943
    in pregnancy and breast feeding, 968
    prevalence, 956
    recommended regimens, 968
Chlamydia Screening Studies (ClaSS), 951
Chlorambucil, 549
Choice of operation, 93
Cholesterol, origins and intracellular
        transport of, 145–147
Cholinergic agents, 844
Choriocarcinoma
    clinical features, 655–656
    epidemiology and aetiological factors, 653
    genetic factors, 653
    genetics and pathology, 652
    imaging of, 74–75, 74f
    infantile, 656
    see also Gestational trophoblastic tumours
        (GTTs)
Chromatography, 138
Chromogenic in-situ hybridization
        (CISH), 727

Chromosomal abnormalities
    miscarriage
        recurrent, 342–343
        sporadic, 336–337, 336t
    premature ovarian failure, 418
Chromosome 5 mutations, Lynch type 2
        syndrome, 679
Chromosome analysis, male reproductive
        disorders, 305
Chronic pelvic pain (CPP), 929–941
    adhesions, 935
    chronic pelvic inflammatory disease, 935
    definition, 930
    diagnosis and treatment
        adhesions, 935
        chronic pelvic inflammatory disease, 935
        hernias, 937
        nerve entrapment, 935–937
        neuropathic and postsurgical pelvic pain,
            937
    diagnostic overlap/lack of diagnosis,
        937–938
    endometriosis, 492, 935
    hernias, 937
    management settings and strategies,
        938–939
    nerve entrapment, 935–937
    neuropathic and postsurgical, 937
    non-cyclic, 492
    ovarian cysts, 669
    ovarian point tenderness, 933
    pelvic inflammatory disease, 950
    prevalence, 930–931
    special features, 929
    trigger point tenderness, 933
    see also Pain; Pelvic pain
Cigarette smoking
    breast infections, 700
    cervical cancer, 511, 583
    dysmenorrhoea, 457
    ectopic pregnancy, 365
    fibroids, 474
    in menopause, 407
    and miscarriage, 338–339
    and ovarian cancer, 517
    Zuska's disease (recurring subareolar
        abscess), 701
    see also Smoking cessation
Cimetidine, 869–870
Ciprofloxacin, 700, 965, 967
Circulating tumour cells (CTCs), breast
        cancer, 730
Circumcision, female, 610
Cisplatin chemotherapy, 540, 549–550, 592,
        661, 684
    intraperitoneal, 548–549
    nephrotoxicity, 552
Citalopram, 412
Civil Partnership Act 2004, access to health
        care, 1013
Clam cystoplasty, overactive bladder
        syndrome, 829
Clamps
Claus model, breast cancer risk, 711
Clean intermittent self-catheterization (CISC),
        voiding difficulties, 843–845
Clear cell adenocarcinoma, 625
Clear cell carcinoma, ovarian cancer, 681

Clear cell (mesonephroid) tumours, 675
Cleveland Clinic Incontinence Score, 907, 908t, 912
Climacteric transition/syndrome, 406
Clindamycin/clindamycin cream, 609, 700, 974
Clinical assays, hormones, 138–139
Clinical target volume (CTV), radiotherapy, 541
Clips, sterilization, 430
Clitoris
  anatomy, 6, 599
  damage to, 929
Cloacal anomalies, 193
Clobetasol, 603–604
Clomiphene citrate (CC), 236–237, 261
  adjuvant treatment, 237
  indications for treatment, 236
  mechanism of action, 236
  results of treatment, 237
  risks of treatment, 237
  side-effects of treatment, 237
  treatment regimes/monitoring, 236
Clomipramine, 445
Clonidine, 412
Cloning, reproductive/therapeutic, 163, 274–275
Cluster analysis, 158–159
Clustering, lateral migration, 132, 133f
CMF (adjuvant chemotherapy for breast cancer), 728
Coadjuvants, tubal disease, 356
Coagulation cascade, 451
Coagulation disorders, 455
Co-amoxiclav, 700
Coccygeus muscles, pelvis, 10
Cochrane Library, 1019
COCP see Combined hormonal contraceptives
Codeine, 552, 938
Coelomic epithelium, transformation in endometriosis, 489
Cognitive behavioural therapy (CBT), 395, 443, 446, 938–939
Cognitive decline, and menopause, 408, 412
Coital disorders, male infertility, 301
Colectomy, 916
Collaborative Group on Hormonal Factors in Breast Cancer study, 425–426, 709
Colles' fracture, 407–408
Colony-forming units (CFUs), UTIs, 896–897
Colorectal cancer, 410, 630
  see also Hereditary non-polyposis colorectal cancer (HNPCC)
Colostomy, 914
Colpography, fistulae, 884
Colposcopically-directed punch biopsy (CDB), 573–574
Colposcopy
  abnormalities, 571–572, 572f–573f
  biopsy, 573–574, 573f
  diagnosis, 572, 573f, 573t
  examination, 571, 571f–572f
  forensic gynaecology, 992
  of vulva, 600–601

Columnar cell lesions, in breast, 696
Combined oral contraception (COCP)
  acute myocardial infarction, 425
  benefits, 426
  breakthrough bleeding, 426
  cancers, 425–426
  contraindications, 423–424, 424b
  fibroids, 474
  human immunodeficiency syndrome, 984
  hypertension, 426
  mode of action, 423
  preoperative care, 99, 102–103
  sexual problems, 920
  side-effects, 424–426
  stroke, 425
  venous thrombosis/thromboembolism, 424–425
Common iliac artery, laparoscopic damage to, 40
Comparative genomic hybridization (CGH), 529–530, 533
Competitive protein-binding assays, 138
Complementary and alternative medicine
  mastitis, 700
  osteoporosis, 416–417
Complete androgen insensitivity syndrome (CAIS), 213–214
Complete hydatidiform mole (CM), 650–651, 651f
Complications
  hysteroscopy procedures, 31–32
    late complications, 33
  laparoscopy, 40–41, 45, 45b
  postoperative
    bowel, 124–125
    cardiovascular, 125–126
    haematoma formation, 121
    haemorrhage, 120–121
    infection and pyrexia, 121–122
    pulmonary, 125
    urinary tract injuries, 123–124
    venous thromboembolism, 122–123
  vaginoplasty, 177
  see also Surgical injury
Compression stockings, 99–100
Computer database systems, ultrasound, 81
Computerized tomography (CT scanning)
  breast cancer, 716
  cervical cancer, 70–71, 71f
  endometrial cancer, 73, 638
  endometriosis, 500
  fistulae, 884
  gestational trophoblastic tumours, 657
  and miscarriage, 343
  ovarian cancer, 75, 682
  ovarian cysts, 670
  radiotherapy planning, 541
  techniques, 60–61
  urinary tract infections, 900–901
  urogram, 789
Comu, uterus, 3
Conception, time to, 278
Condylomata accuminata see Genital warts
Conformal radiotherapy, 541–542, 542f
Congenital adrenal hyperplasia (CAH)
  3β-dehydrogenase deficiency, 171
  endocrine control of steroid synthesis, 151–152, 152f

21-hydroxylase deficiency, 170–171
11-hydroxylase deficiency, 171
  late-onset, 188
    and hirsutism, 385
  pathophysiology, 169
  precocious puberty, 188
  steroid synthesis defects, 152–153
  surgical correction, in 21-hydroxylase deficiency, 171
Congenital anomalies
  androgen insensitivity syndrome, 193
  assisted reproduction treatments risks, 327–328
  cloacal anomalies, 193
  Müllerian abnormalities, 192–193
  urogynaecological disorders, 768
Congenital hypogonadotrophic hypogonadism, 191
Conization, cervical cancer, 588
Conjugated equine oestrogen cream, 409
Consent
  additional consents, 94
  for additional procedures, 94
  case law, 96
  duration of, 94
  forensic examination, 990–991
  hysteroscopy complications, 33
  and operative risks, 94
  persons obtaining, 94
  of special groups of patients, 94–96
  valid, 93–94
Constipation
  defined, 915
  obstructive defaecation, 916
  Rome criteria, 915–916
Contact tracing, 88–89, 904, 977
Continence
  anal, mechanisms, 779–780, 779f
  bladder/bowel comparison, 781
  central nervous control, 773–774, 774f
  effect of surgery on mechanisms of, 776, 781
  urinary, 7f
  see also Faecal incontinence; Incontinence; Urinary incontinence
Contraception/contraceptive advice, 422–439
  barrier methods, 429–430, 951
  birth control methods, pregnancy rates, 424t
  cervical cancer, 583
  combined hormonal contraceptives see Combined oral contraception (COCP)
  condom use, 961
  emergency, 430, 993
  gestational trophoblastic tumours, 663–664
  and HIV, 984
  infertility, 985
  IUCDs see Intrauterine devices (IUDs)
  lactational amenorrhoea method, 429
  natural family planning, 429
  planning of pregnancy, 984–985
  premature ovarian failure, 419
  progestogen-only contraceptives, 427–428
  reproductive dysfunction, 226–227
  termination of pregnancy, 984
  see also Abortion; Sterilization
Contrast studies, 59
Copper IUDs, 428

Cornual occlusion, tubal disease, 356
Cornual polyps, removal, 356
Cornual pregnancy, 378
Coronary heart disease (CHD), 407, 411–412
Coronary vascular disease (CVD), 411
Corpora albicantes, ovary, 1
Corpora lutea, ovary, 1, 64
Corpus, uterus, 3
Corpus luteum, 345
Corpus luteum cysts, 673
Cortical granules, 268
Corticosteroids
  chronic pelvic pain, 935–937
  hirsutism, 388
  vulval conditions, 601–602
Corticotrophin-releasing hormone (CRH),
    204, 217–218
Cortisol, 131, 140–141
Cortisol replacement therapy, long-term
    (21-hydroxylase deficiency), 171
Cough stress test, pelvic organ prolapse,
    853–854
Counselling, 433
  abortion, 434
  fistulae management, 886
  miscarriage, 347
  for OHSS, 246
  referral to counselling services, 993
  sterilization, 431
CpG dinucleotides (CpGs), 525–526
CpG islands (CGIs), 525–526
Cranberries, UTI prevention, 902
CREB (cAMP response element binding
    protein), 135–136
Critical body fatness, 185
Crohn's disease, 606, 878, 910–911
Cryoablation, 29
Cryopreservation of embryo see Embryo
    cryopreservation
Cryotherapy, 604, 970–971
Cryptorchidism, 299, 309
CT2103 (paclitaxel agent), 560
C-terminal cytoplasmic domain, 131
Culdocentesis, ectopic pregnancy, 370
Cusco's speculum, hysteroscopy, 22
Cushing's disease, 455
Cyclic adenosine monophosphate, second
    messenger pathways, 135–136
Cyclophosphamide, 549, 684, 870
CYP17 enzymes, 147–148
CYP19 gene mutations, 153–154
CYP21 activity, 152f, 153
Cyproterone acetate, 260, 387–388
Cystadenomas, 674
Cystitis
  chronic, 870
  defined, 864
  differential causes, 864, 865f
  drug-induced, 870
  eosinophilic, 871
  granulomatous, 871
  interstitial, 869–870
  radiation, 870
  recurrent bacterial, 864
  see also Bladder disorders
Cystitis cystica, 871
Cystodistension, 868–869
Cystography, fistulae, 882–884

Cystometry, 786–788
  abnormal, 787–788
  cystometric trace, 788f–789f
  equipment, 786–787
  indications, 786–787
  measurements, 787
  method, 787
  normal, 787
  overactive bladder syndrome, 817–818,
      817f–819f
  pressure lines, 787f
Cystosarcoma phyllodes, 691–692
Cystoscopy
  cervical cancer, 584
  endometriosis, 500
  eosinophilic cystitis, 871
  fistulae, 884–885
  urinary tract infections, 901
Cystourethroscopy, 793–794
  bladder disorders, 868–869
  indications, 793–794
  overactive bladder (OAB) syndrome, 819
  technique, 794
  voiding difficulties, 842
Cysts
  breast, 695, 695f, 702–703
  laparoscopic procedures, 42–44
  ovarian see Ovarian cysts
  urethral, 792
Cytochrome P450 enzymes, 147–148, 149t
Cytokines and growth factors
  endometriosis, 491
  implantation, 272
  obesity, 629–630
Cytologic examination, menstrual
    abnormalities, 459
Cytology, cervical
  detection, 569–570, 570f
  and HPV, 570, 583

D

Daily Record of Severity of Problems
    (DRSP), premenstrual syndrome, 396f
Danazol, 399, 462, 503, 694, 870
Darifenacin, 824, 829
Dark ground microscopy (DGM),
    963, 963f
DAX1 gene, 167–168
Day surgery, assessing suitability for, 97
Deep vein thrombosis (DVT), 99, 122
Defaecation cycle, 778–779, 778f
Dehydroepiandrosterone, osteoporosis, 417
3β-dehydrogenase deficiency, congenital
    adrenal hyperplasia (CAH), 171
Delayed ejaculation, 445
Delayed puberty, 189–191
  congenital hypogonadotrophic
      hypogonadism, 191
  constitutional delay of growth and
      puberty, 189–190
  and fertility, 191
  idiopathic, 219
  management of, 191
  polyglandular autoimmune
      syndromes, 191
  premature ovarian failure, causes,
      190–191

  and pubertal development, 191
  Turner's syndrome, 190
  see also Amenorrhoea
Delorme's procedure, faecal incontinence,
    915
Dementia, 408, 412
Deoxycorticosterone (DOC), 153
Deoxycorticosterone acetate (DOCA), 171
Depilatory creams, hirsutism, 386–387
Depolarization, diathermy, 48
Depo-provera, 427
Depot medroxyprogesterone acetate (DMPA),
    427
Depression, pelvic pain, 931
Dermatitis artefacta, 606
Dermoid cysts, 673–674
Dermovate, 601–602
Desipramine, 306–307
20, 22 desmolase deficiency, 173
17, 20 desmolase deficiency, 173
Desmopressin, 825–826
Desogestrel (Marvelon), 388
Desvenlafaxine, 412
Detrusor instability, 813
Detrusor muscle, bladder, 771
Detrusor myectomy, overactive bladder
    syndrome, 829
Detrusor overactivity, overactive bladder,
    813–815
Detrusor-stimulating drugs, 844
DHEA, congenital adrenal hyperplasia,
    152–153
DHT (5α-dihydrotestosterone), 152–153, 169
Diabetes, 606, 840
Diabetic fibrous mastopathy, 697
Diacylglycerol, second messenger pathways,
    136
Diagnostic catetory, unexplained infertility,
    289
Dianette, 260, 387–388
Diarrhoea, 552
Diathermy
  bipolar, 48, 49f, 50
  capacitative coupling, 51
  conclusions, 58
  current, 48–49
  current flow to adjacent organs, 51
  cutting and coagulation, 49, 49f
  damage, 115
  direct coupling, 51
  disposable and reusable instruments, 51
  duration of application, 50
  electrosurgical equipment set-up, 52
  electrosurgical unit, 51
    changes to, 51–52
  factors influencing effect of, 48–50
  fire/explosion risk, 52
  heat and tissue injury, 50
  insulation failure, 50–51
  joint prostheses, 52
  keloid scarring, 52
  laparoscopic ovarian, 263t
  monopolar, 48, 49f
    avoiding in pacemaker users, 52
  neuromodulators, 52
  and pacemakers, 52
  safety factors, 50–52
  short-wave, 50

size and shape of electrode, 50
surgical clothing, 51
tissue effects, 48, 49f
tissue type, 50
use of, 48–52
see also Lasers
Dicer enzyme, ovarian cancer, 163
Dietary factors
  bladder disorders, 869
  breast cancer risk, 710
  constipation, 915
  fistulae, 886
  haemorrhoids, 910
  irritable bowel syndrome, 916–917
  osteoporosis, 414–415
  polycystic ovary syndrome, 258–259
  premenstrual syndrome, 395
Dietary fibre, 415
Diethylstilboestrol exposure
  ectopic pregnancy, 365
  uterus, malformations of, 179
  vaginal cancer, 519
Digitally reconstructed radiograph (DRR),
    virtual simulation, 542
Dihydropyrimidine dehydrogenase (DPD),
    550–551
Dihydrotestosterone (DHT), 152–153, 169
Dihydroxyphenylalanine (DOPA), 201
Dilation and curettage (D&C), 436, 637–638,
    651–652
Diltiazem ointment, 911
Dimethyl sulfoxide, 869–870
Direct coupling, diathermy, 51
Disability, sexual assault, 998
Disseminated tumour cells (DTCs), breast
    cancer, 730
Distension medium, 20, 32, 50
DMSA nuceotide, nuclear medicine scanning,
    901
DNA (deoxyribosenucleic acid)
  binding dyes, 160
  gynaecological cancers, 525–528,
    525f, 535
  methylation, 534
  topoisomarase inhibitors, 551
Docetaxel, 551
Doctor-patient relationship, 1013
Doderlein's bacillus, 5
Domestic violence, 1002
  see also Violence against women
Dong quai, 416
Donovanosis, 965–966, 966f
Dopamine, 130–131, 201–202, 203f
Dopamine agonists, 238–239
Doppler ultrasound
  chronic pelvic pain, 934
  colour scanning, 60, 67
  continuous wave Doppler, 60
  ectopic pregnancy, 369
  endometrial cancer, 72
  gestational trophoblastic tumours (GTTs),
    656–657
  and miscarriage, 345
  operation of, 60
  ovarian varices, 64–65
  pelvic inflammatory disease, 947f
  postnatal assessment, 85–86
  pulsed Doppler, 60

three-dimensional power, 72
  venous thrombosis, 67
Double strand break (DSB), 527
Downregulation, 200
Down's syndrome, 405, 418
Doxorubicin, 551–552, 870
Doxycycline, 949, 965, 968
Drains, 106–107, 118
Drisperonone, 388
Drosha enzyme, 162–163
Drospirenone, 423
Drug resistance, chemotherapy, 549
Drug sensitivity, gene expression signatures as
    predictors of, 731
Drug treatments
  antiobesity drugs, 259
  dopamine agonists, 238–239
  premenstrual syndrome, 397–400
  preoperative care
    additional medications prior to
      gynaecological surgery, 102
    pre-existing medications, 102–103
  progestogens *see* Progestogens
  sexual problems, 446
  stimulatory drugs, 245
Drug-induced cystitis, 870
Drug-induced sexual differentiation disorders,
    172
Drugs, non-prescription *see* Substance abuse
Duct ectasia, 693
Duct of Gartner, 2
Ductal carcinoma in situ (DCIS), 700, 713,
    717
Ductal hyperplasia, 696
Ductoscopy, nipple discharge, 692
Duloxetine, 803
Dydrogesterone, 502
Dye hydrotubation, 283–285
Dye studies, fistulae, 882
Dynamic imaging, intestinal tract disease,
    908–909
Dynamic Spectral Imaging System, 573f
Dysfunctional uterine bleeding (DUB),
    453–454
Dysmenorrhoea
  chronic pelvic pain, 930
  endometriosis, 491–492
  magnetic resonance imaging, 65
  puberty/menstrual disorders, 194,
    455–456, 467
Dyspareunia
  chronic pelvic pain, 930
  endometriosis, 492
  lateral fusion disorders, 175
  sexual problems, 444, 920, 923–924
  vaginal dryness, 926
  vaginismus, 442
  vaginoplasty, 177
Dysplasia, 871
Dyssynergic detrusor dysfunction, 768, 813
Dysuria, 864

E

E. coli
  antibiotic prophylaxis, 100
  salpingitis, 353–354
  UTIs, 897, 901

E. vermicularis, 608
Early Breast Cancer Trialists' Collaborative
    Group (EBCTCG), 724–726
Ectopic pregnancy, 363–381
  abdominal pain, 366
  acute presentation, 367
  aetiology and risk factors, 363–365
  amenorrhoea, 366–367
  ampullary implantation, 366
  anti-D immunoglobulin use, 376
  and assisted conception, 365
  assisted reproduction treatments, 365
  assisted reproduction treatments risks,
    325–326
  biochemical tests, 368–369
  controlled expectant management,
    375–376
  cornual, 85f, 378
  culdocentesis, 370
  definitions, 363
  diagnosis, 366–368, 367t
  diethylstilboestrol exposure, 365
  differential diagnosis, 370
  fimbrial evacuation, 373
  β-hCG (biochemical test)
    quantitation of subunit, 368
    serial measurements, 368
    single measurement, 368
  heterotopic pregnancy, 378–379
  histological changes, 366
  imaging of, 67, 67f
  incidence, 363
  interstitial implantation, 366
  intrauterine device users, current,
    364–365
  investigations
    biochemical tests, 368–369
    ultrasonography, 369–370
  isthmic implantation, 366
  and laparoscopic surgery, 360
  laparoscopy, 370–371
    history, 36
    vs methotrexate, 375
  linear salpingotomy, 372–373
  medical treatment (methotrexate)
    see under Methotrexate
  non-tubal pregnancies
    abdominal, 377
    caesarean scar, 376–377
    cervical, 376
    interstitial, 378
    intraligamentous, 378
    ovarian, 377
  pathology, 365–366
  pelvic inflammatory disease, 364
  physical examination, 367
  pregnancy of unknown location, 85, 86f,
    370, 371f–372f
  presentation, 367–368
  progesterone, serum, 368
  protein and steroid markers, 369
  salpingectomy, 371–372
  salpingitis isthmica nodosa, 365
  segmental resection, 373
  sites, 365, 365t
  smoking, 365
  sterilization, 432
  subacute presentation, 367–368

surgical treatment, 370–376
  reproductive outcome, 373
symptoms and signs, 366–367, 367t
and termination of pregnancy, 365
tubal pregnancy
  image of, 85f
  natural progression, 365–366
  previous, 364
  time of rupture at various sites, 366
tubal surgery, previous, 364
ultrasonography, 369–370
ultrasound, 84–85, 369–370
Edward's syndrome, and partial hydatidiform
      mole, 651
Efavirenz, 984
Eflornithine, 259
Ejaculatory duct obstruction, male infertility,
      307
Ejaculatory failure, treatment, 306–307
Elastography ultrasound, 718
Elderly patients, breast cancer in, 735
Electrocautery, 48, 105–106, 430, 970
Electrolysis, 387
Electrolyte imbalance, 117
Electromagnetic radiation, 539
Electromyography, 794, 842
Electrons, 539
Electrophysiological tests, 794
Electrosurgical unit, 51–52
Embolization
  angiographic, 81
  chronic pelvic pain, 936f
  haemorrhage, 69
  see also Uterine artery embolization
Embryo cryopreservation, 324–325, 328,
      733–734
Embryo transfer, assisted reproduction
      treatments, 320–321, 324
Embryological development of reproductive
      system
  gonadal, genetic control, 167–168, 168f
  normal, 166–168, 167f
  ovary, 166
  sex chromosome anomalies, 168, 168b
  testis, 166
Embryonic aneuploidy and preimplantation
      genetic screening, 273
Embryonic development, 268–270
Embryonic genome activation (EGA), 270
Emergency contraception, 430
Emergency Gynaecological Unit (EGU),
      80–82, 90
Emollients, 602–604
Encephalins, 828
Endocervix, 4
Endocrine control, 150–152
Endocrine disorders
  anovoluation/amenorrhoea, 214–215, 223
  recurrent miscarriage, 344–345
Endocrine profile, polycystic ovary syndrome,
      253–254
Endocrine tests, hirsutism, 384–386
Endocrine therapy
  breast cancer, 725–727
  male infertility, 306
Endogenous infections, prevention, 952
Endogenous opioids, and GnRH secretion,
      203–204

Endometrial ablation techniques
  abnormal menstrual bleeding, 463–466
  menorrhagia, 93
Endometrial cancer, 514–516, 629–649
  adenoacanthoma, 632, 633f
  adenosquamous carcinoma, 632–633
  advanced disease, 640
  ASTEC trial, 641
  biopsy, 637–638
  chemotherapy, 644–645, 645t
  classification of endometrial carcinomas,
      632t
  clinical examination, 637
  diagnosis
    investigations, 637–638
    presenting symptoms, 636–637
  early-stage, surgery for, 638–639
  endometrial hyperplasia, 635
  endometrioid adenocarcinoma, 632
  epidemiology, 629–630
  FIGO staging, 631–632, 635–636, 658–659
  follow-up, 647
  future trends, 647
  genetic factors, 679
  hereditary non-polyposis colorectal cancer,
      630
  histopathological reporting, 633–634
  histopathology, 631–632, 632t
  hormonal therapy, 645
  hormones, 630
  HRT risks, 411
  hysteroscopy, 23, 33, 638
  imaging techniques, 72–74, 72f–73f
  immunohistochemical markers, useful,
      634–635
  laparoscopic surgery, 639
  lymphadenectomy, role of, 639
  mixed, 633, 634f
  molecular genetics, 534
  non-surgical treatment, 640–645
  obese patients, 515, 629–630
  obesity, 629–630
  one-stop postmenopausal bleeding clinic,
      638
  papillary serous/clear cell adenocarcinomas,
      633, 634f
  pathology, 630–635, 631f–633f, 632t
  polycystic ovary syndrome, 257
  in postmenopausal patient, 637–638
  in premenopausal patient, 637
  preoperative evaluation, 638
  prevalence, 629
  primary tumour, imaging, 72–74, 72f–73f
  prognosis, 629, 646
  radiotherapy, 640–644, 640t, 642f–644f
  recurrent disease, 74, 644
  sarcomas, 633–634, 634f, 645–646
  screening for, 638
  spread of disease, 635
  stages IA and 1B, grade 3 or high-risk
      histology, 640–641
  stages IA and 1B, grades I and II, 640
  stages IC, IIA and IIB, 641–642
  stages IIIA, IIIB and IIIC, 642
  stage IVA, 642
  stage IVB, 642
  surgical treatment, 638–640
  survival rates, 629

symptoms presented, 636–637
tamoxifen, 630
targeted therapies, 646–647
and thecomas
  treatment, 638–645
  ultrasound, 72f
  uterine sarcomas, 645–646
Endometrial destruction, hysteroscopy, 27–28
Endometrial hyperplasia, 25f, 635
  atypical, 577–579
  clinical presentation, 578
  granulosa cell tumours
  investigation, 579
  management of, 579
  non-atypical (simple or complex), 579
  polycystic ovary syndrome, 257–258
Endometrial intraepithelial carcinoma (EIC),
      577
Endometrial premalignancy
  aetiology and molecular pathology, 578
  endometrial hyperplasia see Endometrial
      hyperplasia
  histopathology, 578
  screening for, 578
  terminology, 577–578
Endometrial repair, 452–453
Endometrial resection, 27f, 463, 466
Endometrial sampling, 23
  menstrual abnormalities, 459
Endometrial thickness, assisted reproduction
      treatments, 324
Endometrioid adenocarcinoma, 632
Endometrioid carcinoma, 632f
  ovarian cancer, 678, 681
Endometrioid tumours, clear cell carcinoma
      association, 681
Endometrioma, 87, 497, 497f–498f, 505
Endometriosis, 488–508
  Additive Diameter of Implants score, 500
  analgesia, 501
  aromatase inhibitors, 504
  assisted reproduction treatments, 313
  and benign endometrioid tumours,
      674–675
  black lesions, morphology, 495, 495f
  CA125 serum markers, 499, 670
  café-au-lait spots, 496
  classification systems, 500
  clear cell carcinoma association, 681
  clinical examination, 494–495
  coelomic epithelium, transformation in,
      489
  computerized tomography, 500
  correlation of symptoms and severity of,
      492–493, 493t
  cystoscopy, 500
  cytokines and growth factors, 491
  danazol, 503
  definitions, 488
  as disease of theories, 489
  dysmenorrhoea, 455, 491–492
  dyspareunia, 492
  endometrial disease theory, 490
  and endometrioid carcinoma, 681
  entrapelvic, 497–499
  gastrointestinal tract, 498
  genetic and immunological factors,
      489–490

gestagen/antigestagen, 501–502
gestrinone, 503–504
gonadotrophin-releasing hormone agonists, 502–503
Halban's theory, 490
hysterectomy, 505
iatrogenic dissemination, 490
imaging, 499–500, 499f
imaging of, 66, 66f
and infertility, 493–494, 493t
laparoscopic uterosacral nerve ablation, 504–505
levonorgestrel intrauterine system, 502
macrophages, peritoneal, 490–491
magnetic resonance imaging, 66, 500
markers, diagnostic, 499
menstrual problems, 492
menstrual regurgitation and implantation, 489
metastatic theory, 489
molecular biology, application to, 163
monocyte chemotactic protein-1, 499
new therapies, 504
non-invasive diagnostic methods, 499
oophrectomy, 505
oral contraception, 502
origin of pain, 492
ovarian, 496–497, 497f–498f
and ovarian cancer, 678
pathogenesis, 489–490, 490f
pelvic, 495–496
pelvic pain, 87, 935
peritoneal, 489
peritoneal fluid environment, 490–491
presentation, 491–493, 492t–493t
prevalence, 488–489
prostaglandin synthetase inhibitors, 501
prostaglandins, 491
prostanoids, 491
pulmonary and thoracic, 499
recurrent, 505–506
red lesions, 495–496, 495f–496f
subovarian adhesions, 496
subtle appearances, classification and morphology, 495–496, 495f–496f
superficial, 496, 497f
surgical scars, involvement in, 498
surgical treatment, 504–505
symptomatic pointers, 492t, 494, 494b
treatment
    general principles, 500–501
    medical, 501–504
    surgical, 504–505
tubal damage, 354
tubal factor infertility, 287–288
ultrasound, 499–500, 499f
urinary tract, 497–498
vaginal, 498–499
vascular and lymphatic metastasis, 490
vascular damage, 113
white lesions, 496, 496f
Endometrium, 4, 448–449
cystic glandular hyperplasia of, 454
trancervical resection, 26–27
Endorphins, 203–204
Endoscopy
fistulae, 884–885, 885f
hysterectomy, 467

Endothelins, idiopathic (primary) dysmenorrhoea, 455
Entrapelvic endometriosis, 497–499
Entry inhibitors, 979–980
Enzastaurin, 559
Enzyme deficiencies, in POF, 418
Enzyme immunoassays, chlamydia, 968
Enzyme-labelled immunosorbent assay, 139
Enzymoimmunoassay, 139
Enzymoimmunometric assay, 139
Eosinophilic cystitis, 871
Ephedrine, 306–307
Epidermal growth factor (EGF), 452, 531
Epidermal growth factor receptor (EFFR), 556–557, 727
Epilepsy, 218
Epinephrine, 484
Epispadias, 769
Epithelial hyperplasia, 696
Epithelial ovarian cancer (EOC), 555
Epithelium, 5, 8, 452
Epitheloid trophoblastic tumours (ETTs), 652, 656
Epoophoron, ovarian anatomy, 2
Epothilones, 560
Epstein-Barr virus, 601, 691
Erectile dysfunction, 444–445
    treatment of erectile failure, 306
Ergometrine, 341
Erlotinib (Tarceva), 557
Erythromycin, 965, 968
Essure system, hysteroscopic sterilization, 31, 31f, 431
Ethamsylate, 460
Ethinyl oestradiol, 409
Ethnic factors
    accessory breast tissue and supernumerary nipples, 690
    cancers, 509–511
    fibroadenomas, 691
    hydatidiform mole, 652
    inflammatory breast cancer, 714
    menopause, 405, 407
    ovarian cancer, 678
    pelvic organ prolapse, 849
    phyllodes tumour of breast, 691–692
    pubertal development, 184–185
Etidronate, 413
Etoposide, 551, 660–661
Euprolactinaemia, 238
Evening primrose oil (RPO), 396, 416, 694
Evidence-based medicine (EBM), 1017–1024
    2 x 2 table, 1022t
    appraising diagnostic article, 1021
    appraising systematic reviews/meta-analysis, 1021–1022, 1022t
    benefit and harm, balance between, 1023
    definition, 1017
    five 'As', 1018f
    forest plot, example, 1023f
    formulation of structured question, 1017, 1018t
    fundamental elements, 1017, 1018f
    generalizability of results, 1023
    interpretation of findings, 1022–1024
    likelihood ratios, 1022t
    literature evaluation, 1020–1022
    PICOD, 1017, 1018t

Pubmed 'clinical queries', 1020
Pubmed 'related articles', 1020
Pubmed 'SLIM', 1020
randomized controlled trials, 1020, 1021t
search of literature, 1017–1020
sources of evidence, 1019t
sources of guidelines and evidence summaries, 1019t
thoughts of patient, 1023–1024
urethral sphincter incompetence, 803–804
Excimer lasers, 56
Excision
    cervical premalignancy, 574–575, 574t
    total duct, in nipple discharge, 694
Excretion urography, fistulae, 882
Exemethstane, 726
Exercise see Physical activity
Expert witnesses, sexual assault, 999–1000
External beam radiotherapy see Teletherapy (external beam radiotherapy)
External iliac artery and branches, pelvis, 11–12
External sphincter, 8–9
Extracellular matrix (ECM), 452–453
Extracellular matrix protein 1 (ECM1), 603
Eyes, laser hazards, 57

F

Factor VII deficiency, 455
Faecal fistula, 125
Faecal incontinence, 911–915
    Altemeier operation, 915
    assessment, 911–912
    Cleveland Clinic Incontinence Score, 907, 908t, 912
    defaecation cycle, 778–779, 778f
    definitions, 776
    Delorme's procedure, 915
    graciloplasty and artificial bowel sphincter, 913–914
    initial management, 912
    injectable bulking agents, 914
    mechanism of anal continence, 779–780, 779f
    neurogenic cause, 781
    NICE guidelines, 911
    pathophysiology, 780–781
    pelvic organ prolapse, 853
    prevalence, 776
    rectal prolapse surgery, 914–915
    rectopexy, 914–915
    sacral nerve stimulation, 912–913
    stoma, 914
    urge incontinence, 912
    Vaizey score, 907
    Wexner score, 776, 778t
    see also Anal sphincter mechanisms; Intestinal tract disease; Urinary incontinence
Fallopian tubes
    anatomy/anatomical relations, 3
    blocked, 285f
    blood supply, 3
    cancer, 535
    carcinoma of, 535, 684–686
    imaging of, 63–64
    reproductive roles, 353

structure, 3
tubal disease *see* Tubal disease
Falope ring, female sterilization, 430
Famciclovir, 960–961
Familial adenomatous polyposis (FAP), 526
Family history *see* Genetic factors
Family planning *see* Contraception/
    contraceptive advice
Farnesyl transferase inhibitors, 561
Fascial ligaments, pelvis, 10
Faslodex (Fulvestrant/ICI 182,780), breast
    cancer, 726
Fat necrosis, breast, 702
[18]FDG, positron-emitting tracer, 62
FDG-PET/FDG-PET/CT scanning, breast
    cancer, 720–721
Feeding, postoperative, 119–120
Female circumcision, 610, 876–877
Female genital tract
    congenital anomalies, 191–193, 266
      androgen insensitivity syndrome, 193
      cloacal anomalies, 193
      Müllerian duct abnormalities, 174, 192
      Müllerian/uterine anomalies, 192–193
      vagina, 192
    transport of gametes in, 266
Female pseudohermaphroditism, steroid
    synthesis defects, 152
Female reproductive disorders, 278–291
    appropriate initial investigations, 280t, 281
    assisted conception, 289
    diagnostic categories, 279
    epidemiology, 278–279
    history, 280
    infertility *see* Infertility
    initial assessment, 279–280
    integrated care, 280
    ovulation *see* Ovulation disorders
    prevalence, 278–279
    tubal factor infertility *see* Tubal factor
      infertility
    unexplained infertility, 288–289
    when to refer, 279–280
    see also Male reproductive disorders;
      Reproductive dysfunction
Female sexual dysfunction (FSD), 919–920
    definition, 920b
    management, 924
    and menopause, 407
    treatment, 925
Femoral nerve, 14
Fenamates, prostaglandin synthetase
    inhibitors, 460
Fenfluramine, 870
Fentanyl, 81
Fertility issues
    delayed puberty, 191
    molecular biology, application to, 163
    ovarian cancer treatment, 683
    premature ovarian failure, 419
    preservation of fertility in breast cancer,
      733–734
    reproductive dysfunction, 226
    see also Contraception/contraceptive advice
Fertilization
    adhesion molecules and mucins, 271–272
    capacitation, 266
    clinical and scientific correlates, 273

commencement, 266–267
cumulus penetration, 267
cytokines and growth factors, implantation,
    272
description, 265
egg activation, 268
embryo-endometrial synchronization, 273
embryonic aneuploidy and preimplantation
    genetic screening, 273
formation of pronuclei and syngamy, 268
implantation, 270–273
matrix metalloproteinases and
    prostaglandins, 272
maturation, 266
molecular cross-talk during implantation,
    271
morphologic changes and window of
    implantation, 270–271
preimplantation, 268–270
prelude to, 265–266
sperm-egg binding and fusion, 268
sperm-zona interaction, 267–268
stem cell technology, 273–275
see also Assisted reproduction treatments
Fertiloscopy, 355
Fesoterodine, 824
Fetus, 142–143
Fibre, dietary, 415
Fibrin formation, 451
Fibroadenolipoma, 701
Fibroadenoma of breast, 691–692, 691f
Fibroblast growth factor (FGF), 452
Fibroblast growth factor receptor 1 (FGFR1),
    215–216
Fibrocystic change in breast, 695–697, 695f
Fibroids, 473–487
    abnormal bleeding/menorrhagia, 477–478,
      478f
    aetiology, 473–474
    antiprogesterone treatment, 481–482
    assisted reproduction treatments, 313–314
    cervical, 476
    clinical classification, 475–477
    clinical presentation, 477–479
    common nature of in women, 473
    cytogenetic changes, 473–474
    degeneration, 88
    epidemiology, 474
    hysteroscopic resection, 483–484
    hysteroscopy techniques, 28
    incidence, 473–474
    infertility/miscarriage, 478–479
    intramural, 475
    investigations, 479–480
    laparoscopic myomectomy, 484
    laparoscopic procedures, 42–44
    macroscopic appearance, 474–475
    malignant transformation in, evidence
      issues, 479
    menorrhagia, treatment, 481
    microscopic appearance, 476–477,
      476f–477f
    myometomy, abdominal, 482–483
    and ovarian cysts, 669
    pelvic pain and pressure symptoms, 478
    pregnancy complications, 479
    pseudocapsule/false capsule, 475
    recurrent, following surgery, 485

reproductive outcomes, 478–479
submucosal, 475, 483–484
subserosal, 475
surgical injury, 7
treatment
    aromatase inhibitors, 481
    expectant management, 480
    future directions, 486
    gonadotropin-releasing hormone
      analogues, 481
    medical management, 480–486
    menorrhagia associated with fibroids,
      481
tubal factor infertility, 288
uterine artery embolization, 485–486
vascular supply, 476
Fibromas, 608, 676
Fibroplant (IUD), 428
Fibrosis, 701
Filshie clip (sterilization), 430
Fimbriae, fallopian tubes, 3
Fimbrial evacuation, ectopic pregnancy, 373
Finasteride, 388
Fine needle aspiration cytology (FNAC), 71,
    721
Fish oil, 694
Fissurectomy, anal fissures, 911
Fistulae
    abdominal procedures, 890
    aetiology and epidemiology, 874–878,
      875t, 876f, 878t, 879f
    anaesthesia, examination under, 884, 884f
    antimicrobial therapy, 886
    barium enema/meal, 884
    bladder, 8
    bladder drainage, 891
    bowel management, 891
    bowel preparation, 886
    cervical cancer, 596
    classification, 880–881, 881f
    colpography, 884
    computerized tomography, 884
    congenital, 874
    counselling, 886
    cystography, 882–884
    cystoscopy, 884–885
    definitions, 874
    dissection, 887–889
    endoscopy, 884–885, 885f
    excretion urography, 882
    faecal, 125
    fistulography, 884
    fluid balance, 891
    genital, 877
    hysterosalpingography, 884
    imaging, 882–884
    immediate management, 885–886
    inflammatory bowel disease, 878
    interposition grafting, 890–891
    intestinal, 882
    investigations, 882
    magnetic resonance imaging, 884
    malignancy, 878
    management, 885–891
    miscellaneous causes, 878
    nutrition, 886
    obstetric, 874–877, 885–886, 892–893
    obstructed labour, 876f

palliation and skin care, 886
physiotherapy, 886
postfistula stress incontinence, 892
postoperative management, 891
presentation, 881–882, 883f
prevalence, 879–880
prevention, 893–894
proctoscopy, 885
prognosis, 891–893
radiation as cause of, 878
results of treatment, 891–892
retrograde pyelography, 882
risk factors, 880t
saucerization, 889–890
sigmoidoscopy, 885
subsequent management, 891
subsequent pregnancy, 892–893
surgical, 877–878, 877f, 880t, 886–887
surgical treatment
    abdominal procedures, 890
    dissection, 887–889, 888f–889f
    general principles, 886–889
    instruments, 887, 887f
    interposition grafting, 890–891
    outcome, 892t
    repair in layers, 889
    route of repair, 887, 887t
    saucerization, 889–890
    suture materials, 889
    testing repair, 889
    timing of repair, 886–887
    transperitoneal repair, 890
    transvesical repair, 890
    vaginal procedures, 889–890
suture materials, 889
transperitoneal repair, 890
transvesical repair, 890
ultrasound, 884
ureteric, 881–882
ureterovaginal, 885
urethrovaginal, 881
urogenital, 879f
vaginal procedures, 889–890
Fistulography, fistulae, 884
Fitz–Hugh–Curtis syndrome, 354, 354f,
    967–968
5-fluorouracil (5-FU), 550–551, 555–556,
    970–971
Flavonoids, 415
Flow cytometry, 651
Flucloxacillin, 607, 700
Fluconazole, 606, 975
Fluid retention, premenstrual syndrome, 394
Fluids and electrolyte management,
    postoperative care, 116–117
Fluorescence in-situ hybridization (FISH),
    727
18f-fluorodeoxyglucose (FDG), 718
Fluoroquinolones, 901–903
Fluoxetine, 412, 870
Flutamide, 388
Folinic acid rescue, methotrexate, 374, 550
Follicle aspiration equipment, 319f
Follicle-stimulating hormone (FSH),
    139, 140f, 197
    and amenorrhoea
        endocrine control of steroid synthesis, 150
        follicular development, 231–232

gonadotrophins, 240
male reproductive disorders, 294
ovarian function and menopause, 406
ovarian reserve, assessment, 314
paracrine and autocrine control, 205f
peptide hormones, 128
receptor gene polymorphism, in POF, 418
recombinant, 240
threshold/window, 232f
urinary, 240
Follicular development
    failure of, 454
    monitoring, 318
    and ovulation induction, 231–232
Folliculogenesis, normal, 316
Follistatin, 205
Footwear, operating theatre, 51
Foreign bodies, 18, 701
Forensic gynaecology, 988–1001
    colposcopic examination, 992
    communication with forensic science
        laboratory, 993
    consenting to medical/forensic
        examination, 990
    court proceedings
        cross-examination, 999
        doctor in court, 999
        examination-in-chief, 999
        expert witness statement, 999–1000
        expert witnesses in sexual assault, 999
        pretrial conference, 999
        re-examination, 999
        victim in court, 998
    documentation, 991–994
    emergency contraception, 993
    examining doctor, 991
    HIV testing and hepatitis screening,
        993–994
    injuries
        clinical injury extent scoring, 994
        genital, 994
        non-genital, 994, 996
        patterns of, 997–998
        photographs, 993
    interpretation of findings, 996
    medical witness statement, 996
    odontological examination, 994
    persons undertaking examination, 990
    photographs of injuries, 993
    police officer, role, 991
    postexamination arrangements, 993
    record of forensic examination, 991–994
        account of event, 992
        colposcopic examination, 992
        consent, 991
        emergency contraception, 993
        forensic sampling, 992–993
        general medical examination, 992
        genital examination, 992
        HIV testing and hepatitis screening,
            993–994
        medical details, 991–992
        postexamination arrangements, 993
        referral to counselling services, 993
        severely injured patient, 992
        sexually transmitted infections, 993
    re-examination, 993
    references, relevant, 997

referral to counselling services, 993
sampling, 992–993
sexual assault see Sexual assault
sexually transmitted infections, 993
statement preparation, 996–997
Forest plot, example, 1023f
46XX embryo
    complete hydatidiform mole, 650–651
    sex reversal, 172–173
46XY embryo, 166
46XY sexual development disorders, 172–174
    3β-hydrosteroid dehyogenase deficiency,
        173
    17, 20 desmolase deficiency, 173
    17-ketosteroid reductase deficiency, 173
    20, 22 desmolase deficiency, 173
    46XX sex reversal, 172–173
    46XY true hermaphroditism, 172
    androgen insensitivity at target site,
        173–174, 173t
    errors in testosterone biosynthesis, 173
    failure of testicular development, 172
    17α-hydroxylase deficiency, 173
    Leydig cell hypoplasia, 172
    partial gonadal dysgenesis, 172
    true gonadal dysgenesis, 172
Fourchette, labia minora, 6
Fractionation, radiation dose and scheduling,
    540–541
Fracture, 996
Fragile histidine triad (FHIT), 583
Fragile X gene, 283, 418
FRAX algorithms, osteoporosis, 408
Free fluid ablation, hysteroscopy, 30, 30f
FTZ1 gene, 167
Functional electrical stimulation, stress
    incontinence, 803
Functional foods, osteoporosis, 415
Fundocervical contractions, 453
Fundus, uterus, 3
Fungal infections
    chemotherapy, 551–552
    vulva, 606

G

GABAergic system, premenstrual syndrome,
    394, 395t
Gabapentin, 412, 606, 938
Gadopenate dimeglumine, contrast
    enhancement with, 718
Gail model, breast cancer risk, 711
Galactocele, benign breast disease, 698, 699f
Galactorrhoea, 693
Galactosaemia, 418
Gallbladder disease, HRT risks, 411
Gametes, transport of, 266
Gametogenesis, sexual dimorphism in,
    265–266
Gamma-rays, 539
Gangrene of skin, 607
Gardasil, 583
Gas chromatography, 138
Gastrointestinal tract endometriosis, 498
Gefitinib, 557
Gemcitabine, chemotherapy, 550–551, 661
Gender factors, pain perception, 930
Gender identity, 440–441

Gender Recognition Act 2004, 440–441
Gene cloning, 163, 274–275
Gene expression signatures, 730–731
  invasiveness gene signature, 731
  oncotype DX, 731
  as predictors of drug sensitivity, 731
  as predictors of recurrence, 730–731
  70-gene prognostic signature, 730–731
  76-gene prognostic signature, 731
  wound response signature, 731
  see also Breast cancer
Gene therapy, gynaecological cancers,
    535–536
General Medical Council (GMC), 990
Genetic factors
  assisted reproduction treatments, 329
  benign breast disease (BBD), 689–690,
    690f
  breast cancer risk, 711
  endometriosis, 489–490
  fibroids, 473–474
  gestational trophoblastic tumours, 650–653
  gonadal development, 167–168, 168f
  hereditary non-polyposis colorectal cancer,
    630
  human papilloma virus, 582
  incontinence, 769
  male infertility, 299
  miscarriage, recurrent, 342–343
  and molecular biology, in gynaecological
    cancers, 522–538
  ovarian cancer see under Ovarian cancer
  pain susceptibility, 930
  preimplantation, 269–270
Genetic screening, and preimplantation, 273
Genital arousal disorder, 920
Genital cancers, assisted reproduction
    treatments risks, 327
Genital examination, forensic
    examination, 992
Genital herpes, 958–961
  aetiology, 958–959
  clinical features, 959, 959f
  diagnosis, 959–960
  differential diagnosis, 960t
  first episode, 959
  HSV-1 and HSV-2, differentiating, 959–960
  recurrent, 959–961
  serology, 960
  suppressive antiviral therapy, 960–961
  third-trimester acquisition, 961
  treatment
    first episode, 960–961
    in pregnancy/neonatal herpes
      prevention, 961
    recommended regimens, 960
    recurrent, 960–961
    short-course therapies, 960
    suppressive antiviral therapy, 960–961
  ulcers, 959, 959f, 960t
  virus detection and characterization,
    959–960
Genital mutilation, 610
Genital prolapse, 769
Genital tract
  female see Female genital tract
  male see Male genital tract
Genital tract obstruction, male infertility, 300

Genital ulceration, and HIV, 982
Genital virilization, steroid synthesis
    defects, 152
Genital warts
  aetiology, 969
  cervical, 970f
  diagnosis, 969
  and HIV, 982
  in immunosuppressed patients, 971
  laser treatment, 970
  physical ablation, 970
  in pregnancy, 970–971
  prevention, 969
  surface applications, 969–970
  treatment, 969–971
  vulval, 970f
  vulval infections, 606–607
Genito-ano-rectal syndrome,
    lymphogranuloma venereum, 964
Genitourinary medicine (GUM) clinics,
    956–958, 993
Genome-wide association studies
    (GWAS), 161–162
Gentamicin, 965
Geographical variation, breast cancer risk,
    708
Germinal epithelium, ovary, 1
Gestagen/antigestagen, endometriosis,
    501–502
Gestational and secretory hyperplasia,
    benign breast disease, 697
Gestational choriocarcinoma, 650
Gestational trophoblastic tumours (GTTs)
  acute disease-induced complications,
    management of, 662
  cerebral metastases, management, 662
  chemotherapy, 658–660, 663
  choriocarcinoma see Choriocarcinoma
  clinical features, 655–656
  contraceptive advice, 663–664
  drug-resistant, 657, 661–662
  epidemiology and aetiological factors,
    652–653
  epitheloid trophoblastic tumour,
    652, 656
  experimental imaging techniques, 657
  following hydatidiform mole, complete
    or partial, 654
  see also Hydatidiform mole
  genetic analysis, 657
  genetic factors, 653
  genetics and pathology, 650–652
  haemorrhage complication, 662
  high-risk patients, 660–662
  human chorionic gonadotrophin,
    654–657
  hydatidiform mole
  see also Hydatidiform mole
  investigations, 656–657
  long-term complications of therapy, 664
  low-risk patients, 660–661
  molar evacuation, 657–658
  placental-site trophoblastic tumour see
    Placental-site trophoblastic tumour
  prognosis, 664
  registration and follow-up following
    uterine evacuation, 658
  respiratory failure complication, 662

  scoring versus International Federation of
    Gynaecology and Obstetrics Staging,
    658–659, 659t–660t
  terminology
  timing of pregnancy after treatment, 663
  twin pregnancies, 655, 658
  see also Cancers; Gynaecological cancers
Gestational trophoblastic tumours (GTTs)
    (GTTs), 650
Gestrinone, endometriosis, 503–504
Gigantomastia, benign breast disease, 698
'Gillick competence', consent issues, 96
Gingko biloba, 416
Ginseng, 416
Glandular hyperplasia, 635
Glomerular filtration rate, 899
Glucocorticoids, 145, 151, 552–553
Glucose tolerance, polycystic ovary syndrome
    (PCOS), 255t
Glucosuria, 606
Glyceryl trinitrate, 911
Glycine-lycine-arginine (GLY-LYS-ARG), 200
B1-Glycoprotein, 652
Glycoprotein hormones, 133
Glycoproteins, 128
GnRH see Gonadotrophin-releasing hormone
    (GnRH)
Gonadal development, genetic control,
    167–168
Gonadoblastoma, 676
Gonadotrophin deficiency, male infertility,
    301
Gonadotrophin resistance, 220–221, 418
Gonadotrophin-associated peptide
    (GAP), 200
Gonadotrophin-releasing hormone
    (GnRH), 28, 199, 462
  agonist, 474, 477
  analogues, 481, 734
    assisted reproduction treatments, 317
    hypothalamic-pituitary-ovarian function,
      control, 201
    menstrual disorders, 450, 462
  assisted reproduction, 317
  endometriosis, 502–503
  fibroids, 481
  genetic control, 168f
  hypothalamic-pituitary dysfunction,
    214–215
  hypothalamic-pituitary-testicular axis,
    294–295
  hysteroscopy, 20–21
  mechanism of action on pituitary cells,
    200–201
  modulatory control of monoamines, other
    neurotransmitters and second
    messengers on secretion of, 201–204
  corticotrophin-releasing hormone, 204
  dopamine, 201–202
  endogenous opioids, 203–204
  leptin, 204
  neuropeptide Y, 203
  noradrenaline, 202–203
  prolactin, 204
  serotonin, 203
  neural connections, 198
  neurone system, 199–200
  overview of secretion, 205

ovulation failure, 282
premenstrual syndrome, 393, 399, 400f
preoperative preparation, 102
pubertal development, 182–183
pulsatile nature of gonadotrophin release,
   207–208, 234
regulation of gonadotrophin secretion
   by, 200
regulation of secretion and action, 129
schematic representation, 201f
self-priming of pituitary gonadotroph by,
   206–207, 207f
see also Gonadotrophin-releasing hormone
   agonists
Gonadotrophins
concomitant use of gonadotrophin-
   releasing hormone agonist
   results, 242
deficiency, management of, 306
hypogonadotrophic hypogonadism, 241
indications for ovulation induction with,
   241–242
ovulatory patients undergoing intrauterine
   insemination, 241–242
peptide hormones, 128
polycystic ovary syndrome, 241, 261–262,
   384
preparations, 240–241
recombinant follicle-stimulating
   hormone, 240
recombinant human chorionic, 240–241
recombinant luteinizing hormone, 240
regimens and monitoring, 242
risks, 242
sequential protocol, 242
step-up protocol/step-down protocol, 242
steroid hormones, regulation of
   synthesis, 151
urinary follicle-stimulating hormone, 240
urinary human chorionic, 240
urinary human menopausal, 240
see also Gonadotrophin-releasing
   analogues
Gonadotrophin-secreting tumours, 189
Gonococcal cervicitis, 966f
Gonococcal PID, 944
Gonorrhoea
clinical features, 966
diagnosis, 966, 966f
management, 967
in pregnancy and breast feeding, 967
treatment, 967
G-protein coupled hormone receptors,
   135, 136f
Graafian follicles, ovary, 1
Graciloplasty and artificial bowel sphincter,
   913–914
Granular cell tumour, 608, 702
Granulocyte colony-stimulating factor,
   551–552, 660–661
Granuloma inguinale, 965–966, 966f
Granulomatous cystitis, 871
Granulomatous mastitis, 700
Granulosa cell tumours, 670, 675
Grief, 763–764
Growth hormone (GH), 131, 140
'G-spot', 443
Gynaecological cancers, 522–538

'bad news', breaking *see* 'Bad news',
   breaking
bladder, 866
BRCA 1 and *BRCA 2* genes, 527
carers, needs of, 750
cervical *see* Cervical cancer
children, talking to about, 759–760
   aged 3-7 years, 760
   aged 7-11 years, 760
   teenagers, 760
clinical aspects, 535–536
cross-country differences in types, 509
DNA, 525–528, 525f, 535
early detection, 535
effects, 751–752
   on partners, 752
   on patients, 751–752
   sexuality and psychosexual issues,
   754–755
endometrial *see* Endometrial cancer
epidemiology, 509–521
epigenetics and DNA methylation,
   525–526, 525f
fallopian tubes, 535, 684–686
familial
   family history inconsistent with
     familial syndrome, 529
   genetics of, 526–528
   management of, 528–529
   prevention, 528
   risk assessment, 528
   screening for, 528–529
genetics of familial cancer, 526–528
germline and somatic genetic alterations,
   526
HNPCC-associated, and DNA repair
   genes, 527–528
molecular basis of carcinogenesis,
   523–526, 523f–525f
needs of dying woman, 763
novel therapies, 554–565
   alpha folate receptor, 560
   angiogenesis inhibition, 554–556
   CA125, 559
   epidermal growth factor receptor,
     556–557
   epothilones, 560
   mammalian target of rapamycin,
     558–559
   miscellaneous, 560–561
   for ovarian cancer, 684
   poly (ADP-ribose) polymerase
     inhibitors, 557–558
   protein kinase C (PKC), 559
   Src, 559–560
   taxanes, 551, 560
   vascular endothelial growth factor,
     554–556
oncogenes, 523, 524f
ovarian *see* Ovarian cancer
partners, effects on, 752
prevention, 535
prognostic and predictive indicators, 535
psychological effect on patient, 750
psychosocial issues/returning to
   normality, 754
quality of life *see* Quality of life
radionucleides used in, 544

recurrence of disease and cessation of
   therapy
fear of symptoms in advanced stage,
   761–762
reactions of partner, family and close
   friends, 761
symptom control, 762–763
route/frequency of drug administration,
   763
sexuality and psychosexual issues, 754–756
   background, 754
   behavioural therapy, 756
   effects of gynaecological cancer, 754–755
   goal of intervention, 755
   information requirements, 755
   intervention, 755–756
   listening and asking, 755
   preserving sexual identity, 756
spiritual and emotional pain caused by,
   750–751
sporadic, molecular genetics, 529–535
strategies for gene therapy, 535–536
supportive care for patients, 750–766
symptom control, 761–763
terminal illness *see* Terminal illness
tumour suppressor genes, 524–525, 525f
vaginal, 517–519, 518f
variation in rates *see* Ovarian cancer
vulval, 517–519
vulval cancer, 534–535
WHO, on sexual health, 754
see also Chemotherapy; Radiotherapy
Gynecologic Oncology Group (GOG) study,
   ovarian cancer, 683

H

Hadfield's operation, nipple discharge, 694
Haematoma
   forensic gynaecology, 995
   postoperative care, 121
Haematometra, hysteroscopy
   complications, 33
Haematuria, 864
Haemodynamic shock, ectopic pregnancy,
   367
Haemolysis-elevated liver enzymes-low
   platelets syndrome, 983–984
Haemophilus ducreyi, 965
Haemorrhage
   cervical cancer, 595
   ectopic pregnancy, 367
   gestational trophoblastic tumours, 662
   hysteroscopy, 32
   imaging techniques, 68–69, 69f–70f
   ovarian cysts, 668–669
   see also Bleeding
Haemorrhoidectomy, 910
Haemorrhoids (piles), 909–910
Hailey-Hailey disease, 606
Hair bleaching/plucking, hirsutism, 386–387
Halban's theory, endometriosis, 490
Hamartoma, of breast, 701
Hand-eye coordination exercises, laparoscopy
   training, 41
Harmonic Scalpel, laparoscopic
   procedures, 44
Hasson entry technique, laparoscopy, 40

B-hCG (ectopic pregnancy biochemical test)
quantitation of subunit, 368
serial measurements, 368
single measurement, 368
Health Protection Agency Centre for
Infections, 943
Heart, chemotherapy effects, 552
Heavy menstrual bleeding (HMB), 448,
453–455
pelvic pathology, 454–455
Height, breast cancer risk, 710
Heparin, 100, 102
Hepatitis, viral
characteristics of known viruses, 971t
hepatitis A, 971–972
hepatitis B, 972–973
hepatitis C, 973
hepatitis D, 973
hepatitis E, 973
and HIV, 985
screening, following rape, 993–994
serology, 972, 972t
HER dimerization inhibitors, 557
HER-2 (c-erbB2) gene
breast cancer, 716, 727
endometrial cancer, 647
Herbal medicine, menopause, 416
Herceptin (trastuzumab), 727–728
metastatic disease, 732
Hereditary non-polyposis colorectal cancer
(HNPCC), 630
genetics of familial cancer, 526–527
management of familial cancer, 528–529
Hermaphroditism, 46XY true, 172
Hernias, 937
Heroin use, 1006
Herpes simplex, 337–338, 607, 982
Herpesviridae, 958–959
Heterotopic pregnancy, 378–379
Heterozygosity, loss of see Loss of
heterozygosity (LOH)
Hidradenitis, vulva, 607
Hidradentitis suppurativa, 700
Highly active antiretroviral therapy (HAART),
979–980, 983–986
High-performance liquid chromatography,
138
Hilar cell tumours
Hip protectors, osteoporosis, 414
Hirschsprung's disease, 779
Hirsutism, 382–390
biochemical monitoring of androgen-
suppressive therapy, 388–389
definition problems, 382
diagnostic approach, 383–384
electrolysis, 387
endocrine tests, usefulness of, 384–386
hair growth pattern in hirsuties, 382
hypertrichosis, hirsuties distinguished, 382
investigation recommendations, 386
investigations, 383–384
laser depilation, 387
metabolic factors, evaluation, 385–386
ovarian cysts, 669
polycystic ovaries, diagnostic investigations,
384–385
polycystic ovary syndrome, 259–260
postmenopausal women, 386

psychological factors, 386
scoring scale, 382
synacthen test, late-onset congenital
adrenal hyperplasia, 385
systemic antiandrogen therapy, 387–388
therapy, 386–387
topical/cosmetic procedures, 386–387
weight reduction, 387
Histiocytosis X, 606
Histone deacetylase (HDAC) inhibitors, 561
HIV see Human immunodeficiency
syndrome (HIV)
HNPCC-associated gynaecological cancer,
and DNA repair genes, 527–528
Homeopathic treatment, osteoporosis, 417
Homocysteine, 257
Hormonal therapy, endometrial cancer, 645
Hormone receptors, 131–138, 132f
see also Cell surface receptors; Nuclear
receptors
Hormone replacement therapy (HRT),
709
androgens, 409
atrophy, 609
bioidentical hormones, 409
breast cancer risk, 411, 709–710
CHD primary prevention, 411
CHD secondary prevention, 412
colorectal cancer, 410
CVD risk, 411
dementia and cognition, 412
endometrial cancer risk, 411, 630
gallbladder disease risk, 411
hysterectomized women, 409
menopause options, 408–409
non-hysterectomized women, 409
oestrogen-based, 408–409
benefits, 410
libido loss, 443
risks, 411
uncertainties, 411–412
osteoporosis, 410
ovarian cancer, 412
premature ovarian failure, 418–419
progestogens, 409
quality of life, 412
stroke, 412
tibolone, 409
urogenital symptoms and sexuality, 410
vasomotor symptoms, 410
venous thromboembolism risk, 411
in young women, 552
Hormones
adrenal, 140–141
amino acid derivatives, 128
availability of to a cell, 131
bioidentical, 409
and chemotherapy, 552–553
clinical assays, 138–139
communication, 129f
endocrine rhythms, 131
endogenous, breast cancer risk, 710
endometrial cancer, 630
follicle-stimulating see Follicle-
stimulating hormone (FSH)
growth, 140
inhibitory control, 130–131
luteinizing, 139–140

measurement and action of individual,
139–143
anterior pituitary, 139–140
measurement of in male reproduction
disorders, 305
metabolic, regulating reproductive function,
218
negative feedback, 129, 205–206
ovarian, 141–142
peptide, 128
placenta, 142
positive feedback, 130, 206
premenstrual syndrome, 393, 394f
prolactin, 140
receptors see Hormone receptors
regulation of secretion and action,
129–131, 130f
role, 128
simple control, 129
steroid see Steroid hormones
steroids, 128–129
thyroid see Thyroid hormones/thyroid-
stimulating hormone (TSH)
tissue distribution, 131
types and action, 128–129
Hot flushes, 407
HPV see Human papilloma virus (HPV)
HRT see Hormone replacement therapy (HRT)
HSD enzymes, 148–150
Hulka-Clemens clip (sterilization), 430
Human chorionic gonadotrophin, hormones,
placenta, 142
B-human chorionic gonadotrophin (β-hCG)
assays, 82–83
Human chorionic gonadotrophin (hCG)
and beta-human chorionic gonadotrophin
assays, 654
gestational trophoblastic tumours (GTTs),
654–657
in GTTs, 650
hyperglycosylated, 654
luteal phase deficiency, 345
ovarian cysts, 669
peptide hormones, 128
polycystic ovary syndrome, 262
Human Fertilization and Embryology Act
1990, 312
Human Fertilization and Embryology
Authority (HFEA), 312, 325
Human Genome Project (HUGO), 148, 156
draft version, 156
sequence data produced by, 161
Human immunodeficiency syndrome (HIV),
979–987
antiretroviral therapy, 983–984
background, 979–981, 980f
breast infections, 700
CD4 count, 979–980, 982–983, 985
and cervical cancer, 511–512, 983
cervical intraepithelial neoplasia, 982–983
deaths from, 981
delivery route, in labour, 984
epidemic of, 981
fourth-generation assays, 981
genital neoplasias, 983
genital warts, 982
gynaecological symptomology, 981–983
herpes simplex and genital ulceration, 982

IUD use, 429
male-to-female transmission, 980
menstrual cycle, 981–982
and miscarriage, 337–338
molluscum contagiosum, 971
mother-to-child transmission, 981
natural history, 979
nosocomial transmission, 985–986
occupational transmission to healthcare
    workers, 985
pelvic sepsis, 982
and PID, 949
postexposure prophylaxis, 985, 993–994
in pregnancy, 983–984
pregnancy control, 984–985
preparation for gynaecological surgery, 985
reverse transcriptase, use of, 957f
syphilis, 982
testing, 981, 993–994
transmission, 980–981, 984
    to healthcare workers, 985
    HIV-infected healthcare workers, 985
    nosocomial, 985–986
    postexposure prophylaxis, 985,
        993–994
    rates of, in pregnancy, 984
treatment, 979–980
vaginitis, 982
see also Sexually transmitted infections
    (STIs)
Human leukocyte antigen (HLA), 170
Human menopausal gonadotrophin (hMG),
    191, 317
Human papilloma virus (HPV)
aceto-white epithelium, 601
and cervical cancer, 509, 511, 570,
    582–583, 1011
prevalence in lesbian and bisexual women,
    1011
transmission between women, 1011
vaccines, 513–514, 583
vulval cancer, 613
Human placental lactogen (jPL), 652
Hydatidiform mole, 651
age factors, 652–653
complete and partial
    clinical features, 655
    genetics and pathology, 650–651
    risk of gestational trophoblastic
        tumours (GTTs) following, 654
genetic factors, 653
incidence/ethnic origin, 652
invasive, 651–652, 655
pregnancies mistaken for, 651–652
previous pregnancies, 653
see also Gestational trophoblastic tumours
    (GTTs)
Hydration and early mobilization,
    thromboprophylaxis, 99
Hydrosalpinges, tubal disease, 357–358, 360
Hydrosalpinx, 313
Hydrothermal ablation (fluid-filled thermal
    endometrial ablation), 466
17α-hydroxylase deficiency, 46XY sexual
    development disorders, 173
21-hydroxylase deficiency, aetiology, 170
11-hydroxylase deficiency, congenital adrenal
    hyperplasia (CAH), 171

21-hydroxylase deficiency
    epidemiology, 170
    investigation, 170–171
    prenatal diagnosis, 171
    presentation, 170
    treatment, 171
Hydroxymethylglutaryl-coenzyme A
    reductase, 146
3β-hydroxysteroid dehyogenase deficiency,
    173
Hydroxysteroid dehyogenase (HSD)
    enzymes, 148–150
Hyfrecator, 970
Hymen, 5
    torn, 609
Hyperandrogenism, 253f, 254, 259–260
Hypergonadotrophic hypogonadism,
    234–235
Hyperhomocysteinaemia, 346
Hyperinsulinemia, 153, 254–255, 385–386
Hyperplactinaemic amenorrhea, 238
Hyperprolactinaemia, 219–220
    amenorrhoea, 223–224
    causes
    and male infertility, 305
    management, 225–226
    mechanism of action
    ovulation disorders, 234
    ovulation failure, 282
    placental-site trophoblastic tumour, 656
    polycystic ovary syndrome, 345
Hypersensitivity tests, 97
Hypertension, 426, 556
Hypertrichosis, hirsuties distinguished, 382
Hypnotherapy, 444, 828
Hypoactive sexual desire order, 443
Hypoglycaemic agents, pre-existing
    medications, 102
Hypogonadotrophic hypogonadism, 191,
    224–225, 241
Hypokalaemia, 117
Hypothalamic opioidergic neurones, 203–204
Hypothalamic regulation of pituitary
    secretion, 198–201
    antagonist analogues, 201
Hypothalamic-pituitary axis, 197–198
Hypothalamic-pituitary dysfunction, 212–230
    see also Amenorrhoea; Oligomenorrhoea
Hypothalamic-pituitary-ovarian axis (HPO),
    194, 204
    amenorrhoea and oligomenorrhoea, 212,
        216, 223
Hypothalamic-pituitary-ovarian function,
    control, 197–211
    follicular phase, 209
    hypothalamic-pituitary axis, 197–198
    integrative control during menstrual cycle,
        208–210
    luteal phase, 210
    mechanisms for preovulatory
        gonadotrophin surge, 209–210
    modulatory control of monoamines, other
        neurotransmitters and second
        messengers on GnRH secretion,
        201–204
    corticotrophin-releasing hormone, 204
    dopamine, 201–202
    endogenous opioids, 203–204

    leptin, 204
    neuropeptide Y, 203
    noradrenaline, 202–203
    prolactin, 204
    serotonin, 203
    other neurotransmitters and second
        messengers, 204–205
    ovarian steroids, modulatory effect,
        205–206
    pulsatile nature of gonadotrophin release,
        207–208
    self-priming of pituitary gonadotroph by
        GnRH, 206–207, 207f
    see also Hypothalamic regulation of
        pituitary secretion
Hypothalamic-pituitary-testicular axis,
    294–295
Hypothalamus, anatomy, 198f
Hypothyroidism, 455
Hypovolaemia, ovarian cysts, 670
Hysterectomy
    abdominal or vaginal approach for, 105
    abnormal menstrual bleeding, 466–467
    cervical cancer, 70–71, 588
    complications of, 590–591
    damage avoidance, 109
    endometrial destruction methods
        compared, 27–28
    endometriosis, 505
    fibroids, 482
    and fistulae, 879–880
    heavy bleeding, 462–463
    laparoscopic, 36
    menopause, 409
    ovarian cancer, 682
    pain following, 937
    and pelvic organ prolapse, 849–850
    pelvic organ prolapse, 856
    radical, for cervical cancer, 589–591
    secondary premature ovarian failure, 418
    surgical injury, 7
    vaginal vault brachytherapy following, 545
    without oophorectomy/uterine artery
        embolization, 418
Hysterosalpingo contrast sonography
    (HyCoSy)
    reproductive dysfunction, 285, 285t, 287
    tubal disease, 355
Hysterosalpingogram/hysterosalpingography,
    63–64
    fibroids, 478f
    fistulae, 884
    imaging, 63f
Hysteroscopic resection, fibroids, 483–484
Hysteroscopic sheaths, 20, 20f
Hysteroscopy, 17–35
    Adiana procedure, 31, 31f
    anaesthesia, 21
        complications of, 32
    arcuate deformity, 20
    Bettochi hysteroscope, 19f, 28f
    bipolar electrosurgery, 27, 28f
    bleeding
        benign disease, 25
        complications, 33
        contraindicated for, 18
        diagnostic indications, 17
    camera and stack system, 19f, 20

cancer
  complications, 33
  as contraindication, 18
cardiopulmonary disorders, contraindicated
    for, 18
cervical stenosis, contraindicated for, 18
choice of equipment, 22, 23f
choice of technique, 105
complications of
  abnormal menstrual bleeding, 33
  cancer, 33
  consent issues, 33
  distension medium, 32
  haematometra and pyometra, 33
  haemorrhage, 32
  infertility, 33
  late, 33
  postablation sterilization syndrome, 33
  pregnancy, 33
  surgeon related, 31
contraindications, 18
cryoablation, 29
Cusco's speculum, 22
diagnostic indications, 17–18
distension medium, 20, 32
endometrial ablation techniques, 463
endometrial cancer, 638
endometrial cavity without intracavity
    lesions, treatment, 29–31
endometrial destruction, 27–28
endometrial preparation, 20–21
endometrial sampling, 23
Essure system, sterilization, 31, 31f
fibroids, 18, 480
foreign body, 18
free fluid ablation, 30, 30f
haemorrhage complication, 32
historical development, 17
hysteroscopic sheaths, 20, 20f
hysteroscopic sterilization, 31, 31f
image recording equipment, 20
impedance bipolar radiofrequency, 30
infection
  complications of hysteroscopic
      procedures, 32
  contraindicated for, 18
infertility
  complications, 33
  diagnostic indications, 17–18
  tubal factor, 285
instrumentation, 18–20, 25–28, 26f
intrauterine synaechiae, 18
light lead, 20
light source, 20
malignancy, contraindicated for, 18
mechanical instrumentation, 25
menstrual abnormalities, diagnostic
    indications, 459
microwave endometrial ablation, 30
and miscarriage, 343
miscarriage, diagnostic indications, 18
monitor, 20
monopolar electrical instrumentation,
    25–27, 26f
Müllerian anomalies, diagnostic
    indications, 18
myomectomy, 28
Nd-YAG radiation, 56

newer developments, 33–34
ocal intracavity lesions, identification, 25
operative, indications for, 25
outpatient management, 21–23
pathology sean, 23, 23f–25f
pelvic pain, diagnostic indications, 18
polypectomy, 28
polyps, 18, 22f, 23, 24f
positioning, 21
postoperative care, 22
pregnancy, contraindicated for, 18
procedure, 21
second-generation ablation devices,
    complications, 29–31
skills, 23–29, 25b
surgeon related complications, 31
technique, 22
telescopes, 19–20
therapeutic strategy, benign disease, 25
thermal balloon ablation, 29
training and learning curve, 25
trauma, 32
uterine adhesion and septa, 28–29, 29f
uterine perforation, 32
  reduction of risk, 19–20
Versascope system, 22

I

Iatrogenic dissemination, endometriosis, 490
Ibandronate, 413
Ice packs, haemorrhoids, 910
ICSI (intracytoplasmic sperm injection) see
    Intracytoplasmic sperm injection
    (ICSI)
Idiopathic (primary) dysmenorrhoea,
    455–456
Idiopathic bladder neck obstruction, voiding
    difficulties, 841
Idiopathic delayed puberty, 219
Idiopathic hypogonadotropic hypogonadism,
    218
Ifosfamide, 549–550
Iliac artery, 11–13
Iliohypogastric nerves, 13–14
Ilioinguinal nerves, 13–14
Iliolumbar artery, 12
Iliorectal anastomosis, 916
IMAGE (Integrated Molecular Analysis of
    Genomes and their Expression), 157
Image recording equipment, hysteroscopy, 20
Image-guided biopsy, breast cancer, 721
Imaging, 59–79
  adenomyosis, 65–66, 65f–66f
  angiography, 62
  bladder disorders, 867–868
  cervical cancer, 584, 585f
  of cervical carcinoma, 69–72, 71f
  choriocarcinoma, 74–75, 74f
  conclusions, 77
  contrast studies, 59, 70
  ectopic pregnancy, 67, 67f
  of endometrial cancer, 72–74, 72f–73f
  endometriosis, 66, 66f
  experimental techniques, in GTTs, 657
  of fallopian tubes, 63–64
  fistulae, 882–884
  haemorrhage, 68–69, 69f–70f

hysterosalpingogram see
    Hysterosalpingogram
  infections, 67, 67f
  inferior vena cava filter insertion, 68,
      68b, 68f
  leiomyomas, 66–67
  of ovarian carcinoma, 75–76, 75f–76f
  of ovaries/ovarian varices, 64–65, 64f
  pelvic inflammatory disease, 946–947
  radionuclide, 61–62, 62f
  safety factors, 76–77
  urinary tract infections, 900–901
  of uterus, 62–63, 63f
  venous thrombosis, 67–68
  x-ray techniques, 59
  see also Computerized tomography (CT
      scanning); Magnetic resonance
      imaging (MRI); Positron emission
      tomography (PET); Transvaginal
      ultrasonography (TVUS)/transvaginal
      ultrasound (TVS); Ultrasound
Imidazole therapy, topical, 606, 975
Imiquimod, 970
Immune factors, implantation, 272–273
Immune tolerance, 272
Immunization, cervical cancer, 569
Immunoassays, 138–139
Immunocompromised patients, genital
    herpes, 959
Immunodeficiency, cervical cancer, 583
Immunological factors, endometriosis,
    489–490
Immunosuppressed patients, 971, 979
Impedance bipolar radiofrequency, 30
Impetigo, 607
Implanon (contraceptive implant),
    428, 984
Implantation, 270–273, 489
  ectopic pregnancy, 366
Implants, progestogen-only, 428
Incapacitated adults, consent issues, 96
Incessant ovulation theory, 678
Incisions, 995
  abdominal, 106
Incontinence, 768–769
  faecal see Faecal incontinence
  overflow, 837
  possible effects on female sexual r
      esponse cycle, 922f
  prevalence, 798
  quality of life assessment, 784
  urge, 815–816, 912
  urinary see Urinary incontinence
  see also Stress incontinence
Induced menopause, 406
Infantile choriocarcinoma, 656
Infections
  ductal, 700
  endogenous, prevention, 952
  hysteroscopy complications, 32
  hysteroscopy contraindicated for, 18
  iatrogenic, prevention, 952
  imaging techniques, 67, 67f
  male accessory gland, 300–301
  miscarriage, 337–338, 344
  postoperative care, 121–122
  reducing transmission risk, in
      ultrasound, 81

sexually transmitted see sexually transmitted infections (STIs)
surgical site, risk factors for, 100t
of vulva, 601
wound care, 119
Infective endocarditis, antibiotic prophylaxis, 101
Inferior mesenteric artery, 11
Inferior vena cava, 11, 68, 68b, 68f
Infertility
    abortion, 437
    causes, 322–323
    chemotherapy treatment, 552
    diagnostic indications, 17–18
    duration, 323
    and endometriosis, 493–494, 493t
    fallopian tube carcinoma, 684–685
    fibroids, 478–479
    hysteroscopy complication, 33
    investigations, 65
    and ovarian cancer, 516, 678
    pregnancy control, 985
    primary, uterus, malformations of, 178
    substance abuse, 1006
    tubal factor see Tubal factor infertility
    unexplained, 288–289, 360–361
    vaginismus, 442
Inflammatory bowel disease (IBD)
    fistulae, 878
    male infertility, 306
Inflammatory breast cancer, 714–716
Infundibulopelvic ligament, ureter
Infundibulum
    contents, 201
    fallopian tubes, 3
    hypothalamic-pituitary axis, 197
Inhibin
    hypothalamic-pituitary-ovarian function, control, 204–205
    ovarian hormones, 141
Inhibin B
    assessment of ovarian reserve, 314
    mutation, in POF, 418
Inorgasmia, 443
Insulation failure, diathermy, 50–51
Insulin, pubertal development, 183
Insulin resistance, polycystic ovary syndrome, 256–257, 282–283
Insulin-like growth factors (IGFs)
    amenorrhoea, 217–218
    breast cancer, 728
    pubertal development, 183
    steroid synthesis, 151
Insulin-sensitizing agents
    ovulation induction, 239
    polycystic ovary syndrome, 262
Integrase inhibitors, 979–980
Intensity-modulated radiotherapy (IMRT), 543
Interferons, 970
Internal iliac artery and branches, pelvis, 12–13
Internal mammary nodes (IMN), 724
International Federation of Gynaecology and Obstetrics (FIGO), staging systems
    cervical cancer, 584–586
    endometrial cancer, 631–632, 635–636

gestational trophoblastic tumours, 658–659
    vulval/vaginal cancer, 623, 624t
International Pelvic Pain Society, 933
International Society for the Study of Vulvovaginal Disease (ISSVD), 600
Interposition grafting, fistulae
Intersex disorders
    androgen-secreting tumours, 171
    associated multiple congenital abnormalities, 172
    congenital adrenal hyperplasia see Congenital adrenal hyperplasia (CAH)
    drugs, 172
    female (46XX), 169
    management, 194
    see also Puberty disorders
Interstitial brachytherapy, 545–546
Interstitial cystitis, 869–870
Interstitial implantation, ectopic pregnancy, 366
Interstitial pregnancy, 378
Intestinal tract disease, 907–918
    anal fissures, 910–911
    anorectal manometry, 907–908
    Bristol stool chart, 917f
    cancer, 670
    constipation see Constipation
    dynamic imaging, 908–909
    faecal incontinence see Faecal incontinence
    haemorrhoids, 909–910
    independence of pathology, 907
    investigations, 907–909
    irritable bowel syndrome, 916–917
    shapes study, 909
    solitary rectal ulcer syndrome, 915
    thrombosed external haemorrhoids, 910
    ultrasound, 908–909
    see also Anal sphincter and mechanisms; Bowel
Intracavitary brachytherapy, 545, 545f
Intracavitary receiver coils, 69–70
Intracytoplasmic sperm injection (ICSI), 273, 305, 320
    with epididymal spermatozoa, 308
    introduction for male infertility, 323
    pregnancy following, 328
    problems with, 273
    with testicular spermatozoa, 308–309
Intraligamentous pregnancy, 378
Intramural fibroids, 475
Intraperitoneal therapy, ovarian cancer, 684
Intrapituitary paracrine-autocrine system, 204, 205f
Intrauterine devices (IUDs), 422, 428–429
    ectopic pregnancy, 364–365
    emergency contraception, 430
    as foreign body, removal under hysteroscopy, 18, 23, 25
    heavy bleeding, 454
    and PID, 949
    systems, 428–429
Intrauterine gestation sac, 82–83, 83f
Intrauterine insemination, 241–242
Intrauterine synaechiae (Asherman's syndrome) see Asherman's syndrome
Intravenous urography, 789, 900–901
Intravesical therapy, 827
Invasive ductal carcinoma (IDC), 714

Invasive lobular carcinoma (ILC), 714
Invasive mole, 650
Invasiveness gene signature, breast cancer, 731
In-vitro fertilization (IVF), 65, 419, 478–479, 678, 1010–1011
In-vitro fertilization-embryo transfer (IVF-ET), 356–359
Ionizing radiation exposure, breast cancer risk, 709
Irritable bowel syndrome (IBS), 916–917, 933
Ischaemic heart disease, polycystic ovary syndrome, 256
Ischiocavernosus, pelvic musculature, 11
Ischiocavernous muscle, clitoris, 6
Ischiorectal fossa, pelvic musculature, 11
Isoflavones, 415
Isotretinoin, oral, 260
Isthmic implantation, ectopic pregnancy, 366
Isthmus
    fallopian tubes, 3
    uterus, 3
Itraconazole, 606
IUDs see Intrauterine devices (IUDs)
IVF (in vitro fertilisation), problems with, 273

J

JAK-STAT signalling, 135
Janus-associated kinase (JAK1-4), 135
Jehovah's witnesses, consent issues, 94
Joint prostheses, diathermy, 52
Junctional zone (JZ), myometrium, 449–450
Juvenile hypertrophy, 690–691

K

Kallman's syndrome, 191, 198, 215–216, 282, 303
Kartagener's syndrome, 302–303
Kava kava, 416–417
Kegel exercises, pelvic organ prolapse, 855
Keloid scarring, diathermy, 52
Keratinizing squamous metaplasia of bladder, 871
Ketobemidone, 805
Ketoconazole, 388
17-ketosteroid reductase deficiency, 46XY sexual development disorders, 173
Kidneys, chemotherapy effects, 552
Kinetic energy, 539
Kisspeptins, 218
Kleinfelter's syndrome, 168
Kleneprep, 886
Klinefelter's syndrome (47XXY), 299
Knudson's 'two-hit' hypothesis, 524–525
Krukemberg tumour

L

Labia majora, vulva, 5–6, 599, 614–615
Labia minora, vulva, 6–7, 599
Lacerations, 995
Lactating adenoma, 701
Lactational amenorrhoea method (LAM), contraception, 429

Lactogenesis, benign breast disease, 697
Lamina propria, 871
Laminaria, 102
Laparoscopes, 38
Laparoscopic myomectomy, fibroids, 484
Laparoscopic ovarian drilling (LOD),
    243–244
Laparoscopic uterosacral nerve ablation,
    endometriosis, 504–505
Laparoscopy, 36–47
  blood vessels, damage to, 114–115
  bowel damage, 114
  Burch colposuspension, 805
  camera system, 38, 38f
  chronic pelvic pain, 934
  closed, 39–40
  complications, 40–41, 45, 45b
  diagnostic uses, 45
  diathermy contrasted, 50–51
  diathermy damage, 115
  direct entry, 40
  dysmenorrhoea, 456
  ectopic pregnancy, 370–371, 375
  Endo-catch bag, 42
  endo-loop, 41
  endometrial cancer, 639
  energy sources, 44
  equipment, 37–39, 38f
    handles, 39
    jaws, 39
    safety devices, 37–39
    shaft, 39
  fallopian tube carcinoma, 685
  fibroids, 480
  gasless, 44
  Hasson entry technique, 40
  history, 36
  insufflators, 38–39, 44
  intra-abdominal adhesions, 41
  laparoscopes, 38
  laparoscopic ovarian drilling, 243–244
  laparoscopic para-aortic lymph node
      sampling, 584
  light source and lead, 38
  mechanical morcellators, 44
  and miscarriage, 343
  open, 39–40
  operating instruments, 39
  or methotrexate (ectopic pregnancy), 375
  ovarian diathermy, laparoscopic, 263t
  pelvic floor repair, 859–860
  pelvic inflammatory disease, 947, 948f, 950
  pneumoperitoneum, 40
  port entry, 39–41
  RCOG training guidelines, 36
  recording equipment, 38
  robotic techniques, 44
  Roeder knot, 41, 41f
  scissors, 39f
  site of entry, 39–40
  specimen removal, 42–44
  stapling, 41–42, 42f–43f
  surgical team, 37
  suturing, 41, 43f, 114
  teaching and learning, 41–44
  television monitor, 36, 38
  theatre set-up, 36–37, 37f
  therapeutic, 45–46, 46b
  trocars, 37–38, 37f
  tubal disease, 355, 359–360
  tubal factor infertility, 283–285
  umbilicus as site of entry, 39
  uses, 45–46
  Veress needle, 36, 40, 40f
Laparotomy
  ectopic pregnancy, 370–371
  fallopian tube carcinoma, 685
  gestational trophoblastic tumours, 662
  minilaparotomy technique, 114, 430
  uterine perforation and false passage, 114
Lapatinib, 727
Large bowel, 112, 124–125, 670
Large loop excision of transformation zone
    (LLETZ), cervical premalignancy, 575
L-arginine, 926
Larmor frequency, magnetic resonance
    imaging, 61
Lasers
  ablation, 463
  acronym, 52
  argon, 56
  basic physics, 52–53, 53f
  carbon dioxide, 54–55, 55f
  common systems, 53f, 54–56
  conclusions, 58
  control of hazard, 57
  definitions, 52
  female sterilization, 430–431
  genital warts, 970
  helium-neon, 55
  hirsutism, 387
  laparoscopic surgery, 359
  light-tissue interaction, 53–54, 54f
  metal vapour, 56
  nature of hazard, 57
  neodymium:yttrium aluminium garnet,
      55–56
  photodynamic therapy, 56
  pulse repetition rate, 54
  Q-switched, 54, 56
  safety factors, 57
  ultraviolet, 56
  zoom optics, 55
  see also Diathermy
Lasofoxifene, 414
Lateral migration, cell surface receptors, 132,
    133f
Laxatives, 891, 915–916
Leak point pressure, urodynamic
    investigations, 793
Leiomyoma of uterus, 66–67, 476f
Leiomyomata see Fibroids
Leiomyosarcoma, 635f
Leptin, 204, 218
Lesbian and bisexual women, 441,
    1009–1016
  access to maternity services, 1011
  advice from healthcare professionals, 1012
  aetiology of lesbianism, 1010
  and assumption of heterosexuality, 1010,
      1012–1013
    avoiding, 1014
  attitudes in health care, 1010
    improving, 1014
  breast cancer, 1012
  cervical screening and cancer, 1011–1012
  communication with, 1014
  discriminatory treatment less common in
      health care, 1009
  education and research, 1013–1014
  experiences of health care, 1012–1013
  facilitating access to health care, 1013
  good practice, 1014
  health issues, 1009–1016
  improving attitudes and behaviours to,
      1013
  legislation, 1009–1010
  medical model, 1010
  recommendations towards, 1014–1015
  reproductive health, 1010–1011
  research into health of, 1013–1014
  sexual problems, 444
  sexually transmitted infections, 1012
  and social change, 1009–1010
  undergraduate medical education, 1013
  welcoming environment towards,
      1014–1015
Letrozole, 237–238, 261
Leukaemia, chronic myeloid, 523
Leukaemia inhibitory factor (LIF), 272
Levator ani, pelvis, 10, 801
Levatoroplasty, 781
Levonorgestrel, 409
Levonorgestrel intrauterine system (LNG-
    IUS), 28, 462, 502
Leydig cell hypoplasia, 172
Leydig cells, 167–168, 294
LGV see Lymphogranuloma venereum (LGV)
LH:FSH ratio, 153–154, 208
LH-releasing hormone (LHRH), 199
Libido loss
  in female, 443, 755
  in male, 445
Lichen planus, vulva, 600, 604–605
Lichen sclerosus, vulva, 603–604
  cause, 603
  description of lesions, 603
  histology, 603
  prevalence, 603
  treatment, 603–604
  and vulval squamous cell carcinoma, 604
Lidocaine (lignocaine) ointment, 926, 960
Lifestyle modification
  pelvic organ prolapse, 855
  premenstrual syndrome, 395, 398t
Ligaments, pelvic, 9–10
Ligasure system, laparoscopic procedures, 44
Ligation, female sterilization, 430
Likelihood ratios, 1022t
Lipofibroadenoma, 701
Lipoid cell tumours
Lipomas, 608, 701–702
Lipoproteins, low-density, 132
Liposarcoma, of breast, 701–702
Liquorice root, 417
Lithotomy, 884
Lithotomy poles, hysteroscopy, 21
Lloyd Davies supports, hysteroscopy, 21
Lobular hyperplasia, 696
Lobular in-situ neoplasia (LISN), 713–714
LOD (laparoscopic ovarian diathermy), 263t
Long-acting reversible contraception (LARC),
    422
Loperamide hydrochloride, 552, 912

Loss of heterozygosity (LOH), 527, 529–530
Low compliance, 768
Lower intestinal tract disease *see* Intestinal tract disease
Lower urinary tract disorders
  calculi, 871
  cystitis *see* Cystitis
  evaluation, 783
  non-infective sensory conditions, 866b
  non-malignant conditions, 866
  quality of life assessment, 784
  and sexual dysfunction, 929
  tumours, 871
  urinary symptoms, 783–784
  see also Bladder disorders; Urinary tract infections
Low-molecular-weight heparin (LMWH), preoperative prophylaxis, 100
L-selectin, 271f
Lumbosacral trunk, 14
Lungs, chemotherapy effects, 552
Luteal phase, 210, 345
Luteinized thecoma
Luteinizing hormone (LH), 139–140, 197
  anovulatory dysfunctional uterine bleeding, 454
  and beta-human chorionic gonadotrophin assays, 654
  endocrine control of steroid synthesis, 150
  follicular development, 232, 318
  hypersecretion, in recurrent miscarriage, 345
  menstrual cycle, 208, 208f
  ovarian function and menopause, 406
  peptide hormones, 128
  recombinant, 240
Luteomas
Lyell's syndrome, 606
Lymph nodes
  benign breast disease, 703
  bilateral groin lymph node dissection, vulval cancer, 617–619
  breast disease, benign, 703
  cervical cancer, 592
  elective regional node dissection, in malignant melanoma, 622
  in ILC, 714
  inguinal, 15–16
  laparoscopic para-aortic lymph node sampling, 584
  para-aortic dissection, 11
  sentinel lymph node detection, vulval cancer, 617
  vulval cancer, 592, 616–617
Lymphadenectomy
  role in endometrial cancer, 639
  superficial inguinal/pelvic (in vulval cancer), 619–620
Lymphadenitis, 964
Lymphadenopathy, 964
Lymphatic drainage, to pelvis, 14–16, 15f, 15t
Lymphoedema, 620, 722–723
Lymphogranuloma venereum (LGV)
  aetiology, 964
  clinical features, 964–965
  diagnosis, 965
  genito-ano-rectal syndrome, 964

long-term complications, 965
  lymphadenitis, 964
  lymphadenopathy, 964
  and PID, 944
  primary lesion, 964
  secondary lesion, 964
  tertiary stage, 964
  treatment, 965
Lynch syndrome, 515, 527–528, 679

M

M. contagiosum, 971
M. tuberculosis, 354
Macrophages, peritoneal, 490–491
Magnesium, premenstrual syndrome, 397
Magnesium hydroxide, 915–916
Magnetic resonance defaecography, 916
Magnetic resonance imaging (MRI)
  adenomyosis, 65–66
  breast cancer, 717–719, 719f
  cervical cancer, 69–71, 584, 585f
  chronic pelvic pain, 934
  endometrial cancer, 73–74, 73f, 638
  endometriosis, 66, 500
  female pelvis suitable for, 61
  fibroids, 480
  fistulae, 884
  gastrointestinal tract endometriosis, 498
  gestational trophoblastic tumours, 657
  infertility, 65
  interventional, 61
  intestinal tract disease, 908–909, 909f
  invasive lobular carcinoma, 714
  leiomyomas of uterus, 63
  and miscarriage, 343
  ovarian cancer, 75, 76f
  ovarian cysts, 670
  P nuclear spectroscopic studies, 449–450
  pelvic organ prolapse, 851f, 855
  pelvis, 253f
  pituitary macroadenoma, 225f
  pituitary microadenoma, 224f
  radiotherapy planning, 541
  techniques, 61
  urinary tract infections, 900–901
  uterine artery embolization, 485–486
Malaria, and miscarriage, 344
Malathion, 977
Male genital tract
  congenital malformations of, 309
  infection management, 306
  obstruction, 300
Male infertility
  accessory gland infection, 300–301
  aetiology, 298–299, 298f
  and assisted conception, 307–309
  coital disorders, 301
  cryptorchidism, 299, 309
  definition/epidemiology, 297
  genetic causes, 299
  genital tract obstruction, 300
  gonadotrophin deficiency, 301
  iatrogenic, 300
  immunological causes, 301
  micromanipulation techniques, 307–309
  occupational and environmental factors, 300

orchitis, 299
  pathophysiology, 297–298
  semen *see* Semen
  varicocoele, 299
Male reproductive ageing, 297
Male reproductive disorders, 292–311
  changes in male reproductive health, 309–310
  chromosome analysis, 305
  clinical management, 302–309
  examination, 303
  history, 302–303
  hormone measurements, 305
  infertility *see* Male infertility
  obstruction
    ejaculatory duct, 307
    epididymal, 307
    relief of, 307
    vasal, 307
  physiology, 292–294
  testicular biopsy, 305
  treatment
    antisperm antibodies, management, 306
    ejaculatory failure, 306–307
    erectile failure, 306
    general measures, 306
    genital tract infection, management, 306
    gonadotrophin deficiency, management, 306
    medical, 306–307
    surgical, 307
    varicocoele treatment, 307
  see also Female reproductive disorders
Malignancy *see* Cancers
Malignant melanoma, 621–622, 625
Malnutrition, 185
Mammalian target of rapamycin (mTOR), 558–559
Mammographic density, breast cancer risk, 710
Mammography, 717–718
  high-resolution, 718
Marshall-Marchetti-Krantz (MMK) procedure, Burch colposuspension, 804–805, 805f
Martius graft, fistulae
Mass closure technique, incisions, 106
Massive oedema, 673
Mast cells, 869–870
Mastalgia, 694
Mastectomy
  breast reconstruction, 735
  inflammatory breast cancer, 716
  Paget's disease, 714
  prophylactic, 712
Masters and Johnson sexual response model, 441, 443, 446
Mastitis
  granulomatous, 700
  of infancy, 701
  puerperal, 698–700
Maternal age, 338, 591–592
Matrix metalloproteinases (MMPs), 272, 450, 453
Maturation inhibitors, 979–980
Mature cystic teratoma, 673–674
Mature solid teratomas, 674
Mayer-Rokitansky-Kuster-Hauser syndrome, 192–193

Maylard incision, abdominal procedures, 106
McCune–Albright syndrome, 189
McGill Short Form pain questionnaire, 933
McIndoe-Reed operation, absent vagina, 176–177
Mechanical prophylaxis, preoperative preparation, 99–100
Medical students, consents for, 94
Medicines and Healthcare Products Regulatory Agency, laser safety, 57
Medroxyprogesterone acetate, 502, 934–935
Mefenamic acid, 460
Meigs syndrome
Melatonin, 128
Melphalan, 549
Menarche, 187
  delayed, 186
Menopausal transition, 406
Menopause, 405–421
  anatomical changes, 2
  cardiovascular disease, 407
  chemotherapy-related, in breast cancer, 733
  chronic conditions, 407–408
  definitions/physiology, 405–407
  dementia and cognitive decline, 408
  discharge, in endometrial cancer, 637
  hysterectomized women, 409
  libido loss, 443
  Million Women Study, UK, 410
  natural, 405
  non-hysterectomized women, 409
  non-oestrogen-based treatments for symptoms, 412–413
    hormonal, 412
    non-hormonal, 412
    osteoporosis see under Osteoporosis
  osteoporosis, 407–408
  and ovarian function, 406
  premature ovarian failure see POF (premature ovarian failure)
  psychological symptoms, 407
  sexual dysfunction, 407
  stages of reproductive ageing, 406
  surgical, 418
  see also Hysterectomized women
  symptoms, 407
  therapeutic options, 408–409
  ultrasound, clinical conditions, 89–90
  urinary human menopausal gonadotrophins, 240
  urinary incontinence, 408
  urogenital atrophy, 408
  uterus, changes to, 5
  vaginal lubricants and moisterisers, 413
  vasomotor symptoms, 407
  Women's Health Initiative, US, 409–410
  see also Postmenopausal women
Menorrhagia
  choice of operation, 93
  endometrial cavity, treatment, 29
  fibroids, 477–478, 481
  HIV, 981–982
  IUD use, 429
  magnetic resonance imaging, 65
  puberty disorders, 194

Menstrual cycle/menstruation
  abnormal, 453–456
    anovulatory dysfunctional uterine bleeding, 454
    coagulation disorders, 455
    dysfunctional uterine bleeding, 453–454
    dysmenorrhoea, 455–456, 467
    epidemiology, 456–457
    examination, 457
    failure of follicular development, 454
    heavy bleeding, 453–455
    investigations, 457–459
    medical problems, 455
    ovulatory dysfunctional uterine bleeding, 454
    presentation, 457
    quantification of menstrual blood loss, 459
    treatment see Treatment of abnormal bleeding below
    uterus, malformations of, 178
  angiopoietins, 452
  distribution of menstrual intervals, 213f
  endometrial ablation techniques, 463–466
  endometrial repair, 452–453
  endometriosis, 492
  haemostasis, 451
  heavy bleeding, 453–455
  history of menstrual intervals, 213f
  and HIV, 981–982
  integrative control of hypothalamic-pituitary unit during, 208–210
  matrix, 452–453
  normal, 212, 450–453
  ovarian cysts, 669
  pelvic pathology, heavy bleeding, 454–455
  proliferative phase, 449, 450f
  quantification of menstrual blood loss, 459
  sterilization problems, 432
  treatment of abnormal bleeding
    antifibrinolytics, 460
    danazol, 462
    ethamsylate, 460
    general management principles, 459
    gonadotrophin-releasing hormone analogues, 462
    hormonal, 460–462, 462b
    non-hormonal, 460
    oestrogen/progestogen regimes, 462
    progestogens, 460–462
    prostaglandin synthetase inhibitors, 460
    surgical, 462–467
    uterine artery embolization, 466
  vasculature, endometrial repair, 452–453
  vasoconstriction, 451–452
Menstrual irregularity, polycystic ovary syndrome, 259
Mental Capacity Act 2005, consent issues, 96
Mental health problems, sexual assault, 998
Mesothelin level, ovarian cancer, 679
Mesovarium, ovary, 1–3
Metabolic factors, hirsutism, 385–386
Metal vapour lasers, 56
Metaplasia, 696
Metformin, 239, 258, 262
Methadone treatment, 1006
Methicillin-resistant S.aureus (MRSA), 101

Methotrexate
  chemotherapy, 550
  contraindications, 374
  ectopic pregnancy, 67, 373–375
  folinic acid rescue, 374, 550
  gestational trophoblastic tumours, 660–661
  liver toxicity, 374
  and mifepristone, 375
  mode of action/pharmacokinetics, 373
  myeolosuppression, 374
  or laparoscopic surgery (ectopic pregnancy), 375
  persons benefiting from, 374
  renal function, 374
  routes of administration/dose, 374–375
  side-effects, 373–374
Metoclopramide, 81
Metronidazole
  bacterial vaginosis, 609
  pelvic inflammatory disease, 949
  sexually transmitted infections, 974, 976
  vulval infections, 607–608
MIAME (Minimum Information About a Microarray Experiment), 159
Microadenosis, 695–696
Microarrays
  cDNA, 157, 533
  limitations, 159
  practical aspects, 157, 158f
  technology, 156–157
  validation of data, 159–161
  Watson-Crick base pairing, 157
  see also Molecular biology
Microcalcifications, 697
Microdocectomy, 694
Microglandular adenosis, 695–696
Micromanipulation techniques, male infertility, 307–309
Microprolactoma, 238
MicroRNAs, ovarian cancer, 534
Microsurgical epididymal sperm aspiration (MESA), 308
Microsurgical treatment, tubal disease, 356–359
Microwave endometrial ablation (MEA)
  endometrial ablation techniques, 463–466
  hysteroscopy, 30
Micturition cycle, normal, 775–776
Midazolam, 81
Midstream urine (MSU), collection, 784, 816
  UTIs, 866, 896, 900
Midurethral sling procedures, 845
Mifepristone, 341, 435–436, 481
  and methotrexate, 375
Migraines, 218
Migrant women, sexual assault, 998
Milk stasis, 699–700
Million Women Study (MWS), UK, 410, 710
Mineralcorticoids, 145
Mineralocorticoid receptors, 137
Minilaparotomy technique, female sterilization, 114, 430
Mirena (IUD), 428
Miscarriage, 335–352
  in abused women, 1003
  alloimmune factors, 346–347
  aneuploidy, recurrent, 343
  antiphospholipid syndrome, 346

and assisted reproduction treatments
  autoimmune disease, 345–346
  cervical incompetence, 344
  chromosomal abnormalities, 336–337,
    336t
  complete, 84, 340
    tubal pregnancy, 366
  counselling, 347
  definitions, 335
  early fetal demise, 340, 342
  endocrine disease, systemic, 344–345
  fetal malformations other than
    chromosomal anomaly, 337
  fetal sex, 338
  fibroids, 478–479
  hypersecretion of luteinizing hormone, 345
  incomplete, 340–342
    tubal pregnancy, 366
  inevitable, 339
  infections, 337–338, 344
  investigations, 347
  luteal-phase deficiency, 345
  maternal age, 338
  maternal health, 338–339
  missed (early fetal demise), 83–84
  multiple pregnancy, 338
  parental chromosomal abnormalities,
    342–343
  and partial hydatidiform mole, 651
  placental abnormalities, 337
  rate, 240, 335–336, 336t
  recurrent
    anatomical factors, 343–344
    autoimmune and thrombophilic factors,
      345–346
    diagnostic indications, 18
    endocrine factors, 344–345
    genetic factors, 342–343
    investigations, 347
  sepsis, 340
  sporadic
    aetiology, 336–339
    epidemiology, 335–336
    pathophysiology, 339
    presentation, 339–340
    problems of definition/ascertainment,
      335
    psychological aspects, 342
    rate, 335–336, 336t
    treatment, 341–342
  threatened, 339, 341
  treatment
    sporadic miscarriage, 341–342
    unexplained miscarriage, 347
  trophoblastic tumours, 340
  ultrasound, role, 83–85
  unexplained, 347
  uterine anomalies, 343–344
  uterus, malformations of, 178
Misoprostol, 102, 436
MISTLETOE study, endometrial destruction,
  27, 32
Mitochondria, 146–147
Mitomycin, 870
Mixed androgen insensitivity syndrome
  (MAIS), 213–214
MLH1 mismatch repair gene, 630
Mobilization, postoperative care, 120

Modified intention-to-treat (MITT) analysis,
  513–514
Molar evacuation, gestational trophoblastic
  tumours, 657–658
Molecular biology
  applications to reproductive biology, 163,
    533
  exploratory data analysis and data models,
    158–159
  fluorescent chemistry, quantitative reverse
    transcriptase polymerase chain
    reaction, 160, 160f
  genetic factors, 522–538
  genome-wide association studies, 161–162
  global screening and analysis, 156–157,
    157t
  mapping of single nucleotide
    polymorphisms/links to complex
    diseases, 161–162
  microarrays
    cDNA, 533
    limitations, 159
    practical aspects, 157, 158f
    technology, 156–157
    validation of data, 159–161
  microRNA, role, 162–163, 162f
  ovarian cancer, 679
  polymerase chain reaction, quantitative,
    159–160
    data analysis and interpretation,
      160–161
  post-transcriptional repression and
    regulation, 162–163, 162f
  premature ovarian failure, 220–221
  principles and new developments, 156–165
  quantitative polymerase chain reaction,
    159–160
  short, interfering RNA, role, 162–163, 162f
  statistical analysis, 158
  t-test, 158
Molecular genetics
  cervical cancer, 529–530
  endometrial cancer, 534
  fallopian tube cancer, 535
  ovarian cancer, 530–534
  sporadic gynaecological cancers, 529–535
  vulval cancer, 534–535
  see also Molecular biology
Molecular genetics, sporadic gynaecological
  cancers, 529–535
Molluscum contagiosum, 971
Mondors's disease, breast, 702
Monoclonal antibodies, 61, 557, 559
Monocyte chemotactic protein-1, 499
Monopolar diathermy, 48, 49f, 52
Monopolar electrical instrumentation,
  hysteroscopy, 25–27, 26f
Monosomy X, 336
Montgomery's glands, benign breast disease,
  702
MORAb-003 (monoclonal antibody), 560
Mosaicism, sex chromosome anomalies, 168
Movicol, 915–916
Moxifloxacin, 949
MRI *see* Magnetic resonance imaging (MRI)
MSH2 mismatch repair gene, 630
Mucinous carcinoma, 681
Mucositis, 552

Müllerian abnormalities/anomalies, 18,
  192–193
Multicystic ovary, transabdominal scan, 253f
Multiple sclerosis, voiding difficulties, 840
Muscarinic receptors, 814
Mustine, 300
Mycoplasma genitalium, 968–969
Myocardial infarction, combined hormonal
  contraceptives, 425
Myomas *see* Fibroids
Myometomy, 28, 482–483
Myometrium, 3, 448–450

N

Nalidixic acid, 901–902
Naloxone, 828
NALP7 gene, hydatidiform mole, 653
Naproxen, 456
National Breast Screening Programme
  (NHSBSP), 717
National Cancer Database, 714
National Cancer Guidance Group, 759
National Chlamydia Screening Programme
  (NCSP), 943, 967
National Health Service Breast Screening
  Programme, 409–410
National Institute for Health and Clinical
  Excellence Guidelines, 97, 99, 101
National Service Framework for Children,
  Young People and Maternity Services,
  90
Natural family planning (NFP), 429
Nausea and vomiting, chemotherapy, 552
Nd-YAG radiation, lasers, 55–56, 463
Necrotizing fasciitis, 119
Needle core biopsy, 697, 721
Negative feedback, 129, 205–206, 205f
Negative p-mesons, 539
Neisseria gonorrhoeae, 353–354, 958
Neodymium:yttrium aluminium garnet lasers,
  55–57, 463
Nephrotoxicity, 552
  cisplatin chemotherapy, 552
Nerve entrapment, chronic pelvic pain,
  935–937
Nerve stimulation, voiding difficulties,
  844–845
Nerve supply, to pelvis, 13–14
Nervous system, chemotherapy effects, 552
Neuroendocrine cervical carcinomas, 587
Neuroendocrine systems, premenstrual
  syndrome, 393
Neurohypophysis, hypothalamic-pituitary
  axis, 198
Neurological disease, voiding difficulties, 840
Neuromodulators, diathermy, 52
Neuropeptide Y, 203, 218
Neurosurgery, electrosurgery in, 48
Neutrons, 539
Neutropenia, 551–552
Neviripine, 983
Newborn infants, risk of malignancy in
  assisted reproduction treatments
  treatment, 191
Nifedipine, 911
Night sweats, 407
Nipple areola complex, 690

Nipple discharge
  benign disease, 692–694, 693f
  in pregnancy, 697–698
Nitrofurantoin, 306, 901–902
Nocturia, 864
Node of Cloquet, 15–16
Non-nucleoside reverse transcriptase
    inhibitors (NNRTIs), 979–980
Non-steroidal anti-inflammatory drugs
    (NSAIDs), 455, 460, 870–871
Noradrenaline, 201–203
Norethisterone, 20–21, 409, 502
Normogonadotrophic anovulation, 225
Normogonadotrophic hypogonadism, 235
Norplant, 428
No-scalpel vasectomy (NSV), 432
Nottingham Prognostic Index (NPI), breast
    cancer, 729
NovaSure system, endometrial ablation, 466
Nuclear medicine scanning, urinary tract
    infections, 901
Nuclear receptors, 136–138, 137f
  hormone specificity of, 136–137
  nuclear localization, DNA binding and
    transcriptional activation, 137–138
  target cell conversion of hormones destined
    for, 136
  see also Cell surface receptors; Hormone
    receptors
Nuclear reprogramming, 275
Nucleic acid amplification technique (NAAT),
    946, 965–966, 968
Nucleoside reverse transcriptase inhibitors
    (NRTIs), 979–980
Nulliparity, as breast cancer risk, 708
Numbers needed to treat (NNT), 1020

O

Obese patients
  and assisted reproduction treatments, 322
  endometrial cancer, 515, 629–630
  hirsutism in, 387
  ovulation induction, 261
  polycystic ovary syndrome, 254–255,
    258–259
  risk assessment, 97–99
  stress incontinence, 800
  see also Body weight
Obstetric risk, pelvic organ prolapse, 855–856
Obstructive defaecation, 915–916
Obturator nerve, 14
Ocal intracavity lesions, identification, 25
Odontological examination, forensic
    gynaecology, 994
Oedema
  leg, 594–595, 620
  massive, in ovarian cysts, 673
Oestradiol, 141, 150, 451–452
Oestrial cream, 902
Oestrogen receptors (ER), 634–635
Oestrogen-secreting tumours, ovarian cysts,
    669, 675
Oestrogens/oestrogen treatment
  atrophy, 609
  deficiency of oestrogen, 225
  and endometrial cancer, 515
  menopause, 409

oestrogen/progestogen regimes, 462
overactive bladder (OAB) syndrome,
    826–827
positive feedback, 206, 206f
premenstrual syndrome, 397–399
synthetic, 409
thyroid hormones, 140
tissue distribution, 131
voiding difficulties, 844
Ofloxacin, 949, 967–968
Oil cysts, breast, 702–703
Oligomenorrhoea, 212
  definitions, 212–213
  diagnosis and management, 223–225
Oliguria, 117
Omega-3 fatty acids, 415
Omental pedicle grafts, fistulae
Omentectomy, ovarian cancer, 682
Oncogenes, gynaecological cancers,
    523, 524f, 531–532
Oncotype DX, breast cancer, 731
Oncovin, 660–661
One-stop postmenopausal bleeding clinic,
    638
Oocyte banking, 734
Oocyte donation, assisted reproduction
    treatments, 325
Oocyte retrieval, assisted reproduction
    treatments, 318–319
Oocytes, 232
Oophorectomy
  breast cancer risk, 712
  endometriosis, 505
  and family history inconsistent with
    familial syndrome, 529
  laparoscopic procedures, 42
  ovarian cancer risk, 679
  premenstrual syndrome, 400
  secondary premature ovarian
    failure, 418
  and sexual dysfunction, 929
Operation, choice of, 93
Ophthalmology, ultraviolet lasers, 56
Opioid analgesia, postoperative care, 119
OPRM1 gene, 930
Oral contraception
  antiandrogen therapy, systemic,
    387–388
  breast cancer risk, 709
  combined see Combined oral
    contraception (COCP)
  combined hormonal contraceptives,
    fibroids, 474
  dysmenorrhoea, 456, 467
  endometriosis, 502
  and ovarian cancer, 678
  pre-existing medications, 102–103
  premenstrual syndrome, 399
  vulval infections, 606
Orchitis, 299
Organ rupture, 996
Orgasmic disorder, 920
Orlistat, 243
Ospemifene, 414
Osteoporosis
  dietary factors, 414–415
  HRT benefits, 410
  menopause, 407–408

non-oestrogen-based therapy
  complementary and alternative medicine,
    416–417
  exercise, 415–416
  non-pharmacological interventions,
    414–415
  pharmacological interventions,
    413–414
Outer mitochondrial membrane (OMM),
    146–147
Outpatient management
  hysteroscopy, 21–23
  pelvic inflammatory disease, 947, 949b
Ovarian ablation, breast cancer, 726
Ovarian cancer, 678–688
  aetiology, 678
  anaplastic tumours, 680
  application of molecular biology to, 163,
    533
  borderline tumours
    epithelial, 681–682
    surgery for, 683
  CA125 (surface antigen), 559
  carcinogenesis, early events, 530–531
  cDNA microarrays, 533
  chemotherapy, 684
  classification of ovarian tumours,
    679–680
  clear cell carcinoma, 678, 680–681
  comparative genomic hybridization, 533
  debulking, optimum, 682–683
  descriptive epidemiology, 516
  diagnosis, 682
  DNA methylation, 534
  endometrioid carcinoma, 681
  and endometriosis, 678
  epidemiology, 678
  epithelial, 555
  exogenous hormones, 516–517
  family history, 517
  fertility-sparing procedures, 683
  genetic factors, 653, 679
  growth factor receptors, 531–532
  growth signals, 531
  heterozygosity, loss of, 532–533
  and HRT, 412
  imaging of, 75–76, 75f–76f
  and infertility, 516, 678
  intraperitoneal therapy, 684
  microRNAs, 534
  molecular genetics, 530–534, 679
  mucinous carcinoma, 681
  novel approaches, 684
  oncogenes, 531–532
  other factors, 517
  ovulation induction risks, 247–248
  pathology of epithelial tumours, 680–682
  pelvic and abdominal spread, 75–76
  polycystic ovary syndrome, 258
  in premenopausal patient, 516
  prevention and screening, 517
  prophylactic surgery, 679
  relapse, 554
    surgery at, 684
  risk factors, 516
  screening, 517
  second-look surgery, 683
  serous carcinoma, 678, 680–681

sporadic
  oncogenes, 531
  tumour suppressor genes, 532
Src (non-receptor tyrosine kinase),
  559–560
subclassification, 680
surgery, 682–684
survival rates, 516
TLK-286, 561
transitional cell tumours, 681
trials, 683
tumour suppressor genes, 532
see also Ovarian cysts
Ovarian cysts, 668–677
  abdominal examination, 670
  abdominal swelling, 669
  adrenal-like tumours, 676
  androgen-secreting tumours, 675–676
  aspiration of, ultra-sound guided, 81
  asymptomatic patient, 671
  benign epithelial tumours, 674–675
  benign germ cell tumours, 673–674
  bimanual examination, 670
  bloating, 669
  CA125 serum markers, 670–671
  clear cell (mesonephroid) tumours, 675
  conservative treatment, 81
  corpus luteum, 673
  dermoid (mature cystic teratoma),
    673–674
  differential diagnosis, 669
  endometrioid, benign, 674–675
  general history and examination, 670
  gonadoblastoma, 676
  granulosa cell tumours, 675
  gynaecological history, 669
  hormonal effects, 669
  investigations, 669–671
  less than 8 cm in diameter, 671
  management of, 671–672
  massive oedema, 673
  mature solid teratomas, 674
  morphology U score
  mucinous cyst adenoma, 674
  normal CA125 levels, 671
  oestrogen-secreting tumours, 669, 675
  in older women, 671
  and other cysts, 672
  pain, 668–669
  pathology, 672–677, 672b
  patient with symptoms, 672
  physiological, 672–673
  physiological ovarian cysts, 668
  in pregnancy, 672
  pressure effects, 669
  risk of malignancy index, 670–671
  risk of malignancy index (RMI), 670–671
  serous, benign, 674
  Sertoli cell tumours, pure, 675
  Sertoli-Leydig tumours, 675–676
  serum tumour markers, 670
  sex cord stromal tumours, benign, 675–676
  simple, 671
  simple follicular cyst, 673
  'somatic-type' tumours, 674
  surgical injury, 7
  symptomatic, clinical presentation,
    668–669

symptoms and signs, 670
theca lutein, 657
thecomas/thecoma-fibroma tumour group,
  675–677
transitional cell (Brenner) tumours, 675
ultrasound, 670
ultrasound-guided diagnostic aspiration,
  671
see also Ovarian cancer
Ovarian endometriosis, 496–497, 497f–498f
Ovarian failure, 283, 733
  premature *see* POF (premature ovarian
    failure)
Ovarian hormones *see* Anti-Müllerian
  hormone (AMH); Inhibin;
  Progesterone; Testosterone
Ovarian hyperandrogenism, steroid synthesis
  defects, 153
Ovarian hyperstimulation syndrome, risk
  factors, 245
Ovarian hyperstimulation syndrome
  (OHSS)
  assisted reproduction treatments risks,
    326–327, 326f
  counselling, 246
  description, 244–246
  diagnosis/classification, 244
  inpatient management, 246
  management, 245
  outpatient management, 245–246
  pathophysiology, 244
  pituitary downregulation, 317
  prevention, 245
  response to ovulation stimulation, 245
  risk factors, 244–245
  types of stimulatory drugs, 245
Ovarian pregnancy, 377
Ovarian reserve, 315
  assessment, 314–315
  and chemotherapy
  measuring, 222
  tests, 315
Ovarian reserve tests (ORTs), 419
Ovarian steroid synthesis, control,
  150–151
Ovarian steroids, modulatory effect,
  205–206
Ovarian stimulation, controlled, 317–318
Ovarian varices, imaging of, 64–65
Ovarian wedge resection, 243
Ovaries
  age-related changes, 2
  anatomy/anatomical relations, 1–3
  androgen-secreting tumours, 171
  blood supply, 2–3, 3f
  cancer of *see* Ovarian cancer
  development, 166
  functions of, 231
  imaging of, 64, 64f, 75
  multicystic, 253f
  premalignant disease, 579–580
  see also Ovarian cancer
  prevention of premalignancy, 580
  structure, 1, 2f
  type I and II pathways, 579–580
  vestigial structures, 2
  see also Vulval intraepithelial neoplasia
    (VIN)

Overactive bladder (OAB) syndrome, 769,
  813–835
  acupuncture, 828
  α-Adrenoreceptor antagonists, 826
  aetiology, 814, 815b
  ambulatory urodynamics, 818, 820f
  antidiuretic agents, 825–826
  antimuscarinic drugs, 821–824
  behavioural therapy, 827–828
  biofeedback, 828
  and bladder pain syndrome, 869
  calcium-channel antagonists, 825
  characteristics of, 864
  clam cystoplasty, 829
  clinical presentation, 815–816
  conclusions, 830
  cystometry, 817–818, 817f–819f
  cystourethroscopy, 819
  darifenacin, 824
  desmopressin, 825–826
  detrusor myectomy, 829
  detrusor overactivity, 813
  epidemiology, 813–814
  fesoterodine, 824
  frequency/volume chart, 816–817,
    816f
  general management, 820
  hypnotherapy, 828
  incidence, 813–814
  intravesical therapy, 827
  investigations
    cystometry, 817–818
    cystourethroscopy, 819
    frequency/volume chart, 816–817,
      816f
    urine culture, 816
    uroflowmetry, 817
  Multicentre Assessment of Transdermal
    Therapy in Overactive Bladder with
    Oxybutinin study, 930
  muscarinic receptors, 814
  National Institute for Health and Clinical
    Excellence Guidelines, 829–830
  neuromodulation, 828–829
  oestrogens, 826–827
  OPERA study, 823
  oxybutynin, 824
  pathophysiology, 814–815
  peripheral neuromodulation, 829
  pharmacology, 820–826, 822t
    antidiuretic agents, 825–826
    drugs with mixed action, 824–825
  potassium-channel-opening drugs, 825
  propiverine, 824–825
  prostaglandin synthetase inhibitors, 826
  sacral neuromodulation, 828–829
  and sexual dysfunction, 929–930
  solifenacin, 823
  surgery, 829
  symptoms and signs, 815–816
  technique for bladder drill, 828
  terminology, 813
  tolterodine, 821–823
  treatment, 819–820
  tricyclic antidepressants, 825
  trospium chloride, 823
  urinary diversion, 829
  urine culture, 816

videocystourethrography, 819, 821f
voiding difficulties, 841
Overflow incontinence, 837
Overlap anterior sphincteroplasty, 781
Oviductal transport and nutritional support, preimplantation, 269
Ovolutory cycles, breast cancer risk, 708
Ovregovomab, 559
Ovulation
 assessing, 232
 failure of, 282–283
 induction *see* Ovulation induction
 presumptive signs of, 281
 and progesterone, 141
Ovulation disorders, 232–234, 281–283
 classification, 232–233
 diagnosis and treatment, 234–235
 history, 233
 investigations, 233–234
 ovarian failure, 283
 ovulation failure, 282–283
 physical examination, 233
 serum progesterone measurement, 281
 ultrasound follicle tracking, 281–282
Ovulation induction, 231–250
 aim, 231
 dopamine agonists, 238–239
 drug pharmacology/mechanism of action, dopamine agonists, 238
 gonadotrophins, indications for induction with, 241–242
 see also Gonadotropins
 indications for treatment, dopamine agonists, 238
 insulin-sensitizing agents, 239
 laparoscopic ovarian drilling, 243–244
 medical, 236
 multiple pregnancy, risk of, 246–247
 polycystic ovary syndrome, 260–263
 principles, 231–232
 pulsatile gonadotrophin-releasing hormone, 239–240
 regimens and monitoring
  dopamine agonists, 238
  gonadotrophins, 242
  pulsatile gonadotrophin-releasing hormone, 239–240
 results of treatment, dopamine agonists, 238
 risks of treatment
  cancers, 247–248
  gonadotropins, 242
  multiple pregnancy, 246–247
  ovarian cancer, 247–248
  ovarian hyperstimulation syndrome *see* Ovarian hyperstimulation syndrome (OHSS)
  prion disease, 248
  pulsatile gonadotrophin-releasing hormone, 240
 side-effects of treatment
  dopamine agonists, 238–239
  pulsatile gonadotrophin-releasing hormone, 240
 surgical, 262–263
 weight loss, 242–243
Oxybutynin, 823–824, 828, 869–870
Oxytocin, 128

P

*P*53 gene mutations, in cancer, 526, 529–531
 gene therapy strategies, 535–536
 ovarian cancer, 532
Pacemakers, and diathermy, 52
Paclitaxel, chemotherapy, 551, 561, 661, 684
Pad tests
 urethral sphincter incompetence, 801
 urodynamic investigations, 785
Paget's disease
 of breast, 714
 nipple adenoma mimiking, 701
 of vulva, 577, 577f–578f, 605, 622
Pain
 abdominal, ectopic pregnancy, 366
 assessment in cancer patients, 762–763
 biology of, 929–930
 bladder, 864
 cervical cancer, 595
 childbirth, 926
 chronic and visceral, special features, 929
 definition, 929
 endometriosis, 492
 genetic variation in susceptibility to, 930
 organic, 931
 ovarian cysts, 668–669
 pelvic
  absence of pathology on scan, 88–89
  chronic *see* Chronic pelvic pain (CPP)
  hysteroscopy, 18
  with negative pregnancy test, 86
  with positive pregnancy test, 83
 postoperative management, 118–119, 118t
 psychogenic, 931
 relief of *see* Analgesia
 sex differences, 930
 sexual pain disorders, 920
 see also Dyspareunia; Vaginismus
 total, 761
 vascular, and pelvic congestion, 929–930
 vulval *see* Vulvodynia
Painful bladder syndrome, 869–870
Palliative care, 761
 vulval cancer, 621
Palmar-plantar erythrodysethesia (PPE), 550–551
PAP7 (PBR-associated protein 7), 146–147
Papaverine, 306
Papillomas
 intraductal, 693–694, 693f
 serous surface, 674
Papillomatosis, 693–694, 693f
Paracrine control, ovarian steroid synthesis, 151
Paraffin, 701
Paralytic ileus, 124
Paramedian incision, abdominal procedures, 106
Parametrium
 anatomy, 4
 cervical cancer, 70–71
 imaging, 70–71
Parasympathetic nerves, 13
Parathyroid hormone peptides, 414

Parenteral administration of drugs, 548
Parkinson's disease
 neuromodulators, 52
 voiding difficulties, 840
Paroophoron, ovarian anatomy, 2
Parovirus B19, and miscarriage, 338
Paroxetine, 412
Partial androgen insensitivity syndrome (PAIS), 213–215
Partial hydatidiform mole (PM), 650–651
Particulate radiation, 539
Passive drains, 118
Patient-controlled analgesia (PCA), 119
Patupilone, 560
PCOS *see* Polycystic ovary syndrome (PCOS)
PEACH (Pelvic Inflammatory Disease Evaluation and Clinical Health), 947
Pediculosis pubis (*Phthirus pubis*), 976–977, 977f
Pegylated liposomal doxorubicin (PLDH), 551
Pelvic congestion, and vascular pain, 929–930
Pelvic congestion syndrome, 64–65, 933–935, 936f, 937–938
Pelvic endometriosis, 495–496
Pelvic floor
 anatomy, 10, 10f, 771–772, 772f
 dysfunction *see* Pelvic floor dysfunction
 ultrasound and dynamic imaging, 908, 908f
Pelvic floor dysfunction
 effect on sexual function, 921–922
 laparoscopic/robotic repair, 859–860
 muscle training, 416, 856, 912
 physiotherapy, 444
 and sexual dysfunction, 920–922
  aetiology, 920–921
  effect of treatment on sexual function, 922–924
Pelvic floor muscle training (PFMT), 802–803, 856
 devices, 803
Pelvic inflammatory disease (PID), 942–954
 aerobic and anaerobic agents, 944
 analgesia, 948
 antibiotics, 948–949
 biochemical tests, 946
 chlamydia, 943f, 944, 967–968
 chronic, 935
 compliance and partner screening, 949–950
 contact prevention, 951
 definitions, 942
 diagnosis, 944–946
 ectopic pregnancy, 364
 epidemiology, 942–943
 evidence-based management, 946–950
 gonococcal, 944
 and HIV, 949
 iatrogenic infections, prevention, 952
 identifying populations at risk, 951–952
 imaging tests, 946–947
 inpatient management, 947–948
 investigations, 946–947, 949
 and IUCDs, 949
 laparoscopy, 947, 948f

long-term societal and global health impact, 950
outpatient management, 947, 949b
ovarian cysts, 669
pathogenesis and pathogens, 943–944
in pregnancy, 949
prevalence estimates, 942–943
prevention, 950–952
risk assessment, 946
screening, 951–952
sexually transmitted infections, prevention, 950–951
sources of entry, 944
specific tests, 946
symptoms and signs, 944–946, 945b
treatment, 947–950
tubal pathology, 88
Pelvic musculofascial support, 9–11
ligaments, 9–10
musculature, 10–11, 10f
peritoneum, 9
Pelvic organ prolapse see Pelvic organ prolapse (POP)
Pelvic organ prolapse (POP), 849–863
aetiology, 849–850
anterior compartment, surgery for, 858–859
apical, treatment for, 857–858
bowel symptoms, 853
CARE trial, 854–855
classification, 850–851
clinical presentation, 852–854
grading systems, 852f, 853–854
investigations, 854–855
laparoscopic/robotic pelvic floor repair, 859–860
lifestyle modification, 855
management, 850
non-surgical treatment, 856–857
obliterative surgical procedure, 860
pelvic anatomy, 851–852
pelvic floor muscle training, 856
physical examination, 853–854
posterior compartment, surgery for, 859
prediction of symptoms, 853
prevalence, 849, 850f
preventive surgery/natural history, 855–856
sexual problems, 853, 923
surgical treatment, 857–860, 929
urinary symptoms, 852–853
vaginal pessaries, 856–857
voiding difficulties, 841
weight loss, 856
Women's Health Initiative, 849
Pelvic Organ Prolapse Quantification (POP-Q) system, 850–851, 852f
Pelvic pain
absence of pathology on scan, 88–89
abuse and somatization, 931–932
chronic see Chronic pelvic pain (CPP)
clinical assessment, 933–934
consulting patterns, 930–931
depression, 931
diagnosis and treatment, 934–938
endometriosis, 935
pelvic congestion syndrome, 934–935, 936f
endometrial cancer, 637

endometriosis, 935
epidemiology, 930–931
fibroids, 478
history, 933
impact on quality of life, 933
investigations, 934
with negative pregnancy test, 86
pelvic congestion syndrome, 934–935, 936f
pelvic mass association, 87
physical examination, 933–934
with positive pregnancy test, 83
problems with, 929
psychological factors, 931–932
referral patterns, 931
sexual and physical abuse, 933
Short Form-36 (SF-36) questionnaire, 931
sociocultural factors, 932
studies, 931
systems review, 933
women, prevalence in, 930
see also Pain; Pelvis
Pelvic sepsis, and HIV, 982
Pelvis
anatomy, 2f, 851–852
blood supply to, 11–13, 12f–13f, 12t
cervical cancer, recurrent, 594–595
lymphatic drainage to, 14–16, 14f–15f, 15t
median sagittal section through, 4f
MRI examination, suitability for, 61
musculofascial support see Pelvic musculofascial support
nerve supply to, 13–14
pathology, heavy bleeding, 454–455
Penicillin
side-effects, 97
urinary tract infections, 901–902
vulval infections, 607
Peptide hormones, 128, 129f
Percutaenous epididymal sperm aspiration (PESA), 308
Perimenopause, 405
Perineal body, vulva, 6
Perineal ultrasound, 791–792
Perineum, dissection, 6f
Peripheral benzodiazepine receptor (PBR), 146–147
Peripheral blood lymphocytes (PBLs), 561
Peripheral neuromodulation, overactive bladder syndrome, 829
Peripheral tumours, puberty disorders, 188–189
Peristeen pump, rectal irrigation, 912
Peritoneal flap grafts, fistulae
Peritonealization, 358–359
Peritoneum
anatomy, 8–9
closure of, 107, 107t
ovarian anatomy, 1
rectum, 8
uterus, 3
Periurethral injection therapy, 809–810, 809f
Permethrin cream, 977
Pertuzumab, 557, 727
Pessaries, pelvic organ prolapse, 856–857, 923
Petechiae, 995
Peutz-leghers syndrome
Peyronie's disease, 303

Pfannenstiel incision, abdominal procedures, 106
Pharmacodynamics, 548
Pharmacokinetics, 548
Pharmacological prophylaxis, preoperative preparation, 100, 102
Phenothrin, 977
Phentolamine, 202, 926
Philadelphia chromosome, chronic myeloid leukaemia, 523
Phosophdiesterases (PDEs), 136
Phosphatidylinositol-3-kinase (PI3K)/AKT pathway, 558
Phosphorylation, tyrosine kinase hormone receptors, 135
Photodynamic therapy, 56, 871
Photons, 52, 539
Phyllodes tumour of breast (PT), 691–692
Physical activity, 217–218, 415–416, 710
Physiochemical assays, 138
Physiotherapy, 120, 444, 886
Phytoestrogens, 416
Phytosterols, 415
PICOD (Population, Intervention, Comparison, Outcome and Design), 1017, 1018t
Picolax, 886
PID see Pelvic inflammatory disease (PID)
Piles see Haemorrhoids (piles)
Pioglitazone, 239
Pipelle sampler, endometrial sampling, 459
PISQ questionnaire, sexual problems, 924
Pituitary downregulation, 317
Pituitary gland
anatomy, 198f
hypothalamic regulation of pituitary secretion, 198–201
Placenta
hormones, 142
miscarriage, abnormalities causing, 337
Placental-site trophoblastic tumour (PSTT), 650
clinical features, 656
epidemiology and aetiological factors, 653
genetics and pathology, 652
management of, 662–663
see also Gestational trophoblastic tumours (GTTs)
Planning target volume (PTV), radiotherapy, 541
Plasma protein A, pregnancy-associated, 142
Platinum agents, ovarian cancer, 516, 682–684
P-LI-SS-IT model, 756, 756b
PMS see Premenstrual syndrome (PMS)
Podophyllin, 969–971
Podophyllotoxin, 969–971
POF (premature ovarian failure) see Premature ovarian failure (POF)
POF1(X chromosome), 418
Poland syndrome, 690, 690f
Poly (ADP ribose) polymerase inhibitors, 557–558, 684
Polycystic ovaries, diagnostic investigations, 384–385
Polycystic ovary syndrome (PCOS), 251–264
causes, 668
characteristics, 239, 263–264

clinical manifestations, 252t
clomiphene-resistant, 241
endocrine profile, 253–254
familial, 418
glucose tolerance definitions, 255t
health consequences, 256–258
heterogeneity of, 255–256
hirsutism, 383–384
hyperprolactinaemia, 345
investigations, 234, 253–255
morphology, 251
national and racial differences in
    expression, 256
non-fertility aspects, management,
    258–260
obesity, 258–259
and OHSS, 245
ovarian hyperandrogenism, 153
ovulation failure, 282
ovulation indicators, 260–263
and ovulation induction, 241
pathogenesis, 251–253
prevalence, 251
psychological support/quality of life, 258
transabdominal scan
    multicystic ovary, 253f
    polycystic ovary, 252f
transvaginal ultrasound scan, three-
    dimensional, 253f
ultraviolet lasers, 56
Polyethylene glycol, 886
Polyglandular autoimmune syndromes, 191
Polymerase chain reaction (PCR),
    quantitative, 159–160
absolute quantification, 161
choriocarcinoma, 652
data analysis and interpretation, 160–161
DNA-binding dyes, 160
hydrolysis, 160
normalization, 161
quantitative reverse transcriptase,
    fluorescent chemistry, 160, 160f
relative quantification (delta delta C_1
    method), 161
Polypectomy, hysteroscopy, 28
Polypoidy, 337
Polyps, hysteroscopy, 18, 22f, 23, 24f
Positive feedback, 130, 206
Positron emission tomography (PET)
breast cancer, 716, 719–721, 720f
cervical cancer, 72, 584
gestational trophoblastic tumours, 657
radiotherapy planning, 541
techniques, 62f
Postablation sterilization syndrome, 33
Postcoital testing, unexplained infertility,
    288–289
Posterior tibial nerve stimulation (PTNS),
    829, 844
Postmenopausal women
bleeding, 637–638
cervix in, 50
discharge, 637
hirsutism, 386
libido loss, 443
ovarian cancer, 678
ovarian cysts, 671
sexual assault, 997

tamoxifen use, 725–726
ultrasound, 89–90
UTI prevalence, 902
Postmenopause, 405–406
Postnatal assessment, ultrasound, 85–86
Postoperative care, 116–127
breast cancer, 725
complications, recognition and
    management
    bowel, 124–125
    haematoma formation, 121
    haemorrhage, 120–121
    infection, 121–122
    pulmonary, 125
    pyrexia, 121–122
    urinary tract injuries, 123–124
fistulae, 891
hysteroscopy, 22
routine
    bladder care, 117–118
    drains, 118
    feeding, 119–120
    fluid and electrolyte management,
        116–117
    mobilization and physiotherapy, 120
    pain management, 118–119, 118t
    wound care, 119
venous thromboembolism, 122–123
Postpartum voiding difficulty, 840
Post-tubal sterilization syndrome, 432
Postvasectomy syndrome, 433
Potassium chloride, ectopic pregnancy, 67
Potassium-channel-opening drugs, 825
Prebiotics, 415
Precocious puberty
androgen receptor blockade, 189
congenital adrenal hyperplasia, 188
definitions, 187–189
gonadotrophin-secreting tumours, 189
inhibition of puberty, 189
management, 189
McCune–Albright syndrome, 189
ovarian cysts
premature adrenarche, 188
premature thelarche, 188
sex-steroid-secreting tumours, 188–189
thelarche variants, 188
true, 188
Precursor hormones, 406
Prednisolone, 300
Pregabalin, 606
Pregnancy
abdominal, 377
benign breast disease
    bloody nipple discharge, 694, 697–698
    galactocele, 698, 699f
    gestational and secretory hyperplasia,
        697
    gigantomastia, 698
    lactogenesis, 697
    pseudohamartoma, 698
    pseudolipoma, 698
    puerperal mastitis, 698–700
caesarean scar ectopic, 376–377
cervical, 376
cervical cancer in, 596
chlamydia treatment, 968
cornual, 378

cyst aspiration in, 81
early
    anatomical landmarks, 83
    assessment of viability, 84f
    gestational sac, 82–83
    pain or bleeding in, 82
ectopic, 84–85
fibroids, complications due to, 479
first
    age at for breast cancer risk, 708
    displacement of ovary, 1
first trimester, abortion in, 435–436
fistulae surgery, 892–893
genital herpes in, 961
genital warts, treatment of, 970–971
gonorrhoea treatment, 967
heterotopic, 378–379
HIV in, 983–984
human chorionic gonadotrophin in, 654
and hydatidiform mole, 651–652
hydatidiform mole mistaken for, 651
hysteroscopy
    complications, 33
    contraindications, 18
interstitial, 378
intraligamentous, 378
lesbian mothers, access to maternity
    services, 1011
mid trimester, abortion in, 436
multiple
    miscarriage, 338
    ovulation induction, 246–247
negative test
    and acute bleeding, 89–90
    with pelvic pain, 86
and OHSS, 245
ovarian, 377
ovarian cysts in, 672
pelvic inflammatory disease in, 949
pelvic organ prolapse, 855–856
positive test, bleeding and/or pain
    with, 83
postpartum voiding difficulty, 840
previous, and hydatidiform moles, 653
timing of after gestational trophoblastic
    tumours treatment, 663
twin pregnancies, 655, 658
ultrasound, role, 83–85
of unknown location, 85, 86f, 370,
    371f–372f
violence against women in, 1002–1003
see also Abortion; Fetus; Miscarriage;
    Placenta
Pregnancy-associated breast cancer (PBAC),
    734–735
Pregnancy-associated plasma protein A
    (PAPP-A), 142
Pregnenes, 145
Preimplantation, 268–270, 273
Preimplantation genetic screening (PGS),
    273, 329
Premalignant disease of genital tract,
    566–581
cervical premalignancy see Cervical
    premalignancy
endometrial premalignancy see Endometrial
    premalignancy
ovaries, 579–580

vaginal intraepithelial neoplasia, 575–576, 575f
vulval intraepithelial neoplasia, 576–577, 577f–578f
see also Cancers
Premature adrenarche, 188
Premature ejaculation, 441, 445
Premature ovarian failure (POF)
    aetiological classification, 218b
    age definition
    as cause of amenorrhoea, 220–222
    causes, 190–191
    consequences, 418
    diagnosis and management of oligomenorrhoea and amenorrhoea, 223
    fertility/contraception issues, 419
    incidence
    management, 418–419
    primary, 417–418
    secondary, 418
Premature thelarche, 188
Premenopause, 405
Premenstrual dysphoric disorder (PMDD), 391–394
Premenstrual syndrome (PMS), 391–404
    aetiology and pathophysiology, 391–394, 393f
    agnus castus, 396
    alternative therapies, 397, 398t
    antidepressants, 399–400, 401t
    anxiolytic agents, 400
    bromocriptine, 397
    calcium, 395–396
    Daily Record of Severity of Problems, 396f
    danazol, 399
    diagnostic criteria, 391
    differential diagnoses, 397b
    evening primrose il, 396
    GABAergic system, 394, 395t
    gonadotrophin-releasing hormone agonists, 399, 400f
    lifestyle modification, 395, 398t
    magnesium, 397
    management of, 394–395
    neuroendocrine systems, 393
    oestrogen, 397–399
    oral contraception, 399
    ovarian hormones, 393, 394f
    pharmacological treatments, 397–400
    progesterone, 397, 398f
    prolactin, 394
    psychological interventions, 395
    serotonergic system, 394
    sodium/fluid retention theories, 394
    spironolactone, 400
    SSRIs, 399–400, 401t
    St John's Wort, 397
    surgery for, 400
    symptoms, 391, 392b, 392t
    vitamin B6 and pyridoxine, 395–397
    vitamin D, 397
Preoperative care
    additional medications prior to gynaecological surgery, 102
    antibiotic prophylaxis, 100–101
    assessment see Assessment, preoperative
    bowel preparation, 102

choice of operation, 93
consent see Consent
pre-existing medications, 102–103
risks and benefits of common procedures, 95t
smoking cessation, 102
thromboprophylaxis, 99–100
weight loss, 101
Preovulatory cervicofundal contractions, 453
Pressure-flow studies, voiding difficulties, 842
Primary breast lymphoma (PBL), 716
Primary dysmenorrhoea, 194
Primary ovarian insufficiency, 221
Primer design, PCR reaction, 160
Principal components analysis, 158–159
Prion disease, 248
Probenecid, 967
Probiotics, 415
Procarbazine, 300
Proctoscopy, fistulae, 885
Progesterone
    in early pregnancy, 341
    ectopic pregnancy test, 368
    in menopause, 409
    ovarian hormones, 141
    positive feedback, 206, 207f
    premenstrual syndrome, 397, 398f
    serum progesterone measurement, 281
    therapeutic option, menopause, 409
    tissue distribution, 131
    transdermal creams, osteoporosis, 417
Progesterone receptors (PR), 634–635
Progestins, 145, 552–553
Progestogen challenge test, 223–224
Progestogen-only contraceptives (POCs), 427–428
Progestogens
    continuous, 460–462
    cyclical, 460
    intrauterine, 462
    and masculinization of female fetus, 172
    menopause treatments, 412
    menstrual bleeding, abnormal, 460–462
    oestrogen/progestogen regimes, 462
    receptors, 137
Prolactin, 140
    endocrine rhythms, 131
    and GnRH secretion, 204
    hyperprolactinaemia, 219
    premenstrual syndrome, 394
Prolactinomas, 693
Prolapse, pelvic organ see Pelvic organ prolapse (POP)
Propiverine, 824–825, 829
Prostaglandin synthetase inhibitors (PGSIs)
    abnormal menstrual bleeding, 460
    dysmenorrhoea, 456, 467
    endometriosis, 501
    overactive bladder (OAB) syndrome, 826
Prostaglandins
    endometriosis, 491
    idiopathic (primary) dysmenorrhoea, 455–456
    and matrix metalloproteinases, 272
    ovarian steroid synthesis, control, 151
    sexual problems, 926
    vasoconstriction, 451
    voiding difficulties, 844

Prostanoids, endometriosis, 491
Prostheses, joint, 52
Prostitution management, 1005–1006
Protease inhibitors, 979–980
Protein binding, 548
Protein kinase A (PKA), 146–147
Protein kinase C (PKC), 136, 559
Proton beam radiotherapy, 539
Proto-oncogenes, 523
Protoscopy, 909
Psammocarcinoma, 680
Pseudoangiomatous stromal hyperplasia (PASH), of breast, 697
Pseudohamartoma, benign breast disease, 698
Pseudolipoma, benign breast disease, 698, 701–702
Pseudomyxoma peritonei, 674
Psoas hitch procedure, 109, 111f
Psychodynamic treatment methods, sexual problems, 445–446
Psychological factors
    abortion, 437
    Emergency Gynaecological Unit, 82
    hirsutism, 386
    miscarriage, 342
    polycystic ovary syndrome, 258
    voiding difficulties, 840–841
    vulval cancer, 620
Psychological interventions, premenstrual syndrome, 395
Psychological support/quality of life, congenital adrenal hyperplasia, 171
Psychosexual therapy, 440, 443
Psychosomatic circle of sex, 441
Pubertal development, 182–187
    breasts, 689
    corpus, changes to, 5
    and delayed puberty, 191
    labia minora, 6
    menarche, 187
    ovarian and uterine, 187
    precocious puberty, 187–189
    tempo of, 183–187
    vagina, 5
Puberty disorders, 182–196
    androgen receptor blockade, 189
    congenital adrenal hyperplasia, 188
    congenital anomalies of genital tract see under Female genital tract
    delayed puberty see Delayed puberty
    gynaecological complaints, 193–194
    inhibition of puberty, 189
    McCune–Albright syndrome, 189
    peripheral tumours, 188–189
    precocious puberty, 187–189
    premature adrenarche, 188
    premature thelarche, 188
    thelarche, 188
Pubic hair development, 184–185, 185f–186f
Puborectalis muscle
    and anorectal angle, 779
    and external anal sphincter, 776–778
Pudendal nerve, 14, 781
    terminal motor latencies, 908
Puerperal mastitis, 698–700
Puerperium, pelvic floor dysfunction, 923–924

Pulmonary complications, postoperative care, 125
Pulmonary embolism
  definitive diagnosis, 122
  diagnosis, 122
  incidence, 99
  screening for, 122
Pulmonary endometriosis, 499
Pulsatile gonadotrophin-releasing hormone, ovulation induction, 239–240
Purpura, 995
Pyelonephritis, 903
Pyoderma gangrenosum, 606
Pyometra
  endometrial cancer, 637
  hysteroscopy complications, 33
Pyrexia, postoperative care, 121–122
Pyridium pad test, 801
Pyridoxine, premenstrual syndrome, 395–397

Q

Quality of life
  changing focus of need, 752–753
  defined
  effects of gynaecological cancer, 751–752
  goals to achieve, 752–754
  healthcare professionals, requirements for, 753–754
  and HRT, 412
  incontinence, 784
  needs assessment, 752
  pelvic pain, impact on, 933
  polycystic ovary syndrome, 258
Queen Square bladder stimulator, voiding difficulties, 845
Quinacrine pellet, sterilization, 431
Quinagolide, 238
Quinolone, 901–902

R

RAD001 (everolimus), 559
Radial arteries, 448–449
Radiation
  fistulae, 878
  laser physics, 53
  primary angiosarcoma of breast, induced by, 716
Radiation cystitis, 870
Radiobiology, 539–540
Radiology
  bladder neck position, 791
  computerized tomography urogram, 789
  general, 789
  intravenous urography, 789
  micturating cystogram, 791
  postmicturition urine estimation, 791
  ultrasound, 791, 791f
    bladder neck position, 791
    perineal
    postmicturition urine estimation, 791
    transvaginal see Transvaginal ultrasonography (TVUS)
    urethral
  videocystourethrography, 790–791, 790f
Radiology, interventional, 81
Radionuclide imaging, 61–62, 62f

Radiotherapy
  accelerated, 540–541
  adjuvant, 594
  axillary, 725
  brachytherapy see Brachytherapy
  breast cancer, 716, 724–725
  cerebral metastases, 662
  cervical cancer, 592–595
  concomitant chemoradiation, 540
  conformal, 541–542, 542f
  conventional, 543
  dose prescription, 541
  electromagnetic radiation, 539
  emergency and palliative, 594
  endometrial cancer, 640–644, 640t, 642f–644f
  external beam, 541–543, 592
  fractionated, 540
  hyperfractionation, 540–541
  hypofractionation, 540–541, 725
  intensity-modulated, 543
  and miscarriage, 339
  normal tissue tolerance, 540
  palliative, 541
  particulate radiation, 539
  planning/planning procedures, 541, 542f
  primary, 592–594
  proton beam, 539
  radiation dose and scheduling, 540–541
  radiation morbidity, 547, 548t
  radiation physics, 539
  radiobiology, 539–540
  radionucleides used in gynaecological malignancies, 544
  secondary premature ovarian failure, 418
  simulator-based planning, 541
  techniques, 541
  vaginal cancer, 624
  virtual simulation, 542
  vulval cancer, 620–621
Radium-226, 544
Raloxifene, 414, 727
Randomized controlled trials
  breast cancer treatment, 726
  cervical cancer, 592
  endometrial cancer, 641
  evidence-based medicine, 1020, 1021t
  mastalgia, 694
  ovulation induction, 238
  pelvic inflammatory disease, 951–952
RANKL, 414
Rapamycin, 558, 728
RASSF1A, growth factor receptors, 531–532
Receptor assays, 138
Receptor-mediated endocytosis, 132, 134f
Recombinant follicle-stimulating hormone, 240
Recombinant human chorionic gonadotrophin, 240–241
Recombinant luteinizing hormone, 240
Reconstructive surgery
  breast cancer, 736b, 737
  nipple-areola reconstruction, 735, 737
  oncoplastic techniques, 736b, 737
  tubal disease, 356
Rectal compliance, 780
Rectal irrigation, 912

Rectal prolapse surgery, faecal incontinence, 914–915
Rectoanal inhibitory reflex (RAIR), 779–780
Rectopexy, 914–915
Rectosigmoidoscopy, cervical cancer, 584
Rectosphincteric reflex (RAIR), 779–780
Rectum
  anal canal, 9
  anatomy/anatomical relations, 8–9, 9f
  dynamic imaging, 908
  palpation of, haemorrhoids, 909
  structure, 9
Recurrent implantation failure (RIF), 288
5α-Reductase deficiency, androgen insensitivity, 173
ReeTrakt retractor, POP surgery, 857
Regenerative medicine, 275
Rehabilitation, 753
Remonabant, 243
Renal failure, cervical cancer, 595
Reproductive cloning, 274–275
Reproductive dysfunction, 212–230
  amenorrhoea see Amenorrhoea
  chemotherapy effects, 552
  contraceptive advice, 226–227
  definitions, 212–213
  fertility issues, 226
  management of hyperprolactinaemia, 225–226
  metabolic causes, 218
  oestrogen deficiency, 225
  oligomenorrhoea see Oligomenorrhoea
  therapeutic issues, 225–226
  see also Female reproductive disorders; Male reproductive disorders
Resiniferatoxin, 827
Respiratory failure, gestational trophoblastic tumours, 662
Respiratory infections, antibiotic prophylaxis, 101
Resuscitation equipment, ultrasound, 81
Retained products of conception, 85–86
Retinoblastoma, 524
Retrograde pyelography, fistulae, 882
Retroperitoneal lymph node sampling, ovarian cancer, 682
Retroversion/retroflexion, uterus, 4–5
Retroviruses, oncogenes, 523
Rhadbomyosarcoma (sarcoma botryoides), 624
Rhesus-D-negative women, anti-D immunoglobulin use, 82
Ringer's lactate solution, 356
Risedronate, 413
Risk assessment, preoperative, 97–99
  allergic patients, 97
  day surgery suitability, 97
  obese patients, 97–99
  purpose, 97
Risk of malignancy index (RMI)
  ovarian cancer, 682
  ovarian cysts, 670–671
Risk-reducing mastectomy (RRM), breast cancer, 712
Robertsonian translocations, parental chromosomal abnormalities, 342–343

Robotic techniques
  laparoscopy, 44
  pelvic organ prolapse, 859–860
Rokitansky syndrome, 175, 192
Rosiglitazone, 239
Royal College of Obstetricians and
    Gynaecologists
  on evidence-based care, 1017–1019
  oral contraception advice, 103
Rubber band ligation, haemorrhoids, 910
Rubella infection, 337–338
Rutherford-Morrison incision, abdominal
    procedures, 106

S

Sacral nerve stimulation
  faecal incontinence, 912–913, 914f
  voiding difficulties, 844–845
Sacral neuromodulation, overactive bladder
    syndrome, 828–829
Sacral reflexes, 794
Sacrocolpopexy, abdominal, apical prolapse,
    857–858
Sacrospinous ligament suspension, apical
    prolapse, 858
Safe sex, 951
Sagittal plane, 74
Saline distension medium, bipolar diathermy,
    50
Salpingectomy
  chronic pelvic inflammatory disease, 935
  ectopic pregnancy, 371–372
Salpingitis, 353–354
Salpingitis isthmica nodosa (SIN), 365
Salpingoscopy, tubal disease, 355
Salpingostomy, 360
Salpingotomy, linear, 372–373
Salt-losing crisis, acute (21-hydroxylase
    deficiency), 170–171
Sampling
  endometrial, 23, 459
  forensic, 992–993
  lymph node, 584
  ovarian cancer, 682
Sarcomas
  endometrial cancer, 633–634, 634f,
    645–646
  vulval cancer, 623
Saucerization technique, fistulae, 889–890
Scabies, 977–978
Scanning electron microscopy (SEM), 898f
Schwann cells, granular cell tumour, 702
Sciatic nerve, 14
Sclerosing adenosis, 695–696
Sclerosing stromal tumours, 676
Screening
  abnormal vaginal bleeding, 90
  breast cancer, 712, 716–717
    lesbian and bisexual women, 1012
  cervical cancer, 513, 1011–1012
  endometrial cancer, 638
  endometrial premalignancy, 578
  familial cancers, 528–529
  fertilization/assisted reproduction
    treatments, 273, 329
  forensic gynaecology, 993–994
  hepatitis, 993–994

hereditary non-polyposis colorectal cancer,
    529
  molecular biology, 156–157, 157t
  ovarian cancer, 517
  pelvic inflammatory disease, 951–952
  pulmonary embolism, 122
  sexually transmitted infections, 956–957
Sebaceous cysts, breast, 703
Seborrhoeic keratosis, 608
Second messenger pathways, hormone
    receptors, 135–136
Secondary vulval vestibulitis, 932
Second-look surgery (SLL), ovarian
    cancer, 683
Segmental resection, ectopic pregnancy, 373
Selective serotonin reuptake inhibitors
    (SSRIs)
  menopausal symptoms, 412
  premature ejaculation, 445
  premenstrual syndrome, 394, 399–400,
    401t
  sexual problems, 443
  see also Antidepressants
Selective transcervical salpingography,
    355–356, 359
Self-image, and sexual problems, 442
Self-priming, 206–207, 207f
Semen
  additional diagnostic tests, 305
  analysis of, 303–305
  antisperm antibodies, 304
  changing quality, 309–310
  idiopathic impairment of quality, 301–302
  microscopic evaluation, 304
  morphology, 304
  motility, 304
  sample collection/delivery, 304
  sperm concentration, 304
Semen analysis, 304
Seminal fluid allergy, 609–610
Sentinel lymph nodes
  cervical cancer, 592
  lymphatic drainage, 614
  vulval cancer, 617
Sepsis, 340, 982
Septrin, 983–984
Serotonergic system, premenstrual syndrome,
    394
Serotonin, and GnRH secretion, 203
Serotonin and noradrenaline reuptake
    inhibitors, menopausal symptoms, 412
Serous carcinoma, ovarian cancer, 680–681
Serous coat, uterus, 448
Serous tumours, benign, 674
Sertoli cell function, 293–294
Sertoli cells, 141, 166–168
Sertoli-Leydig tumours, 675–676
Sertraline, 931
70-gene prognostic signature, breast cancer,
    730–731
76-gene prognostic signature, breast cancer,
    731
Sex chromosome anomalies, 168, 168b
Sex cord stromal tumours, benign, 675–676
Sex steroids, 306
Sex-hormone-binding globulin (SHBG), 131,
    183, 254
Sex-steroid-secreting tumours, 188–189

Sexual activity, prevention of STIs, 950–951
Sexual arousal disorder, 920
Sexual assault
  abrasions, 995
  adolescent victims of, 997–998
  alcohol- and drug-facilitated, 994–995
  attrition, 989
  bruises, 995
  conviction rates, 988
  definition of intimate violence, 988
  on disabled women, 998
  escalating epidemic of rape, 988
  examination of complainant, 990
  expert witnesses in, 999–1000
  fracture, 996
  haematoma, 995
  HIV and hepatitis screening following,
    993–994
  Home Office cross-government action plan
    on, 988
  incisions, 995
  injuries
    clinical injury extent scoring, 994
    genital, 994
    non-genital, 994, 996
    patterns of, 997–998
    photographs, 993
  lacerations, 995
  legal aspects, 988–989
  mental health problems, 998
  migrant women, 998
  organ rupture, 996
  petechiae, 995
  postmenopausal women, 997
  purpura, 995
  reasons for failure to report, 989
  Sexual Assault Referral Centres, 989–991
  stab wounds, 995–996
  terminology, 988
  thermal injury, 996
  training in sexual assault examination,
    990–991
  trauma, 609
  vulnerable women, 998
  in war, 1006–1007
  see also Forensic gynaecology
Sexual Assault Referral Centres (SARCs),
    989–991
Sexual differentiation, 166–181
  anomalous vaginal development
    aetiology, 174
    classification, 174
    complications of, 177
    epidemiology, 174
    investigation, 175–176
    lateral fusion disorders, 174–177, 175f
    pathophysiology, 174
    presentation, 174–175
    transverse vaginal septum, 176
    treatment, 176–177
    vertical fusion defects, 174–175, 175f,
      177
  46XY sexual development disorders,
    172–174
    3β-hydroxysteroid dehyogenase
      deficiency, 173
    17, 20 desmolase deficiency, 173
    17α-hydroxylase deficiency, 173

17-ketosteroid reductase deficiency, 173
20, 22 desmolase deficiency, 173
46XX sex reversal, 172–173
46XY true hermaphroditism, 172
  androgen insensitivity at target site,
    173–174, 173t
  errors in testosterone biosynthesis, 173
  failure of testicular development, 172
intersex disorders
  androgen-secreting tumours, 171
  associated multiple congenital
    abnormalities, 172
  congenital adrenal hyperplasia see
    Congenital adrenal hyperplasia (CAH)
  drugs, 172
  female (46XX), 169
normal embryological development of
    reproductive system, 166–168, 167f
  ovary, 166
  sex chromosome anomalies, 168, 168b
  testis, 166
sex chromosome anomalies, 168, 168b
Sexual Offences Act (SOA) 2003 (UK),
    988–989
Sexual orientation, 441
Sexual problems, 440–447, 919–928
  aversion disorder, 920
  behavioural treatment methods, 446
  combined genital and subjective arousal
    disorder, 920
  conditions affecting female sexual function
  definitions of sexual dysfunction, 441–442
  drug treatments, 446
  evaluation, 924–925
  expression of sexuality, 919
  in female
    definition of female sexual dysfunction,
      919–920, 920b
    dyspareunia, 444
    female sexual response cycle, 920f, 922f
    gynaecological cancer-related see below
    inorgasmia, 443
    lesbian and bisexual women, 444
    libido loss, 443
    pelvic floor dysfunction, 920–921
    research into female sexuality, 919
    with urogynaecological problems,
      prevalence, 920
    vaginismus, 442–443
  function or desire, problems of, 442
  genital sexual arousal disorder, 920
  gynaecological cancer-related
    background, 754
    behavioural therapy, 756
    effects of cancer, 754–755
    information requirements, 755
    intervention, 755–756
    intervention goal, 755
    listening and asking, 755
    preserving sexual identity, 756
  gynaecology, relevant to, 442
  laboratory testing, 925
  libido loss
    in female, 443
    in male, 445
  in male
    delayed ejaculation, 445
    erectile dysfunction, 444–445

    libido loss, 445
    premature ejaculation, 445
  menopause, 407
  orgasmic disorder, 920
  pelvic floor dysfunction, 920–922
  pelvic organ prolapse, 853
  persistent sexual arousal disorder, 920
  physical examination, 925
  P-LI-SS-IT model, 756b
  population prevalence, 441
  prevalence, 919
  psychodynamic treatment methods,
    445–446
  role of gynaecologist, 440
  service provision, 446
  sexual interest/desire disorder, 442, 920
  sexual pain disorders, 920
  see also Dyspareunia; Vaginismus
  specialized diagnostic testing, 925
  subjective sexual arousal disorder, 920
  treatment, 445–446, 925–926, 926f
  vaginal dryness, 444, 925–926
  WHO on sexual health, 754
Sexual response, 441
Sexuality, human, 440–441
Sexually transmitted infections (STIs), 952
  chancroid, 965
  chlamydia see Chlamydia
  clinical presentations, 958
  condom use, 961
  ectoparasitic infestations, Pediculosis pubis,
    976–977, 977f
  epidemiology, 956–957
  examination, 958
  excluding HIV, 955–978
  forensic gynaecology, 993
  genital herpes see Genital herpes
  genital warts see Genital warts
  gonorrhoea see Gonorrhoea
  granuloma inguinale, 965–966, 966f
  hepatitis, viral see Hepatitis, viral
  history, 957–958
  lesbian and bisexual women, 1012
  lymphogranuloma venereum see
    Lymphogranuloma venereum
  management principles, 957–958
  molluscum contagiosum, 971
  mycoplasma genitalium, 968–969
  prevalence, 955
  prevention, 950–951
  recommendations for at-risk groups,
    956–957
  recommendations for patients with, 957
  salpingitis, 354
  scabies, 977–978
  screening, 956–957
  specialist clinic tests, 958
  swabs, 958
  syphilis see Syphilis
  tubal factor infertility, 283
  ureaplasma urealyticum, 968–969
  vaginal see Vaginal infections
  see also Human immunodeficiency
    syndrome (HIV)
SH2/SH3 domains, tyrosine kinase hormone
    receptors, 135
Short Form-36 (SF-36) pain questionnaire,
    931

Short-wave diathermy, 50
Sibutramine, 243
Side-effects of treatment, ovulation induction,
    238–239
Sigmoid colon
  anatomy/anatomical relations, 8
  insulation failure, diathermy, 51
  structure, 8
Sigmoidoscopy, fistulae, 885
Signet ring stromal tumours, 676–677
Significance Analysis of Microarrays (SAM),
    158
Sildenafil (Viagra), 306, 443, 926
Silicone granulomas, 701
Sim's speculum, pelvic organ prolapse,
    853–854
Simulators, laparoscopy training, 41
Simvastatin, 870
Sinography, 884
Sjogren's syndrome, 610
Skene's tubules, urethra, 8
Skin, chemotherapy effects, 552
Skin tags, 608
Small bowel
  leak, 125
  repair of, 112f
Smoking cessation
  preoperative care, 102
  see also Cigarette smoking
SNB use, breast cancer, 723–724
Socioeconomic status, breast cancer risk, 710
Sodium, premenstrual syndrome, 394
Sodium picosulphate (Picolax), 886
Solifenacin, 823, 829
Solitary rectal ulcer syndrome, 915
Somatic nerves, 13–14
Somatic-cell nuclear transfer (SCNT),
    273–275
Sonohysterography, 85–86, 459
Sonohysteroscopy, 480
Sorafenib, 556
SOX9 gene, 167–168
Spectinomycin, 967
Sperm granulomas, 433
Spermatogenesis, 292–293
  hormonal control, 294–297
Spermatozoon, 295–296
Spermicides, 984
Sperm/spermatozoa
  antisperm antibodies, 304, 306, 433
  concentration, 304
  electron microscopy picture, 266f
  epididymal, with ICSI, 308
  testicular, with ICSI, 308–309
  transport/maturation, 296–297
  see also Semen
Sphincterotomy, anal fissures, 911
Spiral arterioles, 448–449
Spironolactone, 260, 388, 400
Squamous cell carcinomas, 587, 604
Squamous metaplasia, 871
Squamous papillomata, 608
Src (non-receptor tyrosine kinase), 559–560
SSRIs see Selective serotonin reuptake
    inhibitors (SSRIs)
St John's Wort, 397, 417
Stab wounds, 995–996
Staff pain, 751

Staging of cancers *see under individual cancers*
Standardized uptake value (SUV), 62
Stanols, 415
Staphylococcus aureus, 100, 698–699
Staphylococcus saprophyticus, 866, 897
Stapling, laparoscopy, 41–42, 42f–43f
START (short-term antiretroviral therapy), 983
Stem cell technology, 273–275
Stem cell transplantation, 662
Sterilization
  clips, 430
  Collaborative Review, 431
  complications of
    female sterilization, 431–432
    vasectomy, 432–433
  counselling for, 431
  efficacy, 431
  electrocautery, 430
  Essure system, 31, 31f
  falope ring, 430
  female, 430–432
  and HIV, 984
  hysteroscopic, 31, 31f
  laser, 430–431
  ligation, 430
  previous tubal surgery, 364
  reversal, 364, 431
  success of reversal, 360
  vasectomy *see* Vasectomy
  see also Abortion; Contraception/
    contraceptive advice
Steroid hormones
  biosynthesis, 145–155
  classification, 145, 146f, 147t, 148f
  definitions, 145
  origins and intracellular transport of
    cholesterol, 145–147
  ovarian function and menopause, 406
  ovarian steroid synthesis, control, 150–151
  physiology, 145–149
  regulation of steroid synthesis, 149–152
  steroidogenic enzymes, 147–149
  see also Hormones
Steroid synthesis
  defects, 152–154
  regulation, 149–152, 150f
Steroidogenesis, 145
Steroidogenic acute regulatory (StAR) protein, 146–147
Steroids, 128–129, 130f, 170f
Stevens-Johnson syndrome, 606
STIs *see* Sexually transmitted infections (STIs)
Stoma, faecal incontinence, 914
Streptococcus pyogenes, antibiotic prophylaxis, 100
Stress incontinence, 768–769, 798–812
  aetiology, 799–800
  assessment, 800
  bladder neck sling procedures, 807–809, 808f
  Burch colposuspension, 804–805, 806f
  conservative treatment, 802–803
  cough stress test, 801
  DIAPERS mnemonic, 799
  epidemiology, 798–799
  evidence-based practice, importance, 803–804

examination, 800–801
  genuine, 768
  investigations
    pad tests, 801
    urodynamics, 801–802
  minitape procedures, 807, 807f
  Modified Oxford System, 801, 804b
  obesity, 800
  origin of term, 767–768
  pad tests, 801
  pathophysiology, 799
  pelvic floor muscle training, 802–803
  pelvic organ prolapse, 852–855
  periurethral injection therapy, 809–810, 809f
  pharmacotherapy, 803
  postfistula treatment, 892
  pyridium pad test, 801
  and sexual dysfunction, 929
  sign, 798
  surgical treatment, 803–810
    bladder neck sling procedures, 807–809, 808f
    Burch colposuspension, 804–805, 805f–806f
    evidence-based practice, importance, 803–804
    minitape procedures, 807
    periurethral injection therapy, 809–810
    tension-free vaginal tape procedure *see*
      Tension-free vaginal tape procedure *below*
    transobturator tape procedure, 806, 807f
    urethral bulking agents, 809–810, 809f
  symptom questionnaires, 800
  tension-free vaginal tape procedure, 805–806, 807f
  transobturator tape procedure, 806, 807f
  terminology, 798
  terminology and definitions, 798, 799b
  urethral bulking agents, 798, 809–810
  urodynamic, 768–769
  urodynamics, 801–802
  voiding difficulties caused by surgery for, 838–839
  see also Stress incontinence; Urethral
    sphincter incompetence; Urinary
    incontinence
Stroke
  combined hormonal contraceptives, 425
  and HRT, 411–412
Stromal cell tumour, minor sex cord elements, 676
Strontium ranelate, 413–414
Stuart's transport medium, 958
Sublingual apomorphine, 926
Submucosal fibroids, 475, 483–484
Subserosal fibroids, 475
Substance abuse, 1003, 1006
Suction drains, 118
Sulphasalazine, 306, 870
Sunitinib, 556, 728
Surgical clothing, diathermy treatment, 51
Surgical injury, 105
  bladder, 8
  bowel
    delayed presentation of injury, 124
    faecal fistula, 125

incidence, 124
    intraoperative detection of injury, 124
    large bowel leak, 124–125
    management, 125
    minor laceration, 124
    obstruction, 124
    paralytic ileus, 124
    small bowel leak, 125
    Veress needle puncture, 124
  ureter, 7
  urinary tract
    bladder, 123
    ureter, 123–124
    vaginal wall, 875–876
  see also Complications; Postoperative care
Suturing
  fistulae, 889
  laparoscopic, 41, 43f, 114
  pre-tied sutures, 41
'Swiss cheese disease', 693–694
Synacthen test, late-onset congenital adrenal hyperplasia, 385
Syntocinon, 341
Syphilis, 961–964
  aetiology, 962
  clinical features, 962–963
  diagnosis, 963
  guidelines, 964b
  and HIV, 982
  late sequelae, 963
  latent, 962
  management, 963–964
  and miscarriage, 338, 344
  primary, 962, 962f
  secondary, 962, 962f
  swabs, 963
Systemic antiandrogen therapy, hirsutism, 387–388

T

T. pallidum venereum, 962, 965
T. vaginalis, 608, 958, 975
Taeniae coli, rectum, 9
Tamoxifen
  breast cancer, 712, 725–726
  dysmenorrhoea, 456
  endometrial cancer risk, 515, 630, 638
  mastalgia, 694
  ovulation induction, 237
  side-effects, 552
Taq polymerase, 159
Taqman chemistry, 160
Tarceva, 557
Targeted Intraoperative Radiotherapy Trial (TARGIT), 725
Taxanes, chemotherapy, 551–552, 560, 661, 716
Taxol, 551, 661, 684
T-cells, HIV, 979
Teenage Pregnancy Independent Advisory Group, 433
Telescopes, rigid or flexible, (hysteroscopy), 19–22, 23f
Teletherapy (external beam radiotherapy), 541–543
  brachytherapy compared, 544
  cervical cancer, 592

vaginal cancer, 624
vaginal vault brachytherapy following, 545
Telomeric shortening, 551
Temozolomide, chemotherapy, 661
Temsirolismus, 728
Tension-free vaginal tape procedure (TVT)
    urethral sphincter incompetence, 805–806,
        807f
    voiding difficulties, 845–846
Teratozoospermia, 302
Terminal illness
    'bad news', breaking see 'Bad news',
        breaking
    bereavement, 763–764
    common symptoms in last 48 hours of life,
        763b
    needs of dying woman, 763
    recurrence of disease and cessation of
        therapy see under Gynaecological
        cancers
    sources of support, 764
Testicular biopsy, 305
Testicular cancer, 309
Testicular development, 46XY disorders, 172
Testicular-determining factor (TDF), 167–168
Testis, development, 166
Testosterone, 141, 173, 406
Testosterone replacement therapy, 925–926
Tetracycline, 700
Tetralodotyronine (T4), 140
Theca cell tumours, 676
Thecafibromas, 676
Thecomas/thecoma-fibroma tumour group,
        675
    fibroma, 676
    sclerosing stromal tumours, 676
    signet ring stromal tumours, 676–677
    stromal cell tumour, minor sex cord
        elements, 676
    theca cell tumours, 676
Thelarche, 188
Therapeutic cloning, 274–275
Thermal balloon ablation, 29, 463
Thermal injury, 996
Thiazolidinedione hypoglycaemic drugs, 239
Thoracic endometriosis, 499
Threadworms, 608
Thrombocytopenia, 551–552
Thrombocytopenic purpura, 455
Thromboprophylaxis, preoperative
        preparation, 99–100
Thrombosis see Venous thrombosis/
        thromboembolism
Thyroid disease, 457–458
Thyroid hormones/thyroid-stimulating
        hormone (TSH), 140
    and beta-human chorionic gonadotrophin
        assays, 654
    peptide hormones, 128
    tissue distribution, 131
Thyrotoxicosis, 669
Tiaprofenic acid, 870
Tibolone, 409, 412
Tinea cruris, 606
TLK-286, ovarian cancer, 561
Toll-like receptor (TLR) family, 899
Tolterodine, 821–823, 829
Topoisomarase inhibitors, 551

Topotecan, 551, 661
Torsion, ovarian cysts, 668–669
Total pain, 761
Toxic shock syndrome, 609
TP53 gene mutations, vulval cancer, 534–535
Trabectedin, 560–561
Trachelectomy
    cervical cancer, 588
    and maternal age at childbirth, 591–592
    procedure/technique, 591
    radical vaginal
        follow-up, 592
        outcome following, 591–592
        selection criteria, 591
Trancervical resection of the endometrium
        (TCRE), 26–28, 30
Transcutaneous electrical nerve stimulation
        (TENS), 938
Transforming growth factor-beta (TGF-β),
        450–451
Transitional cell tumours, 675
Translabial pelvic floor ultrasound, 850f
Translocator protein (TSPO), 146–147
Transobturator tape (TOT) procedure
    and sexual dysfunction, 930
    urethral sphincter incompetence, 806, 807f
    voiding difficulties, 839, 845–846
Transperineal ultrasound (TPUS), pelvic
        organ prolapse, 855
Transsexuality, 440–441
Transvaginal ultrasonography (TVUS)/
        transvaginal hydrolaparoscopy, 355
Transvaginal ultrasonography (TVUS)/
        transvaginal ultrasound (TVS), 791
    ectopic pregnancy, 369
    endometrial hyperplasia, 579
    as extension of bimanual examination, 82
    high-resolution, 82–83
    infertility, 65
    as non-invasive procedure, 81
    pelvic inflammatory disease, 946–947
    three-dimensional, 253f
    uterine leiomyomas, 88
    value of, 80–83, 85–86
Transverse colon, laparoscopic damage to, 40
Trastuzumab, breast cancer, 727–728
    metastatic, 732
Treitz's muscle, haemorrhoids, 909
Trendelenberg position, laparoscopy, 37, 45
Treosulfan, 549
Trichloroacetic acid (TCA), 969–970
Trichomoniasis
    aetiology and clinical features, 975–976,
        976f
    diagnosis, 975–976
    management and treatment, 976
Tricyclic antidepressants, 825, 869–870, 917
Trigone, bladder, 7–8, 109
Trimethoprim, 901–902
Triodothyronine (T3), 140
Triploidy, 651
Tripolar instruments, bipolar diathermy, 50
Trisomies, 336
Trocars, laparoscopy, 37–38, 37f
Troglitazone, 239
Trophinin, 271f
Trophoblastic tumours, miscarriage, 340

Trospium chloride, 823, 829
Tryptophan, 128
Tubal anastomosis, 356–357
Tubal blood mole, 366
Tubal disease, 353–362
    aetiology, 353–354
    assessment of tubal function, 360–361
    diagnosis, 354–355
    infertility see Tubal factor infertility
    proximal, 359–360
    reconstructive surgery, 356
    results of treatment, 359–360
    salpingitis, 353–354
    treatment
        adhesions, 358–359
        coadjuvants, 356
        cornual occlusion, 356
        cornual polyps, removal, 356
        hydrosalpinges, 357–358
        laparoscopic surgery, 359
        microsurgical, 356–359
        reconstructive tubal surgery, 356
        selective transcervical salpingography,
            356
        tubal anastomosis, 356–357
Tubal factor infertility, 283–287
    diagnostic tests, evaluation, 285–287
    endometriosis, 287–288
    fibroids, 288
    hysterosalpingo contrast sonography, 285,
        285t, 287
    hysteroscopy, 285
    laparoscopy and dye hydrotubation,
        283–285
    potential endometrial abnormalities, 288
    X-ray hysterosalpingography, 283–287,
        283f
    see also Tubal disease
Tubal pathology, ultrasound, 88
Tubal pregnancy
    complete miscarriage, 366
    image of, 85f
    incomplete miscarriage, 366
    natural progression, 365–366
    previous, 364
    rupture, 365–366
    spontaneous involution, 366
    time of rupture at various sites, 366
    unruptured, 365
    see also Ectopic pregnancy
Tubal reconstruction and repair, 364
Tubal surgery, previous, 364
Tuberculosis of breast, 701
Tubular adenoma, 701
Tubular adenosis, 695–696
Tumour markers, 654–655, 670
    see also CA125 serum markers
Tumour suppressor genes, 524–525, 525f,
        532
Tumour vascular proteins, 679
Tumours
    androgen-secreting
        intersex disorders, 171
        ovarian cysts, 675–676
    gonadotrophin-secreting, 189
    granular cell see Granular cell tumour
    granulosa cell, 670, 675
    multicentric, 713

multifocal, 713
ovarian subtypes, 679–681
see also Ovarian cancer; Ovarian cysts
parenchymal, 900
Phyllodes tumour of breast, 691–692
sex-steroid-secreting, 188–189
trophoblastic, in miscarriage, 340
urothelial, 871, 900
see also Cancers
Tunica albuginea, 1, 166
Turner's syndrome, 168, 190–191
   amenorrhoea, 216
   chromosome abnormalities, 418
   ovarian failure, 283
   and partial hydatidiform mole, 651
   premature ovarian failure, 220–221
TVT procedure *see* Tension-free vaginal tape
   procedure (TVT)
Twin pregnancies, 650–652, 655, 658
Twin-twin transfusion syndrome, 56
Tyrer-Cuzick model, breast cancer risk,
   711–712
Tyrosine derivatives, 128
Tyrosine kinase hormone receptors, 135

U

Ulcerative colitis, 878
Ultrasound
   amenorrhoea
   analgesia, 81
   bladder, 117
   breast cancer, 718, 719f
   cervical pregnancy, 376
   chronic pelvic pain, 934
   clinical conditions, 83–90
      acute bleeding and negative pregnancy
         test, 89–90
      acute urinary retention, 88
      adnexal pathology, 87
      bleeding and/or pain with positive
         pregnancy test, 83
      coexistent pathology, 85
      ectopic pregnancy, 84–85
      endometriosis, 87
      miscarriage, 83–85
      non-gynaecological pathology, 89
      pain with mass, 87, 88f
      pelvic pain and negative pregnancy test,
         86
      in postmenopausal patient, 89–90
      postnatal assessment, 85–86
      pregnancy of unknown location, 85, 86f
      in premenopausal patient, 86–90
      terminology, 83–84
      tubal pathology, 88
      uterine leiomyomas, 88
   computer database systems, 81
   Doppler *see* Doppler ultrasound
   echoes, 59
   ectopic pregnancy, 369–370
   Emergency Gynaecological Unit, 81–82
   endometriosis, 499–500, 499f
   fibroids, 479–480
   fistulae, 884
   follicle tracking, 281–282
   frequency choice, 59–60
   high-frequency, 718

infection transmission, reduction
   of risk, 81
interactivity of, 60
interventional radiology, acute
   gynaecology, 81
intestinal tract disease, 908–909
lactogenesis, 697
machinery, 81
menstrual abnormalities, 458–459
and miscarriage, 343
ovarian and uterine development, 187
ovarian cancer, 75, 682
ovarian cyst aspiration, ultrasound-
   guided, 81
ovarian cysts, 668, 670
   ultrasound-guided diagnostic aspiration,
   671
perineal, 791–792
postmicturition urine estimation, 791
radiology, 791, 791f
resources for services, 81
resuscitation equipment, 81
role, 80–92
techniques, 59–60, 60f
three-dimensional ultrasonography
   ectopic pregnancy, 369–370
   polycystic ovary syndrome (PCOS), 253f
transvaginal *see* Transvaginal
   ultrasonography (TVUS)/transvaginal
   ultrasound (TVS)
urethral, 792
urinary tract infections, 900–901
Ultraviolet lasers, 56
Undescended testis, 299
Unexplained infertility, 288–289, 360–361
Unstable bladder, 768
Ureaplasma urealyticum, 968–969
Ureter
   anastomosis, 109
   anatomy/anatomical relations, 5, 7, 107
   damage to, 107–109
   divided, 109f
   duplex
   lower, 107–108
   at pelvic brim/ovarian fossa, 107
   postoperative complications, 123–124
   reimplantation, 110f
   relations and course, 7
   repairing, 108–109
   structure, 7
   surgical injury, 7
   ureteric tunnel, 1
Urethra
   anatomy/anatomical relations, 8, 771
   extrinsic striated muscles, 774
   hermetic seal, 774
   innervation, 772–774
   intrinsic smooth and striated muscles, 774
   structure, 8
   urethral support, 775
   urinary incontinence, mechanism, 774–775
   see also Urinary incontinence
Urethral diverticulum, 871–872
Urethral function investigations, 792–793
Urethral pain syndrome, 865
Urethral pressure measurement, 792–793
Urethral sphincter incompetence *see* Stress
   incontinence

Urethral syndrome, 872
Urethral ultrasound, 792
Urge incontinence, 815–816, 912
Urinalysis, 88–89, 900
Urinary diary, 784–785, 866
Urinary diversion, 829, 845
Urinary fistulae, 769
Urinary follicle-stimulating hormone,
   240
Urinary human chorionic
   gonadotrophin, 240
Urinary human menopausal
   gonadotrophins, 240
Urinary incontinence, 771–776
   anatomy of lower urinary tract
      bladder, 771
      pelvic floor, 771–772, 772f
      urethra, 771
   bladder, anatomy, 771
   classification, 768f
   extraurethral conditions, 769
   fistulae, 876f
   innervation of bladder and urethra,
      772–774
   mechanism, 774–775, 777f
      bladder, 774
      urethra, 774–775
   menopause, 408
   normal micturition cycle
      filling and storage phase, 775
      initiation phase, 775
      voiding phase, 775–776
   pathophysiology, 776
   pelvic floor
      anatomy, 771–772
      dysfunction and sexual function,
         922–923
   pelvic organ prolapse, 852–853
   see also Pelvic organ prolapse (POP)
   striated muscle, innervation, 773
   surgery for, 803, 845, 929
   urethra, anatomy, 771
   urethral conditions, 768–769
   see also Faecal incontinence; Stress
      incontinence; Urethral sphincter
      incompetence
Urinary retention, 769
   acute, 88, 837
   chronic, 837
   genital herpes, 960
   herpes simplex, 607
   see also Voiding difficulties
Urinary tract
   endometriosis, 497–498
   infections *see* Urinary tract infections
   injuries, postoperative care, 123–124
   lower *see* Lower urinary tract disorders
   tuberculosis of, 904
Urinary tract infections, 896–906
   acute pylonephritis, 903
   antibiotic prophylaxis, 101
   antimicrobial therapy, 901–902
   asymptomatic bacteriuria, 903
   bacterial virulence factors, 897, 898f
   blood tests, 901
   catheter-associated, 903–904
   classification of urogynaecological
      disorders, 769

complicated, conditions associated with, 897, 897b
computed tomography, 901
cystitis *see* Cystitis
cystoscopy, 901
and fistulae, 882
functional abnormality, 897
future approaches, 902–903
general measures, 901
history and examination, 899–900
hospital-acquired, 897
host factors, 897–899
imaging studies, 900–901
intravenous urography, 900
investigations, 900–901
magnetic resonance imaging, 901
microbiology, 897
micturating cystogram, 901
natural history, 899
nuclear medicine scanning, 901
obstruction/structural, 897
pathogenesis, 897–899, 898f
physical signs, 899
plain abdominal radiograph, 900–901
presentation, 899
prevalence, 896
prevention, 902
recurrent, 837, 867, 896, 903
specific clinical situations, 903–904
terminology/definitions, 896–897
tuberculosis of urinary tract, 904
ultrasound, 900
urinalysis, 900
urine microscopy and culture, 900
urolithiasis, 904
vaginal oestrogen replacement, 410
see also Bladder disorders; Lower urinary tract disorders
Urine
midstream collection *see* Midstream urine (MSU), collection
monitoring of output, 117
Urine culture, overactive bladder (OAB) syndrome, 816
Urodynamics/urodynamic investigations, 783–797, 866–867
ambulatory monitoring, 788–789, 790f
cystometry, 786–788, 787f–789f
cystourethroscopy, 793–794, 868
electrophysiological tests, 794
leak point pressure, 793
midstream urine specimen, 784
pad test, 785
radiology *see* Radiology; Ultrasound
urethral function, 792–793
urethral sphincter incompetence, 801–802
urinary diary, 784–785, 866
urodynamic stress incontinence, 768–769
uroflowmetry, 785–786, 785f–786f
Uroflowmetry, 785–786
abnormal flow rates, 785–786, 786f
equipment, 785, 785f
indications, 785
measurements, 785
overactive bladder (OAB) syndrome, 817
voiding difficulties, 841–842
Urogenital atrophy, 408, 410
Urogenital diaphragm, 11, 11f

Urografin filling medium, 790
Urography, intravenous, 789, 900
Urogynaecological disorders, 767–770
bladder neuropathy, 769
classification, 768–769
bladder neuropathy, 769
congenital anomalies, 768
genital prolapse, 769
incontinence *see* Below
urgency and frequency, 769
urinary fistulae, 769
voiding difficulties, 769
congenital anomalies, 768
genital prolapse, 769
incontinence
extraurethral conditions, 769
urethral conditions, 768–769
terminology, 767–768
urgency and frequency, 769
urinary fistulae, 769
urinary tract infections, 769
see also Urinary tract infections
voiding difficulties, 769
Urokinase-type plasminogen activator (uPA), 451
Urolithiasis, 904
USPIO (ultrasmall particles of iron oxide), 71–72
Uterine artery, anatomy, 5, 13, 448–449
Uterine artery embolization
clinical outcomes, 485
complications of, 485
fibroids, 485–486
menstrual abnormalities, 466
MRI-focused, 485–486
technique, 485
Uterine cavity, assessment, 458–459
Uterine corpus, premalignancy *see* Endometrial premalignancy
Uterine leiomyomas, 88
Uterine perforation, hysteroscopy, 32
Uterine ultrasound (US), invasive hydatidiform mole, 651–652
Uterovesical pouch, bladder, 8
Uterus
with absent vagina, 177
age-related changes, 5
anatomy/anatomical relations, 3–5, 19f, 20, 448
anomalies, recurrent miscarriage, 343–344
anovulatory dysfunctional uterine bleeding, 454
bleeding, diagnostic indications, 17
blood supply, 448–449
cervix, 4
dysfunctional uterine bleeding, 453–454
fibroids *see* Fibroids
gravid, 669
histology, 449–450
hyperactivity, in dysmenorrhoea, 455
imaging of, 62–63, 63f
interior divisions, 4f
layers, 3
leiomyoma of, 476f
malformations
classification, 177–178, 178f
diethylstilboestrol exposure, 179
incidence, 178

infertility, primary, 178
investigations, 179
menstrual disorders, 178
pathophysiology, 177–178, 178f
pregnancy loss, recurrent, 178
presentation, 178
treatment, 179
urological abnormalities, 178
malignant disease *see* Endometrial cancer
non-functioning, with absent vagina, 176–177
ovulatory dysfunctional uterine bleeding, 454
perforation of and false passage, 114
position, 4–5
structure, 3–4
uterine natural killer cells, 272–273
see also Endometrial cancer; Menstrual cycle/menstruation; Pregnancy
UTIs *see* Urinary tract infections

V

Vabra curette, endometrial sampling, 459
Vaccines, cervical cancer, 513–514, 583
Vacuum aspiration, early abortion, 435
Vacuum-assisted mammotome, breast cancer, 721
Vagina
absent
with coexistent functional uterus, 177
with non-functioning uterus, 176–177
age-related changes, 5
anatomy/anatomical relations, 5, 599–600
atrophy, 609
benign disease, 599–612
congenital absence, 192
development, 599–600
fusion abnormalities, 192
hymen, 5
pathology
seminal fluid allergy, 609–610
Sjogren's syndrome, 610
structure, 5
toxic shock syndrome
trauma, 609
Vaginal artery, 12
Vaginal atresia, 174–176
Vaginal cancer, 517–519, 518f
aetiology, 623
clinical assessment, 623
incidence, 623
interstitial brachytherapy, 545–546
pathology, 623
pattern of spread, 623–624
prognosis, 624
staging, 623
treatment, 624
uncommon tumours, 624–625
see also Vulval cancer
Vaginal cones, stress incontinence, 802, 803f
Vaginal development, anomalous
aetiology, 174
classification, 174
complications of, 177
epidemiology, 174
investigation, 175–176
lateral fusion disorders, 174–177, 175f

monozygotic twins, evidence, 174
Müllerian duct development, failure, 174, 192
pathophysiology, 174
presentation, 174–175
transverse vaginal septum, 175–176
treatment, 176–177
vertical fusion defects, 174–175, 175f, 177
Vaginal dryness, 444, 925–926
Vaginal endometriosis, 498–499
Vaginal flora, healthy, 897
Vaginal infections
    bacterial vaginosis see Bacterial vaginosis
    candidiasis, 974–975, 975f
    differential diagnosis, discharge, 973t
    trichomoniasis, 975–976
Vaginal intraepithelial neoplasia (VAIN), 518–519, 575–576, 575f
Vaginal lubricants and moisturisers, 413
Vaginal smear, gram-stained, 974
Vaginal vault brachytherapy, 545
Vaginal vault prolapse surgery, 923
Vaginismus, 442–444, 920
Vaginitis, and HIV, 982
Vaginoscopy, 22
Valaciclovir, 960–961
Valerian root, 417
Valsalva manoeuvre, voiding difficulties, 836
Valsalva test, pelvic organ prolapse, 853–854
Vaniqa, 259
Varicocoele, 299, 307
Vasal obstruction, male infertility, 307
Vascular damage, 112–113
Vascular dementia, 408
Vascular endothelial growth factor (VEGF)
    breast cancer, 728
    endometrial repair, 452
    fibroids, 476
    gynaecological cancers, 554–556
Vascular medulla, ovary, 1
Vascular pain, and pelvic congestion, 929–930
Vascular smooth muscle cells (VSMCs), 452
Vasectomy
    antisperm antibodies, 433
    and cancers, 433
    cardiovascular and autoimmune disease, 433
    chronic intrascrotal pain and discomfort, 433
    complications of, 432–433
    late recanalization, 433
    postvasectomy syndrome, 433
    reversal, 307, 433
    sperm granulomas, 433
Vasomotor symptoms, HRT benefits, 410
Vasopressin, idiopathic (primary) dysmenorrhoea, 456
VATER syndrome, 172
Vault haematoma formation, 121
Vecchetti procedure, 192
Vector analysis, anal manometry, 908t
Venlafaxine, 412
Venography, ovarian varices, 64–65
Venous thrombosis/thromboembolism
    cervical cancer, 595
    combined oral contraception risk, 424–425
    deep vein thrombosis, 122

definitive diagnosis of pulmonary embolism, 122
diagnosis, 67
diagnosis of pulmonary embolism, 122
HRT risks, 411
imaging of, 67–68
postoperative care, 122–123, 122t
preoperative care, 99
screening for pulmonary embolism, 122
treatment, 122–123
Veress needle
    blind insertion of, 114
    blood vessels, damage to, 114–115
    laparoscopy, 36, 40, 40f
    puncture, bowel complications, 124
Verrucous carcinoma, 622–623
Vertical fusion defects, anomalous vaginal development, 174–175, 175f, 177
Vesicovaginal fistula, bladder, 8
Vestibule, vulva, 6
Vestigial structures, ovarian anatomy, 2
Viagra, 926
Videocystourethrography (VCU)
    functions of, 867
    overactive bladder syndrome, 819, 821f
    urethral sphincter incompetence, 790–791, 790f
Villous trophoblast, vs placental-site trophoblastic tumour, 652
VIN see Vulval intraepithelial neoplasia (VIN)
Vinca alkaloids, chemotherapy, 551
Vincristine, 300, 551–552
Violence against women, 1002–1008
    abuse, 1003, 1005
    background, 1002–1003
    British Crime Survey (1992), 988, 1002–1003
    Home Affairs Select Committee Report, 1003
    identification, 1004–1005
    intimate violence, 988
    management of abuse, 1005
    in pregnancy, 1002–1003
    presentation, 1004
    prevalence, 1002–1003
    prostitution management, 1005–1006
    reproductive health consequences, 1003–1005
    sexual assault, 988
    WHO study, 1003
    see also Forensic gynaecology; Sexual assault
Virilism, 669
Virtual simulation, radiotherapy, 542
Visual analogue scale (VAS)
    chronic pelvic pain, 933
    postoperative pain, 118
Vitamin B6, premenstrual syndrome, 395–397
Vitamin C, voiding difficulties, 843
Vitamin D
    in menopause, 414
    osteoporosis, 414
    premenstrual syndrome, 397
Vitamin E, menopausal symptoms, 412
Voiding difficulties, 769, 836–848
    causes, 838–841, 838b
        bladder overdistension, 841
        diabetes, 840

effects of age on voiding function, 838
idiopathic bladder neck obstruction, 841
lumbar intervertebral disc prolapse, 840
neurological disease, 840
obstruction following colposuspension, 842f
others, 841
pelvic organ prolapse, 841
postoperative, 838–839
postpartum voiding difficulty, 840
psychological factors, 840–841
cystourethroscopy, 842
definitions
    acute retention of urine, 837
    chronic retention of urine, 837
    voiding difficulty, 836–837
detrusor contraction
    voiding with, with abdominal straining, 837f
    voiding without, 839f
diabetes, 840
drug therapy, role, 844
electromyography, 842
idiopathic bladder neck obstruction, 841
incidence, 837
investigations
    cystourethroscopy, 842
    electromyography, 842
    pressure-flow studies, 842
    uroflowmetry, 841–842
    videourodynamics, 842
long-term management, 843–844
lumbar intervertebral disc prolapse, 840
multiple sclerosis, 840
nerve stimulation, role, 844–845
neurological disease, 840
normal voiding, 837f
obstruction
    following colposuspension, 842f
    urethral diverticulum, 845–846
Parkinson's disease, 840
pelvic organ prolapse, 841
pelvic surgery, 838
postoperative, 117, 838–839
    pelvic surgery, 838
    stress incontinence surgery, 838–839
postpartum, 840
postvoid residuals, 837
pressure-flow studies, 842
prevention, 845–846, 846b
prolapse surgery, 839
psychological factors, 840–841
Queen Square bladder stimulator, 845
short-term management, 843
stress incontinence surgery, 838–839
surgery, role, 844
symptoms and clinical effects, 837–838
urinary diversion, 845
uroflowmetry, 841–842
videourodynamics, 842
see also Urinary retention
Volociximab, 561
Von Willebrand's disease, 455
Vulva
    age-related changes, 6–7
    anatomy/anatomical relations, 5–7, 6f, 599–600
    bartholinitis, 607

benign disease, 599–612
    classification, 600
    corticosteroids, 601–602
    dermatoses, 602–605
    examination of patient, 600–601
    lesions, prevalence, 601
    Paget's disease, 605
    presentation, 600
    tumours, 608
clitoris, 6
dermatoses, 602–605
    dermatitis, contact and irritant, 602
    lichen planus, 604–605
    lichenoid lesions/vulval intraepithelial
        neoplasia, 602–605
development, 599–600
hidradenitis, 607
infections
    bacterial, 607
    fungal, 606
    genital warts, 606–607
    herpes simplex, 607
    protozoal/parasitic, 608
    streptococcal, 607
labia majora, 5–6
labia minora, 6
lichen sclerosus, 603–604
lichenoid lesions/vulval intraepithelial
    neoplasia, 602–605
malignant disease see Vulval cancer
Paget's disease, 605
pain/vulvodynia, 444, 605–606
perineal body, 6
protozoal/parasitic infections, 608
squamous cell carcinoma, 604
staphylococcal infections, 607
streptococcal infections, 607
threadworms, 608
trichomonas vaginalis, 608
tumours
    benign, 608
    cancerous, 517–519, 534–535
ulceration, 606
vestibule, 6
Vulval cancer, 517–519, 613–628
    advanced disease, 621
    aetiology, 613–614
    assessment, 615
    basal cell carcinoma, 623
    bilateral groin lymph node dissection,
        617–619
    'butterfly' incision, 618–620
    chemotherapy, 621
    depth of invasion, 616
    diagnosis, 615
    examination, 615
    grading, 615
    groin morbidity, 620
    groin recurrences, 615t
    Groningen International Study, 617
    histology, 614
    interstitial brachytherapy, 545–546
    lymph node status, 616–617
    lymphatic drainage, 614
    lymphovascular space permeation, 616
    malignant melanoma, 621–622
    molecular genetics, 534–535
    neoadjuvant therapy, 620–621

non-squamous, 614
Paget's disease, invasive, 622
palliation, 621
presentation, 614
primary treatment, 621
prognostic factors, 614–615
psychological morbidity, 620
radiotherapy, 620
recurrent, 621
risk factors, 613–614
sarcoma, 623
sentinel lymph node detection, 617
sexual problems, 754
site of tumour, 617–618
squamous, 614
    natural history, 614
staging, 615–616
subtypes, 613, 614f
superficially invasive disease, 614
surgical treatment, 618–620
    modified radical vulvectomy/wide local
        excision, 619
    morbidity, 620
    pelvic lymphadenectomy, 619–620
    postoperative adjuvant therapy, 620
    separate incisions, 618–619
    superficial inguinal lymphadenectomy,
        619
    unilateral inguinofemoral
        lymphadenectomy, 619
tumour size, 616
verrucous carcinoma, 622–623
of vulva, invasive, 622
vulvar morbidity, 620
see also Vulva; Vulval intraepithelial
    neoplasia (VIN)
Vulval intraepithelial neoplasia (VIN),
    518–519, 576–577, 577f–578f,
    602–605
    carbon dioxide laser, 577
    diagnosis and assessment, 576
    incidence, 534
    medical therapy, 576–577
    natural history, 576
    Paget's disease, 577, 577f–578f, 605
    pathology, 576
    subtypes, 576
    surgical treatment, 577
    treatment, 576–577
    see also Vulval cancer
Vulval pain syndrome see Vulvodynia
Vulval squamous cell carcinomas (VSCCs),
    534–535
Vulval warts, 970f
Vulvar intraepithelial neoplasia (VIN), 601,
    613
Vulvar vestibulitis, 444
Vulvectomy, radical, 442, 619, 619f, 622
Vulvodynia, 444, 605–606
Vulvovaginal vestibule, 600

W

War time, sexual violence in, 1006–1007
Weaning, 689
Weight loss
    and amenorrhoea, 217
    hirsutism, 387

ovulation induction, 242–243
pelvic organ prolapse, 856
preoperative care, 101
see also Body weight/BMI; Obese patients
Wertheim's hysterectomy, 7
Western blot diagnosis, genital herpes, 960
Wexner score, faecal incontinence, 776, 778t
WHO (World Health Organization)
    on osteoporosis, 408
    on sexual health, 754
Wild yam cream, 417
Williams vulvovaginoplasty, absent vagina,
    177
Wilms' tumour gene (WT1), 167
Women's Health Initiative (WHI) , US,
    409–410
World Health Organization (WHO)
    analgesic ladder, 763
    on breast cancer, 712
    on gestational trophoblastic disease, 650
    International Classification of Diseases,
        1010
    on miscarriage, 335
    Multi-Country Study on Women's Health
        and Domestic Violence Against
        Women (2005), 1003
    on osteoporosis, 408, 408t
    on ovarian cancer, 679–680
    on ovulation disorders, 232–233, 282t
    on ovulation failure, 282
    on phyllodes tumour, 691–692
    on PID, 942
    on sexual health, 754
    on sexually transmitted infections,
        955–956, 962
Wound response signature, breast cancer, 731
Wounds
    classification, infection risk, 101t
    haematoma formation, 121
    postoperative care, 119, 995–996
    stab, sexual assault, 995–996
WTI gene, 167

X

X chromosomes, structural abnormalities,
    168, 169f
X-ray hysterosalpingography, 285–287
X-ray hysterosalpingography (HSG)
    miscarriage, 343
    reproductive dysfunction, 283–285, 283f
    tubal disease, 355
X-ray techniques, 59
X-rays, 539
XXX syndrome, 168
XYY syndrome, 168

Y

Yaws, 962
Young's syndrome, 302–303

Z

Zoledronic acid, 413
Zona pellucida, 232, 267
Zuska's disease (recurring subareolar
    abscess), 701